Comprehensive Gynecology

Comprehensive Gynecology

Expert Consult – Online and Print

6th Edition

Gretchen M. Lentz, MD

Professor of Obstetrics and Gynecology
Adjunct Professor of Urology, Division Director for Urogynecology
University of Washington School of Medicine
Seattle, Washington

Roger A. Lobo, MD

Professor of Obstetrics and Gynecology
Columbia University College of Physicians and Surgeons
New York, New York

David M. Gershenson, MD

Professor and Chairman, Gynecologic Oncology
The University of Texas MD Anderson Cancer Center
Houston, Texas

Vern L. Katz, MD

Clinical Professor, Department of Obstetrics and Gynecology
Oregon Health Sciences University
Director of Perinatal Services, Sacred Heart Medical Center
Center for Genetics and Maternal-Fetal Medicine
Eugene, Oregon

ELSEVIER
MOSBY

1600 John F. Kennedy Blvd.
Ste 1800
Philadelphia, PA 19103-2899

COMPREHENSIVE GYNECOLOGY: EXPERT CONSULT ONLINE AND PRINT

ISBN: 978-0-323-06986-1

Notices

Knowledge and best practice in this field are constantly changing. As new research and experience broaden our understanding, changes in research methods, professional practices, or medical treatment may become necessary.

Practitioners and researchers must always rely on their own experience and knowledge in evaluating and using any information, methods, compounds, or experiments described herein. In using such information or methods they should be mindful of their own safety and the safety of others, including parties for whom they have a professional responsibility.

With respect to any drug or pharmaceutical products identified, readers are advised to check the most current information provided (i) on procedures featured or (ii) by the manufacturer of each product to be administered, to verify the recommended dose or formula, the method and duration of administration, and contraindications. It is the responsibility of practitioners, relying on their own experience and knowledge of their patients, to make diagnoses, to determine dosages and the best treatment for each individual patient, and to take all appropriate safety precautions.

To the fullest extent of the law, neither the Publisher nor the authors, contributors, or editors, assume any liability for any injury and/or damage to persons or property as a matter of products liability, negligence or otherwise, or from any use or operation of any methods, products, instructions, or ideas contained in the material herein.

ISBN: 978-0-323-06986-1

Content Strategist: Stefanie Jewell-Thomas
Content Development Specialist: Deidre Simpson
Publishing Services Manager: Julie Eddy
Project Manager: Marquita Parker
Designer: Lou Forgione

Printed in the United States

Last digit is the print number: 9 8 7 6 5 4 3 2 1

Contributors

Diane C. Bodurka, MD, FAGOC, FACS
Professor and Fellowship Director
Department of Gynecologic Oncology
and Reproductive Medicine
The University of Texas MD Anderson
Cancer Center
Houston, Texas

Edith Cheng, MD, MS
Adjunct Professor
Medical Genetics Department of Internal Medicine
University of Washington
Seattle, Washington

Robert L. Coleman, MD, FACOG, FACS
Professor
Department of Gynecologic Oncology
Vice-Chairman, Clinical Research
Ann Rife Cox Chair in Gynecology
The University of Texas MD Anderson
Cancer Center
Houston, Texas

Allan L. Covens, MD, FRCSC
Professor
Obstetrics and Gynecology
Division of Gynecologic Oncology
University of Toronto
Toronto, Ontario

Ann Jeannette Davis, MD
Professor
Department of Obstetrics and Gynecology
Dartmouth University School of Medicine
Hanover, New Hampshire

Deborah J. Dotters, MD
Director, Gynecologic Oncology
Northwestern Gynecologic Oncology
Eugene, Oregon

Linda O. Eckert, MD
Associate Professor
Department of Obstetrics and Gynecology
Adjunct Associate Professor
Department of Global Health
University of Washington
Seattle, Washington

Michel Ferin, MD
Professor
Obstetrics and Gynecology
Columbia University
New York, New York

Michael Frumovitz, MD, MPH, FACO, FACS
Associate Professor
Gynecologic Oncology
The University of Texas MD Anderson
Cancer Center
Houston, Texas

David M. Gershenson, MD
Professor and Chairman, Gynecologic Oncology
The University of Texas MD Anderson Cancer Center
Houston, Texas

Jeffrey T. Jensen, MD, MPH
Leon Speroff Professor and Vice Chair
Research Department of Obstetrics and Gynecology
Oregon Health and Science University
Portland, Oregon

Anuja Jhingran, MD
Professor, Radiation Oncology
The University of Texas MD Anderson
Cancer Center
Houston, Texas

Vern L. Katz, MD
Clinical Professor
Department of Obstetrics and Gynecology
Oregon Health Sciences University
Clinical Professor
Department of Human Physiology
University of Oregon
Director of Perinatal Services
Sacred Heart Medical Center
Center for Genetics and Maternal-Fetal Medicine
Eugene, Oregon

James Michael Kelley, III, JD
Shareholder and Partner
Elk and Elk Co. Ltd
Cleveland, Ohio

Gretchen M. Lentz, MD
Professor of Obstetrics and Gynecology
Adjunct Professor of Urology
Division Director for Urogynecology
University of Washington School of Medicine
Seattle, Washington

Charles F. Levenback, MD
Professor and Deputy Chairman for Patient Care
Gynecologic Oncology and Reproductive Medicine
The University of Texas MD Anderson
Cancer Center
Houston, Texas

Roger A. Lobo, MD
Professor of Obstetrics and Gynecology
Columbia University College of Physicians and Surgeons
New York, New York

Karen H. Lu, MD
Professor of Gynecologic Oncology
H.E.B. Professor of Cancer Research
Department of Gynecologic Oncology
The University of Texas MD Anderson
Cancer Center
Houston, Texas

Jacob McGee, MD
Gynecologic Oncology
London Health Sciences Centre
University of Western Ontario
London, Ontario

Daniel R. Mishell, Jr., MD
Professor
Department of Obsetrics and Gynecology
Keck School of Medicine
University of Southern California
Los Angeles, California

Kenneth L. Noller, MD
Louis E. Phaneuf Professor and Chair
Department of Obstetrics and Gynecology
Director of Evaluation
American Board of Obsetrics and Gynecology
Dallas, Texas

Pedro T. Ramirez, MD
Professor
Department of Gynecologic Oncology
The University of Texas MD Anderson
Cancer Center
Houston, Texas

Kathleen M. Schmeler, MD
Assistant Professor
Department of Gynecologic Oncology
The University of Texas M.D. Anderson
Cancer Center
Houston, Texas

Judith Ann Smith, Pharm.D., BCOP, FCCP, FISOPP
Associate Professor and Director of
Pharmacology Research
Gynecologic Oncology and Reproductive Medicine
Director, Translation Reserch Fellowship Division
of Pharmacy
The University of Texas MD Anderson
Cancer Center
Houston, Texas

Pamela T. Soliman, MD, MPH
Assistant Professor
Department of Gynecologic Oncology
The University of Texas MD Anderson
Cancer Center
Houston, Texas

Anil K. Sood, MD
Betty Asche Murray Professor and Vice Chair for
Translational Research
Departments of Gynecologic Oncology
and Reproductive Medicine
Cancer Biology Director, Center for RNA Interference
and Non-Coding RNA
The University of Texas MD Anderson
Cancer Center
Houston, Texas

Premal H. Thaker, MD, MS
Assistant Professor
Gynecologic Oncology
Washington University School of Medicine
St. Louis, Missouri

Preface

In the 25 years since the first edition of *Comprehensive Gynecology*, many scientific advances have occurred in medical practice. The first four editions were largely the work of the original four editors: Drs. William Droegemueller, Arthur L. Herbst, Daniel R. Mishell, Jr., and Morton A. Stenchever. Once again we wish to acknowledge our mentors for their vision, support, and professional guidance.

With the staggering volume of medical literature published and the complexities of the gynecologic subspecialties, we have collaborated with additional experts for the sixth edition. We've "examined disease" and added a new chapter on the interaction of medical diseases and female physiology. We've "investigated discord" with new authors to completely rewrite the emotional and psychological issues in gynecology and the legal issues for obstetrician-gynecologists. Other chapters have delved into the controversies in breast cancer screening, vitamin D use, the ongoing debates in hormone therapy, and vaginal mesh use for pelvic organ prolapse surgery.

Specifically, I wish to highlight some of the more drastic changes in this edition. Chapter 6 on medical-legal risk management was rewritten with a new author who is a practicing attorney in malpractice claims. There is much practical advice to avoid malpractice suits. As has been found in all specialties and in the patient safety literature, communication with the patient and the team members, as well as in the medical record, is critical. Chapter 9 on emotional and psychological issues was completely rewritten with a practicing psychiatrist. The sections on depression, anxiety, substance abuse, and eating disorders will be very helpful in our practice. Maybe the single most relevant new topic in the entire textbook is the section on dealing with the "difficult patient." Our day can be disrupted and upsetting because of this. This section helps us understand this problem and how we can be effective in helping the woman and not become frustrated ourselves.

Chapter 15 has significant updates on breast disease with emphasis on the gynecologist's role in managing breast problems, both benign and malignant. Due to the increasing complexity of the women we care for, Chapter 7 is a completely new chapter on the interaction of medical disease and female physiology. This chapter discusses how a woman's physiology affects diseases such as migraines, epilepsy, and autoimmune phenomenon, and how treatments are affected. On the flip side, this chapter explores how disease states affect the menstrual cycle.

The entire gynecologic oncology section has been revamped to cover the important changes in this field. Chapter 26 explores details of the molecular biology of specific gynecologic malignancies. With the new targeted chemotherapeutic agents, Chapter 27 adds information on hormonal agents as well as bevacizumab, which is a monoclonal antibody that inhibits angiogenesis. A global overview of the latest clinical trials and strategies for systemic treatment includes considerations of the addition of biologic or targeted agents. Work is presented on research into drug resistance and how new agents are developed and evaluated. Other chapters highlight the new FIGO staging for uterine cancers, minimally invasive surgery for the treatment of early stage ovarian cancer, and cytoreductive surgery for advanced ovarian cancer. Last but certainly not least, an entirely new Chapter 34, with new authorship is presented on Fallopian Tube and Primary Peritoneal Cancer.

Discord is good for the advancement of medical knowledge. This edition hopefully brings more harmony of understanding in both basic science and outcomes research that covers the wide breadth of gynecologic conditions. We believe that the sixth edition will be a valuable resource for the resident in training and the busy practicing gynecologist. As a specialty, we remain committed to the comprehensive medical needs of women, the care of their complex diseases, and in promoting wellness through education, counseling, and early detection of disease.

Gretchen M. Lentz, MD
Roger A. Lobo, MD
David M. Gershenson, MD
Vern L. Katz, MD

ACKNOWLEDGMENTS

The editors of this edition wish to acknowledge a few of the many scientists, clinicians, and mentors who have contributed to past editions on which we have built and also to this edition. Drs. William Droegemueller, Arthur L. Herbst, Daniel R. Mishell, Jr., and Morton A. Stenchever top the list. In addition, thanks to Marta Abrams, Jan Hammanishi, Phillip Patton, and Carolyn Westoff.

We also wish to express our deepest thanks and love to our families, who have lent incredible support and encouragement during the long hours of work on this edition.

Contents

Part IV GYNECOLOGIC ONCOLOGY

Part V REPRODUCTIVE ENDOCRINOLOGY AND INFERTILITY

GLOSSARY (available online at expertconsult.com*)

*To access your account, look for your activation instructions on the inside front cover of this book.

1

Fertilization and Embryogenesis
Meiosis, Fertilization, Implantation, Embryonic Development, Sexual Differentiation

Edith Cheng and Vern L. Katz

Several areas of medical investigation have brought increased attention to the processes of **fertilization** and embryonic development, including teratology, stem cell research, immunogenetics, and assisted reproductive technology. The preimplantation, **implantation**, and embryonic stages of development in the human can now be studied because of the development of newer techniques and areas of research. This chapter considers the processes of oocyte meiosis, fertilization and early **cleavage**, implantation, development of the genitourinary system, and sex differentiation. Chapter 2 (Reproductive Genetics) continues with a discussion of closely related issues of genetics.

THE OOCYTE AND MEIOSIS

The oocyte is a unique and extremely specialized cell. Initially, during the process of oocyte meiosis, the genetic variability of the species is ensured. Later, the oocyte develops the ability to facilitate fertilization and to provide the energy system to support early embryonic development.

The primordial germ cells in both males and females are large eosinophilic cells derived from endoderm in the wall of the yolk sac. These cells migrate to the germinal ridge by way of the dorsal mesentery of the hindgut by ameboid action by 6 weeks. In the human female, **oogenesis** begins with the multiplication of the diploid oogonia through multiple rounds of mitosis to produce primary oocytes, reaching a peak number of 6 to 7 million during the first 10 to 12 weeks of gestation. The numbers then rapidly decline to 2 to 4 million by birth, and at menarche, only about 400,000 remain in the ovary. The meiotic process begins as mitosis is ending in the fetal ovary. Oocytes in the early stage (prophase) of meiosis may be seen at 10 to 12 weeks' gestation. Meiosis is the mechanism by which diploid organisms reduce their gametes to a haploid state so that they can recombine again during fertilization to become diploid organisms. In humans, this process reduces 46 chromosomes (or 23 pairs) to 23 chromosome structures in the gamete. The haploid gamete contains only one chromosome for each homologous pair of chromosomes, so that it has either the maternal or paternal chromosome for each pair, but not both. Meiosis is also the mechanism by

which genetic exchange is completed through **chiasma** formation and crossing over between homologous chromosome pairs. In humans, all of this is completed during fetal life of the yet-to-be-born female.

Two meiotic cell divisions are required to produce haploid gametes. The first, known as the reduction division, division I, or meiosis I, is complicated, and in the human female occurs over a time span from fetal life to menarche. Of the five stages, prophase I lasts the longest, occurs exclusively during fetal life, and sets the stage for genetic exchange that ensures genetic variation in our species.

The oocytes complete prophase before entering a quiescent period. Reentry into meiosis is signaled by the endocrine changes of puberty. In the mature cycle, usually one oocyte each month will complete meiosis I as a function of ovulation and meiosis II if fertilization occurs. Thus, it is in fetal life that the ovary makes all of the oocytes that the adult women will have for reproduction.

In the human female, oogonia enter meiosis in "waves" (**Fig. 1-1**)—that is, not all oogonia enter meiosis at the same time. The initiating signal or signals are unknown, but cytologic evidence suggests that oocytes represent the first substage of prophase, leptotene, in the human fetal ovary as early as 10 weeks' gestation. With increasing **gestational age**, greater proportions of oocytes in later stages of meiosis may be observed, and by the end of the second trimester of pregnancy, the majority of oocytes in the fetal ovary have cytologic characteristics that are consistent with the diplotene/dictyotene substages of prophase I of meiosis I (the stage at which the oocytes are arrested until ovulation) (**Fig. 1-2**).

The structural characteristics of the chromosomes in prophase of meiosis I in human oogenesis are seen in **Figure 1-3**. Interphase I has not yet been observed in the fetal ovary cytologically. It is a time when DNA replication takes place, thus transforming the diploid oogonia with a DNA content of $2N$ to an oocyte with a DNA content of $4N$. Each chromosome is duplicated, and the identical copies, called sister chromatids, of each chromosome are tightly held together along their length. Leptotene is proportionately the most abundant of all the prophase I substages in the early gestations. Cells in this meiotic phase are

1

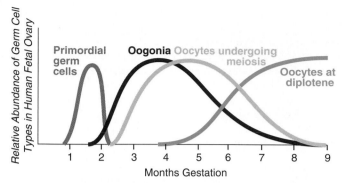

Figure 1-1 Diagrammatic representation of the different meiotic cell types and their proportions in the ovary during fetal life. (Courtesy of Edith Cheng, MD.)

characterized by a large nucleus with fine, diffuse, stringlike chromatin evenly distributed within the nucleus. Chromatin of homologous pairs occupies "domains" and does not occur as distinct linear strands of chromosomes. By this stage each chromosome has replicated, and the DNA content is now 4*N*. The zygotene substage (**Fig. 1-3A**) is defined by the initiation of pairing, which is characterized by the striking appearance of the synaptonemal complex formation in some of the chromosomes (**Fig. 1-3B**). There is cytologic evidence of chromosome condensation and linearization, and the chromatin is seen as a fine, stringlike structure. The pachytene substage is the most easily recognizable period of the prophase and is

characterized by clearly defined chromosomes that appear as continuous ribbons of thick beadlike chromatin. By definition, this is the substage in which all homologues have paired. In this substage, the paired homologues are structurally composed of four closely opposed chromatids and are known as a tetrad. The frequency of oocytes in pachytene increases with gestational age and peaks in the mid-second trimester of pregnancy (about 20–25 weeks' gestation). The diplotene substage is a stage of desynapsis that occurs as the synaptonemal complex dissolves and the two homologous chromosomes pull away from each other. However, these **bivalents**, which are composed of a maternally and a paternally derived chromosome, are held together at the centromere and at sites of chiasma formation that represent sites where crossing over has occurred. In general, chiasma formation occurs only between chromatids of homologous pairs and not between sister chromatids. Usually, one to three chiasma occur for each chromosome arm. Oocytes at this stage of prophase I constitute the majority of third-trimester fetal and newborn ovaries. Diplotene merges with diakinesis, the last substage of meiosis I, and is a stage of transition to metaphase, lasting many years in the humans. Oocytes are arrested at this stage until puberty, when sometime before ovulation, metaphase, anaphase, and telophase are completed. The result is two daughter cells, which are diploid (2 *N*) in DNA content but contain 23 chromosome structures, each containing two closely held sister chromatids. One daughter cell, the oocyte, receives the majority of the cytoplasm, and the other becomes the first **polar body** when ovulation occurs. Both the oocyte and the polar body are present within the **zona pellucida**.

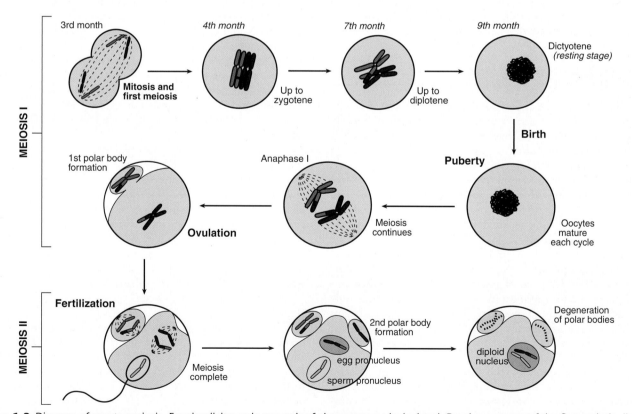

Figure 1-2 Diagram of oocyte meiosis. For simplicity, only one pair of chromosomes is depicted. Prophase stages of the first meiotic division occur in the female during fetal life. The meiotic process is arrested at the diplotene stage ("first meiotic arrest"), and the oocyte enters the dictyotene stages. Meiosis I resumes at puberty and is completed at the time of ovulation. The second meiotic division takes place over several hours in the oviduct only after sperm penetration. (Courtesy of Edith Cheng, MD.)

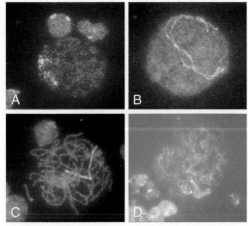

Figure 1-3 Fetal ovary with fluorescent in situ hybridization. The first three images are meiotic cells from a 21-week fetal ovary. **A,** Fluorescent in situ hybridization (FISH) with a whole chromosome probe for chromosome X was completed to visualize the pairing characteristics of the X chromosome during leptotene. **B,** Zygotene. **C,** Pachytene. **D,** Image of a meiotic cell from a 34-week fetal ovary that underwent dual FISH with probes for chromosomes 13 (*green signal*) and 21 (*red signal*) to illustrate the pairing characteristics of this substage of prophase in meiosis I. (Courtesy of Edith Cheng, MD.)

In contrast to the long and complex process of meiosis I, meiosis II is rapid, and the oocyte advances immediately to metaphase II where the sister chromatids for each chromosome are aligned at the equatorial plate, held together and on the spindle fibers by the centromere of the chromosome. If sperm penetration occurs, then meiosis II is completed in the oviduct with union of the sperm and oocyte nucleus and extrusion of the first and second polar bodies. In the male, meiosis generates four haploid gametes of equal reproductive potential, whereas in the female, only one oocyte is generated for reproduction (**Fig. 1-4**).

FERTILIZATION AND EARLY CLEAVAGE

In most mammals, including humans, the egg is released from the ovary in the metaphase II stage (**Fig. 1-5**). When the egg enters the fallopian tube, it is surrounded by a cumulus of granulosa cells (**cumulus oophorus**) and intimately surrounded by a clear zona pellucida. Within the zona pellucida are both the egg and the first polar body. Meanwhile, spermatozoa are transported through the cervical mucus and the uterus and into the fallopian tubes. During this transport period the sperm undergo two changes: **capacitation** and **acrosome reaction**. These changes activate enzyme systems within the sperm head and make it possible for the sperm to transgress the cumulus oophorus and the zona pellucida (**Fig. 1-6**).

The sperm are attracted to an egg through the process known as **chemotaxis**, which is related to capacitation of the sperm. The process is aided by the binding of progesterone to a surface

Figure 1-4 Diagram of oocyte meiosis. For simplicity, only three pairs of chromosomes are depicted (1-4). Prophase stages of the first meiotic division, which occur in most mammals during fetal life. The meiotic process is arrested at the diplotene stage ("first meiotic arrest"), and the oocyte enters the dictyate stages (5-6). When meiosis is resumed, the first maturation division is completed (7-11). Ovulation occurs usually at the metaphase II stage (11), and the second meiotic division (12-14) takes place in the oviduct only after sperm penetration. (From Tsafriri A: Oocyte maturation in mammals. In Jones RE [ed)] The Vertebrate Ovary. New York, Plenum, 1978. With kind permission of Springer Science and Business Media.)

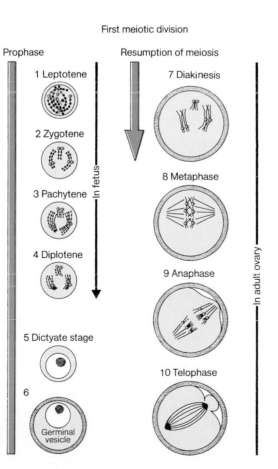

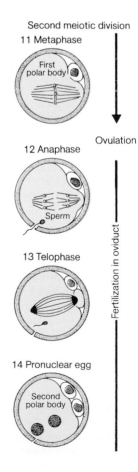

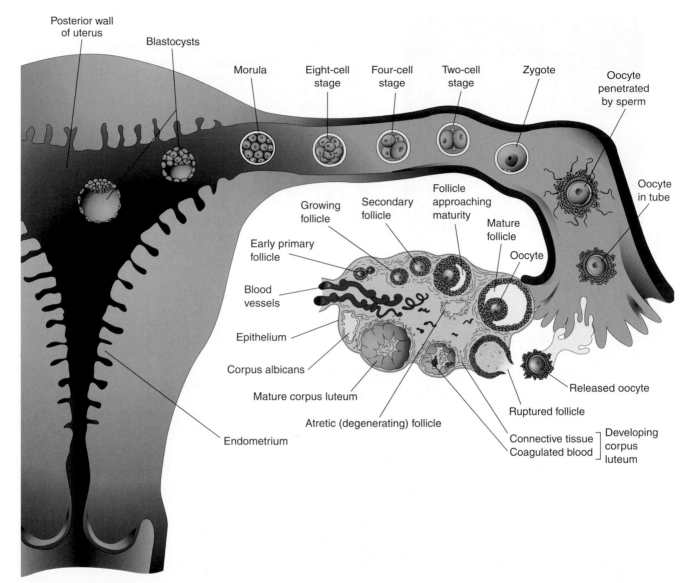

Figure 1-5 Summary of the ovarian cycle, fertilization, and human development during the first week. Stage 1 of development begins with fertilization in the uterine tube and ends when the zygote forms. Stage 2 (days 2–3) comprises the early stages of cleavage (from 2 to about 32 cells, the **morula**). Stage 3 (days 4–5) consists of the free (unattached) blastocyst. Stage 4 (days 5–6) is represented by the blastocyst attaching to the posterior wall of the uterus, the usual site of implantation. The blastocysts have been sectioned to show their internal structure. (From Moore KL, Persaud TVN: The Developing Human: Clinically Oriented Embryology, 7th ed. Philadelphia, WB Saunders, 2003.)

receptor on the sperm. This allows an increase in intracellular calcium ion concentration, which increases sperm motility (**chemokinesis**). Once the sperm has passed the barrier of the zona pellucida, it attaches to the cell membrane of the egg and enters the cytoplasm. When the sperm enters the cytoplasm, intracytoplasmic structures, the coronal granules, arrange themselves in an orderly fashion around the outermost portion of the cytoplasm just beneath the cytoplasmic membrane, and the sperm head swells and gives rise to the male pronucleus. The egg completes its second meiotic division, casting off the second polar body to a position also beneath the zona pellucida. The female pronucleus swells as well. In most mammals the male pronucleus can be recognized as the larger of the two. The pronuclei, which contain the haploid sets of chromosomes of maternal and paternal origin, do not fuse in mammals. However, the nuclear membranes surrounding them disappear, and the chromosomes contained within each membrane arrange themselves on the developing spindle of the first mitotic division. In this way the diploid complement of chromosomes is reestablished, completing the process of fertilization.

Cell division (cleavage) then occurs, giving rise to the two-cell **embryo** (Fig. 1-7). The first division takes about 20 hours to complete, and the actual phase of fertilization generally occurs in the ampulla of the fallopian tube. A significant number of fertilized ova do not complete cleavage for a number of reasons, including failure of appropriate chromosome arrangement on the spindle, specific gene defects that prevent the formation of the spindle, and environmental factors. Importantly, **teratogens** acting at this point are usually either completely destructive or cause little or no effect. Twinning may occur by the separation of the two cells produced by cleavage, each of which has the potential to develop into a separate embryo. Twinning may occur at any

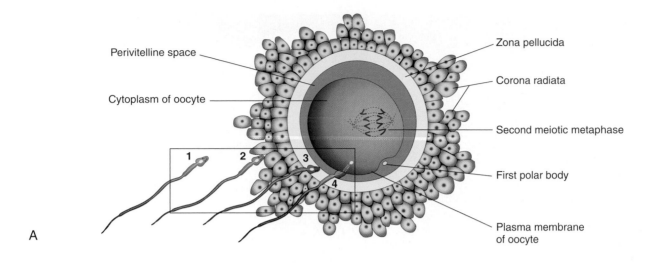

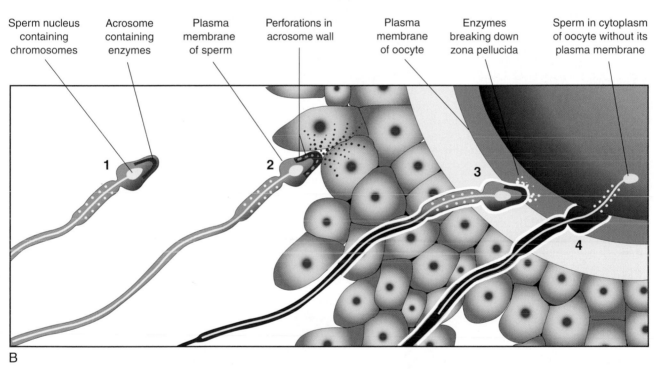

Figure 1-6 Acrosome reaction and a sperm penetrating an oocyte. The detail of the area outlined in **A** is given in **B**. 1, Sperm during capacitation, a period of conditioning that occurs in the female reproductive tract. 2, Sperm undergoing the acrosome reaction, during which perforations form in the acrosome. 3, Sperm digesting a path through the zona pellucida by the action of enzymes released from the acrosome. 4, Sperm after entering the cytoplasm of the oocyte. Note that the plasma membranes of the sperm and oocyte have fused and that the head and tail of the sperm enter the oocyte, leaving the sperm's plasma membrane attached to the oocyte's plasma membrane. (From Moore KL, Persaud TVN: The Developing Human: Clinically Oriented Embryology, 7th ed. Philadelphia, WB Saunders, 2003.)

stage until the formation of the **blastula**, because each cell is totipotential. Both genetic and environmental factors are probably involved in the causation of twinning.

MORULA AND BLASTULA STAGE: EARLY DIFFERENTIATION

After the first mitotic division, the cells continue to divide as the embryo passes along the fallopian tube and enters the uterus. This process takes 3 to 4 days after fertilization in the human,

and the embryo may arrive at the uterus in any form, from 32 cells to the early blastula stage. In the human, implantation generally takes place 3 days after the embryo enters the uterus.

Implantation depends on the development of early trophoblastic cells during the blastula stage. These cells digest away the zona pellucida and allow the embryo to fix to the wall of the uterus and subsequently to burrow within the endometrium. The development of the blastula and the separation of the embryonic disk cells from the developing trophoblastic cells together make up the first stage of differentiation in the

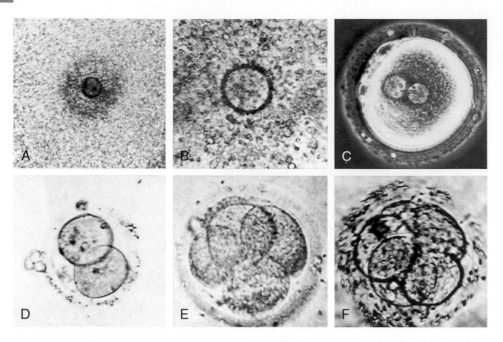

Figure 1-7 Six photomicrographs of fresh, unmounted human eggs and embryos. **A,** Early maturing oocyte. **B,** Mature oocyte surrounded by granulosa cells, zona pellucida visible. **C,** Fertilized oocyte demonstrating male and female pronuclei and both polar bodies. **D,** Two-cell zygote. **E,** Four-cell embryo. **F,** Eight-cell embryo. (Courtesy of Edith Cheng, MD.)

embryo. Again, at this stage of development, teratogens are generally either completely destructive or have little or no effect, as each of the cells of the early embryonic disk is pluripotent. Differentiation within the embryonic disk, however, proceeds fairly rapidly, and if separation of cells and twinning occur at this point, the twins are frequently conjoined in some fashion.

Advances in assisted reproductive technology and genetics now provide practitioners assess to the early embryo for preimplantation genetic diagnosis (PGD) of single-gene or chromosome disorders (**Fig. 1-8**). This technique, initiated in the United Kingdom in the late 1980s, involves the removal of one or two cells at the cleavage stage (six to eight cells) at day 2 to 4 after fertilization using highly sophisticated micromanipulation techniques. For PGD of single-gene disorders, DNA is extracted from the cell(s), amplified by polymerase chain reaction (PCR), and tested for the gene mutation in question. Embryos containing the mutation are discarded (not transferred), and embryos in which the mutation in question is not detected are saved. Some of these may be transferred into the primed uterine cavity as in any in vitro fertilization (IVF) cycle. For PGD of chromosomal defects such as aneuploidy or structural rearrangements, fluorescent in situ hybridization (FISH) is completed on the one or two cells removed from each embryo for only the chromosomal abnormality in question. PGD must be completed within 12 to 24 hours of embryo biopsy in order to transfer appropriate embryos into the uterus.

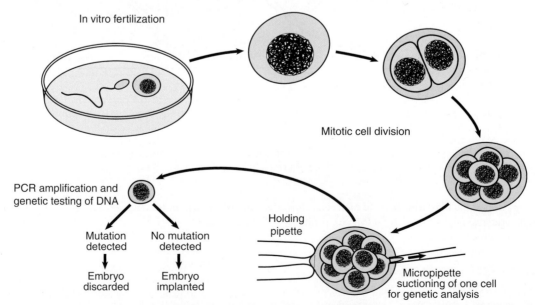

Figure 1-8 Schematic illustration of preimplantation diagnosis. PGD requires in vitro fertilization technology to achieve pregnancy. After fertilization, one or two blastomeres are removed at the six- to eight-cell stage from each embryo. For gene mutational analysis, the DNA is extracted and amplified several hundredfold. Embryos without the mutation are kept and transferred. (Courtesy of Edith Cheng, MD.)

IMPLANTATION

Implantation has been noted to occur in the human embryo as early as day 6 after ovulation (**Table 1-1**). For implantation to take place, the zona pellucida must be removed from the developing **blastocyst**, which occurs because of enzyme action produced either by cells of the blastocyst or by some endometrial enzymes. Endometrial capillaries in contact with the invading syncytiotrophoblast are engulfed to form venous sinuses at or about 7½ days after conception and are seen abundantly by day 9. Endometrial spiral arteries are not invaded at this point. The endoplasmic reticulum of the syncytiotrophoblast is probably responsible for the synthesis of human chorionic gonadotropin (HCG), which is well developed by 11 days after ovulation. Transfer is most likely through the venous sinuses before intact circulation to the developing embryo has been established. HCG must be transmitted to maternal circulation because it is responsible for maintaining the corpus luteum. HCG has been detected in the peripheral blood of the mother as early as 6 days after ovulation, but it is always seen by day 12. The concentration doubles every 1.2 to 2 days, reaching its highest point at 7 to 9 weeks of pregnancy.

EARLY ORGANOGENESIS IN THE EMBRYONIC PERIOD

During the third week after fertilization, the primitive streak forms in the caudal portion of the embryonic disk, and the embryonic disk begins to grow and change from a circular to a pear-shaped configuration. At that point the epithelium facing superiorly is considered ectoderm and will eventually give rise to the developing central nervous system, and the epithelium facing downward toward the yolk sac is endoderm. During this week the neuroplate develops with its associated notochordal process. By the sixteenth day after conception the third primitive germ layer, the intraembryonic mesoderm, begins to form between the ectoderm and endoderm. Early mesoderm migrates cranially, passing on either side of the notochordal process to meet in front in the formation of the cardiogenic area. The heart soon develops from this area. Later in the third week extraembryonic mesoderm joins with the yolk sac and the developing amnion to contribute to the developing membranes.

An intraembryonic mesoderm develops on each side of the notochord and neural tube to form longitudinal columns, the paraxial mesoderm. Each paraxial column thins laterally into the lateral plate mesoderm, which is continuous with the extraembryonic mesoderm of the yolk sac and the amnion. The lateral plate mesoderm is separated from the paraxial mesoderm by a continuous tract of mesoderm called the intermediate mesoderm. By the twentieth day, paraxial mesoderm begins to divide into paired linear bodies known as somites. About 38 pairs of somites form during the next 10 days. Eventually a total of 42 to 44 pairs will develop, and these will give rise to body musculature.

Angiogenesis, or blood vessel formation, can be seen in the extraembryonic mesoderm of the yolk sac by day 15 or 16. Embryonic vessels can be seen about 2 days later and develop when mesenchymal cells known as angioblasts aggregate to form masses and cords called blood islands. Spaces then appear within these islands, and the angioblasts arrange themselves around these spaces to form primitive endothelium. Isolated vessels form channels and then grow into adjacent areas by endothelial budding. Primitive blood cells develop from endothelial cells as the vessels develop on the yolk sac and allantois. However, blood formation does not begin within the embryo until the second month of gestation, occurring first in the developing liver and later in the spleen, bone marrow, and lymph nodes. Separate mesenchymal cells surrounding the primitive endothelial vessels differentiate into muscular and connective tissue elements. The primitive heart forms in a similar manner from mesenchymal cells in the cardiogenic area. Paired endothelial channels, called heart tubes, develop by the end of the third week and fuse to form the primitive heart. By the twenty-first day, this primitive heart has linked up with blood vessels of the embryo, forming a primitive cardiovascular system. Blood circulation starts about this time, and the cardiovascular system becomes the first functioning organ system within the embryo. All the organ systems form between the fourth week and seventh week of gestation.

A teratogenic event that takes place during the embryonic period gives rise to a constellation of malformations related to the organ systems that are actively developing at that particular time. Thus, cardiovascular malformations tend to occur because of teratogenic events early in the embryonic period, whereas genitourinary abnormalities tend to result from later events. Teratogenic effects before implantation often cause death but not malformations. The effects of a particular teratogen depend on the individual's genetic makeup, other environmental factors in play at the time, the embryonic developmental stage during which the teratogenic exposure occurred, and in some cases the dose of the teratogen and the duration of exposure. Some teratogens in and of themselves are harmless, but their metabolites cause the damage. Teratogens may be chemical substances and their by-products, or they may be physical phenomena, such as temperature elevation and irradiation. Teratogen exposure after the forty-ninth day of gestation may injure or kill the embryo or cause developmental and growth retardation but usually will not be responsible for specific malformations. The period of embryonic development is said to be complete when the embryo attains a crown–rump length of 30 mm, corresponding in most cases to day 49 after conception.

DEVELOPMENT OF THE GENITOURINARY SYSTEM

The development of the genital organs is intimately involved with the development of the renal system.

Table 1-1 Events of Implantation

Event	Days after Ovulation
Zona pellucida disappears	4-5
Blastocyst attaches to epithelial surface of endometrium	6
Trophoblast erodes into endometrial stroma	7
Trophoblast differentiates into cytotrophoblastic and syncytial trophoblastic layers	7-8
Lacunae appear around trophoblast	8-9
Blastocyst burrows beneath endometrial surface	9-10
Lacunar network forms	10-11
Trophoblast invades endometrial sinusoids, establishing a uteroplacental circulation	11-12
Endometrial epithelium completely covers blastocyst	12-13
Strong decidual reaction occurs in stroma	13-14

RENAL DEVELOPMENT

Nephrogenic cords develop from the intermediate mesoderm as early as the 2-mm embryo stage, beginning in the more cephalad portions of the embryo. Three sets of excretory ducts and tubules develop bilaterally. The first, the pronephros, with its pronephric ducts, forms in the most cranial portion of the embryo at about the beginning of the fourth week after conception. The tubules associated with the duct probably have no excretory function in the human. Late in the fourth week, a second set of tubules, the mesonephric tubules, and their accompanying mesonephric ducts begin to develop. These are associated with tufts of capillaries, or glomeruli, and tubules for excretory purposes. Thus, the **mesonephros** functions as a fetal kidney, producing urine for about 2 or 3 weeks. As new tubules develop, those derived from the more cephalad tubules degenerate. Usually about 40 mesonephric tubules function on either side of the embryo at any given time.

The **metanephros**, or permanent kidney, begins its development early in the fifth week of gestation and starts to function late in the seventh or early in the eighth week. The metanephros develops both from the metanephrogenic mass of mesoderm, which is the most caudal portion of the nephrogenic cord, and from its duct system, which is derived from the metanephric diverticulum (ureteric bud). It is a cranially growing outpouching of the mesonephric duct close to where it enters the cloaca. The metanephric duct system gives rise to the ureter, the renal pelvis, the calyces, and the collecting tubules of the adult kidney. A critical process in the development of the kidney requires that the cranially growing metanephric diverticulum meets and fuses with the metanephrogenic mass of mesoderm so that formation of the kidney can take place. Originally the metanephric kidney is a pelvic organ, but by differential growth it becomes located in the lumbar region.

The fetus produces urine throughout all the periods of gestation, but the placenta handles the excretory functions of the fetus. The urine produced by the fetus contributes to the amniotic fluid. The fetus may swallow the amniotic fluid and recirculate it through the digestive system. This seems to be an important factor in regulating the amount of amniotic fluid present in the fetus. Congenital abnormalities that impair normal development or function of the fetal kidneys generally result in little or no amniotic fluid (oligohydramnios or anhydramnios), whereas structural abnormalities of the gastrointestinal tract or neuromuscular conditions that prevent the fetus from swallowing can lead to excess amniotic fluid (polyhydramnios).

BLADDER AND URETHRA

The embryonic cloaca is divided by the urorectal septum into a dorsal rectum and a ventral urogenital sinus. The urogenital sinus, in turn, is divided into three parts: the cranial portion (the vesicourethral canal), which is continuous with the allantois; a middle pelvic portion; and a caudal urogenital sinus portion, which is covered externally by the urogenital membrane. The epithelium of the developing bladder is derived from the endoderm of the vesicourethral canal. The muscular layers and serosa of the bladder develop from adjacent splanchnic mesenchyme. As the bladder develops, the caudal portion of the mesonephric ducts is incorporated into its dorsal wall. The portion of the mesonephric duct distal to the points where the metanephric duct is taken up into the bladder becomes the trigone of the bladder. Although this portion is mesoderm in origin, it is probably epithelialized eventually by endodermal epithelium from the urogenital sinus. In this way the ureters, derived from the metanephric duct, come to open directly into the bladder.

In the male the mesonephric ducts open into the urethra as the ejaculatory ducts. Also in the male, mesenchymal tissue surrounding the developing urethra where it exits the bladder develops into the prostate gland, through which the ejaculatory ducts traverse. **Figure 1-9** demonstrates graphically the development of the male and female urinary systems. The epithelium of the female urethra is derived from endoderm of the vesicourethral canal. The urethral sphincter develops from a mesenchymal condensation around the urethra after the division of the cloaca in the 12- to 15-mm embryo. Following the opening of the anal membrane at the 20- to 30-mm stage, the puborectalis muscle appears. At 15 weeks' gestation, striated muscle can be seen, and a smooth muscle layer thickens at the level of the developing bladder neck, forming the inner part of the urethral musculature. Thus the urethral sphincter is composed of both central smooth muscle and peripheral striated muscle. The sphincter develops primarily in the anterior wall of the urethra in a horseshoe or omega shape.

SEX DIFFERENTIATION

Genetic sex is determined at the time of conception. A Y chromosome is necessary for the development of the testes, and the testes are responsible for the organization of the sexual duct system into a male configuration and for the suppression of the **paramesonephric (Müllerian) system**. In the absence of a Y chromosome or in the absence of a gonad, development will be female in nature. General phenotypic development of the female seems to be a neutral event, only slightly related to maternal estrogen activity. Sex differentiation occurs from genes that are coded on the Y chromosome. The primary determinant is the *SRY* gene, sometimes called the testis-determining factor. The *SRY* gene is found on the short arm of the Y chromosome. The *SRY* gene influences Sertoli cell differentiation, development of cells in the mesonephric ridge, and male architectural development of the gonad, including blood vessels and other structures of the testes. Several other genes, including those that express steroidogenic factor-1, WT1, DAX1, on other chromosomes are also necessary for normal testicular development. Male gonadal development precedes female development (**Fig. 1-10**). The secretion of testosterone and **anti-Müllerian hormone (AMH)** from the testes steers the further development of the rest of the genital tracts.

An interesting bit of evidence for the importance of the *SRY* gene in the development of male sexual differentiation is seen in the 45,X/47,XYY mosaics. Hsu reviewed the phenotypes of 15 postnatally diagnosed cases and found that 8 were female, 3 male, and 4 intersex. She postulated that the sex reversal occurred because of deletion or mutation of the *SRY* gene. To date, multiple mutations of the *SRY* gene have been reported, and all are associated with sex reversals (female phenotype). In very rare male individuals, a Y chromosome may be absent, but the *SRY* gene may be located on another chromosome, most commonly the X chromosome. Other rare genetic causes of gonadal dysgenesis may occur from mutations or deletions in a number of other genes that influence hormonal and cellular differentiation.

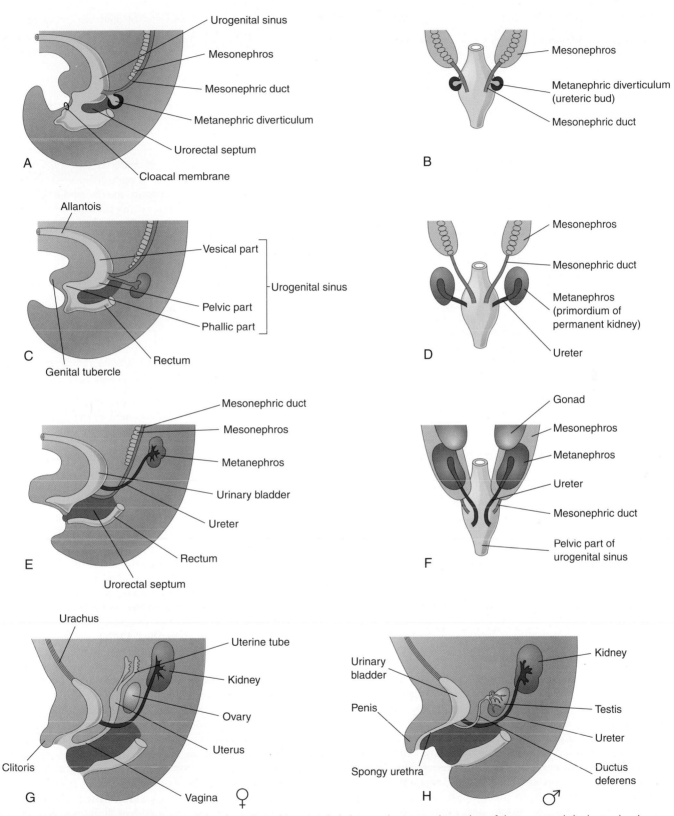

Figure 1-9 Diagrams showing division of the cloaca into the urogenital sinus and rectum; absorption of the mesonephric ducts; development of the urinary bladder, urethra, and urachus, and changes in the location of the ureters. **A,** Lateral view of the caudal half of a 5-week embryo. **B, D,** and **F,** Dorsal views. **C, E, G,** and **H,** Lateral views. The stages shown in **G** and **H** are reached by the twelfth week. (From Moore KL, Persaud TVN: The Developing Human: Clinically Oriented Embryology, 7th ed. Philadelphia, WB Saunders, 2003.)

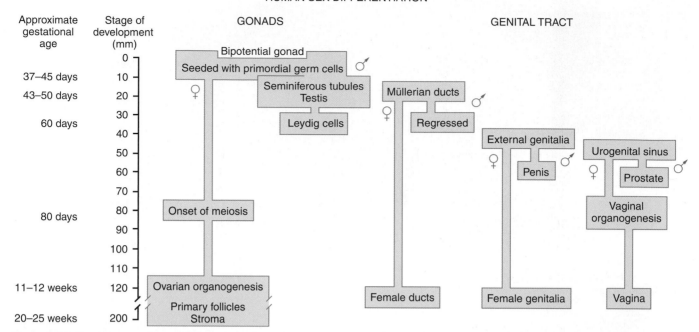

Figure 1-10 Development of sexual differentiation in the human. Note the lag from male to female development. (Modified from Grumbach MM, Hughes IA, Conte FA: Disorders of sex differentiation. In Larsen PR, Kronenberg HM, Melmed S, Polonsky KS [eds]: Williams Textbook of Endocrinology, 10th ed. Philadelphia, WB Saunders, 2003, p 870.)

During the fifth week after conception, coelomic epithelium, later known as germinal epithelium, thickens in the area of the medial aspect of the mesonephros. As germinal epithelial cells proliferate, they invade the underlying mesenchyme, producing a prominence known as the gonadal ridge. In the sixth week the primordial germ cells, which have formed at about week 4 in the wall of the yolk sac, migrate up the dorsal mesentery of the hindgut and enter the undifferentiated gonad. These cells may differentiate into the testes or ovaries. For the formation of a testis, the H-Y antigen must be activated. The somatic cells of the primitive gonadal ridge then differentiate into interstitial cells (Leydig cells) and Sertoli cells. As they do so, the primordial germ cells and Sertoli cells become enclosed within seminiferous tubules, and the interstitial cells remain outside these tubules. The H-Y antigen can be demonstrated in Sertoli cells at this stage but not in the developing germ cells. Sertoli cells are encased in the seminiferous tubules in the seventh and eighth weeks. In the eighth week Leydig cells differentiate and begin to produce testosterone. At this point the mesonephric (Wolffian) duct differentiates into the vas deferens, epididymis, and seminal vesicles, while the paramesonephric duct is suppressed because of the secretion and action of AMH.

Primary sex cords, meanwhile, have condensed and extended to the medullary portion of the developing testes. They branch and join to form the rete testis. The testis therefore is primarily a medullary organ, and eventually the rete testis connects with the tubules of the mesonephric system and joins the developing epididymal duct.

In specific androgen target areas, testosterone is converted to 5-α-dihydrotestosterone by the microsomal enzyme Δ-4-5-α-reductase. Data suggest that two androgens—testosterone and its metabolite, dihydrotestosterone—are involved in sexual differentiation in the male fetus, with selective roles for each hormone during embryogenesis; that is, dihydrotestosterone

stimulates the testes and scrotum, and testosterone stimulates the prostate gland.

Androgen action must be initiated at the target areas. Testosterone enters the cell and either is bound to a cytoplasmic receptor or, in certain target tissue, is converted to dihydrotestosterone. Dihydrotestosterone in such cells would then bind to a cytoplasmic receptor. Afterward, the androgen-receptor complex gains access to the nucleus, where it binds to chromatin and initiates the transcription of messenger ribonucleic acid. This leads to the metabolic process of androgen action.

For normal male development in utero, the testes must differentiate and function normally. At a critical point, AMH, produced by Sertoli cells, and testosterone, secreted by Leydig cells, must be produced in sufficient amounts. AMH acts locally in suppressing the Müllerian duct system, and testosterone acts systemically, causing differentiation of the mesonephric duct system and affecting male development of the urogenital tubercle, urogenital sinus, and urogenital folds. Thus, the masculinization of the fetus is a multifactorial process under a variety of genetic controls. Genes on the Y chromosome are responsible for testicular differentiation. Enzymes involved in testosterone biosynthesis and conversion to dihydrotestosterone are regulated by genes located on autosomes. The ability to secrete AMH is a recessive trait coded on either an autosome or the X chromosome, and genes for development of cytoplasmic receptors of androgens seem to be coded on the X chromosome.

Development of the ovary occurs at about the eleventh or twelfth week, though the primordial germ cells have migrated several weeks earlier to the germinal ridge (Fig. 1-11). Two functional X chromosomes seem necessary for optimal development of the ovary. The effect of an X chromosome deficiency is most severe in species in which there is a long period between the formation and use of oocytes (i.e., the human). Thus in 45,X and 46,XY females, the ovaries are almost invariably devoid of

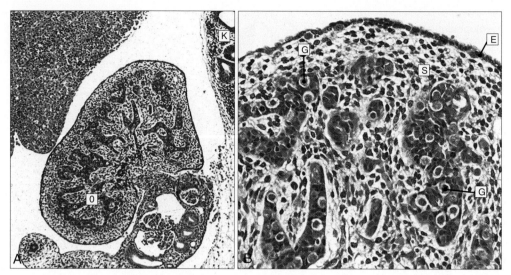

Figure 1-11 Ovary in embryo. **A,** The developing ovary (O) in a 9-week-old embryo is shown close to the developing kidney (K). **B,** At this stage of development, the columns of primordial germ cells (G) are embedded in a mesenchymal stroma (S) covered by a layer of cuboidal surface cells (E). (From Stevens A, Lowe J: Human Histology, 3 rd ed. Philadelphia, Elsevier Mosby, 2005, p 357.)

oocytes. On the other hand, germ cells in the testes do best when only one X chromosome is present; rarely do they survive in the XX or XXY condition.

When non-Y-bearing oocytes enter the differentiating gonad, the primary sex cords do not become prominent but, instead, break up and encircle the oocytes in the cortex of the gonad (in contrast to the structure of the XY gonad). This occurs at about 16 weeks' gestation, and the isolated cell clusters derived from the cortical cords that surround the oocytes are called primordial follicles. No new oogonia form after birth, and many of the oogonia degenerate before birth. Those that remain grow and become primary follicles to be stimulated after puberty. The processes of gonadal development are schematically summarized in **Figure 1-12.**

GENITAL DUCT SYSTEM

Early in embryonic life, two sets of paired genital ducts develop in each sex: the mesonephric (Wolffian) ducts and the paramesonephric (Müllerian) ducts. The mesonephric duct development precedes the paramesonephric duct development. The paramesonephric ducts develop on each side of the mesonephric ducts from the evaginations of the coelomic epithelium. The more cephalad ends of the ducts open directly into the peritoneal cavity, and the distal ends grow caudally, fusing in the lower midline to form the uterovaginal **primordium.** This tubular structure joins the dorsal wall of the urogenital sinus and produces an elevation, the Müllerian tubercle. The mesonephric ducts enter the urogenital sinus on either side of the tubercle.

Male Genital Ducts

Some seminiferous tubules are produced in the fetal testes during the seventh and eighth weeks after conception. During the eighth week, interstitial (Leydig) cells differentiate and begin to produce testosterone. At this point the mesonephric duct differentiates into the vas deferens, epididymis, and seminal vesicles, and the Müllerian **anlage** is suppressed by the action of AMH, previously called Müllerian-inhibiting factor (MIF), produced by the Sertoli cells of the testes. The development of the

prostate gland was referred to earlier. The bulbourethral glands, which are small structures that develop from outgrowths of endodermal tissue from the membranous portion of the urethra, incorporate stroma from the adjacent mesenchyme. The most distal portion of the paramesonephric duct remains, in the male, as the appendix of the testes. The most proximal end of the paramesonephric duct remains as a small outpouching within the body of the prostate gland, known as the prostatic utricle. Rarely, the prostatic utricle is developed to the point where it will excrete a small amount of blood and cause hematuria in adult life.

Female Genital Ducts

In the presence of ovaries or of gonadal agenesis, the mesonephric ducts regress, and the paramesonephric ducts develop into the female genital tract. This process begins at about 6 weeks and proceeds in a cephalad to caudal fashion. The more cephalad portions of the paramesonephric ducts, which open directly into the peritoneal cavity, form the fallopian tubes. The fused portion, or uterovaginal primordium, gives rise to the epithelium and glands of the uterus and cervix. Endometrial stroma and myometrium are derived from adjacent mesenchyme.

Failure of development of the paramesonephric ducts leads to agenesis of the cervix and the uterus. Failure of fusion of the caudal portion of these ducts may lead to a variety of uterine anomalies, including complete duplication of the uterus and cervix or partial duplication of a variety of types, which are outlined in Chapter 11 (Congenital Anomalies of the Female Reproductive Tract).

Peritoneal reflections in the area adjacent to the fusion of the two paramesonephric ducts give rise to the formation of the broad ligaments. Mesenchymal tissue here develops into the parametrium.

Pietryga and Wózniak studied the development of uterine ligaments, documenting the development of the round ligament at the eighth week, the cardinal ligaments at the tenth week, and the broad ligament at week 19. From weeks 8 to 17, the round ligament is connected to the uterine tube. Beginning at week 18, it comes to arise from the edge of the uterus.

The vagina develops from paired solid outgrowths of endoderm of the urogenital sinus—the sinovaginal bulbs. These grow

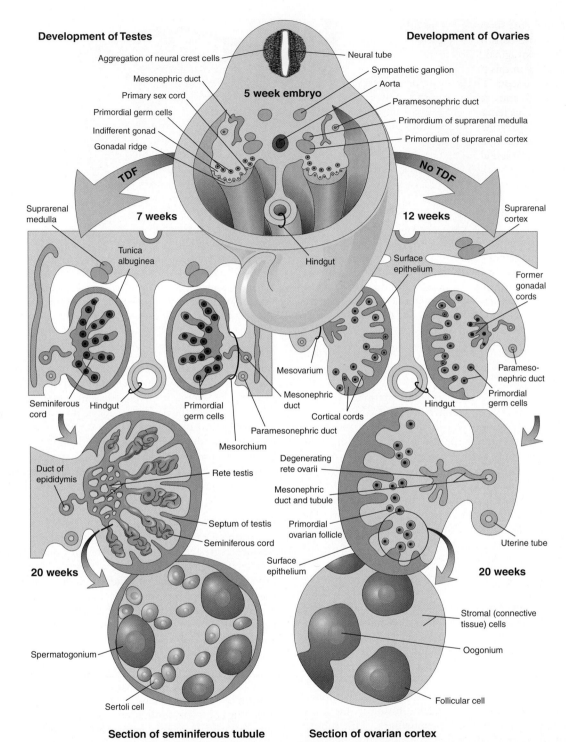

Figure 1-12 Schematic illustration showing differentiation of the indifferent gonads of a 5-week embryo *(top)* into ovaries or testes. Left side shows the development of testes resulting from the effects of the testis-determining factor (TDF), also called the SRY gene, located on the Y chromosome. Note that the gonadal cords become seminiferous cords, the primordium of the seminiferous tubules. The parts of the gonadal cords that enter the medulla of the testis form the rete testis. In the section of the testis at the bottom left, observe that there are two kinds of cells: spermatogonia derived from the primordial germ cells and sustentacular (Sertoli) cells derived from mesenchyme. Right side shows the development of ovaries in the absence of TDF. Cortical cords have extended from the surface epithelium of the gonad, and primordial cells have entered them. They are the primordia of the oogonia. Follicular cells are derived from the surface epithelium of the ovary. (From Moore KL, Persaud TVN: The Developing Human: Clinically Oriented Embryology, 7th ed. Philadelphia, WB Saunders, 2003.)

caudally as a solid core toward the end of the uterovaginal primordium. This core constitutes the fibromuscular portion of the vagina. The sinovaginal bulbs then canalize to form the vagina. Abnormalities in this process may lead to either transverse or horizontal vaginal septa. The junction of the sinovaginal bulbs with the urogenital sinus remains as the vaginal plate, which forms the hymen. This remains imperforate until late in embryonic life, although occasionally, perforation does not take place completely (imperforate hymen).

Failure of the sinovaginal bulbs to form leads to agenesis of the vagina. The precise boundary between the paramesonephric and urogenital sinus portions of the vagina has not been established.

Auxiliary genital glands in the female form from buds that grow out of the urethra. The buds derive contributions from the surrounding mesenchyme and form the urethral glands and the paraurethral glands (Skene glands). These glands correspond to the prostate gland in males. Similar outgrowths of the urogenital sinus form the vestibular glands (Bartholin glands), which are homologous to the bulbourethral glands in the male.

The remnants of the mesonephric duct in the female include a small structure called the appendix vesiculosa, a few blind tubules in the broad ligaments (the epoophoron), and a few blind tubules adjacent to the uterus (collectively called the paroöphoron). Remnants of the mesonephric duct system are often present in the broad ligaments or may be present adjacent to the uterus and/or the vagina as **Gartner duct** cysts. The epoophoron or paroöphoron may develop into cysts. Cysts of the epoophoron are known as paraovarian cysts (Chapter 18, Benign Gynecologic Lesions).

Remnants of the paramesonephric duct in the female may be seen as a small, blind cystic structure attached by a pedicle to the distal end of the fallopian tube—the hydatid of Morgagni.

Table 1-2 categorizes the adult derivatives and residual remnants of the urogenital structures in both the male and the female. Figure 1-13 outlines schematically the development of the internal sexual organs in both sexes.

EXTERNAL GENITALIA

In the fourth week after fertilization, the genital tubercle develops at the ventral tip of the cloacal membrane. Two sets of lateral bodies—the labioscrotal swellings and urogenital folds—develop soon after on either side of the cloacal membrane. The genital tubercle then elongates to form a phallus in both males and females. By the end of the sixth week, the cloacal membrane is joined by the urorectal septum. The septum separates the cloaca into the urogenital sinus ventrally and the anal canal and rectum dorsally. The point on the cloacal membrane where the urorectal septum fuses becomes the location of the perineal body in later development. The cloacal membrane is then divided into the ventral urogenital membrane and the dorsal anal membrane. These membranes then rupture, opening the vulva and the anal canal. Failure of the anal membrane to rupture gives rise to an imperforate anus. With the opening of the urogenital membrane, a urethral groove forms on the undersurface of the phallus, completing the undifferentiated portion of external genital development. Differences between male and female embryos can be noted as early as the ninth week, but the distinct final forms are not noted until 12 weeks' gestation (**Fig. 1-14**).

Androgens (testosterone and dihydrotestosterone), produced by the testes and by peripheral conversion of testosterone in target cells, respectively, are responsible for the masculinization of the undifferentiated external genitalia in males. The phallus grows in length to form a penis, and the urogenital folds are pulled forward to form the lateral walls of the urethral groove

Table 1-2 Male and Female Derivatives of Embryonic Urogenital Structures

	Derivatives	
Embryonic Structure	**Male**	**Female**
Labioscrotal swellings	Scrotum	Labia majora
Urogenital folds	Ventral portion of penis	Labia minora
Phallus	Penis	Clitoris
	Glans, corpora cavernosa penis, and corpus spongiosum	Glans, corpora cavernosa, bulb of the vestibule
Urogenital sinus	Urinary bladder	Urinary bladder
	Prostate gland	Urethral and paraurethral glands
	Prostatic utricle	Vagina
	Bulbourethral glands	Greater vestibular glands
	Seminal colliculus	Hymen
Paramesonephric duct	Appendix of testes	Hydatid of Morgagni
		Uterus and cervix
		Fallopian tubes
Mesonephric duct	Appendix of epididymis	Appendix vesiculosis
	Ductus of epididymis	Duct of epoophoron
	Ductus deferens	Gartner's duct
	Ejaculatory duct and seminal vesicle	—
Metanephric duct	Ureters, renal pelvis, calyces, and collecting system	Ureter, renal pelvis, calyces, and collecting system
Mesonephric tubules	Ductuli efferentes	Epoophoron
	Paradidymis	Paroöphoron
Undifferentiated gonad	Testis	Ovary
Cortex	Seminiferous tubules	Ovarian follicles
Medulla	—	Medulla
	Rete testis	Rete ovarii
Gubernaculum	Gubernaculum testis	Round ligament of uterus

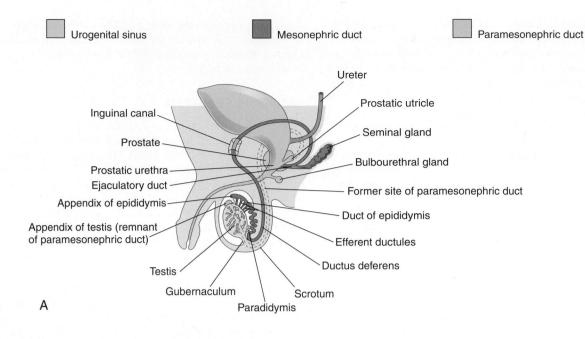

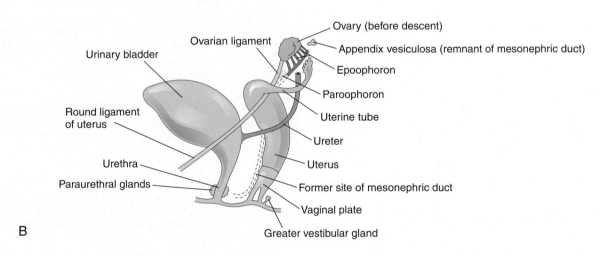

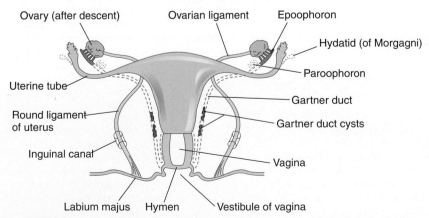

Figure 1-13 Schematic drawings illustrating development of the male and female reproductive systems from the genital ducts and urogenital sinus. Vestigial structures are also shown. **A,** Reproductive system in a newborn male. **B,** Female reproductive system in a 12-week fetus. **C,** Reproductive system in a newborn female. (From Moore KL, Persaud TVN: The Developing Human: Clinically Oriented Embryology, 7th ed. Philadelphia, WB Saunders, 2003.)

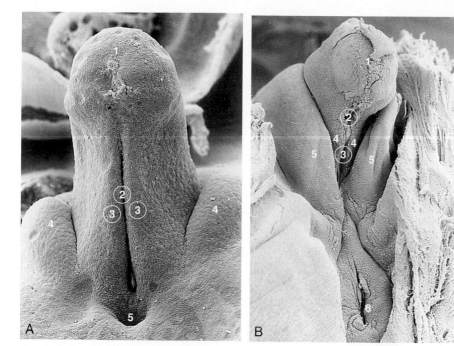
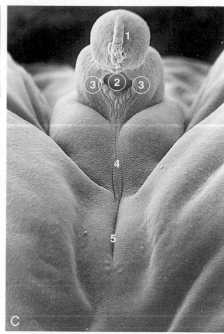

Figure 1-14 Scanning electron micrographs (SEMs) of the developing male external genitalia. **A,** SEM of the perineum during the indifferent state of a 17-mm, 7-week embryo (×100). 1, Developing glans of penis with the ectodermal cord. 2, Urethral groove continuous with the urogenital sinus. 3, Urogenital folds. 4, Labioscrotal swellings. 5, Anus. **B,** External genitalia of a 7.2-cm, 10-week female fetus (×45). 1, Glans of clitoris. 2, External urethral orifice. 3, Opening into urogenital sinus. 4, Urogenital folds (labia minora). 5, Labioscrotal swelling (labia majora). 6, Anus. **C,** SEM of the external genitalia of a 5.5-cm, 10-week male fetus (×40). 1, Glans of penis with ectodermal cord. 2, Remains of urethral groove. 3, Urogenital folds in the process of closing. 4, Labioscrotal swelling fusing to form the raphe of the scrotum. 5, Anus. (From Moore KL, Persaud TVN: The Developing Human: Clinically Oriented Embryology, 7th ed. Philadelphia, WB Saunders, 2003.)

on the undersurface of the penis. These folds then fuse to form the penile urethra. Defects in fusion of various amounts give rise to various degrees of hypospadias. The skin at the distal margin of the penis grows over the glans to form the prepuce (foreskin). The vascular portion of the penis (corpora cavernosa penis and corpus cavernosum urethrae) arises from the mesenchymal tissue of the phallus. Finally, the labioscrotal swellings grow toward each other and fuse in the midline to form the scrotum. Later in embryonic life, usually at about the twenty-eighth week, the testes descend through the inguinal canal guided by the gubernaculum.

Androgen receptors have been found in the fetus in the corpus cavernosum and the stroma of the inner prepuce, scrotum, and periphery of the glans penis. The periurethral mesenchyme, the early progenitor of the corpus spongiosum, is also rich in androgen receptors. The epithelium of the preputial skin, penile shaft skin, and scrotal skin are initially androgen-receptor-negative. No estrogen receptors have been noted in these regions, suggesting that maternal estrogen has no direct influence on male genital development. Female external genital structures also contain androgen receptors, and the distribution of androgen receptors resembles that of the male. This would explain why female genitalia can be masculinized if exposed to high androgen levels early in gestation. Diseases of incomplete or absent masculinization of a male (XY karyotype) fetus may occur for three reasons: (1) inadequate or deficient secretion of androgens or peripheral conversion of testosterone to dihydrotestosterone, (2) absence or deficient receptors, or (3) deficient or absent AMH.

Feminization of the undifferentiated external genitalia occurs in the absence of androgen stimulation. The embryonic phallus does not demonstrate rapid growth and becomes the clitoris. Urogenital folds do not fuse except in front of the anus. The unfused urogenital folds form the labia minora. The labioscrotal folds fuse posteriorly in the area of the perineal body but laterally remain as the labia majora. Beyond 12 weeks' gestation, the labioscrotal folds will not fuse if the fetus is exposed to androgens, though masculinization may occur in other organs of the external genitalia. The labioscrotal folds fuse anteriorly to form the mons pubis. A portion of the urogenital sinus between the level of the hymen and the labia develops into the vestibule of the vagina, into which the urethra, the vagina, and the ducts of Bartholin glands enter. The work of Kalloo and coworkers demonstrated that female external genitalia are intensely estrogen-receptor-positive compared with the genitalia of the male. These receptors may be seen primarily in the stroma of the labia minora and in the periphery of the glans and interprepuce. The presence of such receptors suggests that there may be a direct role of maternal estrogens in the development of female external genitalia. This is in contrast to the long-held belief that female genital development was passive and occurred in the absence of androgens. Virilization, masculinization, of a female (karyotype XX) fetus may occur from exposure to androgens, either from the mother or through fetal androgens as a result of genetic deficiencies in the steroid biosynthetic pathway such as occurs in congenital adrenal hyperplasia.

The ovaries do not descend into the labioscrotal folds. A structure similar to the gubernaculum develops in the inguinal canal, giving rise to the round ligaments, which suspend the uterus in the adult. **Figure 1-15** summarizes the development of the external genitalia in each sex.

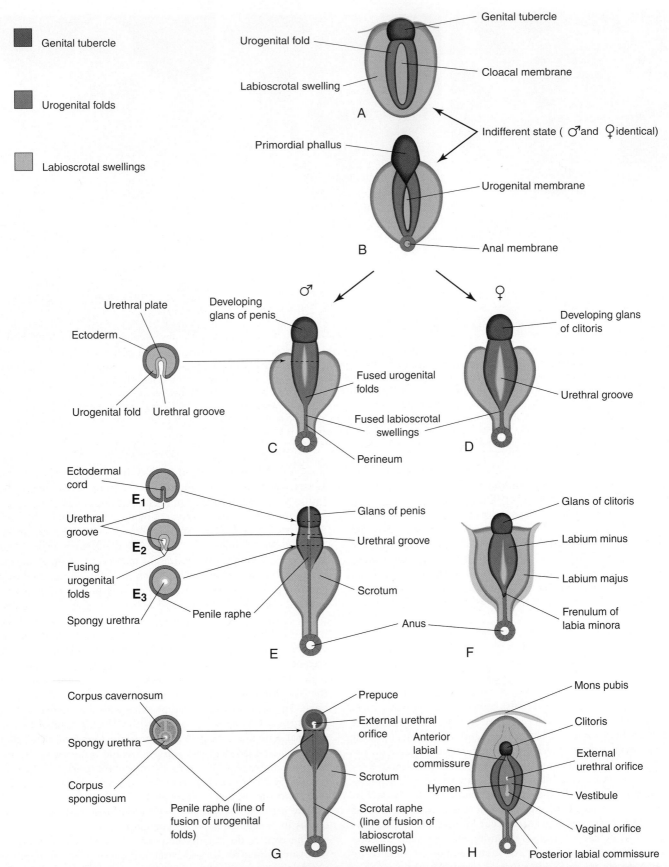

Figure 1-15 Development of the external genitalia. **A** and **B,** Diagrams illustrating the appearance of the genitalia during the indifferent state (fourth to seventh weeks). **C, E,** and **G,** Stages in the development of male external genitalia at 9, 11, and 12 weeks, respectively. To the left are schematic transverse sections of the developing penis, illustrating formation of the spongy urethra. **D, F,** and **H,** Stages in the development of female genitalia at 9, 11, and 12 weeks, respectively. (From Moore KL, Persaud TVN: The Developing Human: Clinically Oriented Embryology, 7th ed. Philadelphia, WB Saunders, 2003.)

KEY POINTS

- Oocyte meiosis is arrested at prophase I from the fetal period until the time of ovulation.
- Fertilization occurs in the ampulla of the fallopian tube before the second polar body is cast off.
- After fertilization, first cell division leading to the two-cell embryo takes 20 hr.
- The human embryo enters the uterus somewhere between 3 and 4 days after conception. Preimplantation genetic diagnosis in conjunction with IVF techniques could be accomplished at this time. By the time the embryo enters the uterus, it will be between the 32-cell and blastocyst stages of development.
- Implantation occurs when trophoblastic cells contact endometrium and burrow beneath the surface by enzymatic action. This generally takes place 3 days after the embryo enters the uterus.
- Twinning may occur at any time until the formation of the blastula, after which time each cell is no longer pluripotent.
- The earliest fetal epithelium to develop is the ectoderm, the second is the endoderm, and the third is the mesoderm.
- HCG is secreted by the syncytiotrophoblast at about the time of implantation. It doubles in quantity every 1.2 to 2 days until 7 to 9 weeks' gestation.
- Angiogenesis is seen by day 15 or 16. Embryonic heart function begins in the third week of gestation.
- Organogenesis is complete by postconception day 49.

- The mesonephric duct system gives rise in the male to the epididymis, vas deferens, and seminal vesicles. Remnants of the mesonephric duct system in the female remain as parovarian cysts and the Gartner duct.
- The paramesonephric duct system develops in the female to give rise to the fallopian tube, uterus, and cervix. Remnants give rise to the hydatid of Morgagni at the end of the fallopian tubes. Remnants in the male remain as the appendix of the testes and prostatic utricle. This duct system is suppressed in the male by the action of AMH.
- The vagina develops from the sinovaginal bulbs, which are outgrowths of the urogenital sinus. Failure of these bulbs to form leads to agenesis of the vagina.
- The adult kidney develops from the metanephros, and its collecting system (ureter and calyceal system) develops from the metanephric (ureteric) bud from the mesonephric duct.
- The urinary bladder develops from the urogenital sinus.
- A Y chromosome is responsible for the development of testes. Without the presence of a Y chromosome, the gonadal development is usually that of an ovary or is undifferentiated. If no testicular tissue is present, the paramesonephric duct system develops into a phenotypic female configuration, and the mesonephric duct system is suppressed.
- The genital tubercle elongates to form the penis in the male and the clitoris in the female.
- Two functional X chromosomes are necessary for optimal development of the ovary.

RECOMMENDED READING

Delhanty JD, Harper JC: Pre-implantation genetic diagnosis, *Baillieres Best Pract Res Clin Obstet Gynaecol* 14(4):691, 2000.

Feckner P: The role of Sry in mammalian sex determination, *Acta Paediatr Jpn* 38:380, 1996.

MacLaughlin DT, Donahoe PK: Sex determination and differentiation, *N Engl J Med* 150:367–378, 2004.

Moore KL, Persaud TVN: *The Developing Human: Clinically Oriented Embryology*, ed 8, Philadelphia, 2008, WB Saunders.

REFERENCES CAN BE FOUND ON
EXPERTCONSULT.com

2

Reproductive Genetics
Gene Structure, Mutation, Molecular Tools, Types of Inheritance, Counseling Issues, Oncogenes

Edith Cheng and Vern L. Katz

A number of illnesses and conditions have a genetic basis. In some cases the problem arises from a single-point **mutation** within a **gene**, whereas others may involve changes in multiple genes or in an interreaction of genes and environmental factors. Finally, some conditions are the result of **chromosome** abnormalities of a variety of types. Although this chapter cannot provide a complete course in genetics, it attempts to offer an understanding of the genetic basis of conditions of particular interest to the gynecologist.

GENE STRUCTURE, EXPRESSION, AND MUTATION

Genetic information is stored in the form of deoxyribonucleic acid (DNA) molecules, which are made up of a linear sequence of nucleotides intertwined together as a double helix. The backbone of the linear DNA molecule is composed of a phosphate and a pentose sugar (deoxyribose) to which is attached a nitrogen base. Four such bases are found in a DNA molecule: two purines (adenine [A] and guanine [G]) and two pyrimidines (thymine [T] and cytosine [C]). Purine and pyrimidine occur in equal amounts; A is always paired with T in the two strands of the double helix, and G is always paired with C. These associations allow for accuracy both in the replication of the DNA molecule and in the translation of a genetic message from the DNA molecule to a single-strand **ribonucleic acid (RNA)** molecule known as *messenger RNA* (mRNA). The message is transmitted in such a fashion that a configuration with three bases in sequence (**codon**) represents a code, known as the *genetic code,* for an amino acid. With the message of the gene encoded on the mRNA, the latter leaves the nucleus of the cell, attaches to a cytoplasmic structure (the ribosome), and then attracts amino acids by means of smaller RNA molecules known as *transfer RNA (tRNA).* Transfer RNA molecules each carry a specific amino acid and have three bases, which match the code of the mRNA, following the A-to-T and G-to-C pairings. In the RNA molecule, uracil (U) is substituted for thymine. When all segments of the message are covered, the amino acids are spliced together, and the protein determined by the message is complete and free for use in the cell and for transport from the cell. **Figure 2-1** schematically demonstrates this process.

In its simplest form, a gene is a sequence of codons that, when transcribed and translated, will become a functional product. However, with the exception of a few organisms, the sequences of base pairs that actually form a gene in eukaryotes are complex and provide many opportunities for different types of mutations to occur. **Figure 2-2** illustrates the structure of a typical human gene. Most genes have a promoter region and transcriptional start point, both of which are necessary to begin transcription. Within the gene itself, regions of coding sequences (**exons**) are interspaced with noncoding regions (**introns**). At the end of the gene, there is a termination site and other regulatory elements that end the transcriptional process for that gene.

Transcription occurs through both intron and exon portions of the gene and beyond the position on the chromosome that corresponds to the most distal part of the gene. The resulting primary RNA transcript then undergoes many posttranscriptional modifications, including splicing out the introns and splicing together the exons, placing a "chemical cap" on the 5′ end and a "tail" of adenosine nucleotides (poly A) at the 3′ end. The poly A tail appears to stabilize the mature mRNA, which is now ready for transport into the cytoplasm for translation. In the cytoplasm, after translation, the resultant protein often undergoes further posttranslational modifications.

A gene mutation occurs when there has been a change in the genetic code; these changes are the source of genetic variation. The mutation may involve changing a single base, known as a point mutation, or a larger segment, in which bases are removed, duplicated, or inserted. Mutations occur as a result of environmental damage to DNA, through errors during DNA replication or repair, and through uneven crossing over and genetic exchange during meiosis. The loss or gain of bases may disrupt the reading frame of the triplet codons. The consequences depend on the location of the mutation: In a promoter region, it may enhance or prevent transcription; in splice site junctions between introns and exons, there may be duplications or **deletions** of those sequences such that the resulting mRNA cannot be translated into a functional product; or mutations could affect the poly A tail and thus the stability of the mRNA. The position of the mutation in the gene is also important; a mutation at the beginning of the gene can be so disruptive that transcription ceases at the site of the mutation. No mRNA is generated and, therefore, no gene product. Conversely, a mutation at the end of the gene may result in a truncated but still translatable mRNA, leading to a partially

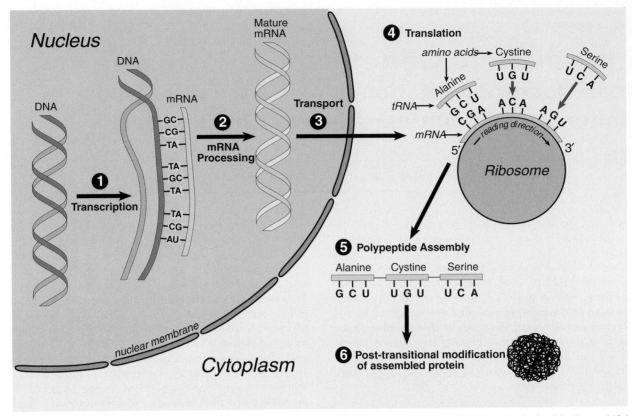

Figure 2-1 Schematic representation of polypeptide production from genetic message to final product. (Courtesy of Edith Cheng, MD.)

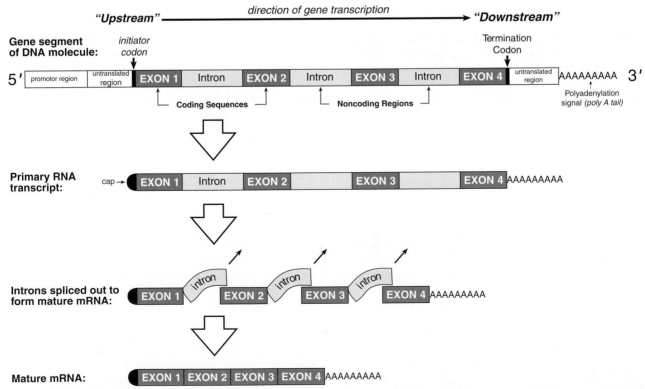

Figure 2-2 Structure of typical human gene and its processing to become a mature mRNA transcript for translation. Mutations can affect any of these steps. (Courtesy of Edith Cheng, MD.)

Hemoglobin-Binding Protein	DNA Triplet Codons		Amino Acid
HgbA (normal)	CTT	CTC	→ Glutamic acid
HgbS	CAT	CAC	→ Valine
HgbC	TTT	TTC	→ Lysine

Figure 2-3 A single base pair substitution in the same DNA triplet codon for glutamic acid at amino acid position 6 for normal hemoglobin results in hemoglobin S (valine in sickle cell disease) or hemoglobin C (lysine in Hgb C disease). (Courtesy of Edith Cheng, MD.)

functional gene product. Point mutations within the gene could result in an amino acid substitution, leading to different products with altered functions. **Figure 2-3** demonstrates such an occurrence for sickle cell anemia caused by the substitution of a single base at a single point. The cystic fibrosis transmembrane conductance regulator (CFTR) gene is an example of a gene for which more than 1000 mutations or **alleles** have been described to date. Some genes also have regions that are more prone (hot spots) to mutational events.

In spite of the potential clinical importance of mutations, only a small fraction of the **genome**, about 2% to 5%, actually encodes protein or has regulatory significance. In addition, most base pair changes in coding sequences do not lead to a change in amino acid substitution. These mutations are known as silent substitutions. These benign substitutions are generally passed on from generation to generation and are referred to as **polymorphisms**. The term *mutation,* then, is generally reserved for new changes in the genetic code that lead to altered function and clinical consequences.

MOLECULAR TOOLS AND DIAGNOSIS IN HUMAN GENETICS

Technical advances in molecular genetics have made it possible to study mutations either directly or indirectly. The use of **polymerase chain reaction (PCR)** permits rapid amplification of a sequence of DNA or multiple different sequences simultaneously for analysis. This section covers common molecular techniques of which the gynecologist should have a basic understanding.

POLYMERASE CHAIN REACTION

PCR has essentially revolutionized DNA diagnostics and medicine. Our daily laboratory assessment of the subject's medical issues now relies heavily on material amplified by PCR. This is essentially a form of cloning, because PCR can selectively amplify a single sequence of DNA or RNA several billion-fold in only a few hours. By taking advantage of the double-stranded complimentary pairing characteristics of DNA, the PCR reaction separates (denatures) the two strands and uses each strand as a template to synthesize two more copies (**Fig. 2-4**). Target sequences of DNA flanked by primers undergo repeated cycles of heat penetration, hybridization with primers, and DNA synthesis, resulting in an exponential amplification of the target DNA sequence.

RESTRICTION ENDONUCLEASES AND RESTRICTION FRAGMENT LENGTH POLYMORPHISMS

The key to the analysis of DNA sequences has been the discovery of a group of more than 1000 bacterial enzymes, called **restriction endonucleases**, that recognize and cut specific nucleotide sequences in the double-stranded DNA molecule. The sites of their action are known as restriction sites. Each enzyme recognizes a unique sequence of nucleotides, usually a palindrome of four to eight base pairs (bp) in length, and will cut the double-stranded DNA molecule wherever the specific site is recognized. For example, *Hind*III cuts the palindromic site 5'-AAGCTT-3' at A and T. **Table 2-1** lists some of the more commonly used restriction endonucleases and their cut sites. Restriction endonucleases are used to digest a sample of DNA (e.g., extracted from a subject for carrier testing) into a collection of DNA **fragments** in varying sizes. These fragments are then separated by gel electrophoresis according to size and denatured into single strands, which are then transferred (blotted) onto a nitrocellulose or nylon filter. The single-stranded DNA sequences of interest are then hybridized with the known sequence, which has been radioactively labeled (probe). The hybridized sequences are then detected. This method, known as Southern blotting, permits identification of specific DNA fragments of interest and, in some cases, the number of copies of the fragment. **Figure 2-5** is an example of how Southern blotting is used to detect the sickle cell gene. Some cut sites of restriction endonucleases result in "sticky ends," such as those generated by *Eco*RI. This property of *Eco*RI is used to create recombinant DNA. Benign base pair changes at cut sites that alter the recognition site of a restriction endonuclease will result in a change in the fragment size generated. Mutations within a gene or near a gene can also alter the recognition sites of restriction endonucleases, which will generate an altered length of DNA fragment containing the gene of interest. These **restriction fragment length polymorphisms (RFLPs)** can be used to follow the transmission of a gene in a family.

MICROARRAY TECHNOLOGY

Microarray technology, first introduced in 1995, permits the expression and analysis of thousands of genes simultaneously. Initially it was used to understand the molecular basis of cancer and the biologic behavior of tumors (**Fig. 2-6**). This powerful tool can provide a "molecular fingerprint" of an individual's disease and is referred to as gene expression profiling (GEP). Molecular differences revealed by gene expression patterns of individuals with the same condition, such as type 2 diabetes, may give insights into the mechanisms contributing to the disease, to its prognosis, and to more specific treatments, such as individualized drug therapy. More recently, this technology has expanded into genome-wide microarrays designed to cover the entire human genome. These microarrays, known as array comparative genomic hybridization (aCGH), can detect duplications and deletions across the human genome. Array CGH has resolution at less than 3 Mb compared with conventional cytogenetics, which detects chromosomal deletions or duplications at 3 to 10 Mb. Genomic imbalances have been identified in as many as 10% of individuals with unexplained mental retardation with normal **karyotypes**. The increasing use of aCGH in clinical genetics has generated interest in applying this technology to prenatal

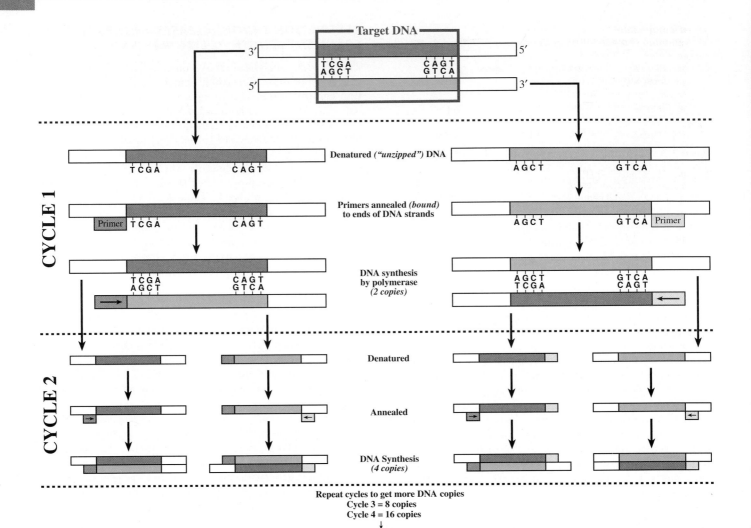

Figure 2-4 Schematic representation of the polymerase chain reaction (PCR). (Courtesy of Edith Cheng, MD.)

Table 2-1 Examples of Common Restriction Endonucleases, Their Source, and Their Recognition Sequence

Restriction Enzymes	Recognition Sequence	Source
BamHI	Bacillus amyloliquefaciens H	5'-G^GATC C-3' 3'-C CTAG^G-5
EcoRI	Escherichia coli RY 13	G^AATT C C TTAA^G
HaeIII	Haemophilus aegyptius	GG^CC CC^GG
HindIII	Haemophilus influenzae R_d	A^AGCT T T TCGA^A
NotI	Nocardia otitidis-cavarium	GC^GGCC GC CG CCGG^CG
Sau3A	Staphylococcus aureus 3A	^GATC CTAG^
SerII	Streptomyces stanford	CC GC^GG GG^CG CC

^ = cleavage sites.
From Thompson MW, Thompson HFV: Genetics in Medicine, 6th ed. Philadelphia, WB Saunders, 1991.

diagnosis. However, because of the limitations of this technology in detecting balanced chromosome rearrangements and the detection of copy number variations of uncertain clinical significance, the American Congress of Obstetricians and Gynecologists issued a committee opinion (Number 446, November 2009) with guidelines for the use of aCGH in prenatal diagnosis.

GENETIC TESTING: DIRECT AND INDIRECT METHODS

For many genetic conditions, the gene and its mutations (e.g., cystic fibrosis) responsible for the condition have been molecularly characterized. In these conditions, direct testing for the actual mutation in an affected individual to confirm the clinical diagnosis or to provide presymptomatic diagnosis or prenatal diagnosis would be possible by obtaining DNA from the subject. Direct testing or typing of the disease causing the mutation can be accomplished by sequencing the gene itself or through analysis of RFLPS. As is the case with sickle cell anemia, the mutation within the gene itself leads to an alteration that removes a cut site, resulting in a larger fragment that is associated with

Figure 2-5 Schematic representation of the Southern blot procedure—in this case, for diagnosis of sickle cell disease. Genomic DNA from the carrier parents, an unaffected daughter, and the affected son is extracted from a sample of peripheral blood. The DNA samples are digested with restriction enzymes and fragmented into smaller pieces. In this case, the restriction enzyme *Mst*II is used specifically because it recognizes the normal sequences that encompass the codons for glutamic acid at position 6 of the hemoglobin A polypeptide. The DNA fragments are separated based on size by gel electrophoresis, then they are transferred (blotted) onto a nitrocellulose filter. The DNA of the filter paper is then hybridized with a specifically labeled DNA probe containing the sequences of interest. The fluorescent or radioactive probe is visualized as bands at sites where the genomic DNA has hybridized with the labeled DNA. (Courtesy of Edith Cheng, MD.)

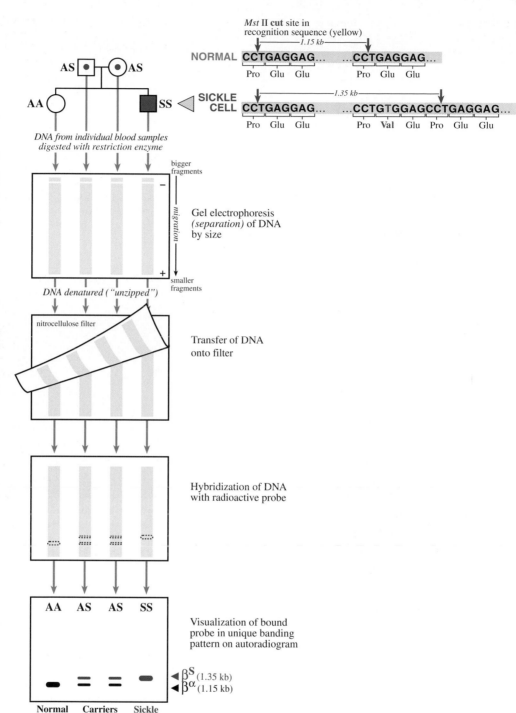

the mutation. This example also illustrates that the entire hemoglobin gene does not have to be analyzed to identify the mutation responsible for sickle cell anemia.

When "direct testing" is not possible, as is the case when the disease-causing gene has not been isolated, when the gene is too large to sequence, or when a mutation cannot be directly found, indirect testing using linkage analysis is the alternative strategy. This approach does not involve direct examination of the disease-causing mutation. The simplest explanation for this concept is that DNA markers located (or tightly linked) to the presumptive disease-causing gene/mutation are used as road maps to identify the travel or passage of the gene from an affected parent to an at-risk offspring. This strategy requires that the affected individual has markers that are informative—in other words, unique or distinctive from markers of the non-affected individual. Multiple family members, both affected and unaffected, must have DNA available for analysis in order for this approach to be informative. The "markers" are often RFLPs. **Figure 2-7** uses autosomal dominant breast cancer as an example of how linkage studies are used to predict the inheritance of a gene for which direct mutational analysis is not possible.

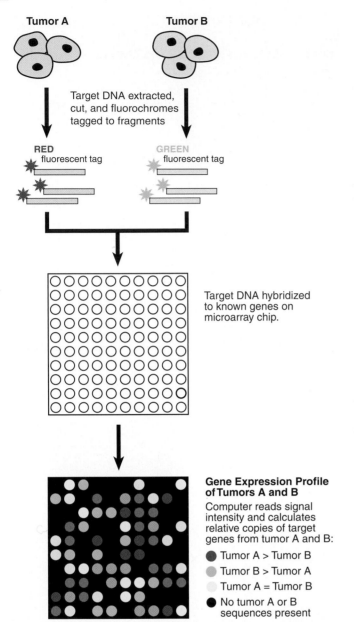

Figure 2-6 Schematic example of how microarray technology can be used to study or compare gene expression patterns from different sources. Here, it is used to compare the gene expression profiles of two different tumors. However, one can easily substitute DNA from two individuals with diabetes. (Courtesy of Edith Cheng, MD.)

MOLECULAR CYTOGENETICS

Molecular cytogenetic technology is a powerful tool to analyze chromosome abnormalities (deletions, additions, rearrangements) that are not visible using traditional karyotyping and microscopy. The most widely used procedure is fluorescent in situ hybridization (FISH). Like PCR and Southern blotting, FISH takes advantage of the complimentary nature of DNA. In this approach, denatured DNA sequences labeled with a fluorescent dye are hybridized onto denatured chromosomes that have been immobilized onto a slide. The chromosomes are then viewed with a wavelength of light that excites the fluorescent dye (**Fig. 2-8**). FISH is used commonly to screen for chromosome aneuploidy in amniotic fluid cells in prenatal diagnosis

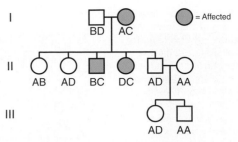

Figure 2-7 Hypothetical autosomal dominant condition illustrating the principle of indirect mutational analysis. Genetic markers A, B, C, D are used. In this pedigree, it appears that the condition segregates (travels) with marker C. Therefore, the male and female in generation III, who did not inherit marker C, are not expected to manifest the condition. (Courtesy of Edith Cheng, MD.)

WCP: Chromosomes 1 and 4

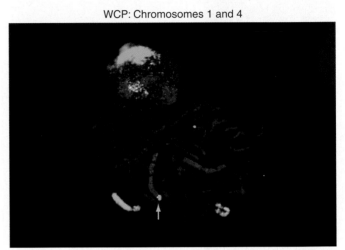

Figure 2-8 Example of fluorescent in situ hybridization (FISH) with whole-chromosome DNA (whole-chromosome paint [WCP] from chromosomes 1 (*red signal*) and 4 (*green signal*) hybridized onto a metaphase nucleus containing all 46 chromosomes. This FISH study revealed a translocation of a piece of material from chromosome 4 onto chromosome 1. (Courtesy of Lisa Shaffer, PhD, Washington State University).

(**Fig. 2-9**). FISH is also a powerful tool to confirm or diagnose syndromes that are due to microdeletions of segments of chromosome material (**Fig. 2-10**). FISH is also used to identify the actual physical location of a gene or to order a series of DNA sequences or genes on a chromosome.

Two other powerful diagnostic and investigational tools for human chromosome analysis directly expanded from FISH technology are comparative genome hybridization (CGH) and spectral karyotyping (SKY). CGH is used to measure differences in copy number or dosage of a particular chromosome segment. Its widest application has been in the study of gene dosage in normal and cancer cell lines. Currently, aCGH has replaced conventional cytogenetics as the first-line test of an individual with unexplained birth defects or mental retardation. The second technique, SKY, uses the FISH principle to visualize all 24 chromosomes by "painting" with chromosome-specific probes in different colors simultaneously. Because each chromosome probe emits its own unique wavelength of fluorescence, and therefore color, structural rearrangements and chromosome fragments can be identified (**Fig. 2-11**). However, array CGH has essentially replaced SKY.

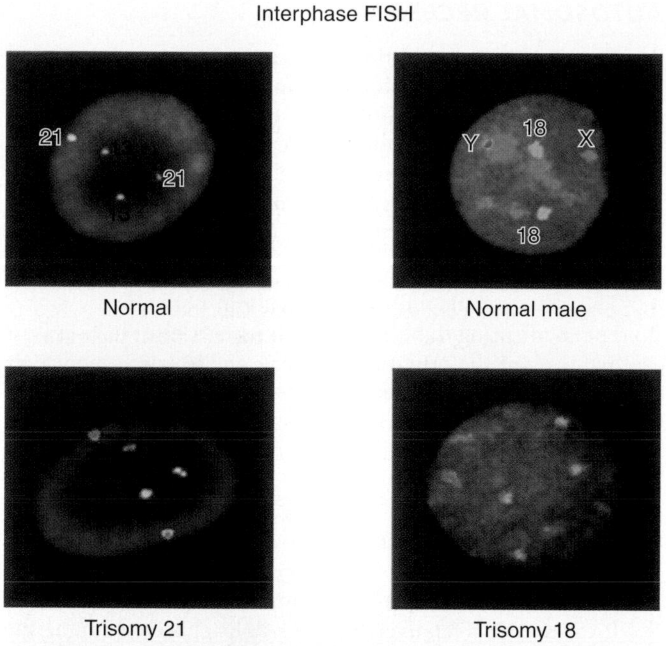

Interphase FISH

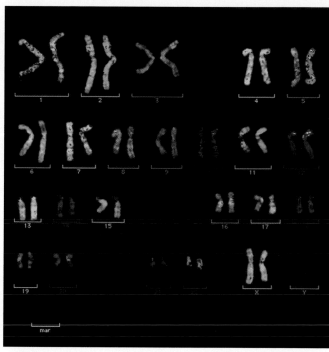

Figure 2-9 Interphase FISH on amniotic fluid cells to screen for aneuploidy. (Courtesy of Edith Cheng, MD.)

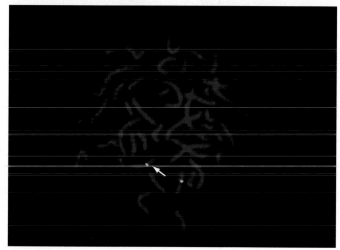

Deletion of 11p

Figure 2-10 Example of FISH technology in the diagnosis of microdeletion syndromes. Here, standard karyotyping appears to be normal. However, using FISH microdeletion probes, this child was discovered to have a submicroscopic deletion (*arrow*) of the terminal section of the long arm of chromosome 1. The other chromosome containing the red signal is the normal chromosome (Courtesy of Lisa Shaffer, PhD, Washington State University).

PATTERNS OF INHERITANCE

Any evaluation of the segregation pattern of a trait or disease in a family requires the development of a pedigree (**Fig. 2-12**). This graphic representation of family history data assists in determining the transmission pattern of the gene. In some conditions, the pattern of transmission and the constellation of clinical characteristics of affected individuals in the pedigree provides the diagnosis, which otherwise would not be evident if only one individual were evaluated.

24-color painting probes

Figure 2-11 Example of spectral karyotyping (SKY) on standard metaphase chromosomes (Courtesy of Lisa Shaffer PhD, Washington State University).

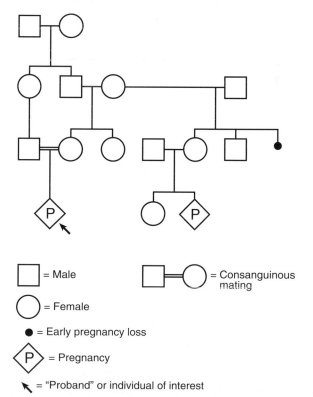

☐ = Male   ☐═◯ = Consanguinous mating

◯ = Female

● = Early pregnancy loss

⬦P⬦ = Pregnancy

↖ = "Proband" or individual of interest

Figure 2-12 Standard figures and nomenclature for a pedigree. (Courtesy of Edith Cheng, MD.)

AUTOSOMAL DOMINANT

In an autosomal dominant mode of inheritance, only one copy of the mutated gene is required for expression of the trait, and the individual is said to be heterozygous for the trait. There are more than 4000 known autosomal dominant conditions, and most occur in the heterozygous form in affected individuals. With a few exceptions, autosomal dominant conditions occurring in the homozygous form (two copies of the affected gene) are rare, the **phenotype** is more severe, and they are often lethal.

The general characteristics of autosomal dominant inheritance are illustrated in **Figure 2-13** and summarized as follows:

1. Every affected individual has an affected parent (unless this is a new mutation—to be discussed later). The inheritance pattern is vertical.
2. If reproductively fit, the affected person has a 50% risk of transmitting the gene with each pregnancy.
3. The sexes are affected equally.
4. There is father-to-son transmission.
5. An individual who does not carry the mutation will have no risk of transmission to his or her offspring.

Three additional properties associated with, but not exclusive to, autosomal dominant traits are variable **expressivity**, **penetrance**, and new mutations. Variable expressivity describes the severity of the phenotype in individuals who have the mutation. Some autosomal dominant conditions have a clear clinical demarcation between affected and unaffected individuals. However, some conditions express the clinical consequences of the mutation in varying degrees among members of the same family and between different families. These differences in expression are modified by age, sex of the affected individual, the individual's genetic background, and by the environment. Variable expression of a condition can lead to difficulties in diagnosis and interpretation of inheritance pattern. Penetrance refers to the probability that a gene will have any clinical manifestation at all in a person known to have the mutation. A condition is 100% penetrant if all individuals with the mutation have any clinical feature of the disease (no matter how minor). A number of autosomal dominant conditions are the result of new mutations. For example, about 70% of achondroplasia cases occur as new mutations. Because this condition has 100% penetrance, the recurrence risk in subsequent pregnancies in the normal parents of an affected child is not 50%, but the risk to the offspring of the affected is 50%. If an autosomal dominant condition is associated with poor reproductive fitness, then the likelihood that the cases occurred because of new mutation is greater.

AUTOSOMAL RECESSIVE

Autosomal recessive conditions are rare and require the affected individual to have two copies of the mutant allele (homozygous) in order to manifest the condition. In the heterozygote carrier, the product of the normal allele is able to compensate for the mutant allele and prevent occurrence of the disease. **Figure 2-14** is a typical pedigree illustrating autosomal recessive inheritance. The following general statements can be made about an autosomal recessive trait:

1. The characteristic will occur equally in both sexes.
2. For an offspring to be at risk, both parents must have at least one copy of the mutation.
3. If both parents are heterozygous (carriers) for the condition, 25% of the offspring will be homozygous for the mutation and manifest the condition, and 50% will be carriers and unaffected. The remaining 25% will not have inherited the mutation at all, will be unaffected, and will not be at risk of transmitting the mutation to any offspring.
4. Consanguinity is often present in families demonstrating rare autosomal recessive conditions.
5. If the disease is relatively rare, it will be clustered among the siblings and will not be seen among other family members such as ancestors, cousins, aunts, and uncles.

Because autosomal recessive conditions require two copies of the mutant allele, and because most matings are not consanguineous, counseling couples about the risk for an autosomal recessive condition requires knowledge of the carrier frequency of the condition in the general population. Cystic fibrosis exemplifies the importance of knowing the population in which screening/counseling is being provided (**Table 2-2**). Depending on the ethnic group of the mother and father, the risk for a child having

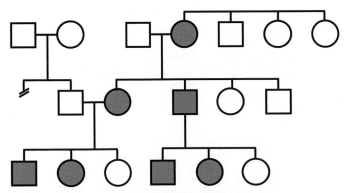

Figure 2-13 Example of autosomal dominant inheritance. (Courtesy of Edith Cheng, MD.)

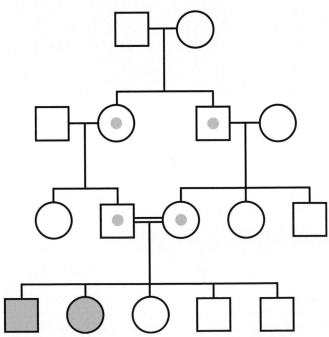

Figure 2-14 Pedigree illustrating autosomal recessive inheritance. Here the parents of the affected children are first cousins, as denoted by the double line connecting them. (Courtesy of Edith Cheng, MD.)

Table 2-2 Carrier Frequencies for Cystic Fibrosis in Different Populations

Ethnicity	Chance of Being Carrier	Chance Both Carriers*
European descent	1 in 29	1 in 841
Hispanic American	1 in 46	1 in 2,116
African American	1 in 65	1 in 4,225
Asian American	1 in 90	1 in 8,100

*The chance for an affected child being born to these couples is the chance that both are carriers times ¼.

cystic fibrosis could be as high as 1 in 1936 (1/22 × 1/22 × ¼) if they are of Caucasian (European) descent or negligible if they are of Asian descent.

X-LINKED TRAIT

The human X chromosome is quite large, containing about 160 million base pairs, or about 5% of the nuclear DNA. Of the 500 genes that have been mapped to the X chromosome, 70% are known to be associated with disease phenotypes. Diseases caused by genes on the X chromosome are said to be X-linked, and most are recessive. In contrast, the Y chromosome is quite small, about 70 million base pairs, and contains only a few genes.

The expression of genes located on the X chromosome demonstrate a unique characteristic known as dosage compensation, which was put forth by Mary Lyon in the 1960s to explain the equalization of X-linked gene products in males and females. Achievement of dosage compensation is through the principles of X inactivation, also known as the Lyon hypothesis. The tenets of the Lyon hypothesis are as follows:

1. One X chromosome in each cell is randomly inactivated in the early female embryo (soon after fertilization).
2. The inactivation process is random: either the paternally or maternally derived X chromosome is chosen. The female is thus a mosaic for genes located on the X chromosome.
3. All descendants of the cell will have the same inactive X chromosome.

The Lyon hypothesis is supported by clinical evidence derived from animal and human observations of traits located on the X chromosome, such as the calico cat pattern of red and black patches of fur on female cats but not on male cats. In humans, male and females have equal quantities of the enzyme glucose-6-phosphate dehydrogenase (G6PD), which is encoded by a gene on the X chromosome. Barr bodies, or sex chromatin, which are condensed, inactive X chromosomes found only in females, are cytogenetic evidence that only one X chromosome is transcriptionally active in females. The mechanism for X inactivation is unknown at this time, but clearly requires the presence of the X inactivation center, which has been mapped to the proximal end of the long arm of the X chromosome (Xq). This center contains an unusual gene call XIST (X-inactive specific transcript), which seems to control X inactivation, which cannot occur in its absence.

The principles of the Lyon hypothesis remain true for the majority of genes located on the X chromosome. The silencing of these genes appears to occur as a function of DNA methylation at the promoter regions of these genes. However, several regions remain genetically active on both chromosomes. They include the pseudoautosomal regions located at the tips of the long and short arms, which are the regions that contain the genes for steroid sulfatase, the Xg blood group, and Kallman syndrome (hypogonadism and anosmia). The pseudoautosomal region on the short arm shares extensive homology with the Y chromosome and is the region involved in the pairing of the X and Y chromosome at meiosis.

Another exception to the Lyon hypothesis is that one X chromosome is nonrandomly, preferentially inactivated. This is observed for most cases of **translocations** between an X chromosome and an autosome. If the translocation is balanced, the structurally normal X chromosome is preferentially inactivated. If the translocation is unbalanced, then the structurally normal X chromosome is always active. These nonrandom patterns of inactivation are an attempt to minimize the clinical consequences of the chromosomal rearrangement. Studies can be done to look at patterns of inactivation, as in the case of prenatal diagnosis, to predict the clinical consequences of a de novo X/autosome translocation in the fetus.

Random inactivation confers a mosaic state for the carrier female. The normal allele is able to compensate for the abnormal allele (as in autosomal recessive traits), and carrier females of X-linked recessive conditions usually do not have clinical manifestations of the disease. Occasionally, however, there is skewed or less than 50-50 chance of inactivation such that the X chromosome carrying the normal allele is inactivated more frequently. In such cases, carrier females display some features of the condition and are referred to as manifesting heterozygotes. Manifesting heterozygotes have been described for hemophilia A, Duchenne muscular dystrophy, and X-linked color blindness. Genetic counseling of recurrent risks for X-linked recessive condition depends on the sex of the affected parent and of the offspring. **Figure 2-15** is a pedigree illustrating X-linked recessive inheritance, the characteristics of which are the following:

1. Affected individuals are usually males unless X chromosome activation is skewed in the carrier female or the female is homozygous for the trait.
2. The affected males in a kindred are related through females.
3. The gene is not transmitted from father to son.
4. All daughters of affected males will be carriers.
5. Daughters of carrier females have a 50% chance of being carriers; sons of carrier females have a 50% chance of being affected.

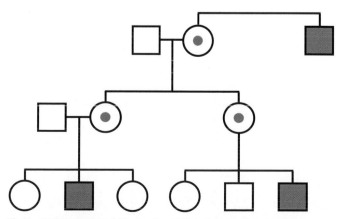

Figure 2-15 Pedigree illustrating X-linked recessive condition. (Courtesy of Edith Cheng, MD.)

X-LINKED DOMINANT INHERITANCE

The major feature of X-linked dominant inheritance is that all heterozygotes, both male and female, manifest the condition. Although the pedigree may resemble autosomal dominant inheritance, the distinguishing feature is that affected males never have affected sons, and all daughters of affected males are affected. There are usually more affected females than males, and the majority of the females are heterozygotes.

ATYPICAL PATTERNS OF INHERITANCE

Trinucleotide-Repeat Disorders: Unstable Mutations

In the early 1990s a new class of genetic conditions was recognized as being due to unstable dynamic mutations in a gene. In the previous section, the diseases and their inheritance patterns were due to mutations that were passed on from generation to generation in a stable form. That is, all affected members in a family had the identical inherited mutation. In 1991, however, a number of reports began to describe a new class of genetic conditions in which the gene mutation was dynamic and would change with different affected individuals within a family. The most common group of disorders is known as triplet, or trinucleotide-repeat, disorders. More than a dozen diseases are now known to be associated with unstable trinucleotide repeats (**Table 2-3**).

These conditions are characterized by an expansion of variable size, within the affected gene, of a segment of DNA that contains a repeat of three nucleotides such as CAGCAGCAG (CAG)n, or CCGCCG(CCG)n. These triplet repeats are unstable in that they tend to expand as the gene is passed on from generation to generation. The molecular mechanism is most likely misalignment at the time of meiosis. The result of increasing triplet expansion is progressively earlier onset or more severe manifestation of disease with each successive generation. This phenomenon is known as anticipation and is generally characteristic of genetic conditions caused by unstable repeats.

The commonality of this group of genetic condition stops at the shared molecular mechanism. Each disease, otherwise, has its own features. Some, such as myotonic dystrophy, are inherited in an autosomal dominant pattern, but others, such as Friedrich's ataxia, are autosomal recessive conditions. The susceptibility of the triplet repeat to expand also depends on the parent of origin, paternal in Huntington's disease, and exclusively maternal in fragile X syndrome.

Fragile X Syndrome

Fragile X syndrome, although a disease within the unstable triplet group, is discussed in this section because of its unique molecular and clinical characteristics. This is the most common heritable form of moderate mental retardation and is second to Down syndrome among the causes of mental retardation in males. In women, a mild carrier state may present as premature menopause. The gene is located on the X chromosome at Xq27.3 and causes a pattern of abnormalities, including mental retardation and characteristic facial features in at least 1 in 4000 male births. The condition is due to an expansion of the triplet repeat CGG located in the untranslated region of the first exon of the gene called *FMR1* (fragile X mental retardation 1). The triplet expansion blocks normal function of the *FMR1* gene, thus causing the syndrome.

Normal individuals have about 8 to 50 copies of the CGG triplet, whereas affected individuals have from 200 to more than 1000 copies. Individuals with an intermediate number of copies (52–200) are known as premutation carriers; this level of "expansion" renders the triplet-repeat segment unstable. These carriers are generally unaffected but are at risk for having affected children or descendants if the premutation expands in successive generations. The premutation, however, can be passed on without expanding.

Long-term follow-up of premutation carriers has revealed that these individuals are not necessarily "unaffected." Premature ovarian failure has been associated with female premutation carriers, and in men, a syndrome of atypical adult-onset ataxia has now been described.

Although the unstable triplet is transmitted in an X-linked pattern, the probabilities of the different phenotypes are far from traditional X-linked inheritance. Understanding of this feature of the fragile X syndrome is crucial to genetic counseling and assessing recurrence risks. The possible outcomes of the offspring of a premutation carrier female are the following:

1. Male offspring: Three possibilities:
   a. Unaffected by not having inherited the X chromosome with the premutation.
   b. Unaffected by inheriting the X chromosome with the premutation, which did *not* expand (about 20% of the time); this male, however, is at risk for passing the premutation to his daughters, who in turn will be at risk for having affected children. Therefore, for this male, his grandchildren will be at risk for the fragile X syndrome.
   c. Affected by having inherited the abnormal X chromosome, in which the premutation also expanded to a full mutation.
2. Female offspring: Four possibilities:
   a. Unaffected by not having inherited the X chromosome with the premutation.

Table 2-3 Some Commonly Known Disorders Associated with Unstable Triplet Repeats

Disease	Inheritance Pattern	Triplet Repeat	Location of Expansion	Normal	Unstable	Affected
					Repeat Number	
Huntington's disease	Autosomal dominant	CAG	Exon coding region	<36	29-35	>35
Fragile X	X-linked	CGG	5' untranslated region	<55	56-200	>200
Myotonic dystrophy	Autosomal dominant	GTG	3' untranslated region	<35	50-100	>100
Spinal cerebellar ataxias*	Autosomal dominant	CAG	Exon	<40	Different for each subtype	>40
Friedrich's ataxia	Autosomal recessive	GAA	Intron of gene	<33	34-65	>65

*Spinal cerebellar ataxias are a heterogeneous group of conditions, all of which appear to be associated with a CAG repeat. Each subtype has its own specific range of normal, unstable, and affected repeat sizes.

b. Unaffected by inheriting the X chromosome with the premutation that did *not* expand.

c. Unaffected, but inherited the X chromosome *with* an expansion—about 50% of females with the expansion appear to be clinically unaffected.

d. Affected by inheriting the X chromosome with an expansion.

Genomic Imprinting and Uniparental Disomy

Genomic imprinting and uniparental disomy refers to the differential activation or expression of genes depending on the parent of origin. In contrast to Mendel's hypothesis that the phenotype of a gene is no different if inherited from the mother or the father, there is now a group of diseases in which the parent of origin of a gene or chromosome plays a role in the phenotype of the affected individual. The best-studied examples of this mechanism are molar pregnancies and Prader–Willi syndrome (PWS) and Angelman syndrome (AS). PWS is characterized by obesity, hyperphagia, small hands and feet, hypogonadism, and mental retardation. In about 70% of cases, cytogenetic deletion of the proximal arm of the paternally inherited chromosome 15 is observable at 15q11-q13. In contrast, the same deletion of the maternally inherited chromosome 15 results in a different phenotype (AS) of severe mental retardation, short stature, spasticity, and seizures. More interestingly, 30% of subjects with PWS do not have a cytogenetic deletion but rather inherit two intact chromosomes 15 from the mother. No genetic information on chromosome 15 is inherited from the father. This is referred to as maternal uniparental disomy. As expected, individuals with Angelman syndrome without a cytogenetic deletion have two copies of the paternally derived chromosome 15 and no chromosome 15 from the mother—a condition termed paternal uniparental disomy. These findings indicate that at least for the region of 15q11-q13, the expression of the PWS phenotype is brought on by the absence of a paternal contribution of the genes in this region. Likewise, the expression of Angelman syndrome is due to the absence of the maternal contribution of genes located at 15q11-q13. The genes in this region are said to be "imprinted" because their parent of origin has been "marked."

Many regions of the human genome have now demonstrated evidence of imprinting. Knowledge of diseases that occur as a result of imprinting has implications in prenatal diagnosis, especially when **mosaicism** is encountered.

Germline Mosaicism

Mosaicism is defined as the presence of two or more genetically different cell lines in the same individual or tissue derived from a single zygote. Females, because of X inactivation, are mosaics for genes on the X chromosome. Mosaicism, however, is not necessarily evenly or randomly distributed throughout the body. In other words, using the entire body as the whole organism, an individual is mosaic either because different organs or tissues have genetically different cells, but each organ or tissue has the same cell line, or because the genetically different cell lines are dispersed throughout many tissues in the body. The distinction between these two types of mosaicism is particularly important in making a prenatal diagnosis in cases in which mosaicism is identified in amniotic fluid cells. One cannot be confident that a trisomy 21 phenotype, such as mental retardation, would be less severe because of mosaicism. The brain cells could be all trisomy 21, but the cells of the skin could all be normal diploid. In germline mosaicism, the implication is that the mutation is present in only one parent and arose during embryogenesis in all or some of the germ cells but few or none of the somatic cells of the embryo. This concept was developed to explain recurrence of a genetic condition in a sibship (usually autosomal dominant) in which incorrect diagnosis, autosomal recessive inheritance, reduced penetrance, or variable expression could not be the reason for the recurrence. The best example of germline mosaicism is osteogenesis imperfecta type II (lethal form). At the molecular level, the mutation causing the condition is dominant—that is, only one copy of the abnormal gene is necessary to cause this perinatal lethal condition. Yet there are families in which multiple affected pregnancies are seen in the same couple or one parent has recurrences with different partners. If the spontaneous mutation rate for an autosomal dominant mutation is 1 chance in 10^5, then the probability of two independent spontaneous mutations for the same lethal autosomal dominant condition is $(1/10^5)^2$, a highly unlikely event. Germline mosaicism is now well documented for about 6% of cases of osteogenesis imperfecta type II. Unfortunately, the exact recurrence risk is difficult to assess because the proportion of gametes containing the mutation is unknowable.

MITOCHONDRIAL INHERITANCE—MATERNAL INHERITANCE

Most inherited conditions occur as a result of mutations in the DNA of the nucleus (nuclear genome). However, a growing number of conditions resulting from abnormalities of the mitochondria have now been identified. Because the mitochondrial apparatus and its function are under the control of both nuclear and mitochondrial genes, diseases affecting the mitochondria do not follow the typical Mendelian pattern of inheritance. Each human cell contains a population of several hundred or more mitochondria in its cytoplasm. Most of the subunits that make up the mitochondrial apparatus are encoded by the nuclear genome. However, mitochondria have their own DNA molecules, which contain a small fraction of genes whose product are vital to the function of the cell. Mitochondrial DNA (mtDNA), which was completely sequenced in 1981, is small, about 16.5 kilobase pairs (kbp) in size, and is packaged as a circular chromosome located in the mitochondria. The replication process is self-sufficient, with the molecule coding for 37 genes. These genes code for two types of rRNA, 22 tRNAs, and 13 of 87 polypeptides that are subunits of the oxidative phosphorylation pathway (OXPHOS). Nuclear DNA encodes the other 74 polypeptides. Therefore, mitochondrial diseases can be caused by mutations in the mtDNA or in the nuclear genes that code for components of the OXPHOS system.

Because the primary function of the OXPHOS complex is to provide energy (ATP) for the cell, mutations that affect the OXPHOS complex will likely result in cell dysfunction and death. The organs most affected would be those that depend heavily on mitochondria. The diseases that result are generally neuromuscular in nature, such as encephalopathies, myopathies, ataxias, and retinal degeneration, but the mutations have **pleiotropic** effects.

The first pathogenic mutations in mtDNA were identified in the early 1990s. They include mutations in the coding regions of genes that alter the activity of an OXPHOS protein, mutations in tRNA or rRNA genes that impair mitochondrial protein synthesis, or rearrangements that result in deletions or duplications of the mtDNA molecule. The lack of mtDNA repair mechanisms and constant exposure to oxygen free radicals may explain the high mutation rate of mtDNA (10 times that of nuclear DNA, which has a spontaneous mutation rate of 1 in 10^5).

The most significant characteristic of mitochondrial diseases caused by mutations in mtDNA is that they are all maternally inherited. Leber's hereditary optic neuropathy (LHON) is a well-known mitochondrial disease in which rapid, bilateral loss of central vision occurs. Males and females are affected equally, and all affected individuals are related through maternal lineage. This is because the cytoplasm of the ovum is abundant with mitochondria, but the sperm contain very few mitochondria. Therefore, an individual's mitochondria (and its DNA) is essentially all inherited from the mother. If the mother has an mtDNA mutation, then all of her children will inherit that mutation. When a mutation arises in the DNA of a mitochondrion in the cytoplasm of the ovum, it is at first one mutation in one mitochondrion. However, as replication and division of this mutated mitochondrion occurs, they become randomly distributed among the normal mitochondria and between the daughter cells. One daughter cell by chance may contain a large population of mitochondria with the mutation, but the other has none or very little. Fertilization of the egg with a large proportion of mitochondria containing the mutation would result in an offspring that is at risk for manifesting a mitochondrial disease.

A second feature is that of variable expression. Within each cell and tissue, there is a threshold for energy production below which the cells will degenerate and die. Organ systems with large energy requirements will be most susceptible to mitochondrial abnormalities. Thus, if there is an mtDNA mutation, the severity of the mitochondrial disease will depend on the proportion of mitochondria with the mutation that the individual inherited from his or her mother and the susceptibility of different tissues to altered ATP metabolism.

Abnormalities of mitochondrial function caused by mutations in the nuclear genome will, however, exhibit traditional Mendelian inheritance patterns with autosomal dominant and recessive, as well as X-linked conditions now being observed. A few conditions occur as sporadic, somatic mutations and have little or no recurrence risk. **Table 2-4** lists some of the currently known mitochondrial diseases and their inheritance patterns. However,

mitochondrial dysfunction has now been found to be associated with many conditions, including diabetes, Alzheimer's disease, Parkinson's disease, and human oocyte aging.

MULTIFACTORIAL INHERITANCE

Multifactorial inheritance is defined as traits or characteristics produced by the action of several genes, with or without the interplay of environmental factors. A number of structural abnormalities occurring as isolated defects and not part of a syndrome, such as cleft lip with or without cleft palate, open neural tube defect (including anencephaly and spina bifida), and cardiac defects are examples of such conditions. When both parents are normal and an affected child is produced, the chance of recurrence is generally between 2% and 5% for any given pregnancy. Because the underlying mechanisms by which the genes and the environment interact to cause these conditions are unknown, genetic counseling of recurrent risks must measure the observed recurrence risks in collections of families to gene-rate a population-based empiric risk. These risk rates, however, are modified by ethnicity, the sex of the carrier parent, the sex of the affected parent and at-risk offspring, the presence of the defect in one or both parents, the number of affected family members, and by consanguineous parentage.

CHROMOSOME ABNORMALITIES

A variety of chromosome abnormalities may occur during meiosis or mitosis (see Chapter 1, Fertilization and Embryogenesis). They fall into several general categories, and many clinical conditions are associated with each type. Although it is impossible within the scope of this chapter to discuss every clinical condition associated with a known chromosome abnormality, an attempt is made to categorize the specific types of anomalies and the more common problems seen by obstetricians and gynecologists that relate to these anomalies. Several conditions are dealt with in more detail in other chapters of this book.

Numerical Chromosomal Abnormalities

Two terms are used in the description of numerical chromosomal abnormalities: *aneuploidy* refers to an extra or missing chromosome, such as in trisomy 21 (Down syndrome) or monosomy X (Turner syndrome), respectively; *polyploidy* refers to

Table 2-4 Some Mitochondrial Disorders and Their Features

	Disease	Features	Inheritance Pattern
Mitochondrial DNA mutations	Leber's hereditary optic neuropathy (LHON)	Blindness, rapid optic nerve death in young adulthood	Maternal
	Leigh disease (NARP)	Neuropathy, ataxia, retinitis pigmentosa, mental retardation, lactic acidosis	Maternal
	MERRF	Myotonic epilepsy, ragged red fibers in muscle, ataxia, sensorineural deafness	Maternal
	MELAS	Mitochondrial encephalopathy, lactic acidosis, strokelike episodes, sensorineural deafness	Maternal
Nuclear DNA mutations	Friedreich's ataxia	Limb movement abnormalities, dysarthria, absent tendon reflexes, triplet repeat affecting gene that codes for mitochondrial protein (Frataxin)	Autosomal recessive
	Barth syndrome	Dilated cardiomyopathy, cyclic neutropenia, skeletal myopathy, growth deficiency, abnormal mitochondria	X-linked
	Wilson disease	Copper accumulation in brain and liver leading to cirrhosis, parkinsonism, and dystonia	Autosomal recessive

numerical chromosome abnormalities in which there is an addition of an entire complement of haploid chromosomes, such as in triploidy, in which three haploid sets occur (69, XXX or XXY or XYY). Numerical or aneuploid chromosome abnormalities involve either autosomes or sex chromosomes. Most occur as the result of **nondisjunction** during meiosis or mitosis in which homologous chromosome pairs fail to disjoin. The result in meiosis is that one daughter cell receives two copies of the homologs and the other receives none. Fertilization with a gamete containing a normal chromosome complement will result in a zygote that is either trisomic or monosomic (**Fig. 2-16**). Molecular studies for the parent of origin have identified that the majority of autosomal aneuploidies result from nondisjunctional errors in maternal meiosis I.

The majority of trisomic conceptions are nonviable, and autosomal trisomies have been seen in abortus material in all but chromosomes 1 and 17. However, trisomies 21, 18, 13, and 22 result in live births and are associated with advanced maternal age (**Fig. 2-17**). Trisomy 13 (Patau syndrome) occurs in approximately 1/10,000 live births. The syndrome is characterized by gross multiple structural defects involving the midline (holo-proencephaly, cleft lip/palate, cardiac defects), and postaxial polydactyly. Trisomy 18 (Edwards syndrome) is found in 1/6000 live births and is associated with prenatal growth restriction, rocker bottom feet, and cardiac and renal defects. Trisomy 21 is the most common viable autosomal trisomy and has an incidence of 1/800 live births. The majority (95%) of individuals with Down syndrome have trisomy 21—that is, three separate copies of chromosome 21 because of maternal nondisjunction. However, about 2% to 3% of individuals with clinical Down syndrome have a structural rearrangement (robertsonian translocation—to be discussed in the next section), and another 1% to 3% are mosaic for trisomy 21. Trisomy 22 has been seen in a few live-born individuals and is associated with severe neurologic impairment. Monosomic states involving autosomes are extremely rare and generally lethal.

Sex chromosome aneuploidy usually occurs in the trisomic state. Monosomy Y is lethal and has never been seen in a clinical situation or even in an abortus. Monosomy of the X chromosome (45,X), however, is the typical finding in the condition known as Turner syndrome. However, because most 45,X conceptions are lethal, the actual incidence of live female births is about 1/5000. At birth, Turner syndrome is characterized by lymphedema, hypotonia, and webbed neck. Girls with Turner syndrome have short stature, a broad chest with wide spaced nipples, cubitus valgus (widened carrying angle of the arms), and gonadal dysgenesis resulting in lack of secondary sex characteristics, amenorrhea, and infertility (**Fig. 2-18**). Other features include congenital heart disease (coarctation of the aorta is the most common), kidney disease, and hypertension in later life. Intelligence is normal although spatial perception abnormalities are common. Hormonal supplementation during puberty allows girls with Turner syndrome to develop secondary sex characteristics.

Unlike autosomal trisomies in which the majority are maternally derived, the 45,X karyotype occurs through paternal nondisjunction and is not associated with advanced maternal or paternal age. There is no increased recurrence for 45,X, which accounts for 50% of women with Turner syndrome. Another 30% to 40% of individuals are mosaic for the 45,X cell line and another cell line (usually 46,XX) because of postzygotic nondisjunction during mitosis. The clinical features of these women will vary depending on the proportion of normal 46,XX cell lines present. However, females who are mosaic with a 45,X/ 46,XY karyotype are at an increased risk for gonadoblastoma. Therefore, women suspected of having Turner syndrome should have a chromosomal analysis, not only for diagnosis but for exclusion of mosaicism for a 46,XY cell line. The remaining 10% to 20% of individuals with Turner syndrome have a structural abnormality of the X chromosome (**Table 2-5**). Occasional correlation between phenotype and the type of structural abnormality has led investigators to examine the genes responsible for ovarian development and function and other features associated with Turner syndrome. For example, women with 46,X,i(Xq) are indistinguishable from women with 45,X, whereas women with a deletion of the long arm of X (Xq) often only have gonadal dysfunction, and women with deletions of the short arm of X (Xp) have short stature and congenital malformations.

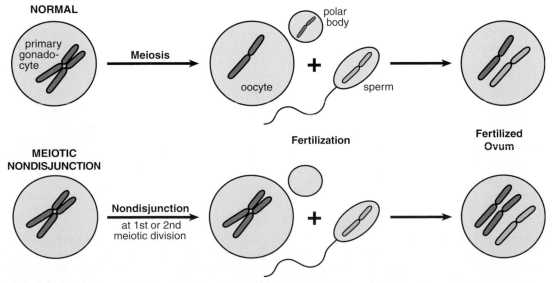

Figure 2-16 Graphic representation of meiotic nondisjunction. (Courtesy of Edith Cheng, MD.)

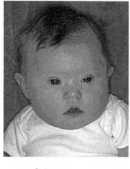

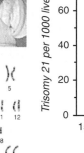

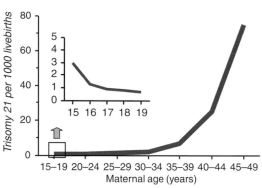

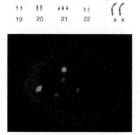

◀ FISH *(Fluorescent In Situ Hybridization)*
2 green signals are X chromosomes
3 red signals are chromosome 21

Figure 2-17 Trisomy 21 infant with karyotype demonstrating three separate chromosomes 21. Interphase FISH illustration of screening for trisomy 21. Graph illustrating the maternal age association and increasing risk for aneuploidy. Note that there is an increased risk at the peripubertal ages as well. (Courtesy of Edith Cheng, MD.)

Other trisomies involving the sex chromosomes are seen in 47,XXX, 47,XXY (Klinefelter syndrome), and 47,XYY karyotypes. The incidence of 47,XXX is approximately 1/1000 live female births and is due to maternal nondisjunction associated with increasing maternal age. Most women are phenotypically normal with the exception of possible mild developmental delay; fertility is normal and there may be a slightly increased risk for offspring with aneuploidy involving the sex chromosomes and autosomes. Klinefelter syndrome, 47,XXY, is a common sex chromosome abnormality associated with maternal age and occurs in 1/1000 live male births. Clinical features include tall gynecoid stature, gynecomastia (with an increased risk for breast cancer), and testicular atrophy. Mental retardation is not a typical feature, but affected individuals may have IQ scores that are lower than those of their siblings. Nondisjunction during spermatogenesis involving the Y chromosome leads to 47,XYY. These males may be taller than average, but they are otherwise phenotypically normal. Contrary to previous and outdated observational studies, this sex chromosome aneuploidy is not associated with violent crime. However, behavioral problems such as attention deficit disorder may be observed.

Nondisjunctional events during mitosis in the early embryo (after fertilization) will produce individuals with cell populations containing different chromosome numbers. This condition, known as *mosaicism,* may involve the autosomes or the sex chromosomes. The actual phenotype depends on the proportion of aneuploid and euploid cells in the embryo and in the specific organs or tissues involved.

Structural Chromosome Abnormalities

Chromosome breaks and rearrangements may lead to no obvious phenotypic consequences (genetically balanced), loss or gain of chromosomal material (genetically imbalanced) that produces abnormalities, or abnormalities resulting from the interruption of a critical gene at the breakpoint site on the chromosome. Types of structural rearrangements include translocations (reciprocal and robertsonian), **insertion**s, **inversions**, **isochromosomes**, duplications, and deletions. The rate of formation of balanced rearrangements is generally very low, 1.6×10^{-4}, although some chromosomal segments are more prone to breakage (hot spots) than others. This section discusses the clinical and reproductive implications of some of these structural rearrangements.

Balanced Reciprocal Translocations

Translocations occur as a result of a mutual and physical exchange of chromosome (genetic) material between nonhomologous chromosomes. Balanced reciprocal translocations are found in about 1/11,000 newborns. **Figure 2-19** is an example of a hypothetical balanced translocation between the short arms (p arm) of two chromosomes. The carrier of a reciprocal balanced translocation is usually phenotypically normal. However, the carrier is at an increased risk for producing offspring who are chromosomally abnormal. In meiosis, the two pairs of nonhomologous chromosomes involved in the translocation resolve their pairing difficulties by forming a quadriradial. Three segregation possibilities are illustrated in **Figure 2-19**, but only one segregation (alternative) pattern will result in genetically balanced gametes. Of the six possible gametes, four are partially monosomic and trisomic, one has a normal complement of chromosomes, and the other contains a pair of reciprocally balanced translocation chromosomes (like its parent). The viability of the genetically unbalanced gametes depends on the chromosomes involved in the reciprocal translocation, the size of the translocated chromosome material, and the sex of the carrier. In addition, most reciprocal translocations are unique to a family, and, consequently, the reproductive fitness of the carrier depends on the

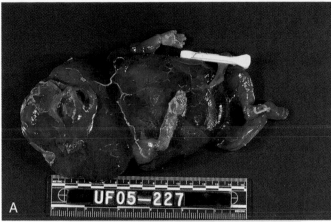

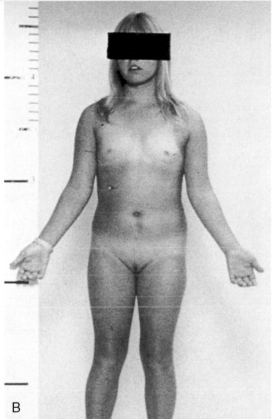

Figure 2-18 A, Photo of a 20-week fetus with Turner syndrome, 45, X. This fetus was diagnosed during a routine 20-week ultrasound for anatomy and growth and was found to have a large cystic hygroma and hydrops. The autopsy revealed a complex cardiac defect, abnormal kidneys, streaked ovaries, and malrotation of the gut with the appendix in the left lower quadrant. **B,** A 17-year-old woman with Turner syndrome. Note the short stature, poor sexual development, and increased carrying angles at elbows. Subject also has webbing of the neck. (**A,** Courtesy of Drs. W. Tony Parks and Corrine Fligner, Department of Pathology, University of Washington.)

Table 2-5 Karyotypes discovered in Subjects with Phenotypic Characteristics of Turner Syndrome

Karyotype	Error
45,X	Deletion X
45,Xi(Xq)	Deletion Xp, Isochromosome Xq
45,X,Xq	Deletion Xp
45,X/46,XX	Mosaicism
45,X/46,XX/47,XXX	Mosaicism
45,X/46,XY	Mosaicism
45,X/46,XY/47,XYY	Mosaicism
45,XringX	Ring chromosome
46,XX	Phenotype with normal karyotype

the acrocentric chromosomes: chromosome pairs 13, 14, 15, 21, and 22. In this structural rearrangement, the short arms (p arms) of two nonhomologous chromosomes are lost, and the long arms fuse at the **centromere**, forming a single chromosome structure. **Figure 2-20** is an example of a robertsonian translocation involving chromosomes 14 and 21. The phenotypically normal carrier of a robertsonian translocation has 45 chromosomes in each cell because the two acrocentric chromosomes involved in the translocation have formed into one chromosome structure. This person is genetically balanced—that is, he or she has two copies of each chromosome. However, the gametes are at risk to be unbalanced. As in reciprocal translocations, the chromosomes involved in the rearrangement resolve the pairing of homologous segments at meiosis by forming a triad as seen in **Figure 2-21.** The chromosomes can segregate into gametes in one of three patterns. Only one segregation pattern (alternate) results in normal offspring, one gamete will have a normal chromosome complement, and the other will be a balanced carrier with 45 chromosome structure, like its parent. The other two segregation patterns result in chromosomally unbalanced gametes that are monosomic for chromosome 21 or 14 (both lethal), or trisomic for chromosome 14 (lethal). In addition, one of the gametes will have the robertsonian (14q;21) translocation, and, if fertilized, the resultant offspring will have Down syndrome. The risk for recurrence of translocation Down syndrome depends on parent of origin (10% to 15% for maternal carriers, and 1% to 2% for paternal carriers).

One very important exception in translocation Down syndrome is that associated with a 21q21q translocation. Here, the chromosome structure is composed of two chromosomes 21. Although this chromosome rearrangement is extremely rare, this translocation confers a 100% risk that the carrier will have abnormal gametes and 100% of viable gametes will result in a conception with Down syndrome.

Chromosome inversions occur when two breaks occur on a chromosome followed by a 180-degree turn of the segment and reinsertion at its original breakpoints. Thus, if a sequence of markers on a chromosome is ABCDEFGHIJ, but an inversion occurs between markers D and H, the sequence of markers becomes ABCHGFEDIJ. If the centromere is included in the inverted segment, it is called a *pericentric inversion.* If the centromere is not involved, then the inversion is called a *paracentric inversion.* Chromosome inversions are generally considered balanced and usually do not confer an abnormal phenotype unless one of the breakpoints disrupts a critical gene. Inversions, however, do interfere with pairing at meiosis and can result in gametes with chromosome abnormalities.

carrier's sex and nature of the translocation. In general, however, the recurrence for an unbalanced conception is 3% to 5% for male carriers and 10% to 15% for female carriers of reciprocal balanced translocations.

A second and important type of translocation is the robertsonian translocation. This is a structural rearrangement between

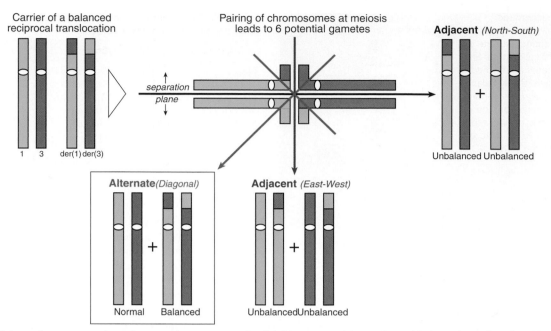

Figure 2-19 Schematic representation of segregation patterns of a diploid gamete with a reciprocal balanced translocation. Here, exchanges have occurred between the short arms of chromosomes 1 and 3. The two pairs of chromosomes pair in a quadriradial fashion. There are three potential axes in which the cell can divide. Only two of the six potential gametes will be genetically balanced. (Courtesy of Edith Cheng, MD.)

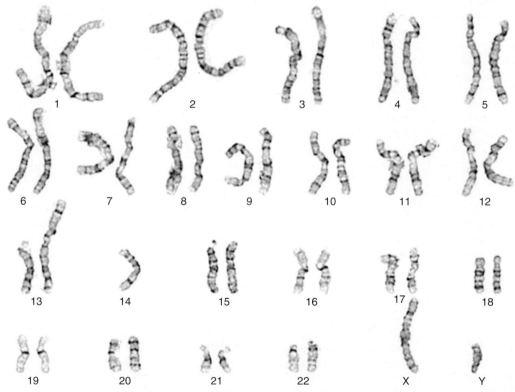

Figure 2-20 Karyotype demonstrating a robertsonian translocation between chromosomes 13 and 14. Notice that there are only 45 chromosome structures, but this male is genetically diploid. (Courtesy of Edith Cheng, MD.)

Isochromosomes occur as a result of the chromosome dividing along the horizontal axis rather than the longitudinal axis at the centromere. The result is a chromosome that has two copies of one arm and no copies of the other. Isochromosomes involving autosomes are generally lethal because the resultant conception will be both trisomic and monosomic for genetic information. However, an isochromosome involving the long arm of the X chromosome (iso Xq) is compatible with life.

Finally, deletions and duplications of chromosome segments arise from unequal crossing over at meiosis or from crossing over

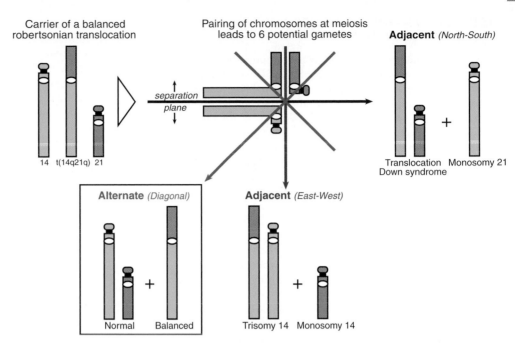

Figure 2-21 Schematic representation of the segregation patterns of a diploid gamete with a robertsonian translocation. Six potential gametes are formed, but only two are genetically balanced. One of the six gametes containing the 14/21 translocation and the free chromosome 21 will result in a conception with Down syndrome. (Courtesy of Edith Cheng, MD.)

during pairing of inversions or reciprocal translocations. Breaks resulting in loss of chromosome material at the tip are called *terminal deletions,* and loss of chromosome material between two breaks within a chromosome is called an *interstitial deletion.* There are several well-documented terminal deletion syndromes, including cri-du-chat (5p-) syndrome, characterized by microcephaly, profound mental retardation, growth retardation, a unique facial appearance, and a distinctive catlike cry. Most cases occur as a de novo chromosome deletion of the tip of the short arm (p arm) of chromosome 5, but approximately 10% to 15% arise as a consequence of a parental reciprocal translocation involving chromosome 5 and another chromosome.

Microdeletion/Duplication or Contiguous Gene Syndromes

The discussion in the previous section described only phenotypes that were associated with chromosome abnormalities visible with traditional cytogenetic techniques and light microscopy that imply involvement of large segments of chromosomes containing a large number (hundreds) of genes. In the past decade, high-resolution chromosome banding and advances in molecular cytogenetics technology have revealed a new class of chromosome syndromes known as microdeletion, or contiguous gene, syndromes in which the involved chromosome region(s) are submicroscopic and so

small that a molecular cytogenetic technique such as fluorescent in situ hybridization (FISH) is necessary to localize the affected region. **Table 2-6** lists some of the more commonly recognized syndromes, most of which are due to deletions although some duplication syndromes have now been identified. The phenotypes of these conditions are due to the absence (or duplication) of multiple contiguous genes within the involved region. These regions are small, usually about 1.5 to 3 Mb (compared with traditional chromosome banding and microscopy, which has a resolution requirement of at least 5 Mb). Fine mapping of the breakpoints in some of these conditions has implicated unequal or abnormal recombination between low-copy repetitive DNA sequences in the area of the deleted or duplicated regions. The discovery of microdeletion/duplication or contiguous gene syndromes has been important in clinical genetics and genetic counseling in that it finally provides a diagnosis, recurrence risk, and prenatal diagnosis for a large group of syndromes that previously had no cytogenetic confirmation. Moreover, these "naturally occurring" sequestered small regions of contiguous genes have provided a powerful tool for developmental geneticists to decipher the critical genes for normal human development. For example, the 22q11 region appears to be rich in genes responsible for specific congenital heart defects and craniofacial anomalies.

Table 2-6 Common Microdeletion/Contiguous Gene Syndromes

Syndrome	Incidence	Location	Abnormality	Size (Mb)
		Chromosome		
Sotos	Rare	5q35	Deletion	2.2
Smith–Magenis	1/25,000	17p11.2	Deletion and duplication	4
Williams	1/20,000–1/50,000	7q11.23	Deletion	1.6
Charcot-Marie-Tooth (*CMTIA/HNLPP*) h	1/10,000	17p12	Duplication and deletion	1.5
DiGeorge/ Velocardiofacial	1/4,000		Deletion	1.5
Cat's eye	Rare	22q11	Duplication	3
der(22)	Rare			3
Neurofibromatosis	1/40,000–1/80,000	17q11	Deletion	1.5

CHROMOSOME ABNORMALITIES AND PREGNANCY OUTCOME

The incidence and types of chromosome abnormalities differ between spontaneous abortions, stillbirths, and live births. Experience from pregnancies achieved by assisted reproductive technology indicates that 15% of fertilized ova fail to divide. Another 15% fail to implant, and 25% to 30% are aborted spontaneously at previllous stages. Of the roughly 40% of fertilized ova that survive the first missed menstrual period, as many as one fourth are aborted spontaneously, so that only about 30% to 35% of fertilized ova actually result in live-born infants. Chromosome and lethal genetic abnormalities play a major role in early losses. Thirty to 60% of first-trimester abortuses are found to have a chromosome abnormality of which approximately 50% are due to autosomal trisomies. Certain chromosomes are more commonly involved than others; for example, trisomy 16 accounts for one third of trisomic abortuses. Autosomal monosomies are extremely rare, accounting for less than 1% of chromosomally abnormal abortuses. This may reflect selection at the gametic level in that the gamete with monosomy is not viable. Triploidy accounts for 16% of spontaneous abortions. Turner syndrome due to 45,X is by far the most common chromosome abnormality, accounting for 20% of spontaneous abortions that are chromosomally abnormal. This topic is discussed further in Chapter 16 (Spontaneous and Recurrent Abortion).

Molar Gestations

Molar gestations comprise two clinical entities: the syndrome of associated triploidy, also known as partial moles, and the hydatidiform, or complete, mole. Each has a distinctive chromosome abnormality and different clinical consequences. Triploidy (three chromosome complements) is found in 16% of abortuses with chromosome abnormalities (**Fig. 2-22**). They occur as a consequence of errors in meiosis or from double fertilization of a single ovum. The clinical features of a triploid pregnancy depend on the parent of origin of the extra set of chromosomes. In two thirds of cases, there is one maternal set and two paternal sets of chromosomes, resulting in poor embryonic development but a large hydropic placenta, the partial mole. Conversely, if there is an extra maternal set, an anomalous and growth-restricted fetus and a small fibrotic placenta are seen. Thus, triploidy is an example of imprinting in which the parent of origin of genetic information is marked and important for development.

In contrast to the triploid, partial mole, the complete mole is diploid with a 46,XX karyotype. The chromosomes are all paternally derived. When genetic markers are used to characterize the two sets of paternal chromosome, all of the markers are homozygous. Complete moles arise through the fertilization of an anucleated oocyte and subsequent duplication of the haploid chromosome complement (23,X) of the sperm. The absence of maternal contribution results in the development of abundant, hydropic trophoblastic tissue, and no recognizable embryonic tissue.

The clinical features of molar gestations indicate that normal pregnancies require both maternal and paternal genetic contributions, with the paternal genome being important for extraembryonic development and the maternal genome necessary for fetal development. Molar gestations and trophoblastic disease are discussed further in Chapter 35 (Gestational Trophoblastic Disease).

CANCER GENETICS

All cancer is genetic. However, most cancer is not inherited. To the patient and her family, this is a difficult concept to explain. Listening to the plethora of news reports, it is no wonder that the

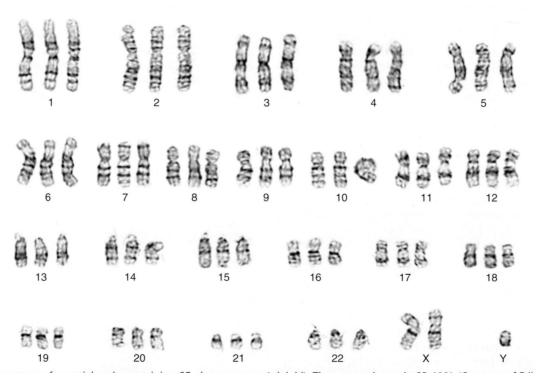

Figure 2-22 Karyotype of a partial mole containing 69 chromosomes (triploid). The nomenclature is 69, XXY. (Courtesy of Edith Cheng, MD.)

nonmedical world believes that any history of cancer in the family implies an inherited risk, and an absence of cancer in the family constitutes a protective effect. Helping patients reach an appropriate level of understanding through communicating accurate information and forging a partnership will likely help them understand and accept our recommendations. This discussion focuses on mechanisms of inheriting a susceptibility to cancer. Discussions of specific cancer syndromes are addressed in the chapters dealing with the specific cancers and organ systems.

For a normal cell line to be transformed into a malignant cell line, several genetic mutations in that somatic cell line must occur that alter cell growth and differentiation. All cells have mechanisms to either repair a mutation or inhibit growth and replication if errors in DNA occur. Thus, before malignancy can arise, most cancer cells have to "escape" those repair functions. The first mutations must occur in either DNA repair genes or genes that suppress growth of abnormal cells (the genes that maintain the integrity of the genome). Subsequent mutations are then passed on to daughter cells. Increasing cell replications occur, and as mutations build up, some will allow the cell line to grow abnormally and often confer biologic advantages over surrounding normal cells. When "enough" DNA change occurs, the resulting abnormal cells are capable of metastasizing, thereby usurping resources of vital organs, and without treatment, eventually lead to death. This process of multiple sequential mutations is called the "multistep process of cancer." In a small percentage of families with cancer, approximately 5% to 10%, there is a germline (inherited) mutation that predisposes certain tissues to begin to move through the multistep series of mutations more easily. More than 200 inherited cancer syndromes have been described, although most are quite rare. These inherited cancer genes do not cause cancer; rather they allow cancer to happen more easily. Inherited cancer syndromes that affect female organs are listed in **Table 2-7**.

Carefully regulated cellular processes, such as differentiation, proliferation, and programmed cell death, are altered in cancer cells. The stages of carcinogenesis are termed *initiation* (single initial proliferative cell), *promotion* (acquired selective growth advantage), *progression* (tumor characteristics become irreversible), and *metastasis* (process by which cells are displaced). Types of genes and genetic mechanisms involved in malignancy may be grouped into four categories: **oncogenes**, tumor suppressor genes, DNA repair genes, and epigenetic mechanisms.

Oncogenes (gain of function) behave as growth-promoting genes, and they act in a genetically dominant manner. They originate from normal cellular genes called proto-oncogenes. The proto-oncogenes have normal functions within a cell to control and enhance cell growth. Oncogene activation (through mutation) can lead to either increased expression of proteins or changes in structure and function of a proto-oncogene's product. For example, the HER 2/neu receptor may be overexpressed on by an oncogene. Only a few inherited cancer syndromes involve oncogenes. Examples include the RET, CDK4, and KIT oncogenes. The RET oncogene is the underlying cause of multiple endocrine neoplasia (MEN type 2). These individuals have an increased risk to develop endocrine tumors.

Tumor suppressor genes restrain cell growth in damaged cells; therefore, loss of the tumor suppressor gene through mutation leads to increased cell proliferation of abnormal cells and cancer development. They account for the majority of autosomal dominant cancer syndromes. Some examples include BRCA1

Table 2-7 Inherited Cancer Syndromes affecting Gynecologic Organ Systems

Body Part	Cancer Syndrome	Gene Name
Breast	**Inherited breast-ovarian cancer** (autosomal dominant; tumor suppressor gene, involved in the maintenance of genomic stability)	BRCA1, 17q21
	Inherited breast-ovarian cancer (autosomal dominant; tumor suppressor gene, involved in the maintenance of genomic stability)	BRCA2, 13q12.3
	Li-Fraumini (autosomal dominant; regulates the cell-cycle arrest that is required to permit repair of DNA damage)	p53, 17p13.1
	Cowden	PTEN
	Peutz-Jeghers	LKB1
	p16^{INK4a}	p16^{INK4a}
	p14^{arf}	p14^{arf}
Endometrium	Chordoma	
	Cowden	
	Lynch syndrome (HNPCC)	
	Peutz-Jegher	
Fallopian tube	Inherited breast-ovarian cancer	BRCA1
	Inherited breast-ovarian cancer	BRCA2
Ovarian	Basal cell nevus	
	Inherited breast-ovarian cancer	BRCA1
	Inherited breast-ovarian cancer	BRCA2
	Lynch syndrome (HNPCC)	
	Peutz-Jegher	
Vulva	Fanconi	

and BRCA2 genes, and the p53 gene (Li-Fraumini syndrome). Tumor suppressor genes are dominantly inherited. However, on the cellular level, they are recessive. In other words, a cell must have two genetic hits (one hit to each copy of the gene in question) before the cell can head down the multistep process to cancer. The first hit is inherited, and the second hit is acquired.

DNA repair genes identify and mend DNA replication errors made during replication. When they are nonfunctional, replication errors can lead to cancer development. Lynch syndrome (HNPCC) has four mismatch repair genes (MLH1, MSH2, MSH6, and PMS2) that predispose an individual to colon cancer and uterine cancer. One could imagine these genes as editors that find and correct spelling errors. Loss of their function allows mutations to accumulate and leads the daughter cells down the path of the multistep process of cancer. There are other genes that concentrate on repairing DNA sequences that were damaged by and external source such as radiation. Some examples include Fanconi anemia, Bloom syndrome, ataxia-telangiectasia, and xeroderma pigmentosum. These are the few cancer syndromes that follow and autosomal recessive pattern of inheritance.

The last genetic concept to consider is epigenetic mechanisms in which growth regulating genes are activated or silenced. An epigenetic modification of gene expression does not involve alteration of the gene's DNA sequence. Two major mechanisms of gene silencing are genomic imprinting (a process by which the gender of the parental allele determines whether or not the gene is silenced) and methylation (the addition or removal of a methyl group to the gene, usually in the promoter region, which blocks the initiation of the gene). Thus, if a gene like the tumor suppressor gene becomes inappropriately methylated, it is turned off. Abnormal epigenetic syndromes are not yet known to be part of the inherited cancer syndromes.

When considering a family history of cancer, one should first obtain a complete history including who has and who has not had cancer in the family. This information will help determine to which group the family likely belongs: *average risk* (sporadic—somatic cell changes), *moderate risk* (common exposures—somatic cell changes or low penetrance genes), or *high risk* (inherited cancer genes—germline mutations). For certain cancer syndromes, computer models are available to help determine the chance a family has an inherited cancer syndrome. It is important to note that taking a detailed family history involves more than asking who has had cancer. One important factor to be cognizant of is the difference between primary cancers, recurrences, and metastatic disease. Patients rarely understand the subtleties of these important distinctions and inadvertently report inaccurate information. It is quite common for a woman to tell her physician about a family member who was treated for uterine cancer. Upon detailed history taking the physician finds that the woman had a procedure for cervical dysplasia. This type of information is critical to sort this out in order to provide a risk estimate. Once it is determined to which group the person belongs, then an estimation of that person's risk to develop cancer can be determined, and, finally, an individualized cancer screening recommendations can be agreed upon.

KEY POINTS

- Base pairing in DNA molecules is always A–T and G–C, and in RNA molecules it is always A–U and G–C.
- Endonuclease enzymes cleave specific nucleotide pairs, making DNA fragment evaluation and gene cloning possible. More than 200 different endonucleases exist.
- Through a process known as polymerase chain reaction (PCR), small fragments of DNA may be cloned to produce larger amounts of the same material suitable for analysis.
- When a heterozygous individual who has an autosomal dominant trait mates with a normal individual, 50% of their offspring will have the trait.
- When two individuals who carry an autosomal recessive trait mate, 25% of their offspring will demonstrate the trait and 50% will be carriers.
- X-linked recessive characteristics are transmitted from maternal carriers to male offspring and will affect 50% of such male offspring.
- In general, if a couple produces an offspring with a multifactorial defect and the problem has never occurred in the family, it can be expected to be repeated in 2% to 5% of subsequent pregnancies.
- The findings always present in 45,X Turner syndrome are shortness of stature and sexual infantilism.
- A variety of different karyotypes have been discovered in individuals with the phenotype of Turner syndrome.
- Nondisjunctional events have been described in every autosome except chromosomes 1 and 17. The risk of producing a second conceptus with a nondisjunctional event is approximately 1%.

- Conditions always seen in individuals with Klinefelter syndrome (47,XXY) are tallness of stature and azoospermia. One third of these individuals have gynecomastia.
- Of ova penetrated by sperm, 15% fail to implant, and 25% to 30% are aborted spontaneously at a previllous stage. Of the 40% that survive the first missed menstrual period, as many as one fourth abort spontaneously. From 30% to 35% of ova penetrated by sperm end in live-born individuals.
- Between 30% and 60% of known aborted conceptuses have chromosome abnormalities. Half of these have autosomal trisomies; 20% have 45,X; 14% to 19% have triploidy; 3% to 6% have tetraploidy; and 3% to 4% have chromosome rearrangements.
- Of live-born infants with chromosome abnormalities, about 0.8% to 1% have 45,X; 36.8% have other sex chromosome abnormalities; 21% have autosomal trisomies; and balanced chromosome translocations occur in 32.4%. About 3.2% have unbalanced translocation abnormalities.
- One in 200 women has recurrent (three or more) abortions, with chromosome abnormalities occurring in about 4.8% of the mothers and 2.4% of the fathers.
- When chromosome 21 is present as part of a robertsonian translocation with a D group chromosome, the chance of transmission of an unbalanced karyotype (leading to an offspring with Down syndrome) is 10% to 15% if the mother is the carrier and 1% to 2% if the father is the carrier.
- Hydatidiform moles are either diploid (46,XX or 46,XY) or triploid. The chromosomes of the diploid type, usually seen in true moles, are completely derived from paternal chromosomes. Triploid moles have at least two haploid sets derived from paternal origin.

REFERENCES CAN BE FOUND ON EXPERTCONSULT.com

3

Reproductive Anatomy
Gross and Microscopic, Clinical Correlations

Vern L. Katz

The organs of the female reproductive tract are classically divided into the external and the internal genitalia. The external genital organs are present in the perineal area and include the mons pubis, clitoris, urinary meatus, labia majora, labia minora, vestibule, Bartholin's glands, and periurethral glands. The internal genital organs are located in the true pelvis and include the vagina, uterus, cervix, oviducts, ovaries, and surrounding supporting structures. This chapter integrates the basic anatomy of the female pelvis with clinical situations.

Embryologically the urinary, reproductive, and gastrointestinal tracts develop in close proximity. This relationship continues throughout a woman's life span. In the adult, the reproductive organs are in intimate contact with the lower urinary tract and large intestines. Because of the anatomic proximity of the genital and urinary systems, altered pathophysiology in one organ often produces symptoms in an adjacent organ. The gynecologic surgeon should master the intricacy of these anatomic relationships to avoid surgical complications. The clinician must also appreciate that wide individual differences in anatomic detail exist among patients. Understanding these variations is one of the greatest challenges of clinical medicine.

This chapter focuses on the norms of human anatomy; it does not duplicate the completeness of an anatomic text or surgical atlas.

EXTERNAL GENITALIA

VULVA

The vulva, or pudendum, is a collective term for the external genital organs that are visible in the perineal area. The vulva consists of the following: the mons pubis, labia majora, labia minora, hymen, clitoris, vestibule, urethra, Skene's glands, Bartholin's glands, and **vestibular bulbs** (Fig. 3-1).

The boundaries of the vulva extend from the mons pubis anteriorly to the rectum posteriorly and from one lateral **genitocrural fold** to the other. The entire vulvar area is covered by keratinized, stratified squamous epithelium. The skin becomes thicker, more pigmented, and more keratinized as the distance from the vagina increases.

MONS PUBIS

The mons pubis is a rounded eminence that becomes hairy after puberty. It is directly anterior and superior to the symphysis pubis. The hair pattern, or escutcheon, of most women is triangular. Genetic and racial differences produce a variety of normal hair patterns, with approximately one in four women having a modified escutcheon that has a diamond (malelike) pattern.

LABIA MAJORA

The labia majora are two large, longitudinal, cutaneous folds of adipose and fibrous tissue. Each labium majus is approximately 7 to 8 cm in length and 2 to 3 cm in width. The labia extend from the mons pubis anteriorly to become lost in the skin between the vagina and the anus in the area of the **posterior fourchette**. The skin of the outer convex surface of the labia majora is pigmented and covered with hair follicles. The thin skin of the inner surface does not have hair follicles but has many sebaceous glands. Histologically the labia majora have both sweat and sebaceous glands (**Fig. 3-2**). The **apocrine glands** are similar to those of the breast and axillary areas. The size of the labia is related to fat content. Usually the labia atrophy after menopause. The labia majora are homologous to the scrotum in the male.

LABIA MINORA

The labia minora, or nymphae, are two small, red cutaneous folds that are situated between the labia majora and the vaginal orifice. They are more delicate, shorter, and thinner than the labia majora. Anteriorly, they divide at the clitoris to form superiorly the prepuce and inferiorly the frenulum of the clitoris. Histologically they are composed of dense connective tissue with erectile tissue and elastic fibers, rather than adipose tissue. The skin of the labia minora is less cornified and has many sebaceous glands but no hair follicles or sweat glands. The labia minora and the breasts are the only areas of the body rich in sebaceous glands but without hair follicles. Among women of reproductive age, there is considerable variation in the size of the labia minora. They are relatively more prominent in children and postmenopausal women. The labia minora are homologous to the penile urethra and part of the skin of the penis in males.

HYMEN

The hymen is a thin, usually perforated membrane at the entrance of the vagina. There are many variations in the structure and shape of the hymen. The hymen histologically is covered by stratified squamous epithelium on both sides and consists of

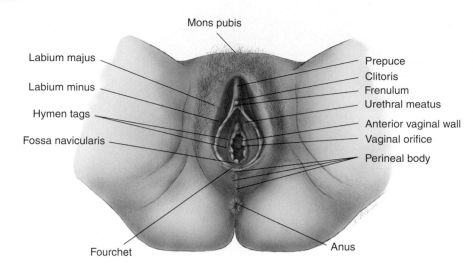

Mons pubis

Labium majus

Labium minus

Hymen tags

Fossa navicularis

Fourchet

Prepuce
Clitoris
Frenulum
Urethral meatus

Anterior vaginal wall
Vaginal orifice
Perineal body

Anus

Figure 3-1 The structures of the external genitalia that are collectively called the vulva. (Redrawn from Pritchard JA, MacDonald PC, Gant NF: Williams' Obstetrics, 17th ed. New York, Appleton-Century-Crofts, 1985, p 8.)

fibrous tissue with a few small blood vessels. Small tags, or nodules, of firm fibrous material, termed **carunculae myrtiformes**, are the remnants of the hymen identified in adult females.

CLITORIS

The clitoris is a short, cylindrical, erectile organ at the superior portion of the vestibule. The normal adult glans clitoris has a width less than 1 cm, with an average length of 1.5 to 2 cm. Previous childbearing may influence the size of the clitoris, but age, weight, and oral contraceptive use do not change the anatomic dimensions. Usually, only the glans is visible, with the body of the clitoris positioned beneath the skin surface. The clitoris consists of a base of two crura, which attach to the periosteum of the symphysis pubis. The body has two cylindrical corpora cavernosa composed of thin-walled, vascular channels that function as erectile tissue (**Fig. 3-3**). The distal one third of the clitoris is the glans, which has many nerve endings. The clitoris is the female homologue of the penis in the male.

VESTIBULE

The vestibule is the lowest portion of the embryonic urogenital sinus. It is the cleft between the labia minora that is visualized when the labia are held apart. The vestibule extends from the clitoris to the posterior fourchette. The orifices of the urethra and vagina and the ducts from Bartholin's glands open into the vestibule. Within the area of the vestibule are the remnants of the hymen and numerous small mucinous glands.

URETHRA

The urethra is a membranous conduit for urine from the urinary bladder to the vestibule. The female urethra measures 3.5 to 5 cm in length. The mucosa of the proximal two thirds of the urethra is composed of stratified transitional epithelium, whereas the distal one third is stratified squamous epithelium. The distal

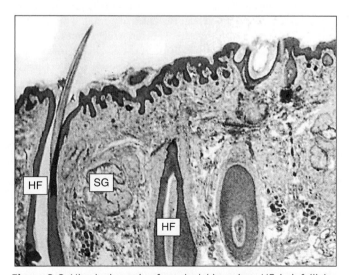

Figure 3-2 Histologic section from the labia majora. HF, hair follicles; SG, sebaceous glands. Note the **eccrine glands** and ducts. (From Stevens A, Lowe J: Human Histology, 3 rd ed., Philadelphia, Elsevier, 2002, p 346.)

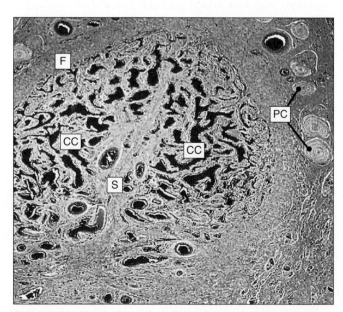

Figure 3-3 A histologic section of the clitoris. Note the two corpus cavernosa (CC), the septum (S), and the fibrous-collagenous sheath (F). Multiple nerve endings may be seen surrounding the clitoris. PC, pacinian touch corpuscles. (From Stevens A, Lowe J: Human Histology, 3 rd ed. Philadelphia, Elsevier, 2002, p 346.)

orifice is 4 to 6 mm in diameter, and the mucosal edges grossly appear everted.

SKENE'S GLANDS

Skene's glands, or paraurethral glands, are branched, tubular glands that are adjacent to the distal urethra. Usually Skene's ducts run parallel to the long axis of the urethra for approximately 1 cm before opening into the distal urethra. Sometimes the ducts open into the area just outside the urethral orifice. Skene's glands are the largest of the paraurethral glands; however, many smaller glands empty into the urethra. Skene's glands are homologous to the prostate in the male.

BARTHOLIN'S GLANDS

Bartholin's glands are vulvovaginal glands that are located immediately beneath the fascia at about 4 and 8 o'clock, respectively, on the posterolateral aspect of the vaginal orifice. Each lobulated, racemose gland is about the size of a pea. Histologically the gland is composed of cuboidal epithelium (**Fig. 3-4**). The duct from each gland is lined by transitional epithelium and is approximately 2 cm in length. Bartholin's ducts open into a groove between the hymen and the labia minora. Bartholin's glands are homologous to Cowper's glands in the male.

VESTIBULAR BULBS

The vestibular bulbs are two elongated masses of erectile tissue situated on either side of the vaginal orifice. Each bulb is immediately below the bulbocavernosus muscle. The distal ends of the vestibular bulbs are adjacent to Bartholin's glands. They are homologous to the bulb of the penis in the male.

CLINICAL CORRELATIONS

The skin of the vulvar region is subject to both local and general dermatologic conditions. The intertriginous areas of the vulva remain moist, and obese women are particularly susceptible to chronic infection. The vulvar skin of a postmenopausal woman is sensitive to topical cortisone and testosterone but insensitive to topical estrogen. The most common large cystic structure of the vulva is a Bartholin's duct cyst. This condition may become painful if the cyst develops into an acute abscess. Chronic infections of the periurethral glands may result in one or more urethral diverticula. The most common symptoms of a urethral diverticulum are similar to the symptoms of a lower urinary tract infection: urinary frequency, urgency, and dysuria.

Vulvar trauma such as straddle injuries frequently results in large hematomas or profuse external hemorrhage. The richness of the vascular supply and the absence of valves in vulvar veins contribute to this complication. The abundant vascularity of the region promotes rapid healing, with an associated low incidence of wound infection in episiotomies or obstetric tears of the vulva. The subcutaneous fatty tissue of the labia majora and mons pubis are in continuity with the fatty tissue of the anterior abdominal wall. Infections in this space such as cellulites and necrotizing fasciitis are poorly contained, and may extend cephalady in rapid fashion.

INTERNAL GENITALIA

VAGINA

The vagina is a thin-walled, distensible, fibromuscular tube that extends from the vestibule of the vulva to the uterus. The potential space of the vagina is larger in the middle and upper thirds. The walls of the vagina are normally in apposition and flattened in the anteroposterior diameter. Thus, the vagina has the appearance of the letter H in cross section (**Fig. 3-5**).

The axis of the upper portion of the vagina lies fairly close to the horizontal plane when a woman is standing, with the upper portion of the vagina curving toward the hollow of the sacrum. In most women an angle of at least 90 degrees is formed between the axis of the vagina and the axis of the uterus (**Fig. 3-6**). The vagina is held in position by the surrounding endopelvic fascia and ligaments.

The lower third of the vagina is in close relationship with the urogenital and **pelvic diaphragms**. The middle third of the vagina is supported by the levator ani muscles and the lower portion of the cardinal ligaments. The upper third is supported by the upper portions of the cardinal ligaments and the **parametria**. The vagina of reproductive-age women has numerous transverse folds, vaginal **rugae**. They help provide accordion-like distensibility and are more prominent in the lower third of the vagina. The cervix extends into the upper part of the vagina. The spaces between the cervix and attachment of the vagina are called *fornices*. The posterior fornix is considerably larger than the anterior fornix; thus, the anterior vaginal length is approximately 6 to 9 cm in comparison with a posterior vaginal length of 8 to 12 cm. Vaginal length is increased slightly by a woman's weight and height. Age, conversely, leads to a shortening of vaginal length. A study by Tan et al. noted a decrease of 0.08 cm per 10 years. Menopause leads to a shortening of 0.17 cm of length.

Histologically the vagina is composed of four distinct layers. The mucosa consists of a stratified, nonkeratinized squamous epithelium (**Fig. 3-7**). If the environment of the vaginal mucosa is modified, as in uterine prolapse, then the epithelium may become keratinized. The squamous epithelium is similar microscopically to the exocervix, although the vagina has larger and more frequent papillae that extend into the connective tissue.

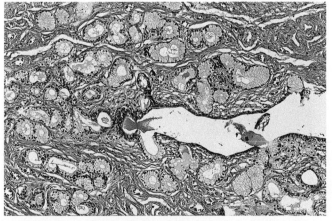

Figure 3-4 A histologic section of a Bartholin's gland. Note the multiple alveoli draining into a central duct. (From Shea CR, Stevens A, Dalziel KL, Robboy SJ: Vulva. In Robboy SJ, Anderson MC, Russell P [eds]: Pathology of the Female Reproductive Tract. Edinburgh, Churchill Livingstone, 2002, p 36.)

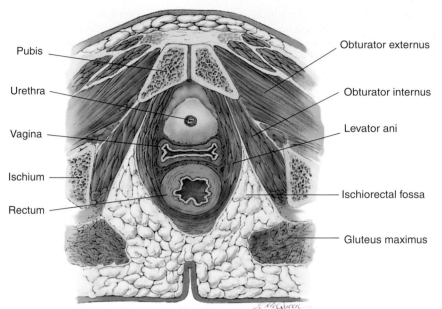

Pubis

Urethra

Vagina

Ischium

Rectum

Obturator externus

Obturator internus

Levator ani

Ischiorectal fossa

Gluteus maximus

Figure 3-5 A schematic drawing of a cross section of the female pelvis, demonstrating the H shape of the vagina. Note the surrounding levator ani muscle. (Redrawn from Pritchard JA, MacDonald PC, Gant NF: Williams' Obstetrics, 17th ed. New York, Appleton-Century-Crofts, 1985, p 12.)

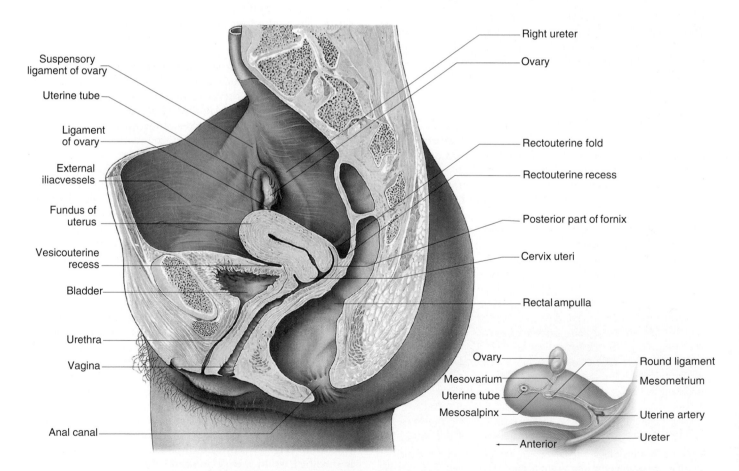

Suspensory ligament of ovary

Uterine tube

Ligament of ovary

External iliacvessels

Fundus of uterus

Vesicouterine recess

Bladder

Urethra

Vagina

Anal canal

Right ureter

Ovary

Rectouterine fold

Rectouterine recess

Posterior part of fornix

Cervix uteri

Rectal ampulla

Ovary

Mesovarium

Uterine tube

Mesosalpinx

Round ligament

Mesometrium

Uterine artery

Ureter

Anterior

Figure 3-6 A median sagittal section through the pelvis. The peritoneum is shaded blue. Note the proximal vagina at a diagonal axis and in a near 90-degree juxtaposition to the uterus. In this woman, the uterus is anteflexed. (From Standring S [ed]: Gray's Anatomy, 39th ed. Edinburgh, Elsevier Churchill Livingstone, 2005, p 1321.)

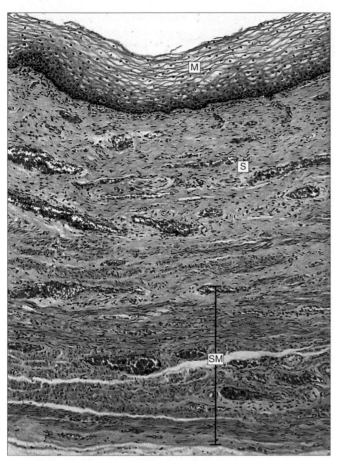

Figure 3-7 Histologic section of the vaginal squamous epithelium (M). Submucosa (S) is well vascularized. (Lamina propria). SM, smooth muscle. (From Stevens A, Lowe J: Human Histology, 3 rd ed. Philadelphia, Elsevier, 2002, p 347.)

The nerve supply of the vagina comes from the autonomic nervous system's vaginal plexus, and sensory fibers come from the pudendal nerve. Pain fibers enter the spinal cord in sacral segments two to four. There is a paucity of free nerve endings in the upper two thirds of the vagina.

The lymphatic drainage is characterized by its wide distribution and frequent crossovers between the right and left sides of the pelvis. In general the primary lymphatic drainage of the upper third of the vagina is to the external iliac nodes, the middle third of the vagina drains to the common and internal iliac nodes, and the lower third has a complex and variable distribution, including the common iliac, superficial inguinal, and perirectal nodes.

CLINICAL CORRELATIONS

In clinical practice anatomic descriptions of pelvic organs are derived from Latin roots, such as the word *vagina*, which is derived from the Latin word for sheath. In contrast, the names for surgical procedures of pelvic organs are derived from Greek roots. *Colpectomy, colporrhaphy,* and *colposcopy* are derived from *kolpos* (fold), the Greek word for the vagina, or hysterectomy (Greek) versus uterus (Latin).

Clinicians should consider the H shape of the vagina when they insert a speculum and inspect the walls of the vagina. The posterior fornix is an important surgical landmark, because it provides direct access to the **cul-de-sac of Douglas**. The distal course of the ureter is an essential consideration in vaginal surgery. Ureteral injury has occurred as a result of vaginally placed sutures to obtain hemostasis with vaginal lacerations. The anatomic proximity and interrelationships of the vascular and lymphatic networks of the bladder and vagina are such that inflammation of one organ can produce symptoms in the other. For example, vaginitis sometimes produces urinary tract symptoms, such as frequency and dysuria.

Gartner's duct cyst, a cystic dilation of the embryonic mesonephros (**Fig. 3-8**), is usually present on the lateral wall of the vagina. However, in the lower third of the vagina these cysts are present anteriorly and may be difficult to distinguish from a large urethral diverticulum.

An interesting phenomenon is the source of vaginal lubrication during intercourse. For years there was speculation on how an organ without glands is able to "secrete" fluid. Vaginal lubrication occurs from a transudate produced by engorgement of the vascular plexuses that encircle the vagina. This richness of vascularization allows many drugs to readily enter the systemic circulation when placed in the vagina. Medications that are absorbed vaginally go directly into the systemic circulation, bypassing the liver and its metabolism on the first round through the circulation.

The anatomic relationship between the long axis of the vagina and other pelvic organs may be altered by pelvic relaxation resulting primarily from the trauma of childbirth. Atrophy or weakness of the endopelvic fascia and muscles surrounding the vagina may result in the development of a cystocele, rectocele, or enterocele. One of the popular operations for vaginal vault prolapse is fixation of the apex of the vagina to the sacrospinous ligament. A rare complication of this operation is massive hemorrhage. The arterial bleeding is usually from the inferior gluteal or pudendal arteries.

The normal vagina does not have glands. The next layer is the lamina propria, or tunica. It is composed of fibrous connective tissue. Throughout this layer of collagen and elastic tissue is a rich supply of vascular and lymphatic channels. The density of the connective tissue in the endopelvic fascia varies throughout the longitudinal axis of the vagina. The muscular layer has many interlacing fibers. However, an inner circular layer and an outer longitudinal layer can be identified. The fourth layer consists of cellular areolar connective tissue containing a large **plexus** of blood vessels.

The vascular system of the vagina is generously supplied with an extensive anastomotic network throughout its length. The vaginal artery originates either directly from the uterine artery or as a branch of the internal iliac artery arising posterior to the origin of the uterine and inferior vesical arteries. The vaginal arteries may be multiple arteries on each side of the pelvis. There is an anastomosis with the cervical branch of the uterine artery to form the azygos arteries. Branches of the internal pudendal, inferior vesical, and middle hemorrhoidal arteries also contribute to the interconnecting network and the longitudinal azygos arteries.

The venous drainage is complex and accompanies the arterial system. Below the pelvic floor, the principal venous drainage occurs via the pudendal veins. The vaginal, uterine, and vesical veins, as well as those around the rectosigmoid, all provide venous drainage of the venous plexuses surrounding the middle and upper vagina.

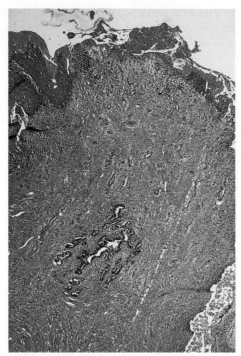

Figure 3-8 Mesonephric duct remnant in the vaginal wall. (From Robboy SJ, Anderson MC, Russell P [eds]: Pathology of the Female Reproductive Tract. Edinburgh, Churchill Livingstone, 2002, p 77.)

CERVIX

The lower, narrow portion of the uterus is the cervix. The word *cervix* originates from the Latin word for neck. The Greek word for neck is *trachelos,* and when the cervix is removed, the surgical procedure is termed *trachelectomy.* The cervix may vary

in shape from cylindrical to conical. It consists of predominantly fibrous tissue in contrast to the primarily muscular corpus of the uterus.

The vagina is attached obliquely around the middle of the cervix; this attachment divides the cervix into an upper, supravaginal portion and a lower segment in the vagina called the *portio vaginalis* (**Fig. 3-9**). The supravaginal segment is covered by peritoneum posteriorly and is surrounded by loose, fatty connective tissue—the parametrium—anteriorly and laterally.

The canal of the cervix is fusiform, with the widest diameter in the middle. The length and width of the endocervical canal varies; it is usually 2.5 to 3 cm in length and 7 to 8 mm at its widest point. The width of the canal varies with the parity of the woman and changing hormonal levels. The cervical length increases in pregnancy, with maximal length in the second trimester. The cervical canal opens into the vagina at the external os of the cervix. In the majority of women, the external os is in contact with the posterior vaginal wall. The external os is small and round in nulliparous women. The os is wider and gaping following vaginal delivery. Often lateral or stellate scars are residual marks of previous cervical lacerations.

The mucous membrane of the endocervical canal of nulliparous women is arranged in longitudinal folds, called **plicae palmatae**, with secondary branching folds, the arbor vitae (**Fig. 3-10**). These folds, which form a herringbone pattern, disappear following vaginal delivery.

A single layer of columnar epithelium lines the endocervical canal and the underlying glandular structures. This specialized epithelium secretes mucus, which facilitates sperm transport. An abrupt transformation usually is seen at the junction of the columnar epithelium of the endocervix and the nonkeratinized stratified squamous epithelium of the portio vaginalis (**Fig. 3-11**). The stratified squamous epithelium of the exocervix is identical to the lining of the vagina.

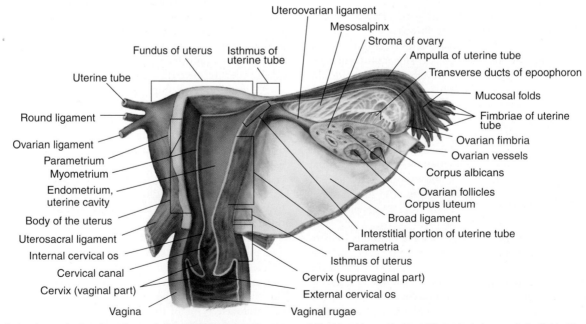

Figure 3-9 A schematic drawing of a posterior view of the cervix, uterus, fallopian tube, and ovary. Note that the cervix is divided by the vaginal attachment into an external portio segment and a supravaginal segment. Note that the uterus is composed of the dome-shaped fundus, the muscular body, and the narrow isthmus. Note the fimbria ovarica, or ovarian fimbria, attaching the oviduct to the ovary. (Redrawn from Clemente CD: Anatomy: A Regional Atlas of the Human Body, 3 rd ed. Baltimore-Munich, Urban & Schwarzenberg, 1987.)

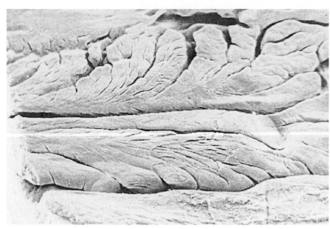

Figure 3-10 An electron micrograph of the endocervical canal, demonstrating the arbor vitae. These folds and crypts provide a reservoir for sperm. (From Singer A, Jordan JA: The anatomy of the cervix. In Jordan JA, Singer A [eds]: The Cervix. Philadelphia, WB Saunders, 1976, p 18.)

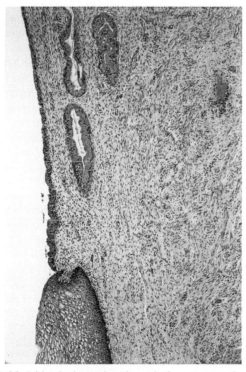

Figure 3-11 A histologic section through the squamocolumnar junction of the cervix. Note the abrupt transformation from squamous to columnar epithelium. (From Standring S [ed]: Gray's Anatomy, 39th ed. Edinburgh, Elsevier Churchill Livingstone, 2005, p 1335.)

The dense, fibromuscular cervical stroma is composed primarily of collagenous connective tissue and mucopolysaccharide ground substance. The collagen framework and ground substance are sensitive to hormonal effects. The connective tissue contains approximately 15% smooth muscle cells and a small amount of elastic tissue (**Fig. 3-12**). However, there are few muscle fibers in the distal portions of the cervix.

It is not surprising that the cervical and uterine vascular supplies are interrelated. The arterial supply of the cervix arises from the descending branch of the uterine artery. The cervical arteries

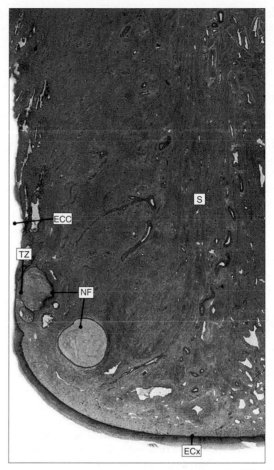

Figure 3-12 A low-power histologic section of the cervix. The stroma (S) has a small amount of smooth muscle. The ectocervix (Ecx) is covered in stratified squamous epithelium. The endocervix (ECC) is lined by tall columnar cells. NF-nabothian follicles, a normal finding, and TZ-transformation zone. (From Stevens A, Lowe J: Human Histology, 3 rd ed. Philadelphia, Elsevier, 2002, p 349.)

run on the lateral side of the cervix and form the coronary artery, which encircles the cervix. The azygos arteries run longitudinally in the middle of the anterior and posterior aspects of the cervix and the vagina. There are numerous anastomoses between these vessels and the vaginal and middle hemorrhoidal arteries. The venous drainage accompanies these arteries. The lymphatic drainage of the cervix is complex, involving multiple chains of nodes. The principal regional lymph nodes are the obturator, common iliac, internal iliac, external iliac, and visceral nodes of the parametria. Other possible lymphatic drainage includes the following chains of nodes: superior and inferior gluteal, sacral, rectal, lumbar, aortic, and visceral nodes over the posterior surface of the urinary bladder. The stroma of the endocervix is rich in free nerve endings. Pain fibers accompany the parasympathetic fibers to the second, third, and fourth sacral segments.

CLINICAL CORRELATIONS

The major arterial supply to the cervix is located on the lateral cervical walls at the 3 and 9 o'clock positions, respectively. Therefore, a deep figure-of-eight suture through the vaginal mucosa and cervical stroma at 3 and 9 o'clock helps to reduce blood loss during procedures such as cone biopsy. If the gynecologist is overzealous in placing such a hemostatic suture high in the vaginal fornix, it is possible to compromise the course of the distal ureter.

The transformation zone of the cervix is an important anatomic landmark for clinicians. This area encompasses the transition from stratified squamous epithelium to columnar epithelium. Dysplasia of the cervix develops within this transformation zone. The position of a woman's transformation zone, in relation to the long axis of the cervix, depends on her age and hormonal status.

The endocervix is rich in free nerve endings. Occasionally, women experience a vasovagal response during transcervical instrumentation of the uterine cavity. Serial cardiac monitoring during insertion of intrauterine devices demonstrates a reflex bradycardia in some women. The sensory innervation of the exocervix is not as concentrated or sophisticated as that of the endocervix or external skin. Therefore, usually the exocervix may be cauterized by either cold or heat without major discomfort to the patient.

UTERUS

The uterus is a thick-walled, hollow, muscular organ located centrally in the female pelvis. Adjacent to the uterus are the urinary bladder anteriorly, the rectum posteriorly, and the broad ligaments laterally (**Figs. 3-6** and **3-13**). The uterus is globular and slightly flattened anteriorly; it has the general configuration of an inverted pear. The short area of constriction in the lower uterine segment is termed the **isthmus** (**Fig. 3-14**). The dome-shaped top of the uterus is termed the **fundus**. The lower edge of the fundus is described by an imaginary line drawn between the site of entrance of each oviduct. The size and weight of the normal uterus depend on previous pregnancies and the hormonal status of the individual. The uterus of a nulliparous woman is approximately 8 cm long, 5 cm wide, and 2.5 cm thick and weighs 40 to 50 g. In contrast, in a multiparous woman, each measurement is approximately 1.2 cm larger, and normal uterine weight is 20 to 30 g heavier. The upper limit for weight of a normal uterus is 110 g. The capacity of the uterus to enlarge during

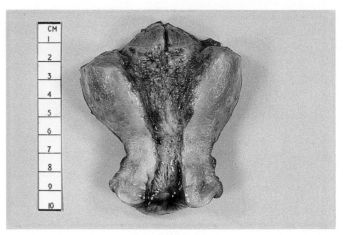

Figure 3-14 A surgical specimen of a uterus that has been opened. (From Robboy SJ, Anderson MC, Russell P [eds]: Pathology of the Female Reproductive Tract. Edinburgh, Churchill Livingstone, 2002, p 241.)

pregnancy results in a 10- to 20-fold increase in weight at term. After menopause the uterus atrophies in both size and weight.

The cavity of the uterus is flattened and triangular. The oviducts enter the uterine cavity at the superolateral aspects of the cavity in the areas designated the **cornua**. In the majority of women, the long axis of the uterus is both anteverted in respect to the long axis of the vagina and anteflexed in relation to the long axis of the cervix. However, a retroflexed uterus is a normal variant found in approximately 25% of women.

The uterus has three layers, similar to other hollow abdominal and pelvic organs. The thin, external serosal layer comprises the visceral peritoneum. The peritoneum is firmly attached to the uterus in all areas except anteriorly at the level of the internal os of the cervix. The wide middle muscular layer is composed of three indistinct layers of smooth muscle. The outer longitudinal layer is contiguous with the muscle layers of the oviduct and vagina. The middle layer has interlacing oblique, spiral bundles of smooth muscle and large venous plexuses. The inner muscular layer is also longitudinal. The endometrium is a reddish mucous

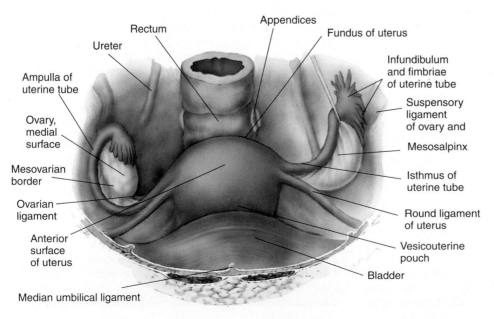

Figure 3-13 The organs of the female pelvis. The uterus is surrounded by the bladder anteriorly, the rectum posteriorly, and the folds of the broad ligaments laterally. (Redrawn from Clemente CD: Anatomy: A Regional Atlas of the Human Body, 3rd ed. Baltimore-Munich, Urban & Schwarzenberg, 1987.)

Day of Cycle		Before 14	15-16	17	18	19-22	23	24-25	26-27	28+
Post-ovulatory day		-	1-2	3	4	5-8	9	10-11	12-13	14+
Cycle phases		Proliferative	'Interval'	Early secretory		Mid-secretory			Late secretory	Menstrual
Key feature		Mitoses	Mitoses and subnuclear vacuoles	Maximum subnuclear vacuoles	Subnuclear vacuoles present	Stromal edema	Focal decidua around spiral arteries	Patchy decidua	Extensive decidua	Stromal crumbling
Microscopic features of functional zone	Stroma	Loose stroma. Mitoses	Same as proliferative	Loose stroma, scanty mitoses	Loose stroma	Stromal edema	Focal decidua around spiral arteries. Edema prominent	Decidua throughout stroma. Some edema	Extensive decidua. Prominent granulated lymphocytes	Stromal crumbling. Hemorrhage
	Glands	Straight to tightly coiled tubules. Mitoses	Some subnuclear vacuoles, otherwise as prolifertaive	Extensive subnuclear vacuoles	Dilated glands. Some subnuclear vacuoles	Dilated glands with irregular outline. Luminal secretion		'Saw tooth' glands	Prominent 'saw tooth' glands	Disrupted glands. Secretory exhaustion. Regeneraing epithelium
Appearances		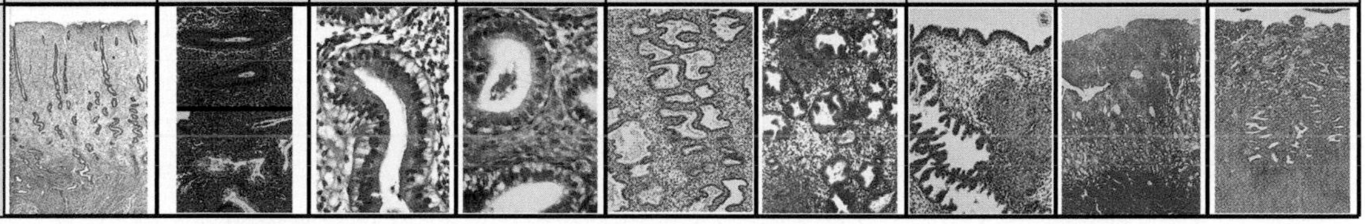								

Figure 3-15 The endometrium is responsive to the hormonal changes of the menstrual cycle. Glands and stroma change activity and thus histologic appearance throughout the cycle. (From Robboy SJ, Anderson MC, Russell P [eds]: Pathology of the Female Reproductive Tract. Edinburgh, Churchill Livingstone, 2002, p 248.)

membrane that varies from 1 to 6 mm in thickness, depending on hormonal stimulation (**Fig. 3-15**). The uterine glands are tubular and composed of tall columnar epithelium. The cells of the endometrial stroma resemble embryonic connective tissue with scant cytoplasm and large nuclei (**Fig. 3-16**). The endometrium may be divided into an inner stratum basale and an outer stratum functionale. The stratum functionale may be further subdivided into an inner compact stratum and a more superficial spongy stratum. Only the stratum functionale responds to fluctuating hormonal levels.

The arterial blood supply of the uterus is provided by the uterine and ovarian arteries. The uterine arteries are large branches of the hypogastric arteries, whereas the ovarian arteries originate directly from the aorta. The veins of the pelvic organs accompany the arteries. Therefore, venous drainage from the fundus goes to the ovarian veins and blood from the corpus exits via the uterine veins into the iliac veins. The lymphatic drainage of the uterus is complex. The majority of lymphatics from the fundus and the body of the uterus go to the aortic, lumbar, and pelvic nodes surrounding the iliac vessels, especially the internal iliac nodes. However, it is possible for metastatic disease from the uterus to be found in the superior inguinal nodes transported via lymphatics in the round ligament.

In contrast to other pelvic organs, the afferent sensory nerve fibers from the uterus are in close proximity to the sympathetic nerves. Afferent nerve fibers from the uterus enter the spinal cord at the eleventh and twelfth thoracic segments. The sympathetic nerve supply to the uterus comes from the hypogastric and ovarian plexus. The parasympathetic fibers are largely derived from the pelvic nerve and from the second, third, and fourth sacral segments.

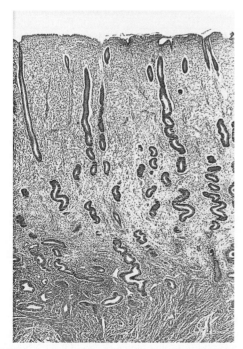

Figure 3-16 Low-power histologic section of proliferative endometrium. (From Robboy SJ, Anderson MC, Russell P [eds]: Pathology of the Female Reproductive Tract. Edinburgh, Churchill Livingstone, 2002, p 248.)

CLINICAL CORRELATIONS

Removal of the uterus is termed *hysterectomy*, which is derived from the Greek word *hystera*, meaning womb. The symptoms of primary dysmenorrhea are treated successfully in most women by prostaglandin synthetase inhibition. Usually a woman's pain is controlled by oral medication. However, it is possible to alleviate uterine pain by cutting the sensory nerves that accompany the sympathetic nerves. This operation is termed a *presacral neurectomy.* During the operation, the gynecologist must be careful to avoid injuring the ureters and also careful to control hemorrhage from vessels in the retroperitoneal space.

The position of the fundus of the uterus in relation to the long axis of the vagina is quite variable. Not only are there differences among individual women, but also in the same woman differences occur secondary to normal activity. In some women the uterus is anteflexed or anteverted, whereas in others the normal position is retroflexed or retroverted. In the 1930s and 1940s, a retroflexed uterus was believed to be one of the primary causes of pelvic pain. To alleviate this condition, many women underwent an anterior uterine suspension. Modern gynecologists have abandoned the suspension operation as a treatment for pelvic pain.

The arterial blood supply enters the uterus on its lateral margins. This relationship allows morcellation of an enlarged uterus to facilitate removal of multiple myomas without appreciably increasing blood loss during vaginal hysterectomy.

Methods of transcervical female sterilization designed to occlude the tubal ostia at the uterine cornua have been attempted for many years. Procedures that blindly inject caustic solutions into the uterine cornua have a high percentage of failure. Individual differences in the size and shape of the uterine cavity and muscular spasm of this region are the primary reasons that sufficient amounts of the caustic chemicals do not reach the fallopian tubes in up to 20% of patients.

OVIDUCTS

The paired uterine tubes, more commonly referred to as the *fallopian tubes* or *oviducts,* extend outward from the superolateral portion of the uterus and end by curling around the ovary (**Fig. 3-17**). The oviducts are also referred to using the prefix "salpingo," from the Greek *salpinx,* meaning a tube. The tubes are contained in a free edge of the superior portion of the broad

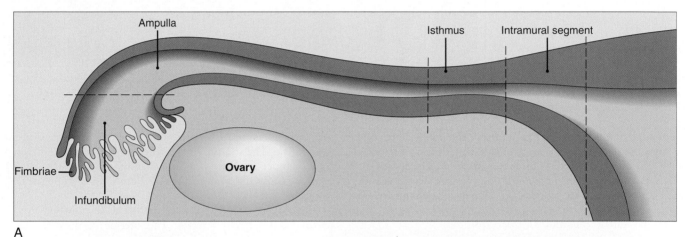

A

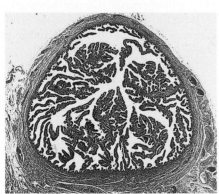

B

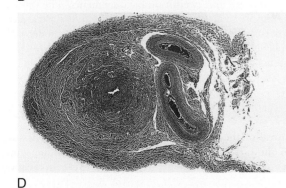

D

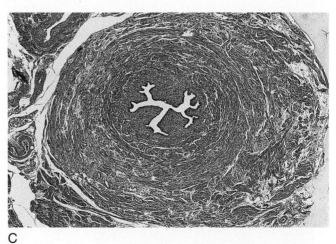

C

Figure 3-17 The fallopian tube. **A.** Schematic representation. Note that the intramural segment is within the uterine body. **B,** Low-power histologic section from the ampulla. **C,** Section from the isthmus of the tube. **D,** Section from the isthmus. Note the thick muscular wall. (**A, B,** and **D,** from Stevens A, Lowe J: Human Histology, 3 rd ed. Philadelphia, Elsevier, 2002, p 354; **C,** from Robboy SJ, Anderson MC, Russell P [eds]: Pathology of the Female Reproductive Tract. Edinburgh, Churchill Livingstone, 2002, p 416.)

ligament. The mesentery of the tubes, the mesosalpinx, contains the blood supply and nerves. The uterine tubes connect the cornua of the uterine cavity and the peritoneal cavity. The ostia into the endometrial cavity are 1.5 mm in diameter, whereas the ostia into the abdominal cavity are approximately 3 mm in diameter.

The oviducts are between 10 and 14 cm in length and slightly less than 1 cm in external diameter. Each tube is divided into four anatomic sections. The uterine intramural, or interstitial, segment is 1 to 2 cm in length and is surrounded by myometrium. The isthmic segment begins as the tube exits the uterus and is approximately 4 cm in length. This segment is narrow, 1 to 2 mm in inside diameter, and straight. The isthmic segment has the most highly developed musculature. The ampullary segment is 4 to 6 cm in length and approximately 6 mm in inside diameter. It is wider and more tortuous in its course than other segments. Fertilization normally occurs in the ampullary portion of the tube. The infundibulum is the distal trumpet-shaped portion of the oviduct. From 20 to 25 irregular finger-like projections, termed *fimbriae,* surround the abdominal ostia of the tube. One of the largest fimbriae is attached to the ovary, the **fimbria ovarica**.

The tube contains numerous longitudinal folds, called plicae, of mucosa and underlying stroma. Plicae are most prominent in the ampullary segment (see **Fig. 3-17**). The mucosa of the oviduct has three different cell types. Columnar ciliated epithelial cells are most prominent near the ovarian end of the tube and overall compose 25% of the mucosal cells (**Fig. 3-18**). Secretory cells, also columnar in shape, compose 60% of the epithelial lining and are more prominent in the isthmic segment. Narrow peg cells are found between secretory and ciliated cells and are believed to be a morphologic variant of secretory cells. The stroma of the mucosa is sparse. However, there is a thick lamina propria with vascular channels between the epithelium and muscular layers. The smooth muscle of the tube is arranged into inner circular and outer longitudinal layers. Between the peritoneal surface of the tube and the muscular layer is an adventitial layer that contains blood vessels and nerves.

The arterial blood supply to the oviducts is derived from terminal branches of the uterine and ovarian arteries. The arteries anastomose in the mesosalpinx. Blood from the uterine artery supplies the medial two thirds of each tube. The venous drainage runs parallel to the arterial supply. The lymphatic system is separate and distinct from the lymphatic drainage of the uterus. Lymphatic drainage includes the internal iliac nodes and the aortic nodes surrounding the aorta and the inferior vena cava at the level of the renal vessels. The tubes are innervated by both sympathetic and parasympathetic nerves from the uterine and ovarian plexuses. Sensory nerves are related to spinal cord segments T11, T12, and L1.

CLINICAL CORRELATIONS

The majority of ectopic pregnancies occur in the oviduct. The acute abdominal and pelvic pain that women with an ectopic pregnancy experience is believed to be caused by hemorrhage. The most catastrophic bleeding associated with ectopic pregnancy occurs when the implantation site is in the intramural segment of the tube.

The isthmic segment of the oviduct is the preferred site to apply an occlusive device, such as a clip, for female sterilization. The right oviduct and appendix are often adjacent. Clinically it may be difficult to differentiate inflammation of the tube from acute appendicitis. Accessory tubal ostia are discovered frequently and always connect with the lumen of the tube. These accessory ostia are usually found in the ampullary portion of the tube.

The wide mesosalpinx of the ampullary segment of the tube allows torsion of the tube, which occasionally results in ischemic atrophy of the ampullary segment. Paratubal or paraovarian cysts can reach 5 to 10 cm in diameter and occasionally are confused with ovarian cysts before surgery.

Although a definitive anatomic sphincter has not been identified at the uterotubal junction, a temporary physiologic obstruction has been identified during hysterosalpingography. Sometimes clinicians may alleviate this temporary obstruction by giving the patient intravenous sedation, a paracervical block, or intravenous glucagon.

OVARIES

The paired ovaries are light gray, and each one is approximately the size and configuration of a large almond. The surface of the ovary of adult women is pitted and indented from previous ovulations. The ovaries contain approximately 1 to 2 million oocytes at birth. During a woman's reproductive lifetime, about 8000 follicles begin development. The growth of many follicles is blunted in various stages of development; however, approximately 300 ova eventually are released. The size and position of the ovary depend on the woman's age and parity. During the reproductive years, ovaries weigh 3 to 6 g and measure approximately 1.5 cm × 2.5 cm × 4 cm. As the woman ages, the ovaries become smaller and firmer in consistency.

In a nulliparous woman who is standing, the long axis of the ovary is vertical. The ovary in nulliparous women rests in a depression of peritoneum named the ovarian fossa. Immediately adjacent to the ovarian fossa are the external iliac vessels, the ureter, and the obturator vessels and nerves.

Three prominent ligaments determine the anatomic mobility of the ovary (**Fig. 3-19**). The posterior portion of the broad ligament forms the mesovarium, which attaches to the anterior border of the ovary. The mesovarium contains the arterial anastomotic branches of the ovarian and uterine arteries, a plexus of veins, and the lateral end of the ovarian ligament. The ovarian ligament is a narrow, short, fibrous band that extends from

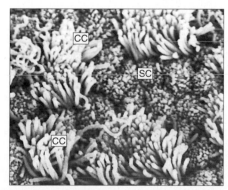

Figure 3-18 Electron micrograph of the tubal mucosa from the ampulla. CC, ciliated cells; SC, secretory cells. (From Stevens A, Lowe J: Human Histology, 3 rd ed. Philadelphia, Elsevier, 2002, p 354.)

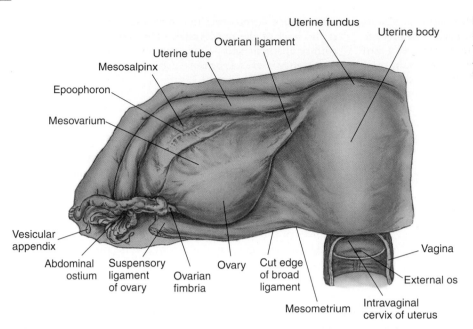

Uterine fundus
Ovarian ligament
Uterine tube
Uterine body
Mesosalpinx
Epoophoron
Mesovarium
Vesicular appendix
Abdominal ostium
Suspensory ligament of ovary
Ovarian fimbria
Ovary
Cut edge of broad ligament
Mesometrium
Intravaginal cervix of uterus
Vagina
External os

Figure 3-19 The posterior aspect of the broad ligament-spread out to demonstrate the ovary. (From Standring S [ed]: Gray's Anatomy, 39th ed. Edinburgh, Elsevier Churchill Livingstone, 2005, p 1322.)

the lower pole of the ovary to the uterus. The infundibular pelvic ligament, or suspensory ligament of the ovary, forms the superior and lateral aspect of the broad ligament. This ligament contains the ovarian artery, ovarian veins, and accompanying nerves. It attaches the upper pole of the ovary to the lateral pelvic wall.

The ovary is subdivided histologically into an outer cortex and an inner medulla (**Fig. 3-20**). The ovarian surface is covered by a single layer of cuboidal epithelium, termed the *germinal epithelium.* This term is a misnomer because the cells are similar to those of the coelomic mesothelium, which forms the

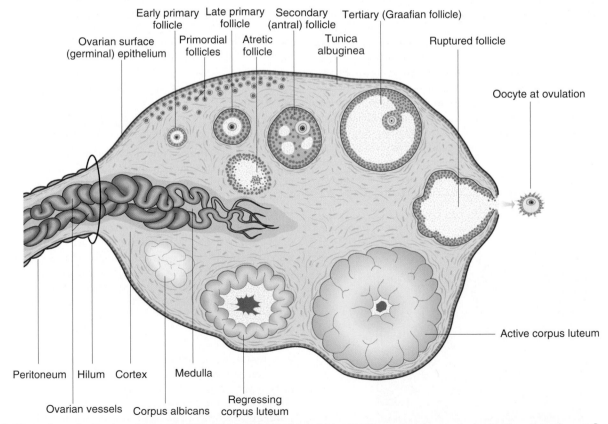

Early primary follicle
Late primary follicle
Secondary (antral) follicle
Tertiary (Graafian follicle)
Ovarian surface (germinal) epithelium
Primordial follicles
Atretic follicle
Tunica albuginea
Ruptured follicle
Oocyte at ovulation
Active corpus luteum
Peritoneum
Hilum
Cortex
Medulla
Ovarian vessels
Corpus albicans
Regressing corpus luteum

Figure 3-20 A schematic drawing of the ovary. Note the single layer of cuboidal epithelium called the *germinal epithelium.* Note the graafian follicles in different stages of development. (From Standring S [ed]: Gray's Anatomy, 39th ed. Edinburgh, Elsevier Churchill Livingstone, 2005, p 1324.)

peritoneum, and because the germinal epithelium is not related to the histogenesis of graafian follicles. If the ovary is transected, numerous transparent, fluid-filled cysts are noted throughout the cortex. Microscopically these are graafian follicles in various stages of development, active or regressing corpus luteum, and atretic follicles. The stroma of the cortex is composed primarily of closely packed cells around the follicles. These specialized connective tissue cells form the theca. The medulla contains the ovarian vascular supply and a loose stroma. The specialized polyhedral hilar cells are similar to the interstitial cells of the testis.

Each of the ovarian arteries arises directly from the aorta just below the renal arteries. They descend in the retroperitoneal space, cross anterior to the psoas muscles and internal iliac vessels, and enter the infundibulopelvic ligaments, reaching the mesovarium in the broad ligament. The ovarian blood supply enters through the hilum of the ovary. The venous drainage of the ovary collects in the pampiniform plexus and consolidates into several large veins as it leaves the hilum of the ovary. The ovarian veins accompany the ovarian arteries, with the left ovarian vein draining into the left renal vein, whereas the right ovarian vein connects directly with the inferior vena cava.

The lymphatic drainage of the ovaries is primarily to the aortic nodes adjacent to the great vessels at the level of the renal veins. Metastatic disease from the ovary occasionally takes a shorter course to the iliac nodes. The autonomic and sensory nerve fibers accompany the ovarian vasculature in the infundibulopelvic ligament. They connect with the ovarian, hypogastric, and aortic plexuses.

CLINICAL CORRELATIONS

The size of the "normal" ovary during the reproductive years and the postmenopausal period is important in clinical practice. Before menopause a normal ovary may be up to 5 cm in length. Thus, a small physiologic cyst may cause an ovary to be 6 to 7 cm in diameter. In contrast, the normal atrophic postmenopausal ovary usually cannot be palpated during pelvic examination.

It is important to emphasize that the ovaries and surrounding peritoneum are not devoid of pain and pressure receptors.

Therefore, it is not unusual for a woman during a routine pelvic examination to experience discomfort when normal ovaries are palpated bimanually.

Attempts have been made to alleviate chronic pelvic pain by performing an ovarian denervation operation by cutting and ligating the infundibulopelvic ligaments. This operation has been abandoned because of the high incidence of cystic degeneration of the ovaries, which resulted from the interruption of their primary blood supply that was associated with the neurectomy procedure.

The close anatomic proximity of the ovary, ovarian fossa, and ureter is emphasized in surgery to treat severe endometriosis or pelvic inflammatory disease. It is important to identify the course of the ureter to facilitate removal of all of the ovarian capsule that is adherent to the peritoneum and surrounding structures so as to avoid immediate ureteral injury and residual retroperitoneal ovarian remnants in the future. Prophylactic oophorectomy is performed at the time of pelvic operations in many peri- and postmenopausal women. Sometimes bilateral oophorectomy is technically more difficult when associated with a vaginal procedure in contrast to an abdominal hysterectomy. Vaginal removal of the ovaries may be facilitated by identifying the anatomic landmarks similar to the abdominal approach and separately clamping the round ligaments and infundibular pelvic ligaments.

VASCULAR SYSTEM OF THE PELVIS

Several generalizations should be made in describing the network of arteries that bring blood to the female reproductive organs. The arteries are paired, are bilateral, and have multiple collaterals (**Fig. 3-21**). The arteries enter their respective organs laterally and then unite with anastomotic vessels from the other side of the pelvis near the midline. There is a long-standing teaching generalization that the pelvic reproductive viscera lie within a loosely woven basket of large veins with numerous interconnecting venous plexuses. The arteries thread their way through this interwoven mesh of veins to reach the pelvic reproductive organs, giving off numerous branching arcades to provide a rich blood supply.

Figure 3-21 The arteries of the reproductive organs. Note the paired arteries entering laterally and freely anastomosing with each other. (Redrawn from Clemente CD: Anatomy: A Regional Atlas of the Human Body, 3 rd ed. Baltimore-Munich, Urban & Schwarzenberg, 1987.)

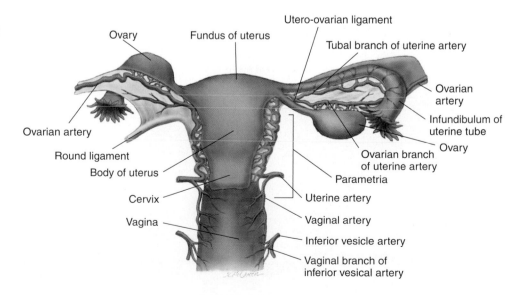

ARTERIES

Inferior Mesenteric Artery

The inferior mesenteric artery, a single artery, arises from the aorta approximately 3 cm above the aortic bifurcation. It supplies part of the transverse colon, the descending colon, the sigmoid colon, and the rectum and terminates as the superior hemorrhoidal artery. The inferior mesenteric artery is occasionally torn during node dissections performed in staging operations for gynecologic cancer. Because of the rich collateral circulation from the middle and inferior hemorrhoidal arteries, the inferior mesenteric artery can be ligated without compromise of the distal portion of the colon.

Ovarian Artery

The ovarian arteries originate from the aorta just below the renal vessels. Each one courses in the retroperitoneal space, crosses anterior to the ureter, and enters the infundibulopelvic ligament. As the artery travels medially in the mesovarium, numerous small branches supply the ovary and oviduct. The ovarian artery unites with the ascending branch of the uterine artery in the mesovarium just under the suspensory ligament of the ovary.

Common Iliac Artery

The bifurcation of the aorta occurs at the level of the fourth lumbar vertebra, forming the two common iliac arteries. Each common iliac artery is approximately 5 cm in length before the vessel divides into the external iliac and hypogastric arteries.

Hypogastric Artery (Internal Iliac Artery)

The hypogastric arteries are short vessels, approximately 3 to 4 cm in length. Throughout their course they are in close proximity to the ureters, which are anterior, and to the hypogastric veins, which are posterior. Most commonly (variations are frequent), each hypogastric artery branches into an anterior and a posterior division (or trunk). The branching is usually 2 cm from the common iliac. The posterior trunk gives off three parietal branches: the iliolumbar, lateral sacral, and superior gluteal arteries. The anterior trunk has nine branches. The three parietal branches are the obturator, internal pudendal, and inferior gluteal arteries. The six visceral branches include the umbilical, middle vesical, inferior vesical, middle hemorrhoidal, uterine, and vaginal arteries. The superior vesical artery usually arises from the umbilical artery. The individual branches of the hypogastric artery may vary from one woman to another.

Uterine Artery

The uterine artery arises from the anterior division of the hypogastric artery and courses medially toward the isthmus of the uterus. Approximately 2 cm lateral to the endocervix, it crosses over the ureter and reaches the lateral side of the uterus. The ascending branch of the uterine artery courses in the broad ligament, running a tortuous route to finally anastomose with the ovarian artery in the mesovarium (**Fig. 3-22**). Through its circuitous route in the parametrium, the uterine artery gives off numerous branches that unite with arcuate arteries from the other side. This series of arcuate arteries develops radial branches that supply the myometrium and the basalis layer of the endometrium. The arcuate arteries also form the spiral arteries of the functional layer of the endometrium. The descending branch of the uterine artery produces branches that supply both the cervix and the vagina. In each case the vessels enter the organ laterally and anastomose freely with vessels from the other side.

VAGINAL ARTERY

The vaginal artery may arise either from the anterior trunk of the hypogastric artery or from the uterine artery. It supplies blood to the vagina, bladder, and rectum. There are extensive anastomoses with the vaginal branches of the uterine artery to form the azygos arteries of the cervix and vagina.

Internal Pudendal Artery

This artery is the terminal branch of the hypogastric artery and supplies branches to the rectum, labia, clitoris, and **perineum**.

VEINS

The venous drainage of the pelvis begins in small sinusoids that drain to numerous venous plexuses contained within or immediately adjacent to the pelvic organs. Invariably there are numerous anastomoses between the parietal and visceral branches of

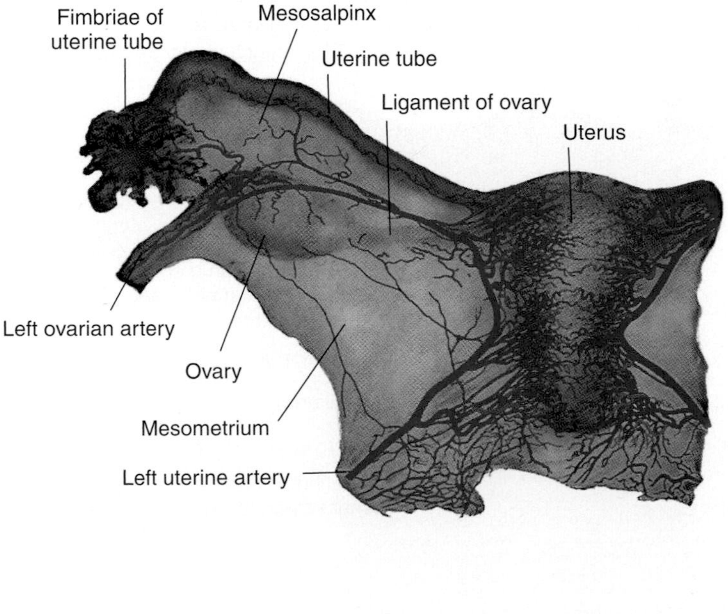

Fimbriae of uterine tube
Mesosalpinx
Uterine tube
Ligament of ovary
Uterus
Left ovarian artery
Ovary
Mesometrium
Left uterine artery

Figure 3-22 A photograph of an injected specimen demonstrating the rich anastomoses of the uterine and ovarian arteries. (From Warwick R, Williams PL: Gray's Anatomy, 35th ed. Edinburgh, Churchill Livingstone, 1973, p 1361.)

the venous system. In general the veins of the female pelvis and perineum are thin walled and have few valves.

The veins that drain the pelvic plexuses follow the course of the arterial supply. Their names are similar to those of the accompanying arteries. Often multiple veins run alongside a single artery. One special exception is the venous drainage of the ovaries. The left ovarian vein empties into the left renal vein, whereas the right ovarian vein connects directly with the inferior vena cava.

CLINICAL CORRELATIONS

Although the external iliac artery and its branches do not supply blood directly to the pelvic viscera, they are important landmarks in surgical anatomy. The fact that the external iliac artery gives rise to the obturator artery in 15% to 20% of women must be considered in radical cancer operations with associated node dissections of the obturator fossa. The external iliac artery also gives rise to the inferior epigastric artery. The inferior epigastric artery should be avoided when performing laparoscopic operative procedures.

In certain clinical situations associated with profuse hemorrhage from the female pelvis, hypogastric ligation is performed. Because of the extensive collateral circulation, this operation does not produce hypoxia of the pelvic viscera but reduces hemorrhage by decreasing the arterial pulse pressure. The extent of collateral circulation after hypogastric artery ligation depends on the site of ligation and may be divided into three groups (Table 3-1).

In cases of intractable pelvic hemorrhage, it may be necessary to supplement the effects of bilateral hypogastric artery ligation with ligation of the anastomotic sites between the ovarian and uterine vessels. Ligation of the terminal end of the ovarian artery preserves the direct blood supply to the ovaries, and there is no fear of the subsequent cystic degeneration of the ovaries that may occur after ligation of the vessels in the infundibulopelvic ligaments. Arterial embolization provides an alternative approach to ligation. A catheter is advanced under fluoroscopic visualization, and small particulate material is injected to produce hemostasis in the bleeding vessels. This less invasive technique, when appropriate, may preserve fertility. A rare condition that presents an interesting challenge to the clinician is a congenital arteriovenous (A-V) malformation in the female pelvis. Most of these A-V

fistulas are treated with preoperative embolism and subsequent operative ligation.

One of the treatments for repetitive embolization arising from thrombosis is the placement of a vascular umbrella into the inferior vena cava. Collateral circulation exists between the portal venous system of the gastrointestinal tract and the systemic venous circulation through anastomosis in the pelvis, especially in the hemorrhoidal plexus. The pelvic veins also anastomose with the presacral and lumbar veins. Thus, though rare, patients may develop trophoblastic emboli to the brain without the trophoblast being filtered by the capillary system in the lungs.

LYMPHATIC SYSTEM

EXTERNAL ILIAC NODES

The external iliac nodes are immediately adjacent to the external iliac artery and vein (**Figs. 3-23** and **3-24**). There are two distinct groups, one situated lateral to the vessels and the other posterior to the psoas muscle. The distal portion of the posterior group is enclosed in the femoral sheath. Most of the lymphatic channels to this group of nodes originate from the vulva, but there are also channels from the cervix and lower portion of the uterus. The external iliac nodes receive secondary drainage from the femoral and internal iliac nodes.

INTERNAL ILIAC NODES

The internal iliac nodes are found in an anatomic triangle whose sides are composed of the external iliac artery, the hypogastric artery, and the pelvic sidewall. Included in this clinically important area are nodes with special designation, including the nodes of the femoral ring, the obturator nodes, and the nodes adjacent to the external iliac vessels. This rich collection of nodes receives channels from every internal pelvic organ and the vulva, including the clitoris and urethra.

COMMON ILIAC NODES

The common iliac nodes are a group of nodes located adjacent to the vessels that bear their name and are between the external iliac and aortic chains. Most of these nodes are found lateral to the

Table 3-1 Collateral Arterial Circulation of the Pelvis

Branches from Aorta
Ovarian artery—anastomoses freely with uterine artery
Inferior mesenteric artery—continues as superior hemorrhoidal artery to anastomose with middle and inferior hemorrhoidal arteries from hypogastric and internal pudendal
Lumbar and vertebral arteries—anastomose with iliolumbar artery of hypogastric
Middle sacral artery—anastomoses with lateral sacral artery of hypogastric
Branches from External Iliac Artery
Deep iliac circumflex artery—anastomoses with iliolumbar and superior gluteal of hypogastric
Inferior epigastric artery—gives origin to obturator artery in 25% of cases, providing additional anastomoses of external iliac with medial femoral circumflex and communicating pelvic branches
Branches from Femoral Artery
Medial femoral circumflex artery—anastomoses with obturator and inferior gluteal arteries from hypogastric
Lateral femoral circumflex artery—anastomoses with superior gluteal and iliolumbar arteries from hypogastric

Reprinted with permission from Mattingly RF, Thompson JD: Te Linde's Operative Gynecology, 6th ed. Philadelphia, JB Lippincott, 1985.

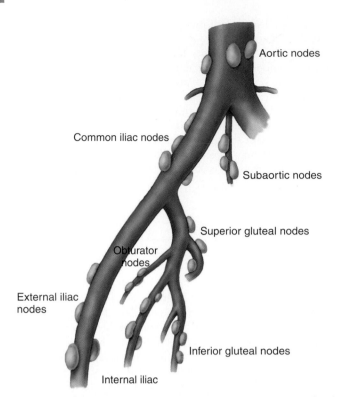

Figure 3-23 Schematic view of the pelvic lymph nodes. (From Plentl AA, Friedman EA: Lymphatic System of the Female Genitalia. Philadelphia, WB Saunders, 1971, p 13.)

vessels. To remove this chain, it is necessary to dissect the common iliac vessels away from their attachments to the psoas muscle. This group receives lymphatics from the cervix and the upper portion of the vagina. Secondary lymphatic drainage from the internal iliac, external iliac, superior gluteal, and inferior gluteal nodes flows to the common iliac nodes.

INFERIOR GLUTEAL NODES

A small group of lymph nodes, the inferior gluteal nodes, are located in anatomic proximity to the ischial spines and are adjacent to the sacral plexus of nodes. It is difficult to remove these nodes surgically. The nodes receive lymphatics from the cervix, the lower portion of the vagina, and Bartholin's glands. This group of nodes secondarily drains to the internal iliac, common iliac, superior gluteal, and subaortic nodes.

SUPERIOR GLUTEAL NODES

The superior gluteal nodes are a group of nodes found near the origin of the superior gluteal artery and adjacent to the medial and posterior aspects of the hypogastric vessels. The superior gluteal nodes receive primary lymphatic drainage from the cervix and the vagina. Efferent lymphatics from this chain drain to the common iliac, sacral, or subaortic nodes.

SACRAL NODES

The sacral nodes are found over the middle of the sacrum in a space bounded laterally by the sacral foramina. These nodes receive lymphatic drainage from both the cervix and the vagina. Secondary drainage from these nodes runs in a cephalad direction to the subaortic nodes.

SUBAORTIC NODES

The subaortic nodes are arranged in a chain and are located below the bifurcation of the aorta, immediately anterior to the most caudal portion of the inferior vena cava and over the fifth lumbar vertebra. The primary drainage to this chain of nodes is from the cervix, with a few lymphatics from the vagina. This group is the first secondary chain to receive the efferent lymphatics as lymph flow progresses in a cephalad direction from the majority of other pelvic nodes.

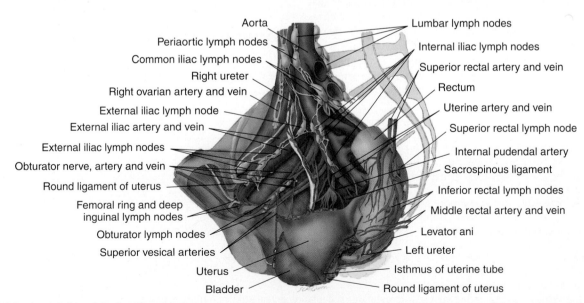

Figure 3-24 A lateral view of the female pelvis demonstrating the extensive lymphatic network. Note that most of the lymphatic channels follow the courses of the major vessels. (Redrawn from Clemente CD: Anatomy: A Regional Atlas of the Human Body, 3 rd ed. Baltimore-Munich, Urban & Schwarzenberg, 1987.)

AORTIC NODES

The many aortic nodes are immediately adjacent to the aorta on both its anterior and lateral aspects, predominantly in the furrow between the aorta and inferior vena cava. Primary lymphatics drain from all the major pelvic organs, including the cervix, uterus, oviducts, and especially the ovaries. The aortic chain receives secondary drainage from the pelvic nodes. In general, primary afferent lymphatics drain into the nodes over the anterior aspects of the aorta, whereas secondary efferent drainage from other pelvic nodes is found in those nodes situated lateral and posterior to the aorta.

RECTAL NODES

The rectal nodes are found subfascially and in the loose connective tissue surrounding the rectum. Primary drainage from the cervix flows to the superior rectal nodes, and drainage from the vagina appears in the rectal nodes in the anorectal region. Secondary drainage from the rectal nodes goes to the subaortic and aortic groups.

PARAUTERINE NODES

The number of lymph nodes in the group of parauterine nodes is small; most frequently there is a single node immediately lateral to each side of the cervix and adjacent to the pelvic course of the ureter. Though anatomists frequently do not comment about the parauterine nodes, the group receives special attention in radical surgical operations to treat uterine or cervical malignancy. Primary drainage to this node originates in the vagina, cervix, and uterus. Secondary drainage from this node is to the internal iliac nodes on the same side of the pelvis.

SUPERFICIAL FEMORAL NODES

The superficial femoral nodes are a group of nodes found in the loose, fatty connective tissue of the femoral triangle between the superficial and deep fascial layers. These lymph nodes receive lymphatic drainage from the external genitalia of the vulvar region, the gluteal region, and the entire leg, including the foot. Efferent lymphatics from this group of nodes penetrate the fascia lata to enter the deep femoral nodes (**Fig. 3-25**).

DEEP FEMORAL NODES

The deep femoral nodes are located in the femoral sheath, adjacent to both the femoral artery and the vein within the femoral triangle. The femoral triangle is the anatomic space lying immediately distal to the fold of the groin. The boundaries of the femoral triangle are the sartorius and adductor longus muscles and the inguinal ligament. Each space contains, from medial to lateral, the femoral vein, artery, and nerve. This chain receives the primary lymphatics for the lower extremity and receives secondary efferent lymphatics from the superficial lymph nodes and thus the vulva. This group of lymph nodes is in direct continuity with the iliac and internal iliac chains.

CLINICAL CORRELATIONS

A precise knowledge of pelvic lymphatics is important for the gynecologic oncologist who is surgically determining the extent of spread of a pelvic malignancy. Aortic and pelvic lymphadenectomy operations require precise knowledge of normal anatomy and possible anomalies in both the urinary and vascular systems. The fact that most lymphatic metastatic spread from ovarian carcinoma occurs in a cephalad direction should be

Figure 3-25 A lymphangiogram of the pelvis and lumbar areas. This x-ray film shows the course of the lymphatics from the deep femoral nodes into the iliac nodes. Note the extensive network of nodes in the inguinal region. (From Clemente CD: A Regional Atlas of the Human Body, 3 rd ed. Baltimore-Munich, Urban & Schwarzenberg, 1987.)

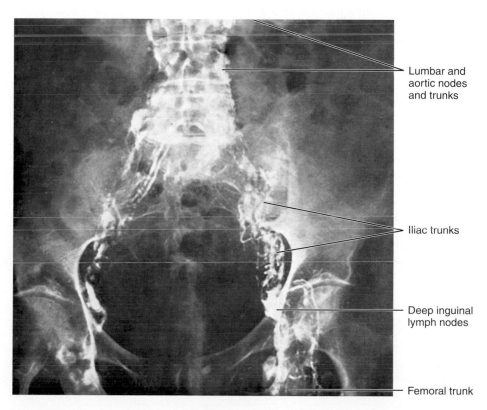

Lumbar and aortic nodes and trunks

Iliac trunks

Deep inguinal lymph nodes

Femoral trunk

emphasized. This explains the importance of sampling periaortic nodes in staging operations for ovarian and uterine malignancy. In carcinoma of the vulva, lymphatic drainage may occur to either side of the pelvis. Thus, bilateral node dissections are important. Pelvic hemorrhage is the most common acute complication of a lymph node dissection because most pelvic lymph nodes are in anatomic proximity to major pelvic vessels. Lymphocysts in the retroperitoneal space are the most common chronic complication associated with radical node dissections.

For many years it was believed that all the superficial femoral nodes drained to a sentinel node called *Cloquet's node.* Cloquet's node, by the present classification system, would be one of the most proximal and medial of the nodes in the external iliac chain. Cloquet's node is only of historical interest, because the assumption is neither anatomically nor clinically correct.

INNERVATION OF THE PELVIS

INTERNAL GENITALIA

The innervation of the internal genital organs is supplied primarily by the autonomic nervous system. The sympathetic portion of the autonomic nervous system originates in the thoracic and lumbar portions of the spinal cord, and sympathetic ganglia are located adjacent to the central nervous system. In contrast, the parasympathetic portion originates in cranial nerves and the middle three sacral segments of the cord, and the ganglia are located near the visceral organs. Although the fibers of both subdivisions of the autonomic nervous system frequently are intermingled in the same peripheral nerves, their physiologic actions are usually directly antagonistic. As a broad generalization, sympathetic fibers in the female pelvis produce muscular contractions and vasoconstriction, whereas parasympathetic fibers cause the opposite effect on muscles and vasodilation.

The semantics of pelvic innervation are confusing and imprecise. A *plexus* is a mixture of preganglionic and postganglionic fibers; small, inconsistently placed ganglia; and afferent (sensory) fibers. Throughout both the anatomic and surgical literature, a plexus may also be termed a *nerve.* For example, the superior hypogastric plexus is also called the *presacral nerve.*

Although autonomic nerve fibers enter the pelvis by several routes, most are contained in the superior hypogastric plexus, which is a caudal extension of the aortic and inferior mesenteric plexuses. The superior hypogastric plexus is found in the retroperitoneal connective tissue. It extends from the fourth lumbar vertebra to the hollow over the sacrum. In its lower portion the plexus divides to form the two hypogastric nerves, which run laterally and inferiorly. These nerves fan out to form the inferior hypogastric plexus in the area just below the bifurcation of the common iliac arteries. The nerve trunks descend farther into the base of the broad ligament, where they join with parasympathetic fibers to form the pelvic plexus. Both motor fibers and accompanying sensory fibers reach the pelvic plexus from S2, S3, and S4 via the pelvic nerves, or nervi erigentes. The pelvic plexus is found adjacent to the coccygeus muscle and sacrospinous ligaments. This "complex" is richly vascularized. The motor fibers to the levator ani (**levator ani nerve**) arise from the S2 to S4 nerve roots (primarily S3 and S4), traversing perpendicular to the muscle bundles and branching out to innervate the muscle fibers. The levator ani nerve does not innervate the anal sphincter, but the nerve is responsible for pelvic floor support. The pudendal nerve fibers also originate from the sacral plexus, with nerve fibers from S2 to S4. From the pelvic plexus, secondary plexuses are adjacent to all pelvic viscera, namely, the rectum, anus, urinary bladder, vagina, and **Frankenhäuser's plexus** in the uterosacral ligaments. Frankenhäuser's plexus is extensive and contains both myelinated and nonmyelinated fibers passing primarily to the uterus and cervix, with a few fibers passing to the urinary bladder and vagina. The ovarian plexus, like the blood supply to the ovaries, is not part of the hypogastric system. The ovarian plexus is a downward extension of the aortic and renal plexuses.

It is impossible to separate afferent, sensory fibers from pelvic organs into morphologically independent tracts. Most fibers accompany the vascular system from the organ and then enter plexuses of the autonomic nervous system before eventually entering white rami communicates to the cell bodies in dorsal root ganglia of the spinal column. The major sensory fibers from the uterus accompany the sympathetic nerves, which enter the nerve roots of the spinal cord in segments T11 and T12. Thus, referred uterine pain is often located in the lower abdomen. In contrast, afferents from the cervix enter the spinal cord in nerve roots of S2, S3, and S4. Referred pain from cervical inflammation and uterine irritation is characterized as low back pain in the lumbosacral region.

EXTERNAL GENITALIA

The pudendal nerve and its branches supply the majority of both motor and sensory fibers to the muscles and skin of the vulvar region. The pudendal nerve arises from the second, third, and fourth sacral roots. It has an interesting course in which it initially leaves the pelvis via the greater sciatic foramen. Next, it crosses beneath the ischial spine, running on the medial side of the internal pudendal artery. The pudendal nerve then reenters the pelvic cavity and travels in Alcock's canal, which runs along the lateral aspects of the ischial rectal fossa. As the nerve reaches the **urogenital diaphragm**, it divides into three branches: the inferior hemorrhoidal, the deep perineal, and the superficial perineal (**Fig. 3-26**). The dorsal nerve of the clitoris is a terminal branch of the deep perineal nerve.

The skin of the anus, clitoris, and medial and inferior aspects of the vulva is supplied primarily by distal branches of the pudendal nerve. The vulvar region receives additional sensory fibers from three nerves. The anterior branch of the ilioinguinal nerve sends fibers to the mons pubis and the upper part of the labia majora. The genital femoral nerve supplies fibers to the labia majora, and the posterior femoral cutaneous nerve supplies fibers to the inferoposterior aspects of the vulva.

CLINICAL CORRELATIONS

An unusual but troublesome postoperative complication of gynecologic surgery is injury to the femoral nerve. During abdominal hysterectomy, the femoral nerve may be compromised by pressure from the lateral blade of a self-retaining retractor in the area adjacent to where the femoral nerve penetrates the psoas muscle. During vaginal surgery, the femoral nerve may be injured from exaggerated hyperflexion of the legs in the lithotomy position, because hyperflexion produces stretching

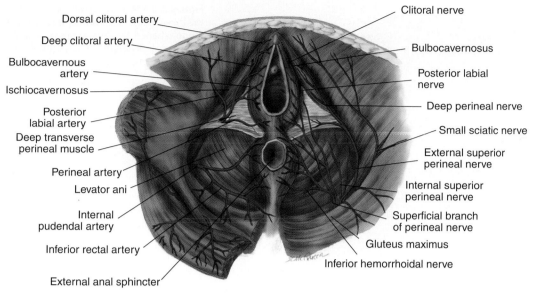

Dorsal clitoral artery
Deep clitoral artery
Bulbocavernous artery
Ischiocavernosus
Posterior labial artery
Deep transverse perineal muscle
Perineal artery
Levator ani
Internal pudendal artery
Inferior rectal artery
External anal sphincter

Clitoral nerve
Bulbocavernosus
Posterior labial nerve
Deep perineal nerve
Small sciatic nerve
External superior perineal nerve
Internal superior perineal nerve
Superficial branch of perineal nerve
Gluteus maximus
Inferior hemorrhoidal nerve

Figure 3-26 A posterior view of the female perineum demonstrating the pudendal nerve emerging externally. The nerve divides into three segments as it passes out of the pelvis: the inferior hemorrhoidal nerve and the deep and superficial perineal nerves. The clitoral nerve is the terminal branch of the deep perineal nerve. (Redrawn from Mattingly RF, Thompson JD: Te Linde's Operative Gynecology, 6th ed. Philadelphia, JB Lippincott, 1985, p 49.)

and compression of the femoral nerve as it courses under the inguinal ligament.

Because of the low density of nerve endings in the upper two thirds of the vagina, women are sometimes unable to determine the presence of a foreign body in this area. This explains how a "forgotten tampon" may remain unnoticed for several days in the upper part of the vagina until its presence results in a symptomatic discharge, abnormal bleeding, or odor. Infrequent but serious complications of pudendal nerve block are hematomas from trauma to the pudendal vessels and intravascular injection of anesthetic agents. The vessels or nerves are in close anatomic proximity to the ischial spine.

The fallopian tube is one of the most sensitive of the pelvic organs when crushed, cut, or distended, a fact that is appreciated in performing tubal ligations with the patient under local anesthesia. Damage to the obturator nerve during radical pelvic operations does not affect the pelvis directly. Although the nerve has an extensive pelvic course, its motor fibers supply the adductors of the thigh, and its sensory fibers innervate skin over the medial aspects of the thigh. Stitches placed during sacrospinous ligament fixation for pelvic support may interfere with neural roots S2 to S4 and the muscle pudendal and levator ani nerves.

DIAPHRAGMS AND LIGAMENTS

PELVIC DIAPHRAGM

The pelvic diaphragm is a wide but thin muscular layer of tissue that forms the inferior border of the abdominopelvic cavity. Composed of a broad, funnel-shaped sling of fascia and muscle, it extends from the symphysis pubis to the coccyx and from one lateral sidewall to the other. The primary muscles of the pelvic diaphragm are the levator ani and the coccygeus (**Fig. 3-27**). This structure is the evolutionary remnant of the tail-wagging muscles in lower animals. The *endopelvic fascia* is another term often used

interchangeably with the pelvic diaphragm. The pelvic diaphragm and endopelvic fascia are terms to characterize the connective tissue, the support for the pelvis, and the pelvic floor. The pelvic diaphragm is composed of collagen, elastic tissue, and muscle.

The muscles of the pelvic diaphragm are interwoven for strength, and a continuous muscle layer encircles the terminal portions of the urethra, vagina, and rectum. The levator ani muscles constitute the greatest bulk of the pelvic diaphragm and are divided into three components, which are named after their origin and insertion: pubococcygeus, puborectalis, and iliococcygeus. Recent studies using magnetic resonance imaging (MRI) and three-dimensional ultrasound validate the change in terminology from pubococcygeus muscle to a more accurate name—the *pubovisceral muscle*. This grouping of the intermediate component of the levator ani muscle lies posterior to the pubic bone and may be visualized as pubovaginalis, puboanalis, and puboperinealis muscle bundles. These three bundles constitute the pubovisceralis. Cadaveric dissection has also validated the imaging studies. The puborectalis component of the levator ani muscle is dorsal to the rectum and helps form the sling supporting the rectum. The coccygeus is a triangular muscle that occupies the area between the ischial spine and the coccyx.

The paired levator ani muscles act as a single muscle and functionally are important in the control of urination, in parturition, and in maintaining fecal continence. The pelvic diaphragm is important in supporting both abdominal and pelvic viscera and facilitates equal distribution of intraabdominal pressure during activities such as coughing.

UROGENITAL DIAPHRAGM

The urogenital diaphragm, also called the *triangular ligament,* is a strong, muscular membrane that occupies the area between the symphysis pubis and ischial tuberosities (**Fig. 3-28**) and stretches across the triangular anterior portion of the pelvic outlet. The urogenital diaphragm is external and inferior to the pelvic

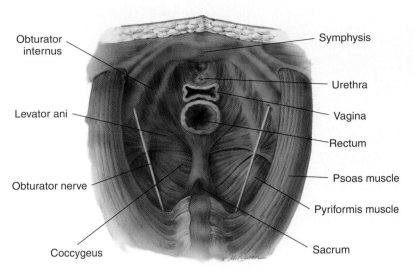

Obturator internus

Symphysis

Levator ani

Urethra

Vagina

Obturator nerve

Rectum

Psoas muscle

Coccygeus

Pyriformis muscle

Sacrum

Figure 3-27 A superior view of the pelvic diaphragm and the pelvic floor. The primary muscles that compose this funnel-shaped sling are the coccygeus and the levator ani. (Redrawn from Mattingly RF, Thompson JD: Te Linde's Operative Gynecology, 6th ed. Philadelphia, Lippincott, 1985, p 41.)

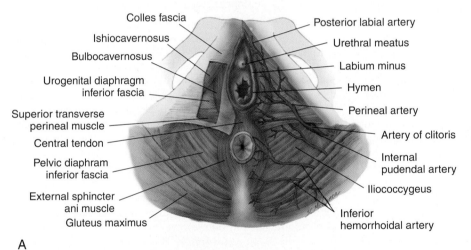

Colles fascia

Posterior labial artery

Ishiocavernosus

Urethral meatus

Bulbocavernosus

Labium minus

Urogenital diaphragm inferior fascia

Hymen

Superior transverse perineal muscle

Perineal artery

Central tendon

Artery of clitoris

Pelvic diaphram inferior fascia

Internal pudendal artery

External sphincter ani muscle

Iliococcygeus

Gluteus maximus

Inferior hemorrhoidal artery

A

Figure 3-28 A, Schematic views of the perineum demonstrating superficial structures. Note the two layers of the urogenital diaphragm enfolding the deep transverse perineal muscle. **B,** Schematic views of the perineum demonstrating superficial structures and deeper structures. (Redrawn from Pritchard JA, MacDonald PC, Gant NF: Williams' Obstetrics, 17th ed. New York, Appleton-Century-Crofts, 1985, p 14.)

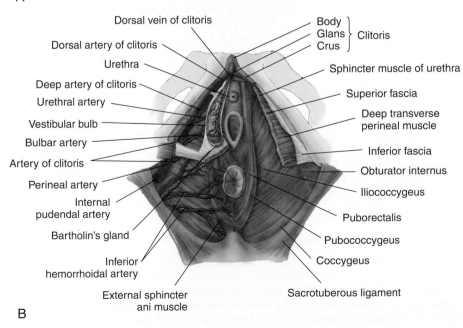

Dorsal vein of clitoris

Body
Glans   Clitoris
Crus

Dorsal artery of clitoris

Urethra

Sphincter muscle of urethra

Deep artery of clitoris

Superior fascia

Urethral artery

Deep transverse perineal muscle

Vestibular bulb

Bulbar artery

Inferior fascia

Artery of clitoris

Obturator internus

Perineal artery

Iliococcygeus

Internal pudendal artery

Puborectalis

Bartholin's gland

Pubococcygeus

Inferior hemorrhoidal artery

Coccygeus

External sphincter ani muscle

Sacrotuberous ligament

B

diaphragm. Anteriorly, the urethra is suspended from the pubic bone by continuations of the fascial layers of the urogenital diaphragm. The free edge of the diaphragm is strengthened by the superficial transverse perineal muscle. Posteriorly, the urogenital diaphragm inserts into the central point of the perineum. Situated farther posteriorly is the ischiorectal fossa. Located more superficially are the bulbocavernosus and ischiocavernosus muscles.

The urogenital diaphragm has two layers that enfold and cover the striated, deep transverse perineal muscle. This muscle surrounds both the vagina and the urethra, which pierce the diaphragm. The pudendal vessels and nerves, the external sphincter of the membranous urethra, and the dorsal nerve to the clitoris are also found within the urogenital diaphragm. The deep transverse perineal muscle is innervated by branches of the pudendal nerve. The major function of the urogenital diaphragm is support of the urethra and maintenance of the urethrovesical junction.

LIGAMENTS

The pelvic ligaments are not classic ligaments but are thickenings of retroperitoneal fascia and consist primarily of blood and lymphatic vessels, nerves, and fatty connective tissue. Anatomists call the retroperitoneal fascia *subserous fascia,* whereas surgeons refer to this fascial layer as *endopelvic fascia.* The connective tissue is denser immediately adjacent to the lateral walls of the cervix and the vagina.

Broad Ligaments
The broad ligaments are a thin, mesenteric-like double reflection of peritoneum stretching from the lateral pelvic sidewalls to the uterus (**Fig. 3-29**). They become contiguous with the uterine serosa, and thus the uterus is contained within two folds of peritoneum. These peritoneal folds enclose the loose, fatty connective tissue termed the *parametrium.* The broad ligaments afford minor support to the uterus but are conduits for important anatomic structures. Within the broad ligaments are found the following structures: oviducts; ovarian and round ligaments; ureters; ovarian and uterine arteries and veins; parametrial tissue; embryonic remnants of the mesonephric duct, Wolffian body, and secondary two ligaments; the mesovarium; and the mesosalpinx. The round ligament is composed of fibrous tissue and muscle fibers. It attaches to the superoanterior aspect of the uterus, anterior and caudal to the oviduct, and runs via the broad ligament to the lateral pelvic wall. It, too, offers little support to the uterus. The round ligament crosses the external iliac vessels and enters the inguinal canal, ending by inserting into the labia majora in a fanlike fashion. In the fetus a small, finger-like projection of the peritoneum, known as *Nuck's canal,* accompanies the round ligament into the inguinal canal. Generally, the canal is obliterated in the adult woman.

Cardinal Ligaments
The cardinal, or Mackenrodt's, ligaments extend from the lateral aspects of the upper part of the cervix and the vagina to the pelvic wall. They are a thickened condensation of the subserosal fascia and parametria between the interior portion of the two folds of peritoneum. The cardinal ligaments form the base of the broad ligaments, laterally attaching to the fascia over the pelvic diaphragm and medially merging with fibers of the endopelvic fascia. Within these ligaments are found blood vessels and smooth muscle. The cardinal ligaments help to maintain the anatomic position of the cervix and the upper part of the vagina and provide the major support of the uterus and cervix.

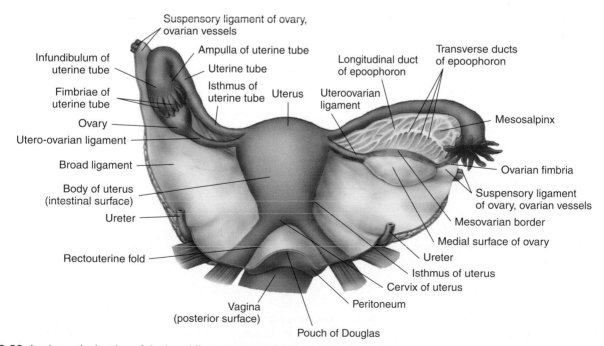

Figure 3-29 A schematic drawing of the broad ligament, posterior view. Note the many structures contained within the broad ligament. Note the posterior aspect of the rectouterine fold, called the cul-de-sac, or pouch, of Douglas. (Redrawn from Clemente CD: Anatomy: A Regional Atlas of the Human Body, 3 rd ed. Baltimore-Munich, Urban & Schwarzenberg, 1987.)

Uterosacral Ligaments

The uterosacral ligaments extend from the upper portion of the cervix posteriorly to the third sacral vertebra. They are thickened near the cervix and then run a curved course around each side of the rectum and subsequently thin out posteriorly. The external surface of the uterosacral ligaments is formed by an inferoposterior fold of peritoneum at the base of the broad ligaments. The middle of the uterosacral ligaments is composed primarily of nerve bundles. The uterosacral ligaments serve a minor role in the anatomic support of the cervix.

CLINICAL CORRELATIONS

The posterior fibers of the levator ani muscles encircle the rectum at its junction with the anal canal, thereby producing an abrupt angle that reinforces fecal continence. Surgical repair of a displacement or tear of the rectovaginal fascia and levator ani muscles resulting from childbirth is important during posterior colporrhaphy. Normal position of the female pelvic organs in the pelvis depends on mechanical support from both fascia and muscles. Vaginal delivery sometimes results dysfunction of the anal sphincter. The etiology of this problem may be direct injury to the striated muscles of the pelvic floor or damage to the pudendal and **presacral nerves** (levator ani nerves) during labor and delivery.

The round ligament is an important surgical landmark in making the initial incision into the parietal peritoneum to gain access to the retroperitoneal space. Direct visualization of the retroperitoneal course of the ureter is an important step in many pelvic operations, including dissections in women with endometriosis, pelvic inflammatory disease, large adnexal masses, broad ligament masses, and pelvic malignancies. A cyst of Nuck's canal may be confused with an indirect inguinal hernia. When a large amount of fluid is placed in the abdominal cavity, postoperative bilateral labial edema may develop in some women because of patency of the **canal of Nuck**.

During pelvic surgery, traction on the uterus makes the uterosacral and cardinal ligaments more prominent. There is a free space approximately 2 to 4 cm below the superior edge of the broad ligament. In this free space there are no blood vessels, and the two sides of the broad ligament are in close proximity. Often gynecologic surgeons utilize this area to facilitate clamping of the anastomosis between the uterine and ovarian arteries.

NONGENITAL PELVIC ORGANS

URETERS

The ureters are whitish, muscular tubes, 28 to 34 cm in length, extending from the renal pelves to the urinary bladder. The ureter is divided into abdominal and pelvic segments. The diameters vary. The abdominal segment is approximately 8 to 10 mm in diameter. The pelvic segment is approximately 4 to 6 mm. A congenital anomaly of a double, or bifid, ureter occurs in 1% to 4% of females. Ectopic ureteral orifices may occur in either the urethra or the vagina. The abdominal portion of the right ureter is lateral to the inferior vena cava. Four arteries and accompanying veins cross anterior to the right ureter. They are the right colic artery, the ovarian vessels, the ileocolic artery, and the

superior mesenteric artery. The course of the left ureter is similar to its counterpart on the right side in that it runs downward and medially along the anterior surface of the psoas major muscle.

The iliopectineal line serves as the marker for the pelvic portion of the ureter. The ureters run along the common iliac artery and then cross over the iliac vessels as they enter the pelvis (**Fig. 3-30**). There is a slight variation between the two sides of the female pelvis. The right ureter tends to cross at the bifurcation of the common iliac artery, whereas usually the left ureter crosses 1 to 2 cm above the bifurcation.

The ureters follow the descending, convex curvature of the posterolateral pelvic wall toward the perineum. Throughout its course, the ureter is retroperitoneal in location. The ureter can be found on the medial leaf of the parietal peritoneum and in close proximity to the ovarian, uterine, obturator, and superior vesical arteries (**Fig. 3-31**). The uterine artery lies on the anterolateral surface of the ureter for 2.5 to 3 cm. At approximately the level of the ischial spine, the ureter changes its course and runs forward and medially from the uterosacral ligaments to the base of the broad ligament. There the ureter enters into the cardinal ligaments. In this location the ureter is approximately 1 to 2 cm lateral to the uterine cervix and is surrounded by a plexus of veins. A cross-sectional study by Hurd and colleagues, using computed tomography of women with normal anatomy, evaluated the distance from the ureter to the lateral aspect of the cervix. The measurement of the closest distance in any individual woman was (median of all subjects) 2.3 cm ± 0.8 cm. However, the authors noted that in 12% of women, the ureter was less than 0.5 cm from the cervix (**Fig. 3-32**). This finding emphasizes the caution needed in surgery to prevent ureteral injury. This close proximity also underscores the fact that ureteral injury may be unavoidable in some women. The ureter then runs upward (ventral) and medially in the vesical uterine ligaments to obliquely pierce the bladder wall. Just before entering the base of the bladder, the ureter is in immediate contact with the anterior vaginal wall and the inferolateral aspect of the **space of Retzius**.

The ureter has a rich arterial supply with numerous anastomoses from many small vessels that form a longitudinal plexus in the adventitia of the ureter. Parent vessels that send branches to this arterial plexus surrounding the ureter include the renal, ovarian, common iliac, hypogastric, uterine, vaginal, vesical, middle hemorrhoidal, and superior gluteal arteries. The ureter is resistant to injury resulting from devascularization unless the surgeon strips the adventitia from the muscular conduit.

URINARY BLADDER

The urinary bladder is a hollow muscular organ that lies between the symphysis pubis and the uterus. The size and shape of the bladder vary with the volume of urine it contains. Similarly, the anatomic proximity to other pelvic organs depends on whether the bladder is full or empty. The superior surface of the bladder is the only surface covered by peritoneum. The inferior portion is immediately adjacent to the uterus. The **urachus** is a fibrous cord extending from the apex of the bladder to the umbilicus. The urachus, which is the adult remnant of the embryonic allantois, is occasionally patent for part of its length. The base of the bladder lies directly adjacent to the endopelvic fascia over the anterior vaginal wall. The **bladder neck** and connecting urethra are attached to the symphysis pubis by fibrous ligaments. The prevesical or retropubic space

Figure 3-30 Photograph taken during a dissection of the lateral pelvic wall at the time of a radical hysterectomy. Note the ureter coursing over the common iliac artery in close proximity to the bifurcation. The ureter then drops under and very close to the uterine artery. The retractor is lifting the internal iliac vein. (Courtesy Deborah Jean Dotters, MD, Eugene, OR.)

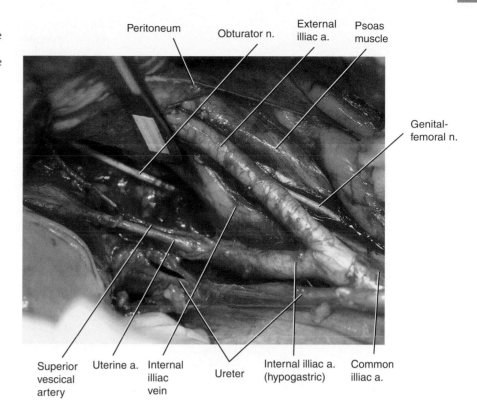

Peritoneum · Obturator n. · External iliac a. · Psoas muscle · Genital-femoral n. · Superior vescical artery · Uterine a. · Internal iliac vein · Ureter · Internal iliac a. (hypogastric) · Common iliac a.

Figure 3-31 A schematic drawing of the female pelvis, lateral view, demonstrating the ureter's relation to the major arteries. Note the uterine artery crossing over the ureter. (From Buchsbaum HJ, Schmidt JD: Gynecologic and Obstetric Urology. Philadelphia, WB Saunders, 1978, p 24.)

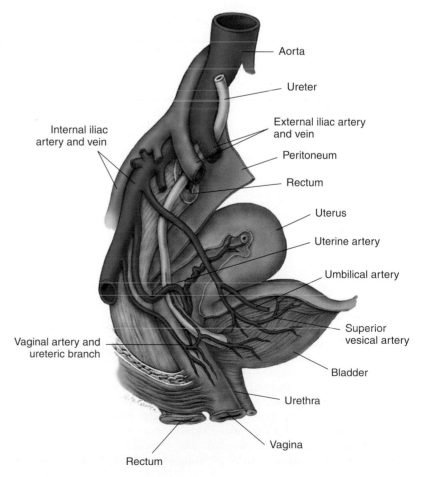

Internal iliac artery and vein · Aorta · Ureter · External iliac artery and vein · Peritoneum · Rectum · Uterus · Uterine artery · Umbilical artery · Superior vesical artery · Bladder · Urethra · Vaginal artery and ureteric branch · Vagina · Rectum

The arterial supply of the bladder originates from branches of the hypogastric artery: the superior vesical, inferior vesical, and middle hemorrhoidal arteries. The nerve supply to the bladder includes sympathetic and parasympathetic fibers, with the external sphincter supplied by the pudendal nerve.

RECTUM

The rectum is the terminal 12 to 14 cm of the large intestine. The rectum begins over the second or third sacral vertebra, where the sigmoid colon no longer has a mesentery. After the large intestine loses its mesentery, its anatomic posterior wall is in close proximity to the curvature of the sacrum. Anteriorly, peritoneum covers the upper and middle thirds of the rectum. The lowest one third is below the peritoneal reflection and is in close proximity to the posterior wall of the vagina. The rectum empties into the anal canal, which is 2 to 4 cm in length. The anal canal is fixed by the surrounding levator ani musculature of the pelvic diaphragm (see **Fig. 3-5**). The external sphincter of the anal canal is a circular band of striated muscle. Recent studies of the cross-sectional anatomy of the external anal sphincter by both ultrasound and magnetic resonance imaging have identified two distinct layers of the external anal sphincter. With MRI with 3-D reconstruction, Hsu and colleagues noted three separate components to the external sphincter: a main muscle body, a separate encircling subcutaneous band of muscles, and bilateral wing-shaped muscle bands that attach near the ischiopubis. They are a subcutaneous and a deep layer. The rectum, unlike other areas of the large intestine, does not have teniae coli or appendices epiploicae. The arterial supply of the rectum is rich, originating from five arteries: the superior hemorrhoidal artery, which is a continuation of the inferior mesenteric, the two middle hemorrhoidal arteries, and the two inferior hemorrhoidal arteries. Approximately 10% of carcinomas of the large bowel occur within the rectum. Therefore, during rectal examination special emphasis to palpate the entire circumference of the rectum, not just the area of the rectovaginal septum, is an important part of screening for colon cancer.

CLINICAL CORRELATIONS

The anatomic proximity of the ureters, urinary bladder, and rectum to the female reproductive organs is a major consideration in most gynecologic operations. Surgical compromise of the ureter may occur during clamping or ligating of the infundibulopelvic vessels, clamping or ligating of the cardinal ligaments, or wide suturing in the endopelvic fascia during an anterior repair, even with apparent normal anatomy and utmost surgical care. Particular attention to the proximity of the distal ureter to the anterior vagina is very important. Operative injuries to the bladder or ureter occur in approximately 1 out of 100 major gynecologic operations. Bladder injuries are approximately five times more common than ureteral injuries. Two of the classic ways to differentiate a ureter from a pelvic vessel are (1) visualization of peristalsis after stimulation by a surgical instrument and (2) visualization of **Auerbach's plexuses**, which are numerous, wavy, small vessels that anastomose over the surface of the ureter. Injury to the ureter or bladder during urethropexy operations for genuine stress incontinence is common. Therefore, many urogynecologists routinely inject indigo carmine and

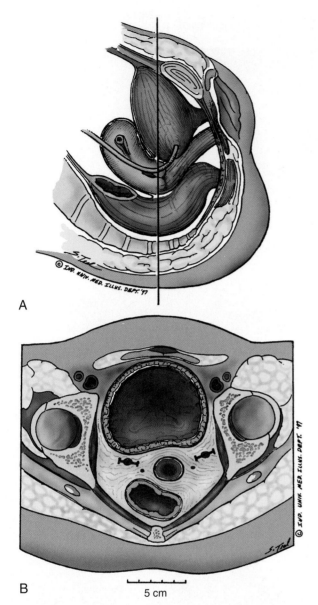

A

B   5 cm

Figure 3-32 Average location of the ureters in relation to the cervix. **A,** Sagittal view representing the plane from the CT cut noted in **B.** The most proximal point from the ureter to the cervix. Bars represent standard deviation. (From Hurd WW, Chee SS, Gallagher KL, et al: Location of the ureters in relation to the uterine cervix by computed tomography. Am J Obstet Gynecol 184:338, 2001.)

of Retzius is the area lying between the bladder and symphysis pubis and is bounded laterally by the obliterated hypogastric arteries. This space extends from the fascia covering the pelvic diaphragm to the umbilicus between the peritoneum and transversalis fascia.

The mucosa of the anterior surface of the bladder is light red and has numerous folds. The inferoposterior surface delineated by the two ureteral orifices and the urethral orifice is the trigone. The trigone is a darker red than the rest of the bladder mucosa and is free of folds. When the bladder is empty, the ureteral orifices are approximately 2.5 cm apart. This distance increases to 5 cm when the bladder is distended. The muscular wall of the bladder, the detrusor muscles, is arranged in three layers.

either open the bladder or perform cystoscopy near the end of the operative procedure.

For years, gynecologic teachers have referred to the area in the base of the broad ligament near the cervix where the uterine artery crosses the ureter as the area where "water flows under the bridge."

The urinary bladder, if properly drained, will heal rapidly after a surgical insult if the blood supply to the bladder wall is not compromised. This capacity allows the gynecologist to use suprapubic cystostomy tube without fear of fistula formation.

One of the surgical approaches for urinary stress incontinence is to suspend the periurethral tissue to either the symphysis pubis or Cooper's ligaments. Occasionally, this surgical approach is complicated by a significant amount of postoperative venous bleeding. A subfascial hematoma may extend as high as the umbilicus in the space of Retzius. One of the most common causes of female urinary incontinence is defective connective tissue, especially in the periurethral connective tissue, the pubourethral ligaments, and pubococcygeus muscles.

Rectal injury may occur during vaginal hysterectomy with associated posterior colporrhaphy. In the middle third of the vagina the distance between vaginal and rectal mucosa is only a few millimeters, and usually the connective tissue is densely adherent and should be separated by sharp dissection. The rectum bulges anteriorly into the vagina in this area, producing a further challenge during the operative procedure.

OTHER STRUCTURES

CUL-DE-SAC OF DOUGLAS

The cul-de-sac of Douglas is a deep pouch formed by the most caudal extent of the parietal peritoneum. The cul-de-sac is a potential space and is also called the *rectouterine pouch* or *fold* (**Figs. 3-29** and **3-33**). It is anterior to the rectum, separating the uterus from the large intestine. The parietal peritoneum of the cul-de-sac covers the cervix and upper part of the posterior vaginal wall then reflects to cover the anterior wall of the rectum.

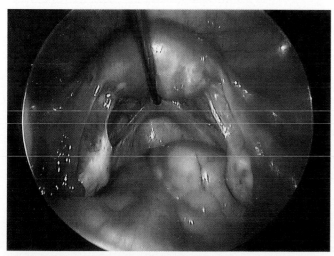

Figure 3-33 Laparoscopic visualization of a normal pelvis. The probe is elevating the uterus to expose the cul-de-sac of Douglas. (Courtesy of Burke Beller.)

The pouch is bounded on the lateral sides by the peritoneal folds covering the uterosacral ligaments.

PARAMETRIA

The parametria are the coats of extraperitoneal fatty and fibrous connective tissues adjacent to the uterus. The parametria lie between the leaves of the broad ligament and in the contiguous area anteriorly between the cervix and bladder. This connective tissue is thicker and denser adjacent to the cervix and vagina, where it becomes part of the connective tissue of the pelvic floor. The parametria may also thicken in response to radiation, pelvic cancer, infection, or endometriosis.

PARAVESICAL AND PARARECTAL SPACES

The paravesical and pararectal spaces are actually potential spaces that become true spaces when developed by the surgeon. Development of these spaces is very useful in pelvic lymph node dissection and in radical pelvic surgery because it makes the anatomic landmarks so clear. The paravesical space is bordered medially by the bladder and upper vagina and is contiguous with, but lateral to, the space of Retzius. Laterally, it is bordered by the obturator fossa and the external iliac vessels. Inferiorly, it is bordered by the pubic ramus, and superiorly by the cardinal ligament.

The pararectal space is developed by dissecting the adventitial tissue within the broad ligament, between the ureter (medially), and the internal iliac vessels (laterally). More deeply, the medial border is the rectum. Superiorly, the pararectal space is limited by the sacral hollow. Inferiorly, it is limited by the cardinal ligament, containing the uterine artery. The paravesical and pararectal spaces are actually potential spaces that become true spaces when developed by the surgeon. Development of these spaces is very useful in pelvic lymph node dissection and in radical pelvic surgery because the anatomic landmarks become so clear.

CLINICAL CORRELATIONS

The parametria and cul-de-sac of Douglas are important anatomic landmarks in advanced pelvic infection and neoplasia. Intrauterine infection, cervical carcinoma, and endometrial carcinoma may penetrate the endocervical stroma or the myometrium and secondarily may invade the loose connective tissue of the parametria.

The pouch of Douglas is easily accessible in performing transvaginal surgical procedures. Posterior colpotomy is frequently chosen for drainage of a pelvic abscess occurring in the cul-de-sac of Douglas.

When the paravesical and pararectal spaces have been developed and the uterus is held on traction medially, the pelvic anatomy, including the ureter, internal and external iliac vessels, obturator fossa, and the cardinal ligament, with the uterine artery crossing the ureter, can be clearly and readily identified.

Many women with uterine prolapse have an associated enterocele, which is a hernia that protrudes between the uterosacral ligaments. Occasionally the cul-de-sac of Douglas is obliterated by the inflammatory process associated with either endometriosis or advanced malignancy.

- The labia majora are homologous to the scrotum in the male. The labia minora are homologous to the penile urethra and a portion of the skin of the penis in males.
- The clitoris is the female homologue of the penis in the male. Skene's glands are homologous to the prostate gland in the male.
- The average length of the clitoris is 1.5 to 2 cm. Clinically, in determining clitoromegaly width is more important and should be less than 1 cm, for it is difficult to actually measure the length of the clitoris.
- The female urethra measures 3.5 to 5 cm in length. The mucosa of the proximal two thirds of the urethra is composed of stratified transitional epithelium, and the distal one third is stratified squamous epithelium.
- When a woman is standing, the axis of the upper portion of the vagina lies close to the horizontal plane, with the upper portion of the vagina curving toward the hollow of the sacrum.
- The vaginal length increases with weight and height, and decreases with age.
- The lower third of the vagina is in close anatomic relationship to the urogenital and pelvic diaphragms.
- The middle third of the vagina is supported by the levator ani muscles and the lower portion of the cardinal ligaments.
- The primary lymphatic drainage of the upper third of the vagina is to the external iliac nodes, the middle third of the vagina drains to the common and internal iliac nodes, and the lower third has a wide lymphatic distribution, including the common iliac, superficial inguinal, and perirectal nodes.
- Descriptive terms for pelvic organs are derived from the Latin root, whereas terms relating to surgical procedures are derived from the Greek root.
- The length and width of the endocervical canal vary. The width of the canal varies with the parity of the woman and changing hormonal levels. It is usually 2.5 to 3 cm in length and 7 to 8 mm at its widest point.
- The fibromuscular cervical stroma is composed primarily of collagenous connective tissue and ground substance. The connective tissue contains approximately 15% smooth muscle cells and a small amount of elastic tissue.
- The major arterial supply to the cervix is located in the lateral cervical walls at the 3 and 9 o'clock positions.
- The pain fibers from the cervix accompany the parasympathetic fibers to the second, third, and fourth sacral segments.
- The transformation zone of the cervix encompasses the border of the squamous epithelium and columnar epithelium. The location of the transformation zone changes on the cervix depending on a woman's hormonal status.
- The uterus of a nulliparous woman is approximately 8 cm long, 5 cm wide, and 2.5 cm thick and weighs 40 to 50 g. In contrast, in a multiparous woman each measurement is approximately 1.2 cm larger and normal uterine weight is 20 to 30 g heavier. The maximal weight of a normal uterus is 110 g.
- In the majority of women, the long axis of the uterus is both anteverted in respect to the long axis of the vagina and anteflexed in relation to the long axis of the cervix. However, a retroflexed uterus is a normal variant found in approximately 25% of women.
- The uterine and ovarian arteries provide the arterial blood supply of the uterus. The uterine arteries are large branches of the anterior division of the hypogastric arteries, whereas the ovarian arteries originate directly from the aorta.
- Afferent nerve fibers from the uterus enter the spinal cord at the eleventh and twelfth thoracic segments.
- The oviducts are 10 to 14 cm in length and are composed of four anatomic sections. Closest to the uterine cavity is the interstitial segment, followed by the narrow isthmic segment, then the wider ampullary segment, and distally the trumpet-shaped infundibular segment.
- The right oviduct and appendix are often anatomically adjacent. Clinically it may be difficult to differentiate inflammation of the upper portion of the genital tract and acute appendicitis.
- During the reproductive years, the ovaries measure approximately 1.5 cm × 2.5 cm × 4 cm.
- The ovary in nulliparous women rests in a depression of peritoneum named the *fossa ovarica*. Immediately adjacent to the ovarian fossa are the external iliac vessels, the ureter, and the obturator vessels and nerves.
- Three prominent ligaments determine the anatomic mobility of the ovary: the mesovarian, the ovarian ligament, and the infundibulopelvic ligament.
- The arterial supply of the pelvis is paired, bilateral, and has multiple collaterals and numerous anastomoses.
- The extent of collateral circulation after hypogastric artery ligation depends on the site of ligation and may be divided into three groups: branches from the aorta, branches from the external iliac arteries, and branches from the femoral arteries.
- The internal iliac nodes are found in an anatomic triangle whose sides are composed of the external iliac artery, the hypogastric artery, and the pelvic sidewall. This rich collection of nodes receives channels from every internal pelvic organ and the vulva, including the clitoris and urethra.
- The femoral triangle is the anatomic space lying immediately distal to the fold of the groin. The boundaries of the femoral triangle are the sartorius and adductor longus muscles and the inguinal ligament.
- The pudendal nerve and its branches supply the majority of both motor and sensory fibers to the muscles and skin of the vulvar region.
- The femoral nerve may be compromised by pressure on the psoas muscle during abdominal surgery and by hyperflexion of the leg during vaginal surgery.
- The pelvic diaphragm is important in supporting both abdominal and pelvic viscera and facilitates equal distribution of intraabdominal pressure during activities such as coughing. The levator ani muscles constitute the greatest bulk of the pelvic diaphragm.
- The major function of the urogenital diaphragm is to support the urethra and maintain the urethrovesical junction.

- Contained within the broad ligaments are the following structures: oviducts, ovarian and round ligaments, ureters, ovarian and uterine arteries and veins, parametrial tissue, embryonic remnants of the mesonephric duct and Wolffian body, and two secondary ligaments.
- The cardinal ligaments provide the major support to the uterus.
- A congenital anomaly of a double, or bifid, ureter occurs in 1% to 4% of females.
- When the urinary bladder is empty, the ureteral orifices are approximately 2.5 cm apart. This distance increases to 5 cm when the bladder is distended.
- The distal ureter enters into the cardinal ligament. In this location the ureter is approximately 1 to 2 cm lateral to the uterine cervix and is surrounded by a plexus of veins. In approximately 12% of women, the cervix will be less than 0.5 cm from the cervix.
- Two ways of distinguishing the ureter from pelvic vessels are (1) identification of peristalsis after stimulation with a surgical instrument and (2) identification of Auerbach's plexuses.
- Surgical compromise of the ureters may occur during clamping or ligating of the infundibulopelvic vessels, clamping or ligating of the cardinal ligaments, or wide suturing in the endopelvic fascia during an anterior repair.
- The following three important axioms should be in the forefront of decision making during difficult gynecologic surgery: (1) do not assume that the anatomy of the left and right side of the pelvis are invariably identical mirror images; (2) during difficult operations with multiple adhesions, operate from known anatomic areas into the unknown; and (3) from the sage advice of a distinguished Canadian gynecologist, Dr. Henry McDuff:

  If the disease be rampant and the anatomy obscure,
  And the plans of dissection not pristine and pure,
  Do not be afraid, nor faint of heart,
  Try the retroperitoneum, it's a great place to start.

REFERENCES CAN BE FOUND ON EXPERTCONSULT.com

4

Reproductive Endocrinology
Neuroendocrinology, Gonadotropins, Sex Steroids, Prostaglandins, Ovulation, Menstruation, Hormone Assay

Michel Ferin and Roger A. Lobo

The endocrine regulation of the reproductive system is very complex. Much information has been obtained in the past three decades, and new information is constantly becoming available. It would be impossible to include all of it in a single chapter. Thus, this chapter presents only the basic information required to understand this complex subject. More detailed and in-depth information is found in the several books that have been dedicated to this subject.

Successful function of the reproductive system requires the involvement of several organs, none of which acts independently. In this chapter, we discuss the physiology of the hypothalamic-pituitary-ovarian (HPO) axis. For ease of understanding, each organ will be discussed first as an individual unit; information will include the central nervous system control of gonadotropin-releasing hormone (GnRH), the primary neurohormone controlling the whole reproductive endocrine axis, the GnRH action on the anterior pituitary and the resultant secretion of the gonadotropins, the gonadotropins action on the ovaries and the release of gonadal steroids, and finally the action of these sex steroids on the uterus and cervix. Although it is fair to state that the HPO axis is driven by the hypothalamus and its release of GnRH, it is important to point out that normal function of the hypothalamic-pituitary-ovarian endocrine axis requires a remarkable information flow and coordination between each of these organs, as exemplified by the existing inhibitory and stimulatory feedback loops. Their relevance will become obvious in the discussion of the menstrual cycle, which will close the chapter.

THE HYPOTHALAMUS AND GnRH

The reproductive process starts in the brain, through the activation of the initial hormonal signal that will release the gonadotropins from the pituitary gland. This hormone released by the hypothalamus is **gonadotropin-releasing hormone (GnRH)**, a decapeptide (10 amino acids) (**Fig. 4-1**). The GnRH gene (situated on the short arm of chromosome 8) encodes for a 92 amino acids precursor molecule, comprised of a signal peptide sequence, the GnRH sequence itself, a posttranscriptional processing signal (3 amino acids long), and a 56-amino acid peptide known as GnRH-associated peptide (GAP). (Several forms of the GnRH decapeptide have been identified, the principal of

which is GnRH-2, which differs from GnRH by 3 amino acids. It is found in several areas of the body, where it may subserve functions unrelated to those of GnRH. Its role in fertility, if any, remains to be determined.)

ANATOMY

The Relationship of the Olfactory and GnRH Systems in Early Fetal Life

Surprisingly, GnRH-synthesizing neurons do not originate within the brain, like the majority of all neurons. Rather, GnRH neurons derive from progenitor cells in the embryonic olfactory placode where they develop. In a particular journey unique for a neuron, GnRH neurons migrate toward the brain during early fetal life to reach the locations that they will occupy during adult life. This migration of GnRH neurons over long distances and through changing molecular environments suggests that numerous factors, local and possibly external, influence this process at its different stages. Such factors play critical roles, such as mediating the adhesion of GnRH neurons to changing surfaces along their voyage, promoting cytoskeleton remodeling, or modulating axonal guidance.

Functional connections between GnRH neurons and the hypophyseal portal system that will transport GnRH to the anterior pituitary gland are established by about 16 weeks of fetal life. Migration failure of GnRH neurons and the resultant lack of the establishment of functional connections are characteristic of patients with the **Kallmann syndrome,** who show hypogonadotropic hypogonadism accompanied by anosmia. In the 19-week old fetus with X-linked Kallmann syndrome, the GnRH neurons accompanying the olfactory nerves have been shown to be arrested in their voyage within the meninges, and therefore contact with the brain and the hypophyseal portal system is not established.

The GnRH Neuronal System

In the adult, neurons producing GnRH are present in several hypothalamic nuclei as well as other parts of the brain. However, the majority of GnRH neurons controlling the HPO axis are located within the anterior hypothalamus and primarily within the medial basal hypothalamus, with the greatest number in the primate within the **arcuate nucleus**. The 92 amino acid GnRH precursor is released into the axons of these neurons and cleaved

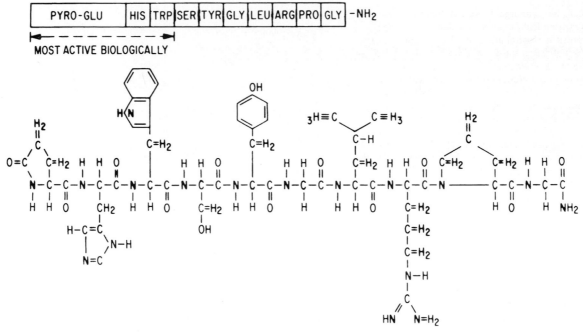

Figure 4-1 The 10-amino acid sequence of gonadotropin releasing hormone (GnRH). (From Klerzky OA, Lobo RA: Reproductive neuroendocrinology. In Mishell DR, Davajan V, Lobo RA [eds]: Infertility, Contraception and Reproductive Endocrinology, 3 rd ed. Cambridge, MA, Blackwell Scientific, 1991.)

during transport to yield GnRH and GAP. (The biologic function of GAP or fragments thereof remains to be clarified.)

A substantial number of GnRH axons terminate within the external zone of the **median eminence** (infundibulum) where GnRH is released. This area is the site of an important capillary plexus, with a fenestrated epithelium similar to that of peripheral capillaries, which allows passage of large molecules. (These capillaries differ from brain capillaries, which are not fenestrated. Thus, the median eminence is viewed as an area outside the blood-brain barrier.) This pathway is the most relevant one in regard to the control of the pituitary-ovarian axis (**Fig. 4-2, A**). Another substantial projection of GnRH axons is through circumventricular organs, the major of which is the organum vasculosum of the lamina terminalis (OVLT). These areas are also outside the blood-brain barrier. (The function of GnRH release into these areas remains somewhat unknown. One role may be to enable the release of GnRH into cerebrospinal fluid [CSF], perhaps to facilitate actions of GnRH in other areas of the brain. GnRH levels have been found to be elevated in CSF as opposed to being minimal in peripheral blood.) Another possible route of GnRH release may involve specialized ependymal cells, referred to as **tanycytes**. These have been found to extend from the lumen of the third ventricle to the external zone of the median eminence.

Transport of GnRH to the Anterior Pituitary
The capillary plexus of the external median eminence, into which GnRH is released, collects into several **hypophyseal portal vessels,** which descend along the pituitary stalk to terminate within another capillary plexus (hence the term portal) within the anterior lobe of the pituitary (**Fig. 4-2, *right***). (Unlike the posterior lobe of the pituitary, also referred to as the neurohypophysis, the anterior lobe has no direct blood supply and receives all of its vascularization from this portal system.) The vascular arrangement

whereby GnRH as well as other neurohormones reach the anterior pituitary is very important to the proper function of the endocrine system: it allows for the rapid (within minutes) and undiluted transport of relatively small amounts of neurohormones to the pituitary. This is especially crucial to GnRH, because this neurohormone has a short half-life of about 2 to 4 minutes (it is rapidly degraded by peptidases in blood; as a consequence, GnRH is not measurable in peripheral blood) and because of its pulsatile mode of release (discussed later).

PHYSIOLOGY

The GnRH Pulse Generator
Studies have shown that GnRH is characteristically released intermittently, in a pulsatile fashion. Hence comes the concept of the "**GnRH pulse generator**" responsible for the pulsatile release of the hormone. GnRH pulses occur at about hourly intervals (**Fig. 4-3**). The rising edge of each GnRH pulse is abrupt, such that GnRH can increase by a factor of 50 within 1 minute. Each GnRH pulse is preceded by an increase in multiunit activity within the area of the arcuate nucleus.

Mechanisms Responsible for GnRH Pulsatility
The cellular basis and the mechanisms that determine the timing of the increase in multiunit activity resulting in pulsatile GnRH activity are still under study. First, there is a growing consensus that pulsatile activity originates from an inherent pace-making activity of the GnRH neuron itself: in vitro data have shown that individual neurons have the capacity of spontaneous oscillations in activity. In this case, such activity would also require a synchronized action from enough neurons to provide a discrete GnRH pulse. Intercommunication between GnRH neurons may occur through gap junctions between such neurons, which have been demonstrated, and through synaptic forms of interaction

Figure 4-2 A, Nuclear organization of the hypothalamus, shown diagrammatically in a saggital plane as viewed from the third ventricle. Rostral area is to the left and caudal area is to the right. Fast transport of GnRH pulses released into the median eminence from axons originating from GnRH neurons in the arcuate nucleus occurs through the portal vessels derived from the capillary plexus in the median eminence. **B,** The pituitary stalk and several individual hypophyseal portal veins transporting hypothalamic neurohormones to the anterior pituitary in a nonhuman primate. (**A,** Redrawn from Moore RY: Neuroendocrine mechanisms: Cells and systems. In Yen SSC, Jaffe R [eds]: Reproductive Endocrinology: Physiology, Pathophysiology and Clinical management. Philadelphia, WB Saunders, 1986. **B,** Image courtesy of Drs. Peter Carmel and Michel Ferin.)

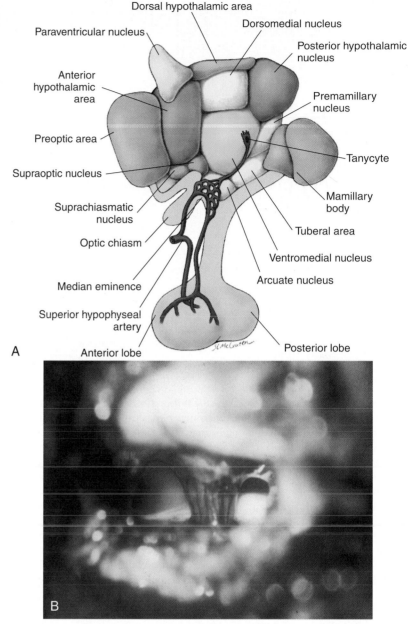

Modulatory influences on GnRH pulsatility

The foremost modulatory influence on the frequency and amplitude of GnRH pulses is exerted by the ovarian steroid hormones through their feedback loop actions. In general, estradiol is known to decrease GnRH pulse amplitude, whereas progesterone decreases GnRH pulse frequency (see the discussion presented later for details).

Numerous other studies suggest that the spontaneous activity of the GnRH pulse generator may also be modulated by a variety of additional stimulatory and inhibitory afferent neural signals. Stimulatory inputs to GnRH release may originate from neurons using the biogenic amine neuroepinephrine (NE), the amino acid glutamate and the peptide neuropeptide Y (NPY). Inhibitory inputs may come from amino acid gamma aminobutyric acid (GABA), the biogenic amine dopamine (DA), the endogenous opioid β-endorphin, and the neurosecretory peptide

between cells. Second, recent evidence suggests a key role of **kisspeptin** (KISS1), a product of the KISS1 gene, and its receptor (GPR54 or KISS1R) in the regulation of GnRH release. KISS1 neurons have been found to directly innervate and stimulate GnRH neurons. In humans, mutations or targeted deletions of KISS1 or of its receptor cause hypogonadotropic hypogonadism. Patients with these mutations, however, do not have anosmia unlike those with Kallmann syndrome, suggesting that there are no major deficits in the embryonic migration of olfactory or GnRH neurons. KISS1 neurons within the arcuate nucleus express the estrogen and the androgen receptors, and KISS1 signaling in the brain is now implicated in mediating sex steroids feedback loops, especially during the preovulatory GnRH/LH surge. KISS1 has also been shown to play a role in the initiation of puberty. Much remains to be studied, however, on how KISS1 neurons interact with other neurotransmitter systems.

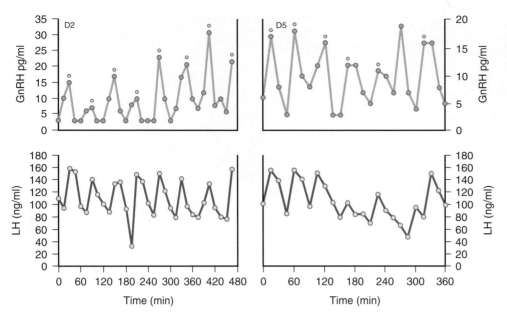

Figure 4-3 GnRH release by the hypothalamus is pulsatile. Shown in the upper panel are hourly GnRH pulses over an 8-hour period in an ovariectomized monkey in the absence of ovarian steroid modulation. Note the concordance of LH pulses *(lower panel).* (From Xia L, Van Vugt D, Alston EJ, et al: A surge of gonadotropin-releasing hormone accompanies the estradiol-induced gonadotropin surge in the rhesus monkey. Endocrinology 131:2812, 1992.)

corticotropin-releasing hormone (CRH) neurons. These systems may affect the GnRH pulse generator either *tonally* or *conditionally.*

In the first category, we find, for example, NE as a potential tonal stimulator and GABA as a tonal inhibitor of GnRH release. Administration of α-adrenergic blockers has been shown to reduce pulse frequency in animals, in accord with the postulated tonal stimulatory role for NE. The role of GABA as a tonal inhibitor may be more prominent during the prepubertal period, at which time a diminishing inhibitory GABA tone may activate puberty and the resumption of GnRH pulsatile release. Glutamate's role is more uncertain, although it also is suspected in the initiation of pulses at puberty. Dopamine infusions in women are associated with a decrease in circulating LH and prolactin (dopamine is also known as the prolactin-inhibitory neurohormone). The effect on LH is thought to be mediated through GnRH because, in patients with hypothalamic amenorrhea in whom there appears to be an excess of dopaminergic tone, administration of a dopamine blocker may return the LH pulse frequency to normal. It should also be remembered that specific effects of neurotransmitters on GnRH neurons may be altered by the administration of certain drugs, which may interfere with the proper synthesis, binding, storage or receptor function of these neurotransmitters. Thus, upon treatment with such drugs (for example, methyl dopa, reserpine, tricyclic antidepressants such as propranolol, phentolamine, haloperidol, and cyproheptadine, selective serotonin reuptake inhibitors [SSRIs] or serotonin-norepinephrine reuptake inhibitors [SNRIs]), patients may develop disorders such as oligomenorrhea or galactorrhea, the result of alterations in GnRH secretion or hyperprolactinemia. Other studies also suggest that hypothalamic prostaglandins may also modulate the release of GnRH; for instance, the midcycle surge of LH (see The Menstrual Cycle, presented later in the chapter) can be abolished in animals by the administration of aspirin or indomethacin, which block the synthesis of prostaglandins. Clinical studies have also shown that inhibition of prostaglandin at midcycle may disrupt ovulation.

In the second category, other systems may affect the GnRH system only *conditionally*—that is, under specific hormonal or physiologic conditions. One example is the endogenous opioid **β-endorphin**, which exerts an inhibitory action on GnRH pulsatile activity that depends largely on the endogenous endocrine milieu. This is related to the fact that ovarian hormones control the release of brain β-endorphin within the brain, which is lowest in the absence of estradiol, such as in the ovariectomized nonhuman primate, and highest in the presence of both estradiol and progesterone, such as during the luteal phase of the menstrual cycle. Experimental administration of the opiate antagonist, naloxone, during the luteal phase increases GnRH/LH pulse frequency, significantly suggesting the reversal of a inhibitory action under the endocrine milieu that characterizes the luteal phase. No effect on LH pulsatility follows naloxone injection in postmenopausal or ovariectomized women, unless they are replaced with an estrogen-progesterone therapy. Another example is corticotropin-releasing hormone (CRH), the main neuropeptide controlling the adrenal endocrine axis, which is released in greater amount during stress. In this condition, increased CRH release impacts negatively on the GnRH pulse generator, which results in a decrease in GnRH pulse frequency. This action is indirect through the release of β-endorphin and is prevented by the administration of the opiate antagonist naloxone, as demonstrated in studies in nonhuman primates and in patients with hypothalamic amenorrhea, many of whom have elevated levels of cortisol.

Metabolic influences and GnRH release

There is good clinical evidence linking energy homeostasis and reproductive function in the human. A functional reproductive system requires an accurate integration of energy balance, and a significant imbalance may lead to reproductive dysfunction and amenorrhea. Nutritional deprivation and abnormal eating habits are known to interfere with the normal reproductive process. Anorexia nervosa is a well-known and extreme example of how alteration in food intake can result in the suppression of the menstrual cycle. Obesity also may contribute to menstrual disorders.

Growing evidence indicates that complex and extensively integrated physiologic mechanisms connect an active reproductive axis to the metabolic state. The brain, and in particular the hypothalamus and the GnRH pulse generator, function as the center for the integrative metabolic response process. The nature of the afferent signals that provide information about energy metabolism to the reproductive axis is presently under intense study, and recent data have shown possible roles for several energy-related proteins.

One such example is leptin, an anorexigenic protein that is the product of the ob gene and that is primarily produced by adipocytes. Leptin levels are reduced when body fat stores are decreased by fasting. Besides conveying metabolic information to several parts of the brain through its own receptors, leptin also appears to function as one of the metabolic cues regulating the GnRH pulse generator. High leptin levels are interpreted as conducive to reproduction, and the administration of leptin stimulates the secretion of GnRH and of the gonadotropins, with the effects most pronounced in individuals showing signs of reproductive impairment. Peripheral injections of leptin can prevent the reduction in GnRH/gonadotropins and the disturbances in cyclicity that accompany caloric reduction. Ob/ob mice, which are leptin deficient because of a mutated leptin gene, besides exhibiting a pronounced obesity, show a complete failure to display normal estrous cycles because of absent GnRH secretion. The latter can be reversed by leptin administration. Another example is the orexigenic peptide, neuropeptide Y (NPY), which is synthesized in the arcuate nucleus. During fasting, expression of NPY mRNA increases in this nucleus and intracerebroventricular injection of NPY stimulates food intake. NPY has been shown to affect pulsatile GnRH/LH activity in the nonhuman primate, but this occurs in two apparently contradictory modes, one excitatory and one inhibitory. It was shown in the ovariectomized monkey and rodent that a pulsatile intracerebroventricular infusion of NPY stimulates GnRH release, whereas a continuous infusion clearly decreases the pulsatile electric activity of GnRH neurons as well as pulsatile LH release. In accord with this observation of an inhibitory effect of NPY is that, whereas fasting decreases LH secretion in normal mice, fasting mice lacking NPY Y1R have a higher pituitary LH content than wild-type ones. What these data suggest is that although a supportive effect of NPY on the GnRH pulse generator may occur within a limited window of normalcy (i.e., within a normal background of basic and pulsatile NPY release), in physiopathologic situations (i.e., in circumstances mimicking increased endogenous NPY activity such as in undernutrition) an inhibitory effect of NPY on the GnRH pulse generator can be observed. Recent evidence suggests a potentially important central role of KISS1 neurons in the regulation of reproduction by metabolic factors.

Overall, in regard to the reproductive system, the GnRH pulse generator actually acts as the link between the environment, the internal milieu, and the reproductive axis. Its overall activity most probably reflects the summation of simultaneous stimulatory and inhibitory inputs. It is evident that events, disorders, or drug administration may tip the physiologic balance, cause disruption or cessation of GnRH pulse activity, and lead to disruptions of the menstrual cycle and to reproductive disorders such as oligomenorrhea and hypothalamic amenorrhea.

THE ANTERIOR PITUITARY GLAND AND THE GONADOTROPINS

ANATOMY

The anterior pituitary (also referred to as the **adenohypophysis**) derives from *Rathke's pouch,* a depression in the roof of the developing mouth in front of the buccopharyngeal membrane. It originates at about the third week of life. Origin of the adenohypophysis contrasts with that of the posterior pituitary (*neurohypophysis*), which develops as a direct extension of the brain. It should also be noted that whereas the neurohypophysis receives a direct arterial blood supply from the hypophyseal arteries, the only vascularization to the adenohypophysis is through the hypothalamic-hypophyseal portal system (into which GnRH and several other neuropeptides are secreted) (discussed earlier).

The gonadotropes are the specialized cells within the adenohypophysis that produce the **gonadotropins**. Upon stimulation of the gonadotropes by GnRH, two gonadotropins are released into the general circulation and regulate endocrine function in the ovaries and testes.

PHYSIOLOGY

The GnRH Receptor

Pulses of GnRH released by the GnRH neurons in the arcuate nucleus reach the gonadotropes in the anterior pituitary via the hypophyseal portal circulation. These GnRH pulses then act on GnRH receptors (**GnRH-R**) on the gonadotropes to stimulate both the synthesis and release of both gonadotropins, LH and FSH. Females with GnRH-R mutations typically present with incomplete or absent pubertal development and primary amenorrhea. Although reproductive function is compromised, conception may be successfully obtained following gonadotropin treatment.

On the cell membranes of the gonadotrope, GnRH interacts with high-affinity GnRH receptors. The gene encoding the GnRH-R is located on chromosome 4q13.2-13.3, spanning 18.9 kb. This receptor belongs to a large family of G protein-coupled receptors. These contain seven transmembrane helices connected by six alternating intracellular and extracellular loops, with the amino-terminus located on the extracellular side. In contrast to other protein receptors (see **Fig. 4-9**, presented later in the chapter), the GnRH-R lacks a carboxyterminus located on the intracellular site.

Activation of the GnRH Receptor

GnRH activation of the receptor requires the release of constraining intramolecular bonds, which maintain the receptor in an inactive configuration. Once activated, the GnRH receptor stimulates cellular production of specific membrane-associated lipid-like diacylglycerols, which, acting as a second messenger, activate several cellular proteins. Among these are the enzyme **protein kinase C (PKC)** and **mitogen-activated protein kinase (ERK)**. Phosphorylated ERK activates transcription factors, the end result being gene transcription of gonadotropin subunits and the synthesis of both gonadotropins.

Binding of GnRH to its receptor also rapidly mobilizes transient intracellular calcium, which triggers a burst of exocytosis to rapidly release LH and FSH. It also provokes a rapid influx of

Ca^{++} into the cell from the extracellular pool, which in turn activates calmodulin, a calcium-binding protein, maintaining gonadotropin release. Diacylglycerols amplify the action of Ca^{++}-calmodulin, thereby synergistically enhancing the release of gonadotropins. Administration of a calmodulin antagonist has been shown to decrease GnRH-stimulated gonadotropin release.

Estrogens and the GnRH Receptor

Pulsatile GnRH increases GnRH-R gene expression and the number of GnRH-R on the gonadotrope's cell surface. The number of GnRH-R also varies with the hormonal environment, with highest number of receptors expressed when high concentrations of estrogens are present. This leads to an increase in the overall $Ca2^{++}$ response and a significantly amplified gonadotropin response to a GnRH pulse. This action explains the variations in the gonadotropin response to GnRH at various times of the menstrual cycle: GnRH pulses of similar amplitude elicit greater gonadotropin responses during the late follicular phase and luteal phase when estradiol levels are highest, but the responses are lower during the early follicular phase when estradiol levels are lowest (**Fig. 4-4**).

GnRH Pulse Frequency and Gonadotropin Release

It is also important to note that varying frequencies of the GnRH pulse signal regulate gonadotropin subunit gene transcription differentially. Overall, a low GnRH pulse frequency favors FSH synthesis, whereas a high GnRH pulse frequency favors LH synthesis. This is well demonstrated experimentally where

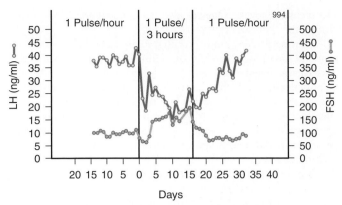

Figure 4-5 Increase in the FSH:LH ratio following a decrease in the GnRH pulse frequency (from 1 pulse/hour; *left and right panels*) to 1 pulse/3 hour *(center panel)*. Experiment was performed in a monkey lacking endogenous GnRH and infused with GnRH. (From Wildt L, Hausler A, Marshall G, et al: Frequency and amplitude of gonadotropin-releasing hormone stimulation and gonadotropin secretion in the rhesus monkey. Endocrinology 109:376, 1981.)

changing a pulsatile infusion from a high to a low pulse frequency results in a matter of days in an increase in the FSH:LH ratio (**Fig. 4-5**). This phenomenon may play a role during the luteal phase of the menstrual cycle and in the changing FSH:LH ratio that occurs during the passage from one menstrual cycle to another (see The Luteal Phase, discussed later). It is also reflected in patients known to have a high GnRH pulse frequency, such as in women with the polycystic ovary syndrome in which a high proportion of patients have a characteristically elevated LH:FSH ratio.

GnRH Receptor Desensitization

Gonadotropin release following a GnRH pulse is rapid: within minutes, both FSH and LH are released. It is important to recognize that the pulsatile release mode of GnRH is essential for the maintenance and control of normal gonadotropin secretion.

In contrast to the response to the normal pulsatile mode of GnRH release, sustained exposure of the GnRH-R to constant GnRH concentrations drastically reduces the response of the gonadotrope to subsequent stimulation with GnRH. This phenomenon is referred to as homologous **desensitization** or **downregulation** of the receptor, which denotes a reduction in the ability of GnRH to elicit gonadotropin release after prior continuous exposure to GnRH. This phenomenon is well illustrated in a classic experiment performed by Knobil and collaborators in ovariectomized monkeys lacking endogenous GnRH secretion following lesion of the arcuate nucleus (**Fig. 4-6**). As illustrated, 6-minute duration pulses administered once an hour restored normal LH levels in these animals. In contrast, when a continuous mode of GnRH infusion was substituted to the pulsatile mode, there occurs a profound inhibition of LH concentrations. This reflects desensitization of the GnRH receptor. This phenomenon, which takes a few days to be established, may reflect a loss of active cell surface receptors and be maintained by a loss of functional Ca^{++} channels. However, the mechanism of desensitization is still under investigation, and additional intermediary changes remain to be characterized.

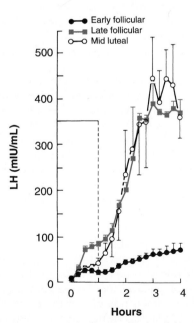

Figure 4-4 GnRH pulses of similar amplitude elicit greater overall gonadotropin responses during the late follicular phase and luteal phase when estradiol levels are highest, but they elicit lower responses during the early follicular phase when estradiol levels are lowest. Note also a greater early response in the late follicular phase, denoting greater LH reserves under the effect of estradiol. (From Hoff JD, Lasley BL, Wang CF, Yen SSC: The two pools of pituitary gonadotropins: Regulation during the menstrual cycle. J Clin Endocrinol Metab 44:302, 1977.)

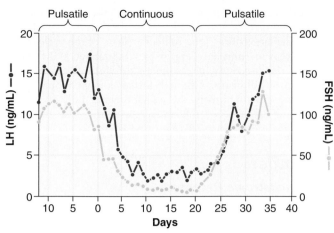

Figure 4-6 GnRH release in a pulsatile mode is required for a normal pituitary gonadotropin response. An experiment was performed in a monkey lacking endogenous GnRH and infused with hourly pulses of GnRH *(left and right panels)* or with a continuous GnRH infusion *(center panel)*. (From Belchetz PE, Plant TM, Nakai Y, et al: hypophyseal responses to continuous and intermittent delivery of hypothalamic gonadotropin-releasing hormone. Science 202:631-633, 1978.)

GnRH Analogues and the GnRH Receptor

The GnRH half-life in the peripheral circulation is very short as peptidases rapidly degrade naturally occurring GnRH by cleaving the decapeptide molecule at the Gly^6 to Leu^7 and at the Pro^9 to Gly^{10} bonds. However, by substituting amino acid 6 in the natural GnRH molecule with a d-amino or replacing amino acid 10 with a N-ethylamide (Na-CH2-CH3) or Aza-Gly (NHNHCO) moiety, gonadotropin-releasing hormone analogues (GnRH analogues) were synthesized and shown to have acquired a greater resistance to enzymatic proteolysis and hence a longer half-life (hours versus 2 to 4 minutes). Following administration of these **GnRH agonists**, there is an initial stimulation of gonadotropin release (flare), followed by the process of desensitization blocking the releasing effect on the gonadotropins. This observation has led to the clinical application of the functional desensitization property of GnRH:GnRH analogues having been used to induce a "medical castration" state by shutting down the pituitary-gonadal axis in a variety of clinical conditions. In contrast to GnRH agonists, **GnRH antagonists** act by competing with GnRH for receptor sites and thereby never activating a stimulatory signal. Many of these result from the substitution of amino acids at the 2 or 3 position. Thus, GnRH antagonists have the advantage over the GnRH agonists of a rapidly decreasing LH and FSH release, without the flare. Clinical applications for both GnRH agonists and antagonists are listed on **Table 4-1**.

The Gonadotropins

There are two distinct gonadotropins: **luteinizing hormone (LH)** and **follicle-stimulating hormone (FSH)**. (A third gonadotropin, chorionic gonadotropin [hCG], is produced in the primate by the placenta.)

Structure

LH and FSH are glycoproteins of high molecular weight. They are heterodimers, containing two monomeric units (**subunits**). Both LH and FSH have a similar α-subunit, the structure

Table 4-1 Clinical Applications of GnRH and Its Agonists

Activation of Pituitary-Gonadal Function (GnRH)
Delayed puberty
Cryptorchidism
Functional hypothalamic amenorrhea
Hypogonadotropic hypogonadism (Kallmann's syndrome)
Pituitary-gonadal inhibition (Agonists)
Precocious puberty
Hormone-dependent tumors
Endometriosis
Uterine leiomyoma
Breast cancer
Prostatic cancer
Suppression of ovarian function in polycystic ovary syndrome and in vitro fertilization
Premenstrual syndrome
Dysfunctional uterine bleeding including clotting disorders
Contraception
Suppression of spermatogenesis
Ovulation inhibition

(92 amino acids) of which is highly conserved. (The same α-subunit is also shared with hCG and thyroid stimulating hormone [TSH].) However, β-subunits have different structures consisting of different amino acids and carbohydrates. These LH and FSH subunits are each encoded by a separate gene. (The hCG subunits are also different and encoded by six genes.)

The α- and β-subunits are joined by disulfide bonds, which are essential to maintain biologic activity. Reducing agents break the disulfides bounds and reduce or remove the biologic activity of the gonadotropin. Highly purified free subunits have little if any biologic activity relative to that of the intact hormone. However, it is the β-subunit that confers the specific biologic activity of each hormone. For instance, LH has a β-subunit of 121 amino acids, a structure that is responsible for the specificity of the interaction with the LH receptor. LH and FSH also differ in the composition of their sugar moieties. The different composition of several different oligosaccharides affects bioactivity and speed of degradation of each gonadotropin. For example, the biologic half-life of LH is 20 minutes, much shorter than that of FSH (3 to 4 hours). (The half-life of hCG is 24 hours.)

Although both gonadotropins act synergistically in the female, FSH acts primarily on the granulosa cells of the ovarian follicles to stimulate follicular growth, whereas LH acts primarily on the theca cells of these follicles as well as on the luteal cells to stimulate ovarian steroid hormone production (see the following discussion).

THE OVARIES

ANATOMY

Ovarian Gametogenesis (Oogenesis)

Oogenesis begins in fetal life when the *primordial* germ cells, or **oogonia**, migrate to the genital ridge. The number of oogonia increases dramatically from about 600,000 by the second month of fetal life to a maximum of about 7 million by the sixth to seventh month. The oogonia then begin meiotic division (they are now referred to as **primary oocytes**) until they reach the diplotene stage of the prophase (the germinal vesicular stage), in which they will remain until stimulation by gonadotropins in adulthood during the menstrual cycle (discussed later). However, by a process of apoptosis and atresia of the enveloping follicle, which starts prenatally and persists throughout childhood, the number of primary oocytes declines drastically from about 2 to 4 million at birth to become 90% depleted by puberty. Further depletion of the pool occurs throughout adulthood, so that by age 37, only about 25,000 and by age 50 only about 1000 oocytes remain.

Ovarian Folliculogenesis

The primary oocyte is surrounded by a single layer of granulosa cells in a unit referred to as the **primordial follicle**. Even in the absence of stimulation by gonadotropins, some primordial follicles will develop into **primary** (or preantral) follicles, at which stage multiple layers of granulosa cells surround them. Development of follicles to this stage appears to be relatively independent of pituitary control but is probably influenced by intraovarian, nonsteroidal processes that remain to be understood. Development to this stage occurs during the nonovulatory stages of childhood, pregnancy, oral contraceptive use, as well as during ovulatory cycles.

With formation of an antrum (cavity), the follicle, now referred to as a **secondary** or **antral follicle**, enters the final stages of folliculogenesis characterized by the transition from intraovarian regulation to a major control by the hypothalamic-pituitary unit. This requires the presence of the characteristic increase in FSH that occurs in the early menstrual cycle (see The Menstrual Cycle, presented later).

The development process from primary follicle (preantral follicle) to secondary or antral follicle, and to a mature preovulatory follicle, the latter during the follicular phase of the cycle, takes about 1 year to complete (**Fig. 4-7**). Only about 400 follicles complete this process, whereas the majority of follicles undergo programmed cell death. Although little is known about factors controlling growth during the earlier stages, more is known about the final stage of folliculogenesis during the follicular phase of the menstrual cycle (discussed later).

PHYSIOLOGY

The Gonadotropin Receptors

Although the two gonadotropins act synergistically in the female, FSH acts primarily on the granulosa cells of the maturing antral follicle to stimulate follicular growth, whereas LH acts primarily on the theca cells of these follicles to induce steroidogenesis. Binding to and activation of their respective receptors at the cell surface membrane is the necessary first step in the hormonal function of both FSH and LH.

Gonadotropin receptors are transmembrane G protein-coupled receptors, which possess seven membrane-spanning domains (**Fig. 4-8**). It is believed that the receptor molecule exists in a conformational equilibrium between active and inactive states, which is shifted by binding of LH or FSH. Upon binding to the gonadotropin, the receptor shifts conformation and mechanically activates the G protein, which detaches from the receptor and activates cyclic AMP-dependent protein kinases. These protein kinases are present as tetramers with two regulatory units and two catalytic units. Upon binding of cyclic AMP

Life history of ovarian follicles

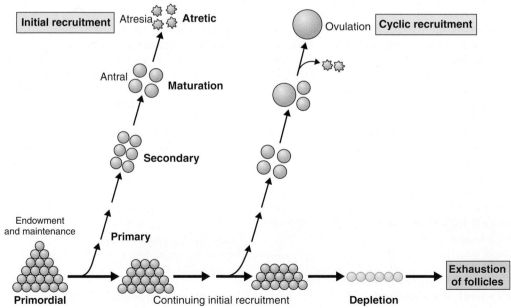

Figure 4-7 Life history of ovarian follicles: endowment, maintenance, initial recruitment, maturation, atresia or cyclic recruitment, ovulation, and exhaustion. A fixed number of primordial follicles are endowed during early life, and most of them are maintained in a resting state. Growth of some of these dormant follicles is initiated before and throughout reproductive life (initial recruitment). Follicles develop through primordial, primary, and secondary stages before acquiring an antral cavity. At the antral stage, most follicles undergo atresia; however, under the optimal gonadotropin stimulation that occurs after puberty, a few of them are rescued (cyclic recruitment) to reach the preovulatory stage. Eventually, depletion of the pool of resting follicles leads to ovarian follicle exhaustion and senescence. (From McGee EA, Hsueh AJW: Initial and cyclic recruitment of ovarian follicles. Endocrine Rev 21:200-214, 2000; with permission.)

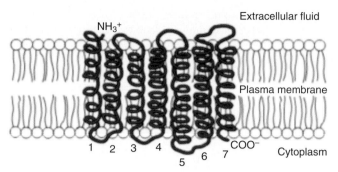

Figure 4-8 The seven transmembrane α-helix structure of a G protein-coupled receptor, such as that for LH or hCG. (The structure for the GnRH receptor is similar, except that the GnRH-R lacks a carboxy-terminus on the intracellular site; see the preceding text.) (From trans-membrane helix of G-protein coupled FSH receptor; from Wikipedia.)

(cAMP) to the regulatory units, the catalytic units are released and initiate the phosphorylation of proteins, which bind to DNA in the cell nucleus, resulting in the activation of genes and leading to the physiologic action (**Fig. 4-9**).

The Ovarian Steroids: Biosynthesis

One primary function of the ovary is the secretion of ovarian steroids, which occurs following binding of both FSH and LH to their respective receptors. The ovary secretes three primary hormones: **estradiol** (the primary estrogen), **progesterone,** and **androstenedione.** These hormones are the chief secretory products of the maturing follicle, the corpus luteum, and the ovarian stroma. The ovary also secretes, in varying amounts, estrone (a less potent estrogen), pregnenolone, 17-hydroxyprogesterone, testosterone, and dehydroepiandrosterone (DHEA). Because of the lack of the appropriate enzymes, the ovary does not synthesize mineralo-or glucocorticoids.

Steroids are lipids that have a basic chemical structure or nucleus (**Fig. 4-10**). The nucleus consists of three six-carbon rings (A, B, and C) joined to a five-carbon atom (D) ring. The carbon atoms are numbered as shown on Figure 4-10. Functional groups above the plane of the molecule are preceded by the β symbol and shown in the structural formula by a solid line, whereas those below the plane are indicated by an α symbol and a dotted line. All steroids, whether secreted by the ovary, testis, or adrenal, are derived from **acetate** (a two-carbon compound), which, in a series of complex reactions, is transformed into **cholesterol** (a 27-carbon steroid) (**Fig. 4-11.**)

The sex steroids (as well as the corticosteroids) are then derived from a stepwise transformation of the cholesterol molecule into steroids with 21 carbon atoms (the corticosteroids, pregnenolone, 17-hydroxy pregnenolone, progesterone, and 17-hydroxyprogesterone), 19 carbon atoms (androgens such as DHEA, androstenedione, and testosterone), and 18 carbon atoms (estrogens such a estradiol and estrone). In the first step, cholesterol is transferred from the outer mitochondrial membrane to the inner membrane where cytochrome P450 enzyme is located. The latter will split off the cholesterol side chain, which is the first enzymatic step in steroid biosynthesis. Being lipophilic, cholesterol is unable to cross the aqueous phase between these two membranes on its own, unless assisted. It is now believed that steroidogenic acute regular protein (StAR)

plays that role. The next steps in steroid biosynthesis require participation of a variety of enzymes, most of which are part of the cytochrome P450 superfamily of heme-based enzymes. First is the transformation of cholesterol into pregnenolone by hydroxylation of C-20 and C-22 and cleavage between these two atoms, reducing the C-27 cholesterol to the C-21 compound pregnenolone. At this point, ovarian steroid biosynthesis proceeds along two major pathways, controlled by specific enzymes at each step: (1) the Δ^5 *pathway* through 17-hydroxypregnenolone and DHEA to Δ^5 androstenediol and (2) the Δ^4 *pathway* via progesterone and 17-hydroxyprogesterone to the androgens, androstenedione and testosterone.

The Aromatase Enzyme

Androgens are converted to the estrogens estrone or estradiol by the enzyme **aromatase,** through the loss of the C-19 methyl group and the transformation of the A-ring to an aromatic state (hence the enzyme's name) through oxidation and subsequent elimination of a methyl group. The aromatic (or phenolic) ring is characteristic of the estrogens (**Fig. 4-12**).

Aromatase is a complex enzyme comprising two proteins. The first, P450arom (also a member of the cytochrome P450 superfamily of genes), catalyzes the series of reactions required for the formation of the phenolic A ring. The second is NADPH-cytochrome P450 reductase, a ubiquitous protein required for transferring reducing equivalents from NADPH to any microsomal form of cytochrome P450 with which it comes into contact. (All microsomal P450 enzymes require this reductase for catalysis. Disruption of this reductase has lethal consequences, as shown in knockout mice.)

The aromatase enzyme is found in many tissues besides the gonads, such as the endometrium, brain, placenta, bone, skin, and others. It is also particularly relevant to note that in humans, in contrast to other species, estrogens are also synthesized in adipose tissue, which in the postmenopausal woman becomes the major site of estrogen biosynthesis. The tissue-specific expression of the CYP19 aromatase gene is regulated by the use of different promoters. For instance, expression in the ovary uses a promoter element proximal to the start of translation, whereas expression in adipose tissue uses distal elements. Overall, the C_{18} estrogen produced in different tissue sites of biosynthesis is rather specific and dependent on the nature of the C_{19} steroid presented to the aromatase enzyme: in the ovary, the main androgen source is ovarian testosterone and thus the main estrogen product from the ovary is estradiol, whereas in adipose tissue the main androgen source is circulating androstenedione (produced by the adrenals) and hence the principal estrogen produced is estrone. (The greater the amount of fat present, the greater the amount of androstenedione that is converted to estrone.)

Mutation of the CYP19 aromatase gene leads to the **aromatase deficiency syndrome,** which is inherited in an autosomal recessive way. In these female patients, accumulation of androgens during pregnancy may lead to virilization at birth. Individuals of both sexes have abnormal pubertal maturation and are tall because of the lack of estrogen to affect epiphyseal closure. Female patients have primary amenorrhea. Aromatase inhibition evidently leads to profound hypoestrogenism. Aromatase inhibitors have become useful in the management of patients with estrogen receptor positive tumors—for example, in breast cancer.

Interconversion between androstenedione and testosterone and estrone and estradiol can occur outside the ovaries.

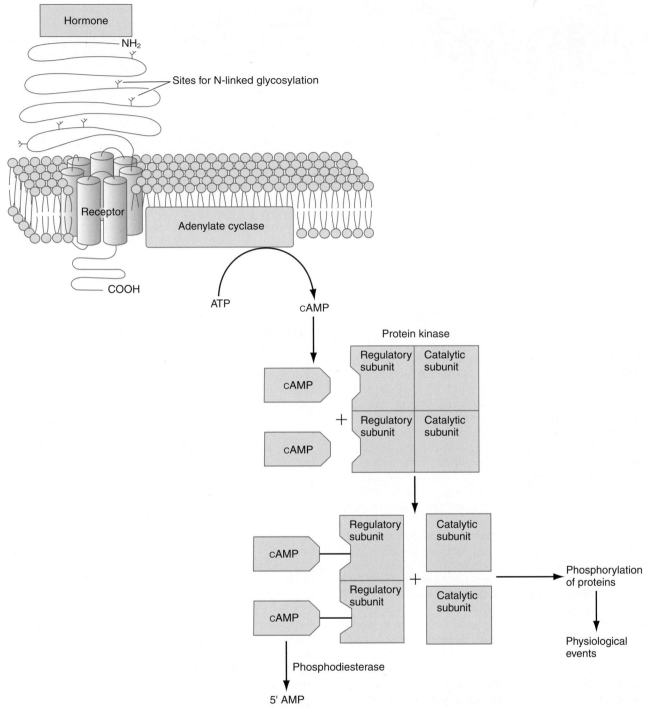

Figure 4-9 Upon binding to their receptor, the gonadotropins activate cyclic AMP-dependent protein kinases (see text). (Adapted from Speroff L, Friz M [eds]: Clinical Gynecologic Endocrinology and Infertility. New York, Lipincott Williams & Wilkins, 2005, pp 71-72.)

Oxidation of the latter to the former reduces biologic potency because both androstenedione and estrone have weaker biologic activity. Estrone is also converted to estrone sulfate, which has a longer half-life and is the largest component of the pool of circulating estrogens. Estrone sulfate is not biologically active; however, sulfatases in various tissues (such as breast and endometrium) can readily convert it to estrone, which in turn can be converted to the more biologically active estradiol. Steroids are in general insoluble in water but dissolve readily in organic solvents. In contrast, steroids that have a sulfate or glucuronide group attached (conjugated steroids)—such as, for example, estrone sulfate, dehydroepiandrosterone sulfate (DHEAS), or pregnanediol glucuronide—are water soluble.

The Ovarian Steroids: Blood Transport and Metabolism
After release into the circulation, sex steroids bind to a steroid-specific transport protein, **sex hormone-binding globulin (SHBG)** (a β-globulin synthesized by the liver), to the

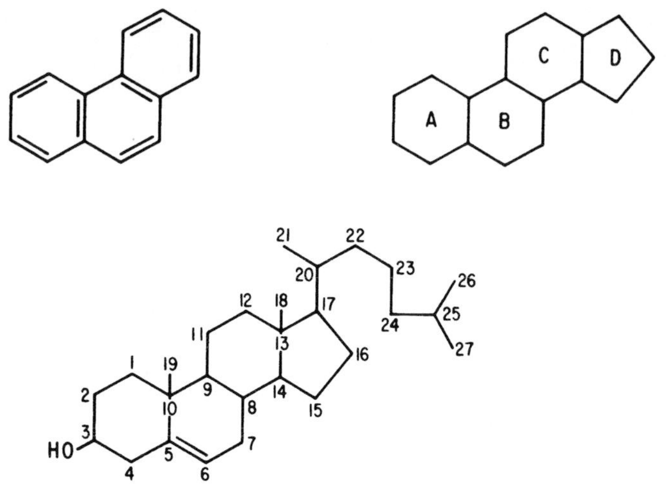

Figure 4-10 Phenantrene *(top left)*.
Cyclopentanoperhydrophenanthrene nucleus *(top right)*, which incorporates the three six-carbon rings of the phenanthrene ring system (**A**, **B**, and **C**) and a five-carbon ring (**D**), which resembles cyclopentane. Cholesterol *(bottom)* is the common biosynthetic precursor of steroid hormones. Numbers 1 to 27 indicate the conventional numbering system of the carbon atoms in steroids. (From Stanczyk FZ: Steroid hormones. In Lobo RA, Mishell DR, Paulson RJ, Shoupe D [eds]: Mishell's Textbook of Infertility, Contraception and Reproductive Endocrinology, 4th ed. Malden, MA, Blackwell Science, 1997.)

non–steroid specific albumin, or circulate in an unbound or "free" form. (There is a separate steroid specific protein, corticosteroid-binding protein [CBG; transcortin], which binds primarily adrenal steroids, and to a lesser degree progesterone.) Both SHBG and CBG have a high affinity (by definition) but low capacity for steroids. Albumin, in contrast, has a high capacity but binds with low affinity; thus, steroids can readily dissociate from its binding and enter target cells.

The free and loosely albumin-bound steroids are believed to be the most biologically important fractions because the steroid is free to diffuse or be actively transported through the capillary wall and bind to its receptor. (There is also evidence, however, that uptake of protein-bound hormone may also play a role.) SHBG binds primarily dihydrotestosterone, testosterone, and estradiol, in order of decreasing affinity. Thus, in premenopausal women, 65% of testosterone is bound to SHBG, 30% to albumin, and 5% is free, whereas 60% of estradiol is bound to SHBG, 38% to albumin, and 2% to 3% is free. The metabolic clearance rate of sex steroids is inversely related to their affinity to SHBG. It is thus important to remember that the level of SHBG, and therefore the level of free active hormone, may be influenced by various clinical conditions. For instance, circulating levels of SHBG are increased by estrogens (oral contraceptives, pregnancy) and by thyroid hormone (hyperthyroidism) and are lowered by androgens and in hypothyroidism.

The major sites of steroid metabolism are the liver and kidney. Steroids are mainly oxidized by cytochrome P450 oxidase enzymes, through reactions that introduce oxygen into the steroid ring allowing a breakdown by other enzymes to form bile acids as final products. These bile acids can then be eliminated through secretion from the liver. In another process, which involves conjugation, the steroids are transformed from lipophilic compounds, which are only sparingly soluble in water, into metabolites that are readily water soluble and can be eliminated in urine. Examples are estradiol-17 glucuronide, estrone sulfate, and pregnanediol-3-glucuronide (the major urinary metabolite of progesterone).

Prostaglandins

Prostaglandins (a subclass of eicosanoids and prostanoids) are in general mediators of inflammatory and anaphylactic reactions. Their most abundant precursor is arachidonic acid, itself formed from linoleic acid supplied in the diet. Their biosynthesis can be inhibited by several groups of compounds, including the nonsteroidal anti-inflammatory drugs (NSAIDs) type 1 (aspirin and indomethacin), which inhibit endoperoxide formation (the immediate precursor of eicosanoids), and type 2 (phenylbutazone), which inhibits the action of endoperoxidase isomerase and reductase. Corticosteroids also can inhibit prostaglandins synthesis.

In contrast to steroid hormones, which are stored and act at targets distant from their source, prostaglandins are produced intracellularly shortly before they are released and generally act locally. Specific prostanoids can have variable effects on different tissues, as well as variable effects on the same organ, even when released at the same concentration, hence the difficulty of studying their actions. One important effect is their ability to modulate the responses of endogenous stimulators and inhibitors, such as ovarian stimulation by LH, which is modulated by prostaglandin F2α (PGF2α), which in turn regulates ovarian receptor availability.

Prostaglandins play an important role in ovarian physiology. They help control early follicular growth by increasing blood supply to certain follicles and inducing FSH receptors in granulosa cells of preovulatory follicles. Both PGF2α and PGE2 are concentrated in follicular fluid of preovulatory follicles and may assist in the process of follicular rupture by facilitating proteolytic enzyme activity in the follicular walls. Many prostanoids are produced in the endometrium. Concentrations of PGE2 and PGF2α increase progressively from the proliferative to the secretory phase of the cycle, with highest levels at menstruation. These prostaglandins may help regulate myometrial contractility and may also play a role in regulating the process of menstruation.

COMMUNICATION WITHIN THE HYPOTHALAMIC-PITUITARY-OVARIAN ENDOCRINE AXIS

THE STEROID RECEPTORS

Gonadal steroids are integrated into every aspect of reproduction, and disruption of their signaling pathways, which obviously require initial binding to their receptors, leads to reduced fecundity and aberrations in multiple organs systems. For the sex steroid feedback loops (discussed later) to be active, there must be steroid receptors in the appropriate regions of the hypothalamus and pituitary gland to respond to the ovarian signals.

As opposed to peptide or protein hormones receptors that reside on the cell membrane (discussed earlier), steroid receptors reside in the nucleus or in the cytoplasm, in between which they may shuttle in the absence of hormone (**Fig. 4-13**). The

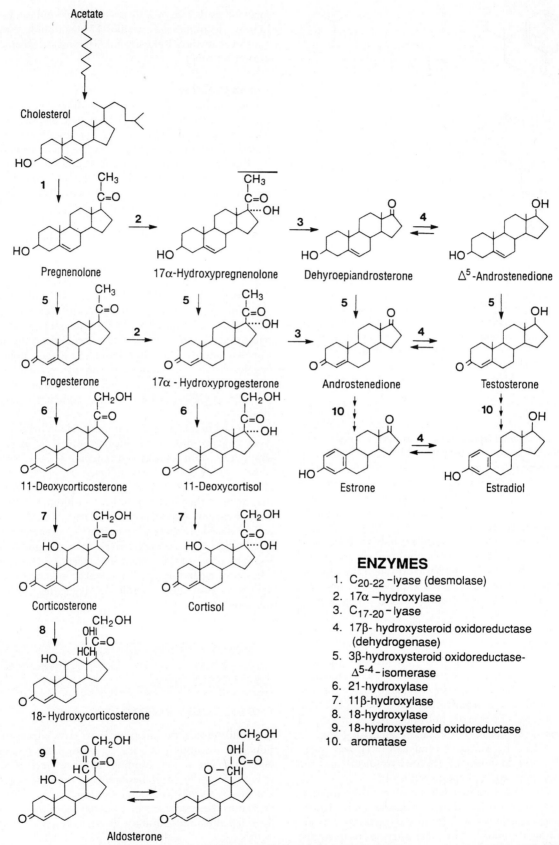

Figure 4-11 Biosynthesis of androgens, estrogens and corticosteroids. (From Stanczyk FZ: Steroid hormones. In Lobo RA, Mishell DR, Paulson RJ, Shoupe D [eds]: Mishell's Textbook of Infertility, Contraception and Reproductive Endocrinology, 4th ed. Malden, MA, Blackwell Science, 1997.)

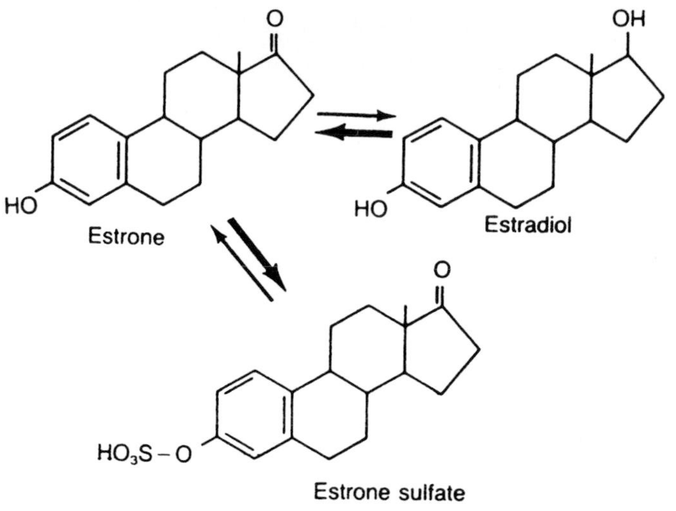

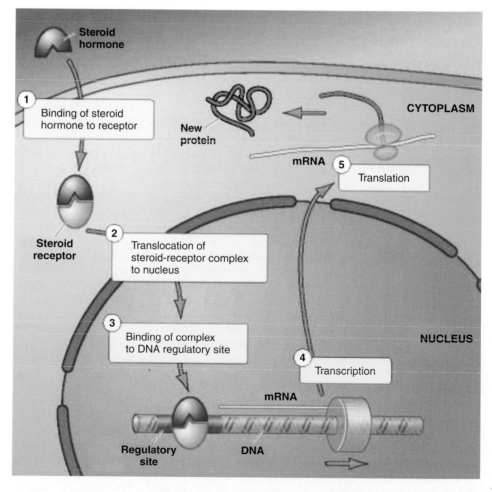

Figure 4-12 Interconversion of the three main circulating estrogens. (From Stanczyk FZ: Steroid hormones. In Lobo RA, Mishell DR, Paulson RJ, Shoupe D [eds]: Mishell's Textbook of Infertility, Contraception and Reproductive Endocrinology, 4th ed. Malden, MA, Blackwell Science, 1997.)

cytoplasmic receptor is sequestered (hence in an "inactive" state) within a multiprotein inhibitory complex that includes heat shock proteins. Hormone binding leads to dissociation from the heat shock proteins. The lipophilic steroids freely diffuse across the nuclear membrane to bind to their cognate receptor. This binding leads to conformational changes that transform the receptor into an "activated" state, which allows it to bind to a **hormone responsive element (HRE),** the specific DNA-binding site to which steroid receptors bind conferring hormone sensitivity within target gene promoters. mRNA is then generated from a segment of nuclear DNA in the process of transcription. Transcription is the most important process regulated by steroid hormones. All genes share a common basic design composed of a structural region in which the DNA encodes the specific amino acids of the protein and a regulatory region that interacts with various proteins to control the rate of transcription. The mRNA migrates into the cytoplasm where it translates information to ribosomes to synthesize the required new protein.

Several alternative receptor mechanisms besides the classic one outlined previously appear to exist. Some are plasma membrane steroid signaling events that are mediated through various kinases and second messengers including cAMP. These are independent of nuclear interactions and do not involve direct steroid

Figure 4-13 The steroid receptor activation process. As opposed to protein hormones receptors, which reside on the cell membrane, steroid receptors reside in the nucleus or in the cytoplasm. See the text for details.

activation of gene transcription (nongenomic). As opposed to the longer time required by the genomic pathway (hours to days), these alternate mechanisms may be responsible for some of the very rapid effects of steroids—for instance, as activated by the negative steroid feedback loop (discussed later), which occurs within minutes.

Members of the steroid receptor superfamily share amino acid homology and a common structure. They contain key structural elements that enable them to bind to their respective ligands with high affinity and specificity and to recognize and bind to discrete response elements within the DNA sequence of target genes with high affinity and specificity. For instance, estrogen receptors will bind natural and synthetic estrogens, but not androgens or progestins. The affinity of a receptor for a steroid also correlates with steroid potency; for example, the estrogen receptor has a greater affinity for estradiol than for estrone and estriol, which are much less potent than estradiol. Overall, the magnitude of the signal to the cell and of the cell response to the steroid depend on the concentration of the hormone and of the receptors, as well as on the affinity of the receptor to the hormone.

In the human, there are actually two estrogen receptors, ER-α and ER-β, which are distinct receptor forms encoded by separate genes. There are also two forms of the progesterone receptor, but these are isoforms (differing only by minor structural differences), which are encoded by the same gene.

THE OVARIAN-HYPOTHALAMIC-PITUITARY FEEDBACK LOOPS

FSH and LH act on the ovaries to induce morphologic changes and ovarian steroid secretion. Morphologic processes include folliculogenesis (i.e., the cyclic recruitment of a pool of follicles to produce a mature follicle ready for ovulation) and the formation of a corpus luteum. These processes occur in sequence, conferring a monthly rhythm to the reproductive cycle. Granulosa and theca cells within the follicle and luteal cells respond to LH by synthesizing and releasing ovarian steroids, mainly estradiol-17β and progesterone. The type and amount of hormone released depend on the status of the follicle and the corpus luteum (see The Menstrual Cycle, presented later).

Feedback communication between the ovaries and the hypothalamic-pituitary unit is an essential component to the physiology of the reproductive cycle. It is important for the brain and pituitary gland to modulate their secretion in response to the minute-to-minute activity status of the ovary. Through their receptors, both in various areas of the hypothalamus and in the anterior pituitary gland, the two ovarian steroids, estradiol and progesterone, play a major role in these feedback communications. More recent evidence shows that several nonsteroidal compounds are also involved in these feedbacks.

The Negative Steroid Feedback Loop

As in other endocrine systems, the major ovarian to brain/pituitary feedback loop is inhibitory (the **negative feedback loop**), whereby the steroid secreted by the target organ (the ovary) regulates the hypothalamic-hypophyseal unit to adjust GnRH and gonadotropin secretion appropriately (**Fig. 4-14**).

Estradiol-17β is a potent physiologic inhibitor of GnRH and of gonadotropin secretion. The threshold for the negative feedback action of estradiol is such that even small increases in

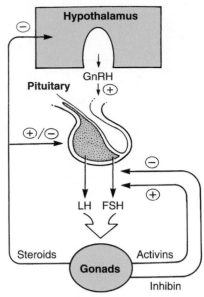

Figure 4-14 The rapidly acting negative feedback loop of steroids on GnRH and both gonadotropins release is supplemented by a slower-acting negative feedback loop by the inhibins. (From Hylka VW, di Zerega GS: Reproductive hormones and their mechanisms of action. In Mishell DR Jr, Davajan V, Lobo RA [eds]: Infertility, Contraception and Reproductive Endocrinology, 3 rd ed. Cambridge, MA, Blackwell Scientific, 1991.)

the levels of the hormone induce a decrease in gonadotropins. Levels of LH and FSH during the follicular phase vary in accord with the changes in estradiol concentrations that accompany maturation of the follicle. Thus, as circulating estradiol levels increase during the follicular phase, gonadotropin concentrations decrease. In postmenopausal women or women who have undergone ovariectomy or have aromatase enzyme deficiency, all of whom lack estradiol secretion, sustained increases in LH and FSH release occur because of the absence of an active negative feedback loop. In these conditions, administration of physiologic doses of estradiol results in a rapid and sustained decrease in LH and FSH to levels equivalent to those seen during the menstrual cycle. The estradiol negative feedback loop acts to decrease LH secretion rapidly, mainly by controlling the *amplitude* of each LH pulse. Most evidence suggests that this action is secondary to inhibitory effects on the GnRH pulse, most probably relayed by estrogen-receptive kisspeptin and possibly GABA neurons. Effects on the pituitary gonadotrope, whereby estradiol decreases the gonadotropin response to GnRH, may also take place.

Progesterone, at high concentrations such as those observed during the luteal phase of the cycle, also exerts an inhibitory effect on gonadotropin secretion. In contrast to estradiol, progesterone affects mainly the GnRH pulse generator by slowing the frequency of pulses. This effect is responsible for the significant decrease in LH pulse frequency observed during the luteal phase of the cycle, when high levels of progesterone are present, and which becomes more pronounced as the luteal phase progresses (discussed later).

There is good evidence that the slowing action of progesterone on GnRH-LH pulse frequency is mediated by central β-endorphin. Indeed, brain levels of this opioid peptide, as measured in hypophyseal portal blood in the nonhuman primate, are

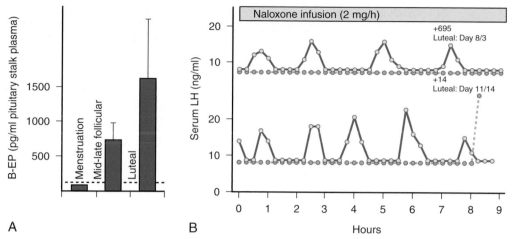

Figure 4-15 The endogenous opiates and the menstrual cycle. **A,** Changes in hypothalamic β-endorphin activity (as determined by its secretion into the pituitary stalk portal vasculature) during the menstrual cycle in the nonhuman primate. In the presence of low ovarian steroids, such as at menstruation, endorphin levels are lowest. They are highest in the presence of progesterone during the luteal phase. **B,** Role of β-endorphin in modulating the negative feedback action of progesterone during the luteal phase; note the dramatic increase in LH pulse frequency after endogenous opiate antagonism by naloxone *(closed circles)* compared with controls receiving saline *(open circles)*. (**A,** Van Vugt DA, Lam NY, Ferin M: Reduced frequency of pulsatile luteinizing hormone secretion in the luteal phase of the rhesus monkey: Involvement of endogenous opiates. Endocrinology 115:1095, 1984. **B,** Ferin M, Van Vugt D, Wardlaw S: The hypothalamic control of the menstrual cycle and the role of endogenous opioid peptides. Rec Prog Horm Res 40:441, 1984.)

elevated during the luteal phase (**Fig. 4-15, A**). Furthermore, naloxone administration (an opiate antagonist) in women during the luteal phase results in a significant acceleration in pulse frequency (**Fig. 4-15, B**).

In view of these estradiol and progesterone inhibitory feedback loops, it is not surprising that the characteristics of pulsatile LH secretion vary greatly with the stage of the menstrual cycle. During the estrogenic stage or follicular phase, pulses of high frequency but of low amplitude are seen, whereas during the progesterone stage or luteal phase, there is a progressive reduction in the frequency of the LH pulse, with pulse intervals reaching 200 minutes or more by the end of the luteal phase. This decreased pulse frequency is accompanied by a significant increase in pulse amplitude.

The Positive Estradiol Feedback Loop

At higher physiologic concentrations, estradiol can also exert a separate stimulatory effect (**positive feedback loop**) on gonadotropin secretion. This positive feedback is dependent on rapidly rising estradiol levels, in combination with a small but significant progesterone rise, both produced by the mature dominant follicle and responsible for the generation of the preovulatory LH and FSH surge. The positive feedback loop is observed in many species: it serves as the critical signal to the hypothalamic-pituitary axis that the dominant follicle is ready to ovulate. In most species, a GnRH surge precedes the LH surge, suggesting that the positive feedback loop acts centrally. However, there is also ample evidence that high levels of estradiol can increase GnRH pituitary receptors and augment the pituitary response to GnRH, suggesting effects at the pituitary site as well.

Experimentally, late follicular phase estradiol levels infused during the early follicular phase are able to activate the positive

feedback loop and release an LH surge, however inappropriate and untimely, because no mature follicle is present at the time (**Fig. 4-16**).

Ovarian Peptides Feedback Loops

In addition to the negative steroid feedback loop, there is also evidence that nonsteroid ovarian factors exert negative feedback effects on the anterior pituitary. Such are the **inhibins,** which are a family of glycoproteins that consist of a dimer with two dissimilar α and β subunits. The two subunits are coded by different genes. Two forms of the β subunit have been identified, and thus inhibin can exist as α-βA (**inhibin A**) and as α-βB (**inhibin B**) (**Fig. 4-17**), both of which are detected in serum in women during the reproductive years. The ovaries are the only source of circulating dimeric inhibins.

The inhibins are characterized by their preferential inhibition of FSH over LH through their own negative feedback loop (see **Fig. 4-14**). This negative feedback loop, however, functions at a significantly slower rate (hours) than that of the steroid negative feedback loop (which is activated within minutes) and is directed mainly at the pituitary gland. It is believed that the decline in FSH after its peak in the early follicular phase of the normal cycle results from a negative feedback action of inhibin B at the pituitary level. At menopause or in premature ovarian failure, data show a decreased secretion of inhibin with reproductive aging, suggesting that inhibin B negative feedback may be an important factor controlling the early monotropic increase in FSH with aging (reflecting the decreasing number of small antral follicles recruited in each cycle and the consequent insufficient inhibin B production).

The circulating patterns of inhibin A and B during the menstrual cycle are different: plasma concentrations of inhibin B rise rapidly on the day after the intercycle FSH rise (discussed later),

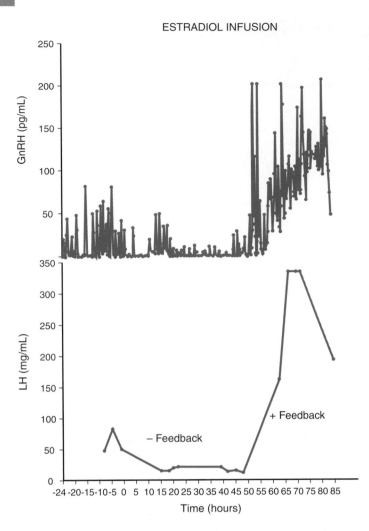

ESTRADIOL INFUSION

Figure 4-16 GnRH and LH responses to a 3.5-hour estradiol infusion mimicking late follicular phase estradiol levels. After a period of suppression (caused by the rapid estradiol negative feedback), note the large increase in both GnRH and LH (caused by the positive estradiol feedback). (From Xia L, van Vugt D, Alston EJ, Luckhaus J, Ferin M: A surge of gonadotropin-releasing hormone accompanies the estradiol-induced gonadotropin surge in the rhesus monkey. Endocrinology 131:2812-2820, 1992.)

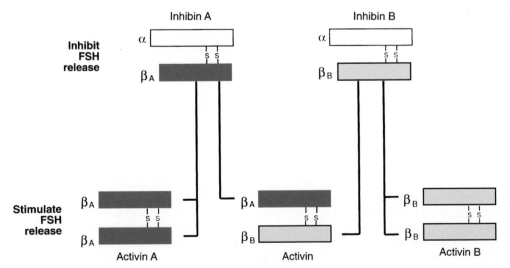

Figure 4-17 Chemical relationships of inhibins and activins. S: disulfide bond. (From Hylka VW, Di Zerega GS: Reproductive hormones and their mechanisms of action. In Mishell DR, Davajan V, Lobo RA [eds]: Infertility, Contraception and Reproductive Endocrinology, 3 rd ed. Cambridge, MA, Blackwell Scientific, 1991.)

remain elevated for a few days, then fall progressively during the remainder of the follicular phase. After a short-lived peak following the ovulatory gonadotropin surge, inhibin B falls to a low concentration during the luteal phase. In contrast, inhibin A concentrations rise only in the later part of the follicular phase and are maximal during the midluteal phase (**Fig. 4-18**.) These different patterns of circulating inhibin B and inhibin A during

the human menstrual cycle suggest different physiologic roles (discussed later).

Other dimers of the β subunit have also been described, such as **activin** A (A-β/ A-β), which in contrast to the inhibins stimulate FSH release from the pituitary (see **Fig. 4-17**). This effect is probably not very significant because of the irreversible binding of activin to follistatin, which neutralizes activin's bioactivity.

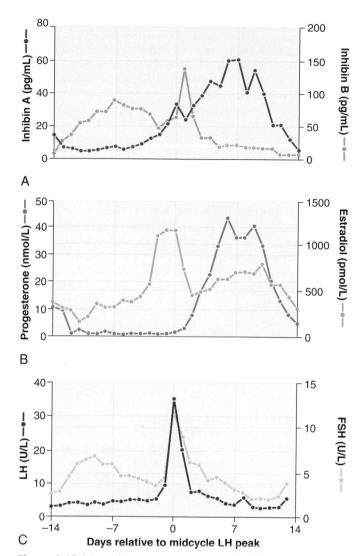

Figure 4-18 Mean plasma concentrations of inhibin A and inhibin B *(upper panel)* compared with estradiol and progesterone *(center panel)*, and LH and FSH *(lower panel)* during the menstrual cycle. Day 0 is the day of the LH surge. (From Groome NP, Illingworth PJ, O'Brien M, et al: Measurement of dimeric inhibin B throughout the human menstrual cycle. J Clin Endocrinol Metab 81:1401-1405, 1996.)

THE MENSTRUAL CYCLE

The menstrual or ovulatory cycle involves a remarkable coordination of morphologic changes and hormonal secretion occurring not only at several levels of the hypothalamic-pituitary-ovarian axis but also in organs outside of this main axis, such as the uterus and the cervix, and expressed in an orderly sequence of events. The initial stimulus from the brain under the form of GnRH pulses is crucial to proper gonadotropin responses, which in turn instigate folliculogenesis, ovulation, and the formation of the corpus luteum. Essential to the coordination of these events is the communication between the ovaries and the hypothalamic-pituitary unit through the hormonal feedbacks, which provide continuous information of the ovarian status to the brain, which in turns responds with the proper

pattern of GnRH pulses and of gonadotropin release. Humans are spontaneous ovulators (as opposed to light or seasonally related) in that the gonadotropin surge, the initiator of ovulation, is triggered by the endogenous changes in estradiol that accompany the maturation of the follicle.

This sequence of events is such that the reproductive process in the human occurs in a cyclic process at about monthly intervals. The primate menstrual cycle is divided into two phases: the follicular phase, followed by the luteal phase. These are separated by the ovulatory period. Mean duration of the menstrual cycle is 28 ± 7 days. The length of the follicular phase is more variable, whereas the life span of the corpus luteum is about 14 days. In many women, the length of the follicular phase usually decreases from about 14 days to about 10 days in women over 40 years old. However, menstrual cycle length also varies in an individual woman: it is most variable in the 2 years following menarche and preceding menopause, times of life during which anovulatory cycles are most frequent. The mean age of menarche (the first menstruation) occurs around age 12, while menopause (the end of the reproductive phase) usually occurs between ages 45 to 55. Endocrine changes during the menstrual cycle are illustrated in **Figure 4-18**.

THE FOLLICULAR PHASE

The follicular phase can be subdivided into three periods; these denote the successive recruitment of a cohort of antral follicles, the selection of a dominant follicle, and the growth of the selected dominant follicle.

Recruitment of a Cohort of Antral Follicles

When cohorts of growing follicles reach the early antral stage (see **Fig. 4-19**; see also **Fig. 4-7**), continuing growth requires a proper gonadotropin stimulatory action. **FSH** provides the critical signal for the recruitment of a **cohort** of preantral follicles. This FSH signal (cyclic recruitment) is the major survival factor that rescues the follicles from their programmed death (atresia) and allows them to start growing, increasing in size and beginning to synthesize steroids. In fact, the start of each follicular phase is characterized by a small but significant increase in the FSH:LH ratio (see **Fig. 4-18**), resulting in the recruitment of a cohort consisting of about three to seven secondary preantral follicles. (Only preantral follicles are able to respond to the FSH signal; follicles at an earlier stage of development lack an independent vascular system so that the signal does not reach them.)

Ovarian reserve is a term that is used to denote the number of antral follicles in the ovaries and therefore to determine the capacity of the ovary to provide oocytes that are capable of being fertilized. The determination of the ovarian reserve is an important tool in the treatment of infertility. Mainly, it can be assessed by the following means: (1) by a measurement of **FSH** on day 2 to 3 of the cycle: higher FSH levels denote ovarian aging (resulting from a decreased activity of the estradiol negative feedback loop), hence fewer recruitable follicles; (2) by a sonographic **antral follicle count**; (3) by the measurement of **inhibin B** on day 2 to 3 of the cycle, the recruitment of the follicle cohort being reflected by an increase in this hormone produced and secreted by these recruited follicles; thus, inhibin B levels provide an early indicator of the number of recruited follicles and of their secretory activity (see **Fig. 4-19**); and (4) by the measurement

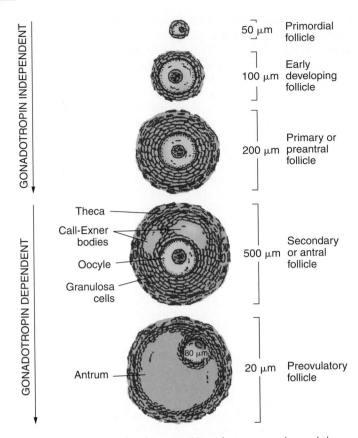

GONADOTROPIN INDEPENDENT

GONADOTROPIN DEPENDENT

50 μm Primordial follicle

100 μm Early developing follicle

200 μm Primary or preantral follicle

Theca
Call-Exner bodies
Oocyle
Granulosa cells

500 μm Secondary or antral follicle

Antrum

80 μm

20 μm Preovulatory follicle

Figure 4-19 Follicle development: Note that progress beyond the primary or preantral follicle stage depends on FSH stimulation. (From Paulson RJ: Oocytes: from development to fertilization. In Mishell DR, Davajan V, Lobo RA [eds]: Infertility, Contraception and Reproductive Endocrinology, 3 rd ed. Cambridge, MA, Blackwell Scientific, 1991.)

of Müllerian inhibiting substance (**MIS**) (also named anti-Müllerian hormone [AMH].) MIS belongs to the transforming growth factor-β superfamily. It is a secretory product of granulosa cells in preantral and in small antral follicles. Together with other factors, MIS appears to inhibit the initiation of premature follicle growth. MIS levels decline with age, in parallel with the reduced follicle pool. Recent data have indicated that in the treatment of infertility, the measurement of MIS in conjunction with sonography offers a more useful assessment of ovarian reserve and a better correlation with the number of oocytes retrieved than that provided by FSH measurement. Unlike FSH, MIS may be measured at any time of the menstrual cycle. (Very high levels of MIS may, however, be misleading as they may reflect conditions such as the polycystic ovary syndrome.)

Selection of a Dominant Follicle

Although several primary preantral follicles are recruited at the start of each cycle as part of a cohort, in the primate usually only one (the **dominant** follicle) is selected to complete growth to maturity (see **Fig. 4-19**), while the other follicles in the cohort become atretic. Although the process of selection is not well

understood, it most probably reflects the competitive advantage of the dominant follicle, characterized by a well-vascularized theca layer allowing a better access of the gonadotropins to their target receptors. This results in a greater local estradiol secretion, which in turn increases the density of gonadotropin receptors and promotes cell multiplication.

At the same time, elevation of peripheral estradiol levels will activate the negative estradiol feedback loop and result in a decrease in circulating FSH to a concentration insufficient to sustain growth in the other follicles of the cohort. Experimentally in the nonhuman primate, this process can be overridden by injecting antibodies to estradiol; this prevents the estradiol negative feedback loop from decreasing FSH secretion and results in the maturation of several follicles at the same time. In addition to estradiol, granulosa cells of the recruited follicles also secrete inhibin B (discussed earlier), the action of which selectively suppresses FSH secretion, further decreasing the stimulus to maturation. The dominant follicle, however, continues to grow because of its greater density of FSH receptors and greater vascularization of its theca cell layer, allowing more FSH to reach its receptors.

The process of selection is completed by day 5 of the follicular phase. At this point, if the dominant follicle is experimentally destroyed, no surrogate follicle is available to replace it during that cycle.

Growth of the Dominant Follicle: The Maturing Secondary or Antral Follicle

GnRH pulse frequency at this time of the follicular phase is at its maximum, at about 1 GnRH pulse/90 minute (**Fig. 4-20, A**). This is the optimal pulse frequency to activate the proper gonadotropin response to increase steroid biosynthesis and the production of estradiol within the ovary. The main role of the gonadotropins and of locally produced estradiol is to continue to stimulate growth of the dominant follicle during the remainder of the follicular phase.

Production of estradiol requires successive events within different locations in the growing follicle (**Fig. 4-21**). **FSH receptors** are located within the avascular **granulosa** cell layer of the antral follicle. Stimulation by FSH of its receptors activates production of the enzyme **aromatase** (responsible for the biosynthesis of estrogens) within these cells. An important change in the structure of maturing follicles is the acquisition of the **theca** cell layer, which surrounds the granulosa layer and rapidly differentiates into the theca interna and the theca externa. The theca layer rapidly becomes well vascularized (in contrast to the granulosa layer, which remains avascular) through an active angiogenesis process, characterized by the presence of several vascular growth-promoting proteins such as vascular endothelial growth factor (VEGF), which stimulates growth of new blood vessels. This allows access of blood, and the hormones and nutrients it carries, to reach the follicle and to diffuse through to the granulosa layer. Circulating FSH now stimulates **LH receptor** synthesis within stromal cells of the **theca interna**. LH, in turn, promotes steroid biosynthesis by theca cells and the production of **androgens**. These androgens, following diffusion into the granulosa layer where the enzyme aromatase is located, are then biotransformed into **estradiol**. This leads to an overall increase in estradiol production, increased intraovarian estradiol

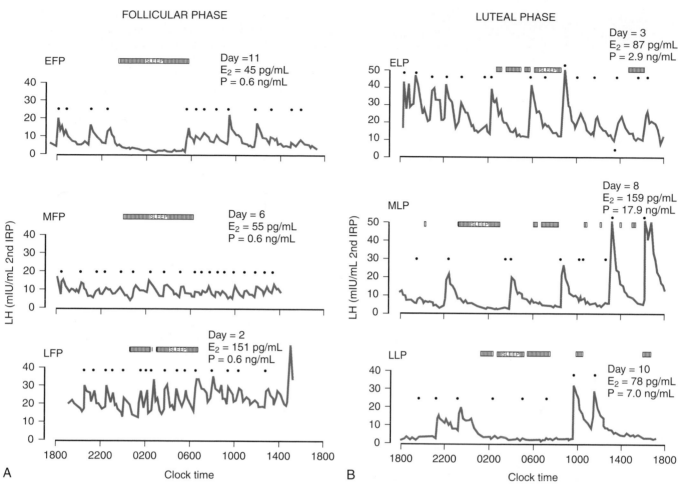

Figure 4-20 Contrasting patterns of pulsatile LH secretion throughout the follicular phase *(left panel)* and luteal phase *(right panel)* of the menstrual cycle. Representative examples of early (EFP), mid (MFP), and late (LFP) follicular phases are shown. LH pulses are indicated by asterisks. E2: estradiol; P: progesterone. (Note that in about 20% of volunteers, there is a suppression of pulsatility during deep sleep in EFP. This does not appear to interfere with the normal cycle.) (From Filicori M, Santoro N, Merriam GR, et al: Characterization of the physiological pattern of episodic gonadotropin secretion throughout the menstrual cycle. J Clin Endicrinol Metab 62:1136, 1986.)

levels, and increased estradiol secretion into the peripheral circulation, which parallels follicular parameter (**Fig. 4-22**).

Thus, the growing dominant follicle generates its own estradiol microenvironment. Estradiol, being a mitogenic hormone, in turn directly promotes its exponential growth. (Testosterone, on the other hand, increases follicular atresia in the absence of adequate aromatase activity, which converts it to estradiol.) Indirectly, estradiol also promotes follicular growth through the activation of several regulatory protein and peptide hormones, such as inhibins, activin, folliculostatins, insulin-like growth factors (IGFs), and others. For instance, various IGFs have been shown to stimulate granulosa cell proliferation and aromatase activity. Most actions of these factors remain, however, to be elucidated in the primate. By the time the follicle reaches the preovulatory stage, the number of granulosa cells has increased from about 50 at the primordial stage to 5×10^7. This is accompanied by an exponential increase in peripheral estradiol levels (see **Fig. 4-21**).

As the dominant follicle grows, an **antrum** (cavity) forms into which follicular fluid accumulates. This fluid contains several steroids, peptide and protein hormones, and nutrients. The growth pattern of the dominant follicle can be documented by ultrasonography, which is well correlated with the endocrine pattern: indeed, increases in both follicle diameter and volume parallel the increase in estradiol levels in blood. At maturation, the dominant follicle reaches a mean diameter range of 18 to 25 mm.

Within the dominant follicle, the oocyte also develops and becomes surrounded by the **zona pellucida**. This is a mucopolysaccharide coat containing specific protein sites that later will allow only spermatozoa to penetrate and fertilize the ovum. Underneath the zona pellucida is the **vitelline membrane** that surrounds the ooplasm. At the end of the follicular phase, the antral follicle contains oocytes that are fully grown but are unable to undergo normal activation if retrieved and fertilized in vitro. Activation will have to await the ovulatory LH surge.

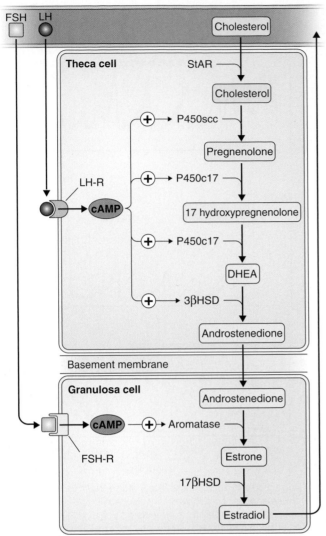

Figure 4-21 Production of estradiol within the growing dominant follicle requires successive events within different locations (see text). **FSH receptors** are located within the avascular **granulosa** cell layer, whereas synthesis of **LH receptors**, stimulated by FSH, occurs within stromal cells of the **theca interna**. The enzyme **aromatase** (responsible for the biosynthesis of estrogens) stimulated by FSH originates within the granulosa cells. LH, in turn, promotes steroid biosynthesis by theca cells and the production of **androgens**. These androgens, following diffusion into the granulosa layer where the enzyme aromatase is located, are then biotransformed into **estradiol**. ATP: adenosine triphosphate; cAMP: cyclic-AMP, which mediates the action of each gonadotropin. A: androgen.

THE OVULATORY GONADOTROPIN SURGE AND OVULATION

Maturation of the dominant follicle is marked by high blood levels of estradiol. When a threshold is reached, estradiol activates the positive feedback loop, thereby signaling to the hypothalamus and anterior pituitary gland that the follicle is ready for ovulation and that a large gonadotropin surge is to be released (see **Fig. 4-16**). (A small but significant increase in progesterone is also secreted by the follicle before the LH surge; because

administration of a progesterone receptor antagonist delays the timing of the surge, it is thought that these low levels of progesterone help to synchronize the surge.)

In the nonhuman primate, the gonadotropin surge has been shown to be preceded by a surge of GnRH, as measured centrally, suggesting a major hypothalamic site for the positive feedback loop. For reasons unknown, this **GnRH surge** significantly outlasts the LH surge. Because GnRH cannot be measured in the human in peripheral blood, the relative importance of the sites of action of estradiol during the spontaneous surge remains to be established. (Studies in GnRH-deficient women receiving exogenous GnRH replacement in an unchanging 60-minute pulse frequency provide evidence for the relevance of pituitary sensitization to GnRH in the presence of high estradiol, as abrupt LH increases can be observed under this experimental protocol.)

During the ovulatory surge, LH levels increase 10-fold over a period of 2 to 3 days, whereas FSH levels increase about 4-fold. This gonadotropin surge is an absolute requirement for the final maturation of the oocyte and the initiation of the follicular rupture.

The LH surge initiates germinal vesicle (or nucleus) disruption, and the fully grown oocyte resumes meiosis (**meiotic maturation**). Thus, it progresses from the diplotene stage of the first meiosis (which was initiated during fetal life; discussed earlier) to metaphase II of the second meiotic division. As the oocyte enters metaphase II, the first polar body appears. (Three haploid polar bodies are produced during the two-step meiosis process, at ovulation and fertilization.) To conserve nutrients, most of the cytoplasm is concentrated into the oocyte or egg. The polar bodies generated from the meiotic events contain relatively little cytoplasm, and the oocyte eventually discards them. At ovulation, meiosis is arrested again (the **second meiotic arrest**). The second meiotic division will only be completed at the time of fertilization. The oocyte's ability to be fertilized coincides with the completion of meiotic maturation and the associated increased secretion of specific proteins such as the IP$_3$ receptor, glutathione and calmodulin-dependent protein kinase II, and others.

Ovulation (follicle rupture) occurs about 32 hours after the initial rise of the LH surge and about 16 hours after its peak (**Table 4-2**). Ultrasonographic pictures of the ovaries at ovulation are shown in **Figure 4-23**. The LH surge induces a cascade of molecular events and changes in the mature follicle that are associated with ovulation. Studies of these have been complex, with the result that the precise mechanisms underlying ovulation remain to be completely understood. Currently, it is postulated that the LH surge induces an acute inflammatory-like reaction; inflammatory cytokines, such as interleukins, and countless genes are also up-regulated. There is an increase in cyclooxygenase, which catalyzes the conversion of arachidonic acid into several prostanoids, which include the **prostaglandins** that are produced intracellularly. Prostaglandins then act locally—for instance, to induce the hyperemia and edema seen in the first hours of the process of ovulation and which result from increased blood flow and vascular permeability. Intense protease activity is generated in the follicle. The resultant **proteolytic cascade**, which among others involves collagenases and plasminogen activator (which converts plasminogen into the proteolytic enzyme plasmin), leads to the degradation of the follicular layers and wall, which plays an essential role in follicle rupture. Plasmin helps in detaching the cumulus cell-enclosed oocyte from the

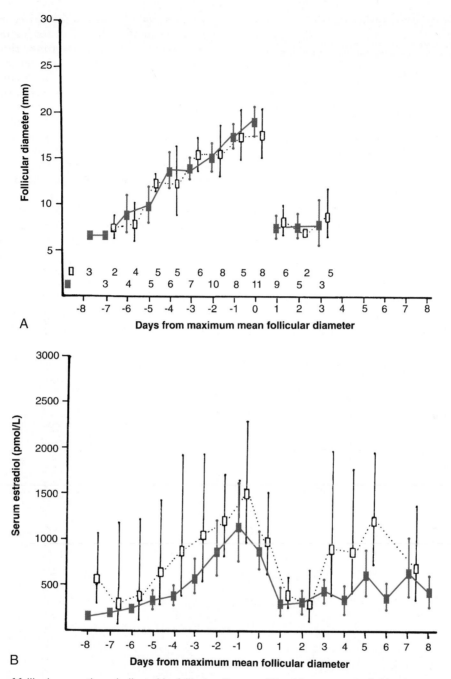

Figure 4-22 Correlation of follicular growth, as indicated by follicular diameter (**A**), with serum estradiol levels (**B**), in spontaneous (black bars) and in induced conception (blue bars) cycles. (Adapted from: Eissa MK, Obhrai Ms, Docker MF et al: Follicular growth and endocrine profiles in spontaneous and induced cycles. Fert Ster 45:191, 1986.)

granulosa cells, which initiates the process of extrusion of the oocyte and cumulus when the follicle ruptures. (It is worthwhile to point out that the LH surge paradoxically stimulates the expression of both proteolytic enzymes and their inhibitors. This allows for a tight regulation of proteolytic activity during both the follicle rupture process and the formation of the corpus luteum out of the remaining follicle.)

THE LUTEAL PHASE

After the oocyte is extruded from the mature dominant follicle, the amount of follicular fluid is markedly reduced, the follicular wall becomes convoluted, and the follicular diameter and volume greatly decrease. As a result, a new ovarian structure evolves from the ovulated follicle, the **corpus luteum**.

Table 4-2 Range of Observed Times from Defined Hormonal Events and Time of Ovulation

	Time of Ovulation (hr) from Rise to Peak			
	First Significant Rise		Peak	
Hormone	Median	Range	Median	Range
17β-Estradiol	82.5	48–168	24.0	0–48
LH	32.0	24–56	16.5	0–48
FSH	21.1	8–24	15.3	8–40
Progesterone	7.8	0–32	—	—

From World Health Organization: Temporal relationships between ovulation and defined changes in the concentration of plasma estradiol-17 beta, luteinizing hormone, follicle-stimulating hormone, and progesterone. I. Probit analysis. World Health Organization, Task Force of Methods for the Determination of the Fertile Period, Special Programme of Research, Development and Research Training in Human Reproduction. Am J Obstet Gynecol 138:383-390, 1980.

The corpus luteum is the result of two important events initiated at ovulation. First, granulosa and theca cells hypertrophy, take up increasing amounts of lipids, and acquire organelles associated with steroidogenesis. Simultaneously, tissue-specific gene transcription results in the activation of new key steroidogenic enzymes; the hallmark of the human corpus luteum is its secretion primarily of **progesterone**. Although there is a significant drop in estradiol and androgen secretion at ovulation, 17-hydroxylase and aromatase are present in the corpus luteum, so that it also secretes 17-hydroxyprogesterone and estradiol. Significant amounts of inhibin A are also produced. Second, the basal lamina, which separated the granulosa and theca cell layers, is disrupted, and capillaries from the theca interna now invade the granulosa layer (which up to now had been avascular) to form an extensive capillary network. The result is that each steroidogenic cell within the corpus luteum is in close proximity to blood vessels.

Like the dominant follicle, growth and development of the corpus luteum occur rapidly. Vascular growth plays a central role in this process. Angiogenic factors, such as vascular endothelial growth factor (VEGF), are present in high quantity in the forming and developing corpus luteum. In nonhuman primates, experimental treatment that interferes with normal VEGF activity in the early and midluteal phase of the cycle suppresses vascular development and hence luteal growth; luteal function is compromised, as indicated by a marked fall in plasma progesterone levels.

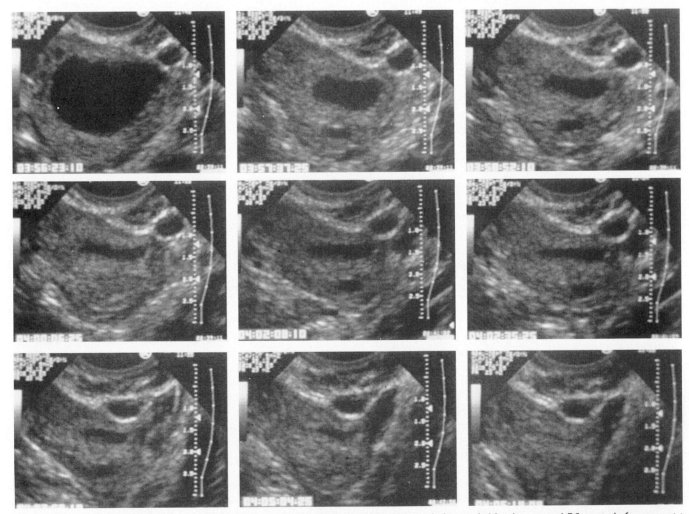

Figure 4-23 Sequence of images recorded during an ovulation research study. This ovulation took 10 minutes and 56 seconds from onset to complete follicular evacuation. Images are shown at intervals of 1 minute and 14.5 seconds. The first half of the follicular fluid was evacuated in 20 seconds; the remainder was evacuated over the next 10 minutes and 36 seconds. Time code values representing hours, minutes, seconds, and video frame are seen in the lower left corner of each image. (Adapted from Hanna MD, Chizen DR, Pierson RA: Characteristics of follicular evacuation during human ovulation. J Ultrasound Obstet Gynecol 4:488, 1994.)

Endocrine Factors and the Corpus Luteum

Normal function of the corpus luteum depends primarily on LH stimulation throughout the luteal phase. This has been demonstrated in hypophysectomized women, in whom ovulation was induced by LH treatment. In these patients, continuing injections of small amounts of LH were essential to maintain the secretory viability of the corpus luteum. Other studies have shown that GnRH antagonist treatment (by interrupting LH secretion) readily disrupts luteal cell morphology and suppresses plasma progesterone levels.

Progesterone dominance in the luteal phase results in a significant activation of the **progesterone negative feedback loop** on the GnRH pulse generator, which acts to decrease GnRH pulse frequency. Thus, during the luteal phase, there is progressive slowing down of LH pulse frequency, from 1 pulse/90 minute at the beginning of the luteal phase to 1 pulse/3 h or even less toward the later luteal phase (**Fig. 4-20**, *right panel*). This negative progesterone feedback effect is not directly exerted on the GnRH pulse generator as it is mediated by central **β-endorphin** (an endogenous opioid peptide). β-endorphin neurons are preferentially concentrated in the arcuate nucleus, in close proximity to GnRH neurons. Studies in the nonhuman primate have shown that β-endorphin release from the hypothalamus is significantly increased in the presence of progesterone, such as in the luteal phase, and lowest in its absence, such as after ovariectomy or at menstruation. Experimental administration of a competitive β-endorphin antagonist, such as naloxone, is particularly effective in accelerating LH pulse frequency when given in the luteal phase (see **Fig. 4-15**, *right panel*).

Progesterone dominance during the luteal phase also affects the hypothalamic thermoregulatory center, such that a small increase in **basal body temperature** (BBT) reflects increased progesterone secretion during the luteal phase. Thus, the typical BBT curve of the ovulatory menstrual cycle is biphasic (i.e., elevated during the duration of the luteal phase). (This small temperature rise does not, however, reflect the quantity of progesterone increase in that it occurs when progesterone reaches the low threshold level of 2 to 3 ng/mL.)

Corpus Luteum Regression (Luteolysis)

In primates, the life span of the corpus luteum is limited to a period of about 14 days. Histologically and biochemically, the corpus luteum reaches maturity 8 to 9 days after ovulation, after which time luteal cells start to degenerate and its secretory capability begins to decline. Thus, after a progressive increase in progesterone, estradiol, and inhibin A levels in the first half of the luteal phase, the period after the midluteal peak is paralleled by a decline in these hormones. (Only rapidly rising concentrations of **chorionic gonadotropin** [hCG] [secreted by the syncytiotrophoblast] following conception can rescue the corpus luteum and maintain the production of progesterone.)

Structural luteolysis is a complex process responsible for the elimination of the corpus luteum, and little progress has been made in defining the factors responsible for luteolysis in the primate. Steroidogenic luteal cells undergo characteristic degenerative changes, with intense cytoplasmic vacuolization and invasion by macrophages. It has been postulated that regression of the corpus luteum may be related to an alteration in age-dependent luteal cell responsiveness to LH and is dictated by various luteotropic and luteolytic agents, the existence and dynamics of which remain to be investigated in the human. (Although uterine prostaglandin $F_{2\alpha}$ seems to be an important luteolytic signal in nonprimate species, the primate uterus is not the source of luteolytic agents because hysterectomy does not result in a prolonged luteal phase in the human.) Degradation of the luteal cells terminates in a perimenstrual apoptotic wave, and menstruation follows ovulation by 13 to 15 days, unless conception has occurred ("the missed menses").

THE LUTEAL-FOLLICULAR TRANSITION

The end of the luteal phase is characterized by a dramatic decrease in progesterone, estradiol, and inhibin A. This is accompanied by a characteristic divergence in the FSH:LH ratio, now favoring a specific rise in FSH (see **Fig. 4-18**). The increase in the FSH:LH ratio heralds a new menstrual cycle and the recruitment of a new cohort of follicles.

The increase in the FSH:LH ratio most probably reflects the following interacting phenomena: (1) A rise in FSH may be the result of the rapid decline in estradiol accompanying the demise of the corpus luteum because FSH seems to be slightly more sensitive to the estradiol negative feedback loop than LH. (2) The end of the luteal phase is also characterized by a decline in inhibin A, a hormone that specifically suppresses FSH. (3) The rise in FSH also reflects the differential effects of GnRH pulse frequency on the synthesis of LH and FSH: the lower GnRH pulse frequency throughout the luteal phase favors FSH β-subunit synthesis over that of the LH β-subunit (discussed earlier), and thus a larger pituitary pool of FSH is available for release at the end of the luteal phase. The naturally occurring slowing of GnRH pulse frequency during the luteal phase is very relevant to a timely passage to a new cycle: indeed, imposed changes in the normal pulse frequency of this hypophysiotropic signal during the luteal phase results in significant disturbances in cyclicity.

The decrease in progesterone levels at the end of the cycle results in decreased activity in central β-endorphin, and consequently there is a resultant increase in GnRH pulse frequency. The return to a 1/pulse/90 minute frequency is essential to create the optimal conditions for the new menstrual cycle.

THE MENSTRUAL CYCLE AND THE ENDOMETRIUM

Integration and synchronization between cyclic changes within the hypothalamic-pituitary-ovarian axis and the endometrium is an essential prerequisite for viable reproduction. The primary goal is to ensure an appropriate environment for the implantation of the developing conceptus.

Human endometrium (the glandular part of the uterus) is made up of two major layers: (1) The stratum basale, which lies on top of the myometrium (the muscle part of the uterus), consists of primordial glands and densely cellular stroma, which change little during the menstrual cycle and do not desquamate at menstruation. (2) The stratum functionale, which lies between the basale and the lumen of the uterus, is composed of two layers. The superficial layer (stratum compactum) consists of the neck of the glands and densely populated stromal cells. The lower layer (stratum spongiosum) consists primarily of glands with less populated stroma and large amounts of interstitial tissue. Differences in structure in the two layers reflect different biologic functions: whereas the upper layer serves as the site of blastocyst implantation and provides the metabolic environment for it,

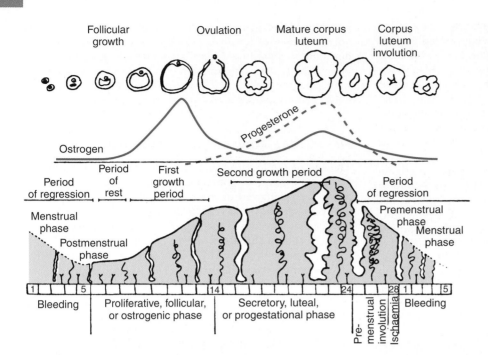

Figure 4-24 Diagram of changes in normal human ovarian and endometrial cycles. (From Shaw ST, Roche PC: Menstruation. In Finn CA [ed]: Oxford Rev Reprod Endocrin, vol 2. London, Oxford University Press, 1980.)

the lower layer maintains the integrity of the mucosa. Changes in hormones during the menstrual cycle affect mainly the *stratum functionale*. A diagrammatic representation of endometrial changes during the menstrual cycle is presented in **Figure 4-24**.

THE ENDOMETRIUM IN THE PROLIFERATIVE (FOLLICULAR) PHASE

Immediately after menstruation, the endometrium is only 1 to 2 mm thick and consists mainly of the *stratum basale* and a few glands. As estradiol levels increase with the growth and maturation of the dominant follicle, the number of estradiol receptors in the endometrium increases and the *stratum functionale* proliferates greatly by multiplication of both glandular and stromal cells. Synthesis of DNA is increased, and mitoses are numerous. Toward the late follicular phase, the straight glands become progressively more voluminous and tortuous. At the time of onset of the LH surge and before ovulation, subnuclear vacuoles appear at the base of the cells lining the glands. This is the first indication of an effect by progesterone, reflecting the small but significant increase in progesterone seen at that time. Sonography during the follicular phase shows that endometrial thickness, including both anterior and posterior layers, increases from a mean of about 4 mm in the early follicular phase to about 12 mm at the time of ovulation. Examples of structural changes of the endometrium during the menstrual cycle are shown in **Figure 4-25**.

THE ENDOMETRIUM IN THE SECRETORY (LUTEAL) PHASE

After ovulation, the proliferative endometrium undergoes a rapid **secretory** differentiation: well-developed subnuclear glycogen-rich vacuoles appear in every cell of a given gland. This correlates with a total lack of mitoses in all glands. Both effects can be

attributed to rising levels of postovulatory progesterone. Progesterone antagonizes the mitotic action of estradiol by decreasing estrogen receptors and by increasing the progesterone-specific enzyme 17 β-hydroxydehydrogenase, which converts estradiol into the much less active estrone.

As progesterone levels increase during the first part of the luteal phase, the glycogen-containing vacuoles ascend progressively toward the gland lumen. Soon thereafter, the contents of the glands are released into the endometrial lumen. The peak of intraglandular content and its release into the lumen coincides well with the arrival of the free-floating blastocyst, which reaches the uterine cavity by about 3.5 days after fertilization. This release of glycogen-rich nutrients is crucial in that it provides energy to the energy-starved free-floating blastocyst. Implantation occurs about 1 week after fertilization.

Several specific proteins are produced by the secretory endometrium. The three major proteins are placental protein 10 (PP10), 12 (PP12), and 14 (PP14). Little is known of their specific role in the endometrium. The better known is **PP14**, also known as **glycodelin** or progestagen-associated endometrial protein. Although it has also been referred to as pregnancy-associated endometrial alpha-2-globulin, it is actually not a placental protein but rather a major secretory product of the glandular endometrial epithelium during the secretory phase. Circulating levels of glycodelin correlate well with serum progesterone levels. Glycodelin is a glycoprotein of which there are three distinct forms, with identical protein backbones but different glycosylation profiles. These glycoproteins appear to have essential roles in producing a uterine environment suitable for pregnancy and in the timing and occurrence of the appropriate sequence of events in the fertilization process.

After the first week of the luteal phase, changes in the stroma rather than in the glands become more important and relevant. The stroma becomes more edematous as a result of increased capillary permeability. Endothelial proliferation results in the

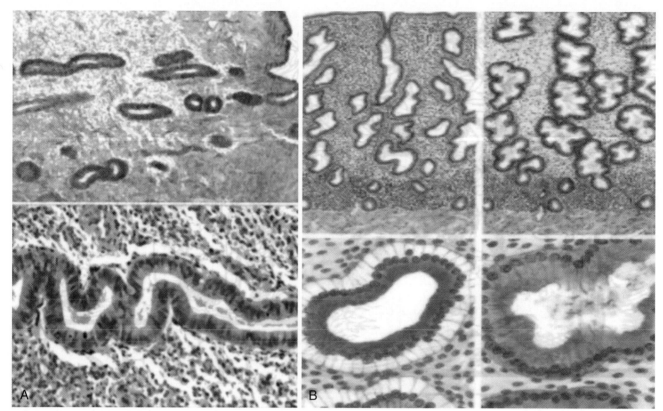

Figure 4-25 Histology of proliferative (**A**), and secretory (**B**) endometrial.

coiling of capillaries and vessels, particularly in the upper functionale level producing vascular clusters. (These changes have been postulated to be mediated by prostaglandin F2α [PGF2α] and prostaglandin E [PGE2], the production of which is stimulated by estradiol and progesterone.) These changes are essential in the steps that will lead to the predecidual transformation of stromal cells.

Predecidual stromal cells are precursor forms of gestational decidual cells. (These cells are not involved in the implantation process because they develop after implantation.) In the nongestational endometrium, predecidual cells are engaged in phagocytosis and digestion of extracellular collagen matrix. These cellular activities may contribute to the breakdown of the endometrium at menstruation. (Predecidual cells also have metabolic functions related to pregnancy; for example, they secrete prolactin, which is related to osmoregulation of amniotic fluid. These cells also play a supportive role to the endometrial mucosa and appear to control the invasive nature of the normal trophoblast: in their absence, the trophoblast may invade the myometrium leading to placenta accreta.) Decidualization succeeds predecidualization if pregnancy occurs.

Clinically, the measurement of hormonal levels in parallel with the use of quantitative morphometric endometrial measurements produce a significant correlation with chronologic dating of the length of the luteal phase. Clinical dating of the endometrium, however, is somewhat subjective and is rarely carried out today. Sonography shows that endometrial thickness remains at the same level reached at ovulation (8 to 14 mm) throughout the luteal phase.

MENSTRUATION

If implantation of the blastocyst does not occur in the late luteal phase and hCG is not produced to maintain the corpus luteum, the endometrial glands begin to collapse and fragment. Subsequently, polymorphonuclear leukocytes and monocytes infiltrate the glands and stroma, autolysis of the stratum functionale occurs, and desquamation begins.

Current data support the contention that cyclic elimination of the endometrium functional layer through menstrual bleeding results from intense tissue breakdown by proteolytic enzymes, mainly members of the matrix **metalloproteinase** family (**MMPs**), and that these enzymes are stimulated by the products of an inflammatory process. A number of MMPs, capable of degrading both interstitial matrix and basement membrane components, have been localized to perimenstrual endometrium, and the focal nature of their production suggests local regulation. There are probably important relationships between cells of the immune system (such as mast cells, eosinophils, neutrophils, and macrophages) and the local production and activation of MMPs.

The degrading actions by MMPs lead to the loss of integrity of blood vessels, destruction of endometrial interstitial matrix, and the resultant bleeding characteristic of menstruation. Regular menstruation lasts for usually 3 to 5 days, but anywhere from 2 to 7 days is considered normal. Menstrual intervals vary depending of age and time of initiation of the premenopause period (**Fig. 4-26**). The average blood loss is 35 milliliters with 10 to 80 mL considered within the normal range. A similar

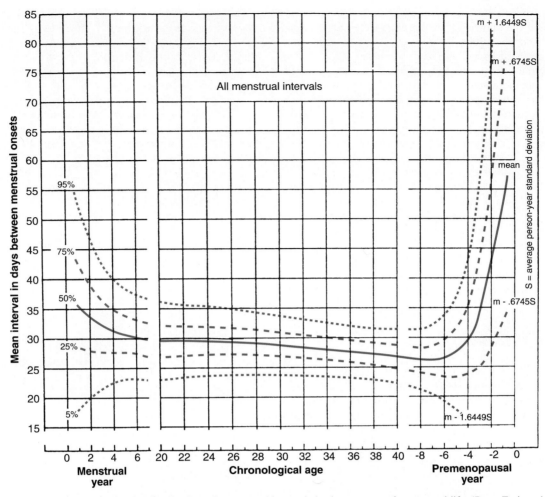

Figure 4-26 Normal curve contours for the distribution of menstrual intervals in three zones of menstrual life. (From Treloar AE, Boynton RE, Brown BW: Variation of the human menstrual cycle through reproductive life. Int J Fert 12:77, 1967.)

volume of nonhematogenous fluid is also shed during menstruation. Many women also notice shedding of the endometrial lining that appears as tissue mixed with the blood. (Sometimes, this may be erroneously thought to indicate an early term miscarriage of an embryo.) The enzyme plasmin tends to inhibit the blood from clotting. Because of the blood loss, premenopausal women have higher dietary requirements for iron to prevent iron deficiency.

THE MENSTRUAL CYCLE AND THE CERVICAL GLANDS

The cervix plays a substantial role in fertility. Changes in the production and property of mucus secreted by the cervical glands are closely correlated to changes in estradiol and progesterone during the menstrual cycle. Enhanced production of cervical mucus and the presence of crypts within the endocervix serve to facilitate the transport and storage of spermatozoa around midcycle. Cervical mucus is produced in copious amounts in response to high estradiol levels at the end of the follicular phase: it has a clear, water-like appearance, which is acellular, takes the aspect of a "fern" when it dries as viewed under the

microscope, and is "stringy," referred to as "spinnbarkeit" (i.e., cervical mucus that can stretch on a slide at least 6 cm). So characteristic are these findings that the appearance of this type of mucus signifies the "fertile period" in women practicing natural family planning methods. In contrast, one of the actions of progesterone (as seen after ovulation during the luteal phase or as used in the "minipill") is to thicken the cervical mucus, thereby making it less conducive for sperm transport, thus providing a contraceptive effect.

From a fertility testing perspective, postcoital tests examining spermatozoa within the cervical canal at midcycle to rule out a cervical factor are seldom used in today's practice. The subjective nature of this testing makes it not highly predictive of the ability to conceive.

HORMONE ASSAY TECHNIQUES

IMMUNOASSAYS

No other method has had such an impact on the measurement of hormones as immunoassay methods. These techniques provide ways of measuring very small amounts of hormone in small quantities of serum or plasma rapidly and relatively specifically.

The use of these techniques, pioneered by Yalow and Berson, has indeed increased the knowledge of reproductive endocrinology exponentially since the 1960s. Immunoassays and their variants have rapidly replaced previously used cumbersome bioassays. They are comparatively much faster and much easier to perform, have a much enhanced sensitivity, and usually require far less than 1 mL of serum or plasma. It should be kept in mind, however, that these techniques measure the immunologic property of a hormone, not its biologic activity (as tested by bioassays). These two effects may differ in magnitude under certain physiologic or pathologic conditions.

The basic principle of an immunoassay involves the competition between an unlabeled antigen (the hormone in the blood sample) and a labeled antigen, both of which are present in excess, for binding sites on a limited amount of antibody. The following is a brief description of the several steps required in the creation of such an assay. Even though the availability of commercial assays for a great number of hormones has greatly facilitated the measurement of hormones, proper interpretation of the generated data requires a general knowledge of these steps.

Preparation of Antibodies

The first step in setting up an immunoassay is the production or availability of an antibody to the analyte (here, the hormone) to be measured. Antibodies used in immunoassays are either polyclonal or monoclonal. **Polyclonal antibodies** are usually produced following the injection of the hormone in larger animals such as sheep or rabbits. For many **protein hormones**, this means injecting the purified hormone, which will be recognized by the host as foreign. In the natural immune reaction that follows, the host will produce polyclonal antibodies against the hormone. In contrast to protein hormones, **steroid hormones** are too small to produce an immune reaction on their own (haptens) and are not recognized as foreign because they are the same in most species. To become antigenic, they need to be attached to a carrier protein (usually bovine serum albumin). This conjugated compound is now perceived as a foreign body to the host animal and large enough to induce antibody formation.

Even with the injection of a purified antigen, polyclonal antibodies may "cross-react" with other closely related hormones and thus in some assays may lack specificity to the concerned hormone. To increase assay specificity, one may now choose to produce **monoclonal antibodies**, which provide unique specificity by recognizing only one epitope (antigenic determinant). These antibodies are produced by first injecting the antigen into a mouse to induce an immunogenic reaction in its spleen. The spleen cells are then screened to identify and separate those clones capable of secreting a single antibody type. These cells are then fused with a myeloma cell from the same species to form a hybrid cell (hybridoma), which can then be maintained in culture. Because of its immortality, the hybridoma continues to produce homogenous antibodies as long as the culture is maintained.

The Choice of Assay Markers

The second step in preparation for an immunoassay is the availability of a **labeled analyte** (hormone) in the competitive immunoassay or a **labeled second antibody** to the analyte in a reagent excess immunoassay. The choice of labels to be attached to the analyte or antibody is multiple.

In the initially developed radioimmunoassays, these labels were radioactive, such as iodine I^{125}. Although these assays were initially the norm, they mostly have been replaced by new types of immunoassays, which do not require the use of radioactive elements and thus avoid the attendant problems related to their use and to radioactivity disposal.

During recent years, major advances in the identification of nonradioactive labels and of new measurement equipment to detect and quantitate these have occurred. Presently, most current assays use nonradioactive labels. Enzyme immunoassays (enzyme-linked immunosorbent assays, or ELISA; immunometric assays) use enzymes as labels, such as, for example, horseradish peroxidase or alkaline phosphatase. Chemiluminescent immunoassays (CIA) use luminol. Fluorimetric immunoassays (FIA) use fluorescent compounds (such as fluorescein) as labels.

The Separation of Bound and Unbound Antigen

The third step requires a method to separate antibody-bound antigen from unbound antigen in order to determine how much antigen is bound to the antibody. In commercial assays, antibodies can be attached to solid surfaces such as to plastic tubes, beads or plates, or cellulose particles. Separation can then be assured by washing off the unbound antigen.

Separation can also be performed by the use of a second antibody-label conjugate, which is directed against an antigenic site different from that recognized by the first antibody (see sandwich ELISA, discussed later).

The Immunoassay Reaction

In step 1, a specific antibody (ab) to the hormone (which served as the antigen, ag) binds in the patient's blood sample to the antigen during a fixed period of incubation. A set amount of labeled form of the hormone (ag^x) is added to compete with the unlabeled hormone to bind to the antibody, resulting in the following reaction:

$$ab + ag + ag^x \rightleftharpoons ab.ag + ab.ag^x$$

In this competitive reaction, the amount of labeled antigen bound to the antibody will be inversely proportional to the amount of antigen (hormone) present in the blood sample. For measurement, the bound antigen is then separated for the free antigen by washing or other approaches.

Immunometric assays (also referred to as "sandwich assays") use a labeled second antibody, which is usually attached to a solid phase, such as the assay tube or assay plate, in the following reactions. The second antibody is directed against an antigenic site different from that recognized by the first antibody:

$$Ab1 + ag \rightleftharpoons ab1.ag$$
$$Ab1.ag + ab^x2 \rightleftharpoons ab1.ag.ab^x2$$

Because the sandwich assay depends on occupancy of the binding sites rather than competition for these sites, an excess of reagents is used.

The Standard Curve

To allow for the actual measurement of the hormone levels in the blood sample, a standard curve must accompany each assay. A standard preparation of the hormone to be measured is used at various increasing or decreasing concentrations, and each concentration is then processed as for the measurement of the sample with unknown concentrations. A standard curve is then constructed by plotting the measured end points. The result for each unknown sample is then located on the ordinate of the standard curve. By drawing a perpendicular line to the abscissa, the amount of hormone present in the unknown sample can be determined. Nowadays, these determinations are rapidly computed.

Standard curves require varying amounts of pure preparations of hormone. This is no problem for steroid hormones, which are available in chemically pure preparations. Thus, the amount added to construct the standard curve to determine the amount in the patient's sample can be expressed in terms of absolute mass or weight, such as nanograms (ng; 10^{-9} gram) or picograms (pg; 10^{-12} gram). Sometimes, the results may be expressed in nanomoles (nmol). For most steroids, 1 ng/mL is equivalent to about 3 nmol/L.

Because proteins have higher molecular weights and are more complex, it is not always possible to obtain these in their pure form. In these cases, the results are usually expressed in terms of the amounts of a standard reference preparation used for the standard curve. Standard preparations are obtained by extracting the hormone from large collections of blood, urine, or tissues (such as the pituitary gland for FSH and LH.) These protein standards are then most often an international reference preparation with the results expressed as international units. However, because of the use of different standard preparations, data obtained from different laboratories or assays may not agree. Thus, clinicians should be aware of the normal levels reported by each laboratory reporting to them. Further complicating interpretation is the observation that protein hormones may also circulate in several forms varying slightly by amino acid or carbohydrate content.

ASSAY EVALUATION

When evaluating the value, accuracy, and relevance of an assay, four items must be examined:

1. **Sensitivity** measures the least hormone that can be measured with accuracy. This will set the lower limit of the assay.
2. **Specificity** is the ability of the assay to measure only the specific hormone of interest. Frequently with polyclonal antibodies, results may be altered by the presence of other cross-reacting substances also recognized by the antibody, although usually at lower levels of detection. This is important to know because cross-reaction may influence the precise measurement of the hormone of interest. In such instance, a preassay separation of the cross-reacting hormones may be necessary.
3. **Accuracy** is the ability to measure the exact amount of the hormone present in the sample. Controls containing varying low and high amounts of the hormone must be always assayed alongside the patient's samples in each assay.
4. **Precision** is the ability of the assay to consistently reproduce the same results. Precision is determined by two measurements. The first, the **intra-assay coefficient of variation (intra-assay CV)** measures the within assay variation. It is calculated by determining the results obtained from measuring a known sample in a number of replicates (usually 10) in the same assay. The second measurement is the **inter-assay coefficient of variation (inter-assay CV)**, which is calculated by measuring known samples in multiple assays.

KEY POINTS

- GnRH analogues are synthesized by substitution of amino acids in the parent molecule at the 6 and 10 positions. The various agonists have greater potencies and longer half-lives than the parent GnRH.
- LH and FSH have the same α subunit of thyroid-stimulating hormone (TSH) and human chorionic gonadotropin (HCG). The β subunits of all these hormones have different amino acids and carbohydrates, which provide specific biologic activity.
- LH acts on the theca cells to produce androgens, which are then transported to the granulosa cells, where they are aromatized to estrogens.
- Pregnenolone, 17-hydroxypregnenolone, progesterone, 17-hydroxyprogesterone, and corticosteroids have 21 carbon atoms; androgens (testosterone and androstenedione) have 19 carbon atoms; estrogens have 18 carbon atoms and a phenolic ring A.
- Kisspeptin (KISS1) plays a key role in the regulation of GnRH release.
- Because the ovaries lack 21-hydroxylase, 11-β-hydroxylase, and 18-hydroxylase reductase activity, they are unable to synthesize mineralocorticoids or glucocorticoids.

- Sex hormone-binding globulin (SHBG) primarily binds dihydrotestosterone, testosterone, and estradiol. About 65% of circulating testosterone is bound to SHBG and 30% to albumin. Approximately 2% remains unbound or free.
- Estrogen stimulates the synthesis of both estrogen and progesterone receptors in target tissues, and progestins inhibit the synthesis of both estrogen and progesterone receptors.
- With ultrasound it has been found that there is a steady increase in follicular diameter and volume that parallels the rise in estradiol. The dominant follicle has a maximal mean diameter of about 19.5 mm, with a range of 18 to 25 m just before ovulation. The mean maximal follicular volume is 3.8 mL, with a range of 3.1 to 8.2 mL.
- Ovulation occurs about 24 hours after the estradiol peak, as well as 32 hours after the initial rise in LH, and about 12 to 16 hours after the peak of LH levels in serum.
- Progesterone levels in serum are less than 1 ng/mL before ovulation and reach midluteal levels of 10 to 20 ng/mL.

KEY POINTS—CONTINUED

- After menstruation, regeneration of the endometrium comes from cells in the spongiosum that were previously a portion of the secretory endometrium and not from the stratum basale as previously believed.
- Enzyme-linked immunosorbent assay (ELISA), or "sandwich," techniques have been developed to measure protein hormones (e.g., LH, FSH, HCG) with the use of monoclonal antibodies against the α and β subunits. The end point is a color reaction and can be read in a spectrophotometer.
- There are four characteristics of hormone assays that establish their reliability: sensitivity, specificity, accuracy, and precision.

REFERENCES CAN BE FOUND ON EXPERTCONSULT.com

SUGGESTED READINGS

Bousfield JR, Jia L, Ward DN: Gonadotropins: chemistry and biosynthesis. In Neill JD, editor: *Physiology of Reproduction*, 2006, Elsevier-Academic Press, pp 1581–1634.

Engel JB, Schally AV: Drug insight: Clinical use of agonists and antagonists of luteinizing-hormone-releasing hormone, *Nat Clin Pract Endocrinol Metab* 3:157–167, 2007.

Ferin M: The menstrual cycle: An integrative view. In Adashi EY, Rock JA, Rosenwaks Z, editors: *Reproductive Endocrinology, Surgery, and Technology*, Philadelphia, 1996, Lippincott-Raven, 103–121.

Ferin M, Van Vugt D, Wardlaw S: The hypothalamic control of the menstrual cycle and the role of endogenous opioid peptides, *Recent Prog Horm Res* 40:441, 1984.

Giudice LC: The endometrial cycle. In Adashi EY, Rock JA, Rosenwaks Z, editors: *Reproductive Endocrinology, Surgery, and Technology*, Philadelphia, 1996, Lippincott-Raven, p 272.

Gross KM, Matsumoto AM, Bremner WJ: Differential control of luteinizing hormone and follicle-stimulating hormone secretion by luteinizing hormone-releasing hormone pulse frequency in man, *J Clin Endocrinol Metab* 64(4):675–680, 1987.

Herbison AE: Physiology of the gonadotropin-releasing hormone neuronal network. In Neill JD, editor: *Physiology of Reproduction*, 2006, Elsevier-Academic Press, p 1415.

Hotchkiss J, Knobil E: The hypothalamic pulse generator: The reproductive core. In Adashi EY, Rock JA, Rosenwaks Z, editors: *Reproductive Endocrinology, Surgery, and Technology*, Philadelphia, 1996, Lippincott-Raven, p 123.

Katges B, Karges W, deRoux N: Clinical and molecular genetics of the human GnRH receptor, *Hum Reprod Update* 9:523–530, 2003.

Krasnow SM, Steiner RA: Physiological mechanisms integrating metabolism and reproduction. In Neill JD, editor: *Physiology of reproduction*, 2006, Elsevier-Academic Press, p 2553.

Liu JH, Yen SS: Induction of midcycle gonadotropin surge by ovarian steroids in women: A critical evaluation, *J Clin Endocrinol Metab* 57:797–802, 1983.

McGee EA, Hsueh AJ: Initial and cyclic recruitment of ovarian follicles, *Endocr Rev* 21:200–214, 2000.

Oakley AE, Clifton DK, Steiner RA: Kisspeptin signaling in the brain, *Endocr Rev* 30:713–743, 2009.

Stenvers KL, Findlay JK: Inhibins: From reproductive hormones to tumor suppressors, *Trends Endocrinol Metab* 21:174–180, 2010.

Stouffer RL: Corpus luteum formation and demise. In Adashi EY, Rock JA, Rosenwaks Z, editors: *Reproductive Endocrinology, Surgery, and Technology*, Philadelphia, 1996, Lippincott-Raven, p 251.

Tasfiri A, Chun SY: Ovulation. In Adashi EY, Rock JA, Rosenwaks Z, editors: *Reproductive Endocrinology, Surgery, and Technology*, Philadelphia, 1996, Lippincott-Raven, p 234.

Tobet SA, Schwarting GA: Minireview: Recent progress in gonadotropin-releasing hormone neuronal migration, *Endocrinology* 147:1159–1165, 2006.

Wheeler MJ: Immunoassay techniques, *Methods Mol Biol* 324:1–23, 2006.

5

Evidence-Based Medicine and Clinical Epidemiology

Vern L. Katz

The ongoing explosion of knowledge in the basic and clinical sciences presents a challenge to clinicians. The fundamental task of medical science is to take the knowledge of embryology, genetics, anatomy, and endocrinology and apply this knowledge to clinical problems. The leap from bench to bedside, however, is vast and uncertain, and the results can be inadequate. Clinical **epidemiology** comprises a set of methods that can help us directly at the bedside as well as inform public health decisions. The results of observational epidemiologic studies, such as case reports, help by generating hypotheses about diseases that can then be tested. Experimental studies in humans, the **randomized clinical trials** (RCTs), test hypotheses to see if they may apply to clinical practice. The main goal of trials is to move from association to the establishment of cause and effect, and then to assess efficacy of treatments and interventions.

This chapter presents the basics of epidemiologic study design and the statistical terminology commonly used to present results of clinical studies; statistical methods per se are not covered here. We also discuss approaches for interpreting study results. Finally, we consider new, explicit approaches to combining data from different studies that are used to prepare evidence reviews and clinical guidelines. The emphasis of the chapter is an approach to help clinicians read and interpret the vast volumes of information referred to as "the literature."

EVIDENCE-BASED MEDICINE

Evidence-based medicine relies on the assessment of our full body of knowledge. The process of evidence-based medicine starts with formulating a specific clinical question and then finding the best and most appropriate research evidence. Research evidence rarely applies exactly to an individual or to her particular clinical problem. Therefore, clinical decisions must be evaluated with specific context, integrated with clinical expertise, and must consider the preferences and values of each woman. The process of making a clinical decision is based on the application of up-to-date and valid information regarding diagnosis, prognosis, therapy, and preventive services. Practicing evidence-based medicine has become possible in large part because of the development of information systems that allow us to search for relevant clinical data and literature. At best, we can look for data using the Internet right at the bedside or clinic to address specific questions that

apply to a current individual. The bedside practice of evidence-based medicine can be efficient and practical if we learn to find and use sources that synthesize and summarize the effects of the interventions we are interested in.

To make the assessment of evidence more uniform, a grading system is often used that rates studies according to quality (**Table 5-1**). This grading system rates blinded randomized clinical trials as the highest level of evidence. Following this are controlled trials without randomization. The next level of evidence comes from **cohort studies** and case-control studies. Although results taken from cross-sectional studies, studies that rely on external control groups, and ecologic studies are a lesser level of evidence, they often remain valuable specifically because of the lack of higher levels of evidence. All of these sources of evidence are more valuable than opinion, regardless of the credentials of the individual, committee, or organization that might publish an opinion. The lowest grade of evidence is the case series. The basic element or unit, as described by Grimes and Schulz, is the case report. This is not to say that case reports are not valuable. It was through a report of a few cases of unusual infections and disturbed immunity that AIDS was first described. Case reports, series, and cross-sectional studies are hypothesis generating. They do not prove causality! One of the difficult roles of the clinician is explaining to patients and families the difference between the associations highlighted in case reports and true causality, given the widespread reporting in the media and on the Internet of **observational studies**.

Individual studies often have imprecise results. Statistical methods to combine results from several studies sometimes can be helpful. Studies may also have insufficient numbers of patients to show a significant effect, particularly if the disease or condition is uncommon. The study of rare diseases may have insufficient **power**. **Metaanalysis** is a collection of techniques to produce a pooled effect estimate from several studies. Metaanalysis at its best involves pooling and reanalyzing raw data from several similar randomized trials to produce a result with a tighter **confidence interval**. Several statistical approaches are used, but the main purpose of any metaanalysis is to improve **precision**. Not all metaanalyses are equal, though. Many metaanalyses combine data from observational studies (rather than randomized trials), but these must be interpreted with extreme caution because the individual studies always vary in population, entry criteria, case definition, and exposure definitions, and these differences make combining the data problematic. This is particularly true if the analysis combines data from

We acknowledge the inspiration of David Grimes in preparing this chapter.

Table 5-1 Categorizing the Level of Evidence

Level	Evidence
I	Blinded randomized controlled trial
II-1	Controlled trials without randomization
II-2	Well-designed cohort and case-control studies
II-3	Cross-sectional studies, studies with external control groups, or ecologic studies
III	Case series evidence-derived from report of an expert committee, which itself used a scientific approach

Modified from The periodic health examination. Canadian Task Force on the Periodic Health Examination. CMAJ 121:1193-1254, 1979.

published tables rather than combining the raw data from the original studies. If the results from individual studies disagree in direction or report very different results, then the metaanalysis is not an appropriate tool to answer the question. Often the main value of a metaanalysis proves to be the rigorous approach to collecting, evaluating, and presenting together all of the relevant data regarding a particular problem. A risk of metaanalysis is taking many published studies that are small and finding a significant effect that is not true. Hennekens and DeMets have suggested that when this occurs, when multiple studies are put together to produce a new finding, that the results should be interpreted with caution and viewed as hypothesis generating until a large RCT with adequate power can be performed. This is particularly true when some of the pooled results were secondary **outcomes**.

Because of the clinical need for good evidence and because of the need for synthesis of evidence that goes beyond opinion, additional approaches to reviews are being developed and used. **Systematic reviews** include a comprehensive review and evaluation of the literature. Systematic reviews are reported using a standardized format that must include a detailed description of the search strategy used to identify the relevant literature and the results of the search. Systematic reviews also carry out critical appraisal of the studies they evaluate. Critical appraisal employs a rigid standardized assessment of the relevance and quality of each study. The goal of systematic reviews is to synthesize the literature regarding a specific clinical question and to use an approach that will minimize **bias** and **random error**.

Journal articles may present a summary of an evidence review, but readers generally have to go to sources on the Web to find complete documentation of these reviews. The major source of systematic reviews is the Cochrane Collaboration (www.cochrane.org). This collaboration is an international organization that aims to help people make well-informed decisions about health care by preparing, maintaining, and promoting the accessibility of systematic reviews of the effects of health care interventions. There are review groups for more than 50 areas of medicine, including several that are relevant to gynecology; the groups in each area prepare and electronically publish systematic reviews. The U.S. Preventive Services Task Force also performs systematic reviews regarding clinical preventive services; these are published in book form and increasingly as electronic publications by the Agency for Healthcare Research and Quality (ARHQ). To help translate these often lengthy reviews into briefer, clinically useful documents, many professional groups have begun to issue practice guidelines to assist clinicians in making patient care decisions. An electronic collection of such guidelines is now available; to be accepted for electronic publication, the guideline must specify the search strategy that was used to obtain the evidence and must specify the methods of data synthesis (www.guidelines.gov). When evaluating these, or any, guidelines for care, the clinician must take into account the date the guidelines were developed.

Recommendations are often graded, but the systems for grading evidence and practice recommendations are continuing to evolve. In general, recommendations for or against clinical interventions need to specify whether they are based on ample or sparse evidence and whether the evidence comes from randomized trials or from lesser studies. Even with recommendations based on ample evidence from RCTs, clinicians will always need to decide individually whether the available evidence applies to their practice setting and whether it applies directly to their specific patient's problem. Guyatt et al. from the American College of Chest Physicians task force recommend several factors that should influence the strength of a recommendation. These include quality of evidence, importance of treatment, risks of treatment, **incidence** of the problem, costs, and value of outcome.

ESSENTIALS OF STUDY DESIGN

The basic purpose of an epidemiologic study is to estimate the relationship between an exposure and an outcome in order to assess causality. An exposure can be a behavior, a genetic factor, a screening program, or any aspect of a treatment. An outcome might be a symptom, a measure of functional status, the development of disease, or a change in the course of an existing disease. Some studies are primarily descriptive, providing statistics about incidence, prevalence, and mortality rates of diseases in particular populations. Descriptive studies are important to the clinician in order to provide a context—the most dramatic new research findings always must be interpreted with respect to the frequency and characteristics of the disease in one's own patient population. Descriptive studies can also help generate new hypotheses, but studies with this design do not test hypotheses or answer etiologic questions. No matter the plausibility, every clinician must read descriptive studies with a cautious interpretation. This fact cannot be emphasized enough; many associations seem incredibly logical and plausible. It does not mean the association is true and causative. Clinicians must remember Leo's law: In the field of medicine, just because a connection seems true and logical, it is not necessarily true until it is proven. The law derives from the understanding that our knowledge of pathophysiology is incomplete.

The most basic element or unit of the descriptive study is the case report. Case reports are valuable initial descriptions of unusual infections and abnormal immune responses.

More valuable to evidence-based medical practice are analytic epidemiologic studies that focus on establishing a cause-and-effect relationship between a particular exposure (e.g., hormone replacement therapy) and the risk of a particular disease or outcome (e.g., reduction in the incidence of osteoporotic fractures). Analytic epidemiologic studies can be classified as experimental or observational. In experimental studies, the clinical investigator controls exposure to the factor of interest—the dependent variable. Experimental studies, or randomized controlled trials, are characterized by the prospective assignment of study participants to a study group (who receive the factor of interest, typically a new treatment) or a placebo, no treatment, or standard care group. Study groups, usually two, but often many more, are then followed over time to evaluate differences in outcomes.

The outcomes may include prevention or cure of a disease, reduction in severity of the condition, or differences in costs, quality of life, or side effects between the treatments. The important feature of RCTs is that, through randomizing participants, the study can equalize other factors that might influence the outcome and leave only the effect of the study treatment itself. RCTs usually provide the best evidence for making clinical decisions. Blinded RCTs are superior to nonblinded efforts because the investigators will not interpret the results with a bias. Despite the theoretic superiority of the RCT approach, these studies provide the best evidence only if the study has been thoughtfully designed, implemented with extraordinary care, and analyzed appropriately.

Subjects recruited for a trial must receive information about the study purpose, its procedures, the likely risks and benefits, and the available alternatives. Both ethical and practical considerations may limit the use of randomized trials to answer clinical questions. It is clearly unethical to expose anyone to a potential cause of disease simply to learn about its cause; thus, patients would not be randomized to smoking in order to learn about the effect of tobacco on the ovary. RCTs are rarely used to address etiologic questions. To study the effect of a treatment, making comparisons with a placebo control group is usually most efficient. However, if an effective and accepted treatment exists, it is not ethical to use a placebo control group for studies of serious conditions in which the subject may experience harm from a lack of effective treatment. If the condition is mild, the treatment period is brief, or effective treatment is not generally available, many investigators believe that a placebo control group is ethical. For a clinician to recruit or refer patients into a clinical trial, it is essential the clinician believe, based on current evidence, that the study treatments may be similar or at least balanced in benefits and harms. This belief state is called **therapeutic equipoise**. If a clinician believes that evidence already exists to indicate a treatment is superior, then it is not ethical to recruit subjects into a comparative trial. In contrast, if the superior treatment is unclear, then a randomized trial is the most ethical approach for all patients because it provides them with an equal chance to undergo the better treatment and also may provide an unbiased answer to the clinical question more quickly so all future patients can benefit. Clearly, it is critical to be honest and humble about our current state of knowledge prior to planning any randomized clinical trial.

One problem is that subjects and controls in RCT are often special populations that may not be *generalizable*. The population may not correspond to a specific patient. This potential weakness of randomized trials is a problem of external validity. Can the results from a specific population with a tightly controlled treatment regimen be generalized to a diverse population in clinical practice—or, as is often stated, "the real world." Often, the more sophisticated and complex the protocol, the greater the difference between RCT results and general clinical outcomes. This has been referred to as the difference between efficacy ("can it work") and effectiveness ("will it work").

Importantly, RCTs often use **surrogate markers** to substitute for clinical outcomes. Surrogate markers are easier to measure in shorter periods of time than the true clinical endpoint. However, surrogate markers may not always equate with the disease process being assessed. For example, the effects of a medication on lowering cholesterol are not necessarily the same as the effects for preventing heart attacks. Another example is bone mineral density. Because osteoporotic fractures are rare and occur over a long

time period, interventions may be assessed by the surrogate marker of bone mineral density. Fractures and bone mineral density change are not the same. Lactation lowers bone mineral density; however, breast-feeding does not necessarily increase the risk of fractures. When interpreting randomized trials, surrogate markers must be used with caution. Additionally, the significant effect on a surrogate marker may not be a significant effect on the true outcome. Studies that control for confounders of a surrogate outcome may not control for confounders that affect the ultimate outcome in question. Grimes and Schulz have emphasized that surrogate markers should, among other characteristics, have similar confounders and influences, and they should show a near identical response to a treatment. They cite the example of fluoride treatments, which improve the surrogate marker-bone density but increase fractures (the valid outcome) by making bones more brittle. Occasionally, authors will use a "combined outcome," which includes a surrogate and valid clinical outcome. This combined outcome should be interpreted cautiously because the relative effect of treatments on the various components is unknown.

Another problem with randomized clinical trials is that authors may report on "secondary outcomes" or subgroup analyses. These outcome values may or may not have similar validity to primary outcomes. Randomized trials are designed to test hypotheses on primary outcomes, and **confounding** variables that affect the primary outcome are controlled for. Often the confounders, randomizations, and study design do not contain the strict control regarding subgroups or secondary outcomes (sometimes they do). Thus, many epidemiologists suggest results of secondary outcomes be interpreted with caution and as hypothesis generating. This is particularly true when secondary outcomes and subgroup analyses are incorporated into metaanalysis.

Practical considerations frequently determine whether a clinical question will be addressed using a randomized trial. Acute clinical problems in which every patient has a relevant outcome in a short period of time are ideal to study using clinical trials. Gynecologic examples include comparisons of short-term pain or febrile morbidity following different surgical approaches, comparisons of cure rates or side effects in the treatment of infections, or pregnancy rates following different infertility treatment regimens. For clinical problems like these, clinicians should be able to rely on RCT data. In contrast, RCTs intended to study long-term or rare outcomes are much more difficult to carry out. If a treatment outcome is rare or takes years to develop (cancer being an excellent example of both), one needs a very large study over years or decades to answer the clinical question. Often **cohort** trials will be used to evaluate rare outcomes. Even when large trials like the Women's Health Initiative are implemented, clinicians usually have to rely on other data for clinical decision making during the many years before study results are available. Finally, because of the time, effort, and expense involved in carrying out an RCT, many questions of great clinical interest have not yet been addressed in this way.

Observational studies, in which the investigator does not control the exposure, provide an alternative approach to answering clinical questions. Depending on the data collection process, observational studies are classified as cross-sectional, cohort, or case-control studies. Cross-sectional studies generate prevalence data by examining the relationship between exposure and the outcomes of interest in a defined population at a single point in time. With reference to only a designated moment in time,

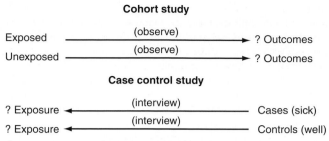

Figure 5-1 Schematic diagram of methodology used to estimate risk of exposure to outcome in cohort and case-control studies.

these studies are not able to provide as strong causal evidence. However, cross-sectional studies can highlight associations that deserve additional evaluation.

Epidemiologic studies that may be used to provide stronger evidence than a cross-sectional analysis are cohort and case-control studies (**Fig. 5-1**). A cohort study selects a group of individuals at risk for the outcome of interest and divides them into subgroups based on the presence or absence of one or more exposures to be studied. Subgroups are then evaluated over time to count the outcomes as they occur. Unlike RCTs, in cohort studies, the individual subject selects the exposure, not the investigator. Most studies of the long-term health effects of contraceptive methods have employed a cohort design where the subjects themselves decided which contraceptive method to use. A particular difficulty of this approach is that the subjects almost certainly differ in many characteristics beyond the main exposure of interest. When these different characteristics are related to both the exposure and the risk of experiencing an outcome, they can confound the results of the study. Age, for instance, is nearly always a confounding variable. Advancing age increases the risk of a heart attack and is associated with a very decreased use of oral contraceptives. If age is not accounted for in a statistical analysis, it might appear that oral contraceptives provide enormous protection against heart attacks because all of the (older) women experiencing heart attacks are not oral contraceptive users.

To the extent that information is collected about known or suspected confounding factors, it is possible to control their effect in the statistical analysis. Adjustment techniques can work only for confounding variables that an investigator knows about and measures. A reason that RCTs provide stronger evidence than observational studies is that randomization balances confounding variables across the study groups, even confounders that are not recognized to be important at the time the study is performed.

A strength of cohort studies is the possibility of assessing many different outcomes over time, but a weakness is often the need to wait many years until enough outcomes occur to allow an analysis. Thanks to computerized databases of medical information, cohort studies can now sometimes be done historically—that is, the research question is formulated and the analyses are done years after the data have been collected and recorded for routine uses. This approach can be quick and very cost effective, but the value of such studies is completely dependent on the quality of the original data. Information from large databases is dependent on exclusions, data entry, and limited input, to name only a few factors.

Case-control studies are always retrospective. Study participants are selected on the basis of already having the outcome of interest (the case group) or of not having that outcome (the control group). Case status needs to be carefully defined and should include all cases of new-onset disease drawn from an identifiable population. Controls should be sampled from the same population; the purpose of the control group is to estimate the frequency in the population of the exposures being studied if there were no relationship with the disease being studied. In the past, investigators often found it convenient to select controls from among other patients found in the same hospital as the cases, but choosing controls from the general population is highly preferable. Similar to all studies (no matter the type) the ability to generalize from the study population to all populations determines the external validity of the study; its generalizability is a key feature. All clinicians evaluating a study should assess the study's "external validity." After identifying the cases and controls, data are then gathered, usually by interview, concerning past exposures. The exposure information from cases and controls is then compared quantitatively to obtain an estimate of risk. Case-control studies are quite useful for evaluating rare occurrences. As with cohort studies, statistical adjustment techniques are needed to account for confounding variables. The quality of the results from these studies is dependent on uniform, meticulous interview techniques when collecting data from cases and controls. Recall bias is a particular problem.

The **case-control study** is often the best approach to study rare diseases. A case-control study including only 8 cases and 31 controls was able to identify the strong association between vaginal adenocarcinoma and in utero exposure to diethylstilbestrol (DES). Although a randomized trial of DES had been performed to evaluate its now-recognized ineffectiveness in preventing spontaneous abortion, that study was not large enough or long enough to identify a rare cancer that was identified in daughters 20 years later.

The best experiment to test causality is the randomized controlled trial. The investigator may control for differences between two groups, except the treatment or exposure. This kind of evidence provides the strongest support for causal relationships. If a **relative risk** is strong, at least greater than 2.0 or less than 0.5, causality is a more likely explanation. Weaker associations can often be explained by confounding variables. However, enthusiastic investigators, worried patients, or sensationalistic media frequently overinterpret weak associations.

Statistical testing is used to detect whether a study's findings are due to a chance occurrence—the traditional p value is the indication of the likelihood that the results of the finding were "accidental." Small sample size, and low study power increase the likelihood of a chance result.

PRESENTATION OF STUDY RESULTS

Epidemiologic studies use a quantitative approach to describing both exposures and outcomes. Whether RCT, cohort study, or case-control study, all of these studies attempt to present their results as a single number, usually referred to as the point estimate, that quantifies the relationship between the exposure and the outcome. This number is an estimate of the truth rather than the truth itself because each study, however large, includes only a sample of all the people who are affected by

Table 5-2 Interpretation of Relative Risk (RR) and Odds Ratio (OR) Values

RRs and ORs < 1.0 indicate protection from outcome.
RRs and ORs > 1.0 indicate risk of outcome.
RRs and ORs = 1.0 indicate no association to outcome.

For both RR and OR, the further away the value is from 1.0 the stronger the relationship.

the exposure-outcome relationship. The point estimate expresses the strength of the association between the exposure and outcome. In an RCT or a cohort study, the point estimate is the relative risk (RR). Risk in the study subjects is the number of cases or outcomes that occur over time. The RR is simply the risk of disease (or other outcome) among the exposed or treated subjects divided by the risk in the unexposed subjects. A case-control study does not measure risk directly but calculates its results as an **odds ratio** (OR), which is generally equivalent to an RR from a cohort study (**Table 5-2**).

If there is no association at all between the exposure and outcome, then the RR or OR would be 1.0. RRs and ORs greater than 1.0 indicate an increased risk of the outcome. RRs and ORs less than 1.0 indicate a decreased risk of the outcome. For both RRs and ORs, the further away the value is from 1.0, the stronger the relationship between the exposure and the outcome (**Fig. 5-2**). Investigators do not limit the presentation of all of their analyses to a single point estimate. Usually RRs are presented separately for different doses (e.g., estrogen levels in the oral contraceptive) or durations of exposure (e.g., pack-years of cigarette smoking) or for subgroups of subjects (e.g., those with or without a family history of the outcome).

The RR is based on results from the people in a particular study and not the entire population possible, thus there is always a possibility of sampling error. The quantitative description of the study results needs to include a measure of this uncertainty. The confidence interval is widely used to express the precision of the point estimate; a wide confidence interval indicates less

precision, and a narrow confidence interval indicates more. In general, the larger the study, the narrower the confidence interval. There are several cautions about interpreting confidence intervals correctly. First, the confidence interval indicates only uncertainty that is due to the play of chance; it does not inform us about uncertainty in the results because of other factors, such as confounders that have not been controlled for, or of peculiarities of the population that was studied, or poor study quality. Second, a wide confidence interval does not mean there is no association between the exposure and the outcome; even an imprecise point estimate remains the best explanation of the relationship until a larger or better study is performed. Finally, confidence intervals are often drawn as a straight line around the point estimate to show the width of their range; this might seem to suggest that the location of the true point estimate would be equally likely to fall anywhere within that interval. In fact, the confidence interval could better be shown as a bell-shaped curve centered on the point estimate.

Relative risk estimates do not take into account the incidence or the importance of the problem being evaluated. A relative risk of 4 says that the outcome increases 400% in exposed individuals compared with unexposed individuals. This increase often causes great worry or excitement (particularly in the media). However, the relative risk must be interpreted in the context of the frequency of the outcome. For instance, the incidence of venous thromboembolism (VTE) in young women without using oral contraceptives is about 1 in 10,000, and the incidence while using oral contraceptives is 4 in 10,000; thus, the relative risk is 4. However, the absolute risk of VTE is still low in both groups of women with a difference in risk of 3 in 10,000. The risk in the exposed minus the risk in the unexposed is the risk difference. The *risk difference* describes the size of the effect in absolute terms. This is also called **attributable risk**, and it is very useful for putting large relative risks into a clinically useful perspective. This is also called the *absolute risk reduction* when a benefit is identified, and the *absolute risk increase* when a harm is identified.

For clinicians and patients, even the calculation of absolute risk differences in a population may not be helpful in assessing possible risks or benefits. An alternative calculation looks at the complementary concept: how many patients need to be treated to observe one benefit or one adverse event? The **number needed to treat (NNT)**, the number of patients who need to be treated to achieve an additional positive outcome, is the reciprocal of the absolute risk reduction (the risk difference for good outcomes). If the effect is dangerous, the value is called the number needed to harm (NNH). The number of patients who, if they received the treatment, would lead to one additional patient being harmed, compared with patients not receiving the treatment, is the reciprocal of the absolute risk increase (the risk difference for bad outcomes). Thus, using the example of oral contraceptives, with a risk of VTE of 4 in 10,000, the number needed to harm (NNH)—that is, to experience one extra VTE—is 3333, the reciprocal of 3 in 10,000, which is the absolute risk increase.

The effectiveness of oral contraceptives is extraordinarily high, and because pregnancy is extremely common in the absence of contraception, the NNT of oral contraceptives is 1/0.97 or 1.03 (1/0.97 is the reciprocal of OCP effectiveness, 97%). The NNT is close to 1—that is, one treatment yields one good outcome. One person using OCP will prevent one

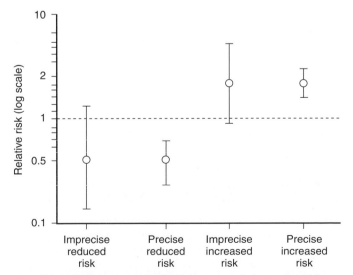

Figure 5-2 Examples of point estimates (*open circles*) and confidence intervals (*between the crossbars*) of two studies with reduced risk and two studies with increased risk. If the confidence interval overlaps 1.0, the change in risk is statistically insignificant.

pregnancy. In contrast, for most preventive services, the outcome being prevented is less common, and the treatment is less effective. Thus, in providing drug therapy to prevent osteoporotic fractures in menopausal women, the NNT is generally greater than 20. Calculations of NNT and NNH are essential to calculate the potential benefits and harms of therapies, preventive services, and screening tests. Another benefit of these calculations is that they allow us to compare benefits and harms across different treatment strategies. A caution about NNT and NNH is that the number may vary over time. The data from which an NNT is calculated are often specific and may not be generalizable to a person's lifetime or the course of a disease. NNT and NNH derived from metaanalysis should be viewed with caution. If the studies are from varied populations or used slightly different methods, the NNT and NNH may not always apply to an individual patient, or be a simple arithmetic summation.

INTERPRETATION OF STUDY RESULTS

Most associations found in a study do not represent a cause-and-effect relationship. We can attempt to assess whether causation is a good explanation of an association based on the quality of the study, the design of the study, and other specific criteria. Making these assessments is a critical part of evidence-based medicine. Studies must be free of bias or, in other words, have internal validity. Grimes and Schulz have described three main categories of bias that distort the internal validity of a study: selection, information, and confounding bias.

Selection bias is an error due to systematic differences in characteristics between those selected to participate in the study and those who are not selected. For instance, women without health insurance might never have a chance to enter a study because they cannot be seen at the center where the study is offered; women who are very busy with work and home responsibilities might not have the time to meet study requirements; study results thus may only apply to the subset of women who have an opportunity to enter a study. Biases may also be due to diagnostic testing. For instance, women who take oral contraceptives may see their physician more often than women who have undergone tubal ligation. Consequently, women using oral contraceptives may undergo more screening and diagnostic tests, and diseases may be uncovered more often in this group.

Information bias may occur when data about subjects are obtained differently in the different study groups. An example is recall bias. This occurs because recall of information is affected by illness, which can be a major problem for retrospective studies. Women (or their families) with an illness may recall in great detail all events they believe might be associated with the illness, whereas healthy controls may not remember similar exposures. Sometimes information in case-control studies is obtained by chart review for the "case" group, but in the control group, interviewers or mail surveys are used to collect data. Several other factors can bias the assessment of information. First is the intense surveillance of patients who are placed on a new therapy compared with those taking an older, conventional therapy. This often leads to more complete identification of adverse events among those using newer therapy. Conversely, the long-term users of any treatment tend to be unusually healthy and free of side effects because all those who don't tolerate the treatment will have stopped using it. These biases tend to make new treatments appear more dangerous and old treatments safer than they really are.

Confounding biases exist when the exposure creates associated conditions that may affect outcomes. For example, women who have undergone surgery for cervical cancer will usually have general anesthesia, but women being treated with radiation don't. In theory the anesthesia may produce side effects unrelated to the specific outcomes of surgery versus radiation. Confounding biases are one of the most common problems of observational studies. Often statistical techniques, such as multivariate analysis and logistic regression, are used to help eliminate confounders.

Distinguishing whether findings in a study are associations or are causal is essential to clinical care. If an association is strong (i.e., the relative risk is far from 1.0) and precise (i.e., narrow confidence intervals) and if the risk or benefit is clinically important based on the context, then it is particularly important to assess causality. The Bradford-Hill criteria offer a valuable approach to differentiate causality from association (**Table 5-3**). In the United States these criteria are often referred to as the surgeon general's criteria because of their initial use in interpretation of evidence regarding cigarette smoking and lung cancer. Most of the principles of causality are intuitive.

The presence of a dose-response effect or duration-response effect also supports a causal association as when a higher dose or a longer treatment is associated with a better treatment response. In contradistinction, peculiar dose-response effects indicate the need for more study to understand the effect. Biologic plausibility also needs to be considered in evaluating results, especially from observational studies; our knowledge of physiology can often support, refute, or indicate a need for more data. The notion of **specificity** can be more challenging to apply. One exposure to one outcome is an appealing and parsimonious approach to scientific explanation, and when a relationship is that specific, causality is likely. Conversely, when an exposure is related to a wide range of bad outcomes—or good ones—one must suspect a placebo effect is operating or an unsuspected bias. As a caution against dismissing such relationships too easily: One early argument rejecting the adverse health effects of cigarette smoking was that the very wide range of adverse effects was too nonspecific to be true! It seems obvious that an exposure causes an outcome only if it precedes the outcome. An important weakness of cross-sectional studies is that they often cannot establish the temporality of the relationship being evaluated.

Table 5-3 Bradford-Hill Criteria for Causation

Experiment	Investigator control or laboratory experiments
Strength	Size of RR (>2.0 or <0.5)
Consistency	Similar RR in several studies
Gradient	Dose-response relationship
Biologic plausibility	Physiologic explanation for association
Specificity	Outcome only associated with intervention
Temporality	Exposure precedes outcome
Analogy	Similar association in other related diseases or exposures
Coherence	Evidence from different sources fits together

RR, relative risk.

From Bradford-Hill A: Principles of Medical Statistics, 9th ed. New York, Oxford University Press, 1971, p 309.

Even with stronger study designs, our lack of knowledge about the timing of the preclinical onset of a condition can make it difficult to obtain exposure information for the biologically important interval. Seeking analogies can help clarify a possible cause-and-effect relationship. We need to consider whether similar agents or drugs are known to have similar effects. We also need to consider whether the same exposure is known to cause similar diseases. Finally, coherence of the evidence demands that the previously listed criteria be considered in conjunction with all of our other knowledge.

KEY POINTS

- Epidemiologic studies link laboratory bench research to the bedside.
- Randomized controlled trials (RTCs) provide the strongest level of evidence to link cause and effect and are used to test hypotheses.
- Randomized trials may not be practical to study outcomes that are extremely rare or take many years to develop.
- Cohort studies are often excellent for studying a single exposure that may lead to a wide range of outcomes.

- Case-control studies are excellent for studying rare diseases and for evaluating a wide range of exposures.
- Descriptive studies, including cross-sectional and ecologic studies, help generate hypotheses and also can illuminate the size and context of a health problem.
- Evidence-based medicine helps provide firm basis for clinical decisions.

REFERENCES CAN BE FOUND ON EXPERTCONSULT.com

6

Medical-Legal Risk Management

James M. Kelley, III and Gretchen M. Lentz

The word *malpractice* evokes a guttural response in physicians and health care providers. This is perhaps more true in the areas of obstetrics and gynecology, where the physical damages are often catastrophic and the economic damages are often in the millions of dollars. The fear of being unjustly involved in litigation and judged by nonphysicians as liable—despite having provided reasonable and appropriate care—seems unavoidable to many conscientious health care providers. The little-known reality, however, is that the growing consensus of empirical data on outcomes of malpractice actions shows that the legal system works for the provider in the end far more often than it does not. Understanding how the system works and making minor practice modifications to minimize risk are essential to avoiding claims and adverse outcomes.

A medical negligence case comprises three basic elements: a deviation from the standard of care, proximate causation, and damages. Each of these elements is required to be proved by way of "competent" expert testimony. The definition of *competent* varies state to state, but all states are uniform in requiring a physician to agree that malpractice occurred, and that it directly resulted in injury. A deviation from the standard of care, although a cumbersome legal phrase, is simply a failure to act reasonably as compared with another health care provider in the same or similar clinical circumstance. A deviation from the standard of care can be an act (intraoperative perforation, administration of the wrong medication, etc.) or an omission (failure to run the bowel intra-op or failure to timely review laboratory results).

Proximate causation is often a more medically complex component. The law requires that the deviation from the standard of care be *a* direct, proximate cause of injury to the plaintiff. It is important to note that the deviation does not have to be the exclusive cause of injury but rather need only be *a* direct proximate cause. Proximate cause, legally, just means that with appropriate or reasonable treatment, the injury would not have occurred.

The final element is damages. Damages are economic and noneconomic. Economic damages include such items as past and future medical bills and past and future wage loss. Noneconomic damages contemplate such things as past and future physical pain, emotional suffering, and, in certain instances, wrongful death. To be successful, the plaintiff must prove each of these elements to a probability, through expert testimony, in order to win. A failure on any of the elements will result in a verdict for the defendant.

As mentioned, many health care providers will be surprised to learn what the growing consensus of empirical data reflects regarding medical claims. A review of approximately 1400 closed malpractice claims from five different liability carriers showed that only 3% of claims that were filed had no verifiable medical injuries. Additionally, 37% of those did not involve errors, but rather would be what a physician would commonly refer to as "frivolous." Despite common perceptions about runaway juries and lottery verdicts levied against faultless physicians, the study demonstrated that 84% of the claims that did not involve errors resulted in nonpayment. Conversely, approximately six times that rate of claims resulted in nonpayment to the plaintiff, despite the presence of medical errors and verifiable injuries.

Box 6-1   What Constitutes Medical Malpractice?

To successfully maintain a medical malpractice action, a plaintiff must be able to establish three distinct elements of his or her case by way of expert testimony:

1. *Deviation from the standard of care.* The health care provider deviated from what a reasonable provider would have done in the same or similar circumstances.
2. *Causation.* The deviation was a direct cause of the injury suffered.
3. *Damages.* Economic and noneconomic damages were suffered as result of the injury.

Although these data should be heartening for health care providers, they do little to eliminate burdens of excessive litigation costs, time away from practice and families, and the stress of participating in litigation. The goal for conscientious providers must be one focused on risk management: balancing improved patient care and minimizing medical legal risk. Realizing lawsuits will inevitably occur, the following are practical insights aimed at helping you enhance patient care and communication, minimize the risk of involvement in meritless litigation, and provide your best defense in the event a claim is made.

COMMUNICATION

Medical-legal risk management, at its core, centers on communication in both the written and verbal form. Awareness of the common pitfalls in the processes employed in communicating information to patients—as well as concurrent and subsequent care providers—will be invaluable if problems or litigation arise. The medical record, institutional policies and guidelines, and information communicated to patients (prospective plaintiffs) will be the only information attorneys, claim representatives, and reviewing expert physicians have available to judge the validity of a potential malpractice claim. The following examines good practices to improve communications with patients (both before and after treatment), improve the accuracy of the medical records, and provide useful information about navigating the litigation process to your best outcome.

COMMUNICATION WITH THE PATIENT

Physicians well understand that the relationship with their patient is in large measure a relationship of trust. More often than not, a perceived breach of that trust is the impetus for a patient to seek the advice of an outsider for explanations about unfortunate medical outcomes. It must become a routine practice for physicians to thoroughly and carefully discuss potential problems with their patients prior to treatment. Taking the time necessary to assess a patient's understanding of the procedures and possible outcomes, and answering all questions the patient may have, are critical to managing and controlling expectations. Concurrent notations in the record that you have, in fact, reviewed all risks and benefits of a potential treatment, thoroughly explained alternative treatments or procedures, and answered all patient questions will provide important evidence of careful and appropriate treatment should it later become necessary.

Box 6-2 Practice Tip

Sample Progress Note
Risks/Benefits/Alternatives (R/B/A's) discussed w/patient.
   All ?'s answered in full.

The abbreviations and words in **Box 6-2** are an invaluable resource in the event of a complication or litigation.

In the unfortunate event of a poor outcome, it is imperative you communicate more, not less, with your patient or the patient's family where appropriate. Health care providers often dramatically change—or end entirely—their relationship with patients following a maloccurrence. For example, in situations where the patient may have ongoing care issues but is transferred to a tertiary center or a different specialist, there is often minimal or no ongoing relationship. Despite what may be the urge to distance yourself from an unpleasant or uncomfortable interaction, keep in mind that your patient and his or her family members will begin assessing whether or not you are forthcoming with them at this very time. If there is an attempt to avoid interaction it can, and likely will, be misperceived as an attempt to avoid explaining the cause or causes of the bad outcome. It is important that your trust relationship with the patient and the patient's family continues at this crucial time and that they feel you are willing to answer all questions.

When discussing the outcome or problem, revisit the discussion of risks and outcomes at the time of the informed consent. Reiterate the information you previously provided, and explain how this result is related to the risks previously discussed, if appropriate. Finally, it is also important that you are involved in establishing the plan for care going forward, even if it is outside of your specialty. Remaining involved preserves the physician-patient relationship. Patients are far less likely to file claims against physicians with whom they have an ongoing, trusting relationship. It is therefore important to make yourself available as long as is necessary to assure the patient and his or her family that you are answering all of their questions. Absence or avoidance will make the patient or another family member suspicious and can ultimately lead them to seek answers to their questions from an outside source—most often an attorney.

Once again, it is imperative that you write contemporaneous and accurate notes. The timing of such notes, combined with their detail and clarity, will begin to establish good defense in the event the records are reviewed for a possible claim. It is easy to defend conscientious care, regardless of outcome, if the record supports you.

Box 6-3 Practice Tip

Communication with the patient when a problem occurs is an opportunity to explain how the poor outcome happened, despite vigilance. Patients will naturally have questions, and most who contact a malpractice attorney are doing so to get answers to questions they feel were not sufficiently answered by the health care provider.

COMMUNICATION THROUGH MEDICAL RECORDS

Once the litigation process has commenced, a plaintiff attorney's best friend is inaccurate or inconsistent documentation of the care provided. Inaccurate documentation can stem from a genuine standard-of-care issue; however, inaccuracies can also arise from the use of inappropriate nomenclature. In either situation, the health care provider will be in the untenable position of attempting to defend a narrative note or deposition testimony that is factually inconsistent with literature, policies, or objective data in the medical record. Needless to say, in a courtroom, inconsistencies never favor the inconsistent party. Careful attention to recordkeeping will not only demonstrate attentive care and rationally based treatment decisions, but it will ultimately become a provider's best defense in a courtroom.

Within your hospital, facility, office, and charts, you must use nomenclature designed to standardize the verbiage utilized between providers. Unfortunately, despite the attempts at standardization, many health care providers have been slow to adapt. This is often based on variable levels of education by authors, and it is also generational. This increases not only the risk of inaccurate communication among health care providers, but also the risk of a medical record replete with inconsistencies. Inconsistencies can be easily used to portray a provider as incompetent or disingenuous.

From a medicolegal risk management standpoint, it is critical to keep in mind when a plaintiff's counsel attempts to determine whether or not medical malpractice may have occurred; the medical record is the primary (and often the only) source of information available to evaluate the potential claim. Any narrative notes supplied will be read against subsequent health care providers' notes and the objective data such as lab results and imaging. As stated earlier, clearly noted and accurate recognition and description of reassuring and nonreassuring findings in the record will demonstrate attentive and competent care. However, inaccurate terminology, when read against the objective data, could result in the commencement of litigation.

Beyond the initial review phase of a potential claim, inconsistent and inaccurate nomenclature and recordkeeping will continue to present obstacles to a favorable resolution of the claim during the testimonial phase of trial. When a witness employs modified or nonstandardized nomenclature, other health care providers, including expert medical witnesses, do not necessarily understand the full extent of what is meant. This unclear communication can result in actual medical errors between providers or, at a minimum, the appearance of errors within a medical record.

Box 6-4 Factual Scenario

In a previous deposition, a physician was questioned regarding a nursing narrative note.

Q. Dr. Doe, do you expect the nurse to relay to you if there are any postoperative changes?

A. Any relevant postoperative changes should be relayed to me, particularly if there are more than one.

Q. By relevant change do you mean if any vital signs manifest persistent change?

A. I do not understand what that means; however, if a nurse sees vitals change, I want to know about it immediately, especially if it persists.

The narrative notes within the case included the nurse describing labile blood pressures. Utilizing charting terminology such as *labile* created a scenario where the physician had expectations of being told immediately, and a medical record suggesting the call should have been made. Further testimony demonstrated that no information regarding these changes was relayed. The nurse testified as follows:

Q. Did you relay to Dr. Doe that the blood pressures were labile?

A. No.

Q. Why not?

A. Because I felt it was not necessarily significant and may be routine postop fluctuations.

Q. So you felt it was unstable but not labile?

A. Yes.

Q. So when you chart the word *labile*, you want the jury to believe it doesn't mean labile?

A. I guess.

The preceding example shows how the inappropriate and inconsistent nomenclature forced the physician to be critical of the nurse's actions, while the nurse attempted to separate herself from her own charting. This is not only a difficult posture to defend, but also it reflects poorly on the competency and truthfulness of the parties involved. Simply employing appropriate, consistent nomenclature would have provided an easy defense.

Box 6-5 Practice Tip

The consistent use of appropriate nomenclature not only minimizes risk in the defense of a medical legal action. It will also allow the physicians and nurses to communicate clearly by ensuring they are discussing the same findings and placing the same significance.

COMMUNICATION CONSISTENT WITH INSTITUTIONAL POLICIES

Published institutional policies and procedures should be reviewed regularly and integrated into your daily practice. The purpose of the policies or protocols is not merely for JCAHO, or to fill shelf space, but to effectuate patient care and create a consistent safe administration of the medication and care to patients. However, each individual patient obviously deserves individual care and modifications to the policy or protocol as may be necessary. Policies and protocols relevant to the issues that are the bases of any litigation should be familiar to you *before* you provide sworn testimony under oath. Because these written policies can form the basis of an accepted standard of care in your institution, any testimony or records inconsistent with these policies can be viewed by a jury as being outside the standard of care, or negligent.

Box 6-6 Factual Scenario

Many gynecologic cases involve the failure to recognize perforations or bleeds. Total abdominal hysterectomy usually carries with it a specific physician's postoperative order or, more commonly, a hospital's postoperative policy or protocol. It is of critical importance that the nurse and physician both have an understanding of the specific details of the policy or protocol prior to executing care and prior to testifying regarding these issues. The following example highlights why this is important:

Q. Are you aware as to whether or not there is a postoperative policy at this facility?

A. I don't know. I guess there probably is.

Q. Do you agree that you as a reasonable nurse have a duty to follow the policy here at the facility?

A. I don't really know what the policy says, but I'm sure it's reasonable and yes I should probably follow it.

Q. If you failed to follow the policy, can we agree that you would have been acting unreasonably and beneath the accepted standards of care?

A. I probably should follow a policy if it exists. I guess if I didn't, I was beneath the standard of care.

The nurse went on to define terms differently from the definition contained in the policy and testified that the physician with whom she was working was aware of her actions. When the physician was questioned he testified as follows:

Q. Do you expect the nurses to follow your specific orders and, when orders are not present specific to the chart, to follow policies or protocols that are in place for the delivery of health care to patients?

A. Absolutely.

Q. For this patient did you write a specific postoperative order?

A. No.

Q. Your order says, "post TAH protocol"?

A. Yes.

Q. Does that mean the nurse should follow the hospital's policy or protocol?

A. Absolutely.

Q. Is a reasonable nurse allowed to deviate from that policy or protocol without calling you first?

A. No.

Here, a lack of familiarity with the standard policy within the hospital created a scenario where the physician and nurse were uncertain as to what was expected by the hospital. Compounding matters, the lack of familiarity with the policy and protocol prior to deposition created a scenario where not only did the nurse provide testimony that she deviated from the policy, but also she was forced to acknowledge a total lack of familiarity with the same. In short, knowledge of and compliance with institutional policies, guidelines, and resources can demonstrate the implementation of appropriate care, and documentation can be the shield of your defense; or ignorance of and deviation from such policies can provide a documented deviation from the standard of care that will become the plaintiff's sword.

WHEN A CLAIM IS MADE

The institution of a claim varies from state to state and is defined differently among various insurance policies. It is imperative that you have an understanding through your institution, insurance policy, and within your state as to what constitutes knowledge or notice of a claim. When notice of a claim is received, it is imperative that you immediately notify your hospital or group administrator and your insurance company. A failure to timely notify individuals can jeopardize insurance coverage or compromise your defense, and in a worst-case scenario it may potentially result in a default judgment for failure to timely respond. Although the legal system does move slowly, there are certain parameters, and timely responses are mandatory at the beginning of litigation.

Participation in a claim is aggravating, frightening, and an imposition upon your professional or personal time. However, it is of critical import to avoid procrastination or de-prioritization of the claim regardless of the level of merit or damages you perceive. A lawsuit is typically commenced by the filing of a legal pleading known as a *complaint*. Thereafter, there will be a statutory amount of time for an *answer* to be filed on your behalf. Thereafter, the first portion of litigation is referred to as *discovery*. This is where each side exchanges information either through documents or sworn testimony between the sides—first regarding factual information, then regarding expert opinions in the claim. A deposition is simply the opposing attorney's opportunity to ask questions under oath that are reasonably calculated to lead to relevant discoverable evidence.

Your deposition is an obligation, not an opportunity. In that regard, it is critical that you meet with your attorney in advance of your deposition so you can be prepared for the relevant issues. A critical review of your care with your attorney is important so that you can anticipate all areas of questioning and avoid being surprised under oath. The answers you give under oath are sworn testimony in the case, and oftentimes depositions circulate even after the closure of the file. It is recommended that you meet at least 1 week in advance of your deposition with counsel for a preparatory session—which will allow you adequate time in the event your practice requires a delay or cancellation to reschedule that meeting—before you actually give your testimony at deposition. Additional techniques include a mock deposition, where another attorney questions you in a practice session to prepare you for the format. This can be very useful for pointing out medically complex issues and for enhancing your preparation for giving sworn testimony.

Your deposition testimony, along with the other factual witnesses, will then become a supplement to the medical record for the expert witnesses to utilize and, ultimately, jurors to judge which position they deem more reasonable. Accordingly, just as accurate, concise, and consistent communication in your medical record is a priority, so too should it be within your deposition.

Following discovery, cases are usually scheduled for jury trials based on individual court docket systems. You should plan on attending each day of your trial and participating in the same. While it is no physician's desire to take time away from his or her practice to be in a courtroom, it is imperative that when you arrive there, you have an accurate medical record and deposition to support the reasonableness of the decisions you made at the time that you made them.

> **Box 6-7** Practice Tip
>
> 1. Secure and isolate the patient's complete medical record.
> 2. Make no additions, modifications, or alterations to that chart.
> 3. Notify either your institutional administrative or insurance representative of the claim, in order to preserve coverage.
> 4. Participate fully—and as a priority—in the defense of the quality of your care.

PHYSICIAN'S DEFENSIVE STRATEGIES

ABANDONMENT

Unilateral dismissal of the patient by the physician without proper notice to the patient is popularly conceived of as being the entire tort of abandonment. However, failure to keep an express promise (being present for a delivery, making a house call, or treating with a particular modality are common examples), failure to give proper discharge instructions, or abrogating your authority to a less qualified individual are much more likely to result in charges of abandonment. This is particularly true in the case of the obstetrician/gynecologist, in which the courts consider the physician/patient relationship to be particularly personal and private.

Physician's Defense Strategy

Explain your coverage arrangements in a patient brochure and document that the patient has received it. Do not sign out to family practitioners or partially trained gynecologists. If house officers are going to be involved in the patient's care, explain their role and do not allow them to exceed the stated role. Do not make express promises if there is even a minimal chance a change of circumstances will prevent you from keeping your promise.

ABORTION

See the preceding discussion. Two subsequent Supreme Court cases (*Webster v. Reproductive Health Services*, 109 S. Ct. 1759 [1989]; *Planned Parenthood v. Casey*, 112 S. Ct. 2791 [1992]) have greatly expanded the local control of abortion, and preabortion procedures.

Physician's Defense Strategy

Seek local legal counsel. Make sure all aspects of your abortion practice conform to local, state, and federal law. Insist on an opinion letter that covers preabortion, abortion, and postabortion issues. Do not do the procedure without "on advice of counsel" protection. Get timely legal reviews.

CANCELLATIONS AND "NO SHOWS"

Cancellations and "no shows" of follow-up patients appointments are often ignored in the busy clinic or office. They can be, and are, frequently responsible for subsequent malpractice suits.

Physician's Defense Strategy

Each cancellation or no show should be documented in the chart. The chart should then be reviewed by the treating physician and, where appropriate, a letter or phone call made to the patient. All efforts to communicate with the patient should be documented.

COVERAGE ARRANGEMENTS

As mentioned earlier improper coverage arrangements may lead to charges of abandonment. Poor communication among coverage groups frequently leads to offended patients and can be the first step on the path to a malpractice suit.

Physician's Defense Strategy

The previously mentioned strategy applies here:

1. List your coverage arrangements in your new patient brochure.
2. Sign out to qualified individuals.
3. Do not make specific promises as to your presence or procedures.
4. In addition, coverage groups should meet regularly to exchange information and maintain protocols.
5. Problem patients should be known to the entire group.
6. All after-hours care should be carefully documented and entered in the medical record either contemporaneously or at the latest, the next business day.
7. All medical records should be available to all members of the group.

When you have the coverage:

1. Don't put geographic barriers between you and the patient (although it is not written in stone, The Emergency Medical treatment and Active Labor Act and other federal regulations and cases based thereon would indicate that you should be able to reach your patient's bedside within **thirty** (30) minutes).
2. Do not drink alcohol or take drugs (even prescription drugs) that can affect your cognition or cause somnolence.
3. Document all phone calls. Err on the side of caution.
4. Emergency physicians are great, but emergency departments are often overworked and slow and you are inserting an intervening opinion between you and the patient. An "I will meet you at the emergency room!" has been a great relief to many a patient and many a physician.

CONTRACEPTION AND STERILIZATION

Contraceptive methods and sterilization procedures can involve the physician in multiple issues of informed consent, treatment of minors, emancipation of minors, and court-ordered procedures, wrongful pregnancy as well as wrongful life and wrongful birth suits.

Physician's Defense Strategy

There is no escaping the necessity of researching your state's requirements. However, no where in obstetrics/gynecology practice is the communication with the patient more important. A thorough, unbiased informed consent is required. In addition, be careful of your terms. A tubal transection should be truly a tubal transection and a piece of tube sent as a pathology specimen is a splendid proof that the tube was sectioned. A clamped, crushed, or cauterized tube signed out as a tubal transection is a much less satisfactory form of evidence at a subsequent trial.

FRAUD AND ABUSE

In 1972, as part of the first amendments to the Medicaid and Medicare rules and regulations, Congress passed antifraud and abuse regulations. The first such laws were hardly more than "a slap on the wrist." However, in 1977 Congress made those laws draconian. False statements, which include:

1. Knowingly and willfully making or causing to be made any false statement or representation of a material fact in seeking to obtain any benefit or payment
2. Fraudulently concealing or failing to disclose information affecting one's rights to a payment
3. Converting any benefit or payment rightfully belonging to another, and
4. Presenting or causing to be presented a claim for a physician's service knowing that the individual who furnished the service was not licensed as a physician.

These also encompass false claims, bribes, kickbacks, rebates or "any remuneration" and are felonies with a maximum of 5 years in jail and a $25,000.00 fine possible for **each** such offense. (The law states that any provider who knowingly and willfully solicits, pays, offers, or receives, any remuneration, in cash or in kind, directly or indirectly, overtly or covertly, to induce or in return for arranging for or ordering items or services that will be paid for by Medicare or Medicaid will be guilty of a felony). These rules and regulations essentially made it impossible to practice without violating some aspect of the fraud and abuse laws. It was, however, 10 years before the laws were refined in the Medicaid–Medicare Patient Protection Act of 1987 which provided some "safe harbors" to free normal course of business procedures. Since 1987, the government has pursued fraud and abuse cases with ever-increasing vigor. In 2003, settlements in fraud and abuse cases netted the government close to $2 billion (*Wall Street Journal*, A1, Friday, June 11, 2004). The real danger to the physician is not the fine that may force him or her into bankruptcy or the unusual imposition of jail time (to date, the government has seemed more interested in recovering cash and calling a halt to illegal practices than it has in jailing doctors), but the felony conviction that may result in the automatic loss of the license to practice. Thus Medicare/Medicaid fraud and abuse is a far more dangerous hazard than is malpractice.

Physician's Defense Strategy

Have your patients sign in whether they have come for an office visit or just a procedure. If you are worried about privacy issues, use a privacy sign in sheet that prevents subsequent signers from seeing who has signed in before (Colwell Publishing provides several styles of such sheets and they are very likely supplied by local firms as well.)

Don't unbundle procedures that are supposed to be bundled on a physician's visit. Don't unbundle surgical procedures. Don't charge for procedures done by another licensed provider or charge for physician's services if the physician is not physically present. Send your personnel to an accredited coding course and make sure your coding is being done in an accurate manner. Do not be tempted to code up. Time studies and statistics are against you. Finally, beware of the "coding consultant" who promises to increase your accounts receivable.

INFORMED CONSENT

Physicians continually ask for a foolproof informed consent form. Informed consent has little to do with a form. Informed consent has to do with the physician's fiduciary duty to his or her patient. As the patient's fiduciary, it is the physician's duty to give the patient all the information needed for the patient to make an intelligent decision about the therapies suggested. The information given must be accurate for published studies and compared with the physician's own figures, unbiased by the physician's privileges or other agenda, and presented in language the patient in question can understand in view of her education, intelligence, experience, and social standing. The information should include the diagnosis; a description of the suggested treatment; an explanation of what the treatment is thought to accomplish; the hoped for prognosis with the treatment; the possible side effects and possible adverse happenings with treatment; the therapeutic alternatives, their benefits, and possible adverse and side effects; and the patient's prognosis with the alternative and no therapy.

Physician's Defense Strategy

Give the woman all the information called for and document it in the medical record. Ask her is she has any questions. Answer the questions, and document both the questions and the answers. Use diagrams when necessary. Add the diagrams to the medical record and ask the patient to initial the diagrams. Have the patient sign the consent form—use the statutory form if your state has one—if not, use one approved by your clinic or local medical organization and approved by your attorney. After the patient signs again ask her if she has any questions. Answer those questions, and again document both the questions and answers. Before the surgery, procedure, or therapy covered by the form, again go over the same material, answer any last-minute questions, and document the entire episode. Remember, the duty to secure informed consent is the *physician's* duty, not the nurse's duty or a hospital admission clerk's duty. It is still questionable whether the physician is legally able to delegate that duty elsewhere.

LABORATORY TESTS

One of the most common reasons for malpractice suits is the unreported abnormal laboratory or X-ray finding. The usual story is that the pathologist or radiologist returns the report and the super efficient clerk, receptionist, or nurse staples it in the medical record and then files the record. The alternative story is that the report is never sent and there is no follow-up. Of course, normal clerical errors do occur in any business; nevertheless, the physician's fiduciary duty extends to communicating the results and meanings of all abnormal tests to the patient. Therefore, the failure to communicate the results of an abnormal pap smear, glucose tolerance test, or mammogram to a patient can have disastrous legal consequences.

Physician's Defense Strategy

A gynecologist must have a system to track and document all laboratory and diagnostic tests and imaging studies ordered. There is no totally satisfactory way to do this. Old-fashioned "tickler" files are the least efficient, but better than nothing. Some office-generated computer programs have been highly successful, and some of the commercially available programs even generate an automatic notification letter. In any case, the physician must track all ordered tests and make every reasonable effort to notify the patient. The notification and follow-up must be documented. Telling the patient to call for the test results does not relieve the physician of his or her duty to notify. Finally, use the information you secure. Do not order laboratory or other diagnostic tests and then ignore or belittle those results.

MEDICAL HIGH-RISK PATIENTS

Elderly, frail women with or without serious concomitant conditions and women of any age with serious gynecologic or concomitant conditions are legally and medically at high risk.

Physician's Defense Strategy

Treat these women as being at high risk. Question all of your routine procedures. Check what medications (prescription, over-the-counter, and health food store) they are taking. Watch the dosages you prescribe. Make sure your staff assists them from the moment they enter the door until they are safely over the doorstep and into someone else's capable hands. To let one of these patients get on or off an examining table by herself is courting disaster. A premises liability suit can be just as expensive as a malpractice suit, and it is much easier and cheaper to bring.

MEDICAL RECORDS

The 1930s wag who came up with the saying, "Medical records are the malpractice witness that never dies!" offered a truism that has only increased in value over time. The world of judges and juries of 2012 expects much more than the hand-written scribbles on a 4 × 6 inch card that marked the medical record of 1930s.

Physician's Defense Strategy

If at all possible, all your records should be typed. Even the best penmanship can be misinterpreted. All records should be written or dictated contemporaneously with the event described. All records should be in English, as objective as possible, clear without confusion or ambivalence, dated, timed, signed legibly, and kept in chronological order. Chart by the subjective, objective, assessment, plan (SOAP) method whenever possible. Do not use abbreviations! (That includes abbreviations "approved" by the institution or organization. Even the most common abbreviations have multiple meanings. There will always be an expert that interprets the abbreviation in a manner contrary to your interest.) Scrivener's errors may be corrected en page. Errors of fact or substance should be corrected as a new entry placed in the chart chronologically. Do not obliterate, destroy, change, or "lose" any portion of a medical record. Such activities are termed *spoliation of evidence*. At best they may call for civil penalties at trial and at worst may constitute malpractice per se or invoke criminal penalties. In any case such spoliation of evidence makes any subsequent suit almost impossible to win. If your state or hospital or the American College of Obstetrics and Gynecology (ACOG) has a standard form that is widely used in the community, use that form or one even more extensive. Do not leave blanks on your form. If the question is worth asking it is worth recording. Although many sources advise keeping medical records for a period of 10 years after the last contact with the patient, a safer approach is to keep the record for a period that would allow a conception at the date of last visit to reach maturity and expire its statutory limitations or statute of repose in states where there is a discovery rule.

PRESCRIPTIONS

Adverse drug events are among the most common medical errors, and although physicians are loathe to admit it, more than two thirds of all adverse drug events are caused by physician error. Transmission errors and compounding (filling the prescription) errors make up the remaining third of the errors. Proper prescribing amounts to several simple basics, the appropriate drug, the appropriate dose, the appropriate directions, the appropriate time of administration, the appropriate termination, and the appropriate refill directions. Today the appropriate drug category can preclude prescribing a drug ineffective or marginally effective for the patient's diagnosis, a drug the patient is allergic to, or a drug with adverse interactions with another drug that the woman is taking. The prescription of a drug can no longer be thought of as something a physician does "off the top of his head." He needs help from an information base that can explore the medical chart, drug interactions, recorded allergies, drug doses, and the most effective therapy, and then must transmit a legible prescription for compounding. Therefore, the best approach lies in an extensive electronic medical record and database system that is updated at least monthly and that controls prescription writing. Absent such a system we can only offer homilies.

Physician's Defense Strategy

Type or block print all orders and prescriptions.

1. Prescriptions should always be written in duplicate or triplicate (one for the patient, one for the medical record, and one as your personal permanent record.) The patient's copy should always be on safety paper.
2. Do not issue oral phone orders or call prescriptions to pharmacies; use the fax line.
3. Clear, unabbreviated syntax works best. **Never use abbreviations for drugs.**
4. Always use the leading zero; never use the trailing zero (0.4 = yes; .40 = no)
5. Spell out "units" never use the symbol "U."
6. Always specify drug strength and route of administration.
7. Avoid decimals whenever possible (1500 mg rather than 1.5 g).
8. Think carefully before you sign on the "substitution permitted" line. (Generics may have blood levels that vary as much as $\pm 20\%$ from the original. Therefore, if blood level is important, the potential variation of up to 40% from one refill to another should rule against a generic equivalent.)
9. Use reasonable prescription pad security. Do not leave your prescription pad exposed on your desk or in your examining rooms.
10. Be careful of multipharmacy especially in the high-risk patient, and be alert to the use of multiple psychoactive drugs including opiates.
11. Give your patients printed instructions (Several good systems are on the market, don't ignore the AMA Patient Medicinal Instructions or the USP Dispensing Information), do not depend on the nurse or pharmacist.
12. Finally, check each prescription or order you write for clarity, legibility, appropriateness of drug and dosage in relation to the information available on the drug, the patient, and the diagnosis.

Addendum: A caution about drug samples. Samples should be stored properly and with reasonable security. (Neither the patient, nor nonmedical personnel should be able to gain access to samples.) Rotate the samples appropriately, and dispose of out-of-date samples safely and legally. **Samples should be distributed by personnel with prescriptive authority only.** (Some states may permit others to do so under supervision and written protocols.) **Do not distribute samples without issuing full oral and written instructions.**

WHEN THINGS ARE NOT GOING AS EXPECTED

Physicians are used to seeing cases progress in a somewhat predictable manner. Some patients progress more rapidly than others, but, in general, the course of disease and treatment follows a course that physicians are used to. When things take an unusual turn, physicians are prone to take one or both of two destructive courses. First, they irrationally get angry at the patient, or they lose perspective on the important issues.

Physician's Defense Strategy

Hold your temper in check. A woman who is not progressing as expected is the patient you need to have the best relations with. Go out of your way to let her know that something unusual is happening and what you are doing to solve the problem. **Do not blame her!** Reevaluate your diagnostic reasoning and differential diagnosis early. Check the chart, medication orders, nurses' notes, and medications given for possible errors. Request those cultures, chemistries, and imaging studies you thought you could short cut. Do **not** reject the patient's suggestions out of hand. If it will do no harm, the expense is not overwhelming, and it is neither unethical or illegal, concede to her wishes. Do not let your ego get in your way. **Get help early!** Get a formal consultation, don't just talk to someone in the doctor's dressing room. **Get the best help available!** Don't just ask a friend because he will concur with what you are doing. Establish good relationships with quality consultants early; do not wait until you need them to help in a disaster.

CONCLUSION

In the broadest sense, medical malpractice is defined by whether or not conduct and decisions were reasonable. The fear of all physicians is that they will be judged ultimately by lesser-trained individuals, who identify more with the patient than the provider. The tests of reasonableness they will utilize are often as simple as asking the question, based on the care and testimony you provided, would the jurors be comfortable being treated by you? If the answer to that is yes, regardless of the complications, decision making, and outcomes, the most likely jury verdict will be in favor of the defendant physician. However, if the care appears to be inattentive or inconsistent and the records or depositions are inaccurate, the chance to explain your decision and the reasonableness you feel is behind it may be lost through no one's fault but your own.

Breakdowns in the systems of communication—with patients, care providers, or through the medical records—can create a host of problems for physicians, nurses, and health care institutions in the event of an unfavorable treatment outcome. By focusing attentively on both system-wide and individual best practices for accurate and contemporaneous communications, many problems can be avoided or quickly resolved. Awareness that your patients will have serious questions about unexpected, often life-altering outcomes is integral to avoiding legal problems. Only when a patient feels that he or she has not received satisfactory answers from care providers will the patient seek those answers elsewhere—most likely from an attorney.

REFERENCES CAN BE FOUND ON EXPERTCONSULT.com

SUGGESTED READINGS

American College of Obstetricians and Gynecologists: Expert testimony: ACOG Committee Opinion No. 374: American College of Obstetricians and Gynecologists. Washington, DC, *Obstet Gynecol* 110(2 Pt 1):445–446, 2007.

Baker T: *The Medical Malpractice Myth,* Chicago, 2005, University of Chicago Press.

Charles SC, Frish PR: *Adverse Events, Stress and Litigation: A Physician's Guide,* New York, 2005, Oxford University Press.

Coping with the stress of medical professional liability litigation. ACOG Committee Opinion No. 406, ACOG, *Obstet Gynecol* 111:1257, 2008.

Erickson TB, Buys EA, DeFrancesco MS: *Report of the Presidential Task Force on Patient Safety in the Office Setting,* Washington, DC, March 20 2010, ACOG.

Mann S, Pratt S: Role of clinician involvement in patient safety in obstetrics and gynecology, *Clin Obstet Gynecol* 53(3):559–575, 2010.

Nygaard I: What does "FDA approved" mean for medical devices? *Obstet Gynecol* 111(1):4–6, 2008.

Richardson DA: Ethics in gynecologic surgical innovation, *Am J Obstet Gynecol* 170:1–6, 1994.

Wall LL, Brown D: The perils of commercially driven surgical innovation, *Am J Obstet Gynecol* 202 (1):30, e1-e4, 2010.

7

History, Physical Examination, and Preventive Health Care
General, Gynecologic, and Psychosocial History and Examination, Health Care Maintenance, Disease Prevention

Gretchen M. Lentz

The first contact a physician has with a patient is critical. It allows an initial bond of trust to be developed on which the future relationship may be built. The patient will share sensitive medical, reproductive, and psychosocial information. The physician will gain her confidence and establish rapport by the understanding and nonjudgmental manner in which he or she collects these data. Open communication with awareness of diverse cultural backgrounds and sensitivity to the needs of the disabled woman will aid in obtaining a through history and will enable accurate diagnosis and appropriate counseling.

The first contact generally involves taking a complete history, performing a complete physical examination, and ordering appropriate initial laboratory tests. In such a way the physician gains impressions of the patient's problems and needs and develops a plan for solutions. A gynecologic history includes a complete general history and adds information of gynecologic importance. In like manner, the physical examination should be complete; no corners should be cut. The physician practicing obstetrics and gynecology should not assume that others are caring for the patient's general medical needs. It may be appropriate to assume the role of her primary physician, with your care including attention to preventive health services, depending on the physician's training and skills.

This chapter focuses on the appropriate manner that a gynecologic physician should use to conduct a history and physical examination and discusses the appropriate ingredients of ongoing health maintenance. An accurate, legible, and complete medical record is an important component of the patient's care.

DIRECT OBSERVATIONS BEFORE SPEAKING TO THE PATIENT (NONVERBAL CLUES)

When meeting a patient, it is important to *look* at her even before speaking. Differing cultural backgrounds and belief systems may greatly affect the information transfer and challenge effective communication. The general demeanor of the patient should be evaluated. Five general impressions can be transmitted both by facial expression and by posture, including happiness, apathy, fear, anger, and sadness.

A patient who is happy, self-assured, and in good personal control generally has a relaxed face with a smile. Many new patients are apprehensive about meeting a new physician and the pelvic examination, and this apprehension may modify their usual expression of good spirits.

Apathetic patients generally have a blank facial expression. The eyes lack sparkle, there is little muscular movement of the face, and the mouth is generally thin and in a neutral position, neither turned up nor down. The posture may be somewhat slouched, the handshake may be weak, and answers to verbal questions are short and unemotional. Although apathetic patients may have severe emotional illness, they may also be demonstrating resignation to an imagined or serious condition or they may be responding to multiple problems, which make them feel overwhelmed.

The frightened patient frequently has a tense expression on her face; her mouth is tight and the eyes are darting and narrow. She may be perspiring but have a dry mouth. She is leaning forward, and there is often endless hand activity. When she reacts, it may be grossly out of proportion to offered stimuli.

The angry patient frequently has narrowed eyes, furrowed brows, and narrow, tight lips. She may be sitting on the edge of her chair, leaning forward as if to pounce. Unlike the frightened patient, whose pose may be defensive, the angry patient radiates aggression. Her voice is usually harsh, and her overreaction to questions usually involves short, threatening phrases.

The sad patient generally sits with slouched shoulders; large, sad eyes; and a turned-down mouth. The eyes may glisten, there may be tears, and she may not make eye contact. This patient is most likely depressed, and her speech reflects remorse and hopelessness.

Be culturally sensitive
Establish rapport
Listen and respond to the woman's concerns (empathy)
Be nonjudgmental
Include both verbal and nonverbal communication
Engage the woman in discussion and treatment options (partnership)
Convey comfort in discussing sensitive topics
Abandon stereotypes
Check for understanding of your explanations
Support—help the woman to overcome barriers to care and compliance with treatment

Box 7-2 History Outline

I. Observation—nonverbal clues
II. Chief complaint
III. History of gynecologic problem(s)
   A. Menstrual history—LMP, PMP
   B. Pregnancy history
   C. Vaginal and pelvic infections
   D. Gynecologic surgical procedures
   E. Urologic history
   F. Pelvic pain
   G. Vaginal bleeding
   H. Sexual status
   I. Contraceptive status
IV. Significant health problems
   A. Systemic illnesses
   B. Surgical procedures
   C. Other hospitalizations
V. Medications, habits, and allergies
   A. Medications taken
   B. Medication and other allergies
   C. Smoking history
   D. Alcohol usage
   E. Illicit drug usage
VI. Bleeding problems
VII. Family history
   A. Illnesses and causes of death of first-order relatives
   B. Congenital malformations, metal retardation, and reproductive loss
VIII. Occupational and avocational history
IX. Social history
X. Review of systems
   A. Head
   B. Cardiovascular
   C. Respiratory
   D. Gastrointestinal
   E. Genitourinary
   F. Neuromuscular
   G. Psychiatric
     1. Depression/anxiety
   H. Physical abuse
     1. Sexual abuse
       a. Incest
       b. Rape

LMP, last menstrual period; **PMP**, previous menstrual period.

By observing these nonverbal clues, the physician determines the appropriate style for conducting the interview. The act of greeting the woman by name, making eye contact, and shaking hands is a formal, but friendly start to the visit. Often an opening remark appropriate to the patient's demeanor may be useful, such as "You seem sad today, Ms. Jones" or "I detect a note of anger in your voice, Ms. Smith. Can you tell me why that is?" By so doing, the physician projects sensitivity to the patient's feelings and genuine care with respect to her circumstances.

Four qualities have been recognized as potentially important in caring communication skills: comfort, acceptance, responsiveness, and empathy. Despite the busy demands of clinical practice, effective communication skills enhance patient satisfaction and patient safety and decreases the likelihood of medical liability litigation. **Box 7-1** lists some components of effective physician communication.

ESSENCE OF THE GYNECOLOGIC HISTORY

CHIEF COMPLAINT

The patient should be encouraged to tell the physician why she has sought help. The chief complaint is a concise statement describing the woman's problem in her words. Questions such as "What is the nature of the problem that brought you to me?" or "How may I help you?" are good ways to begin.

HISTORY OF THE PRESENT ILLNESS (HPI)

The patient should be able to present the problem as she sees it, in her own words, and should be interrupted only for specific clarification of points or to offer direction if she digresses too far. During the interview the physician should face the patient with direct eye contact and acknowledge important points of the history, either by nodding or by offering a word or two. This approach allows the physician to be involved in the problem and demonstrates a degree of caring to the patient. When the patient has completed the history of her current problem, pertinent open-ended questions should be asked with respect to specific points. This process allows the physician to develop a more detailed database. Directed questions may be asked where pertinent to clarify points. In general, however, the patient should be encouraged to tell her story as she sees it rather than to react with short answers to very specific questions. Under the latter circumstance, the physician may get the answers he or she is looking for,

but they may not be accurate answers. When the HPI is written up for the medical record, it represents a chronologic history of the current problem.

A general outline for a gynecologic and general history is given in **Box 7-2**. The outline is given in a specific order for general orientation. The information, however, may be collected through any comfortable discussion with the patient that seems appropriate in the circumstances. It is important that all aspects be covered.

PERTINENT GYNECOLOGIC HISTORY

A pertinent gynecologic history can be divided into several parts. It begins with a menstrual history, in which the age of menarche, duration of each monthly cycle, number of days during which menses occurs, and regularity of the menstrual cycles should be noted. The dates of the last menstrual period and previous menstrual period should be obtained. In addition, the characteristics of the menstrual flow, including the color, the amount of flow, and accompanying symptoms, such as cramping, sweating, headache, or diarrhea, should be noted. In general, menstruation that occurs monthly (range 21 to 40 days), lasts 4 to 7 days, is bright red, and is often accompanied by cramping on the day preceding and the first day of the period is characteristic of an ovulatory cycle. Menstruation that is irregular, often dark in color, painless, and frequently short or very long may indicate lack of ovulation. The first few cycles in teenagers or cycles in premenopausal women are frequently **anovulatory cycles** and as a result may come at irregular intervals. Any vaginal bleeding not related to menses (intermenstrual bleeding) should be noted, as well as its relationship to the menstrual cycle and to other events, such as coitus (postcoital bleeding), the use of tampons, or the use of a contraceptive device. For the postmenopausal woman, the age at last menses, menopausal symptoms such as vasomotor complaints, history of hormone replacement therapy, and postmenopausal bleeding should be noted.

The second pertinent point in the gynecologic history is that of previous pregnancies. The woman should be asked specifically to list pregnancies, including the year of the pregnancy; the duration; the type of delivery; the size, sex, and current condition of the baby; any complications that may have occurred; and whether the infant was breast-fed and, if so, for how long. Elective terminations of pregnancy and spontaneous abortions should also be noted, including the time of gestation at termination and the circumstances under which they took place. Ectopic or molar pregnancies should also be noted, including the type of therapy that was given. When such events have occurred, obtaining old records for review is appropriate. Any pregnancy should be discussed with respect to excessive bleeding, chills, fever, known infection, diabetes mellitus, hypertension, or other complicating events. It is also appropriate to ask the woman about the individual who fathered each of these pregnancies so that the physician may start determining the number of sexual partners the woman has had. Women with multiple sexual partners are at increased risk for acquiring the human papillomavirus (HPV) and risk of cervical dysplasia and cancer as well as contracting sexually transmitted diseases (STDs).

A history of vaginal and pelvic infections should be obtained. The patient should be asked what types of infection she has had, what treatment she received, and what complications she experienced. Risk factors for human immunodeficiency virus (HIV) infection, such as intravenous drug abuse or coitus with drug abusers or bisexual men, should be sought by direct questioning and HIV screening offered where appropriate. All hospitalizations should be reviewed as to cause and outcome.

The physician should obtain a Pap smear screening history, including the date of the last Pap smear, the frequency of screening, and any abnormal tests and the treatment. The patient's HPV vaccination status should be checked. The woman's contraceptive history should be investigated, including methods used, length of time they have been used, effectiveness, and any complications that may have arisen.

All instances of gynecologic surgical procedures should be noted, including minor operations, such as endometrial biopsies; dilation and curettage; vulvar, vaginal, or cervical biopsies; cervical conization or cryotherapy; laparoscopic examinations; and any major procedure that the patient may have undergone. When such data are elicited, dates, types of procedures, diagnoses, and significant complications should be noted.

Box 7-3 Important Points of Sexual History

1. Sexual activity (presence of)
2. Types of relationships
3. Individual(s) involved
4. Satisfaction? Orgasmic? Desire/Interest?
5. Dyspareunia
6. Sexual dysfunction
   a. Patient
   b. Partner

In cases where pertinent, past records, particularly operative and pathology reports, should be sought.

A complete sexual history should be obtained (**Box 7-3**), and specific problems should be evaluated. The history should include whether the patient is sexually active, the types of relationships she has, whether she is orgasmic, whether she experiences pain or discomfort with coitus (**dyspareunia**), and whether she or her partner is experiencing problems with sexual performance (**sexual dysfunction**). It is important that the physician review or rehearse the types of questions that will be asked and consider the response he or she will give to less typical answers (e.g., responses concerning homosexuality or less common sexual practices). This helps to prevent the physician from demonstrating surprise and thus transmitting an attitude of disapproval. Counseling women to practice safe sex to avoid contracting sexually transmitted diseases may be relevant.

Symptoms of pelvic pain or discomfort should be discussed fully. Six common questions should be asked about the pain: location of the pain; timing of pain; quality of the pain such as throbbing, burning, colicky; radiation of pain to other body areas; intensity of pain on a scale of 1 to 10, with 10 being the worse pain imaginable; and duration of pain symptoms. Additional questions about what causes the pain to worsen or subside; the context of the pain symptoms; and associated triggers, signs, and symptoms may be helpful. The pain should be described, noting the presence or absence of a relationship to the menstrual cycle and its association with other events, such as coitus or bleeding and bladder and bowel symptoms.

GENERAL HEALTH HISTORY

The woman should be asked to list any significant health problems that she has had during her lifetime, including all hospitalizations and operative procedures. It is reasonable for the physician to ask about specific illnesses, such as diabetes, hepatitis, tuberculosis, or heart disease, that seem likely based on what is known about the woman or about her family history. Many physicians use a history checklist of the most common conditions.

Medications taken and reasons for doing so should be noted, as should allergic responses to medications. The woman should be encouraged to bring all medications, both prescription and over-the-counter drugs, including herbal preparations, to subsequent health maintenance visits. Most women who use complementary and alternative medicines do not offer this information to physicians.

The woman should be questioned for evidence of a bleeding or clotting problem, such as a history of hemorrhage with minor procedures, easy bruisability, or bleeding from mucous membranes.

A history of smoking should be obtained in detail, including amount, length of time she has smoked, and attempts at quitting smoking. She should be questioned about the use of illicit drugs, including marijuana, heroin, methamphetamines, cocaine, and prescription drug abuse like narcotics. Any affirmative answers should be followed by specific questions concerning length of use, types of drugs used, and side effects that may have been noticed. Her use of alcohol should be detailed carefully, including the number of drinks per day and any history of binge drinking or previous therapy for alcoholism.

FAMILY HISTORY

A detailed family history of first-order relatives (mother, father, sisters, brothers, children, and grandparents) should be taken and a family tree constructed (**Fig. 7-1**). Serious illnesses or causes of death for each individual should be noted. Also, an inquiry should be made about any congenital malformations, mental retardation, or pregnancy loss in either the woman's or her spouse's family. Such information may offer clues to hereditarily determined causes of reproductive problems.

OCCUPATIONAL AND SOCIAL HISTORY

The woman should be asked to detail her and her spouse's occupational histories, including jobs held and work performed. It is also useful to elicit a history of hobbies and other avocations that might affect health or reproductive capacity.

A social history should be obtained. This involves where and with whom the woman lives, other individuals in the household, areas of the world where the woman has lived or traveled, and unusual experiences that might affect her health.

SAFETY ISSUES

The patient should be questioned about safety matters. She should be asked about the use of seat belts and helmets (if she rides a bicycle or motorcycle or rides a horse). She should be asked whether there are firearms in her household and, if so,

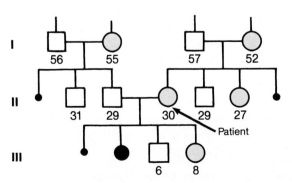

- ● Spontaneous miscarriage
- ◯ Living females
- ☐ Living males
- ● Female who died neonatally because of prematurity (30 weeks)

Figure 7-1 Family tree of typical gynecologic patient.

whether appropriate safety precautions are taken. A question about intimate partner violence is appropriate and can be asked in a nonthreatening manner, such as, "Has anyone in your household threatened or physically hurt you?"

A discussion regarding whether the patient's hearing is adequate to ensure safety while she goes about her usual activities is important, especially in older women who may be suffering hearing loss, but also in younger women who may use MP3- or iPod-type music players while they walk or jog. Appropriate footwear should be encouraged, taking into consideration the woman's usual activities, physical capabilities, and age.

REVIEW OF SYSTEMS

A complete review of systems is necessary to uncover symptoms from other areas that relate to reproduction and gynecologic problems (e.g., serious headaches, epileptic seizures, dizziness, or fainting spells) or other important medical conditions. Such a history also may indicate exposure to medications that may be injurious should a pregnancy occur. The general organ systems review includes asking about constitutional systems; eyes, ears, nose and throat; skin problems; and musculoskeletal problems. Questions on dieting habits may be relevant to unmask potentially serious disorders such as anorexia, bulimia, or binge/purge cycles. Early counseling to avoid **obesity** may be relevant.

It is important to obtain a good cardiovascular/respiratory history, as well as a history of hypertension, heart disease, rheumatic fever, or chest problems, such as asthma and lack of exercise and smoking. Each of these may have an immediate effect on the patient and may also influence a future pregnancy.

Of importance to the gynecologist is a history of gastrointestinal disorders, such as functional bowel problems, diverticulitis, diverticulosis, or hepatitis. Patients should be asked about any anal incontinence of gas or stool that they may be experiencing or have experienced in the past. Affirmative answers should be fully investigated with respect to specific illnesses that may affect the patient's current health or well-being.

Questions about the genitourinary system are important both from the standpoint of bladder function and as an indication of whether renal function has been or is impaired. A history of bladder dysfunction, **dysuria**, loss of urine (incontinence), acute or chronic bladder or kidney infections, bladder pain, urinary frequency, nocturia, or other urologic problems, such as hematuria or the passage of kidney stones, should be noted.

Neurologic or neuromuscular impairment may be important from the standpoint of the ability of the patient to carry and deliver a child without difficulty. Similarly, asking about endocrine symptoms of diabetes mellitus and thyroid disease are relevant. Menstrual abnormalities may be symptomatic of endocrine problems that affect the hypothalamic-pituitary-ovarian axis.

A history of vascular disease, including thrombophlebitis with or without pulmonary embolism, varicose veins, or other vascular problems, should be sought. If a positive history of thrombophlebitis is obtained, possible relationship to a hormonal exposure, such as pregnancy or oral contraceptive use, should be determined.

The psychiatric history should be detailed carefully for any emotional or mental disease processes. Specifically, evidence for depression and suicidal ideology should be sought. In addition, the patient should be asked specifically whether she has been sexually abused in adult life, in childhood, by a stranger or incestuously, or raped. This topic is further discussed in Chapter 9 (Emotional Aspects of Gynecology). Finally, she should be questioned about the possibility of physical abuse, neglect, or intimidation, and elder abuse must not be forgotten.

ESSENCE OF COMPLETE PHYSICAL EXAMINATION

The gynecologist should perform a complete physical examination on every patient at the first visit and at each annual checkup, particularly if the gynecologist is the primary physician caring for the patient. Physical examination is a time both to gather information about the patient and to teach the woman information she should know about herself and her body.

The patient should disrobe completely and cover herself with a hospital gown that ensures warmth and modesty. During each step of the examination she should be allowed to maintain personal control by being offered options whenever possible. These options begin with the presence or absence of a chaperone. The chaperone, a third party, usually a woman, serves a variety of purposes. She may offer warmth, compassion, and support to the patient during uncomfortable or potentially embarrassing portions of the examination. She may help the physician to carry out procedures, such as the Papanicolaou (Pap) smear, and in some cases she offers the physician protection from having his or her intentions misunderstood by a naïve or suspicious individual. Although the presence of a chaperone is not absolutely imperative in every physician-patient relationship, the availability of one for the specific instance where it is deemed advisable should be ensured. Many clinics insist on the presence of a chaperone, and it is wise for the physician to follow local custom.

The examination should begin with a general evaluation of the patient's appearance and affect. Her weight, height, and blood pressure should be taken initially. A **body mass index (BMI)** can be calculated by the following formula: weight in pounds divided by the height squared in inches and times 700. Online calculators are readily available. Postmenopausal women should have their height measured routinely to document evidence of osteoporosis, which causes loss of height from vertebral compression fractures. Some institutions require a pain scale reporting at each visit and consider it a fourth vital sign.

The patient's eyes, ears, nose, and throat should be examined. Funduscopic examination should be performed at least annually to inspect the blood vessels of the retina and to observe the lens for evidence of early cataract formation. Although few gynecologists perform this exam, reminding the woman to have regular eye exams is important. The patient should be inspected for evidence of upper lip or chin hair, which may indicate increased androgen activity.

The thyroid gland should be palpated for irregularities or increase in size (goiter). Discrete areas of enlargement, hardness, and tenderness should be described. The patient's neck should be palpated for evidence of adenopathy along the supraclavicular and posterior auricular chains.

The chest should be inspected for symmetry of movement of the diaphragm, percussed for areas of consolidation, and auscultated bilaterally for breath and adventitious sounds. Wheezing or rales should be noted.

The heart should be examined by palpation for points of maximum impulse, percussed for size, and auscultated for

Table 7-1 Clinical Breast Examination Elements

1. Examination of each breast with the patient sitting with arms raised, and with the patient supine
2. Attention to the entire breast mound from midsternum to the posterior axillary line and from the costal margin to the clavicle
3. Inspection and palpation to assess:
    Skin flattening or dimpling
    Skin erythema
    Skin edema
    Nipple retraction
    Nipple eczema
    Nipple discharge
    Breast fixation
    Tissue thickening
    Palpable masses
4. Evaluation for axillary and supraclavicular lymphadenopathy

irregularities of rate and evidence of murmurs and other adventitious sounds. An older woman's neck should be auscultated for evidence of vascular bruits. The patient's heart should be auscultated in both the lying and the sitting positions.

A careful breast examination should be carried out in a systematic fashion. To summarize a detailed clinical breast examination, refer to **Table 7-1**. Research has shown the following factors are associated with a high-quality breast examination: longer duration, thorough coverage of the breast, a consistent exam pattern, use of variable pressure with the finger pads, and use of the three middle fingers. Recommending breast self-examination has been controversial as two trials, from Russia and China, do not suggest benefit. More research is needed on both breast self-examination and clinical breast examination. Although there is lack of definitive data to support or refute the usefulness of breast self-examination, it is reasonable to teach the exam so the woman becomes familiar with her own breast irregularities and texture.

The abdomen should be systematically examined as detailed in the following sections.

ABDOMINAL INSPECTION

The abdomen should be inspected for symmetry; scars, protuberance, or discoloration of the skin; and striations, which may suggest previous pregnancies or adrenal gland hyperactivity. The hair pattern should be noted. The typical female escutcheon is that of an inverted triangle over the mons pubis. A male escutcheon involves hair growth between the area of the mons pubis and the umbilicus, also known as a diamond pattern, and may indicate excessive androgen activity in the patient (**Fig. 7-2**).

ABDOMINAL PALPATION

The abdomen should be palpated for organomegaly (enlarged organs), particularly involving the liver, spleen, kidneys, and uterus, and for adnexal masses, which may be palpated abdominally, if large. Palpation also affords the possibility of noting a fluid wave, which would suggest either ascites or hemoperitoneum. Palpation also yields evidence for rigidity of the abdomen, which would imply spasm in the rectus muscles secondary to intraabdominal irritation. Where the irritation is caused by intraabdominal hemorrhage or infection, this rigidity is often evidence of an acute abdomen. During the palpation of the

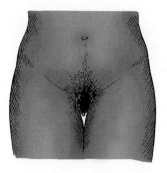 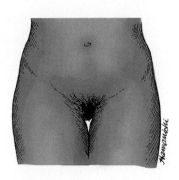

Figure 7-2 Normal female pubic hair pattern (right) and hair pattern of female showing male (androgenized) pattern (left).

abdomen, the physician should elicit the phenomenon of *rebound,* which also signifies intraabdominal irritation, by gently pressing the abdomen and then releasing. The release may cause pain either under the spot (direct rebound) or in a different portion of the abdomen (referred rebound). It should be noted, however, that sudden, rough pressure may cause pain even in a normal patient. Gentle pressure carried out systematically may elicit painful "trigger points." With the woman straining or simulating an abdominal sit-up, an abdominal or incisional hernia may be visualized and the fascial defect palpated.

ABDOMINAL PERCUSSION

Percussion affords the ability to differentiate fluid waves and to outline solid organs and masses.

ABDOMINAL AUSCULTATION

The physician should listen for bowel sounds. Hypoactive or absent bowel sounds may imply an ileus caused by peritoneal irritation of the bowel. Hyperactive bowel sounds may imply intrinsic irritation of the bowel or partial or complete bowel obstruction.

The groin should be palpated for adenopathy and inguinal hernias. The physician should also elicit the femoral pulses beneath the groin in the femoral triangles, and when these are present, the differences that may exist between the two femoral areas should be noted.

Legs should be examined for evidence of varicose veins, edema, venous stasis changes or ulcers (particularly in diabetics), and other lesions. In addition, it is reasonable to judge arterial circulation to the extremities by palpating pedal pulses on the dorsum of the foot.

PELVIC EXAMINATION

The pelvic examination is conducted with the patient lying supine on the examining table with her legs in stirrups. The patient may or may not desire to be draped with a sheet. Because the physician should be pointing out aspects of the patient's pelvic anatomy where possible, many patients prefer to have the head of the table elevated and to use a small hand mirror to follow the examination with the physician. In such instances, a sheet may be cumbersome. The physician should be sure the patient is as relaxed as possible and should take a few minutes to describe the procedure and allow the shy or nervous patient to prepare herself. Suggesting that the patient allow her legs to fall wide apart and concentrate on relaxing her abdominal muscles may be helpful.

INSPECTION

The perineum should be carefully inspected beginning with the mons pubis. The quality and pattern of the hair on the mons and the labia majora should be noted. Areas of alopecia should be noted because they may imply a skin abnormality. In general, as a woman ages, the pubic hair becomes less dense and may turn gray. During the inspection of the pubic hair the physician should look for evidence of body lice (pediculosis). Next, the skin of the perineum is inspected for redness, excoriation, discoloration, or loss of pigment and for the presence of vesicles, ulcerations, pustules, warty growths, or neoplastic growths. In addition, pigmented nevi or other pigmented lesions should be noted, as should varicose veins. Skin scars denoting previous episiotomy or other obstetric lacerations should be noted.

Next, the specific structures of the perineum should be systematically evaluated. The clitoris should be noted and its size and shape described. Normally it is 1 to 1.5 cm in length. Any irregularities or abnormalities of the labia majora or minora should be noted and carefully described. At times these areas are injured by trauma related to coitus, accidental injury, or childbearing. The patient should be questioned about evidence of trauma when appropriate.

The introitus should be observed closely. Whether the hymen is intact, imperforate, or open and whether the perineum gapes or remains closed in the usual lithotomy position should be noted.

The perineal body, the area at the posterior aspect of the labia where the muscles of the superficial perineal compartment come together, should be inspected. It represents the focal point of support for the perineum and is between the vagina and the rectum. The perianal area is then inspected for evidence of hemorrhoids, sphincter injury, warts, and other lesions (**Fig. 7-3**).

PALPATION

The next step in the examination of the perineum involves palpation. With the second and fourth fingers of the gloved hand separating the labia minora, the urethra is inspected and the length of the urethra is palpated and "milked" with the middle finger. In this way, irregularities and inflammation of Skene's glands (periurethral glands), pus or mucus expressed, or a suburethral diverticulum can be noted. Any pus expressed from the urethra should be submitted for Gram stain and cultured, because it is frequently found to contain gonococci. The gloved

Figure 7-3 Normal female perineum. (Redrawn from Krantz KE: Anatomy of the female reproductive system. In Benson RC [ed]: Current Obstetric and Gynecologic Diagnosis and Treatment, 5th ed. Los Altos, CA, Lange Medical, 1984.)

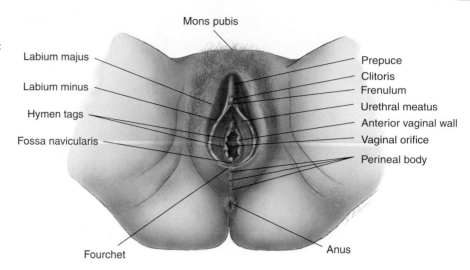

Mons pubis

Labium majus

Labium minus

Hymen tags

Fossa navicularis

Prepuce

Clitoris

Frenulum

Urethral meatus

Anterior vaginal wall

Vaginal orifice

Perineal body

Fourchet

Anus

hand then palpates the area of the posterior third of the labia majora, placing the index finger inside the introitus and the thumb on the outside of the labium. In this way, enlargements or cysts of Bartholin's glands are noted. This exercise should be performed on each side.

With the gloved hand holding the labia apart, the opening of the vagina should be inspected. The presence of a cystocele or a cystourethrocele should be noted. This would be seen as a bulging of vaginal mucosa downward from the anterior wall of the vagina. The presence of this abnormality may be noted either by simply observing or by asking the patient to bear down (**Fig. 7-4**). Likewise, the posterior wall should be observed for a bulging upward, which would represent a rectocele (**Fig. 7-5**). A cystic bulge in the cul-de-sac may represent an enterocele (**Fig. 7-6**). Also, with the patient bearing down, the cervix may become visible, indicating prolapse of the uterus (**Fig. 7-7**). Each of these observations is evidence for relaxation of the pelvic supports. Accurate evaluation of pelvic organ prolapse is improved by examining the woman standing with her legs spread apart and with a Valsalva maneuver.

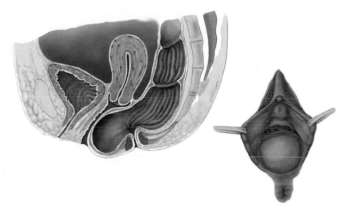

Figure 7-5 Side and direct views of rectocele. (Redrawn from Symmonds RE: Relaxations of pelvic supports. In Benson RC [ed]: Current Obstetric and Gynecologic Diagnosis and Treatment, 5th ed. Los Altos, CA, Lange Medical, 1984.)

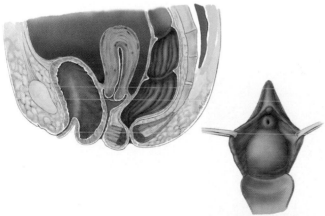

Figure 7-4 Side and direct views of cystocele. (Redrawn from Symmonds RE: Anatomy of the female reproductive system. In Benson RC [ed]: Current Obstetric and Gynecologic Diagnosis and Treatment, 5th ed. Los Altos, CA, Lange Medical, 1984.)

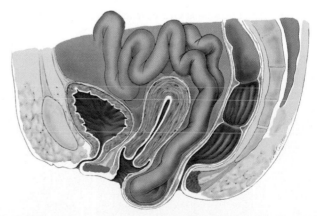

Figure 7-6 Lateral view of enterocele. (Redrawn from Symmonds RE: Relaxations of pelvic supports. In Benson RC [ed]: Current Obstetric and Gynecologic Diagnosis and Treatment, 5th ed. Los Altos, CA, Lange Medical, 1984.)

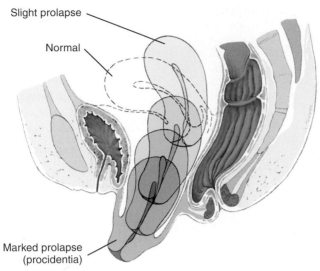

Slight prolapse

Normal

Marked prolapse
(procidentia)

Figure 7-7 Depiction of prolapse of uterus. (Redrawn from Symmonds RE: Relaxations of pelvic supports. In Benson RC [ed]: Current Obstetric and Gynecologic Diagnosis and Treatment, 5th ed. Los Altos, CA, Lange Medical, 1984.)

The descriptions, definitions, and staging of pelvic organ prolapse have been used in many variations but were not standardized until 1996. The International Continence Society Committee of Standardization of Terminology, Subcommittee on Pelvic Organ Prolapse and Pelvic Floor Dysfunction has been collaborating with the American Urogynecology Society and the Society of Gynecologic Surgeons to develop a standardized site-specific system for describing, quantitating, and staging pelvic support in women. Its purpose is to enhance clinical and academic communication with respect to individual patients and populations of patients. In 1996, these organizations adopted this system. Basically, stages I to IV are recognized for pelvic organ prolapse with stage II being within 1 centimeter above or below the hymen and an easy reference point to remember. It is discussed and defined in Chapter 20 (Anatomic Defects of the Abdominal Wall and Pelvic Floor).

SPECULUM EXAMINATION

After palpation, the physician chooses the appropriate speculum for the patient. The typical Graves speculum generally is of three sizes: small, which is used in young children, women who have undergone tight perineal repair, or in the aged patient who has undergone severe involution; medium, used for most women; and large, which is often useful in large or obese women or those who are grand multiparas. Also available is the Pederson speculum, which is the length of the Graves speculum but narrower, for women who have not become active sexually, have never been pregnant, or have not used tampons. It is also of value for women who have undergone operations that have narrowed the vaginal diameter. For the majority of women the length of the vagina is similar, approximately 6 to 8 cm, and the Pederson or medium Graves speculum is appropriate (**Fig. 7-8**) for them.

The speculum should be warmed, either by a warming device or by being placed in warm water, and then touched to the patient's leg to determine that she feels the temperature is appropriate and comfortable. The speculum is then inserted by placing the transverse diameter of the blades in the anteroposterior position and guiding the blades through the introitus in a downward motion with the tips pointing toward the rectum. Because the anterior wall of the vagina is backed by the pubic symphysis, which is rigid, pressure upward causes the patient discomfort. This is avoided by following the described method of introducing the speculum. Also, in the resting state the vagina lies on the rectum and actually extends posteriorly from the introitus. The procedure may be facilitated by placing two fingers into the introitus and pressing down.

Once the blades are inserted, the speculum should be turned so that the transverse axis of the blades is in the transverse axis of the vagina. The blades should be inserted to their full length and then opened so that the physician may inspect for the position of the cervix. The cervix generally fits into the open blades with ease. If this does not occur, the physician should inspect for the position of the cervix with his or her finger and then reinsert the speculum accordingly. Once the blades are inserted and the cervix is visualized, the speculum should be opened and the introitus widened so that the cervix can be adequately inspected and a Pap smear taken. This can be done by using the screw adjustment on the base of the speculum. When inserted properly, the speculum generally stays in place.

The physician then inspects the vagina and cervix. The vaginal canal is inspected during the insertion of the speculum or on its removal. The vaginal epithelium should be noted for evidence of erythema or lesions. Fluid discharge should be evaluated for pH and on slides prepared by placing one drop of vaginal secretion in one drop of sodium chloride solution, placing a cover slip over the specimen, and inspecting it for unicellular flagellated

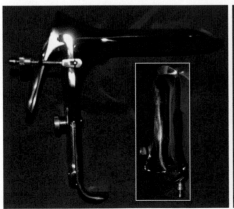

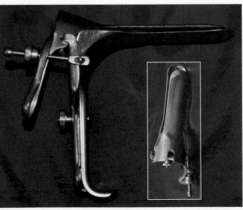

Figure 7-8 (NEW) Graves *(left)* and Pederson *(right)* specula.

protozoa, *Trichomonas vaginalis.* The vaginal epithelial cells should also be inspected. The cells should have sharp borders and normal-appearing nuclei. Any variation from the normal appearance of cells may imply infection (see Chapter 23, Infections of the Upper and Lower Genital Tract). A drop of potassium hydroxide is placed on another slide, and a drop of vaginal secretion is placed within this. The potassium hydroxide causes lysis of the epithelial cells and trichomonads but leaves intact the mycelium of *Candida.* Thus, the presence of mycelium is helpful in diagnosing vaginal candidiasis. Vaginal lesions, such as areas of adenosis (see Chapter 11, Congenital Abnormalities of the Female Reproductive Tract), clear cystic structures (Gartner's cysts), or inclusion cysts on the lines of scars or episiotomy incisions, should be noted.

The cervix is inspected next. It should be pink, shiny, and clear. In a nulliparous individual, the external os should be round. When a woman is parous, the external os takes on a fishmouth appearance, and if there have been cervical lacerations, healed stellate lacerations may be noted (**Fig. 7-9**). Normally, the transformation zone (i.e., the junction of squamous and columnar epithelium) is just barely visible inside the external os. Occasionally, glandular epithelium may be present on the **portio vaginalis**, moving the transformation zone onto the portio. This is common in teenage girls, women who have been exposed to diethylstilbestrol in utero, some women with vaginitis, or women immediately postpartum or postabortion. Generally, this is cleared by a process of **metaplasia**, in which squamous epithelium covers the columnar epithelium. This process, however, may leave small areas of irregularities and inclusion cysts, called **nabothian cysts**, which may be seen in various sizes and shapes. They are of no clinical significance. Often after a woman has delivered a baby, there is lateral scarring at the 3 o'clock and 9 o'clock positions, causing an eversion of the external os so that the reddened columnar epithelium is visible on the anterior and posterior lips of the cervix. If the observer looks closely, the transitional zone can be seen along the edges of this area of eversion and may be perfectly healthy. This is called an **ectropion** and is not evidence of a pathologic condition.

Any lesions of the cervix should be noted and, where appropriate, a biopsy should be performed. In a patient with acute herpes simplex, vesicles or ulcers may be noted. In a patient infected with human papillomavirus, warts (condylomata acuminata) on the cervix may also be observed.

PAPANICOLAOU SMEAR

At this point in the examination a Pap smear is usually taken. In 1943, Papanicolaou and Trout published their now classic monograph demonstrating the value of vaginal and cervical cytology as a screening tool for cervical neoplasm. With the use of the Pap smear in screening programs, the incidence of invasive cervical cancer has been reduced 50%. The 2009, the American College of Obstetricians and Gynecologists (ACOG) Practice Bulletin guidelines now advise that initial screening should begin at age 21 regardless of when sexual activity began. The Pap cytology screening interval may be extended from the usual 1 year to 2 years in women ages 21 to 29 and every 3 years in certain low-risk individuals after age 30 if three consecutive Pap smears are negative. High-risk women, including HIV seropositive women, immunosuppressed women, women exposed to DES in utero, and women previously treated for dysplasia or cervical cancer should be screened annually. A case-control study by Shy and colleagues questioned the wisdom of extending the screening interval beyond 2 years. Although no significant increase was noted in the incidence of cervical cancer in women screened every 2 years compared with those screened annually, the risk increased 3.9 times if the interval was 3 years and 12.3 times in women not screened for 10 years. The presence of risk factors did not influence these results. Pap smear screening may stop between the ages of 65 and 70, although various organizations (ACOG, the United States Preventive Services Task Force [USPSTF], and the American Cancer Society) differ on the exact age. But certain criteria should be met, including having three consecutive negative screens in the prior decade. This recommendation may be altered depending on a history of new sexual partners or a history of prior dysplasia where 20 years of yearly screening is advised. It is important to remember that 50% of cervical cancer cases develop in women who have never had a Pap test or very infrequent testing. So if a woman is 65 years old and has never been screened, the provider may wish to continue screening. No Pap smear screening is necessary after a hysterectomy done for benign conditions. A 2007 study reported that 15% of Pap tests were performed in hysterectomized women, most of whom, according to current guidelines, should not be screened. However, if a supracervical hysterectomy was performed, the same screening guidelines pertain as if there had been no hysterectomy, since the cervix remains in situ.

A Pap smear can be performed in a number of ways. The major objective is to sample exfoliated cells from the endocervical canal and to scrape the transitional zone. It is also useful to sample the vaginal pool, although this does not usually yield as high an incidence of cervical disease as does sampling of the canal and the transitional zone. One way of performing the Pap smear is as follows:

1. After excess mucus is gently removed (routine swabbing may cause insufficient cells to be sampled), the endocervical canal is sampled with either a cotton-tipped applicator or a Cytobrush, which is placed into the canal and rotated. Although both instruments generally dislodge adequate numbers of cells for study, the Cytobrush appears to give more accurate results and higher yields of positive findings. The material obtained is then smeared thinly on a microscope slide by rotation of the swab or brush on the glass surface. This is labeled *endocervix* and fixed immediately either by use of a spray fixative or by immersion of the slide into a fixative solution (**Fig. 7-10**).

2. With an Ayres spatula or some variation thereof, the entire transformation zone is scraped and the sample smeared thinly on a second slide, which is immediately fixed. If the physician wishes a sample of the vaginal pool, this may be taken with the reverse side of the Ayres spatula and smeared on a third

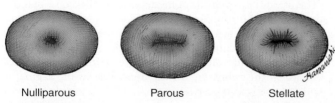

Nulliparous   Parous   Stellate

Figure 7-9 Nulliparous, parous, and stellate lacerations of cervix.

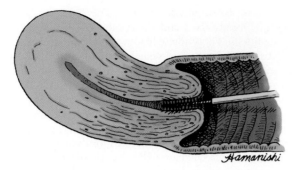

Figure 7-10 Obtaining cells from endocervix using a Cytobrush.

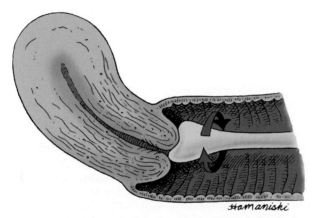

Figure 7-11 Obtaining cells from transformation zone using Ayers spatula.

slide or on a second portion of the slide containing the transformation zone material (**Fig. 7-11**). Recent data suggest an extended-tip spatula is better for collecting endocervical cells. The best results come from using both the Cytobrush and an extended-tip spatula.

A number of fixatives are available, but it is important that they be applied immediately before drying and distortion of the cells takes place. Newer liquid-based, thin-layer Pap smear preparations are available. No slides are needed. The Cytobrush and spatula are used to obtain cervical cells as described earlier, and they both are placed in a liquid jar of fixative and gently rotated to dislodge cells in the liquid. Evidence-based data show both a Pap slide prepared in a conventional manner and liquid-based methods for cervical cytology screening are acceptable. Pap smears may be reported using the following descriptive system (2001 Bethesda system):

Negative for Intraepithelial Lesion or Malignancy
Epithelial Cell Abnormality
Squamous cell

- Atypical squamous cells (ASC)
- Low-grade squamous intraepithelial lesions (LSIL)
- High-grade squamous intraepithelial lesions (HGSIL)
- Squamous cell carcinoma

Glandular cell

- Atypical glandular cells (AGC)
- Atypical glandular cells, favor neoplastic

- Endocervical adenocarcinoma in situ (AIS)
- Adenocarcinoma

Interpretation/Result
Other nonneoplastic findings:

- Reactive
  - inflammation
  - radiation
  - intrauterine contraceptive device
- Glandular cells status posthysterectomy
- Atrophy

Organisms

- Cellular changes consistent with herpes simplex
- *Trichomonas vaginalis* infection
- Bacteria consistent with *Actinomyces* infection
- Fungal organisms
- Shift in flora suggestive of bacterial vaginosis

In most instances, particularly with new patients and women younger than 25, it is appropriate to screen for chlamydia and gonorrhea using swabs that sample secretions from the endocervical canal. This step may be performed after the Pap smear. The gold standard now is nucleic acid amplification testing (**NAAT**) of the urine or endocervix (not vaginal secretions), rather than a culture. Yearly chlamydia testing is recommended for all sexually active women up to age 25.

BIMANUAL EXAMINATION

The bimanual examination allows the physician to palpate the uterus and the adnexa. The lubricated index and middle fingers of the dominant hand are placed within the vagina, and the thumb is folded under so as not to cause the patient distress in the area of the mons pubis, clitoris, and pubic symphysis. The fingers are inserted deeply into the vagina so that they rest beneath the cervix in the posterior fornix. The physician should be in a comfortable position at this point, generally with the leg on the side of the vaginal examining hand on a table lift and the elbow of that arm resting on the knee. The opposite hand is placed on the patient's abdomen above the pubic symphysis. The flat of the fingers are used for palpation. The physician then elevates the uterus by pressing up on the cervix and delivering the uterus to the abdominal hand so that the uterus may be placed between the two hands, thereby identifying its position, size, shape, consistency, and mobility. In the normal and nonpregnant state, the uterus is approximately 6 cm × 4 cm and weighs about 70 g. It may be somewhat larger in a woman who has had children (**Fig. 7-12**).

Enlargement of the uterus should be described in detail. Size may be estimated in centimeters or by comparing with weeks of normal gestational age.

The uterus in two thirds of instances is anteflexed so that the abdominal hand is palpating the posterior wall of the uterus and the vaginal fingers the anterior wall. The uterus may be retroverted. If it is positioned in a straight line with the vagina, it is said to be midposition or first-degree retroverted; if it lies backward in the cul-de-sac off the direct line of the vagina, it is said to be second-degree retroverted; if it is flexed deeply into the cul-de-sac pressing toward the rectum, it is third-degree retroverted. A third-degree retroverted uterus that cannot be

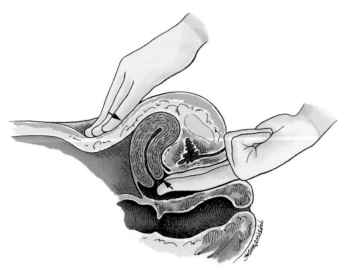

Figure 7-12 Bimanual examination of uterus.

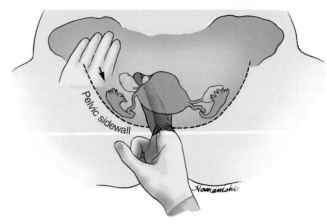

Figure 7-13 Bimanual examination of adnexa.

brought forward by manipulation is best examined by rectovaginal examination, which is described later in the chapter. The general shape of the uterus is that of a pear, with the broadest portion at the upper pole of the fundus. Generally, the uterus is mobile, and if it fails to move, it may be fixed by adhesions. The surface should be smooth; irregularities may indicate the presence of uterine leiomyomas (fibroids).

The shape of the uterus should also be described in detail. The consistency of the uterus is generally firm but not rock hard, and this should be noted in the examination. Any undue tenderness caused by palpation or movement of the uterus should be noted, because it may imply an inflammatory process.

Attention is then turned to examination of the adnexa. If the right hand is the pelvic hand, the first two fingers of the right hand are then moved into the right vaginal fornix as deeply as they can be inserted. The abdominal hand is placed just medial to the anterior superior iliac spine on the right, the two hands are brought as close together as possible, and with a sliding motion from the area of the anterior superior iliac spine to the introitus, the fingers are swept downward, allowing for the adnexa to be palpated between them. A normal ovary is approximately 3 cm × 2 cm (about the size of a walnut) and will sweep between the two fingers with ease unless it is fixed in an abnormal position by adhesions. When the adnexa is palpated, its size, mobility, and consistency should be described. However, this portion of the examination should be brief, because it causes the patient a mild to moderate sickening sensation. When the right adnexa has been palpated, the left adnexa should be palpated in a similar fashion by turning the vaginal hand to the left vaginal fornix and repeating the exercise on the left side (**Fig. 7-13**). Adnexa are usually not palpable in postmenopausal women because of involution and retraction of the ovary to a position higher in the pelvis. A palpable organ in such an individual may need further investigation for ovarian pathology if enlarged, although mostly benign or no disease is found.

RECTOVAGINAL EXAMINATION

After completing the vaginal portion of the bimanual examination, the middle finger is relubricated with a water-soluble lubricant and placed into the rectum. Many physicians think the glove

should be changed so as not to contaminate the rectum with vaginal organisms or HPV. The index finger is reinserted into the vagina. In this fashion the rectovaginal septum is palpated between the two fingers, and any thickness or mass is noted. The finger should also attempt to identify the uterosacral ligaments, which extend from the posterior wall of the cervix posteriorly and laterally toward the sacrum. Any thickening or beadiness of these structures may imply an inflammatory reaction or endometriosis. If the uterus is retroverted, that organ should be outlined for size, shape, and consistency at this point. It may be examined appropriately using the fingers inserted into the vagina and the rectum, as well as using the abdominal hand (**Fig. 7-14**).

RECTAL EXAMINATION

The rectum is then palpated in all dimensions with the rectal examining finger. It should be possible to palpate as many as 70% of distal bowel lesions with the rectal finger. Because bowel

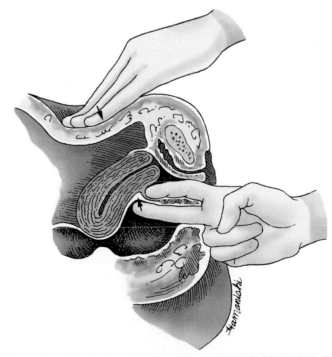

Figure 7-14 Rectovaginal examination.

cancer is common in women, particularly after the age of 50, this part of the examination should not be overlooked. The physician should also note the tone of the anal sphincter and any other anal abnormalities, such as hemorrhoids, fissures, or masses. A stool sample taken on the rectal examining finger and tested for occult blood is no longer recommended for office screening. A recent large trial found this technique missed 95% of polyps and cancers that were found at subsequent colonoscopy. Better screening for colorectal cancer is described later in this chapter. This is particularly important in women past the age of 50 who may be at risk for bowel cancer.

At the end of the examination the physician should give the patient some facial tissue so that she may remove the lubricating jelly from her perineum before she dresses.

It is important that each step of the examination be explained to the patient and that she is reassured about all normal findings. Wherever possible, abnormal findings should be pointed out to the patient either by allowing her to palpate the pathologic condition or by demonstrating it to her using a hand mirror. It is also appropriate to demonstrate normal structures to the patient, such as the cervix and portions of the vagina that she may be able to see with her hand mirror. The physician should use the examination as a vehicle for teaching the patient about her body.

THE ANNUAL VISIT

The annual visit is important for both health maintenance and preventive medicine reasons. Although the visit varies in emphasis depending on the patient's age, the long-term goals should be to maintain the woman in the best health and functional status possible, to promote high-quality longevity, and to aid in early detection of disease. Long-term continuity of care may improve health status. Major preventable problems must be discussed because patient behavior can make a difference. Various medical groups update recommendations for primary and preventive screening services regularly. Much of this chapter utilizes guidelines from the United States Preventive Services Task Force (USPSTF), American College of Obstetricians and Gynecologists (ACOG), Centers for Disease Control and Prevention (CDC), Morbidity and Mortality Weekly Report (MMWR), other subspecialty guidelines, and the Agency for Healthcare Research and Quality. The latter is a clearinghouse of evidence-based guidelines that allows comparison of differing recommendations, as many societies do not always agree on these guidelines. Their websites can be checked for updates.

Is it important not to confuse screening with diagnosis. Screening is looking for a condition in an asymptomatic woman. Diagnostic tests are performed to clarify the etiology of a woman's complaints (symptoms) and are not screening. So when one of the organizations like the USPSTF makes a recommendation for screening for chlamydia yearly up to age 25, it does not mean you should not test a 26-year-old woman who has symptoms of vaginal discharge. Furthermore, screening recommendations need to be considered in light of local prevalence of disease and additional risk factors an individual patient might present. The USPSTF also makes recommendations that are qualified by a grade: A = strongly recommends; B = recommends; C = no recommendation for or against; D = recommends against; and I = insufficient evidence to recommend for or against.

A 2004 article published in the *Journal of the American Medical Association* estimated the root causes of American deaths and attributed 18% to tobacco, 15% to poor diet and physical inactivity, 3.5% to alcohol, 4% to microbial agents, 1% to illicit drug use, 2% to toxic agents, 1.2% to firearms, 1.8% to motor vehicles, and 1% to sexual behavior. Obviously, much of this can be altered by patients taking an active role in changing their behavior, and physicians have the opportunity to advise them at the annual visit.

Although the gynecologist is generally the primary physician for women during their reproductive years, until recently this was not necessarily the case for postmenopausal women. However, it has become clear that the gynecologist with appropriate training and motivation can continue being the primary physician for older women as well. In 1618, an English clergyman observed, "Prevention is so much better than healing because it saves the labor of being sick." In 1973, Belloc reported that in a study of women past the age of 45, the life expectancy was 7 years greater for those who routinely practiced six of seven important health habits as compared with those who practiced three or fewer (**Box 7-4**). These recommendations hold true today according to a 2009 report from the Agency for Healthcare Research and Quality (AHRQ). During the annual visit, physicians should therefore discuss nutrition regarding (1) proper caloric intake to maintain the patient's weight near her optimum and avoid obesity, (2) restricting saturated fat and cholesterol, and (3) understanding the need for adequate calcium and vitamin D in the diet.

At each checkup the physician should also encourage the patient to develop an exercise program appropriate for her abilities and to avoid smoking and excessive alcohol use (if she has these habits). The physician should discuss possible stressors in the patient's life, such as her relationship with her husband or partner and other family members, her satisfaction or dissatisfaction with her job, and other social problems that she may be experiencing. It is appropriate to ask questions that assess her sexual activity and gratification and questions that detect abuse or intimidation in her life. It is also appropriate to discuss the physical and emotional implications of loss and grief. Everyone suffers loss during his or her lifetime, and the older the patient the more likely that this is the case. Grief may be the result of a loss of a spouse or loved one, a pet, a job, a body part, or the ability to perform activities the patient has enjoyed (see Chapter 9, Emotional Aspects of Gynecology).

The patient should be asked to bring all medications that she is taking. Prescription and over-the-counter drugs, as well as any dietary or herbal supplements, should be included. This will give

---

Box 7-4   Good Health Habits

Eat moderately
Eat a healthy diet focusing on fruits, vegetables, whole grains, and foods low in saturated fats*
Eat breakfast
Be tobacco free
Exercise regularly; 30 minutes or more on most days of the week
Use alcohol in moderation or not at all
Sleep 7 to 8 hours per night
Stay at a healthy weight†

*Modified from original according to AHRQ recommendations.
†Added to original according to AHRQ recommendations.

the physician the opportunity to review with the patient why she is taking each one and also to assess for possible potential adverse drug interactions. It may also be possible to tie specific drug use to an undesirable symptom the patient may be experiencing.

The annual visit is an opportunity for the physician to screen for a variety of illnesses affecting not only the reproductive organs but all of the organ systems. The visit should include an interim health history and a complete physical examination. The weight, height, and blood pressure measurements and the breast, pelvic, and rectal examinations should all be performed and recorded so that comparisons may be made from year to year. A gross assessment of the patient's hearing ability and visual acuity should be performed annually in women over 65 years of age.

The American College of Obstetricians and Gynecologists Task Force on Primary Preventive Health Care recommended screening laboratory tests for the annual visit for women in different age groups (**Table 7-2**). It is recommended that an annual Pap smear be begun at age 21, which was a significant change in the guidelines in 2009. For women younger than 18 who are in specific high-risk groups, hemoglobin, urine testing for bacteriuria, testing for sexually transmitted diseases (chlamydia yearly if

sexually active and gonorrhea and human immunodeficiency virus (HIV), if high risk; **Box 7-5**) and genetic testing, rubella titer, tuberculosis skin test, lipid profile, and hepatitis C virus testing may be appropriate.

For women age 19 to 39, Pap smear screening intervals were discussed earlier in this chapter under "Papanicolaou Smear." Human papillomavirus (HPV) typing and use for screening for cervical disease is discussed in Chapter 28 (Intraepithelial Neoplasia of the Lower Genital Tract [Cervix, Vulva, Vagina]). Women with diabetes, positive family history of heart disease, hypertension, or tobacco abuse should have a fasting cholesterol and high-density lipoprotein (HDL) cholesterol test. The United States Preventive Services Task Force (USPSTF) only recommends screening for type 2 diabetes in individuals with hypertension (sustained blood pressure greater than 135/80 mm Hg) in asymptomatic women. The American College of Obstetricians and Gynecologists and Center for Disease Control recommend routine human immunodeficiency virus (HIV) screening for women aged 19 to 64 years at least once in their lifetime and targeted screening for women with risk factors outside of that age range. For women in this age group who are at high risk,

Table 7-2 Suggested Laboratory Studies for Annual Health Maintenance Visit

Age	Routine	High Risk
13–18	HPV vaccine (one series between ages 9 and 26) Hepatitis B vaccine (if not immunized) Tdap booster (once between 11 and 18 years)	Hgb Urinalysis, STD, HIV testing, genetic testing, Rubella titer, TB skin test, FBS (if hypertension)
19–39	Pap test (start at age 21) Tdap once and Td (every 10 years) HPV vaccine (one series between ages 9 and 26) Fasting lipid profile (every 5 years starting age 20) HIV once between 19 and 64 (more if at risk)	Consider additional immunizations in high-risk groups Hepatitis C virus testing Urinalysis Mammography (if strong family history or BRCA-1/BRCA-2 genetic mutations) FBS (if hypertension) Lipid profile more often[†] STD, HIV testing Genetic testing Rubella titer TB skin test TSH Hepatitis C virus testing
40–64	Pap test per text recommendations Mammography per text recommendations Fasting lipid profile (every 5 years) Colorectal screening (≥50) Tdap once and then Td (every 10 years)* TSH (every 5 years beginning at 50)	Consider additional immunizations in high-risk groups Hbg Urinalysis FBS (if hypertension) STD, HIV testing TB skin test Lipid profile more often[†] Hepatitis C virus testing
65 and older	Pap test (depends on prior screening and risk factors) Mammography (continue >70 years if no serious comorbid disease) Fasting lipid profile (every 3-5 years) Colorectal cancer screening Bone density screening (≥every 2 years) TSH (every 5 years) Influenza vaccine yearly	Consider additional immunizations in high-risk groups (i.e., Herpes zoster vaccine at age 60) Hgb FBS (if hypertension) Urinalysis STD, HIV testing Lipid profile more often[†] Hepatitis C screening

*Tdap should be given for one booster dose. Td should be used for later doses every 10 years.
[†]Lipid profile appropriate for family history of hyperlipidemia or premature cardiovascular disease (men <50 years, women <60 years), diabetes, and multiple coronary heart disease risk factors (hypertension, smoking, obesity).
FBS, fasting blood sugar; Fasting lipid profile includes total cholesterol, LDL, HDL and triglycerides; Hgb, hemoglobin; HIV, human immunodeficiency virus; STD, sexually transmitted disease; TB, tuberculosis; Td, tetanus–diphtheria vaccine; Tdap, tetanus toxoid, reduced diphtheria toxoid and acellular pertussis vaccine; TSH, thyroid-stimulating hormone.

Box 7-5 United States Preventive Services Task Force*
Definitions of High Risk for HIV and Gonorrhea

Gonorrhea risk
  History of previous gonorrhea infection
  Treatment or presence of other STDs†
  New or multiples sexual partners
  Inconsistent condom use
  Sex trade work
  Drug use
HIV risk
  Men and women having unprotected sex with multiple partners
  Past or present injection drug use
  Women who exchange sex for money or drugs or who have partners who do
  Women whose past or present partners were/are HIV-infected, bisexual or IV drug users
  Women being treated for STDs
  Women with a history of blood transfusion between 1978 and 1985
  Women receiving health care in a high prevalence or high-risk clinical setting.

*USPSTF – United States Preventive Services Task Force.
†STDs – Sexually transmitted diseases.
Modified from: Campos-Outcalt D: US Preventive Services Task Force; The gold standard of evidence-based prevention. J Fam Pract 54:517-519, 2005.

hemoglobin, urinalysis, mammography (family history of premenopausal breast cancer), testing for sexually transmitted diseases (chlamydia annually for women 25 and under and at risk) and HIV, rubella titer, tuberculosis skin test, thyroid-stimulating hormone (TSH), and hepatitis C virus testing may be indicated. Routine serologic screening for herpes simplex virus in asymptomatic women is not recommended in adolescents or adults. The USPSTF and ACOG recommend referral for genetic counseling and evaluation for the breast cancer susceptibility gene (BRCA) for women whose family history is associated with an increase risk for deleterious mutations in the BRCA1 or BRCA2 genes. Ninety percent of breast cancers are sporadic, but 10% are due to inherited disorders. The prime findings in the history include multiple family members with breast or ovarian cancer, breast and ovarian cancer in a single individual, and early age of breast cancer onset. With women having a one out of eight chance of developing breast cancer in their lifetime, it makes sense to counsel even low-risk women about healthy lifestyle interventions that can lower their risk of cancer, including eating a healthy diet, exercising, and maintaining a normal body weight.

For women between the ages of 40 and 64, the Pap smear testing interval was discussed earlier. In 2009, the USPSTF published substantial changes in the mammography recommendations that have been extremely controversial. Routine screening mammography was no longer recommended in women 40 to 49 years old. Instead, the decision about when to begin regular screening should be individualized with each woman. This received a "C," which means the organization did not recommend for or against. Reasons for this change are that while breast cancer mortality does decrease with screening in this age group, it is a small net benefit. Furthermore, there were concerns about the potential harm of mammography in terms of excess radiation exposure, excess need for additional imaging and breast biopsies (false positive tests), and patient worries and

anxiety about the testing. The recommendation does leave room for an open a discussion with the individual woman and ACOG's recommendations have not changed with screening mammography every 1 to 2 years being appropriate from 40 to 50 years of age.

In 2009, screening for ages 50 to 74 was also changed from annual to biennial with a "B" recommendation by USPSTF. ACOG still recommends yearly mammograms for women 50 and older. Also, ACOG still recommends breast self-exam for all women, but the USPSTF recommends against with "D" grade. Mammograms are reported with the Breast Imaging Reporting and Data System (**BI-RADS**), which classifies abnormalities identified by mammography with standardized reporting (see Chapter 15, Breast Diseases).

Other screening for 50- to 64-year-olds includes cholesterol levels every 5 years. Fasting glucose testing is not recommended routinely unless the woman has a sustained blood pressure of 135/80 mm Hg or higher. The USPSTF found convincing evidence that screening in this population and lowering blood pressure below conventional targets reduced the incidence of cardiovascular events and cardiovascular mortality. For women in this age group who are considered high risk, hemoglobin, urinalysis, testing for sexually transmitted diseases and HIV, tuberculosis skin test, lipid profile, TSH, colonoscopy, and hepatitis C virus testing should be considered. Women age 50 and older should be offered screening for colorectal cancer. The 2008 American College of Gastroenterology guidelines suggest the preferred test is colonoscopy every 10 years. The other alternatives are for people unwilling or unable to undergo colonoscopy or if colonoscopy services are not available in that community. The alternatives include flexible sigmoidoscopy every 5 years, an annual cancer detection test that replaced low-sensitivity fecal occult blood testing (FOBT) with a higher-sensitivity fecal immunochemical test for blood (FIT), computed tomography (CT), and colonography every 5 years. These guidelines recommend African Americans begin routine screening at age 45. A family history of polyps does not evoke earlier onset of screening unless the polyps were advanced adenomas. If a single first-degree relative had colorectal cancer diagnosed after age 60, routine screening is recommended. Otherwise, 10 years before the age at which the family member developed colorectal cancer is the time to begin screening. Some women in other high-risk groups, such as those who are obese or who smoke heavily, should consider screening earlier than age 50. TSH screening is recommended every 5 years beginning at age 50. The USPSTF recommends routine use of combined estrogen and progestin for the prevention of chronic conditions in postmenopausal women and the routine use of unopposed estrogen for the prevention of chronic conditions in postmenopausal women who have had a hysterectomy.

For women who are 65 and older, Pap smear screening was discussed earlier. Urinalysis, mammography, cholesterol (every 3 to 5 years), colorectal cancer screening as noted earlier, and TSH every 5 years should be ordered. For women in particular high-risk groups, hemoglobin, fasting glucose for sustained blood pressure elevation over 135/80 mm Hg, testing for sexually transmitted diseases and HIV, tuberculosis skin testing, and hepatitis C virus testing should be considered. Bone density screening tests for osteoporosis detection can be offered at age 65 and not more frequently than every 2 years. High-risk women should be screened earlier than age 65 (those who fall into the following categories: steroid use chronically, family history, fracture history, physically inactive, tobacco or abuse alcohol, **underweight**, dementia, European or Asian ancestry, history of falls, estrogen deficiency, or poor nutrition). Effectively reducing bone fractures among older people involves both preventing falls and increasing bone strength. The USPSTF recommends against screening women for an abdominal aortic aneurysm or peripheral arterial disease and with spirometry for chronic obstructive pulmonary disease.

Cancer screening besides breast, cervix, and colorectal are more symptom based. Endometrial cancer recommendations for early detection consist of advising women at menopause of their risk factors and the symptoms of endometrial cancer. Those symptoms include unexpected vaginal bleeding or spotting. Even in women known to be at increased risk of endometrial cancer, there is insufficient evidence to recommend screening (unopposed estrogen treatment, tamoxifen therapy, late menopause, nulliparity, infertility or anovulation, obesity, hypertension, and diabetes). Women at very high risk should have annual endometrial biopsy starting at age 35 (known HNPCC, genetic mutation carrier, or strongly suspected carrier). Regular health exams to include thyroid, ovaries, lymph nodes, oral cavity, and skin should be offered, but no special recommendations have been made.

The best source of updated recommendations for adult immunization schedules is the CDC's MMWR website. Women in the youngest age group should be given tetanus-diphtheria and acellular pertussis vaccine (Tdap) booster shots once between the ages of 11 and 18. Measles/mumps/rubella (MMR), hepatitis B vaccine, and fluoride supplementation to prevent tooth decay should be offered to those at risk. Susceptible adolescents *and* adults should be offered varicella vaccination. The meningococcal vaccine is now recommended once before entry to high school if not done at ages 11 to 12 years. For women age 19 to 39, a Tdap booster is indicated once. Then, every 10 years the regular Td (tetanus-diphtheria) booster is given.

Two highly efficacious human papillomavirus (HPV) are available. The quadrivalent vaccine was first licensed in 2007. It became approved for use in 10- to 25-year old females in the United States in 2009. A second bivalent HPV vaccine has been licensed recently. Ideally, the vaccine should be administered before the onset of sexual activity to prevent cervical dysplasia and cancer and other diseases caused by certain strains of HPV. Both have excellent safety profiles and contain virus-like particles (VLPs), but no infectious virus, and are given in a three-dose series. The bivalent vaccine contains VLPs for HPV types 16 and 18, which protect against 70% of cervical cancer. The quadrivalent vaccine contains VLPs for HPV types 16, 18, 6, and 11. HPV types 6 and 11 cause 90% of genital warts. Because both vaccines prevent new infection against the vaccine containing VLP types, but are not effective in preventing disease in individuals already exposed to these types, every effort should be made to target HPV-naïve individuals. See the discussion of intraepithelial neoplasia of the cervix in Chapter 28 for further details.

For women between the ages of 40 and 64, the Tdap booster should be given once and then Td every 10 years. The influenza vaccine should be offered annually beginning at age 50 and any younger person wishing to decrease her risk for influenza. Specifically, the influenza vaccine should be offered to women younger than 50 with chronic medical conditions (e.g., cardiovascular or respiratory disease, diabetes, or immunosuppression, asplenia, chronic liver disease, kidney failure). In addition, health care workers in direct patient care and caretakers of children younger than 6 months of age should be immunized. For women in high-risk groups, MMR, hepatitis B vaccine should be given if indicated. Pneumococcal vaccine should be offered to women with chronic lung, liver, or cardiovascular disease; diabetes; asplenia; cochlear implants; and immunocompromising conditions. Herpes zoster vaccine (for shingles) can be offered to women age 60 and over.

For women who are 65 and older, the Tdap booster once and Td every 10 years should be continued, the influenza vaccine should be given annually, and the pneumococcal vaccine should be given once.

In addition, women in all age groups should be offered appropriate immunizations and vaccinations when they travel to other countries. The hepatitis A vaccine is available and should be offered to women of all ages. In particular the hepatitis A vaccine should be given to women who are traveling to areas with a high or intermediate endemicity of hepatitis A, use injection drugs, have chronic liver disease, receive clotting factor concentrates, or work with HAV-infected primates.

Physicians should discuss risk behavior annually with their patients. In line with injury prevention, the patient should be reminded about the use of seat belts and helmets and other safety concerns mentioned earlier in this chapter. Fall precautions can be discussed with elderly patients.

Exposure of the skin to ultraviolet radiation and proper precautions to avoid overexposure should be discussed. Regular dental checkups should be encouraged. Adequate calcium and vitamin D intake for proper bone health and age-appropriate intake recommendations should be reviewed at the annual visit (**Table 7-3**). Destructive habits such as the use of tobacco, excessive alcohol, or drugs should be addressed, and possible remedial suggestions should be given. Tobacco use is the leading preventable cause of death in the United States. It is the most important modifiable risk factor associated with adverse pregnancy outcomes, and pregnancy is often a time when a woman will be motivated to quit smoking. The nonreproductive effects of smoking include cancer, coronary artery disease, peripheral vascular disease, respiratory disorder, peptic ulcer disease, and osteoporosis. The five "A"s of smoking cessation are important for providers to know: ask (about use), advise (about use), assess (willingness to quit), assist (in plan and counseling), and arrange (regular contact and follow-up). Counseling strategies have been published and show that 5 to 15 minutes of motivational interviewing and problem-solving strategies results in a 5% to 10% quit rate. More intensive options to aid in smoking cessation include pharmacotherapy with nicotine replacement or bupropion.

Table 7-3 Recommended Intakes of Calcium and Vitamin D

Age (years)	Intake Calcium (mg)	Intake Vitamin D (IU)
14–18	1300	200
19–50	1000	200
51+	1200	400
71+	1200	600

From http://ods.od.nih.gov/factsheets/calcium; http://ods.od.nih.gov/factsheets/vitamind.

Many women will ask their physician about prophylactic aspirin use. Although randomized trials in men have shown that low-dose aspirin decreases the risk of a first myocardial infarction, this was not so for women in a large trial in 2005. Ridker and coworkers randomly assigned 38,876 healthy women older than 45 years of age to 100 mg of aspirin on alternate days or placebo and followed them for 10 years. Aspirin did reduce the risk of ischemic stroke in women by 17%, but it had no significant effect on the risk of fatal or nonfatal myocardial infarction. A subgroup analysis of the 4097 women older than 65 years of age did show a significant reduction in the risk of myocardial infarction but at the cost of more gastrointestinal hemorrhages requiring transfusion. Therefore, the use of aspirin as primary cardiovascular prevention in women must be carefully weighed between the risks and benefits for each individual. A 2009 systematic review of the USPSTF recommendations upheld these findings. The organization also highlighted that the dose of aspirin varied in the RCTs, which leaves the appropriate dose for primary prevention unclear if it is deemed appropriate.

Promoting good health is a continuing responsibility for both the physician and the patient. It represents a challenge that includes education and observation on the physician's part and motivation on the patient's part. The U.S. Department of Health and Human Services has a division devoted to women's health titled the Office on Women's Health. Its website (www.womenshealth.gov and girlshealth.gov) offers accurate patient information on screening recommendations for both healthy and at-risk women. Furthermore, the website lists symptoms of serious health conditions for heart attack, stroke, reproductive, breast, lung, digestive, bladder, skin, mental health, and muscle or joint problems.

SPECIAL POPULATIONS

The 2004 United States Census data estimate there are almost 4 million noninstitutionalized women with a self-care disability. Women with disabilities have some unique barriers to gynecologic care. Aside from communication obstacles and nonavailability of facilities with exam tables to make routine pelvic exams easily performed, there may be ignorance or negative attitudes about a woman's life with disabilities. Women with disabilities undergo screening for cervical and breast cancer less often than recommended. Contraception, sexuality issues, childbearing plans, and abuse issues might all need to be addressed.

Lesbian and bisexual women may encounter misinformation, inadequate care, and discrimination when presenting for care. Physicians should not assume all women are heterosexual, and asking about sexual activity can be done in a sensitive manner. Physicians sometimes conclude lesbian women do not need STD or Pap screening because they are considered low risk. However, most lesbians have been sexually active with men at some time in their lives, so appropriate questions need to be asked. Fertility services should not be influenced by sexual orientation.

Other populations that might encounter problems accessing gynecologic care include transgendered individuals and incarcerated, abused, or drug-addicted women.

KEY POINTS

- Strive to become a culturally sensitive and aware physician with a nonjudgmental approach to women regardless of race or ethnicity, age, faith, disabilities, profession, sexual orientation, or activities.
- Menstrual history includes age of menarche, number of days of cycle, number of days of flow, presence of bleeding between menstrual periods, the date of the last menstrual period, and the date of the previous menstrual period.
- Menstrual cycles occurring just after puberty and just before menopause are frequently anovulatory and may be irregular in frequency.
- A complete gynecologic evaluation should always include a sexual history, contraceptive history, and history of physical or sexual abuse.
- Occupational and avocational activity should be investigated for the presence of potential hazards to the patient's health.

- Annual cervical cytology screening should begin at age 21 regardless of the onset of sexual activity.
- Pap smears should be performed every 1 to 3 years, depending on the patient's risk level, age, and Pap test history.
- Sexually active women should be evaluated at appropriate intervals for sexually transmitted diseases, with annual chlamydia screening for women age 25 and under. Counseling women on safe sex practices to avoid contracting sexually transmitted diseases is important.
- Goals of preventive medicine include maintaining good health and function and promoting high-quality longevity.
- The physician should maintain an immunization record for each patient and offer appropriate vaccinations as recommended by public health guidelines.

REFERENCES CAN BE FOUND ON
EXPERTCONSULT.com

8

The Interaction of Medical Diseases and Female Physiology

Vern L. Katz

This chapter highlights the interactions and influences of female physiology on major medical disease processes. The chapter also reviews how medical diseases impact female physiology. Many disease processes act directly; for example, renal disease commonly induces abnormal bleeding. Other disease act not only directly but indirectly through their therapies, such as cancer chemotherapy, which may induce ovarian failure. Multiple chapters in this text discuss important aspects of female physiology. This chapter serves as an addendum to those discussions. Because the science of medicine is always improving and treatments are constantly evolving, we will limit our review of pharmacologic therapies. When considering specific drug interactions and doses, the clinician is encouraged to review current pharmacologic literature.

In general, the impact of female physiology on medical disease is primarily via the effects of estrogen and to a lesser extent progesterone. Other hormones such as prolactin, oxytocin, and gonadotropins play minor roles. Estrogen and progesterone affect almost all major organ systems in both tonic and cyclic modes. For example, estrogen plays a role as a B-cell enhancer in antibody production as a tonic mode. Whereas the withdrawal of progesterone at the end of the luteal phase leads to increased seizures in a cyclic fashion. The effects of the female hormones are mediated directly through receptors (estrogen alpha, estrogen beta, progesterone) as well as indirectly through their effects on other organ systems, such as smooth muscle relaxation and changes in prostaglandin levels. In the central nervous system, estrogen acts primarily through the GABA system, whereas progesterone acts through its metabolite allopregnenalone.

The responses induced by estrogen and progesterone may be theorized, in a teleologic sense, as promoting successful reproduction. For example, a blunted cellular immune response, as well as improved thrombus formation may improve pregnancy outcomes. Disease occurs when the normal hormonal effects overlap a disease already present. The upregulation of humoral immunity is a good example. Estrogen enhances B-cell activity and women have an improved survival from infection compared with men, but women have more problems with the antibodies of autoimmune disease such as Graves' disease. When the physiologic response occurs in the presence of another disease process or coupled with an inherent predisposition for disease, then pathology develops.

On the flipside, medical diseases affect female physiology at all aspects of the hypothalamic-pituitary-ovarian-genital axis, from anovulation to vaginal stenosis. Medical diseases also affect female physiology in a horizontal manner, throughout a woman's life. Thus, medical diseases must be seen in both a vertical and horizontal context (i.e., a three-dimensional manner).

The gynecologist acts as a consultant to other health professionals. As such, we are frequently asked to help with complications stemming from gynecologic issues. Though different clinicians direct the treatment of lupus, multiple sclerosis, or epilepsy, modulating the effects of female physiology is the role of the gynecologist.

PULMONARY DISEASE

Asthma is more common in boys up until puberty. After puberty, the ratio reverses with women more prone to asthma until menopause. Asthma is one of several major diseases in which the severity of symptoms is increased around the time of menses (Table 8-1). Premenstrual asthma is well described, affecting up to 40% of reproductive-age women who have asthma. The symptoms in these women will exacerbate, with large series documenting increasing cough, wheezing, and shortness of breath around the time of menses. Up to 50% of hospitalizations for asthmatic women in their 20s will occur around the time of their menstrual periods.

There are several mechanisms that lead to the hormonal effects. Estrogen and progesterone increase both serotonin and histamine release from granulocytes, potentially leading to increased symptomatology during reproductive years. Estrogen also increases eosinophilic adhesion to the bronchial lining. Progesterone has a significant smooth-muscle relaxing effect and the perimenstrual withdrawal of estrogen and progesterone has been theorized to lead to increased bronchial reactivity. The effect of estrogen and progesterone withdrawal on prostaglandin levels has also been suggested as one of the mechanisms of increasing premenstrual asthma.

Dratva et al. measured bronchial hyperreactivity in reproductive-age women during different times of their menstrual cycles. Most women had a decline in respiratory function with the end of the cycle; 13% of women had greater than a 20% decline in FEV1 from 3 days before their period until 2 days after menses began. In their large study, women who were on oral contraceptives seemed to have a blunting of this effect. Other studies have

We acknowledge the help of Deborah Dotters in preparing this chapter.

Table 8-1 Major Diseases in Which Menstrual Hormonal Changes Affect Disease Symptoms

Asthma
Atopic reactions
Epilepsy
Eating disorders
Irritable bowel syndrome
Menstrual migraines
Mental health disorders
Multiple sclerosis

also shown oral contraceptives to be mildly protective in decreasing the severity of asthma, in addition to confirming significant variations in FEV1, peak flow, as well as an increase in clinical symptoms in the premenstrual time period. As might be expected, because hormonal levels fluctuate from one cycle to the next, investigators have noted variability in symptoms from one cycle to the next as well.

In respect to the effects of asthma on female physiology, small series have noted a later menarche and an increased incidence of abnormal menstrual cycles in women with severe asthma. Whether this is due to glucocorticoid medications or whether this is a direct effect from severe pulmonary disease on the hypothalamus is unclear. Women who are taking inhaled glucocorticoids who are postmenopausal are noted to have decreased bone mineral density, but this effect is not seen in women who are still menstruating. Clinicians who care for women with asthma beyond their third decade should obtain vitamin D levels and council the women about adequate calcium intake.

It is now common for women with cystic fibrosis (CF) to reach reproductive age. Tsang et al., in a review of reproductive problems, noted that women with cystic fibrosis tend to have shorter stature and often delayed puberty with delayed growth spurts and delayed menarche. The degree of delay is related to the severity of the disease. Girls with cystic fibrosis tend to be as sexually active as their peers; however, they tend to have less counseling regarding contraception than their peers. Whether this is due to the fact that nongynecologists are taking care of them is unclear. The pediatric literature has emphasized how important it is to counsel young women with CF about contraception. Estrogen-based contraceptives are acceptable for women with cystic fibrosis as long as they do not have pulmonary hypertension or a history of thromboembolism. Progesterone intrauterine devices (IUDs) are also reasonable. These women do not have an increased risk of pelvic inflammatory disease (PID), but they do need counseling concerning safe sex. Cervical mucus is thicker in women with cystic fibrosis and may be problematic as a fertility issue, although most women with cystic fibrosis have appropriate fertility. Oligomenorrhea and amenorrhea are increased in adolescents with cystic fibrosis, again related to the degree of severity of disease. Issues of sexuality may be problematic for young women with severe cystic fibrosis because of poor body image secondary to chronic disease, infections, gastrointestinal disturbances from pancreatic problems, and chronic antibiotics, as well as sometimes enlarged rib cages from chronic hyperventilation. Thus, counseling on sexuality may be indicated in conjunction with contraceptive counseling.

Progesterone has a mild stimulatory effect on the central nervous system (CNS) respiratory center. Progesterone has been used in patients with severe sleep apnea and Pickwickian syndrome. Men suffer more commonly from sleep apnea than women prior to menopause.

THE EFFECTS OF ESTROGEN ON INFLAMMATION, ALLERGY, AND THE IMMUNE SYSTEM

The profound effect that female physiology has on immunity is best exemplified by the remarkably increased survival of women compared with men from infectious causes. Estrogen and progesterone have multiple affects on the immune processes, through numerous cellular sites. This is manifest in multiple disease processes (**Tables 8-2** and **8-3**). In most women the effects are mild, but in women constitutionally or genetically predisposed to atopic reaction or autoimmune disease, the effects can be significant. Estrogen and progesterone are immune modulators. The immune system is arguably the most complex physiologic system in the body. By necessity, several cell lines with multiple regulatory cytokines help produce measured, specific responses to fine-tune each reaction. Estrogen affects most of the cytokines in different manners, even within similar groupings of cytokine families. A detailed review of these relationships is beyond the scope of this text. However the specifics of those estrogen-immune relationships is an area of much research with far-reaching implications both experimentally and for a variety of therapies.

Estrogen effects are mediated through both estrogen alpha and estrogen beta-receptors. The overall effect may be grossly simplified in noting estrogen's effect on the B cell as an immune enhancer. In contrast, on T cells estrogen tends to act as an inhibitor. Importantly, estrogen effects vary by the level of estrogen. At lower levels, as in most of the menstrual cycle, estrogen

Table 8-2 Effects of Estrogen and Progesterone on Cellular Processes of the Immune System

B cell
Inhibited bone marrow B-cell lines with high concentrations of estrogen
Increased antibody production through inhibition of T-cell suppression
Enhanced IL-10 response

T cell
Lower doses of estrogen are stimulatory, higher doses of estrogen are inhibitory, primarily through TNF
Stimulation of inhibitory T-cell pathways and T-cell cytokines
Low-level stimulation of interleukins

Monocytes
Increased monocyte apoptosis inhibiting differentiation
Inhibited dendritic cell differentiation (in vitro)
Inhibited migration of inflammatory cells with decreased migration at higher estrogen levels

Mast Cells and Granulocytes
Estrogen increases serotonin and histamine release through estrogen alpha-receptors
(Tamoxifen inhibits this effect)
Progesterone promotes IgE production

General Inflammation
Increased presence of estrogen beta-receptors over estrogen alpha receptors with generalized inflammation
Increased sensitization of sensory neural tissue leading to increased neurogenic inflammation
Increased fibroblast activity and improved wound healing
Increased stimulation of the HPA axis

Adapted from Chen et al 2004, Lang et al 2008, Straub 2007.

Table 8-3 Effects of Estrogen and Progesterone on General Immunity

Allergy—increased in women*
Atopic problems (eczema)—increased in women*
Anaphylaxis—increased in women *
Drug-induced anaphylaxis and reactions
Radiologic contrast media–induced anaphylaxis
Anesthetic medication increased angioedema
Asthma—increased in women

Generalized IgM response—increased in women
Autoimmune disease*
Increased incidence and severity of SLE 1
Increased incidence of severity of myasthenia gravis[†]
Increased IgA nephropathy
Increased celiac disease
Myasthenia gravis*,[†]
Multiple sclerosis
Increased mixed connective tissue disorder*
Increased Sjögren syndrome
Increased autoimmune thyroid disease

Infection
Increased survival at all ages
Decreased severity of infection
Increased male childhood rhinitis changing in sex ratio after menarche
Men increased sepsis associated with trauma

Hepatic Disease
Women with greater autoimmune hepatitis than men
Men worse liver fibrosis, equal after menopause

Rheumatoid Arthritis
Increased susceptibility with equal susceptibility in severity of disease after menopause

Wound Healing
Improved wound healing
Hormone replacement therapy improves healing

*After menarche.
[†]Biphasic response with pregnancy levels of estrogen inhibiting disease states.
Data from Chen 2008, Lang 2004, Straub 2002.

stimulates immune responses. However, at high estrogen levels such as with pregnancy, estrogen generally inhibits immune cellular responses. Reviews by Straub and Chen et al. have emphasized the immune modulating characterization of estrogen. Much of the B-cell enhancement is derived from suppression of the T-cell inhibition of the B cells. Thus, when estrogen inhibits T cells, B cells are able to produce more antibody and stronger reactions. At all ages women, have less morbidity as well as lower mortality from infection than men.

B-cell–dominated autoimmune diseases, such as autoimmune thyroiditis, have a higher incidence and severity in women. Estrogen also enhances the hypersensitivity responses from both B-cell activity and granulocyte action in allergic responses. Women are more prone than men to eczema, atopic irritations, hypersensitivity, and anaphylaxis from foods, medications, radiologic contrast media, and anesthesia. Granulocytes, eosinophils, mast cells, and basophils are enhanced by estrogen. Estrogen also enhances serotonin and histamine release.

In contrast to humoral immunity, cellular-mediated immune mechanisms, primarily controlled through T cells, tend to be functionally inhibited by estrogen. At low to moderate levels of estrogen, there is both a mild stimulation of some T-cell activity, a through effect on the interleukin system and other cytokines, and a stimulation of other aspects of T cells. Depending on the aspect of the T-cell system that is being invoked, mild stimulation or mild inhibition at the functional level may occur. At high, pregnancy levels of estrogen, there is functional inhibition of T-cell function, leading to improvement of T-cell–mediated autoimmune diseases during pregnancy such as rheumatoid arthritis or multiple sclerosis.

During periods of estrogen withdrawal, late luteal phase, menstruation, postpartum, and early menopause, there are often clinical rebounds and an increase in disease flares with the release of T-cell suppression. Thus, rheumatoid arthritis worsens in menopause. Straub, in his review, theorized that the long-term effect of low-level stimulation of some T-cell activities primes those diseases for a "breakout" in later decades with exacerbation of cellular-based immune diseases as estrogen levels wane. He theorized that the cell-mediated autoimmune diseases smolder until estrogen levels drop, and then those diseases flare with clinical severity.

The effects of estrogen on inflammation have important consequences for wound healing. Estrogen stimulates fibroblast activity and nerve growth. Women heal much better than men. Estrogen's positive effect on reepithelialization lasts until several years after menopause. Interestingly, hormone replacement therapy improves wound healing.

Several studies have evaluated the impact of oral contraceptives and hormone-containing contraceptives on autoimmune diseases. Oral contraceptives are acceptable for women with systemic lupus erythematosus (SLE) if they do not have thrombophilic problems. Two randomized controlled trials found oral contraceptives to be safe in the setting of SLE. Estrogen-containing contraceptives do not increase the severity of disease or the number of flares in premenopausal women. Hormone replacement therapy (HRT) has been shown to increase the number of mild flares in lupus patients, but HRT does not increase the number of severe flares.

SLE does not seem to affect menses or the timing of menopause. However, some anti-inflammatory medications, including glucocorticoids and antineoplastic agents, will affect the hypothalamic-pituitary-ovarian (HPO) axis as well as ovarian follicles (Table 8-4). Women with severe end-organ disease from lupus may develop downregulation of the HPO axis (see Chapter 37).

Table 8-4 Antineoplastic and Chemotherapeutic Agents That May Produce Ovarian Failure

Major Risk to the Ovaries
Cyclophosphamide
Melphalan
Busulfan
Chlorambucil
Procarbazine
Nitrogen mustard
Moderate Risk
Cisplatin
Adriamycin
Paclitaxel (unquantified risk at this time)
Minimal Risk
Methotrexate
5-fluorouracil
Vincristine
Bleomycin
Actinomycin

Modified from Sonmezer et al 2006.

Table 8-5 Antibiotics Interacting with Oral Contraceptives

Ampicillin
Doxycycline
Fluconazole
Metronidazole
Quinolone
Tetracycline

Adapted from the American College of Obstetricians and Gynecologists (ACOG) Practice Bulletin #72, 2006, Use of Hormonal Contraception in Women with Coexisting Medical Conditions.

For the gynecologist asked to consult on women with autoimmune diseases, important strategies include assuring that any pregnancy is planned. The best pregnancy outcomes occur at times when autoimmune diseases are inactive. Thus, effective contraception is essential. In general, most of the chronic autoimmune diseases are not worse around the time of menses. However, a small proportion of women with multiple sclerosis (MS) will have menstruation-related changes in symptoms. For the women with menstrual exacerbation, oral contraceptives may help to decrease periodic variability. For severe disease, some authors have reported using gonadotrophin-releasing hormone (GnRH) agonists with low-dose estrogen added back to inhibit flares. In general, women with severe multiple sclerosis have an increased risk of sexual dysfunction, primarily related to brain stem lesions, which affect bowel and bladder function.

Systemic antibiotics may affect the metabolism of oral contraceptives (**Table 8-5**). This needs to be taken into account, and women should be counseled about considering using supplemental forms of contraception during antibiotic use.

GASTROINTESTINAL DISEASE

Estrogen and progesterone affect symptoms of irritable bowel syndrome (IBS). Up to half of women with IBS will have exacerbations of symptoms with menses. Progesterone, through smooth muscle relaxation, produces mild constipation. Among women with irritable bowel syndrome, that can be problematic. With rapid progesterone withdrawal at the end of the luteal phase, there is the increase in systemic prostaglandins in addition to the withdrawal of the smooth muscle relaxation, both of which lead to exacerbations of diarrhea. For women in whom menstrual affects become debilitating, the use of GnRH agonists has been suggested. Continuous use of oral contraceptives to minimize the number of periods is also reasonable. Similarly, women with celiac disease have more problems with menstrual hormone fluctuations.

Estrogen has beneficial effect on hepatitis-related liver fibrosis because of the inhibition of T-cell function. Thus, women who have chronic hepatitis with subsequent liver fibrosis do much better than men. Some reports have also detailed the use of hormone replacement in postmenopausal women to inhibit liver fibrosis.

VASCULAR AND HYPERTENSIVE DISEASES

In general, estrogens have a positive effect on the vascular system through improved lipid profiles. However, women who have preexisting thrombophilias and women with dyslipidemias may have problems with estrogen because of its procoagulant effects. This is rarely a problem for women in their second and third decades, but it becomes more problematic later in life. Women with a dyslipidemia should avoid estrogen-based contraceptives and hormone replacement therapy. However, progesterone-based contraceptives, or the progestin-based IUD, are very reasonable.

In contrast, vascular and hypertensive diseases have important effects on women. Studies indicate that women with hypertension have much higher than expected levels of sexual dysfunction with impaired genital congestion and decreased arousal. Women who are taking antihypertensive medicines have a compounding affect. Most of the antihypertensive medications induce decreased genital blood flow as well as decreased arousal. Thus, during yearly examinations, it is helpful for gynecologists to inquire about sexual issues in women on these medications.

Hormonally based contraceptives are mildly problematic in women who are taking antihypertensive medications. If there is not associated thrombosis, guidelines of the American College of Obstetricians and Gynecologists (ACOG) suggest that women may take oral contraceptives as long as their blood pressures are well controlled. Seeing women back in 2 or 3 months, after they have started oral contraceptives, is appropriate. Studies have shown a small increase in stroke and myocardial infarction in women on oral contraceptives with hypertension, but the risk is quite small. As long as women are not smoking and/or do not have other aspects of vascular disease besides mild hypertension, oral contraceptives are reasonable. Progesterone-based IUDs may be preferable in many situations if appropriate for the patient. Certainly, after age 35, progesterone-based contraceptives may be more appropriate.

RENAL DISEASE

Women with advanced and end-stage renal disease have problems with abnormal bleeding, both menorrhagia and metrorrhagia. Some investigators theorize that this is due to abnormal platelet function or potential changes in thrombotic activity. The precise etiology is unclear. The effects of chronic disease (see Chapter 37) may downregulate the HPO axis, leading to an increased likelihood of anovulatory bleeding. Investigations have documented that women with end-stage renal disease have an increase in endometrial hyperplasia, as well as an increased incidence of cervical dysplasia. The cervical dysplasia is most likely increased because of reduced immunity with increased susceptibility to human papillomavirus (HPV) infection. During surgery, some case series have documented a higher risk of surgical complications in these patients.

Women who are on hemodialysis, with chronic renal disease, and those who have had renal transplants also suffer from an increased incidence of sexual dysfunction. Studies have documented that up to 70% of women have higher levels of sexual dysfunction, including arousal disorders, decreased libido, and decreased genital blood flow, with lubrication and orgasm problems. Women in their childbearing years who receive antineoplastic agents to suppress autoimmune nephritides may develop problems with premature ovarian failure.

HEMATOLOGIC AND THROMBOTIC DISEASES

Estrogen affects hematologic diseases primarily through its prothrombotic effects. Progesterone decreases smooth muscle venous tone, which leads to increased clotting potential. Estrogen increases the levels of several clotting factors and decreases elements of the fibrinolytic pathways. Women with a history of thrombosis, either personal or familial, should be offered testing for thrombophilias prior to receiving estrogen-based medications. Routine screening for thrombophilias in women without a history of thrombosis, prior to the use of oral contraceptives or hormone replacement, is not indicated. Women with known thrombophilias can use progesterone-based contraceptives and medications, including the progesterone-based IUD.

Because supplemental estrogen is contraindicated in women with thrombophilias, these women may be more prone to osteoporotic problems over time. These women should be regularly screened for a dietary history of calcium intake as well as serum levels of vitamin D, with appropriate supplementation given.

Women with sickle cell disease may benefit from progesterone. Progesterone stabilizes red-cell membranes and significantly decreases the frequency of sickling crises. Women with frequent crises have been given injectable medroxyprogesterone acetate as an adjunct therapy with very good results. The effects of progesterone-based IUDs have not yet been well documented. Oral contraceptives and hormone replacement therapies do not improve sickling but are not contraindicated.

Women who receive oral anticoagulants, for either treatment or prophylaxis, experience increased vaginal bleeding, menorrhagia, and metrorrhagia. One series of women on oral anticoagulants noted that 30% sought medical therapy for excess vaginal bleeding. Anovulatory cycles may be particularly troublesome for these women. Progesterone-based IUD or progesterone supplementation for the 14 days at the end of the cycle may be necessary to decrease heavy bleeding.

The most common inherited bleeding diathesis is von Willebrand disease. This is caused by inadequate or dysfunctional von Willebrand factor. The association of von Willebrand disease and vaginal bleeding is discussed in Chapter 37. Both combination and continuous oral contraceptives, as well as other hormonally based contraceptives, may be helpful in women with von Willebrand disease, because estrogen increases von Willebrand factor. Progestin-based IUDs are also acceptable. For women who have problems with excess bleeding or ovarian cysts, hormonal contraceptives may be particularly advantageous. Women with rare bleeding disorders fall into similar categories, and oral contraceptives may be helpful for them. James et al., in a consensus report, have discussed other therapies including endometrial ablation or hysterectomy as potential options in appropriate women with bleeding disorders who do not desire fertility.

ENDOCRINE DISEASE

Many endocrinopathies have an autoimmune basis, with a higher incidence and severity in women compared with men. The interaction of endocrinopathies on the hypothalamic-pituitary-ovarian axis is straightforward and is an inhibition of normal function, producing anovulation.

Women with type 2 diabetes, and those who are obese, have increased anovulation, infertility, and potential problems with endometrial hyperplasia. Estrogen and progesterone mildly promote insulin resistance and worsen carbohydrate intolerance. Oral contraceptives are acceptable in women with diabetes, as are progesterone-based contraceptives. The need for protection of the endometrium in an anovulatory environment makes combined hormonal contraceptives very helpful. Because many women with diabetes have coexisting vascular disease or hyperlipidemia, the American College of Ob/Gyn has suggested that oral contraceptives be limited to women who are nonsmokers and less than 35 with no other significant pathology.

Obese women have a higher failure rate from hormone-based contraceptives and progesterone-based contraceptives. They may need higher doses of medication. Thus, caution should be used in women with a body mass index over 35. Given the increased incidence of anovulation with obesity, a progestin-based IUD is often helpful. Obese women undergoing bariatric surgery should also be counseled about contraception. Sexual activity often increases as body image improves. With rapid weight loss, pregnancy may be problematic with reports of higher risks of fetal structural defects. After surgery, women may transition from being anovulatory to regular ovulation with improved glucose control. Thus, discussions of contraception with all women who are undergoing bariatric surgery are important.

Studies of sexuality in women with diabetes have noted increased sexual dysfunction, particularly for type 1 diabetics and those with long-standing disease. Sexual dysfunction is due to end-organ disease, with decreased genital blood flow, and decreased lubrication and orgasm problems.

Thyroid disease (discussed in Chapter 37) affects the hypothalamic-pituitary-ovarian axis, with an increased risk of anovulation and infertility. The incidence of sexual dysfunction is not well described in the literature, though increased levels of depression with low thyroid levels has been noted. Women with thyroid disease may take oral contraceptives and other hormonally based treatments.

Women with congenital adrenal hyperplasia are usually treated with glucocorticoid replacement. These women are exposed to an increased androgen environment throughout their lives. They tend to have problems similar to women with Cushing's disease. For women with increased androgens, hormonally based contraceptives, including oral contraceptives, are a good form of birth control. Many of these women have increased problems with hirsutism. This should not be treated with spironolactone because it may affect the mineralocorticoid regulation. Infertility is common, secondary to chronically increased progesterone and androgen levels. These women tend to have a marked decrease in sexual activity, which has been theorized to be due to vaginal stenosis and dyspareunia from congenital deformations, as well as poor self-image. Sexual counseling for these women is helpful.

CENTRAL NERVOUS SYSTEM DISEASE

SEIZURE DISORDERS

Estrogen and progesterone have significant effects on a woman's susceptibility to seizures. Estrogen is a pro-convulsant, decreasing seizure threshold. Estrogen increases neuronal excitability directly on nerve cells, as well as secondarily through inhibition of the GABA system. The GABA receptor network is the primary neural inhibitory system within the CNS.

More potent than the estrogen effects are those of progesterone. Progesterone acts primarily via its metabolite

allopregnenalone, which is a **neurosteroid**. Allopregnenalone acts rapidly and directly on the GABA receptors to enhance their activity, producing a potent neural inhibition throughout the CNS. Withdrawal of progesterone (even in small amounts such as periovulatory) leads to a significant decline in seizure threshold and an increase in seizure frequency and severity.

More than 1 million women in the United States are affected with seizure disorders. Over 20% of these women have increased seizure activity related to changes in menstrual hormones. **Catamenial** epilepsy (from the Greek *katomenios,* meaning "monthly") has been defined as seizures that occur from 3 days prior to 4 days after the onset of menses. Pure catamenial epilepsy affects 10% of all women with epilepsy. However, a much higher percentage of women will have an increase in seizure activity related to declines in progesterone levels. When gynecologists care for women with coexistent seizure disorders, they should inquire about seizure periodicity. Progesterone-based contraceptives or a small amount of progesterone add-back during menses has been used to decrease seizure frequency. Continuous oral contraceptives with an every-3-month withdrawal may also be helpful.

Though hormonal contraception is acceptable for women with seizure disorders, estrogen may affect metabolism of some anticonvulsants (**Table 8-6**). Women who experience menstrual-related seizures should have serum levels of their anticonvulsant medications checked during menses. Some of these women will benefit from perimenstrual adjustments of their medications. In contrast, some seizure medications affect metabolism of hormonal contraception, and adjusting the type and dose of estrogen may be indicated.

Migraine Headaches

A **menstrual migraine** may be defined as a migraine headache, without aura, occurring within the last 2 days of the menstrual cycle and the first 3 days of menses. Additionally, it should affect two of every three cycles. Fourteen percent of all women with migraines have pure menstrual migraines, and 46% have exacerbation of severity and frequency of their migraines during menses. Because more than 25 million American women have migraine headaches, approximately 17 million women are affected by this problem. In general, women have three times more migraines than men. After menopause, the incidence of migraines decreases by two thirds, and women and men have equal frequencies.

The etiology of menstrual migraines is related to estrogen withdrawal. Migraines are primarily vascular headaches, and the withdrawal of the estrogen leads to a relative vascular instability. The mechanisms by which estrogen withdrawal induces the headache are multifactorial. Estrogen affects the CNS serotonin receptors. The change in serotonin metabolism as estrogen is withdrawn affects the brainstem, which controls cerebral blood flow. Serotonin uptake is blocked by triptans, and triptans are noted to be extremely effective for menstrual migraines. Changes in prostaglandin metabolism, melatonin, and opioid activity are also other contributing etiologies. Continuous use of oral contraceptives has been somewhat effective in ameliorating this problem. When menstrual migraines and menstruation-related migraines are diagnosed, therapeutic choices include modifying estrogen withdrawal with therapies such as the continuous use of oral contraceptives, patches, or small amounts of estrogen add-back in the appropriate time window. Prophylactic triptans and antiprostaglandins may be coordinated with the primary care provider. Long-term therapies have included tricyclic antidepressants, beta-blockers, and other medications, which in themselves may affect sexuality.

Women who have migraines with aura are more susceptible to stroke, and thus the use of oral contraceptives in women with migraines with aura is contraindicated.

MENTAL HEALTH ISSUES

Changes in estrogen and progesterone levels have profound effects on psychiatric and psychological symptomatology and on psychiatric diseases (**Tables 8-7** and **8-8**). Estrogen and progesterone affect multiple psychologic symptoms, including anxiety, vulnerability, mood lability, depression, and appetite changes. In most women these symptoms are well controlled. However, women who have a predisposition to mental health disorders may be strongly affected by the hormonal fluctuations.

Premenstrual dysphoric disease (PMDD) affects up to 5% of women and is discussed in Chapter 9. Pinkerton et al., in a recent review, noted the cyclic exacerbation of symptoms in multiple psychiatric diseases (see **Table 8-8**). As discussed previously, estrogen and progesterone are neuromodulators, so exacerbation in almost any mental health disease may occur with menstrual hormonal fluctuations. Mental health disorders are best managed by mental health providers with clinical expertise. However, the gynecologist may be helpful in providing hormonal stability. Continuous oral contraceptives with add-back estrogen, either through a patch or oral medications, can help improve depression that occurs around the time of menses. If hormone-based contraceptives are not desired or not appropriate, other types of contraception should be provided. Additionally, women with depression commonly have sexual dysfunction as part of their disease. Many antidepressants, including the selective serotonin reuptake inhibitor (SSRI) class of drugs, decrease libido.

Table 8-6 Interactions of Anticonvulsants and Oral Contraceptives

Anticonvulsants That Strongly Affect Oral Contraceptive Levels
Barbiturates
Carbamazepine
Phenytoin
Topiramate
Vigabatrin
Anticonvulsants That Have Minimal Interaction with Oral Contraceptive Metabolism
Gabapentin
Lamotrigine
Valproic acid
Ethosuximide

Adapted from the American College of Obstetricians and Gynecologists (ACOG) Practice Bulletin #72, 2006, Use of Hormonal Contraception in Women with Coexisting Medical Conditions.

Table 8-7 Changes in Mental Health Disease Symptomatology Related to Menstrual Cycle Changes

Panic disorder
Generalized anxiety disorder
Obsessive compulsive disease
Bipolar disease
Eating disorders
Severe PMS
Premenstrual dysphoric disease—PMDD
Schizophrenia

Adapted from Pinkerton et al 2010.

Table 8-8 Emotional Symptoms Affected by Changes in Estrogen and Progesterone

Anxiety
Feelings of phobia
Vulnerability
Mood lability
Depression
Appetite change
Temperature fluctuations
Anger
Irritability
Inhibited control of limbic system sensations
Increased sense of fatigue
Decreased self-esteem
Loss of pleasure
Memory problems

Adapted from Pinkerton et al 2010.

CANCER

Cancer affects all areas of health. However, the gynecologist can play a valuable role in improving quality of life. Sexuality in cancer patients should be addressed from the beginning of cancer therapy. Cancer chemotherapy and pelvic radiation are toxic to the ovaries and often produce ovarian failure, sterility, and premature menopause. The issues of depression and sexual dysfunction are enhanced by the ovarian failure, the loss of hair, and the change in relationships. Abnormal vaginal bleeding in the first few cycles of chemotherapy is very frightening, and the role of the gynecologist is important at this phase of treatment.

Chemotherapy produces toxic effects on ovarian function that are related to dose, duration, and type of chemotherapy. Agents that are particularly toxic to the ovary are listed in **Table 8-4**. Of these, alkylating agents are the most toxic to the ovaries. Importantly, women who receive antineoplastic agents for control of severe autoimmune disease can also develop ovarian failure. Radiation to the ovaries greater than or equal to 20 Gy (which is well within the dose for childhood cancers) may also produce ovarian failure.

Young women, often wishing to preserve ovarian function and fertility, need consultation prior to treatments. Mature oocytes are the most susceptible to chemotherapy, whereas immature oocytes in the prepubertal females are somewhat resistant. Thus, investigators have used GnRH antagonists to suppress follicular maturity and preserve ovarian function. The results are mixed, and in many patients this would be inappropriate. Currently, large studies are under way to evaluate GnRH antagonists as a treatment modality for women who desire fertility and ovarian preservation. Authors have addressed other potential options to save oocyte function and preserve fertility. These treatments include in vitro fertilization with freezing embryos, harvesting of mature oocytes after ovarian stimulation (which is problematic in itself prior to chemotherapy), and experimental ovarian cryopreservation. All of these are problematic. All have specific risks and benefits and varied efficacy. The options should be reviewed in light of the patient's needs, fertility desires, and clinical situation. Early referral to a reproductive endocrinologist with expertise in potential therapies to preserve fertility is important. This is obviously difficult given the much higher priority of dealing with the cancer. That priority dominates the concerns of the family and the patient.

SUMMARY

The interaction of female physiology and medical disease is complex. The gynecologist has several roles in the treatment of these women. All providers who address women's health should regularly discuss issues of sexual function, particularly in the setting of coexisting disease. Additionally, the exacerbation of symptoms around the time of menses should be reviewed. Hormonal changes that increase the symptoms of women will change over the course of a woman's reproductive life. Disease manifestation in a woman's 20s will not be the same as symptoms in her 40s. There are many treatment options that can improve quality of life. Though gynecologists may not be the primary providers for nongynecologic diseases, they are best suited to act as a consultant for adjunctive therapy, which may enhance the efficacy and treatment of medical disease.

KEY POINTS

- The severity of asthma symptoms increases around the time of menses.
- Estrogen's effect on the B cell as an immune enhancer, whereas in contrast, estrogen tends to act as an immune inhibitor to T cells.
- Up to half of women with IBS will have exacerbations of symptoms with menses.
- Women who are on hemodialysis, with chronic renal disease, and those who have had renal transplants suffer from an increased incidence of sexual dysfunction.
- Women with chronic renal disease often experience menorrhagia.
- Progesterone stabilizes red-cell membranes and significantly decreases the frequency of sickling crises.
- Allopregnenalone acts rapidly and directly on the GABA receptors to enhance their activity, producing a potent neural inhibition throughout the CNS. Withdrawal of progesterone (even in small amounts such as periovulatory) leads to a significant decline in the seizure threshold and an increase in seizure frequency and severity.
- Fourteen percent of all women with migraines have pure menstrual migraines, and 46% have exacerbation of severity and frequency of their migraines during menses.
- Women who have migraines with aura are more susceptible to stroke, and thus the use of oral contraceptives in women with migraines with aura is contraindicated.
- Radiation to the ovaries greater than or equal to 20 Gy (which is well within the dose for childhood cancers) may produce ovarian failure.
- Early referral of women with cancer to a reproductive endocrinologist with expertise in potential therapies to preserve fertility is important.

REFERENCES CAN BE FOUND ON
EXPERTCONSULT.com

SUGGESTED READINGS

American College of Obstetricians and Gynecologists (ACOG): Use of hormonal contraception in women with coexisting medical conditions, 106:1453, 2006.

Basson R, Weijmar Schultz W: Sexual sequelae of general medical disorders, *Lancet* 369:409, 2007.

Case AM, Reid RL: Menstrual cycle effects on common medical conditions, 27:65, 2001.

Dratva J, Schindler C, Curjuric I, et al: Perimenstrual increase in bronchial hyperreactivity in premenopausal women: Results from the population-based SAPALDIA 2 Cohort. American Academy of Allergy, *Asthma Immunol* 125:823, 2009.

Jeruss JS, Woodruff TK: Preservation of fertility in patients with cancer, *N Engl J Med* 360:902, 2009.

Lang TJ: Estrogen as an immunomodulator, *Science Direct* 113:224, 2004.

Lay CL, Payne: Recognition and treatment of menstrual migraine, *Neurologist* 13:197, 2007.

Murphy VE, Gibson PG: Premenstrual asthma: Prevalence, cycle-to-cycle variability and relationship to oral contraceptive use and menstrual symptoms, *J Asthma* 45:696, 2008.

Pinkerton JV, Guico-Pabia CJ, Taylor HS: Menstrual cycle-related exacerbation of disease, *Am J Obstet Gynecol* 202:221, 2010.

Reddy DS: Pharmacology of catamenial epilepsy, *Methods Find Exp Clin Pharmacol* 26:547, 2004.

Schmidt KT, Larsen EC, Andersen CY, et al: Risk of ovarian failure and fertility preserving methods in girls and adolescents with a malignant disease, *BJOG* 117:163, 2009.

Straub RH: The complex role of estrogens in inflammation, *The Endocrine Society* 28:521, 2007.

Tsang A, Moriarty C, Towns S: Contraception, communication and counseling for sexuality and reproductive health in adolescents and young adults with CF, *Paediatr Respir Rev* 11:84, 2010.

Wax JR, Pinette MG, Cartin A, et al: Female reproductive issues following bariatric surgery, *CME Review Article* 62:595, 2007.

Emotional Aspects of Gynecology
Depression, Anxiety, PTSD, Eating Disorders, Substance Abuse, "Difficult" Patients, Sexual Function, Rape, Intimate Partner Violence, and Grief

Deborah Cowley and Gretchen M. Lentz

Gynecologists follow women across the life cycle, from puberty through old age. The gynecologist may be a woman's primary health care provider for much of this time and thus is in an important position to help her to navigate normal developmental stages and challenges, to share in critical life events from adolescence to late life, and to provide or obtain counseling for her as she works her way through emotional adjustments and problems. Normal development includes challenges such as building an identity and self-esteem; dealing with sexuality and sexual development; forming meaningful relationships; pregnancy and motherhood; life roles and transitions; and inevitable losses, such as loss of relationships, loss of important career and life roles, loss of physical or mental abilities through illness or accident, and loss of loved ones through separation or death. In addition to these normal developmental transitions and challenges, a woman may have to deal with trauma related to difficult early childhood experiences, **abuse**, incest, **rape**, or domestic violence. Psychiatric disorders such as depression, anxiety, posttraumatic stress disorder, and eating disorders are common in women, and conditions such as alcohol and drug abuse and dependence often have a different presentation and course in women compared with men.

This chapter reviews common psychiatric disorders occurring in gynecologic patients, sexual function and disorders, and psychosocial issues and traumas that may arise during a woman's lifetime, and it offers suggestions as to how the physician can aid the patient.

DEVELOPMENTAL ISSUES IN CHILDHOOD AND ADOLESCENCE

Self-esteem begins to develop in early childhood and is affected by the positive efforts of parents and others in the child's immediate environment. Continuous reinforcement of a child's worth as an individual, by verbal and nonverbal means, should be encouraged. Touching, talking to the child in gentle ways, positively praising the child's positive actions, and, as the child becomes older, setting consistent, predictable limits that are socially acceptable within the framework of the family are all reasonable steps. Punishment should be limited to reinforcing the needs for the limits that have been set. Intimidation by verbal or physical means should be avoided. The physician may have the opportunity to suggest help for parents by offering reading material, discussing issues directly with them, or referring them to parenting classes. In general, positive reinforcement of the child's worth as an individual, mixed with appropriate warmth and love, tends to build self-esteem, whereas negative statements or actions tend to tear it down. A child has little basis for comparison, and if she is given negative information about herself, she will tend to believe it.

Girls and women, starting in childhood, often are highly invested in maintaining relationships, caring for others, not being "selfish" in pursuing their own goals and desires, and striving for ideal standards of appearance and behavior. These characteristics make it difficult, throughout life, to effectively and constructively express anger, be appropriately assertive, and know or pursue individual goals, and they may predispose girls and women to conditions such as depression and eating disorders, which are discussed later in the chapter. The physician can help by recognizing these characteristics and conditions early and providing support and referrals for mental health treatment as needed.

Physical, sexual, or emotional abuse in childhood and adolescence can have serious consequences for the child's development. Evidence for abuse must be addressed vigorously. The health care professional should communicate to the child or adolescent that she is a victim and is in no way responsible for what has happened. Reporting to child protective services may be legally mandated. Issues of abuse are discussed more fully later in this chapter.

DEPRESSION

Major depression is common in women, with a lifetime prevalence of 20% to 25%. Although boys and girls are equally likely to experience depression, major depression is about twice as common in women as in men, starting in adolescence. Major depression refers to persistent sadness or lack of interest or pleasure in usual activities, lasting for at least 2 weeks, and accompanied by symptoms such as changes in eating habits, trouble sleeping, lack of energy and motivation, poor memory or concentration, and feelings of guilt, worthlessness, hopelessness, and despair.

In severe cases, depression may lead to suicidal thoughts and attempts. The diagnostic criteria for major depression are listed in **Table 9-1**. The PHQ-9 (**Table 9-2**) is a useful screening tool for major depression, can be filled out quickly by the woman in the waiting room or in the office prior to a visit, and helps in identifying depression, monitoring effects of treatment, and educating the woman about her own characteristic symptoms of depression. Scores of 5, 10, 15, and 20 are cutoff scores indicating mild, moderate, moderately severe, and severe depression, respectively.

The cause of major depression is unclear. It may occur without a clear stress or precipitant, especially in women with a strong family history of depression who are genetically predisposed. Having a family history of depression, having had a prior depressive episode, and older age are all risk factors for depression. In addition, environmental stressors such as loss of relationships and loved ones, divorce, role transitions, interpersonal conflicts, medical illness, or feelings of being trapped in a stressful situation without a way to escape or cope can precipitate depression. The cause of depression in a particular person may be uniquely determined by individual factors, such as family relationships while growing up and past experiences that are highly meaningful and evoke negative feelings and memories triggered by current situations or events.

Loss of a parent during childhood is an important factor predisposing to later depression. Although there is conflicting literature—confounded by other consequences of parental loss such as financial problems, the nature of substitute care giving, and potential family disruption—it appears that both boys and girls are at heightened risk for later depression if they lose their primary caregiver in childhood. That risk is higher if the lost caregiver is of the same gender as the child. A 2009 prospective, longitudinal study by Coffino of 164 children who lost their primary caregiver between infancy and sixth grade found elevated levels of depression at age 26, especially if the loss occurred when the child was between age 5 and second grade.

The increased rate of depression in women starting at menarche has also been thought to result from hormonal factors. There are clear increases in risk for depressive symptoms premenstrually, with some women only experiencing mood symptoms at this time and others noting a worsening of underlying depression in the week or two prior to menses (for a discussion of premenstrual dysphoric disorder, see Chapter 36). The postpartum period is a high-risk time for depression and is the highest risk time in a woman's life for psychiatric hospitalization. There is also an increase in depressive symptoms at the time of menopause and the menopausal transition.

There is increasing evidence for gene-environment interactions in risk for depression. For example, Caspi et al. demonstrated that individuals carrying one or more copies of the S allele of the serotonin transporter gene linked polymorphic region (5HTTLPR) were more likely to develop depression

Table 9-1 Diagnostic Criteria for Major Depressive Episode

Five or more of the following symptoms have been present during the same 2-week period and represent a change from previous functioning; at least one of the symptoms is either (1) depressed mood or (2) loss of interest or pleasure.

1. Depressed mood most of the day, nearly every day, as indicated by either subjective report (e.g., feels sad or empty) or observation made by others (e.g., appears tearful)
2. Markedly diminished interest or pleasure in all, or almost all, activities
3. Significant weight loss (when not dieting) or weight gain, or decrease or increase in appetite
4. Insomnia or hypersomnia
5. Psychomotor agitation or retardation observable by others
6. Fatigue or loss of energy
7. Feelings of worthlessness or excessive or inappropriate guilt
8. Diminished ability to think or concentrate, or indecisiveness
9. Recurrent thoughts of death (not just fear of dying), recurrent suicidal ideation, or a suicide attempt or specific suicide plan

Adapted from American Psychiatric Association: Diagnostic and Statistical Manual of Mental Disorders, 4th ed, Text Revision, DSM-IV-TR. Washington, DC, American Psychiatric Association, 2000, p 356.

Table 9-2 PHQ-9

Over the past 2 weeks, how often have you been bothered by any of the following problems?	Not at all	Several days	More than half the days	Nearly every day
1. Little interest or pleasure in doing things	0	1	2	3
2. Feeling down, depressed, or hopeless	0	1	2	3
3. Trouble falling or staying asleep, or sleeping too much	0	1	2	3
4. Feeling tired or having little energy	0	1	2	3
5. Poor appetite or overeating	0	1	2	3
6. Feeling bad about yourself—or that you are a failure or have let yourself or your family down	0	1	2	3
7. Trouble concentrating on things, such as reading the newspaper or watching television	0	1	2	3
8. Moving or speaking so slowly that other people could have noticed, or the opposite—being so fidgety or restless that you have been moving around a lot more than usual	0	1	2	3
9. Thoughts that you would be better off dead or of hurting yourself in some way	0	1	2	3
Total Score ___ = ___ + ___ + ___				

If you checked off any problems, how difficult have these problems made it for you to do your work, take care of things at home, or get along with other people?

____ Not difficult at all   ____ Somewhat difficult   ____ Very difficult   ____ Extremely difficult

The PHQ was developed by Drs. Robert L. Spitzer, Janet B.W. Williams, Kurt Kroenke, and colleagues. PRIME-MD® is a trademark of Pfizer Inc. Copyright© 1999 Pfizer Inc. All rights reserved.

Spitzer RL, Kroenke K, Williams JBW: For the Patient Health Questionnaire Primary Care Study Group. Validation and utility of a self-report version of PRIME-MD: The PHQ Primary Care Study. JAMA 282:1737-1744, 1999; Spitzer RL, Williams JBW, Kroenke K, et al: Validity and utility of the Patient Health Questionnaire in assessment of 3000 obstetrics-gynecologic patients. Am J Obstet Gynecol 183:759-769, 2000.

and suicidality after experiencing stressful life events and childhood abuse.

The differential diagnosis of major depression includes adjustment disorder, dysthymic disorder, minor depression, depression related to drugs and alcohol or secondary to a medical condition, and bipolar disorder. Adjustment disorder is a stress-related, short-term emotional or behavioral response to a stressful life circumstance. Depressive symptoms begin within 3 months of the onset of the stressor and resolve within 6 months once the stressful circumstance ends. The symptoms do not meet criteria for major depression. The physician can help a woman with an adjustment disorder by helping her to problem solve and cope with the situation she is in or by referring her for short-term therapy or counseling.

Dysthymic disorder is a chronic, low-grade depression, with symptoms present more than half the time for at least 2 years. The best treatment is antidepressant medication and psychotherapy, but this condition is often harder to treat than major depression because of its chronicity. Minor depression refers to a depressive episode that does not quite meet criteria for major depression that may be best treated with psychotherapy. Major depression can also be caused by alcohol or drug use, or by medical conditions, such as hypothyroidism, vitamin B_{12} deficiency, anemia, or cancer (most classically pancreatic cancer). Women presenting with depression should be screened for medical disorders and asked about use of alcohol and drugs.

Probably the greatest dilemma in deciding to prescribe antidepressants is the concern that if the woman has bipolar disorder, antidepressants can cause a "switch" into a manic episode. Manic episodes are characterized by feelings of euphoria or irritability, decreased need for sleep, increased energy, increased activity or agitation, talkativeness, racing thoughts, grandiose and unrealistic plans, and impulsive and risky behavior. If a woman has been hospitalized for **mania** or has had such symptoms for a week or more in the past, the diagnosis may be clear. However, people often do not recall their manic symptoms or have little insight into them, or they may have had briefer periods of a few days (hypomania) that still predispose them to mania with antidepressants. It is often difficult to make the diagnosis of bipolar disorder, especially just from the woman's report. Any suspicion of this condition is an indication for psychiatric consultation, because bipolar depression requires treatment with a mood stabilizer instead of, or combined with, an antidepressant.

> A history of manic or hypomanic symptoms increases the risk for a "switch" into mania with antidepressant treatment.

Treatment of major depression can include antidepressant medication, psychotherapy, or both. Because both antidepressant medication and psychotherapy are effective, the initial choice of treatment can be made according to the woman's preference, although for more severe depression medication is indicated. Commonly prescribed antidepressant medications and dosages are listed in **Table 9-3** (and for a review of medication treatment of depression, see **Mann, 2005**). A 2009 metaanalysis by Cipriani et al. suggested that the best combination of efficacy and tolerability is for sertraline or escitalopram. Because of their more benign side effect profiles, it is reasonable to start a selective serotonin reuptake inhibitor

Table 9-3 Commonly Prescribed Antidepressants

Antidepressant	Dose Range (mg/day)
Serotonin reuptake inhibitors (SSRIs)	
Citalopram	20-60
Escitalopram	10-20
Fluoxetine	20-80
Paroxetine	20-50 (25-62.5 controlled release)
Sertraline	50-200
Serotonin and norepinephrine reuptake inhibitors (SNRIs)	
Duloxetine	60-120
Venlafaxine	75-375
Other	
Bupropion	300-450
Mirtazapine	15-45
Trazodone	25-100 (for insomnia)

(SSRI) as the first antidepressant in most cases. SSRI side effects include gastrointestinal side effects (nausea, diarrhea, vomiting), which are minimized by taking the medication with a meal. Other common side effects include initial dizziness and headaches, as well as **sexual dysfunction**, most commonly delayed orgasm or anorgasmia. Serotonin and norepinephrine reuptake inhibitors (SNRIs) include venlafaxine and duloxetine. Venlafaxine is associated with a dose-related risk for gradual onset of hypertension, and blood pressure should be monitored carefully on this medication. SNRI side effects include gastrointestinal side effects, headaches, dizziness, anorgasmia, activation, and anxiety. Bupropion appears to exert its therapeutic effect by enhancing effects of dopamine and norepinephrine. It increases energy and can cause insomnia, increased anxiety, headaches, and gastrointestinal side effects. Bupropion also lowers the seizure threshold and should not be used in women with a history of a seizure disorder or bulimia. Mirtazapine is an alpha$_2$-adrenergic, 5-HT2, and 5-HT3 receptor antagonist, which also has antihistaminic effects. Its common side effects include sedation and weight gain. Trazodone is a highly sedating serotonergic antidepressant that is used primarily at low doses (25 to 100 mg at bedtime) for insomnia. Tricyclic and MAO inhibitor antidepressants are infrequently prescribed currently because of the side effects, the dietary restrictions, and the risk of hypertensive crisis with MAO inhibitors. It is important to warn women that antidepressant medication can take up to 4 to 6 weeks to work, and to schedule a follow-up visit within that time to monitor treatment adherence, side effects, and therapeutic response. Recently, the Food and Drug Administration (FDA) has required black box warnings regarding increases in suicidal ideation with antidepressants, especially in adolescents and young adults. The mechanism for this is unclear but may be in part an increase in energy and motivation before improvement in mood. Women should be warned of this potential phenomenon and instructed to stop the medication and call the provider if this occurs. Overall, antidepressants reduce depression and risk for suicide, but this potentially serious side effect is another indication for close follow-up early in treatment.

> Close follow-up, in 1 to 2 weeks, is recommended to monitor for increases in suicidal thoughts with antidepressants, especially in adolescents and young adults.

Effective psychotherapies for depression include **cognitive behavioral therapy (CBT)** and **interpersonal therapy (IPT)**. Cognitive behavioral therapy addresses the negative, distorted thinking characteristics of depression, such as the belief that things are bad now, have always been bad, and will always be bad, or thoughts of worthlessness. In addition, behavioral activation, or scheduling activities that provide a sense of accomplishment, mastery, or pleasure, is helpful in depression, and exercise has been shown to be an effective treatment. Interpersonal therapy addresses the life changes and interpersonal challenges that contribute to depression, especially in women. These include grief, conflicts in interpersonal relationships including marital conflict, transitions in roles within work or the family, and social isolation with a lack of supportive relationships. These therapies are usually weekly for an hour for 3 to 4 months. In cases of clear-cut couple's issues, couples therapy may be indicated, especially after the woman has recovered from depression sufficiently to participate in such therapy. Other nonmedication treatments for depression include morning light for seasonal or winter depression and electroconvulsive treatment (ECT) or repetitive transcranial magnetic stimulation (rTMS) for depression that does not respond to medication and psychotherapy.

Both medication and psychotherapy are significantly more effective than placebo for treatment of major depression, with response rates varying between about 50% to 70%, depending on the patient population. Combined treatment with both psychotherapy and medication is more effective and is indicated for more severe depression. In adolescents, who are more at risk of suicidal thoughts with antidepressants, March et al. reported that combined treatment, adding cognitive behavioral therapy to fluoxetine, may reduce the risk of suicidal ideation.

Suicide is a feared and tragic outcome of depression and other mental health conditions as reviewed by Hawton and van Heeringen in 2009. In the United States, there were 33,300 suicide deaths in 2006, 4.5 per 100,000 women and 17.7 per 100,000 men committed suicide, and suicide was the third highest cause of death in young people aged 15 to 24. There are 12 to 25 suicide attempts per every suicide death. Risk factors for suicide include depression or other mental health disorders, **substance abuse** or **substance dependence**, a prior suicide attempt, a family history of psychiatric or substance use disorders, family violence including physical or sexual abuse, access to means such as firearms in the house, and exposure to suicidal behavior by others such as family members, peers, or celebrities. All depressed women should be asked about suicidal thoughts. This can include asking about whether the woman feels hopeless, has had thoughts that life is not worth living, or thoughts of ending her life, followed by more specific questions about whether she has made specific plans and how far she has gone to carry these out. Active suicidal thoughts and plans are a psychiatric emergency. The woman should not be left alone. The physician or staff should call 9-1-1 to have her taken to the nearest emergency room. Even in less acute cases, it is important to engage family members and other supportive people as possible, to remove firearms and other means of suicide from the home, to have someone else supervise the woman's medication, and to seek psychiatric or other mental health consultation as soon as possible.

> Active suicidal thoughts and plans are a psychiatric emergency.

EATING DISORDERS

Anorexia nervosa, **bulimia nervosa**, and **binge eating disorder** are the major eating disorders and have a lifetime prevalence of 0.6%, 1%, and 3%, respectively. Eating disorders primarily affect younger people and have their peak onset between the ages of 10 and 19. In fact, a study of children in the United States aged 9 to 14 found disordered eating behaviors in 7.1% of boys and 13.4% of girls. Eating disorders are more common in women than in men. Many young women with eating disorders are secretive about their disorder, do not view it as a problem, and do not seek treatment for it. Gynecologists may see such girls or women for related problems, such as amenorrhea, menstrual dysfunction, low bone density, sexual dysfunction, infertility, anxiety, depression, hyperemesis gravidarum, or other pregnancy complications. Because the woman may not volunteer information about disordered eating, it is important to have a high index of suspicion for eating disorders. A simple, five-question self-rating scale, the "SCOFF" (**Table 9-4**), is highly sensitive and specific in detecting eating disorders in primary care settings, and thus is a useful screening tool. The DSM-IV diagnostic criteria for anorexia nervosa and bulimia nervosa are listed in **Table 9-5**. Binge eating disorder (discussed later) is currently included as Eating Disorders Not Otherwise Specified, but is likely to be a separate diagnosis in DSM-V.

> Girls or women presenting with amenorrhea, menstrual dysfunction, low bone density, sexual dysfunction, infertility, anxiety, depression, or hyperemesis gravidarum should be screened for eating disorders.

Anorexia nervosa is characterized by a disturbed body image; fears of becoming fat or gaining weight, even though the woman's body weight is 85% or less than expected; and amenorrhea. Weight loss is achieved by restricting food intake, over-exercising, self-induced vomiting, or use of laxatives, emetics, and diuretics. Anorexia is most common in Caucasian teenage girls in industrialized Western societies. Societal pressures and standards of attractiveness for women, which emphasize thinness, have long been considered to increase the risk for anorexia nervosa, and a preoccupation with dieting is common in girls at menarche. Increasing evidence indicates, however, that there is clearly a significant genetic contribution to anorexia nervosa and other eating disorders, with heritability estimates of 50% to 80%. Other risk factors include a history of childhood sexual

Table 9-4 SCOFF Screening Questionnaire for Eating Disorders

1. Do you make yourself sick because you feel uncomfortably full?   _____ Yes _____ No
2. Do you worry you have lost control over how much you eat?   _____ Yes _____ No
3. Have you recently lost more than one stone (14 pounds) in a 3-month period?   _____ Yes _____ No
4. Do you believe yourself to be fat when others say you are too thin?   _____ Yes _____ No
5. Would you say that food dominates your life?   _____ Yes _____ No
Two or more "yes" answers indicate that the patient may have an eating disorder.

Adapted from Morgan JF, Reid F, Lacey JH. The SCOFF questionnaire: assessment of a new screening tool for eating disorders. BMJ 319:1467-1468, 1999.

Table 9-5 Diagnostic Criteria for Eating Disorders

Anorexia Nervosa
A. Refusal to maintain body weight at or above a minimally normal weight for age and height (body weight less than 85% of that expected).
B. Intense fear of gaining weight or becoming fat, even though underweight.
C. Disturbance in the way one's body weight or shape is experienced, undue influence of body weight or shape on self-evaluation, or denial of the seriousness of the current low body weight.
D. In postmenarcheal females, amenorrhea (i.e., the absence of at least three consecutive menstrual cycles).

Type
Restricting type: During the current episode of anorexia nervosa, the person has not regularly engaged in binge-eating or purging behavior (i.e., self-induced vomiting or the misuse of laxatives, diuretics, or enemas).
Binge-eating/purging type: During the current episode of anorexia nervosa, the person has regularly engaged in binge-eating or purging behavior (i.e., self-induced vomiting or the misuse of laxatives, diuretics, or enemas).

Bulimia Nervosa
A. There are recurrent episodes of binge eating. An episode of binge eating is characterized by both of the following:
   Eating, in a discrete period of time (e.g., within any 2-hour period), an amount of food that is definitely larger than most people would eat
   A sense of lack of control over eating during the episode
B. There is recurrent, inappropriate compensatory behavior in order to prevent weight gain, such as self-induced vomiting; misuse of laxatives, diuretics, enemas, or other medications; fasting; or excessive exercise.
C. The binge eating and inappropriate compensatory behaviors both occur, on average, at least twice a week for 3 months.
D. Self-evaluation is unduly influenced by body shape and weight.
E. The disturbance does not occur exclusively during episodes of anorexia nervosa.

Adapted from American Psychiatric Association: Diagnostic and Statistical Manual of Mental Disorders, 4th ed, Text Revision, DSM-IV-TR. Washington, DC, American Psychiatric Association, 2000, pp 589 and 594.

abuse and psychological traits of low self-esteem, perfectionism, and obsessive thinking.

Medical signs and symptoms associated with anorexia nervosa include bradycardia, hypotension, hypothermia, leukopenia, hair loss, skin changes, and constipation. Vomiting or laxative use may cause hypokalemia. Endocrine changes include low estrogen and testosterone levels, amenorrhea, decreased libido, hypercortisolemia, and low bone density. Prolonged QT interval is a serious sequela of anorexia nervosa and has been associated with sudden death. The mortality rate of anorexia nervosa from all causes is 5% to 6% per decade of illness.

Psychiatric symptoms associated with anorexia nervosa include depression, anxiety, social difficulties, sleep disturbance, agitation, poor emotion regulation, rigidity, obsessional thinking, and compulsive behaviors. Interestingly, these symptoms occur in individuals without anorexia nervosa during starvation and resolve with weight gain and so are most likely caused, or at least exacerbated, by the illness.

Anorexia nervosa is difficult to treat. Women do not usually seek help themselves, but instead they are brought to treatment by concerned family members. They fear gaining weight, do not see their illness as a problem, are frequently nonadherent to treatment, feel isolated and do not engage with treatment providers,

and may have multiple relapses. About one third recover completely, but this may take a number of years. Early recognition and treatment improve outcome. Family members often become frustrated with the woman's multiple relapses, lack of insight, and apparent lack of cooperation with treatment, and may need support themselves in dealing with her illness.

The best treatment for anorexia nervosa involves referral to a multidisciplinary team, with medical, nutritional, psychological, and psychiatric expertise in this area. The focus is on gradual refeeding to achieve weight gain, and outpatient treatment, with hospitalization only for acute, dangerous medical or psychiatric complications. In adolescents, family therapy or, in nonintact families, adolescent-centered individual psychotherapy is most effective according to Lock and colleagues' report in 2010. There is little evidence supporting any specific type of psychotherapy in adults, but treatment by a therapist with expertise in anorexia nervosa is more effective than support from a nonspecialist. There is no clear evidence supporting treatment with psychotropic medications. An early study showing efficacy of fluoxetine to maintain weight gain has not been replicated. Preliminary trials of atypical antipsychotics, with the goal of addressing distorted thinking about weight and body shape, have shown initial promise.

Bulimia nervosa is characterized by binge eating, combined with inappropriate compensatory mechanisms to avoid weight gain, such as self-induced vomiting, misuse of laxatives or diuretics (purging type), or fasting or excessive exercise (nonpurging type). Binge eating and compensatory behaviors occur an average of twice a week for 3 months (see **Table 9-5** for full diagnostic criteria). Bulimia, like anorexia, is most common in young women, has a significant genetic component, may follow teasing or criticism about the woman's weight or shape, and is thought to involve disturbances in hunger-satiety pathways, the drive system and rewarding characteristics of food, or self-regulation. Comorbidity with mood and anxiety disorders, addictions, and suicidal thoughts and behaviors is common. All-cause mortality rates, including suicide rates, are elevated, with a mortality rate of 3.9% over 8 to 25 years of follow-up.

Women with bulimia nervosa and purging may develop hypokalemia, hyponatremia, hypochloremia, a metabolic alkalosis as a result of vomiting, or a metabolic acidosis with laxative abuse. Recurrent self-induced vomiting can result in loss of dental enamel, parotid gland enlargement, or calluses and scars on the dorsal aspect of the hand. Rare but serious complications include esophageal tears, gastric rupture, rectal prolapse, and cardiac arrhythmias.

There is strong evidence for the efficacy of cognitive behavioral therapy for bulimia nervosa, although complete remission of binging and purging occurs in only 30% to 40%. Other therapies that have some evidence for efficacy are interpersonal therapy, dialectical behavior therapy focusing on emotion regulation, and family therapy in adolescents. Antidepressants are superior to placebo in treatment of bulimia, with the agent of choice being fluoxetine 60 mg daily. Of note, the antidepressant bupropion is contraindicated in women with a history of bulimia because of an elevated risk of seizures, presumably because of electrolyte abnormalities. The outcome of bulimia overall, based on a review of 27 studies, is full recovery in 45%, significant improvement in 27%, and a chronic, protracted course in about 23%.

In binge eating disorder, the woman binge eats (as in bulimia nervosa) at least 2 days a week for at least 6 months, but she does not engage in compensatory behaviors such as purging, fasting, or excessive exercise. As a result, she may also develop **obesity** but does not develop the medical complications associated with purging or low weight.

There is strong evidence for the efficacy of cognitive-behavioral therapy in binge eating disorder. Medications have moderate effects, with one metaanalysis showing remission rates with antidepressants of 49%, versus 29% on placebo. Weight loss agents and topiramate may also be effective.

OBESITY

The prevalence of obesity has dramatically increased in the United States. The World Health Organization (WHO) definitions for body weight are shown in **Table 9-6**. Weight classification by body mass index (BMI) is outlined in **Table 9-7**. Based on this definition, 33.9% of U.S. adults are obese. Twenty-two percent of non-Hispanic white women were classified as obese during the period 2006-2008, with non-Hispanic black women at a higher rate (39%), and Hispanic women at 29%. From a 2005 report on the Framingham cohort studied from 1971 to 2001, the long-term risk for becoming overweight was 50% and for obesity, 25%. WHO also describes a global epidemic of obesity, which is a major burden to worldwide chronic disease and disability.

There is a strong relationship between mortality and increased BMI above 25 kg/m^2 (and below 20 kg/m^2) (**Fig. 9-1**). Increased central adiposity is associated with increased risk of morbidity and mortality as well as BMI, so waist circumference can easily be measured. Using a tape measure at the level of the iliac crest, the waist circumference is taken. For women with a BMI of 25 to 34.9 kg/m^2, a waist circumference of over 35 inches is associated with heart disease and diabetes mellitus. Because of these risk factors, many organizations, including the American College of Obstetricians and Gynecologists, recommend screening for obesity.

Severe obesity is a health hazard that carries a 12-fold increase in mortality. Often these individuals suffer complicating factors, such as hypertension, diabetes mellitus, dyslipidemias, heart disease, stroke, arthritis, increased operative morbidity and mortality, and compromised pulmonary function (sleep apnea). Obesity has been linked to multiple obstetric and gynecologic problems, including spontaneous abortion, endometrial hyperplasia, and endometrial and breast cancer, to name a few. Renehan et al.'s 2008 metaanalysis of increased BMI and cancer risk found a strong association between a five-point BMI increase and endometrial cancer (RR 1.59, p < 0.0001), gall bladder cancer (RR 1.59, p = 0.04), esophageal adenocarcinoma (RR 1.51, p < 0.0001), and renal cancer (RR 1.34, p < 0.0001). A weaker positive association was found with postmenopausal breast, pancreatic, thyroid and colon cancer plus leukemia, multiple myeloma, and non-Hodgkin lymphoma. The mechanisms of cancer association with obesity may be linked to hormone systems like insulin, insulin-like growth factor, sex steroids, adipokines, and other substances.

Diet, exercise, and behavior modification provided by lay supervision is appropriate for those suffering from mild obesity; diet, exercise, and behavior modification under medical supervision is appropriate for those suffering from moderate obesity; and operative intervention is appropriate for those suffering from severe obesity if conservative measures have failed. Patients suffering from severe obesity almost always have medical complications, and these often improve with weight reduction.

Craighead and associates pointed out that unless behavior is modified, weight loss is usually not maintained. These workers studied 145 patients who were approximately 60% overweight and divided them into three groups. Treatment continued for 6 months, and there was at least 1 year of follow-up in 99% of those who completed the therapy. Group 1 underwent behavior modification using Ferguson's *Learning to Eat* manual. They lost an average of 11.4 kg and regained only 1.8 kg during the follow-up year. Group 2 received medication therapy with an appetite suppressant, fenfluramine hydrochloride (Pondimin). They lost an average of 14.5 kg but regained 8.6 kg during the follow-up period. The third group was treated with a combination of behavior modification and medication and lost an average of 15 kg but regained 9.5 kg during the follow-up period. The authors concluded that behavior modification without medication was the most appropriate therapy for moderate obesity. Setting goals is important in behavior therapy, and a 5% to 10% loss of total body weight is realistic over 6 months and can decrease the severity of comorbid diseases.

Mild obesity seems to respond best to dieting, exercise, and behavior modification under lay supervision. Such individuals will generally embrace fad diets and look for magic cures. However, if placed on a nutritionally appropriate limited-caloric diet, they will generally do well if their attitudes toward eating and response to various stimuli are modified. Lay groups, such as Weight Watchers or Take Off Pounds Sensibly (TOPS), may be successful for motivated individuals, although there are no direct comparisons of the variety of different commercial weight loss programs. One study suggested that if these structured weight loss programs could be provided free of charge to participants, both retention in the program and average weight loss outcomes might be far better than when participants must pay for these programs. Currently, many commercial diet centers are available for referral. Most prescribe or sell low-fat foods in an attempt to achieve a diet containing about 20% to 30% fat. Because fat represents 9 Cal/g and protein and carbohydrate represent 4 Cal/g, it is possible by changing eating habits to allow a patient a considerable quantity of food without high numbers of calories. Low-carbohydrate diets have become popular, but comparison studies have not proved better long-term results with these over other diets. The use of portion-controlled servings has been demonstrated to be effective for weight loss because obese persons tend to underestimate the amount of food they consume. Educating patients to change eating habits in this fashion is the key not only to losing weight but to maintaining the weight loss. Moderately obese patients will lose weight on diets of 1200 to 1500 calories (Cal). However, weight loss under these circumstances takes a long time. A weight loss of 5% of initial body weight is realistic over 6 months. The major problem with such individuals is maintaining weight loss, and, in fact, most do not maintain the weight loss.

Exercise is a useful addition to diet regimens. Several studies have demonstrated that although similar weight loss can be obtained by both diet alone and diet plus exercise programs, the latter will allow for a greater loss of fat stores while maintaining muscle mass. To maintain this advantage, exercise programs must be maintained. Although exercise alone is not a good method for losing weight, studies indicate exercise is very beneficial for long-term weight management and overall health.

Table 9-6 Body Mass Index Table

BMI	19	20	21	22	23	24	25	26	27	28	29	30	31	32	33	34	35
Height (inches)									Body Weight (pounds)								
58	91	96	100	105	110	115	119	124	129	134	138	143	148	153	158	162	167
59	94	99	104	109	114	119	124	128	133	138	143	148	153	158	163	168	173
60	97	102	107	112	118	123	128	133	138	143	148	153	158	163	168	174	179
61	100	106	111	116	122	127	132	137	143	148	153	158	164	169	174	180	185
62	104	109	115	120	126	131	136	142	147	153	158	164	169	175	180	186	191
63	107	113	118	124	130	135	141	146	152	158	163	169	175	180	186	191	197
64	110	116	122	128	134	140	145	151	157	163	169	174	180	186	192	197	204
65	114	120	126	132	138	144	150	156	162	168	174	180	186	192	198	204	210
66	118	124	130	136	142	148	155	161	167	173	179	186	192	198	204	210	216
67	121	127	134	140	146	153	159	166	172	178	185	191	198	204	211	217	223
68	125	131	138	144	151	158	164	171	177	184	190	197	203	210	216	223	230
69	128	135	142	149	155	162	169	176	182	189	196	203	209	216	223	230	236
70	132	139	146	153	160	167	174	181	188	195	202	209	216	222	229	236	243
71	136	143	150	157	165	172	179	186	193	200	208	215	222	229	236	243	250
72	140	147	154	162	169	177	184	191	199	206	213	221	228	235	242	250	258
73	144	151	159	166	174	182	189	197	204	212	219	227	235	242	250	257	265
74	148	155	163	171	179	186	194	202	210	218	225	233	241	249	256	264	272
75	152	160	168	176	184	192	200	208	216	224	232	240	248	256	264	272	279
76	156	164	172	180	189	197	205	213	221	230	238	246	254	263	271	279	287

BMI	36	37	38	39	40	41	42	43	44	45	46	47	48	49	50	51	52	53	54
58	172	177	181	186	191	196	201	205	210	215	220	224	229	234	239	244	248	253	258
59	178	183	188	193	198	203	208	212	217	222	227	232	237	242	247	252	257	262	267
60	184	189	194	199	204	209	215	220	225	230	235	240	245	250	255	261	266	271	276
61	190	195	201	206	211	217	222	227	232	238	243	248	254	259	264	269	275	280	285
62	196	202	207	213	218	224	229	235	240	246	251	256	262	267	273	278	284	289	295
63	203	208	214	220	225	231	237	242	248	254	259	265	270	278	282	287	293	299	304
64	209	215	221	227	232	238	244	250	256	262	267	273	279	285	291	296	302	308	314
65	216	222	228	234	240	246	252	258	264	270	276	282	288	294	300	306	312	318	324
66	223	229	235	241	247	253	260	266	272	278	284	291	297	303	309	315	322	328	334
67	230	236	242	249	255	261	268	274	280	287	293	299	306	312	319	325	331	338	344
68	236	243	249	256	262	269	276	282	289	295	302	308	315	322	328	335	341	348	354
69	243	250	257	263	270	277	284	291	297	304	311	318	324	331	338	345	351	358	365
70	250	257	264	271	278	285	292	299	306	313	320	327	334	341	348	355	362	369	376
71	257	265	272	279	286	293	301	308	315	322	329	338	343	351	358	365	372	379	386
72	265	272	279	287	294	302	309	316	324	331	338	346	353	361	368	375	383	390	397
73	272	280	288	295	302	310	318	325	333	340	348	355	363	371	378	386	393	401	408
74	280	287	295	303	311	319	326	334	342	350	358	365	373	381	389	396	404	412	420
75	287	295	303	311	319	327	335	343	351	359	367	375	383	391	399	407	415	423	431
76	295	304	312	320	328	336	344	353	361	369	377	385	394	402	410	418	426	435	443

Evidence Report of Clinical Guidelines on the Identification, Evaluation, and Treatment of Overweight and Obesity in Adults, 1998, www.nhlbi.nih.gov/guidelines/obesity/bmi_tbl.pdf

Table 9-7 Weight Classification by Body Mass Index (BMI)

Weight	BMI*
Normal weight	18.5-24.9
Overweight	25.0-29.9
Obesity	>30
Class I	30.0-34.9
Class II	35.0-39.9
Class III	>40

*BMI calculation = weight in kilograms/height in square meters.

A 2010 study by Lee et al. looking at amount of physical activity and weight gain in women concluded that physical activity is inversely related to weight gain in women of normal weight, but not in women who are overweight.

The FDA has approved medications for weight loss, although there have been many concerns about safety. Generally the medication must be continued for sustained benefit or weight gain recurs. Medications are mainly recommended for BMI > 30 kg/m^2 or BMI > 27 kg/m^2 when comorbid conditions are present. Orlistat inhibits dietary fat absorption and is considered first-line treatment because of its better safety profile than other medications. It has side effects of fecal urgency, flatulence, and oily stools. Sibutramine inhibits reuptake of neurotransmitters and affects satiation. Adverse effects include increases in heart rate and blood pressure, so sibutramine was removed from the market. These drugs cause modest weight loss (2.8 to 4.8 kg) compared with placebo. Other pharmacologic options include phentermine and diethylpropion, or metformin for women with type 2 diabetes. A guide to selecting treatment for obesity is given in **Table 9-8**.

Eligible candidates for bariatric surgery include those with a BMI > 40 kg/m^2 or a BMI > 35 kg/m^2 if serious comorbid conditions are present, if nonsurgical weight loss measures have failed, if the woman is motivated and well-informed, and there is acceptable surgical risk. A 2004 metaanalysis found the majority of postsurgical obesity patients have resolution or improvement in comorbid conditions such as diabetes, hypertension, dyslipidemia, and obstructive sleep apnea. A 2005 metaanalysis on surgical treatment of obesity found only a few controlled trials, but again, surgery was more effective for weight loss and control of some comorbid medical conditions when a patient BMI was 40 kg/m^2 or greater. Surgical options can provide long-term weight loss but are not without complications. Bariatric procedures used (gastric bypass, laparoscopic gastric band, vertical banded gastroplasty, and biliopancreatic diversion and switch) result in a 20% complication rate and 1% mortality. A patient with a BMI of 35 to 39 kg/m^2 appears to do better with surgery as well as the morbidly obese. In fact, there is even one randomized trial on laparoscopic adjustable gastric banding in adults with a BMI of 30 to 35 kg/m^2. The surgery was significantly more effective at reducing weight, resolving the metabolic syndrome, and improving quality of life at 2 years after the intervention.

Obesity in adolescence is a variant of the problem in the general population. The percentage of young people who are overweight has more than tripled since 1980. Sixteen percent of young people (6 to 19 years old) are overweight. Being overweight in adolescence is a more powerful predictor of morbidity from cardiovascular disease than being overweight in adulthood. Because the risk for progression with increasing morbidity and mortality is great, prompt support and behavior modification are most important. School and parental involvement are important aspects of controlling the problem. Where an obese parent is also present, best results seem to be achieved when both the parent and the child undergo therapy but in separate counseling sessions. Brownell and colleagues studied 42 obese adolescents, ages 12 through 16, divided into three groups, and using 16 weeks of treatment. When the child alone attended group therapy, there was an average 3.3-kg weight loss; when the child and mother were treated together, there was an average 5.3-kg weight loss; and when the child and mother were both treated but separately,

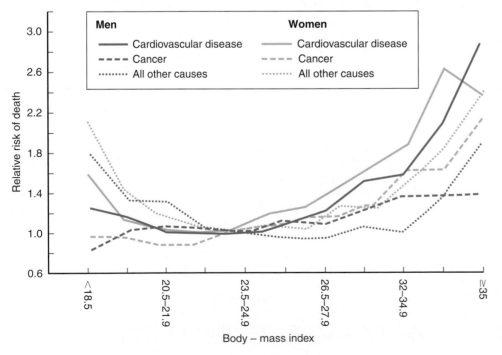

Figure 9-1 Relation between mortality and body mass index in men and women who have never smoked. (Data from Calle EE, Thun MJ, Petrelli JM, et al: Body-Mass Index and mortality in a prospective cohort of U.S. adults. N Eng J Med 341:1097, 1999.)

Table 9-8 Guide to Selecting Treatment

Body Mass Index Category					
Treatment	25-26.9	27-29.9	30-34.9	35-39.9	>40
Diet, physical activity, and behavior therapy	With comorbidities	With comorbidities	+	+	+
Pharmacotherapy		With comorbidities	+	+	+
Surgery			With comorbidities	With comorbidities	With comorbidities

The + represents the use of indicated treatment regardless of comorbidities.
From The Practical Guide: Identification, Evaluation, and Treatment of Overweight and Obesity in Adults. National Heart, Lung, and Blood Institute and North American Association for the Study of Obesity. Bethesda, MD, National Institutes of Health, 2000.

there was an 8.4-kg weight loss. After 1 year of follow-up, the group in which the mother and child were treated separately maintained their weight loss at a mean of 7.7 kg, whereas the other two groups had regained their previous baseline levels. The Cochrane Collaboration reviewed interventions for treating obesity in children in 2009, and although 64 randomized controlled trials were found, the data quality was limited. However, combined behavior lifestyle modifications with dietary changes, physical activity, or behavioral therapy were favored over standard or self-care for meaningful weight control. In obese adolescents, pharmacologic treatment warranted consideration in addition to the combined lifestyle modifications.

The Centers for Disease Control and Prevention (CDC) mentions the following promising approaches for preventing obesity: (1) breast-feeding, which is associated with a reduced risk of overweight children; (2) regular physical activity; (3) increasing physical activity in overweight people to prevent the complications associated with obesity; and (4) decreasing children's time watching television.

ANXIETY DISORDERS AND POSTTRAUMATIC STRESS DISORDER

Anxiety disorders are the most common psychiatric disorders in the general population. They usually have their onset in childhood, adolescence, or early adulthood and are more common in women than in men. Anxiety is a normal, adaptive response to danger or threat and is associated with physical symptoms (e.g., increased heart rate, sweating, shaking) and cognitive symptoms (e.g., worry, fear). Increases in anxiety are common with life stressors, including medical appointments, diagnoses, and procedures. In addition, anxiety may result from a number of drugs (e.g., caffeine, cannabis, cocaine, methamphetamine, withdrawal of alcohol or opiates), medications (e.g., theophylline, steroids), or medical conditions (e.g., asthma, arrhythmias, temporal lobe epilepsy). Some people experience primary anxiety disorders, involving excessive anxiety that interferes with daily functioning, without apparent explanation or out of proportion to any stressor. Primary anxiety disorders include **panic disorder**, **generalized anxiety disorder (GAD)**, **social anxiety disorder**, specific phobias, **obsessive compulsive disorder (OCD)**, and posttraumatic stress disorder (PTSD).

Panic disorder is characterized by sudden, intense attacks of fear. The symptom criteria for a panic attack are shown in **Table 9-9**. People with panic disorder have recurrent, unexpected panic attacks, with at least a month of persistent concern about having additional attacks, worry about the implications or

Table 9-9 Criteria for a Panic Attack

A discrete period of intense fear or discomfort, in which four (or more) of the following symptoms develop abruptly and reach a peak within 10 minutes.
1. Palpitations, pounding heart, or accelerated heart rate
2. Sweating
3. Trembling or shaking
4. Sensations of shortness of breath or smothering
5. Feeling of choking
6. Chest pain or discomfort
7. Nausea or abdominal distress
8. Feeling dizzy, unsteady, lightheaded, or faint
9. Derealization (feelings of unreality) or depersonalization (being detached from oneself)
10. Fear of losing control or going crazy
11. Fear of dying
12. Paresthesias (numbness or tingling)
13. Chills or hot flushes

Adapted from American Psychiatric Association: Diagnostic and Statistical Manual of Mental Disorders, 4th ed, Text Revision, DSM-IV-TR. Washington, DC, American Psychiatric Association, 2000, p 432.

consequences of panic attacks (e.g., losing control, having a heart attack, going crazy), or changes in behavior because of panic attacks (e.g., going to the emergency room, avoiding certain situations for fear of having an attack). About one third of people in the general population have at least one panic attack during their lives, so that a woman presenting with a single panic attack can be reassured that this is very common. Panic attacks can be precipitated by frightening situations or heightened stress, in which case they are called situational panic attacks. People with only situational panic attacks are not diagnosed with panic disorder. Panic attacks without apparent precipitant are called spontaneous.

Panic disorder occurs in 1% to 2% of the population and is about twice as common in women than in men. Risk factors include a family history of panic disorder and significant life stress in the year before the development of symptoms. The disorder has a genetic component, with a heritability of about 30%. Complications include depression in about two thirds of people, and one third are depressed at the time of clinical presentation. Especially as panic attacks are unpredictable, they frequently lead to **anticipatory anxiety** (anxiety about having the next panic attack) and **phobic avoidance**, or avoidance of situations in which the person has had or would fear having a panic attack. These situations commonly include crowds, being in lines or in the middle of an audience, driving (especially in tunnels, over bridges, or in freeways), or other situations in which the woman would feel trapped, unable to get out, or publicly embarrassed.

With time, the fear and avoidance surrounding panic attacks often become significantly more distressing and disabling than the attacks themselves and may lead to agoraphobia, or avoidance of multiple situations and activities. Panic disorder, like other anxiety disorders, is also associated with an increased rate of alcohol abuse as a form of self-medication. Finally, panic and other anxiety disorders are associated with an increased risk for suicide attempts. Thus, even though a woman presents with anxiety and does not endorse depression, she should be asked about hopeless or suicidal thoughts.

> Women with anxiety disorders, especially panic disorder and posttraumatic stress disorder, are at increased risk for suicide and should be asked about suicidal thoughts or plans.

The treatment of panic disorder includes reassurance, education, general measures, medication, and psychotherapy. Fortunately, treatment response rates are high, so it is possible to be optimistic that the woman has a highly treatable condition. She may fear that she is dying, has a life-threatening or serious medical illness, or that she is "going crazy," and she can be reassured that, although panic attacks are terrifying, none of these fears is true. Presenting a model of panic attacks as being the body's natural, healthy "alarm system" that is malfunctioning and being triggered for no reason is often helpful. As general measures, the woman should be counseled to avoid exacerbating factors, such as caffeine, alcohol, stimulants, or other illicit drugs and to examine possible modifiable sources of increased life stress.

> Anxiety disorders respond well to reassurance, education, and treatment with psychotherapy and medications (especially SSRI antidepressants).

Panic disorder responds well to both medication and psychotherapy. In more severe cases or with significant comorbid phobic avoidance, a combination of both treatments is preferable. However, because both are effective, the approach to treatment can be determined by the woman's preference. The first-line medication treatment for panic disorder is serotonin reuptake inhibitor antidepressants (SSRIs). There are two important differences in prescribing these medications for panic disorder versus for depression. First, people with panic disorder are frequently very sensitive to medication side effects. Because panic attacks involve feeling out of control of physical sensations and one's own body, side effects can initially increase anxiety and panic. Thus, although ultimately doses need to be similar to antidepressant doses, it is wise to start treatment at a low dose (e.g., a daily dose of 12.5 mg sertraline, 5 mg citalopram), increasing the dose rapidly after a few days if the woman has no side effects. Second, whereas antidepressants take 4 to 6 weeks or less to relieve depression, they can take up to 12 weeks to have their full effect on panic and anxiety, with some effect expected by 6 weeks. It is important to educate the woman about this delayed and gradual onset of action. Many women present in distress and ask about something that will act more rapidly. In cases of disability resulting from panic attacks (e.g., inability to function, work, or go to school), it is reasonable to prescribe a benzodiazepine along with an SSRI, with the expectation that the SSRI will be the long-term treatment and the benzodiazepine will be tapered after at most 12 weeks. A benzodiazepine such as clonazepam, which

has a longer half-life, requires only twice a day dosing, and maintains more constant blood levels, is preferable to shorter-acting agents such as alprazolam. For women with a history of substance use disorders or who need to avoid the potential slowed reflexes, psychomotor impairment, and cognitive slowing associated with benzodiazepines, other alternative adjuncts to reduce anxiety and panic quickly could include hydroxyzine or gabapentin. Buspirone has not been proved effective for panic disorder. In women who do not tolerate SSRIs, most other antidepressants (e.g., venlafaxine, mirtazapine) are also effective for long-term treatment of panic disorder, with the exception of bupropion, which increases anxiety symptoms.

Psychotherapy is a highly effective treatment for panic disorder. The best established therapy treatment is cognitive behavioral therapy (CBT), which focuses on addressing the catastrophic thoughts associated with panic attacks (e.g., "I'm dying," "I'm going to crash my car and kill myself and other people"), learning coping and anxiety reduction strategies (e.g., relaxation, paced breathing to combat hyperventilation), and gradual approach to feared situations to decrease disability. CBT is a weekly therapy for about 12 to 16 weeks, has significant improvement rates equal to or better than the 70% response rate with medication, yields long-term benefits after therapy is over, and increases the patient's sense of mastery and control, which is valuable in a disorder that makes people feel out of control. CBT can also help patients tolerate medication side effects and benzodiazepine withdrawal symptoms. Overall, of the varied symptoms of panic disorder, panic attacks are the easiest to treat and quickest to resolve with both medication and therapy. Phobic avoidance and anticipatory anxiety usually linger for a longer time, because of the unpredictability of panic attacks. People with panic disorder in most cases have a relapsing and remitting condition that requires long-term medication treatment (at least a year and frequently longer) and may recur in periods of increased stress.

In contrast with the sudden attacks of fear in panic disorder, generalized anxiety disorder (GAD) is characterized by excessive anxiety and worry about a number of life situations (e.g., work, school, family members) occurring more days than not for at least 6 months. The patient experiences her worries as excessive and difficult to control and as causing significant distress or trouble functioning. In addition, she has three symptoms of restlessness, insomnia, muscle tension, fatigue, trouble concentrating, or irritability. GAD usually begins early in life, is about twice as common in women than in men, has a genetic component, and has a lifetime prevalence of 5%. This is often a chronic disorder, with other lifetime psychiatric diagnoses (depression, other anxiety disorders, substance use disorders) superimposed in up to 90% of people. The restlessness and trouble concentrating associated with GAD and anxiety in general may lead to a misdiagnosis of attention deficit disorder.

The treatment of GAD often depends on the need to treat comorbid psychiatric conditions, which may have actually led the woman to seek medical help. In general, though, GAD responds to general measures such as avoiding caffeine, alcohol, and illicit drugs; medication; and psychotherapy. Antidepressants are effective for GAD, and the first-line long-term medication treatment is an SSRI. Buspirone 30 to 60 mg daily is effective for GAD and has few side effects. Hydroxyzine and beta-blockers have been shown to be effective, as are benzodiazepines. However, given the chronic, often lifelong course of

Table 9-10 Diagnostic Criteria for Social Phobia (Social Anxiety Disorder)

A. A marked and persistent fear of one or more social or performance situations in which the person is exposed to unfamiliar people or to possible scrutiny by others. The individual fears that she will act in a way (or show anxiety symptoms) that will be humiliating or embarrassing.

B. Exposure to the feared social situation almost invariably provokes anxiety, which may take the form of a situational panic attack.

C. The person recognizes that the fear is excessive or unreasonable.

D. Feared social or performance situations are avoided or endured with intense anxiety or distress.

E. The avoidance, anxious anticipation, or distress in the feared social or performance situation(s) interferes significantly with the person's normal routine, occupational or academic functioning, or social activities or relationships, or there is marked distress about having the phobia.

Adapted from American Psychiatric Association: Diagnostic and Statistical Manual of Mental Disorders, 4th ed, Text Revision, DSM-IV-TR. Washington, DC, American Psychiatric Association, 2000, p 456.

GAD, benzodiazepines are not recommended. Psychotherapy for GAD focuses on addressing and coping with worry ("What if" thoughts).

Social anxiety disorder (or social phobia) refers to anxiety in and avoidance of social situations, where the woman is or feels the center of attention and fears humiliation, embarrassment, or being judged negatively by other people (for diagnostic criteria, see **Table 9-10**). Symptoms of social anxiety disorder can include full-blown panic attacks, but these are provoked by social situations and are not spontaneous. In many cases, social anxiety disorder is restricted to specific situations, most often public speaking or other public performances. Generalized social anxiety disorder refers to a more pervasive form of this disorder, in which fears and avoidance relate not just to public performance but to most social situations and interactions, such as meeting new people, parties, initiating and maintaining conversations, dating, group projects, speaking with authority figures, or asserting oneself.

In epidemiologic studies, the lifetime prevalence of social anxiety disorder ranges from 3% to 13%. Age of onset is usually early in life, and women are more commonly affected than men. In Asian cultures, social anxiety disorder also includes fears of giving offense to other people—for example, through making inappropriate eye contact, body odor, flatulence, or blushing. There is evidence for a genetic or familial risk for this condition. Women with social anxiety disorder may have associated poor self-esteem, difficulty asserting themselves, depression, or alcohol abuse. Social anxiety disorder exists on a continuum with, and may be difficult to differentiate from, normal shyness, although by definition social anxiety disorder involves marked distress or impairment in functioning.

Treatment of social anxiety disorder also includes medication and psychotherapy. Serotonin reuptake inhibitors (SSRIs) are the first-line medication treatment and, as in other anxiety disorders, may take up to 12 weeks to have their full therapeutic effect. MAO inhibitors, though effective, bring with them dietary restrictions and risk of hypertensive crisis. Beta-blockers are helpful for performance anxiety but not for more generalized social anxiety disorder. Benzodiazepines are effective but should be used with caution because of the chronicity of this disorder

and the comorbidity with alcohol abuse and dependence. There is some evidence for efficacy of gabapentin.

Women with social anxiety restricted to public speaking may benefit from attending Toastmasters and thus practicing public speaking in a safe setting. Cognitive behavioral therapy (CBT) for social anxiety disorder is very effective. CBT includes individual treatment focusing on distorted thoughts about social situations (e.g., thoughts that the patient will make a fool of herself, has embarrassed herself, and that this will have catastrophic consequences) and on problem solving around and role-playing feared situations. Surprisingly, group cognitive behavioral therapy is also effective for social anxiety disorder.

Specific phobias occur in up to 20% of the general population and include fears of specific animals (e.g., snakes, spiders), phenomena (e.g., lightning), or situations (e.g., heights, flying in airplanes, driving, medical or dental procedures). People usually come to medical attention for specific phobias when these interfere with daily life or with their medical treatment. For example, people may develop specific phobias related to repeated medical events like chemotherapy treatments or to necessary aspects of their daily life, such as driving or traveling by plane. The best treatment for a specific phobia is desensitization, or gradually confronting the feared situation with the aid of an anxiety reducing strategy such as relaxation or imagery. In an acute situation, a benzodiazepine may help the woman to get through the particular event, but this will not reduce her future fear of the same situation.

Obsessive-compulsive disorder (OCD) is a specific anxiety disorder characterized by persistent, repetitive thoughts, ideas, or images that the patient finds irrational and intrusive (obsessions), with repetitive behaviors or rituals (compulsions) designed to decrease the anxiety caused by obsessions. Common obsessions include fears of contamination, dirt, germs, and illness; doubts (e.g., about having locked the door, turned off the oven, run over someone in one's car); needing to have things in order; and sexual or religious images or preoccupations. Compulsions include repetitive and excessive washing, cleaning, checking, putting things in order, or asking for reassurance. These obsessions and compulsions are distressing, take more than an hour a day, or interfere with functioning. The full diagnostic criteria are shown in **Table 9-11**.

Obsessive-compulsive disorder has a lifetime prevalence of 2% to 3% and is more common in monozygotic than dizygotic twins and in first-degree relatives of affected individuals than in the general population. Unlike other anxiety disorders, rates are similar in men and women. However, males have an earlier peak age of onset than females (6 to 15 years old versus 20 to 29 years old) and a higher comorbidity with Tourette's syndrome and tic disorders. In people with OCD, the incidence of Tourette's is 5% to 7% and of tics is 20% to 30%. Other conditions commonly associated with OCD, in both genders, include major depression, other anxiety disorders, hypochondriacal concerns, and excessive use of alcohol and sedatives.

Treatment of OCD includes both medications and psychotherapy. The first-line treatment is serotonergic antidepressants, specifically SSRIs, and clomipramine, which is a highly serotonergic tricyclic antidepressant. People with OCD may require higher doses of these medications than do depressed patients and take about 12 weeks for a full response. Response rates tend to be lower than in other anxiety disorders and are generally 40% to 60%. It is uncommon for a patient with OCD to have

Table 9-11 Diagnostic Criteria for Obsessive Compulsive Disorder

A. Either obsessions or compulsions:
Obsessions as defined by (1), (2), (3), and (4):
(1) Recurrent and persistent thoughts, impulses, or images that are experienced at some time during the disturbance as intrusive and inappropriate and that cause marked anxiety or distress
(2) The thoughts, impulses, or images are not simply excessive worries about real-life problems
(3) The person attempts to ignore or suppress such thoughts, impulses, or images, or to neutralize them with some other thought or action
(4) The person recognizes that the obsessional thoughts, impulses, or images are a product of his or her own mind (not imposed from without as in thought insertion)
Compulsions as defined by (1) and (2):
(1) Repetitive behaviors (e.g., hand washing, ordering, checking) or mental acts (e.g., praying, counting, repeating words silently) that the person feels driven to perform in response to an obsession or according to rules that must be applied rigidly
(2) The behaviors or mental acts are aimed at preventing or reducing distress or preventing some dreaded event or situation; however, these behaviors or mental acts either are not connected in a realistic way with what they are designed to neutralize or prevent or are clearly excessive
B. At some point during the course of the disorder, the person has recognized that the obsessions or compulsions are excessive or unreasonable.
C. The obsessions or compulsions cause marked distress, are time consuming (take more than 1 hour a day), or significantly interfere with the person's normal routine, occupational (or academic) functioning, or usual social activities or relationships.

Adapted from American Psychiatric Association: Diagnostic and Statistical Manual of Mental Disorders, 4th ed, Text Revision, DSM-IV-TR. Washington, DC, American Psychiatric Association, 2000, pp 462-463.

Table 9-12 Diagnostic Criteria for Posttraumatic Stress Disorder (PTSD)

A. The person has been exposed to a traumatic event in which both of the following have been present:
(1) The person has experienced, witnessed, or been confronted with an event or events that involve actual or threatened death or serious injury, or a threat to the physical integrity of oneself or others.
(2) The person's response involved intense fear, helplessness, or horror.
B. The traumatic event is persistently reexperienced in at least one of the following ways:
(1) Recurrent and intrusive distressing recollections of the event, including images, thoughts, or perceptions
(2) Recurrent distressing dreams of the event
(3) Acting or feeling as if the traumatic event were recurring (includes a sense of reliving the experience, illusions, hallucinations, and dissociative flashback episodes, including those that occur upon awakening or when intoxicated)
(4) Intense psychological distress at exposure to internal or external cues that symbolize or resemble an aspect of the traumatic event.
(5) Physiologic reactivity upon exposure to internal or external cues that symbolize or resemble an aspect of the traumatic event
C. Persistent avoidance of stimuli associated with the trauma and numbing of general responsiveness (not present before the trauma), as indicated by at least three of the following:
(1) Efforts to avoid thoughts, feelings, or conversations associated with the trauma
(2) Efforts to avoid activities, places, or people that arouse recollections of the trauma
(3) Inability to recall an important aspect of the trauma
(4) Markedly diminished interest or participation in significant activities
(5) Feeling of detachment or estrangement from others
(6) Restricted range of affect (e.g., unable to have loving feelings)
(7) Sense of foreshortened future (e.g., does not expect to have a career, marriage, children, or a normal life span)
D. Persistent symptoms of increasing arousal (not present before the trauma), indicated by at least two of the following:
(1) Difficulty falling or staying asleep
(2) Irritability or outbursts of anger
(3) Difficulty concentrating
(4) Hypervigilance
(5) Exaggerated startle response
E. Duration of the disturbance (symptoms in B, C, and D) is more than 1 month.
F. The disturbance causes clinically significant distress or impairment in social, occupational, or other important areas of functioning.
Specify if:
Acute: if duration of symptoms is less than 3 months
Chronic: if duration of symptoms is 3 months or more
Specify if:
With delayed onset: if onset of symptoms at least 6 months after the stressor

Adapted from American Psychiatric Association: Diagnostic and Statistical Manual of Mental Disorders, 4th ed, Text Revision, DSM-IV-TR. American Psychiatric Association, Washington, DC, American Psychiatric Association, 2000, pp 467-468.

complete resolution of symptoms, and this is usually a chronic, relapsing, and remitting disorder requiring ongoing treatment. The specific psychotherapy treatment most helpful in OCD is exposure and response prevention. This treatment involves gradually increasing exposure to the feared situation, without performing the compulsive ritual (e.g., exposure to dirt without the ability to wash one's hands). Patients who agree to this treatment must tolerate significant anxiety, which, however, subsides with time after each exposure and diminishes over the course of treatment.

Posttraumatic stress disorder (PTSD) refers to a characteristic set of responses to a traumatic situation that involves direct personal experience of, witnessing, or being confronted with an event involving actual or threatened death or harm to oneself or someone else. The trauma provokes a response of helplessness, fear, horror, or (in children) disorganized or agitated behavior. The characteristic responses include symptoms of reexperiencing the event, emotional numbing and avoidance, and increased arousal. The full diagnostic criteria and lists of symptoms are given in **Table 9-12**. It is common for people to experience symptoms like this in the first month following a major trauma, in which case the diagnosis is acute stress disorder. After a month, when most people would have recovered, persistent symptoms are then diagnosed as PTSD.

PTSD has an estimated lifetime prevalence of 8% in adults in the United States. Rates of PTSD vary from one third to over half of people exposed to specific traumas, such as combat, rape, or captivity. Risk factors for development of PTSD in people exposed to a specific trauma include female sex, younger age, severity and duration of the event, lack of social support, history of prior trauma, or history of preexisting psychiatric disorders.

There is also evidence that people with greater autonomic arousal (higher heart rate and blood pressure) following the trauma are at increased risk. Although PTSD would appear to be a quintessentially environmentally determined disorder, the risk of development of PTSD following trauma appears to be heritable. PTSD is associated with depression, panic attacks and anxiety, substance abuse and dependence, suicidal thoughts and attempts, and, in severe cases, psychotic symptoms such as hallucinations or paranoia.

Several types of individual and group psychotherapy are effective in the treatment of PTSD. These therapies include coping with current life problems and triggers, gradual exposure and reexperiencing of the trauma with desensitization, and examining any distorted thoughts about the trauma, such as guilt that the woman brought this upon herself or could have done more to prevent or stop it. It is important to recognize that many people are retraumatized and their symptoms worsened by retelling the story of the trauma, especially if this is not in the context of a structured, ongoing psychotherapeutic treatment.

Medications are frequently used to address symptoms of PTSD. For example, SSRIs are effective in reducing depression, anxiety, and emotional numbing. Medications such as valproate may help with impulsivity and anger. Hypnotics may be helpful for insomnia. Prazosin, an alpha-adrenergic antagonist, has been shown to be helpful in reducing trauma-related nightmares and more general PTSD symptoms. Benzodiazepines should be used with caution, given the comorbidity with substance use disorders and reports of increased impulsivity in patients with PTSD given these medications. Acute management immediately following a rape is discussed further later in the chapter.

PSYCHOTROPIC MEDICATIONS AND ORAL CONTRACEPTIVES

The gynecologist frequently sees women who are taking psychotropic medications, for one of the disorders described earlier or for other less common psychiatric disorders such as bipolar disorder or schizophrenia, and may be called upon to advise them about options for birth control. There are several psychotropic medications that alter the metabolism and efficacy of oral contraceptives (OCs) or whose metabolism is in turn altered by OCs.

Induction of the hepatic cytochrome P450 3A4 enzyme can increase OC metabolism and cause contraceptive failure. Psychotropic medications that induce 3A4 and that have been associated with spotting, breakthrough bleeding, or unwanted pregnancy include the mood stabilizers carbamazepine (Tegretol) and oxcarbazepine (Trileptal), topiramate (Topomax; at doses above 200 mg daily), and the wakefulness enhancing agent modafinil (Provigil). St. John's wort, commonly used over the counter as an antidepressant, also induces 3A4 and can cause contraceptive failure. OC activity may be increased or prolonged by 3A4 inhibitors such as the antidepressants fluoxetine (Prozac) and possibly fluvoxamine (Luvox).

Oral contraceptives are themselves moderate 1A2 and 2C19 inhibitors and mild 2B6 and 3A4 inhibitors. Thus, OCs can increase levels and effects of amitriptyline (Elavil), bupropion (Wellbutrin), chlordiazepoxide (Librium), chlorpromazine (Thorazine), clozapine (Clozaril), diazepam (Valium), imipramine (Tofranil), and possibly olanzapine (Zyprexa). Drugs whose clearance is increased, and that therefore have lower levels, with OCs include nicotine, and with the mood stabilizers lamotrigine (Lamictal), and valproic (Depakote) acid. Lamotrigine levels have been found to be 84% higher in the week of the cycle off ethinyl estradiol. Given the risk of Stevens-Johnson syndrome with fluctuating levels of lamotrigine, and the likelihood of worsening mood symptoms with variations in blood levels of mood stabilizers such as lamotrigine and valproic acid, it may be best to advise women taking these medications to use a continuous daily OC or another form of birth control.

SUBSTANCE ABUSE AND DEPENDENCE

Women have lower rates of alcohol and drug abuse and dependence than men, except in adolescence, when the rates are similar. However, substance use disorders are common in women and the rates are increasing. In 2006, 41% of women 12 years of age or older had tried an illicit drug during their lifetimes; currently, 6% reported use of illicit drugs, 23% tobacco use, and 45% alcohol use (3% heavily, 15% binge drinkers). Six percent of women (versus 12% of men) met criteria for substance abuse or dependence in the past year as published by Albright and Rayburn in 2009. In contrast to a male: female ratio for alcohol use disorders of 5:1 in the 1980s, a 2010 survey by Greenfield shows a ratio of about 3:1. Alcohol, tobacco, and other drug use in women are of particular concern to gynecologists, not only because of the risks to the woman but also because of the risks to her children, through teratogenic risks and effects on parenting abilities.

Women consistently have been noted to have an accelerated progression of substance use disorders, with a shorter time between first use of a substance to onset of dependence and then first treatment. This phenomenon is known as **telescoping** and is best established for alcohol, cannabis, and opiates. Women generally present for treatment with a more severe form of the disorder and more social, behavioral, and medical complications than men, despite a shorter period of heavy use. They are more likely than men to suffer psychosocial consequences, such as violence and victimization, and to have psychiatric comorbidity, especially depression, anxiety, eating disorders, and posttraumatic stress disorder; 72% of women, as opposed to 57% of men, have coexisting psychiatric disorders, and in women these other disorders are more likely to have preceded, and to exacerbate, the substance use disorder. Thus, it is important to recognize and treat other mental health problems in women with alcohol and drug abuse and dependence. Heavy drinking in women increases general health risks, as it does in men, but also is associated with amenorrhea, anovulation, luteal phase dysfunction, and early menopause.

> Women have a more accelerated progression of substance use disorders, present for treatment with a more severe form of the disorder, and have more social, behavioral, and medical complications than men.

The DSM-IV criteria for substance abuse and dependence are shown in **Table 9-13**. Whereas abuse is characterized by adverse life consequences of substance use, dependence also carries with it escalation of use or physiologic or psychological dependence.

Patients frequently do not report excessive alcohol or drug use or may not recognize their use as excessive. As in primary care

Table 9-13 Diagnostic Criteria for Substance Abuse and Dependence.

Substance Abuse

A maladaptive pattern of substance use leading to clinically significant impairment or distress, as manifested by at least one of the following, occurring within a 12-month period:

(1) Recurrent substance use resulting in a failure to fulfill major role obligations at work, school, or home (e.g., repeated absences or poor work performance related to substance use; substance-related absences, suspensions, or expulsions from school; neglect of children or household)

(2) Recurrent substance use in situations in which it is physically hazardous (e.g., driving an automobile or operating a machine when impaired by substance use)

(3) Recurrent substance-related legal problems (e.g., arrests for substance-related disorderly conduct)

(4) Continued substance use despite having persistent or recurrent social or interpersonal problems caused or exacerbated by the effects of the substance (e.g., arguments with spouse about consequences of intoxication, physical fights)

Substance Dependence

A maladaptive pattern of substance use, leading to clinically significant impairment or distress, as manifested by at least three of the following, occurring at any time in the same 12-month period:

(1) Tolerance, as defined by either of the following:
  (a) A need for markedly increased amounts of the substance to achieve intoxication or desired effect
  (b) Markedly diminished effect with continued use of the same amount of the substance

(2) Withdrawal, as manifested by either of the following:
  (a) The characteristic withdrawal syndrome for the substance
  (b) The same, or a closely related, substance is taken to relieve or avoid withdrawal symptoms

(3) The substance is often taken in larger amounts or over a longer period than was intended

(4) There is a persistent desire or unsuccessful efforts to cut down or control substance use

(5) A great deal of time is spent in activities necessary to obtain the substance (e.g., visiting multiple doctors or driving long distances), use the substance (e.g., chain smoking), or recover from its effects

(6) Important social, occupational, or recreational activities are given up or reduced because of substance use

(7) The substance use is continued despite knowledge of having a persistent or recurrent physical or psychological problem that is likely to have been caused or exacerbated by the substance (e.g., current cocaine use despite recognition of cocaine-induced depression, or continued drinking despite recognition that an ulcer was made worse by alcohol consumption)

Specify if "With Physiological Dependence" if evidence of tolerance or withdrawal (i.e., if either item (1) or (2) is present).

Adapted from American Psychiatric Association: Diagnostic and Statistical Manual of Mental Disorders, 4th ed, Text Revision, DSM-IV-TR. Washington, DC, American Psychiatric Association, 2000, pp 197, 199.

and mental health settings, patients seeing gynecologists are far less likely to be recognized as having a substance use disorder based on physician assessment and documentation. There are several screening tests that can help identify these disorders (**Table 9-14**). The CAGE is a very brief and widely used screening test. Although it is generally helpful in detecting alcohol dependence, it appears to be less sensitive in white than in black women, and in heavy drinking as opposed to dependence. The T-ACE is a variation on the CAGE, which replaces the "guilt" about drinking item with a question about tolerance. The T-ACE was developed specifically for use in pregnant women, given the high rate of guilt in women who consume any alcohol during pregnancy. The AUDIT is a longer, 10-item screening test that has been well validated and includes self-reports of quantity and frequency of drinking. Probably the best screening test in detecting heavy alcohol use as well as dependence in groups of women of mixed ethnicity is the TWEAK. Women who score at or above the cutoff score on any of these screening tests, or who endorse use of an illicit drug or tobacco, should be questioned further about the frequency, amount, and consequences of their use of alcohol and illicit drugs. Although women with severe alcohol dependence may have abnormalities in laboratory tests such as hepatic enzymes (ALT, AST, GGT) or mean corpuscular volume (MCV), questionnaires provide a significantly more sensitive method of detecting heavy drinking.

The gynecologist is frequently a woman's primary care provider and is in an ideal position to help the patient seek help for a substance use disorder. The patient may not realize that her use is problematic or dangerous. It can be useful to educate her about "safe" levels of alcohol use, for example. Consuming more than two drinks per day on average is considered heavy drinking for a woman and has been linked to increases in mortality, cirrhosis, and breast cancer. Women may benefit from education about adverse effects of alcohol, tobacco, and drugs to the fetus and newborn.

> More than two drinks per day on average is considered heavy drinking for a woman.

Once the patient has been educated, her motivation to engage in behavior change or specific substance abuse treatment can be enhanced using **motivational interviewing**, an efficient and highly effective brief counseling technique that aims to accomplish behavior change by helping people explore and resolve ambivalence. Advice alone is often not sufficient to bring about behavior change, and patients vary in their stage of "readiness to change" (**Table 9-15**). The goal of motivational interviewing is to move people through the stages of change listed in this table. Motivational interviewing was developed for substance use disorders but is also highly effective in promoting weight reduction, exercise, safe sex practices, and regular use of contraception.

Motivational interviewing emphasizes reflective listening, rather than advice giving. In the context of a trusting relationship, the physician expresses empathy and understanding of the patient's ambivalence and the obstacles to change, avoids arguments, points out discrepancies between the patient's behavior and her goals, helps problem solve ways to succeed in meeting goals, and supports the patient's own motivation and efforts to change. Training in motivational interviewing is readily available. Motivational interviewing has been shown to be a highly effective intervention, and practicing this technique adds an average of only 3 minutes to a clinic visit. Resources and videos are listed in the 2009 American College of Obstetricians and Gynecologists (ACOG) Committee Opinion regarding motivational interviewing.

> Motivational interviewing is a highly effective, brief intervention that increases women's engagement in substance abuse treatment and other behavior change.

Table 9-14 Substance Use Disorder Screening Tests

Audit

The following questions pertain to your use of alcoholic beverages during the past year. A "drink" refers to a can or bottle of beer, a glass of wine, a wine cooler, or one cocktail or shot of hard liquor.

1. How often do you have a drink containing alcohol? (never, 0 points; monthly or less, 1 point; 2-4 times per month, 2 points; 2-3 times per week, 3 points; 4 or more times a week, 4 points)
2. How many drinks containing alcohol do you have on a typical day when you are drinking? (1-2 drinks, 0 points; 3-4 drinks, 1 point; 5-6 drinks, 2 points; 7-9 drinks, 3 points; 10 or more drinks, 4 points)
3. How often do you have 6 or more drinks on one occasion? (never, 0 points; less than once a month, 1 point; monthly, 2 points; weekly, 3 points; daily or almost daily, 4 points)
4. How often during the past year have you found that you were not able to stop drinking once you had started? (same scoring as question 3)
5. How often during the past year have you failed to do what was normally expected from you because of drinking? (same scoring as question 3)
6. How often during the past year have you needed a first drink in the morning to get yourself going after a heavy drinking session? (same scoring as question 3)
7. How often during the past year have you had a feeling of guilt or remorse after drinking? (same scoring as question 3)
8. How often during the past year have you been unable to remember what happened the night before because you were drinking? (same scoring as question 3)
9. Have you or someone else been injured as a result of your drinking? (no, 0 points; yes, but not in the past year, 2 points; yes, during the past year, 4 points)
10. Has a relative or friend, or a doctor, or other health care worker been concerned about your drinking or suggested you cut down? (same scoring as question 9)

Scoring: Add up points; score 0-40; score of 4 or above indicates possible alcohol abuse or dependence for women.

CAGE	C	Have you ever felt you ought to cut down on your drinking?
	A	Have people annoyed you by criticizing your drinking?
	G	Have you felt bad or guilty about your drinking?
	E	Have you ever had a drink in the morning (eye opener) to steady your nerves or get rid of a hangover?
		Scoring: 1 point for each "yes"; any yes response warrants further assessment.
TWEAK	T	Tolerance: How many drinks can you hold (6 or more indicates tolerance) or how many drinks does it take before you begin to feel the first effects of the alcohol? (3 or more indicates tolerance)
	W	Worried: Have close friends or relatives worried or complained about your drinking in the past year?
	E	Eye opener: Do you sometimes take a drink in the morning when you first get up?
	A	Amnesia: Has a friend or family member ever told you about things you said or did while you were drinking that you could not remember?
	K	Kut down: Do you sometimes feel the need to cut down on your drinking?
		Scoring: 2 points each for Tolerance or Worried; 1 point each for others; total Possible = 7 points; 2 points or more warrants further assessment in women.
T-ACE	T	Tolerance: How many drinks does it take to make you feel high? (3 or more indicates tolerance)
	A	Annoyed question from CAGE
	C	Cut down question from CAGE
	E	Eye opener question from CAGE
		Scoring: 2 points for tolerance, 1 point each for "yes" on other items; 1 or more points warrants further assessment in women.

Adapted from Bradley KA, Boyd-Wickizer J, Powell SH, Burman ML: Alcohol screening questionnaires in women: a critical review. JAMA 280:166-171, 1998.

Table 9-15 Stages of Readiness for Change

- Precontemplation—The patient does not believe a problem exists. ("I won't get pregnant!")
- Contemplation—The patient recognizes a problem exists and is considering treatment or behavior change. ("Maybe I could get pregnant and there are things I could do to prevent this.")
- Action—The patient begins treatment or behavior change. ("I'll take that prescription for birth control pills.")
- Maintenance—The patient incorporates new behavior into daily life. ("I'm taking the pill every day.")
- Relapse—The patient returns to the undesired behavior. ("The pill makes me sick. I think I'll stop.")

From ACOG Committee Opinion: Motivational interviewing: a tool for behavior change. Obstet Gynecol 113:243-246, 2009.

Once a patient has expressed interest in cutting down use of drugs or alcohol, she may be able to do this on her own. If not, treatments include Alcoholics Anonymous, Women for Sobriety, Cocaine Anonymous, or Narcotics Anonymous; psychotherapy; or outpatient and inpatient substance abuse treatment centers. The Substance Abuse and Mental Health Services Administration (SAMHSA) provides a convenient list of drug and alcohol treatment programs by state and local area at http://dasis3.samhsa.gov.

Specific substances of abuse are associated with particular gender differences in patterns of use and treatment success. Alcohol use in women is associated with the phenomenon of telescoping, or an accelerated course from onset of use to significant alcohol-related problems. There are several biologic factors that may contribute to this more rapid course, including the lower percentage of body water in women, lower levels of alcohol dehydrogenase in the gastric mucosa and thus decreased first pass metabolism, and slower rates of alcohol metabolism. Women also appear to have different motives for drinking, with a higher likelihood of drinking in response to stress, negative emotions, and underlying primary coexisting psychiatric disorders. Women are less likely to seek treatment, perhaps related to childcare responsibilities, financial resources, and greater stigma related to women's use of alcohol. Female patients may benefit from women-only treatment settings or groups addressing women's issues. Effective pharmacologic treatments for alcohol dependence in both genders include naltrexone, topiramate, and baclofen, whereas acamprosate has yielded mixed results, with some negative and some positive treatment trials. Alcohol use during pregnancy is associated with fetal alcohol syndrome and fetal alcohol effects, and most women avoid alcohol once they know that they are pregnant.

In 2008, 28% of people in the United States reported using nicotine currently. Although rates are higher in men than in women, women are at increased risk for heart attacks, chronic obstructive pulmonary disease, and lung cancer secondary to nicotine. Nicotine also is associated with early menopause and with spontaneous abortion, low birth weight, and preterm birth with in utero exposure. Only 3% of smokers are able to quit in any given year, and women appear to have more difficulty quitting than men. Women have more success quitting in the follicular versus the luteal phase of their cycle, but they are more likely to relapse because of weight gain associated with smoking cessation and have a high rate of relapse (about 65%) even if they have quit during pregnancy. Specific smoking cessation treatments, such as the nicotine patch, bupropion, and Varenicline, show equal efficacy in men and women in short-term treatment trials. Bupropion may be particularly useful in women who have comorbid depression.

Cannabis abuse is more common in men, but it has a more rapid progression in women. Cannabis is associated with impaired memory, attention, and motivation; increases risk for onset of panic attacks; may increase vulnerability to depression and psychotic disorders; and has been associated with shorter gestation, decreased birth weight, and possible impairments in executive functioning with in utero exposure. Treatments such as cognitive behavioral therapy and therapeutic communities appear equally effective for both genders.

Women may be more vulnerable than men to the reinforcing effects of stimulants, especially during the follicular phase when estrogen levels are high. The diagnosis of attention deficit disorder is increasingly being made in women, with a corresponding increase in therapeutic use of stimulants. Illicit use of stimulants more than doubled in the general population in the decade between 1995 and 2005, and in 2006, 24% of pregnant women admitted to federally funded substance abuse treatment had methamphetamine dependence. The literature regarding stimulant effects during pregnancy is conflicting, but growth restriction, decreased birth weight, decreased gestational age, and maternal hypertension have been reported.

Use of heroin and ther intravenous drugs is less frequent in women than in men, and women are more likely to inject drugs if their partner uses IV drugs and introduces them to injection. In contrast, overuse of prescription narcotics is more common in women than in men. Use of opiates, including methadone, during pregnancy is associated with neonatal abstinence syndrome, respiratory depression, preterm delivery, premature rupture of membranes, fetal growth restriction, and meconium-stained amniotic fluid.

"DIFFICULT" PATIENTS

In a study of more than 500 adult patients seen in a primary care clinic, Jackson and Kroenke found that physicians described more than 15% of their patients as "difficult." "Difficult" patients were more likely to have a depressive or anxiety disorder, poor level of functioning, unmet expectations, low levels of satisfaction, and higher use of health care services. It is always possible for a physician to have a personality clash with an individual patient, but "difficult" patients are a subset of patients who evoke negative feelings in many, if not most, physicians. These patients may be angry, argumentative, threatening, mistrustful, demanding, dissatisfied; may misuse habit-forming prescribed medications or appear "drug seeking"; may challenge the physician's approach and not comply with treatment recommendations; or may be very difficult to engage in a productive treatment alliance. In a classic 1978 paper, Groves described "hateful patients" as people who "kindle aversion, fear, despair, or even downright malice in their doctors." These are challenging people to interact with, and feeling frustration, anxiety, or dislike in seeing them significantly reduces a physician's satisfaction with providing medical care.

A woman may not comply with treatment because of denial and fear of illness; cultural factors; having a different explanatory model of the symptoms, their cause, and their optimal treatment; or a misunderstanding of the diagnosis, treatment, or the physician's instructions and expectations. In these cases, education, reassurance where appropriate, use of a skilled interpreter, or gaining a better understanding of the woman's culture and view of her symptoms and illness may be very helpful. In some cases, a formal cultural consultation may be needed. Although such situations may be challenging, their health care providers do not generally experience these women as being "difficult" or "hateful."

Groves grouped "hateful patients" into four different categories—"dependent clingers," "entitled demanders," "manipulative help-rejecters," and "self-destructive deniers"—and described their behavior patterns and ways in which the physician can intervene to work with them more effectively. In a more recent paper, Strous et al. revisited Groves' original categories and suggested an overall framework for approaching these people based on empathy and an understanding of the physician's own responses. Empathy refers to understanding another person's feelings, motives, and point of view. It is not synonymous with sympathy, because empathy does not involve pity. Understanding what a woman is experiencing and where the woman is coming from allows the physician to more calmly take a nonblaming, problem-solving approach. In addition, the physician can use his or her own responses to understand the woman better. For example, a woman who is feeling helpless and angry may, by complaining or demanding, evoke similar responses of helplessness or anger in her health care provider, allowing the provider insight into the woman's state of mind.

Groves's first group of "hateful patients," which he called "dependent clingers," appears insatiable in their escalating demands for medical care and to represent a "bottomless pit." They require constant reassurance and inordinate amounts of time and attention, interfering with the rest of the physician's personal as well as professional life. These women may frequently and intrusively page, e-mail, call the physician at home or on the physician's cell phone, feeling unable to cope on their own. The physician cannot possibly fulfill all of the woman's demands, feels overwhelmed and angry, and tries to withdraw from caring for her. Groves suggested intervening as the woman's demands escalate and setting firm but reasonable limits (e.g., not giving out personal contact information, limiting visits or calls). The physician can empathically understand that the woman feels overwhelmed and unable to cope, but in order to preserve an effective treatment relationship the physician needs to be clear about what he or she realistically can and cannot do for the woman.

The second group, which Groves called "entitled demanders," is similarly dependent and needy but displays a sense of entitlement, aggressively makes demands of the physician (e.g., for controlled substances, expensive diagnostic tests), and may make implicit or explicit threats, such as threats of litigation. This often leads the physician to feel angry and resist complying with the demands, even if some are reasonable. Groves has recommended validating the woman's entitlement to good medical care but focusing on a shared therapeutic goal and the woman's role in working with the treatment team to accomplish that goal. Empathically recognizing the woman's fear of loss of control may allow the physician to respectfully point out destructive patterns of behavior and attempt to establish a more collaborative decision-making process.

"Manipulative help-rejecters" seek care but do not improve despite extensive workups and multiple attempts at treatment. Groves has suggested that these patients are afraid of losing the relationship with the physician if they improve. He recommended setting up a schedule of regular appointments that do not depend on having acute symptoms, much as one would do with a patient with chronic somatization and multiple physical symptoms of unclear etiology.

Finally, "self-destructive deniers" persist in self-destructive behavior such as drinking, smoking, risky sexual behavior, and use of drugs, despite obvious and significant medical problems that have resulted from this behavior. Groves conceptualized these people as having a form of chronic suicidal behavior and recommended ruling out depression, if needed with the help of a psychiatric consultation. In general, in cases where the physician feels angry or overwhelmed and does not wish to treat the woman, consultation with colleagues, consultation with a psychiatrist, and having the woman see a psychiatrist, if she is willing to do so, can be very helpful in better understanding and managing the woman and the physician-patient relationship.

Women with the diagnosis of borderline personality disorder are often challenging for physicians to treat, given their chronic suicidal thoughts, self-harm behavior such as suicide attempts and cutting, intense and rapidly changing emotions, anger, and difficulty regulating and controlling their emotions rather than acting on them. Women with borderline personality disorder may also see one or more members of the treatment team as wonderful and other members of the team as being punitive or bad. This can lead to "splitting" within the treatment team, with team members having quite different views of and responses to the woman and resulting disagreements within the team about how to best manage the woman's care. It is important in these cases for the members of the team to have a unified approach, focusing on the best care of the woman and avoiding being overly punitive or gratifying. Psychiatric consultation can be very helpful, and there are well-validated, effective psychotherapies

for people with this condition (for a review of borderline personality disorder, see Lieb et al., 2004).

Women who seek and misuse habit-forming prescription medications are another class of "difficult" patients and may evoke feelings of anger, helplessness, and confusion in providers. Such women may be quite skilled in presenting plausible reasons for their needing the medication, or they may present as "entitled demanders" and make actual or veiled threats. It is important to have clear limits regarding the circumstances under which the physician will or will not be willing to continue prescribing the medication and to convey these to the woman empathically and with the woman's best interests in mind. It may be necessary to establish a formal treatment agreement with her, spelling out how the medication will be prescribed, in what amounts, and what will happen in the case of lost prescriptions or early refill requests. In an institutional setting, such as a hospital or clinic with multiple providers, it is important to include this treatment agreement in the medical record and make sure that it is consistent with institutional policies and values. Psychiatric consultation and addressing substance abuse or dependence issues directly may be necessary.

> In cases of misuse of potentially habit-forming medications, a formal treatment agreement may be necessary.

An understanding of **attachment styles** can be very useful in interacting with "difficult patients" as well as less extreme problems in delivering the best possible medical care. Attachment theory was first elaborated by John Bowlby, a British psychiatrist, in the 1950s, and it posits that early interactions with caregivers in the first years of life influence an individual's later interpersonal relationships. These relationships include those with health care providers. When people become ill, often they "regress," become more vulnerable and childlike, and are less able to use more effective coping strategies. The position of being ill, with associated worries about loss of control, loss of health, needing to depend on others, and uncertainty about the future, amplifies any maladaptive patterns of attachment and interpersonal interactions stemming from relationships with early caregivers.

Thompson and Ciechanowski in 2003 described the application of attachment theory to primary care settings. Most people have secure attachment styles and assume both that they themselves are deserving of care and that others can be trusted. There are three insecure attachment styles that affect relationships with medical providers and the quality of medical care: dismissing, preoccupied, and fearful attachment styles.

People with a dismissing attachment style have not been able to rely on early caregivers, have had to fend for themselves, and are compulsively self-reliant. They deny their own needs, tend to minimize symptoms or disability, have difficulty seeking and complying with medical care, and avoid seeking help or support. Women with this attachment style are hard to engage in regular care, especially for chronic illnesses, and may have worse health outcomes. In a study of 4095 patients with diabetes treated in primary care, 35.8% had a dismissing attachment style. This group, compared with people with other attachment styles, had significantly lower levels of exercise, foot care, and adherence to oral hypoglycemic medications. Such patients may either fall through the cracks in a busy practice or be frustrating for the physician who tries to engage them in more active treatment. Engaging such women requires respecting their need for autonomy and respect, being flexible about appointment frequency and duration, giving them control over their care where possible, and using tracking systems and appointment reminders to make sure that they are being followed appropriately.

A preoccupied attachment style is characterized by compulsive care seeking. These people have received inconsistent responses to their needs in the past and feel they must exaggerate their symptoms and distress to evoke consistent care and support. In a study of 701 female primary care patients, those with a preoccupied attachment style reported more physical symptoms, despite comparable medical morbidity, and had the highest health care costs and utilization. Such women respond best to brief, frequent, regularly scheduled appointments and to a physician who is responsive, but calm, consistent, and unflappable.

The main feature of a fearful attachment style is mistrust of oneself and others, usually based on a history of mistreatment or abuse in the past. The woman seeks help, but she mistrusts and may reject it. She seems anxious, demanding, and highly distressed on the one hand, but she misses appointments and is nonadherent on the other. For example, in the 2002 study by Ciechanowski et al. of 701 female primary care patients mentioned previously, women with a fearful attachment style reported considerable distress and symptoms but had the lowest health care costs and utilization. A major challenge in treating these women is to be patient, accept them as they are and not withdraw from care. Thompson and Ciechanowski in 2003 recommended providing care through a number of different clinic providers or a treatment team if possible, so that the woman can develop a relationship with the clinic rather than needing to trust a single person.

> Understanding patients' attachment styles, consultation with colleagues, and collaboration and discussion with other members of the treatment team can help in effectively managing and providing the best possible health care for "difficult" patients.

Understanding attachment styles, and that women's interactions with the health care system reflect earlier formative relationships, can be helpful in maintaining a nonpejorative stance toward the woman and in achieving the best health care outcome possible. In general, seeking an empathic understanding of the woman's point of view can allow the physician not to become caught up in the negative feelings these women can evoke. Understanding the woman's fears and wishes does not mean that the physician needs to or should do what the woman wishes. However, it may help the physician to be able to set reasonable limits and expectations and pursue an approach that is in the woman's ultimate best interests, without feeling cruel, withholding, or intimidated. All physicians find some of their patients to be "difficult." Each physician can also increase his or her ability to manage these situations and reduce personal feelings of frustration, anger, or guilt, through consultation with colleagues, participating in a Balint group to discuss the psychological aspects of patient care, collaborating with other team members in discussing and making a plan for dealing with a patient, or consulting with a mental health specialist for or about the patient.

SEXUAL FUNCTION AND DYSFUNCTION

Sexual satisfaction is one of the more important human experiences, yet it has been estimated that as many as 50% of all married couples experience some sexual dissatisfaction or dysfunction. Although there is a strong physiologic basis for sexual function, it is impossible to separate sexual response from the many emotional and other contributing factors that may influence a relationship. Cultural or religious beliefs have influence on sexual function and dysfunction. For example, many African and some Asian and Middle Eastern countries practice female circumcision to varying degrees. The more extreme genital cutting or the trauma from the experience can result in reduced sexual activity, pain, and lowered frequency of orgasm.

In 1966, Masters and Johnson published their now famous book *Human Sexual Response,* which was a discussion of observations made on the sexual cycles of 700 subjects. It is on this important work that our early understanding of the female sexual response was based. Masters and Johnson described four phases of the sexual response: excitement, plateau, orgasm, and resolution (**Fig. 9-2**).

The excitement or seduction phase may be initiated by a number of internal or external stimuli. As shown in **Box 9-1**, physiologically this phase is associated with deep breathing, an increase in heart rate and blood pressure, a total body feeling

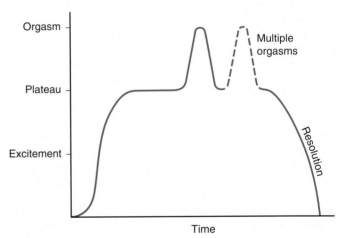

Figure 9-2 Sexual response cycle defined by Masters and Johnson. (From Masters WH, Johnson VE: Human Sexual Response. Boston, Little, Brown, 1966.)

Box 9-1 Characteristics of the Excitement Phase of Sexual Response Cycle in the Female

Deep breathing
Increased pulse
Increased blood pressure
Warmth and erotic feelings
Increased tension
Generalized vasocongestion
Skin flush
Breast engorgement
Nipple erection
Engorgement of labia and clitoris
Vaginal transudation
Uterine tenting

of warmth associated often with erotic feelings, and an increase in sexual tension. There is generalized vasocongestion, which leads to breast engorgement and the development of a maculopapular erythematous rash on the breasts, the chest, and the epigastrium, which is called the sex flush. There is also engorgement of the labia majora (seen particularly in multiparous women) and of the labia minora. The clitoris generally swells and becomes erect because of increased genital blood flow and the neurotransmitter nitric oxide, causing it to be tightly applied to the clitoral hood. The vagina "sweats" a transudative lubricant, and the Bartholin glands may secrete small amounts of liquid. With the increasing deep breathing, the uterus may tent up into the pelvis, perhaps as a result of the Valsalva maneuver. There is also a myotonic effect, which is most notable in nipple erection. Much of the response in the excitement phase is caused by stimulation of the parasympathetic fibers of the autonomic nervous system. Dynamic genital magnetic resonance imaging (MRI) studies enable the visualization of the physiologic arousal response that provides the direct observation of the time course and magnitude of this response, along with the variability that appears to occur in women with **sexual arousal disorder**. In some cases, anticholinergic drugs may interfere with a full response in this stage. A diabetic woman with peripheral neuropathy might complain of poor arousal because of lack of sensation.

Next is the plateau stage, which is the culmination of the excitement phase and is associated with a marked degree of vasocongestion throughout the body. Breasts and their areolae are markedly engorged, as are the labia and the lower third of the vagina. The vasocongestion in the lower third of the vagina is such that it forms what has been called the orgasmic platform, causing a decrease in the diameter of the vagina by as much as 50% and thus allowing for greater friction against the penis. At this stage, the clitoris retracts tightly against the pubic symphysis, and the vagina lengthens, with dilation of the upper two thirds. Uteri in the normal anteflex position tend to tent up more. Retroverted uteri do not.

The next stage is orgasm, in which the sexual tension that has been built up in the entire body is released. Characteristics of orgasm are listed in **Box 9-2**. A myotonic response involves muscle systems of the entire body. Individuals may experience carpal spasm. Rarely, a grand mal–type seizure may be observed. There is contraction of the muscles surrounding the vagina, as well as the anal sphincter. The uterus also contracts. Muscle contraction occurs 2 to 4 seconds after the woman begins to experience the orgasm and repeats at 0.8-second intervals. The actual number and intensity of contractions vary from woman to woman. Some women observed to have orgasmic contractions are not aware that they are having an orgasm. Masters and Johnson feel that prolonged stimulation during the excitement phase, during masturbation, or in conjunction with the use of a vibrator may lead to more pronounced orgasmic activity. Whereas the excitement phase is under the influence of the parasympathetic portion of the autonomic nervous system, orgasm seems to be related to

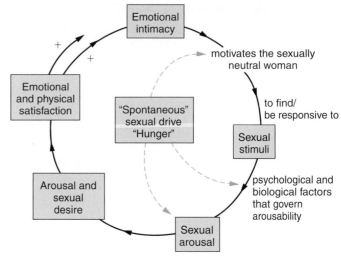

Figure 9-3 Blended intimacy-based and sexual drive-based cycles. (From Basson R: Female sexual response: The role of drugs in the management of sexual dysfunction. Obstet Gynecol 98:350, 2001.)

the sympathetic portion. Medication such as antihypertensive or antidepressant drugs, particularly SSRIs, may affect orgasmic response. A spinal cord injury might result in orgasmic disorder.

The resolution stage is last and represents a return of the woman's physiologic state to the preexcitement level. Although a refractory period is typical of the sexual response cycle in the male, no such refractory periods have been identified in women. Therefore, new sexual excitement cycles may be stimulated at any time after orgasm. During the resolution phase, the woman generally experiences a feeling of personal satisfaction and well-being.

Alternative models of the human sexual response have been proposed that differ from the linear progression of Masters and Johnson's model and also incorporate women's motivations and reasons for engaging in sex. Basson proposed that the phases overlap and may even occur in a different order. Women in established relationships may engage in sex, not because of sexual desire but because of a desire for intimacy with their partner (**Fig. 9-3**). Masters and Johnson identified the clitoris as the center of sexual satisfaction in the female. Recently, several lay publications have suggested that the cervix plays a role in sexual response, basing this theory on the fact that the cervix has a rich nerve supply. To date, no scientific data support this theory. Sexual gratification and orgasmic behavior definitely seem to be associated with nerve endings in the clitoris, mons pubis, labia, and possible pressure receptors in the pelvis. In a study by Andersen and coworkers, 42 women ages 31 to 81 (average 50.3) who had been treated for in situ vulvar carcinoma were compared with a group of comparable women ages 30 to 61 (average 44.3) with respect to sexual function. Six of the women had undergone local therapy with laser or chemotherapy, 26 had wide excision of lesions, 9 had undergone simple vulvectomy, and 1 had undergone a radical vulvectomy. Sexual behavior patterns and desires were maintained after therapy, but a specific disruption of the phases of excitement and resolution, and to a lesser extent orgasm, were noted. The incidence of sexual dysfunction was two to three times greater in the patient group, and 30% became sexually inactive. Loss or disruption of the clitoris seemed to be the single most important factor.

Box 9-2 Characteristics of Orgasm in the Female

Release of tension
Generalized myotonic contractions
Contractions of perivaginal muscles and anal sphincter
Uterine contractions

SEXUAL RESPONSE AND MENOPAUSE

Many factors contribute to sexual changes as a woman enters menopause. Aging in general is associated with the slowing of sexual response and decreases in the intensity of response. Specifically, arousal may be slower and orgasms may be less intense and less frequent. Aging may also lead to psychosocial changes affecting self-esteem in relation to desirability. Of course, hormonal changes are a factor. The postmenopausal woman who is not on hormone replacement therapy (HRT) experiences progressive atrophy of vaginal epithelium, a change in vaginal pH, a decrease in quantity of vaginal secretions, and a decrease in the general circulation to the vagina and uterus. Although estrogen clearly plays a role in maintaining the integrity of the vaginal mucosal epithelium and promotes lubrication, there is no direct link between estrogen levels and sexual desire or symptoms. If quality of life is poor from menopausal vasomotor symptoms and poor sleep, then estrogen can improve well-being overall without directly impacting sexual desire complaints. Testosterone is the predominant androgen in women. Both the ovaries and adrenal gland produce androgens, even after the menopause and the ovarian production ceases with oophorectomy, which may lead to lower circulating levels of testosterone. Decreased testosterone levels are associated with decreased sexual desire, arousal, sensation and orgasm, but levels of endogenous androgens do not predict sexual function.

A postmenopausal woman may experience other sexual problems relating to her partner, or if she is single, widowed, or divorced, to her lack of availability of male partners. In addition, her general health and the general health of her partner will play a role in her ability to respond sexually in a satisfactory manner. Pelvic organ prolapse and poor levator muscle function may contribute to poorer sexual function. Couples with marital or communication problems may find that menopause is an appropriate excuse to cease sexual activities. A concerned physician can help a couple sort out their needs and desire for sexual compatibility at this stage of life. Frequently, counseling aimed at dealing with problems of the relationship will alleviate sexual response difficulties.

Male partners of older women may suffer from medical conditions or be affected by medications they must take, with resultant decrease in arousal, difficulties in maintaining an erection, or complete impotence. The physician should ask women about sexual function and if male dysfunction is evident, they should make suggestions for appropriate referral to physicians or other health care workers who may deal with the male sexual dysfunction problems.

SEXUAL DYSFUNCTION

Sexual dysfunction is quite common. Masters and Johnson estimated that it exists in 50% of marriages. Higher percentages of dysfunction are seen in couples presenting for marital therapy. That sexual dysfunction is not necessarily incompatible with a happy marriage was noted in a study by Frank and associates, who surveyed couples felt to be well adjusted who were selected from general community groups. Of these couples, 83% rated their marriages as happy or very happy, but 63% of the women and 40% of the men gave a history of sexual dysfunction. A total of 48% of the women stated that they had difficulties becoming sexually excited, and 33% found difficulty in maintaining

excitement. Of the total group, 46% of the women experienced difficulty in reaching orgasm, and 15% had never had an orgasm. Finally, 35% of the women expressed disinterest in sex. These workers' experience implies that physicians caring for women should make a special effort to uncover sexual dysfunction or poor sexual response in their patients even when the patients demonstrate general marital satisfaction. Many studies around the world have reported female sexual dysfunction population prevalence rates of 45% to 71%. However, lower rates are reported when actual personal distress is added into the definition. The 2008 Prevalence of Female Sexual Problems Associated with Distress and Determinants of Seeking Treatment (PRESIDE) study found low sexual desire accompanied by personal distress to be 10% in women aged 30 to 39 years, 11% in women aged 40 to 49 years, 13% in women aged 50 to 59 years and 10% in women aged 60 to 69 years. A 2009 report with the PRESIDE data of 31,581 respondents found the prevalence of a desire disorder was 10%, but reduced to 6.3% for those without concurrent depression. Overall, 40% of those respondents with sexual disorder of desire, arousal, or orgasm have concurrent depression.

Obviously, assembling a careful history by asking general and directed questions is appropriate when dealing with a patient in a gynecologic visit. The patient should be asked if she is sexually active, if intercourse is comfortable and enjoyable (if heterosexual), and if she experiences orgasm. If she answers no to any of these questions, more specific questioning should follow with the objective of outlining the extent of the problem and the basis for it.

Sexual response problems may be the result of a previous negative sexual experience or may be secondary to emotional or physical illness. Primary medical conditions causing female sexual dysfunction can be hormonal, anatomic, vascular, or neurologic. The problem may also be related to difficulties in the current relationship or to alcohol or drug abuse. Although an occasional alcohol drink may decrease inhibitions and improve sexual response, in general, alcohol is a depressant and decreases the woman's ability to become sexually aroused and to become vaginally lubricated. Drugs with antihypertensive and anticholinergic activity, as well as those active at the α- and β-adrenergic receptors, may decrease arousal or inhibit sexual interest. Narcotics, sedatives, and antidepressant drugs, such as SSRIs, may also depress sexual responsiveness. Finally, decreased arousal or ability to remain aroused may be due to distractions in the woman's life such as concerns for children, job, or other problems that may enter her consciousness during arousal.

Decreased sexual desire is the most common sexual dysfunction and is reported by 10% to 43% of women surveyed. Because each individual has his or her own libidinal drive, it is not surprising that couples may have some incompatibility of needs. It is important, however, that these needs and desires be discussed openly and that reasons for lack of sexual desire that may involve experiences or problems inherent in the relationship be resolved. At times the problem may be merely a failure to set aside appropriate time and effort for intimacy. The couple should be encouraged to give sexual activity a high priority within their relationship rather than leaving it last on the list after the 11 o'clock news. Couples should be encouraged to use arousal and seduction techniques that are appropriate for their relationship. Satisfactory foreplay of a mutually enjoyable nature should be encouraged. Lack of sexual arousal is characterized by a persistent inability to attain adequate lubrication and swelling response of sexual excitement. The prevalence of this disorder is uncertain and often coexists with decreased sexual desire.

Hormonal levels are frequently obtained in evaluating desire disorders. However, there is no evidence that low testosterone levels distinguish women with sexual desire disorder from others. Davis and colleagues reported on 1021 women who had androgen levels drawn from a random recruitment in Australia. Neither total nor free testosterone nor dehydroepiandrosterone sulfate (DHEAS) levels discriminated between the women with and those without low sexual function. Testosterone testing in women is not recommended because the commonly available tests are not sensitive enough to detect the low concentrations in women and the normal range in women has not been established.

There are no FDA-approved medications to treat desire disorders other than estrogen for vaginal atrophy. Estrogen may improve sexual desire if hypoestrogenism is causing an overall lack of well-being from nighttime hot flashes and poor sleep or genital discomfort from atrophy. The risks of estrogen are discussed elsewhere. Androgen therapy is not at present FDA approved in women, but randomized, controlled trials have noted some benefits in postmenopausal women with **hypoactive sexual desire disorders** and arousal disorders. Levels of endogenous androgens therapy that increases serum concentrations to the upper limit of normal has consistently been shown to improve female sexual function in selected populations of postmenopausal women. The group that has the most response to testosterone is women who have had surgical menopause. However, long-term safety and efficacy data are not available and testosterone use remains controversial. Phosphodiesterase inhibitors have not been found to be effective. Bupropion has shown some effectiveness, but further studies are needed. At present, a sound approach to female sexual dysfunction is complex and needs to assess sexual education knowledge, all forms of abuse including emotional abuse, depression, concerns about sexually transmitted diseases, pain, other medical problems, and everyday fatigues and stresses. Exercise to improve blood flow to the pelvis and decrease fatigue, changing SSRI medication for depression if negative sexual side effects occur, and psychotherapy/sex therapy can all be beneficial.

Sexual arousal disorders have received relatively little scientific inquiry. Masters and Johnson taught women sensate focus using masturbation training and working with the partners with apparently good results. Vaginal or systemic estrogen therapy improves arousal disorder by improving vaginal blood flow and lubrication in postmenopausal women. The FDA-approved EROS–CTD (Clitoral Therapy Device, UroMetrics, Inc., St. Paul, MN) is a cup that sits over the clitoris and a gentle vacuum is applied via a battery-powered device. The EROS-CTD has been reported to improve clitoral blood flow, engorgement, and genital sensation, which is effective in the ability to reach orgasm.

Sexual pain disorders include **dyspareunia** and **vaginismus**. Vaginismus is a condition that is secondary to involuntary spasm of vaginal introital and levator ani muscles. Because of this spasm, penetration is either painful or impossible. Lamont has attempted to classify the degrees of vaginismus and, in a group of 80 patients, noted that 27 (34%) had first-degree vaginismus, defined as perineal and levator spasm relieved by reassurance during pelvic examination. Another 21 (26%) had second-degree vaginismus, defined as perineal spasm maintained throughout the pelvic examination. Another 18 (22.5%) demonstrated third-degree vaginismus, defined as levator spasm and elevation of the buttocks. A total of 10 (12.5%) had fourth-degree vaginismus, defined as levator and perineal spasm with withdrawal and retreat. Four of the 80 patients refused pelvic examination. These patients frequently complain not only of pain or fear of pain with coitus or pelvic examination but also of difficulty in inserting a tampon or vaginal medication. The condition may be primary, in which case the individual has never experienced successful coitus. This problem is generally based on either early sexual abuse or aversion to sexuality in general. This leads to a form of conversion disorder or to a lack of appropriate learning about sex secondary to cultural or familial teaching that sex is evil, painful, or undesirable. Vaginismus may also occur in patients who have been sexually active when an injury or vaginal infection has led to vaginal pain with attempted coitus. This has been seen in rape victims and in women who have had painful episiotomy repairs, severe yeast vaginitis, or vulvar vestibulitis. When the underlying cause for the vaginismus is understood, the matter may be discussed frankly with the patient and her partner to effect a relearning process that is conducive to relieving the symptoms. Psychotherapy is encouraged, and then desensitization treatment can begin. The actual vaginal spasm then may be relieved by teaching the patient muscle relaxation, then self-dilation techniques, using fingers or dilators, in which she and her partner can participate. The period of therapy is usually short and the results good. There are little data from controlled trials, although one trial compared two desensitization techniques which were both effective.

Dyspareunia is a sexual dysfunction where genital pain occurs before, during, or after intercourse that frequently has an organic basis. The physician should obtain a careful history of when the dyspareunia occurs (i.e., on insertion of the penis, at the midvagina during thrusting, or with deep penetration of the vault), because facts obtained by this history may point to organic causes, such as poor lubrication and vaginal atrophy, a painful bladder disorder, vulvodynia and vulvar vestibulodynia, poorly healed vaginal lacerations or episiotomy, and diseases such as pelvic inflammatory disease, pelvic congestion syndrome, or endometriosis. **Table 9-16** lists some causes of dyspareunia. Vulvodynia is chronic pain and burning in the vulva and affects 6 million women and the cause is largely unknown. When no organic cause can be found for the dyspareunia, techniques similar to those used in evaluating and managing vaginismus are appropriate. Pelvic floor physical therapy may be beneficial for vaginismus, vulvar vestibulitis, and dyspareunia as well as sex therapy. With all the sexual pain disorders, it is not uncommon to treat the underlying organic cause with success and find the pain continues. It is often muscle tension problems from the pain-tension-pain cycle that remain (**Fig. 9-4**). Specific pathologic conditions should, of course, be treated. At times, changing coital position can relieve dyspareunia. Couples should be encouraged to experiment with female-dominant and side-by-side positions to see if the pain can be prevented. An algorithm for thinking about sexual dysfunction is shown in **Figure 9-5**.

Orgasmic dysfunction is quite common and often situational. As many as 10% to 15% of women have never experienced an orgasm through any form of sexual stimulation, and another 25% to 35% will have difficulty reaching an orgasm

Table 9-16 Causes of Dyspareunia

Vulvodynia
Vulvar vestibulitis
Dysesthetic, generalized
Vaginitis
    Yeast or other infectious agents
    Desquamative inflammatory vaginitis
Skin conditions
    Contact dermatitis (eczematous or contact)
Lichen sclerosis
Lichen planus
Urologic
    UTI
    Interstitial cystitis
    Urethral diverticulum
Episiotomy
Pelvic floor myalgia (hypertonus)
Endometriosis
Leiomyomata
Pelvic inflammatory disease
Adnexal pathology
Postradiation in pelvis

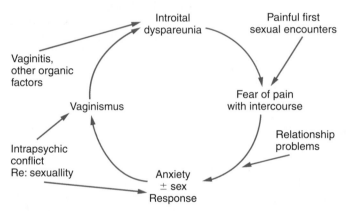

Figure 9-4 Dyspareunia and vaginismus cycle. (From Steege JF: Dyspareunia and vaginismus. Clin Obstet Gynecol 27:750, 1984.)

on any particular occasion. Many women may be orgasmic secondary to masturbation or oral sex but may not be orgasmic with penile intercourse. It is important to discern by history the extent of the patient's problem and to place it into proper perspective. If the patient is anorgasmic during intercourse but has experienced orgasms, communication with her partner may aid in bringing about an orgasm during intercourse by allowing her or her partner to stimulate her clitoral area with the intensity and timing necessary to bring about an orgasm. If the woman is anorgasmic, she may be taught masturbatory techniques to demonstrate an orgasm to her, and then these techniques may be applied to the coital situation, thereby developing the desired response during coitus. Couples should be encouraged to communicate their sexual needs so that appropriate stimulation is offered during the arousal period and during intercourse. For situation orgasmic disorder, the focus of dialogue should be the relationship. Developing this type of dialogue is often difficult but can be aided by counseling with a sensitive physician or sex therapist.

Sexual response is a complex problem involving physiologic responses and psychosocial influences, which makes research studies hard to control. Although physicians and women may

desire a pharmacologic solution, at present there is a paucity of good quality evidence. In fact, in the clinical trials of drug treatments for female sexual dysfunction, the placebo responses have been substantial. Whether attention to sexual function or changes in sexual behavior during a trial result in the marked placebo response, this definitely complicates the study and needs to be considered in any treatment offered. Psychosexual counseling is often appropriate, as well as a comprehensive medical evaluation.

LESBIAN HEALTH CARE

Before 1990, there was little information in the literature regarding lesbian health care or health issues. In 1994, Bradford et al. conducted a survey of 1925 lesbians from all 50 states. Over half of the sample had considered suicide at some point, and 18% had attempted suicide; 37% had been physically abused, 32% had been raped or sexually attacked, and 19% had been involved in incestuous relationships during childhood; 30% drank alcohol more than once a week, and 6% daily. About three fourths had been in counseling, half for sadness or depression. Most had significant support within the lesbian community, but few had come out to family and coworkers.

This survey was not a population-based study and had no comparison group. However, the observations of significant levels of mental health problems have been borne out by subsequent studies. A recent systematic review and metaanalysis found an increased rate of depression, anxiety disorders, and substance abuse and dependence in lesbian, gay, and bisexual individuals. The risk for suicide attempts was twofold, in comparison with heterosexuals. Lesbian and bisexual women had a particularly high rate of alcohol and drug dependence. A number of studies have now documented that lesbian women use mental health services at high rates, with 70% to 80% having been in therapy, primarily for depression and relationship problems. The rate of depression is significantly higher than that in heterosexual women, as is the rate of suicide attempts, which is particularly elevated in lesbian and bisexual adolescents. Elevated rates of substance use disorders are particularly pronounced in lesbian and bisexual, versus heterosexual, adolescents. The reasons for the higher rates of mental health and substance use disorders are unclear but may include a higher rate of childhood sexual abuse, being a member of a stigmatized minority group, and dealing with conflict and secrecy regarding sexual orientation.

> Lesbian and bisexual women have an elevated rate of mental health problems, substance use disorders, and suicide attempts, especially during adolescence.

Lesbians not only have a higher rate of mental health and substance use disorders, but they also have a higher rate of cardiovascular risk factors, such as obesity and smoking. Smoking rates are especially high in lesbian adolescents. Over the past two decades, lesbian women have become increasingly willing to disclose their sexual orientation to health care providers and to seek routine physical examinations. Nonetheless, their rates of routine physicals and pap smears are lower than national guidelines and lower than those of their heterosexual peers, and adolescents in particular have difficulty disclosing their sexual orientation to physicians. In a recent survey of lesbian, gay,

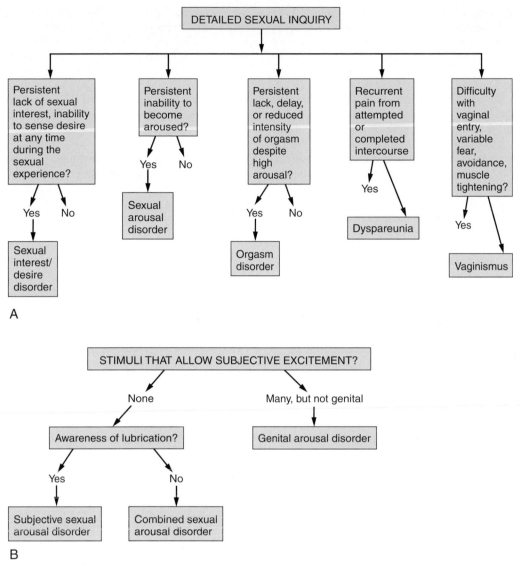

Figure 9-5 A, Detailed sexual inquiry. **B,** Further assessment of arousal disorder. (From Basson R, Althof D, Davis S: Summary of the recommendations on sexual dysfunctions in women. J Sex Med 1:29, 2004.)

and bisexual (LGB) youth, most said that they thought their health care provider should know their sexual orientation to provide the best possible care, but two thirds had not disclosed this information. Lesbians prefer female and preferably lesbian health care providers and frequently use alternative health care providers such as nonphysicians, acupuncturists, and massage therapists. The low rate of pap smears has been thought to be due to lack of concern and a belief that lesbian women were at low risk for cervical cancer. However, recent studies show human papillomavirus (HPV) in lesbian women and that Pap smear frequency should be the same as in heterosexual women. Sexually transmitted diseases also occur in lesbian women, particularly those who have had male partners.

> Lesbian women have the same need for routine gynecologic care as heterosexual women but are less likely to seek routine medical care, have Pap smears, or disclose their sexual orientation to health care providers.

Lesbians are increasingly having children through artificial insemination and adoption. Couples wishing to have children through donor insemination have concerns about coming out to their obstetrician, involving the nonpregnant partner, legal issues, family support, and parenting issues. Obstetrician-gynecologists need to be comfortable treating and advising lesbian women and couples, not just for pregnancy but for general health issues, or should refer them to an appropriate provider.

RAPE, INCEST, AND DOMESTIC VIOLENCE

RAPE

Rape, or the sexual assault of children, women, and men, is a common act. Sexual violence is defined as any sexual act performed by one person on another without that person's consent. Unfortunately, this is a common problem all over the world.

In a 2007 nationally representative survey of 9684 adults, 10.6% of women reported a sexual assault at some time in their lives. Another study reported one in six women reported experienced attempted or completed rape. In separating out by female age groups, 11% of high school adolescents reported having been forced to have sex. The percentage increases the younger the adolescent is for involuntary first intercourse. Twenty to 25% of women in college have been victims of actual or attempted sexual assault during college. Among women 18 years of age or older, 31.5% who were raped sustained physical injury, and 36% of injured female victims received medical treatment. This type of crime, however, is often underreported, and the actual incidence may be much higher. Victims are often reluctant to report sexual assault to the authorities because of embarrassment, fear of retribution, feelings of guilt, assumptions that little will be done, or simply lack of knowledge of their rights. Homeless women and women with mental illness are particularly vulnerable to sexual assaults compared with the general population.

In the past, society has held many misconceptions about the rape victim, particularly female victims. These included the notion that the individual encouraged the rape by specific behavior or dress and that no person who did not wish to be raped could be raped. Furthermore, the feeling that rape was an indication of basic promiscuity was widely held. To some extent many of these societal misconceptions are held today.

Sexual assault happens to people of all ages and races in all socioeconomic groups. The very young, the mentally and physically handicapped, and the very old are particularly susceptible. While men can be victims of sexual violence, most victims are female. Sexual violence can be unwanted touching and rape, but it also includes nonphysical distressing acts of sexual harassment, threats, peeping, and taking nude photos without consent. The Centers for Disease Control reported in 2006 that high school black (9.3%) and Hispanic (7.8%) students had higher rates of forced sexual intercourse than white students (6.9%). Although the perpetrator may be a stranger, he or she is often an individual well known to the victim. In fact, for first rape experience in women, 30.4% of the time the perpetrator was known to be an intimate partner, 23.7% a family member, and 20% of the time an acquaintance.

Some situations have been defined as variants of sexual assault. These include marital rape, which involves forced coitus or related acts without consent but within the marital relationship, and "date rape." In the latter situation the woman may voluntarily participate in sexual play, but coitus is performed, often forcibly, without her consent. Date rape is often not reported because the victim may believe she contributed by partially participating. This, however, can be a traumatic event and scar her self-esteem.

Almost all states have statutes that criminalize coitus with females under certain specified ages. Such an act is referred to as statutory rape. Consent is irrelevant because the female is defined by statute as being incapable of consenting.

During a rape, the victim loses control over his or her life for that period and frequently experiences anxiety and fear. When the attack is life threatening, shock with associated physical and psychological symptoms may occur. Burgess and Holmstrom identified two phases of the rape-trauma syndrome. The immediate, or acute, phase lasts from hours to days and may be associated with a paralysis of the individual's usual coping mechanisms. Outwardly, the victim may demonstrate manifestations ranging from complete loss of emotional control to a well-controlled behavior pattern. The actual reaction may depend on a number of factors, including the relationship of the victim to the attacker, whether force was used, and the length of time the victim was held against his or her will. Generally, the victim appears disorganized and may complain of both physical and emotional symptoms. Physical complaints include specific injuries or general complaints of soreness, eating problems, headaches, and sleep disturbances. Behavior patterns may include fear, mood swings, irritability, guilt, anger, depression, and difficulties in concentrating. Frequently, the victim will complain of flashbacks of the attack. Medical care is often sought during the acute period, and at this point it is the physician's responsibility to assess the specific medical problems and also to offer a program of emotional support and reassurance.

The second phase of the rape-trauma syndrome involves long-term adjustment and is designated the reorganization phase. During this time, flashbacks and nightmares may continue, but phobias may also develop. These may be directed against members of the offending sex, the sex act itself, or nonrelated circumstances, such as a newly developed fear of crowds or heights. During this period the victim may institute a number of important lifestyle changes, including job, residence, friends, and significant others. If major complications such as the contraction of a sexually transmitted disease (STD) or a pregnancy occur, resolution may be more difficult. The reorganization period may last from months to years and generally involves an attempt on the part of the victim to regain control over his or her life. During this time medical care and counseling must be nonjudgmental, sensitive, and anticipatory. When the physician realizes that the patient is contemplating a major lifestyle change during this period, it is probably appropriate to point out to the patient why the change is being contemplated and the complicating effects it may have on the patient's overall well-being.

In some women, rape, like other trauma, can lead to ongoing, persistent posttraumatic stress disorder (PTSD; see earlier section in this chapter), with disabling nightmares, flashbacks, hyperarousal, avoidance, depression, anxiety, and panic. Individuals with a prior history of trauma before the rape; greater severity, duration, and life-threatening nature of the assault; poor social support; and a past history of depression or anxiety are more susceptible to developing PTSD. Approximately 15% to 20% of women ages 18 to 50 have chronic pelvic pain of more than a year's duration. An estimated 40% to 50% of those women have a history of physical or sexual abuse.

Physician's Responsibility in the Care of a Rape Victim

Although any individual may become a rape victim, this discussion will be limited to the care of a female, as is appropriate for a gynecology textbook. The physician's responsibility may be divided into three categories: medical, medicolegal, and supportive, as shown in **Box 9-3**.

Medical

The physician's medical responsibilities are to treat injuries and to perform appropriate tests for, to prevent, and to treat infections and pregnancies. It is important to obtain informed consent before examining the patient and collecting specimens. In addition to addressing legal requirements, it helps the victim to regain control over her body and her life. After acute injuries have been determined and stabilized, a careful history and physical examination should be performed. It is important to have a chaperone present while taking the history, performing the examination, and collecting the specimen, to reassure the victim and to provide support. The presence of such a third party probably reduces feelings of vulnerability on the part of the victim. She should be asked to state in her own words what happened; if she knew the attacker, and if not, to describe the attacker; and to describe the specific act(s) performed. A history of previous gynecologic conditions, particularly infections and pregnancy, use of contraception, and the date of last menstrual period, should be recorded. It is necessary to determine whether the patient may have a preexisting pregnancy or be at risk for pregnancy. It is also important to ascertain whether she has had a preexisting pelvic infection.

Experience derived at the Sexual Assault Center in Seattle, Washington, demonstrated that between 12% and 40% of victims who are sexually assaulted have injuries. Most of these, however, are minor and require simple reparative therapy. Only about 1% require hospitalization and major operative repair. Nonetheless, the victim will perceive the experience as having been life threatening, as in many cases it may have been. Many injuries occur when the victim is restrained or physically coerced into the sexual act. Thus, the physician should seek bruises, abrasions, or lacerations about the neck, back, buttocks, or extremities. Where a knife was used as a coercive tactic, small cuts may also be found. Erythema, lacerations, and edema of the vulva or rectum may occur because of manipulation of these areas with the hand or the penis. These are particularly common in children or virginal victims but may occur in any woman and should be looked for. Superficial or extensive lacerations of the hymen or vagina may occur in virginal victims or in the elderly. Lacerations may also be noted in the area of the urethra, the rectum, and at times through the vaginal vault into the abdominal cavity.

In addition, bite marks may be noted in any of these regions. Occasionally, foreign objects are inserted into the vagina, the urethra, or the rectum and may be found in situ.

In recent years, some authorities have advised close inspection with a magnifying glass or colposcope of the vulva and vagina of infants and children suspected to be victims of rape. However, in a study of 130 prepubertal girls (mean age 5.5) identified as victims of sexual abuse, Muram and Elias could identify evidence of trauma in 96% with unaided inspection. Four additional cases were identified by colposcopy, but the lesions were obvious on repeat unaided examination. Simple visual examination without the aid of a colposcope should be sufficient to detect signs of trauma in children. Colposcopy is used in women by some sexual assault response teams to enhance detection of subtler genital trauma. Where oral penetration has been effected, injury of the mouth and pharynx should be looked for.

Most victims are concerned about possible infections incurred as a result of the rape, but until recently no careful follow-up studies in victims had been performed. To determine actual risk, it is important to know the prevalence of existing STDs in the victim population. In 1990, Jenny and colleagues examined 204 girls and women within 72 hours of a rape and discovered that 88 (43%) were harboring at least one STD. These included *Neisseria gonorrhoeae* in 13 of 204 (6% of all tested), cytomegalovirus in 13 of 170 (8%), *Chlamydia trachomatis* in 20 of 198 (10.1%), *Trichomonas vaginalis* in 30 of 204 (14.7%), herpes simplex virus in 4 of 170 (2.4%), *Treponema pallidum* in 2 of 199 (1%), human immunodeficiency virus (HIV)-1 in 1 of 123 (0.8%), and bacterial vaginosis in 70 of 204 (34.3%). In 109 patients (53%) who returned for follow-up (excluding those who were found to be infected on the first visit or who were treated prophylactically), there were 3 of 71 (4%) cases of gonorrhea, 1 of 65 (0.02%) of chlamydia, 10 of 81 (12%) of trichomoniasis, and 15 of 77 (19%) of bacterial vaginosis. These authors concluded that women who are raped have a higher than average prevalence of preexisting STDs but are also at a substantial risk of acquiring such disease as a result of the assault.

Reynolds and coworkers presented a review on the risk of infection in rape victims that was the result of a MEDLINE search of the English language journals. They also noted that it was often difficult to separate new from existing infection but placed the prevalence of STDs as follows: *N. gonorrhea* 0 to 26.3%, *C. trachomatis* 3.9% to 17%, *Treponema pallidum* 0 to 5.6%, *Trichomonas vaginalis* 0 to 19%, and HPV 0.6% to 2.3%. Few studies are available to predict the actual risk of acquiring an STD, but *Chlamydia trachomatis* may be the most commonly acquired infection incurred under these circumstances. Most victims fear acquiring HIV as a result of a sexual attack, but current risks are probably not high depending on the population involved and the sexual acts performed. Some studies place the risk for adult rape victims of acquiring syphilis as high as 3% to 10%. These authors did not believe the risk of acquiring STDs can be quantified, but they noted that the acquisition of viral STDs, including HIV, has been reported both in adults and children. In consensual sex, the risk for HIV transmission from vaginal intercourse is 0.1% to 0.2% and for receptive anal intercourse it is 0.5% to 3%.

Commercial "evidence kits" are available. State crime lab testing might include urine or serum for "date rape" drugs when amnesia or sedation is present. A speculum exam is not always necessary, but if bleeding is reported or noted on external vulvar exam, it is appropriate. It must be remembered that infection may not be limited to the vagina but may also include the pharynx or the rectum. Specific history to raise a suspicion of this possibility should be sought. Urine or nonculture nuclear amplification tests (NAATs) for *Neisseria gonorrhoeae* and *Chlamydia trachomatis* are preferred according to the Centers for Disease Control 2010 guidelines. In addition, conventional cultures of the rectum and of the oral pharynx are indicated when the history suggests that this would be productive. A wet mount for *Trichomonas vaginalis* and bacterial vaginosis and a potassium hydroxide mount for *Candida albicans* are also useful (**Box 9-4**). Investigation for syphilis (RPR) is not routinely recommended at the Sexual Assault Center in Seattle, Washington, but may be done in follow-up.

Because the victim is also at risk for infection by the herpes virus, hepatitis B virus, cytomegalovirus, HIV, condyloma acuminatum, and a variety of other STDs, the physician may wish to screen for those that seem appropriate at the time the victim is seen in the acute stage. Hepatitis B vaccine is appropriate if the victim is not previously vaccinated. Tetanus prophylaxis is appropriate in some cases as well. At follow-up visits the patient should again be investigated for signs and symptoms of the STDs, and appropriate repeat cultures and serologies should be obtained. Be aware that compliance with follow-up visits is poor. Prophylactic antibiotics are useful in acute rape management when the patient is concerned about contracting an STD or knows the assailant to be high risk. The CDC recommends the woman can be given a single dose of cefixime 400 mg PO or ceftriaxone 250 mg IM, for gonorrhea prophylaxis plus single dose azithromycin, 1 g PO or doxycycline 100 mg orally twice a day for 7 days, for chlamydia prophylaxis plus metronidazole 2 grams orally in a single dose for trichomonas. If the patient is pregnant, consider giving no medications, and follow-up screening should be done in 2 weeks. If prophylaxis is desired, these antibiotics are class B drugs in pregnancy (except doxycycline which should not be given and is class D). This should prevent gonorrhea and *Chlamydia* infection but will have no effect on herpes, condylomata, or many of the other problems mentioned. Postexposure therapy with zidovudine is controversial for HIV prevention as the benefit is unknown and extrapolated from needle-stick injuries in health care workers.

Box 9-4 Sexually Transmitted Diseases and Tests Available to Physicians Caring for a Rape-Trauma Victim

Should Perform
NAATs for *Neisseria gonorrhoeae*
NAATs for *Chlamydia trachomatis*

Could Perform
Herpes simplex—culture lesion or serology
Hepatitis B—screening serology
HIV—serology
Cytomegalovirus—serology
Condyloma virus—study lesion
Trichomonas—saline wet mount preparation and culture or point-of-care testing
Bacterial vaginosis—pH, saline wet mount preparation
Candida—potassium hydroxide wet mount preparation
Syphilis—rapid plasma regain (RPR)

Centers for Disease Control website, www.cdc.gov/std/treatment/2010/STD-Treatment-2010-RR5912.pdf; Harborview Sexual Assault Center.

Pregnancy

The patient's menstrual history, birth control regimen, and pregnancy status should be assessed. If the patient is at risk for pregnancy at the time of the assault, an appropriate emergency contraception or "morning after" prophylaxis can be offered as long as the pregnancy test was negative. This is discussed more fully in Chapter 13 (Family Planning). In the experience of most sexual assault centers, the chance of pregnancy occurring is quite low. It has been estimated to be approximately 2% to 4% of victims having a single, unprotected coitus. However, if the patient has been exposed at midcycle, the risk will be higher. Holmes and associates estimated the national rape-related pregnancy rate at 5% and stated that among adult women 32,101 pregnancies resulted from rape each year in the United States. Many of these pregnancies occurred in women who did not receive immediate medical attention.

Medicolegal

To be meaningful, medicolegal material must be collected shortly after the assault takes place and definitely within 96 hours. The woman can be reassured that laws in all 50 states strictly limit use of past STDs or past sexual history during a trial so as not to discredit her testimony. Commercially manufactured "evidence kits" are available and may help with preserving the "chain of evidence" for a legal case. Victims should be encouraged to come immediately to a center where they can be evaluated before bathing, urinating, defecating, washing out their mouths, changing clothes, or cleaning their fingernails. The United States Department of Justice, Office of Victims of Crime, supports Sexual Assault Nurse Evaluation (SANE) programs, which have models for acute care for sexual assault. Some institutions have Sexual Assault Response Teams (SARTs) so experts are available to do the appropriate psychological, medical, and legal evaluation. You should know the resources available in your community.

In general, evidence for coitus will be present in the vagina for as long as 48 hours after the attack, but in other orifices the evidence may last only up to 6 hours. Appropriate tests should document the patient's physical and emotional condition as judged by her history and physical examination and should include data that document the use of force, evidence for sexual contact, and materials that may help identify the offender. To document that force was used, the physician should carefully describe each injury noted and illustrate with either drawings or photographs. Detail is important, because injuries suffered by sexual assault victims have common patterns. Because rape and sexual assault are legal terms, they should not be stated as diagnoses; rather the physician should report findings as "consistent with use of force." Documentation of sexual contact must begin with a history of when the patient had intercourse before the attack. If sperm or semen is found in the vagina or cervix of a victim, it must not be confused with such substances deposited during the victim's prior consenting sexual acts. Sexual contact will be verified by analysis of secretions from the vagina or rectum by identifying motile sperm. Nonmotile sperm may be present as well if the attack occurred 12 to 20 hours previously. In some instances, motile sperm will be noted for as long as 2 to 3 days in the endocervix. Vaginal wet mount is no longer recommended for identifying sperm as it lacks reproducibility. Manufactured "evidence kits" are available.

Table 9-17 Survival Time of Sperm

Source	Motile Sperm	Sperm	Acid Phosphatase
Vagina	Up to 8 hr	Up to 7 to 9 days	Variable (up to 48 hr)
Pharynx	6 hr	Unknown	100 IU*
Rectum	Undetermined	20 to 24 hr	100 IU*
Cervix	Up to 5 days	Up to 17 days	Similar to vagina

*Minimum detectable.
From Anderson S: Sexual assault—medical-legal aspects. An unpublished training packet for pediatric house staff. Harborview Medical Center, Seattle, WA, 1980.

It is difficult to ascertain whether ejaculation occurred in the mouth, because residual seminal fluid is rapidly destroyed by bacteria and salivary enzymes, making documentation of such an event difficult after more than a few hours have passed. Seminal fluid may be found staining the skin or the clothing several hours after the attack, and this should be looked for. Because acid phosphatase is an enzyme found in high concentrations in seminal fluid, substances removed for analysis should be tested for this enzyme. **Table 9-17** demonstrates the survival time of sperm in the pharynx, rectum, and cervix.

In addition to documenting that intercourse has taken place, an attempt should be made to identify the perpetrator. In this regard, all clothing intimately associated with the area of assault should be collected, labeled, and submitted to legal authorities. In addition, smears of vaginal secretions or a Pap smear should be made to permanently document the presence of sperm. Vaginal secretions needed for DNA typing should be collected by wet or dry swab and refrigerated until a pathologist can process them. In the near future tests may also be available to identify prostate-specific antigen and seminal vesicle–specific antigen in vaginal secretions. DNA fingerprinting is now readily available in all areas and is admissible in many jurisdictions. Pubic hair combings should be performed in an attempt to obtain pubic hair of the assailant. Saliva should be collected from the victim to ascertain whether she secretes an antigen that could differentiate her from substances obtained from the perpetrator. Finally, fingernail scrapings should be obtained for skin or blood if the victim scratched the perpetrator. Specific blood or DNA typing may be conducted to help identify the attacker. All materials collected should be labeled and turned over to the legal authority or pathologist, depending on the system used by the medical unit. A receipt should be obtained, and this should be documented in the patient's chart.

Emotional Support of the Victim

After the physical needs of the patient have been met and after the physician has carefully documented the information concerning the sexual contact, he or she should discuss with the victim the degree of injury, probability of infection or pregnancy, general course that the victim might be expected to follow with respect to these, and how follow-up to aid prevention will be carried out. The physician must allow the victim to give vent to anxieties and to correct misconceptions. The physician should reassure her, insofar as possible, that her well-being will be restored. In doing this, the physician may call on other health personnel, such as individuals trained to help rape-trauma victims, to facilitate counseling and follow-up. The patient should not be released until specific follow-up plans are made and the patient understands what they are. A follow-up visit should be planned

within 1 to 4 weeks to reevaluate the patient's medical, infectious disease, pregnancy, and psychological status. At this point, follow-up counseling should be encouraged. It is important at each visit to emphasize to the patient that she was a victim and holds no blame. At each step she must be allowed to vent her feelings and to discuss her current conceptions of the problem. It is important that the physician realize that some patients will appear to have excellent emotional control when seen immediately after a rape. This is an acute expression of the patient's defense mechanisms and should not be misinterpreted to indicate that the patient is coping with the circumstances. All the recommendations just listed should be followed *regardless* of the patient's apparent condition. Specific plans for follow-up are equally important in such an individual, because it must be anticipated that she will follow the same post-rape emotional process as anyone else. Finally, it is important to emphasize and reemphasize that at no time during the management or follow-up care of the rape victim should any comments be made by health care professionals suggesting that the patient was anything other than a victim. These women are sensitive to any accusations and insinuations and may even believe that they may have in some way been responsible for the rape. Their future well-being may be severely affected by creating such an impression.

Female Circumcision

A form of sexual abuse only recently observed in the Western world is female circumcision or genital cutting. It is a practice growing out of cultural and traditional beliefs dating back several thousand years. The World Health Organization estimates that between 85 and 200 million women undergo these procedures each year. Although they are often performed in parts of Africa, the Middle East, and Southeast Asia, they are rarely performed in the United States or the rest of the western world. About 168,000 women who have undergone such procedures currently live in the United States, and physicians may see the results of these procedures in patients who emigrate from countries where they are practiced.

The various forms of female genital mutilation include removal of the clitoral prepuce, excision of the clitoris, or removal of the clitoris and labia minora. Occasionally, the labia majora is also partially removed and the vagina partially sutured closed. The procedures are often performed between early childhood and age 14 and frequently without anesthesia under unsterile conditions by untrained practitioners. Therefore, a variety of complications often occur, including infection, tetanus, shock, hemorrhage, and death. Long-term problems include chronic infection, scar formation, local abscesses, sterility, and incontinence. In addition, depression, anxiety, sexual dysfunction, obstetric complications, and the psychosomatic conditions associated with sexual abuse may be seen. Physicians who care for women with this condition must develop an understanding of the cultural mores that lead to the performance of the procedure and the current implications on these cultural beliefs that remedial surgery may imply. Certainly the patient and her sexual partner should be involved in all decisions concerning intervention.

INCEST

Incest must be placed within the context of child sexual abuse. The actual overall incidence of such abuse is difficult to estimate, although several authorities claim that about 10% of all child abuse cases involve sexual abuse. Sarafino estimated that roughly 336,000 children are sexually abused each year in the United States. Retrospective historical data derived from adults imply that incestuous activity may be experienced by as many as 15% to 25% of all women and approximately 12% of all men. These figures seem appropriate for the population in general but vary from group to group, being higher in young prostitutes.

Sexual abuse of children may be divided into two types: the first in which the child is victimized by a stranger and the second in which a family member or friend is the perpetrator. It has been estimated that about 80% of all sexual abuse cases of children involve a family member. Rimsza and Niggemann found that only 18% of 311 children and adolescents who were evaluated for sexual abuse were assaulted by strangers. In the case of child sexual abuse involving a stranger, the act is usually a single episode and is usually reported to the authorities. The child is capable in most instances of clearly stating what happened, and the act may involve any form of sexual activity and may have taken place because of enticement, coercion, or physical force. In such instances the child should be interviewed carefully and allowed to tell what happened. The police or protective services should be notified, and, where appropriate, the techniques used in evaluating a rape victim should be applied. Appropriate prophylaxis against infection should be employed, and counseling should be arranged with a mental health care worker, who should see the child immediately and also take the responsibility for planning long-term follow-up. The molester should be apprehended, and if it is an individual living in the home, he or she should be made to leave. Most communities have sexual abuse crisis intervention centers, and these are appropriate in such circumstances. In each case the child should be carefully told that he or she was a victim of a wrongful act and that in no way was he or she to blame. Statements that imply the child might in some way have enticed the perpetrator into performing the act are inappropriate and may lead to serious compromise in the development of the child's self-esteem in the future. The welfare of siblings or other children in the household must also be considered, and an effort to discover their status should be made.

About 80% of child sexual abuse involves a parent, guardian, other family member, mother's partner, or some other person known to the family. Father-daughter incest accounts for about 75% of reported cases, with mother-son, father-son, mother-daughter, brother-sister, or incest involving another close family member constituting the remaining 25%. Brother-sister incest may be the most common form but may not be reported often. Different states define incest in different legal terms. In some, intercourse is required; in others, it is not. Incest is noted to occur in all social groups, including cultures in which it is a stated taboo.

Families in which incestuous activity is taking place may appear normal, but family members frequently have limited contact with the outside world. Family relationships are often chaotic, including problems such as alcohol and drug abuse and severe mental illness. In father-daughter incestuous relationships, the father is frequently a passive, introspective person who experiences a weak sexual relationship with the child's mother. He may therefore turn his attentions to his daughter or daughters out of loneliness and the sexual activity may be quite affectionate. Frequently, the mother is aware of the situation, but both parents agree consciously or subconsciously that the incestuous

relationship is more acceptable than an extramarital one. In such situations the daughter may assume more of the role of the wife around the house, fulfilling many homemaker duties.

Children who have been victimized by incest often feel guilty during adolescence. Many may be afraid to withdraw from the relationship out of fear that in so doing they would destroy the family and the security it provides. Such victims frequently feel humiliated and develop poor self-esteem. Because of this, these women may have difficulty in developing appropriate relationships with members of the opposite sex and may make poor choices in their interpersonal relationships in the future. They frequently choose chaotic family existences after they leave home. Fewer than 10% of children involved in incestuous relationships have normal psychological development at the time of evaluation. Usually, they exhibit guilt, anger, behavioral problems, unexplained physical complaints, lying, stealing, school failure, running away, and sleep disturbances. Gynecologists may see such individuals as teenagers or young adults and may note that some or all of these complaints have been fully developed. When such a profile occurs, the gynecologist should investigate the possibility of a history of incest to fully understand the psychopathology of the patient. Appropriate questions such as, "Were you physically or sexually abused or raped as a child or adolescent?" should be asked as part of a routine history. Affirmative answers to any of these questions require specific detailed and discreet questioning about the individual involved and the circumstances of the incestuous act. The physician should assess the kinds of counseling the patient may already have experienced. Questioning should be nonjudgmental, clear, and specific. For example, the patient should be questioned about the sexual activity experienced and whether it included touching, genital manipulation, or intercourse. Often the individual is relieved to tell the health professional about her experience, because it may be something that she has never previously discussed. The knowledge that this is a common human experience and that the individual is blameless can be very helpful. The physician must then determine the necessity for an appropriate referral to a mental health worker.

Incest victims as adults frequently choose partners capable of physical and sexual violence. Several studies have looked at the long-term follow-up of incest victims. Two separate studies in the 1970s, one by Lukianowicz and the other by Meiselman, found that daughters in father-daughter incestuous relationships demonstrated difficulties in sexual adjustment, including promiscuity and homosexuality. In 28 cases, 11 girls became promiscuous, as well as delinquent, and 4 of these became prostitutes. Of the 11, 5 married and had problems with sexual arousal and 4 demonstrated psychiatric symptoms of depression, anxiety, and suicidal ideology. Six, however, demonstrated no specific ill effects. In another study by Browning and Boatman, a gradual improvement in symptomatology occurred with time, regardless of whether treatment plans were followed. In specific instances of incestuous relationships with uncles, however, there was great anxiety over the possibility of repeat incest when the uncles were left at large. In this same study, violence was reported, including suicides in fathers and one murder of a mother by her son.

Earlier studies had suggested that the degree of emotional disturbance was greater the closer the relationship of the relative and that the degree was also related to whether genital contact actually took place. In a 1980 study of 796 college students,

Finkelhor reported that about one third of the incestuous activity occurred only once, but that in 27% the activity continued with varying frequency for more than a year. Of the involved individuals, 30% considered their experience positive, 30% negative, and the rest did not feel strongly one way or the other. In this series, women students who had sexual incestuous experiences as children were more likely to be sexually active. Experiences with siblings seemed to have a more positive effect on sexual development as long as the overall experience with the sibling was positive. Men who had sibling sexual experiences did not seem to have a higher current level of frequency of intercourse and seemed to have lower self-esteem. Thus, it is difficult to predict what overall long-term potential problems may occur in victims of incestuous experiences.

Whatever the effect childhood sexual abuse and incest may have on the development of psychological well-being and self-esteem in the victim, it is more and more clear that at least a subset of such victims develops physical complaints involving several organ systems including respiratory, gastrointestinal, musculoskeletal, and neurologic, as well as a variety of chronic pain syndromes. Forty percent to 50% of women with chronic pelvic pain report a history of abuse, either physical or sexual. Recently, chronic fatigue syndrome and bladder problems have been added to the list of problems associated with childhood sexual abuse. Therefore, physicians who have patients with such chronic problems should consider childhood sexual abuse and incest as a possible contributor and should offer counseling where appropriate as part of the treatment program.

ABUSE

Intimate Partner Violence

Domestic violence, partner abuse, **intimate partner violence** (IPV), the battered woman, and spouse abuse are terms that refer to violence occurring between partners in an ongoing relationship even if they are not married. A battered woman is defined as any woman over the age of 16 with evidence of physical abuse on at least one occasion at the hands of an intimate male partner. The battered wife syndrome is defined as a symptom complex occurring as a result of violence in which a woman has at any time received deliberate, severe, or repeated (more than three times) physical abuse from her husband or significant male partner in which the minimal injury is bruising. Intimate partner violence is the CDC's currently preferred term because it allows for males or females to be the victim and intimate partners can be the same or opposite sex. Actual or threatened physical, sexual, or psychological abuse by a current or former spouse (including common-law spouses), dating partner, boyfriend, or girlfriend is considered intimate partner violence. The American Medical Association has treatment guidelines and defines IPV as a "pattern of coercive behaviors that may include repeated battering and injury, psychological or emotional abuse, sexual assault, progressive societal isolation, economic deprivation, intimidation and stalking." The actual physical abuse may vary from minimal activity, such as verbal abuse or threat of violence, to throwing an object, throwing an object at someone, pushing, slapping, kicking, hitting, beating, threatening with a weapon, or using a weapon. These acts may be spontaneous or intentionally planned. Most such violence is accompanied by mental abuse and intimidation. Partner abuse is often seen in conjunction with abuse of children and elderly persons in the same

household. A 2008 study by Breiding et al. investigated risk factors for IPV in noninstitutionalzed adults and found the victims to be female, of ethnic/racial minority, to have a lower income, to be less educated, and to be older. There remain significant societal, cultural, and economic barriers for victims to seek help.

It is difficult to ascertain the specific incidence of domestic violence, but it has been estimated that 4.5 million cases of IPV occur in the United States each year, and some authors have stated that at least 50% of family relationships are violent. In a 1984 U.S. Department of Justice study, 57% of 450,000 annual acts of family violence were committed by spouses or ex-spouses, and the wife was a victim in 93% of cases. In at least one fourth of these cases the violent acts had occurred at least three times in the previous 6 months. In 1990, FBI statistics reported similar findings. A 2008 phone survey of noninstitutionalized adults provided some of the best IPV prevalence data to date. Nineteen percent of women reported threatened physical violence over their lifetime, 14.5% reported attempted physical violence, and 20.2% completed physical violence. The frequency of unwanted sex for an intimate partner was 10.2%. Within the last 12 months, 1.4% of women reported completed physical or sexual violence.

In addition, it has been estimated that between one third and one half of female homicide victims are murdered by their male partners, whereas only 12% of male homicide victims are killed by their female partners. In 1992, the American Medical Association (AMA) published guidelines for the diagnosis and treatment of domestic violence. The association noted that 47% of husbands who beat their wives do so three or more times per year, that 14% of ever-married women reported being raped by their current or former husbands, and that rape is a significant or major form of abuse in 54% of violent marriages. The AMA guidelines also summarized various studies noting that battered women may account for 22% to 35% of women seeking care for any reason in emergency departments (the majority of whom are seen by medical or nontrauma services) and 19% to 30% of injured women seen in emergency departments. This was confirmed in a 2005 study where 17% of women seeking care in an emergency department reported current abuse. Nine to 14% of women seen in ambulatory care internal medicine clinics currently suffer IPV, and 26% to 28% of such women have been battered at some time. The study states that 25% of women who attempt suicide, 25% who are receiving psychiatric services, and 23% of pregnant women seeking prenatal care have been victims of domestic violence. In addition, 45% to 59% of mothers of abused children have been abused, and 58% of women older than 30 who have been raped have been abused. In a gynecologic clinic in England, John and colleagues surveyed a cohort of 825 women. Twenty-one percent reported physical abuse, and of those, 48% also had forced sexual activity. A 2005 report confirmed the prevalence rates in health care facilities with 35% of obstetrics and gynecology patients reporting IPV and 13% of women seeking care reporting current abuse. Therefore, it can be seen that domestic violence and battered women are common in our society today.

The most common sites for injury are the head, neck, chest, abdomen, breast, and upper extremities. Minor injuries such as scratches, bruises, sore muscles, and welts are common. The upper extremities may be fractured as the woman attempts to defend herself. Broken teeth, burns, laceration, head injury, and strangulation are also frequently observed. In a study from Yale,

84% of the injuries were severe enough to require medical treatment, and in 81% of the cases patients stated that the assailant had beaten them with the fists. In an English study of 100 women brought to a hostel for battered women, 44% suffered from lacerations and 59% stated that they had been kicked repeatedly. All women stated that they had been hit with a clenched fist. Fractures occurred in 32, and 9 of the women had been beaten and taken to the hostel unconscious. A 2006 study also found significant injury among victims; of 519,031 cases, 41% of assaults caused observable injuries and 28% required medical treatment.

Murder and suicide are frequent components of the domestic violence problem. In a large study from Denver, Walker reported that three quarters of the battered patients felt that the batterer would kill them during the relationship, and almost half felt that they might kill the batterer. Of these victims, 11% stated that they had actually tried to kill the batterer, and 87% believed that they themselves would be the ones to die if someone were killed. This is not an exaggeration, as IPV resulted in 1544 deaths in 2004. One third of these women stated that they seriously considered committing suicide. Walker noted that victims and their attackers frequently are depressed and may move rapidly between suicidal and homicidal intent.

There is a strong relationship between spouse battering and child abuse. In Walker's study, 53% of men who abused their partners were noted also to abuse their children. Another one third had threatened to abuse their children. Interestingly, in the same relationship, 28% of the wives who themselves were abused stated that they had abused their children while living in the violent household, and an additional 6% thought that they might abuse their children at the time they were evaluated.

Physical abuse in pregnancy is common and may be referred to as prenatal child abuse. The incidence is somewhere between 1% and 20% depending on the study population. In one study, 81 of 742 (10.9%) patients visiting a prenatal clinic stated that they had been victims of abuse at some time in the past, and 29 of these women stated that the abuse had continued into the pregnancy. Violence may increase postpartum. One fifth of these noted an increase in abuse during pregnancy, and one third noted a decrease. In a study of a group of Medicaid-eligible postpartum women, a constellation of factors associated with violence during pregnancy was noted. Of the patients in this study, 7% suffered battering, and significant correlates including anxiety, depression, housing problems, inadequate prenatal care, and drug and alcohol abuse were identified. The women in the study who were battered during pregnancy suffered a more severe constellation of symptoms than did those who were battered only prior to pregnancy. In the case of pregnant patients, most studies note that battering is frequently directed to the breasts and abdomen.

It is important that physicians increase their ability to recognize the signs of domestic violence and spouse abuse. A study by Hilberman and Monson demonstrated that 25% of women treated for injuries in an emergency room were victims of wife battering. The physicians who were treating these patients made the correct diagnosis originally in only 3% of cases. Viken has listed a profile of the characteristics of the abused wife. These include a history of having been beaten as a child, raised in a single-parent home, married as a teenager, and pregnant before marriage. Such women frequently visit clinics and emergency rooms with a variety of somatic complaints, including headaches, insomnia,

Box 9-5 Somatic Complaints in Abused Women
Headaches
Insomnia
Choking sensation
Hyperventilation
Chest, back, or pelvic pain
Other Signs and Symptoms
Shyness
Fright
Embarrassment
Evasiveness
Jumpiness
Passivity
Frequent crying
Often accompanied by male partner
Drug or alcohol abuse (often overdose)
Injuries

From ACOG Technical Bulletin Number 124: *The battered woman.* January 1989.

choking sensation, hyperventilation, gastrointestinal symptoms, and chest, pelvic, and back pain. Noncompliance with the advice of physicians with respect to these complaints is frequent (**Box 9-5**).

In visits to the physician's office or emergency room, the patient often appears shy, frightened, embarrassed, evasive, anxious, or passive and often cries. The batterer may accompany the patient on such visits and stay close at hand to monitor what she says to the physician. Thus, the woman may be hesitant to provide information about how she was injured, and the explanation given may not fit the injuries observed. Alcohol or other drug abuse is common in such individuals.

Physicians should become comfortable in asking the patient whether she has been physically abused. Every pregnant woman should be screened for intimate partner violence. Questions such as, "Has anyone hurt you or tried to injure you?" "Has an intimate partner ever threatened you with physical violence?" and, "Have you ever been physically abused either recently or in the past?" are appropriate introductory questions. The physician should follow up on any positive answers in a nonjudgmental manner in an attempt to learn what is happening. Physical examinations should be complete with particular attention to bruises, lacerations, burns, improbable injury, and other signs of injury. If the patient is wearing sunglasses, she should be asked to remove them so the physician can determine whether there are eye injuries. If the patient is pregnant, bruises seen on the breasts or abdomen should always be discussed. Physicians should carefully note evidence for abuse in the patient's record.

Battering acts tend to run in cycles consisting of three phases. The first phase is tension building, in which tension between the couple gradually escalates, manifested by discrete acts that cause family friction. Name calling, intimidating remarks, meanness, and mild physical abuse such as pushing are common. The batterer often expresses dissatisfaction and hostility in a somewhat chronic form. The victim may attempt to placate the batterer in hopes of pleasing him or calming him. She may actually believe at this point that she has the power to avoid aggravating the situation. She may not respond to his hostile actions and may even be successful from time to time in apparently reducing tensions. This, of course, will reinforce her belief that she can control the situation. As the tension phase builds, the batterer's anger is less controlled, and the victim may withdraw, fearing that she will inadvertently set off explosive behavior. Often this withdrawal is the signal for the batterer to become more aggressive. Anything may spark the hostile act, and the acute battering then takes place. This is the cycle's second phase and is represented by an uncontrollable discharge of tension that has built up through the first phase. The attack may take the form of both verbal and physical abuse, and the victim is often left injured. In self-defense the victim may actually injure or kill the batterer. In approximately two thirds of cases reported by Walker, alcohol abuse was involved. However, the alcohol use may have been the excuse rather than the reason for the battering. After the abuse has taken place, the third phase generally follows. In this situation, the batterer apologizes, asks forgiveness, and frequently shows kindness and remorse, showering the victim with gifts and promises. This gives the victim hope that the relationship can be saved and that the violence will not recur. Batterers are often charming and manipulative, offering the victim justification for forgiveness. The cycles, however, do repeat themselves, with the first phase increasing in length and intensity, the battering becoming more severe, and the third phase tending to decrease in both duration and intensity. The batterer learns that he can control the victim without obtaining much forgiveness. The victim becomes more demoralized and loses her ability to leave the situation even if she has the means and opportunity to do so.

Batterers, too, tend to have a specific profile in most cases. They are men who refuse to take responsibility for their behavior, blaming their victims for their violent acts. They often have strong controlling personalities and do not tolerate autonomy in their partners. They have rigid expectations of marriage and sexual behavior and consider their wives or partners as chattel. They wish to be cared for in their most basic needs, frequently make unrealistic demands on their wives, and show low tolerance for stress. Depression and suicide attempts are often a part of their behavior pattern, but in general they are aggressive and assaultive in most of their behavior, generally using violence to solve their problems. On the other hand, they are often charming and manipulative, especially in their relationships outside the marriage. They often exhibit low self-esteem, feelings of inadequacy, and a sense of helplessness, all of which are generally made worse by the prospects of losing their wives. It is typical behavior for male batterers to exhibit contempt for women in their usual activities. Therapy is usually ineffective and seems to work only when the man can be made to give up violence as his primary means of solving problems.

Once the physician discovers that a woman is living in an abusive relationship, it is important to acknowledge to the patient the seriousness of the situation. To do otherwise is to give the impression that the physician approves or at least accepts the violent condition. It is important to attend to the patient's injuries and to assess the patient's emotional status from the standpoint of a psychiatric condition such as a suicidal ideation, depression, anxiety, or signs of abuse of drugs, alcohol, or other medications. The physician should also attempt to estimate the woman's ability to assess her own situation and her readiness to take appropriate action. If problems involving mental illness are present, a referral to an appropriate mental health worker who is sensitive to the issues of domestic violence should be made. Physicians should determine community resources available for handling family violence. The police department, crisis hotline, rape relief centers, domestic violence programs, and legal aid services

for abused women can offer help in the acute situation. Hospital emergency rooms and shelters for battered women and children are also excellent resources. Health care workers in these organizations or private practitioners who specialize in the care of battered women, their spouses, and their children can offer counseling and follow-up care. Such individuals may be social workers, psychologists, psychiatrists, or other mental health workers trained specifically for this purpose. The physician's job is to recognize the problem and either offer counseling or get counseling for the patient so that she understands her rights and alternatives and learns to protect herself and her children from future harm. The victim of abuse very likely will not wish to leave her home because of economic concerns and a fear that the batterer may continue to pursue her. Although she may have the batterer arrested and served with restraining orders, she may be convinced that she and her children cannot be protected from the batterer. She may also believe that there is a possibility of reconciliation and of change in behavior on the part of the batterer. It is therefore reasonable to discuss an exit plan with the victim to be used should the violence recur. This exit plan should include the following:

1. Have a change of clothes packed for both her and her children including toilet articles, necessary medications, and an extra set of keys to the house and car. These can be placed in a suitcase and left with a friend or family member.
2. Keep some cash, a checkbook, and a savings account book with the friend or family member.
3. Other identification papers, such as birth certificates, social security cards, voter registration cards, utility bills, and driver's license, should be kept available, because children will need to be enrolled in school and the woman may have to seek financial assistance.
4. Have something special, such as a toy or book, for each child.
5. Have financial records available, such as mortgage papers, rent receipts, and an automobile title.
6. Determine a plan on exactly where to go regardless of the time of day or night. This may be to a friend or relative's house or to a shelter for battered women and children.
7. Ask neighbors to call police if violence begins.
8. Remove weapons.
9. Teach children to call 9-1-1.

Rehearsing an exit plan as one would conduct a fire drill makes it possible for the battered woman to respond even under the stress of the battering. Long-term aid and referral of the patient, her children, and the batterer to the appropriate resources is an important aspect of the care of such patients. The American College of Obstetricians and Gynecologists has prepared a patient education brochure that physicians can keep in their offices and give to individuals who suffer from this problem. Making the brochures available in the office waiting room may encourage women with these needs to get help.

These women often suffer from severe psychiatric problems, such as anxiety, depression, posttraumatic stress disorder (PTSD), and other pathologic conditions that may require psychotherapy. Women who are both physically and sexually assaulted have significantly higher levels of PTSD compared with women who are physically abused only. However, women who suffer any abuse, including emotional abuse without physical or sexual abuse, have a higher rate of mental health problems, including postpartum depression. Group counseling or individual counseling may also help them to rebuild their lives as single individuals or single parents. It is frequently necessary to help them develop a skill that will enable them to be employable. Counseling programs take these things into consideration. Children of victims who may be victims as well also require counseling to avoid behavior patterns that will lead to aggressive behavior in their later lives.

Intimate partner violence is a common problem that affects the family unit in particular and society in general. It can occur in all segments of society and reflects the violence that is a part of life today and the behavior of many. Physicians should learn to detect its presence in their patients and offer ways the victim can seek help. The help may include counseling for the victim, batterer, and children or constructing a plan for the woman to exit the relationship and rebuild her life in safety. There are many possible barriers for physicians screening for IPV and acting on their suspicions (**Table 9-18**). **Ferguson's 2010** presidential address about IPV gave multiple recommendations regarding clinical practice, education and training, and research needs in this area in hopes of "ending this blight against women."

If the male batterer has not undergone anger management therapy, family counseling or intervention can be extremely dangerous, as it often raises issues that exacerbate the violence and increase the risk of serious harm to the woman and her children. Therefore, this should not be advised until such time as the male batterer has addressed and eliminated his violent behavior. In general, success in such attempts with respect to the male partner is usually minimal.

Although all states have requirements for reporting child abuse, not all states require the reporting of domestic violence. However, many states have aggressive programs for intervening in domestic violence cases, and physicians should become aware of the programs in effect in their area. The patient should always be encouraged to leave a violent situation and may need community resources to help with economic and social adjustment, as well as protection for herself and her children from the violent partner. The American College of Obstetricians and Gynecologist's

Table 9-18 Possible Barriers to Physician Screening for Intimate Partner Violence (IPV)

Belief that "someone else will take care of it"
Forgetfulness
Not a physician's responsibility/role
IPV "should be private"
"Can not offer much"
Lack of scientific evidence that screening improves outcomes
Cynicism: "nothing will happen"
Legal entanglement
Worry about offending/angering patients
Screening will take too much time
Insufficient training
Uncertainty about training requirements
Uncertainly about legal implications if screen is positive
Uncomfortable discussing issues of IPV
"Do not need to ask; the patient will volunteer the information"
Beliefs about victims of spouse abuse
Fear of retaliation against patient
Frustration over lack of patient disclosure
Not scientific, "sexy"

From Ferguson JE II: Why doesn't SOMEBODY do something? Am J Obstet Gynecol 202(6):635-643, 2010.

website has a page on resources for violence against women and lists each state's coalitions for sexual assault and domestic violence (www.acog.org/departments/dept_web.cfm?recno=17).

The Elderly

The Select Committee on Aging, in investigating domestic violence against the elderly, held hearings before the Subcommittee of Human Services of the House of Representatives in 1980. The committee noted that approximately 500,000 to 2.5 million cases involving abuse of the elderly occur per year in the United States. The committee documented that abuse of the elderly may be as large a nationwide problem as child abuse. Usually, the abused person is a woman older than age 75, often with a physical impairment. She is generally white, widowed, and living with relatives. The abuser is generally an adult child living within the family but may also be a spouse. Counseling issues involve the entire family but particularly the individual causing the abuse. Physicians who care for geriatric patients should be alert for signs and symptoms of this type of domestic abuse; when it is found, community resources should be activated. All 50 states have passed legislation protecting the elderly from domestic violence and neglect. Forty-two states have mandatory reporting laws.

GRIEF AND LOSS

The term *grief* is usually used to refer to the emotional, behavioral, and functional response to the death of a loved one. However, many people experience grief in response to losses other than death, such as losing a marriage, a job, one's health, or hope of having children, as in infertility. Such losses—in addition to losses resulting from spontaneous abortion; the death of a parent, child, friend, or other loved one; or the death of a pet—occur throughout a woman's life. Gynecologists are likely to see women at times of uncomplicated grief, **complicated grief**, or grief-related major depression. Recognizing when a grief reaction is following an expectable course, as opposed to being complicated or involving major depression, is important in ensuring that the woman receives needed treatment.

Uncomplicated or "normal" grief has been postulated to follow defined stages, including initial numbness or shock, then sadness and depression, reorganization, and recovery. However, the literature suggests that grief experiences vary significantly among different cultures, people, and individual losses, often with intermingling of different "stages" of grief at the same time. Grief is currently thought to be a process with a wide spectrum of individual responses and a variable course, including not only painful feelings but also positive emotions and memories.

The nature of uncomplicated grief, complicated grief, and grief-related depression has been reviewed recently by **Zisook and Shear (2009)**. Acute grief occurs early after the loss, is intensely painful, and includes sadness, crying, preoccupation with thoughts of the deceased or of the loss, disturbed sleep and appetite, trouble concentrating, and separation from and lack of interest in other people and usual activities. Within a few months, acute grief gives way to integrated grief, a state in which the deceased or what has been lost is thought of often with sadness, but the woman is not preoccupied and can once more participate in pleasurable and meaningful activities and relationships. Triggers, including birthdays, anniversaries, or situations that remind her of the loss, may precipitate waves of grief, which gradually become less intense and less frequent over time. Uncomplicated grief may include hallucinations (seeing or hearing the deceased) early after bereavement. Uncomplicated grief does not require formal treatment, but instead gradually lessens with the support of family, friends, and community such as church and clergy; reassurance; information about the expected course of grief; and sometimes the help of support groups.

Complicated grief occurs in about 10% of bereaved people, represents a failure to move from acute to integrated grief, and is associated with significant difficulty functioning. Symptoms include intense pain and longing, difficulty accepting the loss, anger, intrusive thoughts, guilt, feelings of estrangement from other people, and suicidal thoughts. Risk factors include a history of mood and anxiety disorders, multiple losses, adverse life events, and other stressors reducing the woman's ability to cope. Complicated grief requires treatment to avoid becoming chronic and unremitting. Treatment should include psychotherapy and often also antidepressant medication.

> Complicated grief requires specific treatment, including psychotherapy and antidepressant medication.

Acute grief is commonly associated with symptoms that meet the criteria for major depression; 40% to 50% of bereaved people meet criteria at 1 month, about 20% to 25% at 2 months, and about 16% at 1 year. There is considerable controversy about when to treat major depression occurring in the context of bereavement, especially because bereavement-related depression is similar in clinical characteristics, course, and treatment response to major depression occurring after a range of other stressors or without any identifiable trigger. Women with a past history of depression, or severe depressive symptoms as part of grief, should probably be treated aggressively, even in the first month or two after the loss, with antidepressant medication and psychotherapy, whereas those with milder depression can be monitored or referred for psychotherapy alone.

Obstetricians and gynecologists may need to counsel patients experiencing grief related to several areas of reproduction, including spontaneous abortion, perinatal loss, and infertility. About 15% of pregnancies end in miscarriage. Following a miscarriage, a woman may experience sadness, guilt, anger, posttraumatic stress disorder (PTSD) symptoms, and anxiety about future pregnancies. Men are also affected, although they tend to talk less about their feelings and may feel that they need to be strong to support their partner. In most cases, there is little discussion within the couple about the loss. A miscarriage most commonly represents the loss not of an established relationship but of hopes and expectations for the future, including pregnancy and motherhood. Despite this difference in the nature of the loss, the feelings of grief after miscarriage resemble those that may arise after losing a loved one, and the course of recovery is similar to that of other types of grief. Acute symptoms usually lessen significantly within about 6 months or sooner if the woman becomes pregnant again.

Several studies have examined the psychological interventions after miscarriage. For example, **Swanson et al. (2009)** studied 341 couples, randomized to four different interventions at 1, 5, and 11 weeks after the miscarriage. Interventions were couples-focused counseling by a nurse in the couple's home for three sessions, a set of three video and workbook modules, a combination of one nurse counseling session with the three video and workbook modules, and no intervention. All interventions used previously established models, Swanson's Caring Theory and the Meaning of Miscarriage Model, took a supportive approach and focused on discussing the miscarriage, losses and gains resulting from the miscarriage, sharing the loss and rejoining public life, "getting through it," and trying again. The most effective intervention overall, for both depression and grief, was the three sessions of counseling by the nurse. In the absence of this resource, the obstetrician-gynecologist can help the patient and couple by normalizing feelings of depression and grief, giving the expectation that these will resolve, but also monitoring carefully for more severe or persistent symptoms of depression, PTSD, or suicidal thoughts indicating a need for referral for mental health treatment.

Perinatal loss, or stillbirth, occurs in 1% or less of pregnancies. In the weeks following a stillbirth, women commonly experience sadness, irritability, feelings of guilt, physical symptoms, depression, and anxiety, characteristic of grief; 20% continue to have symptoms a year later. Women with poor social support or preexisting mental health problems are at higher risk for more intense and prolonged grief. PTSD is reported in about 20% of women during the next pregnancy, and women who hold their dead baby are at higher risk. Fathers also experience similar symptoms of grief after a stillbirth, experience anxiety and PTSD with the next pregnancy, and are also reported to have a higher risk of subsequent PTSD if they hold the dead baby. Loss of a baby may cause relationship strain or breakup, especially if the intensity or timing of grief differs significantly between the two parents. In addition, siblings may, depending on their age, be confused about what has happened, feel that they are to blame, or feel loss. Parents preoccupied by their own grief may have difficulty recognizing or helping their other children with these feelings.

Recommendations for clinicians include giving the woman and her partner clear information about what is going wrong and what is being done, involving the parents in decision making as possible, ensuring that the woman has access to postpartum medical care (e.g., suppression of lactation, contraception, help with gynecologic and sexual problems), and holding a meeting 1 to 2 months later to review what is known about the cause of the baby's death and to answer questions regarding future pregnancies. Couples are commonly advised, at the time of the loss, to create memories of the child, including holding the dead baby, giving the baby a name, taking photographs, and having a funeral. Many parents may want this and find it very important. However, especially holding the dead baby has been associated with poorer psychological outcome, increased rates of PTSD in the next pregnancy, and poor attachment to the subsequent baby. Couples may benefit from support groups, and those women or their partners who experience more severe or persistent depression, grief, anxiety, PTSD, or suicidal thoughts should be referred for mental health treatment with psychotherapy and medication, as indicated.

A special counseling challenge involves the care of a woman with an unplanned pregnancy. Such individuals often suffer conflicting feelings, which may include shame and guilt, a genuine desire to have a child, fear of social and family consequences, and fear for their own future and physical well-being. In addition, they may suffer from guilt about the termination of pregnancy if abortion is considered. Although many such women have good social support (e.g., family, significant other, friends, and religious counselors), others will rely on the physician for advice and direction. The physician should discuss all possible options with the woman, including having and raising the child, offering the child for adoption, or terminating the pregnancy. Issues involving the role of the baby's father, the effect of any decision on the future life of the woman, and the risks of procedures should be considered. The woman should be aided in reaching the most appropriate decision for her circumstances and supported in carrying out her decision. When necessary, appropriate referrals to social agencies (e.g., adoption, abortion counseling, or welfare services) should be made. The woman may experience depression, anxiety, or grief in this situation, even when making what she thinks is the best decision possible.

The inability to have a child, or infertility, affects about 1 in 10 couples and can precipitate feelings of isolation, inadequacy, poor self-esteem, guilt, anger, loss of control over one's life, depression, difficulty being around pregnant women or couples with young children, changes in one's identity and sense of meaning, and relationship strain. Infertility treatment involves significant cost, medical treatments and procedures, and psychological stress. Among women presenting for infertility treatment in one study, 40% met criteria for a psychiatric disorder, including 23% with an anxiety disorder and 17% with major depression. Failed infertility treatment engenders further stress and depression. Psychological distress has been reported to be the primary reason for dropout from infertility treatment, and pretreatment depression is predictive of dropout after one IVF cycle. There is some evidence that higher levels of psychological stress are associated with lower success rates of infertility treatment. Only about 50% of couples have a child as a result of infertility treatment, and those not succeeding commonly experience a grief reaction.

Many infertile women gain information and support from the Internet, although using this as one's sole source of support has been linked with higher levels of psychological distress. Women and their partners may benefit from support groups or individual or group psychotherapy. Interventions proved effective in reducing distress, and in some studies in improving conception rates, include cognitive behavioral therapy, ongoing counseling and education throughout the infertility treatment process, relaxation, stress management, coping skills, and group support. Again, women with severe depression, grief, or suicidal thoughts should also be referred for evaluation for antidepressant or other psychotropic medication treatment.

> Women suffering losses as a result of miscarriage, perinatal loss, unplanned pregnancy, or infertility benefit from support, counseling, and screening for depression and posttraumatic stress disorder.

DEATH AND DYING

Gynecologists, especially gynecologic-oncologists, care for women who are dying. There are several challenges for physicians caring for dying patients. First, physicians have been shown to be optimistic and inaccurate in their prognoses for terminally ill patients and to overestimate their ability to combat disease. This makes it difficult to know when to shift the conversation with a patient from a focus on cure or fighting the disease to a focus on palliative care. Making this transition may be difficult for the physician, who does not wish to give up hope prematurely. On the other hand, most patients are very concerned about issues of quality of life in confronting dying and hope for a process in which they can retain dignity, feel like themselves as much as possible, have adequate time and opportunity to put their "house in order," and have maximal possible comfort and pain relief. It is important for physicians to help women by discussing with them issues of DNR orders, treatment of pain, referral to hospice, and other end-of-life issues. In fact, introducing palliative care discussions earlier in treatment appears to be helpful. For example, in a study of 151 patients with metastatic non-small-cell lung cancer, patients randomized to early palliative care integrated with oncologic care had a better quality of life and mood, less aggressive care at the end of life, and longer survival.

> Women with terminal illness benefit from an engaged, genuine relationship with physicians and other health care providers, treatment of depression and anxiety states, psychological interventions and psychotherapy, and early integration of palliative care into treatment.

Psychological issues for dying patients are highly variable, depending on the person's stage of life, sense of the meaning of her life and of the illness, coping style, relationships and family support, spiritual beliefs, and economic circumstances. Feelings of grief, sadness, despair, fear, anxiety, and loneliness are present at some stage for nearly all dying patients, but some are able to achieve a high degree of equanimity and acceptance.

Developmentally, young adults with terminal illness commonly struggle with anger about the unfairness of the illness, grief and loss about life experiences they will not have, and issues related to being dependent on their parents for care. Parents of young children are concerned about the impact of their illness and death on their children, losing the opportunity to see their children grow up, and how to maintain a normal life and routine for their children and family in the face of their illness. For women in later stages of life, feelings about death depend on the degree of satisfaction and meaning that they feel with their life and what they have done, the kinds and quality of attachments they have, whether they feel robbed of retirement and later life, and whether they have lost their spouse or intimate partner already.

Block provided a comprehensive overview of psychological issues faced by dying patients and ways to explore with them issues related to the meaning of the illness, meaning of their life and achievements, spirituality, relationship issues, other life stressors, maintaining a sense of self, and fears and hopes that the patient has. Terminally ill patients benefit from the treatment of depression or anxiety states, in order to improve the quality of the remainder of their lives. Dying patients also benefit from psychological interventions, including listening, the opportunity to share feelings, and the chance to reflect on past experiences and future hopes. The gynecologist can help a dying woman by maintaining an engaged, genuine relationship with the woman as an individual throughout the dying process, helping the woman and family to anticipate and address practical issues such as enrolling in hospice and other palliative care services, and maximizing comfort and pain control.

KEY POINTS

- Depression and anxiety disorders are treatable with medications or psychotherapy.
- Eating disorders are life-threatening conditions that are often unrecognized.
- Many substance use disorders, such as alcoholism, have a more rapidly progressive course in women than in men ("telescoping").
- Understanding attachment styles can help providers to work effectively with "difficult" patients.
- Nonpharmacologic treatments for hypoactive sexual desire disorder include lifestyle changes for reducing stress and fatigue, recognizing and treating depression, increasing quality time with the partner, improving body image, and bringing novelty into the sexual repertoire.
- Lesbian and bisexual women require routine gynecologic care, have a high rate of mental health and substance use problems, and prefer female, preferably lesbian, health care providers.
- Intimate partner violence crosses all ethnic, racial, educational, age, and socioeconomic lines and has a large burden of social, physical, mental, and public health implications.
- The physician has a responsibility to screen and acknowledge intimate partner violence and abuse, identify the community resources for immediate referrals, assess safety, assist with reporting if necessary or desired, document appropriately using medicolegal tools, and provide ongoing clinical care.
- Gynecologists are often called on to provide or refer women for counseling related to grief; losses such as miscarriage, perinatal loss, infertility; and end-of-life issues.
- Complicated grief and grief accompanied by symptoms of depression benefit from antidepressant medication treatment.

REFERENCES CAN BE FOUND ON EXPERTCONSULT.com

BIBLIOGRAPHY

ACOG Committee on Health Care for Underserved Women: ACOG Committee Opinion. Motivational interviewing: A tool for behavior change, *Obstet Gynecol* 113(1):243–246, 2009.

Basson R: Sexual desire and arousal disorders in women, *N Engl J Med* 354: 1497, 2006.

Benowitz NL: Nicotine addiction, *N Engl J Med* 362:2295–2303, 2010.

Berrington de Gonzalez A, Hartge P, Cerhan JR, et al: Body-mass index and mortality among 1.46 million white adults, *N Engl J Med* 2 363(23):2211–2219, 2010.

Block SD: Psychological issues in end-of-life care, *J Palliat Med* 9:751–766, 2006.

Breiding MJ, Black MC, Ryan GW: Prevalence and risk factors of intimate partner violence in eighteen US states/territories, *Am J Prev Med* 34: 112–118, 2008.

Brier N: Grief following miscarriage: A comprehensive review of the literature, *J Womens Health* 17: 451–464, 2008.

Cipriani A, Furukawa TA, Salanti G, et al: Comparative efficacy and acceptability of 12 new-generation antidepressants: A multiple-treatments meta-analysis, *Lancet* 373:746–758, 2009.

Clinical updates in women's health care, *Eat Disord* 7(1):1–81, 2008 Washington, DC, American College of Obstetricians and Gynecologists.

Ferguson JE II: Why doesn't SOMEBODY do something? *Am J Obstet Gynecol* 202(6): 635–643, 2010.

Greenfield SF, Back SE, Lawson K, et al: Substance abuse in women, *Psychiatr Clin North Am* 33: 339–355, 2010.

Hawton K, van Heeringen K: Suicide, *Lancet* 373: 1372–1381, 2009.

Jenike MA: Obsessive compulsive disorder, *N Engl J Med* 350:259–265, 2004.

Katon WJ: Panic disorder, *N Engl J Med* 354: 2360–2367, 2006.

King M, Semlyen J, Tai SS, et al: A systematic review of mental disorder, suicide, and deliberate self-harm in lesbian, gay, and bisexual people, *BMC Psychiatry* 70: doi:10.1186/1471-244X-8-70.

Lieb K, Zanarini MC, Schmahl C, et al: Borderline personality disorder, *Lancet* 364:453–461, 2004.

Mann JJ: The medical management of depression, *N Engl J Med* 353:1819–1834, 2005.

Oesterheld JR, Cozza K, Sandson NB: Oral contraceptives, *Psychosomatics* 49:168–175, 2008.

Schneier FR: Social anxiety disorder, *N Engl J Med* 355:1029–1036, 2006.

Shifren JL, Monz BU, Russo PA, et al: Sexual problems and distress in United States women prevalence and correlates, *Obstet Gynecol* 112(5): 970–978, 2008.

Strous RD, Ulman AM, Kotler M: The hateful patient revisited: Relevance for 21st century medicine, *Eur J Intern Med* 17:387–393, 2006.

Swanson KM, Chen HT, Graham JC, et al: Resolution of miscarriage and grief in the first year after miscarriage: A randomized controlled clinical trial of couples focused interventions, *J Womens Health* 18:1245–1257, 2009.

Thompson D, Ciechanowski PS: Attaching a new understanding to the patient-physician relationship in family practice, *J Am Board Fam Pract* 16: 219–226, 2003.

Treasure J, Claudino AM, Zucker N: Eating disorders, *Lancet* 375:583–593, 2010.

Zisook S, Shear K: Grief and bereavement: What psychiatrists need to know, *World Psychiatry* 8: 67–74, 2009.

10
Endoscopy: Hysteroscopy and Laparoscopy
Indications, Contraindications and Complications

Gretchen M. Lentz

This chapter presents an overview of frequently used endoscopic procedures in gynecology. Indications, contraindications, and complications are included for each procedure. For those unfamiliar with the procedures, the diagnostic uses are described. Therapeutic uses and pitfalls are introduced, but complex surgical procedures are covered in gynecologic surgical textbooks.

Since the 1960s, there have been significant changes in the use of endoscopy in gynecologic practice. The fiberoptic bundle and more versatile light sources, as well as the incorporation of advances in technology, have dramatically increased the diagnostic and therapeutic capabilities of the hysteroscope and laparoscope.

The tremendous advances in technology have led to the emergence of more office-based procedures. Many gynecologic surgeries done by laparotomy in years past have been converted to ambulatory, outpatient procedures. Other cases previously completed by laparotomy have been converted to complex laparoscopic or robotic surgeries with shorter recovery time and hospital stays. This chapter serves as an introductory overview of gynecologic endoscopy.

HYSTEROSCOPY

Hysteroscopy is the direct visualization of the endometrial cavity via the cervix using an endoscope and a light source. The earliest hysteroscope was nothing more than a hollow tube with an alcohol lamp and mirror for a light source. In 1869, Pantaleoni reported the successful removal of an endometrial polyp through the scope. Modern hysteroscopes are modifications of cystoscopes with channels to introduce light via fiberoptics. Various infusion media are used for uterine cavity distention, which is necessary for inspection. Many surgical instruments and devices are available for diagnostic biopsy and pathology removal and therapeutic procedures. Office and operating room hysteroscopy requires knowledge of instrumentation, techniques, indications, contraindications, and complication management. If office hysteroscopy is used, proper office safety protocols are needed.

Inserting a hysteroscope for diagnostic purposes only is not a risky procedure. The key is predicting ahead of time which diagnostic procedures might be very challenging from severe cervical stenosis or which complex operative hysteroscopic procedures might be more safely accomplished in the operating room setting. Office hysteroscopy saves time for both the patient and physician, saves money, and is convenient. It makes sense to gain experience with the simpler hysteroscopic procedures in the

office. Judgment is necessary, as a 1-cm pedunculated polyp or myoma might be easily removed in the office; however, a 3-cm sessile polyp or 3-cm myoma with 50% of the myoma intramyometrial would require more expertise and might be more safely attempted in the operating room. Once expertise has been gained from sufficient operative hysteroscopic procedural volume, the more involved and challenging procedures can be moved from the operating room to the office setting.

HYSTEROSCOPIC INDICATIONS AND CONTRAINDICATIONS

The popularity of hysteroscopy has been enhanced because it is a simple technique that can be performed in the office. Office indications include diagnosing abnormal uterine bleeding, for both pre- and postmenopausal women. Women with recurrent abnormal uterine bleeding, particularly if abnormal perimenopausal or postmenopausal bleeding recurs or persists following a negative endometrial biopsy, are good candidates for hysteroscopy. Endometrial biopsy and dilatation and curettage (D&C) procedures frequently miss focal lesions, particularly pedunculated structures. Feldman and colleagues evaluated 286 women with perimenopausal bleeding who had had a D&C or an endometrial biopsy. Nine of 86 (10.5%) who had negative findings initially, but continued to bleed, had carcinoma or complex hyperplasia on follow-up biopsy. Hysteroscopy with directed biopsy can be useful in this setting, although controversy exists regarding the spread of endometrial cancer with hysteroscopy. Hysteroscopy is ideal for directly visualizing and removing intrauterine foreign bodies like a partially perforated or broken intrauterine device (IUD) or retrieving an IUD with missing strings. Other indications include performing hysteroscopic sterilization, evaluation of recurrent miscarriage, uterine synechiae, abnormal hysterosalpinography (HSG), and infertility. More involved operative procedures for correcting an abnormality, which might require local, regional, or general anesthesia, include resection of submucous myomas, lysis of synechiae, incision of uterine septa, and removal of endometrial polyps or ablation of the endometrium. **Table 10-1** lists common indications.

There are few contraindications to hysteroscopy. Absolute contraindications include acute pelvic or vaginal infections including genital herpes, because of the potential of spreading the disease by the media used for uterine distention. One exception might be for the retrieval of an IUD if the pelvic infection is related to the IUD. Pregnancy is a contraindication, as is recent

Table 10-1 Possible Hysteroscopic Indications

Abnormal uterine bleeding
    Premenopausal
    Postmenopausal
Persistent abnormal uterine bleeding after negative endometrial biopsy
Postmenopausal endometrial thickening and negative endometrial biopsy
Endometrial polyp
Submucosal myoma or possibly <50% intramural
Uterine septum
Uterine synechiae
Retained IUD
Sterilization
Endocervical lesions

uterine perforation. Active bleeding is a relative contraindication. If the bleeding is brisk, the hysteroscopic view might be unsatisfactory. Other relative contraindications include extensive adhesions and leiomyomata that are largely (>50%) intramyometrial rather than submucous. Cervical and uterine cancers are cited as absolute contraindications. There continues to be debate over risking endometrial cancer dissemination into the peritoneal cavity by pushing endometrial cancer cells out the fallopian tubes with the distending media. A 2010 systematic review by Polyzos et al. found hysteroscopy resulted in a significantly higher rate of malignant peritoneal cytology (odds ratio 1.78) when done before surgery and therefore disease upstaging, although it is unclear if the outcome is adversely affected. Unfortunately, gynecologists are often doing hysteroscopy, endometrial biopsy, and polyp resection for abnormal bleeding before the diagnosis of endometrial cancer is made in order to make the diagnosis. This is considered acceptable management, however.

HYSTEROSCOPIC EQUIPMENT AND TECHNIQUES

Rigid hysteroscopes vary in diameter. The smaller caliber scopes, 3 to 5 mm in diameter, are used for diagnostic purposes. Several are available that have views from 0 to 70 degrees, but those with views of 12 to 30 degrees are most commonly used. Similar to a cystoscope, the outer sleeve of a rigid hysteroscope contains several channels that extend the full length of the instrument. **Figure 10-1** shows the anatomy of a hysteroscope and names of the various sections. For office hysteroscopy, often a 4-mm telescope with a 7-mm outer sheath is used, so there is a channel for seven French flexible or semirigid instruments such as scissors, biopsy or grasping forceps. The outer sheath also allows for inflow of the distending media. Although a 5-mm hysteroscope often passes without cervical dilation, a 7-mm diameter scope often does not. Large scopes, with diameters of 8 to 10 mm, may be used for high flow of distending media and have a second channel for outflow of blood and fluid. These are used for moderate to complex procedures. Flexible minihysteroscopic instruments and microendoscopes are convenient and very well tolerated in the office for diagnosis and simple operative procedures such as directed biopsies. There is generally less pain with the small flexible hysteroscopes, but the visual quality is poorer. They do allow more ease when lysing intrauterine adhesions in difficult locations (**Fig. 10-2**).

The cavity of the uterus is a potential space. The success of hysteroscopy depends on the media used to expand this space. Many distending media are available, including 32% dextran 70, which is highly viscous; 5% dextrose and water (D_5W), which has low viscosity; 1.5% glycine; Ringer's lactate; normal saline; and carbon dioxide gas. The surgeon must know which is ideal for the particular case and instrumentation and the potential risks (**Table 10-2**). High-molecular-weight dextran (average molecular weight, 70,000 Da in 10% glucose) is extremely viscous fluid and is biodegradable, nontoxic, nonconductive, and has good optical qualities. Most important, dextran is immiscible with blood, which helps to keep the field clear during intrauterine surgery, especially when there is active bleeding. Dextran has two drawbacks: it is antigenic, and anaphylaxis has been reported. It also rapidly crystallizes; thus, endoscopic instruments must be cleaned shortly after the procedure. It is sticky to work with and can lock the valves. Rare cases of pulmonary edema and coagulopathies from intravascular dextran have been reported. Dextran can osmotically draw fluid many times its own volume into the intravascular space if extravasation occurs. A different distention media is recommended if one predicts that greater than 500 mL of dextran will be needed. Carbon dioxide must be infused with special equipment

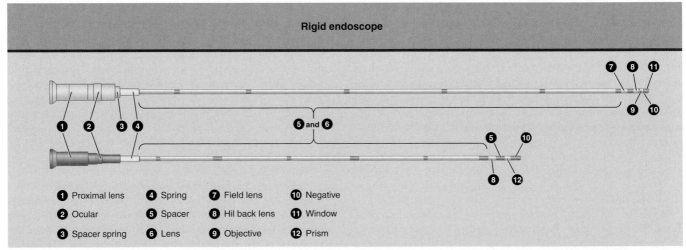

Rigid endoscope

1. Proximal lens
2. Ocular
3. Spacer spring
4. Spring
5. Spacer
6. Lens
7. Field lens
8. Hil back lens
9. Objective
10. Negative
11. Window
12. Prism

Figure 10-1 Anatomy of a rigid endoscope. (Figure 35-3 from Beiber EJ, Sanfilippo JS, Horowitz IR: Clinical Gynecology. Philadelphia, Elsevier, 2006.)

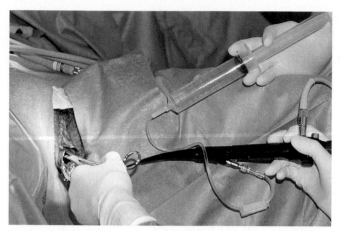

Figure 10-2 Flexible hysteroscopy. Uterine distention is maintained with normal saline or lactated Ringer's solution injected through intravenous extension tubing. (From Goldberg JM, Falcone T: Atlas of Endoscopic Techniques in Gynecology. London, WB Saunders, 2000, p 185.)

(not a laparoscopic insufflator) that carefully limits flow to less than 100 mL/min and maintains the pressure at approximately 60 to 70 mm Hg. Because no fluid is involved, there is no mess. If the patient has patent fallopian tubes, the CO_2 gas can cause diaphragmatic irritation and discomfort. The major precaution with D_5W is the monitoring of total fluid intake so as not to produce water intoxication. In contrast, office hysteroscopy with the smaller flexible scopes most commonly incorporates the use of saline or lactated Ringer's solution because either is easier to use, causes less pain, and avoids the risk of electrolyte and osmolar imbalances. For operative hysteroscopy, carefully and frequently monitoring the intake and outflow of distention media is required. Fluid management systems are available that calculate these values continuously. Guidelines exist for terminating a procedure when fluid deficits reach a set amount. For nonelectrolyte media, the recommended cutoff is 1000 to 1500 mL; and for an electrolyte media it is 2500 mL, but other factors should be considered such age, comorbid conditions, cardiovascular disease, and patient body mass index. For operative procedures with electrocautery, saline or isotonic solutions cannot be used because they conduct electricity (except bipolar cautery).

Hysteroscopy techniques are fairly similar whether performed as an office procedure or in an operating room. A list of general equipment needed for office hysteroscopy is given in **Table 10-3**. A complete history and physical exam is needed; in particular, a relevant allergies and medication list needs to be confirmed. Appropriate tests might include a Papanicolaou smear, pregnancy test, hemoglobin or hematocrit testing, and gonorrhea or chlamydia testing. Hysteroscopy can be performed at any time during the menstrual cycle, but it is best scheduled in the early to middle proliferative phase. A bimanual examination is performed to note the size of the uterus and direction of the uterine fundus. Knowing whether the uterus is anteverted or retroverted is important to avoid uterine perforation, and a rectovaginal exam can aid in determining position. It is helpful to explain to the patient that she will experience discomfort if cervical dilation is needed and uterine cramping during the short time that the hysteroscope is inside the uterus. A single-toothed tenaculum may be used to secure the anterior cervical lip. Gentle traction on the tenaculum straightens out the uterine axis to facilitate endocervical passage of the instruments. Techniques have been described for diagnostic hysteroscopy with a small scope diameter than do not utilize a tenaculum and thus avoid causing that pain. The exocervix is then cleaned of mucus and bacteria. Many physicians will cleanse the cervical os with an iodine solution prior to introducing the scope. The most frequent problem in performing hysteroscopy is cervical stenosis or spasm. When this is encountered, the optimal method to obtain pain relief and overcome resistance is a paracervical block with 1% lidocaine (Xylocaine). Liberal use of paracervical block in difficult procedures allows the physician to be successful in obtaining endometrial biopsy tissue in more than 95% of cases, so this is likely true for hysteroscopy as well. Subsequently, the cervix can be dilated with tapered plastic or metal dilators, and the hysteroscopy can be completed. Unlike with larger rigid scopes, most patients will not require anesthesia for diagnostic procedures in the office. The infusion line should be flushed through the scope prior to insertion, otherwise bubbles will be introduced and obscure the view.

When inserting the hysteroscope, it is useful to wait a few seconds to let the distending media open the internal cervical os so the uterine cavity can be entered more easily by following the fluid flow. Then angle of the telescope view is opposite

Table 10-2 Comparison of Hysteroscopic Distention Media

Medium	Advantage	Disadvantage	Risks
CO_2	Safe Ease of use Rapidly absorbed	Poor visibility in the presence of bleeding	
Normal saline Lactated Ringer's	Isotonic	Not suitable for monopolar electrosurgery	Fluid overload
Glycine 1.5% Sorbitol Mannitol 5%	Electrolyte free Nonconductive	Hypotonic	Hypotonic fluid overload Hyponatremia
Hyskon (32% dextran)	Nonconductive Immiscible with blood	Difficult to deliver	Hypertonic fluid overload Anaphylactic reaction

From Beiber EJ, Sanfilippo JS, Horowitz IR: Clinical Gynecology. Philadelphia, Elsevier, 2006.

Table 10-3 Equipment for Office Hysteroscopy

Procedure table that elevates to 46 to 48 inches
Comfortable behind-the-knee padded stirrups
Open-sided speculum
Paracervical block equipment
Tenaculum
Hysteroscope with 4-mm diameter and fore-oblique 25- to 30-degree lens
Diagnostic sheath of 5 mm
Operative sheath of 7 mm
Flexible or semirigid scissors and biopsy and grasping forceps
Rigid scissors and biopsy and grasping forceps
Ring forceps
Myoma grasping forceps
Emergency kit
Foley catheter with 30-mL balloon

the direction of the light post. This point needs to be remembered in the context of viewing an anteverted versus retroverted uterus. If the light post is pointing upward, the view is downward. If uterine cavity vision is obscured, it may be due to insufficient distention fluid, bleeding, or being up against the uterine wall or pathology. Withdraw the hysteroscope slowly while slightly increasing the distention fluid. Never advance the hysteroscope without good visualization because perforation can occur. The cavity should be inspected thoroughly and systematically. First, an overall view can be seen on entry looking for the general cavity shape, polyps, myomas, and foreign bodies. As the hysteroscope is advanced, it is rotated clockwise and counterclockwise to see the cornua and tubal ostia. On removal, endocervix is viewed. Overzealous cervical dilation can create a poor seal between the cervix and scope allowing the fluid to run out of the cervix and poor uterine distention. Short-term complications are listed in **Table 10-4**.

Vaginal misoprostol (prostaglandin E₁), in dosages of 200 to 400 micrograms, has also been used to aid in the transcervical passage of the hysteroscope. It is usually given the night before the procedure, but administration 4 to 12 hours preoperatively has been described for cervical softening. This can be particularly helpful if cervical stenosis is present or suspected. Women at risk for cervical stenosis include those with prior cervical surgery such as cone biopsy or postmenopausal status, particularly nulliparous women. It acts on the extracellular matrix of the cervix, leading to water absorption, collagenase release, and cervical softening. Women should be warned of the side effects of misoprostol, including diarrhea, cramping, uterine bleeding, and fever. Concomitant nonsteroidal anti-inflammatory (NSAID) agents can reduce side effects. Anxious patients may be pretreated with alprazolam, diazepam, or some other anxiolytic. Many clinicians pretreat women with NSAIDs to decrease the pain associated with this procedure, but studies suggest this only helps for postoperative pain, which is still an advantage. For more involved procedures, intravenous analgesia and conscious sedation may be needed, and proper protocols are needed to ensure patient safety. If extensive resections are anticipated via hysteroscopy, then the procedure is better performed on an outpatient basis in the surgical suite.

For the severely stenotic cervix, having the right instruments available is critical. Lacrimal-duct dilators (from ophthalmologic surgery) come in sizes down to 1-mm diameter and in graduated sizes. This can lead to cervical access when barely a dimple is seen in the external cervical os. Then, the usual tapered metal or plastic cervical dilators can facilitate complete dilation. Also, real-time ultrasonography can help the surgeon to visualize the tip of the dilator, direct the surgeon along the right track into the endometrial cavity, and prevent the surgeon from making a false cervical path or uterine perforation.

OPERATIVE HYSTEROSCOPY TECHNIQUES

The variety and extent of surgery performed transcervically with the hysteroscope have expanded significantly with technologic advances. Endoscopic procedures have progressed from snaring small polyps to hysteroscopic tubal sterilization to complex myomectomies and ablating the entire endometrial lining. The ability to detect, biopsy, or remove focal lesions is extremely useful for abnormal bleeding workup over blind endometrial sampling. Approximately 50% of all Essure hysteroscopic tubal occlusions performed in the United States are done in an office setting, and the percentage is rising. Operative hysteroscopy may be performed with mechanical devices such as small operating scissors, electrocautery, and modified resectoscopes and lasers. Laser hysteroscopy with carbon dioxide or neodymium:yttrium-aluminum-garnet (Nd:YAG) or argon lasers requires more expensive equipment and expertise. With the development of the second-generation technology for uterine ablation and polyp and fibroid resection, the laser and resectoscope equipment is significantly less popular and less advantageous than simpler techniques.

Women with repetitive miscarriages should have a diagnostic hysteroscopic procedure, which often leads to an operative procedure. Congenital abnormalities that interfere with the success of early pregnancies, such as septa of the uterus, may be seen and removed (**Fig. 10-3**). Often endometrial polyps or submucous myomas are discovered and may be removed with a resectoscope wire (**Fig. 10-4**) or a newer morcellator type device (**Fig. 10-5**). The uterine synechiae of a woman with Asherman's syndrome can be cut with microscissors, reestablishing the endometrial cavity. Because adhesions interfere with the configuration of the cavity, it can be difficult for the surgeon to identify usual landmarks. Simultaneous **laparoscopy** guidance is often used to avoid perforation when cutting the intrauterine adhesions. Hysteroscopic metroplasty of intrauterine septa has replaced abdominal metroplasty, as it is safer and has fewer complications than laparotomy. Simultaneous laparoscopy is often used with this procedure as well to gauge the end point of cutting the septum.

Hysteroscopy is superior to hysterosalpingogram (HSG) in discovering intrauterine disease. In comparative studies, the use of hysteroscopy revealed synechiae, polyps, or myomas in 40% of patients with normal HSGs. These abnormalities were undetected and unsuspected using radiographic techniques. The false-positive rate of HSG is 33% compared with hysteroscopy. One in three women diagnosed as having an intrauterine filling defect by x-ray imaging will have a normal cavity directly visualized with the hysteroscope. Women with amenorrhea and

Table 10-4 Short-Term Complications of Hysteroscopy

Complication	Rate (%)
Overall Complication Rate	
Diagnostic hysteroscopy	0.95%
Operative hysteroscopy	2% to 3%
Hysteroscopic myomectomy	1% to 5%
Uterine Perforation	
Operative hysteroscopy	1%
Endometrial ablation—resectoscope	2% to 2+%
Endometrial ablation—nonresectoscope	1%
Fluid overload	0.06% to 2%
Bleeding	0.03% to 3%
Pelvic Infection	0.01%
Death—fluid overload or septicemia	0.01%
Embolism; gas, air	*
Cervical laceration	*
Creation of false cervical passage	*
Failure to complete the procedure	*
Electrocautery injury	*
Urinary tract or bowel injury	*
Pulmonary and cerebral edema	*
Dissemination of cervical or endometrial cancer	*

*Rare complication or exact rate of complication unknown.

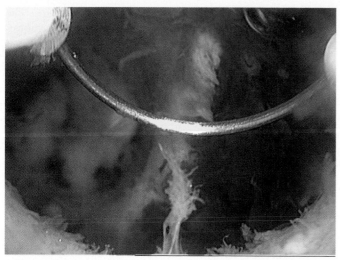

Figure 10-3 The loop is placed at the center of the apex of the septum. As the current is activated, the loop is advanced toward the fundus in small increments, always staying in the center of the septum. The septum separates, as it is divided so that no tissue needs to be excised. (There are small endometrial fragments in the right cornua and a small clot adherent to the left aspect of the septum.) (From Goldberg JM, Falcone T: Atlas of Endoscopic Techniques in Gynecology. London, WB Saunders, 2000, p 194.)

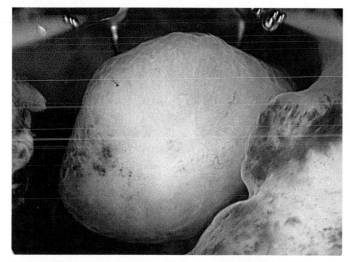

Figure 10-4 A uterine polyp with the hysteroscopic resection tool behind the polyp. (From Goldberg JM, Falcone T: Atlas of Endoscopic Techniques in Gynecology. London, WB Saunders, 2000, p 187.)

Figure 10-5 Intrauterine polyp before **(A)** and after **(B)** hysteroscopic morcellation. (Images courtesy of Dr. Howard Topel and Smith & Nephew.)

a history of curettage who do not respond to a hormonal challenge should have an HSG or hysteroscopy. Uterine synechiae are identified by slowly injecting a water-soluble medium on HSG or by the inability to visualize the uterine cavity on hysteroscopy. If a woman has synechiae, tubal obstruction on HSG, and pelvic calcifications, a diagnosis of pelvic tuberculosis should be strongly suspected.

Submucous myomas were initially removed with a modified urologic resectoscope using a cutting 40-watt electric current and a 90-degree wire loop for shaving the myoma until it was flat with the surrounding endometrial lining. The electrocautery led to bubbles obscuring the view and the potential risk of gas or air emboli. If unsuspected perforation occurred, the risk of thermal injury was present. Greatly improved instrumentation is available with a hysteroscopic rotary or reciprocating morcellator blade for removing polyps and fibroids. It does not use electrocautery and continuously suctions out the pathology so there are no bubbles and no pieces of shaved pathology floating in the cavity. This problem with the resectoscope required frequent interruption of the procedure to remove the chips. The device is simple, and the morcellator is placed against the polyp or fibroid and activated. The morcellator simultaneously aspirates and cuts the polyp or fibroid. Saline is used as the infusion media as no cautery is used, which lessens the electrolyte imbalance risk. The drawback without electrocautery is that more bleeding can occur. Studies have shown successful removal of the submucous myoma at the initial hysteroscopy being 85% to 95%. The success rate of complete resection at the initial surgery is higher with myomas that are nearly completely submucous versus fibroids with a significant intramural portion. Another surgery is needed in approximately 5% to 15% of cases, although most are another hysteroscopic surgery. Polena's 2007 study of 235 patients reported a success rate of 94.6% at 1 year, which decreased to 76.3% at 5 years. The pregnancy rate is as good as or better with hysteroscopic myomectomy than with transabdominal myomectomy.

In women with abnormal bleeding or menorrhagia who are poor surgical candidates, desire a minimally invasive procedure, or wish to preserve their uterus, the endometrial lining may be ablated or resected through the hysteroscope. It is not indicated if there is endometrial cancer or if the woman still desires pregnancy. Sterilization or contraception needs should be addressed. One of the early techniques for **endometrial ablation** utilized a roller ball electrode to coagulate and thus destroy the endometrium (**Fig. 10-6**) or a wire loop as described previously to resect the endometrium. Although lasers may also be used to produce ablation of the endometrium by photovaporizing the

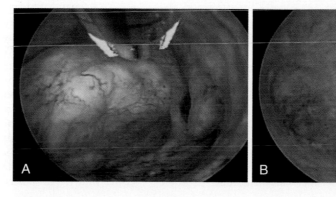

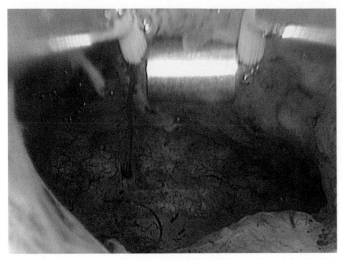

Figure 10-6 Endometrial cavity prior to ablation with a roller-ball. (From Goldberg JM, Falcone T: Atlas of Endoscopic Techniques in Gynecology. London, WB Saunders, 2000, p 197.)

epithelium, laser photovaporization takes longer than electrode resection, and the equipment is more expensive. Hysterograms following treatment have demonstrated contraction, scarring, and dense adhesion formation. Long-term follow-up has documented that endometrial carcinoma may develop in residual foci of endometrium. The newer second-generation devices for endometrial ablation offer safer and simpler options. These new devices are nonresectoscope types. The Food and Drug Administration (FDA) has approved five global endometrial ablation devices: thermal balloon endometrial ablation (ThermaChoice, Ethicon Inc., Menlo Park, California), radiofrequency endometrial ablation (NovaSure, Cytyc Surgical Products, Palo Alto, California), hydrothermal endometrial ablation (HydroTermAblator, Boston Scientific, Natick, Massachusetts), cryoablation (Her Option, CryoGen Inc., San Diego, California), and microwave endometrial ablation (Microsulis, Hampshire, England). The 2009 Cochrane database review concluded that endometrial ablation techniques offer a less invasive alternative to hysterectomies. All of the currently available nonresectoscopic endometrial ablation devices have limitations on acceptable endometrial cavity size and endometrial surface irregularities like myomas. No gold standard system exists yet. The second-generation devices compare favorably with the resectoscope technique. Similar rates of intrauterine adhesions and contracture have been found in about one third of women. This does not seem to cause problems unless obstructed bleeding occurs (see the Complications section presented later in the chapter).

Selective salpingography is an extension of hysteroscopy to evaluate the lumen of the fallopian tubes. The tube can be cannulized and contrast instilled for confirming proximal tubal obstruction observed on HSG.

Hysteroscopic sterilization may be accomplished with insertion of coils in the tubal ostia or radiofrequency and plugs. This is desirable, as no incision is needed as for laparoscopic sterilization and it can be performed in the office. Two devices are FDA approved in the United States: Essure in 2002 and Adiana in 2009. Under hysteroscopic viewing, the Essure coil is placed in the proximal portion of the fallopian tube. Chronic inflammation around the coil leads to tubal blockage. The Adiana system uses hysteroscopic guidance to utilize radiofrequency energy to disrupt the proximal tubal endothelium and then a silicone matrix, which also causes tubal obstruction by tissue ingrowth. Neither technique works immediately, and a follow-up HSG is needed in 3 months to make sure the tubes are indeed blocked. No procedure is of yet reversible. Short-term efficacy studies suggest a rate equal to or greater than other tubal sterilization methods.

In summary, hysteroscopy is a simple technique for the diagnosis and treatment of intrauterine pathology. The indications for intrauterine surgery via the hysteroscope are expanding, and many laparotomies can be avoided. Operative hysteroscopic costs vary depending on the time involved and the specific procedure performed.

COMPLICATIONS

Complications following diagnostic hysteroscopy are exceedingly rare. The major complication is uterine perforation, and office hysteroscopy has an incidence of 1 or 2 cases per 1000. Infection and postprocedure hemorrhage are very rare. Some women develop a severe vasovagal reflex from instrumentation of the uterine cavity. Symptoms include dizziness, nausea, sweating, and fainting. The woman may be pale, diaphoretic, and bradycardic. Syncope can occur with none of the symptoms reported. This reflex can be diminished by giving the patient intravenous atropine (0.5 to 1 mg IV), IV fluids or by performing a paracervical block. Use of the Trendelenburg position or having the patient lie supine with the legs raised can be beneficial in recovery. If bleeding is excessive, electrocautery coagulation at the bleeding point may be sufficient. If not, others have reported injecting dilute vasopressin at the bleeding point with caution to avoid intraarterial injection, which can result in hypertension, bradycardia, cardiovascular collapse, and even death. An inflatable 30-cc Foley balloon can be inserted into the uterine cavity, inflated, and left for 12 to 24 hours, facilitating hemostasis.

Complications of hysteroscopy in general are noted in less than 2% of the procedures. Jansen and coworkers, using a large database of 136,000 hysteroscopies, noted the significant complication rate to be 0.28%. Complications include uterine perforation (0.12%), pelvic infection (0.01%), bleeding (0.03%), fluid overload (0.06%) from absorption of distending media, and bladder or bowel injury (0.02%). Diagnostic hysteroscopy has a significantly lower complication rate than operative hysteroscopy (0.95%). Uterine perforation can be midline or lateral. Midline perforation rarely results in significant complications unless electrocautery or laser energy is used. Lateral perforation is risky in terms of bleeding complications, as the uterine artery and vein can be punctured. Suspect uterine perforation if the operative view suddenly disappears, the fluid deficit suddenly increases, or the hysteroscope suddenly inserts farther than the fundus. Thermal injury to surrounding organs may occur with deep resections or perforations with the electrocautery instrument. If injury or perforation is suspected during hysteroscopy, then an intraperitoneal evaluation should be performed either by laparoscopy or by laparotomy. Unrecognized uterine perforation might result in postoperative abdominal or pelvic pain beyond what is normally expected; abdominal distention heavy vaginal bleeding, hypotension, nausea or vomiting or hematuria, or bowel injury, particularly thermal injuries, may present with delayed onset of symptoms and often go unrecognized. **Table 10-4** summarizes the complications with diagnostic and operative hysteroscopy.

The potential complications of the distending media include anaphylaxis to dextran, circulatory overload with D_5W, pulmonary and cerebral edema, hyponatremia, seizure, coagulopathies, and the potential of air or gas embolism with carbon dioxide. Monitoring of the patient's fluid status is important because of problems with absorption of distending media, leading to volume overload and electrolyte imbalance. Cardiac arrest has been reported with uterine insufflation with carbon dioxide when unmonitored amounts of gas were used.

For in-office hysteroscopy, an emergency kit is needed. Medication should be readily available to treat vasovagal reactions. A Foley catheter with a 30-cc balloon is useful for persistent bleeding. The catheter is inserted via the cervix, and the balloon is filled to tamponade bleeding. The catheter acts as a drain so bleeding can be monitored.

A note is indicated about patient safety during procedures. The American College of Obstetricians and Gynecologists (ACOG) published guidelines in 2010 that contain a section on free-standing surgical units where many operative hysteroscopy procedures are performed. Care must be taken to ensure adequate training of personnel, knowledge, uses, maintenance and cleaning of equipment, and safety protocols for sedation or anesthesia complications or surgical complications. Emergency care and hospital transfer protocols are required in writing in many states when more than minimal sedation or local anesthetic infiltration in peripheral nerves is required.

Some long-term complications exist after endometrial ablation, including recurrent or persistent abnormal bleeding. The 2007 ACOG Practice Bulletin states that hysterectomy rates after both resectoscopic and the second-generation nonresectoscopic ablations are at least 24%. Older women have a higher success rate, because menopause occurs before the recurrent bleeding problems or obstructive symptoms occur. The inability to evaluate the endometrium if bleeding recurs and the risk of a delay in diagnosis of endometrial cancer are added concerns. Pregnancy following an endometrial ablation can occur and is often complicated by the intrauterine scarring and contracture. This can result in abnormal placentation including placenta accreta or percreta, uterine rupture, higher spontaneous abortion rates, preterm delivery, ectopic pregnancy, and fetal limb malformations. Residual areas of endometrium that are not ablated or regrown can lead to trapped bleeding within the uterine cavity, leading to retrograde bleeding or cornual or uterine hematometra. (Additional risks are listed in **Table 10-5**.)

Table 10-5 Long-Term Complications of Endometrial Ablation Devices

Persistent bleeding
Central hematometra
Cornual hematometra
Postablation tubal sterilization syndrome (PATSS)
Retrograde bleeding
Inability to evaluate the endometrium if bleeding recurs
Delay in diagnosis of endometrial cancer
Pregnancy
Postablation cornual endosalpingoblastosis

LAPAROSCOPY

Laparoscopy has radically changed the clinical practice of gynecology. As an often outpatient surgical technique, laparoscopy provides a window to directly visualize pelvic anatomy as well as a technique for performing many operations with less morbidity than laparotomy (**Fig. 10-7**). Operative laparoscopy for complex surgeries is associated with an easier recovery and a shorter hospital stay.

The first human laparoscopy was first performed in 1910 in Sweden. Two events of the early 1960s renewed interest in this surgical technique, the first being the development of fiberoptic cables for better illumination and the second the change in society's attitude toward sterilization procedures. Patrick Steptoe is considered the father of modern laparoscopy for his work in the mid-1960s with laparoscopic sterilization. By the mid-1970s, laparoscopy had been adopted as the method of choice for female sterilization. Once laparoscopic cholecystectomy was embraced and new instrumentation developed, the way was paved for laparoscopic hysterectomy.

The advantages of less postoperative pain, shorter recovery time, and shorter hospital stays are obvious when laparoscopy is compared with laparotomy. This is particularly true in the obese woman who has increased risk of wound infection, thromboembolic events, and other complications from laparotomy. These events are significantly less with a laparoscopic approach. Laparoscopic visualization is excellent because the video camera and endoscope magnify the image.

LAPAROSCOPIC INDICATIONS AND CONTRAINDICATIONS

There are multiple indications for laparoscopy, both diagnostic and therapeutic. The most common indication used to be female sterilization but is now diagnostic laparoscopy, and this includes the evaluation of pelvic pain. In the past decades, gynecologists have progressed from using the laparoscope to perform such

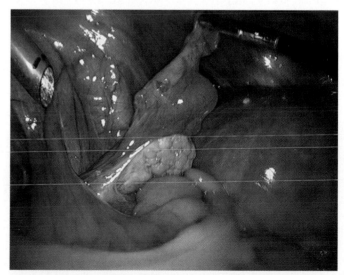

Figure 10-7 Laparoscopic view of left pelvis viewing left lower quadrant port and right atraumatic grasper holding left fallopian tube with paratubal cyst and normal ovary. (Courtesy of Dr. Seine Chiang, University of Washington.)

simple surgical tasks as tubal ligation to more complicated surgery such as hysterectomy with pelvic and paraaortic lymph node dissection for endometrial cancer. The present indications for laparoscopy are almost identical to those for laparotomy, and the laparoscope is utilized for numerous diagnostic and therapeutic indications. Some indications include removal of ectopic pregnancies, resection or ablation of endometriosis, ovarian cystectomy or salpingo-oophorectomy, myomectomy, hysterectomy, lymph node dissections, and urogynecologic procedures. Intraperitoneal intrauterine devices are best retrieved with the laparoscope. Laparoscopic ovarian biopsy (for karyotyping in certain endocrine disorders) is possible. Laparoscopic lysis of adhesions might be done for pain or to transform an abdominal hysterectomy into a vaginal hysterectomy or laparoscopically assisted vaginal hysterectomy. The limits and indications of surgical procedures via the laparoscope depend on the experience and judgment of the gynecologist. At some point, laparotomy is the more reasonable decision. We believe that a procedure should be performed through the laparoscope only if the gynecologist is prepared for the complications that might arise if that procedure were performed through a laparotomy.

Absolute contraindications to laparoscopy include intestinal obstruction, hemoperitoneum that produces hemodynamic instability, anticoagulation therapy, severe cardiovascular or pulmonary disease, and tuberculous peritonitis. Relative contraindications, in which each case must be individualized, include morbid obesity, large hiatal hernia, advanced malignancy, generalized peritonitis or peritonitis following previous surgery, inflammatory bowel disease, and extensive intraabdominal scarring. Even with these relative contraindications, the surgeon may attempt laparoscopy. Failure to achieve a pneumoperitoneum should signal the potential for bowel injury. Open laparoscopy might allow safe entry or avoidance of complications, but the surgeon and patient should be prepared to convert to a laparotomy.

LAPAROSCOPIC EQUIPMENT AND TECHNIQUES

Laparoscopy may be performed under local, regional, or general anesthesia. For simple procedures, many prefer local anesthesia for its safety, with the addition of conscious sedation by intravenous medication. Regional anesthesia is possible, but the Trendelenburg position needed for gravity to keep the bowels in the upper abdomen can be bothersome to the patient and restrict respiration. The risks associated with general anesthesia are one of the major hazards of laparoscopy. However, when operative laparoscopy is contemplated, general anesthesia is recommended and ensures adequate muscle relaxation, patient comfort, and the ability to manipulate intraabdominal organs. The standard diagnostic laparoscope is 10 mm in diameter, but they come in sizes varying from 2 to 10 mm. The microlaparoscopes are used primarily for diagnostic evaluation. The 5-mm and 10-mm forms are widely utilized. Laparoscopic telescopes come in 0-degree to 30-degree lens angles, but the 0-degree type is most commonly used. Most laparoscopes are 30 cm long and provide a field of vision of 60 to 75 degrees. The inferior margin of the umbilicus is the preferred site of entry, as this is the thinnest area of the abdominal wall. Alternative sites are detailed in **Figure 10-8**. The choice of gas to develop the pneumoperitoneum depends on the choice of anesthesia. Nitrous oxide is preferable with local anesthesia, but carbon dioxide is the choice with general anesthesia. Nitrous oxide is

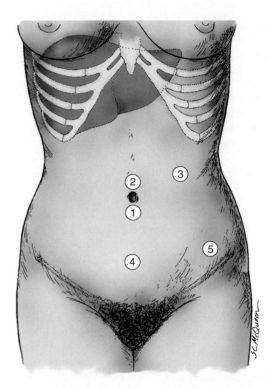

Figure 10-8 Usual sites for insertion of insufflating needle in laparoscopy: (1) infraumbilical fold, (2) supraumbilical fold, (3) left costal margin, (4) midway between umbilicus and pubis, and (5) left McBurney's point. (From Corson SL: Operating room preparation and basic techniques. In Phillips JM (ed): Laparoscopy. Baltimore, Williams & Wilkins, 1977. ©Copyright 1977 by the Williams & Wilkins Co, Baltimore.)

nonflammable but does support combustion. Carbon dioxide quickly forms carbonic acid on the moist parietal peritoneal surface, which results in considerable discomfort to a patient without regional or general anesthesia.

A **Veress needle** (**Fig. 10-9**; radially dilating **trocar** with Veress type needle) has a retractable cutting point that is used for entry into the abdominal cavity for the purpose of insufflating the abdomen with gas for laparoscopy. A trocar is a blunt, bladed, or optical device for entering the abdominal cavity for laparoscopy and is the cannula for holding the laparoscope or laparoscopic instruments (**Fig. 10-10**). Secondary puncture trocars vary from 5 mm (bipolar forceps, 5-mm telescope, suction/irrigation device, vessel sealing, cutting or coagulation devices), 7 or 8 mm in width (Filshie clips for sterilization), to 10 to 12 mm for pouches to remove specimens, or a morcellating device for removing fibroids or a uterus.

There are three techniques to access the abdomen. First, Veress needle insertion is used to create a pneumoperitoneum followed by trocar placement. Second, direct trocar placement in a noninsufflated abdomen has been described. Third, an open or **Hasson technique** can be used when adhesions are expected, particularly under the umbilicus. When using the Veress technique, a skin incision is made large enough to hold the planned trocar, which is usually 10 mm if using the umbilical site. The angle of the Veress needle insertion should vary according to the body mass index of the woman from 45 degrees in a normal weight woman to 90 degrees in an obese woman. Veress intraperitoneal pressure of ≤ 10 mm Hg is a reliable indicator of correct intraperitoneal needle placement, and insufflation of the carbon dioxide gas can begin. Left upper quadrant (Palmer's

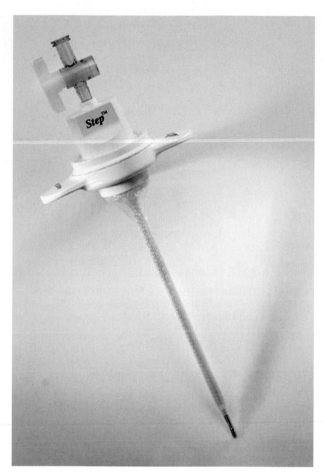

Figure 10-9 Radially dilating trocar with Veress type needle. (Figure 34-7 from Beiber EJ, Sanfilippo JS, Horowitz IR: Clinical Gynecology. Philadelphia, Elsevier, 2006.)

point) laparoscopic entry should be considered in patients with suspected or known periumbilical adhesions, presence of an umbilical hernia, or after three failed insufflation attempts at the umbilicus.

Once the abdomen is insufflated to 15 mm Hg, the primary trocar can be inserted. Because it has been recognized that primary trocar placement leads to the majority of vascular and bowel injuries, many surgical products are available to potentially lessen these injuries, but none has proved safer than another. A bladed, blunt, or radial dilating trocar can be passed. A bladed cutting trocar may come with automatic blade retraction or a shield for safety. These require significantly less force to

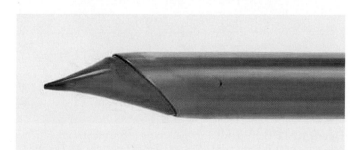

Figure 10-10 Blunt-tip trocar for primary port. (Figure 34-8 from Beiber EJ, Sanfilippo JS, Horowitz IR: Clinical Gynecology. Philadelphia, Elsevier, 2006.)

insert through the abdominal wall compared with blunt trocars. The resulting fascial defects are larger for cutting trocars than radial dilating trocars. The port may not be as fixed in this case. It is recommended that bladed port sites $\geqq$ to 10 mm should have fascial closure at the conclusion of the surgery to avoid postoperative hernia formation. Blunt trocars require more force for passage into the abdomen but theoretically cause fewer vascular and bowel injuries. This has yet to be proved. Radially dilating blunt trocars are available, and one of the touted advantages is that even 10-mm port sites do not need fascial closure because hernias are rare in nonbladed port sites.

Direct trocar entry has been proposed to alleviate the difficulties with preperitoneal or intestinal gas insufflation with the Veress needle and to reduce operative time. There are studies supporting this technique. Disposable optical trocars are available to use a cannula that allows the laparoscope to visualize passing through the abdominal wall. They do not seem to reduce vascular and **visceral injury**, however, but do save time.

Open laparoscopy, often called the Hasson technique, may be used as an alternative to the Veress needle option. Instead of blind entry into the peritoneal cavity, a small incision is made in the fascia and parietal peritoneum. The cone is placed in the abdominal cavity under direct visual control. The fascia is secured to the sleeve of the cone to obtain an airtight seal. Open laparoscopy has not been proved to reduce the rate of bowel injury, but that is the theoretic benefit. Also, if the Veress needle technique fails to result in pneumoperitoneum, open laparoscopy is often an option. It is the procedure of choice if the patient has a history of multiple abdominal operations.

Once the primary trocar is in place, the telescope and camera can be attached and the pelvis visualized. Secondary trocars can be placed under direct visualization, which is why there are fewer vascular and bowel injuries with these trocars. Third and fourth puncture sites are often required for complex cases. Because each puncture site is a potential gas leak, high-flow insufflation equipment is necessary. In addition, several video monitoring screens are employed so that both the surgeon and assistant can work effectively. Unlike the short time needed for diagnostic laparoscopy, operative laparoscopy may require several hours.

Operative laparoscopy may be performed with mechanical instruments, including an extensive variety of scissors, scalpels, endoscopic syringes, myoma screws, suture devices, electrocautery instruments (both unipolar and bipolar), harmonic and vessel sealing devices for hemostasis and cutting, suction, irrigation, stapling devices, endoscopic clips, and laser instruments. During operative laparoscopy, stabilization of the pelvic organs is essential, such as traction and countertraction on the edges of an adhesion. This is why multiple trocar sites are needed so that the primary surgeon and assistant can use both hands. Uterine manipulators are particularly useful in laparoscopic hysterectomy. They are designed to aid in stabilizing and manipulating the uterus and identifying the cervicovaginal junction for cervix amputation.

The FDA approved robotic-assisted laparoscopy for use in gynecology in 2005. The only currently available system in the United States is the daVinci Surgical System. The equipment is bulky and consists of a robot with three or four arms that hold the camera and surgical instruments, the camera and vision system, the console where the surgeon sits away from the patient bedside, and the wristed instruments that insert through the robotic arms and are controlled by the surgeon at the console. The camera is actually two cameras and allows for three-dimensional visualization via the computer image integrator. Other advantages include the added dexterity with the wristed instruments and ergonomic benefits for the surgeon. This can aid in surgeries that require a lot of suturing such as myomectomies or abdominal sacral colpopexy and complex gynecologic oncology or severe endometriosis procedures. Disadvantages include the high cost of the system and maintenance, lack of haptic feedback for the surgeon at the console, and increased operative time for docking the robot and the actual procedure.

LAPAROSCOPIC PROCEDURES

Laparoscopy has made outpatient sterilization available to women throughout the world. Cumulative 10-year pregnancy rates vary between 8/1000 and 37/1000. Sterilization is accomplished with electrocautery, titanium, or spring-loaded clips. Because of the serious complications with unipolar cautery, most cautery sterilization procedures are performed with bipolar coagulation of approximately 3 cm of the isthmic portion of the fallopian tube without division. Use of a current meter is recommended to indicate when complete coagulation has occurred, as visual inspection is not an accurate indication. Mechanical occlusion devices commonly used in the United States include the silicone rubber band (Falope ring), the spring-loaded clip (Hulka-Clemens clip), and the titanium clip lined with silicone rubber (Filshie clip). The ring or clip should be placed on the narrow isthmus so the size of the appliance conforms to the diameter of the fallopian tube. Special equipment is needed for each of these techniques.

There are both diagnostic and therapeutic indications for laparoscopy in infertile women. Tubal patency and mobility can be directly observed via the laparoscope. Laparoscopy is a more sophisticated and accurate method of diagnosing tubal problems during an infertility investigation than HSG. Chromopertubation with an innocuous dye, such as indigo carmine, demonstrates tubal patency during laparoscopy. Comparative studies have documented that HSG discovers only 50% of the peritubal disease diagnosed by direct visualization via the laparoscope. Laparoscopy is able to confirm or rule out intrinsic pelvic disorders, such as endometriosis or chronic pelvic inflammatory disease with adhesions. It is possible not only to describe and stage the extent of endometriosis or pelvic adhesions but also to treat them. Adhesions can be lysed, endometrioma cysts can be removed, and areas of endometriosis can be ablated by electrocautery, laser, or completely excised, which is necessary for deep endometriotic implants (**Fig. 10-11**).

The management of pelvic pain has been dramatically changed by the laparoscope. The differential diagnosis of acute pain may be defined by direct visualization of the fallopian tubes, ovaries, and appendix. Laparoscopy may be used in the management of acute pelvic infection, taking direct bacterial cultures of purulent material from the tubes, draining a tubo-ovarian abscess, or removing a tubo-ovarian abscess complex with unilateral salpino-oophorectomy. These direct transabdominal cultures have changed our opinions concerning the clinical management of polymicrobial pelvic infections. The classic violin string adhesions between the liver and the abdominal wall are sometimes noted by directing the laparoscope into the upper right quadrant in women with prior pelvic inflammatory disease (**Fig. 10-12**). Sometimes the enigma of chronic pelvic pain may be solved by the findings at laparoscopy. Following the procedure, a plan for

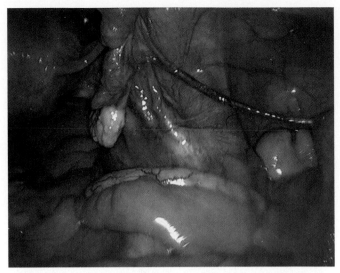

Figure 10-11 Laparoscopic view of a woman with right lower quadrant pain and an adhesion stringing between the fallopian tube and the bowel near the cecum. Normal appearing appendix inferiorly. (Courtesy of Dr. Seine Chiang, University of Washington.)

long-term management of the pain can be discussed with the patient.

Laparoscopic treatment of ectopic pregnancy most often involves salpingotomy but also may include salpingectomy (**Fig. 10-13**). HCG titers must be followed after conservative surgery (salpingotomy) until the titers fall to zero (usually 3 to 4 weeks) to ensure that all trophoblastic tissue has been removed. Tubal patency and subsequent pregnancy rates are comparable between laparoscopic techniques and laparotomy.

Laparoscopic hysterectomy is one area of considerable research. If vaginal hysterectomy cannot be done (which has lower complication rates, lower costs, and better outcomes), then laparoscopic hysterectomy should be considered over abdominal hysterectomy. Many considerations need to go into this decision

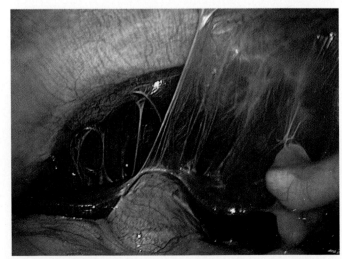

Figure 10-12 Fitz-Hugh-Curtis syndrome in a patient with previous pelvic inflammatory disease. (From Goldberg JM, Falcone T: Atlas of Endoscopic Techniques in Gynecology. London, WB Saunders, 2000, p 71.)

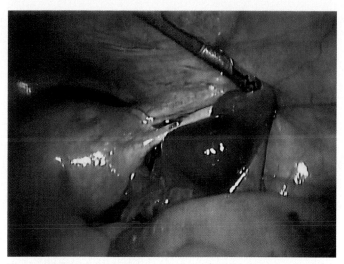

Figure 10-13 Ectopic pregnancy in the right fallopian tube. (Courtesy of B. Beller, MD, Eugene, OR.)

such as the size of the uterus, adnexal disease with risk for ovarian cancer, severe endometriosis, or adhesions. The Cochrane Database of Systematic Reviews considered 34 randomized trials of hysterectomy route. Laparoscopic hysterectomy compared with abdominal hysterectomy was associated with faster return to normal activity, shorter hospital stay, lower intraoperative blood loss, fewer wound infections, longer operating time, and a higher rate of bladder and ureter injuries. **Figure 10-14** shows the beginning of a laparoscopic hysterectomy for uterine fibroids with creation of the bladder flap.

Laparoscopic myomectomy has been studied in two randomized controlled trials with comparison with myomectomy by minilaparotomy. This can be technically challenging laparoscopically because of the dissection and suturing required. The laparoscopic approach resulted in less blood loss, reduced length

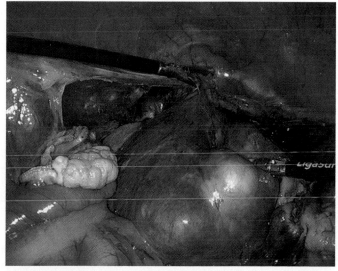

Figure 10-14 The beginning of a laparoscopic hysterectomy for uterine fibroids showing the creation of the bladder flap with the left grasper elevating the bladder peritoneum and a bipolar/cutting device in the right hand. (Courtesy of Dr. Seine Chiang, University of Washington.)

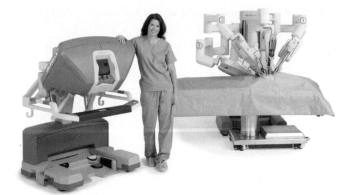

Figure 10-15 DaVinci robot (intuitive surgical).

of postoperative ileus, shorter hospital stay, reduced use of pain medications, and more rapid return to normal activities, but a longer operative time. For unexplained infertility, both approaches improved reproductive outcomes similarly.

Operative laparoscopy has additionally been used for laparoscopic assisted hysterectomy, salpingo-oophorectomy, salpingostomy and fimbrioplasty, tubal reanastomosis, appendectomy, uterosacral ligament transection, presacral neurectomy, retropubic bladder neck suspensions, and complex urogynecologic procedures. Laparoscopy may be used for major cancer staging, including paraaortic and pelvic lymphadenectomy.

Newer laparoscopic equipment using robotics has increased the ease at which minimally invasive major pelvic surgery can occur (**Fig. 10-15**). Cases that can be extremely challenging with traditional laparoscopy are being done with increasing frequency with robotics. Most of the published studies to date are nonrandomized and retrospective case series comparing robotic cases with historical controls. There are data showing safety and feasibility of robot-assisted surgery for numerous procedures, including tubal reanastomosis, myomectomy, hysterectomy, adnexectomy, pelvic, and paraaortic lymph node sampling and abdominal sacral colpopexy for pelvic organ prolapse. A 2010 metaanalysis of 22 controlled but not-randomized studies in gynecologic robotic surgery found robotic surgery patients had a shorter hospital stay and less blood loss than laparotomy. Compared with conventional laparoscopic surgery, robotic surgery achieved reduced blood loss and fewer conversions to laparotomy during the staging of endometrial cancer. No other clinically significant differences were found in the gynecologic procedures published to date. Randomized controlled trials are ongoing that will hopefully clarify the role this expensive technology holds for gynecology.

Advantages of operative laparoscopy over laparotomy include decreased postoperative adhesion formation, decreased postoperative pain, shorter recovery time, and less, if any, hospital stay. Surgical risks from cardiac, pulmonary, and thromboembolic disease should be treated with the same cautions as a corresponding open procedure. These are presented in Chapter 24 (Preoperative Counseling and Management).

LAPAROSCOPIC COMPLICATIONS

The major categories of complications with laparoscopy are laceration of blood vessels, intestinal and urinary tract injuries including trocar and thermal injuries, incisional hernias, and cardiorespiratory problems arising from the pneumoperitoneum

Table 10-6 Intraoperative and Delayed Laparoscopic Surgery Risks

Bleeding
  Laceration of major blood vessels; epigastric, obturator, iliac, vena cava, aorta
  Surgical site bleeding
Trocar or Veress needle injury
Intestinal injury; thermal or direct instrument
Urinary tract injury; thermal or direct instrument
Anesthetic complication
Equipment malfunction
Other endoscopic instrument injury
Other thermal injury
Subcutaneous emphysema

(Table 10-6). One complication has remained unchanged for 25 years. At least 50% of the major laparoscopic complications arise before the planned surgery starts and occur with accessing the abdomen. Most of these injuries are with the primary trocar placement at the umbilicus and involve major vascular injuries or the bowel.

Several studies have evaluated the incidence of complications with operative laparoscopy. A large, multicenter French study of 29,966 laparoscopies showed a high frequency of trocar injuries with a total complication rate of 4.64 per thousand laparoscopies. Complications increase with the age of the patient and the complexity of the procedure. The overall rate of complications from large series of operative laparoscopy varies from 0.2% to 2%. Chandler and coworkers compiled data from a series of injuries resulting from abdominal entry and laparoscopic access injuries reported to large insurance data banks. The series included general surgery as well as gynecology from both the United States and other countries. Over a 20-year period, the data bank collected 594 reports of organ injury, 33% in gynecology patients. Importantly, 50% of bowel injuries were unrecognized for 24 hours or more. Sixty-five deaths were reported. Age older than 59 years and delayed diagnosis of injury were independently associated with mortality in this series. A metaanalysis of 27 randomized controlled trials compared laparoscopy and laparotomy for benign gynecologic procedures. The overall risk of complication was 8.9% with laparoscopy compared with 15.2 with laparotomy (relative risk 0.6). The risk of major complications was the same at 1.4%, so the risk of minor complication was higher in the laparotomy group.

Laceration of the aorta, inferior vena cava, or iliac vessels is a surgical emergency. Because abdominal wall hematomas are usually subfascial in location, care must be taken to avoid the epigastric vessels. For safety, Hurd and colleagues have recommended that lateral trocars be placed at least 5 cm above the symphysis and at least 8 cm from the midline. The Veress needle or the trocar may produce intestinal injuries. Thermal injuries may be recognized at the time of surgery, but if they are not recognized intraoperatively, significant delays in recognition can lead to septicemia and death. The incidence of ureteral injuries varies from 1% to 4% with laparoscopic dissection of the cardinal ligaments.

The risk of incisional hernia is increased for port sites of 12 mm or greater and extraumbilical sites (0.17 to 0.23%). Many of these herniations occur despite fascial closure at the initial surgery. Clinical symptoms include a bulge at the incision site, which may be painful to a bowel obstruction or infarction.

Complications directly related to the pneumoperitoneum include pneumothorax, diminished venous return, gas embolism, and cardiac arrhythmias. It is important not to develop pressures greater than 20 mm Hg in establishing the pneumoperitoneum. High pressures impede venous return and limit excursion of the diaphragm. A rare but life-threatening complication of laparoscopy is gas embolism, which produces hypotension and the classical "mill wheel" murmur, which can be heard over the entire precordium. The patient with this complication should be turned on her left side and the frothy blood aspirated by a central venous catheter directed into the right side of the heart. Other rare complications include incisional hernias at the site of the 10- to 12-mm trocar sites. This has been estimated to occur in 1 in 5000 procedures. Metastases from ovarian malignancies to the laparoscopic wound site are also a rare but real problem.

In summary, laparoscopy, more than any other advance, has changed the clinical practice of gynecology since the 1970s. Today's OB/Gyn residents have a difficult time contemplating the practice of the specialty prior to the introduction of the "silver tube." Laparoscopy provides a window for the diagnosis of infertility, pelvic pain, ectopic pregnancy, abdominal and pelvic trauma, staging the extent of pelvic disease, and the visual diagnosis of abnormal anatomy. Therapeutic uses of the laparoscope vary from female sterilization to hysterectomy and node sampling. The role of robotics is still being established, but benefits exist over laparotomy in nonrandomized but controlled trials, particularly in the gynecologic oncology population.

PATIENT SAFETY IN THE SURGICAL ENVIRONMENT

Many regulatory agencies, hospitals, medical societies and organizations, physicians, and staff have been striving for improvements in patient safety. Wrong-site surgery, wrong-patient surgery, wrong-side surgery, wrong-part surgery, and retained foreign objects have all been reported. Many factors have been associated with wrong-site surgery, including multiple surgical teams being involved in a case, multiple procedures being done during a single case, time pressures, and morbid obesity. In 2003, the Joint Commission for Hospital Accreditation published a universal protocol for improving surgical safety. The protocol recommended a preprocedure verification process, marking the operative site and performing a "time out." A time out promotes patient safety by checking items such as confirming correct patient, correct surgical site, and procedure(s). The World Health Organization published a suggested **surgical safety checklist** to further improve care. Before induction of anesthesia, the first checklist set is done and might include items for team review like patient allergies, airway risks, and estimated blood loss. Before the skin incision, another team review occurs with introductions of all personnel and roles, antibiotic prophylaxis infused if indicated, deep vein thrombosis prophylaxis given or in place if indicated, any equipment issues or concerns voiced, and essential imaging displayed. Before the conclusion of the procedure, the third part of the checklist is completed and includes the name of the procedure, the correct instrument, and sponge and needle counts; the checklist also ensures that specimens are properly labeled and key concerns for the patient recovery are discussed. Good communication between team members appears to be another important factor in patient safety.

KEY POINTS

- The most frequent problem in performing endometrial sampling is cervical stenosis or spasm; it is also a problem for hysteroscopy, and this increases the risk of uterine perforation.

- Major indications for hysteroscopy include abnormal uterine bleeding, removal of endometrial polyps or submucous myomas, endometrial ablations, retained IUD, desire of no incision sterilization, intrauterine adhesions diagnosis and treatment, infertility, resection of a uterine septum, and recurrent pregnancy loss.

- The endometrial lining may be ablated through the hysteroscope in women with abnormal bleeding or menorrhagia who have a normal uterine cavity and are poor surgical candidates, those who wish to retain their uterus, and those who do not desire further childbearing.

- Older resectoscopic and second-generation nonresectoscopic endometrial ablation devices appear to be equivalent with respect to successful reduction in menstrual flow and patient satisfaction at 1 year.

- Vaginal misoprostol administration the night before the hysteroscopic procedure can aid in cervical softening.

- A paracervical block with local anesthetic is the best method of pain control for outpatient hysteroscopy compared with topical or intracervical anesthesia.

- Complications of hysteroscopy include uterine perforation with risk of injury to the surrounding vascular and visceral structures, pelvic infection, bleeding, and absorption of the distending media.

- The primary laparoscopic trocar placement leads to the > 50% of vascular and bowel injuries in gynecologic laparoscopy.

- Absolute contraindications to laparoscopy include a hemoperitoneum that has produced hemodynamic instability, bowel obstruction, anticoagulation therapy, advanced malignancy, large abdominal masses, severe cardiovascular disease, and tuberculous peritonitis.

- The incidence of complications with operative laparoscopy varies from 0.2% to 2%. Thermal bowel injuries often go unrecognized intraoperatively, and diagnostic delays can be life threatening.

REFERENCES CAN BE FOUND ON EXPERTCONSULT.com

SUGGESTED READINGS

Ahmad G, Duffy JMN, Phillips K, et al: Laparoscopic entry techniques, *Cochrane Database Syst Rev* (2), 2008. Art. No. CD006583. doi:10.1002/14651858.CD006583.pub2.

American College of Obstetricians and Gynecologists: Hysteroscopy. ACOG Technology Assessment No. 4, *Obstet Gynecol* 106:439–442, 2005.

Azevedo JL, Azevedo OC, Miyahira SA, et al: Injuries caused by Veress needle insertion for creation of pneumoperitoneum: A systematic literature review, *Surg Endosc* 23(7):1428–1432, 2009.

da Costa AR, Pinto-Neto AM, Amorim M, et al: Use of misoprostol prior to hysteroscopy in postmenopausal women: A randomized, placebo-controlled clinical trial, *J Minim Invasive Gynecol* 15(1):67–73, 2008.

Istre O: Managing bleeding, fluid absorption and uterine perforation at hysteroscopy, *Best Pract Res Clin Obstet Gynaecol* 23:619–629, 2009.

Lethaby A, Shepperd S, Farquhar C, et al: Endometrial resection and ablation versus hysterectomy for heavy menstrual bleeding, *Cochrane Database Syst Rev* (2), 1999. Art. No. CD000329. doi:10.1002/14651858.CD000329. Update 2009.

Nieboer TE, Johnson N, Lethaby A, et al: Surgical approach to hysterectomy for benign gynaecological disease, *Cochrane Database Syst Rev* (3), 2009. Art. No. CD003677. doi:10.1002/14651858.CD003677.pub4.

Rahn DD, Phelan JN, Roshanravan SM, et al: Anterior abdominal wall nerve and vessel anatomy: Clinical implications for gynecologic surgery, *Am J Obstet Gynecol* 202(3):234.e1–234.e5, 2010.

Vilos GA, Ternamian A, Dempster J, et al, The Society of Obstetricians and Gynaecologists of Canada: Laparoscopic entry: A review of techniques, technologies, and complications, *J Obstet Gynaecol Can* 29(5):433–465, 2007.

World Health Organization: *Surgical safety checklist*, Geneva, 2009, WHO. Available at http://whqlibdoc.who.int/publications/2009/9789241598590_eng_Checklist.pdf. Retrieved November 2010.

11

Congenital Abnormalities of the Female Reproductive Tract
Anomalies of the Vagina, Cervix, Uterus, and Adnexa

Vern L. Katz and Gretchen M. Lentz

Congenital abnormalities of the female reproductive tract are common. They can be caused by genetic errors or by teratologic events during embryonic development. Minor abnormalities may be of little consequence, but major abnormalities may lead to severe impairment of menstrual and reproductive functions and affect operative management as well as being associated with anomalies of the urinary tract. This chapter categorizes a number of such abnormalities and discusses diagnosis and treatment. Most studies find the incidence of Müllerian anomalies to occur in 1% to 3% of women. Anomalies present at varying times in a woman's life, at birth, before puberty, with the onset of menses, and during pregnancy with adverse pregnancy outcomes. Because of the profound psychological effects such abnormalities can cause, the gynecologist must approach the problems of genital and Müllerian anomalies with sensitivity and with a wide perspective of the effects they have on the woman and her family. Most tertiary centers involve a multidisciplinary team including medical genetics, cytogenetics, gynecology, pediatric urology, endocrinology, and psychiatry for the evaluation, treatment, and support of the patient with a serious disorder of sex development.

EXAMINATION OF THE NEWBORN FOR AMBIGUOUS GENITALIA

The first major diagnostic decision of the obstetrician with respect to the newborn is gender assignment. In most cases the designation is clear. However, in approximately 1 in 14,000 newborns, **ambiguous genitalia** will be found. This is a serious problem for the infant, the physician, and the parents. Females (individuals with XX karyotypes) with masculinized external genitalia are identified as female **pseudohermaphrodites** (**Table 11-1**). The most common cause is congenital adrenal hyperplasia. The timing of antenatal (embryonic) exposure to androgen influences the degree of masculinization (**Fig. 11-1**). The vaginal septum separates from the urogenital sinus at about 12 weeks. Androgen exposure after that point presents primarily with clitoral hypertrophy. The female who has been

androgenized may appear similar to the male pseudohermaphrodite suffering from incomplete **androgen resistance syndrome**. Also, some vulvar abnormalities may resemble partial androgenization. It is therefore appropriate to systematically evaluate the newborn's genitalia to make the appropriate gender assignment, and when necessary perform imaging studies, chromosomal evaluations, serum electrolytes, and steroid assessment. Until recently, gender was assigned primarily on the principal of "phallic adequacy," with neonates with ambiguous phallus being assigned female gender. This principle is now inappropriate and full evaluation with chromosomal studies and appropriately timed corrective measures is now the desired approach.

The first and probably most important aspect of the examination of the neonate is inspection. The physician should systematically observe the newborn's perineum, beginning with the mons pubis. The clitoris should be noted for any obvious enlargement, the opening of the urethra should be identified, and the labia should be gently separated to see if the introitus can be visualized. If the labia are fused, this maneuver will be impossible. Palpation of the inguinal area and labia for testes is important at this point. At times the labia are joined by filmy adhesions; these generally separate in later childhood or respond to the application of estrogen cream when necessary. If it is possible to separate the labia, the hymen may be observed. Generally, it is partially perforate, revealing the entrance into the vagina. Posteriorly the labia fuse in the midline at the posterior fourchette of the perineum. Posterior to the perineal body the rectum can be visualized, and it should be tested to be sure that it is perforate. Meconium staining about the rectum is evidence for perforation. If there is doubt, the rectum may be penetrated with a moistened cotton-tipped swab.

If the labia are fused and the clitoris is not enlarged, other abnormalities may also be present, such as abnormalities of the abdominal wall or skeletal system. Thus, the infant should be carefully assessed for other anomalies with imaging and karyotype. An enlarged clitoris and fused labia are evidence of androgen effect and may imply congenital adrenal hyperplasia, maternal ingestion of androgens, or increased natural androgen production. A bifid clitoris may be present; this anomaly is

Table 11-1 Classification of Female Pseudohermaphroditism

I. Androgen-Induced
  A. Fetal Source
    1. Congenital adrenal hyperplasia
      a. Virilism only, defective adrenal 21-hydroxylation (CYP21)
      b. Virilism with salt-losing syndrome, defective adrenal 21-hydroxylation (CYP21)
      c. Virilism with hypertension, defective adrenal 11β-hydroxylation (CYP11B1)
      d. Virilism with adrenal insufficiency, deficient 3β-HSD 2 (HSD3B 2)
    2. P450 aromatase (CYP19) deficiency
    3. Glucocorticoid receptor gene mutation
  B. Maternal source
    1. Iatrogenic
      a. Testosterone and related steroids
      b. Certain synthetic oral progestagens and rarely diethylstilbestrol
    2. Virilizing ovarian or adrenal tumor
    3. Virilizing luteoma of pregnancy
    4. Congenital virilizing adrenal hyperplasia in mother*
  C. Undetermined source
    1. Virilizing luteoma of pregnancy
II. Non-Androgen-Induced Disturbances in Differentiation of Urogenital Structures

*In pregnant patient whose disease is poorly controlled or who is noncompliant, especially during the first trimester.
From Grumbach MM, Hughes IA, Conte FA: Disorders of sex differentiation. In Larsen RP, Kronenberg HM, Melmed S, Polonsky KS (eds): Williams Textbook of Endocrinology, 10th ed. Philadelphia, Saunders, 2003.

usually associated with extrophy of the bladder. In such cases, anterior rotation and shortening of the vagina with fused labia is usually present.

In most instances, inspection is all that is necessary. On the rare occasions when the physician needs to examine the vagina or see the cervix of the newborn, an endoscope, such as a pediatric cystoscope, may be used. The hymen is generally perforate and will accept this instrument. If there is any difficulty, ultrasound may be preferable.

If **labial fusion** is noted, the physician should palpate the groins and labial folds for evidence of gonads. Gonads palpable in the inguinal canal, labioinguinal region, or labioscrotal folds are almost always testes. Thus, such a finding implies a male with ambiguous genitalia rather than a virilized female. Conversely, an infant with ambiguous genitalia but without palpable testes in the scrotum is likely to be a virilized female, most often the result of congenital adrenal hyperplasia. Rectal examination may make it possible to palpate a cervix and uterus, thus helping in the sex assignment. Ultrasound should be strongly considered for verification and evaluation.

PERINEAL AND VAGINAL DEFECTS

Clitoral Anomalies

The clitoris is generally 1 to 1.5 cm long and 0.5 cm wide in the nonerect state. The glans is partially covered by a hood of skin. The urethra opens near the base of the clitoris. Abnormalities are unusual, although the clitoris may be enlarged because of androgen stimulation. In such circumstances the shaft of the clitoris may be quite enlarged and partial development of a penile urethra may have occurred (**Fig. 11-2**). Extreme cases of androgen stimulation are generally associated with fusion of the labia. These findings occur in infants with congenital adrenal hyperplasia and in those exposed in utero to exogenous or endogenous androgens (**Fig. 11-3**). Similar in appearance, males with androgen insensitivity syndrome have underdeveloped male external genitalia and a very small phallus that appears as clitoral hypertrophy (**Fig. 11-4**).

Bifid clitoris (**Fig. 11-5**) is usually seen in association with extrophy of the bladder. Extrophy of the bladder occurs rarely (1 per 30,000 births) and has a male predominance (3:1). However, when it occurs in females, it is often associated with bifid clitoris. Stanton noted that 43% of 70 female patients with bladder extrophy had associated reproductive tract anomalies. These included vaginal anomalies and Müllerian duct fusion problems. In such cases, an anterior rotation and a shortening of the vagina with labial fusion are quite common.

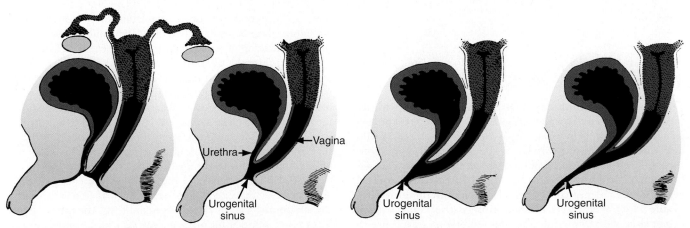

Figure 11-1 Female pseudohermaphroditism induced by prenatal exposure to androgens. Exposure after 12th fetal week leads only to clitoral hypertrophy *(left)*. Exposure at progressively earlier stages of differentiation *(from left to right)* leads to retention of the urogenital sinus and labioscrotal fusion. If exposure occurs sufficiently early, the labia fuse to form a penile urethra. (From Grumbach MM, Hughes IA, Conte FA: Disorders of sex differentiation. In Larsen RP, Kronenberg HM, Melmed S, Polonsky KS [eds]: Williams Textbook of Endocrinology, 10th ed. Philadelphia, WB Saunders, 2003, p 916.)

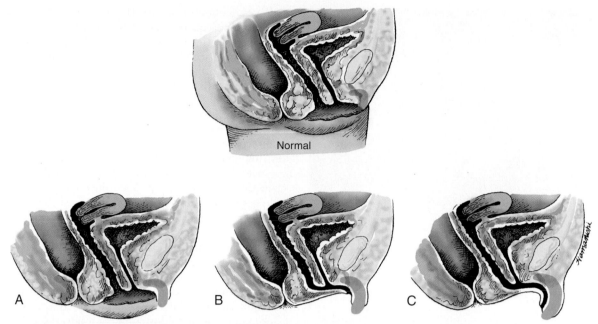

Figure 11-2 Sagittal views of genital deformities seen in female infants who are masculinized. **A,** Minimal masculinization with slight enlargement of the clitoris. **B,** Labial fusion and more marked enlargement of the clitoris. **C,** Complete labial fusion, enlargement of the clitoris, and formation of a partial penile urethra. (Modified from Verkauf BS, Jones HW Jr: Masculinization of the female genitalia in congenital adrenal hyperplasia: Relationship to the salt losing variety of the disease. South Med J 63:634, 1970.)

Labial Fusion

Labial fusion may occur without clitoromegaly. The resultant ambiguous genitalia will imply a form of hermaphroditism. The term **hermaphrodite** is derived from the child of the Greekgods Hermes and Aphrodite, Hermaphroditus, who was part female and part male. A true hermaphrodite has both ovarian (including follicular elements) and testicular tissue, either in the same or opposite gonads. The term *pseudohermaphroditism* applies to individuals with a pure XX or XY karyotype but with the external genitalia of the opposite sex of the karyotype or ambiguous genitalia. True hermaphroditism is extremely rare in North and South America but more common (though still very rare) in Africa.

Although labial fusion may result from exposure to exogenous androgens or be associated with defects of the anterior

Figure 11-3 Clitoromegaly with posterior labial fusion in a child with congenital adrenal hyperplasia. (From McKay M: Vulvar manifestations of skin disorders. In Black M, McKay M, Braude P, et al [eds]: Obstetric and Gynecologic Dermatology, 2nd ed. Edinburgh, Mosby, 2003, p 120.)

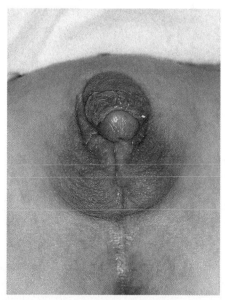

Figure 11-4 Ambiguous genitalia in an XY child with partial androgen insensitivity. (From McKay M: Vulvar manifestations of skin disorders. In Black M, McKay M, Braude P, et al [eds]: Obstetric and Gynecologic Dermatology, 2nd ed. Edinburgh, Mosby, 2003, p 121.)

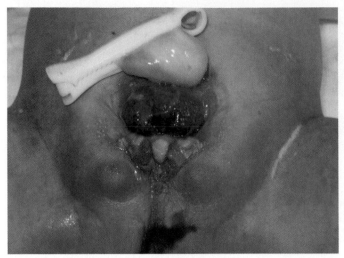

Figure 11-5 An example of a bifid clitoris in an infant with extrophy of the bladder. (Courtesy of Richard Grady, MD.)

abdominal wall, by far the most common cause is congenital adrenal hyperplasia. The most common form of congenital adrenal hyperplasia is caused by an inborn error of metabolism involving deficiency of the enzyme 21-hydroxylase (**Fig. 11-6**). This condition is transmitted as an autosomal recessive gene coded on chromosome 6. Because of the absence of 21-hydroxylase, the major biosynthetic pathway to cortisol is blocked; 17-OH-progesterone is produced instead, which is converted to the

StAR   ACTH
        ↓ ↓
    Cholesterol
CYP11A1 │
        │   CYP 17   CYP 17
  Pregnenolone → 17-OH-Pregnenolone → DHEA
3β-HSDII │   │
         │   │
  Progesterone → 17-OH-Progesterone → Androstenedione
         │   │
    (Blocked at) (Blocked at)
    CYP 21A2   CYP 21A2
         │   │
        DOC   11-Deoxycortisol
CYP11B1 │   CYP11B1 │
        │   │
  Corticosterone   Cortisol
CYP11B2 │
        │
   Aldosterone

MINERALOCORTICOID   GLUCOCORTICOID   ANDROGENS

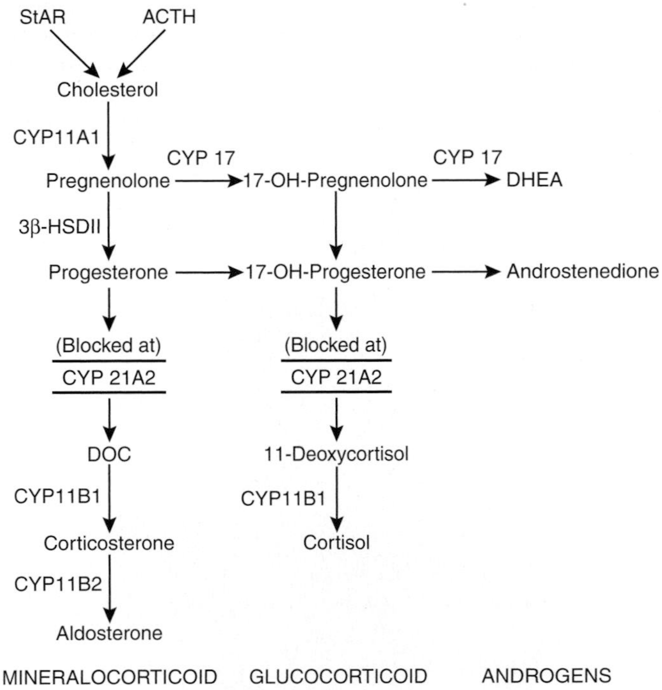

Figure 11-6 Steroid pathway in congenital adrenal hyperplasia with absence of 21 hydroxylase. ACTH, adrenocorticotropic hormone; 3β-HSDII, 3β-hydroxysteroid dehydrogenase; DHEA, dehydroepiandrosterone; DOC, deoxycorticosterone. (From Grumbach MM, Hughes IA, Conte FA: Disorders of sex differentiation. In Larsen RP, Kronenberg HM, Melmed S, Polonsky KS [eds]: Williams Textbook of Endocrinology, 10th ed. Philadelphia, WB Saunders, 2003, p 533.)

androgen androstenedione. The fetal hypothalamic-pituitary axis senses inadequate levels of cortisol and secretes excess adrenocorticotropic hormone (ACTH), which leads to increasing levels of androstenedione from the female adrenal and subsequent masculinization of the external genitalia. Homozygous individuals occur with an incidence as much as 1 per 490, depending on the geographic location. Screening programs have noted the incidence to be approximately 1 in 14,000 births. Carriers of the gene, heterozygotes are present in the population in a frequency ranging from 1 per 20 to 1 per 250. Two other less common enzyme defects, also transmittable as autosomal recessive traits, may produce similar abnormal findings: the 11-hydroxylase deficiency and the 3β-hydroxysteroid dehydrogenase deficiency. These two as well as 21-hydroxylase deficiency may cause ambiguous genitalia with masculinized females.

Congenital adrenal hyperplasia (CAH) may be demonstrated at birth by the presence of ambiguous genitalia in genetic females or present later in childhood. Significant proportions (≤75%) of newborns with this condition are also at risk for the development of life-threatening neonatal adrenal crises as a result of sodium loss because of absent aldosterone. In milder disease, delayed diagnosis may result in abnormalities of accelerated bone maturation, leading to short stature. The development of premature secondary sexual characteristics in males and further virilization in females may also occur (**Fig. 11-7**). At the time of this publication, most states in the United States have mandatory neonatal screening for 17-OH progesterone levels, to screen for CAH.

Treatment of congenital adrenal hyperplasia involves replacement of cortisol. This suppresses ACTH output and therefore decreases the stimulation of the cortisol-producing pathways of the adrenal cortex. For women known to be at risk, those with

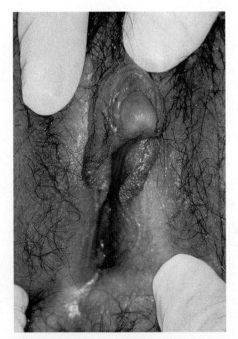

Figure 11-7 Eleven-year-old girl with clitoromegaly and thick genital hair, who presented with facial hair and was found to have 21-hydroxylase deficiency. (From McKay M: Vulvar manifestations of skin disorders. In Black M, McKay M, Braude P, et al [eds]: Obstetric and Gynecologic Dermatology, 2nd ed. Edinburgh, Mosby, 2003, p 120.)

diagnoses of CAH and those with previously affected children, in utero therapy may be offered. Dexamethasone given daily after a positive pregnancy test will suppress fetal adrenal glands until the child's gender can be verified with prenatal diagnosis. Many of the infants affected with in utero androgenization may need corrective surgery. Initial corrective surgeries on the children may need follow-up vaginoplasty as teenagers because of vaginal stenosis. Almost all females with ambiguous genitalia should have ongoing psychological support and counseling because of the profound issues raised about identity with this diagnosis. Even beyond women with ambiguous genitalia, all women with other intersex disorders and genital anomalies, which are collectively termed disorders of sex development, may need multidisciplinary team support throughout their lives for gynecologic, urologic, endocrinologic, and psychological help.

Imperforate Hymen

The hymen represents the junction of the sinovaginal bulbs with the urogenital sinus and is composed of endoderm from the urogenital sinus epithelium. The hymen opens normally during embryonic life to establish a connection between the lumen of the vaginal canal and the vestibule. If this perforation does not take place, the hymen is imperforate (**Fig. 11-8**). The incidence is thought to be approximately 1 in 1000 live-born females. Several variations exist of partial hymeneal perforation (**Fig. 11-9**), many of which require surgical correction.

It is rare to make the diagnosis of imperforate hymen before puberty, at which point primary amenorrhea is the major symptom. Occasionally in childhood a **hydrocolpos** or **mucocolpos** may occur. This is caused by a collection of secretions behind the hymen, which in rare cases may build up to form a mass that obstructs the urinary tract. If discovered, the hymen should be incised to release the buildup. At puberty the patient may experience cyclic cramping but no menstrual flow. Over time the patient may develop a **hematocolpos** and a hematometrium. In more advanced cases the fallopian tubes may be distended with menstrual flow, and the flow may back up through the tubes and form endometrial implants in the peritoneal cavity. Quite surprisingly, many patients are free of symptoms.

The diagnosis can be determined by history and by the presence of a bulging membrane at the introitus. Therapy consists of a cruciate incision into the hymen extending to the 10, 2, and 6 o'clock positions. In the rare case of a thick and dense hymen, a triangular section may be excised. Hemostasis is secured by fine suture, and evolution to normal usually occurs rapidly. A less common technique involves an oval incision with placement of a Foley. This disease is thought to be a sporadic anomaly, though familial cases as well as a case of autosomal dominant inheritance have been noted.

Vaginal Agenesis

Vaginal agenesis, also known as Müllerian agenesis or Müllerian aplasia, is usually associated with the **Mayer–Rokitansky–Küster–Hauser (MRKH) syndrome** (**Fig. 11-10**). This syndrome is characterized by congenital absence of the vagina and uterus, although small masses of smooth muscular material resembling a rudimentary **bicornuate uterus** are not uncommon. The syndrome occurs in approximately 1 in 4,000 to 1 in 10,000 women. These individuals have a 46,XX karyotype. The disorder seems to be an accident of development and not an inherited condition, unless it is associated with other endocrinopathies.

Complete vaginal agenesis is discovered in 75% of patients with Mayer–Rokitansky–Küster–Hauser syndrome. Approximately 25% of patients have a short vaginal pouch. Some women may have **rudimentary uterine horns** and may have myomas as well as adenomyosis in the rudimentary uterus. Many of the

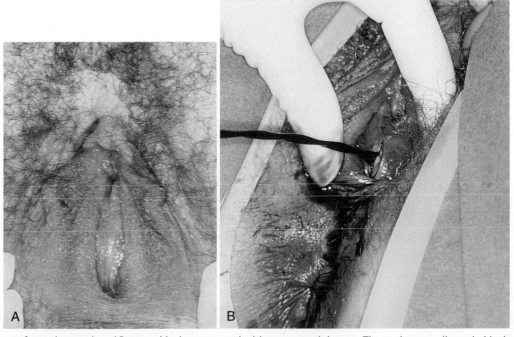

Figure 11-8 A, Imperforate hymen in a 13-year-old who presented with an acute abdomen. The vagina was distended by hematocolpos, with surgical incision **(B)** old blood was released. (From McKay M: Vulvar manifestations of skin disorders. In Black M, McKay M, Braude P, et al [eds]: Obstetric and Gynecologic Dermatology, 2nd ed. Edinburgh, Mosby, 2003, p 122.)

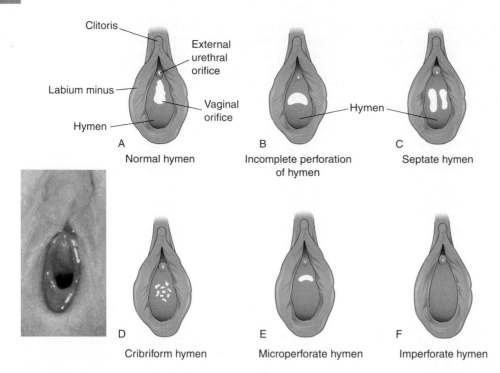

Figure 11-9 Congenital anomalies of the hymen. (From Moore KL, Persaud TVN: The Developing Human, 7th ed. Philadelphia, WB Saunders, 2003, p 322.)

A Normal hymen

B Incomplete perforation of hymen

C Septate hymen

D Cribriform hymen

E Microperforate hymen

F Imperforate hymen

Clitoris
External urethral orifice
Labium minus
Vaginal orifice
Hymen
Hymen

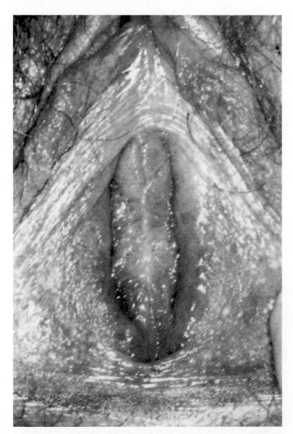

Figure 11-10 External genitalia of patient with congenital absence of vagina. (From Baramki TA: Treatment of congenital anomalies in girls and women. J Reprod Med 29:376, 1984.)

uterine horns will contain small amounts of endometrium with an epithelial lining, and rarely menstruation occurs, giving rise to monthly cyclic cramping. A recent study by Fedele et al. noted that 92 of 106 women had small Müllerian remnants. The ovaries in women with MRKH are normal, and the fallopian tubes are usually present. The differential diagnosis of vaginal agenesis includes transverse vaginal septum, cervical agenesis, and androgen insensitivity syndrome.

The androgen insensitivity syndrome comprises several genetic abnormalities centering on faulty androgen receptors. The syndrome until recently was termed *testicular feminization syndrome.* These individuals have a 46,XY karyotype. Because the developing fetus cannot sense any testosterone, the external genitalia are feminized, and vaginal agenesis or the presence of a short pouch vagina is usually found. These patients have undescended testicles. The Müllerian structures have resolved because the testes make anti-Müllerian hormone. Wolffian duct tissue exists instead. The individuals usually exhibit minimal pubic hair after puberty. After the growth spurt, the testes should be removed to prevent the development of gonadoblastoma. The ovaries of the patient with MRKH syndrome are normal and should not be removed.

Up to 50% of women with Müllerian agenesis have concurrent urinary tract anomalies. Phelan and coworkers reported that of 72 patients with vaginal agenesis, 25% had urologic abnormalities noted on intravenous pyelography. A later study by Baramki demonstrated that 40% of 92 patients had urologic abnormalities. One study described a 12% incidence of skeletal anomalies, usually involving congenital fusion or absence of vertebrae in these patients. These and other studies indicate the need for imaging of the urinary tract in women with MRKH.

MRKH syndrome presents as primary amenorrhea at the time of puberty. Physical examination demonstrates the absence of a vaginal opening or the presence of a short vaginal pouch, and there is an inability to palpate a uterus on rectal examination, coupled with the finding of a normal karyotype. Although ultrasound examination may verify the presence of normal ovaries and the absence of the uterus, magnetic resonance imaging offers an excellent alternative for visualizing congenital anomalies of the internal reproductive organs and is currently the modality of choice for women with Müllerian agenesis. Laparoscopic examination may be performed when the diagnosis is not clear or when there is some concern over the presence of functioning uterine tissue. In most cases, however, laparoscopic diagnosis is not necessary.

Treatment

Therapy involves the creation of a vagina when the patient wishes to become sexually active. There are multiple therapeutic choices, and a detailed review is beyond the scope of this chapter. In overview, the first therapy is time consuming but nonsurgical and requires the use of progressive vaginal dilators. This can best be accomplished in a well-motivated, mature patient over a period of several months. Functioning vaginas have been achieved in many patients in this manner.

Using the concept of vaginal dilators, Ingram devised a useful technique. He used three sets of Lucite dilators. The first set contains 10 that are 1.5 cm in diameter and that increase in length from 1.5 to 10 cm; the second set contains 5 dilators that are 2.5 cm in diameter and that increase in length from 3 to 10 cm; and the third set has 8 dilators, 3.5 cm in diameter and from 3 to 10 cm long. A racing bicycle seat is mounted on a stool and is used to maintain dilator pressure on the introital dimple just posterior to the urethra. The patient holds the dilators in place with a pad or girdle and works through the three sets in progressive fashion, considering length and width as tolerated. The bicycle seat allows continuing pressure against the dilator; pressure is continued for 15 to 30 minutes at a time for a total of at least 2 hours a day. The patient may read or do other activities while sitting. It generally takes 4 to 6 months to develop an adequate neovagina by this technique. Subsequent researchers have validated this technique.

Surgical reconstruction of the vagina has many variations. The operations, for the most part, develop the potential space between the bladder and the rectum and replaced this space with a stent utilizing tissue, most commonly a split-thickness skin graft or synthetic materials. The latter procedure, developed by Abbe-McIndoe, is easy to perform but must be done only when the patient will use the vagina frequently. If she does not or fails to leave a plastic mold in place, the neovagina will frequently shrivel, scar, and become nonfunctional. Early and regular postoperative coitus is important for long-term success and is superior to the wearing of a stent. Thus, the timing of the operation to coincide with the opportunity for coitus is important.

An alternative procedure, to build a neovagina, was devised by Williams. This procedure utilizes labial skin and results in a vaginal pouch whose axis is directly posterior. Although it is not as anatomically similar to a normal vagina as is the result of the McIndoe procedure, it does produce a functioning vaginal pouch and is well received by patients. Eventually, a normal vaginal axis is reported to develop. Other types of skin grafts, including sigmoid lining for a neovaginal pouch, are less popular.

Vecchietti developed a laparoscopic procedure for producing a neovagina. Sutures are placed laparoscopically in the peritoneal folds between the bladder and rudimentary uterus. A cutting edge needle then perforates the pseudohymen, and an olive is attached to the suture and pulled tightly against the perineum. The sutures (two) are then fixed to a traction device on the anterior abdominal wall and graduated traction applied for 6 to 8 days. The olive is then removed and the patient uses vaginal dilators until sexual intercourse begins 10 to 15 days later. Several authors have reported good success with this procedure.

Transverse Vaginal Septum

The Müllerian ducts join the sinovaginal bulb at a point known as the *Müllerian tubercle.* Canalization of the Müllerian tubercle and sinovaginal bulb is necessary to give a normal vaginal lumen. If the area of junction between these structures is not completely canalized, a transverse vaginal septum will occur (**Fig. 11-11**). This may be partial or complete and generally lies at the junction between the upper third and lower two thirds of the vagina (**Fig. 11-12**). Transverse vaginal septum occurs in about 1 per 75,000 females. Partial transverse vaginal septa have been reported in diethylstilbestrol (DES)-exposed females. In the prepubertal state, diagnosis is generally not made unless there is the

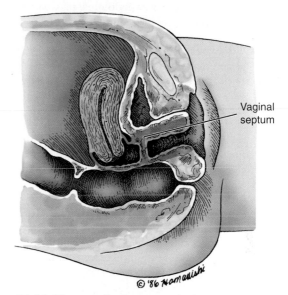

Figure 11-11 Diagram of transverse vaginal septum.

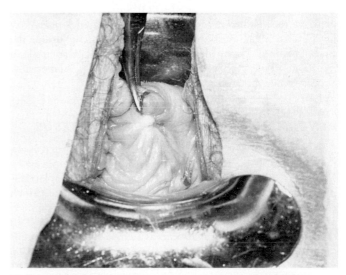

Figure 11-12 Patient with complete transverse vaginal septum.

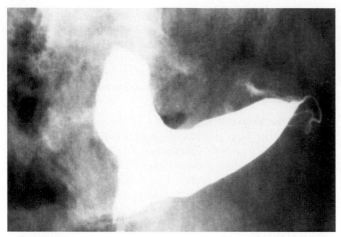

Figure 11-13 Hysterosalpingogram of bicornuate uterus seen in patient with repetitive abortions.

development of a mucocolpos or mucometrium behind the septum. In these girls an unexplained abdominal mass forms. At puberty, however, if the septum is complete, hematocolpos and hematometrium may occur in a fashion similar to that seen in the imperforate hymen, except that there is no bulging at the introitus. The patient complains of primary amenorrhea with cyclic cramping. The patient with an incomplete transverse septum may bleed somewhat but will still develop hematocolpos and hematometrium over time and may also complain of foul-smelling vaginal discharge. The septum is often thin, generally less than 1 cm thick; however, many septa will be as thick as 2 cm. If an opening is noted, it may be expanded by manual dilation or simple incision, with suturing of the edges of the vagina on either side. In cases of a thick septum, the two areas of the vagina may be quite distant. In such cases excision may require the implantation of a split-thickness skin graft in a fashion similar to the Abee-McIndoe procedure. Most all women with congenital Müllerian anomalies should have psychological counseling made available. Longitudinal septa of the vagina will be discussed with duplication of the uterus and cervix.

Vaginal Adenosis

In the female who was exposed to DES in utero, the junction between the Müllerian ducts and the sinovaginal bulb may not be sharply demonstrated. If Müllerian elements invade the sinovaginal bulb, remnants may remain as areas of adenosis in the adult vagina. They are generally palpated submucosally, although they may be observable at the surface.

ABNORMALITIES OF THE CERVIX AND UTERUS

Abnormalities of the cervix and uterus may be categorized as abnormalities of Müllerian duct fusion. Anomalies of duplications may be classified as didelphic, which may involve a complete duplication of the vagina, uterus, and cervix; bicornuate, which consists of a single-chamber vagina and cervix with a complete or partial **septate uterus** and two uterine bodies (**Fig. 11-14**); septate, in which the uterus appears as a single organ but contains a midline septum that is either partial or complete; or arcuate, which demonstrates a small septate indentation at the upper end of the fundus. Additionally, loss or absent development of

one side includes **unicornis (unicornuate) uterus** in a further subclass of these anomalies.

Between the third and fifth weeks of gestation the metanephric ducts develop and join the cloaca. By the fifth week, two bilateral ureteric buds develop from the mesonephric ducts near the distal ends (see Chapter 1, Fertilization and Embryogenesis). These grow cephalad toward the mesonephric mass. The Müllerian, or paramesonephric ducts, form from clefts between the mesonephros and the newly forming gonad. These ducts develop caudally immediately lateral to the mesonephric ducts. The fate of all of these various embryonic elements is closely entwined. Damage or abnormal development of one usually affects the others. The paramesonephric ducts grow caudally, meet in the midline, and descend into the pelvis, reaching the urogenital sinus at an elevation known as the *Müllerian tubercle*.

Musset analyzed 133 cases of genitourinary malformation and described a three-stage process for fusion of the two Müllerian ducts into the uterus and cervix. The first stage is described as short, taking place at the beginning of the tenth week. The medial aspects of the more caudal portions of the two ducts fuse, starting in the middle and proceeding simultaneously in both directions. In this way a median septum is formed. The second stage continues from the tenth to the thirteenth week and occurs because of a rapid cell proliferation and the filling in of the triangular space between the two uterine cornua. In this way a thick upper median septum is formed. This is wedge like and gives rise to the usual external contour of the fundus. At the same time the lower portion of the median septum is resorbed, unifying the cervical canal first and then the upper vagina. The third stage lasts from the thirteenth to about the twentieth week. In this stage the degeneration of the upper uterine septum occurs, starting at the isthmic region and proceeding cranially to the top of the fundus. In this way a unified uterine cavity is formed.

The vagina develops from a combination of the Müllerian tubercles and the urogenital sinus. Cells proliferate from the upper portion of the urogenital sinus to form solid aggregates known as the *sinovaginal bulbs*. These cell masses develop into a cord, the vaginal plate, which extends from the Müllerian ducts to the urogenital sinus. This plate canalizes, starting at the hymen, which is where the sinovaginal bulb attaches to the urogenital sinus, and proceeding cranially to the developing cervix, which has by this time already canalized. The process is completed at about the 21st week of intrauterine life.

Toaff and colleagues noted that the type of abnormality of the uterus depends on a teratogenic process active at a specific stage in the embryonic development. Most symmetrical communicating uteri such as uterine didelphys are associated with a normal urinary system, indicating that normal growth of the two mesonephric ducts had taken place before the fusion problem occurred. Interestingly, almost all patients with communicating uteri with atretic hemivagina have ipsilateral renal agenesis. Similarly, in patients with anomalies in which a hemicervix is absent, ipsilateral renal agenesis occurs. Toaff and colleagues inferred that an early teratogenic process active during the fourth week of gestation resulted in arrested growth of one mesonephric duct, agenesis of the ureteric bud, and therefore renal agenesis.

Genetic Studies of Müllerian Fusion Difficulties

Reviews of the genetics of 24 women with known Müllerian fusion abnormalities suggest that the major genetic transmission mechanism is most likely polygenic or multifactorial, though

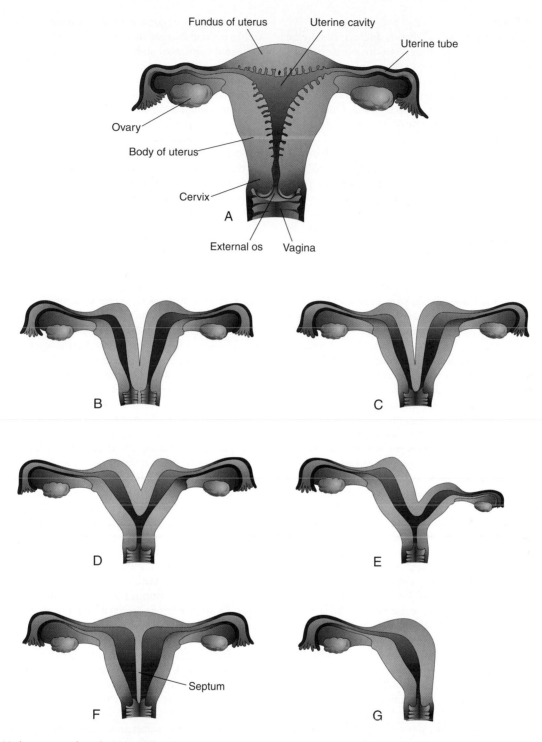

Figure 11-14 Various types of uterine anomalies. **A,** Normal uterus and vagina. **B,** Double uterus (uterus didelphys) and double vagina. **C,** Double uterus with single vagina. **D,** Bicornuate uterus. **E,** Bicornuate uterus with a rudimentary left horn. **F,** Septate uterus. **G,** Unicornuate uterus. (From Moore KL, Persaud TVN: The Developing Human, 7th ed. Philadelphia, WB Saunders, 2003, Figure 13-43, p 321.)

familial clusters have been reported. In a series by Hammoud et al. of 1397 cases, there were 27 family clusters comprising 10% of cases.

It is difficult to estimate the incidence of uterine fusion anomalies because the data in most reports are derived from case studies rather than from evaluation of the general population. The incidence is reported as 0.1% in retrospective studies and from 2% to 3% in observations of uteri at the time of delivery. Most uteri in the latter study, however, fit into the category of **arcuate uterus** or subseptate uterus. Lin and coworkers, summarizing the literature, reported the distribution of congenital uterine abnormalities to be bicornuate uterus 37%, arcuate and incomplete septum 28%, complete septum 9%, **didelphic uterus** 11%, and unicornuate 4%.

Symptoms and Signs

Complete duplication of the vagina, uterus, and cervix may be asymptomatic until the woman begins to menstruate. Frequently, the earliest symptom brought to the attention of the gynecologist is the fact that tampons do not obstruct menstrual flow. What occurs is that the patient inserts a tampon into one vagina but the other vagina is still open. The second most common way the diagnosis is made is by observation at the time of the first pelvic examination.

Obstructive vaginal anomalies often lead to cyclic pain at the time of menstruation or to the presence of a mucus-filled or blood-filled mass in the vagina. This may be mistaken for a paravaginal tumor. A noncommunicating uterine horn becomes symptomatic in one of two fashions. The first may be a mass or pain that is exacerbated at the time of menses. This may be occasionally associated with symptoms and signs of endometriosis in a teenage woman. Along these lines, the early onset of signs and symptoms of endometriosis should alert the physician to the possibilities of uterine malformation. A mass is often noted on physical examination or seen with ultrasound.

The second way such a problem may present is as an ectopic pregnancy. Because sperm may migrate through the patent horn and because the rudimentary horn may have a normal tube attached to it, pregnancy can occur in a rudimentary horn. Because such horns are frequently small, the pregnancy usually leads to pain or rupture. In a review of rudimentary uterine horns, Jayasinghe et al. reviewed 366 published cases, of which 92% were noncommunicating. Functional noncommunicating horns may present with catastrophic rupture in pregnancy.

Another common presenting symptom is repetitive reproductive loss, particularly in the early second trimester. Interestingly, didelphic uteri are usually not associated with this problem. Uterine anomalies and **recurrent miscarriage** is discussed in Chapter 16 (Spontaneous and Recurrent Abortion). Makino and colleagues studied 1200 women with recurrent loss with hysterosalpingography and found that 188 had congenital uterine anomalies (15.7%). Most patients with pregnancy loss, however, had a variation of septate uterus. Metroplasty may lead to successful pregnancy outcomes in as much as 80%. A review by Homer and associates found a total of 658 women experiencing 1062 pregnancies, of which 88% ended in miscarriage and 9% in preterm delivery prior to treatment. Of the 491 pregnancies experienced by these women after hysteroscopic metroplasty, 80% ended in full-term deliveries, and only 14% were aborted and 6% were preterm. It is important to thoroughly evaluate such patients before exposing them to an operative procedure, since other problems may cause pregnancy loss.

Uterine dysfunction and abnormal uterine activity are complicating problems seen in labor in women with septate and bicornuate uteri. Likewise, breech presentations and transverse lies occur more commonly in women with such abnormal uteri as well.

Diagnosis

Diagnosis of a uterine anomaly may be indicated by a history, suggested by physical examination and confirmed with imaging. Several imaging modalities may be used, including sonohysterography, hysterosalpingography, and hysteroscopy (**Fig. 11-13**). Ultrasound is a reasonable diagnostic procedure but should not be considered diagnostic until supplementary studies are performed. Magnetic resonance imaging is also appropriate and recent studies have demonstrated its accuracy. Many radiologists feel it is the modality of choice since the urinary tract may be evaluated simultaneously. Laparoscopy or laparotomy may be useful in some cases.

Evaluation of the urinary tracts is indicated in most cases of Müllerian fusion anomalies to identify any concurrent urinary tract anomalies.

Specific Anomalies

Absence of Cervix and Uterus

As discussed earlier, in many women with Müllerian agenesis, the cervix and uterus are often not completely absent; the fallopian tubes and possibly some fibrous tissue are usually present. Absence is associated with urinary tract anomalies up to 50% of the time.

Unicornuate Uterus

Destruction of one Müllerian duct may occur for various reasons in the embryonic period. It is often related to lack of development of the mesonephric system on one side. When this is the case, there is almost always a missing kidney and ureter on the same side. A single cervix and a single horn of the uterus with the fallopian tube of the side entering it are seen. The ovary may be present on the opposite side.

Historical reviews have noted significant problems with pregnancy loss. In one series, Moutos and colleagues studied 29 women with unicornuate uteri and 25 women with didelphic uteri. Twenty of the 29 women with unicornuate uteri produced a total of 40 pregnancies, and 13 of 25 women with didelphic uteri produced a total of 28 pregnancies. There was a 33% spontaneous abortion rate in the unicornuate group and a 23% rate in the didelphic group. The unicornuate group produced 9% preterm deliveries, 58% full-term deliveries, and 61% had living children. The didelphic group produced 32% preterm deliveries, 45% full-term deliveries, and 60% had living children. None of these differences were statistically different. Other series have noted similar trends. In practice, women with a history of pregnancy losses should be evaluated for Müllerian anomalies.

Toaff and colleagues reviewed the subgroup of malformed uteri that includes duplication of the vagina, cervix, and uterus with communication between the horns. Nine subcategories have been described and are depicted in **Figure 11-15**. Some involve septate uteri and others didelphic uteri. Some involve obstructive areas of the vagina. Because of the structural differences the clinical findings may be quite different from patient to patient. Rarely, uterine diverticula may form.

Management

For patients with unobstructed abnormalities, therapy may not be needed. This is particularly true for women with unicornuate and didelphic uteri. On the other hand, septate uteri are often associated with miscarriage problems, and correction may be necessary. A number of surgical corrective procedures are available. Patton and coworkers have emphasized that thorough evaluation is necessary prior to deciding on surgical treatment to establish the optimal strategy. Misdiagnosis of the anomaly is not uncommon.

Metroplasty was classically described by Strassman and involved the removal of the septum by a wedge incision and the reunification of the two cavities during laparotomy. However, a number of other means have been devised to eliminate the

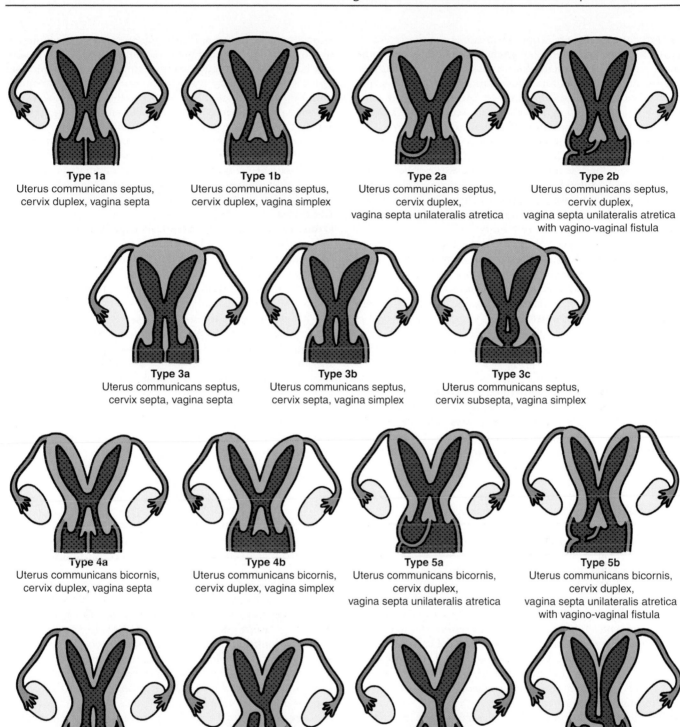

Type 1a
Uterus communicans septus,
cervix duplex, vagina septa

Type 1b
Uterus communicans septus,
cervix duplex, vagina simplex

Type 2a
Uterus communicans septus,
cervix duplex,
vagina septa unilateralis atretica

Type 2b
Uterus communicans septus,
cervix duplex,
vagina septa unilateralis atretica
with vagino-vaginal fistula

Type 3a
Uterus communicans septus,
cervix septa, vagina septa

Type 3b
Uterus communicans septus,
cervix septa, vagina simplex

Type 3c
Uterus communicans septus,
cervix subsepta, vagina simplex

Type 4a
Uterus communicans bicornis,
cervix duplex, vagina septa

Type 4b
Uterus communicans bicornis,
cervix duplex, vagina simplex

Type 5a
Uterus communicans bicornis,
cervix duplex,
vagina septa unilateralis atretica

Type 5b
Uterus communicans bicornis,
cervix duplex,
vagina septa unilateralis atretica
with vagino-vaginal fistula

Type 6
Uterus communicans bicornis,
cervix septa, vagina simplex

Type 7
Uterus communicans bicornis,
cervix septa unilateralis atretica,
vagina simplex

Type 8
Uterus communicans bicornis,
hemicervix una, vagina simplex

Type 9
Uterus bicornis, cervix
communicans septa,
unilateralis atretica,
vagina septa

Figure 11-15 Morphologic classification of communicating uteri. All have an isthmic communication except type 9, which has a low cervical communication. (Reprinted from Toaff ME, Lev-Toaff AS, Toaff R: Communicating uteri: Review and classification with introduction of two previously unreported types. Fertil Steril 41:661, 1984. Copyright 1984, with permission from The American Society for Reproductive Medicine.)

septum. Hysteroscopic resection, the treatment of choice, is easier and in many cases safer. Concurrent laparoscopy is used commonly to visualize the uterus during the procedure. Concurrent laparoscopy also allows for differentiation of a septate uterus from a bicornuate or didelphic uterus. An operating hysteroscope is then used to progressively cut the septum until a cavity with normal-appearing contour is achieved.

After surgical repair, some surgeons may insert an IUD for 30 days, and the patient may be treated with a conjugated estrogen (1.25 mg/day) for 1 month; other physicians prescribe slightly higher doses. This step has not been proved necessary and often can be withheld. This vaginal approach eliminates the need for an abdominal procedure and thus limits the risk of pelvic adhesions, which may interfere with fertility.

The surgical treatment of uterine septa, because of primary infertility, is controversial. Prophylactic cerclage of women with anomalies is not indicated. However, many clinicians recommend transvaginal ultrasound evaluation of the cervix in the second trimester in women with uterine anomalies for the evaluation of cervical competence.

OVARIAN ABNORMALITIES

Accessory Ovary and Supernumerary Ovary

In 1959, Wharton defined **accessory ovary** and **supernumerary ovary**. The former term is used when excess ovarian tissue is noted near a normally placed ovary and connected to it. Supernumerary ovary occurs when a third ovary is separated from the normally situated ovaries. Printz and associates pointed out that such ovaries may be found in the omentum or retroperitoneally, and Hogan and colleagues reported the presence of a dermoid cyst in a supernumerary ovary that occurred in the greater omentum. Wharton estimated that the occurrence of either accessory ovary or supernumerary ovary is quite rare, finding approximately 1 case of accessory ovary per 93,000 patients and 1 case of supernumerary ovary in 29,000 autopsies. In Wharton's review, three of four patients with supernumerary ovary and 5 of 19 patients with accessory ovary had additional congenital defects, most frequently abnormalities of the genitourinary tract.

Ovotestes

Ovotestes are present in individuals with ovaries that have an SRY antigen present. The majority are true hermaphrodites (quite rare). The degree to which Müllerian and mesonephric development occurs depends on the amount of testicular tissue present in the ovotestes and the proximity to the developing duct system. When considerable amounts of testicular tissue are present within the organ, there is a tendency for descent toward the labial scrotal area. Thus, palpation of the gonad in the inguinal canal or within the labial scrotal area is fairly common. Ovulation and menstruation may occur if the Müllerian system is appropriately developed. In a similar fashion, spermatogenesis may occur as well. Where testicular tissue is present, there is an increased risk for malignant degeneration, and these gonads should be removed after puberty. Germ cell tumors, such as gonadoblastomas and dysgerminomas, have been reported in the ovarian portion of ovotestes.

KEY POINTS

- Gender identification in a newborn infant has tremendous emotional influence and should be performed prior to hospital discharge and as accurately as possible.
- Congenital adrenal hyperplasia is an autosomal recessive condition, most commonly the result of an inborn error of metabolism involving the enzyme 21-hydroxylase. Homozygous individuals occur in 1 of every 490 to 67,000 births, averaging 1 in 14,000. Heterozygote carriers are present in 1 in 20 to 1 in 250 individuals. Differences depend on ethnic background of people tested.
- Up to 75% of females with ambiguous genitalia may develop a sodium-wasting adrenal crisis.
- The hymen is the junction of the sinovaginal bulb with the urogenital sinuses and is derived from endoderm.
- Vaginal agenesis is most often associated with Mayer–Rokitansky–Küster–Hauser syndrome. Up to 50% of these women will have urologic abnormalities. Approximately one eighth will have skeletal abnormalities as well.
- Abnormalities of the uterus and cervix may be transmitted as a polygenic or multifactorial pattern of inheritance. They occur in about 2% to 3% of the female population.
- Up to 15% of women with histories of recurrent miscarriage may be found to have anomalies of the uterus.
- Pretherapy pregnancy wastage rates in women with some types of Müllerian anomalies may be as high as 85% to 90%. After surgical repair, the pregnancy efficiency rate may be as high as 80%.
- Accessory ovaries occur in approximately 1 per 93,000 patients. Supernumerary ovaries occur in approximately 1 of every 29,000 women.

REFERENCES CAN BE FOUND ON EXPERTCONSULT.com

12

Pediatric and Adolescent Gynecology
Gynecologic Examination, Infections, Trauma, Pelvic Mass, Precocious Puberty

Ann Jeanette Davis and Vern L. Katz

Gynecologic diseases are uncommon in children, especially compared with the incidence and prevalence of diseases in women of reproductive age. This chapter considers gynecologic diseases of children from infancy through **adolescence**. Congenital anomalies, precocious development, and amenorrhea are covered in more detail in other chapters.

The evaluation of children's gynecologic problems involves considerations of physiology, psychology, and developmental issues that are different from those of adult gynecology. The evaluation of young females is age dependent. For example, the physical presence of the mother often may facilitate examining a 4-year-old girl but may inhibit the cooperation of a 14-year-old adolescent. Thus, the gynecologic physical examination is performed differently in a prepubertal child than in an adolescent of reproductive age or a mature reproductive woman.

An outpatient visit by a prepubertal child to a gynecologist should be structured differently from a gynecologic visit by an adolescent or a reproductive age woman. Considerable effort should be devoted to gaining the child's confidence and establishing rapport. Young girls should feel that they are participating in their examination, not that they are being coerced or forced to have a gynecologic exam. If the interaction is poor during the first visit, the negative experience will detract from future physician-patient interactions.

The pediatric gynecologic visit may be unique to both the child and the parent. Most pediatric visits are preventive in nature. However, the pediatric gynecologic visit is problem oriented. This may create considerable and understandable anxiety in the child and parent. The majority of children's gynecologic problems are treated by medical rather than surgical means.

The most frequent gynecologic disease of children is **vulvovaginitis**. Vulvitis is generally the primary presenting problem, with vaginitis of secondary importance and symptomatology. Other common reasons for a pediatric gynecology visit include **labial adhesions**, vulvar lesions, suspicion of sexual abuse, and genital trauma.

Adolescence is the period of life during which an individual matures physically and begins to transition psychologically from a child into an adult. This period of transition involves important physical and emotional changes. Before **puberty**, the girl's reproductive organs are in a resting, dormant state. Puberty produces dramatic alterations in both the external and the internal female genitalia and hormonal milieu. Because the pubertal changes are frequently a cause of concern for adolescent females and their parents, the gynecologist must offer the adolescent female an empathetic, kind, knowledgeable, and gentle approach. These interactions between the physician and the adolescent female will allow the physician an opportunity to educate the pubertal teenager about pelvic anatomy and reproduction.

GYNECOLOGIC EXAMINATION OF A CHILD

GENERAL APPROACH

A successful gynecologic examination of a child demands that the physician adapt an exam pace that conveys both gentleness and patience with the time spent and not seem to be hurried or rushed. One excellent technique is for the physician to sit, not stand, during the initial encounter. This conveys an unhurried approach. The ambiance of the examining room may decrease the anxiety of the child if familiar and friendly objects such as children's posters are present. Interruptions should be avoided. Speculums and instruments that might frighten a child or parent should be within drawers or cabinets and out of sight during the evaluation. If a child is scheduled to be seen in the middle of a busy clinic, the staff needs to be alerted that the pace and general routine will be different during her visit.

PERFORMANCE OF THE GYNECOLOGIC EXAM IN A CHILD

The components of a complete pediatric examination include a history; inspection with visualization of the vulva, vagina, and cervix; and, if necessary, a rectal examination.

Obtaining a history from a child is not an easy process. Children are not skilled historians and will often ramble, introducing many unrelated facts. Much of the history must be obtained from the parents. However, young children can help define their exact symptomatology on direct questioning. While obtaining a history, an opportunity exists to educate the child on vocabulary to describe the genital area. One way to describe genital area and breasts is to call them "private areas" and define this term as meaning areas that are covered by a bathing suit. The exam also allows a period of opportunity to counsel children, in an age-appropriate manner, about potential sexual abuse.

After the history has been obtained, the parents and the child should be reassured that the examination will not hurt. It is important to give the child a sense that she will be in control of the examination process. A helpful technique is to place the child's hand on top of the physician's hand as the abdominal examination is being performed and to give her some choices such as would she like a doll or toy with her. This will give the child a sense of control as well as divert the child's attention if she is ticklish or is squirming. Emphasize that the most important part of the examination is just "looking" and there will be conversation during the entire process. To successfully examine a child, one needs the cooperation of the patient and a medical assistant.

A child's reaction will depend on her age, emotional maturity, and previous experience with health care providers. She should be allowed to visualize and handle any instruments that will be used. Many young children's primary contact with providers involves immunizations; children should be counseled and assured that this visit does not involve any "shots." It is also helpful to assure the adult that has accompanied the child that adult speculums are not part of the examination.

Occasionally it is best to defer the pelvic examination until a second visit. This is a difficult decision and is based on the extent of the child's anxiety in relation to the severity of the clinical symptoms. Physicians may elect to treat the primary symptoms of vulvovaginitis for 2 to 3 weeks, realizing that on rare occasions they could be missing something more serious. In the field of pediatric gynecology, many errors are errors of omission rather than of commission.

A child should never be restrained for a gynecologic examination. Often reassurance and sometimes delay until another day are the best approach. Sometimes after performing the other elements of the general exam enough rapport has been established that the child will feel safe enough to allow a gynecologic examination. In very rare circumstances, it may be necessary to use continuous intravenous conscious sedation or general anesthesia to complete an essential examination. The most important technique to ensure cooperation is to involve the child as a partner and assure her that shots are not involved. Children should ideally feel they are part of the exam rather than having an "exam done to them."

Draping for the gynecologic examination may produce more anxiety than it relieves and is unnecessary in the preadolescent child. A handheld mirror may help in some instances when discussing specifics of genital anatomy. It is critical to have all tools, culture tubes, and equipment within easy reach during a pediatric genital examination. Children often cannot hold still for long intervals while instruments are being located.

The first aspect of the pelvic examination is evaluation of the external genitalia. An infant may be examined on her mother's lap. Pads should be placed in the mother's lap, as examination often is associated with urination. Young children may be examined in the frog leg position, and children as young as 2 to 3 years of age may be examined in lithotomy with use of stirrups. Lithotomy is generally used for girls 4 to 5 years of age and older.

Once the child is positioned, the vulvar area and introitus should be inspected (**Figs. 12-1** and **12-2**). Many gynecologic conditions in children may be diagnosed by inspection. The introitus will gape open with gentle pressure downward and outward on the lower thigh or undeveloped thigh or labia majora area (**Fig. 12-3**). Asking the child to pretend to blow out candles on a birthday cake may facilitate the process.

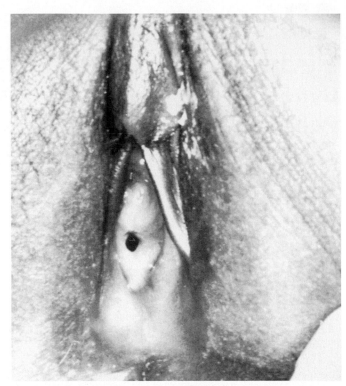

Figure 12-1 Appearance of normal external genitalia of a prepubertal female in the supine position using the lateral spread technique. (From Pokorny SF: Pediatric gynecology. In Stenchever MA [ed]: Office Gynecology, 2nd ed. St. Louis, Mosby, 1996.)

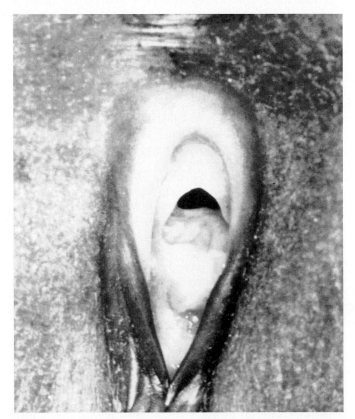

Figure 12-2 The same child shown in Figure 12-1 but in the knee-chest position. (From Pokorny SF: Pediatric gynecology. In Stenchever MA [ed]: Office Gynecology, 2nd ed. St. Louis, Mosby, 1996.)

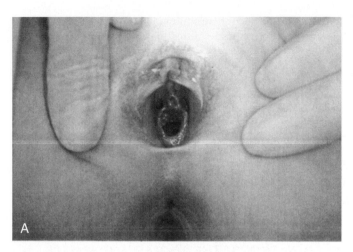

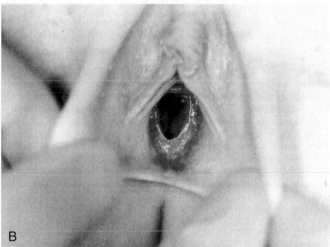

Figure 12-3 Examination of the vulva, hymen, and anterior vagina by gentle lateral retraction **(A)** and gentle gripping of the labia and pulling anteriorly **(B)**. (From Emans SJ: Office evaluation of the child and adolescent. In Emans SJ, Laufer MR, Goldstein DP [eds]: Pediatric and Adolescent Gynecology, 4th ed. Philadelphia, Lippincott-Raven, 1998.)

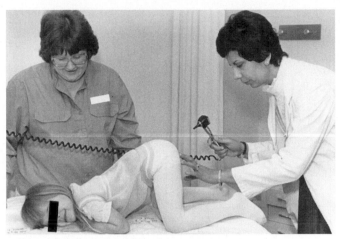

Figure 12-4 Knee-chest position used to examine child to visualize cervix and vagina. The otoscope head is usually longer than one shown in photograph. (From Gidwani GP: Approach to evaluation of premenarchal child with a gynecologic problem. Clin Obstet Gynecol 30:643, 1987.)

The second phase of the examination involves evaluation of the vagina. This can be accomplished without the use of any insertion of instruments. One method is to utilize the knee chest position (**Fig. 12-4**). The child lies prone and places her buttocks in the air with legs wide apart. The vagina will then fill with air, aiding the evaluation. The child is told to have her abdomen sag into the table. An assistant pulls upward and outward on the labia majora on one side while the examiner does the same with the nondominant hand on the contralateral labia. Then an oto ophthalmoscope is used as a magnifying instrument and light source in the examiner's dominant hand. The oto ophthalmoscope *is not* inserted into the vagina.

The light source from the oto ophthalmoscope can be aided by a bright light, which helps to illuminate the vulvar area. The light from the oto ophthalmoscope is shone into the vagina as the examiner evaluates the vaginal walls. The cervix appears as a transverse ridge or flat button that is redder than the vagina. This technique is generally successful in cooperative children unless there is a very high crescent-shaped hymen, in which case it is too difficult to shine the light into the small aperture at the

vaginal introitus. A foreign object and the cervix may be visualized using this technique. Following inspection of the vagina and cervix, vaginal secretions may be obtained for microscopic examination and culture.

NORMAL FINDINGS: HYMEN AND VAGINA OF A PREPUBERTAL CHILD

The hymen of a prepubertal child exhibits a diverse range of normal variations and configurations (**Fig. 12-5**). Hymens are often crescent-shaped but may be annular or ring-like in configuration. There are no reported cases of congenital absence of the hymen. A mounding of hymeneal tissue is often called a bump. Bumps are usually a normal variant and are often attached to longitudinal ridges within the vagina. Hymens in newborns are estrogenized, resulting in a thick elastic redundancy. Older unestrogenized girls will have thin nonelastic hymens.

Prospective studies of hymens in children have demonstrated that complete transactions of the hymeneal tissue between 3 o'clock and 9 o'clock are not congenital but likely acquired. Noncongenital "bumps" may be present near hymeneal transections. The subject of hymens in relation to sexual abuse is covered later in this chapter.

The vaginal epithelium of the prepubertal child appears redder and thinner than the vagina of a woman in her reproductive years. The vagina is 4 to 6 cm long, and the secretions in a prepubertal child have a neutral or slightly alkaline pH. Recurrent vulvovaginitis, persistent bleeding, suspicion of a foreign body or neoplasm, and congenital anomalies may be indications for vaginoscopy. Some clinicians have used very small hysteroscopes in office settings to evaluate these types of problems in children. Introduction of any instrument into the vagina of a young child takes skillful patience. The prepubertal vagina is narrower, thinner, and lacking in the distensibility of the vagina of a woman in her reproductive years.

Vaginoscopy often requires a brief inhalation-anesthesia, but can be performed in the office in very cooperative children in some circumstances. There are many narrow-diameter endoscopes that will suffice, including the Kelly air cystoscope,

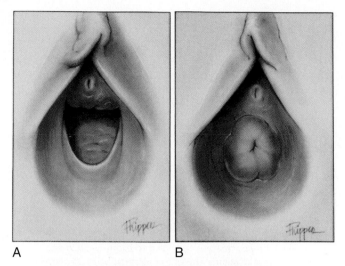

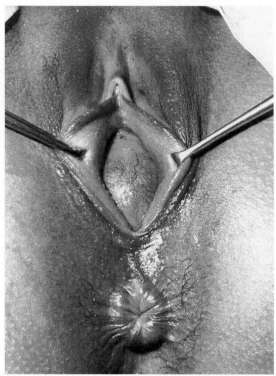

Figure 12-5 Types of hymens in prepubertal girls. **A,** Posterior rim of crescent-shaped hymen. **B,** Fimbriated, or redundant, hymen. **C,** Imperforate hymen. (From Pokorny SF: Configuration of the prepubertal hymen. Am J Obstet Gynecol 157:950, 1987.)

contact hysteroscopes, pediatric cystoscopes, small-diameter laparoscopes, plastic vaginoscopes, and special virginal speculums designed by Huffman and Pederson. The ideal pediatric endoscope is a cystoscope or hysteroscope because the accessory channel facilitates lavage of the vagina. A nasal speculum or otoscope is usually too short for older girls, but it has the advantage of having built-in light sources. Local anesthesia of the vestibule may be obtained with 2% topical viscous lidocaine (Xylocaine) or longer-acting products such as lidocaine/prilocaine. The physician can divert the child's attention from the endoscope in the vagina by simultaneously gently compressing one of the patient's

buttocks, an extinction technique. Vaginal evaluation should never be performed under duress or by force.

The last step in the pelvic examination may be a rectal examination. This is often the most distressing aspect of the examination and may be omitted, depending on the child's symptoms. Common reasons to perform a rectal examination include genital tract bleeding, pelvic pain, and suspicion of a foreign body or pelvic mass. The child should be warned that the rectal examination will feel similar to the pressure of a bowel movement. The normal prepubertal uterus and ovaries are nonpalpable on rectal examination. The relative size ratio of cervix to uterus is 2 to 1 in a child, in contrast to the opposite ratio in an adult. Except for the cervix, any mass discovered on rectal examination in a prepubertal exam should be considered abnormal.

EXAMINATION OF THE ADOLESCENT FEMALE

The critical factors surrounding the pelvic examination of a female adolescent are different from those of examinations of children 2 to 8 years old. Many female adolescents do not want their mother, guardian, or other observers in the examining room. In many adolescent gynecology visits, a full pelvic exam is unnecessary.

Adolescents often come for examinations with preconceived ideas that it will be very painful. Slang terminology for speculums among teens includes the threatening label "the clamp." Teens should be assured that although the exam may include mild discomfort, it is not painful. Providers can counsel patients that they will inform them of each step in the process and then ask the teen if she is ready before performing each step. This places the teen in control of the tempo and allows her to anticipate the next element of the examination. Use of the "extinction phenomenon" may be helpful. The examiner provides pressure lateral to the introitus on the perineum prior to insertion of the speculum.

PROBLEMS IN PREPUBERTAL CHILDREN

Vulvovaginitis

Vulvovaginitis is the most common gynecologic problem in the prepubertal female. It is estimated that 80% to 90% of outpatient visits of children to gynecologists involve the classic symptoms of vulvovaginitis: introital irritation (discomfort/pruritus) or discharge (Table 12-1).

Table 12-1 Clinical Features of Children Presenting with Vulvovaginitis

Features	Number	Percentage
Symptoms		
Itch	81	40
Soreness	108	54
Bleeding	37	19
Discharge	104	52
Signs		
Genital redness	167	84
Visible discharge	66	33
Perianal soiling	35	18
Specific skin lesion	28	14
None	5	2-4

From Pierce AM, Hart CA: Vulvovaginitis: Causes and management. Arch Dis Child 67:509, 1992.

The prepubertal vagina is neutral or slightly alkaline. With puberty the prepubertal vagina becomes acidic under the influence of bacilli dependent on a glycogenated estrogen-dependent vagina. Breast budding is a reliable sign that the vaginal pH is shifting to an acidic environment.

The severity of vulvovaginitis symptoms varies widely from child to child. The pathophysiology of the majority of instances of vulvovaginitis in children involves a primary irritation of the vulva, which may be accompanied by secondary involvement of the lower one third of the vagina. Most cases involve an irritation of the vulvar epithelium by normal rectal flora or chemical irritants. This is referred to as nonspecific vulvovaginitis. In cases that appear to be irrigation of the vulvar epithelium by normal rectal flora, there often are predisposing vulvar irritations from perfumed soaps, tight seams of blue jeans, and the like, which creates denudation, allowing the rectal flora to easily infect the irritated epithelium. Cultures from the vagina return as normal rectal flora or *Escherichia coli*. In a primary care setting, nonspecific vulvovaginitis accounts for the majority of vulvovaginitis cases.

There are both physiologic and behavioral reasons why a child is susceptible to vulvar infection. Physiologically, the child's vulva and vagina are exposed to bacterial contamination from the rectum more frequently than are the adult's. Because the child lacks the labial fat pads and pubic hair of the adult, when a child squats, the lower one third of the vagina is unprotected and open. There is no significant geographic barrier between the vagina and anus. The vulvar and vaginal epithelium lack the protective effects of estrogen and thus are sensitive to irritation or infection. The labia minora are thin and the vulvar skin is red because the abundant capillary network is easily visualized in the thin skin. The vaginal epithelium of a prepubertal child has a neutral or slightly alkaline pH, which provides an excellent medium for bacterial growth. The vagina of a child lacks glycogen, lactobacilli, and a sufficient level of antibodies to help resist infection. The normal vagina of a prepubertal child is colonized by an average of nine different species of bacteria: four aerobic and facultative anaerobic species and five obligatory anaerobic species.

A major factor in childhood vulvovaginitis is poor perineal hygiene (**Table 12-2**). This results from the anatomic proximity of the rectum and vagina coupled with the fact that following toilet training, most youngsters are unsupervised when they defecate. Many youngsters wipe their anus from posterior to anterior and thus inoculate the vulvar skin with intestinal flora. A minor vulvar irritation may result in a scratch-itch cycle, with the possibility of secondary seeding because children wash their hands infrequently. Children's clothing is often tight fitting and nonabsorbent, which keeps the vulvar skin irritated, warm, moist, and prone to vulvovaginitis.

In some cases, nonspecific vulvovaginitis may be caused by carrying viral infections from coughing into the hands directly to the abraded vulvar epithelium. Similarly, a child with an upper respiratory tract infection may autoinoculate her vulva, especially with specific organisms (see **Table 12-2**). Vulvovaginitis in children may also be caused by a variety specific pathogens such as group A or group B β-hemolytic streptococci, *Haemophilus influenzae*, *Neisseria gonorrhoeae*, *Trichomonas vaginalis*, *Chlamydia trachomatis*, and *Shigella boydii*, which result in specific vulvovaginitis (see **Table 12-2**).

Pinworms are another cause of vulvovaginitis in prepubertal children. Approximately 20% of female children infected with pinworms (*Enterobius vermicularis*) develop vulvovaginitis.

Table 12-2 Etiologic Factors of Premenarcheal Vulvovaginitis

Bacterial
A. Nonspecific
 1. Poor perineal hygiene
 2. Intestinal parasitic invasion with pruritus
 3. Foreign bodies
 4. Urinary tract infections with irritation
B. Specific
Bacterial
 1. Group A: β-hemolytic streptococci
 2. *Streptococcus pneumoniae*
 3. *Haemophilus influenzae/parainfluenzae*
 4. *Staphylococcus aureus*
 5. *Neisseria meningitides*
 6. *Escherichia coli*
 7. *Shigella flexneri/sonnei*
 8. Other enterics
 9. *Neisseria gonorrhoeae*
 10. *Chlamydia trachomatis*
Protozoal—*Trichomonas*
Mycotic
 1. *Candida albicans*
 2. Other
Helminthiasis—*Enterobius vermicularis*
Viral/Bacterial Systemic Illness
 1. Chicken pox
 2. Measles
 3. Pityriasis rosea
 4. Mononucleosis
 5. Scarlet fever
 6. Kawasaki disease
Other Viral Illnesses
 1. Molluscum contagiosum in genital area
 2. Condylomata acuminata
 3. Herpes simplex type II
Physical/Chemical Agents
 1. Sandbox
 2. Trauma
 3. Bubble bath
 4. Other
Allergic/Skin Conditions
 1. Seborrhea
 2. Lichen sclerosus
 3. Psoriasis
 4. Eczema
 5. Contact dermatitis
Tumors
Other
 1. Prolapsed urethra
 2. Ectopic ureter

From Blythe MJ, Thompson L: Premenarchal vulvovaginitis. Indiana Med 86:237, 1993.

The classic symptom of pinworms is nocturnal vulvar and perianal itching. At night the milk-white, pin-sized adult worms migrate from the rectum to the skin of the vulva to deposit eggs. They may be discovered by means of a flashlight or by dabbing of the vulvar skin with clear cellophane adhesive tape ideally before the child has arisen in the morning. The tape is subsequently examined under the microscope.

Mycotic vaginal infections are *not* common in prepubertal children, as the alkaline pH of the vagina does not support fungal growth. Mycotic vaginal infections may be seen in immunosuppressed prepubertal girls such as HIV patients or patients on chronic steroid therapy. Other specific causes of vulvovaginitis may include systemic diseases, chicken pox, and herpes simplex infection.

There is nothing specific about the symptoms or signs of childhood vulvovaginitis. Often the first awareness comes when the mother notices staining of the child's underwear or the child complains of itching or burning. There is a wide range in the quantity of discharge, from minimal to copious. The color ranges from white or gray to yellow or green. A discharge that is both bloody and purulent is likely not from vulvovaginitis but from a foreign body (see Prepubertal Bleeding without Signs of Puberty), although patients infected with some pathogens, particularly *Shigella boydii*, often present with a bloody or blood-tinged discharge. The signs of vulvovaginitis are variable and not diagnostic, but they include vulvar erythema, edema, and excoriation.

The differential diagnosis of persistent or recurrent vulvovaginitis not responsive to treatment should include considerations of a foreign body, primary vulvar skin disease, ectopic ureter, and child abuse. If the predominant symptom is pruritus, then pinworms or an irritant/nonspecific vulvitis are the most likely diagnosis.

The vulvar skin of children may also be affected by systemic skin diseases, including lichen sclerosus, seborrheic dermatitis, psoriasis, and atopic dermatitis. The classic perianal "figure-8" or "hourglass" rash is indicative of lichens scleroses with white patches and in some cases blood blisters. An ectopic ureter emptying into the vagina may only intermittently release a small amount of urine; thus, this rare congenital anomaly should be considered in the differential diagnosis in young children.

Treatment of Vulvovaginitis

The foundation of treating childhood vulvovaginitis is the improvement of local perineal hygiene. Both parent and child should be instructed that the vulvar skin should be kept clean, dry, and cool, and irritants should be avoided. For acute weeping lesions, wet compresses of Burrow's solution may be prescribed. The child should be instructed to void with her knees spread wide apart and taught to wipe from front to back after defecation. Loose-fitting cotton undergarments should be worn. Chemicals that may be allergens or irritants, such as bubble bath, must be discontinued. Harsh soaps and chemicals should be avoided.

Most episodes of childhood vulvovaginitis are cured solely by improved local hygiene. The majority of symptoms improve with hygienic changes and sitz baths. Relief of vulvar irritation may be facilitated by using a bland cream, such as zinc oxide creams or cod liver oil creams, both of which are readily available in the infant's sections of drugstores, although studies have not proved this approach. These bland creams should be applied several times per day. Another approach is to utilize very low potency steroid creams, which are available over the counter, or in more severe cases low or medium potency prescription steroid creams. These low-potency steroids, or oral antibiotics given for 10 to 14 days, are often reserved for recalcitrant cases. If, however, the problem is hygiene, then broad-spectrum antibiotics will only offer temporary relief, and the problem is likely to recur.

Vaginal cultures may help to determine the choice of an oral antibiotic. However, cultures usually will not show a specific pathogen. In recurrent cases, a broad spectrum may be appropriate to decrease the *E. coli* inoculums. Dosage of the selected antibiotic depends on the child's weight. One method of obtaining a vaginal culture in children is to use a nasopharyngeal small swab moistened with nonbacteriostatic saline. Pokorny has described another method for collecting fluid from a child's vagina using a catheter within a catheter. This easily assembled adaptation uses a No. 12 red rubber bladder catheter for the outer catheter and the hub end of an intravenous butterfly catheter for the inner catheter (**Fig. 12-6**). The outer catheter serves as an insulator, and the inner catheter is used to instill a small amount of saline and aspirate into the vaginal fluid. The results of the vaginal culture may demonstrate a single organism that is a respiratory, intestinal, or sexually transmitted disease pathogen. The presence of sexually transmitted organisms in a child is usually a strong indication that sexual abuse may have taken place and appropriate referral and follow-up is necessary (see the Sexual Abuse section).

OTHER PREPUBERTAL GYNECOLOGIC PROBLEMS

Labial Adhesions (Sometimes Referred to as Adhesive Vulvitis)

Labial adhesions literally mean the labia minora have adhered or agglutinated together at the midline. Another term sometimes used to describe this condition is *adhesive vulvitis*. Denuded epithelium of adjacent labia minora agglutinates and fuses the two labia together, creating a "flat appearance" of the vulvar surface. A tell-tale somewhat translucent vertical midline line is visible on physical exam at the site agglutination. This thin, narrow line in a vertical direction is pathognomonic for labial adhesions (**Fig. 12-7**). Labial adhesions are often partial and only involve the upper or lower aspects of the labia. Small adhesions are quite common in preschool children, and perhaps as many as 20% will have some degree of labial adhesions on routine examination.

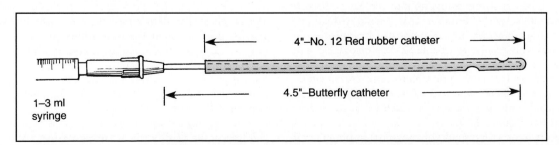

Figure 12-6 Assembled catheter within a catheter, as used to obtain samples of vaginal secretions from prepubertal patients. (Redrawn from Pokorny SF, Stormer J: Atraumatic removal of secretions from the prepubertal vagina. Am J Obstet Gynecol 156:581, 1987.)

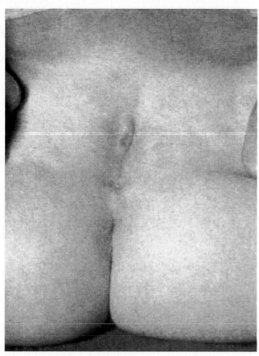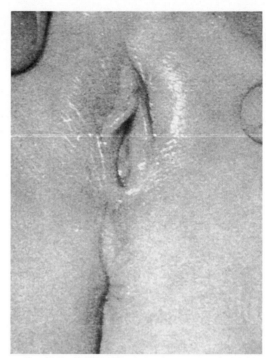

Figure 12-7 A, Labial adhesions in 2½-year-old girl. Two tiny openings exist: one beneath the clitoris and another near the middle of the line of fusion. **B,** Appearance in same child after 10 days of local application of estrogen ointment. (From Dewhurst CJ: Gynaecological Disorders of Infants and Children. Philadelphia, FA Davis, 1963.)

Inexperienced examiners may confuse labial adhesions for an imperforate hymen or vaginal agenesis. Although the physical exam findings are significantly different, all of these conditions may occlude the visualization of the vaginal introitus. In the patient with an imperforate hymen, the labia minora normally appear like an upside down V, and no hymeneal fringe is visible at the introitus. In vaginal agenesis, the hymeneal fringe is typically normal, but the vaginal canal ends blindly behind the hymeneal fringe.

Labial adhesions are most common in young girls between 2 and 6 years of age. Estrogen reaches a nadir during this time, predisposing the nonestrogenized labia to denudation (see **Fig. 12-7**). In one large study, the average age of a child with agglutination of the labia was 2½ years; 90% of cases appeared before age 6.

There is considerable variation in the length of agglutination of the two labia minora. In the most advanced cases, there is fusion over both the urethral and the vaginal orifices. It is extremely rare for this fusion to be complete, and most children urinate through openings at the top of the adhesions, even when the urethra cannot be visualized. However, the partially fused labia may form a pouch in which urine is caught and later dribbled, presenting as incontinence. Associated urinary infections have been reported.

No treatment is absolutely necessary or mandatory for labial adhesions unless the child is symptomatic. Symptoms include voiding difficulties, recurrent vulvovaginitis, discomfort from the labia pulling at the line of adhesions, and in rare cases bleeding from the line of adhesion pulling apart. Jenkinson and Mackinnon published results of a series of 10 girls who had no therapy and noted spontaneous separation of the adhesive vulvitis within 6 to 18 months.

Attempts to separate the adhesions apart in the office by pulling briskly on the labia minora should not be done. It is very painful, and the raw edges are likely to readhese as the child will be reticent to allow application of medication after being subjected to this degree of pain. Some clinicians have also recommended placing local anesthetics on the adhesions and using swabs to tweeze them apart. Many adhesions that would resolve with this therapy are not symptomatic and may not require treatment. However, in rare cases, with small adhesions, this may be appropriate if the local anesthesia (either lidocaine jelly or lidocaine/prilocaine) is completely successful in preventing discomfort. However, it is difficult to predict when and if the pulling will cause discomfort. If discomfort occurs, it is difficult for the child to cooperate with medical intervention.

The most commonly utilized treatment of this condition is topical estrogen cream dabbed onto the labia two times per day at the site of fusion. This will usually result in spontaneous separation, usually in approximately 2 to 8 weeks. In cases when resolution takes longer than several weeks, the clinician can reexamine the patient. If increased pigmentation is noted lateral to the midline line of agglutination, the caregiver should be reinstructed to apply the cream to the line, as the lateral pigmentation indicates the estrogen is being applied lateral to the actual adhesion.

Recurrent labial adhesions occur in one of five children. Once the condition has been resolved, reagglutination can often be prevented by applying a bland ointment (such as zinc oxide cream or petroleum jelly) to the raw epithelial edges for at least one month.

Several authors have reported familial form of true posterior labial fusion. Analysis of the pedigrees of these children suggests that this congenital defect may be an autosomal dominant trait with incomplete penetrance.

McCann and colleagues reported the association between injuries of the posterior fourchette and labial adhesions in sexually abused children. Labial agglutination alone is so common that immediate suspicion of child abuse based solely on this finding in 2- to 6-year-olds is unwarranted. However, the combination of labial adhesions and scarring of the posterior fourchette, especially in children with new-onset labial adhesions after age 6, should prompt the clinician to consider sexual abuse in the differential diagnosis.

Physiologic Discharge of Puberty

In the early stages of puberty, children often develop a physiologic vaginal discharge. This discharge is typically described as having a gray-white coloration, although it may appear slightly yellow but is not purulent. The physiologic discharge represents desquamation of the vaginal epithelium. The estrogenic environment allows acid-producing bacilli to become part of the normal vaginal ecosystem. The acids the bacilli produce cause a desquamation of the prepubertal vaginal epithelium. When the physiologic discharge is examined with the microscope, sheets of vaginal epithelial cells are identified.

Clinically there is usually very little symptomatology associated with this discharge. Occasionally the thickness of the discharge causes the vulva to be "pasted" to undergarments and causes some symptoms of irritation and erythema. Usually the only treatment necessary is reassurance of both mother and child that this is a normal physiologic process that will subside with time. Symptomatic children may be treated with sitz baths and frequent changing of underwear.

Urethral Prolapse

Prolapse of the urethral mucosa is not a rare event in children. The most common presentation is not urinary symptomatology but prepubertal bleeding. Often a sharp increase in abdominal pressure, such as coughing, precedes the **urethral prolapse**. On examination, the distal aspect of urethral mucosa may be prolapsed along the entire 360 degrees of the urethra (**Fig. 12-8**).

This forms a red donut-like structure. The prolapse may be partial or incomplete, presenting as a ridge of erythematous tissue. It is critical to distinguish this from grapelike masses of sarcoma botryoides that originate from the vagina. Occasionally the prolapse becomes necrotic and blue-black in color.

Treatment is conservative and noninteventional. Many experts recommend the application of various medications including estrogen creams and antibiotic ointments. Although such interventions appear appropriate, well-designed prospective studies have not been done to confirm they are therapeutic. Surgery is seldom necessary, except in rare cases where necrosis is obviously present.

Lichen Sclerosus

Lichen sclerosus (LS) or **lichen sclerosus atrophicus**, is a skin dystrophy most commonly seen in postmenopausal women and prepubertal children. The cause is unclear, although there is some evidence that it may be associated with autoimmune phenomena. This has not been confirmed by prospective studies. Histologically there is thinning of the vulvar epithelium with loss of the rete pegs. The most common symptoms are pruritus and vulvar discomfort. Other presentations may include prepubertal bleeding, constipation, and dysuria.

The appearance of LS varies, but lesions are always limited by the labia majora. If lesions go beyond the labia majora, the condition is unlikely to be LS. The lesion often appears in an hourglass or figure-8 formation involving the genital and perianal area (**Fig. 12-9**). The skin may be lichenified with a parchment-like appearance. Parents may note that the genital area appears whitened. Pruritus is typical but not inevitable. In some cases the pruritus is so severe that patients have used hairbrushes

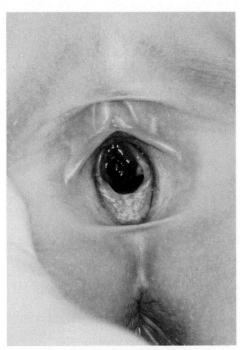

Figure 12-8 Prepubertal urethral prolapse with high crescent-shaped hymen.

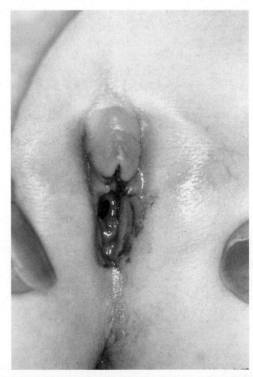

Figure 12-9 Lichen sclerosus atrophicus in prepubertal child with lichenification limited by labia majora and breaks in integument presenting as prepubertal bleeding.

to scratch the area in an attempt to stop the pruritic sensation. Secondary changes may occur subsequent to the patient excoriating the area. When this occurs, there are often blood blisters and breaks in the integument. Patients with blood blisters may present with prepubertal bleeding.

Given the abnormal appearance of LS with secondary changes, clinicians unfamiliar with this skin dystrophy often arrive at the misdiagnosis of sexual abuse. However, clinicians experienced in pediatric or postmenopausal gynecology will usually have no difficulty arriving at the correct diagnosis. In cases where the diagnosis is unclear, a small punch biopsy may confirm the diagnosis. Performing a biopsy in prepubertal children is often difficult. Many children will not tolerate a local injection, and holding down children to perform a biopsy is clearly not acceptable. General anesthesia is preferable in this situation. Rare children will tolerate a biopsy using local anesthesia.

The treatment of LS in children should always start with avoiding irritation or trauma to the genital epithelium. LS is a skin disorder in which lesions are most likely to occur in epithelium that is irritated. Children should be encouraged to avoid straddle activities such as bicycle or tricycle riding when symptomatic. Patients should clean the labia by soaking in sitz baths. Parents sometimes may assume lack of cleanliness is contributing to the disorder and scrub the area with soap, which may actually exacerbate the disease. Tight clothing such as blue jeans may also abrade and irritate the vulva.

In mature reproductive women, clobetasol has become the treatment of choice. This powerful steroid is used for a short duration, given the serious complication of adrenal suppression. The safety of this medication has not been established in children younger than 12 years of age, and use in children is outside product labeling. However, clinicians have had success in treating LS with clobetasol in prepubertal children. Adrenal suppression with clobetasol is likely to be more common in diseases such as psoriasis and atrophic dermatitis in which larger surface areas of skin require treatment. If the clinician elects to use clobetasol in pediatric LS patients, the parents should be counseled regarding the labeling. Tapering the steroid level should be considered as soon as a response is seen or within a 2-week interval. The parents should apply the drug sparingly and, especially given the adrenal suppression issues, not use this on other pediatric skin disorders. Another approach is to reserve this potent steroid for patients in whom the conservative treatment of avoiding trauma and irritation with medium-potency local steroids has not cleared symptomatology.

Previously, many authors have asserted that LS improves with puberty. Though improvement and resolution occur sometimes, many patients will continue to have symptoms or physical findings.

PREPUBERTAL BLEEDING WITHOUT SECONDARY SIGNS OF PUBERTY

Puberty in the female is the process of biologic change and physical development after which sexual reproduction becomes possible. This is a time of accelerated linear skeletal growth and development of secondary sexual characteristics, such as breast development and the appearance of axillary and pubic hair. The usual sequence of the physiologic events of puberty begins with a somatic change: an increase in growth velocity followed by either breast development (thelarche) or the appearance of pubic

hair (adrenarche), followed by the period of maximal growth velocity (approximately 9 cm/year), and, lastly, menarche. Onset of thelarche typically precedes adrenarche in Caucasian girls. In contrast, African American girls often have adrenarche prior to thelarche.

A cross-sectional study of more than 1700 American girls provided contemporary data on pubertal timing (the Pediatric Research in Office Settings [PROS] study). In this study approximately one third of the African-American girls had thelarche or adrenarche at age 7 and almost 50% by age 8. Approximately 15% of Caucasian girls had initiated puberty by age 8 and almost 40% by age 9. Mean ages for thelarche and adrenarche were 8.9 and 8.8 for African-American girls and 10 and 10.5 years for Caucasian girls, respectively. The mean age of menarche was almost 12.2 years for the African-American girls compared with 12.8 years in the Caucasian girls. It should be noted that these ages of pubertal onset were significantly earlier, and sequences somewhat different, than previous, much older, classic descriptions of British children published by Marshall and Tanner.

Recommendations from the PROS have included a new guideline regarding the definition of precocious development. They propose that precocious puberty should be defined as thelarche or adrenarche prior to age 6 in African-American girls or 7 in Caucasian girls. These recommendations are controversial, as some serious pathologic causes (endocrine or CNS) could be overlooked if these guidelines were strictly upheld. Certainly in girls younger than 8 with CNS or behavioral issues, a pathologic etiology of development should be entertained. A common clinical problem that is sometimes mistaken for precocious puberty is prepubertal bleeding in children without any other signs of puberty such as breast development (**Table 12-3**).

Vaginal Bleeding

The normal sequence of puberty is that thelarche precedes menarche. In children with prepubertal bleeding without breast budding, there is almost never an endocrinologic cause, with the exception being a very rare presentation of **McCune-Albright syndrome (polyostotic fibrous dysplasia)**.

The differential diagnosis of vaginal bleeding without pubertal development includes foreign body, vulvar excoriation, lichen sclerosus, shigella vaginitis, separation of labial adhesions, trauma (abuse and accidental), urethral prolapse, and friable genital warts (see **Table 12-2**). Rare causes include malignant

Table 12-3 Differential Diagnosis of Prepubertal Bleeding without Any Breast Development

Foreign object
Genital trauma
Sexual abuse
Lichen sclerosus
Infectious vaginitis (especially from *Shigella*)
Urethral prolapse
Breakdown of labial adhesions
Friable genital warts or vulvar lesions
Vaginal tumor
Rare presentation of McCune–Albright syndrome (typically have breast development)
Isolated menarche (controversial)
Dermatologic conditions with secondary excoriation
Nongenital bleeding; mistaken as genital: rectal and urinary

tumors (sarcoma botryoides and endodermal sinus tumors of the vagina) and an unusual presentation of McCune–Albright syndrome. Lists of the differential diagnosis of prepubertal bleeding often also include accidental estrogen exposure (for example, from ingestion of a mother's birth control pills). However, in reality such exposure would rarely provide enough endometrial stimulation to produce a withdrawal bleed without breast budding. Neonates may develop a white mucoid vaginal discharge or a small amount of vaginal spotting because of the withdrawal of maternal estrogens. The discharge and vaginal spotting are self-limited.

It should be remembered that although the differential diagnosis of prepubertal bleeding includes sexual abuse, most sexually abused children do not have prepubertal bleeding. In some settings, such as emergency departments, it is more likely that prepubertal bleeding is due to sexual abuse than in primary pediatric office or a tertiary referral practice.

Foreign Bodies

Symptoms secondary to a vaginal foreign body are responsible for approximately 4% of pediatric gynecologic outpatient visits. The majority of foreign bodies are found in girls between 3 and 9 years of age. The history is usually not helpful because an adult has not witnessed, nor does the child remember, putting a foreign object into the vagina. Many types of foreign bodies have been discovered; however, the most common are small wads of toilet paper. Other common foreign objects include small, hard objects such as hairpins, parts of a toy, tips of plastic markers, crayons, and sand or gravel. Some of these objects are not radiopaque. When small swabs are used to perform vaginal cultures, the examiner may note an odd sensation of touching something other than vaginal mucosa. Objects such as coins and plastic toys are often easily visible on vaginal examination, especially in the knee-chest position. Foreign bodies may be inserted by children because the genital area is pruritic or when naturally curious children are exploring their bodies.

The classic symptom is a foul, bloody vaginal discharge. However, the discharge is often purulent and without blood. The natural history probably reflects the object initially causing irritation, creating a purulent discharge, and then as the object imbeds itself into the vaginal epithelium, bleeding and spotting may occur. There is often a lag between insertion of the object and the vaginal bleeding. Over time, the foreign body may become partially "buried" or imbedded within the vaginal wall. These imbedded objects are often difficult to remove without discomfort and may require a brief anesthesia.

The presence of unexplained vaginal bleeding is an indication for a vaginoscopy. Especially in children younger than 6 years of age this should be done expeditiously to rule out malignant vaginal tumors. If an object is seen on exam, the clinician may be able, in a cooperative child, to either grasp the object with a forceps or wash the object out by irrigation. The catheter technique described previously may be utilized (see **Fig. 12-6**). Often this is not possible because the child cannot cooperate or because a solid object is imbedded into the vaginal wall. In these cases the object can be removed at vaginoscopy.

Children who insert foreign objects often are "repeat performers." This may be secondary to pain or pruritus in the genital area, and the child uses the object (solid or toilet paper) to rub or scratch the genital area. If the foreign object is toilet paper, then repeat performance may be reduced by having the child use wipes instead of toilet paper.

Shigella Vaginitis

Approximately half of all cases of shigella vaginitis present with prepubertal bleeding. There is generally no concurrent gastrointestinal symptomatology. Cultures for *Shigella* should be strongly considered in any child with no obvious cause for prepubertal bleeding. Rarely, vaginitis caused by other organisms can also present with prepubertal bleeding.

Rare Causes: Vaginal Tumors and McCune–Albright Syndrome

McCune–Albright syndrome is a rare somatic mutation that occurs during embryogenesis in neural crest cells. Because the mutation does not occur in the germline, it is not inherited. The mutation affects G protein receptors and has a quite variable expression, depending on how many early cells are affected (an example of mosaicism). The *GNAS1* gene is the affected area. The syndrome may be manifested by the classic triad of café-au-lait spots, abnormal bone lesions, and precocious puberty. Most McCune–Albright patients present with prepubertal bleeding along with thelarche. Rarely a child may present with bleeding and no breast budding. Examination of the child with prepubertal bleeding should include examination of the skin for café-au-lait spots, and the historical intake should include queries about frequent bone fractures. In cases of unexplained prepubertal bleeding, the possibility of McCune–Albright should be considered, and serial breast examinations may reveal breast budding.

Sarcoma Botryoides and Endodermal Sinus Tumors of the Vagina

Almost all cases of sarcoma botryoides of the vagina in prepubertal children occur prior to age 6 (although cases up until age 8 have been reported), and endodermal sinus tumors occur prior to age 2. Although these tumors are extremely rare causes of prepubertal bleeding, they must be considered in every young child. Both are aggressive malignancies and prompt diagnosis is critical. In young children with no evident cause of prepubertal bleeding, a vaginoscopy should be done to rule out these malignancies.

Vaginoscopy for Prepubertal Bleeding without Signs of Puberty

Many times no clear cause of prepubertal bleeding is defined at vaginoscopy. In these cases there likely was a small foreign object that has been expelled from the vagina or disintegrated. Even though many vaginoscopies are negative, it is especially important for clinicians to perform them promptly in young prepubertal bleeders to exclude the rare but very aggressive vaginal malignancies.

ACCIDENTAL GENITAL TRAUMA

The usual cause of accidental genital trauma during childhood is a fall. Seventy-five percent of accidental trauma to the vulva and vagina involves straddle injuries. Obviously, sexual abuse is an important consideration in the differential diagnosis. Sexual abuse is discussed later in this chapter.

VULVAR TRAUMA: LACERATIONS AND STRADDLE INJURY

One of the most common causes of genital trauma in a child is a straddle injury. This problem occurs when a child stands, or hovers, with her legs apart over a hard object and then falls with the perineum against the object. Common straddle injuries in children occur on playground climbing structures, such as a monkey bar, or fence rails. A straddle injury generally results in unilateral and superficial injury and very rarely involves the hymen. In two separate series involving more than 130 children with straddle injuries, only 3 had hymeneal transection.

In cases of hymeneal transection with a history of straddle injury, sexual abuse should be strongly considered. In the rare cases where the hymen is transected from accidental trauma, there is usually a history of a penetrating injury such as falling onto a stick horse or broom. If hymeneal transection has occurred, the examiner must confirm that the object has not penetrated into the vaginal wall, which could result in a dangerous hematoma, perforation into the cul-de-sac, or perforation of the abdominal cavity with potential visceral damage. A vaginoscopy or laparoscopy (or both) is generally required to rule out these possibilities. Perforations into the abdomen may not result in significant vaginal bleeding.

In children presenting with trauma and genital bleeding, the examiner must first ascertain the site, extent, and amount of bleeding. Viscous lidocaine or a longer-acting topical agent such as lidocaine/prilocaine can be applied and allowed appropriate time to provide anesthesia. Then the area can be gently washed by irrigating with sterile warmed water onto the labial area. Typical lacerations may involve denudation around the urethra or labia. The posterior fourchette is less commonly involved. In children with vulvar trauma, considerations should be given to giving a booster injection of tetanus toxoid if the last immunization was more than 5 years before the trauma.

Lacerations that are superficial (equivalent to first-degree obstetric lacerations) generally do not require repair in contrast to deeper lacerations. Often, superficial lacerations can be adequately treated by applying oxidized cellulose or similar products to stop the bleeding. Slightly deeper lacerations can be repaired with small Steri-Strips. In some deeper lacerations, one well-placed suture will stop substantial bleeding. This scenario is typical of lacerations on the inferior aspect of the labia minora. Placement of the suture may be aided by injection of lidocaine in cooperative children.

General anesthesia is usually required for diagnosis and treatment of extensive lacerations and deep lacerations or in children who are unable to tolerate repair in the office or emergency department. During this anesthesia, the laceration should be irrigated and débrided, the vessels ligated, and the injuries repaired. Occasionally it is necessary to perform laparoscopy or an exploratory celiotomy for a suspected retroperitoneal hematoma or intraabdominal injury.

Vulvar Hematomas

If the vulva strikes a blunt object, a hematoma usually results. The lack of the mature reproductive woman's fat pad in the vulvar area predisposes a young child to bleeding from trauma. If the object is sharp, such as a fence post or skating blade, the injury may be a laceration with the potential for penetration of the perineum and injury to internal pelvic organs. Other common

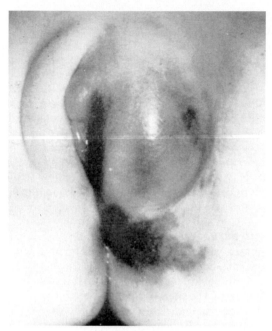

Figure 12-10 Vulvar hematoma resulting from a kick in a 2-year-old child. (From Huffman JW: The Gynecology of Childhood and Adolescence, 2nd ed. Philadelphia, WB Saunders, 1981.)

causes of vulvar and vaginal trauma include sexual abuse, automobile and bicycle accidents, kicks sustained in a fight, and self-inflicted wounds (**Fig. 12-10**).

The size of vulvar and vaginal hematomas varies widely. Initially there is bleeding into the loose connective tissue. When the pressure from the expanding hematoma exceeds the venous pressure, in most cases the hematoma will stop growing. In the majority of cases, surgical exploration should be avoided. It is rare to find a specific vessel to ligate except in cases where the hematoma is quickly expanding over 1 to 2 minutes of observation, which likely represents a rare arterial laceration. The extent of the hematoma should be determined by both visualization and palpation. The treatment of nonexpanding vulvar hematomas is observation by serial examinations and the use of an ice pack or cool sitz bath and pain medications. Patients may have difficulty voiding secondary to urethral injury or because they are anxious to void onto abraded vulvar surfaces or secondary to urinary obstruction or a urinary injury.

SEXUAL ABUSE

Sexual abuse in reproductive women is covered in Chapter 10 (in the section titled Rape, Incest, and Domestic Violence). This chapter contains information specifically related to sexual abuse in the prepubertal child. For a detailed and complete description of evaluation and treatment of the potentially sexually abused child, practitioners should refer to the American Academy of Pediatrics guidelines (published in 2005) and the Sexually Transmitted Diseases Treatment Guidelines from the Center for Disease Control. These documents also contain a detailed table that describes the implications of commonly encountered sexually transmitted or sexually associated infections in the diagnosis and reporting of sexual abuse in children.

Scope of the Problem

Unfortunately, the sexual abuse of children is extremely common in the United States. Estimates indicate that approximately 20% of girls are involved in some type of sexual activity during childhood. Globally this number is even higher, with approximately one fourth of all girls victimized sexually during childhood. Although abduction cases with subsequent sexual abuse by a person unknown to the family attract national media coverage, this scenario is rare. Most perpetrators are male acquaintances known and trusted by the families. Fathers are responsible approximately 21% of the time and other male relatives 19% of the time. It is often not appreciated that mothers are involved 4% to 8% of the time. Babysitting is a common modus operandi for abusers to gain access to children.

History in Sexual Abuse

There are two situations in which health care providers need to garner information regarding potential sexual abuse. One is the child or family that presents with potential sexual abuse as the chief complaint. The other situation is when the child is seen for another complaint, such as a purulent discharge, but the provider considers the possibility of sexual abuse based on historical information or physical examination.

Telephone calls regarding potential sexual abuse are a challenge for practitioners. Urgent evaluation is necessary if the abuse has occurred within 72 hours (for forensic evidence), if the child is currently in a danger of repeated abuse or self-harm, or for obvious injuries such as lacerations require treatment. If none of these criteria are encountered, the child and her family can be evaluated on a nonurgent basis. This is important, because specially trained personnel should become involved as soon as possible in these situations. In many settings these children can be referred to a sexual abuse team on a nonemergency basis. In settings where teams are not available, it is critical that practitioners are aware of other community resources. If at all possible, it is usually ideal that the child and family be interviewed separately by a qualified mental health provider (such as a social worker or psychologist) who is experienced in evaluating sexual abuse. Guidelines have been published on appropriate methods of interviewing children who may be victims of sexual abuse. Often state departments of children's services or the social work department of the community hospital can refer providers to appropriate mental health providers.

Unless there are compelling medical reasons, this interview should be performed prior to a genital examination. There are several reasons for this recommendation. First, latency age children may not be able to separate the exam from touching involved in abuse, making the history more difficult to obtain. Second, in the majority of abused children the exam is completely normal. It is important that families not rely on an exam to decide whether to seek counseling or intervention that would keep their child safe. Although providers should ask relevant questions, the more complete interview by an experienced mental health provider minimizes repetitive questioning of the child. The interview may also allow rapport to begin between the mental health professional doing the interview and the family so that the relationship can transit into therapy if indicated.

Practitioners may also consider sexual abuse based on historical complaints or physical examination findings. In this situation it is critical for the provider to query the guardian or parent in a nonthreatening manner. The approach should be "we are all on the same team and we both want to ensure the safety of your child." Queries directed to the child should be open ended and nonjudgmental. Leading questions should be avoided.

Legal Issues in Reporting Possible Sexual Abuse

Providers must be aware of their state's laws and how to file a report alleging sexual abuse. Every state requires that suspected and known child abuse be reported. The word *suspected,* however, deserves definition. *Isolated* complaints that may be associated with sexual abuse (e.g., nightmares or genital bleeding) often do not require a report. Clinicians may suspect sexual abuse based on a variety of historical complaints and physical exam findings. Consideration to other causes of these complaints and findings is also critical. For example, in children who present with genital bleeding, the differential diagnosis may also include urethral prolapse, foreign bodies, and lichen sclerosus, vaginal tumors, or nonabusive trauma.

If a provider is unsure if a report is required, he or she should discuss the situation with local child protective services or a social worker. These professionals can help providers avoid filing vague unnecessary reports, which clog the services of overburdened state agencies. They can also aid in filing reports in borderline cases that justify exploration to obtain safety of children. In addition, discussion with agencies may help protect providers from prosecution for failure to report. It is important to document discussions in patient charts. Guidelines have been developed by the American Academy of Pediatrics regarding appropriate filing of abuse reports. Providers should not be hesitant to file because of fear of liability for an alleged false report. Although suits have been filed against physicians, states generally ensure immunity, and as of 2005, no such suits have been successful. It should, however, be noted that there have been successful malpractice actions against providers who have failed to diagnose or report sexual abuse.

Physical Examination and Evaluation for Sexually Transmitted Infections

The exam of a potentially sexually abused child should include a general exam. Attention should be directed at evaluating skin for bruising, lacerations, or trauma. Parents or concerned adults should be counseled that a genital exam in children who have been abused is usually normal. Physical evidence is present in less than 5% of children. The genital exam should be carried out as described earlier in this chapter. In addition, a thorough physical exam looking for signs of physical abuse must be documented in the chart.

In situations in which abuse has occurred within 72 hours, careful collection of forensic evidence is important. Collection of all clothing and undergarments is critical. Approximately two thirds of forensic evidence is obtained from linens and clothing. Motile sperm will be present in the prepubertal vagina for approximately 8 hours, and nonmotile sperm for approximately 24 hours. Since prepubertal children do not have cervical mucous, sperm do not exist for the longer durations seen in reproductive females within the cervical canal. "Rape" kits will also often include testing for a protein specific to the prostate. Vaginal specimens may be obtained by using small swabs within the vagina, similar to the method described for obtaining vaginal cultures.

Given that only approximately 5% of abused children acquire a sexually transmitted infection (STI), providers must decide when STI testing is indicated. Both gonorrhea and chlamydia cause a vaginitis not a cervicitis in prepubertal children, so a vaginal culture should be done. In the United States, a vaginal *culture* for gonorrhea and chlamydia, not DNA testing, should be performed as recommended by the Centers for Disease Control and Prevention. There are several issues with the nucleic-acid amplification tests that are commonly used in reproductive females. Because nonculture methods are not labeled for use in children, positive testing may not be admissible in court. The prevalence of gonorrhea and chlamydia in children is usually lower than in appropriately screened adolescents and adults; therefore, the actual positive predictive values of a positive test are lower.

Testing in prepubertal children is also influenced by typical incubation intervals of STIs. If a child was abused in an isolated incident, an STI may not be found on testing immediately after the abuse. However, a purulent discharge would prompt testing and be a red flag for possible ongoing abuse rather than an isolated incident.

In children presenting in nonacute presentations, the provider must decide whether to perform testing for STIs. It is rare for a child to have gonorrhea or chlamydia without a vaginal discharge. Standards of care regarding this issue may differ in various locations.

Hymens in the Evaluation of Sexual Abuse

There is a general misunderstanding regarding the significance of hymeneal changes. The transverse diameter of the hymen was previously used as a marker of abuse. However, it is now clear that there is significant variation in children, and the state of the hymen it is not a reliable marker of abuse. Complete transections of the hymen and clefts that extend to the junction of the hymen between 3 o'clock and 9 o'clock are not congenital, but if present they could be from abuse or a child inserting an object. Controversies exist as to the significance of incomplete transections (**Fig. 12-11**).

Genital Warts

Human papillomavirus (HPV), the causative agent of genital warts, may be transmitted to children from the maternal genital tract at delivery or by sexual or nonsexual transmission after

birth. The incubation interval from transmission to the presence of visible genital warts has not been defined in children; however, it appears likely that most warts appearing prior to approximately 3 years of age are from maternal-child transmission. If the child is 3 years of age or older, serious consideration should be given to the possibility of sexual transmission (see the previous section on sexual abuse in this chapter). However, genital warts "discovered" in a 4-year-old may have been present for some time prior to being noticed. This is particularly a problem in the perianal area, which may not be examined carefully even in children undergoing a cursory genital exam as part of well-child annual care.

Approximately half of lesions will regress over 5 years. Expectant management is reasonable, but parents may prefer treatment. Treatment in children is difficult. Caustic treatments such as trichloroacetic acid are painful even if children are pretreated with local anesthesia. Topical imiquimod cream is labeled for use in children 12 years and older and can cause significant vulvar irritation. If the child accidentally carries imiquimod cream to the cornea, it could cause damage to the eye. Laser treatment is an option for significant wart tissue but must be performed under an inhalation anesthesia and can be associated with significant postoperative pain.

THE OVARY AND ADNEXA IN PEDIATRIC AND ADOLESCENT GYNECOLOGY: CYSTS, TUMORS, AND TORSION

Most ovarian masses in this age group are functional ovarian cysts, and if a tumor is present it most often is a benign teratoma (dermoid). Malignancies can, however, occur and are most often of germ cell origin, but they can also be sex cord tumors such as a granulosa cell malignancy.

Physiologic and functional cysts of the ovaries are from gonadotropin stimulation of the follicles. They may present in the fetus, newborn, infant, at puberty, and in adolescence. The appropriate management may depend on the age and on the appearance of the cyst on ultrasound. Cysts of follicular development will be clear without significant solid components and almost always are less than 7 to 10 cm in size in reproductive adolescents. Management of adolescent functional cysts is essentially the same as the management in reproductive females. Cysts in neonates can generally be observed with resolution. Neonates and children can be observed for any signs of torsion and told to seek immediate medical attention, unless they have exceptionally large cysts. Torsion can certainly occur and is not rare. Many neonatal cysts were initially identified on antenatal ultrasound. There are few studies, all with small numbers, regarding the natural history of antenatal or neonatal ovarian cysts. Cysts during the preschool and early grade school years are unusual, reflecting that gonadotrophins are low.

Corpus luteum cysts are often more complex than other follicular cysts. Management is similar to that in mature reproductive women, and observation is warranted unless signs of malignancy are present. Consideration should be given to dermoids and the possibility of germ cell tumors if a mass has both solid and cystic components. In rare cases of intersex such as mixed gonadal dysgenesis, suspicion of malignancy should be high. A rare presentation of hypothyroidism is pediatric ovarian cysts.

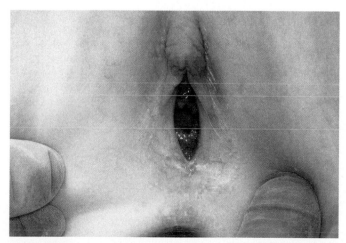

Figure 12-11 Hymenal bump alongside of an incomplete transection of the hymen at approximately 7 to 8 o'clock.

Prenatal Ovarian Cysts

Obstetric ultrasound of a female fetus occasionally demonstrates a simple abdominal cyst. Before a diagnosis of an ovarian cyst is made, it is critical to exclude urinary or gastrointestinal anomalies. Fetal malignancy is quite rare.

There is controversy regarding the management of large antenatal cysts. Antenatal aspiration for the large antenatal cyst (4 centimeters or more) has been proposed by some to avoid potential antenatal torsion. The obvious disadvantage is the risk of the antenatal surgery and the fact that resolution is a typical clinical course. Size and appearance enter heavily into management decisions; for example, if the cyst seems to be wandering about the abdomen on repetitive ultrasounds, it may be of greater risk of torsion. Also, very large cysts (probably greater than 9 cm) would require cesarean sections.

The natural history of both antenatal and neonatal cysts is difficult to define. Data generated from a few small series may be misleading, as the outcome may be dependent on size, mobility, and how the cyst first presented. Presence of what appears to be torsion may not result in the loss of an ovary. The relative rarity of congenital absence of one ovary makes it likely that untwisting occurs. The incidence of congenital unilateral ovarian agenesis is quite rare, perhaps as rare as 1 in approximately 10,000 females. Ovarian malignancy is extremely rare in this age group and is not a consideration in the therapeutic approach.

Neonatal Ovarian Cysts

Simple cystic ovarian masses in newborns and neonates can be followed expectantly. Parents should be given ovarian torsion warnings, and if the infant presents with acute vomiting or abdominal pain, she should be immediately evaluated for ovarian torsion. Repeat serial ultrasonography should be performed approximately monthly until the cyst resolves. Almost all will resolve if they do not undergo torsion. Malignancy is not a consideration in newborns in the therapeutic approach. Aspiration is a possibility for large cysts.

Ovarian Cysts in Children and Adolescents

The management of cystic ovarian structures in children and adolescents should also be expectant unless they are extremely large, in which case the possibility of functional cysts becomes more unlikely. Many times physiologic and functional cysts are discovered on an abdominal ultrasound performed for complaints such as abdominal pain. Often the presence of a cyst is incidental and unrelated to the complaint. However, in patients with pain, the possibility of ovarian torsion should be entertained. Pain from ovarian cysts generally stems from three sources: (1) expansion of the ovarian cortex (which is typically during the growth phase of follicles and lasts less than 72 hours), (2) peritoneal bleeding from rupture (particularly common in bleeding disorders and patients on warfarin, and (3) ovarian torsion. These causes of pain do not typically present as chronic pelvic abdominal pain.

Ovarian Tumors in Childhood and Adolescents

Various tumors, both benign and malignant, can be seen in the childhood and adolescent years. These should always be considered, particularly in patients with solid ovarian masses or cystic and solid components on ultrasound. The diagnosis should also be considered in patients with presumed functional ovarian cysts that do not resolve during serial monitoring.

Germ cell tumors are the most common gynecologic neoplasm in this age group, and fortunately most are benign ovarian teratomas. The most common malignant germ cell tumor is the dysgerminoma followed by endodermal sinus tumors. These tumors are covered in detail in Chapter 33 (Neoplastic Diseases of the Ovary), but several issues are especially pertinent to children and adolescents.

Bilaterality is seen in 10% to 15% of dysgerminomas, but it is rare in all of the other germ cell tumors of the ovary except for immature teratomas. Sex cord tumors, such as granulosa and thecal cell tumors, can also be seen in this age group and often produce steroids. Rare tumors such as gonadoblastomas, a germ cell and sex cord tumor, are seen in patients with intersex disorders such as mixed gonadal dysgenesis.

Recurrent abdominal pain is a frequent complaint of grammar school–age children, and this common symptom occasionally is the presenting problem with ovarian neoplasia. The young child does not differentiate lower abdominal pain from pelvic pain. Because of the small size of the preadolescent female pelvis, the ovaries are abdominal organs. Thus, increasing abdominal girth is a frequent symptom associated with ovarian enlargement.

The most common clinical manifestation of an ovarian tumor is lower abdominal pain or the presence of a mass. Some ovarian tumors in children produce only vague discomfort, such as abdominal fullness or bloating. However, adnexal masses in children are more frequently associated with acute complications, such as torsion, hemorrhage, and rupture, than are similar tumors in adults.

Ovarian tumors constitute approximately 1% of all neoplasms in premenarcheal children. Ultrasound, abdominal computed tomography (CT), or magnetic resonance imaging (MRI) may be utilized in the evaluation of a possible pelvic mass or abdominal pain of uncertain origin in children. Abdominal ultrasonography may be used to establish that the origin of the mass is in the pelvis, whether the mass is cystic or solid, and the presence of ascites. Calcifications in an ovarian mass may appear tooth-like, indicating a diagnosis of ovarian teratoma.

As part of the preoperative workup, the child may be screened for elevated serum levels of tumor markers such as α-fetoprotein, human chorionic gonadotropin (HCG; both alpha and beta), inhibin, lactate dehydrogenase, estradiol, and testosterone; tumor markers that are associated with various ovarian neoplasms are also seen in girls. HCG may be positive for either the α or the β subunit, so a pregnancy test that only tests for the β subunit is inadequate.

Ovarian tumors in preadolescent females, both benign and malignant, are usually unilateral. Thus, it is imperative to be as conservative as possible in managing the opposite ovary in order to protect potential future fertility. During surgery the opposite ovary should be carefully inspected and palpated. It is generally unnecessary and potentially harmful to perform a biopsy on a normal-appearing contralateral ovary in a preadolescent female. This is especially true in patients with dermoids. Appropriate exceptions to this rule include consideration of performing a wedge biopsy in patients with dysgerminoma or an immature teratoma—malignancies in which bilaterality is not as rare.

Children with suspected ovarian cancer should be referred to specialists who are up to date on current data from the Pediatrics Oncology Group or Gynecologic Oncology Group. First, these groups will be skilled in getting their patients proper staging procedures, including lymph node sampling and omentectomy.

In addition, the standard of care is for patients with nondysgerminomas, with a few exceptions, to receive postoperative adjuvant chemotherapy. Use of tumor markers to help differentiate patients with benign teratoma from malignancies is helpful in triaging appropriate referrals. However, regardless of what the makers show, referral is prudent.

Approximately 75% to 85% of ovarian neoplasms that necessitate surgery in premenarcheal females are benign, and approximately 15% to 25% are malignant neoplasms. The risk is less in young children. In a review of ovarian masses in children, Brown and coworkers reported that the risk of malignancy was only 3% up to age 8.

In summary, even though ovarian neoplasia is rare in children, this diagnosis must be considered in a young girl with abdominal pain and a palpable mass. The surgical therapy should have two goals: first, and most important, the appropriate surgical procedure including lymph nodes as necessary, and, second, preservation of future fertility. The traditional hysterectomy performed in adults with epithelial ovarian cancers is not necessary even in rare cases of bilateral childhood or adolescent ovarian malignancy. The uterus should be retained for fertility, which may be possible through artificial reproductive technology such as the use of donor eggs.

Ovarian Torsion

Ovarian torsion is covered in more detail in Chapter 18 (Benign Gynecologic Lesions). Issues unique to children and adolescents are covered in this discussion. Torsion in prepubertal females may be secondary to a pelvic mass or due to mechanical factors that occur in the peripubertal interval. In early puberty, the ovaries drop from their prepubertal position at the pelvic brim into the pelvis. This drop occurs under the influence of gonadotropins that surge at puberty. Some young women may have longer supportive ligaments, predisposing them to twisting. Approximately two thirds of the time, ovarian torsion occurs on the right side, increasing the likelihood of the process being confused with appendicitis. The sigmoid colon in the left lower quadrant helps prevent the left ovary from twisting.

Although both appendicitis and torsion can present with acute pain and rebound, the gradual progression of appendicitis is quite different from the acute severe pain of torsion. Nausea and emesis often ensue immediately with torsion, owing to the severity of the pain. Appendicitis tends to present with anorexia, which gradually worsens. The young girl with an acute onset of pain and simultaneous emesis likely has ovarian torsion rather than appendicitis.

Approximately one third of ovarian torsion cases in children and adolescents are not associated with a predisposing ovarian mass such as a dermoid, large functional cyst, or malignancy. Nevertheless, even in children without an ovarian mass, after torsion the ovary will become swollen and enlarged as the lymphatic flow is blocked. In children and adolescents, the differentiation between torsion and appendicitis is a common dilemma. Radiologic evaluation to rule out appendicitis may reveal a pelvic mass, and the appropriate diagnosis of torsion is defined. The presence of vascular flow in the ovary does not rule out torsion, and in fact many cases of surgically proved torsion will have had normal vascular flow on ultrasound evaluation.

KEY POINTS

- In the field of pediatric gynecology, most diagnostic errors result from errors of omission during the examination rather than errors of commission.
- It is important to give the child a sense that she will be in control of the examination process. Emphasize that the most important part of the examination is just "looking" and that there will be conversation during the entire process.
- Many gynecologic conditions in children can be diagnosed by inspection alone.
- The vaginal epithelium of the prepubertal child appears redder and thinner than the vaginal epithelium of a woman in her reproductive years. The prepubertal vagina is also narrower, thinner, and lacking in the distensibility of the vagina of a reproductively mature woman. The vagina of a child is 4 to 5 cm long and has a neutral pH.
- During the physical examination and rectal examination of the prepubertal child, no pelvic masses except the cervix should be palpable. The normal prepubertal uterus and ovaries are nonpalpable. The relative size ratio of cervix to uterus is 2 to 1 in a child.
- Many female adolescents do not want other observers, such as mothers, in the examining room.
- It is estimated that 80% to 90% of outpatient visits of children to gynecologists involve the classic symptoms of vulvovaginitis: introital irritation and discharge.
- Positive identification of gonorrhea, or chlamydia in a child with premenarcheal vulvovaginitis is considered diagnostic

of sexual molestation. However, many infants are infected with *Chlamydia trachomatis* during birth and remain infected for up to 2 to 3 years in the absence of specific antibiotic therapy.
- The major factor in childhood vulvovaginitis is poor perineal hygiene.
- A vaginal discharge that is both bloody and foul smelling strongly suggests the presence of a foreign body.
- In the period from 6 to 12 months around the time of puberty, children often develop a physiologic discharge secondary to the increase in circulating estrogen levels.
- The foundation of treating childhood vulvovaginitis is the improvement of local perineal hygiene.
- The majority of cases of persistent or recurrent nonspecific vulvovaginitis respond to improved hygiene and treatment of irritation resulting from trauma or irritating substances.
- The classic symptom of pinworms (*Enterobius vermicularis*) is nocturnal vulvar and perianal itching, the treatment for which is the antihelmintic agent, mebendazole.
- The most common vaginal foreign body in preadolescent females is a wad of toilet tissue.
- Persistent vaginal bleeding is an extremely rare symptom in a preadolescent female. However, it is important to do a thorough workup because of the serious sequelae of some of the causes of vaginal bleeding.
- Labial adhesions do not require treatment unless they are symptomatic or voiding is compromised. If necessary, small

amounts of daily topical estrogen to the labia may be used for treatment.

- The usual cause of genital trauma during childhood is an accidental fall. Most such traumas involve straddle injuries.
- Accidental genital trauma often produces extreme pain and overwhelming anxiety for the child and her parents. Because of compassion and empathy, the gynecologist may underestimate the extent of the anatomic injuries.
- Small follicular cysts in preadolescent females and are usually self-limiting.
- Ovarian tumors constitute approximately 1% of all neoplasms in premenarcheal children. In preadolescent females, both benign and malignant ovarian tumors are usually unilateral. Routine biopsy of the contralateral ovary should be avoided. Possible exceptions to this rule are dysgerminomas and immature teratomas.
- Approximately 75% to 85% of ovarian neoplasms necessitating surgery are benign, with cystic teratomas being the most common.
- The most common malignancy in preadolescent females is a germ cell tumor.
- Even though ovarian neoplasia is rare in children, this diagnosis must be considered in a young girl with abdominal pain and a palpable mass. The surgical therapy should have two goals: foremost, removal of the neoplasm and appropriate staging and, secondly, preservation of future fertility.

REFERENCES CAN BE FOUND ON EXPERTCONSULT.com

SUGGESTED READING

American College of Obstetricians and Gynecologists: *Guidelines for women's health care,* 2007.

Bacon JL: Prepubertal labial adhesions: Evaluation of a referral population, *Am J Obstet Gynecol* 187:327, 2002.

Kellogg, American Academy of Pediatrics Committee on Child Abuse and Neglect: The evaluation of sexual abuse in children, *Pediatrics* 116:506–512, 2005.

Pokorny SF, Pokorny WJ, Kramer W: Acute genital injury in the prepubertal girl, *Am J Obstet Gynecol* 166:1461, 1992.

Valerie E, Gilchrist BF, Frischer J, et al: Diagnosis and treatment of ureteral prolapse in children, *Urology* 54:1082, 1999.

13

Family Planning
Contraception, Sterilization, and Pregnancy Termination

Jeffrey T. Jensen and Daniel R. Mishell, Jr.

Contraception represents a preventive health measure with profound intergenerational importance. Reversible contraception is defined as the *temporary* prevention of fertility and includes all the currently available contraceptive methods except **sterilization**. Sterilization should be considered a *permanent* prevention of fertility control even though both vasectomy and tubal interruption can usually be reversed by a meticulous surgical procedure. The reversible methods are also called *active methods,* and sterilization is also called a *terminal method.*

Unintended **pregnancy** occurs because of nonuse of contraception or the failure of a contraceptive method. A perfect method of contraception suitable for all individuals is not currently available and probably will never be developed. Because each of the currently available methods of contraception has distinct advantages and disadvantages, clinicians should explain to the woman or couple the unique features of each method, so they will be fully informed and can rationally choose the method most suitable for them. Because no reversible male contraceptive method other than condoms has been marketed, the health risks and benefits of contraception largely affect women. The contraceptive provider must evaluate whether medical contraindications to a particular method exist for an individual woman and offer her safe and effective alternatives. However, risks are not confined to contraception use, and the health risks associated with unintended pregnancy resulting from the nonuse of contraception or the use of an ineffective method must always be considered in the medically challenging patient.

CONTRACEPTIVE USE IN THE UNITED STATES

The most recently published vital statistics data from the Centers for Disease Control document about 6.4 million pregnancies in the United States in 2004. The estimated pregnancy rate for U.S. women was 103/1000 women aged 15 to 44 years in 2004, and the overall rate has ranged from 102 to 104/1000 since 1995. About two thirds (4.1 million) of these pregnancies resulted in live births, and about one fifth (1.2 million) were terminated by elective abortion. The remainder ended in spontaneous abortion or ectopic pregnancy. According to Finer and Henshaw's review of the 2002 National Survey of Family Growth, about half of the 6.4 million pregnancies in that year were unintended, with about half (48%) of these occurring in couples that reported using a method of contraception in the cycle in which they conceived. Although not all unintended pregnancies are unwanted, 42% of these are terminated by elective abortion and many result in unwanted or under wanted children. Unintended pregnancies are most likely to occur among young, unmarried, black and Latina women and women with low income. While the pregnancy rate for teenagers fell 40% between 1990 and 2005, rates have increased since 2006.

According to an analysis of the 2002 National Survey of Family Growth (the latest survey to be analyzed), of the 61.5 million women of reproductive age in the United States in 2002, 38 million, 62% were using a method of contraception. Among the group using no method of contraception, about 3% had a prior hysterectomy and 9% were pregnant or trying to conceive. About 18% were either not sexually active or were having infrequent episodes of coitus. A total of 7.4% of women of reproductive age were sexually active and not using a method of contraception, a 2.2% increase from the 1995 survey. Of the reproductive age women, nearly 23% used sterilization as their contraceptive method: 16.7% by female methods and 5.7% by vasectomy (**Table 13-1**). Almost 19% used oral contraceptives, and the partners of 11% used the male condom. The **progestin** injection was used by 3%, the diaphragm by 0.2%, periodic abstinence by 1%, withdrawal by 2.5%, and the intrauterine device by about 1%. Thus, of women using contraception, about 70% used very effective methods, including sterilization, oral contraceptives, injection, and IUD, and 30% used less effective methods.

CONTRACEPTIVE EFFECTIVENESS

It is difficult to determine the actual effectiveness of a contraceptive method because of the many factors that affect contraceptive failure. The terms *method effectiveness* and *use effectiveness* (or *method failure* and *patient failure*) were previously used to describe conception occurring while the contraceptive method was being used correctly or incorrectly. These terms have now been replaced by the terms *typical use* and *perfect use*. In general, methods used at the time of coitus, such as the diaphragm, condom, **spermicides**, and withdrawal, have much lower **typical use effectiveness** than **perfect use effectiveness**. There is less difference between perfect and typical use effectiveness among methods not related to the time of coitus, such as oral contraceptives (OCs), **contraceptive patches**, vaginal rings, **implants**, injections, and **intrauterine devices (IUDs)**. Because less

Table 13-1 Percentage of At-Risk Women Using a Contraceptive Method (2006-2008, National Survey of Family Growth)

Contraceptive Status and Method				Age in Years			
	15-44	15-19	20-24	25-29 Number in Thousands	30-34	35-39	40-44
All women	61,864	10,431	10,140	10,250 Percentage Distribution (standard error)	9,587	10,475	10,982
Total	100.0	100.0	100.0	100.0	100.0	100.0	100.0
Using contraception (contraceptors)	61.8 (1.21)	28.2 (1.91)	54.7 (2.81)	64.2 (1.85)	70.3 (2.32)	75.0 (2.23)	77.8 (1.75)
Female sterilization	16.7 (0.96)	*	1.3 (0.41)	9.6 (1.13)	20.6 (2.35)	28.2 (2.39)	39.1 (2.67)
Male sterilization	6.1 (0.53)	—	0.4 (0.16)	2.1 (0.53)	5.8 (0.97)	12.4 (1.71)	15.3 (2.33)
Pill	17.3 (0.83)	15.2 (1.54)	26.2 (2.02)	22.6 (1.79)	17.4 (1.79)	14.4 (1.81)	8.6 (1.55)
Implant Lunelle or patch	0.7 (0.12)	0.5 (0.20)	0.8 (0.22)	1.3 (0.39)	0.9 (0.44)	0.3 (0.14)	*
3-month injectable (Depo-Provera)	2.0 (0.24)	2.6 (0.49)	2.8 (0.64)	3.3 (0.65)	1.6 (0.36)	0.7 (0.34)	0.9 (0.32)
Contraceptive ring	1.5 (0.22)	1.0 (0.51)	3.4 (0.96)	2.0 (0.46)	1.7 (0.61)	0.7 (0.33)	0.3 (0.14)
Intrauterine device (IUD)	3.4 (0.52)	1.0 (0.58)	3.2 (0.70)	4.0 (0.74)	4.7 (1.19)	4.4 (1.57)	3.2 (0.89)
Condom	10.0 (0.63)	6.4 (0.71)	13.4 (1.29)	13.1 (1.33)	12.0 (1.71)	8.4 (1.50)	6.8 (1.19)
Periodic abstinence—calendar rhythm	0.5 (.10)	*	0.2 (0.09)	0.7 (0.39)	0.7 (0.28)	0.9 (0.40)	0.5 (0.24)
Periodic abstinence/natural family planning	0.1 (0.06)	—	—	—	0.6 (0.33)	*	*
Withdrawal	3.2 (0.33)	1.1 (0.27)	2.8 (0.62)	5.1 (0.82)	3.7 (0.80)	4.3 (1.27)	2.5 (0.75)
Other methods\1	0.3 (0.09)	*	*	0.4 (0.16)	0.7 (0.38)	*	*
Not using contraception	38.2 (1.21)	71.8 (1.91)	45.3 (2.81)	35.8 (1.85)	29.7 (2.32)	25.0 (2.23)	22.2 (1.75)
Surgically sterile—female (noncontraceptive)	0.4 (0.13)	—	—	*	*	0.4 (0.23)	1.7 (0.68)
Nonsurgically sterile—male or female	1.7 (0.28)	0.5 (0.24)	1.5 (0.47)	2.6 (1.15)	1.6 (0.49)	2.2 (0.63)	1.8 (0.38)
Pregnant or postpartum	5.4 (0.37)	3.9 (0.52)	10.0 (1.52)	7.7 (1.27)	8.1 (1.73)	5.1 (0.89)	2.5 (0.63)
Seeking pregnancy	4.1 (0.30)	0.9 (0.48)	4.3 (1.02)	6.3 (1.11)	5.9 (1.18)	5.1 (0.89)	2.5 (0.63)
Other nonuse: Never had intercourse or no intercourse in 3 months before interview	19.2 (1.22)	60.0 (2.12)	20.4 (3.08)	10.6 (1.28)	8.7 (1.14)	7.4 (1.12)	8.0 (1.11)
Had intercourse in 3 months before interview	7.3 (0.5)	6.5 (0.84)	9.1 (1.49)	8.6 (1.32)	5.3 (0.78)	8.0 (1.33)	6.4 (1.23)

*Figure does not meet standard or reliability or precision.
— Quantity zero.
\1 Includes diaphragm (with or without jelly or cream), emergency contraception, female condom or vaginal pouch, foam, cervical cap, Today sponge, suppository or insert, jelly or cream (without diaphragm), and other methods.
Note: Percentages may not add to 100 due to rounding.
From Mosher WD, Jones J: Use of Contraception in the United States: 1982-2008.
National Center for Health Statistics. Vital Health Stat 2(29), 2010.

motivation is required with these latter methods than with coitus-related methods, the noncoitus-related methods have greater typical use effectiveness than coitus-related methods. Among noncoitus-related methods, a group of long acting reversible contraceptive (LARC) methods share the additional quality of being highly effect and having equivalent typical use and perfect use failure (**Box 13-1**). Women should be counseled that these four methods are the most effective reversible methods of contraception currently available. "Forgettable methods" are LARC methods that do not require any action by the woman for at least 3 years. Clinicians should always inform women about perfect use failure rates, so that they know the percentage of contraceptive failure that will occur when each method is used correctly and consistently, but at the same time present information on failure with typical use. Couples should be encouraged to use the most acceptable method with the lowest perfect use failure rates. In some cases, correct and consistent use of a birth control method with a higher perfect failure may result in a lower pregnancy rate than imperfect use of a highly effective method (such as oral contraceptives) dependent on daily compliance. Use of two methods ("dual method") provides added protection by ensuring that at least one method is used. Combining a hormonal

Box 13-1 Comparison of Long-Acting Reversible Contraception (LARC) Methods

	LNG-IUS	Copper IUD	ENG implant	DMPA
Duration	5 years	10 years	3 years	3 months
Estrogen-free	+	+	+	+
Progestogen-free	–	+	–	–
Inhibits ovulation	–	–	+	+
Irregular bleeding	+/–	–	+	+/–
Heavy bleeding	–	+/–	–	–
Amenorrhea	+/–	–	–	+

Note: The levonorgestrel intrauterine system (LNG-IUS), copper (Cu T380A) IUD, and etonogestrel subcutaneous (ENG) implants are "Forgettable" methods that provide multiyear protection. Depo medroxyprogesterone acetate (DMPA) requires the patient to have an injection every 3 months.

method with male condoms provides the additional health benefit of reducing sexually transmitted infection.

The overall value of the various contraceptive methods as used by a couple (correctly or incorrectly) over a specific period, sometimes called *extended use effectiveness,* is determined by calculating the actual effectiveness and the continuation rate. Actuarial methods should be used to determine the various **contraceptive failure rates**.

Even with use of these excellent statistical techniques, it is difficult to determine the effectiveness of a contraceptive method in actual practice. Most contraceptive efficacy studies occur in the setting of carefully monitored clinical trials with defined inclusion and exclusion criteria that favor enrollment of subjects who will be compliant with the method. During these studies, the frequent contact with supportive study personnel likely influences outcomes and results in lower failure rates and higher continuation rates than occur in general use. Furthermore, clinical trials are infrequently performed in a comparative randomized manner. Therefore, clinicians cannot accurately compare results of a trial of one type of contraceptive method with those of another.

Several other factors also influence contraceptive failure rates. One of the most important is motivation. Contraceptive failure is more likely to occur in couples seeking to delay a wanted birth compared with those seeking to prevent any more births, especially for coitus-related methods. The woman's age has a strong negative correlation with failure of a contraceptive method, as does socioeconomic status and level of education. Failure rates for most methods usually are lower among populations of married rather than unmarried women. Failure rates reported in prospective studies are also consistently lower than those of retrospective interview studies because of recall bias. Finally, for all methods, failure rates are greater during the first year of use than in subsequent years, yet most studies report only first-year use failure rates. Thus, many variables must be considered when evaluating the effectiveness of any method of contraception for an individual woman.

Trussell and coworkers calculated percentage failure rates with the first year of use for the various methods of contraceptives available in the United States (**Table 13-2**). The percentage of actual use failure rates for durations more than 1 year is available for certain methods of long-acting contraceptives.

The cumulative failure rate for 5 years of use of the levonorgestrel intrauterine system in clinical trials is 1.1%. The cumulative failure rate of the copper T380 IUD was 1.0, 1.4, and 1.6 per 100 women after 3, 5, and 7 years of use, respectively, in a large World Health Organization (WHO) study and only rises to 1.7 per 100 women after 10 and 12 years of use.

The best estimates of failure rate of all types of tubal sterilization is 1.31 after 5 years and 1.85 per 100 women after 10 years, being highest for tubal fulguration and lowest for segmental resection in the 10 years following the procedure.

CONTRACEPTIVE COST

All contraceptive methods reduce overall health care costs because the costs associated with unintended pregnancy greatly outweigh the costs of contraception. Trussell and colleagues used a 5-year Markov model to examine the cost effectiveness of 16 contraceptive methods (including chance, or use of no method) in the United States from a health care payer's perspective. To determine effectiveness, the model calculated the number of pregnancies avoided with typical use of each method of contraception compared with the number of pregnancies expected to occur if the woman used no contraceptive method. To determine the cost of each contraceptive, the direct medical costs of the method itself—costs caused by mistimed pregnancies, as well as costs incurred or avoided by adverse and beneficial side effects of the contraceptive method—were calculated. The costs of unintended pregnancies caused by method failure included the costs of term deliveries as well as spontaneous and **induced abortion** and ectopic pregnancies. Because the costs of unintended pregnancy when no method of contraception is used are substantial, use of any method was less costly than use of no method. Costs were calculated for contraceptive use for 1 and 5 years' duration. Whereas most of the cost associated with more effective methods is due to acquisition cost, pregnancy-related costs contribute most expense related to use of less effective methods. In this analysis, all contraceptive methods were cost effective when compared to no method. The most cost effective methods are vasectomy, the etonogestrel implant, tubal ligation, the levonorgestrel releasing IUD (LNG-IUS), and the copperT IUD. Although insurance coverage of contraception in the United States has increased in recent years because of state mandates, not all methods are covered and upfront costs remain a barrier to the use of LARC methods. When Kaiser Foundation Health Plan in California changed its coverage policy to include 100% universal coverage for the most effective forms of contraception and for emergency contraceptive (EC), use of intrauterine contraceptives (IUCs) and injectables rose by 137% and 32%, and purchasing of EC rose by 88%. The National Institute for Health and Clinical Excellence (NICE) clinical practice guideline for the British National Health Service (NHS) found LARC methods to be more cost effective than combined oral contraceptives.

In the United States, the cost of a health care visit presents another barrier to use of the more effective methods of contraception. Only male and female condoms, spermicides, and the contraceptive sponge are available over the counter and without a prescription.

Table 13-2 Comparison of LARC methods

Method	Percentage of Women Experiencing an Unintended Pregnancy within the First Year of Use		Percentage of Women Continuing Use at 1 Year[a]
	Typical Use[b]	Perfect Use[c]	
No method[d]	85	85	
Spermicides[e]	29	18	42
Withdrawal	27	4	43
Fertility-awareness-based methods	25		51
Standard days method[f]		5	
Two-day method[f]		4	
Ovulation method[f]		3	
Sponge			
Parous women	32	20	46
Nulliparous women	16	9	57
Diaphragm[g]	16	6	57
Condom[h]			
Female (reality)	21	5	49
Male	15	2	53
Combined pill and progestin-only pill	8	0.3	68
Eva patch	8	0.3	68
NuvaRing	8	0.3	68
Depo-Provera	3	0.3	56
IUD			
ParaGaud (copper T)	0.8	0.6	78
Mirena (LNG-IUS)	0.2	0.2	80
Implanor	0.05	0.05	84
Female sterilization	0.5	0.5	100
Male sterilization	0.15	0.10	100

Emergency contraceptive pills: Treatment initiated within 72 hours after unprotected intercourse reduces the risk of pregnancy by at least 75%.[i]
Lactational amenorrhea method: It is a highly effective, temporary method of contraception.[j]

[a]Among couples attempting to avoid pregnancy, the percentage who continue to use a method for 1 year.
[b]Among typical couples who initiate use of a method (not necessarily for the first time), the percentage who experience an accidental pregnancy during the first year if they do not stop use for any other reason. Estimates of the probability of pregnancy during the first year of typical use for spermicides, withdrawal, fertility awareness—based methods, the diaphragm, the male condom, the pill, and Depo-Provera are taken from the 1995 National Survey of Family Growth (NSFG), corrected for underreporting of abortion; see the reference above for the derivation of estimates for other methods.
[c]Among couples who initiate use of a method (not necessarily for the first time) and who use it perfectly (both consistently and correctly), the percentage who experience an accidental pregnancy during the first year if they do not stop use for any other reason. For the derivation of the estimate for each method, see the reference above.
[d]The percentages becoming pregnant in columns 2 and 3 are based on data from populations where contraception is not used and from women who cease using contraception in order to become pregnant. Among such populations, about 89% become pregnant within 1 year. This estimate was lowered slightly (to 85%) to represent the percentage who would become pregnant within 1 year among women now relying on reversible methods of contraception if they abandoned contraception altogether.
[e]Foams, creams, gels, vaginal suppositories, and vaginal film.
[f]The ovulation and two-day methods are based on evaluation of cervical mucus. The standard days method avoids intercourse on cycle days 8 to 19.
[g]With spermicidal cream or jelly.
[h]Without spermicides.
[i]The treatment schedule is one dose within 120 hours after unprotected intercourse and a second dose 12 hours after the first dose. Both doses of plan B can be taken at the same time. Plan B (one dose is one white pill) is the only dedicated product specifically marketed for emergency contraception. The FDA has, in addition, declared the following 22 brands of oral contraceptives to be safe and effective for emergency contraception: Ogestrel or Ovral (one dose is two white pills); Levlen or Nordetto (one dose is four light orange pills), Cryselle, Levore, Low Ogestrel, Lo/Ovral, or Quansen (one dose is four white pills), Tri Levlen or Triphasil (one dose is four yellow pills), Jolessa, Portia, Seasonale, or Trivora (one dose is four pink pills), Seasonique (one dose is four light blue-green pills), Empresse (one dose is four orange pills), Alesse, Lessira, or Levlite (one dose is five pink pills), Aviane (one dose is five orange pills), and Lutera (one dose is five white pills).
[j]However, to maintain effective protection against pregnancy, another method of contraception must be used as soon as menstruation resumes, the frequency or duration of breast-feeds is reduced, bottle feeds are introduced, or the baby reaches 6 months of age.
From Trussell J, Wynn LL: Reducing unintended pregnancy in the United States. Contraception 77:1-5, 2008.

COITUS-RELATED METHODS

SPERMICIDES: FOAMS, CREAMS, AND SUPPOSITORIES

Spermicides consist of an active agent and a carrier. The carriers include gels, foams, creams, tablets, films, and suppositories. The active agent is a surfactant that immobilizes or kills sperm on contact by destroying the sperm cell membrane. Spermicides need to be placed into the vagina before each coital act. The pregnancy rate with use of these agents in the first year ranges from 18% with perfect use to 29% with typical use. Most spermicides are used in combination with a barrier contraceptive to increase effectiveness. The only spermicide that is currently approved for use as a contraceptive is the surfactant nonoxynol 9.

The contraceptive sponge, a cylindrical piece of soft polyurethane impregnated with 1 mg of nonoxynol 9, must be inserted into the vagina before intercourse, but it is effective for 24 hours so provides protection for additional acts of coitus during this interval. The sponge returned to the U.S. market in 2009 after being withdrawn because of manufacturing compliance problems in 1994. The pregnancy rate in the first year with the sponge ranges from 9% with perfect use to 16% with typical use in nulliparous women and is higher in parous women. This makes the sponge slightly better than a spermicide alone but less effective than a vaginal diaphragm.

Although a few early studies linked the use of a spermicide at the time of conception with an increased risk of some congenital malformations, these studies were probably flawed by recall bias. Subsequent well-designed studies have shown no increased risk of congenital malformation in the newborns or karyotypic abnormalities in the spontaneous abortuses conceived in women using spermicides.

Nonoxynol 9 has been associated with an increased risk of vaginal erosions and HIV transmission. Research efforts to develop new dual protection agents with enhanced spermicidal and antimicrobial (including antiviral) effects are under way.

BARRIER METHODS

DIAPHRAGM

Margaret Sanger introduced the vaginal diaphragm to the United States in 1916, and it became the most widely used female-controlled reversible contraceptive method prior to the introduction of oral contraceptive. The diaphragm is a thin dome-shaped membrane of latex rubber or silicone with a flexible spring modeled into the rim. The spring allows the device to be collapsed for insertion and then allows for expansion within the vagina to seat the rim against the vaginal wall to create a mechanical barrier between the vagina and the cervix. A diaphragm must be carefully fitted by a health care provider. A clinical trial of a one-size diaphragm showed a higher failure rate than observed with fitted devices. To be most effective, the clinician should select the largest size that does not cause discomfort or undue pressure on the vaginal mucosa. After the fitting, the woman should remove the diaphragm and reinsert it herself. She should then be examined to make sure the diaphragm is covering the cervix. The diaphragm should be used with a spermicide and be left in place for at least 8 hours after the last coital act. If repeated intercourse takes place, additional spermicide should be used vaginally. Although use of a spermicide is recommended, studies have not conclusively demonstrated that pregnancy rates are lower when a spermicide is used with a diaphragm. Because a primary reason for failure of the method is nonuse, strategies to ensure consistent use of the diaphragm have been studied. In a nonrandomized study of women who left the diaphragm in place without using spermicide, removing it only once daily to wash it before immediately reinserting it, as well as removing it during menses, the 12-month failure rate was only 2.8%. This rate was lower than the failure rate of 9.8% among a cohort of women who inserted the diaphragm with a spermicide in the usual manner only when having sexual intercourse and then leaving it in for 8 hours thereafter. The lower rate of failure was attributed to more consistent use, and subsequent randomized studies have documented more consistent use of the diaphragm at each act of intercourse with continuous use.

Data from the Oxford/Family Planning Association Contraceptive Study indicate that the diaphragm is an effective method of contraception in married, motivated women and that failure rates decline with increasing age and increasing duration of use. Analyses of data from two large clinical trials comparing use of the diaphragm with that of the cervical cap or sponge indicate that the failure rate during the first year of use for the diaphragm ranged from 12.5% to 17.1% among all users and was reduced to 4.3% to 5.3% with perfect use.

The number of urinary tract infections (UTIs) in women who use diaphragms is significantly higher than in nonusers, probably because of the mechanical obstruction of the outflow of urine by the diaphragm. For this reason, it is recommended that women void after intercourse. Postcoital administration of trimethoprim-sulfamethoxazole has also been shown to reduce the risk of UTI in women with both low (two or fewer times per week) and high (three or more times per week) intercourse frequencies. Although older reports cautioned against leaving a diaphragm in place for more than 24 hours because of concerns of ulceration of the vaginal epithelium with prolonged usage, this has not been reported in studies of continuous use of the method.

CERVICAL CAP

A cervical cap is a cup-shaped silicone or rubber device that fits around the cervix. Various versions of the cap have been used for decades mainly in the United Kingdom and Europe, but these have been less popular than the diaphragm in the United States. There has been a recent resurgence of interest in the use of this older method, because the cervical cap can be left in place longer than the diaphragm and is more comfortable. Like the diaphragm, the various types of caps are manufactured in different sizes and should be fitted to the cervix by a clinician. Unlike the diaphragm, which typically expands to find the correct position within the vagina, the cap must be placed directly over the cervix. Women who find this difficult or uncomfortable are poor candidates for the cap. For women motivated to use a barrier method, particularly those interested in avoiding a hormonal method or IUD, the cap can be an excellent choice.

The Prentif Cervical Cap was a latex device, and is no longer available in the United States. The only cap currently on the U.S. market is the FemCap. This product, made of soft, durable, hypoallergenic, silicone rubber, is shaped like a upside down sailor's hat with an upturned brim designed to contact the vaginal walls as the dome of the device sits over the cervix (**Fig. 13-1**). The device can be placed anytime before intercourse and should be used with spermicide applied to both the cervical and vaginal surfaces. Additional spermicide should be applied vaginally if intercourse is repeated. The FemCap comes in only three sizes, making fitting easier than the either the diaphragm or Prentif cap. Like the diaphragm, the clinician should verify correct position of the device and ensure that the woman can insert, remove, and reinsert the device. The cervical cap should not be left in place for more than 48 hours because of the possibility of ulceration, unpleasant odor, and infection.

While randomized trials of the Prentif cap demonstrated efficacy comparable to the diaphragm, the 6-month Kaplan-Meier unadjusted cumulative pregnancy rates were higher for the FemCap (13.5%) than the diaphragm (7.9%). However, a first-generation version of the FemCap, which was available in only one size, was studied. Small noncomparator studies of

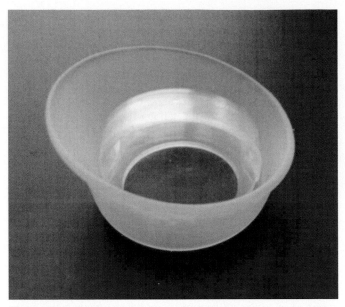

Figure 13-1 The female barrier method Femcap.

the current product approved by the Food and Drug Administration (FDA) suggest that the failure rate may be comparable with, or lower than, the diaphragm.

Because of theoretic concern about a possible adverse effect of the cap on cervical tissue, it has been recommended that cap users not keep the cap in place for more than 48 hours and that they undergo speculum exam and repeat cervical cytologic examination 3 months after starting to use this method. Given our current knowledge that cervical cancer occurs as a result of exposure to high-risk subtypes of the human papilloma (HPV) virus, these cytology recommendations are likely outdated. No difference in Pap smear abnormalities was seen in women randomized to the FemCap compared with those using the diaphragm. Whether prolonged use increases the risk of toxic shock syndrome is not known.

MALE CONDOM

Male condoms are made of three materials: latex, polyurethane, and animal tissue. Clinicians should encourage individuals with multiple sex partners to use a latex or polyurethane male condom either alone, or as part of a dual method strategy. The latex and polyurethane male condoms are the only methods of contraception with FDA-approved labeling that supports use of the product to prevent both pregnancy and the transmission of sexually transmitted infections. Condoms made of animal tissue such as lamb cecum do not prevent transmission of sexually transmitted infections. Although condoms made of polyurethane are thinner and may provide greater sensitivity, randomized studies have documented higher rates of slippage and breakage than latex condoms and higher rates of pregnancy (6-month typical-use pregnancy probabilities are 9% to 10.8% for the polyurethane group and 5.4% to 6.4% for the latex group). For this reason, most experts recommend latex condoms unless sensitivity prevents their use. Clinicians should review proper condom use with both men and women. Excellent instructions are also available at a number of Internet sites (e.g., www.plannedparenthood.org/healthtopics/birthcontrol/condom10187.htm). The condom should be

applied to the erect penis before any contract with the vagina or vulva. Unless a reservoir design is used, the tip should extend beyond the end of the penis by about half an inch to collect the ejaculate. The penis must be removed from the vagina while still somewhat erect, and the base of the condom grasped to ensure the condom is removed intact. Care must be taken upon withdrawal not to spill the ejaculate as the condom is removed and disposed of. When used by strongly motivated couples, the male condom is highly effective. In a U.S. study, the first-year failure rates for male condom use among women wishing no more pregnancies ranged between 3% and 6% when the woman was older than 30 but between 8% and 10% when the woman was younger than 25.

Some condoms come prepackaged with either N9 spermicide or lubricants. A randomized study completed in the Dominican Republic did not demonstrate any additional benefit of N9 over lubricated condoms. Moreover, N9 has been associated with an increase risk of HIV acquisition in high-risk women. Lubrication may reduce condom breakage. Among couples randomized to use condoms alone or with additional vaginal spermicide, there were fewer clinical and nonclinical failures in the additional spermicide arm.

FEMALE CONDOM

A female condom was approved for marketing in the United States in 1994. It consists of a soft, loose-fitting polyurethane sheath with two flexible rings. One ring lies at the closed end of the sheath and serves as an insertion mechanism and internal anchor for the condom inside the vagina. The outer ring forms the external edge of the device and remains outside the vagina after insertion, thus providing protection to the introitus and the base of the penis during intercourse. The female condom is prelubricated and intended for onetime use only. Like male condoms, the device is available over the counter (OTC) and fitting by a health professional is not required.

The female condom offers several advantages over male condoms. It is female controlled and can be inserted prior to the onset of sexual activity and left in place for a longer time after ejaculation has occurred. Because the female condom also partially covers the external genitalia, it should offer greater protection against the transfer of certain sexually transmitted organisms, particularly genital herpes and HPV. Also, because the polyurethane is stronger and thicker than the latex or polyurethane used in male condoms, the female condom is less likely to rupture. Disadvantages include cost (about three times higher for the female condom) and ease of use. The possibility of "bypass" intercourse exists if the penis enters the vagina adjacent to the outer ring. In a randomized study comparing both methods, couples reported mechanical problems during 9% of male and 34% of female condom uses. However, the risk of vaginal exposure to semen (as measured by the presence of prostate specific antigen) did not differ between condom types. Overall, couples using both methods preferred the male condom to the female condom for ease of application or insertion, ease of removal, general fit, feel of the condom during intercourse, and ease of penetration. In a multicenter clinical trial, the cumulative pregnancy rate in U.S. centers at 6 months was 12.4%. The 6-month pregnancy rate with perfect use was 2.6%, indicating that the probable 1-year pregnancy rate with perfect use would be slightly more than 5%. The typical use failure rate at 1 year is estimated to be 21%. At the end of 6 months in the U.S. study, about one third of the women had discontinued use of this method.

Studies assessing the effectiveness of the female condom for reducing sexual disease transmission have not been performed. Because polyurethane does not allow virus transmission, it should reduce the risk of a woman acquiring HIV infection. Still, only male latex and polyurethane condoms contain FDA-approved labeling for duel protection.

The nonprofit Program for Appropriate Technology in Health (PATH) has developed a new female condom that is currently in phase 3 clinical trials. A small randomized study comparing the PATH condom to the current (Reality) female condom found lower rates of condom failure and symptoms of urogenital irritation, and greater acceptability with the new device. A larger-scale study to support product approval is in progress at this writing.

BARRIER TECHNIQUES AND SEXUALLY TRANSMITTED INFECTIONS

Barrier methods have the advantage of reducing the rate of transmission of sexually transmitted infections. Several studies have shown that spermicides reduce the frequency of clinical infection with sexually transmitted infections, both bacterial and viral. Several in vitro studies have demonstrated that latex condoms prevent the transmission of viruses, specifically the herpesvirus and the human immunodeficiency virus (HIV), as well as the *Chlamydia trachomatis* bacteria, a frequent cause of salpingitis. Serial epidemiologic studies, both case control and cohort, indicate that the use of the condom or diaphragm protects both men and women from clinically apparent gonorrheal infection.

An epidemiologic study of women with infertility caused by tubal obstruction found that the past use of barrier techniques protected women against tubal damage. The greatest protection occurred with the use of diaphragms or condoms in conjunction with spermicides. The incidence of cervical neoplasia was also markedly diminished among the female members of couples using condoms or diaphragms, probably because of the decreased transmission of human papillomavirus (HPV). Although epidemiologic studies suggest that spermicides use is associated with a reduction in the risk of cervical cancer, the HPV virus is not inactivated by N9. Other studies have demonstrated that N9 may be associated with an increased risk of HIV transmission. In 2007, the FDA established new warning statements and other labeling information for all OTC vaginal contraceptive products containing N9, advising consumers that these do not protect against infection from HIV or other sexually transmitted diseases and that use of N9 can irritate the vagina and rectum and may increase the risk of getting HIV from an infected partner.

To reduce the risk of sexually transmitted infections (STIs) including HIV, male latex (or polyurethane if latex allergic) condoms are recommended. Unfortunately, the pregnancy failure rates of condom users are highest for persons younger than 25 years, those most likely to become infected with sexually transmitted diseases. Therefore, to prevent the transmission of these diseases as well as prevent unwanted pregnancy in this age group, the use of condoms, together with one of the four most effective reversible methods of contraception, is advisable.

PERIODIC ABSTINENCE

Many highly motivated couples use the avoidance of sexual intercourse during the days of the menstrual cycle when the ovum can be fertilized as a means of preventing pregnancy. Wilcox and colleagues reported that conception can only occur if coitus takes place during the 5 days preceding ovulation or the day of ovulation. Thus, if couples would only avoid coitus on these 6 days each month, conception would not occur. Because a woman cannot precisely determine when she will ovulate, four techniques of periodic abstinence have been utilized. The oldest of these is the calendar rhythm method. With this method, the period of abstinence is determined solely by calculating the length of the individual woman's previous menstrual cycle. The rationale for the rhythm method rests on three assumptions: (1) the human ovum is capable of being fertilized for only about 24 hours after ovulation, (2) spermatozoa retain their fertilizing ability for only about 48 hours after coitus, and (3) ovulation usually occurs 12 to 16 days (13 ± 2 days) before the onset of the subsequent menses. According to these assumptions, the woman records the length of her cycles for several months; she establishes her fertile period by subtracting 18 days from the length of her previous shortest cycle and 11 days from her previous longest cycle. Then, in each subsequent cycle, the couple abstains from coitus during this calculated fertile period.

This method requires abstinence by the majority of women with regular menstrual cycles for nearly half the days of each cycle and cannot be used by women with irregular menstrual cycles. Although calendar rhythm is the most widely used technique of periodic abstinence, pregnancy rates are high, ranging from 13.4 to 47 per 100 woman-years, mainly because most couples fail to abstain for the relatively long periods required. The use of the calendar rhythm method by itself is currently not advocated or taught to couples who are interested in practicing periodic abstinence.

Since the 1990s, new techniques have been developed whereby women rely on physiologic change during each cycle to determine the fertile period and reduce the period of abstinence in the hope of improving compliance. The term **natural family planning** has been used instead of *rhythm* to describe these new techniques. They include the temperature method, the cervical mucus method, and the symptothermal method. Each of these techniques requires a great amount of motivation and training. In most reports, pregnancy rates with use of these methods are relatively high and continuation rates are low.

The temperature method relies on measuring basal body temperature daily. The woman is required to abstain from intercourse from the onset of the menses until the third consecutive day of elevated basal temperature. Because abstinence is required for the entire preovulatory period in ovulatory cycles and for the entire cycle in anovulatory cycles, the temperature method alone is no longer commonly used.

The cervical mucus method requires that the woman be taught to recognize and interpret cyclic changes in the presence and consistency of cervical mucus; these changes occur in response to changing estrogen and progesterone levels. Abstinence is required during the menses and every other day after the menses ends, because of the possibility of confusing semen with ovulatory mucus, until the first day that copious, slippery mucus is observed to be present. Abstinence is required every day thereafter until

4 days after the last day when the characteristic mucus is present (the "peak mucus day"). In two well-designed, randomized clinical trials, the pregnancy rates for new users of this method in the first year, after they completed a 3- to 5-month training period, were 20% and 24% with discontinuation rates between 72% and 74%. In a five-country study of 725 highly motivated couples sponsored by the WHO, the typical use failure rate during the first year after the completion of three cycles of training was 19.6%, with a perfect use failure rate of 3.5%. Three fourths of these pregnancies resulted from conscious deviation from the rules of the method. The mean length of the fertile period in this study was 9.6 days, and abstinence was therefore required for about 17 days of each cycle. In this study the continuation rate after 1 year was high, 64.4%.

Rather than relying on a single physiologic index, the sympto-thermal method uses several indices to determine the fertile period. Most used are calendar calculations and changes in the cervical mucus to estimate the onset of the fertile period and changes in mucus or basal temperature to estimate its end. Because several indices need to be monitored, this method is more difficult to learn than the single-index methods, but it is more effective than the cervical mucus method alone. In two large, randomized studies comparing these methods, the pregnancy rates at the end of 1 year of use, after the training phase, were 10.9% and 19.8% with the symptothermal method, compared with 20% and 24% for the cervical mucus method. In addition, the continuation rate among the women who used the symptothermal method in these studies was higher after 1 year, about 50% in each study, than that among the women who used the cervical mucus method (26% and 40%).

The major reason for the lack of acceptance of natural family planning, as well as the relatively high pregnancy rates among users of these methods, is the need to avoid having sexual intercourse for a large number of days during each menstrual cycle. To overcome this problem, many women use barrier methods, withdrawal, or spermicides during the fertile period. In a study of women who used the symptothermal method with barrier contraceptives or withdrawal during the fertile period, the failure rate during the first year was 9.9%, and the discontinuation rate was 33%.

Because the use of any method of contraception other than abstinence is unacceptable to some couples, simple, self-administered tests to detect hormonal changes have been studied to reduce the number of days of abstinence required in each cycle to a maximum of seven. The development of a low-cost, easy-to-use enzyme immunoassay for urinary estrogen and pregnanediol glucuronide similar to that used for a home pregnancy test could reduce the number of days of abstinence required. It remains to be determined to what extent this aid to natural family planning will be used if it becomes generally available.

COITUS INTERRUPTUS (WITHDRAWAL)

Removal of the penis from the vagina prior to ejaculation to prevent pregnancy is an ancient male-controlled method of contraception. There are no contraindications to its use and the technique involves no devices or cost. The traditional teaching regarding withdrawal is that the method fails because of the small numbers of sperm present in the preejaculate, the fluid produced by the penis during sexual excitement and before climax. The reality is that the millions of sperm deposited in the semen when withdrawal is not performed in a timely or correct fashion are the real agents of fertility.

For some couples, withdrawal is the only acceptable method. Therefore, it is important to stress correct and consistent use with every act of intercourse, not only during suspected fertile times. A major drawback of the method is the lack of any protection against sexually transmitted infections.

LACTATIONAL AMENORRHEA METHOD (LAM)

Because prolactin inhibits gonadotropin pulsatility, nursing women typically remain amenorrheic following giving birth for a variable length of time. Factors associated with menstrual suppression include frequency and duration of nursing. In particular, night nursing is highly correlated with anovulation and amenorrhea. This suppression of fertility likely evolved to increase survival of the infant, as it results in natural spacing of births.

The LAM method was formally defined during the 1988 Bellagio Consensus Conference as the informed use of breast-feeding as a contraceptive method. The criteria for successful use are the presence of amenorrhea, exclusive breast-feeding (no supplements), and performed up to 6 months after delivery. The presence of night nursing is considered highly protective. The method is generally quoted to offer 98% protection from pregnancy in the first 6 months postpartum. In a WHO study published in 1999, 13 pregnancies were reported in about 2900 women-months of use, for a cumulative life table pregnancy rate in fully breast-feeding, amenorrheic women not using any contraceptive method of 0.9 to 1.2 (95% CI 0 to 2.4). However, these rates may underestimate the risk, as rates of sexual activity may be lower in many postpartum women.

Effective use of LAM improves with education regarding the efficacy of the method. Still, many providers may chose to initiate a discussion of a LARC method during the postpartum interval, as a recent birth is a highly motivating experience. Because a variety of factors may influence the duration of breast-feeding, a reliable backup method should be discussed in advance and initiated promptly if the conditions required for success with LAM are no longer in place.

HORMONAL CONTRACEPTION

The most effect strategies of reversible contraception utilize synthetic female hormones. The most widely used methods combine a synthetic estrogen with a synthetic progestin. The major effect of the synthetic progestin component is to inhibit ovulation, but they also contribute other contraceptive actions such as thickening of the cervical mucus. The major effects of the synthetic estrogen are to maintain the endometrium and prevent unscheduled bleeding and to inhibit follicular development. Available combination products include pills (oral contraceptives), a skin (transdermal) patch, injections, and a vaginal ring. A number of progestin-only products are also available for women who prefer not to use an estrogen-containing method or have medical contraindications to estrogens. These delivery systems include injections, implants, pills, and a hormone-releasing intrauterine system.

Progestins are classified according to the steroid from which they were derived. The pregnane and norpregnanes are C21 progestins related to progesterone and derivatives of 17α-acetoxyprogesterone. Medroxyprogesterone acetate (MPA) and megestrol acetate are C21 progestins marketed as tablets for non-contraceptive usage. In the 1960s, studies in animals of a pregnane combination oral contraceptive pill demonstrated an increase in the rate of mammary cancer. Subsequent studies revealed that the animals used (beagle dogs) are a poor model for toxicity, as they metabolize C21 progestins to estrogen; this metabolic pathway does not exist in women. However, concerns about potential carcinogenicity of C21 progestins delayed approval of the depot injectable form of MPA in the United States until 1993. It is expected that an oral contraception containing the pregnane nomegestrol acetate (NOMAc) will be approved in the United States in 2010.

Most hormonal methods use the 19-nortestosterone progestins. Because these molecules are derivatives of testosterone, they have some degree of androgenic activity. The 19-nortestosterone progestins are further classified as either *estranes* or *gonanes*. In comparing formulations, it is important to note that gonanes have greater progestational activity per unit weight than do estranes, and thus smaller doses are required for the same biologic effect. Although the original estrane norethynodrel is no longer used in currently marketed OCs, the estranes norethindrone and its derivatives (with one or two acetates), norethindrone acetate and ethynodiol diacetate, are used in several marketed formulations (**Fig. 13-2**). The parent compound of the gonanes is *dl*norgestrel, a racemic mixture of the dextro and levo isomers. Only the levo form is biologically active. Three less androgenic derivatives of levonorgestrel, desogestrel, norgestimate, and gestodene, have also been synthesized (**Fig. 13-3**). Although formulations with

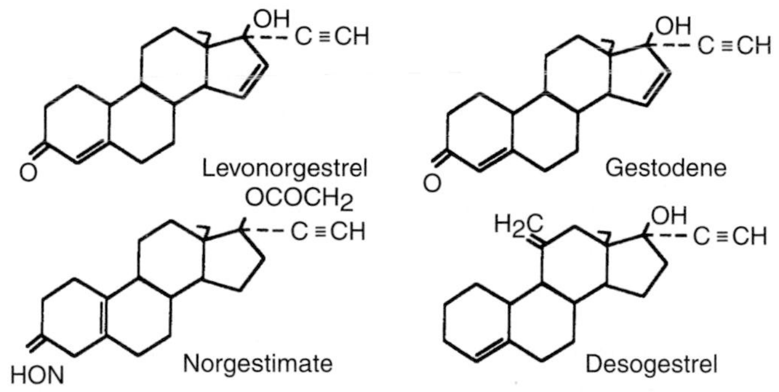

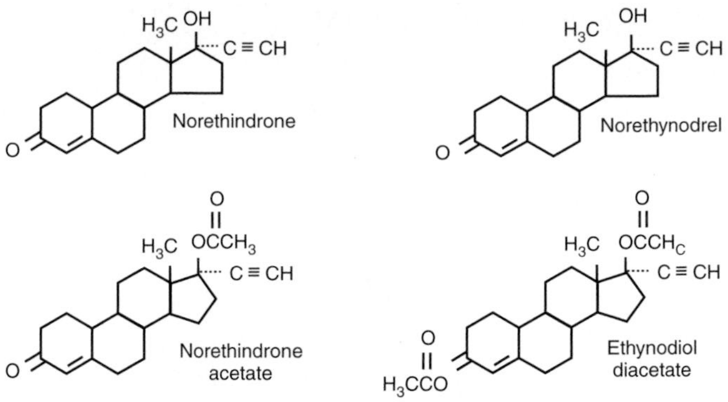

Figure 13-4 Structural formulation of drospirenone.

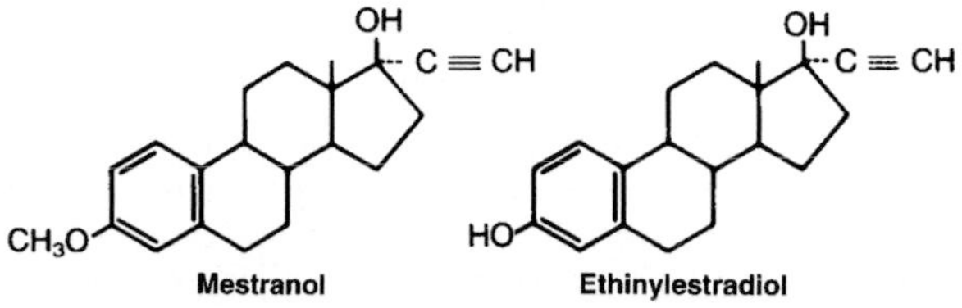

Figure 13-5 Structures of the two estrogens used in combination oral contraceptives.

each of these three newer gonanes have been marketed in Europe, only formulations with desogestrel and norgestimate have been marketed in the United States.

The novel progestin drospirenone is neither a 19-nortestosterone nor 17α-acetoxyprogesterone and is structurally related to spironolactone (**Fig. 13-4**). This progestin has antimineralocorticoid and antiandrogenic activity as well as progestational activity without androgenic activity. Dienogest is a hybrid progestin, derived from the estrane group with a 17 α-cyanomethyl radical. However, it is considered to be closer to the pregnane group as it does not exert the androgenic effects of the testosterone derivatives and in fact has significant antiandrogenic activity.

In combination products, a progestin is delivered along with an estrogen. Because the primary estrogen produced by the ovary, 17 β-estradiol (E_2), is poorly absorbed orally, contraceptive preparations have used the stable, orally active, and highly potent ethinyl estradiol (EE) as the estrogen component. Mestranol, used in the first oral contraceptives, is the biologically inactive 3-methyl-ether of ethinyl estradiol (EE). Because mestranol must undergo demethylation in the liver to become active, it was replaced with EE in subsequent formulations (**Fig. 13-5**). Until recently, attempts to develop an estradiol containing oral contraceptive have been hampered by unsatisfactory cycle control. Considerable efforts with a variety of dosing strategies have led to the development of two new formulations, one containing estradiol valerate in combination with dienogest and another with estradiol and NOMAc (**Fig. 13-6**).

Figure 13-2 Chemical structures of the estrane progestins used in oral contraceptives.

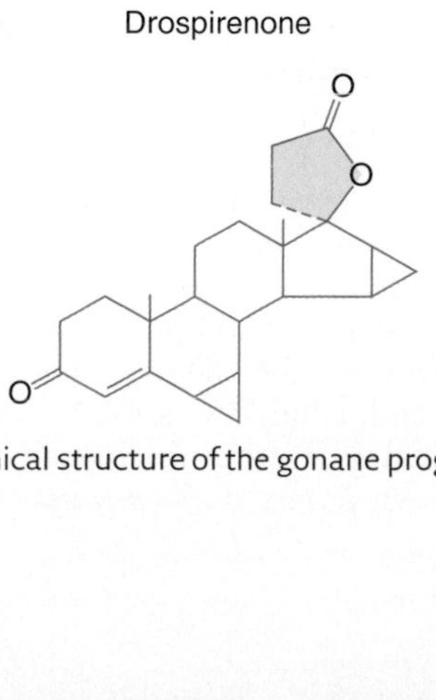

Figure 13-3 Chemical structure of the gonane progestins used in oral contraceptives.

ORAL CONTRACEPTIVES

Combined hormonal contraceptives were first approved in the United States in 1959 and marketed in 1960. The development of an oral contraceptive was based on work by Ludwig

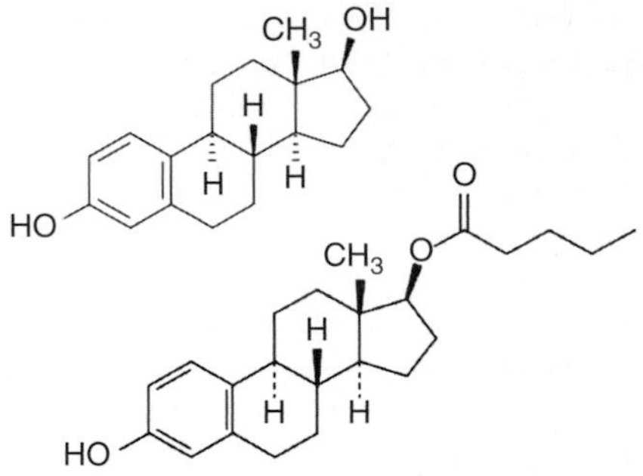

Figure 13-6 Structures of 17-β estradiol and estradiol valerate.

Haberlandt and others that established that ovarian extracts could inhibit ovulation. Inspired by Margaret Sanger, Katherine McCormick provided the financial backing for the early studies by Gregory Pincus and John Rock that led to the approval of the pill. However, an oral contraceptive pill became possible only with the synthesis of the potent synthetic progestogen norethynodrel. The estrogen component of the pill was an afterthought. The initial synthesis of norethynodrel was contaminated with the synthetic estrogen mestranol. However, when this was discovered during early clinical trials and the mestranol was removed, higher rates of breakthrough bleeding were observed. To counter this, mestranol was deliberately added back to Enovid, a combination of 9.85 mg of norethynodrel and 0.15 mg of mestranol, the first oral contraceptive developed by the G.D. Searle Company.

Because of their extremely high rate of effectiveness and ease of administration, OCs became the most widely used method of reversible contraception among both married and unmarried women within a few years of their introduction. The high doses of steroids in the original pill formulations caused minor side effects such as nausea, breast tenderness, and weight gain that frequently led to discontinuation of use and also contributed to some serious health risks. Since that time, many other formulations have been developed and marketed with steadily decreasing dosages of both the estrogen and progestin components. All the formulations marketed after 1975 contain less than 50 mcg of ethinyl estradiol (EE) and 3 mg or less of one of several progestins. Reduction in dose has significantly lowered the incidence of severe adverse cardiovascular effects and minor adverse symptoms without increasing the failure rate.

Because **oral contraceptive steroid** formulations with more than 50 mcg of estrogen were associated with a greater incidence of adverse effects without greater efficacy, they are no longer marketed for contraceptive use in the United States, Canada, and Great Britain. With the exception of women in whom unusually rapid metabolism of synthetic steroids is anticipated (e.g., women on medications that induce the cytochrome P450 system), use of pills containing 50 mcg of estrogen is not recommended.

PHARMACOLOGY

There are three major types of OC formulations: fixed-dose (monophasic) combination, multiphasic combination, and daily progestin-only pills (POPs), also known as minipills. The minipill formulations consist of tablets containing a low dose of progestin without any estrogen and are ingested once every day without a steroid-free interval. The combination formulations are the most widely used and are more effective than the minipill.

Monophasic products contain tablets with the same dose combination of an estrogen and progestin each day. In multiphasic formulations, pills containing several different dose combinations are provided in the same pack. A different tablet color corresponds to each dose. Depending on the number of different dose combinations, these formulations are further classified as biphasic (2), triphasic (3), or four phasic. The rationale given for use of multiphasic formulations is that they lower the total dose of steroid without increasing the incidence of unscheduled uterine bleeding. Although comparative clinical trials have not conclusively demonstrated that multiphasic combinations have significantly fewer adverse effects than monophasic combination formulations, a recent randomized study by Ahrendt documented less bleeding with the four-phasic E2V/DNG pill compared with a monophasic EE/LNG.

Most oral contraceptives regimens revolve around a 28-day (4-week) cycle. Standard combination OC formulations provide active pills continuously for 21 days (3 weeks) followed by a 7-day hormone-free interval (HFI). Most products include inactive spacer (placebo) pills during the HFI to improve compliance. Some formulations provide an iron supplement in the spacer pills. Uterine bleeding occurs secondary to hormone withdrawal during the HFI, typically commencing 1 to 3 days after taking the last active pill. This withdrawal bleeding usually lasts 3 to 4 days and is generally lighter (mean 25 mL) than during menses in a normal ovulatory cycle (mean 35 mL). Two recently introduced formulations provide active tablets for 24 days, reducing the HFI to only 4 days. Another formulation provides a small amount of EE (alone without progestin) during the entire 7-day HFI to reduce symptoms associated with estrogen withdrawal.

Other dosing strategies include extended and continuous cycles. Extended cycle regimens contain 84 days of active pills followed by a 7-day HFI (or 7 days of EE only) that results in withdrawal bleeding four times a year. A continuous daily LNG 90 mcg/EE 20 mcg regimen with 28 active pills in a treatment pack was introduced in 2007 to completely eliminate scheduled withdrawal bleeds. Although this is the lowest dose combination available for continuous dosing, many providers recommend less expensive generic standard monophasic 20 mcg EE OCs, instructing patients to discard the placebo pills and begin a new cycle pack after 21 days. Randomized studies comparing cyclic with continuous dosing regimens have documented a decrease in the overall number of scheduled bleeding days but an increase in irregular bleeding and spotting with extended or continuous use of hormonal contraceptives. Bleeding patterns typically improve over time in most users of continuous OCs, with rates of unscheduled bleeding highest in early cycles of use. Using a continuous dosing regimen of a low-dose (20 mcg EE/100 mcg LNG) oral contraceptive, Miller and colleagues reported rates of amenorrhea of 72% by months 10 to 12, compared with only 16% during the first 3 months of treatment. Women who experience prolonged breakthrough bleeding while taking combined OCs continuously should discontinue the active pills for 3 days and then restart.

All the original higher dosage OC formulations contained mestranol, and this steroid is still present in some 50-mcg pills. All formulations with less than 50 mcg of estrogen contain only the parent compound, ethinyl estradiol. In common usage, formulations with 50 mcg or more of estrogen (ethinyl estradiol or mestranol) have been termed *first-generation* OCs. Those with less than 50 mcg of estrogen (20 to 35 mcg EE) are called *second-generation* products if they contain any progestin except the three newest levonorgestrel derivatives (desogestrel, norgestimate, and gestodene). Those formulations are called *third-generation* formulations. All the synthetic estrogens and progestins in OCs have an ethinyl group at position 17 that enhances the oral activity of these agents by protecting the functional groups from metabolism as they pass through the intestinal mucosa and liver via the portal system. The synthetic steroids have greater oral potency per unit of weight than do the natural steroids. It has been estimated that ethinyl estradiol has about 100 times the potency of an equivalent weight of conjugated equine estrogen or estrone sulfate for stimulating synthesis of various hepatic globulins.

The various modifications in chemical structure of the different synthetic progestins and estrogens also affect their biologic activity. One cannot define the pharmacologic activity of the progestin or estrogen in a particular contraceptive steroid formulation based only on the amount of steroid present. The biologic activity of each steroid also has to be considered. Using established tests for progestational activity in animals, it has been found that a given weight of norgestrel is several times more potent than the same weight of norethindrone. Studies in humans, using delay of menses or endometrial histologic alterations such as subnuclear vacuolization as end points, also determined that norgestrel is about 10 times more potent than the same weight of norethindrone. Norethindrone acetate and ethynodiol diacetate are metabolized in the body to norethindrone and have equivalent potency per unit weight to the parent compound, norethindrone, whereas levonorgestrel is 10 to 20 times as potent. Desogestrel, norgestimate, and gestodene have been shown in animal, but not human, studies to have similar or greater progestogenic potency than an equivalent weight of levonorgestrel, with less androgenic activity. The magnitude of difference in androgenic and progestational effects produced by each progestin is called *selectivity*.

EE is about 1.7 times as potent as the same weight of mestranol, making a 50-mcg mestranol pill approximately as potent estrogenically as a 35-mcg EE pill. Because E2 is less active than EE, the more recently introduced natural estrogen pills must contain much higher doses of estradiol (e.g., 1.5 mg E_2, 2 to 3 mg E_2V) to deliver the same biologic effects. Following oral administration, E_2V is rapidly hydrolyzed and converted to 17 beta estradiol (E_2) during absorption in the gastrointestinal tract (1 mg of E_2V contains 0.76 mg of E_2). Estradiol has a lower hepatic effect than EE (10 mcg EE is equivalent to approximately 2 mg of E_2V 2 mg), but to date clinical studies have not demonstrated an increase in safety.

Brenner and coworkers measured serum levels of levonorgestrel, follicle-stimulating hormone (FSH), luteinizing hormone (LH), estradiol (E_2), and progesterone 3 hours after ingestion of a combination OC containing 0.5 mg of *dl*norgestrel and 50 mcg of ethinyl estradiol in three women during two consecutive cycles, as well as during the intervening pill-free interval. Daily levels of levonorgestrel rose during the first few days of ingestion, plateaued thereafter, and declined after ingestion of the last pill. Nevertheless, substantial amounts of levonorgestrel remained in the serum for at least the first 3 to 4 days after the last pill was ingested. These steroid levels were sufficient to suppress gonadotropin release during the 1-week interval when no steroid was administered, and follicle maturation (as evidenced by rising E_2 levels) did not occur during the HFI.

When lower doses of steroids are administered, follicular growth but not ovulation may occur during the HFI because of initiation of growth of the dominant follicle during the time that no steroid is being ingested. This may represent a mechanism for failure. Detailed studies assessing follicle development and ovulation have documented that shortening or eliminating the HFI reduces the likelihood of reactivation of the hypothalamic-pituitary-ovarian axis. Two formulations with 24 days of hormone pills followed by 4 days of no hormones have recently been marketed, and others are undergoing clinical trials.

Accidental pregnancies occurring during OC use probably do not occur because of failure to ingest one to two pills more than a few days after a treatment cycle is initiated but rather because initiation of the next cycle of medication is delayed for a few days. Therefore, it is important that the pill-free interval is not extended more than 7 days. This is best accomplished by ingesting either a placebo or iron tablet daily during the hormone-free interval. Women should be advised that the most important pill to remember to take is the first one of each cycle. In practice, clinicians should ensure that all patients are able to easily access refills of oral contraceptives. Because many women initiate a pill pack on a Sunday, a request for refill over the weekend is not uncommon. Delaying the start of a new cycle pack is an invitation for unintended pregnancy.

PHYSIOLOGY

Mechanism of Action

Combination oral contraceptives suppress gonadotropins. The estrogen component prevents a rise in follicle stimulating hormone (FSH), while the progestin component inhibits luteinizing hormone (LH). These dual actions lead to inhibition of follicle development and ovulation. The lowest amount of a progestin needed to suppress LH is known as the *ovulation inhibition dose*. Changes in the cervical mucus (which prevent sperm transport into the uterus), the fallopian tube (which interfere with gamete transport), and the endometrium (which reduce the likelihood of implantation) represent other important contraceptive effects of the progestin component. Because doses of a progestin are below the *ovulation inhibition dose* in the minipill, these other mechanisms become the primary mechanism. With both types of formulations, neither gonadotropin production nor ovarian steroidogenesis is completely abolished. Levels of endogenous E_2 in the peripheral blood during ingestion of high-dose combination OCs are similar to those found in the early follicular phase of the normal cycle.

Contraceptive steroids prevent ovulation mainly by interfering with release of gonadotropin releasing hormone (GnRH) from the hypothalamus. Most studies also support that contraceptive steroids directly affect the pituitary. Direct pituitary inhibition occurs in about 80% of women ingesting high-dose combination OCs. Pituitary suppression is unrelated to the age of the woman or the duration of steroid use but is related to the potency of the formulation. The effect is more pronounced with formulations containing a more potent progestin and with those containing 50 mcg or more of estrogen than with 30 to 35 mcg of estrogen. It has not been demonstrated that the amount of pituitary suppression is related to the occurrence of amenorrhea after stopping OC use, but if there is a relationship, lower-dose formulations should be associated with a lower frequency of this entity. Some data show that the mean time to conception after discontinuation of OC use is shorter in women ingesting preparations with less than 50 mcg of estrogen (4.01 cycles) than in those ingesting formulations with 50 mcg of estrogen or more (4.79 cycles).

The daily progestin-only preparations do not consistently inhibit ovulation. They exert their contraceptive action via the other mechanisms listed earlier, but because of the inconsistent ovulation inhibition, their effectiveness is lower than that of the combined pills. Clinicians should counsel their patients using the minipill that preparations should be consistently taken at the same time of day to ensure that blood levels do not fall below the effective contraceptive level.

Although the reported **Pearl Index** of various formulations varies slightly, no significant difference in clinical effectiveness has been demonstrated among the various combination formulations currently available in the United States. As long as no tablets are omitted (perfect use), the pregnancy rate is about 0.3% at the end of 1 year with all marketed combination formulations. In typical use, failure may range as high as 8%.

The balance between estrogen and progestin influences the bleeding profile of a combination OC. Estrogen induces endometrial proliferation. Progestins oppose the mitotic action of estrogen, leading to a stable decidualized endometrium. Even though women taking combined OCs are exposed to both hormones at the same time rather than sequentially, they typically will undergo some endometrial proliferation. The bleeding users of combined OCs experience during the hormone-free interval is called *withdrawal bleeding,* as it occurs upon cessation of the progestin component of the pill. Bleeding that occurs during the time that active pills are ingested is called *unscheduled, intracyclic,* or *breakthrough bleeding.* The dose of progestin used in the minipill is below the ovulation inhibitory dose, therefore estradiol and progesterone produced by the ovary will affect endometrial bleeding. Depending on the influence of the synthetic progestin on the endometrium, withdrawal bleeding will be inhibited and bleeding patterns may be quite irregular.

METABOLIC EFFECTS

The receptor-ligand relationships that involve sex steroids are among the most conserved in vertebrate biology. Therefore, it is not surprising that the synthetic steroids in OC formulations have many metabolic effects in addition to their contraceptive actions (**Table 13-3**). These metabolic effects lead to both inconsequential (but bothersome) side effects and rare potentially life-threatening complications. The magnitude of these effects is directly related to the dosage and potency of the steroids in the formulations. Fortunately, the more common adverse effects are relatively mild. The most frequent symptoms produced by the estrogen component include nausea (a central nervous system effect), breast tenderness, and fluid retention. This latter effect is mediated by increased aldosterone synthesis and decreased sodium and fluid excretion, and it can be a mechanism for weight gain (which usually does not exceed 3 to 4 pounds). Clinically insignificant reductions in circulating levels of the B complex vitamins and ascorbic acid and increases in levels of vitamin A have been reported, but these results have not been consistent across studies, particularly with low-dose formulations. Melasma, a condition where hyperpigmentation of the malar eminences develops, is also related to estrogen. Sunlight accentuates this condition, which may persist for many months

Table 13-3 Metabolic Effects of Contraceptive Steroids

Effects	Chemical	Clinical
Estrogen-Ethinyl Estradiol		
Proteins	↓	None
Albumin	↓	
Amino acids		None
Globulins		
Angiotensinogen		Blood pressure
Clotting factors		Hypercoagulability
Carrier proteins (CBG, TBG, SHBG, transferrin, ceruloplasmin)		None
Carbohydrate		
Plasma insulin	None	None
Glucose tolerance	None	None
Lipids		
Cholesterol		None
Triglyceride		None
HDL cholesterol		? ↓Cardiovascular disease
LDL cholesterol	↓	? ↓Cardiovascular disease
Electrolytes		
Sodium excretion	↓	Fluid retention Edema
Vitamins		
B complex	↓	None
Ascorbic acid	↓	None
Vitamin A		None
Other		
Breast		Breast tenderness
Endometrial steroid receptors		Hyperplasia
Skin	↓	Sebum production Facial pigmentation
Progestins—19-Nortestosterone Derivatives		
Proteins	↓SHBG	None
Carbohydrate		
Plasma insulin		None
Glucose tolerance	↓	None
Lipids		
Cholesterol	↓	None
Triglyceride	↓	None
HDL cholesterol	↓	? ↓Cardiovascular disease
LDL cholesterol		? ↓Cardiovascular disease
Other		
Nitrogen retention		Body weight
Skin-sebum production		Acne
CNS effects		Nervousness, fatigue, depression
Endometrial steroid receptors	↓	No withdrawal Bleeding

CBG, corticosteroid-binding globulin; HDL, high-density lipoprotein; LDL, low-density lipoprotein; SHBG, sex hormone–binding globulin; TBG, thyroxine-binding globulin.

even after OC discontinuation. Reduction in EE dose to below 50 mcg has greatly reduced the incidence of all these estrogenic side effects. Results of the large British Family Planning Association Study and a recent case-control study indicate that the use of OCs does not increase the incidence of gallbladder disease in women. When the data were stratified among women of different body weight or age, no increased risk of gallbladder disease was found in any subgroup. These results indicate that development of gallbladder disease is not a risk factor associated with OC use, even if these agents contain high doses of steroids and are used for more than 8 years.

It was previously postulated that high dosages of the synthetic estrogens could also produce changes in mood and depression brought about by diversion of tryptophan metabolism from its minor pathway in the brain to its major pathway in the liver. The end product of tryptophan metabolism, serotonin, is thus decreased in the central nervous system, and it was postulated that the resultant lowering of serotonin could produce depression in some women and sleepiness and mood changes in others. Analysis of the data from the Royal College of General Practitioners (RCGP) cohort study indicated that OC use was positively correlated with the incidence of depression, which in turn was directly related to the dose of estrogen in the formulation. However, in this study an increased incidence of depression was not found to occur among users of OCs containing less than 50 mcg of estrogen. Data from studies of women using postmenopausal hormone replacement therapy indicate that administration of physiologic doses of estrogen alone improves mood, whereas the addition of a progestin increases the frequency of depression, irritability, tension, and fatigue. Although these observational studies implicate that the progestin component is the major cause of adverse mood changes and fatigue observed in some women after ingestion of OCs, this has not been definitively established.

The structural relationship of the estrane and gonane progestins to testosterone may produce adverse androgenic effects, such as acne. Although estrogens decrease sebum production, progestins increase it, and this can cause acne to develop or worsen. Formulations differ with respect to the effect on skin. The net effect of an OC on acne relates to three qualities: the androgenicity of the progestin component, the extent that endogenous androgens circulate free or are bound to plasma proteins, and the activity of 5 α-reductase, the enzyme that converts testosterone to dihydrotestosterone. For most low-dose OCs, the net effect favors a reduction of acne, but formulations containing norgestimate and drospirenone have been shown in randomized controlled trials to reduce acne to a greater extent than placebo. The treatment of acne is now an approved indication for use of these agents. Weight gain represents a common complaint of women using hormonal contraception, and this may be a dose-related anabolic effect of progestins. However, well-designed cohort and the few randomized studies completed do not demonstrate a significant effect of low-dose OCs on weight. The newer, less androgenic progestins may also prove beneficial with respect to weight. Cagnacci and colleagues randomized postmenopausal women to receive oral nomegestrol acetate (NOMAc) and calcium or calcium alone and found that resting metabolic rate was increased and both body weight and body mass index were reduced after 12 months of NOMAc therapy. Similar findings were observed in postmenopausal women receiving E_2 and norethindrone acetate. Further study is needed to determine if these findings are applicable to users of OCs.

Unscheduled (breakthrough) bleeding and failure of withdrawal bleeding (amenorrhea) occur as a result of insufficient estrogen, too much progestin, or a combination of both. Although neither of these conditions would indicate a significant health concern or increased risk of failure in compliant users, both may contribute to dissatisfaction with the method and discontinuation. Increasing the amount of estrogen in the formulation or changing progestins usually solves the problem. Although many women consider regular withdrawal bleeding to be a reassuring and important signal of the absence of pregnancy, others accept amenorrhea as a health benefit. Absence of withdrawal bleeding is not a reason to change pills if the patient is satisfied.

Many women taking OCs complain of an increased frequency of headaches. This may be related to estrogen withdrawal if it occurs during the HFI. One OC formulation provides a small dose of EE during the last 7 days of the cycle. Menstrual cycle–related symptoms lead many women to seek medical attention and are typically improved on combined OCs. However, Sulak and associates reported that symptoms of pelvic pain, headache, breast tenderness, and bloating were all significantly more prevalent during the hormone-free days than when active hormones were given. Data from prospective and randomized studies indicate that women ingesting OCs with 24 active pills or continuously without a hormone-free interval experience fewer cycle-related symptoms than those using the pill in the standard fashion with a pill-free interval. Surveys suggest that substantial numbers of women would prefer an extended or continuous dosing regimen that reduces or eliminates withdrawal bleeding to reduce symptoms or for convenience.

HEPATIC EFFECTS

The principal health risk of hormonal contraception relates to the effect of synthetic estrogens on the hepatic production of several globulins. Progesterone and androgenic progestins do not affect the synthesis of globulins except that of sex hormone binding globulin (SHBG), which is reduced by androgens and androgenic progestins. Among the principal globulins increased by EE, factors V, VIII, X, and fibrinogen enhance thrombosis, and angiotensinogen (converted to angiotensin) may increase blood pressure in some users. The circulating levels of each of these globulins are directly correlated with the amount of estrogen in the OC formulation. Epidemiologic studies have shown that the incidence of both venous and arterial thrombosis is also directly related to the dose of estrogen.

Although angiotensinogen levels are lower in women who ingest formulations with 30 to 35 mcg of ethinyl estradiol than in those who ingest higher estrogen dosage formulations, a slight but significant increase in mean blood pressure still occurs in women who ingest the lower dosage formulations, and about 1 in 200 OC users will develop clinical hypertension. Thus, blood pressure should be monitored in all OC users. There is some indirect evidence that the progestin component may also raise blood pressure. However, women who receive progestins without estrogen do not have an increase in blood pressure over time, indicating that the estrogen component is the major cause of elevated blood pressure in a few OC users.

SHBG also binds circulating levels of estrogens and androgens. Although progesterone and synthetic pregnancies circulate bound to corticosteroid binding globulin, the androgenic 19-nortestosterone progestins are bound to SHBG. Estrogens increase SHBG levels, but androgens, including 19-nortestosterone derivatives, decrease SHBG levels. Thus, measurement of SHBG is one way to determine the relative estrogenic/androgenic balance of different OC formulations. Van der Vange and colleagues measured SHBG levels before and 6 months following ingestion of several OC formulations containing about the same amount of ethinyl estradiol. The greatest increase occurred with formulations containing cyproterone acetate (not used in OC formulations in the United States), desogestrel, and gestodene. SHBG increases of lesser magnitude occurred following ingestion of formulations containing low doses of norethindrone and levonorgestrel. Because SHBG binds endogenous testosterone and prevents it from acting on the target tissue, formulations causing the greatest increase in SHBG should be associated with the least amount of androgenic effects. These formulations are particularly useful for treating women with symptoms of hyperandrogenism such as polycystic ovarian syndrome. The formulations with the antiandrogenic progestin, drospirenone, are also beneficial in treating women with hyperandrogenism.

Carbohydrate

The effect of OCs on glucose metabolism is mainly related to the dose, potency, and chemical structure of the progestin. Conflicting data exist as to whether the estrogen component affects carbohydrate metabolism. The estrogen may act synergistically with the progestin to impair glucose tolerance. In general, the higher the dose and potency of the progestin, the greater the impairment of glucose metabolism. The magnitude of change appears to be greater with gonanes than with estranes. Several studies have shown that formulations with a low dose of progestin, including one containing levonorgestrel, do not significantly alter levels of glucose, insulin, or glucagon after a glucose load in healthy women or in those with a history of gestational diabetes. However, other studies indicate that the multiphasic formulations with norgestrel, but not those with norethindrone, produce some deterioration of glucose tolerance in normal women, as well as in those with a history of gestational diabetes. Some studies have shown increased levels of both glucose and insulin when glucose tolerance tests were administered to women ingesting desogestrel containing OCs.

Although results from these surrogate marker studies indicate some effect on carbohydrate metabolism, it is important to point out that data from 20 years of experience using mainly high-dose formulations in the large RCGP cohort study indicated that there was no increased risk of diabetes mellitus developing among current OC users (relative risk [RR], 0.80) or former OC users (RR, 0.82), even among women who had used OCs for 10 years or more. More than 1 million woman-years of follow-up of OC users in the large Nurses Health Study cohort, which was initiated in 1976, were analyzed in 1992. Although type 2 diabetes mellitus developed in more than 2000 women, the risk did not increase among current OC users (RR, 0.71) and only marginally increased in past OC users (RR, 1.11). The increased incidence occurred only among women who had used high-dose formulations many years previously and not in those who had used lower-dose formulations. Kjos and coworkers followed a group of women with a history of gestational diabetes mellitus for several years after the end of the pregnancy. Three years after delivery, women ingesting a low-dose norethindrone combination and a low-dose levonorgestrel combination containing OCs had no greater risk of developing diabetes mellitus than the control group not taking OCs. When prescribing oral contraceptives for women with a history of glucose intolerance, it is probably preferable to use formulations with a low dose of a norethindrone-type progestin than a levonorgestrel type and to monitor glucose tolerance periodically.

Current evidence suggests that hormonal contraceptives have limited clinically insignificant effects on carbohydrate metabolism in women without diabetes. Among women with a history of gestational diabetes, anthropometric measures of obesity, gestational age at gestational diabetes diagnosis, and method of glucose control are risk factors for the subsequent development of type 2 diabetes, but current and past OC use is not.

Lipids

The estrogen component of OCs cause an increase in high-density lipoprotein (HDL) cholesterol, a decrease in low-density lipoprotein (LDL) levels, and an increase in total cholesterol and triglyceride levels. The progestin component causes a decrease in HDL and an increase in LDL levels while causing a decrease in both total cholesterol and triglyceride levels.

The original high-dose OCs had adverse effects on the lipid profile. These progestin-dominant formulations produced a decrease in HDL cholesterol levels and an increase in LDL cholesterol levels. They also caused an increase in serum triglyceride because the estrogen effect on triglyceride synthesis exceeded the opposing action of the progestin. Subsequent short-term longitudinal studies of several lower-dose phasic formulations containing levonorgestrel and norethindrone found that a significant increase in triglyceride levels still occurred but there was little change in either HDL cholesterol or LDL cholesterol levels, as well as total cholesterol levels, because the effects of each steroid on lipid synthesis were offset by the other.

In a cross-sectional study in which lipid levels were measured in a large number of women ingesting several OC formulations and compared with non-OC users, Godsland and associates reported insignificant differences in HDL and LDL cholesterol levels in users of low-dose monophasic and triphasic levonorgestrel and norethindrone formulations compared to nonusers. Formulations with only 0.5 mg of norethindrone or 150 mcg of desogestrel had a significant increase in HDL cholesterol levels and a significant decrease in LDL cholesterol levels (**Fig. 13-7**). The three most recently developed progestins derived from levonorgestrel have less androgenic activity than do the older progestins and, as such, when combined with an estrogen would be expected to have a less adverse effect on lipid metabolism than on the older formulations. Speroff and colleagues in 1993 reviewed data from the published studies in which lipid levels were measured in women ingesting formulations with these three less androgenic progestins. They reported that with use of these formulations there was a significant increase in HDL cholesterol levels, a significant decrease in LDL cholesterol levels, little change in total cholesterol levels, and a substantial increase in triglyceride levels (**Table 13-4**). The long-term effect, if any, of these changes in lipid parameters remains to be determined.

The impact of E_2 containing pills on liver proteins and lipids should be lower than that of EE pills. Oral E_2 is subject to first-pass hepatic effect, resulting in conversion to E_1 and estriol (E_3), oxidation to nonestrogens, and conjugation to sulfate and glucuronide conjugates while EE passes through the liver essentially unchanged. Although this first pass effect of E_2 also contributes to the induction of hepatic globulins like SHBG, after the first pass the activation is lower than with EE. At doses of approximate equivalent potency (e.g., EE 10 mcg = E_2V 2 mg), the impacts of E_2V on hemostatic parameters are lower than those induced by EE.

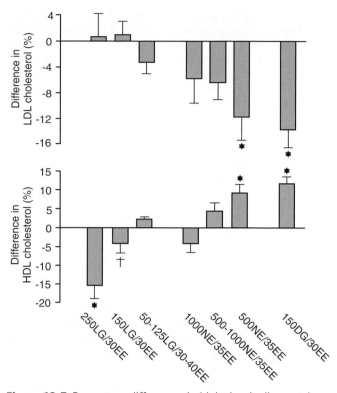

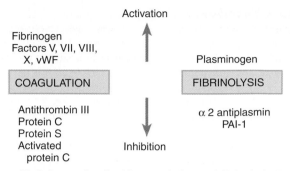

Figure 13-8 Factors involved in coagulation and fibrinolysis. PAI, plasminogen activator inhibitor; vWF, von Willebrand factor.

Figure 13-7 Percentage differences in high-density lipoprotein (HDL) and low-density lipoprotein (LDL) cholesterol levels and in the incremental area for insulin in response to the oral glucose tolerance test (OGTT) between women taking one of seven combination oral contraceptives and those not taking oral contraceptives. The T bars indicate 1 SD. The asterisk (p < 0.001) and dagger (p < 0.01) indicate significant differences between users and nonusers in the mean values for the principal metabolic variables. (Modified from Godsland IF, Crook D, Simpson R, et al: The effects of different formulations of oral contraceptive agents on lipid and carbohydrate metabolism. N Engl J Med 323:1375, 1990. Copyright 1990 Massachusetts Medical Society. All rights reserved. Modified with permission.)

Coagulation Parameters

Epidemiologic studies demonstrate that OCs increase the risk of thrombosis. The effect is related to the estrogen component of the pill and is dose dependent. The estrogen component of oral contraceptives increases the synthesis of several coagulation factors, including fibrinogen, which enhance thrombosis in a dose-dependent manner. The effect of OCs on parameters that inhibit coagulation, such as protein C, protein S, and antithrombin III, is less clear because of the diversity of techniques used to measure these parameters in different laboratories (**Fig. 13-8**). A similar

lack of consistency occurs when parameters that enhance fibrinolysis (e.g., plasminogen) or inhibit fibrinolysis (e.g., plasminogen activator inhibitor-1) are measured in OC users. Changes in most of these coagulation parameters in OC users are very small, if they occur at all, and there is no evidence that these minor alterations in levels of coagulation parameters measured in the laboratory for modern low-dose pills have any effect on the clinical risk of developing venous or arterial thrombosis for most healthy users. Nevertheless, if the woman has an inherited coagulation disorder (e.g., protein C, protein S, or antithrombin III deficiency or the more common activated protein C resistance), which increases her risk of developing thrombosis, her risk of developing thrombosis increases several fold if she ingests estrogen-containing oral contraception. Vandenbroucke and coworkers reported that the relative risk of developing deep venous thrombosis (DVT) among women with activated protein C resistance and OC use was increased 30-fold compared with non-OC users without the mutation. They estimated that the annual incidence of DVT in a woman of reproductive age with this genetic mutation was about 6 per 10,000 women if she did not take OCs and about 30 per 10,000 women if she took them. Currently, it is not recommended that screening for these coagulation deficiencies be undertaken before starting OC use because it is not cost effective unless the woman has a personal or family history of thrombotic events. However, if a woman has a known inherited or acquired thrombophilia, or a family or personal history of idiopathic venous thromboembolism (VTE), she should not take an estrogen-containing contraceptive. Progestins do not affect coagulation parameters.

CARDIOVASCULAR EFFECTS

The cause of the increased incidence of both venous and arterial cardiovascular disease, including myocardial infarction, in users of OCs appears to be thrombosis and not atherosclerosis.

Table 13-4 Lipid Changes with Oral Contraceptives Containing New Progestins

Percentage Change from Baseline							
Progestin	N	TG	C	LDL-C	HDL-C	Apo B	Apo A-1
Desogestrel	608	29.3	2.8	−2.1	12.9	10.5	11.3
Gestodene	296	38.3	3.8	−2.5	8.1	16.0	7.1
Norgestimate	>2550	13.8	4.3	−0.2	9.9	5.3	7.3

Apo, apoprotein; C, total cholesterol; HDL-C, high-density lipoprotein cholesterol; LDL-C, low-density lipoprotein cholesterol; TG, triglyceride.
From Speroff L, DeCherney A, and the Advisory Board for the New Progestins: Evaluation of a new generation of oral contraceptives. Obstet Gynecol 81:1034, 1993.

Venous Thromboembolism

Consistent evidence over the past 40 years has established that the risk of venous and arterial thrombosis increases among users of combined OCs compared with nonpregnant nonusers. Gerstman and colleagues analyzed the effect of OCs with different doses of estrogen on the incidence of VTE in a historical cohort study of more than 230,000 women age 15 to 44 in Michigan between 1980 and 1986. Among users of OC formulations with less than 50 mcg of estrogen, the rate of VTE per 10,000 woman-years was 4.2; among users of formulations with 50 mcg of estrogen, the rate was 7; and among users of formulations with greater than 50 mcg of estrogen, the rate increased to 10 per 10,000 woman-years (**Table 13-5**). These data confirm earlier findings that indicate that the risk of VTE is directly related to the dose of estrogen in the formulation. Comparing the various studies that have assessed thrombosis risks with different OC preparations requires an understanding of the background rate of VTE in women of reproductive age, generally quoted as about 0.8 per 10,000 woman-years. However, a recent review of the literature by Heinemann and Dinger detailed how this figure is derived from database studies, whereas two different VTE incidence rates are reported in the oral contraceptive literature: one for community/cohort studies and one for database studies. The estimated overall VTE incidence rates for women of reproductive age ranges between 0.7-3.8/10,000 woman-years (WY) in database studies, but a much higher background incidence of 5.5-13.5 and 3.8-12.2 per 10,000 WY is reported in community and cohort studies, respectively. This difference is probably attributable to methodological problems associated with some database studies, principally exclusions and selection of controls and verification of disease. Therefore, to interpret the differences in VTE rates observed across studies, it is important to compare rates only across similar study designs. The background rate also varies depending on the prevalence of other risk factors (e.g., smoking, obesity, inactivity) in the population studied.

Another important principle is that while combined oral contraceptives increase the baseline risk of VTE, they offer significant protection against pregnancy, a condition associated with a substantially higher risk of thrombosis roughly twofold higher than that observed with OCs. Recent estimates of the risk of VTE in pregnant women have ranged from 8 to 13/10,000 pregnancies in database studies reported by Liu and Simpson. As expected, the rates seen in the community cohort from Minnesota reported by Heit and colleagues was higher, at almost 20/ 10,000 WYs. An observational database study by Farmer and Preston from nearly 700,000 women ages 13 to 45 years assessed the incidence of VTE events associated with pregnancy and exposure to combined OCs containing more than 20 mcg but less than 50 mcg of estrogen. The incidence of venous thromboembolic events among OC users was 3 per 10,000 woman-years, which was about four times the background rate but half the rate of 6 per 10,000 woman-years associated with pregnancy.

Numerous observational studies have been performed to determine the risk of VTE in users of OCs containing mainly less than 50 mcg estrogen. An analysis of 220 articles published on this subject reported VTE risk was increased two- to threefold among women using combination OCs compared with women not using combination OCs. The increased risk of VTE is similar in women ingesting the same dose of progestin with 30 mcg and 20 mcg of estrogen.

Epidemiologic studies in the early 1990s suggested an increase rate of VTE in users of desogestrel, norgestimate, and gestodene led to a widespread "pill scare" that caused discontinuation of OCs and higher rates of unintended pregnancy and abortion. The U.S. FDA required the inclusion of additional wording in the package insert of desogestrel pills detailing a possible twofold increase in risk of DVT relative to formulations with levonorgestrel. More recently, these same concerns about increased VTE risk have circulated over drospirenone, the most recently introduced progestin. However, important differences in users and nonusers of oral contraceptives create sources of bias caused by confounding factors, not easily adjusted for in epidemiologic studies, including selective prescription of new OCs to high-risk women and the healthy user effect seen in women continuing use of existing products. Large prospective trials completed in both the United States and Europe have contradicted the findings of the observational epidemiologic studies regarding the increase risk of VTE with drospirenone-containing formulations.

The American study was performed using cohorts established to investigate potential hyperkalemic complications possibly related to the potassium-sparing diuretic effects of drospirenone. Women initiating the drospirenone pill, and medically similar initiators of other oral contraceptives were identified and followed, and there was no difference in the rate of thrombosis over an average follow-up of 7.6 months. The European Active Surveillance study (EURAS) was a multinational, prospective, noninterventional cohort study of new users of DRSP, levonorgestrel (LNG), and other progestin-containing OCs. The main clinical outcome of interest was to document the occurrence of uncommon cardiovascular events (e.g., arrhythmias, myocardial infarction, stroke, VTE, and sudden death) and compare the incidence rates between users of DRSP-containing OCs and users of established OCs. Based on the fact that European regulatory authorities considered the progestin LNG to have the least impact on VTE risk, it was decided that the primary cardiovascular outcome of interest should be the VTE hazard ratio (HR) between users of DRSP-containing OCs and users of LNG-containing OCs. To study these rare events, 58,674 study participants were followed up for 132,475 WY of observation. An array of comprehensive multitiered follow-up interventions kept loss-to-follow-up for the entire cohort to an impressively low 2.4% and did not differ between groups. The investigators found no difference in the overall incidence of any serious

Table 13-5 Rates of Deep Vein Thromboembolic Disease in Oral Contraceptive Estrogen Dose-Refined Cohorts

Estrogen Defined-Cohorts (mcg)	No. of Cases	Person-Years (× 10,000)	Rates/10,000 Person-Years
<50	53	12.7	4.2
50	69	9.8	7.0
>50	20	2.0	10.0
All	132	24.5	5.8

From Gerstman BB, Piper JM, Tomita DK, et al: Oral contraceptive estrogen dose and the risk of deep venous thromboembolic disease. Am J Epidemiol 133:32, 1991.

adverse event (SAEs), including VTE among users of any of the oral contraceptive groups. Underlying the health benefits of contraception, the highest rate of SAEs occurred among nonusers, primarily because of pregnancy-related events. Risk of VTE in the EURAS study was highest in the first 3 months of use. Another finding was that obese women (body mass index [BMI], >30.0) had an approximately threefold higher VTE risk compared with women with normal weight (BMI, 20.0 to 24.9).

The interaction of obesity and thrombosis risk was further explored in the Multiple Environmental and Genetic Assessment of risk factors for venous thrombosis (MEGA) study. In this large case-control study, the joint effects of obesity, OC use, and prothrombotic mutations on the risk of VTE were analyzed. Compared with normal weight (BMI < 25 kg/m²), the risk of VTE was increased in both overweight (BMI ≥ 25 and < 30; OR 1.7, 95% CI 1.55 to 1.87) and obese (BMI ≥ 30; OR 2.4, 95% CI 2.15 to 2.78) women. Obese women who used oral contraceptives had a 24-fold higher thrombotic risk than women with a normal BMI who did not use OCs. By comparison, the joint effect of factor V Leiden and obesity led to only a sevenfold increase in risk compared with normal weight women without the mutation. Nightingale and colleagues used the UK MediPlus Database and the General Practice Research Database to explore risk factors for DVT among OC users. The risk was increased with age, being overweight or obese (dramatically with a BMI > 35), smoking, general poor health, and asthma (**Fig. 13-9**).

Because obesity is an independent risk factor for VTE (**Fig. 13-10**), extreme obesity (e.g., a BMI > 40) should be considered a relative contraindication to use of a combined hormonal method. Combined methods are also contraindicated in women with a personal history of VTE, and family history of VTE is a relative contraindication. If a woman has a known thrombophilic mutation, she should not use a combined hormonal method, but it is not cost effective to screen women without a personal or family history of DVT for thrombophilic mutations before prescribing a combined hormonal method. The World Health Organization has established detailed

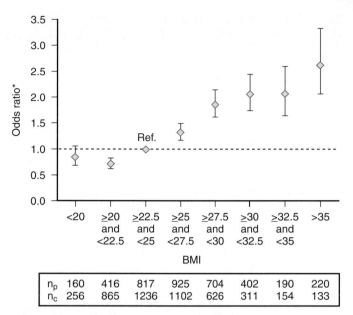

*Adjusted for age and sex.

Figure 13-10 Relative risk (with 95% confidence intervals) of deep vein thrombosis by categories of body mass (BMI). Adjusted for age and sex. (From Pomp ER, le Cessie S, Rosendaal FR, Doggen CJ: Risk of venous thrombosis: Obesity and its joint effect with oral contraceptive use and prothrombotic mutations. Br J Haematol 139:289-296, 2007. By permission.)

recommendations regarding eligibility for different types of contraceptive use in women with all types of medical conditions. The Centers for Disease Control and Prevention has also established medical eligibility criteria for contraceptive use (**Table 13-6**).

Myocardial Infarction

Neither epidemiologic studies of humans nor experimental studies with nonhuman primates have observed an acceleration of atherosclerosis with the ingestion of OCs. Nearly all the published epidemiologic studies indicate that there is no increased risk of myocardial infarction (MI) among former users of OCs. The incidence of cardiovascular disease is also not correlated with the duration of oral contraceptive use. Further data, which indicate that the increased risk of MI in OC users is due to thrombosis, not atherosclerosis, are provided by an angiographic study performed in 1982 by Engel and coworkers of young women who had an MI. In this study only 36% of users of OCs containing 50 mcg of ethinyl estradiol had evidence of coronary atherosclerosis compared with 79% of nonusers. A study with cynomolgus macaque monkeys found that the ingestion of an oral contraceptive containing high doses of norgestrel and ethinyl estradiol lowered HDL cholesterol levels significantly. However, after 2 years of ingesting this formulation and being fed an atherogenic diet, these animals had a significantly smaller area of coronary artery atherosclerosis than did a control group of female monkeys not ingesting OCs but fed the same diet. Another group of monkeys, who received levonorgestrel without estrogen, also had lowered HDL cholesterol levels. In this group, the extent of coronary atherosclerosis was significantly increased compared with that of the controls. The results of this study have since been confirmed in a larger study with two high-dose estrogen-progestin formulations. Both of these

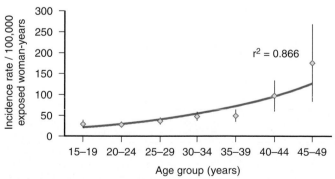

Figure 13-9 Age-specific incidence with 95% confidence intervals for deep vein thrombosis in users of combined oral contraceptives from the MedPlus Database and the General Practice Research database 1992-1997. (From Nightingale AL, Lawrenson RA, Simpson EL, et al: The effects of age, body mass index, smoking and general health on the risk of venous thromboembolism in users of combined oral contraceptives. Eur J Contracept Reprod Health Care 5:265-274, 2000. By permission.)

Table 13.6 Summary Chart of U.S. Medical Eligibility Criteria for Contraceptive Use

Key:

1 No restriction (method can be used)
2 Advantages generally outweigh theoretical or proven risks
3 Theoretical or proven risks usually outweigh the advantages
4 Unacceptable health risk (method not to be used)

Condition	Sub-condition	Combined pill, patch, ring I	C	Progestin-only pill I	C	Injection I	C	Implant I	C	LNG-IUD I	C	Copper-IUD I	C
Age		Menarche to <40=1 ≥40=2		Menarche to <18=1 18-45=1 >45=1		Menarche to <18=2 18-45=1 >45=2		Menarche to <18=1 18-45=1 >45=1		Menarche to <20=2 ≥20=1		Menarche to <20=2 ≥20=1	
Anatomic abnormalities	a) Distorted uterine cavity									4		4	
	b) Other abnormalities									2		2	
Anemias	a) Thalassemia	1		1		1		1		1		2	
	b) Sickle cell disease‡	2		1		1		1		1		2	
	c) Iron-deficiency anemia	1		1		1		1		1		2	
Benign ovarian tumors	(including cysts)	1		1		1		1		1		1	
Breast disease	a) Undiagnosed mass	2*		2*		2*		2*		2		1	
	b) Benign breast disease	1		1		1		1		1		1	
	c) Family history of cancer	1		1		1		1		1		1	
	d) Breast cancer‡												
	i) current	4		4		4		4		4		1	
	ii) past and no evidence of current disease for 5 years	3		3		3		3		3		1	
Breastfeeding (see also Postpartum)	a) <1 month postpartum	3*		2*		2*		2*					
	b) 1 month or more postpartum	2*		1*		1*		1*					
Cervical cancer	Awaiting treatment	2		1		2		2		4	2	4	2
Cervical ectropion		1		1		1		1		1		1	
Cervical intraepithelial neoplasia (CIN)		2		1		2		2		2		1	
Cirrhosis	a) Mild (compensated)	1		1		1		1		1		1	
	b) Severe‡ (decompensated)	4		3		3		3		3		1	
Deep venous thrombosis (DVT)/ Pulmonary embolism (PE)	a) History of DVT/PE, not on anticoagulant therapy												
	i) higher risk for recurrent DVT/PE	4		2		2		2		2		1	
	ii) lower risk for recurrent DVT/PE	3		2		2		2		2		1	
	b) Acute DVT/PE	4		2		2		2		2		2	
	c) DVT/PE and established on anticoagulant therapy for at least 3 months												
	i) higher risk for recurrent DVT/PE	4*		2		2		2		2		2	
	ii) lower risk for recurrent DVT/PE	3*		2		2		2		2		2	
	d) Family history (first-degree relatives)	2		1		1		1		1		1	
	e) Major surgery												
	(i) with prolonged immobilization	4		2		2		2		2		1	
	(ii) without prolonged immobilization	2		1		1		1		1		1	
	f) Minor surgery without immobilization	1		1		1		1		1		1	
Depressive disorders		1*		1*		1*		1*		1*		1*	
Diabetes mellitus (DM)	a) History of gestational DM only	1		1		1		1		1		1	
	b) Non-vascular disease												
	(i) non-insulin dependent	2		2		2		2		2		1	
	(ii) insulin dependent‡	2		2		2		2		2		1	

Table 13.6 Summary Chart of U.S. Medical Eligibility Criteria for Contraceptive Use—cont'd

Condition	Sub-condition	Combined pill, patch, ring		Progestin-only pill		Injection		Implant		LNG-IUD		Copper-IUD	
		I	C	I	C	I	C	I	C	I	C	I	C
DM (cont.)	c) Nephropathy/ retinopathy/ neuropathy‡	3/4*		2		3		2		2		1	
	d) Other vascular disease or diabetes of >20 years' duration‡	3/4*		2		3		2		2		1	
Endometrial cancer‡		1		1		1		1		4	2	4	2
Endometrial hyperplasia		1		1		1		1		1		1	
Endometriosis		1		1		1		1		1		2	
Epilepsy‡§	see drug interactions	1*		1*		1*		1*		1		1	
Gall-bladder disease	a) Symptomatic (i) treated by cholecystectomy	2		2		2		2		2		1	
	(ii) medically treated	3		2		2		2		2		1	
	(iii) current	3		2		2		2		2		1	
	b) Asymptomatic	2		2		2		2		2		1	
Gestational trophoblastic disease	a) Decreasing or undetectable ß-hCG levels	1		1		1		1		3		3	
	b) Persistently elevated ß-hCG levels or malignant disease‡	1		1		1		1		4		4	
Headaches	a) Non-migrainous	1*	2*	1*	1*	1*	1*	1*	1*	1*	1*	1*	
	b) Migraine i) without aura, age <35	2*	3*	1*	2*	2*	2*	2*	2*	2*	2*	1*	
	ii) without aura, age ≥35	3*	4*	1*	2*	2*	2*	2*	2*	2*	2*	1*	
	iii) with aura, any age	4*	4*	2*	3*	2*	3*	2*	3*	2*	3*	1*	
History of bariatric surgery‡	a) Restrictive procedures	1		1		1		1		1		1	
	b) Malabsorptive procedures	COCs: 3 P/R: 1		3		1		1		1		1	
History of cholestasis	a) Pregnancy-related	2		1		1		1		1		1	
	b) Past COC-related	3		2		2		2		2		1	
History of high blood pressure during pregnancy		2		1		1		1		1		1	
History of pelvic surgery		1		1		1		1		1		1	
HIV	High risk or HIV infected‡	1		1		1		1		2	2	2	2
	AIDS (see drug interactions)‡§	1*		1*		1*		1*		3	2*	3	2*
	Clinically well on ARV therapy§	If on treatment see drug interactions							2	2	2	2	2
Hyperlipidemias		2/3*		2*		2*		2*		2*		1*	
Hypertension	a) Adequately controlled hypertension	3*		1*		2*		1*		1		1	
	b) Elevated blood pressure levels (properly taken measurements) (i) systolic 140-159 or diastolic 90-99	3		1		2		1		1		1	
	(ii) systolic ≥160 or diastolic ≥100‡	4		2		3		2		2		1	
Hypertension	c) Vascular disease	4		2		3		2		2		1	
Inflammatory bowel disease	(Ulcerative colitis, Crohn's disease)	2/3*		2		2		1		1		1	
Ischemic heart disease‡	Current and history of	4		2	3	3		2	3	2	3	1	
Liver tumors	a) Benign i) Focal nodular hyperplasia	2		2		2		2		2		1	
	ii) Hepatocellular adenoma‡	4		3		3		3		3		1	
	b) Malignant‡	4		3		3		3		3		1	

Continued

Table 13.6 Summary Chart of U.S. Medical Eligibility Criteria for Contraceptive Use—cont'd

Condition	Sub-condition	Combined pill, patch, ring I	C	Progestin-only pill I	C	Injection I	C	Implant I	C	LNG-IUD I	C	Copper-IUD I	C
Malaria		1		1		1		1		1		1	
Multiple risk factors for arterial cardiovascular disease	(such as older age, smoking, diabetes and hypertension)	3/4*		2*		3*		2*		2		1	
Obesity	a) ≥30 kg/m² body mass index (BMI)	2		1		1		1		1		1	
	b) Menarche to <18 years and ≥30 kg/m² BMI	2		1		2		1		1		1	
Ovarian cancer‡		1		1		1		1		1		1	
Parity	a) Nulliparous	1		1		1		1		2		2	
	b) Parous	1		1		1		1		1		1	
Past ectopic pregnancy		1		2		1		1		1		1	
Pelvic inflammatory disease	a) Past, (assuming no current risk factors of STIs)												
	(i) with subsequent pregnancy	1		1		1		1		1	1	1	1
	(ii) without subsequent pregnancy	1		1		1		1		2	2	2	2
	b) Current	1		1		1		1		4	2*	4	2*
Peripartum cardiomyopathy‡	a) Normal or mildly impaired cardiac function												
	(i) <6 months	4		1		1		1		2		2	
	(ii) ≥6 months	3		1		1		1		2		2	
	b) Moderately or severely impaired cardiac function	4		2		2		2		2		2	
Post-abortion	a) First trimester	1*		1*		1*		1*		1*		1*	
	b) Second trimester	1*		1*		1*		1*		2		2	
	c) Immediately post-septic abortion	1*		1*		1*		1*		4		4	
Postpartum (see also Breastfeeding)	a) <21 days	4		1		1		1					
	b) 21 days to 42 days												
	(i) with other risk factors for VTE	3*		1		1		1					
	(ii) without other risk factors for VTE	2		1		1		1					
	c) >42 days	1		1		1		1					
Postpartum (in breastfeeding or non-breastfeeding women, including post-caesarean section)	a) <10 minutes after delivery of the placenta									2		1	
	b) 10 minutes after delivery of the placenta to <4 weeks									2		2	
	c) ≥4 weeks									1		1	
	d) Puerperal sepsis									4		4	
Pregnancy		NA*		NA*		NA*		NA*		4*		4*	
Rheumatoid arthritis	a) On immunosuppressive therapy	2		1		2/3*		1		2	1	2	1
	b) Not on immunosuppressive therapy	2		1		2		1		1		1	
Schistosomiasis	a) Uncomplicated	1		1		1		1		1		1	
	b) Fibrosis of the liver‡	1		1		1		1		1		1	
Severe dysmenorrhea		1		1		1		1		1		2	
Sexually transmitted infections	a) Current purulent cervicitis or chlamydial infection or gonorrhea	1		1		1		1		4	2*	4	2*
	b) Other STIs (excluding HIV and hepatitis)	1		1		1		1		2	2	2	2
	c) Vaginitis (including trichomonas vaginalis and bacterial vaginosis)	1		1		1		1		2	2	2	2
	d) Increased risk of STIs	1		1		1		1		2/3*	2	2/3*	2

Table 13.6 Summary Chart of U.S. Medical Eligibility Criteria for Contraceptive Use—cont'd

Condition	Sub-condition	Combined pill, patch, ring I	C	Progestin-only pill I	C	Injection I	C	Implant I	C	LNG-IUD I	C	Copper-IUD I	C
Smoking	a) Age <35	2		1		1		1		1		1	
	b) Age ≥35, <15 cigarettes/day	3		1		1		1		1		1	
	c) Age ≥35, ≥15 cigarettes/day	4		1		1		1		1		1	
Solid organ transplantation‡	a) Complicated	4		2		2		2		3	2	3	2
	b) Uncomplicated	2*		2		2		2		2		2	
Stroke‡	History of cerebrovascular accident	4		2	3	3		2	3	2		1	
Superficial venous thrombosis	a) Varicose veins	1		1		1		1		1		1	
	b) Superficial thrombophlebitis	2		1		1		1		1		1	
Systemic lupus erythematosus‡	a) Positive (or unknown) antiphospholipid antibodies	4		3		3	3	3		3		1	1
	b) Severe thrombocytopenia	2		2		3	2	2		2*		3*	2*
	c) Immunosuppressive treatment	2		2		2	2	2		2		2	1
	d) None of the above	2		2		2	2	2		2		1	1
Thrombogenic mutations‡		4*		2*		2*		2*		2*		1*	
Thyroid disorders	a) Simple goiter/hyperthyroid/hypothyroid	1		1		1		1		1		1	
Tuberculosis‡	a) Non-Pelvic	1*		1*		1*		1*		1		1	
	b) Pelvic	1*		1*		1*		1*		4	3	4	3
Unexplained vaginal bleeding	(suspicious for serious condition) before evaluation	2*		2*		3*		3*		4*	2*	4*	2*
Uterine fibroids		1		1		1		1		2		2	
Valvular heart disease	a) Uncomplicated	2		1		1		1		1		1	
	b) Complicated‡	4		1		1		1		1		1	
Vaginal bleeding patterns	a) Irregular pattern without heavy bleeding	1		2		2		2		1	1	1	
	b) Heavy or prolonged bleeding	1*		2*		2*		2*		1*	2*	2*	
Viral hepatitis	a) Acute or flare	3/4*	2	1		1		1		1		1	
	b) Carrier/Chronic	1	1	1		1		1		1		1	
Drug Interactions Antiretroviral therapy (ARV)	a) Nucleoside reverse transcriptase inhibitors	1*		1		1		1		2/3*	2*	2/3*	2*
	b) Non-nucleoside reverse transcriptase inhibitors	2*		2*		1		2*		2/3*	2*	2/3*	2*
	c) Ritonavir-boosted protease inhibitors	3*		3*		1		2*		2/3*	2*	2/3*	2*
Anticonvulsant therapy	a) Certain anticonvulsants (phenytoin, carbamazepine, barbiturates, primidone, topiramate, oxcarbazepine)	3*		3*		1		2*		1		1	
	b) Lamotrigine	3*		1		1		1		1		1	
Antimicrobial therapy	a) Broad spectrum antibiotics	1		1		1		1		1		1	
	b) Antifungals	1		1		1		1		1		1	
	c) Antiparasitics	1		1		1		1		1		1	
	d) Rifampicin or rifabutin therapy	3*		3*		1		2*		1		1	

I = initiation of contraceptive method; C = continuation of contraceptive method

U.S. Medical Eligibility Criteria for Contraceptive Use, 2010. MMWR. Recommendations and reports : Morbidity and mortality weekly report. Recommendations and reports/ Centers for Disease Control, 2010;59(RR-4):1-86. PMID:20559203

*Please see the complete guidance for a clarification to this classification. www.cdc.gov/reproductivehealth/usmec

‡Condition that exposes woman to increased risk as a result of unintended pregnancy.

§Please refer to the US MEC guidance related to drug interactions at the end of this chart compounds lowered the HDL cholesterol levels by half and tripled the cholesterol/HDL cholesterol ratio. In this study, the mean extent of coronary artery plaque formation in the high-risk control group of female animals was more than three times greater than that found in animals ingesting a high-dose norgestrel + ethinyl estradiol compound and more than 10 times greater than that found in animals ingesting a high-dose ethynodiol diacetate + ethinyl estradiol compound. Taken together, these studies suggest that the estrogen component of OCs has a direct protective effect on the coronary arteries, reducing the extent of atherosclerosis that would otherwise be accelerated by decreased levels of HDL cholesterol.

The epidemiologic studies that reported an increased incidence of MI in older users of OCs were published in the late 1970s and reflect a database of women who only ingested formulations with 50 mcg or more of estrogen. In these case-control and cohort studies, a significantly increased incidence of MI was found mainly among older users who had risk factors that caused arterial narrowing, such as preexisting hypercholesterolemia, hypertension, diabetes mellitus, or smoking more than 15 cigarettes a day.

Data accumulated during the first 10 years of the RCGP study (1968 to 1977), in which the majority of users ingested formulations with more than 50 mcg of estrogen and high doses of progestin, showed that a significantly increased relative risk of death from circulatory disease occurred only among women older than 35 years of age who also smoked. A more recent analysis of data obtained during the first 20 years of this study (1968 to 1987) revealed that there was no significant increased relative risk of acute MI among current or former users of oral contraceptives who did not smoke any cigarettes (**Table 13-7**). Women who smoked and did not use OCs had a greater risk of MI than did nonsmokers, whether or not they used OCs; a significantly increased risk of MI with OC use occurred among both mild (<15 cigarettes per day) and heavy cigarette smokers (heavy smokers had a greater relative risk than mild smokers). A case-control study analyzed the relation between OC use and the risk of MI among women admitted to a group of New England hospitals between 1985 and 1988. The overall relative risk of MI among current OC users was not significantly increased compared with nonusers, RR 1.1 (95% confidence interval [CI], 0.4 to 3.1). Significantly, among women who smoked at least 25 cigarettes a day, current OC use increased the risk of MI 30-fold! Smoking alone, without use of OCs, increased the risk of MI about ninefold. The data indicate that cigarette smoking is an independent risk factor for MI, and the use of high-dose OCs by cigarette smokers significantly enhances their risk of

experiencing an MI; the two factors act synergistically. Current or prior OC use is not associated with an increased risk of MI in nonsmokers.

The mechanism whereby cigarette smoking increases the risk of arterial thrombosis in OC users appears to be due to the effect of nicotine on the coagulation process. Although OCs increase the production of prothrombotic factors, they also affect the activity of factors inhibiting coagulation. Notelovitz and colleagues found that smokers who ingested low-dose OCs had a significantly greater decrease in levels of endogenous coagulation inhibitors, mainly antithrombin III, than did OC users who did not smoke. Dynamic tests of coagulation and fibrinolysis by these investigators showed an altered procoagulant activity only among the OC users who also smoked. Mileikowsky and associates reported that platelet aggregation was increased only among OC users who also smoked and not among women who smoked and did not use OCs. This thrombotic effect was probably related to prostacyclin inhibition, as prostacyclin formation was reduced only among the women in the study who smoked and used OCs, altering the usual balance of prostacyclin and thromboxane, producing a relative excess of thromboxane. The results suggest that the synergistic effect of OCs and smoking on arterial thrombosis that leads to MI and cerebral thrombosis is produced by activation of the thromboxane A_2-mediated mechanism of platelet aggregation brought about by reduction of prostacyclin only during nicotine intake. Clinically, this means that former cigarette smokers do not continue to have a risk of enhanced thrombosis and that nicotine administered in any form (including skin patches used in smoking cessation) can increase the risk. Both the RCGP and WHO studies reported that the risk of MI in OC users was several fold greater if they had hypertension than if they did not. Two large case-control studies in the United States have shown no significantly increased risk of MI in OC users. For many years in the United States, OCs have not been prescribed to women with uncontrolled hypertension or those older than age 35 who smoked cigarettes. A WHO technical report stated that women who do not smoke, who have their blood pressure checked, and who do not have hypertension or diabetes are not at increased risk of MI if they use combined oral contraceptives regardless of their age.

Stroke

Although epidemiologic data from studies performed in the 1970s indicated the possibility of a causal relation between ingestion of high-dose OC formulations and stroke, the data were conflicting, with some studies showing a significantly increased risk of ischemic stroke, others an increased risk of hemorrhagic stroke, and still others no significantly increased risk of either entity. Furthermore, as occurred with MI, in studies that demonstrated a significantly increased overall risk of stroke, this occurred mainly in older women who also smoked, were hypertensive, or both. The monkey studies performed by Clarkson and coworkers revealed that the animals ingesting high-dose OCs, which lowered HDL cholesterol, had no greater extent of carotid artery atherosclerosis than did the control group. This is consistent with epidemiologic studies that have consistently reported no increased risk of either ischemic or hemorrhagic stroke in past users of OCs compared to never users.

Data from the epidemiologic studies of OC use and cardiovascular disease performed in the 1960s and 1970s are not relevant to their current use, as the dose of both steroid

Table 13-7 Relative Risk of Myocardial Infarction in Relation to Smoking and Oral Contraceptive Use (RCGP Study, 1968-1987) (*N* = 158)

Smoking	Oral Contraceptive Use		
	Never (CL)	**Previously (CL)**	**Current (CL)**
Never	1.0	1.1 (0.6-2.2)	0.9 (0.3-2.7)
<15 cig./day	2.0 (1.0-3.9)	1.3 (0.6-2.8)	3.5 (1.3-9.5)
≥15 cig./day	3.3 (1.6-6.7)	4.3 (2.3-8.0)	20.8 (5.2-83.1)

CL, confidence limits.
Modified from Croft P, Hannaford PC: Risk factors for acute myocardial infarction in women. BMJ 298:165, 1989.

components in the formulations now being marketed is markedly less, and women with cardiovascular risk factors such as uncontrolled hypertension are no longer receiving these agents. Use of OCs in by women older than age 35 who also smoke is contraindicated.

A nested case-control analysis by Hannaford and associates examined the data obtained between 1968 and 1990 during the RCGP Oral Contraception Study to determine the relationship between OC use and the risk of first-ever stroke, including the diagnosis of subarachnoid hemorrhage, cerebral hemorrhage, or ischemic stroke. Women using OCs containing a high estrogen dose (more than 50 mcg) had a nearly sixfold increase in the risk of stroke, whereas women ingesting OC formulations containing 30 to 35 mcg estrogen did not have an increased risk. Similar data were reported from a WHO study; compared with nonusers, the risk of ischemic stroke among women ingesting OCs with 50 mcg or more of estrogen was 5.3, but it was only 1.5 (insignificant) in women ingesting OCs with less than 50 mcg of estrogen. An analysis by Pettiti and colleagues of strokes occurring in a large health maintenance organization in California from 1991 to 1994 indicated no significant increase of either ischemic or hemorrhagic stroke with OC use. In this study the relative risk of ischemic stroke and hemorrhagic stroke for OC users was 1.18 and 1.13, respectively, compared with never users and past users. Another case study by Schwartz and coworkers analyzed these data as well as data from the state of Washington. The relative risk of ischemic and hemorrhagic stroke in OC users compared with nonusers was 1.4 and 1.3. Neither of these figures was statistically significant.

The results of these recent epidemiologic studies indicate that use of a low-dose estrogen-progestin OC formulation by nonsmoking women without risk factors for cardiovascular disease is not associated with an increased incidence of either MI or ischemic or hemorrhagic stroke. Smoking is a risk factor for arterial but not venous thrombosis. Combination OCs should not be prescribed to women older than the age of 35 who smoke cigarettes or use alternative forms of nicotine.

Return to Fertility

In an attempt to determine whether the reproductive endocrine system recovers normally after cessation of OC therapy, Klein and Mishell measured serum levels of FSH, LH, E_2, progesterone, and prolactin every day for 2 months in six women who discontinued use of high-dose OCs. Except for a variable prolongation of the follicular phase of the first postcontraceptive cycle, the patterns and levels of all of these hormones were indistinguishable from those found in normal ovulating subjects. In these six women, the initial LH peak occurred from 21 to 28 days after ingestion of the last tablet. These results indicate that after a variable, but usually short, interval after the cessation of oral steroids, the suppressive effect on the hypothalamic-pituitary-ovarian axis disappears. After the initial recovery, completely normal endocrine function occurs.

As previously mentioned, the delay in the return of fertility is greater for women discontinuing use of OCs with 50 mcg of estrogen or more than with those containing lower doses of estrogen. However, use of the low-dose formulations still causes a significant reduction in time to conception rates, with a mean of 5.88 cycles for OC users, compared with 3.18 cycles for women discontinuing other contraceptive methods. Among women stopping use of OCs in order to conceive, the reduced probability of conception compared with women stopping use

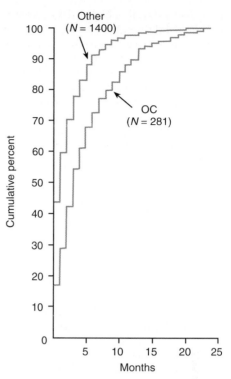

Figure 13-11 Cumulative conception rates for former oral contraceptive and other contraceptive users, Yale-New Haven Hospital 1980-1982. (Reprinted from Bracken MB, Hellenbrand KG, Holford TR: Conception delay after oral contraceptive use: The effect of estrogen dose. Fertil Steril 53:21. Copyright 1990, with permission from The American Society for Reproductive Medicine.)

of other methods is greatest in the first month after stopping their use and decreases steadily thereafter (**Fig. 13-11**). There is little, if any, effect of duration of OC use on the length of delay of subsequent conception. However, the magnitude of the delay to return of conception after OC use is greater among older primiparous women than among others. Thus, for about 2 years after the discontinuation of oral contraceptives, the rate of return of fertility is lower for users of OCs than for women who have used barrier methods, but eventually the percentage of women who conceive after ceasing to use each of these contraceptive methods becomes the same. Thus, the use of OCs does not cause permanent infertility.

Because the resumption of ovulation is delayed for variable periods after OCs are stopped, it is difficult to estimate the expected date of delivery if conception takes place before spontaneous menses return. If conception occurs before resumption of spontaneous menses, gestational age should be estimated by ultrasound. Neither the rate of spontaneous abortion nor the incidence of chromosomal abnormalities in abortuses increases in women who conceive in the first or subsequent months after stopping OCs.

Several large cohort and case-control studies of babies born to women who stopped using OCs have been undertaken. These studies indicate no increase in the risk of any type of birth defect among infants born to women conceived by former OC users compared with nonusers, even if conception occurred in the first month after the medication was discontinued. Further reassurance of the absence of a deleterious effect comes from a large cohort study showing no significant increase in the risk of congenital malformations among offspring of users that continued to ingest OCs after they conceived. Smokers who used OCs after conception had a threefold higher risk of delivering infants with anomalies than did the entire study group, but smoking by itself has been shown to have an adverse effect on reproductive outcome, increasing the risk of abortion. Although an increased risk of certain anomalies has been reported in some case-control studies of women ingesting OCs after conception, recall bias and the confounding effect of smoking may have influenced these results. Statements warning of a possible teratogenic effect of ingestion of OCs during pregnancy have been deleted from current product labeling for OCs.

OBESITY

The rising rates of obesity have heightened concerns about negative interactions with hormonal contraception. The EURAS study documented that women using OCs with a BMI of >30 have a threefold increase risk of venous thrombosis. Obesity may also affect OC efficacy. Holt and colleagues conducted a case-control study of 248 health maintenance organization enrollees who became pregnant while using OCs between 1998 and 2001 and 533 age-matched enrollees who were nonpregnant OC users during the same period. They found that among consistent users (women who missed no pills in reference month), the risk of pregnancy was more than doubled in women with BMI greater than 27.3 (OR 2.17, 95% CI 1.38 to 3.41) or greater than 32.2 (OR 2.22, 95% CI 1.18 to 4.20). A similar increase in risk of OC failure was observed among obese women in South Carolina, but the increase did not remain statistically significant after adjustment for confounders. Burkman and others evaluated a database from a large randomized trial originally designed to compare efficacy between two very low dose OCs (EE 25 mcg norgestimate and EE 20 mcg norethindrone acetate). There were more than 2800 subjects in the study, and the median BMI was 23. Although a small increase in the risk of failure for subjects with a BMI > 25 (RR 1.84, 95% CI 0.98 to 3.45) was observed, this was not statistically significant and there were no differences between the two formulations. Two reports have used the 2002 National Survey of Family Growth (NSFG) database and found no association between obesity and oral contraceptive failure or the overall risk of unintended pregnancy. Moreover, data from the large prospective European Active Surveillance Study (EURAS) cohort surveillance study of 59,510 OC users, found little variation in OC effectiveness by BMI.

Although the results of database and prospective studies do not demonstrate a consistent association between obesity and OC failure, because obesity is also associated with a risk of infertility, any reports of an increase risk of failure of hormonal contraceptives deserves serious consideration. Further studies to determine possible mechanisms for hormonal contraceptive failure in obese women are needed. In the only study that has addressed mechanism, Edelman and colleagues demonstrated that obese women have altered OC pharmacokinetics that lead to greater reactivation of the hypothalamic-pituitary-ovarian axis during the hormone-free interval, compared with normal-weight women.

NEOPLASTIC EFFECTS

OCs have been used for more than 50 years, and numerous epidemiologic studies of both cohort and case-control design have been performed to determine the relation between use of these agents and the development of various types of neoplasms. The most comprehensive of these studies, the Cancer and Steroid Hormone (CASH) study, was performed by the U.S. Centers for Disease Control and Prevention. The study analyzed the exposures of a large number of U.S. women from several geographic areas ages 20 to 54 with cancer initially diagnosed between 1980 and 1983 and an appropriate control group. Further insights have come from the 2007 publication of the findings from the Royal College of General Practitioner's (RCGP) cohort study of oral contraceptive use (**Table 13-8**). This study, begun in 1968, recruited more than 23,000 OC users and 23,000 nonusers over a 13-month period and has followed health outcomes for more than 40 years. The overall risk of cancer was lower in ever users of OCs. Compared with never users, ever users had statistically significant lower rates of cancers of the large bowel or

Table 13-8 Risk of Cancer among Ever and Never Users of Oral Contraceptives in the Main Dataset from the Royal College of General Practitioners Cohort Study

Malignancies	ICD-8 Code	Ever Users Observed Rate (number of women)	Ever Users Standardized Rate	Never Users Observed Rate (number of women)	Never Users Standardized Rate	Relative Risk (95% CI)
Main Dataset*						
Large bowel or rectum	153 and 154	24.65 (188)	26.01	38.56 (135)	36.10	0.72 (0.58 to 0.90)
Gallbladder or liver	155 and 156	1.83 (14)	1.99	3.70 (13)	3.62	0.55 (0.26 to 1.17)
Lung	162	26.97 (206)	27.12	25.94 (91)	25.77	1.05 (0.82 to 1.35)
Melanoma	172	12.58 (96)	12.86	14.28 (50)	13.99	
Breast	174	117.79 (891)	121.53	129.31 (448)	124.20	0.98 (0.87 to 1.10)
Invasive cervix	180	15.48 (118)	14.94	10.28 (36)	11.19	1.33 (0.92 to 1.94)
Uterine body	182	10.61 (81)	11.30	21.41 (75)	19.53	0.58 (0.42 to 0.79)
Ovary	183	12.57 (96)	13.23	26.54 (93)	24.66	0.54 (0.40 to 0.71)
Central nervous system or pituitary	191.1943	4.45 (34)	4.79	4.27 (15)	3.56	1.34 (0.73 to 2.47)
Site unknown	199	7.20 (55)	7.22	12.54 (44)	11.34	0.64 (0.43 to 0.95)
Other cancers		113.93 (863)	119.49	145.20 (504)	135.57	0.88 (0.79 to 0.98)
Main gynecological	180,182,183	38.75 (295)	39.58	58.41 (204)	55.54	0.71 (0.60 to 0.85)
Any cancer	140 to 209	333.68 (2485)	344.91	410.20 (1392)	390.37	0.88 (0.83 to 0.94)

From Hannaford PC, Selvaraj S, Elliott AM, et al: Cancer risk among users of oral contraceptives: Cohort data from the Royal College of General Practitioner's oral contraception study. BMJ 335:651, 2007.

rectum, uterine body, ovaries, tumors of unknown site, and other malignancies. Statistically significant trends of increasing risk of cervical and central nervous system or pituitary cancer and decreasing risk of uterine body and ovarian malignancies were observed with increasing duration of oral contraceptive use. In reviewing studies of risk, the available data support that synthetic steroid hormones are mainly promoters, not initiators, of cancers. Therefore, to be biologically plausible, any adverse (or protective) oncologic effects of these steroids should show a dose response, as demonstrated by an increased risk (or greater protection) occurring with increased duration of use.

Breast Cancer

In 1996 a large, international collaborative group reanalyzed the entire worldwide epidemiologic data that had investigated the relation between the risk of breast cancer and the use of OCs. Analysis was performed on data from 54 studies performed in 25 countries, involving more than 53,000 women with breast cancer and more than 100,000 controls. The analysis indicated that current users of OCs had a slightly increased risk of having breast cancer diagnosed (RR 1.24 [95% CI 1.15 to 1.30]). The magnitude of breast cancer diagnosis risk declined steadily after stopping OCs, so there was no longer a significantly increased risk 10 or more years after stopping their use (RR 1.01 [CI 0.96 to 1.05]). It is of interest that the cancers diagnosed in women taking OCs were less advanced clinically than those that occurred in the nonusers. The risk of having breast cancer that had spread beyond the breast compared with a localized tumor was significantly reduced (RR 0.88 [CI 0.81 to 0.95]) in OC users compared with nonusers. The group concluded that these results could be explained by the fact that breast cancer is diagnosed earlier in OC users than in nonusers or could be due to some biologic effects of the oral contraceptives. It was also found that women who had stopped using OCs more than 10 years earlier and developed breast cancer were significantly less likely to have nonlocalized disease than were women of similar age who had never used OCs. This reanalysis found that the risk of breast cancer diagnosis was not significantly altered by duration of oral contraceptive use, parity, or family history of breast cancer. In this reanalysis, 89% of the women with breast cancer initiated use of oral contraceptives before 1975 when formulations containing less than 50 mcg of estrogen initially became available. Therefore, the data in this reanalysis are not relevant to breast cancer risk with OCs containing a low dose of estrogen. More recent data from the large RCGP cohort study analyzing data from 1968 to 2004 found no association between ever use of OCs and breast cancer (RR 0.98 [0.87 to 1.10] compared to never users). Furthermore, there was no significant risk of breast cancer observed in the RCGP cohort even with increasing duration of use of more than 97 months. Taken together, all of these observations are consistent with the theory that steroid hormones are growth promoters but not initiators of breast cancer.

A population-based case-control study by the National Institute of Child Health and Human Development Women's Contraceptive and Reproductive Experience (Women's CARE) analyzed the effect of OCs on breast cancer in women ages 35 to 64. The investigators interviewed 4575 women with breast cancer and 4682 controls between 1994 and 1998 and found there was no increased risk of breast cancer in current OC users (odds ratio [OR] 1.0, CI 0.8 to 1.3) and past users (OR 0.09, CI 0.8 to 1.0) compared with women who had never used OCs.

There was also no significant difference in OC and breast cancer risk according to duration of OC use, age of first and last OC use, estrogen dose, and family history of breast cancer (**Table 13-9**). Marchbanks and the other investigators concluded

Table 13-9 Risk of Breast Cancer According to the Use of Combination Oral Contraceptives*

Variable	Case Subjects (*N* = 4575)	Controls (*N* = 4682)	Odds Ratio (95% CI)
Number			
No use	1032	980	1.0
Any use	3497	3658	0.9 (0.8-1.0)
Current use[†]	200	172	1.0 (0.8-1.3)
Former use	3289	3481	0.9 (0.8-1.0)[‡]
Duration of use			
<1 yr	782	822	0.9 (0.8-1.1)
1 to <5 yr	1200	1280	0.9 (0.8-1.0)
5 to <10 yr	848	882	0.9 (0.8-1.0)
10 to <15 yr	426	466	0.8 (0.7-1.0)[‡]
≥15 yr	234	202	1.0 (0.8-1.3)
Age at First Use			
<15 yr	72	79	0.9 (0.6-1.2)
15 to 19 yr	1239	1272	1.0 (0.8-1.1)
20 to 24 yr	1260	1369	0.9 (0.8-1.0)[‡]
25 to 29 yr	587	592	0.9 (0.8-1.1)
30 to 34 yr	209	239	0.8 (0.6-1.0)[‡]
35 to 39 yr	84	67	1.2 (0.8-1.6)
≥40 yr	38	35	1.0 (0.6-1.6)
Time Since Last Use			
Current use	200	172	1.0 (0.8-1.3)
7 mo to <5 yr	165	207	0.7 (0.5-0.9)[‡]
5 to <10 yr	244	239	0.9 (0.8-1.2)
10 to <15 yr	426	418	0.9 (0.8-1.1)
15 to <20 yr	650	717	0.9 (0.7-1.0)
≥20 yr	1803	1899	0.9 (0.8-1.0)
High Estrogen Dose[§]			
Any use	1082	1265	0.8 (0.7-0.9)[‡]
Current use	7	10	0.7 (0.2-1.8)
Former use	1074	1255	0.8 (0.7-0.9)[‡]
Low estrogen dose			
Any use	1360	1560	0.9 (0.8-1.0)
Current use	183	160	1.0 (0.8-1.3)
Former use	1267	1398	0.9 (0.8-1.0)

*Odds ratios were derived by conditional logistic regression with the study site, race, and age (in 5-year categories) as conditioning variables and were adjusted for menopausal status, age at menarche, age at menopause, number of term pregnancies, age at first term pregnancy, body-mass index, presence or absence of a family history of breast cancer, and use or nonuse of hormone-replacement therapy. Unknown oral-contraceptive formulations were classified as combination formulations. Missing values not included in one of the specified categories shown in Supplementary Appendix 1 were excluded. The reference group was the group of women who had never used oral contraceptives. Trend tests for the duration of use, age at first use, and time since last use were not significant at the 0.05 level. CI denotes confidence interval.
[†]Current use was defined as use of combination oral contraceptives within 6 months preceding the reference date.
[‡]The confidence interval does not include 1.0; some confidence limits were rounded to 1.0.
[§]A high estrogen dose was defined as 50 mcg or more of ethinyl estradiol or 75 mcg or more of mestranol. A low estrogen dose was defined as less than 50 mcg of ethinyl estradiol or less than 75 mcg of mestranol.
From Marchbanks PA, McDonald JA, Wilson HG, et al: Oral contraceptives and the risk of breast cancer. N Engl J Med 346:2028, 2002. Copyright 2002 Massachusetts Medical Society. All rights reserved.

that these data provide strong evidence that current or former use of OCs does not increase the risk of breast cancer in women ages 35 to 64. Another large case-control study performed in the United States, Canada, and Australia by Milne and colleagues analyzed women with breast cancer diagnosed before age 40 between 1992 and 1998. In this study there were 44 *BRCA-1* carriers, 36 *BRCA-2* carriers, and 1073 noncarriers. Like the Women's CARE study, this analysis showed no increased risk of breast cancer in *BRCA-1* or *BRCA-2* carriers or noncarriers with OC use. The OR for OC ever use more than 1 year and breast cancer in noncarriers was 0.93 (CI 0.6 9 to 1.24), whereas for first OC use after 1975 the OR for OC use and breast cancer was 0.74 (CI 0.55 to 0.99) compared with never use or OC use less than 1 year. The OR for OC use and breast cancer in *BRCA-1* carriers was 0.22 (CI 0.10 to 0.49) and for *BRCA-2* carriers was 1.02 (CI 0.34 to 3.09) compared with no OC use or OC use less than 1 year. The results of these two studies indicate that women who use OCs with less than 50 mcg of estrogen do not have an increased risk of developing breast cancer while taking OCs or after stopping OC use at least up to age 65. The risk of developing breast cancer with OC use is not changed in women with a high risk of developing breast cancer, including women with an immediate family history of breast cancer and those with *BRCA-1* and *BRCA-2* mutations.

Cervical Cancer

The epidemiologic data regarding the risk of invasive cervical cancer as well as cervical intraepithelial neoplasia and OC use are conflicting. Confounding factors, such as the woman's age at first sexual intercourse, number of sexual partners, exposure to human papillomavirus (HPV) (possibly greater among OC users), cytologic screening (probably more frequent among OC users), and the use of barrier contraceptives or spermicides (primarily by women in the control group), as well as cigarette smoking (an independent risk factor for this disease), could account for contrasting results in different studies. In most of these studies, statistical corrections were made for these confounding factors, and in many of them the control group did not use barrier methods of contraception. In 2002, the WHO commissioned a systematic review of published studies to determine the relation of hormonal contraceptives and cervical cancer. This review by Smith and colleagues in 2003 combined data from 28 studies (4 cohort and 24 case-control), published between 1986 and 2002, which included data from 12,531 women with cervical cancer. The combined analysis found that the risk of cervical cancer, both invasive and in situ, for OC users compared with nonusers increased with increasing duration of OC use. The summary relative risks for OC use of less than 5 years, 5 to 9 years, and 10 or more years were 1.1 (CI 1.1 to 1.2), 1.6 (CI 1.4 to 1.7), and 2.2 (1.9 to 2.4), respectively. The results were similar for squamous cell and adenocarcinoma, and in studies that adjusted for risk factors including HPV infection, number of sexual partners, cervical cytology screening, smoking, and use of barrier contraceptives.

The large RCGP cohort study that followed women from 1968 to 2004 found no significant overall increase in the risk of cervical cancer in ever users compared with nonusers (RR 1.33 [0.92 to 1.94]). However, the elevation did become significant when duration of use was considered, with risk estimates varying from 1.10 (0.64 to 1.90) at < 48 months, 1.45 (0.84 to 2.49) between 48 and 96 months, and 2.73 (1.61 to 4.61)

at 97 or more months of exposure. However, these results were not adjusted for barrier contraception use.

There is no evidence that OC use alters the incidence or rate of the progression of cervical dysplasia to invasive cancer. Women with treated cervical dysplasia can use OCs, as can those with newly diagnosed dysplasia awaiting evaluation. A recent case-control study by Harris and others that looked only at women with oncogenic HPV subtypes found no association between OC use and a histologic diagnosis of high-grade dysplasia.

In the past, the inconsistency of these findings led to a recommendation that OC users were at high risk for developing cervical neoplasia and therefore required at least annual screening of cervical cytology, especially if they have used OCs for more than 5 years. Recently published guidelines from the American College of Obstetricians and Gynecologists reflect the current understanding of the relationship of cervical dysplasia and cancer to high-risk subtypes of HPV and not steroid hormones. Pap smear screening should not be initiated until age 21, and done every 2 years if normal. Women over 30 with three consecutive negative pap smears can be screened every 3 years regardless of hormonal contraceptive use.

Endometrial Cancer

Endometrial cancer is the third most common cancer type among U.S. women, after lung and breast cancer. Several case-control studies and cohort studies have examined the relation between OCs and endometrial cancer, and nearly all of these studies have demonstrated a strong protective effect. Compared with nonusers, women who use OCs for at least 1 year have an age-adjusted relative risk of 0.5 for development of endometrial cancer between ages 40 and 55. This protective effect is related to duration of use, increasing from a 20% reduction in risk with 1 year of use to a 40% reduction with 2 years of use to about a 60% reduction with 4 years of use. In Schlesselman's review of 10 studies of more than 1200 women with endometrial cancer, the risk of developing endometrial cancer was decreased by 54% with 4 years' use, 66% with 8 years' use, and 72% with 12 years' use (**Fig. 13-12**). This protective effect persists for at

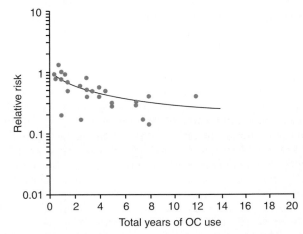

Figure 13-12 Relative risks of endometrial cancer by total years of oral contraceptive use. (From Schlesselman JJ: Net effect of oral contraceptive use on the risk of cancer in women in the United States. Obstet Gynecol 85:793, 1995.)

least 15 years after stopping use of OCs. In the study by Jick and associates of 132 cases of endometrial cancer among women 50 to 64 years of age, prior OC use was associated with a 50% (RR 0.48 [CI 0.26 to 0.84]) reduction in the risk of endometrial cancer risk compared with never users among women 50 to 64 years. Significantly, women at the greatest risk of acquiring the disease—nulliparous women and women of low parity—showed the greatest protective benefit. Voigt and coworkers reported that protection against endometrial cancer occurred with use of both high- and low-dose OC formulations. The RCGP cohort study analyzing data from 1968 to 2004 confirmed this strong protective effect, with an approximately 50% overall reduction in risk (RR 0.58 (0.42 to 0.79)) of uterine body cancer in ever users compared with nonusers.

Ovarian Cancer

Numerous epidemiologic studies have consistently demonstrated that OCs reduce the risk of developing ovarian cancer; more than 1 year of OC use reduces the risk by about 30%, relative to never users. In a review by Hankinson and associates of 20 epidemiologic studies, the summary relative risk of development of ovarian cancer among ever users of OCs was 0.64, a 36% reduction. OCs reduce the risk of the four main histologic types of epithelial ovarian cancer (serous, mucinous, endometrioid, and clear-cell). The risk of both invasive ovarian cancers and tumors of low malignant potential (Borderline) is reduced. The data demonstrate a clear dose response: the magnitude of the decrease in risk is directly related to the duration of OC use, increasing from about a 40% reduction with 4 years of use, to a 53% reduction with 8 years of use, and a 60% reduction with 12 years of use (**Fig. 13-13**). Beyond 1 year there is about an 11% reduction in ovarian cancer risk for each of the first 5 years of use. The protective effect begins within 10 years of first use and continues for at least 30 years after the use of OCs ends. Studies by Ness and colleagues and Royar and coworkers found a similar level of protection (50% reduction in risk) with both low-dose and high-dose formulations.

The RCGP cohort study provides additional evidence of the protective effect of OCs on ovarian cancer risk. The overall risk reduction observed for ever use was 0.54 (0.40 to 0.71). Consistent with biologic plausibility, increasing the duration of use was associated with greater protection, with a RR of 0.58 (0.33 to 1.04) at <48 months, 0.57 (0.30 to 1.07) at 48 to 96 months, and 0.38 (0.16 to 0.88) with 97 or more months of use.

OC use also reduces the risk of ovarian cancer in women with *BRCA-1* and *BRCA-2* mutations and in those with a family history of ovarian cancer to the same extent as in women without these risk factors. Two studies of OC use in women with the *BRCA* mutations found the risk of ovarian cancer is reduced by about 50% with OC use. As with endometrial cancer, the protective effect occurs mainly in women of low parity, who are at greatest risk for this type of cancer.

Liver Adenoma and Cancer

The development of a benign hepatocellular adenoma is a rare occurrence. An increased risk of this tumor was reported in early OC studies of prolonged use of high-dose formulations, particularly those containing mestranol. Two British studies also reported an increased risk of liver cancer among users of OCs, but the number of patients was small and confounding factors could have influenced the results. The rate of death from the disease has remained unchanged in the United States since the late 1980s, a period when millions of women have used these agents. Data from a large, multicenter epidemiologic study coordinated by the WHO found no increased risk of liver cancer associated with OC users in countries with a high prevalence of this neoplasm. This study found no change in risk with increasing duration of use or time since first or last use. In the RCGP cohort study, the RR of liver and gallbladder cancer was reduced in ever users of OCs (0.55 [0.26 to 1.17]), but this was not statistically significant. Women with active liver disease should not use hormonal contraception, as the liver is a major site for the metabolism of synthetic steroids.

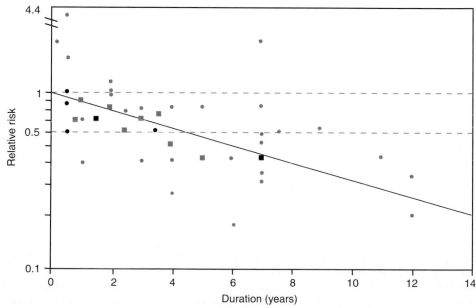

Figure 13-13 Relative risk of ovarian cancer associated with different durations of oral contraceptive use; findings of 15 studies. Study categories, indicating category weights ranging from smallest (weight in bottom 25% of range) to largest (weight in top 25% of range): blue circles = 1 (smallest); blue squares = 2; black circles = 3; black squares = 4 (largest). (From Hankinson SE, Colditz GA, Hunter DJ, Rosner B: A quantitative assessment of oral contraceptive use and risk of ovarian cancer. Obstet Gynecol 80:708, 1992.)

Pituitary Adenoma

OCs can mask the predominant symptoms produced by prolactinoma amenorrhea and galactorrhea. When OC use is discontinued, these symptoms can present, suggesting a causal relation. However, data from three studies indicate that the incidence of pituitary adenoma among users of OCs is not higher than that among matched controls. The RCGP cohort study did not show any overall increase risk of pituitary or central nervous system tumors. However, a trend toward an elevation in risk was seen with increasing duration of OC use, and this only became significant with the longest exposure of more than 96 months (RR 5.51 [1.38 to 22.05]).

Malignant Melanoma

Several epidemiologic studies have been undertaken to assess the relation of OC use and the development of malignant melanoma. An meta-analysis of 10 case-control studies by Karagas and colleagues in 2002 calculated a pooled odds ratio of 0.86 (CI 0.74 to 1.01) among OC users with more than 1 year of exposure compared with never use or use of less than 1 year. Among the 2391 cases of melanoma, there was no association between melanoma incidence and current, former, or prolonged OC use. The RCGP cohort study (initiated in 1968), involving more than 40,000 women, reported no overall increased risk of melanoma in ever users (RR 0.92 [0.65 to 1.29]) and no relationship to duration of exposure. The results of these large studies of long duration and the meta-analysis indicate that OC use does not alter the risk of malignant melanoma.

Colorectal Cancer

Several studies have found that OC use reduces the risk of colorectal cancer. Fernandez and associates performed a meta-analysis of published studies of this relation. OC ever use was associated with a 15% to 20% reduction in the risk of colorectal cancer in the eight case-control studies and four cohort studies. For colon cancer, the summary relative risk from 11 studies was 0.83 (CI 0.74 to 0.95) and for rectal cancer the summary relative risk from 6 studies was 0.74 (CI 0.59 to 0.93). Duration of use did not influence risk. A significant 38% reduction in overall risk was also observed in the RCGP cohort study (RR 0.72 [0.58 to 0.90]), but with no trend for further reduction with duration of use. Thus, OC use decreases the risk of developing both colon and rectal cancer.

ORAL CONTRACEPTIVE USE AND OVERALL MORTALITY

In 1989, Vessey and colleagues reported the causes of mortality (through 1987) among OC users and nonusers enrolled in the Oxford Family Planning Association Cohort Study between 1968 and 1974. During this 20-year follow-up of 17,032 women, there were 238 deaths. The overall risk of death among the OC users was 0.9 (CI 0.7 to 1.2) compared with women of similar age and socioeconomic status who used a diaphragm or condom for contraception. The risk of death from breast cancer in OC users compared with nonusers was 0.9 (CI 0.4 to 1.4), from cervical cancer 3.3 (CI 0.9 to 17.9), and from ovarian cancer 0.4 (CI 0.1 to 1.2). These cancer mortality rates are consistent with the other epidemiologic data reported earlier in this chapter. The death rate for circulatory disease was 1.5 (CI 0.7 to 3.0), and nearly all these deaths in OC users occurred in smokers. Similar mortality rates were reported by Colditz and coworkers in 1994 among the 166,755 women enrolled in the Nurses Health Study in 1976. A total of 2879 deaths occurred in this group of women, and the overall relative risk of death among ever users of OCs compared with never users was 0.93. There was no change in risk of death with long-term use. Among women who had used OCs for 10 or more years, the relative risk of mortality was 1.06 compared with nonusers. There was no change in risk of deaths caused by cardiovascular disease or cancer. The risk of death from ovarian cancer was 0.79, from endometrial cancer 0.33, and from breast cancer 1.07. None of these differences were statistically significant. In 1999, Beral and colleagues reported mortality in the 25-year follow-up of the 46,000 women enrolled in the RCGP study. There were 1599 deaths reported. For current and recent (within 10 years) users, the risk of death from ovarian cancer was 0.2, cervical cancer 2.5, and cerebrovascular disease 1.9. Ten or more years after stopping OCs, mortality rates for all causes, as well as most specific causes, were similar in women who had and those who had not used OCs. The mortality rate for breast cancer was nearly identical in OC users and nonusers. The overall risk of cancer was lower in ever users of OCs observed over almost 40 years in the RCGP cohort study. In 2010, Vessey and colleagues and Hannaford and colleagues updated mortality in the Oxford-Family Planning Association (OFPA) and the Royal College of General Practitioners (RCGP) cohorts. In both studies, even users of OCs had significantly lower rates of death from any cause or from all cancers or all circulatory disease. There is no significant increase in the risk of breast cancer death and a powerful reduction in the risk of death from ovarian cancer. These data provide further reassurance that use of high-dose OCs did not appreciably increase the risk of overall mortality. Because current practice involves exclusive use of low-dose formulations given to women without cardiovascular risk factors who have frequent cervical cytologic screening, an overall beneficial effect on mortality with OC use may be expected.

CONTRAINDICATIONS TO ORAL CONTRACEPTIVE USE

OCs can be prescribed for the majority of women of reproductive age, because these women are young and generally healthy. However, there are certain absolute contraindications, including a history of vascular disease (thromboembolism, thrombophlebitis, atherosclerosis, and stroke) and systemic disease that may affect the vascular system (e.g., lupus erythematosus or diabetes with retinopathy or nephropathy). Cigarette smoking by OC users older than age 35 and uncontrolled hypertension are also contraindications. One of the contraindications listed in the product labeling is cancer of the breast or endometrium; although there are no direct data indicating that OCs are harmful to women with these diseases, these are hormone-sensitive tumors. Two other contraindications are undiagnosed uterine bleeding and elevated triglyceride levels. The World Health Organization has published detailed guidelines listing the medical eligibility criteria for the use of contraceptive methods. The recently revised fourth edition can be downloaded free of charge from the WHO website (www.who.int/reproductivehealth/publications/family_planning/9789241563888/en/index.html). The Centers for Disease Control and Prevention (CDC) Guidelines, specific to practice in the United States, were published in

2010, and are available at http://www.cdc.gov/mmwr/preview/mmwrhtml/rr59e0528a1.htm.

Pregnancy is an obvious contraindication. Whether inadvertant OC use during early gestation is associated with an increase risk of fetal anomalies is controversial. One concern is that the androgenic 19 nortestosterone-derived progestins might have a masculinizing effect on the external genitalia of female fetuses. A meta-analysis of the relevant literature from 1966 to 1992 by Raman-Wilms and colleagues identified seven cohort and seven case-control studies involving 65,567 women calculated an OR of 0.98 (95% CI 0.24 to 3.94) for OC exposure and external genital malformations. As mentioned earlier, concerns that OCs might produce other deleterious fetal effects, such as limb reduction and heart defects, have not proved valid. These concerns were raised by older literature linking ingestion of any progestational agent in pregnancy to an increased incidence of congenital abnormalities. However, in these studies the major use of progestins in pregnancy had been for treatment of threatened abortion. Bleeding in pregnancy is itself associated with an increased incidence of anomalies. The incidence of birth defects has not decreased since the use of progestins for threatened abortion has been discontinued.

Women with functional heart diseases should not use OCs because the mild fluid retention (caused by the increase in aldosterone) they produce could result in congestive heart failure. There is no evidence, however, that individuals with asymptomatic mitral valve prolapse should not use OCs. Women with active liver disease should not take OCs. However, women who have recovered from liver disease, such as viral hepatitis, and whose liver function tests have returned to normal can safely take OCs.

Other relative contraindications to OC use include heavy cigarette smoking younger than age 35, migraine headaches, and undiagnosed causes of amenorrhea or genital bleeding. About 20% of women have migraine headaches, and OC use can worsen their frequency and severity. There is no evidence that the risk of stroke is significantly increased in women with common migraine headaches who use OCs. Some women will also note improvement of headache with OC use. If headache occurs only during the hormone-free interval, continuous dosing might help to control the symptoms. Women that have migraine headache with aura or peripheral neurologic symptoms (classic migraine) should not use oral contraceptives. Women with classic migraine that use combined OCs have an increased risk of ischemic stroke. MacClellan and colleague studied 386 women ages 15 to 49 years with first ischemic stroke and 613 age- and ethnicity-matched controls. Subjects were classified as having no migraine, probable migraine without visual aura, or probable migraine with visual aura (PMVA). Women with PMVA had an increased risk (OR 1.5 [95% CI, 1.1 to 2.0]) of ischemic stroke compared to women with no migraine. Neither current smoking or OC use was an independent risk factor, but the interaction between current cigarette smoking and OC use in women with PMVA greatly increased the risk of stroke (OR 7.0, 95% CI, 1.3 to 22.8). If fainting, temporary loss of vision or speech, or paresthesias develop in an OC user, the use of OCs should be stopped because this could be related to thrombosis.

OC use may mask the symptoms produced by a prolactin-secreting adenoma amenorrhea. Therefore, women with either galactorrhea or amenorrhea women should not receive OCs until a diagnosis is established. If galactorrhea develops during OC use, OCs should be discontinued, and after 2 weeks a serum prolactin level should be measured. If elevated, further diagnostic evaluations are indicated. The presence of a prolactin secreting macroadenoma but not a microadenoma, is a contraindication for OC use. Use of OCs does not cause enlargement of prolactin-secreting pituitary microadenomas or worsen functional prolactinoma as was previously believed. Women with a history of gestational diabetes can take low-dose OC formulations, because these agents do not affect glucose tolerance or accelerate the development of diabetes mellitus. Insulin-dependent diabetes without vascular disease is also not a contraindication for low-dose OC use.

Older literature has suggested a relationship between OC use and depression. An analysis of a large population of female outpatients less than 40 years of age with nonpsychotic major depressive disorder treated in 18 primary and 23 psychiatric care settings across the United States, using data from the Sequenced Treatment Alternatives to Relieve Depression (STAR*D) study, determined that women using combined hormonal contraception demonstrated better physical functioning and less obsessive-compulsive than users of progestin-only products, or women not using hormones. The Australian Longitudinal Study on Women's Health followed more than 9000 women over 3 years and found no association between hormonal contraception and depression. Approximately 5% to 10% of women of childbearing age experience premenstrual symptoms to a degree that disrupts their functioning in the home or workplace and that meet criteria for premenstrual dysphoric disorder (PMDD). Serotonergic antidepressants are approved treatments for PMDD, with about a 60% of patient response rate. A randomized placebo-controlled study demonstrating that an OC with EE and drospirenone was an effective treatment for PMDD led to marketing approval for this indication. Comparator trials with other formulations of OCs have not been performed.

BEGINNING ORAL CONTRACEPTIVES

Adolescents

In deciding whether a sexually active pubertal girl should use OCs for contraception, the clinician should be more concerned about compliance with the regimen than about possible physiologic harm. As long as she has demonstrated maturity of the hypothalamic-pituitary-ovarian axis with at least three regular, presumably ovulatory, menstrual cycles, it is safe to prescribe OCs without concern that their use will permanently alter future reproductive endocrinologic function. It is not necessary to be concerned about accelerating epiphyseal closure in the postmenarcheal female. Endogenous estrogens have already initiated the process a few years before menarche, and use of contraceptive steroids will not hasten this process.

After Pregnancy

There is a difference in the relationship of the return of ovulation and bleeding between the postabortal woman and one who has had a full-term delivery. The first episode of menstrual bleeding in the postabortal woman is usually preceded by ovulation. After a full-term delivery, the first episode of bleeding is usually, but not always, anovulatory. Ovulation occurs sooner after an abortion, usually between 2 and 4 weeks, than after a full-term delivery, when ovulation is usually delayed beyond 6 weeks but may occur as early as 4 weeks in a woman who is not breast-feeding.

Thus, after spontaneous or induced abortion of a fetus of less than 12 weeks' gestation, OCs should be started immediately to prevent conception after the first ovulation. For women who deliver after 28 weeks and are not nursing, the combination pills should be initiated 2 to 3 weeks after delivery. If the termination of pregnancy occurs between 21 and 28 weeks, contraceptive steroids should be started 1 week later. The reason for delay in the latter instances is that the normally increased risk of thromboembolism occurring postpartum may be further enhanced by the hypercoagulable effects of combination OCs. Because the first ovulation is delayed for at least 4 weeks after a full-term delivery, there is no need to expose the woman to this increased risk.

Estrogen inhibits the action of prolactin in breast tissue receptors; therefore, the use of combination OCs (those containing both estrogen and progestin) diminishes the amount of milk produced by OC users who breast-feed their babies. Although the diminution of milk production is directly related to the amount of estrogen in the contraceptive formulation, only one study has been published in which the amount of breast milk was measured by breast pump in women using formulations with less than 50 mcg of estrogen. In this study, the use of this low dose of estrogen reduced the amount of breast milk. No significant health risks are associated with hormones in breast milk for the nursing infant. The major concern is that combined OCs will lower the success of initiation of lactation or lead to poor infant growth or the need for supplemental feeding. Although a small portion of the synthetic steroids circulating in women taking OCs can be detected in breast milk, no long-term effects of this exposure on the infant have been detected to date. A long-term follow-up study comparing breast-fed children from mothers who used 50 mcg EE combined OCs while they were lactating to mothers using nonhormonal contraception revealed no difference in mean body weight or height up to 8 years of age, occurrence of disease, or in intellectual or psychological behavior between the two groups. Women at high risk for unintended pregnancy following delivery should consider the relative advantages of a combination pill over other methods, as well as the effect of the contraceptive on nursing success.

Women who are breast-feeding every 4 hours, including during the night, will not ovulate until at least 10 weeks after delivery and thus do not need contraception before that time. Because only a small percentage of exclusively breast-feeding women will ovulate as long as they continue full nursing and remain amenorrheic, no additional contraception is needed for the first 6 months post partum (see Lactational Amenorrhea Method). For additional protection, either a barrier method or a progestin-only OC can be used until menses resumes. Progestins do not diminish the amount of breast milk, and progestin-only OCs are highly effective in this group of women. Once supplemental feeding is introduced, ovulation can resume promptly and effective contraception is then needed. Combination OCs or another method should be used once supplemental feeding is initiated. If a postpartum woman is exclusively breast-feeding and amenorrheic, OCs can be initiated at any time. If she is more than 6 months postpartum, use of a backup method for 7 days after starting the pill would be recommended. A urine pregnancy test should be performed if amenorrhea persists through the hormone-free interval of the pill pack.

Cycling Women

At the initial visit, after a history and physical examination have determined that there are no medical contraindications for OCs, the woman should be informed about the benefits and risks of the method. This counseling should include a discussion of perfect and typical failure rates and alternative methods. For medicolegal reasons it is best to note on the patient's medical record that the benefits and risks have been explained to her.

To provide protection during the first cycle of use, it is recommended that a pill pack be initiated within 7 days following the onset on menses. With the exception of extended-cycle regimens, oral contraceptives are provided in 28-day cycle packs. Many women find it convenient to start a pill pack on a particular day of the week. Sunday starts have been a popular recommendation, as withdrawal bleeding would be expected to occur midweek rather than on weekends. However, delaying the start of the pill pack will lead to some unintended pregnancies, because some women will fail to initiate the therapy as planned. Westhoff and colleagues recruited 1716 women aged younger than 25 years seeking to initiate the oral contraceptive at three publicly funded family planning clinics and randomly assigned them to conventional initiation of the pill (conventional start) or immediate, directly observed ingestion of the first pill (quick start) during the clinic visit. Although women randomized to "quick start" were more likely to continue to the second OC pack (OR 1.5, 95% CI 1.0 to 2.1.), this did not improve continuation rates at 3 and 6 months. Eighty-one percent of women rated the quick start approach as acceptable or preferable to waiting. Bleeding patterns were similar between groups.

Type of Formulation

Estrogen dose, side effect profile, and cost should guide decisions regarding the type of formulation to prescribe. Because estrogen dose is positively correlated with cardiovascular risk and estrogenic side effects, use of formulations containing 35 mcg or less of EE or one of the new estradiol pills should be recommended. It would also appear reasonable to use formulations with the lowest androgenic potency of progestin, as fewer androgenic metabolic and clinical adverse effects should be associated with their use. The development of multiphasic formulations has allowed the total dose of progestin to be reduced compared with some monophasic formulations, without increasing the incidence of breakthrough bleeding. However, several monophasic formulations have a lower total dose of progestin per cycle than the multiphasic formulations and the incidence of follicular enlargement is more frequent with multiphasic than with monophasic formulations.

The U.S. Food and Drug Administration (FDA) has stated that the product prescribed should be one that contains the least amount of estrogen and progestin that is compatible with a low failure rate and the needs of the individual woman. Because few randomized studies have been performed comparing the different marketed formulations, until large-scale comparative studies are performed, the clinician must decide on the formulation to use based on which has the least adverse effects among women in his or her own practice. Most clinicians pick one or two initial start formulations, and if estrogenic or progestogenic side effects occur with one formulation, a different agent with less estrogenic or progestogenic activity can be given. A logical initial choice would be a generically available 20 to 35 mcg EE pill monophasic combined with one of the lower androgenic progestins.

The progestin-only contraceptive formulations have a lower incidence of adverse metabolic effects than do the combination formulations. Because the factors that predispose to thromboembolism are caused by the estrogen component, the incidence of thromboembolism in women taking the minipill is not increased. Furthermore, blood pressure is not affected, nausea and breast tenderness are eliminated, and milk production and quality are unchanged. Despite these advantages, progestin-only pills have the disadvantages of a high frequency of intermenstrual and other abnormal bleeding patterns (including amenorrhea) than combined formulations. The failure rate of these preparations is also higher than with the combined formulations, and a relatively high percentage of the pregnancies that do occur are ectopic. Because nursing mothers have reduced fertility and are amenorrheic, the major disadvantages of these preparations are minimized for these individuals. Furthermore, because milk production and quality are unaffected in contrast to the changes produced by combination pills, the minipill may be offered to women while they are nursing.

Follow-up

If a healthy woman has no contraindications to OC use, it is unnecessary to perform any laboratory tests, including cervical cytology, unless these are necessary for routine health maintenance. At the end of 3 months, the woman should be seen again; at this time a nondirected history should be obtained and the blood pressure measured. After this visit the woman should be seen annually, at which time a nondirected history should again be taken, blood pressure and body weight measured, and a physical examination (including breast, abdominal, and pelvic examination with cervical cytology) performed. Cervical cytologic screening for OC users should follow American College of Obstetricians and Gynecologists (ACOG) guidelines. The routine use of other laboratory tests is not indicated unless the woman has a family history of diabetes or vascular disease at a younger age. Routine use of these tests in women is not indicated because the incidence of positive results is extremely low. However, if the woman has a family history of vascular disease, such as MI occurring in family members younger than age 50, it would be advisable to obtain a lipid panel before OC use is started, as hypertriglyceridemia may be present and OC use will further raise triglycerides. Because the low-dose formulations do not adversely alter the lipid profile except for triglycerides, it is not necessary to measure lipids, other than the routine cholesterol screening every 5 years, in women with no cardiovascular risk factors, even if they are older than 35. If the woman has a strong family history of diabetes, personal history of gestational diabetes, or evidence of metabolic syndrome, she should be screened for diabetes. If the woman has a history of liver disease, a liver panel should be obtained to make certain that liver function is normal before OCs are initiated.

Drug Interactions

Although synthetic sex steroids can retard the biotransformation of certain drugs (e.g., phenazone and meperidine) as a result of substrate competition, such interference is not important clinically. OC use has not been shown to inhibit the action of other drugs. However, some drugs can interfere clinically with the action of OCs by inducing liver enzymes that convert the steroids to more polar and less biologically active metabolites. Certain drugs (e.g., barbiturates, sulfonamides, cyclophosphamide,

and rifampin) have been shown to accelerate the biotransformation of steroids in humans. Several investigators have reported a relatively high incidence of OC failure in women ingesting rifampin, and these two agents should not be given concurrently. The clinical data concerning OC failure in users of other antibiotics (e.g., penicillin, ampicillin, and sulfonamides), analgesics, and barbiturates are less clear. A few anecdotal studies have appeared in the literature, but reliable evidence for a clinical inhibitory effect of these drugs on OC effectiveness (such as that observed with rifampin) is not available. One study by Murphy and colleagues showed that when 2 g of tetracycline was given daily in divided doses, the levels of both ethinyl estradiol and norethindrone in OC users were similar to those before antibiotic use. In the past, it was recommended that women with epilepsy requiring medication with older first-generation antiepileptic medications (e.g., phenytoin, carbamazepine, barbiturates, primidone, topiramate, and oxcarbazepine) be treated with formulations containing 50 mcg of EE, because a higher incidence of abnormal bleeding had been reported with the use of lower-dose estrogen formulations caused by the increased metabolism brought about by the action of these first-generation antiepileptic medications. Although this interaction is not harmful, it is likely to reduce efficacy. The 2009 WHO medical eligibility criteria state that women using these older agents should use an OC with at least 30 mcg of EE. Use of OCs in women with epilepsy using lamotrigine monotherapy has been associated with an increased risk of seizure in one study. This has not been observed with combined antiepileptic therapy with lamotrigine. Treatment with other newer antiepilepsy drugs does not affect OC efficacy or side effect profiles, and low EE dose OCs can be used.

NONCONTRACEPTIVE HEALTH BENEFITS

In addition to being one of the most effective methods of contraception, OCs provide many other health benefits. Some are due to the fact that in users of combination OCs, there is no time when the estrogenic target tissues are stimulated by estrogens without a progestin (unopposed estrogen). Both natural progesterone and the synthetic progestins inhibit the proliferative effect of estrogen, the so-called antiestrogenic effect. Estrogens increase the synthesis of both estrogen and progesterone receptors, whereas progesterone decreases their synthesis. Thus, one mechanism whereby progesterone exerts its antiestrogenic effects is by decreasing the synthesis of estrogen receptors. Relatively little progestin is needed to exert this action, and the amount present in OCs is sufficient. Another way progesterone produces its antiestrogenic action is by stimulating the activity of the enzyme estradiol-17-α-dehydrogenase within the endometrial cell. This enzyme converts the more potent E_2 to the less potent estrone, reducing estrogenic action within the cell. This enzyme does not bind EE.

Benefits from Antiestrogenic Action of Progestins

As a result of the antiestrogenic action of the progestins in OCs, the height of the endometrium is less than in an ovulatory cycle, and there is less proliferation of the endometrial glands. These changes produce several substantial benefits for the OC user. One is a reduction in the amount of blood loss at the time of endometrial shedding. In an ovulatory cycle, the mean blood loss during menstruation is about 35 mL, compared with 20 mL for women ingesting OCs. This decreased blood loss makes the development of iron deficiency anemia less likely for OC users than for nonusers. Data from the RCGP study showed that OC users were about half as likely to develop iron deficiency anemia as were controls. Moreover, the beneficial effect persisted to a similar degree in women who had previously used OCs and then stopped using them, probably because of an increase in the iron stores that remained for several years after the drug was discontinued.

Because OCs produce regular withdrawal bleeding, it would be expected that OC users would have fewer menstrual disorders than controls. The results of the RCGP study confirmed the fact that OC users were significantly less likely to have menorrhagia, irregular menstruation, or intermenstrual bleeding. Because these disorders are frequently treated by curettage or hysterectomy, OC users require these procedures less frequently than do nonusers. Also, because progestins inhibit the proliferative effect of estrogens on the endometrium, as mentioned earlier, adenocarcinoma of the endometrium is significantly less likely to develop in women who use OCs.

Estrogen exerts a proliferative effect on breast tissue, which also contains estrogen receptors. Progestins may also inhibit the synthesis of estrogen receptors in this organ. Several studies have shown that OCs reduce the incidence of benign breast disease, and two prospective studies have indicated that this reduction is directly related to the amount of progestin in the compounds. Data from the Oxford study indicate that current users of OCs have an 85% reduction in the incidence of fibroadenomas and 50% reductions in chronic cystic disease and nonbiopsied breast lumps, compared with controls using IUDs or diaphragms. The risk of developing these three diseases decreased with increased duration of OC use and persisted for about 1 year after discontinuation of OCs, after which no reduction in risk was observed. A large cohort study showed that long-term use of OCs was associated with a significant reduction in the diagnosis of benign breast disease of the proliferative type.

Benefits from Inhibition of Ovulation

Other noncontraceptive medical benefits of OCs result from their main action: inhibition of ovulation. Some disorders, such as dysmenorrhea and premenstrual syndrome, occur much more frequently in ovulatory than in anovulatory cycles. In fact, inhibition of ovulation by exogenous steroids has been used for decades as therapy for severe dysmenorrhea. The RCGP study showed that OC users had 63% less dysmenorrhea and 29% less premenstrual syndrome than did controls. Another study indicated that OC users were less likely to have variation in the degree of feeling of well-being throughout the cycle than non-OC users.

Another potentially serious adverse effect of ovulatory menstrual cycles is the development of functional ovarian cysts—specifically, follicular and luteal cysts—that occasionally require surgical management because of enlargement, rupture, or hemorrhage. When ovulation is inhibited, functional cysts do not usually develop. In a survey performed by the Boston Collaborative Drug Surveillance Program, less than 2% of women with a discharge diagnosis of functional ovarian cysts were taking OCs, compared with 20% of controls. However, 20% of women with nonfunctional cysts were taking OCs, an incidence similar to that observed in the controls. Although authors of one small case series postulated that the formation of functional ovarian cysts may be increased in users of multiphasic OCs, the rate of hospitalization

Table 13-10 Rate Ratio Estimates for Functional Ovarian Cysts Comparing Each Oral Contraceptive Category with No Oral Contraception

	Rate Ratio*	95% Confidence Interval
No prescription	1.00	Reference category
Active prescription:		
Multiphasic	0.91	0.30-2.31
$\leq$35 mcg estrogen	0.52	0.17-1.33
>35 mcg estrogen	0.24	0.01-1.34

*Rate ratios standardized to age distribution of index (i.e., "exposed") category. From Lanes AF, Birmann B, Walter AM, Singer S: Oral contraceptive type and functional ovarian cysts. Am J Obstet Gynecol 166:956, 1992.

for ovarian cysts in the United States has remained unchanged after the widespread use of multiphasic formulations.

Lanes and colleagues studied the rate of functional cysts more than 2 cm in diameter by ultrasound, which required either hospitalization or outpatient surgery. They found that low-dose monophasic formulations resulted in about a 50% reduction in functional cysts, lower than the 75% reduction with high-dose formulations, whereas use of multiphasic formulations had only a slight reduction of ovarian cyst development (**Table 13-10**).

Another disorder linked to incessant ovulation is ovarian cancer. As mentioned earlier, the development of ovarian cancer is significantly reduced in OC users, with a duration-dependent decrease in risk.

Other Benefits

Several European studies, including the RCGP study, showed that the risk of development of rheumatoid arthritis in OC users was about half that of controls. Women using OCs also have lower rates of ascending genital infection leading to salpingitis, commonly referred to as pelvic inflammatory disease (PID). At least 11 published epidemiologic studies have estimated the relative risk of PID developing among OC users. Seven of these studies compared OC use with nonuse of any other contraception. The relative risk of PID developing among OC users in most of these studies was about 0.5, a 50% reduction. It has been estimated that between 15% and 20% of women with cervical gonorrheal infection will develop salpingitis. In a Swedish study, all women with culture-proven cervical gonococcal infection had a diagnostic laparoscopy 1 day after hospital admission to determine whether salpingitis was present. Of those who used contraception other than the IUD and oral steroids, salpingitis developed in 15%; among OC users the prevalence of salpingitis was about half (8.8%). The results of this study indicate that OCs reduce the clinical development of salpingitis in women infected with gonorrhea. Similarly, although the incidence of cervical infection with *Chlamydia trachomatis* is increased in OC users compared with controls, Wølner-Hanssen and coworkers reported that the incidence of chlamydial salpingitis in OC users was only half that of controls. The mechanism for this protection may be thickening of the cervical mucus and decreased duration of menstrual flow, which reduces the number of organisms that ascend to the upper genital tract and allows the body's defenses to eliminate them more easily. One sequela of PID is ectopic pregnancy. OCs reduce the risk of ectopic pregnancy by more than 90% in current users and may reduce the incidence in former users by decreasing their chance of developing salpingitis.

All of the benefits seen with high-dose pills also occur with low-dose formulations. It is unfortunate that the infrequent adverse effects of OCs have received widespread publicity, but the more common noncontraceptive health benefits have attracted little attention. In a study of women attending a Yale Health Center, about 80% of these well-educated women were unaware of these noncontraceptive health benefits of OCs. Similar low rates of knowledge were seen in a more recent survey of English- and Spanish-speaking clinic patients in Oregon. A nationwide survey sponsored by the American College of Obstetricians and Gynecologists also found limited awareness of the noncontraceptive benefits of OCs by U.S. women, with less than half the women interviewed being aware of any benefit other than contraception.

There is also epidemiologic data that indicate that OCs reduce bone loss, particularly in perimenopausal women with oligomenorrhea. Michaelsson and coworkers reported that OC use by women after the age of 40 decreased the risk of subsequent hip fracture. There are noncontraceptive health benefits associated with continuing OC use beyond age 40 into the perimenopausal years. While there are only limited data regarding metabolic risks of OC use by women older than 40, Godsland and associates reported no changes in cardiovascular risk markers with long-term OC use. Because the dose and type of estrogens (conjugated estrogens and estradiol) given for hormone replacement result in a lower effect on prothrombotic pathways than the EE dose currently used in OCs, it is best to switch therapy at menopause. To avoid discontinuing OC use when the woman is still ovulating, measurement of the FSH and E_2 levels on the last day of the pill-free interval starting at age 50 provides information about ovarian follicular activity. If the FSH level is elevated and the E_2 level low, OCs should be discontinued and hormone therapy considered.

A case-control study by Westhoff and others found a reduction in the risk of endometrioma, a benign ovarian tumor, associated with OC use. A trend toward increased protection was noted with increased duration of use, and this became a significant 50% reduction after 5 years of exposure (OR 0.51, 95% CI 0.29, 0.90).

LONG-ACTING CONTRACEPTIVE STEROIDS

To avoid the contraceptive failure associated with the need to remember to take oral contraceptives daily, methods of administering contraceptive steroid formulations at infrequent intervals have been developed. To date, four types of systemic long-acting steroid delivery systems (injectable suspensions, subdermal implants, a contraceptive skin patch, and intravaginal ring) have been developed and are being used by women in the United States and elsewhere. The patch, ring, and some injections (not available in the United States) are combination methods that contain both an estrogen and a progestin. The implant and progestin injection available in the United States are progestin-only methods. Because these contain no estrogen, endometrial integrity is not maintained and uterine bleeding occurs at irregular and unpredictable intervals. Therefore, to improve long-term acceptability and continuation with these methods, women should undergo extensive counseling about the development of irregular bleeding.

CONTRACEPTIVE PATCH

A contraceptive skin patch with an area of 20 cm² has been marketed for several years (**Fig. 13-14**). Each thin opaque matrix patch consists of three layers. These include an outer protective layer of polyester, an adhesive middle layer containing 75 mcg ethinyl estradiol and 6.0 mg norelgestromin, and a polyester release liner that is removed prior to placement on the skin. Each patch delivers 150 mcg norelgestromin and 20 mcg ethinyl estradiol into the circulation each day at a fairly constant rate for at least 9 days. Norelgestromin is the active metabolite of the gonane progestin norgestimate. The woman applies one patch each week for 3 consecutive weeks and no patch for the following week of a 4-week cycle to allow withdrawal bleeding. The patch may be applied to one of four anatomic sites: buttocks, upper outer arm, lower abdomen, or upper torso excluding the breasts. Following skin application, both steroids appear in the circulation rapidly and reach a plateau within 48 hours. Mean serum levels of norelgestromin are between 600 and 800 pg/mL and for ethinyl estradiol are between 40 and 50 pg/mL. These steroid levels inhibit gonadotropin release and prevent ovulation. Contraceptive effectiveness and metabolic and clinical effects, including irregular bleeding, are similar to combination oral contraceptives. Results from clinical trials suggest that efficacy may be slightly lower in women with body weight more than 90 kg. This observation needs to be placed in context. Most studies of comparator methods such as oral contraceptives exclude obese women from the study population. Furthermore, as discussed previously, some studies have suggested an increase risk of OC failure among obese women. See further discussion in the oral contraceptive section under Obesity.

Rates of complete detachment of the patch from the skin are about 2%. The serum level area under the curve of ethinyl estradiol after patch application is higher than after ingestion of an oral contraceptive containing 30-mcg ethinyl estradiol, but the peak levels of ethinyl estradiol are lower with the patch. The risk of venous thrombosis with this patch has been reported to be similar to that of women ingesting an oral contraceptive containing ethinyl estradiol and norgestimate. However, like with all new methods, initial reports of adverse events have led to "patch scares" and litigation. Highly publicized reports of fatal venous thromboembolism (VTE) in patch users in 2004 led to the addition of a specific package insert warning regarding an increase

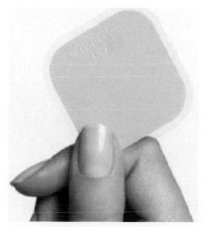

Figure 13-14 The contraceptive skin patch releasing ethinyl estradiol and norelgestromin.

in estrogen exposure (e.g., average steady-state concentrations of EE are 60% higher than in users of a 35-mcg EE OC) in the prescribing information for the product. The results of epidemiologic studies have been inconsistent. A nested case-control study design using an insurance claims database found that the odds ratio for venous thromboembolism was 2.4 (95% CI 1.1 to 5.5) in patch users compared to users of OCs containing norgestimate, the parent compound of the progestin used in the patch. However, Jicks and colleagues used a similar study design and found no increase in risk (OR 1.1 [95% CI 0.6 to 2.1]). In a study of coagulation markers in OC users randomized to use either the patch or the **contraceptive ring**, Jensen and coworkers found that patch users demonstrated unfavorable changes in prothrombotic markers, whereas women switching to the contraceptive ring tended to show values more similar to nonusers.

CONTRACEPTIVE VAGINAL RING

Steroids pass easily through the vaginal epithelium directly into the circulation. A flexible soft colorless ring-shaped device made of ethylene vinyl acetate copolymers with an outer diameter of 54 mm and a cross-sectional diameter of 4 mm has been marketed for several years. Each ring contains 2.7 mg of ethinyl estradiol and 11.7 mg of etonogestrel (**Fig. 13-15**). Etonogestrel (ENG) is the active metabolite of desogestrel. To replicate the standard oral contraceptive regimen, a ring is placed in the vagina for 21 days and then removed for 7 days to allow withdrawal bleeding. After this week, the woman inserts a new ring. Because the steroids act systemically, the ring comes in only one size and does not have to be fitted or placed in a certain location. Following insertion of the ring, the mean daily release of etonogestrel is 120 mcg and ethinyl estradiol is 15 mcg. Serum levels of each steroid rise rapidly and plateau a few days after ring insertion. Mean ENG levels range between 1300 and 1600 pg/mL and mean ethinyl estradiol levels between 17 and 19 pg/mL. Like oral contraceptives, the main mechanism of action is

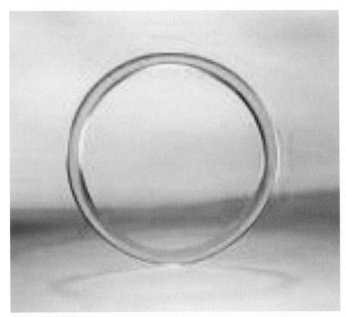

Figure 13-15 The contraceptive vaginal ring releasing ethinyl estradiol and etonogestrel.

inhibition of gonadotropins and prevention of ovulation. Because each ring delivers sufficient steroids to inhibit ovulation for 5 weeks, contraceptive action can be assumed even if the ring is left in place beyond 21 days. Continuous use has been studied, and results are similar to those observed with continuous OCs.

Despite the low amount of ethinyl estradiol delivered each day, bleeding control is good. Irregular bleeding while the ring is in place is uncommon, occurring in 2.6% to 6.4% of cycles. Withdrawal bleeding of 4.7 to 5.3 days duration is initiated a few days after the ring is removed and occurs in 98% of treatment cycles. The area under the curve of EE with the ring is about half that of a combination oral contraceptive containing 30 mcg of ethinyl estradiol, and this likely accounts for the improved profile of thrombosis markers observed in ring users relative to users of the patch or OCs. Contraceptive effectiveness as well as metabolic and clinical effects are similar to combination oral contraceptives. Ring expulsion is uncommon, and both partners typically report high acceptability with use.

INJECTABLE SUSPENSIONS

Three types of injectable steroid formulations are currently in use for contraception throughout the world. These include depomedroxyprogesterone acetate (DMPA), given in a dose of 150 mg intramuscularly (IM) or 104 mg subcutaneously (SC) every 3 months; norethindrone enanthate, given in a dose of 200 mg every 2 months; and several once-a-month injections of combinations of different progestins and estrogens. Only DMPA is currently available in the United States. Although injectable contraceptives are a popular method of contraception worldwide, in the United States they are used by only about 3% of women of reproductive age.

Medroxyprogesterone acetate (MPA) is a 17-acetoxyprogesterone compound and is currently the only progestin used for contraception that is a C-21 progesterone derivative. The 17-acetoxyprogestins, which do not have androgenic activity and are structurally related to progesterone instead of testosterone, were used in oral contraceptive formulations about 30 years ago. Although approved for contraception in many Western countries in the 1960s, regulatory approval for these agents in the United States was stopped when tests on beagle dogs showed that ingestion of oral contraceptives with 17-acetoxyprogestins was associated with an increased risk of mammary cancer. It was discovered later that unlike humans and other animals, the beagle uniquely metabolizes 17-acetoxyprogestins to estrogen, which causes mammary hyperplasia. Thus, when MPA is ingested by the beagle, it behaves differently than it does in the human, where it is not metabolized to estrogen. After epidemiologic studies showed that DMPA does not increase the risk of breast cancer in humans, regulatory approval for marketing this agent as a contraceptive was obtained in the United States in 1992.

Depot Formulation of MPA

MPA is a 17-acetoxy-6-methylprogestin that has progestogenic activity in the human (**Fig. 13-16**). Because MPA is not metabolized as rapidly as the parent compound progesterone, it can be given in smaller amounts than progesterone, with an equivalent amount of progestational activity. DMPA, the long-acting injectable formulation of MPA, consists of a crystalline suspension of this progestational hormone. The original contraceptive dosage with the intramuscular formulation (IM-DMPA) is 150 mg

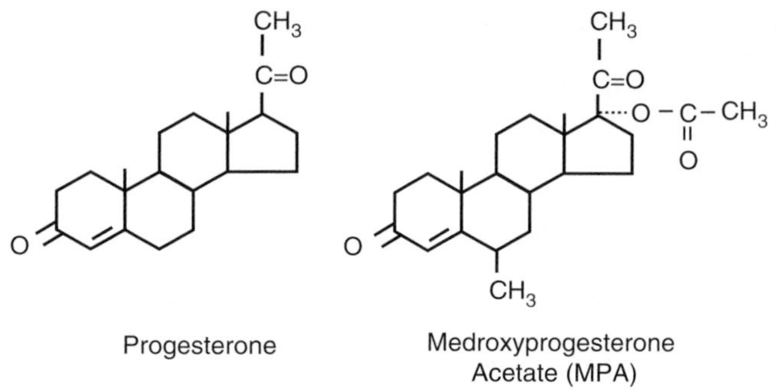

Figure 13-16 Comparative structures of progesterone and MPA.

DMPA, this agent is given by injection deep into the gluteal or deltoid muscle, after which the progestin is released slowly into the systemic circulation. The area should not be massaged, so that the drug is released slowly into the circulation and maintains its contraceptive effectiveness for at least 4 months. The newer subcutaneous formulation contains 104 mg of DMPA in 0.65 mL of diluent and is injected into the subcutaneous tissue of the anterior thigh or abdominal wall.

DMPA is an extremely effective contraceptive. In a large WHO clinical trial studying use of IM-DMPA, the pregnancy rate at 1 year was only 0.1%, and at 2 years the cumulative rate was 0.4%. Jain and colleagues reported the results of two international large open-label phase 3 studies of SC-DMPA in which 1787 women were enrolled. The initial injection was given within 5 days of the onset of menses and every 91 + 7 days. A total of 16,023 woman-cycles of exposure were completed and no pregnancies occurred during the 1 year of the study. This study included a large number of overweight (BMI 25 to 30) and obese (BMI > 30) women. In the American trial, 44% of the women were overweight or obese, and in the European/Asia trial, 27% of women were overweight or obese. Thus SC-DMPA, which delivers a lower total dose of MPA than IM-DMPA, has a similar very high level of contraceptive effectiveness. Three mechanisms of action are involved. The major effect is inhibition of ovulation. Second, DMPA keeps the cervical mucus thick and viscous, so sperm are unlikely to reach the oviduct and fertilize an egg. Third, the endometrium becomes thin and does not secrete sufficient glycogen to provide nutrition for a blastocyst entering the endometrial cavity. With these multiple mechanisms of action, DMPA is one of the most effective reversible methods of contraception currently available.

Pharmacokinetics

MPA can be detected in the systemic circulation within 30 minutes after its IM injection. Although serum MPA levels vary among individuals, they rise steadily to contraceptively effective blood levels (> 0.2 ng/mL) within 24 hours after both IM and SC injection. The pattern of IM-MPA clearance from the circulation varies among different studies according to the type of assay used. After IM-DMPA was administered to three subjects, Ortiz and coworkers assayed blood MPA levels daily for 2 weeks, then three times a week for the next 3 months, and then weekly until MPA was undetectable. In two subjects, MPA levels initially plateaued at 1.0 to 1.5 ng/mL for about 3 months, after which they declined slowly to about 0.2 ng/mL during the fifth

month (**Fig. 13-17**). In a third subject, the blood levels were higher during the first month, then ranged between 1.0 and 1.5 ng/mL for the next 2 months, after which there was a further decline. MPA levels remained detectable in the circulation, above 0.2 ng/mL, for 7 to 9 months in all three subjects, after which it was not detectable. E_2 levels were found to be in the early to midfollicular phase range, but consistently below 100 pg/mL during the first 4 months after injection. After 4 to 6 months, when MPA levels decreased to less than 0.5 ng/mL, E_2 concentrations rose to preovulatory levels, indicating follicular activity, but ovulation did not occur, as evidenced by persistently low progesterone levels. Return of follicular activity preceded the return of luteal activity by 2 to 3 months. This delay in resumption of luteal activity is probably due to the fact that the circulating MPA levels inhibit the positive feedback effect of the rise of E_2 on the hypothalamic-pituitary axis, which in the absence of MPA would stimulate the midcycle release of LH. The return of luteal activity in this study, indicated by a rise in serum progesterone levels, did not occur until 7 to 9 months after the injection, when the MPA levels were less than 0.1 ng/mL.

Following injections of SC-DMPA, absorption of MPA is rapid and rises above 0.2 ng/mL (the contraceptive effective level) within 24 hours. Serum MPA levels peak about 8 days after the injection and gradually decline thereafter, but mean levels remain above the contraceptively effective level of 0.2 ng/mL for about 4 months (**Fig. 13-18**).

Following injections of both IM-DMPA and SC-DMPA, serum levels of FSH, E_2, and progesterone are similar. FSH levels remain in the midfollicular range for 3 months without the midcycle FSH peak. E_2 levels remain suppressed and are similar to the levels on days 1 to 3 of a pretreatment control cycle (40 to 60 pg/mL). Progesterone levels are completely suppressed with both types of formulations. Thus, although low levels of ovarian follicular activity do occur after IM-DMPA and SC-DMPA, ovulation is completely suppressed.

To obtain suppression of ovulation in the initial injection cycle, DMPA has to be administered within several days after the onset of menses. Siriwongse and coworkers reported that when the drug was initially given on days 5 or 7 of the cycle, none of the women ovulated, but when it was given on day 9, 2 of 13 subjects had presumptive evidence of ovulation. The results of this study indicated that DMPA should be given no later than 7 days after the onset of menses to be effective in the first ovulatory cycle. The product labeling states that to ensure the woman is not pregnant at the time of the first injection, it must be given during the first 5 days of the cycle.

Mishell and associates performed a cross-sectional study on 121 women who received 150 mg of DMPA every 3 months for more than 1 year. An assay performed on a serum sample obtained on the day of the next scheduled injection showed marked differences in the E_2 levels, which varied from approximately 15 pg/mL to nearly 100 pg/mL (mean approximately 42 pg/mL) (**Fig. 13-19**). A similar range and mean value were also found among women who had been receiving DMPA for 1 to 2 years and those who had used it for 4 to 5 years. All these women had moist, well-rugated vaginas, and none stated that her breast size had decreased. None of the women complained of hot flushes. These data provide evidence that use of contraceptive doses of DMPA does not decrease endogenous E_2 levels to the postmenopausal range and does not cause symptoms of estrogen deficiency.

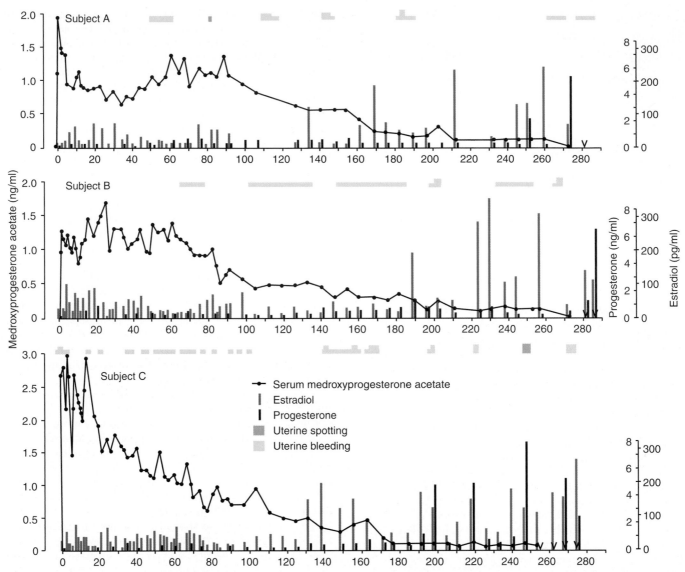

Figure 13-17 Serum MPA concentrations in three subjects during the first 24 hours after intramuscular injection of 150 mg of MPA. (From Ortiz A, Hiroi M, Stanczyk FZ, et al: Serum medroxyprogesterone acetate (MPA) concentrations and ovarian function following intramuscular injection of depo-MPA. J Clin Endocrinol Metab 44:32, 1977.)

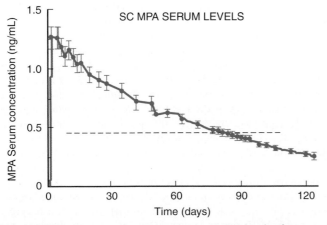

Figure 13-18 Serum medroxyprogesterone (MPA) levels after subcutaneous (SC) injection of depomedroxyprogesterone acetate.

Return of Fertility

Because of the lag time in clearing DMPA from the circulation after both IM-DMPA and SC-DMPA, resumption of ovulation is delayed for a variable period of time, which may last as long as 1 year after the last injection. Results may be different for the two formulations; the median time for return to ovulation was 183 days for IM-DMPA and 212 days for SC-DMPA, a statistically insignificant difference. Women who wish to become pregnant and stop using DMPA should be informed that there will be a delay in the resumption of fertility until the drug is cleared from the circulation. After this initial delay, fecundity resumes at a rate similar to that found after discontinuing a barrier contraceptive (**Fig. 13-20**). Thus, use of DMPA does not prevent return of fertility; it only delays the time at which conception will occur. One year after the last DMPA injection, 94.7% of women receiving IM-DMPA and 97.4% of women receiving SC-DMPA had ovulated.

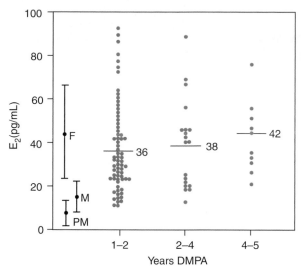

Figure 13-19 Serum estradiol (E2) levels in 121 women who had used depomedroxyprogesterone acetate (DMPA) for contraception for more than 1 year. The horizontal bar in each time period represents the mean value. Vertical bars represent mean (λ) $\pm$ SD of serum estradiol levels in cycling women in the early follicular phase (F), normal males (M), and postmenopausal women (PM). (From Mishell DR Jr, Kharma KM, Thorneycroft IH, Nakamura RM: Estrogenic activity in women receiving an injectable progestogen for contraception. Am J Obstet Gynecol 113:372, 1972.)

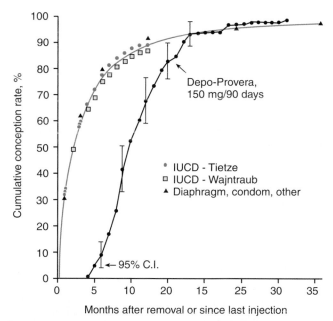

Figure 13-20 Cumulative conception rates of women who discontinued a contraceptive method to become pregnant. IUCD, intrauterine contraceptive device. (From Schwallie PC, Assenzo JR: The effect of depo-medroxyprogesterone acetate on pituitary and ovarian function, and the return of fertility following its discontinuation: A review. Contraception 10[2]:181, 1974.)

Because the half-life of the drug is constant, the return of fertility is not related to the number of injections that a woman receives. Schwallie and Assenzo reported that the median time to conception varied between 9 and 12 months after the last injection but did not differ according to the number of injections.

With 10 or more injections, the median delay to the onset of fertility is similar to that in a woman who received only a few injections. Jain and colleagues reported that BMI and race did not affect the duration until ovulation resumed after an injection of SC-DMPA.

These investigators did find that the median time to conception after DMPA was discontinued varied according to body weight. As body weight increased, there was a similar concomitant increase in the median time to resumption of conception, most likely because the drug had been absorbed into adipose tissue and not cleared as rapidly.

Endometrial Changes

Mishell and coworkers examined the histology of the endometrium at various intervals after starting DMPA. Histologic examination of endometrial biopsies revealed three types of patterns: proliferative, quiescent, and atrophic. Secretory endometrium was not observed. Most of the women had a quiescent pattern, characterized by narrow, widely spaced glands and decidualization of the stroma.

Endometrial biopsies were performed at intervals of 1.5, 3, 6, 9, and 12 months after the first DMPA injection in a group of women receiving DMPA every 3 months. About half the biopsies showed that proliferative endometrium was present 6 weeks after the first injection. The percentage of women with proliferative endometrium then steadily declined, and after the second injection, less than 10% of the biopsy specimens showed proliferative tissue. The majority of the biopsy specimens showed a quiescent type of endometrium, but after 1 year of DMPA, about 40% of the specimens were characterized as atrophic.

Adverse Effects
Clinical

The major side effect of both IM- and SC-DMPA is complete disruption of the menstrual cycle. In the first 3 months after the first injection, about 30% of women are amenorrheic and another 30% to 40% have irregular bleeding and spotting occurring more than 11 days per month. The bleeding is usually light in amount and does not cause anemia to occur. As the duration of therapy increases, the incidence of frequent bleeding steadily declines and the incidence of amenorrhea steadily increases, so that at the end of 1 year, about 55% of women with both SC-DMPA and IM-DMPA are amenorrheic. After 2 years, about 70% of the women treated with IM-DMPA are amenorrheic (**Fig. 13-21**). Women who use this method of contraception should be counseled that with time the irregular bleeding episodes will cease and amenorrhea will most likely occur.

After treatment with IM-DMPA is discontinued, about half of the women resume a regular cyclic menstrual pattern within 6 months and about three fourths have regular menses within 1 year. When bleeding does resume, it is initially regular in about half the women and irregular in the remainder. In a study involving 36 women who stopped using IM-DMPA, Gardner and Mishell reported that in the first 3 months, 27 women were amenorrheic, and 9 had irregular menses, which was usually characterized as spotting. During the next 3 months, about half the women began regular menses. The incidence of regular menses steadily increased, and 2 years after the last injection all the women were having regular menses or were pregnant. In this group of women, amenorrhea did not persist for more than 6 months after the last injection.

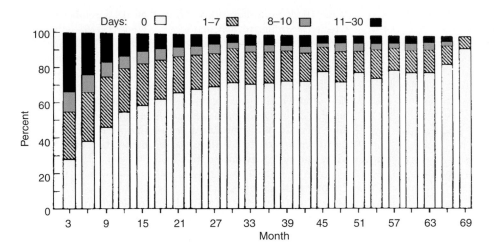

Figure 13-21 Percentage of patients with bleeding or spotting on days 0, 1-7, 8-10, or 11-30 per 30-day cycle while receiving injectable DMPA, 150 mg, every 3 months. (Reprinted from Schwallie PC, Assenzo JR: Contraceptive use: Efficacy study utilizing medroxyprogesterone acetate administered as an intramuscular injection once every 90 days. Fertil Steril 24:331, 1973. Copyright 1973, with permission from The American Society for Reproductive Medicine.)

Weight Changes

In five cross-sectional studies, users of IM-DMPA weighed more than a comparison group not using hormonal contraceptives. Several longitudinal studies have indicated that IM-DMPA users gain between 1.5 and 4 kg in their first year of use and continue to gain weight thereafter. In the studies of SC-DMPA by Jain and colleagues, the median weight change was an increase of 1.7 and 1.0 kg, respectively, after 1 year in the two groups. However, none of these studies included a control group, so the weight could be due to factors other than DMPA use. In one retrospective comparative longitudinal study, Moore and associates found no significant change in mean weight of DMPA, progestin implant, and oral contraceptive users. While the effect among DMPA on body weight remains unclear, the magnitude of weight gain reported is typically higher than with other methods. Le and colleagues followed 240 Texas women starting DMPA every 3 months for 36 months. Early weight gain of more than 5% above baseline within 6 months of DMPA initiation occurred in one fourth of the subjects. However, this group of early weight gainers had a much steeper slope of weight gain over time and significantly more total weight gain (11.08 kg versus 2.49 kg) after 36 months than the regular weight gainers. The risk factors for early weight gain were BMI < 30, parity >1, and self-reported increased appetite. If DMPA users gain weight, they should be counseled to decrease caloric intake and increase their exercise, and those that experience early weight gain should be warned that this may become excessive.

Mood Changes

The product labeling lists depression and mood changes as side effects of DMPA. Several studies, however, indicate that the incidence of depression and mood change in women using this method of contraception is less than 5%. No clinical trials with a comparison group not using DMPA have been performed to determine whether a causal relation between the use of DMPA and the development of depression exists.

Headache

Although the development of headaches is the most frequent medical event reported by DMPA users and a common reason for discontinuation of its use, there are no comparative studies to indicate that use of DMPA increases the incidence or severity of tension or migraine headaches. Therefore, the presence of migraine headaches is not an absolute contraindication for use of DMPA. However, women should be counseled that if the frequency or severity of headaches increases after the injection is given, it may be several months before the drug is cleared from the circulation. For this reason, the presence of migraine headaches may be considered to be a relative contraindication for the use of DMPA. Unlike combined OCs, there is no contraindication to the use of DMPA in women with a history of migraine headache with aura or focal neurologic signs.

Metabolic Effects

Protein

Because DMPA does not increase liver globulin production, as does the estrogen component of oral contraceptives (ethinyl estradiol), no alteration in blood-clotting factors or angiotensinogen levels is associated with its use. Thus, unlike OCs, DMPA has not been associated with an increased incidence of hypertension or thromboembolism and can be safely used in women with these conditions. A WHO study reported that mean blood pressure measurements were unchanged in IM-DMPA users after 2 years of injections. In the 1-year studies of SC-DMPA, there were no significant changes in blood pressure.

Carbohydrate

There have been two studies in which oral glucose tolerance tests have been performed on long-term IM-DMPA users and matched controls not using hormonal contraceptives. The mean glucose levels were slightly greater among the IM-DMPA users than among the controls in one, but not the other, study. Mean insulin levels were also higher. The slight deterioration in glucose tolerance among IM-DMPA users is probably not clinically significant, and it returns to normal after the woman stops using IM-DMPA.

Lipids

Westhoff reviewed the findings of 11 studies that evaluated plasma lipids among groups of women using DMPA. Most of these were cross-sectional studies and compared lipid levels among DMPA users with the levels among women who were not using hormonal methods of contraception. There was little or no change in mean triglyceride and total cholesterol levels, but in all seven studies in which mean HDL cholesterol levels were measured, the levels were lower among the DMPA users. Of the five studies in which LDL cholesterol was measured, three noted an increase among the DMPA users. There are no studies in which the incidence of cardiovascular events among current or former long-term DMPA users was compared with the incidence among controls. Therefore, although the lipid changes with DMPA use are not beneficial, there is no evidence to date that they are associated with an acceleration of atherosclerosis.

Bone Loss

Several observational studies performed in many different countries with women of various ethnic groups indicate that the use of DMPA is associated with some degree of decreased bone mineral density (BMD). The amount and location of the bone loss, as well as the age groups most likely to experience this problem when using DMPA, varied in the different studies. Although there are scant data, the bone loss appears reversible after stopping use of DMPA. Kaunitz and associates observed that the extent of bone loss over 2 years was marginally smaller in women randomized to DMPA-SC than in the DMPA-IM group at both the total hip (-3.3% and -3.6%) and lumbar spine (-4.3% and -5%), respectively. A multivariable logistic regression model developed from a longitudinal study of 240 American women using DMPA for 2 years showed that at least a 5% BMD loss was associated with current smoking (adjusted OR 3.88, 95% CI 1.26 to 11.96), low calcium intake (OR 0.81, 95% CI 0.65 to 0.99 for intake in increments of 100 mg), and low parity (OR 0.49, 95% CI 0.29 to 0.82 for parity as a continuous variable). Age, race or ethnicity, previous contraceptive use, and body mass index were not associated with higher BMD loss (**Fig. 13-22**). However, a recent large study using the Danish national database identified 64,548 cases of fracture among women in the year 2000, and three age-matched controls were randomly drawn from the general population (n = 193,641). After adjustments for confounders, DMPA use was associated with an increased risk of fractures (OR 1.44, 95% CI: 1.01 to 2.06), whereas use of the levonorgestrel IUS showed a decreased risk of fractures (OR 0.75, 95% CI: 0.64 to 0.87). It would appear useful to encourage calcium intake of 1500 mg/day in adolescent DMPA users. Several studies have demonstrated that measurement of bone mineral density is unnecessary because bone density increases after stopping DMPA. There is no need to consider bisphosphonate therapy in DMPA users with low BMD.

Neoplastic Effects

Approval of DMPA for contraceptive use in the United States was delayed for many years because of concern about a causal relation between use of this agent and an increased risk of cervical, breast, and endometrial cancer. These concerns were raised because of studies showing an increased risk of abnormal cervical cytology in women using DMPA and studies reporting an increased risk of breast cancer in beagle dogs treated with DMPA and endometrial cancer in monkeys receiving long-term DMPA. These neoplastic concerns were found to be unwarranted as a result of several large epidemiologic studies, the majority of which were undertaken by the WHO. In the WHO studies the risk of neoplasia development among a large group of DMPA users in three countries (Kenya, Thailand, and Mexico) was investigated.

Breast Cancer

Two large case-control studies, the WHO study and a New Zealand study, indicated that the relative risk of developing breast cancer among all DMPA users was not significantly increased (RR of 1.2 [CI 0.96 to 1.15] and 1.0 [CI 0.8 to 1.3], respectively). When the data from these studies were pooled, the overall breast cancer risk among DMPA users was 1.1 (CI 0.97 to 1.4). In long-term users—that is, in those who had used the drug more than 5 years and those who had started use more than 13 years earlier—the risk of developing breast cancer was also not increased (RR of 1.0 [CI 0.70 to 1.5] and 0.89 [CI 0.6 to 1.3], respectively). However, among those women who had started use within the past 5 years and were mainly younger than age 35, there was a significantly increased risk of having breast cancer diagnosed (RR 2.0 [CI 1.5 to 2.8]), similar to that found with use of oral contraceptives and women with first-term pregnancy at an early age. Thus, DMPA, like other contraceptive steroids, does not appear to change the

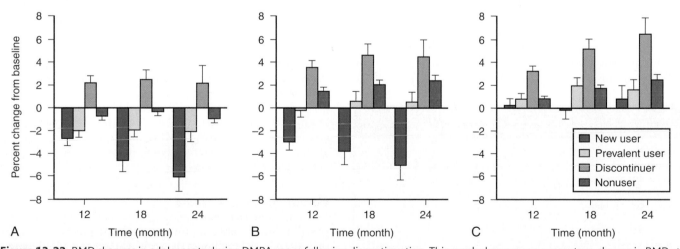

Figure 13-22 BMD changes in adolescents during DMPA use or following discontinuation. This graph shows mean percentage change in BMD at total hip **(A)**, spine **(B)**, and whole body **(C)** for new users (n = 17, 9, and 8 at 12, 18, and 24 months, respectively), prevalent users (n = 26, 18, and 13) and discontinuers (n = 26, 13, and 5) compared with nonuser controls (n = 69, 69, and 59). Results are shown as mean ± S.E., adjusted for baseline covariates (BMD, ethnicity, pregnancy, age at menarche) and time-dependent covariates (age, smoking status, calcium intake, percentage body fat). (Reprinted with permission from Arch Pediatr Adolesc Med 159:139-134, 2005.)

overall incidence of developing breast cancer, and women should be counseled accordingly.

Endometrial Cancer

A WHO case-control study found the risk of developing endometrial cancer to be significantly reduced among DMPA users (RR 0.21 [CI 0.06 to 0.79]). This reduction in risk persisted for at least 8 years after stopping use and was similar in magnitude to the protective effect observed with combination oral contraceptives.

Ovarian Cancer

In a WHO case-control study, the risk of developing ovarian cancer among DMPA users was unchanged (RR 1.07 [CI 0.6 to 1.8]). These findings do not demonstrate a protective effect similar to that observed with oral contraceptives despite inhibition of ovulation with both agents. The lack of a protective effect observed with DMPA was probably due to the fact that in the countries studied, DMPA was given only to multiparous women, women at low risk of developing epithelial ovarian cancer, who differ from the higher risk women of low parity taking oral contraceptives.

Cervical Cancer

In a large WHO case-control study, the risk of developing invasive cancer of the cervix was not increased (RR 1.1 [CI 0.96 to 1.29]), similar to findings observed in a large case-control study in Costa Rica. Long-term use and a long time since first use were also not associated with a significant increase in risk of cervical cancer in these studies. The risk of developing cancer in situ was slightly increased in the WHO study (RR 1.4 [CI 1.2 to 1.7]), but not in the Costa Rica study (RR 1.0 [CI 0.6 to 1.8]) or two New Zealand studies investigating the risk of cancer dysplasia. Thus, the reports in which the neoplastic effects of DMPA on breast and reproductive tract neoplasia have been investigated are very reassuring. A recent case-control study that looked only at women with oncogenic HPV subtypes found no association between DMPA use and a histologic diagnosis of high-grade dysplasia.

Noncontraceptive Health Benefits

Cullins reported that there is good epidemiologic evidence that the use of DMPA reduces the risk of developing iron deficiency anemia, PID, and endometrial cancer. It has a beneficial effect on hematologic parameters in women with sickle cell disease and reduces their incidence of clinical problems (**Box 13-2**).

Box 13-2 Noncontraceptive Health Benefits of Contraceptive Use of DMPA: Reduced Risk of the Following Disorders

Definite
Salpingitis
Endometrial cancer
Iron deficiency anemia
Sickle cell problems

Probable
Ovarian cysts
Dysmenorrhea
Endometriosis
Epileptic seizure
Vaginal candidiasis

DMPA also reduces seizure frequency in women with epilepsy and probably reduces the incidence of primary dysmenorrhea, ovulation pain, and functional ovarian cyst because it inhibits ovulation. DMPA also reduces the symptoms of endometriosis and in two small studies it reduced the incidence of vaginal candidiasis.

Clinical Recommendations

Women should be thoroughly counseled about the occurrence of abnormal bleeding and development of amenorrhea with the use of DMPA prior to receiving the first injection. It has been shown that pretreatment counseling improves continuation rates. In addition, women should be counseled that the action may last as long as 1 year following the last injection if they decide to discontinue use in order to become pregnant or because of side effects.

In cycling women, the initial injection should be given no later than on day 5 of the cycle to be certain to inhibit ovulation in the initial treatment cycle. Because of an absence of thrombogenic effects, the first injection can be given within 5 days postpartum in nonlactating women. For women who exclusively breast-feed their infants, the product labeling states that the first injection should not be given until at least 6 weeks postpartum, but DMPA does not affect the quantity or quality of breast milk or the health of children who breast-feed during its use. If a woman with lactational amenorrhea wishes to commence DMPA use and if a qualitative test for human chorionic gonadotropin (hCG) is negative, it is unlikely she is pregnant and therefore she can receive the injection at any time. A standard strategy for dosing DMPA in an amenorrheic postpartum woman, oligoovulatory woman, or a woman who has previously received DMPA but is delayed beyond 13 weeks in returning for her next injection has been to advise 2 weeks of abstinence or barrier contraception before a return to the clinic for hCG testing and then to administer DMPA if the pregnancy test is negative. However, a recently published extensive review by Paulen and Curtis found that extremely low pregnancy rates for DMPA users were maintained when the drug was administered up to 4 weeks following the missed reinjection date. Since studies of return to ovulation after last injection of DMPA have generally found that the earliest ovulation does not occur until several months after the last injection, it is safe and advisable to provide a reinjection of DMPA to a woman who is up to 16 weeks from her last injection without additional testing. The older protocols that require the patient to return at a later time after a period of abstinence or barrier contraceptive use or to await the onset of spontaneous menses will expose her to an unacceptable risk of unintended pregnancy and should be abandoned in favor of a more liberal reinjection policy. If accidental pregnancy does occur in a woman receiving DMPA, there is no evidence that the agent is teratogenic or that the hormone will adversely affect the outcome of the pregnancy.

Norethindrone Enanthate

Norethindrone enanthate (NET-EN) is another injectable progestagen that has been approved for contraceptive use in more than 40 countries but not in the United States. It is administered in an oil suspension and thus has pharmacodynamics different from those of DMPA. Because of a shorter duration of action, it is recommended that NET-EN be given every 60 days for at least the first 6 months and no less often than every 12 weeks thereafter. The WHO recommends that the drug be given at intervals no shorter than 46 days and no longer than 74 days.

Progestin-Estrogen (Once Monthly) Injectable Formulations

Because the major reason for discontinuance of all progestin injectable contraceptives is menstrual irregularity, several combined progestin-estrogen injectables designed for once-a-month administration and production of regular withdrawal bleeding have been developed. They consist of a low dose of a long-acting progestin plus a small amount of an E_2 ester. Although many different formulations have been developed, currently four of them are most widely used: an injectable formulation containing 17α-hydroxyprogesterone caproate, 250 mg, and estradiol valerate, 5 mg (estimated to be used by at least 1% of all contraceptors in China); a combination of dihydroxy-progesterone acetophenide, 150 mg, plus estradiol enanthate, 10 mg (widely used in Mexico and other Latin American countries marketed under a variety of different brand names); a combination of MPA, 25 mg, and estradiol cypionate, 5 mg (marketed as Cyclofem and also called Cycloprovera); and a combination of norethisterone enanthate, 50 mg, and estradiol valerate, 5 mg (Mesigyna).

Cyclofem is FDA approved and was briefly marketed in the United States under the brand new Lunelle from 2000 to 2003. It is formulated as a microcrystalline suspension given in 0.5 mL of an aqueous solution, and Mesigyna is formulated in 1 mL of an oil solution of castor oil and benzyl benzoate, 60:40. Both of these formulations are administered as deep IM injections into the deltoid, anterior thigh or gluteal muscle every 23 to 33 days (28 ± 5 days), with the first injection being given between 1 to 5 days after the onset of menses. The E_2 levels peak at 250 pg/mL 2 to 7 days after the injection and gradually decline to baseline about 2 weeks after the injection at which time uterine bleeding usually occurs. MPA levels peak about 3 days after injection at 1.25 ng/mL and decline slowly with a half-life of 13.7 days. Nondetectable levels are reached between 63 to 84 days. Steady-state conditions are reached after the first injection. Ovulation is inhibited for 63 to 112 days after the injection, after which there is a prompt return of fertility.

Newton and colleagues summarized the results of clinical trials with these compounds. The combined preparations offered better cycle control and less intermenstrual spotting than did the progestagen-only preparations of MPA and norethisterone enanthate. Amenorrhea rates were also lower with the combination injections, and about 85% of all cycles were regular following the first early bleed about 15 days after the first injection.

The results of five clinical trials with Mesigyna and Lunelle demonstrated a high level of effectiveness, with 12-month pregnancy rates of 0.4% or less for Mesigyna and 0.2% or less for Lunelle. Rates of discontinuation for amenorrhea varied between 0.8% and 4.2% for Mesigyna and 2.1% and 5.2% for Lunelle. For bleeding-related reasons, discontinuations were 5.4% to 12.0% with Mesigyna and 6.3% to 12.7% with Lunelle. The main bleeding disturbances were heavy, prolonged, and irregular bleeding.

Results of a 1-year nonrandomized U.S. study of Lunelle and a combination OC were reported by Kaunitz and coworkers. No pregnancies occurred in the 782 women accumulating 8008 woman-cycles of use with Lunelle. After 3 months, regular menses occurred in women treated with both the injection and OC, but bleeding irregularities were more common with the injection.

Also women receiving the injection had more days of bleeding and spotting than those receiving the OCs as well as greater variability of cycle length. The WHO task force that studied Lunelle found no significant changes in the hemostatic parameters, lipid levels, or carbohydrate metabolism with Lunelle, and in clinical studies involving more than 12,000 women no venous or arterial cardiovascular events were recorded. Indications and contraindications for Lunelle are similar to oral contraceptives.

SUBDERMAL IMPLANTS

Subdermal implants made of polydimethylsiloxane (Silastic) containing levonorgestrel for use as contraceptives were developed by the Population Council and patented with the name Norplant. Clinical trials of this long-acting, effective, reversible method of contraception were initiated in 1975. The FDA approved Norplant in 1990, and marketing in this country began in 1991, but this method of contraception is no longer sold in the United States. As with all steroid-containing Silastic devices, the rate of steroid delivery is directly proportional to the surface area of the capsules, whereas duration of action depends on the amount of steroid within the capsules. To produce effective blood levels of norgestrel, it was found necessary to use six capsules filled with crystalline levonorgestrel. The cylindrical capsules are 3.4 cm long and 2.4 mm in outer diameter, with the ends sealed with Silastic medical adhesive. Each capsule contains 36 mg of crystalline levonorgestrel for a total amount of 215 mg in each six-capsule set.

Insertion is performed in an outpatient setting, and the entire procedure takes about 5 minutes. After infiltration of the skin with local anesthesia, a 3-mm incision is made with a scalpel, usually in the upper arm, although the lower arm, the inguinal, scapular, and gluteal regions have also been used. When the capsules are inserted in any area of subcutaneous tissue, the steroid diffuses into the circulation at a relatively constant rate. The capsules are implanted into the subcutaneous tissue in a radial pattern through a 10- to 12-gauge trocar, and the incision is closed with adhesive. Sutures are not necessary. Because polydimethylsiloxane is not biodegradable, the capsules have to be removed through another incision when desired by the user or at the end of 5 years, which is the duration of maximal contraceptive effectiveness.

The removal process is, like the insertion procedure, performed in the clinic area, using local anesthesia and a small skin incision. Removal of Norplant is a more difficult process than insertion, because fibrous tissue develops around the capsule and must be cut prior to removing the capsules. It is important to insert the capsules superficially to enhance the ease of removal; deeply implanted capsules are more difficult to remove.

The next generation implant developed, Norplant II, used a different technology, a homologous mixture of Silastic and crystalline levonorgestrel extruded as a solid rod and covered with Silastic tubing to limit diffusion of the steroid. The rods are easier to manufacture, insert, and remove than the capsules. Because of different properties of diffusion, higher blood levels of levonorgestrel are achieved with a smaller total surface area, and two 4-cm covered rods achieve the same release rate for levonorgestrel (about 50 mcg/day) as six 3-cm capsules. During a 5-year clinical study comparing rods and capsules, the serum norgestrel levels, bleeding patterns, and incidence of elevated progesterone levels were similar. A multicenter clinical study has confirmed these findings, and the FDA has approved clinical use of the

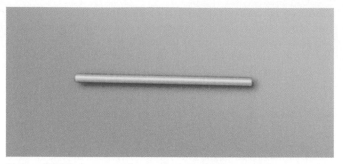

Figure 13-23 Contraceptive implant containing etonogestrel.

two covered rods for 3 years. Although the two-rod system, which is named Jadelle, has never been marketed in the United States, it is available in a number of other countries.

A third generation single implant system is now available and marketed under the trade name Implanon (Merck) (**Fig. 13-23**). This implant is approved for a duration of action of 3 years, is extremely effective, and is much easier to insert and remove than the multiple levonorgestrel-releasing implants. This implant is only 2 mm in diameter and is composed of a solid core of 40% ethylene vinyl acetate (EVA) and 60% crystals (68 mg) of the progestin etonogestrel (ENG, 3-keto desogestrel). The core is surrounded by a thin layer, 0.06 mm thick, of EVA that controls the rate of release of ENG. Etonogestrel is the active metabolite of desogestrel and has high progestational activity but weak androgenic activity. This implant should be inserted in the subcutaneous tissue of the nondominant arm about 6 to 8 cm above the elbow in the crease between the biceps and triceps muscles through the preloaded sterile applicator. No incision is necessary for insertion, but local anesthesia should be used. It is recommended that the implant be inserted during the first 5 days of the cycle. The implant is removed by making a 2-mm incision at the tip of the implant and pushing the rod until it pops out. Etonogestrel is rapidly released from the implant, with about 60 mcg/day being released during the first 2 months, which gradually declines to a release rate of 30 mcg/day at the end of the second year after insertion. Eight hours after insertion, ENG levels rise to a mean of 266 pg/mL, which is sufficient to inhibit ovulation. Maximum ENG levels reach a mean of 813 pg/mL about 4 days after insertion, after which there is a gradual decline to a mean of 196 pg/mL after the first year and 156 pg/mL at the end of 3 years. Mean serum ENG levels are inversely related to body weight. When serum ENG levels are above 90 pg/mL, ovulation is inhibited. Ovulation inhibition is the main mechanism of action of this implant together with thickening of the cervical mucus. Ovulation is inhibited for at least 30 months after insertion, and no pregnancies were reported in clinical trials of nearly 2000 women with 7500 cycles of use. Following removal of the implant, serum ENG levels decline rapidly and are undetectable within 1 week after removal. Ovulation resumes rapidly, and 90% of women ovulate within 1 month after removal and 90% resume regular menses within 3 months.

During the first year after insertion of the implant serum E_2 levels are in the early follicular phase range (60 pg/mL) but rise to late follicular phase levels (80 to 100 pg/mL) in the second and third years after insertion. This implant does not result in a decrease of bone mineral density, even in women with amenorrhea. In clinical trials, continuation rates are high, with 50% to 80% of women continuing use until 2 years in different countries. Bleeding irregularities are the most common reason for discontinuation, accounting for about 60% of early removals. As with all progestin-only methods, nearly all women have disruption of their regular bleeding pattern. Amenorrhea is common, occurring in about 20% of women, and 27% have infrequent bleeding. About 12% of women have prolonged bleeding, and 6% have frequent bleeding. Unlike DMPA or the LNG-IUS, there are no consistencies in the bleeding pattern of individual women. Although an increase in body weight is common in users of this implant, in one study the mean increase in weight was similar to a group of nonmedicated IUD users.

Acne develops in about 13% of women using the implant but accounts for only about 1% of premature removals. No clinically meaningful changes in carbohydrate or lipid metabolism occur with this implant.

According to the labeling for the device, it should not be inserted prior to 6 weeks after delivery. A small pilot study that randomized 40 healthy exclusively breast-feeding women to receive either the ETG-releasing implant 24 to 48 hours after delivery (n = 20) or depot medroxyprogesterone acetate (DMPA group; n = 20) at the sixth week postpartum found that the newborns of implant users showed a trend toward gaining more weight. Although preliminary, these results are reassuring.

EMERGENCY CONTRACEPTION

Various steroids and the copper IUD have been used for **emergency contraception**. The steroids are most effective if treatment begins within 72 hours after an isolated midcycle act of coitus. Their effectiveness is less if more than one episode of coitus has occurred or if treatment is initiated later than 72 hours after coitus. The IUD is effective for 7 days after coitus.

It has been estimated that the clinical pregnancy rate after a single act of midcycle coitus without use of a contraceptive is about 8%. A regimen of four tablets of ethinyl estradiol, 0.05 mg, and *dl*-norgestrel, 0.5 mg, combination oral contraceptive (Ovral), given in doses of two tablets 12 hours apart, was initially tested in Canada by Yuzpe.

Trussell and associates pooled the data from studies that were published between 1977 and 1993 involving 5226 women treated with this regimen. They calculated that the failure rate was 1.5% and that use of this regimen prevented about 75% of the expected pregnancies. The FDA approved a product containing four tablets of these contraceptive steroids (Preven) for emergency contraception, but it is no longer marketed. Nevertheless, combinations of many other oral contraceptives that provide an equivalent dose of ethinyl estradiol and levonorgestrel can also be used. In one large Canadian study, 30% of the subjects treated with this regimen reported having nausea without vomiting and another 20% had nausea with vomiting. These investigators included an antiemetic, a 50-mg tablet of dimenhydrinate, in the package and instructed the women to take it together with the second dose of contraceptive steroid if they experienced nausea after the first dose. They also reported that the time to onset of the subsequent menses was slightly shortened in the users of this regimen.

Ho and Kwan reported results of a randomized trial comparing the use of four tablets of ethinyl estradiol and levonorgestrel taken in divided doses 12 hours apart with a single tablet of 0.75 mg levonorgestrel taken initially and another one 12 hours later. Both regimens were ingested within 48 hours of unprotected intercourse. Failure rates of both regimens, about 2%, were similar, but there was significantly less nausea and vomiting with the progestin alone than with the one combined with estrogen. Subsequently, the WHO performed a randomized trial of the two regimens in about 2000 women in 21 centers. When given within 72 hours after a single act of unprotected sexual intercourse, levonorgestrel alone was more effective, with a pregnancy rate of 1.1%, and had fewer side effects than the estrogen-levonorgestrel combined oral contraceptive, which had a 3.2% pregnancy rate. The authors calculated that levonorgestrel prevented 85% of pregnancies compared with 57% for the combined OC. There were also fewer side effects of nausea and vomiting, dizziness, and fatigue with the levonorgestrel compound. Effectiveness was greater when the agents were given within 24 hours of sexual intercourse than when they were given in the subsequent 48 hours. In this study, the earlier the treatment is initiated after intercourse, the greater the efficacy with a downward gradient of efficacy from treatment within 24 hours to 44 to 72 hours. However, some degree of efficacy is still present when the progestin is given up to 120 hours after unprotected intercourse. A strip of two tablets of 0.75 mg levonorgestrel is marketed in several countries including the United States under a variety of brand names. In the United States it was originally marketed under the name Plan B, but a generic pill (Next Choice) is also available. It is believed that the main mechanism of action of high-dose progestin emergency contraception is inhibition of ovulation, but other mechanisms may be involved. The product was approved as a dose of 0.75 mg given within 72 hours of unprotected intercourse and repeated 12 hours later, but studies have confirmed that it works just as well if both pills (1.5 mg) are taken at the same time. The 1.5-mg dose is now marketed under the name Plan B One-Step and is available without a prescription for women over the age of 17. Studies in new world monkeys have shown that pregnancy is not prevented if high doses of LNG are given after the LH surge.

Novikova and colleagues evaluated 99 women recruited at the time they presented with a request for emergency contraception pills (ECPs). All women took LNG 1.5 mg in a single dose during the clinic consultation, and a blood sample was taken immediately prior to ingestion of the ECP for estimation of serum LH, estradiol and progesterone levels to calculate the day of ovulation. Women were followed up 4 to 6 weeks later to ascertain pregnancy status, and the effectiveness of ECP when taken before and after ovulation was determined. Among 17 women who had intercourse in the fertile period of the cycle and took the ECP after ovulation occurred (on days +1 to +2), three or four pregnancies were expected and three were observed. Based on endocrine data, it was determined that these three subjects had unprotected intercourse between days −1 and 0 (ovulation day) and took the ECP on day +2. Among 34 women who had intercourse on days −5 to −2 of the fertile period and took ECP before or on the day of ovulation, four pregnancies would have been expected, but none were observed. Taken together, these data are highly supportive of the concept that levonorgestrel emergency contraception has little or no effect on postovulation events but is highly effective when taken before ovulation. Levonorgestrel emergency contraception does not affect implantation and is not abortifacient. If the woman has a continuing need for contraception after the cycle in which any of these agents is used, one of the conventional methods should be prescribed.

Intrauterine insertion of a copper IUD within 5 to 10 days of midcycle coitus is a very effective method of preventing continuation of the pregnancy. Fasoli and coworkers summarized the results of four published studies in nine countries involving 879 women using the copper IUD. Only one pregnancy occurred, yielding a pregnancy rate of 0.1%. It is now estimated that more than 9400 postcoital copper IUD insertions have been performed with only 10 pregnancies, yielding a failure rate of less than 0.2%. The LNG-IUS should not be used for emergency contraception.

Glasier and associates have shown that mifepristone (also known as RU-486 and Mifeprex) is extremely effective when used as a postcoital contraceptive and is given as a single 600-mg dosage. Side effects were fewer and efficacy was similar to that with the use of two tablets of oral contraceptives taken 12 hours apart. A study by the WHO reported that use of a single tablet of 10 mg of mifepristone was an effective emergency contraceptive with a pregnancy rate of 1.2%.

Ulipristal, also known as CDB-2913, has been studied as an emergency contraceptive pill. Creinen and coworkers performed a randomized, double-blinded noninferiority trial that enrolled healthy women seeking emergency contraception within 72 hours of unprotected intercourse. Participants were randomly assigned to receive a single dose of 50 mg of CDB-2913, plus a placebo 12 hours later or two doses of 0.75 mg of levonorgestrel taken 12 hours apart. Pregnancies occurred in 7 (0.9%, 95% CI 0.2% to 1.6%) and 13 (1.7%, 95% CI 0.8% to 2.6%) women, respectively. Based on the estimated cycle day of unprotected intercourse, 85% and 69% of anticipated pregnancies, respectively, were averted. Nausea was reported by a somewhat greater percentage of CDB-2913 than levonorgestrel users (29% compared with 24%, P = 0.03), but the distribution of other adverse effects was similar in both groups. Women in both groups experienced considerable variation in menstrual cycle length as compared with their reported individual normal cycle lengths. In 2009, European regulatory approval was granted for a 30-mg tablet of ulipristal (under the brand name of EllaOne) as an emergency contraceptive pill for use up to 5 days after unprotected intercourse. An application for approval in the United States is under review.

INTRAUTERINE DEVICES

The main benefits of IUDs are (1) a high level of effectiveness, (2) a lack of associated systemic metabolic effects, and (3) the need for only a single act of motivation for long-term use. Despite these advantages, only about 1% of women of reproductive age use the IUD for contraception in the United States, compared with 15% to 30% in most European countries and Canada. In contrast to other types of contraception, there is no need for frequent motivation to ingest a pill daily or to use a coitus-related method consistently. These characteristics, as well as the necessity for a visit to a health care facility to discontinue the method, account for the fact that IUDs have the highest continuation rate of all currently available reversible methods of contraception.

Unlike other contraceptives, such as the barrier methods, which rely on frequent use by the individual to be effective and therefore have higher typical failure rates than perfect failure rates, the IUD has similar rates of failure for typical or perfect use. First-year failure rates with the copper T 380A IUD and

Table 13-11 Cumulative Discontinuation Rates in a Randomized Trial of a Copper (Nova T) IUD and the Levonorgestrel-IUS

	Year									
	1		**2**		**3**		**4**		**5**	
Event	**Nova T**	**LNG-IUD**	**Nova T**	**LNG-IUD**	**Nova T**	**LNG-IUD**	**Nova T**	**LNG-IUD**	**Nova T**	**LNG-IUD**
Pregnancy	0.9	0.1	2.2	0.1	3.1	0.2	4.0	0.3	4.2	0.3
Expulsion	3.4	3.4	4.1	4.2	4.8	4.8	5.3	4.9	5.5	4.9
Bleeding problems	5.7	5.8	9.0	8.3	12.0	9.6	14.3	10.3	16.2	10.9
Amenorrhea	0.0	1.5	0.0	2.9	0.0	3.6	0.0	4.2	0.0	4.3
Pain	1.6	1.6	2.6	2.8	3.3	3.4	3.8	3.9	4.2	4.2
Hormonal	0.1	2.3	0.1	4.8	0.6	6.4	0.7	7.6	1.1	8.4
PID	0.4	0.3	1.0	0.5	1.5	0.5	1.5	0.5	1.6	0.6
Other medical	2.4	2.7	3.8	3.6	5.4	4.8	6.4	5.5	7.6	5.8
Planning pregnancy	1.9	1.9	5.5	5.7	8.1	8.2	10.6	10.1	11.8	10.8
Other personal	0.6	0.6	1.0	1.5	1.7	2.0	2.5	2.3	3.3	2.9
Continuation	83.0	79.9	70.7	65.6	59.4	56.7	50.8	50.6	44.5	46.9

Need to request permission.

Net cumulative termination rates per 100 each year in 937 women using Nova T and 1821 women using a 20 micrograms/24 hours levonorgestrel-releasing device (LNG-IUD) during 5 years.

From Andersson K, Odlind V, Rybo G: Levonorgestrel-releasing and copper-releasing (Nova T) IUDs during five years of use: A randomized comparative trial. Contraception 49:56-72, 1994.

the levonorgestrel releasing IUD (LNG-IUS) are less than 1%. Pregnancy rates are related to the skill of the clinician inserting the device. With experience, correct high-fundal insertion occurs more frequently, and there is a lower incidence of partial or complete expulsion. Furthermore, the annual incidence of accidental pregnancy decreases steadily after the first year of IUD use. The cumulative pregnancy rate after 12 years of use of the copper T 380A IUD is only 1.7% and after 5 years of the LNG-IUS is about 1.1%. The incidence of all major adverse events with IUDs, including pregnancy, expulsion, or removal for bleeding or pain, steadily decrease with increasing use (**Table 13-11**). The failure rates associated with IUDs are comparable to those achieved with surgical sterilization. Thus, the IUD is especially suited for older parous women who wish to prevent further pregnancies. The high effectiveness of IUDs make them appropriate choices for women of all ages.

TYPES OF IUDS

Since the early 1980s, many types of IUDs have been designed and used clinically. The devices developed and initially used in the 1960s were made of a plastic, polyethylene, impregnated with barium sulfate to make them radiopaque. In the 1970s, in order to diminish the frequency of the side effects of increased uterine bleeding and pain, smaller plastic devices covered with copper were developed and widely utilized. In the 1980s devices bearing a larger amount of copper, including sleeves on the horizontal arm, such as the copper T 380A and the copper T 220 C, were developed, as well as the Multiload CU 250 and CU 375. These devices have a longer duration of high effectiveness and thus need to be reinserted at less frequent intervals than do the devices bearing a smaller amount of copper. The copper T 380A IUD (**Fig. 13-24**) is the only copper-bearing IUD currently marketed in the United States, but the Multiload CU 375 is widely used in Europe. Because of the constant dissolution of copper, which amounts daily to less than that ingested in the normal diet, all copper IUDs have to be replaced periodically. The copper T 380A is currently approved for use in the United States for 10 years and maintains its effectiveness for at least 12 years. At the scheduled

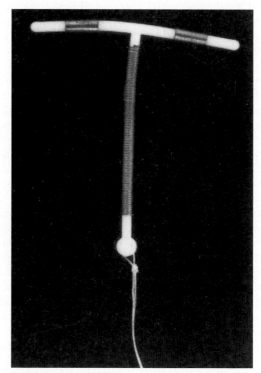

Figure 13-24 Intrauterine device currently being marketed in the United States—copper T 380A.

time of removal, for women desiring continued contraceptive protection, the device can be removed and another inserted during the same office visit.

Adding a reservoir of a progestin to the vertical arm also increases the effectiveness of the T-shaped devices. With the LNG-IUS, about 20 mcg LNG is released into the endometrial cavity each day. This amount is sufficient to prevent pregnancy by thickening the cervical mucus and preventing the transport of sperm into the endometrial cavity and tubes.

A large comparative trial of the copper T 380A and the LNG-IUS found that the effectiveness and continuation rates of both devices were similar. The LNG-IUS has a high level of effectiveness for at least 5 years, with a cumulative pregnancy rate of 1.1%. This IUD also reduces menstrual blood loss and has been used therapeutically to treat excessive uterine bleeding.

MECHANISMS OF ACTION

All intrauterine devices induce a local inflammatory reaction of the endometrium, and the cellular and humoral components expressed in the tissue and the fluid fill the uterine cavity to create an environment that is toxic to sperm, so fertilization of the ovum does not occur. Although this sterile inflammatory reaction is the only mechanism in inert devices, medicated IUDs containing either copper or levonorgestrel produce additional local effects that increase their efficacy in preventing pregnancy. Ortiz and Croxatto recently published a detailed review of the mechanism, which also included some new data. Taken together, these studies indicate that if any embryos are formed in the chronic presence of an IUD, it happens at a much lower rate than in non-IUD users. The common belief that the usual mechanism of action of IUDs in women is destruction of embryos in the uterus is not supported by empirical evidence.

There is an approximate 1000% increase in the number of leukocytes in washings of the human endometrial cavity 18 weeks after the insertion of an IUD compared with washings obtained before insertion. In addition to causing phagocytosis of spermatozoa, tissue breakdown products of these leukocytes are toxic to all cells, including spermatozoa. The amount of inflammatory reaction, and thus contraceptive effectiveness, is directly related to the size of the intrauterine foreign body. Copper markedly increases the extent of the inflammatory reaction, so this metal permitted the development of smaller T-framed devices. The sterile inflammatory products accumulate throughout the uterine lumen and penetrate the cervix and probably the fallopian tubes. This affects the function and viability of gametes at many levels, preventing fertilization and lowering the chances of survival of any embryo that may be formed, before it reaches the uterus. In addition, copper impedes sperm transport and viability in the cervical mucus. Increasing the amount of copper has improved efficacy; the copper T 380 has about twice as much copper surface area as the formerly marketed copper 7 IUD, and it has a significantly lower failure rate. Sperm transport from the cervix to the oviduct in the first 24 hours after coitus is markedly impaired in women wearing IUDs. Because of the spermicidal action of IUDs, very few, if any, sperm reach the oviducts, and the ovum usually does not become fertilized. The small numbers of fertilizations that do occur explain the failure rate of these devices.

Further evidence for this spermicidal action of IUDs was reported by a group of investigators who performed tubal flushing in 56 women wearing IUDs and 45 using no method of contraception who were sterilized by salpingectomy soon after ovulation. These women had unprotected sexual intercourse shortly before ovulation. Normally cleaving, fertilized ova were found in the tubal flushings of about half of the women not wearing IUDs, whereas no eggs that had the microscopic appearance of a normally developing embryo were found in the oviducts of the women wearing IUDs.

Because concern over mechanism of action represents a barrier to acceptance of this important and highly effective method for some women and some clinicians, it is important to point out that there is no evidence to suggest that the mechanism of action of IUDs is abortifacient. A long-term study of women wearing the copper T 380A IUD revealed that although the cumulative intrauterine pregnancy rate gradually increased with duration of IUD use, the ectopic pregnancy rate remained low and constant after the first year of use. If fertilization occurred frequently with IUD use and its main mechanism of action was to prevent uterine implantation of the blastocyst, the ectopic pregnancy rate would be expected to increase at a rate more rapidly than the intrauterine pregnancy rate, and this outcome did not occur. Thus, the principal mechanism of action of the copper T 380A IUD is to interfere with sperm action, preventing fertilization of the ovum.

The LNG-IUS, like the copper device, has a very low ectopic pregnancy rate. Therefore, fertilization does not occur and its main mechanism of action is also preconceptual. Less inflammation occurs within the uterus of LNG-IUS users, but the potent progestin effect thickens cervical mucus to impede sperm penetration and access to the upper genital track. Although the LNG-IUS also produces a thin, inactive endometrium, there is no evidence to suggest that this will prevent implantation, and the device should not be used for emergency contraception. The low levels of circulating steroid do not typically inhibit ovulation. However, as is true with all progestin-only methods, there is an increase in the incidence of persistent functional ovarian cysts. These cysts typically resolve without any intervention and can be followed clinically. In a long-term study where women were randomized to either a copper or levonorgestrel IUD, there was no increase in the number of significant adverse events (hospitalization or surgery) for ovarian cysts among LNG-IUS users. On removal of the IUD, the inflammatory reaction and other changes rapidly disappear. Resumption of fertility following IUD removal is prompt and occurs at the same rate as resumption of fertility following discontinuation of the barrier methods of contraception. The incidence of full-term deliveries, spontaneous abortion, and ectopic pregnancies in conceptions occurring after IUD removal is the same as in the general noncontraceptive-using population.

TIME OF INSERTION

Although it is widely believed that the optimal time for insertion of an IUD is during the menses, there are data indicating that the IUD can be safely inserted on any day of the cycle provided the woman is not pregnant. An analysis was made of 2-month **IUD event rates** of about 10,000 women who had a copper T 200 IUD inserted on various days of the cycle. Differences in event rates with insertion occurring on different days of the cycle were small and of little clinical relevance. Therefore, the IUD can be inserted on any day of the cycle. Because bacteria are introduced into the endometrial cavity at the time of IUD insertion, it is preferable to insert the IUD after the cessation of menses to avoid providing a good environment for bacterial growth.

It has also been recommended that IUDs not be inserted until more than 2 to 3 months have elapsed after completing a full-term pregnancy. Caliskan and coworkers performed ultrasounds on 8343 women in Turkey 1 year after insertion of a copper T-380A IUD. Relative risk estimates and logistic regression analyses were performed to determine the risk factors associated with uterine perforation. The overall incidence of perforation was 2.2 per 1000 insertions with an increased risk seen with insertion 0 to 3 months postpartum (OR 11.7, 95% CI 2.8 to 49.2) and at 3 to 6 months postpartum (OR 13.2, CI 2.8 to 62). However, Mishell and coworkers compared event rates among women who underwent copper T IUDs insertion between 4 and 8 weeks postpartum and at more than 8 weeks postpartum. The 1- and 2-year event rates for all causes were similar for the two groups, indicating that copper T IUDs can be safely inserted at the time of the routine postpartum visit. No uterine perforations occurred in this series. An IUD can be placed at the time of either vaginal or caesarian delivery immediately following delivery of the placenta with acceptable low rates of expulsion. Women randomized to immediate insertion of an IUD after a first trimester surgical abortion by Bednarek and colleagues demonstrated higher rates of IUD continuation, lower rates of repeat unintended pregnancy, and no significant difference in expulsion rates when compared with women randomized to delayed (2 to 4 weeks later) IUD insertion. The effect of breast-feeding on performance of the copper T 380A IUDs was evaluated from data obtained from a large, multicenter, clinical trial in which the device was inserted into 559 breast-feeding women and 590 non–breast-feeding women, all of whom were at least 6 weeks postpartum. There were significantly fewer problems with pain and bleeding at the time of insertion in the group that was breast-feeding. Similar low expulsion rates and high continuation rates were observed both the breast-feeding and non–breast-feeding groups 6 months after insertion. Therefore, insertion of the IUD can be performed in postpartum women who are breast-feeding their infants, as well as in those who are not nursing at the time of the routine postpartum visit.

A number of interventions have been tried to reduce pain with insertion. It is important to remember that most insertions are easy and accomplished on the first attempt. Cervical preparation with misoprostol does not increase the success of insertion and may increase pain. Ibuprofen administered prior to insertion does not reduce insertion pain but may be helpful for the cramping that occurs in the hours immediately following insertion. Clinicians should receive training in correct insertion technique prior to placing an IUD. The correct insertion technique detailed in the product labeling should always be followed. This information should be reviewed prior to each insertion, if the clinician does not routinely place IUDs. If cervical stenosis prevents the passage of a uterine sound, a paracervical block should be placed and direct dilation performed. Dilation to at least 4 mm is desirable, as the insertion tube measures about 4.2 mm. Difficult insertions should be referred to clinicians with expertise in family planning procedures.

ADVERSE EFFECTS

Incidence

In general, in the first year of use, copper IUDs have less than a 1% pregnancy rate, a 6% expulsion rate, and a 12% rate of removal for medical reasons, mainly bleeding and pain. The annual incidence of each of these events, especially expulsion, diminishes steadily in subsequent years.

In an ongoing WHO study of the copper T 380A, termination rates for adverse effects continued to decline annually following the first year after insertion for each of the 12 years in which sufficient data had been accumulated. In this study, the cumulative percentage discontinuation rate for pregnancy, bleeding and pain, and expulsion at the end of 7 years was 1.6, 22.7, and 8.6 per 100 women, respectively, and at the end of 12 years they were 1.7, 35.2, and 12.5 per 100 women. In a large study of the LNG-IUS, Andersson and colleagues reported that termination rates at the end of 1 year for pregnancy, bleeding, and pain and expulsion were 0.1, 7.4, and 3.4 per 100 women, respectively. After 5 years the cumulative discomfort rate for pregnancy, bleeding, and pain and expulsion were 0.3, 15.1, and 4.9 per 100 women, respectively.

Uterine Bleeding

The majority of women discontinuing this method of contraception do so for medical reasons. Nearly all the medical reasons accounting for removal of copper IUDs involve one or more types of abnormal bleeding: heavy or prolonged menses or intermenstrual bleeding. The heavy bleeding may be produced by a premature and increased rate of local release of prostaglandins brought about by the presence of the intrauterine foreign body, as this increase is seen with both inert and copper IUDs. The stimulation of uterine contractions by excessive levels of prostaglandins may prolong the duration of the menstrual flow, which is significantly longer in women wearing copper IUDs than in normally cycling women.

The copper T 380A IUD is associated with about a 55% increase in menstrual blood loss (MBL). Not all women with a copper IUD will experience excessive bleeding. In a study of Swedish women in whom the copper T 380 was inserted, there was no significant change in mean measurements of several hematologic parameters, including hemoglobin, hematocrit, and erythrocyte count at 3, 6, and 12 months after IUD insertion compared with mean values before insertion.

A sensitive indicator of tissue iron stores is the serum ferritin level. In a study of women using the copper T 380A IUD, there was no significant change in mean serum ferritin levels at 3, 6, and 12 months after IUD insertion. None of the women with low ferritin levels had a decrease in hemoglobin levels. An increase in intestinal iron absorption may compensate for the increased MBL, as none of these women developed anemia.

In contrast, there is a significant reduction of MBL, about 60%, during the use of the LNG-IUS. This reduction is seen as early as 3 months after insertion and persists for the duration of use of the device. The amount of blood loss is significantly reduced to about 5 mL/cycle and after 1 year 20% of women using this IUD are amenorrheic. The reduction of MBL results in an improvement of blood hemoglobin levels. Thus, the LNG-IUS is useful in the prevention and the treatment of iron deficiency anemia and the depletion of iron stores by heavy MBL, and it has been approved for this indication in many countries in Europe and throughout the world. In 2009, the FDA granted U.S. labeling approval for a second indication for the LNG-IUS (in addition to contraception) of heavy or prolonged menstrual bleeding.

Excessive bleeding in the first few months following IUD insertion should be treated with reassurance and supplemental oral iron, as well as systemic administration of one of the prostaglandin synthetase inhibitors during menses. The bleeding usually diminishes with time, as the uterus adjusts to the presence of the foreign body. Mefenamic acid ingested in a dosage of 500 mg three times a day during the days of menstruation has been shown to reduce MBL significantly in IUD users. If excessive bleeding continues despite this treatment, the device should be removed. After a 1-month interval, another type of device may be inserted if the woman still wishes to use an IUD for contraception. Consideration should be given to using the LNG-IUS, because this device is associated with less blood loss than the copper-bearing IUDs.

Perforation

Although uncommon, one of the potentially serious complications associated with IUD use is perforation of the uterine fundus. Perforation always occurs at the time of insertion. Sometimes only the distal portion of the IUD penetrates the uterine muscle at insertion. Then uterine contractions over the next few months force the IUD into the peritoneal cavity. IUDs correctly inserted entirely within the endometrial cavity do not migrate or wander through the uterine muscle into the peritoneal cavity. The incidence of perforation is generally related to the shape of the device or to the amount of force used during its insertion, as well as the experience of the clinician performing the insertion. Perforation of the uterus is best prevented by straightening the uterine axis with a tenaculum and then probing the cavity with a uterine sound before IUD insertion.

Perforation rates for the copper T 380A are only about 1 in 3000 insertions. Anderson and colleagues analyzed 50 consecutive perforations occurring with intrauterine devices (IUD) reported to the National Patient Insurance Scheme Register in Sweden during 1990 to 1993. All 50 women were parous and >20 years of age at the time of IUD insertion. Most (84%) of the IUDs were inserted by a midwife, and 90% were inserted <1 year after a full-term pregnancy, with 62% within 12 weeks of delivery. Over half (54%) of the perforations occurred in women who reported that they were breast-feeding at the time of IUD insertion. In most (62%) of the cases of perforation, the women reported severe pain at insertion and during the first 24 hours. Less than one third (28%) of the women had the perforation diagnosed within 1 month of insertion. Lower abdominal pain was the most frequent symptom at early diagnosis, but in two cases, the main symptom was heavy bleeding. Unexpected pregnancy was the most common event leading to a late diagnosis and occurred in 20 women (56%), followed by failure to visualize the threads.

The clinician should always suspect that perforation has occurred if the user did not observe that the device was expelled and cannot feel the threads. One should not assume that an unnoticed expulsion has occurred when the threads are not visualized. Sometimes the IUD is still in its correct position in the uterine cavity, but the threads have been withdrawn into the cavity as the position of the IUD has changed. To assess this, after pelvic examination has been performed and the possibility of pregnancy excluded, a transvaginal ultrasound should be performed to locate the device. Alternatively, if removal is desired, the uterine cavity should be probed.

If the device cannot be felt with a uterine sound or biopsy instrument or the device is not visualized with pelvic ultrasonography, a radiograph visualizing the entire abdominal cavity should be performed. Because IUDs that have been pushed through the uterus may be located anywhere in the peritoneal cavity, even in the subdiaphragmatic area, the x-ray should visualize the entire pelvis and both lung bases.

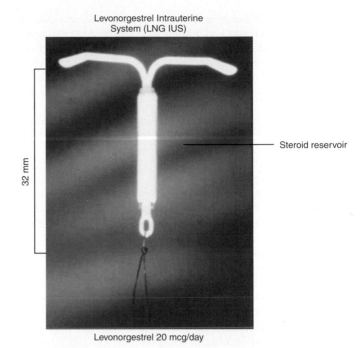

Levonorgestrel Intrauterine System (LNG IUS)

32 mm

Steroid reservoir

Levonorgestrel 20 mcg/day

Figure 13-25 Levonorgestrel intrauterine system.

Any type of IUD found to be outside the uterus, even if asymptomatic, should be removed from the peritoneal cavity because complications such as severe adhesions and bowel obstruction have been reported with intraperitoneal IUDs (**Fig. 13-25**). Therefore, it is best to remove intraperitoneal IUDs shortly after the diagnosis of perforation is made. Unless severe adhesions have developed, most intraperitoneal IUDs can be removed by means of laparoscopy.

Perforation of the cervix has also been reported with devices having a straight vertical arm, such as the copper T. A plastic ball has been added to the distal vertical arm of the copper T 380A to reduce the rate of cervical perforation. When follow-up examinations are performed after IUD insertion, the cervix should be carefully inspected and palpated, because often perforations do not extend completely through the ectocervical epithelium. Cervical perforation is not a major problem, but devices that have perforated downward should be removed through the endocervical canal with uterine packing forceps. Their downward displacement is associated with reduced contraceptive effectiveness.

The common use of transvaginal ultrasound, particularly in emergency departments, has led to the discovery of many IUDs in the lower uterine segment. Faundes and colleagues found no relationship between the IUD position evaluated by ultrasound and complaints of bleeding and pain. In asymptomatic individuals, the device should be left in place regardless of location in the uterine cavity. However, if the stem of the device is visible at the external cervical os, it should be removed.

COMPLICATIONS RELATED TO PREGNANCY

If a woman becomes pregnant with an IUD in place, a pelvic ultrasound should be performed to determine if the pregnancy is intrauterine or ectopic. In the event of an intrauterine pregnancy, the device should be removed as quickly as possible regardless of whether the pregnancy is desired or undesired. As the uterus grows with the pregnancy, the threads will eventually be drawn inside the cervix and become inaccessible. After this time, removal using ultrasound guidance may be possible. Therefore, as there is no benefit to expectant management and the possibility of successful removal will diminish over time, the device should be removed if the threads are visible by the first clinician to examine the patient after a diagnosis of pregnancy is made. Although the miscarriage rate in the first 3 weeks after IUD removal is higher than that in normal pregnancy, after this time the complication rate approaches that of normal pregnancy.

Congenital Anomalies

When pregnancy occurs with an IUD in place, implantation takes place away from the device itself, so the device is always extraamniotic. Although there is a paucity of published data, so far there is no evidence of an increased incidence of congenital anomalies in infants born with a plastic, copper-bearing, or progestin-releasing IUD in utero.

Data from two studies of more than 300 babies conceived with a copper IUD in utero suggest that its presence does not exert a deleterious effect on fetal development or increase the risk of birth defects. Although relatively few infants have been born following gestation in a uterus containing the LNG-IUS, examination of these infants has revealed no evidence of cardiac or other anomalies.

Spontaneous Abortion

In all reported series of pregnancies with any type of IUD in situ, the incidence of fetal death was not significantly increased; however, a significant increase in spontaneous abortion has been consistently observed. If a woman conceives while wearing an IUD that is not subsequently removed, the incidence of spontaneous abortion is about 55%, approximately three times greater than would occur in pregnancies without an intrauterine device.

After conception, if the IUD is spontaneously expelled or if the thread is visible and the IUD is removed by traction, the incidence of spontaneous abortion is significantly reduced. In one study of women who conceived with copper T devices in place, the incidence of spontaneous abortion was only 20% if the device was removed or spontaneously expelled. This figure is similar to the normal incidence of spontaneous abortion and significantly less than the 54% incidence of abortion reported in the same study among women retaining the devices in utero. Thus, if a woman conceives with an IUD in place and wishes to continue the pregnancy, the IUD should be removed if the appendage is visible to significantly reduce the chance of spontaneous abortion. If the appendage is not visible, blind probing of the uterine cavity may increase the chance of abortion, as well as sepsis. However, several recent reports indicate that with sonographic guidance it is possible during early gestation to remove IUDs in the lower uterine cavity without visible threads and not adversely affect the outcome of the pregnancy.

Septic Abortion

If the IUD cannot be removed from the uterine cavity during early gestation, some evidence suggests that the risk of septic abortion may increase if the IUD remains in place. Most of the evidence was based on data from women who conceived while wearing the Dalkon Shield type of IUD. This device, with its multifilament tail, was extensively used in the United States during the 1970s. The structure of the shield's appendage allowed vaginal bacteria to steadily enter the spaces between the filaments of the tail beneath the surrounding sheath. This action differs from the inability of bacteria to enter the monofilament tails or migrate along their surface through the cervical mucus barrier. During pregnancy, when the shield was drawn upward into the uterine cavity as gestation advanced, the bacteria colonizing the tail string could exit into the uterine cavity and cause a severe and sometimes fatal uterine and systemic infection. This infection usually became manifest during the second trimester of pregnancy.

There is no conclusive evidence that modern IUDs with monofilament tail strings can cause sepsis during pregnancy. In a British study, there was no significant difference in the incidence of septic abortion among women who conceived with an IUD in place and those who conceived while using other methods. In another study of 918 women who conceived with the copper T in situ, there were only two instances of septic abortion, both occurring in the first trimester. These data indicate that there is no increase in sepsis in pregnancy caused by the presence of an IUD except for users of the Dalkon Shield. However, about 2% of all spontaneous abortions are septic, and the continued presence of an IUD is associated with about a 50% risk of having a spontaneous abortion. Therefore, the overall incidence of septic abortion may increase with any IUD in place because the incidence of spontaneous abortion increases, not because the presence of the IUD increases the risk of sepsis by itself.

Ectopic Pregnancy

Because copper and levonorgestrel IUDs principally act by preventing fertilization either through a cytotoxic effect on spermatozoa or an effect on cervical mucus, the incidence of both ectopic pregnancy and intrauterine pregnancy decrease with their use. Because the copper T 380A IUD so effectively prevents all pregnancies, the estimated ectopic pregnancy rate is only 0.2 to 0.4 per 1000 woman-years. This rate is one tenth the rate in women using no contraception, 3 per 1000 woman-years. If a woman uses a copper T 380A IUD, her risk of having an ectopic pregnancy is reduced by 90% compared with use of no contraception. However, in the rare circumstances when fertilizations do occur and lead to pregnancy, the risk of the pregnancy being ectopic increases about threefold from 1.4% to 6%. In the 7-year WHO study of the copper T 380A IUD, the cumulative ectopic pregnancy rate at the end of 7 years was only 0.1 per 100 women. These data confirm that the copper T 380A reduces the risk of having both intrauterine and ectopic gestations.

The overall risk of pregnancy with a LNG-IUS is slightly lower (0.5/1000 woman-years after 5 years) than that of copper IUD users. In Andersson's large study of 1821 women using the LNG-IUS, only five pregnancies occurred during 5 years' experience. Only one of these pregnancies was ectopic. Sivin estimated the ectopic pregnancy rate in women using this device was 0.2 per 1000 woman-years. Therefore, about 40% of pregnancies that occur in women wearing a LNG-IUS will be ectopic. The higher proportion of ectopic pregnancy is likely due to effects of levonorgestrel that decrease tubal contractions, thereby slowing the movement of the embryo to the uterine cavity.

The increased risk of ectopic pregnancy for a woman who conceives while wearing an IUD is temporary and does not persist after removal of the IUD. In two large European studies, women wishing to conceive after they had an ectopic pregnancy had a much greater chance of having a subsequent intrauterine pregnancy if they were using an IUD at the time of their ectopic pregnancy than were those who had an ectopic pregnancy and were not using an IUD. A prior ectopic pregnancy is not a contraindication to IUD use.

Prematurity

In the previously cited study of conceptions occurring in the presence of copper T devices, the rate of prematurity among live births was four times greater when the copper T was left in place than when it was removed.

If a pregnant woman has an IUD in place and the device cannot be removed but she wishes to continue her gestation, she should be warned of the increased risk of prematurity, as well as that of spontaneous abortion and ectopic pregnancy. She should also be informed of the possible increased risk of septic abortion and advised to report promptly the first signs of pelvic pain or fever. There is no evidence that pregnancies with IUDs in utero are associated with an increased incidence of other obstetric complications. There is also no evidence that prior use of an IUD results in a greater incidence of complications in pregnancies occurring after its removal.

INFECTION IN THE NONPREGNANT IUD USER

In the 1960s, despite great concern among clinicians that use of the IUD would markedly increase the incidence of salpingitis, or PID, there was little evidence that such an increase did occur. During that decade the IUD was inserted mainly into parous women, and the incidence of sexually transmitted disease was not as high as occurred subsequently. In 1966 a study was performed in which aerobic and anaerobic cultures were made of homogenates of endometrial tissue obtained transfundally from uteri removed by vaginal hysterectomy at various intervals after insertion of a clean but nonsterile loop IUD. During the first 24 hours after IUD insertion, the normally sterile endometrial cavity was consistently infected with bacteria. Nevertheless, in 80% of uteri removed during the following 24 hours, the women's natural defenses had destroyed these bacteria and the endometrial cavities were sterile. In this study, when transfundal cultures were obtained more than 30 days after IUD insertion, the endometrial cavity, the IUD, and the portion of the thread within the cavity were always found to be sterile (**Fig. 13-26**). These findings indicate that development of PID more than a month after insertion of the IUD is due to infection with a sexually transmitted pathogen and is unrelated to the presence of the device.

Results of a large multicenter clinical study coordinated by the WHO confirmed these findings. In this study of 22,908 women inserted with IUDs, the PID rate was highest in the first 3 weeks after insertion but remained lower and constant during the 8 years thereafter at 0.5 per 1000 woman-years (**Fig. 13-27**). An IUD should not be inserted into a woman who may have been recently infected with gonococci or *Chlamydia trachomatis*. Insertion of the device will transport these pathogens from the cervix into the upper genital tract, where the large number of organisms may overcome the host defense and cause salpingitis. If there is clinical suspicion of infectious endocervicitis, cultures should be obtained and

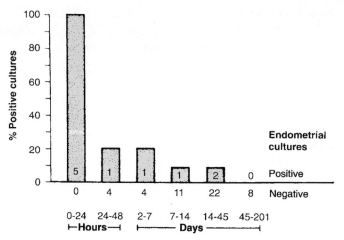

Figure 13-26 Relationship between incidence of positive endometrial cultures and duration of IUD use beyond hysterectomy. (From Mishell DR Jr, Bell JH, Good RG, Moyer DL: The intrauterine device: A bacteriologic study of the endometrial cavity. Am J Obstet Gynecol 96:119, 1966.)

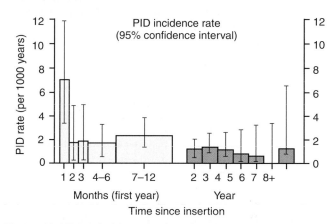

Figure 13-27 PID incidence by time since insertion. Incidence rate was estimated by the number of PID cases and years of exposure in each time interval; 95% confidence intervals were calculated from the Poisson distribution. (From Farley TM, Rosenberg MJ, Rowe PJ, et al: Intrauterine devices and pelvic inflammatory disease: An international perspective. Lancet 339:785, 1992.)

the IUD insertion delayed until the results reveal that no pathogenic organisms are present. To reduce the likelihood of infection, the insertion procedure should be as aseptic as possible. The use of prophylactic antibiotics routinely with every IUD insertion has not been shown to reduce the risk of pelvic infection. A randomized trial comparing use of azithromycin ingested just prior to IUD insertion with a placebo control reported no significant difference in the subsequent rate of pelvic inflammation. The rate was 0.1% in both study arms. In a study of the copper T 380A IUD, the rate of removal because of infection during the first year of use was only 0.3%.

Other epidemiologic studies have shown that the presence of an IUD with monofilament tail strings does not increase the incidence of PID after the insertion interval. One study determined the incidence of tubal infertility among former IUD users. It was reported that nulliparous women with a single

Table 13-12 Use of a Copper IUD, the Presence of Antibodies to Chlamydia, and the Risk of Tubal Occlusion*

IUD Use and Presence of Antibodies to Chlamydia	Infertile Women with Tubal Occlusion (N = 358)	Infertile Controls (N = 953)	Odds Ratio (95% Ci)	Pregnant Controls (N = 584)	Odds Ratio (95% CI)†
		No (%)		No (%)	
No use of a copper IUD					
Antibody-negative	203 (56.7)	583 (61.2)	1.0	420 (71.9)	1.0
Antibody-positive	132 (36.9)	313 (32.8)	1.2 (0.9-1.6)	124 (21.2)	2.4 (1.7-3.2)
Use of a copper IUD					
Antibody-negative	18 (5.0)	33 (3.5)	1.5 (0.8-2.8)	32 (5.5)	1.1 (0.6-2.1)
Antibody-positive	5 (1.4)	24 (2.5)	0.6 (0.2-1.5)	8 (1.4)	1.3 (0.4-4.1)

*For infertile women, data represent the use of a copper intrauterine device (IUD) before the women suspected a fertility problem. Antibody titers of 1:256 or greater were considered positive. For all comparisons, women with no use of a copper IUD and no antibodies resulting from chlamydia served as the reference group. The ratios were adjusted for age, income, number of sexual partners, years of education, and history of sexual intercourse during the teenage years. CI denotes confidence interval.
†The odds ratios are for the comparison with the infertile women with tubal occlusion.

sexual partner who had previously used an IUD had no increased risk of tubal infertility, whereas women with multiple sexual partners who used an IUD did have an increased risk of tubal infertility. Underscoring this relationship, Hubacher and colleagues conducted a case-control study of 1895 women in Mexico, enrolling 358 women with primary infertility who had tubal occlusion documented by hysterosalpingography, as well as 953 women with primary infertility who did not have tubal occlusion (infertile controls) and 584 women who had recently delivered their first child (pregnant controls). They collected information on the women's past use of contraceptives, including copper IUDs, previous sexual relationships, and history of genital tract infections. Each woman's blood was tested for antibodies to *Chlamydia trachomatis*. The odds ratio for tubal occlusion associated with the previous use of a copper IUD was 0.9 (95% CI 0.5 to 1.6) when the primigravid women served as the controls. The presence of antibodies to chlamydia was significantly associated with infertility (**Table 13-12**). Analysis of this large amount of data indicates that PID occurring more than a month following insertion of IUDs with monofilament tail strings is due to a sexually transmitted pathogen and not related to the presence of the IUD.

The increased risk of impairment of future fertility from PID developing in the first month after IUD insertion, as well as the possibility of ectopic pregnancy in the event of contraceptive failure, must be considered when deciding whether to use an IUD in a nulliparous woman, especially if she has multiple sexual partners. The use of male condoms should be advised to reduce the risk of transmission of pathogens in all women with multiple partners. Although the incidence of PID in studies of copper or hormone IUDs is not increased over baseline rates in the general population, subjects in these studies are selected to be of generally low risk. In a large randomized study comparing the copper Nova-T and levonorgestrel IUDs, the rates of PID were low in both groups, but significantly lower among those women wearing the LNG-IUS. Importantly, this effect was largest among women under 25, the group at highest risk of PID (see **Fig. 13-28**). Progestins thicken cervical mucus and reduce the risk of ascending pelvic bacterial infection in women with cervical colonization of gonorrhea or chlamydia. This is the likely mechanism of this observed effect. Symptomatic PID can usually be successfully treated without removing the IUD. A CDC-approved antibiotics regimen for PID should be used until the woman becomes

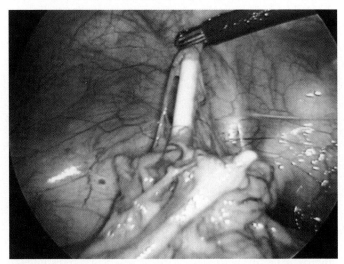

Figure 13-28 Intrauterine device within the peritoneal cavity as a result of perforation during insertion. Note the grasper holding the stem of the device. The T-frame is encased in omentum.

symptom free. If the infection does not improve or if there is evidence of tuboovarian abscess, the device should be removed. For women with clinical evidence of a tuboovarian abscess, the IUD should be removed only after a therapeutic serum level of appropriate parenteral antibiotics has been reached, preferably after a clinical response has been observed. An alternative method of contraception should be substituted if the IUD is removed.

There is evidence that IUD users may have an increased risk for colonizing actinomycosis organisms in the upper genital tract. The relationship of actinomycosis to PID is unclear, as many women without IUDs have actinomycosis in their vagina and are asymptomatic. If actinomycosis organisms are identified on the routine examination of cervical cytology and the woman is asymptomatic, she may be treated with appropriate antimicrobial therapy to eradicate the organisms or she may be followed without therapy. The IUD should not be removed from an asymptomatic woman who is colonized but not infected with actinomycosis. In the rare event that a significant pelvic infection is present, the woman should be treated with antibiotics and the IUD removed (**Fig. 13-29**).

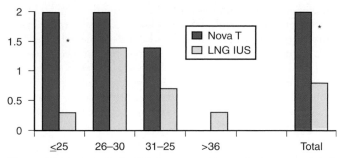

Figure 13-29 Cumulative PID rates over 60 months in an open label, randomized multicenter study comparing the LNG-IUS (n = 1821) to Nova T (n = 937) by age of subject. Asterisks indicate a significant (p < 0.05) difference between groups in the cohort under 25, and in the overall comparison. (Data from Andersson K, Odlind V, Rybo G: Levonorgestrel-releasing and copper-releasing (Nova T) IUDs during five years of use: A randomized comparative trial. Contraception 49:56-72, 1994.)

CONTRAINDICATIONS

It is logical and consistent with good medical practice that IUDs not be inserted into women with any of the following seven conditions, which are listed as contraindications to IUD insertion in the United States: (1) pregnancy or suspicion of pregnancy, (2) acute PID, (3) postpartum endometritis or infected abortion in the past 3 months, (4) known or suspected uterine or cervical malignancy, (5) genital bleeding of unknown origin, (6) untreated acute cervicitis, and (7) a previously inserted IUD that has not been removed. However, little data are available to indicate that the complications of Wilson's disease, allergy to copper, and genital actinomycosis are true contraindications for insertion of copper-bearing IUDs and, because of the infrequency of these conditions, it is unlikely that data will ever become available.

The remaining contraindications for IUD use are listed in the product labeling: abnormalities of the uterus resulting in distortion of the uterine cavity; history of PID; vaginitis, including bacterial vaginosis, until infection is controlled; patient or her partner has multiple sexual partners; and conditions associated with increased susceptibility to infections with microorganisms. These contraindications remain questionable because of the lack of clinical studies of IUD use in women with these conditions.

Why the IUD is stated to be contraindicated in women who have multiple sexual partners or whose partner has multiple sexual partners is unclear. Such women should be counseled to have their partners use condoms to protect against the transmission of diseases and to use the IUD to effectively prevent pregnancy if they so desire. As noted previously, the use of a LNG-IUS may actually reduce the risk of pelvic inflammatory disease.

Conditions previously believed to preclude IUD use but no longer considered to be contraindications include diabetes mellitus, valvular heart disease (including mitral valve prolapse), past history of ectopic pregnancy (except LNG-IUS), nulliparity, treated cervical dysplasia, irregular menses due to anovulation, breast-feeding, corticosteroid use, and age younger than 25. Although women with anovulation will benefit from the progestin effect of the LNG-IUS, they may experience a worsening of bleeding with a copper IUD. HIV-infected women in Zambia

randomized to receive a copper IUD had lower rates of pregnancy and less progression of disease than those randomized to oral contraceptive pills.

The high rate of complication associated with the Dalkon Shield in the early 1970s reduced the confidence and enthusiasm of clinicians and women for all IUDs. It has taken 40 years, considerable research, and excellent modern medicated IUDs to reverse this trend, and IUDs are once again a mainstream method. The method was initially conservatively marketed to only parous women. However, both copper and levonorgestrel IUDs can and should be offered to young or nulliparous women. The high efficacy, favorable bleeding profile, and cervical mucus effects that may reduce the chance of ascending pelvic infection make the LNG-IUS a particularly attractive long-acting method for nulliparous women.

OVERALL SAFETY

Several long-term studies have indicated that the IUD is not associated with an increased incidence of endometrial or cervical carcinoma and may actually be associated with a reduction in risk of developing these neoplasms during and following its use. The IUD is a particularly useful method of contraception for women who have completed their families and do not wish permanent sterilization and have contraindications to, or do not wish to use, other effective methods of reversible contraception. A recent analysis reported that after 5 years of use, the IUD was the most cost-effective method of all methods of contraception, including sterilization. Women in the United States who use an IUD have a higher level of satisfaction with their method of contraception than women using any of the other methods of reversible contraception.

STERILIZATION

In 2002 in the United States, sterilization of one member of a couple was the most widely used method of preventing pregnancy. The popularity of sterilization was greatest if (1) the woman was older than age 30, (2) the couple had been married more than 10 years, and (3) the couple desired no additional children. In contrast to the other methods of contraception, which are reversible or temporary, sterilization should be considered permanent. Although reanastomosis after vasectomy or tubal ligation is possible, the reconstructive operation is much more difficult than the original sterilizing procedure and the results are variable. Pregnancy rates after reanastomosis of the vast range from 45% to 60%, whereas those after tubal reanastomosis range from 50% to 80%, depending on the amount of tissue damage associated with the original procedure, as well as the surgeon's technical competency. If women who have tubal sterilization wish to conceive, in vitro fertilization is now being performed more frequently than tubal reconstructive surgery.

Voluntary sterilization is legal in all 50 states, and the decision to be sterilized should be made solely by the individual in consultation with the provider. Because all currently available sterilization procedures require surgical techniques, individuals who request sterilization should be counseled regarding both the risks and the irreversibility of the procedures. It is advisable to inform the individual fully, and the spouse if possible, of the benefits and risks of these surgical procedures. In addition, it has been

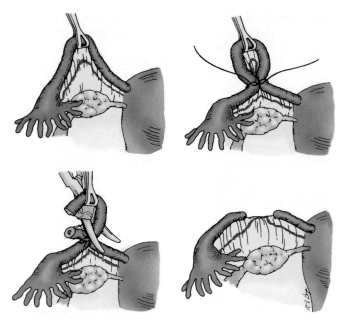

Figure 13-30 Modified Pomeroy technique of female sterilization. (From Sciarra JJ: Surgical procedures for tubal sterilization. In Sciarra JJ, Zatuchni GI, Daly MJ: Gynecology and Obstetrics, vol 6. Philadelphia, Harper & Row, 1984.)

useful to have more than one counselor when a woman younger than age 25 requests sterilization, as well as for all women without children.

The rationale for such careful scrutiny of younger candidates for sterilization is that they tend to change their minds more often, their attitudes may be less fixed, and they face a longer period of reproductive life during which divorce, remarriage, or death among their children can occur.

The most effective, least destructive method of tubal occlusion is the most desirable in younger women, because ovarian dysfunction and adhesion formation diminish and the incidence of successful reversal procedures increases. The effective laparoscopic band techniques or the modified Pomeroy technique (also called partial salpingectomy) (**Fig. 13-30**) should be used in women younger than age 25. Reversal after this method of sterilization is followed by pregnancy in approximately 75% of women, a rate that is higher than that reported after most laparoscopic fulgurations, where more tube is destroyed. However, if pregnancy is desired after tubal occlusion, in vitro fertilization is recommended if there has been extensive tubal destruction by fulguration.

MALE STERILIZATION

Couples considering sterilization should be strongly counseled to accept vasectomy, an outpatient procedure that takes about 20 minutes and requires only local anesthesia. The vas deferens is isolated and cut. The ends of the vas are closed, either by ligation or by fulguration; they are then replaced in the scrotal sac, and the incision is closed. Complications of vasectomy include hematoma (in up to 5% of the subjects), sperm granulomas (inflammatory responses to sperm leakage), and spontaneous reanastomosis. When the last occurs, it usually does so within a short time after the procedure. Vasectomy offers several important advantages over tubal sterilization of women. The procedure is of low cost and can be done in the office with only local

anesthesia, involves no entry into the peritoneal cavity, and there is a simple test to verify efficacy. Usually about 13 to 20 ejaculations are required after the operation before the man is sterile. It is recommended that a semen sample be examined to ensure that no sperm are present before the method is relied on for contraception. Although in the United States reversal requests range from 5% to 7% of men who had a vasectomy, vas reanastomosis is a difficult and meticulous procedure that has an optimal success rate of about 50%.

FEMALE STERILIZATION

Sterilization of the female is more complicated, requiring a transperitoneal incision and usually general anesthesia. Postpartum sterilization is performed by making a small infraumbilical incision and performing either a Pomeroy or modified Irving-type of tubal ligation. These simple and rapid procedures for *postpartum sterilization* can be performed either in the delivery room immediately after delivery or in the operating room the following day without prolonging the hospital stay. Although these same operative techniques can also be rapidly performed through a small suprapubic incision termed *minilaparotomy* for female sterilization at times other than the puerperium, most *interval sterilization* is performed by laparoscopy.

General anesthesia is usually employed for laparoscopic sterilization. This is a day surgical procedure commonly done in outpatient surgery centers. Although both unipolar and bipolar electrosurgical techniques were popular in the early days of laparoscopic sterilization, the most common techniques used today include the Filshie clip and the Silastic band (Falope ring). Both techniques require the surgeon to completely visualize the entire tube. The tube is grasped with the clip applier in the midisthmic portion such that the free end of the clip extends beyond the tube into the mesosalpinx. Pressure on the handle permanently bends the titanium frame to compress a silicone seal, which permanently blocks the tube. Neither material is reactive, and the titanium does not create artifact or otherwise interfere with magnetic resonance imaging (MRI) scans. The Silastic band is pushed over a segment of the midisthmic tube using the specialized applicator that isolates and grasps the tube with a small single tooth forcep specially designed for the purpose. The isolated tubal segment undergoes necrosis similar to a Pomeroy tubal. A Filshie clip applier is also available for postpartum sterilizations via minilap and at the time of caesarian section.

A **microinsert** device that is introduced transcervically through a hysteroscope and placed in the proximal portion of the oviduct to provide occlusion was approved for use as a female sterilization technique in the United States in 2002. The device is 4 cm long and 2 mm in diameter and is made of a flexible stainless steel inner core, a dynamic outer coil made of nickel titanium alloy, and a layer of polyethylene terephthalate fibers (**Fig. 13-31**). The latter material causes tissue ingrowth and

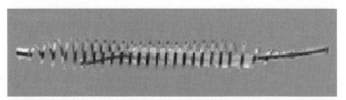

Figure 13-31 Microinsert for transcervical sterilization in women.

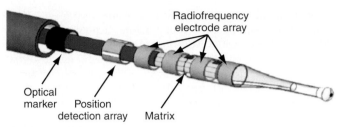

Radiofrequency
electrode array

Optical
marker   Position
detection array   Matrix

Figure 13-32 Tip of catheter used for radiofrequency ablation sterilization procedure and placement of matrix.

permanent tubal occlusion. A large multicenter study by Cooper and colleagues reported that bilateral placement of the microinserts occurred in 86% of initial procedures, which increased to 92% with an additional procedure. Uterine perforation and expulsion of the inserts occur in less than 3% of insertion procedures. A hysterosalpingogram is performed 3 months after insertion to document tubal occlusion. Following this documentation, effectiveness for preventing pregnancy in clinical trials is 99.8% at 3 and 4 years and 99.7% after 5 years of follow-up. Although this is higher than reported with other techniques of female sterilization, the use of a hysterosalpingogram is not routine after laparoscopic or minilaparotomy tubal ligation. A second hysteroscopic sterilization technique was approved in 2009. This approach uses a catheter to apply radiofrequency energy to the intramural portion of the tube to create a superficial lesion and then deploys a small matrix made of silicone comprised of a solid core surrounded by a porous architecture that is 3.5 mm in length and 1.6 mm in diameter into this site (**Fig. 13-32**). During healing, the initial response gives way to a chronic process, which stimulates granulation tissue that ultimately leads to integration fibrous tissue into the matrix and tubal occlusion. In the pivotal trial, bilateral placement success was achieved in 611 of 645 women (95%), and bilateral occlusion was confirmed in 570 of 645 (88.4%). The 1-year pregnancy prevention rate as derived with **life-table methods** was 98.9%.

Female sterilization by surgical removal of a portion of the tube or mechanically occluding a portion of the lumen by clips, bands, or electrocoagulation was previously believed to be the most effective form of pregnancy prevention. This belief was based on studies that reported that failure rates during the first year of use of any type of reversible contraceptive were higher than the first-year failure rate of female sterilization. The results of a long-term study by Peterson and coworkers indicate that pregnancies continue to occur for many years after these sterilization procedures. The failure rate increased from 0.55 per 100 women at 1 year to 1.31 at 5 years, and 1.85 10 years after the operation for all methods of tubal interruption, being higher for bipolar coagulation and spring clips and lower for partial salpingectomy. In women 18 to 27 years of age, 2.8% became pregnant 5 to 10 years after bipolar coagulation of the oviduct. There are several reversible methods of contraception, with failure rates similar to those of tubal sterilization. Cumulative 3-year failure rates with the single implant are less than 0.1%. The 5-year failure of the LNG-IUS is also low, at 0.5%, similar to the 5-year rate seen with postpartum sterilization. The pregnancy rate after 10 years use of copper T 380 IUD is 1.7 per 100 users and is similar to all female sterilization, 1.85 per 100 women. Furthermore, among women who become pregnant after female

sterilization, about one third have ectopic pregnancies compared with 5% with the copper T 380 IUD. Because the copper T 380 IUD has an effective life span of 10 years, with a failure rate comparable to that of female sterilization and a lower ectopic pregnancy rate, as well as being less expensive, rapidly reversible, and more convenient to use, it should be considered as an alternative to tubal sterilization. The favorable bleeding patterns of the LNG-IUS may offer additional health benefits to women considering sterilization, even though it must be replaced after 5 years.

INDUCED ABORTION

Induced abortion is one of the most common gynecologic operations performed in the United States and in many other countries. As determined by the landmark *Roe v. Wade* Supreme Court decision, the state may not interfere with the practice of abortion in the first trimester. In the second trimester, individual states may regulate abortion services in the interest of preserving the health of the woman.

From a public health perspective, safe and legal abortion services are a cornerstone of maternal health care. Worldwide, illegal abortion is one of the leading causes of maternal death. Despite impressive gains in contraceptive safety and use, unintended pregnancy remains a major health and social problem. Half of all pregnancies occurring in the United States are unintended. Although the rate of unintended pregnancy, which excludes miscarriages, dropped from 54 per 1000 women of reproductive age in 1987 to 50 per 1000 in the 2006-2008 National Survey of Family Growth. It remains high, particularly in comparison with other more developed nations. Slightly more than half (53%) of these unintended pregnancies occur in the 94% of sexually active couples who claim to use some method of contraception. The other half come from the approximately 6% of at-risk couples using no method. Clearly, if we wish to meet the goal of all pregnancies being planned and desired, we must improve the use and efficacy of contraceptive methods. However, even if all sexually active couples used a method perfectly, failures would occur. Thus, although we can and should work to reduce the number of unintended pregnancies, failures will continue to occur, and access to safe and legal abortion services will remain a keystone of reproductive health.

From 1973 through 1980, the number of induced abortions performed annually in the United States steadily increased from 750,000 to about 1,600,000. The annual number of abortions stabilized at this figure from 1980 until 1990. Since 1990 there has been a gradual decline in the annual number of abortions performed in the United States, reaching 1.3 million in 2001. In 2005, there were 1.21 million induced abortions, and the abortion ratio (number of abortions per 100 pregnancies) was 18.8, whereas the abortion rate (number of abortions per 1000 women ages 15 to 44) was 19.4. In the United States the abortion rates have declined gradually since 1980 but are higher than in all Western European countries and about one in five pregnancies in the United States are terminated by elective abortion. Approximately one third of abortions are performed in women younger than 20, another third in women age 20 to 24, and the remaining third among women ages 25 and older. Only one fourth of abortions are obtained by married women. Ninety percent of abortions are performed within the first 12 weeks of pregnancy, and about 50% of abortions are performed during the first 8 weeks of pregnancy. In September 2000, the U.S. Food and Drug Administration approved the abortion drug mifepristone to be marketed in the United States as an alternative to surgical abortion. Rates have medication abortion have steadily climbed, and they accounted for 13% of all abortions, and 22% of abortions before 9 weeks' gestation, in 2005.

METHODS

Elective abortion is performed using surgical and medical techniques. Suction curettage, a first-trimester procedure, is the predominant method of performing surgical abortion in the United States, accounting for approximately 75% of all abortion procedures; the remainder are performed by dilation and evacuation, an extraction technique used in the second trimester. Hysterotomy and hysterectomy are major surgical procedures that are rarely used in abortion care. In the early first trimester, medication abortion is an outpatient procedure that mimics miscarriage. Medical termination of pregnancy in the midtrimester mimics labor induction and is performed as an inpatient procedure.

Curettage Methods

Curettage by vacuum aspiration is the predominant method of performing abortion in the first trimester. Very early in pregnancy, *endometrial aspiration,* also termed *menstrual extraction,* can be done with a small, flexible, plastic cannula connected to aspiration syringe. This technique, called *manual vacuum aspiration (MVA),* can typically be performed without dilation or anesthesia. Abortions performed to terminate pregnancies with a gestational age of 8 weeks or more generally require dilation of the cervix and some type of anesthesia, either local or general. The larger volume of material in pregnancies at these gestational ages is more efficiently evacuated with an electric vacuum aspiration system (EVA). In earlier gestations, randomized trials have shown similar efficacy and patient satisfaction with the two techniques.

Following surgical abortion, the tissue must be examined to determine that the gestational sac, placenta, and any fetal parts are completely removed. In very early (under 6 weeks) surgical abortion, it may be difficult to visualize the small gestational sac. MVA produces less disruption of small gestational sacs and may facilitate their identification. If a gestational sac cannot be identified, the women should either be followed by serial hCG evaluation or by repeat ultrasound in 1 week to ensure that pregnancy termination has occurred. The MVA technique is also a low-cost and highly efficient technique to manage threatened, incomplete, or missed abortion in an office setting.

Dilation of the cervix can be facilitated by use of osmotic dilators and administration of prostaglandins. The osmotic dilators are usually placed in the cervical canal for several hours or overnight to produce gradual dilation. Most commonly used are small tents of *Laminaria japonica,* a natural seaweed. These are dried, sorted according to their diameter, and sterilized. Synthetic osmotic dilators include a polyvinyl alcohol sponge impregnated with magnesium sulfate and a hygroscope plastic polymer. By gently opening the cervix over several hours, the osmotic dilators substantially reduce the risk of uterine trauma, such as perforation and cervical injury. Another strategy for cervical preparation is the administration of the prostaglandin and

E_1 analogue misoprostol in a dosage of 400 mcg given orally, vaginally, or buccally a few hours before vacuum aspiration or dilation and evacuation. Misoprostol will soften the cervix and reduce the amount of dilation needed. Although vaginal administration of misoprostol reduces some of the gastrointestinal side effects of the drug, this route of administration has been abandoned because of concerns about infection (see Medication Abortion).

Dilation and evacuation (D&E) is the predominant method of abortion used beyond the first trimester. Because a greater amount of cervical dilation is usually needed, osmotic dilators are usually inserted for several hours or several days before the procedure. Although recent data are lacking, earlier studies indicated that D&E was substantially safer than induction of labor or major operations for abortions of 13 to 16 weeks' gestation. For later abortions, D&E and induction of labor appear to have comparable risks of morbidity and mortality, although the range of complications varies by technique. Disadvantages of D&E include the requirement of technical expertise, the emotional burden for participating physicians and medical personnel, and possible long-term deleterious effects upon the cervix. Advantages include less emotional stress for the woman, avoidance of the need for hospitalization, greater convenience, and lower cost than induction of uterine contractions. Women appreciate the option of choice of procedure.

Medication Abortion

Nonsurgical midtrimester abortion through induction of uterine contractions by instillation of hypertonic solution into the amniotic cavity is an older technique that has been replaced by more effective and less invasive methods. The most common method now used for medical termination in the second trimester is the administration of prostaglandins. The use of prostaglandin E_2 suppositories (which cause significant gastrointestinal side effects) and hyperpyrexia has largely been abandoned in favor of misoprostol. Jain and Mishell reported that the intravaginal placement of two 100-mcg tablets of misoprostol every 12 hours was as successful as prostaglandin E_2, with fewer side effects and less cost. The success rate after 48 hours of treatment was nearly 90%. Dickenson and Evans compared 400 mg of misoprostol intravaginally every 6 hours with 400 mg of misoprostol orally every 3 hours for second-trimester pregnancy termination. Vaginal misoprostol was significantly more effective than oral misoprostol; 86% of women with vaginal misoprostol had delivered within 24 hours and 100% in 48 hours compared with 45% and 79%, respectively, with oral misoprostol. These same investigators compared 400 mg of misoprostol intravaginally every 6 hours with 200 mg intravaginally every 6 hours. The 400-mg dose was more effective and had a shorter induction to delivery interval than the 200-mg dose. At present, the preferred regimen of misoprostol for second-trimester pregnancy terminations is 400 mg intravaginally every 6 hours. This regimen appears to be safe in women with a prior cesarean delivery, as uterine rupture is uncommon.

Early Medical Abortion

In the early 1980s, Healy and coworkers synthesized and tested a progestogenic steroid compound that had weak progestational activity but marked affinity for progesterone receptors in the endometrium. This compound, called RU-486 or mifepristone, is a competitive inhibitor of the progesterone receptor and prevents

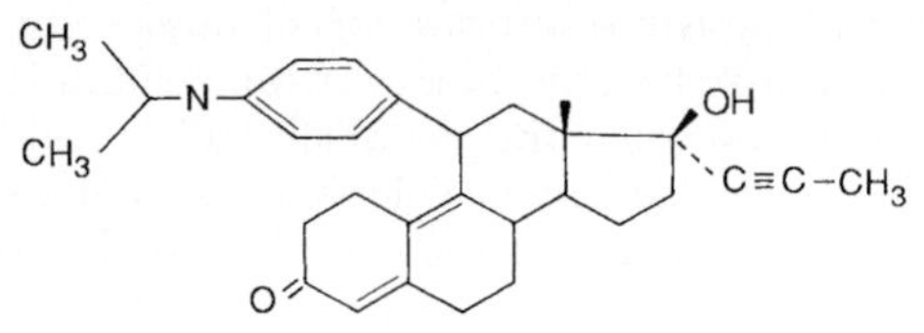

Figure 13-33 Molecular structure of RU-486. Molecular weight is 430, and empirical formula is C29H35NO2. (Reprinted from Healy DL, Baulieu EE, Hodgen GD: Induction of menstruation by an antiprogesterone steroid [RU 486] in primates: Site of action, dose-response relationships, and hormonal effects. Fertil Steril 40:253. Copyright 1983, with permission from The American Society for Reproductive Medicine.)

progesterone from binding to its receptors and thus inhibits the action of circulating progesterone on its target tissue. In clinical trials it was found that if a single 600-mg dose of RU-486 was administered orally in early pregnancy, prior to 7 weeks after the onset of the last menses, about 85% of the pregnancies spontaneously terminated (**Fig. 13-33**). When this treatment was combined with administration of a prostaglandin 36 to 48 hours later, the efficacy increased to 96%. However, side effects include nausea, vomiting, and abdominal pain. Two prostaglandin analogues, intramuscular sulprostone and vaginal gemeprost, were the agents initially used after mifepristone. Sulprostone is no longer marketed for this purpose, as three women who received this agent with mifepristone suffered a myocardial infarction. Gemeprost is much more expensive than misoprostol, a prostaglandin analogue widely used to prevent peptic ulcer disease. The favorable properties of misoprostol (low cost, orally active, highly effective) have led to its widespread adoption as the preferred prostaglandin for medical abortion at all gestational ages. Spitz and associates reported the results of a large multicenter study in the United States of first-trimester abortion using 600 mg mifepristone followed 48 hours later by 400 mcg oral misoprostol. Success rates were 92% for pregnancies less than 49 days gestational age, 83% for pregnancies 50 to 56 days, and 77% for pregnancies 57 to 63 days (**Table 13-13**). The FDA approved this treatment regimen for elective termination of pregnancies of 49 days or less gestational age. The WHO reported that a 200-mg dose of mifepristone was as effective as a 600-mg dose when both doses were followed 48 hours later by 400 mcg of misoprostol orally.

The results of a randomized trial with 400 mcg misoprostol given vaginally or orally found that when misoprostol is given vaginally instead of orally, it is more effective and has fewer side effects. Schaff and colleagues reported that when 200 mg of mifepristone was followed by 800 mg of misoprostol placed intravaginally by the woman at home, 1, 2, or 3 days later in pregnancies of 56 or less days' gestational age, complete abortion rates were 98%, 98%, and 96%, respectively. This regimen reduces the cost of medical abortion, as only one 200-mg tablet of mifepristone is used and one office visit is avoided. This lower-dose mifepristone/misoprostol regimen is called the "evidence-based" protocol to distinguish it from the FDA-approved regimen, and it is the most widely used approach in the United States. Because mifepristone is unavailable in many countries, other pharmacologic agents have been used to terminate early gestation. Studies with 800 mcg of misoprostol tablets used alone and placed in the vagina and moistened with saline for one, two, or three applications 24 hours apart report about a 90% effectiveness when given for a pregnancy of less than 8 weeks' gestational age. Side effects such as vomiting and diarrhea are frequent and can be lessened with use of prophylactic medications. Several investigators have administered methotrexate intramuscularly in a dosage of 50 mg/m² followed 3 to 7 days later by vaginal administration of 800 mcg of misoprostol to groups of women with pregnancies less than 8 weeks' gestational age and found that about 90% of the pregnancies aborted. However, with this regimen only about two thirds of the women aborted within 1 day after receiving misoprostol. The mean time to abortion in the remainder was about 3 weeks. The mean length of time during which uterine bleeding occurred in the entire study group was more than 2 weeks. Because of these problems, as well as the need to determine the true incidence of side effects, this treatment regimen should be considered experimental and only used after an investigative protocol has been approved and the woman has signed an informed consent.

Table 13-13 Results of Mifepristone and Misoprostol in Women Seeking Termination of Pregnancy

Outcome	Pregnant ≤ 49 days (N = 827)	Pregnant 50 to 56 Days (N = 678)	Pregnant 57 to 63 Days (N = 510)
Number (Percentage [95% Confidence Interval])			
Success	762 (92 [90-94])	563 (83 [80-86])*	395 (77 [74-81])*†
After mifepristone alone (0.8)*	40 (5)	12 (2)‡	4
Failure (need for surgical intervention)			
Medical indication for intervention	13 (2)	26 (4)‡	21 (4)‡
Patient's request for intervention	5 (0.6)	13 (2)	
Incomplete abortion	39 (5)	51 (8)‡	12 (2)‡
Ongoing pregnancy	8 (1)	25 (4)*	36 (7)
			46 (9)*§
Total	65 (8)	115 (17)*	115 (23)*†

*p < 0.001 for the comparison with the ≤49-days group.
†p = 0.02 for the comparison with the 50-to-56-days group.
‡0.001 ≤ p < 0.03 for the comparison with the ≤49-days group.
§p < 0.001 for the comparison with the 50-to-56-days group.
From Spitz IM, Bardin CW, Benton L, Robbins A: Early pregnancy termination with mifepristone and misoprostol in the United States. N Engl J Med 338:1243, 1998.

The main disadvantage of medical abortion is prolonged and sometimes heavy uterine bleeding that on occasion can cause anemia and on rare occasion can lead to the need for emergency curettage or even blood transfusion. The mean duration of bleeding after administration of mifepristone is about 12 days when administered alone and 9 days when used with a prostaglandin.

By late 2005, the occurrence of five deaths in the United States and Canada that occurred in otherwise healthy medical abortion patients as a result of infection with an unusual pathogen (but common soil bacterium), *Clostridium sordellii*, shocked the family planning community. In response to these events, the protocol for medical abortion at Planned Parenthood Federation of America (PPFA) was changed. Prior to the switch, PPFA clients received the "evidence-based" protocol (200 mg oral mifepristone followed in 48 hours by 800 mcg of misoprostol dosed vaginally). However, since there had been no reported cases of *C. sordellii* infections in Europe (where medical abortion rates are higher but vaginal administration of misoprostol is uncommon), a link between vaginal administration of misoprostol and *C. sordellii* infection was hypothesized. In response to the deaths, PPFA changed the medical abortion procedure to buccal dosing of misoprostol. The pharmacokinetics of buccal dosing are similar to that for vaginal dosing but with lower gastrointestinal side effects than with oral dosing.

More than 600,000 women had been treated with mifepristone/misoprostol by the time PPFA changed its medical abortion protocol, and the majority of these received misoprostol by the vaginal route. The estimated case-fatality rate for mifepristone abortion (0.8/100,000 procedures) is statistically no different from that of spontaneous abortion (0.7/100,000 miscarriages) and induced abortion (0.7/100,000 procedures). All of these are much lower than the overall risk of death from pregnancy (12.9/100,000 live births). The CDC has continued to investigate reports of toxic shock or death suggestive of *Clostridium* species infection after medical or spontaneous abortion, and the incidence is low.

Because medical abortion does not require instrumentation of the uterine cavity, rates of infection are low. Most serious infections are related to common gynecologic pathogens such as chlamydia. *Clostridium sordellii* is an uncommon cause of infection in humans but can cause toxic shock after pregnancy, injection drug use, trauma, or surgery. A related bacterium, *Clostridium perfringens* can also cause fulminant septic disease in pregnant women after abortion and was a leading cause of death associated with illegal abortion. There have been rare case reports of *C. perfringens* deaths after legal induced abortions, spontaneous abortion, vaginal delivery, cesarean delivery, and amniocentesis. Although approximately 2% to 4% of vaginal cultures reveal *C. perfringens*, the incidence of vaginal carriage of *C. sordellii* is not known. It is likely that both bacteria ascend from colonized vaginal tracts to cause disease after abortion. Because medical abortion typically results in less complete uterine evacuation than suction abortion, colonization may lead to infection.

Even though the absolute risk of death resulting from *C. sordellii* infection is low, avoiding vaginal administration of misoprostol makes sense because buccal administration is well tolerated and provides similar efficacy. Misoprostol suppresses local immunity. Studies using a rat model have demonstrated increased mortality from *C. sordellii* infections with intrauterine

compared with gastric administration of misoprostol. Vaginal administration may be appropriate for some indications (gynecologic procedures) where the potentially lethal combination of retained tissue and *Clostridium* colonization is not a factor.

In addition to abandoning vaginal misoprostol, PPFA health centers provide routine antibiotic treatment (doxycycline 100 mg orally twice daily for 7 days starting the same day as the mifepristone administration) to all medical abortion patients. A large study that tracked outcomes from all PPFA clinics before and after the protocol change determined that the combined approach reduced the number of serious infections (defined as fever accompanied by pelvic pain treated with intravenous antibiotics in an emergency department or inpatient setting) by 93% from 93 to 6 cases in 100,000 medical abortions. Because many more cases of mild uterine infection are treated as an outpatient, the overall significance of this low-cost intervention is impressive. Doxycycline also has in vitro activity against *C. sordellii* and theoretically might prevent an ascending infection from becoming established; the study did not have adequate power to test this association. No cases of *C. sordellii* infection occurred during the study period.

Even clinicians that do not provide abortion care need to be aware of the clinical presentation of *Clostridium* infections during pregnancy and after abortion. Vomiting, diarrhea, and abdominal pain may be the only symptoms before the rapid progress to septic shock seen with *C sordellii* infection. Unfortunately, these are all common symptoms associated with mifepristone and misoprostol. A very high white blood cell count is seen in *C. sordellii* infection. Clinicians should have a high index of suspicion and gather an anaerobic culture of the cervix to aid in diagnosis if they suspect *Clostridium* species infection. The decision to begin intravenous antibiotics and hospitalize a patient may be insufficient to manage a serious infection. *Clostridium* species must have an anaerobic environment to survive and multiply, and the older literature suggested that total hysterectomy or surgical débridement is necessary to remove necrotic tissue and prevent death in cases of *C. perfringens* infection. Early hysterectomy may be life saving. Interestingly, in the only reported case of *C. sordellii* infection after pregnancy where the patient survived, testing at the CDC laboratory indicated that the patient was infected with a strain of *C. sordellii* that did not produce lethal toxin. This patient also did not have a high white blood cell count. Fortunately, no new cases have been reported.

Ancillary Techniques

In the United States, most protocols for both medical and surgical abortion make use of ultrasound to verify gestational age and to confirm that the pregnancy is intrauterine and not ectopic. If a gestational sac is not identified, a serum quantitative β-hCG should be done and the results correlated with the ultrasound findings. Failure to see any evidence of an intrauterine gestation with a serum β-hCG of 1000 mIU or higher is strong evidence for ectopic pregnancy. Increasing numbers of women are seeking surgical or medical abortion at very early gestational ages when diagnosis of intrauterine pregnancy may not be possible. Performing a qualitative pregnancy test 2 weeks later or repeating the ultrasound after the procedure will ensure that the pregnancy has been successfully aborted. In the first trimester, sonography should always be done to determine gestational age when a substantial discrepancy occurs between the menstrual history and clinical examination; when uterine abnormalities, such as leiomyomata, are present; or when the presence of an ectopic gestation is suspected. Sonography should always be performed before initiating second-trimester abortions and has avoided the problem of inaccurate estimation of gestational age, which is an important cause of complications. Performing ultrasonography during a D&E may facilitate the procedure and reduce complications.

Complications

Elective abortion in the United States is a very safe operation. Complications are infrequent, and the overall mortality is less than 1 per 100,000 procedures. Two important determinants of complications are the gestational age and method of abortion chosen. When abortion is performed in pregnancies of 6 weeks' or less gestational age, there are slightly higher complication rates (because of failure to complete the abortion) than when the gestational age is between 7 and 10 weeks. Beyond 10 weeks, abortion complication rates increase progressively with gestational age. Suction curettage is the safest surgical method of abortion, followed by D&E, induction of labor, and major operations.

The most common complication is infection, and the routine use of perioperative antibiotic prophylaxis has been shown to reduce this risk. Other complications include hemorrhage, the consequences of uterine perforation, and anesthetic hazards.

KEY POINTS

- In 2004, there were about 6.4 million pregnancies in the United States. There were 4 million births and about 1.2 million elective abortions. Half of all pregnancies were unintended. About 20% of all pregnancies were electively terminated; the majority of these were unintended at conception.
- Typical and perfect use failure rates in the first year of use range between 5% and 27% for coitus-related methods between 0.3% and 8% for oral contraceptives (OCs) and 0.3% to 3% for the injection. The IUD and implants have typical use failure rates of less than 1%. Contraceptive failure rates increase in inverse relation to the user's age, level of education, and socioeconomic class.
- Most OC formulations in the United States consist of varying dosages of one of the following progestins: estranes: norethindrone, norethindrone acetate, ethynodiol diacetate, or gonanes: norgestrel (or its active isomer, levonorgestrel), desogestrel, norgestimate, or a spironolactone derivative, drospirenone and either of two estrogens, ethinyl estradiol or ethinyl estradiol-3-methyl ether, also called *mestranol*. New formulations containing estradiol or estradiol valerate are in development.
- No significantly increased risk of breast cancer occurs among current or former users of OC or in various high-risk subgroups of OC users. Women with a family history of breast cancer who use OCs do not have an increase risk of developing breast cancer.

- A significantly increased risk of developing myocardial infarction occurs only in current OC users older than age 35 who smoke.
- Users of low-dose OCs do not have a significantly increased risk of developing ischemic or hemorrhagic stroke if they do not smoke or have hypertension.
- The risk of developing endometrial cancer, as well as ovarian cancer, in OC users and former users is only half that in control subjects. OC users also have a 50% reduction in the incidence of benign breast disease.
- Women using injectable DMPA (150 mg every 3 months) intramuscularly or 104 mg subcutaneously have a first-year pregnancy rate of 0.1%.
- The most effective method of emergency contraception available in the United States is ingestion of a single 1.5-mg dose of levonorgestrel taken as soon as possible following an act of unprotected intercourse. Ulipristal acetate, an antiprogestin used in Europe for emergency contraception, is more effective than levonorgestrel.
- The cumulative incidence of accidental pregnancy with the copper T 380A IUD is 1.6% after 7 years of use and 1.7% after 12 years of use. This IUD is approved for 10 years of use.
- After sterilization by tubal interruption, the 1-year failure rate is 0.55 per 100 women, the 5-year failure rate is 1.31 per 100 women, and the 10-year failure rate is 1.85 per 100 women. About one third of the pregnancies are ectopic.

(**REFERENCES CAN BE FOUND ON EXPERTCONSULT.com**)

SUGGESTED READINGS

Andersson K, Odlind V, Rybo G: Levonorgestrel-releasing and copper-releasing (Nova T) IUDs during five years of use: A randomized comparative trial, *Contraception* 49:56, 1994.

Clarkson TB, Shively CA, Morgan TM, et al: Oral contraceptives and coronary artery atherosclerosis of cynomolgus monkeys, *Obstet Gynecol* 75:217, 1990.

Colditz GA: for The Nurses' Health Study Research Group: Oral contraceptive use and mortality during 12 years follow-up: The Nurses' Health Study, *Ann Intern Med* 120:821, 1994.

Collaborative Group on Hormonal Factors in Breast Cancer: Breast cancer and hormonal contraceptives: Collaborative reanalysis of individual data on 53,297 women with breast cancer and 100,239 women without breast cancer from 54 epidemiological studies, *Lancet* 347:1713, 1996.

Cooper JM, Carignan CS, Cher D, et al: Microinsert nonincisional hysteroscopic sterilization, *Obstet Gynecol* 102:59, 2003.

Creasy GW: for the Ortho EVRA/EVRA 004 Study Group: Evaluation of contraceptive efficacy and cycle control of a transdermal contraceptive patch vs an oral contraceptive: a randomized controlled trial, *JAMA* 285:2347, 2001.

Croxatto HB: and the Implanon Study Group: A multicentre efficacy and safety study of the single contraceptive implant implanon, *Hum Reprod* 14:976, 1999.

Doll H, Vessey M, Painter R: Return of fertility in nulliparous women after discontinuation of the intrauterine device: Comparison with women discontinuing other methods of contraception, *Br J Obstet Gynaecol* 108:304, 2001.

El-Rafaey H, Rajasekar D, Abdalla M, et al: Induction of abortion with mifepristone (RU 486) and oral or vaginal misoprostol, *N Engl J Med* 332:983, 1995.

Engel HJ, Engel E, Lichtlen PR: Coronary atherosclerosis and myocardial infarction in young women: Role of oral contraceptives, *Eur Heart J* 4:1, 1983.

Farr G, Gabelnlick H, Sturgen K, et al: Contraceptive efficacy and acceptability of the female condom, *Am J Public Health* 84:1960, 1994.

Gerstman BB, Piper JM, Tomita DK, et al: Oral contraceptive estrogen dose and the risk of deep venous thromboembolic disease, *Am J Epidemiol* 133:132, 1991.

Godsland IF, Crook D, Worthington M, et al: Effects of a low-estrogen, desogestrel-containing oral contraceptive on lipid and carbohydrate metabolism, *Contraception* 48:217, 1993.

La Vecchia C: Oral contraceptives and ovarian cancer: An update, 1998-2004, *Eur J Cancer Prev* 15 (2):117, 2006.

Marchbanks PA, McDonald JA, Wilson HG, et al: Oral contraceptives and the risk of breast cancer, *N Engl J Med* 346:2025, 2002.

Milson I, Anderson K, Jonasson K, et al: The influence of the Gyne-T 380A IUD on menstrual blood loss and iron status, *Contraception* 52:175, 1995a.

Mosher WD, Jones J: Use of Contraception in the United States: 1982-2008, *Vital Health Stat 23* (29):18, May, 2010.

Peterson HB, Xia Z, Hughes JM, et al: The risk of pregnancy after tubal sterilization: Findings from the U.S. Collaborative Review of Sterilization, *Am J Obstet Gynecol* 174:1161, 1996.

Schaff EA, Fielding SL, Westhoff C, et al: Vaginal misoprostol administered 1, 2 or 3 days after mifepristone for early medical abortion: A randomized trial, *JAMA* 284:1948, 2000.

Schwartz SM, Petitti DB, Siscovick DS, et al: Stroke and use of low-dose oral contraceptives in young women: A pooled analysis of two US studies, *Stroke* 29:2277, 1998.

Sidney S, Siscovick DS, Petitti DB, et al: Myocardial infarction and use of low-dose oral contraceptives: A pooled analysis of two US studies, *Circulation* 98:1, 1998.

Smith JS, Green J, Berrington de Gonzalez A, et al: Cervical cancer and use of hormonal contraceptives: A systematic review, *Lancet* 361:1159, 2003.

Sulak PJ, Kuehl TJ, Ortiz M, et al: Acceptance of altering the standard 21-day/7-day oral contraceptive regimen to delay menses and reduce hormone withdrawal symptoms, *Am J Obstet Gynecol* 186:1142, 2002.

Walsh T: for the IUD Study Group: Randomised controlled trial of prophylactic antibiotics before insertion of intrauterine devices, *Lancet* 351:1005, 1998.

Vessey M, Yeates D, Flynn S: Factors affecting mortality in a large cohort study with special reference to oral contraceptive use, *Contraception* 82 (3):221–229, 2010.

14

Menopause and Care of the Mature Woman
Endocrinology, Consequences of Estrogen Deficiency, Effects of Hormone Replacement Therapy, and Treatment Regimens

Roger A. Lobo

Menopause is defined by the last menstrual period. Because cessation of menses is variable and many of the symptoms thought to be related to menopause may occur prior to cessation of menses, there is seldom a precise timing of this event. Other terms used are *perimenopause,* which refers to a variable time beginning a few years before and continuing after the event of menopause, and **climacteric**, which merely refers to the time after the cessation of reproductive function. Although the terms *menopausal* and *postmenopausal* are used interchangeably, the former term is less correct because *menopausal* should only relate to the time around the cessation of menses. As life expectancy increases beyond the eighth decade worldwide, particularly in developed countries, an increasing proportion of the female population is postmenopausal. With the average age of menopause being at 51 years, more than a third of a woman's life is now spent after menopause. Here, symptoms and signs of estrogen deficiency merge with issues encountered with natural aging. As the world population increases and a larger proportion of this population is made up of individuals older than 50, medical care specifically directed at postmenopausal women becomes an important aspect of modern medicine. Between the years 2000 and 2005, the world population older than 60 years is expected to double, from 590 million to 1 billion. In the United States, the number of women entering menopause will almost double in the 30 years between 1990 and 2020 (**Table 14-1**). Age of menopause, which is a genetically programmed event, is subject to some variability. The age of menopause in Western countries (between 51 and 52 years) is thought to correlate with general health status; socioeconomic status is associated with an earlier age of menopause. Higher parity, on the other hand, has been found to be associated with a later menopause. Smoking has consistently been found to be associated with menopause onset taking place 1 to 2 years earlier. Although body mass has been thought to be related to age of menopause (greater body mass index [BMI] with later menopause), the data have not been consistent. However, physical or athletic activity has not been found to influence the age of menopause. There also appear to be ethnic differences in the onset of menopause. In the United States, black and Hispanic women have been found to have menopause approximately 2 years earlier than white women. Although parity is generally greater around the world than in the United States, the age of menopause appears to be somewhat earlier outside the United States. Malay women have menopause at approximately age 45, Thai women at age 49.5, and Filipina women between ages 47 and 48. Countries at higher altitude (Himalayas or Andes) have been shown to have menopause 1 to 1.5 years earlier. Because the average age of menopause in the United States is 51 to 53 years, with an age distribution weighted toward white women, menopause prior to age 40 is considered premature. Conversely, by age 58, 97% of women will have gone through menopause. The primary determinate of age of menopause is genetic. Based on family studies, de Bruin and colleagues showed that heritability for age of menopause averaged 0.87, suggesting that genetics explains up to 87% of the variance in menopausal age. Although other estimates have not been this high, genetic programming remains extremely important.

Other than gene mutations that cause **premature ovarian failure** (explained later in this chapter), no specific genes have been discovered to date that account for this genetic influence. However, several genes are likely involved in aging, including genes coding telomerase activity.

PREMATURE OVARIAN FAILURE INSUFFICIENCY

Premature ovarian failure (POI) or premature ovarian insufficiency (POI), which is the more recently used term, is defined as hypergonadotropic ovarian failure occurring prior to age 40. POI has occurred in 5% to 10% of women who are evaluated for amenorrhea, thus the incidence varies according to the prevalence of amenorrhea in various populations. Estimates of the overall prevalence of POI in the general population range between 0.3% and 0.9% of women. Throughout life, there is an ongoing rate of atresia of oocytes. Because this process is accelerated with various forms of gonadal dysgenesis because of defective X chromosomes, one possible cause of POI is an increased rate of atresia that has yet to be explained. A decreased germ cell endowment or an increased rate of germ cell destruction can also explain POI. Nevertheless, about 1000 (of the original 2 million) primarily follicles may remain. While most of these oocytes are likely to be functionally deficient, occasionally spontaneous

Table 14-1 U.S. Population Entering the Postmenopausal Years, Ages 55 through 64

Year	Population
1990	10.8 million
2000	12.1 million
2010	17.1 million
2020	19.3 million

Adapted from U.S. Bureau of the Census: Current Population Reports: Projections of the Population of the United States 1977 to 2050. Washington, DC, U.S. Government Printing Office, 1993.

Table 14-2 Possible Causes of Premature Ovarian Failure

Genetic
Enzymatic
Immune
Gonadotropin defects
Ovarian insults
Idiopathic

pregnancies occur in young women in the first few years after the diagnosis of POI. There are several possible etiologies of POI (**Table 14-2**).

Defects in the X chromosome may result in various types of gonadal dysgenesis with varied times of expression of ovarian failure. Even patients with classical gonadal dysgenesis (e.g., 45,XO) may undergo a normal puberty, and occasionally a pregnancy may ensue as a result of genetic mosaicism. Very small defects in the X chromosome may be sufficient to cause POI. Familial forms of POI may be related to either autosomal-dominant or sex-linked modes of inheritance. Mutations in the gene encoding the follicle-stimulating hormone (FSH) receptor (e.g., mutation in exon 7 in the gene on chromosome 2p) have been described, but these are extremely rare outside of the Finnish population in which these mutations were originally described. An expansion of a trinucleotide repeat sequence in the first exon on the FMR1 gene (Xq 27.3) leads to fragile X syndrome, a major cause of developmental disabilities in males.

The permutation in fragile X syndrome has been shown to be associated with POI. Type 1 blepharophimosis/ptosis/epicanthus inversus (BPES) syndrome, an autosomal dominant disorder caused by mutations in the forkhead transcription factor FOXL2, includes POI. Triple X syndrome has also been associated with POI. Dystrophic myotonia has also been linked to POI, although the mechanism underlying this relationship is unclear. Under the category of enzymatic defects, galactosemia is a major cause of POI that is related to the toxic buildup of galactose in women who are unable to metabolize the sugar. Even in women with fairly well controlled galactose-free diets, POI tends to occur. Another enzymatic defect linked to POI is 17α-hydroxylase deficiency. This rare condition manifests differently from the other causes discussed here because the defect in the production of sex steroids leads to sexual infantilism and hypertension.

The degree to which autoimmunity may be responsible for POI is unclear but has been suggested to be associated in 17.5% of cases. Virtually all autoimmune disorders have been found to be associated with POI, including autoimmune polyendocrinopathies like autoimmune polyendocrinopathy/candidiasis/ectodermal dystrophy (APECED), which is caused by mutations in the autoimmune (AIRE) gene on band 21 q22. The presence of the thymus gland appears to be required for normal ovarian function as POI has been associated with hypoplasia of the thymus. In patients who have undergone ovarian biopsy as part of their evaluation, lymphocytic infiltration surrounding follicles has been described, as well as resumption of menses after immunosuppression. Immunoassays utilizing antibodies directed at ovarian antigens have been developed and have demonstrated positive findings in some patients with POI, although the relevance of these findings remains unsettled. Ovarian autoantibodies could also conceivably be a secondary phenomenon to a primary cell-mediated form of immunity. Specific enzymes such as 3β-hydroxysteroid dehydrogenase (3βHSD) may also be the target of ovarian autoimmunity.

From a practical standpoint, screening for the common autoimmune disorders is appropriate in women found to have POI. More from a theoretic standpoint, abnormalities in the structure of gonadotropins, in their receptors, or in receptor binding could be associated with POI. Although abnormal urinary forms of gonadotropins have been reported in women with POI, these data have not been replicated. Abnormalities of FSH receptor binding, as mediated by a serum inhibitor, have been described. A genetic defect that may lead to alterations in FSH receptor structure was mentioned previously. Under the category of ovarian insults, POI may be induced by ionizing radiation, chemotherapy, or overly aggressive ovarian surgery. Although not well documented, viral infections have been suggested to play a role, particularly mumps. A dose of 400 to 500 rads is known to cause ovarian failure 50% of the time, and older women are more vulnerable to experiencing permanent failure. A dose of approximately 800 rads is associated with failure in all women. Ovarian failure (transient or permanent) may be induced by chemotherapeutic agents, although younger women receiving this insult have a better prognosis. Alkalizing agents, particularly cyclophosphamide, appear to be most toxic. By exclusion, the majority of women are considered to have idiopathic POI because no demonstrable cause can be pinpointed. Among these women, small mutations in genes lying on the X chromosome or yet to be identified autosomal genes may be the cause.

MANAGEMENT OF PREMATURE OVARIAN INSUFFICIENCY

Evaluation of POI in women younger than 30 should include screening for autoimmune disorders and a karyotype; detailed recommendations for screening of such women are available. In addition, vaginal ultrasound may be useful for assessing the size of the ovaries and the degree of follicular development, which, if present, may signify an immunologic defect. Cases of POI caused by immunologic defects need to be screened carefully for thyroid, adrenal, and other autoimmune disorders. Treatment of all cases usually consists of estrogen replacement. If fertility is a concern, the most efficacious treatment is oocyte donation. Various attempts at ovarian stimulation are usually unsuccessful, and the sporadic pregnancies that may occur are just as likely to occur spontaneously as with any intervention. A spontaneous pregnancy rate as high as 5% has been suggested.

THE MENOPAUSAL TRANSITION (PERIMENOPAUSE)

A workshop was convened in 2001 to build consensus on describing various stages of the menopausal transition. As depicted in **Figure 14-1**, the menopausal transition (perimenopause) is divided into early and late phases according to menstrual acyclicity. These changes signify a varying period of time (years) during which rapid oocyte depletion occurs, followed by hypoestrogenism. The ovary changes markedly from birth to the onset of menopause (**Fig. 14-2**). The greatest number of primordial follicles is present in utero at 20 weeks' gestation and undergoes a regular rate of atresia until around the age of 37. After this time, the decline in primordial follicles appears to become more rapid between age 38 and menopause (**Fig. 14-3**) when no more than a thousand follicles remain. These remaining follicles are primarily atretic in nature.

TYPES OF OVARIAN CHANGES

Although perimenopausal changes are generally thought to be endocrine in nature and result in menstrual changes, a marked diminution of reproductive capacity precedes this period by several years. This decline may be referred to as gametogenic ovarian failure. The concept of dissociation in ovarian function is appropriate. Gametogenic failure is signified by reduced early follicular phase inhibin secretion, rising serum FSH levels, and a marked reduction in fecundity. These changes may occur with normal menstrual function and no obvious endocrine deficiency; however, they may occur in some women as early as age 35 (10 or more years before endocrine deficiency ensues). Although subtle changes in endocrine and menstrual function can occur for up to 3 years before menopause, it has been shown that the major reduction in ovarian estrogen production does not occur until approximately 6 months before menopause (**Fig. 14-4**). There is also a very slow decline in androgen status

(i.e., androstenedione and testosterone), which cannot be adequately detected at the time of the perimenopause. The decline in androgen is largely a phenomenon of aging. Products of the granulosa cell are most important for the feedback control of FSH. As the functional capacity of the follicular units decreases, the secretion of substances that suppress FSH also decreases. Most notably, inhibin B levels are lower in the early follicular phase in women in their late 30s (**Fig. 14-5**). Indeed, FSH levels are higher throughout the cycle in older ovulatory women than in younger women (**Fig. 14-6**). The functional capacity of the ovary is also diminished as women enter into perimenopause. With gonadotropin stimulation, although estradiol (E_2) levels are not very different between younger and older women, total inhibin production by granulosa cells is decreased in women older than 35. From a clinical perspective, subtle increases in FSH on day 3 of the cycle, or increases in the clomiphene challenge test, correlate with decreased ovarian responses to stimulation and decreased fecundability. An excellent marker of ovarian reserve is Müllerian inhibiting substance (MIS) or anti-Müllerian hormone (AMH). Levels decrease throughout life, being undetectable at menopause. Low levels do not vary during the cycle, and when values reach an undetectable range (<0.05 ng/mL), menopause has been found to occur within 5 years (**Fig. 14-7**).

Although there is a general decline in oocyte number with age, an accelerated atresia occurs around age 37 or 38 (see **Fig. 14-3**). Although the reason for this acceleration is not clear, one possible theory relates to activin secretion. Because granulosa cell-derived activin is important for stimulating FSH receptor expression, the rise in FSH levels could result in more activin production, which in turn enhances FSH action. A profile of elevated activin with lower inhibin B has been found in older women (**Fig. 14-8**). This autocrine action of activin, involving enhanced FSH action, might be expected to lead to accelerated growth and differentiation of granulosa cells. Furthermore, activin has been shown to increase the size of the pool of preantral follicles in the rat. At the same time, these follicles become more

Figure 14-1 The Stages of Reproductive Aging Workshop (STRAW) staging system. (Reprinted from Soules MR, Sherman S, Parrott E, et al: Executive summary: Stages of Reproductive Aging Workshop [STRAW]. Fertil Steril 76:874, 2001. Copyright 2001, with permission from The American Society for Reproductive Medicine.)

Stages:	−5	−4	−3	−2	−1	0	+1	+2
Terminology:	Reproductive			Menopausal Transition			Postmenopause	
	Early	Peak	Late	Early	Late*		Early*	Late
				Perimenopause				
Duration of stage:	Variable			Variable		ⓐ 1 yr	ⓑ 4 yrs	Until demise
Menstrual cycles:	Variable to regular	Regular		Variable cycle length (> 7 days different from normal)	≥2 skipped cycles and an interval of amenorrhea (≥60 days)	Amen ? 12 mos	None	
Endocrine:	normal FSH		↑FSH	↑FSH			↑FSH	

Final Menstrual Period (FMP) — at Stage 0

*Stages most likely to be characterized by vasomotor symptoms   ↑ = elevated

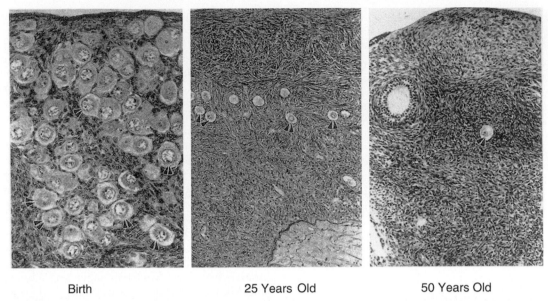

Birth   25 Years Old   50 Years Old

Figure 14-2 Photomicrographs of the cortex of human ovaries from birth to 50 years of age. Small nongrowing primordial follicles *(arrowheads)* have a single layer of squamous granulosa cells. (Adapted from Erickson GF: An analysis of follicle development and ovum maturation. Semin Reprod Endocrinol 4:233, 1986.)

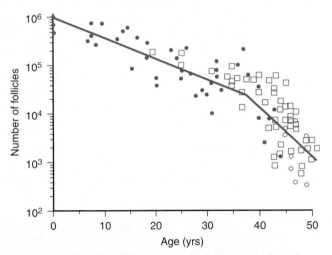

Figure 14-3 The age-related decrease in the total number of primordial follicles (PF) within both human ovaries from birth to menopause. As a result of recruitment (initiation of PF growth), the number of PF decreases progressively from about 1 million at birth to 25,000 at 37 years. At 37 years, the rate of recruitment increases sharply, and the number of PF declines to 1000 at menopause (about 51 years of age). (Adapted from Faddy MJ, Gosden RJ, Gougeon A, et al: Accelerated disappearance of ovarian follicles in mid-life: Implications for forecasting menopause. Hum Reprod 7:1342, 1992.)

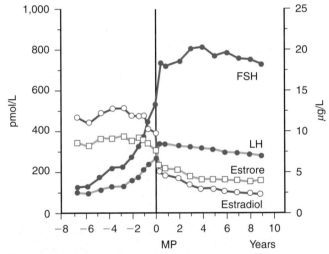

Figure 14-4 Mean serum levels of follicle-stimulating hormone, luteinizing hormone, estradiol, and estrone, showing the **perimenopausal transition**. MP, menopause. (Adapted from Rannevik G, Jeppsson S, Johnell O, et al: A longitudinal study of the perimenopausal transition: Altered profiles of steroid and pituitary hormones-SHBG and bone mineral density. Maturitas 21:103, 1995.)

atretic. Clinical treatment of women in the perimenopause should address three general areas of concern: (1) irregular bleeding, (2) symptoms of early menopause, such as **hot flushes**, and (3) the inability to conceive. Treatment of irregular bleeding is complicated by the fluctuating hormonal status. Estrogen levels may be higher than normal in the early follicular phase and progesterone secretion may be normal, or slightly decreased, although not all cycles are ovulatory. For these reasons, short-term use of an oral contraceptive (usually 20 mcg ethinyl estradiol)

may be an option for otherwise healthy women who do not smoke to help them cope with irregular bleeding. Early symptoms of menopause, particularly vasomotor changes, may occur as the result of fluctuating hormonal levels. In this setting, an oral contraceptive again may be an option if symptoms warrant therapy. Alternatively, lower doses of estrogen used alone may be another option. Reproductive concerns often require more aggressive treatment because of decreased cycle fecundity. Once day 3 FSH levels increase (>15 mIU/mL) and AMH levels decrease (≤0.4 ng/mL), the prognosis for pregnancy is markedly reduced.

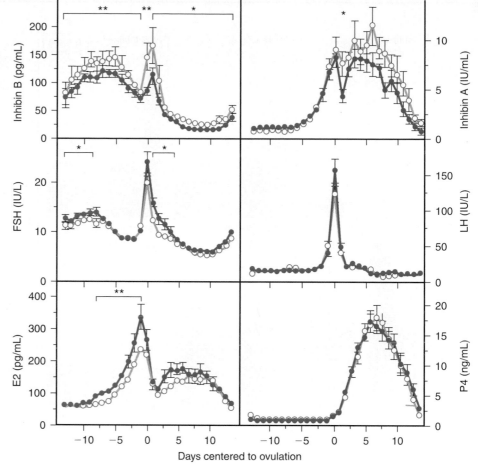

Figure 14-5 An inhibin B, follicle-stimulating hormone (FSH), estradiol (E₂), inhibin A, and progesterone (P₄) levels in cycling women 20 to 34 years old (○) and 35 to 46 years old (●). Hormone levels are depicted as centered to the day of ovulation (*, $p < 0.04$; **, $p < 0.02$) when comparing the two age groups. (Adapted from Welt CK, McNicholl DJ, Taylor AE, Hall JE: Female reproductive aging is marked by decreased secretion of dimeric inhibin. J Clin Endocrinol Metab 84:105, 1999.)

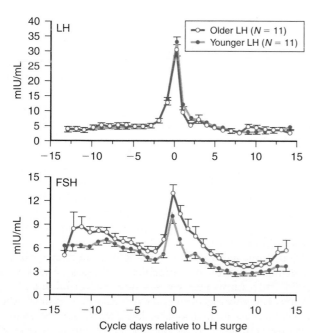

Figure 14-6 The daily serum follicle-stimulating hormone (FSH) and luteinizing hormone (LH) levels throughout the menstrual cycle of 11 women in each group (mean ± SE). The gonadotropin secretion pattern in normal women of advanced reproductive age in relation to the monotropic FSH rise. (Adapted from Klein NA, Battaglia DE, Clifton DK, et al: The gonadotropin secretion pattern in normal women of advanced reproductive age in relation to the monotropic FSH rise. J Soc Gynecol Investig 3:27, 1996.)

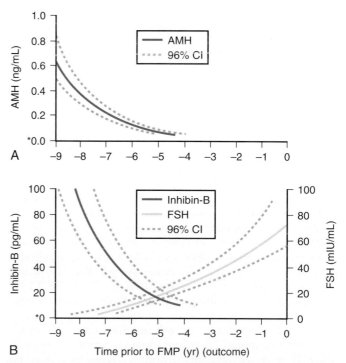

Figure 14-7 AMH decreases to undetectable levels (0.05 ng/mL) 5 years before the final menstrual period, and inhibin B (10 pg/mL) does so 4 years before the last menstrual period. (From Sowers MR. Eyvazzadeth AD, McConnell D, et al: Anti-mullerian hormone and inhibin in the definition of ovarian aging and the menopause transition. J Clin Endocrinol Metab 93[9]:L34768-83, 2008.)

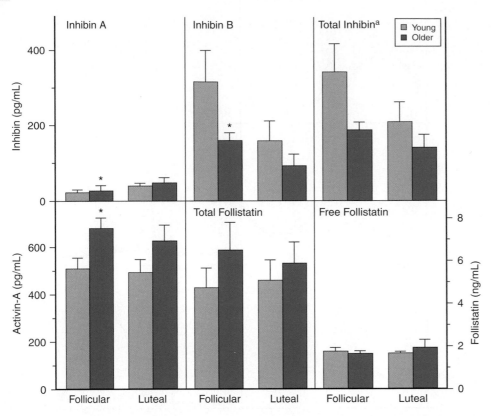

Figure 14-8 Mean concentrations of gonadal proteins from the same subjects. Total inhibin is a derived number from the sum of inhibin A and inhibin B. *Group differences; $p < 0.05$. Net increase in stimulatory input resulting from a decrease in inhibin B and an increase in activin A may contribute in part to the rise in follicular phase follicle-stimulating hormone of aging cyclic women. (Adapted from Reame NE, Wyman TL, Phillips DJ, et al: Net increase in stimulatory input resulting from a decrease in inhibin B and an increase in activin A may contribute in part to the rise in follicular phase follicle-stimulating hormone of aging cyclic women. J Clin Endocrinol Metab 83:3302, 1998.)

HORMONAL CHANGES WITH ESTABLISHED MENOPAUSE

Figure 14-9 depicts the typical hormonal levels of postmenopausal women compared with those of ovulatory women in the early follicular phase. The most significant findings are the marked reductions in E_2 and estrone (E_1). Serum E_2 is reduced to a greater extent than E_1. Serum E_1, on the other hand, is produced primarily by peripheral aromatization from androgens, which decline principally as a function of age. Levels of E_2 average 15 pg/mL and range from 10 to 25 pg/mL but are closer to 10 pg/mL in women who have undergone oophorectomy. Serum E_1 values average 30 pg/mL but may be higher in obese women because aromatization increases as a function of the mass of adipose tissue. Estrone sulfate ($E_1 S$) is an estrogen conjugate that serves as a stable circulating reservoir of estrogen, and levels of $E_1 S$ are the highest among estrogens in postmenopausal women. In premenopausal women, values are usually above 1000 pg/mL; in postmenopausal women, levels average 350 pg/mL. Apart from elevations in FSH and luteinizing hormone (LH), other pituitary hormones are not affected. The rise in FSH, beginning in stage +3 as early as age 38 (see **Fig. 14-1**), fluctuates considerably until approximately 4 years after menopause (stage +1) when values are consistently greater than 20 mIU/mL. Specifically, growth hormone (GH), thyroid-stimulating hormone (TSH), and adrenocorticotropic hormone (ACTH) levels are normal. Serum prolactin levels may be slightly decreased because prolactin levels are influenced by estrogen status. Both the postmenopausal ovary and the adrenal gland continue to produce androgen. The ovary continues to produce androstenedione and testosterone but not E_2, and this production has been shown to be at least partially dependent on LH. Androstenedione and testosterone levels are lower in women who have experienced bilateral oophorectomy, with values averaging 0.8 ng/mL and 0.1 ng/mL, respectively. The adrenal gland also continues to produce androstenedione, dehydroepiandrosterone (DHEA), and dehydroepiandrosterone sulfate (DHEA-S); primarily as a function of aging, these values decrease somewhat (adrenopause), although cortisol secretion remains unaffected. Recent data by Couzinet suggest that much "ovarian" testosterone production may actually arise from the adrenal. Most likely, this production is by indirect mechanisms caused by the adrenal supplying precursor substrate (DHEA and androstenedione). Although DHEA-S levels decrease with age (approximately 2% per year), recent data have suggested that levels transiently rise in the perimenopause before the continuous decline thereafter (see **Fig. 14-9**). This interesting finding from the Study of Women Across the Nation (SWAN) also suggested that DHEA-S levels are highest in Chinese women and lowest in black women.

Testosterone levels also decline as a function of age, which is best demonstrated by the reduction in 24-hour means levels (**Fig. 14-10**). Because of the role of the adrenal in determining levels of testosterone after menopause, adrenalectomy or dexamethasone treatment results in undetectable levels of serum testosterone. Compared with total testosterone, the measurement of bioavailable, or "free," testosterone is more useful in postmenopausal women. After menopause, sex hormone-binding globulin (SHBG) levels decrease, resulting in relatively higher levels of bioavailable testosterone or a higher free androgen index (**Fig. 14-11**). In women receiving oral estrogen, bioavailable testosterone levels are extremely low because SHBG levels are increased. How this

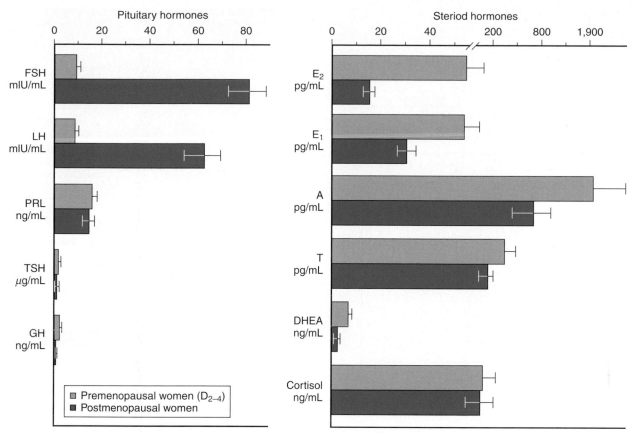

Figure 14-9 Circulating levels of pituitary and steroid hormones in postmenopausal women compared with levels in premenopausal women studied during the first week (days 2 to 4 [D$_{2-4}$] of the menstrual cycle. A, androstenedione; DHEA, dehydroepiandrosterone; E$_1$, estrogen; E$_2$, estradiol; FSH, follicle-stimulating hormone; GH, growth hormone; LH, luteinizing hormone; PRL, prolactin; T, testosterone; TSH, thyroid-stimulating hormone. (Adapted from Yen SSC: The biology of menopause. J Reprod Med 18:287, 1977.)

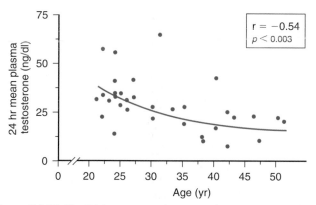

Figure 14-10 The 24-hour mean plasma total testosterone (T) level compared with age in normal women. The regression equation was T (nmol/L) = 37.8 × age (years)−1.12 ($r = -0.54$; $p < 0.003$). (Adapted from Zumoff B, Strain GW, Miller LK, et al: Twenty-four hour mean plasma testosterone concentration declines with age in normal premenopausal women. J Clin Endocrinol Metab 80:1429, 1995.)

relates to the decision to consider androgen therapy in postmenopausal women will be discussed later in this chapter.

Elevated gonadotropin (FSH/LH) levels arise from reduced secretion of E$_2$ and inhibin as described earlier. Although some aging effects of the brain are likely to exist, there is abundant human evidence for menopause in women to be an ovarian-induced event.

EFFECTS OF MENOPAUSE ON VARIOUS ORGAN SYSTEMS

CENTRAL NERVOUS SYSTEM

The brain is an active site for estrogen action as well as estrogen formation. Estrogen activity in the brain is mediated via estrogen receptor (ER) α and ER β. Whether or not a novel membrane receptor (non-ER α/ER β) exists is still being debated. However, both genomic and nongenomic mechanisms of estrogen action clearly exist in the brain. **Figure 14-12** illustrates the predominance of ER β in the cortex (frontal and parietal) and the cerebellum, based on work in the rat. Although 17β E$_2$ is a specific ligand for both receptors, certain synthetic estrogens (e.g., diethylstilbestrol) have greater affinity for ER α, whereas phytoestrogens have a greater affinity for ER β.

There are multiple actions of estrogen on the brain as reviewed by Henderson (**Table 14-3**), thus some important functions linked to estrogen contribute to well-being in general and, more specifically, to cognition and mood. The hallmark feature of declining estrogen status in the brain is the hot flush, which is more generically referred to as a vasomotor episode. The hot flash usually refers to the acute sensation of heat, and the flush or vasomotor episode includes changes in the early perception of this event and other skin changes (including diaphoresis).

Hot flushes usually occur for 2 years after the onset of estrogen deficiency but can persist for 10 or more years. In 10% to

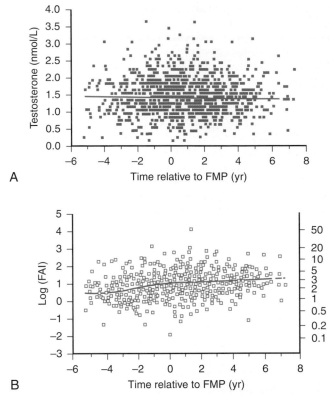

A

B

Figure 14-11 A, Linear regression model: observed testosterone (T) and fitted levels of mean T across the menopausal transition. **B,** Double logistic model: observed free androgen index (FAI) and fitted levels of mean FAI across the menopausal transition. The left and right axes show FAI levels on the log and antilog scales, respectively. The horizontal axis represents time (years) with respect to first menstrual period (FMP); negative (positive) numbers indicate time before (after) FMP. (From Burger HG, Dudley EC, Cui J, et al: A prospective longitudinal study of serum testosterone, dehydroepiandrosterone sulfate, and sex hormone–binding globulin levels through the menopause transition. J Clin Endocrinol Metab 85:2832, 2000.)

15% of women, these symptoms are severe and disabling. In the United States the incidence of these episodes varies in different ethnic groups. Symptoms are greatest in Hispanic and black women, intermediate in white women, and lowest among Asian women (**Fig. 14-13**). The severity of hot flushes decreases with time, but it is known that in some women they may be bothersome for 10 or more years as shown by Oldenhave. As modulated by severity, hot flushes may cause a series of "irregular" symptoms, such as irritability, which may affect quality of life (**Fig. 14-14**). The fall in estrogen levels precipitate the vasomotor symptoms. It has been found that some women who experience hot flushes have a thermoregulatory disruption with a much narrower temperature range between sweating and shivering. Although the proximate cause of the flush remains elusive, the episodes result from a hypothalamic response (probably mediated by catecholamines) to the change in estrogen status. The flush has been well characterized physiologically. It results in heat dissipation as witnessed by an increase in peripheral temperature (fingers, toes); a decrease in skin resistance, associated with diaphoresis; and a reduction in core body temperature (**Fig. 14-15**). There are hormonal correlates of flush activity, such as an increase in serum LH and in plasma levels of pro-opiomelanocortin

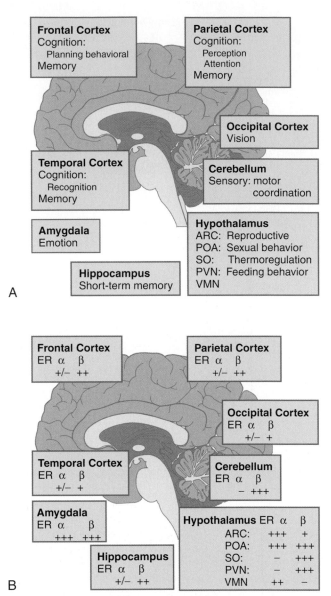

A

B

Figure 14-12 A, Each region of the brain has an important role in specific brain functions. Optimal brain activity is maintained by means of the integration of different areas by neural tracts. ARC, arcuate nucleus; POA, preoptic area; PVN, paraventricular nucleus; SO, supraoptic nucleus; VMN, ventromedial nucleus. **B,** Distribution of estrogen receptors ER α and ER β mRNA in the rat brain. (**B,** adapted from Cela V, Naftolin F: Clinical effects of sex steroids on the brain. In Lobo RA [ed]: The Treatment of the Post-menopausal Woman: Basic and Clinical Aspects, 2nd ed. Philadelphia, Lippincott Williams & Wilkins, 1999, pp 247-262.)

peptides (ACTH, β-endorphin) at the time of the flush, but these occurrences are thought to be epiphenomena that result as a consequence of the flush and are not related to its cause. Freedman has shown that the difference in temperature at which shivering occurs, and when sweating occurs, termed the thermoneutral zone, is wide in asymptomatic women. This zone is substantially more narrowed in symptomatic women, explaining their vulnerability to vasomotor symptoms (**Fig. 14-16**).

One of the primary complaints of women with hot flushes is sleep disruption. They may awaken several times during the night and require a change of bedding and clothes because of

Table 14-3 Effects of Estrogen on Brain Function

Organizational Actions
Effects on neuronal number, morphology, and connections occurring during critical stages of development

Neurotrophic Actions
Neuronal differentiation
Neurite extension
Synapse formation
Interactions with neurotrophins

Neuroprotective Actions
Protection against apoptosis
Antioxidant properties
Antiinflammatory properties
Augmentation of cerebral blood flow
Enhancement of glucose transport into the brain
Blunting of corticosteroid response to behavioral stress
Interactions with neurotrophins

Effects on Neurotransmitters
Acetylcholine
Noradrenaline
Serotonin
Dopamine
Glutamate
Gamma aminobutyric acid
Neuropeptides

Effects on Glial Cells

Effects on Proteins Involved in Alzheimer's Disease
Amyloid precursor protein
Tau protein
Apolipoprotein E

Adapted from Henderson VW: Estrogen, cognition, and a woman's risk of Alzheimer's disease. Am J Med 103(Suppl 3A):11, 1997.

diaphoresis. Nocturnal sleep disruption in postmenopausal women with hot flushes has been well documented by electroencephalographic (EEG) recordings. Sleep efficiency is lower, and the latency to rapid eye movement (REM) sleep is longer in women with hot flushes compared with asymptomatic women. This disturbed sleep often leads to fatigue and irritability during the day. The frequency of awakenings and hot flushes is reduced appreciably with estrogen treatment (**Fig. 14-17**). Sleep may be disrupted even if the woman is not conscious of being awakened from sleep. In this setting, EEG monitoring has indicated sleep disruption in concert with physiologic measures of vasomotor episodes.

In postmenopausal women, estrogen has been found to improve depressed mood regardless of whether or not this is a specific complaint (critics of some of this work point out that mood is affected by the symptomatology and by sleep deprivation). Blinded studies carried out in asymptomatic women have also shown benefit. In an estrogen-deficient state such as occurs after the menopause, a higher incidence of depression (clinical or subclinical) is often manifest. However, menopause per se does not cause depression, and although estrogen does generally improve depressive mood, it should not be used for psychiatric disorders. Nevertheless, very high pharmacologic doses of estrogen have been used to treat certain types of psychiatric depression in the past. Progestogens as a class generally attenuate the beneficial effects of estrogen on mood, although this effect is highly variable.

Cognitive decline in postmenopausal women is related to aging as well as to estrogen deficiency. The literature is somewhat mixed about whether there are benefits of estrogen in terms of cognition. In more recent studies, verbal memory appears to be enhanced with estrogen and has been found to correlate with acute changes in brain imaging, signifying brain activation. Dementia increases as women age, and the most common form of dementia is Alzheimer's disease (AD). **Table 14-3** lists several neurotropic and neuroprotective factors related to how estrogen deficiency may be expected to result in the loss of protection against the development of AD. In addition, estrogen has a positive role in enhancing neurotransmitter function, which is deficient in women with AD. This function of estrogen has particular importance and relevance for the cholinergic system that is affected in AD. Estrogen use after menopause appears to decrease the likelihood of developing or delaying the onset of AD according to several observational studies and meta-analyses. However, once a woman is affected by AD, estrogen is unlikely to provide any benefit. Data from the Women's Health Initiative (WHI), however, suggested a lack of benefit of estrogen or estrogen/progestogen, or even a worsening of cognition in women initiating hormonal therapy after age 65. This suggests that timing of initiation of hormone therapy is critical, and this has also been supported by basic science studies. Here the early exposure to estrogen decreased the possibility of brain damage from free radicals and also promoted maintenance of neuronal and synaptic activity. Unpublished data from WHI also showed

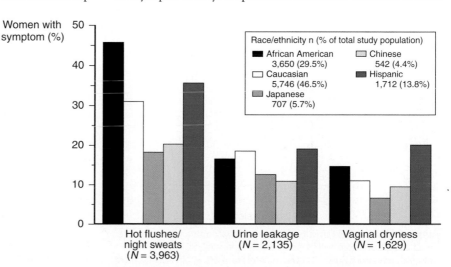

Figure 14-13 A Study of Women's Health Across the Nation (SWAN). Symptom severity. (Adapted from Gold EB, Sternfeld B, Kelsey JL, et al: Relation of demographic and lifestyle factors to symptoms in a multi-racial/ethnic population of women 40 to 55 years of age. Am J Epidemiol 152:463, 2000.)

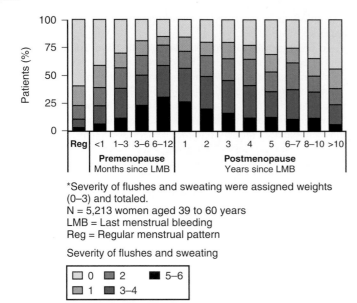

*Severity of flushes and sweating were assigned weights (0–3) and totaled.
N = 5,213 women aged 39 to 60 years
LMB = Last menstrual bleeding
Reg = Regular menstrual pattern

Severity of flushes and sweating

☐ 0	▨ 2	■ 5–6
▨ 1	▨ 3–4	

Figure 14-14 Impact of menopause on well-being. (Adapted from Oldenhave A, Jaszmann LJ, Haspels AA, et al: Am J Obstet Gynecol 168:772, 1993.)

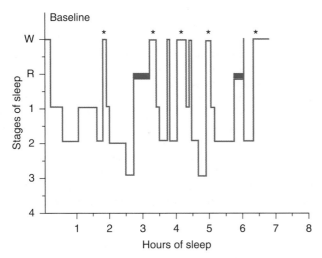

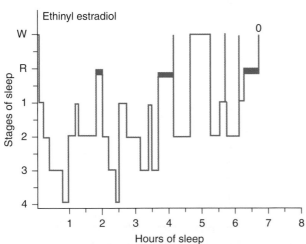

Figure 14-15 Sleep grams measured in symptomatic patient before and after 30 days' administration of ethinyl estradiol, 50 mcg four times daily. (Adapted from Erlik Y, Tataryn IV, Meldrum DR, et al: Association of waking episodes with menopausal hot flushes. JAMA 245:1741, 1981.)

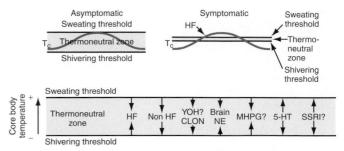

Figure 14-16 Narrowing of the thermoregulatory zone in symptomatic women. HF, hot flush (Data from Freedman RR: Menopausal hot flashes. In Lobo RA[ed]: Treatment of the Postmenopausal Woman, 4th ed., New York, Academic Press, 2007, pp 187-198.)

that prior users of estrogen before entering the WHI trial had less dementia at baseline in the memory study. In summary, while early treatment in younger women at the onset of menopause may be beneficial, (although not proved yet), later treatment (e.g., after age 65) has no benefit and may even be detrimental.

COLLAGEN AND OTHER TISSUES

Estrogen has a positive effect on collagen, which is an important component of bone and skin and serves as a major support tissue for the structures of the pelvis and urinary system. Both estrogen and androgen receptors have been identified in skin fibroblasts. Nearly 30% of skin collagen is lost within the first 5 years after menopause, and collagen decreases approximately 2% per year for the first 10 years after menopause. This statistic, which is similar to that of bone loss after menopause, strongly suggests a link between skin thickness, bone loss, and the risk of **osteoporosis**. Although the literature is not entirely consistent, estrogen therapy generally improves collagen content after menopause and improves skin thickness substantially after about 2 years of treatment. There is a possible bimodal effect with high doses of estrogen causing a reduction in skin thickness. The supportive effect of estrogen on collagen has important implications for bone homeostasis and for the pelvis after menopause. Here, reductions in collagen support and atrophy of the vaginal and urethral mucosa have been implicated in a variety of symptoms, including prolapse and urinary symptoms. Vaginal estrogen has also been shown to reduce recurrent urinary tract infections.

Symptoms of urinary incontinence and irritative bladder symptoms occur in 20% to 40% of perimenopausal and postmenopausal women. Uterine prolapse and other gynecologic symptoms related to poor collagen support, as well as urinary complaints, may improve with estrogen therapy. Although estrogen generally improves symptoms, urodynamic changes have not been shown to be altered. Estrogen has also been shown to decrease the incidence of recurrence of urinary tract infections. Restoration of bladder control in older women with estrogen has been shown to decrease the need for admission to nursing homes in Sweden. Estrogen may also have an important role in normal wound healing. In this setting, estrogen enhances the effects of growth factors such as transforming growth factor-β (TGF-β). Although still not completely settled, it appears that oral estrogen does not improve stress urinary incontinence in postmenopausal women and may even cause such symptoms in previously asymptomatic older women. Estrogen may, however, improve urge and other irritative urinary symptoms.

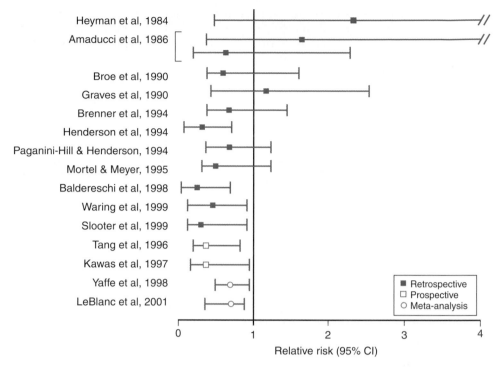

Figure 14-17 Estrogen replacement therapy/hormone replacement therapy use and risk of Alzheimer's disease. References are from the original source. (Adapted from LeBlanc ES, Janowsky J, Chan BK, Nelson HD: Hormone replacement therapy and cognition: Systematic review and meta-analysis. JAMA 285:1489, 2001.)

GENITAL ATROPHY

Vulvovaginal complaints are often associated with estrogen deficiency. In the perimenopause, symptoms of dryness and atrophic changes occur in 21% and 15% of women, respectively. However, these findings increase with time, and by 4 years these incidences are 47% and 55%, respectively. With this change, an increase in sexual complaints also occurs, with an incidence of dyspareunia of 41% in sexually active 60-year-old women. Estrogen deficiency results in a thin, paler vaginal mucosa. The moisture content is low, the pH increases (usually greater than 5), and the mucosa may exhibit inflammation and small petechiae. With estrogen treatment, vaginal cytology changes have been documented, transforming from a cellular pattern of predominantly parabasal cells to one with an increased number of superficial cells. Along with this change, the vaginal pH decreases, vaginal blood flow increases, and the electropotential difference across the vaginal mucosa increases to that found in premenopausal women.

BONE HEALTH

Estrogen deficiency has been well established as a cause of bone loss. This loss can be noted for the first time when menstrual cycles become irregular in the perimenopause from 1.5 years before the menopause to 1.5 years after menopause, spine bone mineral density has been shown to decrease by 2.5% per year, compared with a premenopausal loss rate of 0.13% per year. Loss of **trabecular bone** (spine) is greater with estrogen deficiency than is loss of **cortical bone**.

Postmenopausal bone loss leading to osteoporosis is a substantial health care problem. In white women, 35% of all postmenopausal women have been estimated to have osteoporosis based on bone mineral density. Furthermore, the lifetime fracture risk for these women is 40%. The morbidity and economic burden of osteoporosis is well documented. Interestingly, some data suggest that up to 19% of white men also have osteoporosis. Bone mass is substantially affected by sex steroids through classic mechanisms to be described later in this chapter. Attainment of peak bone mass in the late second decade (**Fig. 14-18**) is key to ensuring that the subsequent loss of bone mass with aging and estrogen deficiency does not lead to early osteoporosis. E_2 together with GH and insulin-like growth factor-1 act to double bone mass at the time of puberty, beginning the process of attaining peak bone mass. Postpubertal estrogen deficiency (amenorrhea from various causes) substantially jeopardizes peak bone mass. Adequate nutrition and calcium intake are also key determinants. Although estrogen is of predominant importance for bone mass in both women and men, testosterone is important in stimulating periosteal apposition; as a result, cortical bone in men is larger and thicker.

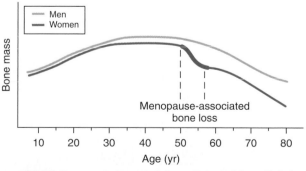

Figure 14-18 Bone mass by age and sex. (Adapted from Finkelstein JS: Osteoporosis. In Goldman L, Bennet JC [eds]: Cecil Textbook of Medicine, 21st ed. Philadelphia, Saunders, 1999, pp 1366-1373; Riggs BL, Melton LJ III: Involutional osteoporosis. N Engl J Med 314:1676, 1986, adapted with permission.)

However, even in men estrogen appears to be important for bone health in that in male individuals with aromatase deficiency (inability to convert androgen to estrogen) osteoporosis ensues.

Estrogen receptors are present in osteoblasts, osteoclasts, and osteocytes. Both ER α and ER β are present in cortical bone, whereas ER β predominates in cancellous or trabecular bone. However, the more important actions of estradiol are believed to be mediated via ER α. Estrogens suppress bone turnover and maintain a certain rate of bone formation. Bone is remodeled in functional units, called bone multicenter units (BMUs), where resorption and formation should be in balance. Multiple sites of bone go through this turnover process over time. Estrogen decreases osteoclasts by increasing apoptosis thus reducing their life span. The effect on the osteoblast is less consistent, but E$_2$ antagonizes glucocorticoid-induced osteoblast apoptosis. Estrogen deficiency increases the activities of remodeling units, prolongs resorption, and shortens the phase of bone formation. It also increases osteoclast recruitment in BMUs, thus resorption outstrips formation. The molecular mechanisms of estrogen action on bone involve the inhibition of production of proinflammatory cytokines, including interleukin-1, interleukin-6, tumor necrosis factor-α, colony-stimulating factor-1, macrophage colony-stimulating factor, and prostaglandin E2, which leads to increased resorption. Estradiol also upregulates TGF-β in bone, which inhibits bone resorption. Receptor activation of nuclear factor kappa (NFκB) ligand (RANKL) is responsible for osteoclast differentiation and action. A scheme for how all these factors interact has been proposed by Riggs (**Fig. 14-19**). In women, Riggs has suggested that bone loss occurs in two phases. With estrogen levels declining at the onset of menopause, an accelerated phase of bone loss occurs which is predominantly of cancellous bone. Here 20% to 30% of cancellous bone and 5% to 10% of cortical bone can be lost in a span of 4 to 8 years. Thereafter a slower phase of loss (1% to 2%/year) ensues during which more cortical bone is lost. This phase is thought to be induced primarily by secondary hyperparathyroidism. The first phase is also accentuated by the decreased influence of stretching or mechanical factors, which generally promotes bone homeostasis, as a result of estrogen deficiency. Genetic influences on bone mass are more important for the attainment of peak bone mass (heritable component, 50% to 70%) than for bone loss. Polymorphisms of the vitamin D receptor gene, TGF-β gene, and the Spl-binding site in the collagen type 1 Al gene have all been implicated as being important for bone mass.

Bone mass can be detected by a variety of radiographic methods (**Table 14-4**). Dual-energy x-ray absorptiometry (DEXA) scans have become the standard of care for detection of **osteopenia** and osteoporosis. By convention, the **T score** is used to reflect the number of standard deviations of bone loss from the peak bone mass of a young adult. Osteopenia is defined by a T score of −1 to −2.5 standard deviations; osteoporosis is defined as greater than 2.5 standard deviations.

Various biochemical assays are also available to assess bone resorption and formation in both blood and urine (**Table 14-5**). At present, serum markers appear to be most useful for assessing changes with antiresorptive therapy having less variability compared to the urinary assessments. Although these biochemical measurements cannot reliably predict bone mass, they may be useful as markers of the effectiveness of treatment. For example, an increased resorption marker may decrease within months into the normal range with an antiresorptive therapy, whereas it takes 1 to 2 years to see a change in BMD with DEXA.

Fracture risk is not only determined by bone mass but by many factors, the most important of which is bone strength. This in turn is determined by bone mass as well as bone turnover for which biochemical assessments may be helpful. A research method employs a high-resolution quantitative computed tomography of bone, which is intended to provide a "virtual" bone biopsy. This may be available in the future. The WHO has made available an algorithm to predict the 10-year fracture risk of men and women living around the world. This model, called FRAX, can be accessed at www.shef.ac.uk/FRAX and is calculated based on individual patient history data and the results from DEXA.

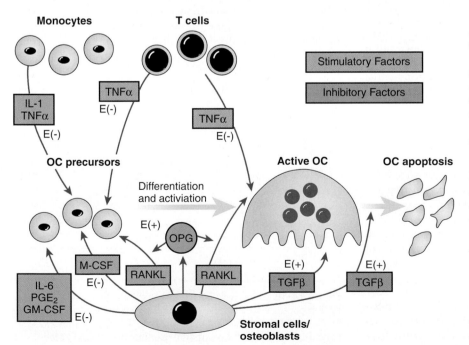

Figure 14-19 Model for mediation of effects of estrogen (E) on osteoclast formation and function by cytokines in bone marrow microenvironment. Stimulatory factors are shown in orange and inhibitory factors are shown in blue. Positive (+) or negative (−) effects of E on these regulatory factors are shown in red. The model assumes that regulation is accomplished by multiple cytokines working together in concert. IL, interleukin; PGE$_2$, prostaglandin E$_2$; GM-CSF, granulocyte macrophage/colony-stimulating factor; M-CSF, macrophage/colony-stimulating factor; RANKL, Receptor activation of B ligand; OC, osteoclast; OPG, osteoprotegerin; TGF-β, transforming growth factor β. (Adapted from Riggs BL: The mechanisms of estrogen regulation of bone resorption. J Clin Invest 106:1203, 2000.)

Table 14-4 Techniques for the Detection of Bone Mass

Effective Technique Equivalent (uSv)	Anatomic Site of Interest	Precision in vivo (%)	Examination and Analysis Time (min)	Estimated Dose
Conventional radiographs	Spine, hip 2000	NA	< 5	2000
Radiogrammetry	Hand	1-3	5-10	< 1
Radiographic absorptiometry	Hand	1-2	5-10	< 1
Single x-ray absorptiometry	Forearm, heel	1-2	5-10	< 1
Dual x-ray absorptiometry	Spine, hip, forearm, total body	1-3	5-20	1-10
Quantitative computed tomography	Spine, forearm, hip	2-4	10-15	50-100
Quantitative ultrasound	Heel, hand, lower leg	1-3	5-10	None

NA, not applicable.

Adapted from van Kuijk C, Genant HK: Detection of osteopenia. In Lobo RA (ed): Treatment of the Postmenopausal Woman: Basic and Clinical Aspects, 2nd ed. Philadelphia, Lippincott Williams & Wilkins, 1999, pp 287-292.

Table 14-5 Bone Turnover Markers

Marker	Specimen
Bone resorption markers	
Cross-linked N-telopeptide of type I collagen (NTX)	Urine, serum
Cross-linked C-telopeptide of type I collagen (CTX)	Urine ($\alpha\alpha$ and $\beta\beta$ forms) Serum ($\beta\beta$ form)
MMP-generated telopeptide of type I collagen (ICTP or CTX-MMP)	Serum
Deoxypyridinoline, free and peptide bound (fDPD, DPD)	Urine, serum
Pyridinoline, free and peptide bound (fPYD, PYD)	Urine serum
Hydroxyproline (OHP)	Urine
Glycosyl hydroxylysine (GylHyl)	Urine, serum
Helical peptide (HelP)	Urine
Tartrate resistant acid phosphatase 5b isoform specific for osteoclasts (TRACP 5b)	Serum, plasma
Cathepsin K (Cath K)	Urine, serum
Osteocalcin fragments (uOC)	Urine
Bone formation markers	
Ostcorcalcin (OC)	Serum
Procollagen type I C-terminal propeptide (PICP)	Serum
Procollagen type I N-terminal propeptide (PINP)	Serum
Bone-specific alkaline phosphatase (bone ALP)	Serum

Many agents are now available for preventing osteoporosis. The use of estrogen will depend on whether there are other indications for estrogen treatment and any possible contraindications. Estrogen has been shown to reduce the risk of osteoporosis as well as to reduce osteoporotic fractures. A dose equivalent of 0.625 mg of conjugated equine estrogens (CEE) was once thought to prevent osteoporosis, but we now know that lower doses (0.3 mg of CEE or its equivalent) in combination with progestogens can prevent bone loss, although there are no fracture data (**Fig. 14-20**). Whether the addition of progestogens by stimulating bone formation increases bone mass beyond that produced by estrogen alone is unclear. The androgenic activity of certain progestogens such as norethindrone acetate (NET) also has been suggested to play a role. **Figures 14-21** and **14-22** provide data on changes in bone mineral density (BMD) at the spine and hip using various agents. **Selective estrogen receptor modulators (SERMs)** such as **raloxifene**, droloxifene, and tamoxifen have all been shown to decrease bone resorption. Raloxifene has been shown to decrease vertebral fractures in a large prospective trial.

However, SERMs such as raloxifene that acts as low-dose estrogen on the skeleton have not been shown to prevent hip fractures (**Fig. 14-23**). **Tibolone** has also been shown to be an effective treatment for osteoporosis. Tibolone (not marketed in the United States) has SERM-like properties, but it is not specifically a SERM because it has mixed estrogenic, antiestrogenic, androgenic, and progestogenic properties. The drug does not seem to cause uterine or breast cell proliferation and also is beneficial for vasomotor symptoms. It prevents osteoporosis and has been shown to be beneficial in treatment of osteoporosis as well at a dose of 2.5 mg daily.

Bisphosphonates have been shown to have a significant effect on the prevention and treatment of osteoporosis. With this class of agents (etidronate, alendronate, risedronate, ibandronate, and zoledronic acid), incorporation of the bisphosphonate with hydroxyapatite in bone increases bone mass. The skeletal half-life of bisphosphonates in bone can be as long as 10 years. These agents reduce both spine and hip fractures (see **Fig. 14-23**). Most data have been derived with alendronate, which, at a dosage of 5 mg daily (35 mg weekly) prevents bone loss; at 10 mg daily (70 mg weekly), alendronate is an effective treatment for osteoporosis, with evidence available that this treatment reduces vertebral and hip fractures Similar data are available for risedronate (35 mg weekly). Ibandronate has been approved as a once-a-month treatment (150 mg), and some data to date support the reduction in vertebral fractures. It can also be injected (3 mg) every 3 months. Zoledronic acid 5 mg is available as an intravenous infusion (over 15 minutes) once a year for the treatment of osteoporosis and every 2 years for prevention.

Some concern has been raised about bisphosphonates and osteonecrosis of the jaw, fractures of long bones such as the

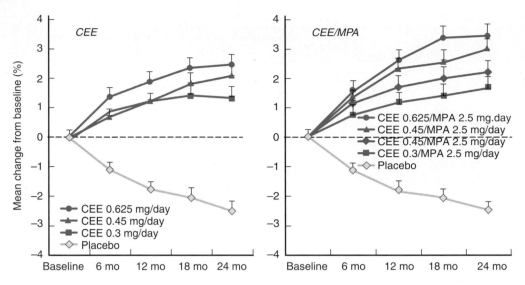

Figure 14-20 Changes in spine bone mineral density (BMD) with hormone therapy (HT). Intent-to-treat population only. The Women's HOPE Study. CEE, conjugated equine estrogens; HOPE, Heart, Osteoporosis, Progestin, Estrogen; MPA, medroxyprogesterone. (From Lindsay R, Gallagher JC, Kleerekoper M, Pickar JH: Effect of lower doses of conjugated equine estrogens with and without medroxyprogesterone acetate on bone in early postmenopausal women. JAMA 287:2668, 2002.)

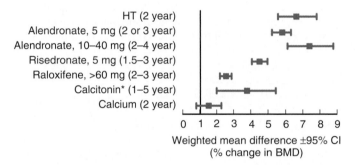

*Doses ranged from 250 to 2800 IU per week; predominantly nasal delivery.

Figure 14-21 Meta-analysis of osteoporosis therapies: Spine bone mineral density (BMD). CI, confidence interval; HT, hormone therapy. (From Cranney A, Guyatt G, Griffith L, et al: Meta-analyses of therapies for postmenopausal osteoporosis. IX: Summary of meta-analyses of therapies for postmenopausal osteoporosis. Endocr Rev 23:570, 2002; Cranney A, Tugwell P, Wells G, et al: Meta-analyses of therapies for postmenopausal osteoporosis. I. Systematic reviews of randomized trials in osteoporosis: Introduction and methodology. Endocrine Rev 23:496, 2002.)

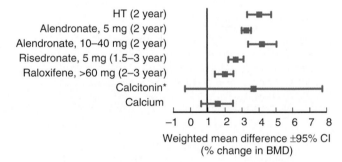

Figure 14-22 Meta-analysis of osteoporosis therapies: Total hip bone mineral density (BMD). CI, confidence interval. (From Cranney A, Guyatt G, Griffith L, et al: Meta-analyses of therapies for postmenopausal osteoporosis. IX: Summary of meta-analyses of therapies for postmenopausal osteoporosis. Endocr Rev 23:570, 2002; Cranney A, Tugwell P, Wells G, et al: Meta-analyses of therapies for postmenopausal osteoporosis. I. Systematic reviews of randomized trials in osteoporosis: Introduction and methodology. Endocrine Rev 23:496, 2002.)

femur with long-term use, and atrial fibrillation. Jaw problems only occur with high doses when poor dentition is present. Femur fractures with long-term use are extremely rare and atrial fibrillation, although statistically increased with bisphosphonate use, is also quite rare. Nevertheless, we do not have very long-term data (>10 yrs), and these drugs should not be used for more than 10 years and not with another antiresorptive agent. Its use in younger postmenopausal women (<60 yrs) should be limited unless there is significant osteoporosis present.

Calcitonin (50 IU subcutaneous injections daily, or 200 IU intranasally) has been shown to inhibit bone resorption.

Vertebral fractures have been shown to decrease with calcitonin therapy. Long-term effects, however, have not been established, and this is not first line therapy today.

Fluoride has been used for women with osteoporosis because it increases bone density. Currently, a lower dose (50 mcg daily) of slow-release sodium fluoride does not seem to cause adverse effects (gastritis) and has efficacy in preventing vertebral fractures.

Intermittent parathyroid hormone (PTH) is an effective agent to increase bone mass in women with significant osteoporosis. In a randomized trial lasting 3 years, average bone density increased in the hip and spine with fewer fractures observed. This

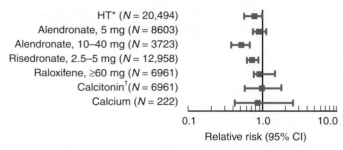

HT* (*N* = 20,494)
Alendronate, 5 mg (*N* = 8603)
Alendronate, 10–40 mg (*N* = 3723)
Risedronate, 2.5–5 mg (*N* = 12,958)
Raloxifene, ≥60 mg (*N* = 6961)
Calcitonin†(*N* = 6961)
Calcium (*N* = 222)

0.1   1.0   10.0
Relative risk (95% CI)

*Includes the Women's Health Initiative (WHI) trial.
†Estimate from the Prevent Recurrence of Osteoporotic Fractures (PROOF) trial.

Figure 14-23 Meta-analysis of osteoporosis therapies: Nonvertebral fractures. CI, confidence interval; HT, hormone therapy. (From Cranney A, Guyatt G, Griffith L, et al: Meta-analyses of therapies for postmenopausal osteoporosis. IX: Summary of meta-analyses of therapies for postmenopausal osteoporosis. Endocr Rev 23:570, 2002; Cranney A, Tugwell P, Wells G, et al: Meta-analyses of therapies for postmenopausal osteoporosis. I. Systematic reviews of randomized trials in osteoporosis: Introduction and methodology. Endocrine Rev 23:496, 2002; Rosen C: Presentation for ASBMR at NIH Scientific Workshop: Menopausal Hormone Therapy, October 23-24, 2002. Available at http//www4.od.nih.gov/orwh/htslides/rosen2.ppt.)

therapy, now available in the United States, is a second tier therapy reserved for severe cases of osteoporosis. Teriparatide 20 mcg needs to be injected subcutaneously on a daily basis for no longer than 18 months. Adjunctive measures for prevention of osteoporosis are calcium, vitamin D, and exercise. Calcium with vitamin D treatment has been shown to increase bone only in older individuals. It will not prevent bone loss in younger women at the onset of menopause. These modalities alone are not thought to be effective for the treatment of osteoporosis. A woman's total intake of elemental calcium should be 1500 mg daily if no agents are being used to inhibit resorption, and 400 to 800 IU of vitamin D should also be ingested. Exercise has been shown to be beneficial for building muscle and bone mass and for reducing falls.

There has recently been the realization that many women in the United States are vitamin D deficient, particularly those in the northern parts of the country, because of less sunlight exposure. Vitamin D may also be important as an antimitotic agent that may prevent certain types of cancer. Although there is some controversy about what a normal vitamin D level should be, a blood level of 25 OH vitamin D under 30 ng/ml warrants more aggressive treatment with Vitamin D.

Although it is clear that women with established osteoporosis (fractures or a T score of −2.5 or greater) should receive an antiresorptive agent (usually a bisphosphonate), there is more controversy with initiating preventative strategies with T scores in the osteopenia range (−1.0 to −2.5). Many women, however, may sustain fractures in this range of T scores. Age and risk factors (thinness, immobilization, nutritional deficiencies, family history, etc.) largely help determine the need to treat those with osteopenia. In this setting, depending on the age of the woman, her family history, and whether she has vasomotor symptoms, she may be offered hormone therapy, a SERM, or a bisphosphonate. The FRAX algorithm may also be useful as a guide to therapy.

DEGENERATIVE ARTHRITIS

Degeneration of intervertebral discs is a process that occurs rapidly after menopause. This is consistent with changes in collagen as noted previously. There is evidence that this is benefited by estrogen after menopause.

Osteoarthritis is a source of significant distress. There is a powerful effect of estrogen in inhibiting damage to chondrocytes. In WHI, estrogen alone (but not combination hormone therapy) significantly decreased osteoarthritis. However, much more work is needed in this area.

CARDIOVASCULAR EFFECTS

Clearly after menopause, the risk of cardiovascular disease in women increases. Data from the Framingham study have shown that the incidence is three times lower in women before menopause than in men (3.1 per 1000 per year in women ages 45 to 49). The incidence is approximately equal in men and women ages 75 to 79 (53 and 50.4 per 1000 per year, respectively). This trend also pertains to gender differences in mortality resulting from cardiovascular disease. Coronary artery disease is the leading cause of death in women, and the lifetime risk of death is 31% in postmenopausal women versus a 3% risk of dying of breast cancer.

Although cardiovascular disease becomes more prevalent only in the later years following a natural menopause, premature cessation of ovarian function (before the average age of menopause) constitutes a significant risk. Premature menopause, occurring before age 35, has been shown to increase the risk of myocardial infarction two- to threefold, and oophorectomy before age 35 increases the risk sevenfold.

When the possible reasons for the increase in cardiovascular disease are examined, the most prevalent finding is an accelerated rise in total cholesterol in postmenopausal women. The changes of weight, blood pressure, and blood glucose with aging, although important, are not thought to be as important as the rate of rise in total cholesterol, which is substantially different in women after menopause versus men. This increase in total cholesterol is explained by increases in levels of low-density lipoprotein cholesterol (LDL-C). The oxidation of LDL-C is also enhanced, as are levels of very low density lipoproteins and lipoprotein (a) lipoprotein. High-density lipoprotein cholesterol (HDL-C) levels trend downward with time, but these changes are small and inconsistent relative to the increases in LDL-C.

Coagulation balance is not substantially altered as a counterbalance of changes occurs. Some procoagulation factors increase (factor VII, fibrinogen), but so do counterbalancing factors like antithrombin III, plasminogen, protein C, and protein S. Blood flow in all vascular beds decreases after menopause; prostacyclin production decreases, endothelin levels increase, and vasomotor responses to acetylcholine are constrictive, reflecting reduced nitric oxide synthetase activity. Most of these latter changes are due primarily to the fairly rapid reduction in estrogen levels in that with estrogen, all these parameters (generally) improve, and coronary arterial responses to acetylcholine are dilatory with a commensurate increase in blood flow.

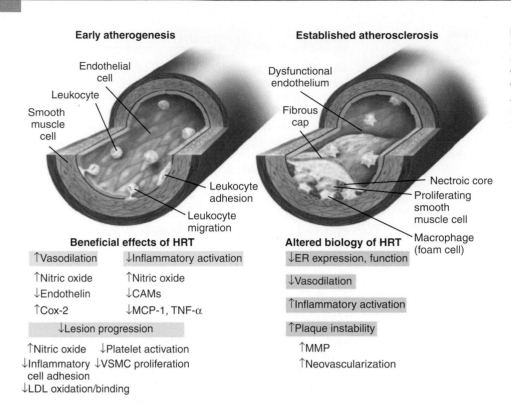

Early atherogenesis

- Endothelial cell
- Leukocyte
- Smooth muscle cell
- Leukocyte adhesion
- Leukocyte migration

Established atherosclerosis

- Dysfunctional endothelium
- Fibrous cap
- Nectroic core
- Proliferating smooth muscle cell
- Macrophage (foam cell)

Beneficial effects of HRT

↑Vasodilation	↓Inflammatory activation
↑Nitric oxide	↑Nitric oxide
↓Endothelin	↓CAMs
↑Cox-2	↓MCP-1, TNF-α

↓Lesion progression

↑Nitric oxide   ↓Platelet activation
↓Inflammatory   ↓VSMC proliferation
cell adhesion
↓LDL oxidation/binding

Altered biology of HRT

↓ER expression, function

↓Vasodilation

↑Inflammatory activation

↑Plaque instability

↑MMP
↑Neovascularization

Figure 14-24 Mechanisms of benefit of hormonal therapy with estrogen in early menopause (relatively clean coronary vessels) and the lack of effect in older women and those with significant atherosclerotic plaque burden. (From Mendelsohn ME, Karas RH: Science 308:1583-1587, 2005.)

Circulating plasma nitrites and nitrates have also been shown to increase with estrogen, and angiotensin-converting enzyme levels tend to decrease. Estrogen and progesterone receptors have been found in vascular tissues, including coronary arteries (predominantly ER β). In addition, some membrane effects are mediated by estrogen, which may or may not relate to either ER α or ER β.

Overall, the direct vascular effects of estrogen are viewed to be as important, or more important, than the changes in lipid and lipoproteins after menopause. Although replacing estrogen has been thought to be beneficial for the mechanisms previously cited, these beneficial arterial effects may only be seen in younger (stage +1) postmenopausal women (**Fig. 14-24**). Women with significant atherosclerosis or risk factors such as those studied in secondary prevention trials do not respond well to this treatment because of coronary plaque burden (see **Fig. 14-24**), which prevents estrogen action. Some of this lack of effect may be accounted for by increased methylation of the promoter region of ER α, which occurs with atherosclerosis and aging. Another mechanism is the significant conversion of cholesterol to 27-0H cholesterol, which also impedes estrogen's production of nitric oxide.

In normal, nonobese postmenopausal women, carbohydrate tolerance also decreases as a result of an increase in insulin resistance. This, too, may be partially reversed by estrogen, although the data are mixed and high doses of estrogen with or without progestogen cause a deterioration in insulin sensitivity. Biophysical and neurohormonal responses to stress (stress reactivity) are exaggerated in postmenopausal women compared with premenopausal women, and this heightened reactivity is blunted by estrogen. Whether these changes influence cardiovascular risk with estrogen deficiency is not known, but clearly estrogen treatment returns many parameters into the range of premenopausal women in early postmenopausal women. Several trials including data from the WHI have shown a reduction in the development of diabetes with hormone therapy.

These consistently strong basic science and clinical data for the protective effects of estrogen on the cardiovascular system, together with strong epidemiologic evidence for a protective effect of estrogen (**Fig. 14-25**) led to the belief that estrogen should be prescribed to prevent cardiovascular disease in women. Recent clinical trial data, however, have refuted this notion in women with established disease as noted previously. Results from several randomized trials in women have failed to show a protective effect in women with established coronary disease. Furthermore, a trend toward increased cardiovascular events (early harm) has been observed in this setting in some women within the first 1 to 2 years. The Women's Health Initiative (WHI) trial, which compared CEE/medroxyprogesterone acetate (MPA) with placebo, came to similar conclusions. This trial was considered to be a primary prevention trial, but it studied a large range of ages (mean age 63). These women did not have vasomotor symptoms and had more risk factors than the healthy women studied in observational cohorts as shown in **Figure 14-25**.

The protective effect of estrogen demonstrated in the observational trials such as the Nurse's Health Study (NHS) (see **Fig. 14-25**) occurred predominantly in young, healthy, symptomatic women. **Table 14-6** compares the demographics of the participants of WHI and the NHS. Trials carried out in the monkey model have shown a 50% to 70% protective effect against coronary atherosclerosis when estrogen is begun at the time of oophorectomy, with or without an atherogenic diet; delaying the initiation of hormonal therapy for even 2 years (in the monkey) prevents this protective effect (**Fig. 14-26**).

Figures 14-25 Estrogen replacement therapy and coronary heart disease. Relationship between relative risk and study type. (Adapted from Stampfer MJ, Colditz GA: Estrogen replacement therapy and coronary heart disease: A quantitative assessment of the epidemiologic evidence. Prev Med 20:47, 1991.)

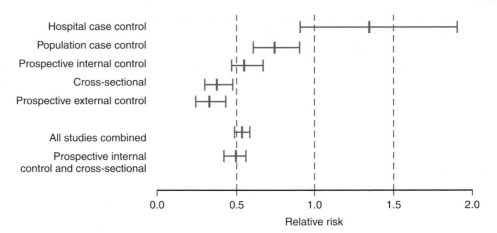

Table 14-6 Demographics of Women in WHI and NHS

	WHI	NHS
Mean age or age range at enrollment (years)	63	30-55
Smokers (past and current)	49.9%	55%
Body mass index (BMI:mean)	28.5 kg/m²	25.1 kg/m²
Aspirin users	19.1%	43.9%
Menopausal symptoms	Rare	Common

Observations in HERS (a secondary prevention trial in older women with established disease) demonstrated that hormone therapy (HT) was ineffective in preventing the progression of coronary heart disease (CHD), particularly if statins and other cardiac medications were already in use. Lack of an effect of estrogen therapy (ET) or HT was also demonstrated in an angiographic end point trial and another secondary prevention trial in the United Kingdom. The differences in types and regimens of HT in these trials suggest that this lack of benefit in secondary prevention is not dependent on the hormonal preparation.

In the WHI, two thirds of the women were older than 60 (at least 10 years postmenopausal). We do not know accurately the age at menopause for participants, but it is likely that women between ages 50 and 59 in WHI, who were largely without menopausal symptoms, were several years postmenopausal. With aging, even in the absence of a documented cardiac event such as myocardial infarction, we know that women have substantial atherosclerosis. Extrapolating from the monkey model, we can estimate that the diminished ability of estrogen to inhibit coronary atherosclerosis can occur as early as 6 years after menopause if no hormones have been administered. This effect, of course, is aggravated if there are cardiovascular risk factors.

In the first year of the HT (CEE + MPA) trial of WHI, more cardiac events occurred. This finding is consistent with the other secondary prevention trials mentioned earlier, including the NHS, in which a subgroup analysis was carried out to examine only those women with documented coronary disease. Here there was an increase in cardiovascular events in the first year in that group (not statistically significant), followed by a reduction in events and mortality with time. No clear explanation exists for what the observed "early harm" may be due to, but these effects were not observed in those women receiving statins

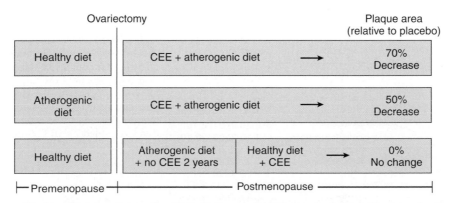

Figure 14-26 Importance of timing of intervention on the effect of estrogens on atherogenesis in nonhuman primates. CEE, conjugated equine estrogen. (Adapted from Clarkson TB, Anthony MS, Jerome CP: Lack of effect of raloxifene on coronary artery atherosclerosis of postmenopausal monkeys. J Clin Endocrinol Metab 83:721, 1998; Adams MR, Register TC, Golden DL, et al: Medroxyprogesterone acetate antagonizes inhibitory effects of conjugated equine estrogens on coronary artery atherosclerosis. Arterioscler Thromb Vasc Biol 17:217, 1997; Clarkson TB, Anthony MS, Morgan TM: Inhibition of postmenopausal atherosclerosis progression: A comparison of the effects of conjugated equine estrogens and soy phytoestrogens. J Clin Endocrinol Metab 86:41, 2001; Williams JK, Anthony MS, Honore EK, et al: Regression of atherosclerosis in female monkeys. Arterioscler Thromb Vasc Biol 15:827, 1995.)

concurrently. This finding suggests that HT (in the doses used) may lead to plaque destabilization and thrombosis in some women with established (although possibly silent) coronary disease. The molecular mechanisms for this may be due to estrogen up-regulating matrix metalloproteinase-9 and inhibiting its natural inhibitor within the mural area of the plaque; the resultant disruption of the gelatinous covering then leads to thrombosis. The anti-inflammatory effects of statins inhibit this process. In women who had been receiving estrogen for a prolonged time, mortality rates decreased in those who sustained a myocardial infarction. No increase in cardiovascular events has been found in young, healthy, symptomatic women during the first 2 years of various ET/HT regimens in clinical trials. In the WHI, the estrogen alone trial did not find any evidence of "early harm," and there was no overall effect over the 6 years of observation in the trial. However, there was a significant trend for a decrease in events with time, and this was also seen in the HT trial. Moreover, with estrogen alone the 50- to 59-year-old group had a reduction in events, which was almost statistically significant, and when global coronary scores were computed for this group there was a statistical beneficial effect. Thus, in younger women, and particularly with estrogen alone, the randomized controlled trial data parallel the findings from the observational studies, all suggesting a beneficial effect. A recent pooled analysis by Salpeter and colleagues, looking at 25 prospective trials, showed that in women within 10 years of menopause who received HT, there was a significant reduction in CHD (**Fig. 14-27**). Newer prospective randomized trials (some of which are underway) will be necessary to prove that young, healthy women receiving hormones at the onset of menopause experience a cardioprotective effect.

Two more areas of cardiovascular disease need to be discussed regarding their interactions with HT, namely stroke and venous thrombosis. Stroke (ischemic, not hemorrhagic) was found to be increased in the WHI trials (both HT and ET). This was approximately a 30% increase over the 5 to 6 years of the trial but was confined primarily to older women in the trial. These data are similar to data from the NHS trial where even younger women had a very small but statistically increased risk of ischemic stroke with standard doses of oral estrogen. Thus, although a rare event, ischemic stroke risk is increased in women taking standard doses

of oral estrogen (women using CEE at 0.625 mg or more) but not with lower doses (e.g., CEE 0.3 mg). Similarly, transdermal therapy has not been associated with an increased risk. These and other data point to a thrombotic risk with oral estrogen (in susceptible women). The mechanism of ischemic stroke risk in younger women is not likely to be due to atherosclerosis as it is in coronary disease in older women (**Fig. 14-28**). The thrombosis risk in younger women, much like the risk of venous thrombosis, is likely due to an aberrant interaction of estrogen with thrombotic factors, at times due to an underlying thrombophilia.

It is now accepted that there is a two- to threefold increase in venous thrombosis risk with oral hormonal therapy. However, the prevalence of this risk is low, particularly in young, healthy women. This two- to threefold risk is similar to that with the use of oral contraceptives. For pulmonary embolism risk, in women at age 50 to 60 years, the background risk is approximately 10 to 20 events/100,000 woman-years. Thus, with HT, the twofold increase may result in 40 events/100,000 woman-years, which is less than the rate in normal pregnancy (approximately 60/100,000 women). This risk is related to age, weight, and dose and route of administration of estrogen. Most events (DVT or pulmonary emboli) occur early (within the first year) and then decrease thereafter, suggesting an aberrant thrombophilic interaction with oral estrogen. The risk has been found not to increase with transdermal estrogen.

In summary, there should be no concern regarding increased cardiovascular risk for young, healthy women at the onset of menopause who are contemplating HT/ET for treatment of symptoms. In this setting there is no evidence of increased risk, and, indeed, these women may be found to benefit from a cardiovascular standpoint.

CANCER RISKS IN POSTMENOPAUSAL WOMEN

Although breast cancer is generally believed to be the leading cause of death in postmenopausal women, in fact it is lung cancer. Indeed, mortality from breast cancer tends to decrease after menopause, on an age-specific basis, but cardiovascular mortality increases, and these lines transect around the time of menopause

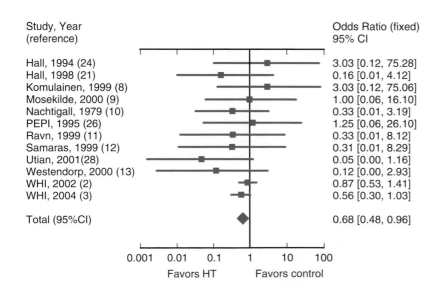

Study, Year (reference)	Odds Ratio (fixed) 95% CI
Hall, 1994 (24)	3.03 [0.12, 75.28]
Hall, 1998 (21)	0.16 [0.01, 4.12]
Komulainen, 1999 (8)	3.03 [0.12, 75.06]
Mosekilde, 2000 (9)	1.00 [0.06, 16.10]
Nachtigall, 1979 (10)	0.33 [0.01, 3.19]
PEPI, 1995 (26)	1.25 [0.06, 26.10]
Ravn, 1999 (11)	0.33 [0.01, 8.12]
Samaras, 1999 (12)	0.31 [0.01, 8.29]
Utian, 2001(28)	0.05 [0.00, 1.16]
Westendorp, 2000 (13)	0.12 [0.00, 2.93]
WHI, 2002 (2)	0.87 [0.53, 1.41]
WHI, 2004 (3)	0.56 [0.30, 1.03]
Total (95%CI)	0.68 [0.48, 0.96]

Figure 14-27 Pooled analysis from 23 randomized trials: younger women (younger than 10 years or younger than 60 years). CI, confidence interval; HT, hormone therapy. References are from the original source. (From Salpeter SR, Walsh JM, Greyber E, Salpeter EE: Brief report: Coronary heart disease events associated with hormone therapy in younger and older women. A meta-analysis. J Gen Intern Med 21:363, 2006.)

Figure 14-28 Mechanisms of Ischemic Stroke risk with estrogen in older women due to atherosclerosis with complicated lesions (left) and due to thrombosis in younger women (right).

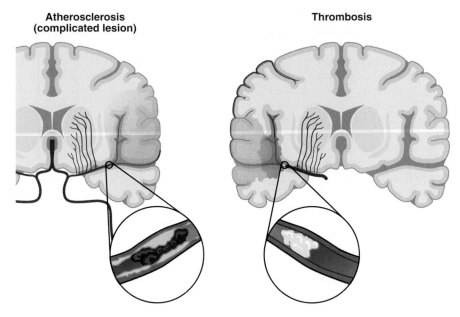

Atherosclerosis (complicated lesion)

Thrombosis

(**Fig. 14-29**). The gynecologist should be well versed in the epidemiology and preventive strategies for breast, lung, cervical, endometrial, ovarian, and colorectal cancer. Further discussions of these cancers may be found in Part IV (Gynecologic Oncology) of this text. What follows is the potential effects of ET and HT on endometrial, breast, ovarian, and colorectal cancer.

Endometrial disease occurs with **unopposed estrogen therapy** in women who have a uterus. Although a woman's risk for endometrial cancer with unopposed estrogen use is twofold to eightfold higher than that for the general population, precursor lesions (primarily endometrial hyperplasia) signal the presence of an abnormality in most patients. Thus, the risk is far less for endometrial cancer than it is for varying degrees of hyperplasia.

One study showed that the risk of endometrial hyperplasia was 20% after 1 year of use of 0.625 mg of oral CEE. In another study, the 3-year postmenopausal Estrogen/Progestin Interventions Trial, this risk was approximately 40% at the end of 3 years. No cancers were reported in either of these two studies, and the addition of a progestogen essentially eliminated the hyperplasia risk. Use of CEE alone at 0.3 mg/day for 2 to 3 years results in a hyperplasia risk of 5% to 10%. With the same dose of esterified estrogens (which is less potent), no hyperplasia was found after 2 years.

The risk for endometrial cancer in women taking estrogen and progestogen is similar to that of women in the general population because combination therapy merely eliminates the excess risk attributed to estrogen; a few studies, however, have suggested a lower risk of endometrial cancer with **continuous combined hormone replacement**. It is important to remember that some endometrial cancers occurring in postmenopausal women are not hormonally related; thus some women may develop a serious type of cancer (poorly differentiated) while on HT, making continuous surveillance important.

Although the risk for endometrial cancer is increased substantially in estrogen users, the risk of death from this type of endometrial cancer does not increase proportionately. Endometrial cancers associated with estrogen use are thought to be less aggressive than spontaneously occurring cancers, in part because tumors in women taking estrogen are more likely to be discovered and treated at an earlier stage, thus improving survival rates.

More controversial is the risk of breast cancer with estrogen use. Several studies and meta-analyses have shown a borderline or small statistical increase in the risk of breast cancer (relative risk [RR] l.2-l.4) after approximately 5 years of use. This risk is related to the dose of estrogen, as well as duration of use. Recent data have pointed to the addition of progestogen as a major contributor to this increased risk of breast cancer. There is some biologic plausibility to this notion in that progesterone in the normal luteal phase increases breast mitotic activity and HT increases mammographic tissue density relative to ET alone. Several recent small case-control studies found no increase with ET alone, but the same studies showed a statistically significant

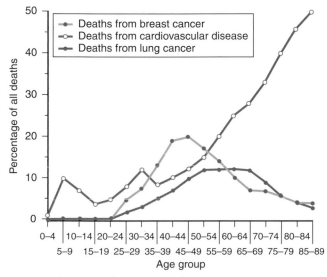

Figure 14-29 Risks of breast cancer and lung cancer versus cardiovascular disease in various age categories. (Adapted from Phillips KA, Glendon G, Knight JA: Putting the risk of breast cancer in perspective. N Engl J Med 340:141, 1999. Copyright 1999 Massachusetts Medical Society. All rights reserved. Adapted with permission.)

increase with progestogen use (in the range of 1.3 or l.4 RR). In the WHI trial, the increase in breast cancer risk was of borderline significance (hazard ratio [HR] 1.24, 1.01-1.54). A re-analysis by Anderson and coworkers found that when correcting for variables known to affect breast cancer risk, the average risk was no longer statistically significant: 1.20 (0.94-1.53). It is important to note that the total duration of therapy is very important for the risk with estrogen/progestogen therapy. In WHI the significant increase over 5 years was only found in prior users of HT, suggesting a longer cumulative effect. A large collaborative case-control study also has shown that continuous combined estrogen-progestogen therapy is associated with increased breast cancer risk over time.

In the estrogen only arm of WHI, after 6½ years there was a *decrease* in breast cancer risk of borderline significance HR = 0.77 (0.59-1.01). In a more complete analysis of these findings, Stefanick and associates found the risk to be significantly decreased for ductal cancer (0.71 [0.52-0.99]), and in a sensitivity analysis among adherent women, the decrease was statistically significant (0.67 [0.47-0.9]) (**Fig. 14-30**). Thus, although it is unclear why there should be a decrease in breast cancer risk, we may conclude that standard dose ET (0.625 mg CEE) is not associated with a risk of breast cancer except for very long-term users. In an analysis from the NHS, Chen and colleagues found that this risk only increases significantly after 20 years (**Table 14-7**). This risk is predominantly seen in lean women because overweight/obese women already have an increased risk of breast cancer, which is not further increased.

Putting these risks into perspective is important for patient counseling. The background risk for breast cancer in a woman between the ages of 50 and 60 is 2.8/100 women. According to data from the WHI, the overall risk for women taking CEE/MPA for 5 years was approximately a relative risk of 1.24. This 24% increase translates into an overall risk of 3.47/100; less than 1% above the background risk. This risk would be less

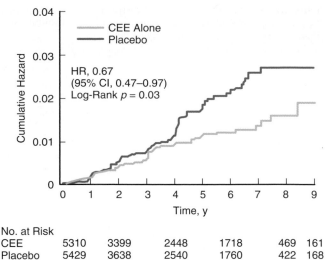

Figure 14-30 Cumulative hazard for invasive breast cancer: sensitivity analysis. CEE, conjugated equine estrogen; CI, confidence interval; HR. (From Stefanick ML, Anderson GL, Margolis KL, et al: Effects of conjugated equine estrogens on breast cancer and mammography screening in postmenopausal women with hysterectomy. JAMA 295:1647, 2006.)

for never users who did not have an increased risk of the 5 years of the trial and possibly may be lower still with low-dose therapy. A relative risk of 1.24 for breast cancer is less than that for obesity alone (3.3) or being a flight attendant (1.87) because of the increase in cosmic radiation. Furthermore, for estrogen alone, there is probably no increased risk at moderate to low doses for up to 20 years of exposure, as noted by Chen and colleagues.

It is generally thought that HT is linked to breast cancer through a promotional effect; that is, by causing the growth of undetectable preexisting small tumors. There is no evidence

Table 14-7 Risk of Invasive Breast Cancer by Duration of ET Use among All Postmenopausal Women Who Had Undergone Hysterectomy and Those with ER+/PR+Cancer Only*

ET Use and Duration (years)	All Postmenopausal Women							
	Who Had Undergone Hysterectomy				ER+/PR+ Cancers Only			
	All		Screened Cohort†		All		Screened Cohort†	
	Cases	Risk	Cases	Risk	Cases	Risk	Cases	Risk
Never	226	1.00	104	1.00	87	1.00	48	1.00
Current								
<5	99	0.96 (0.75-1.22)	59	1.06 (0.76-1.47)	38	1.00 (0.67-1.49)	26	1.04 (0.64-1.70)
5-9.9	145	0.90 (0.73-1.12)	95	0.91 (0.68-1.21)	70	1.19 (0.86-1.66)	50	1.08 (0.72-1.62)
10-14.9	190	1.06 (0.87-1.30)	141	1.11 (0.85-1.44)	85	1.27 (0.93-1.73)	77	1.29 (0.89-1.86)
15-19.9	129	1.18 (0.95-1.48)	95	1.19 (0.89-1.58)	61	1.48 (1.05-2.07)	58	1.50 (1.02-2.21)
≥20	145	1.42 (1.13-1.77)	127	1.58 (1.20-2.07)	69	1.73 (1.24-2.43)	74	1.83 (1.25-2.68)
p for trend for current use		<0.001		<0.001		<0.001		<0.001

BMI, body mass index; CI, confidence interval; ER+/PR+, positive for both estrogen and progesterone receptors; ET, unopposed estrogen therapy.
*All cases are reported as number of cases; risks are reported as multivariate relative risk (95% CI), controlled for age (continuous), age at menopause (continuous), age at menarche (continuous), BMI (quintiles), history of benign breast disease (yes or no), family history of breast cancer in first-degree relative (yes or no), average daily alcohol consumption (0, 0.5-5, 5-10, 10-20, or ≥ 20 g/day), parity/age at first birth (nulliparous; 1-2 children and age at first birth ≤ 22 years; 1-2 children and age at first birth 23-25 years; 1-2 children and age at first birth 25 years; ≥ 3 children and age at first birth ≤ 22 years; ≥ 3 children and age at first birth 23-25 years; ≥ 3 children and age at 1st birth >25 years).
†Screened cohort defined as those women starting in 1988 who reported either a screening mammogram or clinical breast examination in the previous 2 years. All cases before 1988 are excluded.
From Chen WY, Manson JE, Hankinson SE, et al: Unopposed estrogen therapy and the risk of invasive breast cancer. Arch Intern Med 166:1027, 2006.

that estrogen actually causes new cancers. Thus, dose and duration of therapy is important, and particularly the use of a progestogen, which may potentiate growth. The normal time needed for the average breast cancer to be clinically detectable from a microscopic stage is approximately 10 years. Thus, the promotional effect of HT on breast cancer in susceptible women takes several years for clinical detection. With some exceptions in the literature, most reports have shown that the mortality rate in users of ET/HT is improved compared with those women not receiving hormones who are diagnosed with breast cancer. Furthermore, since women on HT/ET are likely (and should) have closer surveillance (exams and mammography) most tumors detected are at an early stage.

Family history and genetic mutations (*BRCA* 1 and 2, etc.) substantially increases the risk of a woman developing breast cancer. However, the literature suggests that the use of ET/HT does not increase this risk further. Nevertheless, for many women it is unacceptable to consider a potentially promotional effect of using HT and they may opt for risk reduction strategies such as use of tamoxifen or other SERMs.

If there is a concern regarding hormones and breast cancer, it is with larger doses, a longer duration, and specifically the use of a progestogen. Accordingly, for longer-term therapy, if warranted (>5 years) lower doses of estrogen should be used, and progestogen exposure should be minimized.

OVARIAN CANCER

Several studies have also suggested an increased risk of ovarian cancer with long duration use of ET/HT. However, the data are inconsistent, and the purported risk is in the range of less than a twofold relative risk. Prospective randomized trials such as WHI have found no statistical increase in risk.

COLORECTAL CANCER

This is the third most frequent cancer in women and is often preventable by the detection and treatment of polyps. Women older than 50 should have a colorectal evaluation by some means (detection of occult blood, sigmoidoscopy, or a colonoscopy). Data have been fairly consistent for a reduction in risk with the use of HT/ET. Several meta-analyses have shown an approximate 33% decrease in risk, as did data from the NHS combined HT arm of WHI. It is unclear why in the ET arm of WHI, a decrease was not observed. No definitive mechanism for this protective effect has been found, although several theories have been advanced (changes in the composition of bile acids, anti-inflammatory effects, etc.).

OTHER CANCERS

There has been more attention paid to lung cancer recently, in part because it is the leading cause of cancer mortality in women. The data on HT, however, has not been consistent, without convincing evidence of any risk of lung cancer with HT use.

THE DECISION TO USE ESTROGEN

Whether hormonal therapy should be considered is an individual decision. The woman must take into account symptoms, risk factors, and individual preferences and needs. The predominant indication for estrogen is for symptoms (vasomotor, vulvovaginal, or urinary). Alternatives should also be considered. If hormonal therapy is chosen, there should be flexibility in prescribing because there is no ideal regimen for every woman, and each woman has individual risks and needs.

RISK-BENEFIT ASSESSMENT

The WHI was conceived in an attempt to determine the overall risks and benefits of ET/HT in a prospective randomized trial. The premise to be tested in an asymptomatic population of postmenopausal women was that ET/HT reduces cardiovascular disease and may increase the risk of breast cancer (primary end points). Several other secondary end points were also assessed: venous thromboembolism, stroke, osteoporotic fracture, colon cancer, and mortality. The HT arm of the trial (CEE 0.625 mg with MPA 2.5 mg) was terminated at 5.2 years because the event rates for breast cancer exceeded a preset monitoring boundary and because there was increased cardiovascular risk encountered (as previously discussed).

A tally of the various end points pointed to overall risks rather than benefit for this group of asymptomatic women, although there was protection from osteoporotic fracture and colon cancer. The ET randomized trial (hysterectomized women) did not have the same risk profile, and data are available for 6½ years of use. Although there have been several analyses and critiques of the WHI data, the size of the trial sheds important light on the decision to use this form of HT in mostly older asymptomatic women. The results of the trial were consistent with observational studies in all areas except for cardiovascular disease and Alzheimer's risk, which have been discussed previously.

The WHI trials computed an arbitrary "global index" adding up various changes in the eight major areas. Although this approach has not been validated, it provides a rough assessment that for older asymptomatic women of these specific regimens, there was more risk than benefit. However, the risk assessment clearly shifts toward benefit in younger symptomatic women as discussed earlier. Also for some women, protection from osteoporotic fractures becomes a significant benefit overriding some other concerns.

It is important that patients understand the "attributable" risk. This is the risk per year for 10,000 women exposed. Thus, an attributable risk of 8/10,000 women/year from cancer with HT is a very small risk and according to WHO terminology has been described as "rare." The media and others who have misinterpreted both relative risk and attributable risk have lost this concept. **Figure 14-31** provides the absolute risk in a 50- to 59-year-old woman using estrogen (E) or estrogen/progestogen (E+P) for 5 years as was witnessed in WHI. One can see clearly that the risk equation is largely favorable. In **Figure 14-32** this is put into the perspective of symptomatic women, although the benefit in terms of vasomotor symptoms overwhelms the other small changes.

In a younger, healthy population, benefits in quality of life predominate over potential risk, and this includes beneficial effects on mood, sleep, and short-term useful memory as well as sexual function. What is key, however, is timing of initiation (probably best within 3 years of menopause). This is most important for cardiovascular health as well as any potential cognitive benefit.

Recently there has been a trend to reduce potential risks and adverse effects by using lower doses of ET/HT, which have been

WOMEN AGES 50–59 OR <10 YEARS OF MENOPAUSAL

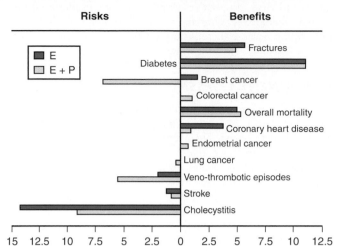

Figure 14-31 Absolute risks in younger women of standard dose therapy with estrogen (E) or estrogen/progestogen (E + P) per 1000 women/year for 5 years. (Adapted from Santen R: JCEM, 95 (7 Suppl 1):s1–s66, 2010.)

shown to be beneficial. The NHS demonstrated a protective effect with a lower dose of CEE (0.3 mg) and no increased risk of stroke. These lower doses have also been found to be sufficient to treat vasomotor symptoms.

CHANGES IN MORTALITY RATES WITH ESTROGEN USE

In several cohort studies, an overall 40% reduction in all-cause mortality has been observed with long-term estrogen use. Two studies have shown that the benefit in mortality is related to

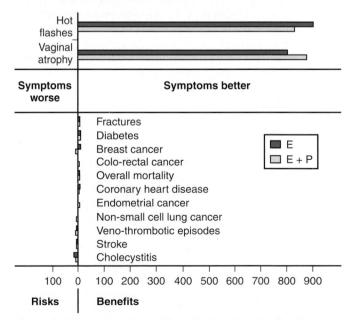

Figure 14-32 Putting risks and benefits in perspective for the 50- to 59-year-old. (Adapted from Santen R: Endocrine Society Position paper, JCEM 2010.)

the duration of use; one study has suggested that the effect is decreased beyond 10 years of use because of an increase in breast cancer mortality (only reported in this cohort and not in the others). Most studies have shown either no change in breast cancer mortality rates with estrogen use or a decrease.

In these observational cohorts looking at all-cause mortality, the overall reduction was found to be attributable to a reduction in cardiovascular mortality, although there was a small effect in cancer mortality as well. It is important to note that the women in these observational (epidemiologic) trials received therapy at the onset of menopause, and the women observed were healthier. In older women (10 or more years after menopause) who may have silent or established cardiovascular disease, there may not be a protective effect on mortality. In the WHI trial, total mortality was similar in HT/ET and placebo groups, but as discussed earlier, in the 50-59-year-old group, there was a statistically significant 30% reduction in all cause mortality (see **Fig. 14-31**), which is consistent with results from observational studies.

OTHER RISKS ASSOCIATED WITH ESTROGEN THERAPY

A discussion of the relationship with cancer was described earlier. One of the concerns of women receiving estrogen is the return of menstrual bleeding. Somatic complaints such as breast tenderness and bloating may also occur with ET/HT, but these can be alleviated by alterations in dose and the type of preparation. Such concerns should be discussed with the patient, and the choice of the regimen should remain flexible.

Idiosyncratic reactions like hypertension and allergic manifestations have been observed in users of estrogen, particularly oral estrogen. Hypertension with estrogen use, the cause of which is not entirely clear, occurs in about 5% of women using the oral route. Otherwise, estrogen usually causes no change in blood pressure; it may actually reduce blood pressure, a finding that has relevance for normotensive as well as hypertensive individuals and is rapidly reversible with discontinuation of the regimen. A different form of estrogen may eliminate the problem, and alterations in the route of estrogen administration have also resulted in normal blood pressure responses in such individuals.

In unsusceptible individuals, ET does not increase procoagulant factors outside the normal range; for many years, ET was not considered to increase the risk of venous thrombosis—unlike oral contraceptive use. However, several recent observational studies and the results of HERS and WHI have suggested a twofold increase in venous thromboembolic phenomena with oral estrogen. This risk has not been definitively related to an unknown thrombophilia, but some women, based on an individual sensitivity, are clearly at increased risk for thrombosis. The observed events all tend to occur in the first 1 to 2 years of estrogen exposure. This increased risk does not increase mortality, however, and the rate is low.

A recent meta-analysis estimated that the absolute increased risk for venous thromboembolic events is small: approximately 15 per 100,000 women per year. Nevertheless, all patients must be informed of these findings. Several reports from France following a large cohort of women found no increased risk with transdermal estrogen therapy and confirmed the increased risk with standard doses of oral hormones. Women who have a family history of thrombosis or have had a thrombotic event linked to oral contraceptives or any prior estrogen use should be counseled carefully and monitored closely. Known and unknown thrombophilias enhance the thrombotic risk manifold. It is unlikely that these other women would ever need any HT or ET.

APPROACH TO THERAPY

In developed countries, much of what women know about health care is gleaned from the mass media. In general, the more sensational an item, the more noteworthy. For example, breast cancer risk is a real and serious concern for all women, but the fear of breast cancer seems to drive all decision making, particularly regarding hormonal options.

American women believe that the leading cause of death in women is breast cancer and attribute only a small percentage of deaths to cardiovascular disease. In reality, the opposite is true. Statistics indicate that one in three women older than 65 has some evidence of cardiovascular disease. Despite public perception, the overall incidence of breast cancer has remained constant in recent years. Nevertheless, what those health care professionals counseling patients do not commonly appreciate is the age-associated relationship in the incidence of breast cancer.

Although it has been widely asserted that the incidence of breast cancer in women is approximately one in eight, this is the lifetime risk. The age-specific data are quite different: 1 of 77 in the fourth decade and 1 of 32 in the fifth decade, rising to 1 of 45 when a woman is in her eighth decade (**Table 14-8**). Misperceptions about the magnitude of cancer risk may lead some women not to consider ET/HT for the prevention of other conditions that actually have greater morbidity and mortality, as well as for the alleviation of menopausal symptoms.

Because the case fatality rate of cardiovascular disease is several times greater than that of breast cancer, many more women would die of cardiovascular disease even if the incidence of these two diseases were similar as mentioned earlier. **Figure 14-29** shows the death rate according to different ages. Soon after menopause, at age 50 to 54, the death rate for breast cancer decreases, but the death rate for cardiovascular disease rises steadily. The leading cause of cancer death in women is lung cancer. By age 55, 20% of all deaths are caused by cardiovascular disease; overall, 30% to 40% of women eventually will die of cardiovascular disease. The rationale for choosing estrogen at the onset of menopause for symptom control is expected to have a minimal effect on breast cancer incidence, particularly if the dose of estrogen is lowered. Whether there is also some cardiovascular benefit in this setting cannot be determined at this time.

HORMONE REGIMENS

The various hormonal preparations available for treatment are listed in **Table 14-9**. A more complete list may be found in the Consumer section of the North American Menopause Society website, www.menopause.org. Also included are the SERM raloxifene and other compounds like bisphosphonates, tibolone, and human parathyroid hormone. For the clinician and patient, the decision to start estrogen therapy need not involve a long-term commitment. For short-term treatment of symptoms, estrogen should be used at the lowest dose that can control hot flushes or can be administered via the vaginal route for symptoms of dryness or dyspareunia.

Oral ET results in higher levels of estrone (E_1) than estradiol (E_2); this is true for oral micronized E_2 as well as E_1 products. CEE is a mixture of at least 10 conjugated estrogens derived from equine pregnant urine. Estrone sulfate is the major component, but the biologic activities of equilin, 17α-dihydroequilin, and several other B-ring unsaturated estrogens, including δ5 dehydroestrone, have been documented. **Table 14-10** compares the standard doses of the most frequently prescribed oral estrogens and the levels of E_1 and E_2 achieved. Much of the following clinical information may be found in systematic reviews.

Synthetic estrogens, given orally, are more potent than natural E_2. Ethinyl estradiol is used in oral contraceptives, with a dose of 5 mcg being equivalent to the standard ET doses used (0.625 mg CEE or 1 mg micronized E_2). Standard ET doses are five or six times less than the amount of estrogen used in oral contraceptives.

Oral estrogens have a potent hepatic "first-pass" effect that results in the loss of approximately 30% of their activity with a single passage after oral administration. However, this results in stimulation of hepatic proteins and enzymes. Some of these changes are not particularly beneficial, for example, an increase in procoagulation factors and an increase in C-reactive protein, whereas other changes are beneficial (an increase in HDL-C and a decrease in fibrinogen and plasminogen activator inhibitor-1).

E_2 can be administered in patches, gels, lotions, sprays, and subcutaneously. These routes of administration are not subject to major hepatic effects as with oral therapy. Accordingly, there is no increase in C-reaction protein and minimal if any change in coagulation factors, but also only a minimal increase in HDL-C. Doses of patches are available from 0.014 mg to 0.1 mg, available for administration once or twice weekly. The ultralow-dose patch of 0.014 mg/day has been marketed for osteoporosis prevention in older women and not for treating hot flushes. Matrix patches are preferable to the older alcohol-based preparations because there is less skin reaction and estrogen delivery is more reliable. Whereas levels of E_2 with oral therapy may vary widely between women and within the day (peaks and valleys) levels with transdermal therapy are more constant within each woman, yet values achieved may vary from woman to woman based on absorption and metabolic characteristics. With the 0.05-mg patch, E_2 levels should be in the 40 to 50-pg/mL range, but an occasional woman can have values as high as 200 pg/mL, or levels that are <20 pg/mL. Note also that many commercial essays for E_2 are not very reliable, and do not accurately reflect estradiol status with oral estrogen therapy.

Table 14-8 Women Who Will Develop Breast Cancer: Risk According to Age

Decade of Life	Incidence
Third	1 of 250
Fourth	1 of 77
Fifth	1 of 42
Sixth	1 of 36
Seventh	1 of 34
Eighth	1 of 45

From Cancer Care Ontario; adapted from Lobo RA: Treatment of the postmenopausal woman: Where we are today. In Lobo RA (ed): Treatment of the Postmenopausal Woman: Basic and Clinical Aspects, 2nd ed. Philadelphia, Lippincott Williams & Wilkins, 1999, pp 655-659.

Table 14-9 Hormonal and Osteoporosis Treatments/Available for Postmenopausal Women

Estrogens
Oral CEE, 0.3, 0.45, 0.625, 0.9, 1.25, and 2.5 mg
Piperazine estrone sulfate, equivalent of 0.625, 1.25, and 2.5 mg
Esterified, 0.3, 0.625, 0.9, 1.25, and 2.5 mg
Micronized estradiol, 0.5, 1, and 2 mg

Transdermal
Estradiol patches, 0.014, 0.025, 0.0375, 0.05, 0.75, and 0.10 mg/d
Estradiol gel, 1.5 and 3 mg

Vaginal
Cream, CEE (0.0625%), estradiol (0.01%)
Estradiol ring, 2 mg; vaginal tablets, 25 mcg
Parenteral
Intramuscular injections should be avoided

Progestins

Oral
Medroxyprogesterone acetate, 2.5, 5, and 10 mg
Norethindrone acetate, 5 mg
Micronized progesterone, 100 and 200 mg
Vaginal
Micronized progesterone, 100 mg
Progesterone gel, 4% and 8%

Combinations

Oral
CEE + MPA (0.625 mg) + MPA (2.5 or 5 mg)
CEE + MPA (0.3 mg + MPA, 1.5 mg)
Micronized estradiol (1 mg) + norethindrone, acetate (0.5 mg)
Micronized estradiol (1 mg) + 0.5 mg drospirenone
Ethinyl estradiol 5 mcg, norethindrone, 1 mg

Transdermal
Patch, 0.05 mg estradiol with 140 mcg or 250 mcg norethindrone acetate
Patch, 0.045 mg estradiol with levonorgestrel 0.05 mg

Androgens

Oral
Esterified estrogen and methyl testosterone (0.625/1/25 mg and 1.25/2.5 mg)

Transdermal
Patch, 150 mcg/300 mcg in development
Bisphosphonates
Alendronate, 5 and 10 mg daily; 35 and 70 mg weekly
Risedronate, 5 mg; 35 mg weekly
Ibandronate, 150 mg monthly and 3l mg IV every 3 months
Zoledronic acid 5 mg once/yr
Etidronate, 200 mg (intermittent)

Selective Estrogen Receptor Modulators
Raloxifene, 60 mg
Others for osteoporosis
Tibolone, 2.5 mg (not approved in the United States)
Human parathyroid hormone 1-34; 20 mcg subcutaneously daily

CEE, conjugated equine estrogens; MPA, medroxyprogesterone acetate.

In women with vulvovaginal or urinary complaints, vaginal therapy is most appropriate. Creams of E_2 or CEE are available, as well as tablets and an estrogen ring. With creams, systemic absorption occurs but with levels that are one fourth of that achieved after similar doses administered orally. Absorption decreases as the mucosa becomes more estrogenized. For CEE, only 0.5 g (0.3 mg) or less is necessary; for micronized E_2, doses as low

Table 14-10 Mean Serum Estradiol (E_2) and Estrone (E_1)

	Level (pg/mL)	Level (pg/mL)
Estrogen dose (mg)	E_2	E_1
CEE (0.3)*	18	76
CEE (0.625)	39	153
CEE (1.25)	60	220
Micronized E_2 (1)	35	190
Micronized E_2 (2)	63	300
E_1 sulfate (0.625)	34	125
E_1 sulfate (1.25)	42	220

*Conjugated equine estrogen (CEE) contains biologically active estrogens other than E_2 and E_1.

as 0.25 mg are sufficient. Other products (tablets and rings) are available that have been designed to limit systemic absorption. A Silastic ring is available that delivers E_2 to the vagina for 3 months with only minimal systemic absorption.

Estrogen may be administered continuously (daily) or for 21 to 26 days each month. If the woman has a uterus, a progestogen should be added to the regimen (see **Table 14-9**). For women who are totally intolerant of progestogens (regardless of the dose and route of administration) and take unopposed estrogen, even at lower doses, periodic endometrial sampling is necessary. In this setting endometrial thickness by ultrasound may be a guide.

USE OF A PROGESTOGEN

There are many ways to administer progestogens. The most commonly used oral progestins are MPA in doses of 2.5 and 5 to 10 mg, NET in doses of 0.3 to 1 mg, and micronized progesterone in doses of 100 to 300 mg. Equivalent doses to prevent hyperplasia when administered for at least 10 days in a woman receiving ET (equivalent to 0.625 mg CEE) are as follows: MPA, 5 mg; NET, 0.35 mg; and micronized progesterone, 200 mg. Larger doses of estrogen may require larger doses and more prolonged regimes of progestins. In the sequential administration of progestogens, the number of days (length of exposure) is more important than the dose. Thus, if a woman is receiving oral ET continuously, a regimen of at least 10 to 12 days exposure is preferable to a 7-day regimen.

When progestogens are administered sequentially (10 to 14 days each month), withdrawal bleeding occurs in about 80% of women. Continuous administration of both estrogen and progestogen (continuous combined therapy) was developed to achieve amenorrhea. In the first 3 to 6 months, breakthrough bleeding and spotting is common. In some women on this regimen, amenorrhea is never completely achieved. The most common combinations in the United States are single tablets containing 0.45 or 0.625 mg CEE with 1.5 and 2.5 mg of MPA, respectively; 5 mcg of E_2 with 1 mg NET and 1 mg micronized E_2 with 0.5 mg NET. A patch with E_2 and NET or E_2 and levonorgestrel is also available.

Progesterone administered vaginally (in low doses) avoids systemic effects and results in high concentrations of progesterone in the uterus. This can be accomplished with capsules, suppositories, or a 4% gel. Intrauterine delivery of progestogens is ideal for targeting the uterus and minimizing systemic effects. However, the only marketed product, the 20-mcg Mirena IUS delivers too high a dose of levonorgestrel for lower doses of estrogen therapy, and the 10-mcg system that was in development has been discontinued by the company, although several studies showed its use to be beneficial.

Progestogens, particularly when taken orally, may lead to problems of continuance or compliance because of adverse effects, including mood alterations and bleeding. This requires flexibility in prescribing habits. Most short-term clinical trials have demonstrated an attenuating effect of progestogens on cardiovascular end points that are improved with estrogen; these effects include lipoprotein changes (an attenuation of the rise in HDL-C) and arterial and metabolic effects. The cardiovascular effects in WHI with CEE alone and CEE with MPA, which generally showed a more favorable effect without MPA also suggests some detrimental effects of added progestogen. However, there were two different populations of women studied in the two WHI trials, which limits any direct comparison. The most inert progestogens, such as micronized progesterone, or vaginal delivery of progesterone should have the least attenuating effects. As noted earlier, it is most likely progestogen exposure that increases the risk of breast cancer with HT. Progestogens should not be used in women who have had a hysterectomy.

ANDROGEN THERAPY

In a subtle way, some women are relatively androgen deficient. Clinicians have proposed adding androgen to ET or HT for complaints or problems relating to libido and energy, which are not relieved by adequate estrogen. Although well-controlled trials using parenteral testosterone have shown benefit in younger oophorectomized women, there have been few data showing benefit using more physiologic therapy, until recently. Recent data using a testosterone patch or pellet (with near physiologic levels) have shown improvement in several scales of well-being and sexual function. An oral preparation (esterified estrogens 0.625 mg with 1.25 mg of methyl testosterone) was shown to improve sexual motivation and enjoyment in women with hypoactive sexual desire who were unresponsive to estrogen alone. The latter findings correlated with an increase in circulating unbound testosterone levels. As newer forms and doses of androgen become available, perhaps more women may benefit from this approach. At present, androgen therapy should be individualized and considered for those women who have symptoms that are not adequately relieved with traditional hormonal therapies. It is important to note that there are no approved products for androgen therapy in the United States.

At lower doses, androgenizing side effects are very infrequent. At present, small doses of methyltestosterone (1.25 and 2.5 mg) added to esterified estrogens are available in tablets, which only have the indication of relief of vasomotor symptoms. As testosterone patches are only available for men, as are gels and creams, considerable dose titration needs to be considered in administering testosterone to women. The low-dose testosterone patch that showed benefit for hypoactive sexual desire in hysterectomized women receiving estrogen has been approved for use in Europe but not in the United States. The U.S. Food and Drug Administration (FDA) has been concerned about long-term cardiovascular and cancer effects, although there are no data in either direction. Administration of dehydroepiandrosterone at 25 to 50 mg/day may also be an option for raising endogenous testosterone.

Another SERM-like compound that is used worldwide but is not yet approved in the United States is tibolone. This progestogen-like compound exhibits estrogenic, antiestrogenic, and androgenic effects by virtue of its structure and metabolites. At 2.5 mg, tibolone suppresses hot flushes, prevents osteoporosis, and has a positive effect on mood and sexual function. There is also limited (or no) uterine stimulation. However, there is suppression of HDL-C, but at the same time a decrease in triglycerides. In the monkey, there is no deleterious effect of tibolone on coronary arteries.

ALTERNATIVE THERAPIES FOR MENOPAUSE

PHYTOESTROGENS

Phytoestrogens are a class of plant-derived estrogen-like compounds conjugated to glycoside moieties. Phytoestrogens are not biologically active in their native forms unless taken orally. After oral ingestion, colonic bacteria cleave the glycosides, producing active compounds that are subject to the enterohepatic circulation. These compounds can produce estrogen-agonistic effects in some tissues, whereas in other tissues they produce antagonistic effects.

Few randomized trials have examined the efficacy of phytoestrogens. For large daily doses (60 mg isoflavone), there appears to be some limited efficacy in relieving hot flushes, although the literature on this issue is mixed in placebo-controlled trials. With doses of 30 to 40 mg, cholesterol levels may be reduced, but this is not a consistent finding. It should be noted that there is an important reduction in hot flushes with any placebo treatment. Phytoestrogens do not appear to have much of an effect on bone loss or on vaginal atrophy.

Estimates are that between 30% and 60% of women use so-called alternative interventions for the symptoms of menopause, including "natural" estrogens, plant estrogens, herbal medicines, and acupuncture. Botanicals, herbals, and many steroid products are sold over the counter, and some do in fact exert significant hormonal activity. The use of botanicals to alleviate the symptoms of menopause is extremely popular. This popularity is fostered by the notion that plant sterols might provide all the benefits of **estrogen replacement therapy (ERT)** without the risks. However, most plant products recommended for menopause have performed poorly in clinical trials. The Dietary Supplement Health and Education Act of 1994 classifies most botanical medicines as food supplements and removes them from regulatory oversight and scrutiny by the FDA. Adulteration, contamination, and poor quality control in their harvesting, manufacture, and formulation yield products of questionable efficacy and safety.

The FDA has determined that more than 25% of Chinese patent medicines are adulterated with hidden pharmaceutical drugs. These kinds of deficiencies make it difficult for consumers and practitioners to employ botanicals with confidence and security. Furthermore, clinical trial data obtained using one brand of herbal product cannot necessarily be extrapolated to other brands using the same plant. DHEA is marketed as a dietary supplement for a variety of purported benefits. There are no data in women to support its role in well-being or immune function. As an androgen, DHEA is converted to androstenedione and testosterone. Doses of 25 to 50 mg raised testosterone and have been mentioned as an option for androgen therapy. However, these doses can reduce HDL-C levels.

KEY POINTS

- The median age of the onset of perimenopause is 47.5 years, and its median length is about 4 years.
- The initial endocrinologic change signaling the onset of menopause is decreased AMH and ovarian inhibin-B production accompanied by an increase in FSH.
- Estradiol does not begin to significantly diminish until 6 months before menopause.
- About 50% of postmenopausal women experience hot flushes, and the incidence decreases to 20% 4 years after menopause; estrogen is the best therapy for the hot flush; other effective therapies are progestogens, selective serotonin reuptake inhibitors (SSRIs), gabapentin, and clonidine.
- Age at menopause is genetically predetermined and is not related to the number of ovulations, race, socioeconomic conditions, education, height, weight, age at menarche, or age at last pregnancy.
- About 1% to 1.5% of bone mass is lost each year after menopause in nonobese white and Asian women. Fractures begin to occur about age 60 to 65 in trabecular bone, such as the vertebral spine, and by age 60, 25% of these women develop spinal compression fractures. Hip fractures begin to increase after age 70.
- Dual-energy x-ray absorptiometry (DEXA) is the most accurate method to measure bone density. The bone mineral density is usually expressed as T scores and Z scores. Bone density does not completely reflect bone strength, which is what determines risk of fracture.
- In addition to estrogen, alendronate, risedronate, ibandronate, zoledronic acid, raloxifene, and calcitonin will reduce postmenopausal bone loss.
- The primary indication for estrogen therapy is symptoms of menopause (hot flushes as well as quality of life issues); bone health may also be an indication in some women.
- In younger postmenopausal women who are receiving hormonal therapy for symptoms, the benefits outweigh risks with standard doses; lowering doses further decreases risks.
- There is no risk of coronary disease and possibly some benefit with early treatment; there are small risks of venous thrombosis and ischemic stroke, which can be minimized or eliminated with lower doses or transdermal therapy.
- Breast cancer risk is related to dose, duration of use, and progestogen exposure. Estrogen alone and possibly the use of natural progestogen does not substantially increase the risk.
- There is no proven cognitive benefit, although this has been shown in observational studies, but there is also no evidence for harm.

REFERENCES CAN BE FOUND ON EXPERTCONSULT.com

SUGGESTED READINGS

Canonico M, Plu-Bureau G, Lowe GD, et al.: Hormone replacement therapy and risk of venous thromboembolism in postmenopausal women: Systematic review and meta-analysis, *BMJ* 336 (7655):1227–1231, 2008.

Chen C-L, Weiss NS, Newcomb P, et al: Hormone replacement therapy in relation to breast cancer, *JAMA* 287(6):734–741, 2002.

Cirillo J, Wallace RB, Wul, et al: Effect of hormone therapy on risk of hip and knee joint replacement in the Women's Health Initiative, *Arthritis Rheum* 54(10):3194–3204, 2006.

Clarkson TB: The new conundrum: Do estrogens have any cardiovascular benefits? *Int J Fertil* 47:61, 2002.

Cooper AR, Baker VL, Sterling EW, et al: The time is now for a new approach to primary ovarian insufficiency, *Fertil Steril* 2010. [Epub ahead of print].

Couzinet B, Meduri G, Lecce MG, et al: The postmenopausal ovary is not a major androgen-producing gland, *J Clin Endocrinol Metab* 86:5060, 2001.

de Bruin JP, Bovenhuis H, van Noord PA, et al: The role of genetic factors in age at natural menopause, *Hum Reprod* 16(9):2014–2018, 2001.

Fournier A, Berrino F, Clavel-Chapelon F: Unequal risks for breast cancer associated with different hormone replacement therapies: Results from the E3N cohort study, *Breast Cancer Res Treat* 107 (2):307–308, 2008.

Freedman RR: Narrowing of the thermoregulatory zone in symptomatic women, HF, hot flush.

Freedman RR: Menopausal hot flashes. In Lobo RA, editor: *Treatment of the Postmenopausal Woman*, ed 3, New York, 2007, Academic Press, pp 187–198 Fig. 14-18.

Grodstein F, Manson JE, Stampfer MJ: Hormone therapy and coronary heart disease: The role of time since menopause and age at hormone initiation, *J Womens Health (Larchmt)* 15(1):35, 2006.

Grodstein F, Newcomb PA, Stampfer MJ: Postmenopausal hormone therapy and the risk of colorectal cancer: A review and meta-analysis, *Am J Med* 106 (5):574–582, 1999.

Henderson BE, Paganini-Hill A, Ross RK: Decreased mortality in users of estrogen replacement therapy, *Arch Intern Med* 151:75, 1991.

Henderson VW: Estrogen, cognition and a woman's risk of Alzheimer's disease, *Am J Med* 103:11, 1997.

Hsia J, Langer RD, Manson JE, et al: Conjugated equine estrogens and coronary heart disease: The Women's Health Initiative, *Arch Intern Med* 166(3):357, 2006.

Hulley S, Grady D, Bush T, et al: Randomized trial of estrogen plus progestin for secondary prevention of coronary heart disease in postmenopausal women, *JAMA* 280:605, 1998.

LeBlanc ES, Janowsky J, Chan BK, et al: Hormone replacement therapy and cognition. Systematic review and meta-analysis, *JAMA* 285:1489, 2001.

Lobo RA: Evaluation of cardiovascular event rates with hormone therapy in healthy postmenopausal women: Results from four large clinical trials, *Arch Intern Med* 164:482, 2004.

Lobo RA, Clarkson TB: Different mechanisms for benefit and risk of coronary heart disease (CHD) and stroke in early postmenopausal women: A hypothetical explanation, *Menopause* 18(2) 2011.

Mendelsohn ME, Karas RH: Molecular and cellular basis of cardiovascular gender differences, *Science (Review)* 308(5728):1583–1587.

Oldenhave A, Jaszmann LJ, Haspels AA, et al: Impact of climacteric on well-being: A study based on 5213 women 39 to 60 years old, *Am J Obstet Gynecol* 168:772, 1993.

Salpeter SR, Walsh JM, Greyber E, et al: Brief report: Coronary heart disease events associated with hormone therapy in younger and older women: A meta-analysis, *J Intern Med* 21(4):363, 2006.

Santen R: Endocrine Society position paper, *JCEM* 95(7 Suppl 1):s1–s66, 2010.

Scarabin PY, Oger E, Plu-Bureau G, the Estrogen and Thromboembolism Risk Study Group: Differential association of oral and transdermal oestrogen-replacement therapy with venous thromboembolism risk, *Lancet* 62(9382): 428, 2003.

Schaiirer C, Lubin J, Troisi R, et al: Menopausal estrogen and estrogen-progestin replacement therapy and breast cancer risk, *JAMA* 283:485, 2000.

Soules MR, Sherman S, Parrott E, et al: Executive summary: Stages of Reproductive Aging Workshop (STRAW), *Fertil Steril* 76:874, 2001.

Sowers MR, Eyvazzadeth AD, McConnell D, et al: Anti-mullerian hormone and inhibin in the definition of ovarian aging and the menopause transition, *J Clin Endocrinol Metab* 93(9):L34768–L34783, 2008.

Stefanick ML, Anderson GL, Margolis KL, et al: Effects of conjugated equine estrogens on breast cancer and mammography screening in postmenopausal women with hysterectomy, *JAMA* 295 (14):1647, 2006.

Writing Group for the Women's Health Initiative Investigators: Risks and benefits of estrogen plus progestin in healthy postmenopausal women: Principal results from the Women's Health Initiative randomized controlled trial, *JAMA* 288:321, 2002.

15

Breast Diseases
Diagnosis and Treatment of Benign and Malignant Disease

Vern L. Katz and Deborah Dotters

The gynecologist's role in managing breast problems is broad and extensive. Our culture attaches great significance to the female breast, as an aspect of sexuality and femininity, as a part of childbearing, and as a symbolic representation of aging. Thus, breast problems may provoke great anxiety for a woman. Women may react to symptoms of breast disease with behaviors that vary from frequent visits to the physician for breast pain to denial of the presence of an obvious mass. The patient's description of her problem and her reactions to diagnoses and treatment must always be considered within the context of this anxiety. At some point in a woman's third or fourth decade, the concerns about breast symptoms change to a fear of cancer. The prognosis and survival of a woman with breast carcinoma improve with early discovery. Thus, every gynecologist has an obligation to educate women concerning self-examination of the breast and to develop a routine for carefully screening women for breast disease. Detailed physical examination of the breast must be an integral step in evaluating every female patient.

This chapter is divided, for organizational purposes, into benign breast problems and breast carcinoma. In practice, though, there is a continuum to the evaluation and differential diagnosis of breast problems. The latter portions of this chapter concentrate on the epidemiology, detection, and management of breast carcinoma with an emphasis on the gynecologist's role.

ANATOMY

Breast development begins in utero from bilateral epithelial mammary ridges. Development into ductal tissue and secretory lobules occurs under the influence of the hormonal changes in puberty (see Chapter 38). True milk production is initiated with hormonal changes during and after pregnancy. The breasts are large, modified sebaceous glands contained within the superficial fascia of the anterior chest wall. A lateral projection of glandular tissue extends from the upper outer portion of the breast toward the axilla and is called the **axillary tail of Spence**. The average weight of the adult breast is 200 to 300 grams during the menstruating years. The mature breast consists of approximately 20% glandular tissue and 80% fat and connective tissue. After menopause, the glandular tissue regresses and is replaced by fatty tissue. Some women will have breasts that are predominately glandular and fibrous. The density of a breast refers to the proportion of fibrous and glandular tissue compared to adipose tissues.

The periphery of breast tissue is predominantly fat, and the central area contains more of the glandular tissue (**Fig. 15-1**).

Each breast is composed of 12 to 20 triangular-shaped lobes varying in size and arranged in a radial fashion around the nipple. Each lobe contains an independent ductal system. The lobes are composed of lobules, from 10 to 100 per lobe. Within the lobules, secretory cells drain into alveoli (acini). These alveoli drain into terminal ducts, which coalesce into larger collecting ducts, finally joining with other ducts from lobules to end in a small series of lactiferous sinuses ending in excretory ducts at the nipple. The ductal cells tend to have two layers, a basal layer, primarily myoepithelial in nature, and a more distal layer, also known as a luminal layer, which faces onto the duct lumen. The organization of the ductal system is stimulated at puberty (**Fig. 15-2**). **Montgomery glands** are accessory glands located around the periphery of the areola. Because they are structurally intermediate between true mammary and sebaceous glands, they can secrete milk but only provide a minor contribution to milk production. Fibrous septa, **Cooper's ligaments**, extend from the skin to the underlying pectoralis fascia (**Fig. 15-3**). They are believed to offer support to the breast. Invasion of these ligaments by malignant cells produces skin retraction, which is a sign of advanced breast carcinoma.

The lymphatic distribution of the breast is complex. Approximately 75% of the lymphatic drainage goes to regional nodes in the axilla. The axilla contains a varying number of nodes, usually between 30 and 60. Other metastatic routes include lymphatics adjacent to the internal mammary vessels. After direct spread into the mediastinum, lymphatic drainage may go to the intercostal glands, which are located posteriorly along the vertebral column, and to subpectoral and subdiaphragmatic areas (**Fig. 15-4**). Lymph drainage usually flows toward the most adjacent group of nodes. This concept represents the basis for sentinel node mapping in breast cancer. In most instances, breast cancer spreads in an orderly fashion within the axillary lymph node basin based on the anatomic relationship between the primary tumor and its associated regional (sentinel) nodes. However, lymphatic metastases from one specific area of the breast may be found in any or all of the groups of regional nodes. In a large multicenter study, Krag and colleagues validated the use of sentinel node biopsy in women with breast cancer. All of the women studied had positive nodes. However, in only 3% of these women did the only positive node occur outside of the axilla. Metastases from one breast across the midline to the other breast or chest wall occur occasionally.

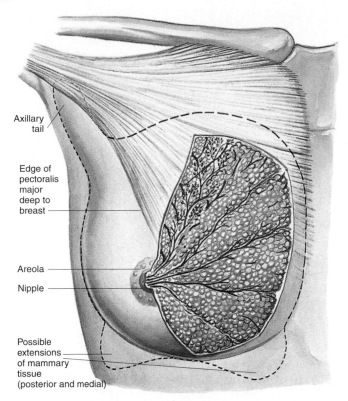

Figure 15-1 The structures of the breast. (From Shah P [ed]: Breast. In Standring S [ed]: Gray's Anatomy. London, Elsevier Churchill Livingstone, 2005, p 969, Figure 58.1A.)

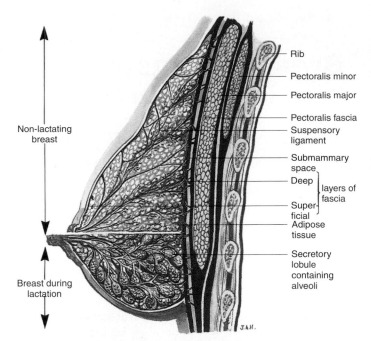

Figure 15-3 Lactating breast. (From Shah P [ed]: Breast. In Standring S [ed]: Gray's Anatomy. London, Elsevier Churchill Livingstone, 2005, p 969, Figure 58.1B.)

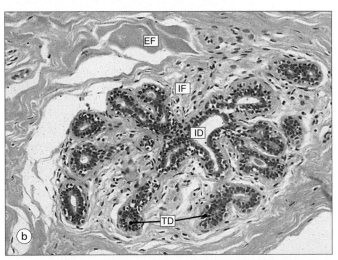

Figure 15-2 Histologic photograph of a mammary lobule. Note the ductal tissue surrounded by fibrous tissue. Terminal ductules (TD) surround the central ductule (ID). EF, extralobular fibrocollagenous tissue. (From Stevens A, Lowe J: Human Histology, 3 rd ed. Philadelphia, Elsevier Mosby, 2005, p 390.)

Breast tissue is sensitive to the cyclic changes in hormonal levels. The epithelium of the breast responds to fluctuating levels of estrogen and progesterone similar to other hormonally sensitive tissue. The stroma of the breasts and the **myoepithelial cells** of the breasts also respond to estrogen and progesterone. Women often experience breast tenderness and fullness during the luteal phase of the cycle. The average increase in volume of the premenstrual breasts is 25 to 30 mL, as measured by water displacement techniques. Premenstrual breast symptoms are produced by an increase in blood flow, vascular engorgement, and water retention. There is a corresponding enlargement in the lumina of ducts and an increase in ductal and acinar cellular secretory activity. During the follicular phase, there is parenchymal proliferation of the ducts. During the luteal phase, there is dilation of the ductal system and differentiation of the alveolar cells into secretory cells. The alveolar elements respond to both estrogen and progesterone. When menstruation begins, there is a regression of cellular activity in the alveoli and the ducts become smaller. Importantly, the breast undergoes normal maturational changes over a woman's lifetime. In addition to the pubertal and pregnancy-induced changes in the lactiferous duct lobule, the fibrous and adipose components will evolve as well. Thus, the findings on breast examination are different in the 20-year-old, the 40-year-old, and the 60-year-old and beyond. The normal maturation is a gradual increase in fibrous tissue around the lobules. With time the glandular elements are completely replaced by fibrous tissue. Women in their 20s and 30s have a gradual increase in nodularity as the lobular tissue increases with repetitive hormonal stimulation of the menses. After pregnancy and lactation, breasts may decrease in size and shape, compared with the prepregnancy state.

The breast also changes throughout each menstrual cycle. This has implications in the evaluation of breast symptoms such as breast pain and breast masses. The changes underscore the value of breast self-awareness as each woman knows the changes in her own body at different times in her cycle. (**Fig. 15-5**).

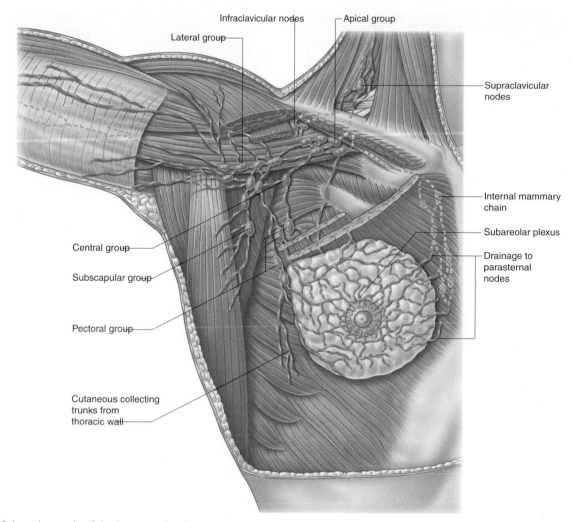

Infraclavicular nodes

Apical group

Lateral group

Supraclavicular nodes

Internal mammary chain

Subareolar plexus

Drainage to parasternal nodes

Central group

Subscapular group

Pectoral group

Cutaneous collecting trunks from thoracic wall

Figure 15-4 Lymph vessels of the breast and axillary lymph nodes. (From Shah P [ed]: Breast. In Standring S [ed]: Gray's Anatomy. London, Elsevier Churchill Livingstone, 2005, p 971, Figure 58.4.)

DEVELOPMENTAL ANOMALIES

Accessory breasts or nipples can occur along the breast or milk lines that run from the axilla to the groin. Supernumerary nipples (**polythelia**) or breasts (**polymastia**) are common anomalies (**Fig. 15-6**), which may be well developed and functional or may be rudimentary. They occur in approximately 1% to 2% of women of European descent and 5% to 6% of women of Asian descent.

Asymmetric breast development is common from adolescence until maturity. In a study of 8408 mammograms, 3% were notable for asymmetric volume differences relative to the contralateral breast. This breast asymmetry represents a benign, normal variation unless an associated palpable abnormality is present. Hypertrophy of the breasts at puberty, juvenile or **virginal hypertrophy of the breasts**, may become extreme. It is a rare occurrence that is often deeply disturbing, affecting a teenager's self-image. Hypertrophy may be asymmetric. This condition may be managed by reduction mammoplasty. Surgery often improves self-image and decreases neck and back pain. This surgery must be done carefully by physicians who have experience to preserve breast-feeding ability. **Poland syndrome** is a unilateral

hypoplasia of the chest muscles and breast tissue that has an incidence of 1 in 20,000 to 30,000 births, with a sporadic inheritance.

BENIGN BREAST PROBLEMS

The most common breast symptoms that women present with are pain, discharge, and breast masses. Less common is mastitis. The symptoms and subsequent physical findings of benign breast disease often cause anxiety and fear. The patient worries that the symptoms are a sign of cancer. However, breast pain is a comparatively late symptom in women with carcinoma and is the sole presenting symptom in less than 10% of women. During the second half of the menstrual cycle, breasts will increase in size, density, and nodularity. These changes are often associated with increased sensitivity or pain. Nipple discharge is even a less frequent of a sign of cancer. The correlation of a mass with malignancy is dependent on the patient's age. Many breast symptoms stem from **fibrocystic changes**, previously termed fibrocystic disease, which are a common and natural maturation of breast tissue over time.

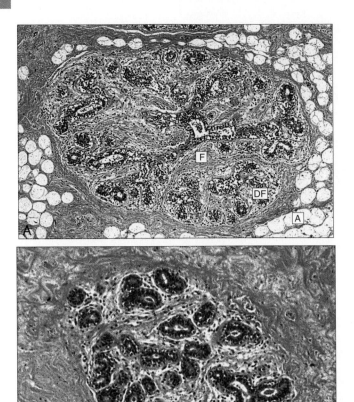

Figure 15-5 A, Micrograph showing normal breast tissue from a 23-year-old woman. At the center is a breast lobule in which the system of terminal ducts and ductules is embedded in loose intralobular fibrocollagenous stroma (F). There is a narrow surrounding zone of dense extralobular fibrocollagenous support tissue (DF), outside of which is the soft adipose tissue (A) that forms the bulk of the breast. **B,** Micrograph showing normal breast tissue from a 43-year-old woman. As women age, the amount of fibrocollagenous tissue (F) in the breast increases, replacing some of the adipose tissue. The mammary lobules become enclosed in dense collagen. (From Stevens A, Lowe J: Human Histology, 3 rd ed. Philadelphia, Elsevier Mosby, p 393.)

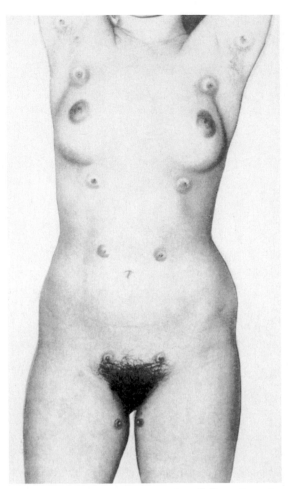

Figure 15-6 Extensive polythelia along the milk lines. (From Degrell I: Atlas of Diseases of the Mammary Gland. Basel, Switzerland, S Karger, 1976, p 41.)

FIBROCYSTIC CHANGES

Fibrocystic changes are the most common of all benign breast conditions. Clinicians use the nonspecific term *fibrocystic change* to describe multiple irregularities in contour and cyclical painful breasts. The term *fibrocystic disease* is a misnomer and should not be used. Fibrocystic changes are a spectrum of change throughout a woman's reproductive age. The changes are different in different patients. Fibrocystic change has a prolific list of synonyms and terminology that includes well over 35 different names and terms.

The exact incidence of fibrocystic changes is difficult to establish. Franz and coworkers found histologic evidence of fibrocystic change in 53% of normal breasts examined in a series of 225 autopsies. Clinical evidence of fibrocystic change is discovered in breast examinations in approximately one in two premenopausal women. Some authors note that 90% of women have some aspect of fibrocystic change, depending again on the definition. Fibrocystic changes in this sense are an exaggeration of normal

physiologic response of breast tissue to the cyclic levels or ovarian hormones. However, no consistent abnormality of circulating hormone levels has been proved. The condition is most common in women between the ages of 20 and 50 and unusual after menopause unless associated with exogenous hormone use. Some postulate the cause to be a subtle imbalance of the ratio of estrogen to progesterone. Other researchers have postulated that fibrocystic changes are secondary to increased daily prolactin production. Some women with fibrocystic changes have enhanced prolactin production in response to thyroid-releasing hormone.

The classic symptom of fibrocystic changes is cyclic bilateral breast pain. The signs of fibrocystic change include increased engorgement and density of the breasts, excessive nodularity, rapid change and fluctuation in the size of cystic areas, increased tenderness, and occasionally spontaneous nipple discharge. Both signs and symptoms are more prevalent during the premenstrual phase of the cycle.

The breast pain of fibrocystic disease is bilateral and is often difficult for the patient to localize. The pain is most frequently located in the upper, outer quadrants of the breasts. Often the pain radiates to the shoulders and upper arms. Severe localized pain may occur when a simple cyst undergoes rapid expansion. The pathophysiology that produces these symptoms and signs

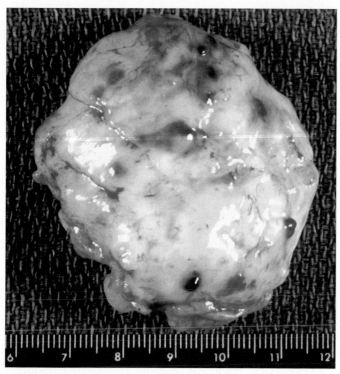

Figure 15-7 Breast biopsy from a 38 year-old woman demonstrating the characteristic gross appearance of fibrocystic changes. Note the multiple cysts interspersed between the dense fibrous connective tissue. (Courtesy of Fidel A Valea, MD.)

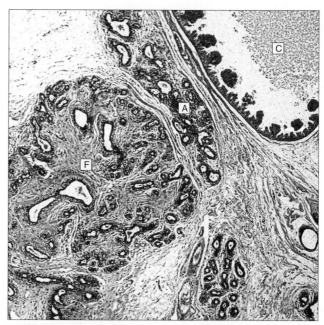

Figure 15-8 Fibrocystic changes from histologic section. Note: Fibrosis (F), adenomatous changes with increased ductal tissue (A), and cysts (C). (From Stevens A, Lowe J: Human Histology, 3 rd ed. Philadelphia, Elsevier Mosby, 2005, p 392.)

includes cyst formation, epithelial and fibrous proliferation, and varying degrees of fluid retention. The differential diagnosis of breast pain includes referred pain from a dorsal radiculitis or inflammation of the costal chondral junction (Tietze's syndrome). The latter two conditions have symptoms that are not cyclic and are unrelated to the menstrual cycle.

On physical examination the findings of excessive nodularity of fibrocystic changes have been described as similar to palpating the surface of a plateful of peas. Multiple solid areas are described as ill-defined thicknesses or areas of "palpable lumpiness" that are rubbery in consistency and may seem more two-dimensional than the three-dimensional mass usually associated with a carcinoma (**Fig. 15-7**). During palpation, the larger cysts have a consistency similar to a balloon filled with water.

There are three general clinical stages of fibrocystic change, with each stage having characteristic histologic findings. Clinically these stages have considerable overlap and variability. The stages are described to allow understanding of the condition's natural history. The first stage occurs in women in their 20s and is termed *mazoplasia* (mastoplasia). Breast pain is noted primarily in the upper, outer quadrants of the breast. The indurated axillary tail is in the most tender area of the breast. During this phase, there is intense proliferation of the stroma.

The second clinical stage of *adenosis* occurs generally in women in their 30s. The breast pain and tenderness are premenstrual but less severe. Multiple small breast nodules vary from 2 to 10 mm in diameter. The histologic picture of adenosis demonstrates marked proliferation and hyperplasia of ducts, ductules, and alveolar cells. The last stage is termed the *cystic* phase and usually occurs in women in their 40s. Breast cysts may occur

at any age. They are usually simple. Complex cysts are worrisome and require core-needle biopsy, whereas simple cysts may be managed with aspiration. There is no severe breast pain unless a cyst increases rapidly in size. In this situation, a woman experiences a sudden pain with point tenderness and discovers a lump. Cysts are tender to palpation and vary from microscopic to 5 cm in diameter. The cysts in fibrocystic changes often regress in size. The fluid aspirated from a large cyst is straw colored, dark brown, or green, depending on the chronicity of the cyst.

Women with a clinical diagnosis of fibrocystic changes have a wide variety of histopathologic findings. The histology of fibrocystic changes is characterized by proliferation and hyperplasia of the lobular, ductal, and acinar epithelium (**Fig. 15-8**). Usually proliferation of fibrous tissue occurs and accompanies epithelial hyperplasia. Many histologic variants of fibrocystic change have been described, including cysts (from microscopic to large, blue, domed cysts), adenosis (florid and sclerosing), fibrosis (periductal and stromal), duct ectasia, apocrine metaplasia, intraductal epithelial hyperplasia, and papillomatosis. Ductal epithelial hyperplasia with atypia and apocrine metaplasia with atypia are the most prominent histologic findings directly associated with the subsequent development of breast carcinoma. If either of these two conditions is discovered on breast biopsy, the chance of breast carcinoma in the future is approximately fivefold greater than in controls.

The management of fibrocystic change depends on a woman's age and includes appropriate imaging techniques. If there is a mass or uncertainty on an examination, then further evaluation for malignancy is indicated. There is a wide range of options for treating this condition, depending on the severity of symptoms, varying from mechanical support of the breast to GnRH therapy. The majority of symptoms can be controlled by medical therapy. Initial therapy of fibrocystic change consists of the patient wearing a sports bra that provides adequate support for the breasts both day and night. Diuretics during the premenstrual phase occasionally relieve breast discomfort. Some authors recommend reducing methylxanthine exposure, a compound found in coffee, tea, cola drinks, chocolate, and many nonprescription medications. However, four case control studies have found no association between caffeine or methylxanthine consumption and benign breast disease. Some patients do find that eliminating caffeine is effective, and trying this option is certainly inexpensive.

Oral contraceptives or supplemental progestins administered during the secretory phase of the cycle have also been used to treat fibrocystic changes. The symptomatology will recur in approximately 40% of women after they have discontinued the use of oral contraceptives. For severe symptoms, danazol is one of the most effective medications, relieving symptoms and decreasing nodularity of the breasts in approximately 90% of patients. Dosages of 100, 200, and 400 milligrams daily for 4 to 6 months have been employed. Therapy should not continue more than 6 months because side effects are common. Danazol should be tapered when it is being discontinued. The effects of danazol last for several months after discontinuation. Patients who do not respond to danazol may receive a trial of bromocriptine or tamoxifen. Bromocriptine is given continuously and works best in women with elevated prolactin levels. Tamoxifen may be given continuously or in the luteal phase. This selective estrogen receptor modifier may be effective but has some significant antiestrogen side effects. Women with cyclic breast pain seem to respond better than do those with chronic mastalgia.

Severe cyclic mastalgia has been associated with abnormal levels of certain essential fatty acids. Gately et al. reported the use of dietary supplementation with alpha linoleic acids and evening primrose oil, with a 58% response in women with cyclical mastalgia. On rare occasions women with severe fibrocystic changes are treated medically with gonadotropin releasing hormone (GnRH) agonists.

Numerous epidemiologic studies have found an increased risk of developing breast carcinoma in women with benign breast disease. Primarily these are women who have proliferative changes found on biopsy. When the proliferative changes are associated with atypical epithelial hyperplasia, the relative risk increases from two- to fivefold (depending on the degree of hyperplasia and the degree of atypia found on biopsy). The pathophysiology of the association between cellular atypia and subsequent carcinoma is straightforward and similar in concept to that seen in endometrial tissue. In a classic cohort study by DuPont and Page, the relationship between benign breast disease and subsequent development of carcinoma was shown in a group of 3000 women followed for 15 years after a benign breast biopsy. The study population was divided into three groups of women according to histology of the original biopsy. The first group, 70%, consisted of women whose biopsies revealed no proliferative changes and no atypia. Their diagnosis included adenosis, apocrine metaplasia, duct ectasia, and mild epithelial hyperplasia without atypia. During the 15 years of follow-up, only 2% of these women developed breast carcinoma. The second group of women, 26%, had breast biopsies that demonstrated varying degrees of epithelial hyperplasia, but no atypia. Of these women, 4% developed breast carcinoma during the 15 years. Their relative risk was increased 1.6. The last group consisted of the 4% of women with histology that demonstrated ductal hyperplasia with atypia or lobular hyperplasia with atypia.

Their relative risk was four to five times greater for developing malignancy. Eight percent of these women developed carcinoma during the 15-year follow-up. It is problematic to convert a relative risk in a study population to a person's lifetime cancer risk. For a woman with ductal hyperplasia with atypia, the lifetime risk increases from a 12% risk to a close to a 15% to 20% lifetime risk.

MASTALGIA (BREAST PAIN)

Breast pain occurs in over two thirds of women at some time in their reproductive years. It is most common in the perimenopausal years. Breast pain may be divided into cyclic pain, related to the menstrual cycle, and noncyclic pain. Cyclic pain is diffuse and bilateral and most commonly associated with fibrocystic changes. Noncyclic breast pain tends to be localized and most commonly is related to a cyst. Noncyclic breast pain should be evaluated, particularly in older women, as there is a small association with malignancy. Imaging, with mammography when indicated, is valuable. The differential diagnosis includes a cyst if the pain is focal, chest-wall pain, radicular pain, costochondritis, mastitis, pregnancy-related pain, prolactinomas, and medication exposure (**Box 15-1**). Laboratory values should include an hCG and prolactin in women prior to menopause. If a mass is detected with imaging, ultrasound is the next step. Breast cysts may be aspirated if they are simple. However, for a more complex cyst, a more detailed workup is necessary. Complex cysts should have a tissue diagnosis with core-needle biopsy. Pain as a presenting symptom of malignancy is uncommon, and without a mass or skin changes it is even more rare. The treatment is directed at the cause. If the pain is idiopathic, nonsteroidal anti-inflammatories are usually prescribed.

MASTITIS AND INFLAMMATORY DISEASE

Any inflammatory process or infectious agent may produce mastitis. Infection of the ductal systems or smaller sebaceous glands is most commonly related to *Staphylococcus aureus*. Empiric treatment when mastitis is found with an agent that covers Gram-positive organisms is appropriate. If there is poor response

---

Box 15-1 Medications Associated with Mastalgia

Antihypertensives
Atenolol and other beta-blockers
Hydrochlorothiazide
Methyldopa
Minoxidil
Spironolactone
Antidepressants and antipsychotic agents
Amitriptyline and other tricyclic antidepressants
Chlorpromazine/promethazine
Fluoxetine
Haloperidol
Hormonal agents
Estrogens
Progestins
Androgens
Ginseng
Clomiphene ditrate
Digoxin
Metochlorpropamide

to the initial course of antibiotics then cultures for methicillin-resistant *Staphylococcus aureus* (MRSA) should be performed and an agent such as a quinine or sulfamethoxazole (trimethoprim) is indicated. These two agents are contraindicated if a woman is pregnant or lactating. Curiously, mastitis in pregnancy usually responds to first-line antibiotics such as a cephalosporin, even in the presence of MRSA. Nonpuerperal mastitis is often associated with breast cysts. Tests for diabetes and HIV may be indicated if yeast is found in nonpuerperal mastitis. Syphilis, tuberculosis, atypical bacterial, and fungal infections may also cause nonpuerperal mastitis. Nipple piercing is associated with mastitis and abscess formation. As with any infection, the foreign body should be removed when treating piercing-related infections. The American College of Obstetricians and Gynecologists recommends counseling women who are planning to have piercing to obtain hepatitis-B vaccine and tetanus vaccine prior.

Inflammatory processes in older women include the possibility of inflammatory carcinoma and are discussed later in the chapter. A rare cause for inflammation is idiopathic granulomatous mastitis (IGM), also called idiopathic granulomatous lobular mastitis (IGLM). This disease may present with a mass, abscess, as well as inflammation and granuloma formation. The granulomas are often found within the lobules and on biopsy are noted to be sterile. Mammography may be equivocal or may be suspicious for malignancy. However, the disease itself, because of the granulomatous formation, is fairly obvious on biopsy. The disease may affect any age group but is most common in women in their fourth to sixth decade. Diagnosis is made by biopsy, preferably core-needle biopsy. The biopsy is often performed after a lack of response to empiric antibiotics. A course of steroids has been used for idiopathic granulomatous mastitis with equivocal results. Sometimes a prolonged course of antibiotics of 3 to 6 months is necessary. The disease is usually self-limited, resolving within months. Skin scarring and residual small abscesses may remain, necessitating surgical treatment. Chronic inflammatory disease, such as lupus, sarcoid, and Wegner's granulomatosis, are rare causes of noninfectious mastitis, and evaluation for these diseases should be performed if antibiotics are not effective. Inflammation not responsive to antibiotics warrants a tissue diagnosis.

NIPPLE DISCHARGE

Nipple discharges are common and represent 7% of physician visits for breast complaints. Nipple discharge is classified as spontaneous or elicited. Elicited discharges arise when the breast is compressed or stimulated. Three quarters of women may have elicited discharge up to 2 years after breast-feeding. Half of premenopausal women have some type of elicited discharge at some time. If the discharge is bilateral and from multiple ducts and is elicited, then it is considered physiologic and does not need further evaluation unless there is a mass or the woman is postmenopausal. In contrast, spontaneous discharge, a discharge that is bloody, or a discharge from one to two ducts does need further evaluation. The evaluation is physical examination and mammography.

Spontaneous discharge from multiple ducts is called galactorrhea and generally represents a systemic rather than a local process. Galactorrhea is discussed in Chapter 39. Many medications and diseases will affect the hypothalamic-pituitary axis and lead to prolactin secretion and galactorrhea. Spontaneous

discharge from one nipple and only a few ducts is also pathologic and needs evaluation with examination and imaging. History may not be adequate to differentiate spontaneous discharge from elicited discharge. When a woman first notices her discharge, she may keep trying to express it and this will cause more fluid to leak.

The first step in evaluation and diagnosis is separating discharges into spontaneous and those that only appear with expression. Expressed discharges that are milky and clearly nonbloody are separated from those that are potentially bloody. Nipple discharges range in color, from white and milky to green, brown, or bloody. Hemoccult testing of the discharge may be used to detect occult blood. Any bloody discharges or any discharge associated with a mass needs further workup to exclude malignancy. Spontaneous discharges are separated into those from both breasts and multiple alveoli. If the discharge is found to come from only one or two adjacent ducts, then further workup is indicated and malignancy must be excluded. Management of discharge from one or two ducts is mammography and ductography, which is employed at this step. The most common cause of a bloody discharge is **intraductal papilloma**.

Intraductal papilloma and fibrocystic changes are the two most common causes of spontaneous nonmilky discharge. Malignancies have been associated with all colors of discharge. However, bloody nipple discharge should be considered to be related to carcinoma until the diagnosis has been excluded. Cytology of the discharge is reasonable to obtain but is rarely diagnostic. Most series document a false negative rate of 20%. Therefore, negative cytology does not help, nor should it deter further imaging and surgical evaluation.

INTRADUCTAL PAPILLOMA

Intraductal papillomas are small papillomas of the glandular tissue of the milk duct. The classic symptom of intraductal papilloma is spontaneous bloody discharge from one nipple and one or a few ducts. Most commonly it presents in women in the perimenopausal age group, but it may present at any age. The discharge from the nipple is spontaneous and intermittent. The consistency of the discharge associated with intraductal papilloma can be watery, serous, or serosanguineous. The amount of discharge varies from a few drops to several milliliters of fluid. Approximately 75% of intraductal papillomas are located beneath the areola. Often these tumors are difficult to palpate because they are small and soft. They typically measure 1 to 3 mm in diameter. During examination of the breast it is important to circumferentially put radial pressure on different areas of the areola. This technique helps to identify whether the discharge emanates from a single duct or multiple openings. When the discharge comes from a single duct, the differential diagnosis involves both intraductal papilloma and carcinoma. Women with these symptoms should have both mammogram and a special study to evaluate the affected duct, called ductography. Ductography, or sonography of the duct, is the most useful diagnostic test for suspected papilloma **Figure 15-9**. The involved duct may be evaluated by cannulation and the injection of contrast material into the duct with a small catheter.

Treatment of intraductal papilloma is excisional biopsy of the involved duct and a small amount of surrounding tissue. Although these tumors tend to regress in postmenopausal women, they should be excised. In one series, women with a solitary

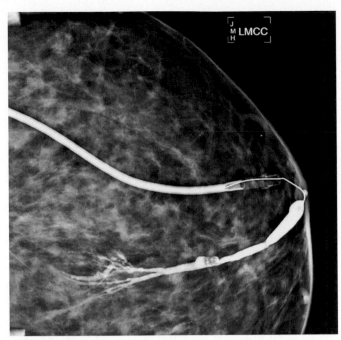

Figure 15-9 Ductogram of an intraductal papilloma. (Courtesy of Cathryn Chicola, MD.)

papilloma showed an approximately twofold increase in subsequent development of breast carcinoma.

FIBROEPITHELIAL TUMORS: FIBROADENOMAS AND PHYLLODES TUMORS

Breast neoplasms, both benign and malignant, may be divided into those arising from ductal and glandular elements, and neoplasias arising from breast stroma and fibrous supporting tissue. The former represent 99% of malignancies, the latter present more commonly in younger women. The stromal or fibroepithelial neoplasms represent a spectrum that includes on one end the very common **fibroadenomas** and on the other end the rare **phyllodes tumors**.

Fibroadenomas are the most common benign neoplasm of the breast. They are firm, freely mobile, solid, and usually solitary breast masses. Fibroadenomas most frequently present in adolescents and women in their 20s. Typically, a young woman discovers a painless mass accidentally while bathing. Growth of the mass is usually slow but may be quite rapid. Fibroadenomas do not change in size with the menstrual cycle and rarely produce breast pain or tenderness. Approximately 30% of fibroadenomas will disappear, and 10% to 12% become smaller when followed for many years. The long-term risk of invasive breast cancer in women with fibroadenomas is approximately twice that for women without fibroadenomas. Women with fibroadenomas should be made aware of this risk and encouraged to maintain annual mammographic screening, commencing at age 40.

The average fibroadenoma is 2.5 cm in diameter. Multiple fibroadenomas are discovered in 15% to 20% of patients. After surgical removal, fibroadenomas recur in approximately 20% of women. Sometimes it is difficult to distinguish a fibroadenoma from a cyst. Complex cysts and any cysts with solid areas should be biopsied or excised. Mammography is rarely indicated in a woman with fibroadenomas younger than 35. However, ultrasound is helpful in differentiating a solid from a cystic mass. If the cause of the mass cannot be established, core-needle biopsy is indicated. Regardless of age, any mass that rapidly increases in size should be surgically evaluated. Any solid mass in women over 35 should be evaluated. Fibroadenomas can be removed without difficulty under local anesthesia. They are rubbery in consistency, well circumscribed, and easily delineated from surrounding breast tissue (**Fig. 15-10**). Nonoperative management is appropriate for small fibroadenomas discovered in women younger than 35 if three separate clinical parameters support the diagnosis of fibroadenoma. The three parameters (the triple test) are clinical exam, imaging evaluation (either mammogram or ultrasound), and biopsy (usually core-needle). The characteristic features of a fibroadenoma are found in approximately 95% of all fibroadenomas. Thus, conservative management can be considered with follow-up every 6 months. The only way to distinguish a fibroadenoma from a malignancy is with a histologic evaluation. Despite the option of conservative management of a fibroadenoma, many women prefer to have the lesion excised.

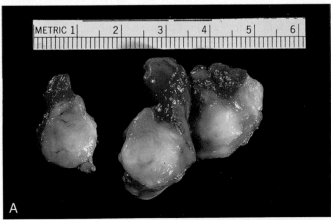
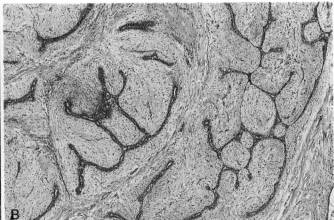

Figure 15-10 A, Fibroadenoma with characteristic tan, well-circumscribed nodule. **B,** Histologic section of fibroadenoma with epithelial cells surrounded by loose mesenchymal fibrous tissue. (From Voet RL: Color Atlas of Obstetric and Gynecologic Pathology. St Louis, Mosby-Wolfe, 1997, p 204.)

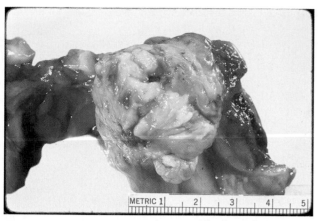

Figure 15-11 Phyllodes tumor with leaflike projections within the fleshy mass. (From Voet RL: Color Atlas of Obstetric and Gynecologic Pathology. St Louis, Mosby-Wolfe, 1997, p 205.)

On the other end of the spectrum of fibroepithelial tumors of the breast are the phyllodes tumors. The old name for these neoplasms was *Cystosarcoma phyllodes*, a misnomer. Phyllodes tumors are divided into benign, borderline, and malignant types. All three types usually present as a mass. Histologically, the stromal elements dominate and will invade the ducts in leafy projection, hence the name phyllodes, or "leaf" (**Fig. 15-11**). The phyllodes tumors may be locally aggressive. The treatment of these tumors is excision with a wide margin of normal tissue. The presence of microscopic tumor at the margins of the excised specimen is the major factor in predicting whether there will be a local recurrence of the tumor. Less than 25% of malignant phyllodes tumors metastasize. However, local recurrence is common, even with benign and borderline tumors. Phyllodes tumors are fibroepithelial breast tumors with hypercellularity of the connective tissue as the distinctive feature. These tumors are rare, representing only 2.5% of fibroepithelial tumors and less than 1% of breast malignancies. They usually present as a mass similar to a fibroadenoma and are most commonly found in the fourth and fifth decades of life. They may grow rapidly and often are larger at diagnosis than fibroadenoma or ductal carcinoma. The differentiation of benign from malignant types is by histologic criteria.

A rare neoplasm of stromal elements of the breast is the myofibroblastoma, which is a benign disease. This is best managed with excisional biopsy rather than needle biopsy.

FAT NECROSIS

Fat necrosis is a rare but important cause of a breast mass or suspicious mammographic finding that is often confused with carcinoma. The patient will most commonly present with a firm, tender, indurated, ill-defined mass that may have an area of surrounding ecchymosis. Sometimes the area of fat necrosis liquefies and becomes cystic in consistency. Mammography may demonstrate fine, stippled calcification and stellate contractions. Occasionally there is skin retraction, which further confuses the prebiopsy diagnosis. The usual cause of fat necrosis is trauma. However, the majority of women do not remember the event that injured the breast. Treatment of fat necrosis is excisional biopsy. There is no relationship between fat necrosis and subsequent breast carcinoma.

BREAST CARCINOMA

Breast carcinoma is the most common malignancy of women and is one of the two leading causes of all cancer deaths in women. One in eight women (12.5% of American women) will develop carcinoma of the breast. The incidence of breast cancer in the United States has been relatively stable since the 1980s. There has been an important reduction in breast cancer mortality in recent years. Since 1989, death rates from breast cancer have declined an average of 1.8% per year. The importance of early detection and diagnosis of breast carcinoma cannot be overemphasized. An increase in public awareness combined with recent improvements in mammography and newer imaging techniques have facilitated earlier detection of breast carcinoma. Earlier detection, combined with improvements with therapy, has resulted in improved survival rates. With the advent of chemoprevention in the high-risk woman, there is an opportunity to alter the natural course of the disease. The majority of women in whom breast cancer is diagnosed will not die of the disease.

Breast carcinoma generally presents in one of two ways. A woman may present with symptoms, usually a mass. The second presentation is when the tumor is found on screening evaluation. Screening includes breast self-examination, examination by a health provider (referred to as clinical breast examination), and imaging. The best time in a woman's life to start imaging, and at what intervals, is individualized for each woman and based on her risk factors. To calculate the risk, it is important to understand the epidemiology of breast cancer. There are several models that help assess a patient's risk. If no risk factors are noted, she is said to be at average or normal risk, corresponding to the 12%, or 1 in 8, risk for a woman of developing breast malignancy over her lifetime. Thus, the message to every woman in the United States is that she is at risk for breast carcinoma. Because a woman's risk may change as her family history evolves and new findings occur on imaging, risk assessment should be ongoing.

This section of the chapter moves from epidemiology and risk assessment to screening and diagnostic modalities, to treatment, and finally to the significant role of the gynecologist.

EPIDEMIOLOGY AND RISKS FOR BREAST CANCER

Like all malignancies, breast cancer is caused by a progressive accumulation of mutations in the cell's DNA. Epidemiologic studies help identify factors that through either exposure or inheritance place a woman at risk for a greater chance of cellular change. Obvious examples are inherited mutations in the DNA repair system, such as the *BRCA* gene, or radiation exposures. The degree of risk is important to know in order to advise women and establish plans for screening or interventions.

Epidemiologic literature, reporting breast cancer risks, usually describes the risk from any given factor as a relative risk, the risk compared with subjects in a control group who do not have the exposure (see Chapter 6). In contrast, clinical and genetic studies usually report results as a woman's lifetime risk. This can become confusing for patients and families. For example, the *BRCA* mutation causes a 10 times increase in relative risk and up to an 85% lifetime risk. The clinician must keep this in mind both when reading the literature and importantly

Table 15-1 Risk Factors for Breast Cancer

Risk Factor	Qualification
Demographic—minor (less than 5 × RR)	
Age	Rare under age 30, common in sixth and eighth decades
Geographic	Common in Western countries
Estrogen exposures—minor	
Age at menarche	Younger than 12 years old
Age at first birth	Over 30 years old
Late menopause	
Hormone replacement therapy	
Lifestyle—minor	
Alcohol use	Dose related (two or more drinks daily)
Sedentary lifestyle	
Obesity	
Postmenopausal weight gain	
Low vitamin D	
Abnormal day/night work patterns (airline attendants and variable shifts)	
Breast characteristics—minor	
Benign breast disease	Very low increase on risk
Hyperplasia without atypia on biopsy	
Breast characteristics—major (increasing a woman's risk > 5 × RR)	Major factors usually push a woman into the high-risk category
Dense breasts	Density proportional to increase in risk Increased fibroglandular elements
Hyperplasia with atypia	
Previous breast cancer	
Familial factors—minor	
Multiple relatives, not first-degree, with breast cancer	
One first-degree relative with breast cancer	First-degree—mother or sister
Family history—major	
Two or more first-degree relatives	Increased risk if the cancers are premenopausal
Inherited breast cancer syndrome such as *BRCA*	Very high risk
Radiation—minor	
Exposure to chest CT	
Radiation—major	
Mantle radiation for treatment of malignancy	Very high risk, which increases with age

Table 15-2 Factors Associated with a Decreased Risk for Breast Cancer

Demographic	Qualification
Born and living outside Western countries	
Estrogen exposures	
Late menarche	After age 14
Oophorectomy	Prior to age 35 without supplemental estrogen
Lactation	Proportional to total cumulative months breast feeding
Age of first birth	Prior to age 20
Parity	5 or greater
Induced abortion	Trend (5 < p < 0.1)
Lifestyle	
Postmenopausal body mass	Minimal postmenopausal weight gain
Physical activity	
Dietary	
Vitamin D	Low levels associated with risk
Intake of vitamin D	Associated with decreased risk
Olive oil/ and omega 3 fatty acids	
Low-fat diet	Results suggestive but not yet conclusive
Medications	
Aspirin	Associated with decreased incidence, recurrence, and mortality

DEMOGRAPHIC ASSOCIATIONS

A woman's age is the strongest risk factor for developing breast cancer. The frequency of breast carcinoma increases directly with the patient's age (**Box 15-2**). Breast carcinoma is almost nonexistent before puberty; the incidence gradually increases during the reproductive years. Eighty-five percent of breast carcinoma occurs after age 40. After menopause the incidence per year increases into the 70s, and then declines.

Variations are found in the incidence of breast carcinoma depending on geographic variables. Women living in the United States have the highest rates of breast carcinoma followed by women in Western Europe and Australia. Women in Eastern Europe, South Africa, Japan, and the Caribbean form a middle group in terms of incidence. The lowest incidences are found in Middle and Eastern Africa, and Central Asia. The incidence of breast carcinoma in American women is six times greater than that for women in Japan. Interestingly, studies of Japanese women who move to the United States demonstrate that their rate of breast carcinoma becomes similar to that of American women after two generations. Epidemiologic studies within the same culture have demonstrated differences in incidences of breast cancer relating directly to the amount of fat in the diet.

In the United States, Caucasians have an increased incidence of breast cancer compared with women of color. Data through 2005 noted a risk in African-American women of 118 per 100,000 for developing malignancy versus 133 per 100,000 for Caucasian women. African-American and Latina women, though, have a higher mortality. This difference may be due to several factors that include both socioeconomic as well the histologic variety of tumors. Black and Latina women tend to have a higher incidence of receptor-negative tumors, which are more aggressive, quicker to metastasize, and usually higher grade.

when counseling patients and their families. In the following discussion, risk refers to relative risk compared with a control group, unless stated as a woman's lifetime or personal risk.

The risk factors for breast cancer may be divided into several categories (**Table 15-1**): demographic, estrogen exposure, lifestyle, personal breast characteristics, familial and inherited genetic mutations, and radiation exposure. Risk is generally grouped as minor and major. Minor risk factors increase a woman's lifetime risk from 12% to approximately 15%. Importantly, epidemiologic studies have also noted factors that decrease a woman's risk (**Table 15-2**).

By Age	
25	1 in 19,608
30	1 in 2525
35	1 in 622
40	1 in 217
45	1 in 93
50	1 in 50
55	1 in 33
60	1 in 24
65	1 in 17
70	1 in 14
75	1 in 11
80	1 in 10
85	1 in 9
Ever	1 in 8

Data from National Cancer Institute. Painter K: Factoring in cost of mammograms. USA Today, p 11D, December 5, 1996.

ESTROGEN-RELATED EXPOSURE RISKS

The relationship between endogenous ovarian hormones and breast cancer has been studied extensively. Estrogens are considered tumor promoters rather than inducers or initiators of carcinoma. Thus, the adverse effects are seen to increase with duration of use, and a dose-response curve can be recognized. There are multiple empiric data indicating that the longer and greater the exposure to estrogens, the higher the risks of breast cancer. Breast cancer is most unusual in the prepubertal female. Bilateral oophorectomy before age 35 without hormone replacement reduces a woman' risk of breast cancer by 70%. Women who have breast cancer and undergo oophorectomy have a lower recurrence rate. Interestingly, the rate of recurrence in oophorectomized women is decreased, even in those women with hormone-receptor-negative cancers. Women have a relative risk of breast cancer 100 times greater than that of men. Obese women are at a higher risk for developing breast cancer during their postmenopausal years, with increased amounts of peripheral conversion of androstenedione to estrone.

Marchant and coworkers described an increased risk associated with prolonged menstrual function. Women with spontaneous menopause before age 45 experienced half the relative risk of developing breast cancer when compared with women who were menstruating at age 54. A similar study documented a twofold increase in the risk of breast cancer for women who menstruated for 40 years or longer, contrasted with women who menstruated for 30 years or less. The age at which a woman delivers her first child is a more important risk factor than parity. If a woman's first term birth occurs before age 20 she has a 50% lower relative risk compared with a nulliparous woman. If her first pregnancy occurs after age 35, the risk is 1.5 times greater than that of a woman whose first birth was before age 26. Nursing offers a protective effect for the future development of breast neoplasia. A systematic review of studies involving 50,300 women with breast cancer and 96,900 controls found a direct correlation between the length of time of lactation and decreasing risk for breast malignancy. Personal risk decreased by 4.3% per 12 months of breast-feeding. This relationship held strongly, even when parity, ethnicity, age of menarche and menopause,

and geographic factors are taken into consideration. Newcomb and colleagues reported that after adjusting for parity, age at first delivery, and other confounding factors, lactation was associated with a slight reduction in the risk of breast cancer among premenopausal women compared with those who had never lactated (RR 0.78 [CI 0.6 to 0.91]). Overall, breast-feeding decreases the risk of breast cancer in a dose-response relationship.

Oral contraceptives and other forms of estrogen-related contraception are a constant source of concern for patients. Multiple studies have noted that the oral contraceptives used since the 1980s do not pose an increased risk compared to the extremely high levels of estrogen used in oral contraceptives in the 1960s and 1970s. Abortion has been shown to not affect breast cancer incidence. A recent prospective cohort by Michels et al. of 105,715 women found no association between induced abortion or spontaneous abortion and the risk of developing breast cancer. A trend for a decreased risk of breast cancer was seen RR 0.89 (CI 0.78 to 1.01). The lack of association held for number of abortions, age at abortion, and timing of abortion.

Epidemiologic studies have produced conflicting results on the effect of hormonal replacement of estrogen and breast cancer risk. Although studies have noted an increased risk with exogenous estrogen, this risk is quantitatively less than that associated with either postmenopausal obesity or alcohol consumption. Shier and colleagues concluded that current and recent users of an estrogen/progesterone regimen had a slightly increased risk of breast cancer compared with that of a woman using estrogen alone. The Women's Health Initiative (WHI), which studied women receiving hormone replacement therapy initiated after menopause, found an increased risk of breast cancer, RR 1.24 (CI 1.02 to 1.5), in women taking both estrogen and progesterone compared with controls. Women who took estrogen without progesterone had a slightly decreased risk of breast cancer, 0.8 (CI 0.62 to 1.04). A summary of the WHI results by Chlebowski et al. noted the increased risk with combined estrogen and progesterone declined quickly after hormone replacement was stopped. The decision to use hormone replacement therapy in patients with and without other risk factors should be individualized and the risks and benefits discussed so that the woman may make an informed decision.

LIFESTYLE AND DIETARY RISK FACTORS

The relationship among diet, weight, and breast cancer is thought to be related to endogenous estrogens. Multiple studies have noted a relationship between dietary fat and malignancy. Studies from Great Britain found an association with decreased incidence of breast cancer associated with decreased meat consumption. High consumption of olive oil modestly reduces breast cancer risk. Overall the affects of dietary fat are mild, and large population based studies do not show major affects. In the WHI study of postmenopausal women, the dietary arm of the study evaluated 48,800 women who tried to reduce fat intake. There was a minimal effect on decreasing malignancy in the breast, RR 0.91 (CI 0.83 to 1.01). The Nurse's Health Study failed to show an association between dietary fat and the risk of breast cancer, but confounders in this study make the data problematic. When studies such as the WHI and the Nurse's Health Study are given systematic review, decreased dietary fat does appear to confer a mildly improved risk for breast cancer.

Increasing BMI confers increased risk. Indeed, the lifestyle modifications that have been shown to induce the greatest risk reduction have been the avoidance of weight gain in adulthood and maintaining a stable weight after menopause. Body fat and weight gain in the perimenopausal period and weight gain after menopause have each been independently associated with an increased risk for breast cancer (see **Table 15-1**). In the Nurse's Health Study, women who gained 10 or more kilograms after menopause increased their personal risk by 18%. The effects of obesity are more pronounced in postmenopausal women when malignancies are overwhelmingly more estrogen-receptor positive, compared with premenopausal women in which tumor types are mixed. Exercise is associated with a decreased risk of breast cancer, but the effect cannot be well quantified because of body mass index (BMI) as a confounder.

Recent studies also have found a significant association with decreased levels of vitamin D and decreased calcium and increased risks of breast cancer and increased morbidity once breast cancer is diagnosed. A large case-control study of 6500 women noted that vitamin D, at least at the level of the adult requirement of 400 IU/day, decreased breast cancer risk by 25%, (CI 0.59 to 0.98). The association of increased bone density and increased breast cancer is again thought to be related to increased exogenous estrogens. Antioxidant supplementation has not been shown to be protective for breast cancer. However, several small studies and a nested study from the WHI noted aspirin to decrease risk for breast cancer, breast cancer recurrence, and breast cancer mortality.

Ingestion of garlic and garlic extracts does not seem to decrease the risk of cancer, despite a flurry of public reports. Caffeine does not affect the risk of breast cancer. Alcohol consumption has been associated with breast cancer risk. Older studies reported a 40% to 50% increase in the relative risk of developing breast cancer related to alcohol consumption. The alcohol effect was primarily in estrogen-receptor–positive tumors. Longnecker showed that the risk of breast cancer was strongly related to the amount of alcohol consumed and that even light drinking was associated with a 10% increase in relative risk. In contrast, Zhang reported that light consumption of alcohol was not associated with an increased risk of breast cancer. At the present time the effects of light consumption of alcohol on breast cancer risk is uncertain.

Phytoestrogens are weak estrogens from plant sources and are a subject of great interest because of the relationship between endogenous estrogen and malignancy. Theoretically, phytoestrogens such as soy proteins might increase breast cancer incidence by stimulating estrogen receptors or may possibly decrease risk by acting as an agonist and inhibiting estrogen binding. Most all phytoestrogens affect estrogen receptors, but soy estrogens, for example, are approximately 1000 times weaker than estradiol. Soy tends to show an agonist activity, whereas most other phytoestrogens show antagonist activity. This is important because some phytoestrogens like *genistein* antagonize tamoxifen. No study has found an increased risk, and some studies (with significant confounders and internal bias) have shown decreased risk with dietary exposure to phytoestrogens. To date, meta-analysis and reports from a National Institutes of Health Consensus Conference have not shown any protective effect, but just as important, no detrimental effect from ingestion of phytoestrogens has been noted either.

Multiple miscellaneous environmental exposures have been studied for possible associations with breast cancer incidence. Breast implants do not increase the risk for breast cancer. Magnetic radiation, power lines, computer terminals, and electric blanket exposure do not increase the risk of breast cancer. Nonsteroidal anti-inflammatory drugs and aspirin may decrease the risk of breast cancer. Megdal et al. found in a meta-analysis that altered day/night exposure, shift work, and increased light exposures to show an increased risk of breast cancer, RR 1.48 (CI 1.36 to 1.61). Thus, airline attendants, for example, with changes in their light exposure as well as variable shifts, are at increased risk for breast cancer.

BREAST HISTORY AND BREAST CHARACTERISTICS

Previous history of breast disease is an important risk factor. Although the risk varies between premenopausal and postmenopausal women with breast cancer, once the patient has developed carcinoma of one breast, her risk is approximately 1% per year of developing cancer in the other breast. Dense breasts, as defined by more fibrous tissue, have been found by Boyd et al. to have a relative risk of 4.7 (CI 2 to 6.2) for breast cancer (**Fig. 15-12**). This finding has been verified in other studies, and the increased risk is not due to a more difficult or later diagnosis but to the biologic characteristics of the breast itself. There is a mild increase in risk when biopsies have shown hyperplasia, but hyperplasia with atypia increases the risk by four to six orders of magnitude. Some studies have found a slight increase in relative risk with benign breast change, but the increase is small.

INHERITED AND FAMILIAL RISKS

Approximately 15% to 20% of breast cancers are associated with a familial or inherited risk. (Thus, 80% to 85% of women who will develop breast cancer have no significant familial risk factors.) About a quarter of familial cancers, 5% to 7% of all breast cancers, are due to a specific inherited gene mutation. There are at least four specific breast cancer syndromes, each associated with a specific mutation. All four of these diseases involve mutations in the proteins that repair DNA, and all are autosomal dominant. By far the most common are the mutations in the *BRCA* 1 and 2 genes. Less common are Li-Fraumeni syndrome, associated with the p53 gene, and Cowden syndrome, associated with the PTEN gene (**Table 15-3**).

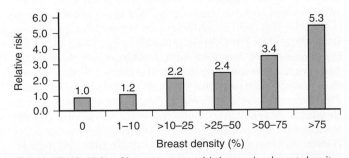

Figure 15-12 Risks of breast cancer with increasing breast density. (Adapted from Santen RJ and Mansel R: Benign breast disorders. N Engl J Med 355:279, 2005.)

Table 15-3 Major Inherited Gene Mutation Syndromes associated with Breast Cancer

Syndrome	Gene	Incidence	Lifetime Breast Cancer Risk	Associated Cancer Risks
BRCA 1	BRCA 1	1/500 to 1/1000	85%	Ovary and pancreas
BRCA 2	BRCA 2	Unclear	85%	Ovary and pancreas
Cowden	PTEN	1/100,000 to 1/200,000	50%	Thyroid and endometrium
Li-Fraumeni	TP53	1/20,000	90%	Sarcoma, brain, and leukemia

Other syndromes, including Petz/Jeghers, Ataxia Telengectasia, CHEK 2, and Fanconi, have much smaller lifetime risks with poorer penetrance.

The *BRCA* genes code for very large tumor suppressor proteins. *BRCA*-1 has 1863 amino acids, with several different functions, the most important of which are DNA repair and control of cell cycle checkpoints. This genomic instability of women with *BRCA* mutations causes them to be more susceptible to further mutations of DNA, which subsequently leads to malignant transformation of breast and ovarian epithelial cells. *BRCA*-1 was mapped at chromosome 17, and in 1994 Miki and colleagues determined the DNA sequence. *BRCA*-1 positivity confers a lifetime risk of breast cancer of approximately 85% and an average lifetime risk of ovarian cancer approaching 40% (but this is variable, depending on the location of the mutation on the *BRCA* gene).

The *BRCA*-2 gene was mapped to chromosome 13, and the DNA sequence determined by Schutte and coworkers in 1995. Women with a *BRCA*-2 gene mutation have up to an 85% lifetime risk of breast cancer and a 15% to 20% lifetime risk of ovarian cancer. The *BRCA*-2 mutations are also associated with male breast cancers, conferring a 5% to 10% risk for a man who has inherited the mutation. Because male breast cancer is so rare, any male with breast cancer should be tested for a *BRCA* mutation. More than 2500 different types of mutations have been described within the large gene, leading to differing penetrance for clinical disease. Women with genetic syndromes tend to develop breast cancer at earlier ages and tend to have more aggressive tumors with a higher prevalence of bilateral disease. Though the incidence of *BRCA* mutation is 1:250 in the United States, the incidence of the mutation is higher in certain ethnic groups. For Ashkenazi Jews, the risk is 2.5%, half of which will be *BRCA*-1 and half of which is *BRCA*-2. In Norwegians, Dutch, and Icelanders, the risk is 6 per thousand for *BRCA*-2.

BRCA-1 mutations are associated with particularly high-grade, hormone-receptor–negative tumors in younger women. In fact one of the considerations for gene testing is the development of a hormone-receptor–negative tumor in a premenopausal woman. *BRCA*-2 associated tumors are more homogenous in cell type and receptor expressivity. Between 65% and 80% are estrogen-receptor–positive, similar to the general population. In addition to the almost 90% lifetime risk for breast cancer in women with *BRCA* genes, there is also a 50% to 64% risk of developing cancer in the contralateral breast prior to age 70. Interestingly, approximately

10% to 30% of women with breast cancer who do not have the *BRCA* gene as an inherited mutation are later found to have developed tumor cells that have mutations in the *BRCA* gene, pointing out its important role in DNA repair.

Other than the inherited cancer syndromes from the specific gene mutations, about 15% of breast cancers are related to familial risk. Women in such families have a combination of low penetrance polygenic inheritance contributing to their personal risk. Familial risk increases a woman's chance of cancer by up to 20%+ over her lifetime when she has several first-degree relatives with cancer. The risk increases for a woman the more relatives she has with breast cancer. Risk increases when the cancers occur in younger women. Models that will predict a woman's breast cancer risk are discussed later.

Studies of breast cancer in twins have produced interesting findings. Verikasale et al., in a cohort study, found monozygotic twins have a decreased risk of breast cancer compared with non-twins, RR 0.76 (CI 0.58 to 1.0), whereas dizygotic twins have similar risks to the general population. What factor leads to protection for identical twins is unknown. Mack et al. found that in dizygotic twins in which one sister had breast cancer, the other twin's risk was similar to the familial risk of a first-degree relative with breast cancer. In their study, that risk was 1.7 (CI 1.1 to 2.6). However, if a monozygotic twin has breast cancer, the other twin's risk is increased 4.4 times (CI 3.6 to 5.6). This is six times higher than first-degree relatives and approaches the relative risk of a woman with a *BRCA* mutation. It is also similar to the risk of a woman who has breast cancer of developing cancer in the contralateral breast.

RADIATION EXPOSURE

Ionizing radiation is an important risk factor, because of the relationship between radiation and malignant transformation of cellular DNA. The first evidence of a radiation effect was noted in Japanese women who survived the atomic bombs. Breast carcinoma developed in a very high incidence when exposed teenagers reached their 30s. Additionally, women who received multiple radiation treatments for postpartum mastitis, irradiation of the thymus in infancy, or multiple fluoroscopic examinations during treatment for tuberculosis were found to have subsequently developed breast carcinoma at an increased rate. Fortunately, those treatments have long since been abandoned. The data associating the increased risk of developing breast carcinoma are consistent with a linear dose-response relationship. Currently, women at highest risk from radiation exposure are those who were treated with radiation for childhood malignancies, in particular Hodgkin's lymphoma. These women are given "mantle" whole upper body radiation therapy. They have over a 30% incidence of breast cancer by age 55. That risk steadily increases as the woman continues to age. This risk is at the same level as that for women with the *BRCA* gene. On the other end of the spectrum are women who have received chest CT scans. One 64-slice chest CT adds to a woman's lifetime risk of breast cancer by a little under 1%.

RISK ASSESSMENT AND PREVENTION

Breast cancer risk should be evaluated on an ongoing basis throughout a woman's life. The 35-year-old woman's risk may be low; however, by the time she is 50, besides her increase

Table 15-4 Risk Levels for the Development of Breast Cancer

Level	Lifetime Risk for Breast Cancer	Recommendations for Screening
Average	12%	Yearly exams and mammograms beginning at age 40
Moderate	12% to 15%	Yearly exams and mammography beginning at age 40
High	15% to 20%	Yearly exams and mammography beginning at age 40; offer chemoprevention
Very high risk	>20%	Exams every 6 months; mammography alternating with MRI should be started on an individualized basis depending on the risk factor (e.g., for women with mantle radiation, imaging should begin at age 30 or 8 years after radiation is finished); offer chemoprevention

Box 15-3 Indications for Referral for Genetic Counseling for *BRCA* Gene Testing

Personal history of both breast and ovarian cancer
Personal history of ovarian cancer or premenopausal breast cancer and Ashkenazi Jewish ancestry
First-degree male relative with breast cancer
Personal history of premenopausal breast cancer, particularly if it is triple negative
Personal history of breast cancer and two first-degree relatives with breast cancer, any ages
Personal history of high grace serous ovarian cancer (also primary peritoneal or fallopian tube cancers)

Adapted and modified from ACOG Practice Bulletin: Hereditary breast and ovarian cancer syndromes. Obstet Gynecol 113:957, 2009.

in age, she may have had an older sister who has developed breast cancer. A woman's risk for developing breast cancer will influence the recommendations for both her screening as well as for preventive measures such as chemoprevention with SERM medications. By evaluating a woman's risk factors, her chances for malignancy may be estimated. The risk factors that influence a woman's chances of developing a malignancy are multifactorial, and thus individualized counseling is the most effective approach to evaluating risk.

Risk factors can be divided into (1) major factors that increase relative risk greater than two times normal and (2) minor factors (see **Table 15-1**). A women's personal risk of developing breast cancer is divided into three levels with the third level, high risk, often subdivided into very high risk for purposes of prophylactic options (**Table 15-4**). Women of average risk have a personal risk of about 12% of developing breast cancer, the risk of the general population. Moderate risk includes women with one or more minor risk factors. These women have personal risks from 12% to 15% of developing breast malignancy over their lifetime. Importantly, women in the moderate risk category do not need any changes from those of the general population in screening recommendations. Women at high risk include those who have greater than a 15% personal risk of developing breast cancer, usually from a major risk factor. Many clinicians further separate out a very high risk category, those women with a personal risk over 25%, such as women with a *BRCA* mutation or women who have had mantle radiation. They are often referred to breast specialists for ongoing evaluation.

Several models have been empirically developed to estimate a woman's risk of breast cancer. The most accepted model is the Gail model, developed by Dr. Mitchell Gail in 1989. He used data from the Breast Cancer Detection and Demonstration Project (BRDDP). The model was developed in Caucasian women, taking into account age, race, age of menarche, number of births, number of first-degree relatives with breast cancer, and number of breast biopsies that have shown atypia. The Food and Drug Administration (FDA) has approved it as a basis to recommend chemoprevention. This model has been modified using data from the surgical adjuvant breast and bowel project and can

be obtained at www.cancer.gov/bcrisktool. The limitations of this model include underestimation of cancer in African Americans and not taking into account *BRCA* mutations, second-degree relatives, or breast density, which are all very important factors.

The Clauss model, developed by Elizabeth Clauss in 1994, uses data from the Cancer and Steroid Hormone Study (CASH). This model uses first- and second-degree relatives, both maternal and paternal, to calculate risk but does not use risk factors beyond family history and also is not as robust in non-Caucasians. The Clauss model provides the lifetime risks for a woman over any given decade of her life. The Tyler-Cuzick model and others are not used in the United States.

There are several risk factors that raise suspicion for an inherited mutation (**Box 15-3**). One of the clinician's roles in evaluating a woman's breast cancer risk is to determine which women should be referred to a genetic counselor for evaluation for the inherited cancer syndromes. If a woman has a 5% to 10% probability of having a BRCA mutation, then she should be referred for counseling for in-depth assessment and workup of the family history. Counseling is best performed by genetic counselors because of the tedious work in determining an accurate family history. Women often equate a family history of biopsies of breast lumps with breast cancers. The counselor is invaluable in discussing the issues and implications of the results, including legal and insurance aspects, noninformative results, and choices for chemoprevention or surgical prophylaxis. The psychological impact for the patient and her family cannot be overemphasized. Reasons for referral include a personal history of cancer at a young age, pre- or perimenopausal breast cancer, a triple receptor negative tumor, women with first-degree (sister, mother, or daughter) relatives with a history, a male first-degree relative, a confirmed mutation in another family member, or women of Ashkenazi Jewish heritage with a family history of ovarian or breast cancer.

Insurance discrimination is a constant concern, and though most states prohibit discrimination in employment based on genetic information (through the nondiscrimination act of 2008), this does not necessarily protect against other types of insurance policies being either denied or placed at a high enough premium that policies are prohibitive. The Genetic Information Nondiscrimination Act (GINA) protects individuals who have had "predisposition testing" in employment and health insurance. Life insurance companies may discriminate as they see fit. Most authors feel that this will change with time with medicines increasing our understanding of genetic diseases. However, at this time there still are areas of intense concern, which the genetic counselor can discuss. Women with negative or noninformative BRCA results may still need screening, as their risks may be greater than that of the average population or they would not have been referred for genetic screening.

In general, women with an average risk, 12%, should have mammographic screening starting at age 40, and every 1 to 2 years after that. The United States Committee on Preventive Task Force recently suggested the consideration of an upper age limit to begin screening at age 50 because of false positive rates and low yields in average-risk women. However, most clinical societies, including the American College of Obstetricians and Gynecologists, have strongly disagreed. Clinical breast exams should be performed every 1 to 3 years up to age 40 and then annually after that. Breast self-examination is more controversial. Most clinical societies recommend monthly breast self-examination. Hormone replacement therapy is acceptable in women with average risk, for the shortest possible time that is clinically appropriate.

Women with moderate risk, those with up to a 15% lifetime risk, should be offered similar screening to women with average risk—annual mammograms beginning at age 40.

Women with high risk, a lifetime risk of 15% or greater to develop breast cancer, should have annual digital mammography and clinical breast exams. These women should also be considered for chemoprophylaxis and offered tamoxifen if they are premenopausal or either raloxifene or tamoxifen if they are postmenopausal.

When the risk is projected to exceed 20% over the woman's lifetime, then a screening every 6 months is recommended, as well as yearly magnetic resonance imaging (MRI) alternating the following 6 months with mammography. Screening should begin 10 years earlier than any affected first-degree family relative. These women should also be offered chemoprevention medications. Women with radiation for malignancy should begin their screening 5 to 10 years after their mantle radiation. Most experts feel that women at the highest risk, very high risk category, should have hormone replacement therapy only if they have had a total abdominal hysterectomy and bilateral salpingo-oophorectomy. Discussion of prophylactic mastectomy is

reasonable in the highest risk patients. The pros and cons of this procedure should be thoroughly explored with both an oncologist and a surgeon knowledgeable in breast cancer prior to a decision being made. See Chapter 33 for more discussion of BRCA management.

CHEMOPROPHYLAXIS AND CHEMOTHERAPEUTIC RISK REDUCTION

Breast cancer risk reduction should be considered throughout a woman's life. Although there is no proved benefit for women with average risk, lifestyle modifications such as weight control, avoidance of smoking, decreased alcohol consumption, and exercise are associated with good general health. Most important, women with a high risk of breast cancer have proved options that can decrease their risk of breast cancer (**Table 15-5**). In the National Surgical Adjuvant Breast and Bowel Project (NSABP) B-14 trial, tamoxifen users had a significant decrease in the incidence of contralateral breast cancers compared with placebo. As a result, the Breast Cancer Prevention Trial (BCPT) was designed to assess whether tamoxifen would decrease the incidence of breast cancer in a high-risk population as determined by the Gail model for breast cancer risk assessment. The trial enrolled 13,388 women in a double-blinded, randomized, placebo-controlled trial to evaluate the effects of tamoxifen on risk reduction. The trial was closed prematurely because of a large discordance between the two groups. Tamoxifen significantly reduced the incidence of breast cancer in this population of patients by 49% compared with controls ($p < 0.00001$). It did not reduce the incidence of estrogen receptor-negative cancers.

Two other trials, the Royal Marsden Hospital trial and the Italian tamoxifen prevention study, failed to confirm this reduction in risk with prophylactic tamoxifen use. However, both studies were smaller and enrolled a lower-risk population than the BCPT. Raloxifene, another selective estrogen receptor modulator, also reduces the relative risk. In a trial designed to test the efficacy of raloxifene on the prevention of bone fractures, 7705 postmenopausal women were treated with either raloxifene or a placebo. There was a 76% reduction in the incidence of breast cancer in the raloxifene group after 40 months of follow-up. As a result, the Study of Tamoxifen and Raloxifene (STAR) trial

Table 15-5 Breast Cancer Chemoprevention

Results	Tamoxifen vs. Placebo[†]	Raloxifene vs. Placebo[†]	Raloxifene vs. Tomoxifea[†]
Benefits			
Invasive breast cancer	0.70 (0.59-0.82)	0.44 (0.27-0.71)	1.02 (0.82-1.28)
Estrogen receptor-positive invasive breast cancer	0.58 (0.42-0.79)	0.33 (0.18-0.61)	0.93 (0.72-1.24)
Estrogen receptor-negative invasive breast cancer	1.19 (0.92-1.55)	1.25 (0.67-2.31)	1.15 (0.75-1.77)
Noninvasive breast cancer	0.85 (0.54-1.35)	1.47 (0.75-2.91)	1.40 (0.98-2.00)
All-cause mortality	1.07 (0.90-1.27)	0.91 (0.81-1.02)	0.94 (0.71-1.26)
Vertebral fracture	0.75 (0.48-1.15)	0.61 (0.54-0.69)	0.98 (0.65-1.46)
Nonvertebral fracture	0.66 (0.45-0.98)	0.97 (0.87-1.09)	Insufficient data
Harms			
Thromboembolic events	1.93 (1.41-2.64)	1.60 (1.15-2.23)	0.70 (0.54-0.91)
Coronary events	1.00 (0.79-1.27)	0.95 (0.84-1.06)	1.10 (0.85-1.43)
Stroke	1.36 (0.89-2.08)	0.96 (0.67-1.38)	0.96 (0.64-1.43)
Endometrial cancer	2.13 (1.36-3.32)	1.14 (0.65-1.98)	0.62 (0.35-1.08)
Cataracts	1.25 (0.93-1.67)	0.93 (0.84-1.04)	0.79 (0.68-0.92)

[†]All values are risk ratio (95% CI). Four trials compared tomoxifen with placebo, 2 trials compared raloxifene with placebo, and 1 trial compared raloxifene with tamoxifen.
Adapted from Nattinger AB: In the clinic breast Cancer screening and prevention. Ann Intern Med, April 6, 2010, Table 1.)

was designed. This study noted that raloxifene and tamoxifen had similar reductions in carcinoma, with less uterine disease in women taking raloxifene. At this time, raloxifene is considered an alternative to tamoxifen in postmenopausal women.

Women with BRCA1 mutations have significantly less benefit from tamoxifen. This is because almost all BRCA1-associated tumors are hormone receptor negative, unlike BRCA2 carriers who should be offered chemoprevention. Though these medications are effective, many women do not want to take them because of the side effects related to premature or perimenopausal symptoms. These women should be offered additional medications to control the side effects.

Surgical prophylaxis is another option for the woman who wants to reduce risk. In a retrospective cohort of 639 patients, Hartmann was able to demonstrate a 90% risk reduction for the patient with a high risk of breast cancer after prophylactic bilateral mastectomy. In a follow-up study, Hartmann was also able to demonstrate a similar risk reduction in a population of women with BRCA gene mutations. Although prophylactic bilateral mastectomy provides the greatest risk reduction, it is usually reserved for the very high-risk patient because of the associated physiologic and complicated psychological consequences. Although most women who have undergone prophylactic bilateral mastectomy do not regret having undergone the procedure, approximately 5% to 20% report dissatisfaction.

DETECTION AND DIAGNOSIS

Breast cancer is usually asymptomatic before the development of advanced disease. Only 10% of women experience breast pain with early breast carcinoma. Nipple discharge is an even less common symptom. The classic sign of a breast carcinoma is a solitary, solid, three-dimensional, dominant breast mass. About 75% of breast cancers present as a breast lump. The borders of the mass are usually indistinct, which makes it difficult to define precisely the size of the mass. Often the mass is not freely mobile. Far-advanced local disease produces changes in the skin and nipples of the breast, including retraction, dimpling, induration, edema (peau d'orange), ulceration, and signs of inflammation. With increased screening, many cancers and in situ lesions are found prior to any symptoms.

The three screening modalities are breast self-examination, clinical breast examination, and imaging with mammography. Clinical breast examination (CBE) and mammography are complementary procedures that must be considered together. Breast self-examination (BSE) has the major advantages of no cost to the patient and convenience. Diagnosis can be established only by biopsy or, sometimes, by fine-needle aspiration. Most important, a negative mammogram does not rule out breast carcinoma. Screening to detect breast carcinoma utilizes tests in asymptomatic women at periodic intervals to discover breast malignancies. Early diagnosis definitively reduces mortality by identifying smaller, more localized lesions and those with a lower percentage of positive node of involvement. Screening decreases mortality in 35% of women between ages 50 and 69 and nearly that much in women age 40 to 49.

The kinetics of growth in breast carcinoma are the basis for the recommendations for screening and detection. The average breast mass doubles in volume every 100 days and doubles in diameter every 300 days. A breast carcinoma grows for 6 to 8 years before reaching a diameter of 1 cm. In slightly less than another year, the carcinoma will reach 2 cm in diameter. The mean diameter of a breast mass discovered by women who perform BSE at monthly intervals is 2 cm.

Greenwald and colleagues studied the results of BSE and of CBE on the stage of breast carcinoma at initial diagnosis. Of 293 women with breast carcinoma, cancer was detected in clinical stage I in 54% when the detection method was routine CBE, in 38% when the detection method was BSE, and in only 27% when the detection of the mass was accidental. In this study, only 50% of women who performed BSE did so on a monthly basis. These authors estimated that the breast cancer mortality rate might be reduced 19% by BSE and 24% by annual CBE. In another study, Foster and Costanza determined the relationship between BSE and survival of breast cancer patients. Their study group included 1004 newly diagnosed cases of invasive breast carcinoma in Vermont from July 1975 to December 1982. During this time, there was not widespread use of screening mammography in that state. The survival rate at 5 years was 75% for women who examined their own breasts versus 57% for women who did not examine their breasts. The authors concluded that in their population, BSE was responsible for earlier detection, improved survival, smaller tumor size, and fewer axillary node metastases. Their findings persisted after controlling the analysis for the potential bias of confounding variables, such as age, length-biased sampling, and lead-time bias.

In summary, present methods of screening for breast carcinoma are not ideal. Nevertheless, screening tests result in a reduction in mortality rate from breast cancer of approximately 25% to 30%.

SELF-EXAMINATION OF THE BREASTS

The majority of breast masses are initially discovered by the patient, either accidentally or during breast self-examination. In a group of women having annual mammography and physical examination by physicians, one of three carcinomas was discovered by the patient in the interval between professional detection methods. Even with widespread national publicity, approximately 50% of women do not perform self-examination of the breast. Although this procedure has long been advocated, breast self-examination in itself does not decrease breast cancer mortality. Several recent studies have failed to show a benefit to breast self-examination because of the increased use of biopsy when masses are felt. Although breast self-examinations may not decrease mortality in research settings, it is important to remember that most women do not get the screening that is recommended by national organizations in terms of annual mammography, and in that sense real life is not a research setting. That is why most clinical societies continue to recommend breast self-examination.

The most effective teaching of BSE occurs in a one-to-one relationship. It is ideal to test the patient's ability to palpate masses in manufactured breast models. These models should contain masses with diameters as small as 0.3 to 0.5 cm. Instructions for the patient concerning the techniques of breast self-palpation should emphasize timing, inspection, and palpation. The few days immediately after a menstrual period are the best time to detect changes in normal lumps or texture of the breasts. Postmenopausal women or women who have had a hysterectomy should be instructed to perform BSE on the same calendar days each month.

Women should be instructed that bilateral soft thickening and nodularity are normal physical findings. Palpation should begin in the shower, because many women have increased tactile sensitivity by using a "wet" technique. After the shower the woman should lie down, initially with one arm at her side and subsequently with the same arm underneath her head. She should be instructed to use the pads of her second, third, and fourth fingers to palpate the contralateral breast. Using the pads of her fingers, in a massaging motion with firm pressure, she should examine the entire breast and surrounding chest wall in a systematic fashion. One of the easier techniques to follow is to palpate the breasts in a clockwise fashion beginning at the nipple and gradually circumscribing larger circles. It is pragmatic not to include specific instructions for the woman to try to express secretions from her nipples.

CLINICAL BREAST EXAMINATION

The ability to detect breast lumps varies widely from physician to physician. Fletcher and coworkers tested the physical examination techniques of 80 different physicians using manufactured breast models. The simulated breasts of the mannequins had a volume of 250 mL and the consistency of the breast tissue of a 50-year-old woman. The ability to detect the mass was directly related to the size of the mass; 87% of 1-cm, 33% of 0.5-cm, and 14% of 0.3-cm masses were discovered. The most disturbing finding was the wide range of detection rates among physicians, from 17% to 83%. In general, physicians with higher discovery rates spent more time performing the examination. The number of masses detected by a physician increased in those who used a consistent geometric pattern of examination with variable pressure exerted by the fingertips. Firmness of a mass and location within the breast (closer to the surface versus deeper) are also factors that influence the sensitivity of the CBE.

Although there has been widespread acceptance of physical exam as part of the screening for breast cancer, for ethical reasons there have not been randomized trials comparing physical exam with no screening. Several studies included the physical exam in addition to mammography, but only the Health Insurance Plan of New York (HIP) study demonstrated a significant reduction in breast cancer. Because 67% of the cancers in the HIP study group were detectable by physical exam, it was postulated that physical exam alone could have contributed to the reduction in breast cancer mortality. One randomized trial that compared physical exam with physical exam plus mammography for women over the age of 50 was the Canadian National Breast Screening Study II. Although there was no difference in mortality between the two groups, it generated interest in screening by physical exam. In a recent meta-analysis of clinical breast exam by Barton, there was indirect evidence of the effectiveness of the clinical exam. Clinical breast exam discovered approximately 15% to 20% of breast cancers that mammography missed.

A thorough breast examination by the physician should take 3 to 5 minutes to complete. This time is also an ideal opportunity to instruct the patient in the technique of BSE. A complete breast examination involves inspecting and palpating the breasts with the patient in the sitting as well as the supine position.

Initially, with a woman sitting on the examining table, the physician inspects the contour, symmetry, and vascular pattern of the breasts and the skin for irritation, retraction, or edema. It is important to have the patient place her arms above her head and subsequently place her hands on her hips. This sequence will contract the pectoralis muscles, which may allow the physician to visualize an abnormality. The patient in the sitting position is in the optimal position for the physician to determine the presence of adenopathy in the axilla.

The woman should subsequently examine her breasts while in the supine position. It is important to examine both nipples for retraction, skin irritation, or a discharge. The areola should be compressed to identify any discharge. The normal breast has a small depression directly below the nipple. The skin of the breast is again carefully inspected for unusual vascular patterns, edema, erythema, or retraction (**Fig. 15-13**).

Palpation is performed with both the woman's arms at her side and raised above her head and should not be limited to the breast tissue alone. A small pillow placed under the shoulder of the breast being examined often improves the examination. The examiner should palpate the axilla, the supraclavicular areas, and the adjacent chest wall. Palpation should use the pads of the first three fingers placed together, exerting firm but gentle pressure. Each physician determines his or her own systematic approach to examining all quadrants of the breast, the majority preferring concentric circles. It is very important that the physician draw a descriptive picture of any positive finding. This picture should include notations concerning the site, shape, size, consistency, and mobility of the mass. Special notation should be made as to whether the mass is tender and whether it is attached to skin or deep structures Physical examination is excellent as a screening procedure, but it is extremely poor in predicting the histopathology of the lesion. Studies have demonstrated that 30% to 40% of breast masses suspected by palpation to be malignant were found after biopsy to be benign. Conversely, 15% to 20% of benign-appearing masses during a physical examination subsequently are discovered by histopathology to be carcinoma.

MAMMOGRAPHY

Mammography is the best method for screening and the most practical method of detecting breast carcinoma at an early and highly curable stage, ideally discovering an occult cancer (< 5 mm in diameter). Most physicians are able to consistently palpate breast masses when they are 1 cm in diameter or greater. The clinical advantages of discovering breast carcinoma during its earliest stage include higher percentage of localized disease, lower incidence of positive regional nodes, and reduced mortality. The 5-year survival rate for women whose breast cancer is believed to be localized to the breast with negative axillary nodes is approximately 85%. In contrast, the 5-year survival rate is only 53% when axillary nodes are positive. Multiple studies have documented a decreased mortality with routine mammography. Mammography is also the most accurate conventional method of detecting nonpalpable breast carcinoma. Therefore, with increasing emphasis on conservative surgery for early carcinomas, mammography will not only save lives but decrease morbidity.

Mammography is not as precise in younger women or in women with dense breasts secondary to fibroglandular tissue. Mammography is most sensitive in older women in which the majority of the breast is composed of fatty tissue. Mammography may discover fine calcifications in breast neoplasms months to years before the carcinoma enlarges to a size that may be palpated on physical examination. Studying the kinetics of growth of breast cancer

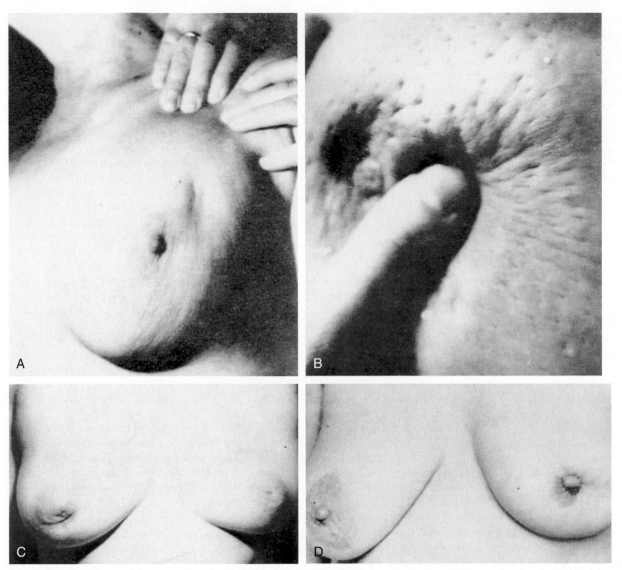

Figure 15-13 Signs of breast carcinoma. **A,** Retraction found during physical examination. **B,** Peau d'orange from underlying carcinoma. **C,** Retraction of right nipple. **D,** Retraction of left nipple from carcinoma. (From Degrell I: Atlas of Diseases of the Mammary Gland. Basel, Switzerland, S Karger, 1976, p 20.)

helps the clinician to appreciate why breast carcinoma is so often a systemic disease. Breast carcinoma must develop neovascularization to grow beyond 1 to 2 mm in diameter. Once neovascularization occurs, the breast carcinoma has the capability of metastasizing via the vascular system. The development of angiogenesis as measured by microvessel density in histopathologic sections is the strongest independent predictor of relapse-free survival in women with node-negative breast cancer. The average breast carcinoma grows for 3 years to enlarge from 1 mm to 1 cm, and that is the threshold of palpation at its best.

Restraints on the optimal use of mammography in identifying early breast carcinoma include a lack of properly trained and committed radiologists and the cost of the test. Mammography is a technically demanding procedure that requires an experienced and meticulous interpretation of the films, as well as correlation of the images with a thorough clinical examination.

Elmore and colleagues reported the diagnostic consistency between pairs of radiologists in interpretation of mammograms. This consistency was moderate, with a median weight for percentage of agreement at 78%. The frequency of the radiologists' recommendations for an immediate workup ranged from 74% to 96% in the woman with cancer and from 11% to 67% in the woman without cancer.

Historically, two landmark studies laid the foundation for the scientific credibility of mammography as a screening procedure. The first large, randomized control study was the HIP study, undertaken in the early 1960s. The HIP investigation involved yearly screening by both mammography and physical examination for 5 years. The women were followed for 10 to 14 years, and the study demonstrated a 30% reduction in mortality from breast carcinoma in the women who had annual mammography compared with the control group.

The second pivotal study was performed in 29 centers throughout the United States during the late 1970s. This immense undertaking was sponsored by the National Institutes of Health and was named the Breast Cancer Detection Demonstration Project (BCDDP). The BCDDP involved screening 275,000 women, and during the 5 years of the project, 3557 breast carcinomas were found, 42% discovered only by mammography.

The definite improvement in mammographic accuracy over the 12-year interval between the two studies is apparent when comparing their results. Cancer detection was approximately two times more frequent in the BCDDP study. In women ages 40 to 49, mammography found 39% of carcinomas in the HIP investigation, compared with 85% identified in the BCDDP project. Most important, in the detection of carcinoma less than 1 cm, the results were 36% in the BCDDP versus 8% in the HIP.

Present studies have demonstrated that screening mammography reduces breast cancer mortality by approximately 33% in women 50 to 70 years of age (**Table 15-6**). However, screening mammography does not show as dramatic a benefit for women 40 to 49 years of age (international randomized trials show about a 17% reduction). This stems from three factors. First, many more women must be screened in this younger age group to detect cancer. Second, mammography is less sensitive with the denser breasts of younger women. Third, tumors in younger

Table 15-6 Breast Cancer Benefit/Risk Ratio for a Woman Having Annual Mammography Beginning at Age 35

Age	Annual Baseline Breast Cancer Incidence/100,000	Fatal Radiation-Induced Cases	Fatal Cases Prevented by Mammography	Benefit/Risk Ratio
35	66	0	1.3	
36	66	0	1.3	
37	66	0	1.3	
38	66	0	1.3	
39	66	0	1.3	
40	129	0	12.9	>400
41	129	0	12.9	
42	129	0	12.9	
43	129	0	12.9	
44	129	0	12.9	
45	187	<0.1	18.7	352
46	187	<0.1	18.7	181
47	187	0.2	18.7	120
48	187	0.2	18.7	91
49	187	0.3	18.7	73
50	229	0.3	22	66
51	220	0.4	22	61
52	220	0.4	22	57
53	220	0.4	22	53
54	220	0.4	22	50
55	268	0.6	26.08	47
56	268	0.6	26.8	44
57	268	0.6	26.8	43
58	268	0.7	26.8	41
59	268	0.7	26.8	39
60	339	0.9	33.9	38
61	339	0.9	33.9	37
62	339	0.9	33.9	36
63	339	1	33.9	35
64	339	1	33.9	34
65	391	1.2	39.1	33
66	391	1.2	39.1	33
67	391	1.2	39.1	32
68	391	1.3	39.1	31
69	391	1.3	39.1	30
70	421	1.4	42.1	30
71	421	1.4	42.1	29
72	421	1.5	42.1	29
73	421	1.5	42.1	28
74	421	1.5	42.1	28
75	421	1.5	42.1	27

Tables assume reduction in mortality from breast cancer as a result of screening as follows: age 35 to 39, 5%; 40 to 49, 15%; and 50 to 75, 25%.
From Mettler FA, Upton AC, Kelsey CA, et al: Benefits versus risks from mammography: A critical reassessment. Cancer 77:903, 1996.

women are often more aggressive and at a higher stage and grade. Thus, the number needed to treat to decrease mortality is higher. In the United States, more than 10,000 deaths occur each year in women who initially developed breast carcinoma between the ages of 40 and 49. In a meta-analysis, Sickles and Kopans demonstrated a 21% mortality reduction in women who had mammographic screening compared with those in the control groups. They felt that screening was at least as beneficial for women who are ages 40 to 49 as for those ages 50 to 64 years.

Many nonscientific factors affect an individual physician's recommendations and an individual woman's decision regarding screening. Among the more important of these are the cost of the test and the patient's anxiety regarding breast cancer. In addition, the anxiety related to false-positive mammograms may be an obstacle to screening. The primary barrier to mammographic screening is the lack of a strong recommendation from the woman's primary care physician. When mammography is used as part of the diagnostic workup of women with breast symptoms, significant occult disease is often identified in another quadrant of the same breast or in the contralateral breast. All patients with breast masses or persistent spontaneous nipple discharge should have mammograms of both breasts before biopsy. Mammography is also indicated in evaluating a breast mass the patient has found but that the physician cannot confirm by palpation. This technique is helpful in difficult clinical situations, such as the evaluation of large breasts or following augmentation mammoplasty. It is important to stress once again that mammography and physical examination are complementary procedures. One procedure does not replace the necessity of carefully performing the other.

Mammographic sensitivity decreases when breasts are classified as dense. Density is not a function of the size of the breasts or the firmness but of the ratio of glandular tissue to fatty elements. Unfortunately, density is also a significant risk factor for the development of breast cancer. When a woman is noted by plain-film mammography to have dense breasts, she should be referred for digital mammography, or if she has dense breasts and a greater than 20% risk of the development of breast cancer, she should be offered an MRI. Hormone replacement therapy (HRT) slightly decreases the effectiveness of mammographic screening. Lundström and coworkers demonstrated that an increase in mammographic density was much more common in women receiving continuous combination hormone replacement (52%) than in women using cyclic (13%) and estrogen-only (18%) treatment. Almost all the changes occurred within the first year of use. Laya and coworkers demonstrated that the specificity of mammography was significantly lower in current users of estrogen replacement therapy (82%) than in women who had never had estrogen replacement therapy (85%). Similarly, sensitivity also was significantly lower in current users (69%) versus 94% for never users.

Optimal identification of early breast carcinoma by mammography depends on a competent technician obtaining excellent images and the radiologist searching for subtle changes. For screening mammography, two views of each breast are performed: the mediolateral oblique (MLO) and the craniocaudal (CC). The MLO is the most effective single view because it includes the greatest amount of breast tissue and is the only view that includes all of the upper outer quadrant and axillary tail. Sickles emphasized the importance of firm breast compression of the breast during mammography for the following reasons

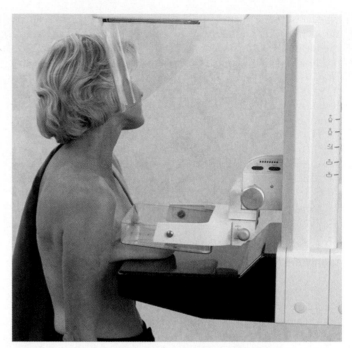

Figure 15-14 Mammography being performed with appropriate compression applied. (Courtesy Hologic Inc.)

(**Fig. 15-14**). First, it holds the breast still to prevent motion artifact. It brings the objects closer into view, thereby reducing the amount of blur. It also separates overlapping tissues that can obscure an underlying lesion. Finally, it decreases the amount of radiation exposure by making the breast thinner and easier to penetrate with less radiation. Attempts to alleviate anxiety and discomfort with radiolucent cushions on the mammogram compression paddles have been found to be helpful.

Breast cancer may be detected by visualizing **clusters** of fine calcifications, spiculations, or poorly defined multinodular masses with irregular contours (**Fig. 15-15**), all characteristic of malignancy. Isolated clusters of tiny calcifications are the most common and important diagnostic sign of an early carcinoma. Calcifications are often smaller than 0.5 mm in diameter and thus must be identified by a magnifying lens. The presence of five or more calcifications within a volume of 1 cm^3 is termed a *cluster*. Subsequent breast biopsies will find 25% of clusters associated with cancer and 75% with benign disease. Conversely, approximately 68% of occult breast carcinomas and 34% of palpable breast cancers demonstrate calcifications on mammographic examination. A side-by-side comparison of old films, evaluating current films with previous ones, facilitates identification of the less classic, indirect signs of breast carcinoma, such as a single dilated duct with intraductal carcinoma, asymptomatic architectural distortion in dense breasts, and a developing density. Multiple experts emphasize the use of comparing old and newer films as a means of increasing accuracy.

Standardized terminology should be used to describe mammographic findings. As a result, the American College of Radiology Breast Imaging Reporting and Data System (BI-RADS) (**Fig. 15-16**) was devised to standardize mammographic terminology, reduce confusing interpretations, and facilitate the monitoring of outcomes. The report includes an overall assessment of the likelihood that the finding represents a malignancy. There

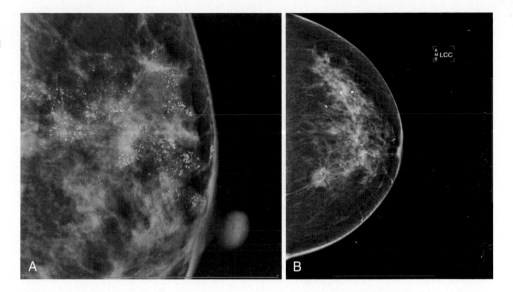

Figure 15-15 A, Mammogram showing multiple small calcifications consistent with DCIS, which was found on biopsy. **B,** Mammogram showing invasive carcinoma *(dotted circle).* (Courtesy of Catherine Chicola, MD.)

BI-RAD class	Description	Probability of malignancy (%)	Follow-up
0	Needs additional evaluation	1	Diagnostic mammogram, ultrasound
1	Normal mammogram	0	Yearly screening
2	Benign lesion	0	Yearly screening
3	Probably benign lesion	<2	Short-interval follow-up
4	Suspicious for malignancy	20	Biopsy
5	Highly suspicious malignancy	90	Biopsy

BI-RAD, Breast Imaging Reporting and Data Systems.

Figure 15-16 BI-RAD classification of mammographic lesions. (From Pazdur R, Coia LR, Hoskins WJ, Wagman LD [eds]: Cancer Management: A Multidisciplinary Approach, 4th ed. Melville, NY, Cligott Publishing Group, p 143, 2006.)

are six assessment categories, each associated with a specific risk of cancer. Category 0 is nondiagnostic. Categories 1 and 2 are nonmalignant. Categories 5 and 6 represent malignancy. In the conclusion of every mammogram report, the final assessment is provided to prevent confusion and to guide the referring health care professional as to a recommended plan of action. Additionally there should be a comment on the density of the breasts.

Computer-aided diagnosis has been an area of active investigation in recent years. Delineation by computer program of microcalcifications and masses gives the radiologist a second opinion of the mammographic films. It has been long established that double reading of a mammographic study by two independent observers improves the breast cancer detection rate tenfold.

The relationship between high levels of radiation and increased risk for breast carcinoma raises questions concerning the relative risk of the carcinogenic effect of mammography. The measured radiation dose to the breast by state-of-the-art mammography equipment is approximately 0.1 rad (0.001 Gy) for a two-view examination. For a woman beginning annual screening at age 50 and continuing until age 75, the benefit exceeds the risk secondary to radiation by a factor of almost 100. For a high-risk woman who begins annual screening at age 35, the benefit-risk in reduced mortality is more than 25-fold. All of the major health societies and professional organizations have emphasized that the benefits of screening far outweigh the very small radiation risk (**Table 15-7**).

DIGITAL MAMMOGRAPHY

Digital mammography is the technique by which x-ray photons are detected after passing through the breast tissue and the radiographic image is recorded electronically in a digital format and stored in a computer. Digital technology has multiple advantages compared with conventional mammography. Image acquisition, display, and storage are much faster, and image manipulation through adjustments in contrast, brightness, and electronic magnification of selected regions enables radiologists to obtain superior views. This technology makes it possible to subtract various layers of computerized imagery in order to examine suspicious areas and improve the ability to detect and diagnose breast carcinoma. Digital mammography is more useful than plain film in screening women with very dense breasts and breast implants. With the ability to manipulate the images, digital mammography reduces the number of women recalled for more images. Computer-aided diagnosis is also possible with this technique as well as the ability to transmit the image electronically. Because of low background "noise" and superior contrast capabilities, the final image is superior to conventional mammography. It also allows the sending of images to other centers for comparison.

The disadvantages of digital mammography include the cost of the equipment and the reduced spatial resolution caused in part by inadequate resolution of current monitors. Digital mammography is associated with a significantly lower recall rate (11.5% versus 14.1%) and a higher rate of positive findings at the time of biopsy (43.3% versus 23.7%).

Table 15-7 Professional Society Recommendations for Screening Mammography

Organization	Age to Initiate Mammography	Age to Conclude Mammography	Interval between Screenings
American Academy of Family Physicians	40 y based on discussion with patient. Routinely at ≥50 y.	Screening recommended to age 74 y. Evidence insufficient for age ≥75 y.	Not stated for age 40–49 y 2 y for age 50–74 y.
American Cancer Society	40 y	While in good health	1 y for all ages.
American College of Obstetricians and Gynecologists	40 y	None stated	1–2 y for age 40–49 y. 1 y for age ≥50 y.
American College of Physicians	40 y, based on benefits, harms, preferences, and risk profile.	Unclear	1–2 y for age. 40–49 y. Unclear for age ≥50 y.
American College of Radiology	40 y	None stated	1 y for all ages.
National Comprehensive Cancer Network	40 y	None stated	1 y for all ages.
U.S. Preventive Services Task Force, 2009	40 y, only based on patient. context. Routinely at ≥50 y	Screening recommended to age 74 y. Evidence insufficient for age ≥75 y.	2 y for all ages.

Adapted from Nattinger AB: In the clinic Breast Cancer Screening and prevention. Ann Intern Med, 152:ITC41, Table 5.

Comparison studies from 2004 through 2008 documented similar sensitivities between plain-film mammography and digital mammography, with a greater specificity for digital. The digital mammography imaging screening trial (DMIST) of 49,528 women demonstrated that digital mammography was superior for women with dense breasts. The earlier Oslo-2 study found a greater sensitivity than plain film, particularly in women in the 45 to 69 age range. This imaging technique will be the screening modality of the future, as it requires less radiation exposure than plain-film mammography because of the increased quantum efficiency of the digital equipment. For the immediate future, the high cost per test will make it financially impractical to implement widespread **digital radiography** for screening purposes. This imaging technique will be gradually phased in. As breast centers convert and the initial expenses are overcome, plain-film mammography will be found less commonly.

The age to discontinue screening in low-risk and moderate-risk women should be individualized based on the health and longevity of the woman. In general, mammography is continued into the late 70s. The United States Preventive Task Force recommends discontinuing mammography after age 74. However, for women with a life span less than 10 years and significant illness, mammography may be discontinued sooner. Conversely, women who are healthy without any major diseases and have a life expectancy beyond age 75 should have consideration for continuing mammograms. The breasts of most women in their 70s will have minimal glandular tissue and in this sense are easier to examine both clinically and with breast self-examination. With the discontinuation of mammogram it is reasonable to talk with women about increasing their own breast self-examination. The decision about when to stop mammography should be discussed with the woman. Some will have a deep fear of breast cancer and will want to continue mammography.

MAGNETIC RESONANCE IMAGING

Magnetic resonance imaging (MRI) is an integral addition for imaging. The ability of MRI to differentiate benign from malignant tissue may reduce the frequency of breast biopsy, especially in women with dense, fibroglandular breasts. MRI has proved effective in detecting new tumors in patients with previous **lumpectomy** because it can accurately distinguish between scar tissue and cancerous lesions. This is best accomplished by the gadolinium-enhanced MRI (**Fig. 15-17**). Other potential uses or indications for MRI are to improve imaging of structures close to the chest wall, to improve imaging of women with breast prosthesis, and to evaluate for prosthesis rupture. It is useful in the patient who presents with axillary adenopathy and no apparent mass in the breast. Because the average examination takes about 45 minutes to an hour, MRI will not be used in mass screening programs. MRI cannot identify microcalcifications. Another limitation of MRI is the loss of image quality with respiratory movements.

Because of higher cost, MRI is used only in specific populations or as an adjunct to nondiagnostic mammography. The specificity is lower than mammography, but the sensitivity is higher. It is especially useful in women with dense fibroglandular breasts. A systematic review by Warner et al. of MRI for screening of high-risk women noted a sensitivity of 0.77 versus 0.39,

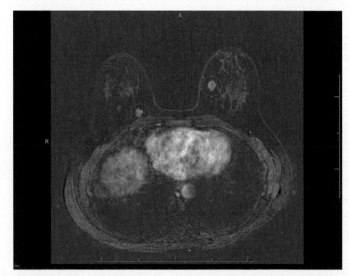

Figure 15-17 MRI of bilateral breast carcinomas. (Courtesy of Catherine Chicola, MD.)

MRI versus plain-film mammography with a specificity of 0.86 versus 0.95, respectively. As tumors increase in size, their growth needs lead to an increased metabolic demand and increased angiogenesis. MRI techniques capitalize on these qualities of tumors and through rapid uptake of gadolinium leading to a better visualization of a neoplasm versus benign mass. This is responsible for the increased sensitivity of this imaging modality.

Current screening recommendations are that women with greater than 20% lifetime risk of breast cancer should be scheduled for regular MRI. Most insurance programs will reimburse for the increased cost of MRI at that level of risk.

ULTRASOUND

Ultrasound has a definite role as a complementary procedure to other imaging techniques in the diagnosis of breast disease, particularly in differentiating cystic from solid masses. Ultrasound should not be used as a "screening test" except for women with very dense breasts who cannot be adequately screened with mammography and those who cannot tolerate an MRI. Ultrasound screening increased the detection of otherwise occult cancers by 37% in a study involving 3626 women age 42 to 67, with dense breasts and no visible abnormalities on mammography. In the general population the effectiveness of ultrasound "screening" is more limited. Sickles and colleagues reported a comparison study using state-of-the-art equipment. Mammography detected 62 of 64 (97%) carcinomas, whereas ultrasound diagnosed only 37 of 64 (58%). Only 8% of carcinomas smaller than 1 cm in diameter were discovered by ultrasound. The conclusion of this study was that the majority of breast carcinomas visualized by ultrasound can be palpated clinically and there was little use for the ultrasound as a screening tool. The primary advantage of ultrasound is the ability to produce images of breast tissue on multiple occasions without harmful effects. It is most useful in evaluating solitary masses greater than 1 cm in diameter. Whether it can distinguish benign from malignant lesions has been a topic of great debate. In one series, Stavros and coworkers described the sonographic evaluation of 750 solid breast nodules (palpable and nonpalpable) all of which had subsequent histologic confirmation. The negative predictive value of sonography was 99.5%. This is a higher negative predictive value than a BI-RAD 3 mammogram for which a 6-month follow-up is recommended. Ultrasound can be used to further evaluate mammographically detected lesions. A low-risk lesion according to strict sonographic criteria can either be aspirated or safely observed.

Ultrasonography of the breast is usually performed by a handheld, real-time, high-frequency probe. It is a highly operator- and reader-dependent test with a great deal of variation among different centers. Breast cancer is usually hypoechoic, and early cancers are difficult to distinguish from surrounding normal hypoechoic breast tissue. The most important use of ultrasound is to differentiate a cystic breast mass from a solid mass. The accuracy rate of ultrasound to diagnose a cystic mass is 96% to 100% and exceeds the combined accuracy of mammography and physical examination.

Ultrasound is frequently used to guide needle aspiration, or direct core-needle biopsy. It has also been used to localize tumors intraoperatively without a guide wire with excellent success rates. In one series, pathologically negative margins were achieved in 97% of the cases by using sonography alone to localize the lesion intraoperatively. This imaging technique also may be useful in women with augmentation mammoplasty, in the differential diagnosis of masses in the dense breast tissue of younger women, evaluating a breast abscess, and possibly determining lymph node status in a woman with carcinoma. Although it can be used to evaluate the integrity of a silicone breast implant, most believe that MRI is better at detecting implant ruptures. Ultrasound is commonly used to increase diagnostic accuracy after a mammogram has demonstrated equivocal findings. In this setting, the increased specificity may help downgrade a BIRAD score, with the identification of a cyst or fibroadenoma. In summary, ultrasound should not be used as a sole imaging technique for breast disease. Because of its lack of sensitivity and specificity for early breast carcinoma, it should not be used in an attempt to detect subclinical disease in the general population at this time.

COMPUTED TOMOGRAPHY

Computed tomography (CT) has limited value when compared with mammography because of higher radiation dose and longer study times. The thickness of cross-sectional slices with CT misses the majority of areas of microcalcification. CT scans have demonstrated some preclinical cancers after injection with radiocontrast media. This imaging technique is excellent for studying the most medial and lateral aspects of the breast. It is sometimes used for preoperative wire location of a mass that is difficult to localize by mammography. However, the increased expense and radiation exposure virtually eliminate CT scans for screening programs.

OTHER IMAGING TECHNIQUES

Thermography is unreliable as a screening technique for breast carcinoma or as a technique to determine women at increased risk for subsequent breast neoplasia. Lawson first described the elevation of skin temperature associated with breast carcinoma in 1956. Although thermography has been used clinically since that time, it has extremely high false-positive and false-negative rates. Thermography is ineffective in detecting occult or preclinical cancers. The major fault of a normal thermography examination is the false sense of security engendered in the symptom-free woman. The addition of thermography to other established diagnostic methods increases costs without providing useful clinical information.

Transillumination, or dynamic optical breast imaging (DOBI), is a radiation-free technique that measures the light transmitted through breast tissue. The breast acts as a filter for the light; the hypothesis is that malignant tissue absorbs more infrared light than does benign tissue. Although this technique is inexpensive, it is still experimental and unproved. To date, results of research studies using transillumination do not compare with results obtained with mammography.

Scintimammography is a radionuclide imaging test for the detection of breast cancer. Technetium-99 m sestamibi is a radiotracer with reported high sensitivity and high negative predictive value for breast cancer. It has a high diagnostic accuracy for the detection of breast cancer in all women, including women who may be unsuitable for conventional mammography. The specificity of scintimammography is better than conventional mammography, 84% and 67%, respectively. The high negative predictive value of this test for breast cancer potentially makes it an important adjunct to mammography by potentially reducing the number of biopsies performed for benign findings. The technique is useful for locating tumors in the lateral areas of dense breasts as well as for detecting metastatic disease in the lymph nodes of the axilla. Additional studies are needed before this test is widely accepted and its utility proved. Because of expense, it is not useful for screening.

Diffraction-enhanced imaging (DEI) is a technique that analyzes the image from a crystal is placed in the x-ray beam between the breast and an image-creating medium such as film or digital detector. The crystal diffracts the x-ray beam and produces two separate images, one based on standard radiograph and the other based on refraction. The result is an excellent quality image with superior tumor visibility. Digital thermal imaging is another technique that uses the principles of thermography as well as digital technology to create an image base determined by temperature differences between the cancer and the normal breast. Microwave radiography is a portable, noninvasive adjuvant diagnostic approach that involves the passive measurement of microwave emissions from breast tissue. None of these techniques have a current role in screening or in the diagnostic algorithm.

CORE-NEEDLE BIOPSY AND EXCISIONAL BIOPSY

When suspicious findings are noted on examination or imaging, then a tissue diagnosis must be obtained. The common indications for tissue biopsy include bloody discharge from the nipple, a persistent three-dimensional mass, or suggestive mammography. Nipple retraction or elevation and skin changes, such as erythema, induration, or edema, are also indications for breast biopsy. Obviously, the suspicious area must be sampled appropriately. Imaging should precede biopsy, as the inflammation and bleeding that may accompany biopsy may significantly impair needed visualization of the breast with imaging. Biopsy may be accomplished in several ways. The best technique is usually core-needle biopsy. Core-needle biopsy will obtain a tissue specimen, which can be used for histologic assessment, gene testing, and hormone receptor assessment. Fine-needle aspiration had been a mainstay in diagnosis and is being replaced with core-needle biopsy. It is difficult to determine the difference between carcinoma in situ and malignancy on fine-needle aspiration because it is a cytologic specimen. Fine-needle aspiration is best used for simple cysts. Tumor markers, grade, angio and lymphatic invasion can all be assessed with core-needle biopsy and definitive surgery can be scheduled in one step rather than two, thus excisional biopsy is becoming less common throughout the United States. Excisional biopsy should be reserved for certain situations when core biopsy cannot be employed. Excisional biopsy is being phased out as a primary tool for diagnosis, and most professional societies have recommended replacing it with core-needle biopsy whenever possible.

Core-needle biopsy is usually performed with a 14- to 16-gauge needle. Sometimes vacuum assistance is also used. Ultrasound-directed core-needle biopsy is extremely accurate and is preferable for all lesions that are seen only by mammography and not palpable. A small amount of material from the biopsy should be sent for evaluation of hormone receptors and for gene profiling. Receptors are heat labile and thus should be frozen within 30 minutes.

Nonpalpable breast lesions are most commonly discovered through screening mammography, and they represent a large proportion of the suggestive areas investigated by biopsy. Although these lesions are relatively easy to identify, localization and subsequent adequate sampling can be challenging. The best available methods are ultrasound guided or occasionally mammographically guided wire-localized excisional biopsy. With this method a wire is placed percutaneously in the vicinity of the abnormality by the radiologist, using imaging guidance. Stereotactic directed biopsy is another technique used to localize lesions. The breast is imaged, and the lesion is localized using computer-assisted positioning and targeting devices. A small nick is made in the skin and the core biopsy needle is advanced into the lesion. The lesion is sampled, and the "cores" of tissue are sent to pathology for histologic evaluation. The false-negative rate for this procedure is less than 2%.

Today the majority of open breast biopsies are performed under local anesthesia on an outpatient basis. In the late 1980s, it was common practice to perform a biopsy, frozen section, and definitive surgery during the same operation. The modern two-step approach significantly decreases anxiety for the patient. The 1- to 2-week interval between biopsy and therapy gives the woman a chance to contemplate alternative choices in therapy.

FINE-NEEDLE ASPIRATION OF SUSPECTED CYSTS

Fine-needle aspiration (FNA) of a breast mass that is thought to be a cyst is a well-established diagnostic test. It is a simple office-based procedure that is well accepted by women because it is sometimes less painful than a venipuncture. FNA is performed after imaging is finished. If the mass is solid or there is suspicion of malignancy, then core-needle biopsy should be performed. Most physicians do not use anesthesia, although some prefer to use a small amount of local anesthetic (1 mL of 1% lidocaine). The skin over the breast is the most sensitive area, but the breast tissue itself has few pain fibers. The anesthetic procedure has more disadvantages than advantages. The major disadvantage is that if excessive amounts of anesthetic are injected into the skin or if a hematoma develops, the mass may be obscured and the accuracy of the FNA is decreased. However, an injection of local anesthesia into a small area of the skin will reduce the patient's anxiety.

The breast mass is secured with one hand and the other hand introduces a 20- or 22-gauge needle attached to a 10- or 20-mL syringe into the mass. If the mass is a cyst, one feels a "give" or reduced resistance after puncturing the cyst wall. It may be technically easier to manipulate the smaller needles without the syringe attached. Complete aspiration of all the fluid from the cyst is facilitated by negative pressure from the syringe and firm pressure on the cyst wall. With withdrawal of the fluid, the cyst wall collapses and a residual mass cannot be palpated. After withdrawal of the needle, firm pressure is applied for 5 to 10 minutes to reduce the possibility of hematoma formation. Complications of needle aspiration are minimal, with hematoma formation being the only substantial one. Infection is very rare. The theoretic risk of spreading cancer along the needle track has not been substantiated.

The color of the fluid obtained via aspiration varies from clear to grossly bloody. It is not uncommon to find yellow, brown, and even green fluid in a cyst. If the aspirated fluid is clear, it is not necessary to submit it for cytologic evaluation. One study documented no breast cancers discovered from almost 7000 consecutive nonbloody cyst aspirates. If the aspirated fluid is turbid or bloody, a sample should be placed on a cover slip and sent for cytologic interpretation and the mass should be further evaluated with a biopsy. Although bloody fluid is usually from a traumatic tap, one must consider the possibility of a carcinoma. FNA is appropriate for new, well-circumscribed, usually tender masses that are thought to be simple (not complex) cysts. Core-needle biopsy is the procedure of choice for all other findings.

No further workup is necessary if the aspirated fluid is clear and no residual mass is palpated immediately after the procedure and again 1 month later. However, if the mass remains after aspiration, a biopsy should be performed even if the cytologic analysis of the fluid was negative. A biopsy should be performed on cysts that recur within 2 weeks or that necessitate more than one repeat aspiration. Slightly less than 20% of cysts recur after a single aspiration and less than 10% recur after two aspirations. The percentage of false-positive, fine-needle aspirations is very rare, usually less than 2%. In the event that no fluid is obtained, the breast mass is probably solid and several passes are made through the mass with continuous suction from the syringe. Moving the needle within a single tract will give a satisfactory cellular yield in the majority of cases. The cellular specimen within the needle should be placed on a slide and fixed for analysis. Definitive diagnosis by core-needle biopsy is the next step.

The "triple test" has been advocated as a reliable alternative to excisional biopsy. According to the National Cancer Institute's committee opinion on FNA, if the physical exam, imaging findings, and cytologic evaluation of the mass all confirm the same benign process, the mass can be followed. Core-needle biopsy is replacing fine-needle aspiration as part of the triple test. However, if any of these assessments indicate cancer, a biopsy should be performed. The false-negative rate of triple test diagnosis approaches that of surgical biopsy, and the false-positive rate is comparable with that for frozen section. Because FNA provides a cytologic specimen, it cannot distinguish invasive from noninvasive breast carcinoma. When suspicion for malignancy exists, core-needle biopsy is preferable. In nonpalpable lesions, found with imaging, false-negative rates approaching 40% have been reported.

CLASSIFICATION

There have been numerous classifications of breast carcinoma that contain mixtures of both clinical and pathologic subgroups. Most carcinomas originate in the epithelium of the collecting ducts (ductal) or the terminal lobular ducts (lobular). The classifications of breast cancer were originally based on histologic appearance or receptor status for estrogen. Currently, gene profiling is used along with histologic appearance. The classifications are useful for further research into etiology, pathophysiology, and, importantly, for prognosis of the various subtypes. For the clinician, breast cancer is evaluated by staging criteria, and treatment decisions begin at that point. The classification may help refine the subsequent treatments. Initially, breast carcinoma may be divided into invasive and in situ lesions (**Table 15-8**). Both in situ and invasive carcinomas have often been described in the same quadrant of the breast. Additionally, multifocal carcinomas are not uncommon, and bilateral breast carcinomas occur in 1% to 2% of newly diagnosed cases.

Intraductal carcinoma in situ (DCIS) is a premalignant lesion in which the cellular abnormalities are limited to the ductal

Table 15-8 Simplified Classification of Breast Carcinoma Based on Histology

Type of Carcinoma	Percentage of All Cases Diagnosed
Ductal carcinoma	
In situ	5
Infiltrating	70
Infiltrating with uniform histologic appearance	10
Medullary, colloid, comedo, tubular, papillary	
Lobular carcinoma	
In situ	3
Infiltrating	9
Inflammatory carcinoma	2
Paget's disease	1

epithelium and have not penetrated the basement membrane. It is most commonly discovered in perimenopausal and postmenopausal women. DCIS is often seen in conjunction with areas of carcinoma. Intraductal carcinoma in situ is not usually detected by palpation because the disease does not produce a definitive mass, although it may rarely produce nipple discharge. Mammography sometimes demonstrates the fine stippling of microcalcifications (**Fig. 15-15A**). Diagnosis is best made with core-needle biopsy, usually ultrasound directed.

The histologic diagnosis of intraductal carcinoma in situ includes a heterogenous group of tumors with varying malignant potential. Literature reviews document carcinoma developing in approximately one third of women with this disease within 10 years of initial diagnosis, usually in the same quadrant of the breast as the original biopsy. Treatment is excision with negative margins, and radiation to the ipsilateral breast. Results of large trials by the NCADP have shown decreased recurrence of cancer if both modalities are used. Additionally, if the DCIS is hormone-receptor–positive, then tamoxifen therapy should be offered. DCIS is a marker for significantly increased breast cancer risk with a lifetime risk of 25%. Lobular carcinoma in situ should not be treated as a cancer. It is a marker for a significantly increased breast cancer, though it does not have the same malignant potential as intraductal carcinoma in situ. It has a greater tendency to be bilateral and to be multifocal. Three of four patients are in the pre- or perimenopausal age group. Lobular carcinoma in situ is not detected by palpation. The latent period for development of malignancy is longer than with intraductal carcinoma in situ; often more than 20 years will elapse before infiltrating carcinoma develops. Approximately 20% of women with this disease will develop invasive breast carcinoma during their lifetime. Interestingly, most of the subsequent carcinomas are ductal, not lobular (**Table 15-9**). If the LCIS is hormone receptor positive, then chemoprevention with an appropriate SERM may be prescribed.

Infiltrating ductal carcinoma is the most common breast malignancy, comprising approximately 75% of malignancies. Histologically, nonuniform malignant epithelial cells of varying sizes and shapes infiltrate the surrounding tissue (**Fig. 15-18**). The degree of fibrous response to the invading epithelial cells determines the firmness to palpation and texture during biopsy. Often the stromal reaction may be extensive.

Table 15-9 Salient Characteristics of In Situ Ductal (DCIS) and Lobular (LCIS) Carcinoma of the Breast

	LCIS	DCIS
Age (years)	44 to 47	54 to 58
Incidence*	2% to 5%	5% to 100%
Clinical signs	None	Mass, pain, nipple discharge
Mammographic signs	None	Microcalcifications
Premenopausal	2/3	1/3
Incidence synchronous		
Invasive carcinoma	5%	2% to 46%
Multicentricity	60% to 90%	40% to 80%
Bilaterality	50% to 70%	10% to 20%
Axillary metastasis	1%	1% to 2%
Subsequent carcinomas:		
Incidence	25% to 35%	25% to 70%
Laterality	Bilateral	Ipsilateral
Interval to diagnosis	15 to 20 years	5 to 10 years
Histology	Ductal	Ductal

*Among biopsies of mammographically detected breast lesions.
From Frykberg ER, Ames FC, Bland KI: Current concepts for management of early (in situ and occult invasive) breast carcinoma. In Bland KI, Copeland EM (eds): The Breast. Philadelphia, WB Saunders, 1991, p 736.

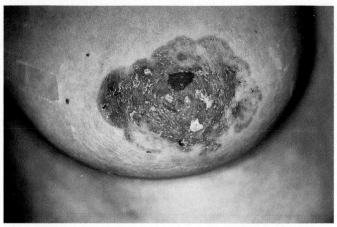

Figure 15-19 Paget's disease of the breast. Note the erythematous plaques around the nipple. (From Callen JP: Dermatologic signs of systemic disease. In Bolognia JL, Jorizzo JL, Rapini RP [eds]: Dermatology. Edinburgh, Mosby, 2003, p 714.)

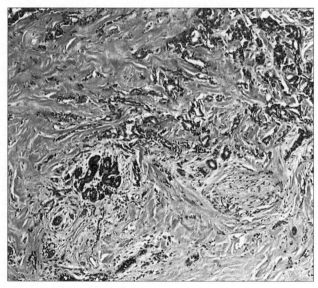

Figure 15-18 Invasive ductal carcinoma of the breast. Malignant cells are invading the fibrous tissue. (From Stevens A, Lowe J: Human Histology, 3 rd ed. Philadelphia, Elsevier Mosby, 2005, p 392.)

Approximately 10% of infiltrating ductal carcinomas are of a uniform histologic picture and are then classified as medullary, colloid, comedo, tubular, or papillary carcinomas. In general the specialized forms are grossly softer, mobile, and well delineated. They are usually smaller and have a more optimistic prognosis than the more common nonhomogeneous variety. Medullary carcinomas are soft, with extensive stromal infiltration by lymphocytes and plasma cells. Colloid carcinomas have a similar soft consistency, with extensive deposition of extracellular mucin. Papillary malignancies tend to have greater fibrovascular elements with a wide spectrum of presentation, between benign and very aggressive.

Approximately 15% of breast carcinomas are lobular. Infiltrating lobular carcinomas are characterized by the uniformity of the small, round neoplastic cells. Often the malignant epithelial cells infiltrate the stroma in a single-file fashion. This neoplasia tends to have a multicentric origin in the same breast and tends to involve both breasts more often than infiltrating ductal carcinoma. Histologic subdivisions of infiltrating lobular carcinoma include small cell, round cell, and signet cell carcinomas.

Inflammatory carcinomas account for approximately 2% of breast cancers. This type is recognized clinically as a rapidly growing, highly malignant carcinoma. Infiltration of malignant cells into the lymphatics of the skin produces a clinical picture that simulates a skin infection (**Fig. 15-19**). There is not a specific histologic cell type, though the tumor is predominantly ductal in origin.

Paget's disease of the breast is rare, comprising slightly less than 1% of breast carcinomas (**Fig. 15-20**). This lesion has an innocent appearance and looks like eczema or dermatitis of the nipple. The clinical picture is produced by an infiltrating ductal carcinoma that invades the epidermis. Paget's disease has a good prognosis.

Breast cancer is a molecularly heterogenous disease. In the past decade, an additional perspective has begun to be understood beyond the simplified histologic classification. This classification is based on gene expression or profiling, including the presence of hormone receptors. The gene microarray analysis of tumors has led to the empiric division of breast cancers into five types. These divisions are detailed in **Table 15-10**.

The lactiferous ducts have two layers: the inner layer closest to the lumen and the outer layer next to the basement membrane with more myoepithelial elements. Cells that appear biochemically with expression of genes similar to luminal cells are usually hormonally estrogen sensitive. Luminal-A breast tumors are generally of good prognosis, low grade, and estrogen and progesterone receptor positive and HER2(Neu) negative. These are more commonly found in older women. Luminal-B have overexpression of HER2(Neu) and have a poorer prognosis. Often they are estrogen and progesterone as well as p53 gene mutation positive (these are acquired p53 mutations as opposed to inherited descriptions, used gene expression information to describe the four different subtypes listed previously: luminal-A, luminal-B, basal, and HER2(Neu) positive.

A fifth type of breast cancer also is triple-receptor negative (estrogen, progesterone, and HER2(Neu). This type represents about 10% of breast cancers but has profiling similar to normal breast tissue and is not basal with respect to expression of the gene profile. This fifth type of breast cancer has a good prognosis. This molecular perspective for classifying breast carcinoma supersedes the histologic classifications. These five subtypes can be found in both carcinoma in situ and invasive carcinomas. Currently, extensive research is being applied to the questions of etiology and differentiation of the different types based on their gene expressions. The classification should become the standard description within the next few years.

MANAGEMENT

The treatment of breast carcinoma is complex, with multiple variables that must be considered. The treatment will obviously vary based on the needs and conditions of the patient. The most important variables for treatment selection are the stage, including the tumor's size; its inherent aggressiveness, as determined by the histology of the initial lesion, and its gene expressions including receptor status; and the presence of positive nodes. The primary direction in the algorithm tree of treatment is the stage. The TNM system is a widely recognized staging system based on both clinical and pathologic criteria (Table 15-11). When generalizations are offered concerning the preferred method of therapy, it is important to remember that breast carcinoma is a heterogeneous group of neoplasms. Unfortunately, neither clinical nor pathologic staging of the disease is nearly as precise as one would postulate in a carcinoma involving an external organ.

Microscopic metastatic disease occurs early via both hematogenous and lymphatic routes. For example, 30% to 40% of women without gross adenopathy in the axilla will have positive nodes discovered during histologic examination. With the additional assessment tools of immunohistochemical staining for the presence of cytokeratin and serial sectioning of axillary nodes, 10% to 30% of women considered to have negative nodes by standard histologic analysis are found to be node positive. Thus, older studies that noted up to 60% of all women with breast carcinoma developing distant metastatic disease regardless of the type of initial therapy are not applicable today with better node evaluation.

It is important to understand the natural history of untreated breast carcinoma. In series of women refusing therapy, 20% will be alive at 5 years and 5% will be alive at 10 years. Breast

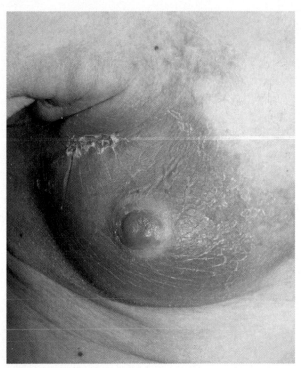

Figure 15-20 Inflammatory breast carcinoma—cellulitic appearing plaque. (From Marks J and Miller J: Lookingbill and Marks' Principles of Dermatology, 4th ed. Philadelphia, Saunders, 2006, an imprint of Elsevier, Figure 23.6.)

mutations). The third type of tumors just express HER2(Neu) but are estrogen and progesterone negative. These tumors have a poor prognosis. They usually have high rates of p53 mutations as well. The fourth type of breast tumor appears to be similar to basal-type duct cells in terms of expression of more myoepithelial gene profiling. These gene profiles include positive expression of cytokeratins 17, 14, 5, and 6, as well as p53, and endothelial growth factor receptors (EGFR).

Basal-type carcinoma results in tumors that tend to be high grade—between 75% and 95% are grade 3—and they act in an aggressive fashion. Unlike hormone receptor positive tumors that metastasize primarily to bone and lymph tissue, basal tumors metastasize primarily to lung and brain. Basal-type tumors are almost always receptor negative and are thus sometimes referred to as triple negative. These types of tumors are disproportionally found in women of color and younger women. BRCA1 tumors are up to 95% basal type. Women with these tumors will usually receive systemic chemotherapy. Dairkee first described these tumors in 1998. Perou, in 2000, building on Dairkee's

Table 15-10 Classification of Breast Carcinoma Based on Gene Profiling and Hormone Receptor

Expression Type	Grade	Characteristic Behavior	Hormone Receptor Status*
Luminal A	Usually low grade	Good prognosis	E and P +
Luminal B	All grades	Mixed prognosis	E and P +, Her 2 (Neu) +
Her 2 (Neu)	Higher grades	Poor prognosis	E and P −, Her 2 (Neu) +
Basal	Usually grade 3	Poor prognosis	Triple negative
Normal breast†	Usually low grade	Good prognosis	Triple negative

*E, estrogen receptor, P, progesterone receptor.
†Normal breast does not express gene profiling of basal elements, myoepithelial gene expression.

Table 15-11 TNM Staging of Breast Cancer

Primary Tumor (T)

TX	Primary tumor cannot be assessed
T0	No evidence of primary tumor
Tis*	Carcinoma in situ; intraductal carcinoma, lobular carcinoma in situ, or Paget's disease of the nipple with no tumor
T1	Tumor is ≤ 2.0 cm in greater dimension
T1a	Tumor is ≤ 0.5 cm in greatest dimension
T1b	Tumor is > 0.5 cm but not more than 1.0 cm in greatest dimension
T1c	Tumor is more than 1.0 cm but not more than 2.0 cm in greatest dimension
T2	Tumor is > 2.0 cm but not more than 5.0 cm in greatest dimension
T3	Tumor is > 5.0 cm in greatest dimension
T4	Tumor of any size with direct extension to chest wall or skin
T4a	Extension to chest wall
T4b	Edema (including peau d'orange) or ulceration of the skin of the breast or satellite skin nodules confined to the same breast
T4c	Both T4a and T4b above
T4d	Inflammatory carcinoma

Regional Lymph Node Involvement (N) (Clinical)

NX	Regional lymph nodes cannot be assessed (e.g., previously removed)
N0	No regional lymph node metastasis
N1	Metastasis to movable ipsilateral axillary lymph node(s)
N2	Metastasis to ipsilateral axillary lymph node(s) fixed to one another or the other structures
N3	Metastasis to ipsilateral mammary lymph node(s)

Distant Metastasis (M)

MX	Presence of distant metastasis cannot be assessed
M0	No distant metastasis
M1	Distant metastasis (includes metastasis to ipsilateral supraclavicular lymph node[s])

Stage Grouping

Stage 0	Tis	N0	M0
Stage I	T1	N0	M0
Stage IIa	T0	N1	M0
	T1	N1*	M0
	T2	N0	M0
Stage IIb	T2	N1	M0
	T3	N0	M0
Stage IIIa	T0	N2	M0
	T1	N2	M0
	T2	N2	M0
	T3	N1, N2	M0
Stage IIIb	T4	Any N	M0
	Any T	N3	M0
Stage IV	Any T	Any N	M1

*The prognosis of patients with pN1a is similar to that of patients with pN0.

Paget's disease associated with a tumor is classified according to the size of the tumor. Chest wall includes ribs, intercostal muscles, and serratus anterior muscle but not pectoral muscle.

From Eberlein TJ: Current management of carcinoma of the breast. Ann Surg 220:121, 1994.

carcinoma is a systemic disease that may recur many years, sometimes decades, after initial diagnosis. However, women with negative nodes have a 10-year survival rate of 75%.

The major changes in management of breast carcinoma since the 1990s have resulted from changing concepts regarding the biology of the disease, with the understanding that many women with breast carcinoma have systemic disease at the time the diagnosis is initially established. The natural history of the majority of developing breast carcinomas results in years of growth of the neoplasm before discovery. Because occult vascular dissemination is likely to occur prior to diagnosis, treatment of breast carcinoma involves both local and systemic therapy. It is beyond the scope of this book to present the details of treatment of breast

carcinoma. Thorough clinical and surgical staging is the cornerstone of any treatment plan.

The three major objectives of treating breast carcinoma are control of local disease, treatment of distant metastasis, and improved quality of life for women treated for the disease. There are several methods for controlling local disease. With multiple therapeutic options in both local and systemic therapy for breast carcinoma, women have an active role in deciding their own treatment regimen. Breast conservation with lumpectomy or quadrantectomy is a frequent choice for the control of local disease. Sentinel node resection is becoming standard practice in the treatment of early-stage breast cancer. Chemotherapy is used not only for patients with proved metastatic disease but also for women at high risk for developing primary or recurrent disease. Emphasis on conservative surgery plus radiation therapy to control multifocal cancer in the same breast and on reconstructive surgery after mastectomy has improved the quality of life for women with breast carcinoma.

Surgical Therapy

The decision concerning appropriate therapy and extent of the surgical operation to treat breast carcinoma should be made by the woman in consultation with the surgeon, radiotherapist, and medical oncologist who will treat her. As emphasized, the size of the tumor, the initial extent of disease, the virulence of the neoplasm, and the presence of estrogen and progesterone receptors are the key medical factors in the decision. The initial size of the breast carcinoma is the single best predictor of the likelihood of positive axillary nodes. The presence and number of axillary node metastasis is the single best predictor of survival. Intensive discussions concerning breast reconstruction or external prostheses are important to help the woman contemplate the effects of surgery on body image. Morris and coworkers have studied the psychological and social adjustments to mastectomy in 160 women, who were followed at intervals of 3, 12, and 24 months after surgery. One in four women was still having problems with depression and associated marital and sexual problems 2 years after the initial therapy.

Until the 1980s, **radical mastectomy** was the standard operation for carcinoma of the breast. Radical mastectomy was designed to control local disease by an extensive en bloc removal of the breast and underlying pectoralis major and pectoralis minor muscles and complete axillary dissection. It is a cosmetically disfiguring operation, leaving a major deformity of the chest wall. With an increased understanding that cancer of the breast is often a systemic disease and prognosis is similar with conservative surgery, the therapeutic emphasis has changed to less radical surgery and increased use of radiotherapy and chemotherapy (**Table 15-12**). Often patients are not cured even with extensive local therapy. Thus, protocols were established for more conservative approaches to local disease. The **modified radical mastectomy** removes the breast and only the fascia over the pectoralis major muscle. The pectoralis minor muscle may be removed to facilitate the axillary dissection. **Simple mastectomy** includes removal of the breast without underlying muscle tissue. Sentinel node biopsy has decreased the need for complete axillary lymphadenectomy.

Increased screening has led to malignancies being found at a time when they are small. Lumpectomy with node sampling is now a common option. The primary therapy for the majority of women with stages I and II breast cancer is conservative surgery, which preserves the breast, followed by radiation therapy. Resection of a wider area of the breast than lumpectomy is referred to as *quadrantectomy*. The latter operation is more effective in preventing local recurrences. However, the cosmetic result is not as satisfactory. In trials with either lumpectomy or quadrantectomy without irradiation, the rate of recurrence in the treated breast was approximately 40% compared with 10% when irradiation was given. Thus, almost all women with conservative surgical therapy for invasive breast carcinoma receive radiotherapy. Radiotherapy may not be necessary in some selected instances in older women.

Veronesi and colleagues published a controlled study of 701 women with carcinomas measuring less than 2 cm in diameter without palpable axillary lymph nodes. The women were randomized preoperatively into two treatment groups. One group of 349 patients had radical mastectomy. The other group included 352 women who had excision of a quadrant of the breast to control the primary lesion, axillary dissection, and radiotherapy involving both external and interstitial sources. Five-year survival rates were virtually identical—90% in both groups. Five-year disease-free survival rates were similar, 83% and 84%. Additional randomized prospective studies have found no difference in therapeutic results contrasting conservative surgery and postoperative irradiation versus radical surgery for stage I or II breast carcinoma. These studies found local recurrence rates of 5% at 5 years and approximately 10% at 10 years. Radiotherapy was begun 1 to 2 weeks postoperatively and given for approximately 5 weeks. The radiotherapeutic dosage was 180 to 200 cGy/day for a total dose of approximately 5000 cGy.

Another conservative approach to the treatment of breast cancer involves the use of sentinel lymph node mapping as an alternative to axillary dissection. Although the presence of axillary node metastasis is an important prognostic factor for patients with breast cancer, there is a high incidence of chronic complications associated with axillary dissection. By injecting the primary tumor with radioactive colloid tracers and dyes, the surgeon can identify the first set of regional lymph nodes that receive lymphatic drainage from the tumor. These are termed *sentinel lymph nodes.* Subsequently, these nodes can be removed and the axillary dissection can be deleted if they are negative. In a large multi-institutional trial, Krag and colleagues were able to identify the sentinel nodes in 93% of the cases. The accuracy of sentinel node mapping in this series for predicting the status of axillary nodes was 97%. The positive predictive value was 100%, and the negative predictive value was 96%.

It is important to offer every woman alternatives in treatment for stages I and II breast carcinoma. The cosmetic result obtained by lumpectomy and radiation therapy depends on the size and shape of the breast and the size of the initial tumor. For some women, mastectomy followed by reconstructive surgery may give a superior cosmetic result. Also, the management of the axillary nodes should be considered and the woman should be informed concerning all of her options.

Many women, depending on their tumor grade and size, will have mastectomy with a primary breast reconstruction at the same time. Again, depending on the tumor, this may be followed by radiation. Primary reconstruction or implants has been shown to be safe and appropriate. Studies have shown that many women benefit with less depression and greater sense of self-esteem and control.

Table 15-12 Ten-Year Disease-Free Survival Rates of Women with Breast Cancer

	Conservation Surgery and Radiation	Radical or Modified Radical Mastectomy Alone
Minimal breast cancer	92%	95%
Stage I	78%	80%
Stage II	73%	65%

Reprinted from Montague ED: Conservation surgery and radiation therapy in the treatment of operable breast cancer. Cancer 53:702, 1984

Medical Therapy

Adjuvant systemic chemotherapy decreases the odds of dying from breast cancer during the first 10 years following diagnosis by approximately 25%. The two major factors in predicting the likelihood of systemic disease in breast carcinoma are the diameter of the primary tumor and the number of positive axillary nodes. Women whose initial tumor is less than 1 cm in diameter and who have negative axillary nodes have excellent chances for disease-free survival, with a 10-year relapse rate of less than 10%.

It is not established whether the response to chemotherapy of specific histologic subtypes differs because women in various chemotherapeutic studies have until recently not been randomized according to histologic type. Current research indicates a significantly increased response of basal tumors to chemotherapy.

The presence and concentration of receptors should be obtained at the initial diagnostic biopsy or surgery, as receptor status may change after radiotherapy or chemotherapy. Estrogen receptors are of two types, ER-alpha and ER-beta. Most laboratories test only for the ER-alpha receptors, and its biology is better understood. ER-beta receptors' role in malignancy is still under investigation. ER-positive is currently not quantified, and women with both low levels of estrogen receptors and high levels of expression of estrogen receptors are all lumped together. Thus, the ones who do not respond to treatment may have lower levels. Additionally, crosstalk between growth factors, such as the estrogen receptors and other cytokine receptors, can lead to phosphorylation of estrogen receptors in some women and not others. Phosphorylated estrogen receptors do not bind as well, thus there is a decreased response to medications like tamoxifen. As tumors mutate and metastasize, the expression of estrogen receptors decreases. Hormonal therapies become less effective in controlling disease. Progesterone receptor positivity is a sign of better differentiation and a greater response to hormonal therapy. Progesterone receptors are often lost as tumors metastasize, as well. In general, luminal type A receptor-positive tumors are usually better differentiated and exhibit a less aggressive clinical behavior, including a lower risk of recurrence and lower capacity to proliferate. When estrogen receptors are positive, approximately 60% of breast cancers will respond to hormonal therapy; an 80% response rate is noted when both estrogen and progesterone receptors are present. If estrogen receptors are negative, less than 10% of tumors respond to hormonal manipulation.

Hormonal therapy may include ablative surgery but is usually accomplished by drugs that change endocrine function by blocking receptor sites or blocking synthesis of hormones. In the past, the most commonly used ablative surgery was bilateral oophorectomy in a premenopausal woman with breast carcinoma. Hormonal therapy is effective in producing a response in advanced metastatic carcinoma for approximately 1 year. Metastatic disease in soft tissue and bone is the most sensitive to hormonal manipulation. Tamoxifen, an oral antiestrogen, is an alternative to surgical castration and presently is the most frequently prescribed hormonal agent for breast carcinoma. The aromatase inhibitor Arimidex is a commonly used agent. Arimidex blocks the peripheral conversion of adrenal androgens to estrone. Because aromatase is primarily found in body fat, Arimidex can be particularly valuable in obese women with ER positive cancers. Medroxyprogesterone (Depo-Provera), androgens, danazol, and gonadotropin hormone-releasing hormone (GH-RH) agonists have also been used to treat breast carcinoma.

Two endocrine agents used simultaneously do not produce better results than a single agent.

Positive receptor expression for HER2(+) is found in 15% to 20% of women with breast cancer. The HER2(Neu) gene is an epithelial growth factor determinant (human epidermal receptor). The HER2(Neu) gene, when overexpressed on tumor cells, is a poor prognostic sign and a marker for aggressive disease. Trastuzumab (Herceptin) is a powerful and remarkably effective agent for treatment of HER2(Neu) tumors. Trastuzumab is a recombinant monoclonal antibody, which is directed against the HER2 protein. Several trials have shown significant improvement in outcome and were stopped because of the improved outcomes compared with placebo. The drug affects multiple steps in the cell cycle and importantly sensitizes cells to other chemotherapy agents. Thus, Herceptin is given concurrent with adjuvant chemotherapy cycles and continued during radiation, because it is also a radiosensitizer. It is usually given for 1 year as a treatment. However, the drug is associated with cardiotoxicity, so caution must be used when patients are also receiving anthracycline-based chemotherapy, such as doxorubicin (Adriamycin).

Adjuvant chemotherapy has produced positive responses and an increase in disease-free survival in many clinical studies. Initially, chemotherapy was selected to treat women with positive axillary nodes or remote disease. Chemotherapy has proved effective in shrinking measurable metastatic disease in both premenopausal and postmenopausal women.

The role for adjuvant therapy in the management of breast cancer continues to expand. Adjuvant chemotherapy has been shown to improve disease-free and overall survival in all patients with operable breast cancer with the exception of select node-negative patients with small (less than 1 cm) tumors that have no high-risk features. A recent update of the National Surgical Adjuvant Breast and Bowel Project (NSABP) B-20 trial indicated a significant advantage in the estrogen receptor-positive, node-negative patient who received chemotherapy in addition to tamoxifen. Even women in the postmenopausal age group with estrogen receptor-positive, node-negative breast cancers that traditionally would be treated with tamoxifen alone have been shown to benefit from the combination of chemotherapy and tamoxifen. Only limited data are available from randomized trials for women over the age of 70. In the absence of other comorbidities, chemotherapy can be considered in this population of older women.

Combination therapy of cytotoxic drugs is vastly superior to single-agent regimens. In the past, combinations included drugs such as cyclophosphamide, methotrexate, doxorubicin (Adriamycin), 5-fluorouracil, and vinblastine. Presently, it is believed that anthracycline-containing combinations are more effective than regimens that do not contain anthracyclines. Paclitaxel therapy has excellent response for breast cancer. The addition of four to five cycles of paclitaxel to four to six cycles of the Adriamycin and cyclophosphamide regimen improved disease-free and overall survival rates in patients with node-positive breast cancer. Other drugs currently under investigation for the treatment of breast cancer include anthra-pyrazoles, liposomal anthracyclines, and gemcitabine. Clinical trials that have investigated the use of extremely intensive chemotherapeutic regimens followed by transplantation of autologous bone marrow in women with advanced or recurrent disease have not found convincing evidence that high-dose chemotherapy is superior to conventional treatment. Its use should be limited to clinical trials.

Tamoxifen has the greatest effect in postmenopausal women. As one would expect, tamoxifen is of greater benefit in women with tumors that have estrogen receptors than in tumors that are negative for estrogen receptors. There is no significant improvement in survival rates in patients with estrogen receptor-negative tumors. However, even in receptor-negative patients, 5 years of tamoxifen use will decrease the risk of a second primary or contralateral breast cancer by as much as 45%. Extending tamoxifen therapy beyond 5 years is not associated with a further reduction in risk. Tamoxifen therapy increases the prevalence of intrauterine polyps and endometrial hyperplasia and carcinoma. However, most tamoxifen-related endometrial cancers are stage I, grade 1 successfully treated with surgery alone.

THE GYNECOLOGIST'S ROLE

Once a suspicious mass has been found, either by screening or by examination, the patient is referred to the multidisciplinary breast cancer team: the oncologist, surgeon, chemotherapist, and radiologist. The further management of her breast cancer is handled in turn by a series of physicians. The primary concerns about treatment are well addressed by these specialists, but for most women, there are myriad of other issues that are better managed by her gynecologist. This is the time when the patient needs her gynecologist as much as any other time in her life. The overwhelming psychosocial issues that breast cancer patients face include changes in body image, fears of loss of femininity, premature menopause and menopausal symptoms, and changes in sexual function. These concerns and issues begin shortly after the diagnosis and continue in varying degrees for several years. Oncologists seldom address with these issues; the patient's gynecologist is trusted and has the most expertise in these areas. These concerns need to be actively brought up in discussion with the patient.

The issues that need addressing are both process issues and content issues. Many authors have documented the psychosocial effects of breast cancer on a woman's self-image. The issue of having cancer affects all people at several levels. Breast cancer is particularly difficult in that it so strongly affects a woman's image of herself as a woman. As expected, younger women have significant problems with this issue, as well as with an early-induced menopause. In general, younger women have increased psychological distress compared with older women. A study by Fobain et al. evaluated 549 women with breast cancer between ages 22 and 50 (the younger population of breast cancer victims). One-half had two or more issues with changes in body image. Half of the sexually active women had issues with sexuality and sexual dysfunction. Researchers have noted the detrimental effect on quality of life in younger women with breast cancer. The effects or breast cancer and its treatments on sexual arousal, vaginal dryness, and decreased libido are well documented. Sexual function should be addressed before, during, and after treatment. The patient needs reassurance that a decrease in sexual functioning during and for a while after treatment are normal. She may need help with lubricants and alternatives to hormones, if her tumor is receptor positive. More than anything else, she needs a safe place to express her concerns and fears and to be reassured. Selective serotonin reuptake inhibitors (SSRIs), used to treat depression, may also decrease libido, and different types of

medication may have to be prescribed to women who are adversely affected by this problem. Studies note that approximately half of couples have significant sexual dysfunction after the diagnosis of breast cancer. However, many clinicians feel that this percentage is closer to 100% of sexually active women. If extended treatment beyond basic counseling is needed, then referral is indicated. Sexual dysfunction may become worse over time, thus it is important to address the issue at least on a yearly basis. These difficulties involve the couple, and it is helpful to involve the partner in counseling and treatment discussions when appropriate. Vaginal dryness may be addressed with vaginal estrogen in several forms, particularly in estrogen receptor–negative tumors. For women with estrogen receptor–positive tumors, vaginal estrogen such as with the Estring give minimal systemic levels; however, use should be discussed with the patient's oncologist.

As therapy finishes, the patient enters into a new phase. An appointment should be set up 4 to 6 weeks after her treatment is finished. A schedule of further appointments at 6 months and then yearly should also be established. It is common for friends and family of patients to ask, "Aren't you glad that your chemotherapy (or radiation) is finished?" However, paradoxically most patients will have a sense of anxiety and dread at this point. The safety of therapy in fighting the cancer has been taken away. The woman's defense mechanism, that the cancer is being destroyed, is taken down. The patient must reorder her reality. At the posttreatment visit, the physician should gently bring this issue up as a natural and normal reaction. Some patients may benefit from support groups or counseling if the anxiety becomes overwhelming. Questions about appetite, sleep, and pleasurable activities are important to ask, as the clinician evaluates for subclinical or overt depression. Fatigue is common after chemotherapy and radiation, and thus this symptom is less helpful in evaluating for depression. Anxiety is common at the anniversary of both finding the tumor and of surgery, and it is helpful to warn patients and their families. In this setting, it is helpful to invite support people/families in, after the initial aspect of the visit is complete. Psychological support for breast cancer patients is one of the most important aspects for the gynecologist to address. Support groups have been shown to be beneficial in several studies. Initially, early reports from the late 1980s found that support groups improved survival. Larger studies have shown that there is no significant effect on survival, but there are psychological benefits.

Depression is common in the first year after the treatment of breast cancer. Approximately 10% to 25% of women will be diagnosed with clinical depression. Baucom et al., in their review of psychosocial issues, described the first year after the diagnosis of breast cancer as marked by "considerable psychological distress including shock, emotional numbness, depression, and anxiety." If a woman with breast cancer is started on antidepressant medication, for treatment of depression or for relief of vasomotor symptoms, it is critical to consider the drug interactions of tamoxifen and certain SSRI medications (**Table 15-13**). Tamoxifen's mechanism of action is through its active metabolites, and the metabolism of tamoxifen is through the cytochrome P450 system, specifically CYP2DP. The change of tamoxifen to its most active metabolite, endoxifen, is inhibited by both fluoxetine and paroxetine. Tamoxifen metabolism is not as affected by sertraline or other SSRIs. Raloxifene metabolism is not affected by SSRI medications.

Table 15-13 Interactions among SSRI, SNRI, and Gabapentin with Tamoxifen Metabolism and CYP2D6 Activity

CYP2D6 Activity and Agent[a]	Efficacy Compared with Placebo for Hot Flashes
Strong CYP2D6 inhibitors	
Fluoxetine	50% vs. 36%, p=0.02
Paroxetine	62% vs. 37%, p=0.007
Moderate CYP2D6 inhibitors	
Duloxetine	Not assessed in placebo-controlled trial
Weak CYP2D6 inhibitors or noninhibitors	
Citalopram	49% vs. 23%, p=0.0021
Escitalopram	Not assessed in placebo-controlled trial
Fluvoxamine	Not assessed in placebo-controlled trial
Gabapentin	46% vs. 15%, p=0.007
Sertraline	36% vs. 27%, p=0.03
Venlafaxine	60% vs. 27%, p<0.0001

[a]Information about the CYP2D6 activity of these agents is from www.drug-interactions.com.
Adapted from Henry NL, Stearns V, Flockhart DA, et al: Drug interactions and pharmacogenomics in the treatment of breast cancer and depression. Am J Psych 165:1253, 2008, Table 2.

Box 15-4 Causes of Chest and Upper Extremity Pain in Women with Breast Cancer

Neuropathies
Myopathies
Tendonitis/rotator cuff inflammation
Costochondritis
Lymphedema
Deep vein thrombosis and superficial thrombosis
Cellulitis
Arthritis
Radiculopathy
Herpes zoster
Intercostal brachial neuralgia (postmastectomy syndrome)
Metastases
Recurrence of breast cancer

Adapted and modified from Stubblefield MD, Custodio CM: Upper extremity pain disorders in breast cancer. Arch Phys Med Rehabil 87:S98, 2006.

Gabapentin, commonly prescribed medication for chronic pain, has some effectiveness for vasomotor symptoms as well. Gabapentin does not affect tamoxifen metabolism.

After a patient's breast cancer treatment is finished, women will usually have residual musculoskeletal effects on their chest and breast on the side of the cancer. These symptoms can involve the shoulder, upper extremity, neck, back, and chest wall. They include pain, decreased sensation, and lymphedema. Within the first year of treatment, approximately 85% of women will experience some type of pain in the ipsilateral upper extremity or chest wall. This symptom is usually rapid in onset, is alarming, and may potentiate anxiety about the issues of recurrence or metastases. Though rapid metastases or recurrence is extremely rare, the patient is usually terrified. She should be invited into the office and given a thorough and appropriate evaluation. Imaging may be necessary. Verbal assurances without a "hands-on" evaluation can be detrimental to the patient's relationship with the gynecologist. It is critical for the patient to feel she is being listened to.

The etiology of upper extremity pain after breast cancer involves issues of radiation, surgery, potential recurrence, as well as issues related to chemotherapy. The differential diagnosis is broad and includes cervical radiculopathy (a pathology which may be related to treatment), neuropathy, rotator cuff injury, tendonitis, phantom breast pain, and a cellulitis that is more rare and usually involves advanced disease, postmastectomy syndrome (burning and sharp pain in the scar, chest, axilla, and sometimes upper arm) (**Box 15-4**). Because so many patients have pain in the first year after treatment, it is a good time, after the pain has been evaluated, to address some of the general issues again, such as anxiety and depression.

Upper extremity pain in the breast cancer patient may be related to lymphedema. Lymphedema has fortunately become less common than in past decades due to sentinel node biopsy replacing the lymphadenectomy and limited surgery such as lumpectomy replacing radical mastectomy. However, it is still a significant problem. Recent estimates have noted between 42% and 54% of breast cancer patients will have lymphedema. Approximately 2.5 million women in the United States currently have the diagnosis. As Fui et al. pointed out, lymphedema is a daily reminder to a woman, long after her cancer is gone and the surgery is over, that she had breast cancer. Women with axillary dissections and larger surgeries, as well as those with radiation, are at most risk, but even women with minimal surgeries and radiation are susceptible. Lymphedema has a detrimental effect on quality of life with symptoms that range from generalized discomfort to pain, heaviness, burning, paresthesias, decreased motility, fibrosis, and potential skin infections. Lymphedema affects both social life and employment. It tends to be progressive and may range from subclinical to massive. Measurements of the severity can be made with both circumferential limb measurements as well as with limb volume displacement.

Though lymphedema is not curable, it is amenable to therapy. Careful attention to infection, avoiding trauma, and weight loss are all helpful. Specific treatments include compression with wrapping bandages and special arm sleeves (garments). These need to be prescribed by therapists trained in lymphedema. Pressures with specially prescribed sleeves can reach up to 50 mm Hg for compression. Unfortunately, there is limited availability of physical therapists and nurses who are trained in lymphedema throughout the United States. Many treatments have been suggested in the past and are lauded on the Internet and in the lay literature. To date, debulking surgery, laser treatments, antioxidants, anticoagulation, and herbs have not been found to be helpful.

Exercise is important, as it improves lymph flow. Exercise with progressive resistance training (PRT) is helpful for the upper body in general and in particular for lymphedema. In a systematic review, Cheema et al. found that progressive resistance training was beneficial for breast cancer survivors and is extremely safe. Traditionally exercise was thought to increase lymphedema; paradoxically, exercise improves lymphedema. Skin care is also important because of the increased risk of infection.

Women with breast cancer are at significantly increased risk for both progressive cardiovascular disease and osteoporosis. Vitamin D metabolism is associated with breast cancer.

An increased incidence of breast cancer as well a worse prognosis have been noted in women who have low levels of vitamin D. Most studies are observational, and it is not known if increasing vitamin D levels will improve outcomes. Because most women with breast cancer will not be receiving estrogen replacement therapy, and many women will be pushed into early menopause, vitamin D supplementation is important to help prevent osteoporosis. Vitamin D levels should be checked in women who have been diagnosed with breast cancer and appropriate vitamin D replacement prescribed. In addition, a basic dietary history and the use of supplemental calcium are appropriate. After a woman has been treated for breast cancer, she should be screened with imaging for osteoporosis and treatment prescribed if she has evidence of decreased bone mineralization. Bisphosphonates are not problematic in women with breast cancer on breast cancer therapy (see Chapter 14).

Women who will be postmenopausal or going into menopause because of treatment will have changes in their lipid profiles. Additionally, obese women are at risk for cardiovascular disease as well. Thus, it is appropriate to obtain lipid profiles after therapy is finished and counsel women about cardiovascular health in terms of weight loss, exercise, and diet. If a patient is on tamoxifen, there is usually a mild improvement in lipid profiles; however, there is an increase in thromboembolic disease. Women who are given aromatase inhibitor therapy usually will have no effect to a slight improvement lipid profiles. As discussed previously in relation to lymphedema, exercise is an important treatment for cardiovascular health as well as being beneficial for lymphedema.

Treatment of breast cancer often involves women who are perimenopausal or may precipitate a rapid transition into menopause. Treatment of vasomotor symptoms is discussed at length in Chapter 14. Other than hormone replacement, SSRI drugs are a reasonable alternative. Given the psychological effects of breast cancer, the rapid transition into menopause further affects women with breast cancer, and symptoms should be addressed. The minimization of hot flushes, sleep disturbance, and vaginal dryness improves psychological well-being in addition to improving quality of life.

Premenopausal women who develop breast cancer may not have finished childbearing. If a woman would like more children, the discussion of fertility preservation needs to be held prior to treatment. There are two major issues that should be addressed in this situation. First, is pregnancy safe after a woman has had breast cancer. Studies evaluating pregnancy after breast cancer treatment have noted an improvement in survival, "the healthy mother effect." These reports, though, have a large selection bias. However, even with this bias, women who have pregnancies after breast cancer are noted to have a decreased risk of recurrence, Maltaris et al. summarized the literature through 2008. In studies of more than 15,000 women with more than 1100 pregnancies, no deleterious effects on survival or relapse were noted in women with a prior diagnosis of breast cancer who became pregnant. Traditional recommendations are to wait 48 to 60 months after treatment before attempting pregnancy.

The second issue involves fertility preservation if a woman wishes to maintain childbearing potential. Because tumors in young women have an increased incidence of being high grade, these women often receive chemotherapy. Breast cancer chemotherapy decreases and sometimes eliminates ovarian function. Up to 60% of women under age 40 will not resume menses after breast cancer chemotherapy, with a higher rate of menopause for women receiving chemotherapy after age 40. Strategies for fertility preservation should be individualized and best coordinated with reproductive endocrinologists prior to beginning treatment with cytotoxic chemotherapy. Cryopreservation of embryos is currently the most effective means of fertility preservation. Cryopreservation of mature follicles, immature follicles, and ovarian tissue, although effective in some cases, in still unproved in terms of its level of efficacy. Obviously, ovarian stimulation to achieve maturation of oocytes requires hormonal manipulation for several weeks prior to treatment. The problematic issue needs to be discussed with the breast cancer team and the family.

Lastly, sensitivity to the constant concern of all cancer patients that they may have a recurrence cannot be overemphasized. Nursing staff and triage staff need to ask a second question when patients call with what seems to be a trivial concern. The second question should be open ended, such as "Are you worried about this?" or "Are things going as expected?" The answer to the second question may reveal a deeper reason for the phone call or inquiry. This patient should then be promptly brought in and her concerns addressed with "the laying on of hands."

ACKNOWLEDGMENTS

We gratefully acknowledge the help of three incredible clinicians and scientists. This chapter is built on the dedicated work of Dr. Fidel Valea. Significant contributions have also been made by Kathryn Murray in genetics and Dr. Cathryn Chicola in imaging and screening.

KEY POINTS

- One out of eight women (12.5% of American females) develops carcinoma of the breast if she lives beyond age 90.
- The breast consists of approximately 20% glandular tissue and 80% fat and connective tissue; increasing proportions of fibroglandular to fatty tissues are the mark of denser breasts. Breast density is associated with increased risks of malignancy.
- Lymph drainage of the breast usually flows toward the most adjacent group of nodes. This concept represents the basis for sentinel node mapping in breast cancer. In most instances, breast cancer spreads in an orderly fashion within the axillary lymph node basin based on the anatomic relationship between the primary tumor and its associated regional (sentinel) nodes.
- Numerous epidemiologic studies have found an increased risk of developing breast carcinoma in women with benign breast disease only if there is associated atypical epithelial hyperplasia.
- The classic symptom of fibrocystic changes is cyclic bilateral breast pain. The signs of fibrocystic changes include increased engorgement and density of the breasts, excessive

- nodularity, rapid change and fluctuation in the size of cystic areas, increased tenderness, and occasionally spontaneous nipple discharge.
- Fibroadenomas are most frequently present in adolescents and women in their 20s.
- Approximately 30% of fibroadenomas will disappear, and 10% to 12% will become smaller after many years.
- The importance of determining the cause of *spontaneous* discharge from the nipple is to rule out carcinoma. The color of the nonmilky discharge does not differentiate a benign from a malignant process. Bloody discharge from the nipple, gross or microscopic, should be considered to be related to carcinoma until this diagnosis has been ruled out.
- Intraductal papilloma and fibrocystic changes are the two most common causes of spontaneous nonmilky nipple discharge.
- Risk factors identify only 25% of women who will eventually develop breast carcinoma.
- Approximately 5% to 10% of breast cancers have a familial or genetic link. Genetic predisposition to develop breast carcinoma has been recognized in some families. In these families, breast cancer tends to occur at a younger age, and there is a higher prevalence of bilateral disease.
- Mutations in *BRCA* family of genes have been identified that confer a lifetime risk of breast cancer that approaches 85%. *BRCA1* and *BRCA2* genes are involved in the majority of inheritable cases of breast cancer. These genes function as tumor suppressor genes, and several mutations have been described on each of these genes.
- Once a woman has developed carcinoma of one breast, her risk is approximately 1% per year of developing cancer in the other breast.
- Women with a high risk of breast cancer have proved options that can decrease their risk of breast cancer. Both tamoxifen and raloxifene significantly decrease the relative risk of developing breast carcinoma.

- Present studies demonstrate that screening mammography reduces breast cancer mortality by approximately 33% in women 50 to 70 years of age.
- Digital technology has multiple advantages compared with conventional mammography. Image acquisition, display, and storage are much faster, and image manipulation through adjustments in contrast, brightness, and electronic magnification of selected regions enables radiologists to obtain superior views.
- The incidence of carcinoma in biopsies corresponds directly with the patient's age. Approximately 20% of breast biopsies in women age 50 are positive, and this figure increases to 33% in women age 70 or older.
- Breast cancer is usually asymptomatic before the development of advanced disease. Breast pain is experienced by only 10% of women with early breast carcinoma. The classic sign of a breast carcinoma is a solitary, solid, three-dimensional, dominant breast mass. The borders of the mass are usually indistinct.
- Microscopic metastatic disease occurs early via both hematogenous and lymphatic routes. For example, 30% to 40% of women without gross adenopathy in the axilla will have positive nodes discovered during histologic examination. With the additional assessment tools of immunohistochemical staining for the presence of cytokeratin and serial sectioning of axillary nodes, 10% to 30% of patients considered to have negative nodes by standard histologic analysis are found to be node positive.
- The initial size of the breast carcinoma is the single best predictor of the likelihood of positive axillary nodes. The presence and number of axillary node metastasis is the single best predictor of survival.
- The primary therapy for the majority of women with stages I and II breast cancer is conservative surgery, which preserves the breast, followed by radiation therapy.
- Gynecologists should actively address the psychosexual problems that breast cancer causes in women, early in the evaluation of the disease and for several years.

REFERENCES CAN BE FOUND ON EXPERTCONSULT.com

SUGGESTED READING

Baines CJ: Breast self-examination, *Cancer* 69:1942, 1992.

Boyd N, Guo H, Martin L, et al: Mammographic Density and the Risk and Detection of Breast Cancer, *NEJM* 356:227, 2009.

Chlebowski R, Kuller L, Prentice R, et al: Breast Cancer after use of Estrogen plus Progestin in Postmenopausal Women, *NEJM* 360:573, 2009.

Colditz GA, Stampher MS, Willett WC, et al: Type of postmenopausal hormone use and risk of breast cancer: 12-year follow-up from the Nurses' Health Study, *Cancer Causes Control* 3:433, 1992.

Gail MH, Brinton LA, Byar DP, et al: Projecting individualized probabilities of developing breast cancer for white females who are being examined annually, *J Natl Cancer Inst* 81:1879, 1989.

Gradishar WJ, Cella D: Selective estrogen receptor modulators and prevention of invasive breast cancer, *JAMA* 295:2784, 2006.

Henderson T, Amsterdam A, Bhatia S, et al: *Systematic Review: Surveillance for Breast Cancer in Women Treated with Chest Radiation for Childhood, Adolescent, or Young Adult Cancer,* 2010.

Kemeny MM, Wellisch DK, Schain WS: Psychosocial outcome in a randomized surgical trial for treatment of primary breast cancer, *Cancer* 62:1231, 1988.

Krag D, Weaver D, Ashikaga T, et al: The sentinel node in breast cancer, *N Engl J Med* 339:941, 1998.

Lu K, Kauff N, Powell C, et al: Hereditary Breast and Ovarian Cancer Syndrome, *Gynecol Oncol* 113:6, 2009.

Rakha E, Reis-Filho J: Basal-like Breast Carcinoma, *Arch Pathol Lab Med* 133:860, 2009.

Santen R, Mansel R: Benign Breast Disorders, *NEJM* 353:275, 2005.

Smith R, Cokkinides V, Brooks D, et al: Cancer Screening in the United States, 2010: A review of current American Cancer Society Guidelines and issues in the Cancer Screening, *Ca Clin J* 60:99, 2010.

Stanton AWB, Modi S, Mellor RH, et al: Recent advances in breast cancer-related lymphedema of the arm: Lymphatic pump failure and predisposing factors, *Lymphat Res Biol* 7:29, 2009.

16

Spontaneous and Recurrent Abortion
Etiology, Diagnosis, Treatment

Vern L. Katz

Spontaneous abortion (SAB) is the loss of a pregnancy prior to 20 weeks' gestation. It has also been defined as the loss of a pregnancy prior to fetal viability outside of the womb. Viability is now in a gray area, beginning at approximately 23 weeks' gestation, although some states have defined viability as 22 weeks. Other definitions of SAB include the loss of a pregnancy less than or equal to 500 g. As medicine progresses, our definitions have evolved, and our terminology has evolved as well. As the word *abortion* has taken on a charged connotation in society, the synonym **miscarriage** has been substituted to an increasing extent for spontaneous abortion. Interestingly, the word *miscarriage* was noted in the *Oxford English Dictionary* to be first used as early as 1615 in the gynecologic context for pregnancy loss. In this chapter the terms *spontaneous abortion* and *miscarriage* will be used interchangeably. Similarly, the term *habitual abortion* has now been almost completely replaced by *recurrent miscarriage*.

Finally, it is important to understand the subtle distinctions between several terms used when discussing genetic issues: *congenital, inherited, genetic,* and *chromosomal.* These words are often used interchangeably; however, that can result in flawed interpretation of the literature. *Congenital* means present at birth. It does not infer whether or not a condition is inherited. *Inherited* means passed on from one or both parents. In other words, one or both parents have a genetic change that can be passed to offspring. *Genetic* means changes in the genes or chromosomes. Genetic changes can be sporadic events that are not inherited such as a "new mutation," or they can be inherited events such as cystic fibrosis. Another example is Down syndrome. If an individual has trisomy 21, it is not inherited. If a person has Down syndrome that resulted from a familial translocation, then it is inherited. *Chromosomal* problems are all genetic, but few are inherited. The only chromosomal problems that are inherited are the result of familial translocations. Current research focuses on an additional source of chromosomal anomalies: microdeletions and microduplications. These problems are in between single gene defects and full chromosomal abnormalities representing small portions of DNA, involving a few genes. These may be inherited or sporadic.

Although common, affecting nearly 20% of all pregnancies, spontaneous abortions are still devastating for both the mother and her partner. The psychological effect of an unintended pregnancy loss cannot be overestimated. The social reaction, in contrast, is often destructive; the response is often societal denial. Some of this reaction may be to avoid the "rubbing off of the bad luck." Seemingly polite responses, such as "You can have another" or "It was for the best," enforce a denial of the couple's natural grieving process. The effect may be quite detrimental and long lasting. It may also serve the purpose to set the couple apart, therefore lessening the perceived risk for others. The denial of a grieving response for a miscarriage may be present unknowingly among medical providers. In this setting, the denial is even worse. The loss of a pregnancy induces a high rate of depression and guilt. The role of the health provider is to assist the woman and the family through the process and, if possible, find a scientific rationale or reason for the pregnancy loss. If appropriate, preventive measures should be offered for the future.

Historically, miscarriage has been treated differently in different cultures. Kueller and Katz described the finding of Greek and Roman burial urns in archeological excavations that were specifically used for the products of conception from miscarriage. Ritual purification has been described in Africa for women after miscarriage to prevent a recurrence of the pregnancy loss. Women in pre-Christian Europe and in the Middle East wore specialized amulets termed *eagle stones.* Eagle stones were hollow rocks with small pebbles inside the hollow that would rattle when shaken, symbolizing the pregnancy. These were worn to prevent pregnancy loss. Southern Asian cultures attributed spontaneous abortion to demons. The demons Con Ranh, Kan Kamiak, and Kaure had to be exorcised to prevent recurrence of a miscarriage. In more modern times, multiple medications, drugs, and vitamins have been suggested as treatment to prevent spontaneous abortion. Vitamin C and vitamin E deficiencies have been postulated to cause miscarriage. Even in the 21st century, magical thinking in the form of superstition persists in every modern subculture regarding the causes of pregnancy loss.

Physicians have often fallen into the medical confusion of mixing up association with cause and effect when working with women with spontaneous and recurrent miscarriage. The classic paradigm of this logic fallacy is the story of diethylstilbestrol (DES). From the 1940s until the early 1960s, women were given the potent synthetic estrogen, stilbestrol (diethylstilbestrol), to prevent pregnancy loss. DES was prescribed as treatment based on the theory that estrogen levels were low in women who were aborting or had aborted. However, the estrogen levels were low as a result of the pregnancy loss, not as its cause. Unfortunately, tens of thousands of women received DES during early pregnancy. The DES did not prevent pregnancy loss, as was well documented, but the medication did cross the placenta and injure the developing genital tracts of both male and female fetuses. The subsequent generation, now almost through their reproductive years, have an excess of pregnancy loss themselves because of their mother's DES exposure.

Treatments such as DES for miscarriage stem from a laudable desire to prevent pain and help our patients. The psychological distress of patients with **recurrent spontaneous abortion** is one of desperation. The desire and the ability to reproduce are central to many couple's identity as well as the feeling of self-worth. Patients and families will go to incredible lengths in hopes for any "miracle cure" to solve the problem of miscarriage.

In this chapter we discuss the epidemiology of pregnancy loss and then review the etiology, diagnosis, and management of spontaneous abortion. Recurrent miscarriage may be caused by any factor that persists from one pregnancy to another, such as a balanced translocation or maternal thrombophilia, but it is unlikely to be caused by an event such as a viral infection. The management of recurrent miscarriage is discussed throughout the chapter.

Spontaneous abortion needs to be viewed as a syndrome, as well as a continuum. Loss in the embryonic period, less than 10 weeks, is in a continuum with a loss in the fetal period. There are multiple causes. The loss at less than 10 weeks is often due to a chromosomal abnormality, compared with a loss at 18 to 20 weeks, which will more often be from structural cervical or uterine problems. Additionally, many women have more than one cause for recurrent miscarriages. Importantly, for women who have miscarriages, a known etiology does not always cause pregnancy loss. Not all women with a particular problem will have a miscarriage, and women who do miscarry will not do so in each pregnancy. For example, a woman who is a carrier of a 14/21 balanced translocation may miscarry with an **embryo** with trisomy 14, give birth to a healthy liveborn, and then have a child with Down syndrome.

In evaluating the medical literature, success of a treatment needs to account for the fact that most patients will have a successful pregnancy, even when there is no medical intervention. Because 90% of spontaneous miscarriages are nonrecurrent, doing nothing, as difficult as this may be from the psychological perspective, will often produce the best outcome. The skill and art of the practitioner must be used to teach and guide families through this difficult time period with gentleness and good medicine based on the best evidence.

About 15% to 20% of all known human pregnancies terminate in clinically recognized spontaneous abortion. However, the incidence of total human embryonic loss is estimated to be much higher. Wilcox and colleagues measured human chorionic gonadotropin (HCG) in daily urine samples of a group of 221 healthy women attempting to conceive. Of the 198 pregnancies that occurred, 22% ended before the pregnancy was clinically recognized and the total pregnancy loss, including clinically recognized abortions, was 31%. Because some fertilized ova do not implant and thus do not secrete detectable HCG and other abnormal pregnancies do not secrete sufficient intact HCG to be detectable by immunoassay, the rate of human pregnancy loss is probably much higher; it has been estimated to be as high as 70% (**Table 16-1**). Therefore, either the process of human reproduction is inefficient or pregnancy loss serves a particular biologic function. Most early pregnancy losses are the result of chromosomal or genetic abnormalities. The high frequency of abortion, as stated by Austin, is "an important and valuable

Table 16-1 Life Table for Intrauterine Mortality in the Human (per 100 Ova Exposed to Risk of Fertilization)

Week after Ovulation	Death (Expulsion of Dead Embryos)	Survivors
—	16 (not fertilized)	100.32
0	15 (failed to cleave)	84 (fertile)
1	27	69 (implanted)
2	5.0	42.32
6	2.9	37.32
10	1.7	34.12
14	0.5	32.42
18	0.3	31.92
22	0.1	31.62
26	0.1	31.52
30	0.1	31.42
34	0.1	31.32
38	0.2	31.32
Live births (including birth defects)		31.32
Natural wastage		69.32

From Léridon H: Intrauterine mortality. In Léridon H (ed): Human Fertility. Chicago, The University of Chicago Press, 1977.

provision of Nature...and...is in the best interests of the race," because "disadvantageous features from gene mutation are prevented from being incorporated into the overall hereditary pattern." However, this benefit does not alleviate the grief that women and their partners and families feel. Thus, the comment "it was for the best" should not be used in comforting or counseling patients.

Obtaining accurate data to determine the true incidence of clinical spontaneous abortion overall, as well as in particular subgroups of women, is difficult because of possible sources of bias produced by the selection process. Probably the most accurate data come from a study by Regan and coworkers. In this study, 630 women who were contemplating pregnancy were interviewed before conception and examined by ultrasonography as soon as pregnancy was suspected and then serially throughout the first trimester. The overall incidence of spontaneous abortion was 12%, and half had occurred before 8 weeks' gestation. The abortion rate in primigravidas was only 5%, whereas it was 14% in multigravidas (**Table 16-2**). Women whose previous pregnancy was successful also had a low abortion rate (5%), whereas women whose previous pregnancy aborted had about a 20% abortion rate. There is not only an increased risk of subsequent miscarriages but also an increased risk of adverse outcomes. In a large, 14-year retrospective study of miscarriages in a couple's first pregnancy, subsequent pregnancies had significantly increased risks for preeclampsia, first trimester bleeding, and low birth weight. The highest rate of abortion (24%) occurred in that group of women who had been pregnant in the past but in whom all the prior pregnancies had terminated in spontaneous abortion. Reproductive history was the most relevant predictive factor for pregnancy outcome in a subsequent pregnancy. More recent large cohorts such as the Danish Copenhagen Cohort (Buss et al.) have substantiated these percentages and epidemiologic predictors.

Warburton and Fraser studied the incidence of abortion over a 10-year period in a group of more than 2000 women who had at least one pregnancy of at least 20 weeks' gestation. The overall

Table 16-2 Effect of Mother's Reproductive History on Risk of Spontaneous Abortion (N = 407)

History	Number of Patients	Number of Patients Aborting	Percentage
Last pregnancy aborted	214	40	19
Only abortions in the past	98	24	24
Only pregnancy aborted	59	12	20
Last pregnancy successful	95	5	5
All pregnancies successful	73	3	4
Only pregnancy successful	62	3	5
Termination of pregnancy	32	2	6
Primigravida	87	4	5
Total	407		

From Regan L, Braude PR, Trembath PL: Influence of past reproductive performance on risk of spontaneous abortion. BMJ 299:541, 1989.

Table 16-4 Overall Risk of Abortion, According to Age of Mother*

Age of Mother	Number of Pregnancies	Spontaneous Abortions (%)
−19	1105	10.8 (9.0-12.7)
20-29	13,173	9.7 (9.2-12.7)
30-34	3900	11.5 (10.6-12.6)
35-39	1299	21.4 (19.2-23.7)
40+	260	42.2 (35.1-47.4)
Overall	19,737	11.3 (10.9-11.8)

*The table is calculated from a 6.6% sample of the study pregnancies. Figures in brackets: 95% confidence limits χ^2 (trend) = 244; df = 1; $p < 0.0001$.
From Knudsen UB, Hansen V, Juul S, Secher NJ: Prognosis of a new pregnancy following previous spontaneous abortions. Eur J Obstet Gynecol Reprod Biol 39:31, 1991.

incidence of clinical abortion was 14.7%, and the risk of a pregnancy terminating in spontaneous abortion increased with increasing parity, maternal age, and paternal age (**Table 16-3**). Each of these parameters was an independent risk factor for abortion, and this information has been confirmed in other studies. These investigators also found that, in this group of women who had previously delivered at least one liveborn infant, the incidence of clinical abortion was 12.3% if they had no prior abortion. After having one or more abortions, there was a 24% to 32% risk of abortion in successive pregnancies that did not vary greatly with the number of abortions. These researchers also reported that a woman with multiple abortions has a tendency to abort at about the same gestational age.

Knudsen and associates reviewed the data for all patients admitted to hospitals in Denmark between 1980 and 1984. There were 33,900 spontaneous abortions during this 5-year period. The overall incidence of spontaneous abortion was 11.3%, which increased in women older than age 35. The abortion risk in women 35 to 40 was 21%, and for women older than 40 it was 42% (**Table 16-4**). The rate of spontaneous abortion also increased with the number of prior abortions. The risk of abortion in women who had no live births with one prior abortion was 13%. With two prior abortions it was 25%, with three it was 45%, and with four prior abortions the risk of abortion increased to 54% (**Table 16-5**). Several other studies have reported the

chance of having a subsequent abortion after three prior abortions to be about 50%. These figures, obtained from clinical studies, are much lower than the theoretic value of 84% for a similar population calculated by Malpas using historical assumptions.

About 80% of clinical abortions occur in the first trimester, with the incidence decreasing with increasing gestational age. Harlap and Shiono reported that the incidence of *clinical* abortion is relatively stable through 12 weeks and declines steadily thereafter (**Fig. 16-1**). Research using serial ultrasounds has noted that once an intrauterine **gestational sac** is visualized sonographically, the rate of pregnancy loss between 4.5 and 8.5 weeks' gestational age is 11.5%. Thus, the majority of pregnancy failure occurs in the embryonic period. Studies note that about two thirds of losses before 10 weeks are due to chromosomal abnormalities.

When embryonic heart activity is present between 8 and 12 weeks' gestational age, the incidence of subsequent pregnancy loss is between 2% and 3%. However, when sonography is performed earlier in gestation, at 6 weeks, the subsequent spontaneous abortion rate after embryonic heart activity varies between 6% and 8%. For women older than 34, compared with younger women, the loss rate after visualization of a heartbeat is two to three times greater.

In the first trimester, if uterine bleeding occurs when embryonic heart activity is present, the risk of abortion increases threefold to about 15%. Although spontaneous expulsion of the

Table 16-3 Relation of Abortion Frequency to Maternal and Paternal Age at Conception

Maternal Age	Percentage Abortion Frequency	Paternal Age	Percentage Abortion Frequency
<20	12.2	<20	12.0
20-24	14.3	20-24	11.8
25-29	13.7	25-29	15.7
30-34	15.5	30-34	13.1
35-39	18.7	35-39	15.8
40-44	25.5	40-44	19.5
44+	23.1		
Mean	14.7	Mean	14.7

From Warburton D, Frazer FC: Spontaneous abortion risks in man: Data from reproductive histories collected in a medical genetics unit. Am J Hum Genet 16:1, 1964.

Table 16-5 Risk of Subsequent Pregnancy Ending in a Spontaneous Abortion*

Number of Previous Abortions	Number of Pregnancies Studied	Abortion Risk (%)
0	18,164	10.7 (10.3-11.2)
1	21,054	15.9 (15.4-16.4)
2	2,231	25.1 (23.4-27.0)
3	353	45.0 (39.8-50.4)
4	94	54.3 (43.7-64.4)
Overall	19,737	11.3 (10.9-11.8)

*The table is calculated from a 6.6% sample of the study pregnancies. Figures in parentheses: 95% confidence limits; χ^2 (trend) = 728; df = 1: $p < 0.001$.
From Knudsen UB, Hansen V, Juul S, Secher NJ: Prognosis of a new pregnancy following previous spontaneous abortions. Eur J Obstet Gynecol Reprod Biol 39:31, 1991.

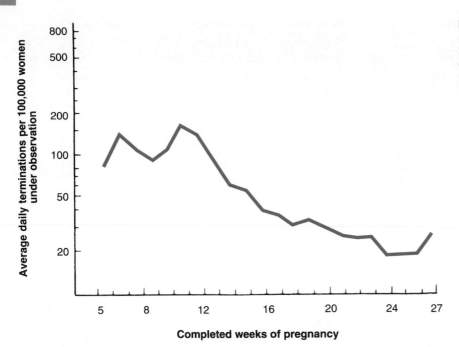

Figure 16-1 Spontaneous abortion by week of pregnancy. (From Harlap S, Shiono PH, Ramcharan S: A life table of spontaneous abortions and the effects of age, parity, and other variables. In Porter IH, Hook EB [eds]: Human Embryonic and Fetal Death. New York, Academic Press, 1980.)

products of conception, clinical abortion, usually occurs between 8 and 12 weeks' gestational age, nearly all **embryonic death**s take place several days or weeks prior to the initiation of uterine bleeding and cramping.

ETIOLOGY

The causes of spontaneous abortion can be divided into intrinsic abnormalities of the **fetus** (chromosomal, genetic, and structural) and those related to maternal conditions, including environmental exposures, diabetes, or thrombophilias. These categories overlap; for example, poorly controlled maternal diabetes may cause a lethal heart defect in the fetus.

CHROMOSOMAL

By far, the major cause of abortion is fetal aneuploidy. Several large cytogenetic studies of tissue expelled from the uterus at the time of abortion confirm that the incidence of chromosomal anomalies varies between 50% and 60% of miscarriages. Samples of chorionic villi or tissue removed by curettage after sonographically confirmed nonviability have documented a 70% to 85% rate of chromosomal abnormalities. The higher incidence of aneuploidy found in these recent studies may be due to several factors, including a greater yield of culturable material. Also, the incidence of chromosomal abnormalities in chorionic villi is higher than in fetal tissue.

The majority of the abnormal karyotypes in the aborted gestational tissue are numeric abnormalities as a result of errors occurring during gametogenesis (chromosomal nondisjunction during meiosis), fertilization (triploidy as a result of digyny or diandry), or the first division of the fertilized ovum (tetraploidy or mosaicism). Only about 5% of the abnormal karyotypes of

the gestations are abnormalities in the structure of individual chromosomes (translocation being the most common).

In most surveys of chromosomal anomalies of abortuses, the relative frequency of the different types of anomalies is similar. The most common type of anomaly is autosomal trisomy, which accounts for about half the abnormal karyotypes when cell cultures were used and about two thirds of the abnormal karyotypes when chorionic villi analysis was performed directly (**Table 16-6**). Trisomies of all autosomes except for autosome 1 have been reported after karyotyping of abortions, with trisomy 16 being the most common. About one third of all autosomal trisomies in abortuses are trisomy 16, with trisomy 22 the next most frequent. Many trisomies occurring in abortions have not been reported in live births, probably because the genotype is incompatible with fetal development.

The second most common chorionic abnormality is polyploidy, most frequently triploidy and less commonly tetraploidy. Studies of chromosomes from miscarriage are derived primarily from placental tissue (chorionic villi) and thus may show more or skewed abnormalities versus embryonic karyotypes. However, these are the best data available, and isolated placental aneuploidy may itself induce pregnancy loss. Polyploidy occurs in about 10% of the chromosome-related abortions, and monosomy 45,X occurs in approximately 7% of the abnormal tissue karyotypes. The survival rate of 45,X gestations is about 1 in 300.

To summarize, autosomal trisomy is the most common abnormal karyotype (50% to 65%), followed in decreasing frequency by monosomy 45,X (20%), triploidy (15%), tetraploidy (10%), and structural abnormalities (5%). The most common single chromosomal abnormality is monosomy 45,X. Karyotypes of abortuses of women who have had more than one abortion tend to be similar if the first abortus had either a normal karyotype or an autosomal trisomy. Except for monosomy, it is possible to estimate the parental origins of the chromosomal abnormalities. Approximately 26% of fetal loss is

Table 16-6 Chromosome Results of 447 Abortuses

	Karyotyped (Banded)	Percentage of All Known Karyotypes
Chromosomally Normal		
46,XY	111	24.8
46,XX	95	21.3
Total	206	46.1
Chromosomally Abnormal		
45,X	44	9.8
Primary autosomal trisomy	138	30.9
Double trisomy	7	1.7
Triple trisomy	1	0.4
Triploidy	29	6.5
Tetraploidy	8	1.8
Mosaicism	1	0.4
Structural rearrangement	11	2.5
Others (XXY, monosomy 21)	2	0.8
Total	241	53.9

From Kajii T, Ferrier A, Niikawa N, et al: Anatomic and chromosomal anomalies in 639 spontaneous abortuses. Hum Genet 55:87, 1980. With kind permission of Springer Science and Business Media.

Table 16-7 Frequency of Cytogenetic Diagnoses in 420 Miscarriages from 285 Couples with Recurrent Miscarriage

Diagnosis	Number of Miscarriages	Frequency (%)
Euploid, female*	120	29
Euploid, male†	105	25
Trisomy 1	0	0
Trisomy 2	4	0.95
Trisomy 3	0	0
Trisomy 4	1	0.24
Trisomy 5	1	0.24
Trisomy 6	3	0.7
Trisomy 7	3	0.7
Trisomy 8	4	0.95
Trisomy 9	4	0.95
Trisomy 10	1	0.24
Trisomy 11	1	0.24
Trisomy 12	1	0.24
Trisomy 13	11	2.6
Trisomy 14	11	2.6
Trisomy 15	22	5.2
Trisomy 16	19	4.5
Trisomy 17	2	0.48
Trisomy 18	4	0.95
Trisomy 19	0	0
Trisomy 20	2	0.48
Trisomy 21	11	2.6
Trisomy 22	16	3.8
Double trisomy	9	2.1
Sex trisomy (47,XXY)	1	0.24
Monosomy X (45,X)	18	4.3
Monosomy X and trisomy 21	1	0.24
Triploidy	27	6.4
Tetraploidy	10	2.4
Unbalanced translocations	8	1.9
Total	420	100

*Consisting of 118 cases of 46,XX and two cases of balanced translocations.
†Consisting of 105 cases of 46,XY.
From Stephenson MD, Awartani KA, Robinson WP: Cytogenetic analysis of miscarriages from couples with recurrent miscarriage: A case control study. Hum Reprod 17:446-451, 2002.

caused by errors of maternal gametogenesis, 5% by errors of paternal gametogenesis, 4% by errors of fertilization, and 4% by errors of zygote division.

Multiple studies have demonstrated no seasonal variability in the incidence of any type of chromosomal abnormality in abortions. Maternal age is directly related to the incidence of trisomies, mainly those in the D and G chromosome group. Maternal age has no effect on the incidence of the other chromosomal anomalies in abortions, although there is evidence that monosomy 45,X is associated with a younger maternal age than other **aneuploid** or **euploid abortuses**. Kleinhaus and associates, reviewing a large cohort, noted paternal age also contributed to miscarriage rates. At a paternal age of 40 years, the risk of abortion was 1.6 (CI 1.3 to 2) compared to men aged 25 to 29.

In contrast to the cause of any specific miscarriage, most recurrent miscarriages are not due to chromosomal abnormalities. Stephenson and colleagues analyzed 420 karyotypes of aborted material from 285 couples with recurrent loss (**Table 16-7**) an found that 66% of recurrent losses had normal cytogenetic evaluations, no different from controls. As would be predicted, advanced maternal age (older than 36) was associated with a significantly higher rate of aneuploidy. When this group of women was separated from the younger group of women, the younger women had a lower rate of aneuploid losses than controls (**Table 16-8**). In other words, in women younger than 36, recurrent loss was due primarily to causes other than chromosomal abnormalities. Other studies by Sullivan and coworkers, Stern and associates, and Carp and colleagues have noted similar results. A small study, $n = 24$, of males from couples with recurrent loss found a slightly higher rate of sperm aneuploidy compared with the general population, RR 1.48. Microdeletions may directly cause recurrent loss. Microdeletions in the Y chromosome are associated with infertility. A recent report of 43 couples with recurrent loss found an association of microdeletions in the Y chromosome with abortion. Larger studies of unexplained recurrent abortion are needed before microarray genetic studies should be ordered on men in this situation. This finding would not necessarily translate into more aneuploid conceptus.

Abortion of chromosomally normal conceptuses tends to occur later in gestation than abortion of chromosomally abnormal embryos. The peak incidence of euploid abortion occurs at about 12 to 13 weeks of gestation. However, expulsion of the products of conception does not necessarily coincide with embryonic or fetal death. This is important because parents will equate the timing of miscarriage with the timing of embryonic or fetal death, and timing of the demise is helpful in evaluating cause.

The incidence of chromosomally normal abortions increases markedly after maternal age 35, rising to more than 30% of clinically recognized conceptions after age 40 (**Fig. 16-2**). Whether this increase in risk of abortion of euploid conceptions is the result of an increase in genetic abnormalities or abnormalities in the maternal environment or both has not been determined, but there is an increased incidence of both first- and second-trimester abortions after age 35, and uterine abnormalities generally are a cause of second-trimester abortion.

Greater than 98% of aneuploidy-related miscarriages occur spontaneously. However, a small proportion is due to balanced translocations in the parents. Tharapel and coworkers reviewed

Table 16-8 Comparison of Cytogenetically Abnormal Miscarriages Stratified by Maternal Age at Time of

Age (years)	Comparative Groups	Cytogenetically Abnormal Miscarriage	Trisomic	45,X	Polyploid	Others*	P
18-29	Recurrent miscarriage	29	16 (55)	5 (17)	8 (28)	0 (0)	NS
	Unselected population†	620	284 (45)	147(24)	135 (22)	54 (9)	
30-35	Recurrent miscarriage	55	27 (49)	7 (13)	18 (33)	3 (5)	NS
	Unselected population†	331	219 (66)	39 (12)	62 (19)	11 (3)	
36-39	Recurrent miscarriage	64	45 (70)	6 (9)	8 (13)	5 (8)	NS
	Unselected population†	109	81 (74)	16 (15)	6 (5.5)	6(5.5)	
≥40	Recurrent miscarriage	47	43 (91)	0 (6)	3 (2)	1	NS
	Unselected population†	55	50 (91)	1 (2)	3 (5)	1 (2)	
Total	Recurrent miscarriage	195	131 (67)	18 (9)	37 (19)	9 (5)	0.008
	Unselected population†	1115	634 (57)	203 (18)	206 (18)	72 (6)	

*Including unbalanced translocations.
†Data from Hassold and Chiu (1985).
Values in parentheses are percentages.
NS, not significant.
From Stephenson MD, Awartani KA, Robinson WP: Cytogenetic analysis of miscarriages from couples with recurrent miscarriage: A case control study. Hum Reprod 17:446-451, 2002.

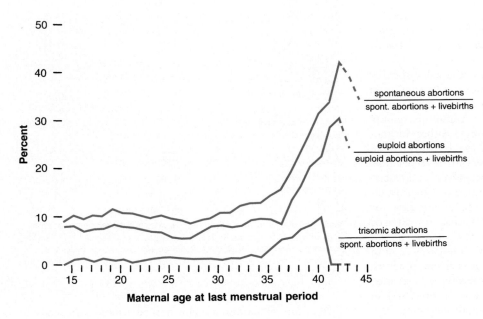

Figure 16-2 Estimated rates (%) of spontaneous abortion, euploid abortion, and trisomic abortion by maternal age for private and public patients combined. (*Broken line*, denominator less than 25.) (From Stein Z, Kline J, Susser E, et al: Maternal age and spontaneous abortion. In Porter IH, Hook EB [eds]: Human Embryonic and Fetal Death, New York, Academic Press, 1980.)

79 studies of couples with two or more pregnancy losses, comprising a total of 8208 women and 7834 men. The composite prevalence of major chromosomal abnormalities in either parent was about 3%, five to six times higher than the general population. Since this review, several large studies, including one from De Braekeleer and Dao, indicate that the prevalence of chromosomal abnormalities in one member of the couple may be as high as 5%. Abnormalities occur in the female parent about twice as frequently as in the male. Chromosomal translocations are more likely to disrupt spermatogenesis than oogenesis, leading to the preponderance of females with chromosomal arrangements having offspring.

About half of all chromosomal abnormalities are balanced reciprocal translocations, and one fourth are Robertsonian translocations. About 12% are sex chromosomal mosaicism in the female, and the rest are inversions and other sporadic abnormalities.

Thus, karyotypes of both members of the couple with two or more spontaneous abortions should be considered. If translocation is found in one parent, one would predict that about 80% of the couple's subsequent pregnancies will abort. In practice, the opposite is closer to the truth! The percentage of liveborn, healthy infants will depend on the translocation. A large study by Carp and colleagues found that the live birth rate was 45% in couples with recurrent loss because of a balanced translocation. Among 99 couples, there were 77 conceptions and 35 live births. If abortion does not occur in a subsequent pregnancy, fetal cytogenetic studies are indicated, because there is about a 5% incidence of unbalanced fetal karyotype in these gestations. Stephenson and Sierra noted a 71% live birth rate in this population without artificial reproductive technology.

There are many possible causes for abortion of chromosomally abnormal conceptions. Simpson postulated that one cause might be a genetic abnormality, a mutation, or set of mutations. He based this assumption on the fact that about 2% of live births have a disorder involving a single gene mutation or polygenic inheritance, whereas only 0.5% of live births have a chromosomal abnormality. Thus, in humans, gene abnormalities are more common than are chromosomal abnormalities. The presumed defect could produce abortion by interfering with fetal metabolism or embryonic structural differentiation. Investigators are beginning to look for genes that induce miscarriage in chromosomally anomalous conceptions. A single abnormal gene that codes for a protein that plays a part in meiosis could play a role.

Another theory involves a gene that may interfere with normal meiotic division. The theory is derived from studies that have identified a small population of women with recurrent pregnancy loss who also have a skewed inactivation of one of their X chromosomes. According to the Lyon hypothesis, X inactivation should occur randomly. These women were noted to have more than 90% of one X chromosome inactivated. Theoretically, a gene on the X chromosome may be either overly suppressed or overly activated, thus affecting chromosomal replication. The women with disproportionate X inactivation have a significantly higher incidence of trisomy conceptuses.

Investigators have reported an increased incidence of histocompatibility locus antigen (HLA) sharing at the A, B, and DR locus among couples with recurrent abortion compared with controls. This has given rise to the theory that one cause of recurrent loss may be the absence of a maternal immunologic blocking factor normally produced in response to paternal antigens. Homozygosity for recessive major histocompatibility complex genes could be the responsible factor for the abortion. In several animal species, genes contributing to spontaneous abortion are located in the region of the chromosome that controls the major histocompatibility complex. In humans the histocompatibility complex is found in the HLA locus on chromosome 6. The sharing of the HLA antigens could be just the detectable marker for the segment of the chromosome that carries recessive genes that are potentially lethal. Some chromosomally normal couples who experience recurrent abortion, in addition to having increased sharing of HLA-A alleles, also have an increased incidence of the transferrin *C3* allele and a decreased frequency of the most common transferrin allele, *C1*, located on chromosome 3.

UTERINE ANOMALIES

Uterine abnormalities, either congenital or acquired, may not provide the optimal environment for nourishment and survival of the embryo and thus may cause the loss of a genetically normal embryo. Congenital uterine abnormalities can be divided into those brought about by abnormal uterine fusion, those produced by maternal DES ingestion, and those caused by abnormal cervical function. The last condition, the **incompetent cervix**, can also be acquired after mechanical cervical dilation. Uterine polyps or submucous myomas may be considered acquired.

ANOMALIES OF UTERINE DEVELOPMENT

Anomalies of uterine development are relatively common, with the incidence reported in the literature ranging from about 1:200 to 1:600 women (Chapter 11). Recent studies have found that some degree of uterine abnormalities, such as small septa, may

occur in as many as 1 in 50 women. Overall, as much as 25% of women with anomalies of uterine fusion have problems with reproduction, recurrent abortion being the most serious. Although it has been stated that bicornuate and septate uteri are the anomalies most frequently associated with abortion, this belief has arisen from the fact that these anomalies can be corrected surgically and thus are more frequently reported as a cause of abortion before surgical correction. Uterine septa tend to cause more difficulties than bicornuate or didelphic uteri. In a study of 182 women with uterine anomalies detected during an 18-year period at a large Finnish hospital, Heinonen and colleagues reported that the least common uterine anomaly, the unicornuate uterus, was associated with the greatest incidence of spontaneous abortion, about 50%. This incidence was higher than the 25% to 30% incidence of abortion that occurred in women with either a septate or bicornuate uterus. Salim and coworkers compared 509 women with unexplained recurrent loss to 1976 controls. Of the subject group, 121 had uterine anomalies. When compared with women in the control group, the uterine distortions in the women with pregnancy loss were more complex, and the uterine volume was smaller.

Surgical correction of bicornuate and septate uteri is possible by using one of the transfundal **metroplasty** techniques originally described by Strassmann, Jones, or Tompkins, or by trans-cervical hysteroscopic resection of the uterine septum. The Strassmann technique of metroplasty was used for a bicornuate uterus, and the Jones and Tompkins techniques were used for resection of a uterine septum. In the series by Heinonen and colleagues, about one fifth of the women with bicornuate and septate uteri had a metroplasty performed, and the abortion rate declined from 84% to 12%. In other series the live birth rate increased from 7% to 76% after metroplastic unification of the uterine cavity. The treatment of uterine anomalies associated with recent pregnancy loss by these major surgical procedures has now been replaced by hysteroscopic resection of the uterine septum. When necessary, cervical **cerclage** may also be used. Sonographic measurements of cervical length help distinguish which patients may benefit from cerclage.

Hysteroscopic incision is the treatment of choice for women with a septate uterus and a history of pregnancy loss, with laparotomy reserved for exceptional and complicated anomalies. March and Israel initially reported that it was possible to incise the septum, even those thicker than 1 cm, of all 82 women with recurrent abortion, using the hysteroscope. After this treatment the abortion rate declined from 95% to 13%. Bider and coworkers reported that when cervical cerclage was used to treat women with a bicornuate uterus and recurrent pregnancy loss, the incidence of viable pregnancies markedly increased. In one series of 41 women with bicornuate uteri and recurrent abortion, 85% had a successful pregnancy outcome after cervical cerclage and the other all 18 women had a term delivery following hysteroscopy.

UTERINE ANOMALIES AFTER DES

DES was prescribed to women throughout the 1950s and early to mid 1960s. Because it was withdrawn from the U.S. market in 1971, it is not a current cause of miscarriage, except in women at the end of their childbearing years. The issues of DES are presented not only for historical interest but as a paradigm of medical management that evolved from the confusion between and association and an assumption of a cause-and-effect relationship.

Comparative studies have shown that women exposed to DES during their fetal life have a significantly greater incidence of spontaneous abortion than do controls. Kaufman and colleagues reported that the percentage of first or all pregnancies in women exposed to DES that ended in spontaneous abortion was similar, whether or not their hysterosalpingogram revealed abnormalities in the shape of the uterine cavity or intrauterine defects. One study noted that the endometrial cavity of women exposed to DES in utero had a significantly smaller surface area than normal, which could perhaps contribute to the increased spontaneous abortion rate in women who had been exposed to DES in utero. No therapy, including cerclage, has been shown to significantly lower the abortion rate in women exposed to DES who have abnormalities of the uterine cavity and recurrent abortion unless they also have cervical incompetence. Because the length of gestation tends to increase with subsequent pregnancies among women who had fetal DES exposure, most of these women ultimately had a viable pregnancy.

CERVICAL INCOMPETENCE (CERVICAL INSUFFICIENCY)

Cervical incompetence is characterized by an asymptomatic dilation of the internal cervical os, leading to dilation of the cervical canal during the second trimester of pregnancy. The consequent lack of support of the fetal membranes leads to their prolapse and rupture, which is usually followed by expulsion of the fetus and placenta. The incidence of this problem was previously estimated to vary from 1 in 57 to 1 in 1730 pregnancies. The huge range of incidence speaks to the difficulty in diagnosis. Although excessive mechanical cervical dilation at the time of dilation and curettage was formerly considered the most common cause of this problem, since recognition of this syndrome, the use of excessive mechanical cervical dilation is now uncommon. Consequently, now the most common cause of cervical incompetence is believed to be a congenital defect in the cervical tissue. Overaggressive LEEP procedures are also associated with cervical incompetence. Cervical incompetence rarely causes recurrent miscarriage, as it is treated after the first occurrence of loss. In a series of 500 consecutive unselected women with recurrent abortion reported by Clifford and associates, none of the 176 women with late abortions had a history of cervical incompetence. Cervical incompetence is associated with the presence of uterine anomalies, particularly uterus didelphys, as well as with anomalies produced by fetal DES exposure.

There is no absolute test for the definitive diagnosis of cervical incompetence. The diagnosis is usually made by obtaining a history of second-trimester pregnancy loss accompanied by spontaneous rupture of the fetal membranes without preceding uterine contractions. Many times the patient will have mild contractions shortly before expelling the pregnancy or before an examination that finds the cervical dilatation to be advanced. Commonly the cervix will be noted to be unexpectedly dilated at the time of a midtrimester ultrasound. If the history is equivocal, ultrasound measurements of cervical length as well as visualization of the internal os should be performed weekly from 16 to 23 weeks' gestation (Fig. 16-3). If the history is suggestive and the cervix shortens to less than 2 cm on transvaginal ultrasound, or a funnel forms in the internal os that measures more than 1 cm, a cerclage should be considered. A cervical length of less than 1.5 cm is considered a strong indication. Normal cervical length is

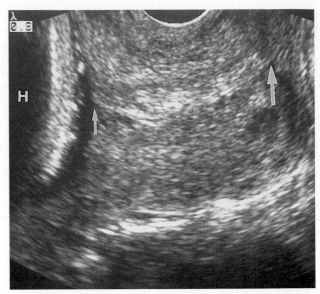

Figure 16-3 Transvaginal ultrasound of a normal appearing cervix. Large arrow to small area denotes canal from external os to internal os, respectively. H, fetal head. (From Fong KW, Farine D: Cervical incompetence and preterm labor. In Rumack CM, Wilson SR, Charboneau JW [eds]: Diagnostic Ultrasound, 2nd ed. St. Louis, Mosby, 1998.)

approximately 3.5 cm or greater. In the second trimester (**Fig. 16-4A and B**). Cerclages performed after the cervix has begun to change, either funneled or dilated, are termed **rescue cerclages**. Their efficacy is less than that of the standard or interval cerclages performed at 11 to 14 weeks.

The best treatment of cervical incompetence is placement of a concentric nonabsorbable suture as close to the level of the internal os as possible. If strict criteria are used to diagnose cervical incompetence, fetal survival rates after cerclage have been reported to increase from 20% to 80%. However, if the criteria for diagnosis are less certain, in several randomized clinical trials, there is only a slight increase in the incidence of term deliveries after cerclage is performed. It is recommended that the suture be placed electively between 11 to 14 weeks' gestation after major embryogenesis has been completed and the incidence of spontaneous abortion caused by genetic abnormalities has markedly lessened. An ultrasound examination should be performed before the cerclage is placed to document that a normal gestation is present. Occasionally, if there is a markedly shortened cervix or placement of a cerclage has failed to maintain the pregnancy, a transabdominal cerclage may be performed. If the suture is placed externally, it is usually removed at 37 to 38 weeks' gestation, and vaginal delivery is permitted to occur. If the suture is buried as in the Shirodkar procedure, then elective cesarean delivery may be considered. Many authors recommend the addition of 250 mg alphahydroxy progesterone in oil be given weekly when a "rescue" cerclage is placed.

ACQUIRED UTERINE DEFECTS

Leiomyomas

Leiomyomas are very common benign uterine tumors that are present in about one third of women of reproductive age. Uterine leiomyomas, especially if they are submucosal, may be

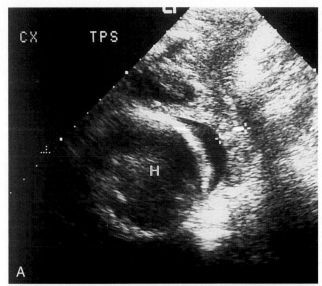

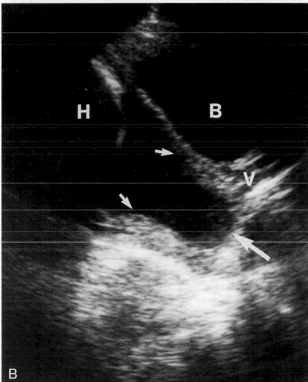

Figure 16-4 A, Cervical shortening, the cervix was measured as 15 mm. Cursors are on the cervix. **B,** Advanced funneling or herniation of the membranes into the canal. This view was seen on transabdominal scan (*small arrows*, internal os; *large arrow,* external os). B, maternal bladder; CX, cervix; H, fetal head; TPS, transperineal scan; V, vagina. (From Fong KW, Farine D: Cervical incompetence and preterm labor. In Rumack CM, Wilson SR, Charboneau JW [eds]: Diagnostic Ultrasound, 2nd ed. St. Louis, Mosby, 1998.)

associated with repetitive abortion but overall are an uncommon cause. Although a causal relationship is difficult to establish, in a review of the literature, Buttram and Reiter reported that when myomectomy was performed for recurrent abortion in a total of 1941 women, the rate of spontaneous abortion was reduced from 41% to 19%. These data indicate that, on occasion, uterine leiomyomas are a cause of pregnancy loss. An important caution exists. Because myomas are present in greater than 30% of women, the presence of a myoma is not verification that the myoma has caused the miscarriage. Much more damage has been done by myomectomy to stop miscarriage than to help the patient. Recurrent miscarriage is a more acceptable indication for myomectomy that a single loss. Hysteroscopic findings of submucous myomas significantly distorting the uterine cavity are much more suggestive as a cause leading to poor implantation. Uterine polyps are a rare cause of abortion and are found and treated hysteroscopically. The presentation is similar to that of submucous myomas. Intermenstrual spotting in this setting is an indication for hysteroscopy.

Intrauterine Adhesions

Adhesions in the uterine cavity can cause partial or complete obliteration of the endometrium, leading to menstrual abnormalities and amenorrhea, as well as being a cause of abortion. The latter is thought to be the result of insufficient endometrium to support adequate fetal growth. The major cause of adhesions is curettage of the endometrial cavity in association with a pregnancy or in the early puerperium (**Table 16-9**). In the series by March and Israel, the most common antecedent factor was curettage for **incomplete abortion**. Curettage after a **missed abortion** or after postpartum hemorrhage is associated with a high

Table 16-9 Definite Causes of IUA in 1856 Cases

	Number of Cases	Percentage
Trauma Associated with Pregnancy		
Curettage after abortion	1237	66.7
Spontaneous	544	
Induced	557	
Unknown	136	
Postpartum curettage	400	21.5
Cesarean section	38	2.0
Evacuation of hydatidiform mole	11	0.6
Trauma without Pregnancy		
Myomectomy	24	1.3
Diagnostic curettage	22	1.2
Cervical manipulation (biopsy, polypectomy, etc.)	10	0.5
Curettage because of menometrorrhagia	8	0.4
Insertion of IUD	3	
Insertion of radium	1	0.3
Without Known Trauma		
Postpartum; after abortion; others	28	1.5
Genital tuberculosis	74	4.0
Total	1856	100.00

IUA, intrauterine adhesion; IUD, intrauterine device.
Reprinted from Schenker JG, Margalioth EJ: Intrauterine adhesions: An updated appraisal. Fertil Steril, 37:593, 1982. Copyright 1982, with permission from The American Society for Reproductive Medicine.

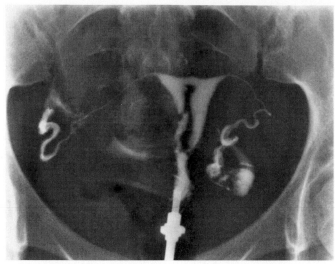

Figure 16-5 Endometrial adhesions. The patient was a 23-year-old gravida 5, para 0, spontaneous abortus 4, ectopic 1, with previous left linear salpingostomy, being evaluated for recurrent abortion. Irregular, linear filling defect represents adhesions between anterior and posterior walls of the endometrial cavity, extending from the internal os to a level near the fundus. (From Richmond JA: Hysterosalpingography. In Mishell DR Jr, Davajan V [eds]: Infertility, Contraception, and Reproductive Endocrinology, 3 rd ed. Oradell, NJ, Medical Economics Books, 1991. Reprinted with permission. All rights reserved.)

incidence of subsequent intrauterine adhesion (IUA) formation. On occasion IUAs develop after a diagnostic curettage, as well as in women with genital tuberculosis. The diagnosis of IUA is usually made by the finding of filling defects seen at the time of hysterosalpingogram. The defects are typically irregular, with sharp contours and homogeneous opacity that persist in a series of films (**Fig. 16-5**). The diagnosis is best confirmed and treated by hysteroscopy (**Fig. 16-6**).

The recommended treatment for IUA is hysteroscopic lysis of the adhesions. After adhesion lysis, an IUD is usually placed in

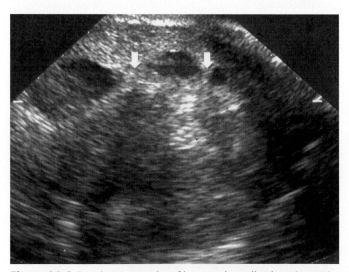

Figure 16-6 Sonohysterography of intrauterine adhesions (*arrows*). (From Goldberg JM, Falcone T: Atlas of Endoscopic Techniques in Gynecology. London, WB Saunders, 2000, p 27.)

the cavity, and high-dose estrogen is administered for 60 days. Medroxyprogesterone acetate 10 mg per day is added for the last 5 to 10 days, and then the IUD is removed. To minimize the chances of developing IUA, curettage of the pregnant or recently pregnant uterus should be gentle and superficial and not extend deep into the muscle. Prophylactic antibiotics should be considered if there is any suggestion of infection or recent infection.

ENDOCRINE CAUSES

Progesterone Deficiency

Maintenance of the endometrium for the first 7 weeks of gestation depends on progesterone produced by the corpus luteum. After this time the corpus luteum regresses, and progesterone synthesized by the trophoblast maintains the decidual tissue. Luteal progesterone synthesis depends on HCG produced by the trophoblast. When progesterone secretion from the corpus luteum is lower than normal or the endometrium has an inadequate response to normal circulating levels of progesterone, endometrial development may be inadequate to support the implanted blastocyst and may lead to spontaneous abortion. Investigators have reported that in conception cycles, midluteal peak progesterone levels in the circulation are always greater than 9 ng/mL.

Diagnosis of luteal insufficiency had historically been made by performing a histologic examination of the endometrium and finding a discrepancy of 3 days or more between the expected and actual endometrial dating pattern in at least two menstrual cycles. Investigators using this method of diagnosis have reported luteal deficiency to occur in as many as one third of women with recurrent abortion, whereas others have reported it to be an uncommon cause of abortion. This discrepancy may have occurred because the precision of endometrial dating by histologic examination varies among different observers, and different criteria are used for determining the day of ovulation. Fadare and Zheng, reviewing multiple studies, advised that diagnosing by endometrial biopsy is of limited accuracy and value because of significant inter- and intraobserver variability. Diagnosis is more commonly made with progesterone levels.

Investigators have treated women with recurrent loss and evidence of luteal deficiency with several progesterone prescriptions including vaginal suppositories 25 mg twice daily and intramuscular progesterone 12.5 mg/day beginning 3 days after ovulation and continuing throughout the first trimester. With this treatment, term pregnancy rates have been reported to range from 80% to 90%. Goldstein and coworkers performed a meta-analysis of randomized control trials of the use of progestational agents given to women in early pregnancy who had a history of two or more abortions without a specific diagnosis of luteal deficiency. There was no significant reduction in the rate of abortion with the use of progestational agents.

Currently most investigators believe that luteal insufficiency is rarely, if ever, the cause of recurrent spontaneous abortion, though it may be a more likely cause of infertility. If it is the cause, then the losses should occur early in the embryonic period, not at 9 to 10 weeks. The Cochrane Collaboration Data Review in 2009 found insufficient evidence to use progesterone to prevent miscarriage, but the researchers also found no adverse effects.

There is no benefit to be derived by initiating progesterone therapy or administering exogenous HCG if the woman develops symptoms of **threatened abortion**. Low progesterone levels at this gestational age are a result, not the cause, of the abortion. When patients inquire about the use of progesterone as a rescue measure, they can be assured that if progesterone deficiency is the cause of a pregnancy loss, the pregnancy is expelled very early in gestation, usually before the sixth week.

Thyroid Disease

Severe hypothyroidism may be associated with abortion; however, three studies with large numbers of women with recurrent abortion found that only a few women have abnormal thyroid function. Currently there is no definitive evidence that hypothyroidism is a cause of recurrent abortion. There are, however, several studies that indicate that the presence of antithyroid antibodies is associated with pregnancy loss.

Stagnaro-Green and associates measured thyroglobulin and thyroid peroxidase antibodies in 552 unselected women in the first trimester of pregnancy. An antithyroid antibody was found in 20% of these women. Among the group of women in whom thyroid antibodies were detected, the spontaneous abortion rate was twice as high, 17% versus 8.4% as that for women without the antibodies. Lejeune and colleagues measured these two antithyroid antibodies in 730 euthyroid women in early pregnancy and reported that one of these antibodies was present in 24% of women who had a first-trimester abortion but in only 5% of those with viable pregnancies.

Stagnaro-Green summarized several studies that have confirmed the association of antithyroid antibodies with recurrent first-trimester loss. The findings of these studies indicate that the presence of significant levels of thyroid antibodies is a risk marker for abortion. Because the antibodies are found in euthyroid women, it is possible that they are a marker for an immunologically mediated factor associated with abortion. Intravenous immunoglobulin, heparin and aspirin, and thyroid supplementation have been used as treatments in women with these antibodies. Treatment with thyroid hormone was more effective than immunoglobulin, heparin, or aspirin in achieving successful pregnancy outcomes in subsequent gestations. In contrast, more recent studies by Stangaro and others have not found associations with antithryroid antibodies and miscarriage. Thus, at this time treatment for clinical thyroid disease is indicated. Treatment that is initiated only for the presence of autoantibodies is discouraged.

Diabetes Mellitus, Insulin Resistance, and Polycystic Ovary Syndrome

Uncontrolled and poorly controlled diabetes mellitus is an accepted cause of miscarriage. The increased miscarriage rate is due in part to structural anomalies in the fetus. Crane and Wahl found the incidence of spontaneous abortion to be similar in a group of women with either gestational diabetes (12.3%) or insulin-dependent diabetes (12.2%) and matched control groups (10.9% and 14.5%). Mills and colleagues performed a prospective study of insulin-dependent diabetic and nondiabetic women enrolled within 3 weeks of conception. The spontaneous abortion rate in both groups was 16%. However, a small group of women whose diabetes was not well controlled and who had elevated blood glucose and glycosylated hemoglobulin levels had a significantly increased risk of spontaneous abortion. Among women with diabetes and good control of blood glucose, diabetes is an unlikely cause of abortion. However, diabetes without good metabolic control is associated with an increased risk of

early pregnancy loss, with a direct correlation between the level of hemoglobin A1C and the rate of abortion.

Recent evidence has supported the association of insulin resistance associated with polycystic ovary syndrome (PCOS) and spontaneous abortion. Some authors cite up to a 50% abortion risk. Women treated with metformin for insulin resistance associated with PCOS have a reduced incidence of pregnancy loss compared with controls. Similarly, Craig and coworkers noted an increased incidence of insulin resistance in a small cohort ($n = 74$) of women being evaluated for recurrent loss, compared with controls. Proposed mechanisms include not only the inherent metabolic problems associated with higher glucose levels and decreased insulin activity such as increased inflammatory mediators, but also increased levels of plasminogen activator inhibitor 1. This protein functions as a strong procoagulant and thrombophilic agent. Insulin resistance also induces a proinflammatory state. Ranidietal reported on a cohort of women with PCOS and procoagulation histories treated with low-molecular-weight heparins and metformin and metformin alone. It was found that the combination of metformin and low-molecular-weight heparin was significantly more effective.

The relationship of PCOS elevated luteinizing hormone (LH) levels and spontaneous abortion is an area of ongoing investigation. Homburg noted that about one third of women with PCOS who conceive after undergoing ovulation induction have a spontaneous abortion—more than twice the incidence of spontaneous abortion of women with hypogonadotropic hypogonadism who conceive after ovulation induction. The incidence of spontaneous abortion was only increased in those women with PCOS who had elevations of follicular phase plasma LH levels, not those in whom the LH levels were in the normal range. Regan and associates prospectively measured follicular phase LH levels in a group of 193 women with regular menstrual cycles who were planning to become pregnant, the majority of whom had a history of one or more previous spontaneous abortions. Within 18 months, 88% of women with normal LH levels (less than 10 IU/L) conceived, compared with 67% of women whose LH levels were elevated. These investigators found that of the women who conceived with elevated LH levels, 65% of the pregnancies ended in abortion, whereas only 12% of the pregnancies in women with normal LH levels aborted. Thus, if the LH levels were elevated on day 8 of the cycle, there was a significantly greater risk of the pregnancy ending in abortion, as well as a greater risk of infertility. These investigators concluded that hypersecretion of LH among women with and without PCOS is a cause of spontaneous abortion.

The mechanism whereby elevated LH levels are associated with miscarriage has not been determined. Clifford and colleagues studied a group of 500 consecutive women with recurrent spontaneous abortion who were referred to a special clinic to study this problem. Sonographic findings of polycystic ovaries were found in 56% of these women, but only 12% of them had elevated follicular phase serum LH levels. However, it was found that nearly 60% of the women with polycystic ovaries had elevated urinary LH levels. Urinary LH may be a more sensitive marker of LH hypersecretion than of serum LH because LH is secreted in a pulsatile manner. Clifford and colleagues performed a randomized controlled trial of women with recurrent abortion and elevated LH levels, comparing therapy of gonadotropin-releasing hormone (GnRH) analogues with no therapy. The viable birth rate was similar in the two groups, indicating that LH suppression with a GnRH analogue is not beneficial for improving live birth rates.

Women with "nonclassical" adrenogenital syndrome from 21 hydroxylase deficiency are known to have decreased fertility. A recent case-control study noted that treatment with glucocorticoids decreased their miscarriage rate from 26.3% to 6.5%.

IMMUNOLOGIC FACTORS

The physiologic mechanism by which the partially foreign fetal tissue is protected from the mother's immunologic system is poorly understood. The foreign antigens produced by the fetus initiate a rejection from the mother. Although progesterone offers some protection from this immunologic effect, in reality a complex biologic network prevents the fetus from being rejected. For five decades, investigators have postulated that abortion, and recurrent abortion in particular, may be associated with a failure of an immunologic suppression. Numerous studies have found differences in the immune mechanisms of couples with recurrent loss. However, to date, immunologic treatments have not been shown to be effective. The immunologic processes are complex, and the potential lesions and differences between the subset of recurrent aborters and controls are specific and very different in different subsets of patients. Some immunologic differences such as specific cytokines may be related to failures in organ systems other than the immunologic system. Treatments such as immunoglobulin or infusions of paternal antigens affect the maternal immunologic system on a broad front. In medicine, the more broad spectrum the treatment, the more numerous the additional affects. With broad-spectrum treatments of the immunologic system to prevent recurrent loss, some beneficial aspects may be affected.

It has also been postulated that if there is sharing of major histocompatibility locus antigens (HLA) between the male and the female in the couple with recurrent abortion, then natural blocking factors would be less likely to develop and abortion would be more likely to occur. Numerous studies have investigated the degree of HLA sharing at several loci in groups of couples with recurrent abortion in whom no cause for the problem could be detected. Bellingard and colleagues, in addition to performing their own study, summarized the results of 23 previously published studies that investigated the degree of HLA sharing between spouses of couples with recurrent abortion. The findings were divided among the studies. HLA-A sharing was reported to be present in 11 and absent in 12 of the 23 studies, and HLA-B sharing was present in 10 but absent in 13 of the 23 studies. In the 17 studies in which HLA-DR sharing was investigated, 11 found sharing of this allele to be more frequent among couples with recurrent abortion of undetected cause than among controls. In their own study of women with three successive spontaneous abortions, Bellingard and colleagues found that the number of couples with HLA sharing in each of the three alleles was not significantly different among women with a known cause for their recurrent abortion and those with unexplained recurrent abortion, as well as a control group of parous women without spontaneous abortion.

In 1985, Mowbray and coworkers performed a randomized treatment trial in a group of women with recurrent abortion and no detectable antibody against paternal lymphocytes. In this study, women injected with paternal white cells had a significantly greater chance of a subsequent successful pregnancy (78%) than did those injected with their own white cells (37%). The investigators concluded that infusion of the foreign leukocytes increased maternal production of the blocking factors that would prevent rejection of the fetal tissues. However, in two subsequent studies performed by Cowchock and Smith and by Hwang and associates, after paternal leukocytes were given to the female the outcome of the subsequent pregnancy was not related to the development of either maternal antipaternal antibodies or blocking factors. After the paternal white cell immunotherapy was performed, neither the formation of antipaternal antibodies nor blocking factors were associated with a decrease in the spontaneous abortion rate or an increase in term pregnancy rate compared with pregnancies after immunotherapy in which these factors did not substantially increase.

Several other aspects of the immune system have been investigated as potential causes of recurrent loss. One line of research involves the populations of lymphocytes in the deciduas compared with the peripheral maternal circulation. Normally, there are few B lymphocytes and neutrophils but a large proportion of natural killer cells in the deciduas. These proportions have been found (in some but not all studies) to be different in patients with unexplained recurrent loss than in controls. The frequency profiles of cytokines, including the interleukins, tumor necrosis factor, tumor necrosis factor, macrophage inhibiting cytokine, and the interferons, are also different in recurrent abortion patients and are influenced by the types of subpopulation of T helper cells in the decidua. These findings have led investigators to propose that immunoglobulin infusion may be helpful in blocking this abnormal immune response and augment a normal response. In a meta-analysis, Scott found no improvement in the miscarriage rate with intravenous immunoglobulin therapy. He also analyzed paternal leukocyte infusion and found no benefits.

Because there are potential risks associated with leukocytic immunotherapy, including the possibility of virus transmission and the development of autoimmune disease, and therapy has not been shown to be effective; it is not cost effective or necessary to perform HLA typing of the couple outside the investigational setting. Infusion of paternal leukocytes should only be performed under research protocols with informed consent, because the procedure has not been proved to be beneficial and has serious potential health risks. Infusions of immunoglobulin are similarly expensive and ineffective and should be used only as part of investigational protocols. Abnormal immune responses may eventually prove for some patients to be a cause of recurrent loss, but which patients and which therapies are as of now unknown.

Celiac Disease

Celiac disease (sprue) is a systemic autoimmune disease caused by an allergy to gluten and is associated with miscarriage. Though its most pronounced symptoms are related to intestinal malabsorption, most patients will have minimal gastrointestinal manifestations. When taking a history, questions of food intolerances are usually not included, and symptoms may be vague and nonspecific. For women with unexplained pregnancy loss, the history should include inquiry with open-ended questions about tolerance to wheat and gluten-containing foods such as pasta, as well as questions about family history of gluten intolerance. A strong association has been documented with adverse pregnancy outcomes, including miscarriage and recurrent miscarriage and the antibodies of celiac disease. Antigliadin antibodies appear to be toxic to trophoblast. Suppression of the antibodies through dietary control has decreased the incidence of miscarriage. In the setting of an evaluation for miscarriage, any woman with a personal or family history of celiac disease or gluten intolerance should be tested for antigliadin and antiendomysial antibodies. The prevalence of celiac disease in first-degree relatives of patients with sprue is 10%. A recent report by Tursi et al. of women with recurrent miscarriage and celiac disease noted a decreased miscarriage rate when women were placed on gluten-free diets.

THROMBOPHILIA

An essential and vital component of a successful gestation is the healthy growth and development of the placental vasculature. The uteroplacental interface receives nearly 20% of maternal cardiac output. A self-protective physiologic adaptation is the increased thrombogenic characteristics of this interface. If the mother has a thrombotic tendency, a thrombophilia, the placenta may develop an overly thrombogenic microenvironment. This may lead to multiple small infarctions at the uteroplacental interface that interfere with placental function. All of the thrombophilias have been associated to varying degrees and strengths of association with miscarriage and adverse pregnancy outcomes, including recurrent miscarriage. Pregnancy, in general, is a time of increased coagulability. Estrogen increases several of the clotting factors (factors VIII, V, and fibrinogen) and induces a decline in thrombolytic factors, including protein S, activated protein C resistance, and plasminogen activator inhibitor 1. The incidence of thrombophilias, both acquired and inherited, is fairly large (>10% of the Caucasian population); thus, it is difficult to equate the presence of a thrombophilia as a definitive cause of a specific adverse pregnancy event. As discussed earlier, miscarriages are frequently multifactorial, particularly recurrent loss. Thrombophilias may be a strong precipitating factor but in most women they are unlikely to be the sole factor. One of the most valuable clues that a thrombophilia led to a pregnancy loss may be found in the placental pathology. The theoretic mechanism that induces pathology in pregnancy is a vasculopathy in the placental bed. If placental vasculopathy is noted, then it is more likely that the thrombophilia is a cause of the miscarriage. Histologic findings include placental infarction, perivillous fibrin deposition, maternal floor infarction, and intervillous thrombosis. The findings, though, are nonspecific and variable. Heparin therapy has been noted to reduce the incidence of vasculopathy. Though the thrombophilias may induce a pregnancy loss at any time in gestation, a loss after a fetal heartbeat has been noted is considered stronger evidence of causality, as so many early first-trimester losses are related to aneuploidy. **Box 16-1** lists thrombophilias that have been associated with pregnancy loss.

Thrombophilias are one of the most common inherited pathologies. Obviously, 10% of the population does not suffer with recurrent pregnancy loss. Thus, there are individual predilections and comorbidities in addition to the thrombophilias that induce pathology. As of yet, most of these cofactors have not been identified. Systematic reviews and meta-analyses of the thrombophilias indicate that there is an association between thrombophilias and miscarriage. Importantly, whether a thrombophilia is the cause of the miscarriage in a specific patient is much more difficult to determine. Cross-sectional and prospective studies show a much weaker association between thrombophilias and

Box 16-1 Thrombophilias Associated with Miscarriage
Antiphospholipid antibodies—anticardiolipin, lupus anticoagulant, and anti-beta-2 glycoprotein
Antithrombin III deficiency
Elevated factor VIII levels
Factor V Leiden mutation
MTHFR mutations*
Plasminogen activator inhibitor-1 deficiency
Protein C deficiency
Protein S deficiency
Prothrombin G2021OA mutation
Thrombocytosis (thrombocythemia—Platelet counts > 750,000)

*Methylenetetrahydrofolate reductase mutations. (Mild hyperhomocysteinemia is technically not a thrombophilia, though it may be associated with thrombosis. Many laboratories include testing for the mutations in thrombophilia panels.)

pregnancy loss. The composite epidemiologic studies to date emphasize the multifactorial nature of the association of thrombophilias (and other causes) and pregnancy loss. For example, insulin resistance increases plasminogen activator 1. In the presence of PCOS with insulin resistance and the presence of factor V Leiden, a woman may have a miscarriage. Similarly, a woman may be exposed to cigarette smoke as a cofactor. The combination of the two or more factors may be the problem. Similarly, studies of patients with multiple and more potent thrombophilias have found a stronger association with pregnancy loss, thus increasing the case for casualty. The essential point to be made with couples is that it is almost impossible to know that a thrombophilia caused their miscarriage. Causation and association are not the same. Antithrombotic treatment of women with one miscarriage and an inherited thrombophilia is problematic.

INHERITED THROMBOPHILIAS

Factor V Leiden is the most common inherited thrombophilia in whites. Up to 8% of some populations are heterozygous for this autosomal dominant mutation. The Leiden mutation is a substitution of glutamine for arginine at position 506 on the factor V protein. This mutation in factor V leads to a defect in binding with the activated protein C (APC) complex. Thus, the factor V cannot be properly inhibited (**Fig. 16-7**). The presence of factor V Leiden may be accessed directly with gene mutation analysis or indirectly by measuring APC resistance. APC resistance decreases in pregnancy as part of the thrombogenic changes. However, an APC resistance of less than 1.8 is pathognomonic for the heterozygous state of factor V Leiden mutation. An APC resistance of less than 1.4 usually indicates the homozygous state. Patients who are homozygous for factor V Leiden have a >80% lifetime risk of thrombosis, as well as a significantly higher risk of adverse pregnancy outcomes, including recurrent miscarriage. Both the heterozygous and the homozygous state have been associated with miscarriage. Meta-analysis by Rey and coworkers noted a 2.01 relative risk (CI 1.13 to 3.58; **Fig. 16-8**) for early recurrent miscarriage and a 7.83 RR (CI 2.83 to 21.67) of late recurrent loss. Kovalevsky and colleagues in their meta-analysis noted an odds ratio of 2.1, (CI 1.6 to 2.7) with factor V Leiden and recurrent pregnancy loss. Homozygosity for factor V Leiden is a greater risk of recurrent loss than the heterozygous state.

THE COAGULATION CASCADE

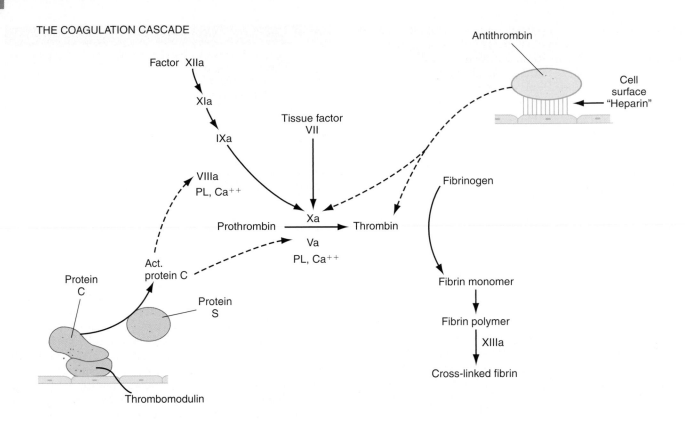

Note: Dashed lines inhibit clotting

Figure 16-7 The coagulation cascade. Inhibitory steps and thrombolytic factor are marked with interrupted lines. The lowercase "a" denotes an activated factor. Ca, calcium; PL, phospholipid.

The second most common thrombophilia is the G20210A mutation in prothrombin. The prothrombin mutation is found in up to 5% of whites. It causes an excess concentration of prothrombin in the circulation. It confers a 2.56 relative risk (CI 1.04 to 6.29) for early pregnancy loss. Kovalesky and colleagues noted a 2.06 relative risk (CI 1.0 to 4.0). The prothrombin mutation is identified by gene analysis.

Less common thrombophilias include deficiencies in protein C (0.5% of the population for the heterozygous state), protein S deficiency (0.5% of the population are heterozygous), and antithrombin-3 deficiency (approximately 0.05% of the population). All three of these proteins contribute to the thrombolytic pathway, and the homozygous states are not compatible with life. All three have been associated in cohort studies with an increased tendency for miscarriage and recurrent loss. Protein C and antithrombin-3 levels may be assessed in pregnancy. However, protein S is an acute-phase reactant, decreasing with pregnancy, trauma, or surgery. Levels are significantly decreased by estrogen in general, and thus they should be measured at least 6 to 8 weeks after a pregnancy. Elevated factor VIII, greater than 180% of normal, and plasminogen activator inhibitor deficiency (PAI-1) have also been associated with early pregnancy loss. Although fewer studies exist at this time, these compounds may be measured directly.

Treatment of the inherited thrombophilias involves subcutaneous heparin. Low-molecular-weight heparin (LMWH) is preferable to unfractionated heparin. LMWH induces less osteoporosis, a much lower (almost absent) incidence of heparin-induced thrombocytopenia, and a decreased number of daily injections. Heparin is metabolized at an increased rate during pregnancy, and to achieve adequate levels of thromboprophylaxis throughout the day, every-8-hour injections are necessary with unfractionated heparin. LMWH, although often given once a day in the nonpregnant state, needs to be given at least every 12 hours during pregnancy. Doses are weight dependent. Adequate prophylaxis to prevent pregnancy loss is an activated partial thromboplastin time (aPTT) of approximately 1.5 times normal for unfractionated heparin. LMWH does not induce changes in the aPTT and is measured with an anti-Xa activity level. Many labs will call this a LMWH level. Because of the increased metabolism in pregnancy, peak levels are not as helpful for LMWH and trough levels may show a greater correlation with the appropriate levels. A trough level should be ordered 1 to 2 hours prior to the next dose. Anti-Xa activity levels of 0.18 to 0.2 are appropriate for thromboprophylaxis. Specific assays are calibrated for each LMWH.

Thus, the assay for dalteparin is different from the assay for tinzaparin or enoxaparin. An antifactor Xa level of 0.2 corresponds approximately to a level of an aPTT of 1.5 times normal. Most investigators check platelets weekly in women on LMWH for 2 to 4 weeks, and then once in each trimester. Women taking unfractionated heparin need platelet levels checked weekly while

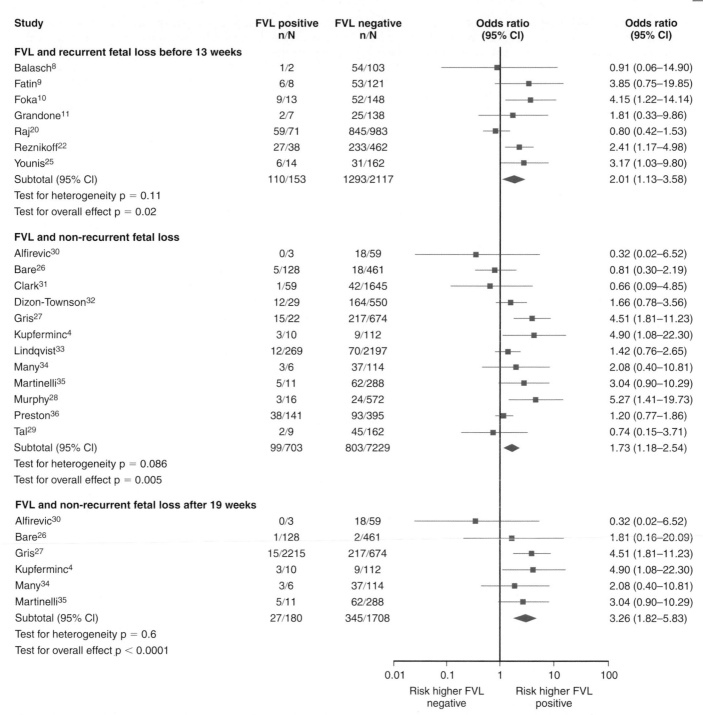

Study	FVL positive n/N	FVL negative n/N	Odds ratio (95% CI)	Odds ratio (95% CI)
FVL and recurrent fetal loss before 13 weeks				
Balasch[8]	1/2	54/103		0.91 (0.06–14.90)
Fatin[9]	6/8	53/121		3.85 (0.75–19.85)
Foka[10]	9/13	52/148		4.15 (1.22–14.14)
Grandone[11]	2/7	25/138		1.81 (0.33–9.86)
Raj[20]	59/71	845/983		0.80 (0.42–1.53)
Reznikoff[22]	27/38	233/462		2.41 (1.17–4.98)
Younis[25]	6/14	31/162		3.17 (1.03–9.80)
Subtotal (95% CI)	110/153	1293/2117		2.01 (1.13–3.58)
Test for heterogeneity p = 0.11				
Test for overall effect p = 0.02				
FVL and non-recurrent fetal loss				
Alfirevic[30]	0/3	18/59		0.32 (0.02–6.52)
Bare[26]	5/128	18/461		0.81 (0.30–2.19)
Clark[31]	1/59	42/1645		0.66 (0.09–4.85)
Dizon-Townson[32]	12/29	164/550		1.66 (0.78–3.56)
Gris[27]	15/22	217/674		4.51 (1.81–11.23)
Kupferminc[4]	3/10	9/112		4.90 (1.08–22.30)
Lindqvist[33]	12/269	70/2197		1.42 (0.76–2.65)
Many[34]	3/6	37/114		2.08 (0.40–10.81)
Martinelli[35]	5/11	62/288		3.04 (0.90–10.29)
Murphy[28]	3/16	24/572		5.27 (1.41–19.73)
Preston[36]	38/141	93/395		1.20 (0.77–1.86)
Tal[29]	2/9	45/162		0.74 (0.15–3.71)
Subtotal (95% CI)	99/703	803/7229		1.73 (1.18–2.54)
Test for heterogeneity p = 0.086				
Test for overall effect p = 0.005				
FVL and non-recurrent fetal loss after 19 weeks				
Alfirevic[30]	0/3	18/59		0.32 (0.02–6.52)
Bare[26]	1/128	2/461		1.81 (0.16–20.09)
Gris[27]	15/2215	217/674		4.51 (1.81–11.23)
Kupferminc[4]	3/10	9/112		4.90 (1.08–22.30)
Many[34]	3/6	37/114		2.08 (0.40–10.81)
Martinelli[35]	5/11	62/288		3.04 (0.90–10.29)
Subtotal (95% CI)	27/180	345/1708		3.26 (1.82–5.83)
Test for heterogeneity p = 0.6				
Test for overall effect p < 0.0001				

0.01   0.1   1   10   100

Risk higher FVL negative | Risk higher FVL positive

Figure 16-8 Prevalence of factor V Leiden in women with fetal loss. From Rey E, Kahn SR, David M, Shrier I: Thrombophilic disorders and fetal loss: A meta-analysis. Lancet 361:9018, 2003. References cited in this figure are from the original source.

they are on therapy. Once adequate dosing is obtained, levels should be checked each trimester. If a woman is being treated with therapeutic levels, for example, for a homozygous state or for deep vein thrombosis (DVT), then levels of an aPTT on unfractionated heparin should be 2.5 to 3 times normal, or an anti-Xa activity trough level of 0.4. Bleeding tends to occur with levels greater than 0.8 to 1.0. Regional anesthesia should not be used within 24 hours of dosing of LMWH because of an increased incidence of epidural hematomas. All women on heparin

should also receive vitamin D and calcium. Importantly for the gynecologist, these women should not be given estrogen-based contraception, nor should they receive estrogen replacement therapy, tamoxifen, raloxifene, or other selective estrogen receptor modulators (SERMs) without specific counseling.

Mild hyperhomocysteinemia is sometimes considered a thrombophilia. Homocysteine is an essential amino acid, which in excess may lead to damage to the vascular endothelium. Hyperhomocysteinemia may induce small clots as the vasculature repairs itself. Estrogen naturally decreases homocysteine levels, thus women with mild hyperhomocysteinemia rarely develop thrombosis prior to menopause. One of the enzyme systems that metabolizes homocysteine is methylenetetrahydrofolate reductase (MTHFR). Mutations in this enzyme can lead to higher levels of homocysteine, and thus blood clots. In the placental bed this is particularly significant, even though systemically it is rare for MTHFR to cause thrombosis during pregnancy. Mutations in the MTHFR enzyme occur in 10% to 15% of the white and Asian populations. With such a common frequency other cofactors, as yet unidentified, will contribute to the well-documented increase in miscarriage and recurrent miscarriage associated with MTHFR. Similar to the other thrombophilias, the MTHFR mutation is much less common in the population of African ancestry. Two mutations are commonly found in the enzyme and either may lead to mild homocystinemia. However, the C677T mutation is significantly more problematic during pregnancy than the A1298C. Mild homocystinemia is autosomal recessive. Even though the A1298C mutation is less of a problem, the compound heterozygous state for the two mutations is also associated with recurrent loss. Some patients refer to MTHFR as the "Monday, Thursday, Friday mutation."

Unlike the thrombophilias, though, mild homocystinemia may also induce pregnancy loss through a teratogenic effect. In some studies, up to 50% of open neural tube defects have been associated with homozygous MTHFR mutation. Complex cardiac disease in the fetus has also been associated with the homozygous state. During the investigation of miscarriage, gene mutation testing of MTHFR is recommended over homocystine levels because these levels vary throughout the menstrual cycle and with dietary influences. Additionally, many studies have evaluated the association of adverse outcomes with the mutation, not with homocysteine levels.

The risk/benefit ratio strongly favors the treatment of this condition when it is found. To bolster enzyme activity, vitamin cofactors (4 mg of folic acid, 500 mcg of vitamin B_{12}) should be given periconceptually and continued until regular menses have resumed. This treatment has been shown to not only decrease the rate of miscarriage but also decrease the risk of pregnancy complications and congenital malformations. The treatment is continued postpartum to decrease the risk of thrombosis in the estrogen deplete puerperium. Women with MTHFR mutations may be given estrogen-based oral contraceptives and hormone replacement therapies, if appropriate, because of the beneficial effects of estrogen on homocysteine levels.

ANTIPHOSPHOLIPID ANTIBODIES AND THE ANTIPHOSPHOLIPID SYNDROME

The first thrombophilias associated with adverse pregnancy outcomes were two antiphospholipid antibodies, the **lupus anticoagulant** (LAC) and the **anticardiolipin antibody** (ACA). Phospholipids are ubiquitous molecules that occur throughout the body and are found in almost all vasculature, particularly the placental vasculature. These antibodies react with proteins on the endothelium and induce platelet activation and thrombosis. The reaction induced by the antibody antigen complexes will induce both arterial and venous thrombosis. Additionally, the antiphospholipid antibodies induce a deleterious effect through a specific reaction to trophoblast in the placental vascular bed, which is cytotoxic. As Meroui et al. have stated, though thrombosis occurs, thrombosis cannot account for all the pathologic

interactions of antiphospholipid disease. Much of the disease is theorized to be caused by inflammatory reactions at the trophoblast interface with activation of complement, cytokine, natural killer (NK) lymphocyte activation, and resultant decreased trophoblast invasion and increased trophoblast apoptosis. Beta 2 glycoprotein is expressed by trophoblast, and higher levels of anti-Beta 2 glycoprotein antibodies are associated with worse outcomes.

Although these antibodies are associated with systemic lupus erythematosus and other collagen-vascular disorders, most women do not have clinical or subclinical lupus. Recurrent pregnancy loss, thrombosis, and the presence of antiphospholipid antibodies are necessary to make the diagnosis of antiphospholipid syndrome. However, most women will just manifest pregnancy loss and not yet have developed thromboses. Between 1% and 3% of the population will have low levels of immunoglobulin (Ig)M for ACA. Moderate to high levels of IgM or IgG are more significant in the setting of a patient with miscarriage. When testing women with miscarriage or recurrent miscarriage, if low levels of IgG or IgM are found we do not prescribe anticoagulation, but we do offer 81 mg of aspirin in subsequent pregnancies.

LAC is paradoxically named because it was first described in women with lupus. And in vitro, due to its binding with phospholipids, it will inhibit coagulation and increase the clotting time. In vivo, LAC is a strong procoagulant. To test for LAC, pathologists use specifically prepared assays, such as the kaolin clotting time or the dilute Russell viper venom test. If blood does not clot, normal serum is added to assess if the result of the clotting is due to a deficiency of clotting factors. If the blood still fails to clot with normal serum being added, then LAC is suspected. Up to 2% of normal women will have low levels of the LAC. Because the Venereal Disease Research Laboratory (VDRL) test for syphilis uses a phospholipid assay, the presence of LAC may induce a false-positive VDRL. When specific tests for syphilis are used, the patient will test negative. Other antiphospholipid antibodies include immunoglobulins that react against β-2 glycoprotein, phosphatidyl serine, phosphatidyl ethanolamine, and annexin-5. These antibodies may also induce pregnancy loss; anti-β-2 glycoprotein is perhaps the most critical.

The treatment of antiphospholipid syndrome in pregnancy is both 81 mg of aspirin daily and prophylactic heparin. Glucocorticoid therapy is not effective. LMWH is given to achieve a trough level of 0.2 anti-Xa activity level. Women with a previous thrombosis and antiphospholipid antibodies are treated with full anticoagulation (trough of 0.4). Women with thrombosis and antiphospholipid antibodies have a near 100% risk of subsequent thrombosis. Thus, the recommendation is anticoagulation for the rest of the woman's life. If a woman is contemplating pregnancy with the antiphospholipid syndrome, warfarin is usually stopped and heparin initiated to prevent warfarin embryopathy. Several studies have evaluated the use of intravenous immunoglobulin (IVIg) in women with refractory cases and antiphospholipid syndrome; this treatment may have value, particularly for those with systemic lupus erythematosus.

INFECTIONS

Numerous infectious agents present in the cervix, uterine cavity, or seminal fluid have been associated with miscarriage. Although there is evidence that clinical endometritis caused by any infectious agent can produce an abortion, the evidence is unclear as to whether subclinical infections with certain microorganisms or viruses are a cause of spontaneous abortion. Histologic studies, of second trimester placenta from women with pregnancies with loss frequently, find evidence of inflammation. Most acute bacterial infections (e.g., *Staphylococcus, Streptococcus, Neisseria gonorrhoeae*) can cause a pregnancy loss. These agents are sporadic causes and are not etiologic agents of recurrent loss.

Although *Listeria monocytogenes* produces abortion in several animal species as well as humans in the second trimester, there is no evidence that it is an abortifacient in women in the first trimester. Rabau and David found no bacteriologic or serologic evidence of *Listeria* infection in 554 women who had aborted, including 74 with recurrent abortions, and Stray-Pedersen and colleagues were unable to isolate this organism from a group of 48 women with recurrent abortion. *Chlamydia trachomatis* is a common sexually transmitted pathogen, but there is no evidence that it causes abortion in asymptomatic women. Primary infections have been associated with pregnancy loss but not recurrent loss.

Several authors have suggested that T strain mycoplasma, both *Ureaplasma urealyticum* and *Mycoplasma hominis,* can cause abortion. Data indicating that the first organism is a cause of abortion are stronger than for the latter. Stray-Pedersen and colleagues found that although the incidence of cervical colonization of *U. urealyticum* was similar in a group of women with recurrent abortion and controls, the incidence of endometrial colonization was significantly more common (28%) in the group with recurrent abortions than in the control group (7%). In this study the cultures were obtained at least 6 months after the last abortion, and there were no clinical or laboratory signs of infection in any of the women. These investigators could not correlate the presence of *M. hominis* in the uterus with an increased frequency of abortion. Stray-Pedersen and Stray-Pedersen reported that eradication of *U. urealyticum* in the endometrium by tetracycline treatment for 10 days resulted in a significantly lower subsequent abortion rate (19%). However, there are no randomized placebo-controlled clinical trials to prove that these organisms cause abortion and that treatment is effective. The parasite *Toxoplasma gondii* may infect the embryo and cause an abortion. However, it is difficult to document the presence of this organism before abortion occurs because there is a lack of correlation between serologic immunoassays for this organism and its detection in the endometrium by immunofluorescence.

Many viral agents may cause abortion if acquired as primary infections. Viral infections have been associated with both first and second trimester loss in cohort and case control studies using histology and PCR. Parvovirus B-19 may be embryotoxic in the first trimester but is not a cause of recurrent loss. Similarly, infection from varicella, cytomegalovirus, and rubella may cause miscarriage but are not a cause of recurrent loss. Primary infection with herpes simplex virus in the genital tract has been reported to cause abortion. Nahmias and coworkers reported that if genital herpes initially occurred in the first half of pregnancy, the abortion rate was about 34%. If pregnancy occurred within 18 months after initial detection of herpes infection, the abortion rate was 55%. Both these rates were significantly higher than the 11.5% abortion rate in the control population. Recurrent infection with herpes simplex does not cause loss. CMV, adenovirus, some types of human papillomavirus (HPV), varicella, and rubella have all been noted to be embryo and feto toxic.

ENVIRONMENTAL FACTORS

SMOKING

In a retrospective study, Kline and associates reported that women who smoked during pregnancy had a significantly greater chance of having a spontaneous abortion than did a control group (**Table 16-10**). For women who smoked more than 14 cigarettes per day, the risk of having an abortion was 1.7 times greater than for women who did not smoke, but smoking less than this amount did not result in a significantly greater incidence of abortion. These investigators found that heavy smokers had an increased risk of aborting chromosomally normal embryos only. There was no increased risk of an aneuploid abortion in smokers. These data indicate that smoking acts as a toxic agent to destroy chromosomally normal fetuses. The data also supports the multifactorial nature of miscarriage, in that most women who smoke do not miscarry. Other researchers have documented increased abortion rates with fewer cigarettes per day. Paternal smoking also increases the risk of miscarriage. When both parents smoke, Blanco-Munoz et al. found a four times increased rate of miscarriage compared with nonsmoking controls.

ALCOHOL

Kline and associates also reported that drinking alcohol, acting independently from smoking, was a risk factor for abortion (**Table 16-11**). Women who drank alcohol at least 2 days a week had an approximate twofold greater risk of having an abortion than women who did not drink during pregnancy. The risk increased to threefold with daily ingestion of alcohol. As with

Table 16-10 Frequency (%) of Smoking among Women Experiencing Spontaneous Abortions (Cases) and Women Delivering at 28 Weeks' Gestation or Later (Controls)

| Number of Cigarettes per Day | Percentage Distribution | | Adjusted Odds Ratio | 95% Confidence Interval |
	Cases	Controls		
None	62.0 ⎫ 37.9	69.8	1.00 ⎫ 1.28	—
1-13	20.5 ⎭	20.5	1.07 ⎭	0.80-1.42
14-80	17.4	10.2 ⎫ 30.2	1.73	1.23-2.43
Total	648	645 ⎭		

From Kline J, Stein Z, Susser M, et al: Environmental influences on early reproductive loss in a current New York City study. In Porter IH, Hook EB (eds): Human Embryonic and Fetal Death. New York, Academic Press, 1980.

Table 16-11 Frequency (%) of Alcohol Consumption among Women Experiencing Spontaneous Abortions (Cases) and Women Delivering at 28 Weeks' Gestation or Later (Controls)

Frequency of Alcohol Consumption during Pregnancy	Percentage Distribution		Adjusted Odds Ratio	95% Confidence Interval
	Cases	Controls		
Never	42.6	43.7	1.00	0.59-0.99
Twice a month and less	28.9	38.0	0.77	0.71-1.52
Less than twice a month	10.8 ⎱	10.4 ⎱	1.04 ⎱	1.30-2.95
2-6 days a week	13.3 ⎰ 17.9	6.5 ⎰ 7.9	1.96 ⎰ 2.36	
Daily	4.5	1.4	3.00	1.39-6.49
Total	648			645

From Kline J, Stein Z, Susser M, et al: Environmental influences on early reproductive loss in a current New York City study. In Porter IH, Hook EB (eds): Human Embryonic and Fetal Death. New York, Academic Press, 1980.

smoking, an increased risk of abortion was confined to chromosomally normal embryos, indicating that drinking alcohol, like smoking, can act as a toxic agent on the normal embryo. Harlap and Shiono found that even moderate drinking of alcohol increased the risk of second-, but not first-trimester pregnancy loss, confirming the toxic effect of alcohol on the embryo.

COFFEE AND CAFFEINE

Some epidemiologic data have suggested that moderate to heavy caffeine ingestion may be an independent risk factor for abortion. Because there may be a causal relation between these agents and abortion, women who become pregnant should limit their intake of caffeine. Studies suggest a threshold effect with more than two cups of coffee or more than a 12-ounce caffeinated soda being problematic. The risk of pregnancy loss increases beyond this limit.

IRRADIATION AND MAGNETIC FIELDS

Animal studies have shown that ionizing radiation can produce congenital malformations, growth retardation, and embryonic and fetal death. These effects are dose related, and there is a threshold dose below which an adverse effect does not occur. Although there is evidence in the human that high-energy radiation exposure is associated with teratogenic effects and growth retardation, there is no conclusive evidence that similar exposure increases the risk of spontaneous abortion. Because studies will never be done, it is presumed that a threshold effect extends from teratogenicity to miscarriage.

Extrapolation from animal data indicates that the embryo is most sensitive to the lethal effect of irradiation during the day of implantation and a few days later (**Table 16-12**). The sensitivity decreases during the period of early embryogenesis, after which the minimum lethal dose (MLD) remains constant to term gestation. Brent reported that the MLD of irradiation to rats is 5 rads on the day of implantation. These data thus indicate that there is little likelihood that irradiation of less than 5 rads

Table 16-12 Estimation of Abortigenic Hazards of X-Irradiation to Human Embryo from Animal Experiments

Stage of Human Gestation (Days)	Lethal Dose/50 (Rads)	MLD (Rads)
1	70-100	10
14	140	25
18	150	25
28	220	50
50	260	50
Late fetus to term	300-400	50

MLD, minimum lethal dose.
From Brent RL: Radiation-induced embryonic and fetal loss from conception to birth. In Porter IH, Hook EB (eds): Human Embryonic and Fetal Death. New York, Academic Press, 1980.

(several-fold greater than the amount used in nearly all diagnostic procedures) will cause an abortion in the human, even if it is administered during the time of implantation. Even exposures greater than 5 rads rarely cause pregnancy loss.

Exposure to magnetic fields induced by electric currents has not been associated with a significantly higher rate of miscarriage. Video display terminals, electric blankets, and power lines are not harmful to a pregnancy.

ENVIRONMENTAL TOXINS

The information that exists concerning the effect of environmental toxins on human pregnancy and abortion is based on case reports and small case-control studies. Recommendations that exist have been developed from data based on effects that cause fetal anomalies. These recommendations are to avoid contact (**Box 16-2**).

Some, but not all, studies have shown an increased risk of abortion among women occupationally exposed to anesthetic gases. Most studies reporting such a relation are retrospective questionnaires. A well-done case-control study by Axelsson and Rylander indicated that the incidence of abortion in women exposed to anesthetic gases was not significantly increased. However, current practice is to adequately ventilate gases in hospitals and physician's and dental offices. Women exposed to anesthetic gases in veterinary offices should inquire about ventilation. Women exposed to chemotherapeutic agents, such as nurses and pharmacy technicians, may have an increased risk of miscarriage.

Information concerning a possible abortifacient effect after increased exposure to other environmental toxins is even less clear. Vianna and Polan reported that the entire population of

---

Box 16-2   Environmental Exposures Associated with Miscarriage

Alcohol
Anesthetic gases
Arsenic
Cadmium
Chemotherapeutic agents
Lead
Mercury
Organic solvents
Pesticides
Radiation
Tobacco smoke

women exposed to toxic chemical wastes in the Love Canal, New York, area had no significant excess of spontaneous abortions, although groups of women living in certain areas with a higher exposure may have had an increased risk of abortion. Heavy metals, lead, cadmium, mercury, and arsenic are embryotoxic. Of these, lead is the most common exposure and most well documented as a cause of miscarriage. If elevated lead levels are found in a patient, then chelation treatment is indicated prior to pregnancy. Chelation treatment may be used if the woman has high levels of lead in pregnancy. Women who drink well water and miscarry may have their water analyzed for minerals and inorganic content. Organic solvents, particularly those used in the computer industry, are particularly worrisome. Organic pesticides are also well-known toxins and may induce miscarriage.

EXERCISE, STRESS, AND DEPRESSION

Severe stress is a well-documented cause of pregnancy loss in the animal model, and anecdotally stress has been associated with pregnancy loss in humans. Older literature, from 75 to 150 years ago, proposed that emotional stress led to adverse pregnancy outcomes. Severe stress may lead to a higher incidence of late pregnancy outcomes, affecting uteroplacental function in some cases. However, stress has not been associated with early pregnancy loss. Women who receive counseling for depression associated with recurrent loss seem to have a higher successful pregnancy rate. Sugiura-Ogasawara and colleagues prospectively evaluated women with a psychological assessment for depression who had experienced two consecutive first-trimester losses. Depression was associated with a greater frequency of subsequent miscarriage. The interaction between stress, depression, and pregnancy outcome is complex. Currently, the relationship with pregnancy loss is equivocal at best. Most all studies have repeatedly shown that employment, work, and exercise are not associated with miscarriage. However, the Danish National Birth Cohort studied 92,671 pregnancies and found that moderate to intense exercise, including "high-impact" exercise in the first trimester, may increase pregnancy loss. This study's design is problematic and affected by recall bias.

DIAGNOSIS

Miscarriage is ultimately diagnosed through confirmation of a nonviable gestation. Originally, the types of abortion were originally described by the appearance of the patient when she presented to the physician. They include (1) threatened—bleeding with a viable pregnancy, (2) missed—nonviable intrauterine gestation less than 20 weeks with the cervical os closed, (3) incomplete—intrauterine gestation less than 20 weeks with the os open and some tissue already passed, (4) inevitable—if the cervix is open but no tissue is passed (this is a misnomer, because in some circumstances a cerclage can be placed), and (5) **complete spontaneous abortion**—passage of all the tissue and an empty uterus. These definitions still remain but are less valuable because of imaging with ultrasound.

The diagnosis of abortion in any of these manifestations is made by physical examination usually augmented with ultrasound and HCG values. Throughout the physician's assessment, the woman should receive the highest levels of care and concern. Studies have found that women who have miscarried and who

had their symptoms treated casually by members of the health care team (technicians, nurses, or physicians) have more difficult recovery. The diagnostic time period is filled with intense anxiety. The caregiver's attitudes are often the most pronounced memory that the patient and her family take away from the experience.

In a healthy pregnancy, in early gestation, the HCG levels should rise in a predictable fashion. Levels may rise to 100,000 IU by week 10, and then fall. The proportionate rate of increase is most pronounced in the first 6 weeks of gestation, and then the rise is less rapid. Barnhart and coworkers performed a longitudinal evaluation of HCG levels. Of 861 observations in 287 subjects, HCG increased a mean of 50% in 24 hours and 124% in 48 hours. In their study, the minimal increase for a viable pregnancy was 24% for a 24-hour period and 53% in 48 hours. The largest increase was 81%, and 330% at 24 and 48 hours, respectively. At a certain point, a viable pregnancy should be visualized by ultrasound in the uterus. The HCG at this point is called the "discriminatory zone" and approximates 1500 IU. After a level of 5000 IU, ultrasound may be used without HCG levels for assessment of viability. A clinical caveat: conception is not always 14 days after the last menstrual period. Because conception is the variable, not last menstrual period, all worrisome ultrasounds should be reconfirmed 1 week later.

The first sonographic finding of a pregnancy is the gestational sac (**Table 16-13**). As Goldstein has stated, this is a sonographic term, not a true anatomic delineation. The sac is an echolucent area in the uterus surrounded by echodense-reactive endometrium (decidualized endometrium; **Fig. 16-9**). Intrauterine lucencies may be first visualized as early as 3 weeks after the last menstrual period, 1 week after conception, and may represent purely fluid in the secretory phase. In the interior of the sac is the developing fluid-filled chorionic sac. With visualization of the chorionic sac with secondary echoes, a true gestational sac may be defined. If the fluid is endometrial secretions, it is considered a pseudogestational sac. The first fetal structure that may be visualized on ultrasound is the yolk sac (**Fig. 16-10**). A distorted or large yolk sac is associated with pregnancy loss. The yolk sac should be seen within 1 week of visualization of the gestational sac and when the yolk sac is 1 cm in diameter.

The embryonic disk is notable as a thickening on the yolk sac as early as a few days after the yolk sac appears. An embryonic disk should be visualized by approximately 5 to 6 weeks'

Table 16-13 Ultrasound Findings in Early Pregnancy

Ultrasound Findings	Gestational Age from LMP (days)	Approximate HCG (IU)	Approximate Risk of Miscarriage*
Gestational sac	23-29	1500	<12%
Yolk sac	32-45	5000	<9%[†]
Embryonic disk	35-45		<8%
Fetal cardiac activity	> 42 with CRL × 5 mm	13,000-15,000	<8%
Embryo 2 cm with heart rate	56		<2%

*If no vaginal bleeding.
[†]If the gestational sac is 10 mm.
CRL, crown-rump length; HCG, human chorionic gonadotropin; LMP, last menstrual period.

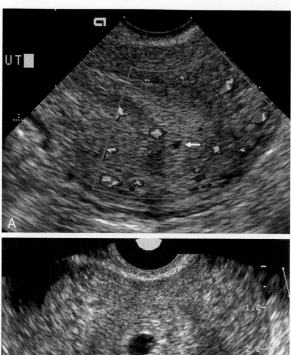

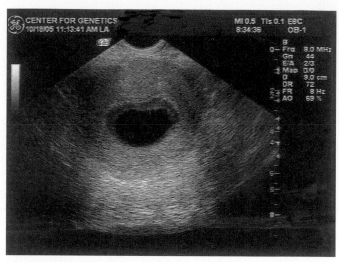

Figure 16-11 Anembryonic gestation in an 8-week pregnancy—empty sac. This has also been referred to as a *blighted ovum*, although the term is a misnomer.

Figure 16-9 A, Ultrasound at 33 weeks with small sac *(arrow).* **B,** Endovaginal ultrasound 6 days after a gestational sac, with mildly increased decidual reaction surrounding the echolucent sac, UT, uterus. (From Lyons EA, Levi CS, Dashefsky SM: The first trimester. In Rumack CM, Wilson SR, Charboneau JW [eds]: Diagnostic Ultrasound, 2nd ed. St. Louis, Mosby, 1998.)

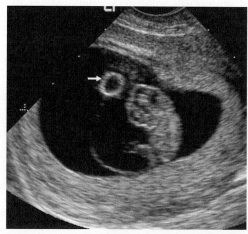

Figure 16-10 Normal yolk sac in a 9-week embryo. Arrow points to yolk sac. (From Lyons EA, Levi CS, Dashefsky SM: The first trimester. In Rumack CM, Wilson SR, Charboneau JW [eds]: Diagnostic Ultrasound, 2nd ed. St. Louis, Mosby, 1998.)

gestational age. Cardiac activity should be seen a few days afterward and any time the embryo is greater than 1 cm in length. When the HCG concentration is more than 13,000 mIU/mL, the gestational sac should be more than 18 mm in diameter and an embryo with embryonic heart activity should be visualized in a normal gestation. If the gestational sac is more than 18 mm in diameter and no embryo is visible, an **anembryonic gestation** is present (**Fig. 16-11**). The earliest cardiac activity has been noted is 5 weeks after the last menstrual period in a 28-day cycle. Cardiac activity should always be noted by 6 weeks (4 weeks after conception). Initially, the fetal heart rate should be in the 80 to 110 beats per minute (bpm) range and will then often increase into the 180 to 220 bpm range for the first few months of pregnancy, but by 12 weeks it should return to 110 to 160 bpm.

If any findings are equivocal, whether gestational sac, yolk sac, or cardiac activity, the exam should be repeated most often in 1 week. Occasionally couples will request rechecking within a shorter time period. For an embryo larger than 1.5 to 2 cm, if there is no heartbeat in 48 hours, it may be adequate to reevaluate in a shorter time. For gestational sacs without embryonic poles, 1 week is preferable.

Several sonographic parameters found in an early gestation are predicators of a viable birth. If embryonic heart activity is seen at 6 weeks' gestational age, the chance of spontaneous abortion is about 7%. If heart activity is still present after 8 weeks' gestation, the chance of spontaneous abortion falls to about 2%. Several studies have noted that an abnormal heart rate, either above or below the expected rate for a gestational age, is a finding associated with a poor outcome.

Sonographic predictors of viable birth have less prognostic value among couples with recurrent spontaneous abortion because the pregnancy loss in those instances is more likely due to maternal disorders instead of problems with the gestation. Many authors have noted that in contrast to the 7% abortion rate found after embryonic heart activity in all gestations, when embryonic heart activity was seen in early gestation, among women with recurrent abortion, the subsequent abortion rate was three times higher, between 22% and 30%.

THREATENED ABORTION

It has been estimated that bleeding occurs during the first 20 weeks of pregnancy in about 30% to 40% of human gestations, with about half of these pregnancies ending in spontaneous abortion. A recent prospective study by Hasan et al. followed 4510 women with apparently viable pregnancies; 27% had first trimester bleeding, 517 miscarried. Most studies find the risk of abortion is greater among those women who bleed for 3 or more days (24%) than among those who bleed only 1 or 2 days (7%). Women with gestational bleeding who do not abort have a minimally increased incidence of complications of pregnancy, including a slightly increased incidence of fetal anomalies and preterm birth. To determine the prognosis of the pregnancy in a woman with threatened abortion, ultrasound is the primary diagnostic modality.

The sonogram of women who present with bleeding in the first trimester may demonstrate a lucency behind the brighter placental disk. Such anomalies can be seen in 20% of women with threatened miscarriage. **Subchorionic hematoma**s have minimal clinical significance, and most women may be assured that things will most likely continue as long as the heart rate appears appropriate.

There have been several reports of ultrasonographic studies of groups of women with threatened abortion. In about two thirds of such pregnancies, a live fetus is present, and about 85% of these fetuses subsequently are delivered and survive. Of the one third of women with a threatened abortion who do not have a live fetus present, about half have an anembryonic gestation, with the remainder being about equally divided between embryonic death and incomplete abortion, with an occasional molar gestation. Siddiqi and colleagues reported that even if embryonic heart activity is visualized early in gestation, the risk of the pregnancy ending in spontaneous abortion was increased about threefold if uterine bleeding occurred, from 5% without bleeding to 16% with bleeding.

In a patient bleeding during the first half of pregnancy, the diagnosis of **inevitable abortion** is strengthened if the bleeding is profuse and associated with uterine cramping pains. Women with threatened abortion who do not abort usually do not have cramps.

MISSED ABORTION

The diagnosis of missed abortion is suspected clinically when the uterus fails to continue to enlarge with or without uterine bleeding or spotting. Typically after an episode of bleeding subsides, a continuous brown vaginal discharge is noted. When a dead fetus is retained in the uterus beyond 5 weeks after fetal death, consumptive coagulability with resultant hypofibrinogenemia may occur. This condition is self-limited, resolving in 1 to 2 weeks. The incidence of this condition is correlated with both the length of gestation and the duration of fetal death: It is uncommon in gestations of less than 16 to 18 weeks. With the use of ultrasonography, the term *missed abortion* is less relevant because the diagnosis of anembryonic gestation or fetal death can be easily determined without delay.

SEPTIC ABORTION

Infection occurs in about 1% to 2% of all spontaneous abortions, with the incidence increasing if a nonsterilized instrument has induced the abortion. All women with uterine bleeding or spotting during the first half of pregnancy accompanied by clinical signs of infection must be considered to have a **septic abortion** if no obvious source of infection outside the genital tract is evident.

Septic abortions can be threatened, inevitable, or incomplete. The infection frequently spreads from the endometrium through the myometrium to the parametrium and sometimes to the peritoneum. Thus, in addition to endometritis, parametritis, and peritonitis frequently occur in women with septic abortions. In addition to an elevated temperature and leukocytosis, lower abdominal tenderness, cervical motion tenderness, and a foul uterine discharge are signs of septic abortion. The cause of the infection is usually polymicrobial, with *Escherichia coli* and other aerobic Gram-negative rods frequently involved. Group B β-hemolytic streptococci, anaerobic streptococci, *Bacteroides* sp., and on occasion *Clostridium perfringens* are other organisms that can cause septic abortion. Because endotoxins can be released from the Gram-negative bacilli, endotoxic shock may accompany septic abortion, particularly if it is caused by insertion of nonsterile agents into the uterine cavity.

TREATMENT

THREATENED ABORTION

Although some physicians recommend that women with threatened abortion restrict their physical activities or stay at bed rest, there is no evidence that these measures or any active medical therapy improves the prognosis of threatened abortion. Nevertheless, restriction of excessive physical activity and avoidance of coitus is commonly suggested until the bleeding ceases. Women should be advised that such measures are primarily for comfort, not for true prevention. Treatment with natural progesterone, synthetic progestins, or HCG was previously advocated, but there is no evidence that such therapy improves the prognosis. Because such treatment may increase the probability of having a missed abortion, the use of this or any type of hormonal therapy is contraindicated. If the woman is Rh negative, Rh immune globulin should be given.

If bleeding increases and is accompanied by uterine cramps, it is likely that the abortion is becoming inevitable and the woman should be examined in a medical facility. Uterine sonography will often aid in predicting the outcome. Once an intrauterine gestation is verified, serial HCG values have minimal value in management.

When the diagnosis of a nonviable pregnancy is made, a thorough discussion with the patient and her support person should be undertaken. If a photograph of the ultrasound can be obtained, it should be offered. The patient's medical history, social history, and physical examination should be obtained. Several factors from the history and physical will influence the next steps in management. The decision of how to proceed further is not only part of the management of the products of conception but is also the first step in grieving and resolution. A patient's personal feelings about the pregnancy, as well as her cultural preferences, will influence whether she chooses an immediate dilation and curettage, expectant management, or opts for medical therapy. If there is no evidence of infection and no medical risk factors, such as cardiac disease, all three options may be acceptable.

Some couples will request combinations of expectant management with an end point at which if there has not been passage of tissue, the woman will have a uterine evacuation. Multiple studies, from several countries, have compared expectant, surgical, and medical management. None of the three options is superior. Surgical complications such as perforation are obviously increased with dilation and curettage. However, heavy bleeding has been shown in some studies to occur more commonly with expectant management. Most all studies document that if women are given the choice of how to deal with the miscarriage, her psychological health is improved. Older texts from the 1940s through the mid-1990s recommend surgical evacuation because of the theoretic risks of infection and bleeding. For most patients with access to health care, these issues are not a problem.

Studies of expectant management show that 50% to 70% of women will initially elect to wait for spontaneous miscarriage after a diagnosis of a missed abortion has been confirmed. In cases of incomplete abortion, up to 95% of women will complete the abortion spontaneously. For a missed abortion, 25% to 85% of women will complete the abortion spontaneously within 2 weeks. de Waard and colleagues noted that 37% of women aborted within 7 days. These authors recommended offering intervention at 7 to 14 days in women who choose expectant management. In their evaluation of 136 women, they found strong preferences by women for whatever choice that woman might make. When expectant management is elected, the patient should be given warnings about infection and severe bleeding, and a return appointment should be made for 10 to 14 days later.

Protocols for medical management commonly employ the prostaglandin E1 analogue, misoprostol. Most patients (80% to 95%) will completely pass an early or mid first-trimester pregnancy loss after one to two doses. Longer gestations are associated with higher rates of incomplete passage, necessitating a sharp curettage. Misoprostol is given orally or vaginally. The vaginal route is preferable, because serum levels peak and drop quickly with an oral route of administration. With vaginal application, serum levels remain higher for a longer period of time. Importantly, gastrointestinal side effects, including nausea, vomiting, and diarrhea, are more common with oral administration. The most common prescription in 600 mcg every 12 hours for four doses, though some authors use 800 mcg with the first dose. Barnhart and coworkers evaluated HCG and progesterone levels in women with pregnancies that aborted prior to 11 weeks who had chosen medical management with E1. The investigators found, as would be expected, that the absolute levels of HCG and progesterone were not related to the success of medical management. Rather, a drop of 80% in hormone levels over the first 48 hours was associated with a 90% success. These authors used 800 mcg of E1. To date, no dosing protocol has been noted to be superior for the medical management of abortion. Many clinicians offer a pretreatment dose of an antiemetic.

Several studies, including that by Chung and associates, have shown that evacuation of retained products of conception after an incomplete abortion can be accomplished with the use of misoprostol. Thus, curettage or vacuum aspiration is not needed. Mifepristone given 24 to 48 hours prior to misoprostol will increase successful passage of a fetus that is 9 to 14 weeks' gestation. Unfortunately, this medication is often difficult to obtain.

Recommendations for surgical versus medical management should be based partially on the size of the intrauterine contents. Many 9- to 10-week pregnancies by gestational age may be only 6 to 8 weeks by size, after ultrasound evaluation. A pregnancy of 11 or more weeks' gestation that presents as a missed or incomplete miscarriage is best handled surgically, because of the increased bleeding. Practitioners skilled in surgical uterine evacuation may perform dilation and evacuation up to 20 weeks. Those practitioners less experienced in uterine surgical evacuation of a second-trimester gestation may opt for induction of labor. Prostaglandin E1 is used in an inpatient setting for patients with larger uteri with pregnancies of later gestations. Prostaglandin E1, 600 to 800 mcg, is administered every 8 to 12 hours. Cervical ripening prior to induction is helpful. Adequate analgesia in these situations is essential.

In all cases of intervention, medical or surgical, prophylactic antibiotics should be considered for patients with cardiac indications. Additionally, women with bacterial vaginosis would receive antibiotics with anaerobic coverage. For the patient with an incomplete abortion and signs of infection, preoperative broad-spectrum antibiotics should be given. Rh immune globulin also should be given to all Rh-negative women.

In the treatment of incomplete abortion with surgical evacuation, deep curettage should be avoided to prevent the subsequent development of **uterine adhesions**. After the procedure, the vital signs and amount of vaginal bleeding should be monitored, after which the woman may be discharged home to remain at rest for 24 hours and avoid intercourse for 2 weeks. Oral ergonovine maleate, 0.2 mg, may be administered every 6 hours for 1 to 2 days. If necessary, iron sulfate, 300 mg, should be administered until hemoglobin levels return to normal and tissue iron stores are replenished. Misoprostol is acceptable for first and early second trimester use in women with previous cesarean deliveries and uterine surgeries.

One of the most commonly asked questions is, "Which method is safest for a future pregnancy?" Studies that have followed women who have had medical, surgical, and expectant management of miscarriage have noted no difference in subsequent pregnancy rates. Smith et al. in the miscarriage treatment trial (MIST) noted that 80% of all women delivered within 5 years.

SEPTIC ABORTION

Septic abortion is a potentially fatal condition, with an estimated fatality rate of 0.4 to 0.6/100,000 spontaneous abortions. All women with the diagnosis of septic abortion should have a complete blood count, urinalysis, chemistry, and electrolyte panel obtained. In addition, a specimen of the uterine discharge should be sent to the laboratory for culture and sensitivity. A Gram stain of the discharge may be performed in the admitting area. If the woman is seriously ill, blood cultures, a chest radiograph, and coagulation and DIC tests should be obtained. Antibiotics should be administered intravenously and the uterine contents evacuated. It is best to use broad-spectrum antibiotic therapy, including an agent that will be effective against anaerobic bacteria. After adequate blood levels of antibiotics are obtained, usually within 2 hours, the uterus should be evacuated as described previously.

If the uterus is larger than 14 weeks' gestation and the cervix is closed (threatened septic abortion), management is more difficult. The uterine cavity needs to be evacuated to provide drainage of the infected material. This can be performed by curettage, dilation and evacuation, or through the administration of oxytocics or prostaglandins. Sometimes it is necessary to perform a hysterectomy if the sepsis is severe and the uterus cannot be evacuated through the cervical canal. All women with septic abortions need to be closely monitored for stability of vital signs and urinary output. If signs of septic shock should develop, a central venous pressure catheter should be placed and additional cardiorespiratory support provided.

FOLLOW-UP CARE

An essential aspect of the care of women with spontaneous miscarriage is the follow-up visit. At this time the patient should be asked open-ended questions about her experience and thoughts. Multiple studies have noted patient's anger and difficulty with the health care system during the time of a miscarriage. Dealing with those frustrations will improve interactions in the future and may also decrease the risk of depression after the loss. Grieving and depression are significant issues after miscarriage. Open-ended questions are the best way to assess a patient's mood and status. Many women experience guilt after miscarriage, believing that the loss was something that they caused by some action that they performed. Counseling regarding this guilt is quite important. The guilt is sometimes brought on by ambivalence, because miscarriage often occurs during the time when the woman is unsure about the pregnancy. Grieving is quite normal and should never be dismissed with rationalizations such as "it is for the best" or "you can always get pregnant again." One study found that 80% of women had some guilt associated with a particular act or habit that is perceived as causing the miscarriage. These issues should be addressed. In addition, an investigation into the cause of miscarriage, whether productive or not, decreases the feelings of self-blame and guilt. Some women develop physical symptomatology with grieving that may mimic symptoms of depression, such as fatigue, anorexia, sleeplessness, and sometimes somatic symptoms such as headache and back pain.

As many as 30% of women will suffer from depression after miscarriage. If symptoms of depression are apparent, then counseling and therapy with antidepressants should be pursued. A patient should be advised that if such symptoms develop, she and her family should return. Staff should be advised that when patients call for advice after a miscarriage, they might be calling with a disguised plea for help. Open-ended questions, such as "Are things going as you expected?" are helpful in assessing a patient's mental state. Any unusual answer should prompt a request for the patient to come in to the office. Gold et al. found that couples experiencing miscarriage are at a 20% increased risk for breaking up compared to couples with live births RR 1.22 (CI 1.08 to 1.38). Cumming et al., in a prospective evaluation of couples after miscarriage, also noted depression and anxiety among couples. In their study, anxiety was more of a problem than depression, and women seemed to adjust faster.

Five percent to 20% of women may develop transient symptoms of thyroid disease after a pregnancy loss. These women have a risk of thyroid disease over the next 5 years. The symptoms should be treated with thyroid replacement for low thyroid and antithyroid medications for hyperthyroid symptoms. Treatment is usually continued for 6 to 9 months, at which point the patient is reevaluated. A free thyroxine level should be obtained.

Also, at the follow-up visit an assessment is given as to potential causes of miscarriage and possible explanations. Any testing can be ordered after two or more miscarriages. Workup is initiated for a cause of recurrent loss. Nikcevic and coworkers noted that an investigation into the cause of the miscarriage decreased the incidence of self-blame.

Future pregnancy planning is also discussed at this visit. Most couples will have resumed sexual activity. If another pregnancy is not desired prior to a year, hormonal-based contraception may be given if appropriate. If pregnancy is desired in less than a year, then barrier methods may be preferable as it is preferable to have two or three normal cycles before trying to conceive again. Couples should wait for at least 3 to 6 cycles after a pregnancy before trying to conceive again, as several studies have noted a slightly increased risk of miscarriage with short interpregnancy intervals. Assessment of general health needs are also performed at this time, including such issues as Pap smear, a mammogram if necessary, iron supplementation, vaccines, and other age-appropriate interventions.

A study by Craig and colleagues found that 7.4% of women with recurrent miscarriage were suffering from severe depression. Thirty-three percent had some aspects of clinical depression and anxiety, and greater than 50% had psychological symptoms that warranted a diagnosis. Treatment for depression is often given for 6 months.

RECURRENT MISCARRIAGE

Recurrent miscarriage has been defined as three spontaneous losses. The calculated probability that a woman will have three consecutive spontaneous abortions is about 0.3% to 0.4%, but the actual incidence is reported to range from 2% to 5% of couples. Approximately 60% of the time, a risk factor for the recurrent losses can be determined. Often this is a factor associated with miscarriages. The remaining couples are said to have "unexplained" recurrent miscarriage.

The abortuses of women who have three or more abortions are more likely to be chromosomally normal (80% to 90%) than those of women with a single spontaneous abortion. Women with recurrent abortions also have a tendency to abort later in gestation, indicating that maternal or environmental factors are a more likely cause of repeated pregnancy loss. Recurrent abortion has been called *habitual abortion*. As well as being pejorative, this term implies that every subsequent pregnancy in these women will end in an abortion; therefore, *recurrent miscarriage* is now the preferred term.

Clifford and associates reported the pregnancy outcome of 201 women with a history of unexplained recurrent abortion who received no pharmacologic therapy for the subsequent pregnancy. The abortion rate in the subsequent pregnancy was 29% and 27% for those with three or four prior abortions, respectively, and 44% and 53% for those with five or six or more prior abortions, respectively. Overall nearly 70% of the women had a viable birth in their subsequent pregnancy without treatment. Brigham and colleagues followed 325 couples with recurrent loss in which thrombophilia and other causes had been excluded. They found that 75% of couples had a successful outcome in the subsequent pregnancy. One conclusion that clearly stands out from such studies is that any potential therapeutic agents should have a placebo control arm to determine true efficacy.

Couples with recurrent abortion require careful, sympathetic care by the practitioner. Psychological counseling is often beneficial. Patients with recurrent loss suffer what has been termed *strain trauma.* The trauma of a single loss produces an emotional shock that is usually healed with grieving. Avoidance behaviors of activities and associations, such as the physician's office, are employed as defenses. However, in situations of repetitive emotional shocks, a strain trauma may develop in which the woman or the couple not only grieve each loss but are constantly afraid of the pain of a new loss. For many women with recurrent miscarriage, this emotional trauma is magnified because they feel helpless to prevent a recurrence. The practitioner needs to express sympathy and continued understanding as counseling is performed and a diagnostic regimen is outlined. The practitioner's staff needs to be attuned to these issues as well.

There is no need to wait for a woman to have three first-trimester abortions with their accompanying emotional trauma before beginning a diagnostic evaluation. Because one early abortion is relatively common, it is recommended that diagnostic evaluation be initiated after a woman has had two first-trimester abortions. Not uncommonly a history may elicit a particular line of investigation that should be initiated even after one loss. If a pregnancy loss occurs in the second trimester, the cause is more likely to recur. Thus, a diagnostic evaluation should be considered after a woman has had only one second-trimester loss.

The evaluation for women with recurrent miscarriage starts with a history and physical examination with pertinent questions regarding cervical incompetence, abnormal exposures, gastrointestinal diseases, family history of miscarriages or birth defects, a family history of unusual thrombosis, and open-ended questions that explore the patient's ideas about causation. Laboratory evaluation should be pointed toward clues from the history. Any history suggestive of thyroid disease may prompt studies for a thyroid-stimulating hormone (TSH) and antithyroid antibodies. Other studies should include a thrombophilia profile, a complete blood count, and or evaluation for PCOS. If all these tests are normal, an evaluation of the uterine cavity by hysterogram, sonohysterography, or hysteroscopy should be considered. Keltz and coworkers, and other investigators have reported that sonohysterography is a sensitive, specific, and accurate screening method for assessing abnormalities in the uterine cavity of women with recurrent miscarriage. If no abnormalities are found, a karyotype of the husband and wife should be performed after three miscarriages to determine if a chromosomal anomaly exists. It is not necessary to obtain endometrial bacteriologic cultures or perform HLA typing of the woman and her partner.

If any of these tests reveals an abnormality, it may be corrected with appropriate surgical or medical therapy. If a chromosomal abnormality is found, genetic counseling is indicated. Some individuals recommend that prophylactic antibiotic treatment be given to the woman and her partner in the conception cycle or that progesterone supplementation be given to all women with recurrent abortion in the first trimester of pregnancy. Neither of these modalities has been demonstrated to improve the outcome of the pregnancy.

If no diagnosis is obtained, the couple should be counseled regarding the probability of abortion in a subsequent pregnancy as described earlier. Pelvic sonography should be performed initially after HCG levels reach 1500 mIU/mL, at which time a gestational sac should be visualized. The sonogram should be repeated 2 weeks later, when an embryo with normal cardiac activity should be seen. These findings are reassuring, both to the woman and to the clinician, but are of less prognostic value to couples with recurrent abortion than to the rest of the population.

Three studies have demonstrated that extensive counseling and emotional support throughout early gestation results in significantly greater live birth rates than when only routine care is given. Stray-Pederson and Stray-Pederson reported that when a group of women with a history of unexplained recurrent abortion were given extensive antenatal counseling and psychological support, the live birth rate was 86%. Liddell and colleagues also reported that when a program of focused emotional support and close supervision was given to a group of 42 women with unexplained recurrent abortion, the live birth rate was 86%. Clifford and associates reported that women with unexplained recurrent miscarriage given supportive care early in pregnancy had a 74% viable birth rate without other therapy. When only routine antenatal care was given to a similar group of women, the live birth rate in these three reports was between 33% and 51%, significantly less. Thus, intensive psychological support during early pregnancy appears to be very beneficial for improving the prognosis of couples with recurrent abortion whose cause remains undetermined.

If a woman does abort, she should be offered cytogenetic evaluation of the conceptus and pathologic examination of the deciduas and placenta. These findings will be informative about the cause of the loss and may direct further management. For example, if pronounced placental vasculopathy is noted, a more extensive workup for the less common thrombophilias could be undertaken. In any case, the possibility of having an explanation is a tool in dealing with the grief of repetitive losses. Couples with unexplained recurrent miscarriage are at even greater levels of anxiety than couples with one loss. That level of anxiety often pushes them toward "any possible cure." The clinician is all too commonly requested to "try anything." Much of the lay press is filled with discussions that inflammation and thrombophilias are associated factors with pregnancy loss. Thus, some couples are offered treatment without evidence of a diagnosis. Large studies and a *Cochrane Review* have shown that heparin, heparin and aspirin, intravenous immunoglobulin and aspirin alone are not, and do not, increase the likelihood of a viable pregnancy. The "give it everything we've got" approach is not helpful and is potentially dangerous. These treatments are appropriate and effective in selected populations of women with proven risks, but not those with recurrent loss that is truly unexplained.

KEY POINTS

- About 15% to 20% of all human pregnancies end in a clinically recognized miscarriage, with 80% occurring in the first trimester; the incidence decreases with increasing gestational age.

- If embryonic cardiac activity is seen sonographically at 6 weeks' gestation, then the subsequent abortion rate is about 6% to 8%. If the embryo is viable at 8 weeks, then the subsequent abortion rate is 2% to 3%.

REFERENCES CAN BE FOUND ON EXPERTCONSULT.com

SUGGESTED READING

Achiron R, Tadmor O, Mashiach S: Heart rate as a predictor of first-trimester spontaneous abortion after ultrasound-proven viability, *Obstet Gynecol* 78:330, 1991.

Bhattacharya S, Townend J, Shetty A, et al: Does miscarriage in an initial pregnancy lead to adverse obstetric and perinatal outcomes in the next continuing pregnancy? *BJOG* 115:1623, 2008.

Bromley B, Harlow BL, Laaboda LA, et al: Small sac size in the first trimester: A predictor of poor fetal outcome, *Radiology* 178:375, 1991.

Buss L, Tolstrup J, Munk C, et al: Spontaneous abortion: A prospective cohort study of younger women from the general population in Denmark, Validation, Occurrence and Risk Determinants 85:467–475, 2006.

Carp H, Feldman B, Oelsner G, et al: Parental karyotype and subsequent live births in recurrent miscarriage, *Fertil Steril* 81(5):1296, 2004.

Carp H, Toder V, Aviram A, et al: Karyotype of the abortus in recurrent miscarriage, *Fertil Steril* 75 (4):678, 2001.

Clifford K, Rai R, Regan L: Future pregnancy outcome in unexplained recurrent first trimester miscarriage, *Hum Reprod* 12:387, 1997.

Duckitt K, Qureshi A: Recurrent miscarriage, 78(8) 2008.

Fadare O, Zheng W: Histologic dating of the endometrium: Accuracy, reproducibility, and practical value, *Adv Anat Pathol* 12:39, 2005.

Frost M, Condon JT: The psychological sequelae of miscarriage: A critical review of the literature, *Aust N Z J Psychiatry* 30:54, 1996.

Gold K, Sen A, Hayward R: Marriage and Cohabitation Outcomes after Pregnancy Loss, 2010.

Goldstein SR: Embryonic death in early pregnancy: A new look at the first trimester, *Obstet Gynecol* 84:294, 1994.

Graham N, Hammond C, Gold M: Caffeine in miscarriages: It's not just in the coffee, 2008.

Hasan R, Baird D, Herring A, et al: Association between first-trimester vaginal bleeding and miscarriage, 114(4) 2009.

Hass DM, Ramsey PS: Progestogen for preventing miscarriage, CD003511, 2008.

Heinonen PK, Saarikoski S, Pystynen P: Reproductive performance of women with uterine anomalies, *Acta Obstet Gynecol Scand* 61:157, 1982.

Hutton B, Sharma R, Fergusson D, et al: Use of intravenous immunoglobulin for treatment of recurrent miscarriage: A systematic review, 2006.

Immunotherapy for recurrent miscarriage, *Cochrane Database Syst Rev* Online (Scott JR: Reviewer) September 2002.

Kaandorp S, Di Nisio M, Goddijin M, et al: Aspirin or anticoagulants for treating recurrent miscarriage in women without antiphospholipid syndrome, CD004734, 2005.

Kaandorp S, Goddijin M, Van der Post J, et al: Aspirin plus heparin or aspirin alone in women with recurrent miscarriage, 10.1056/NEJMoa 1000641 2010.

Kajii T, Ferrier A, Niikawa N, et al: Anatomic and chromosomal anomalies in 639 spontaneous abortuses, *Hum Genet* 55:87, 1980.

Kleinhaus K, Perrin M, Friedlander Y, et al: Paternal age and spontaneous abortion, *Obstet Gynecol* 108:369, 2006.

Laird SM, Tuckerman EM, Cork BA, et al: A review of immune cells and molecules in women with recurrent miscarriage, *Hum Reprod Update* 9:163, 2003.

Pedersen JF, Mantoni M: Prevalence and significance of subchorionic hemorrhage in threatened abortion: A sonographic study, *AJR Am J Roentgenol* 154:535, 1990.

Philipp T, Philipp K, Reiner A, et al: Embryoscopic and cytogenetic analysis of 233 missed abortions:

Factors involved in the pathogenesis of developmental defects of early failed pregnancies, *Hum Reprod* 18:1724, 2003.

Portnoi MF, Joye N, Van Den Akker J, et al: Karyotypes of 1142 couples with recurrent abortion, *Obstet Gynecol* 72:31, 1988.

Rodger M, Paidas M, McLintock C, et al: Inherited thrombophilia and pregnancy complications revisited, 112(2): Part 1 2008.

Sachs ES, Jahoda MGJ, Van Hemel JO, et al: Chromosome studies of 500 couples with two or more abortions, *Obstet Gynecol* 65:375, 1985.

Schumacher A, Brachwitz N, Sohr S, et al: Human chorionic gonadotropin attracts regulatory T cells into the fetal-maternal interface during early human pregnancy, 2009.

Smith L, Ewings P, Quinlan C:Incidence of pregnancy after expectant, medical, or surgical management of spontaneous first trimester miscarriage: Long term follow-up of miscarriage treatment (MIST) randomised controlled trial.

Stern JJ, Dorfman AD, Gutierrez-Najar AJ: Frequency of abnormal karyotypes among abortuses from women with and without a history of recurrent spontaneous abortion, *Fertil Steril* 65:250–253, 1996.

Strobino BA, Pantel-Silverman J: First-trimester vaginal bleeding and the loss of chromosomally normal and abnormal conceptions, *Am J Obstet Gynecol* 157:1150, 1987.

Walker C, Langhome P, Crichton L, et al: SPIN (Scottish Pregnancy Intervention) study: A multicenter, randomized controlled trial of low-molecular-weight heparin and low-dose aspirin in women with recurrent miscarriage, 2010.

Wilcox AJ, Weinberg CR, O'Connor JF, et al: Incidence of early loss of pregnancy, *N Engl J Med* 319:189, 1988.

17

Ectopic Pregnancy
Etiology, Pathology, Diagnosis, Management, Fertility Prognosis

Roger A. Lobo

Ectopic pregnancy was probably first described in 963 AD by Albucasis, an Arab writer. In 1876, before the initiation of surgical therapy, the mortality rate from ectopic pregnancy was estimated to be 60%. The first successful operative treatment of ectopic pregnancy was performed in 1883 by Lawson Tait in England. In 1887, he reported that he had performed salpingectomy on four women with ectopic pregnancy and that they all survived.

EPIDEMIOLOGY

The incidence of ectopic pregnancy has been estimated to be between 1% to 2% of all pregnancies. Although the incidence of ectopic increased sixfold between 1970 and 1992, it has remained stable since then. The incidence varies among different countries, with rates as high as 1 in 28 and 1 in 40 pregnancies reported in Jamaica and Vietnam. In the United States in 1989, the annual ectopic pregnancy rate per 10,000 women age 15 to 44 was 15.5, similar to that in Finland but higher than the rate in France.

Since 1987, there has been an increasing trend toward treating ectopic pregnancy on an ambulatory basis without overnight hospitalization. With earlier detection of ectopic pregnancy, a steadily increasing percentage of women with this problem are now being treated before tubal rupture occurs by outpatient laparoscopic procedures or by medical treatment with methotrexate. An analysis of both hospital discharge data and an ambulatory medical care survey revealed that the estimated number of hospitalizations for ectopic pregnancy in the United States declined from nearly 90,000 in 1989 to about 45,000 in 1994. However, in 1992 about half of all women with ectopic pregnancy in the United States were treated as outpatients, and the estimated number of total ectopic pregnancies in this year was 108,000, for a rate of 19.7 per 1000 reported pregnancies. Thus, in the United States in 1992, about 2 of every 100 women who were known to conceive had an ectopic gestation. This increased incidence of ectopic pregnancy is thought to be due to two factors: (1) the increased incidence of salpingitis, caused by increased infection with *Chlamydia trachomatis* or other sexually transmitted pathogens, and (2) improved diagnostic techniques, which enable diagnosis of unruptured ectopic pregnancy to be made with more precision and earlier in

gestation before asymptomatic resolution of the pregnancy could occur.

There is an increase in the rate of ectopic pregnancy with increasing age. However, because of the lower pregnancy rate in older women, overall only about 11% of ectopic pregnancies in the United States occur in women aged 35 to 44, whereas more than half, 58%, occur in women aged 25 to 34 years. Most ectopic pregnancies occur in multigravid women. Only 10% to 15% of ectopic pregnancies occur in nulligravid women, whereas more than half occur in women who have been pregnant three or more times. In the United States the rates of ectopic pregnancy are similar in each section of the country, but the rates are higher for nonwhite than white women. About 3% of all reported pregnancies in nonwhite women age 35 to 44 in the United States were ectopic.

MORTALITY

Even with the increased use of surgery and blood transfusions and earlier diagnosis, ectopic pregnancy remains a major cause of maternal death in the United States today. In 1988 there were 44, and in 1989 there were 34 deaths from complications related to ectopic pregnancy in the United States. Ectopic pregnancy is the most common cause of maternal death in the first half of pregnancy. Although the percentage of all maternal deaths in the United States that are the result of ectopic pregnancy increased from 8% in 1970 to 13% in 1989, the percentage of ectopic pregnancies that become fatal has decreased. The overall death-to-case rate of ectopic pregnancy has decreased 10-fold, from 35 per 10,000 women with ectopic pregnancy in 1970 to 3.8 in 1989. The death-to-case rate is similar in all age groups but is four times higher in blacks and other nonwhites than in white women. Because the incidence of ectopic pregnancy is also higher in blacks in the United States, a pregnant black woman is about five times more likely to die of ectopic pregnancy than a white woman. Ectopic pregnancy is the most common single cause of all maternal deaths among black women, causing about one fifth of such deaths. Unmarried women of all races have a 1.7 times greater chance of dying of ectopic pregnancy than married women do. Overall risk of death from ectopic pregnancy is about 10 times greater than the risk of childbirth and more than 50 times greater than the risk of legal abortion.

The major cause of mortality from ectopic pregnancy is blood loss. Most cases of mortality (80%) result from gestations in the tube, and the other 20% were interstitial cornual or abdominal gestations. Because the overall incidence of ectopic pregnancy occurring in these latter locations is slightly less than 4%, interstitial and abdominal ectopic pregnancies have about a five times greater risk of being fatal. About three fourths of the women with fatal ectopic pregnancies initially developed symptoms and died in the first 12 weeks of gestation. Of the remaining one fourth who developed symptoms and died after the first trimester, 70% had interstitial or abdominal pregnancies. Patient delay in consulting a physician after development of symptoms accounted for one third of the deaths, whereas treatment delay resulting from misdiagnosis contributed to the death in half.

ETIOLOGY

FACTORS CONTRIBUTING TO THE RISK

The major factor contributing to the risk of ectopic pregnancy is salpingitis. Its morphologic sequelae account for about half of the initial episodes of ectopic pregnancy. However, in about 40% of cases the cause cannot be determined and is presumed to be a physiologic disorder that results in delay of passage of the embryo into the uterine cavity. Ovulation from the contralateral ovary has been implicated as a cause of delay of blastocyst transport, and it has been suggested that contralateral ovulation occurs in about one third of tubal pregnancies, although this has not been confirmed.

Another possibility in the etiology of ectopic pregnancy is a hormonal imbalance; an elevated circulating level of either estrogen or progesterone can alter normal tubal contractility. An increased rate of ectopic pregnancies has been reported in women who conceive with physiologically and pharmacologically elevated levels of progestogens. The latter condition can be produced locally with a progesterone-releasing IUD, as well as systemically with progestin-only oral contraceptives. Iatrogenic, physiologically increased levels of estrogen and progesterone occur after ovulation induction and ART with either clomiphene citrate or human menopausal gonadotropins, and an increased rate of ectopic pregnancies has been reported in women conceiving after each of these treatment modalities.

Another possible cause is an abnormality of embryonic development. Although aneuploidy has been found to be prevalent in ectopic pregnancies, it may not be higher than the normal rate of aneuploidy and is unlikely to be a cause of ectopic pregnancies. Inherited genetic abnormalities are most probably not a cause of ectopic pregnancy either. Also, there is no increased incidence of ectopics among first-degree relatives.

Several epidemiologic studies indicate that cigarette smoking is associated with about a twofold increased risk of ectopic pregnancy, even when the data were controlled for the presence of other risk factors. The risk of ectopic pregnancy was directly related to the number of cigarettes smoked per day, with a fourfold increased risk noted among women who smoked 30 or more cigarettes per day. Known risk factors for ectopic pregnancy, presented as odds ratios and attributable risk, are depicted in Table 17-1.

The major causes of ectopic pregnancy will be discussed in more detail next.

Table 17-1 Odds Ratios for Ectopic Pregnancy (Compared with Women with Recent Successful Pregnancies) and the Attributable Risks Associated with Different Risk Factors

	Odds Ratio	Attributable Risk*
Probable salpingitis	2	
Confirmed salpingitis	3.5	
History of tubal surgery	3.5	0.18[†]
Smoking		0.35
Ex-smoker	1.5	
1-9 cigarettes per day	2	
10-19 cigarettes per day	3	
≥ 20 cigarettes per day	4	
Age (years)		0.14
30-39	1.5	
≥ 40	3	
Spontaneous abortion	3	0.07
Elective abortion	2	0.03
IUD history	1.5	0.05
Previous infertility	2.5	0.18

*From Auvergne registry data (Bouyer J, Coste J, Shojaei T, et al: Risk factors for ectopic pregnancy: A comprehensive analysis based on a large case-control, population-based study in France. Am J Epidemiol 157:185, 2003).
[†]Risk attributable to history of genital infection and tubal surgery together is 0.33. Odds ratios for EP (compared with deliveries) and attributable risks of the principal risk factors.
IUD, intrauterine device.
From Fernandez H, Gervaise A: Ectopic pregnancies after infertility treatment: Modern diagnosis and therapeutic strategy. Hum Reprod Update 10:503, 2004.

TUBAL PATHOLOGY LEADING TO ECTOPIC RISK

The agglutination of the plicae (folds) of the endosalpinx produced by salpingitis can allow passage of sperm, but prevent the normal transport of the larger morula. The morula can be trapped in blind pockets formed by adhesions of the endosalpinx. In their 20-year longitudinal study, Weström and colleagues found that nearly half (45.3%) of the women with ectopic pregnancy had a clinical history or histologic findings of a prior episode of acute salpingitis. This figure is in close agreement with the 40% incidence of prior salpingitis found on histology by several groups of investigators in women with ectopic pregnancy (**Fig. 17-1**).

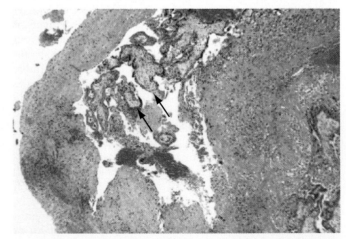

Figure 17-1 Histology of ectopic pregnancy. Note the trophoblastic tissue (*arrows*) in the fallopian tube lumen. (Adapted from www.imaging pathways.health.wa.gov.au.)

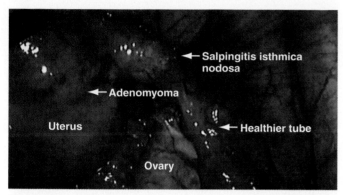

Figure 17-2 Laparoscopic view of salpingitis isthmica nodosa in the isthmic tube and cornual regions of the uterus. Note the normal distal tube. (From www.dan martinmd.com.)

Weström and colleagues prospectively followed 900 women aged 15 to 34 years who had laparoscopically confirmed acute salpingitis and found that the subsequent ectopic pregnancy rate was 68.8 per 1000 conceptions, yielding a sixfold increase in the risk of ectopic pregnancy. The risk of ectopic after acute salpingitis increased both with the number of episodes of infection and with the increasing age of the women at the time of infection.

Salpingitis isthmica nodosa (SIN) (also referred to as **tubal diverticulum**) is defined as the microscopic presence of tubal epithelium within the myosalpinx or beneath the tubal serosa (**Fig. 17-2**). In two histopathologic studies of tubes removed from women with ectopic pregnancy, it was found that about half contained lesions of SIN compared with 5% in a control group. With serial sectioning, it has been determined that SIN is actually a diverticulum or intrauterine extension of the tubal lumen. Associated histologic evidence of chronic salpingitis was seen in only 6% of the tubes, suggesting that SIN was not necessarily the result of infection. It has been found that the **tubal pregnancy** usually implanted in a portion of the tube distal to the SIN, indicating that mechanical entrapment of the morula is not the mechanism whereby SIN causes tubal gestation. It may be that it is SIN itself or associated tubal anomalies that may be responsible for dysfunction of the tubal transport mechanism without anatomic obstruction.

It is likely that adhesions between the tubal serosa and bowel or peritoneum may interfere with normal tubal motility and cause ectopic pregnancy because, as reported, 17% to 27% of women with ectopic pregnancy have had previous abdominal surgical procedures not involving the oviduct. On the other hand, neither endometriosis nor congenital anomalies of the tube have been associated with an increased incidence of ectopic pregnancy.

An operative procedure on the tube itself is a cause of ectopic pregnancy whether the tube is morphologically normal, as occurs with sterilization procedures, or abnormal, as occurs with postsalpingitis reconstructive surgery. The incidence of ectopic pregnancy occurring after salpingoplasty or **salpingostomy** procedures to treat distal tubal disease ranges from 15% to 25%, probably because the damage to the endosalpinx remains. The rate of ectopic pregnancy after reversal of sterilization procedures is lower, about 4%, because the tubes have not been damaged by infection.

Women who have had a prior ectopic pregnancy, even if treated by unilateral salpingectomy, are at increased risk for having a subsequent ectopic pregnancy. Of women who conceive after having one ectopic pregnancy, about 25% of subsequent pregnancies are ectopic. In two large series of women with ectopic pregnancy, 7% had a history of a prior ectopic pregnancy.

The incidence of ectopic gestation is significantly greater (four to five times) in women who have been exposed to diethylstilbestrol (DES) in utero and has been reported at the rate of 4% to 5%. In women exposed to DES whose hysterosalpingograms demonstrated abnormalities in the uterine cavity, the ectopic pregnancy rate was as high as 13%.

CONTRACEPTION FAILURE

For several decades, sterilization has been the most popular method of contraception used by couples in the United States. Since the development of laparoscopic surgery, female tubal sterilization is performed about twice as frequently as vasectomy. In a recent analysis of the long-term risk of pregnancy after tubal sterilization reported by Peterson and coworkers, it was found that within 10 years after the procedure the cumulative life table probability of pregnancy was 1.85%. The 10-year failure rate after bipolar coagulation of the oviducts was 2.48%, which rose to 5.43% if the sterilization procedure was performed when the woman was younger than 28 years of age. These investigators reported that for all 143 pregnancies occurring after tubal sterilization, 43, or 32.9%, were ectopic pregnancies.

Several investigators have reported that if pregnancy occurred after tubal sterilization by laparoscopic fulguration, the ectopic pregnancy rate was as high as 50%. It has been hypothesized that with the extensive tissue destruction caused by electrocoagulation, a uteroperitoneal fistula develops that allows sperm to pass into the distal segment of the oviduct and fertilize the egg (**Fig. 17-3**). Such fistulas can be demonstrated radiographically in about 11% of women after laparoscopic electrocoagulation. Peterson and colleagues reported that within 10 years after the sterilization procedure, twice as many women sterilized by bipolar coagulation had ectopic pregnancies than those sterilized with metal clips or silicone bands. The overall ectopic pregnancy rate after bipolar coagulation sterilization was 1.7%.

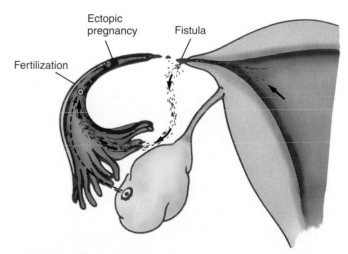

Figure 17-3 Mechanism of ectopic pregnancy after sterilization. (From Corson SL, Batzer FR: Ectopic pregnancy. A review of the etiologic factors. J Reprod Med 31:78, 1986.)

Because about one third of pregnancies that occur after all tubal sterilizations are ectopic, women should be counseled that if they do not experience the expected menses at any time following tubal sterilization before menopause, a test to detect human chorionic gonadotropin (HCG) should be performed rapidly, and if they are pregnant, a diagnostic evaluation to exclude the presence of ectopic pregnancy is necessary. In women who have an ectopic pregnancy after electrocautery sterilization, because the site of the fistula usually cannot be determined clinically, salpingectomies should be carried out.

Although women who become pregnant while using diaphragms or combination oral contraceptives do not have an increased chance of having an ectopic pregnancy and reliable contraception decreases the risk of all pregnancies, including ectopics, women who become pregnant while using a Copper T380 intrauterine device (IUD) or progestin-only oral contraceptives have about a 5% chance of having an ectopic pregnancy. The incidence of ectopic pregnancy in women who become pregnant with the progesterone-releasing IUDs is even higher, about 23%. The progesterone-releasing IUD inhibits tubal contractions and has a higher failure rate than the copper IUD. Women who use this method of contraception have about twice the risk of ectopic pregnancy (7.5 per 1000 woman-years) than women who use no method of contraception (3.5 per 1000 woman-years). Women using IUDs who elect to have their pregnancies terminated should have a histologic examination of the tissue removed from the uterine cavity to be certain the pregnancy was intrauterine.

HORMONAL ALTERATIONS

As occurs with exogenous progesterone administration, if increased levels of exogenous or endogenous estrogens are present shortly after the time of ovulation, the incidence of ectopic pregnancy is increased. Several investigators have reported that the ectopic pregnancy rate is about 1.5% for conceptions that occur after ovulation has been induced with clomiphene citrate. The ectopic rate in pregnancies occurring after ovulation with human menopausal gonadotropins (HMG) has been reported to range between 3% and 4%. Fernandez and colleagues in a case-control study found the risk of ectopic pregnancy was increased about fourfold among ovulatory women treated with controlled ovarian hyperstimulation, either clomiphene citrate, HMG, or a combination of both, for the treatment of unexplained infertility. These reports indicate that increased levels of estrogen, as well as of progesterone, interfere with tubal motility and increase the chance of ectopic gestation. Ectopic gestations occur in about 1% of pregnancies that develop after in vitro fertilization and embryo transfer. The reason for this increased incidence is likely due to one or more of several factors: increased sex steroid hormone levels, the presence of proximal tubal disease (although the ratio is similar in women with normal tubes), and flushing an embryo directly into the tube.

PREVIOUS ABORTION

Although some studies have suggested that a prior induced abortion increases the risk of ectopic pregnancy, there is probably no major association of increased risk.

PATHOLOGY

Most ectopic pregnancies occur in the tube. In Breen's series, 97.7% of the ectopic pregnancies were tubal, 1.4% were abdominal, and less than 1% were ovarian or cervical (**Fig. 17-4**). The majority of tubal gestations, 81%, were located in the ampullary portion of the oviduct, being about equally divided between the distal and middle third of the tube. About 12% of tubal gestations occur in the isthmus and 5% in the fimbrial region. Although Breen considered pregnancies located in the cornual area of the uterus to be uterine in origin, they are in fact pregnancies implanted in the interstitial portion of the tube. About 2% of all ectopic pregnancies are interstitial and are frequently

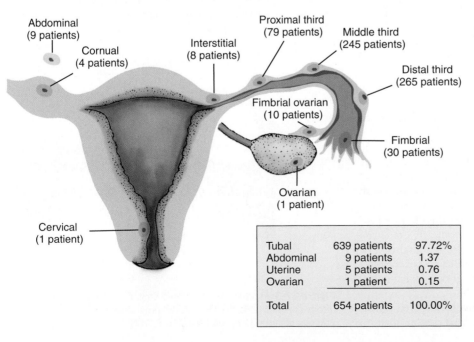

Tubal	639 patients	97.72%
Abdominal	9 patients	1.37
Uterine	5 patients	0.76
Ovarian	1 patient	0.15
Total	654 patients	100.00%

Figure 17-4 Anatomic site of ectopic pregnancy. (From Breen JL: A 21 year survey of 654 ectopic pregnancies. Am J Obstet Gynecol 106:1004, 1970.)

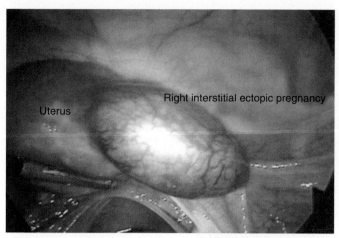

Figure 17-5 Right interstitial pregnancy at laparoscopy. (Adapted from Bolaji I, Gupta S, Medical management of interstitial pregnancy with high beta selective human chorionic gonadotropin. Ultrasound 18[2]:60-67, 2010.)

associated with severe morbidity, because they become symptomatic later in the gestation, are difficult to diagnose, and frequently produce massive hemorrhage when they rupture (**Fig. 17-5**). A true **cornual pregnancy** is one located in the rudimentary horn of a bicornuate uterus, and this occurrence is quite rare. In a review of 240 true cornual pregnancies reported by O'Leary and O'Leary, about 90% of them ruptured with massive hemorrhage.

About 1 in 200 ectopic pregnancies are true ovarian pregnancies that fulfill the four criteria originally described by Spiegelburg:

1. The tube and fimbria must be intact and separate from the ovary.
2. The gestational sac must occupy the normal position of the ovary.
3. The sac must be connected to the uterus by the ovarian ligament.
4. Ovarian tissue should be demonstrable in the walls of the sac.

Many women with ovarian pregnancies are believed to have a ruptured corpus luteum cyst, and the correct diagnosis was made during the surgical procedure only 28% of the time. The hemorrhagic mass (ovarian ectopic) should be located adjacent to the corpus luteum, never within it. **Ovarian pregnancy** is also associated with profuse hemorrhage, with 81% of reported to have a **hemoperitoneum** greater than 500 mL. Nevertheless, most can be successfully treated by ovarian resection and not oophorectomy.

Most abdominal pregnancies occur secondary to **tubal abortion** with secondary implantation in the peritoneal cavity (**Fig. 17-6**). On rare occasions a primary **abdominal pregnancy** may occur. For the latter diagnosis to be made, the following three criteria originally set forth by Studdiford must be present: (1) the tubes and ovaries must be normal, with no evidence of recent or past injury; (2) there must be no evidence of a uteroplacental fistula; and (3) the pregnancy must be related only to the peritoneal surface and early enough in gestation to eliminate the possibility of secondary implantation after primary tubal nidation. An unusual type of primary abdominal pregnancy may implant in the spleen or liver and produce massive intraperitoneal hemorrhage.

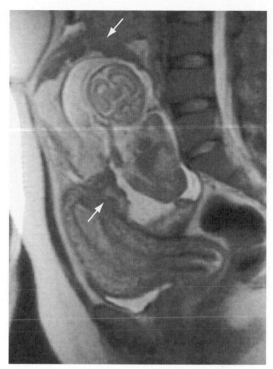

Figure 17-6 MRI of abdominal pregnancy showing placental infarction. Note the distance of the pregnancy from the uterus. (From www.Hmer.ch/selected.)

The prognosis for fetal survival in abdominal pregnancy is poor, found to be 11%, and is difficult to diagnose. Once the diagnosis is established, a laparotomy with removal of the fetus should be performed immediately to prevent a possible fatal hemorrhage. An adjunctive option is to administer methotrexate. On occasion, when the placenta is tightly adherent to bowel and blood vessels, it should be left in the abdominal cavity. In such instances, the placental tissue usually resorbs. However, there may be symptoms of abdominal pain and intermittent fever for many months as well as possible partial bowel obstruction and abscess formation. Thus, it is highly desirable, if it is surgically feasible, to remove the placenta entirely. Partial removal also may result in massive hemorrhage, so the surgical approach and decision making are challenging and critical.

The four pathologic criteria for the diagnosis of **cervical pregnancy** as reported by Rubin and colleagues are (1) cervical glands must be present opposite the placental attachment, (2) the attachment of the placenta to the cervix must be intimate, (3) the placenta must be below the entrance of the uterine vessels or below the peritoneal reflection of the anteroposterior surface of the uterus, and (4) fetal elements must not be present in the corpus uteri (**Fig. 17-7**).

The usual characteristic clinical findings of cervical pregnancy are uterine bleeding after amenorrhea without cramping pain, a softened cervix that is disproportionately enlarged, complete confinement and firm attachment of the products of conception to the endocervix, and a closed internal os.

Most cervical pregnancies occur after the history of having a bad previous sharp uterine curettage. The differential diagnosis is difficult and includes incomplete abortion, placenta previa, carcinoma of the cervix, and a degenerating leiomyoma. Although cervical ectopics previously have been associated with a high

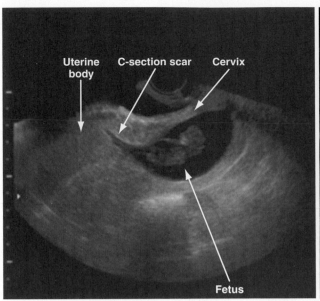

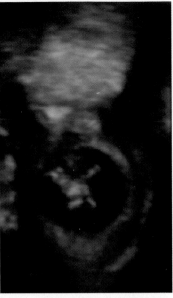

Figure 17-7 Cervical pregnancy as viewed by 2-D ultrasound (*left panel*). Note the normal endometrium to the left of the gestational sac and the larger fetal pole. The right panel shows the same cervical ectopic on 3-D ultrasound. Note the ballooned-out cervix and narrowed uterine isthmus/lower segment above it.

mortality because of massive hemorrhage, currently, with better methods of diagnosis and treatment, death is rare. In the past, more than half of the women with cervical pregnancy required a hysterectomy for treatment, and this was nearly always necessary if the pregnancy had advanced beyond 18 weeks. There have been several case reports in which a cervical pregnancy was successfully treated by systemic methotrexate. Other case reports have shown that after angiographic uterine artery embolization evacuation of the pregnancy can be easily performed transcervically with minimal blood loss. Transvaginal ultrasound-guided injections of potassium chloride directly into the gestational sac have successfully terminated the pregnancies, as has the local injection of methotrexate, with or without uterine artery embolization.

Another uncommon form of ectopic gestation is combined intrauterine and extrauterine (heterotopic) pregnancy (94% tubal and 6% ovarian). It has been calculated that the incidence of **heterotopic pregnancy** should be between 1 in 16,000 or 1 in 30,000 pregnancies. However, a review of the recent experience at one institution by Reece and colleagues revealed that 1 of 8000 pregnancies was combined intrauterine and extrauterine, and 1 of 70 ectopic pregnancies was associated with an IUP. The generally quoted incidence of heterotopic pregnancy in the general population is thought to be 1 in 4000. However, this increases with use of ovulation-inducing agents and may be as high as 1% following in vitro fertilization. The incidence has been reported to be higher when tubal damage was present or four or more embryos were transferred. A **chronic ectopic pregnancy** occurs when the intraperitoneal hemorrhage associated with tubal abortion or rupture is relatively minor and ceases spontaneously, but the ectopic gestation neither resolves completely nor implants and continues to develop as an abdominal pregnancy. The trophoblast continues to secrete HCG in small amounts, with the circulating levels less than 1000 mIU/mL in 50% of cases and less than 100 mIU/mL in 20% of cases. In one series, about 6% of all surgically treated ectopic pregnancies in one institution were classified as chronic. The most common (72%) gross pathologic finding was dense adhesions produced by the inflammatory response to the trophoblast. These adhesions attach omentum and bowel to the site of the ectopic pregnancy. In one third of the cases, a collection of clotted blood or old hematoma was present. It has been reported that because of the extensive disease, it was necessary to perform a hysterectomy in 25% of cases and an oophorectomy in 60% of women with a chronic ovarian ectopic pregnancy.

HISTOPATHOLOGY

When the morula implants in the tube, it does not grow mainly in the tubal lumen as has been assumed for many years. A review of the pathology of tubal gestation found that after implanting on the mucosa of the endosalpinx, the trophoblast invaded the lamina propria and then the muscularis of the tube and grew mainly between the lumen of the tube and its peritoneal covering. Growth occurred both parallel to the long axis of the tube and circumferentially around it. As the trophoblast invaded vessels, retroperitoneal tubal hemorrhage occurred that is mainly extraluminal but may extrude from the fimbriated end and create a hemoperitoneum before tubal rupture (**Fig. 17-8**).

The stretching of the peritoneum covered by this hemorrhage results in episodic pain before the final perforation into the peritoneal cavity. Rupture occurs when the serosa is maximally stretched, producing necrosis secondary to an inadequate blood supply.

Hemoperitoneum is nearly always found in advanced **ruptured ectopic pregnancy** other than that which is cervical in origin. Usually there is a combination of clotted and unclotted blood in the peritoneal cavity. The unclotted blood does not clot on removal from the peritoneal cavity because it originates from lysis of blood that has previously coagulated, similar to what occurs during menstrual bleeding. The hematocrit value of this nonclotting blood is nearly always greater than 15%, such a finding being reported in 98% of specimens obtained by **culdocentesis** in a series of ectopic pregnancies. Historically, at the time of laparotomy for a ruptured ectopic pregnancy, about half of the women have less than 500 mL of hemoperitoneum, one fourth between 500 and 1000 mL, and one fifth more than 1000 mL.

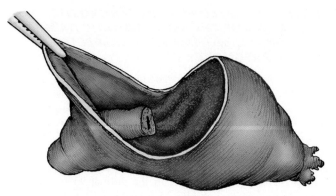

Figure 17-8 Artist's rendition of dissected ampullary ectopic pregnancy showing space between tube and peritoneum, revealed when blood clots and placenta were removed. Toward fimbriated end, no dissection was performed and external appearance is that of dilated tube. (From Budowick M, Johnson TRB, Genadry R, et al: The histopathology of the developing tubal ectopic pregnancy. Fertil Steril 34:169, 1980. Reproduced with permission of the publisher, The American Fertility Society.)

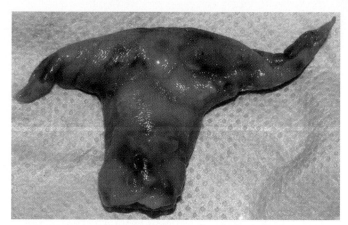

Figure 17-10 Decidual cast. (From www.ispub.com.)

When the tube is removed and examined histologically, inflammatory cells are nearly always seen. These include plasma cells, lymphocytes, and histiocytes. The presence of chorionic villi, which are frequently degenerated or hyalinized, as well as nucleated red cells established the diagnosis of ectopic pregnancy. Decidual reaction in the tube is uncommon.

Because of limited space or inadequate nourishment, the trophoblastic tissue of most ectopic pregnancies does not grow as rapidly as that of pregnancies within the uterine cavity. As a result, HCG production does not increase as rapidly as in a normal pregnancy, and although steroid production of the corpus luteum is initiated, elevated progesterone levels cannot be maintained. Thus, initially the endometrium becomes decidualized because of continued progesterone production by the corpus luteum. Sometimes the secretory cells of the endometrial glands become hypertrophied with hyperchromatism, pleomorphism, and increased mitotic activity, as originally described by Arias-Stella (**Fig. 17-9**). The **Arias-Stella reaction** can be

confused with neoplasia, but it is not unique for ectopic pregnancy, because it can occur with an IUP as well as after ovarian stimulation with clomiphene citrate. In a histologic study of the endometrium in 84 women with ectopic pregnancies, 40% of cases had secretory endometrium, with the remainder being about equally divided among the findings of proliferative endometrium, decidual reaction, and an Arias-Stella reaction. When progesterone levels fall as a result of insufficient HCG, endometrial integrity is no longer maintained and it breaks down, producing uterine bleeding. Sometimes nearly all the decidua is passed through the cervix in an intact way, producing a **decidual cast** that may be clinically confused with a spontaneous abortion (**Fig. 17-10**).

SYMPTOMS

Among women with risk factors for ectopic pregnancy, with the use of early hormonal testing and vaginal sonography, it is now frequently possible to establish the diagnosis of ectopic pregnancy before symptoms develop. However, symptoms often develop when intraperitoneal bleeding occurs from extrusion of blood through the fimbrial end of the tube or from tubal rupture.

The most common symptoms of ectopic pregnancy are abdominal pain, absence of menses, and irregular vaginal bleeding (**Table 17-3**). Abdominal pain is nearly a universal symptom of intraperitoneal bleeding, but its characteristics are similar with different causes of bleeding. Before rupture occurs, the pain may be characterized as only a vague soreness or be colicky in nature. Its location may be generalized, unilateral, or bilateral. Shoulder pain occurs in about one fourth of women with ruptured ectopic pregnancy as a result of diaphragmatic irritation from the hemoperitoneum. During rupture of the tube, the pain usually becomes intense. Syncope occurs in about one third of women with tubal rupture. Other symptoms that occur following tubal rupture include dizziness and an urge to defecate.

The majority of women with ectopic pregnancy fail to have menses at the expected time but have one or more episodes of irregular vaginal bleeding when the decidual endometrial tissue is sloughed. The interval of amenorrhea is usually 6 weeks or more. The bleeding is usually characterized as spotting but may simulate menstrual bleeding. It is rarely as heavy as that

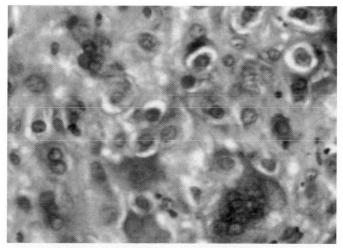

Figure 17-9 Histology of arias stella reaction. Note the enlarged secretory endometrial cells, which are hypertrophied, hyperchromatic, and pleomorphic. (From www.j pathology.com.)

which occurs in spontaneous abortion. About 5% to 10% of women with an advanced ectopic pregnancy will note passage of a decidual cast, as noted previously (**Fig. 17-10**).

SIGNS

The most common presenting sign in a woman with symptomatic ectopic pregnancy is abdominal tenderness, which, together with adnexal tenderness elicited at the time of the bimanual pelvic examination, is present in nearly all women with an advanced or ruptured ectopic pregnancy. It is possible to palpate an adnexal mass in half of the women, and about one third have some degree of uterine enlargement that is nearly always smaller than a normal 8-week intrauterine gestation except when an interstitial gestation is present. Tachycardia and hypotension can occur after rupture if blood loss is profuse, but temperature elevation is an uncommon finding, being present in only about 5% to 10% of women with tubal rupture, and is rarely greater than 38°C.

DIFFERENTIAL DIAGNOSIS OF SYMPTOMATIC ECTOPIC PREGNANCY

The diagnosis is usually obvious for women with the classic symptoms of ruptured ectopic pregnancy: a history of irregular bleeding followed by sudden onset of pain and syncope accompanied by signs of peritoneal irritation. However, before rupture the symptoms and signs are nonspecific and may also occur with other gynecologic disorders. Entities frequently confused with ectopic pregnancy include salpingitis, threatened or incomplete abortion, ruptured corpus luteum, appendicitis, dysfunctional uterine bleeding, adnexal torsion, degenerative uterine leiomyoma, and endometriosis.

In the past, studies have found that women with an ectopic were seen multiple times before a correct diagnosis was made. Because of the possibility of a fatal outcome from undiagnosed ruptured ectopic pregnancy, it is essential that the diagnosis of ectopic pregnancy be considered in any woman of childbearing age with abdominal pain and irregular uterine bleeding even if she has had a previous tubal sterilization procedure or is using an effective method of reversible contraception.

Ectopic pregnancy should be suspected in any woman who develops the symptoms listed earlier, particularly if she has previously had a pelvic operation, especially tubal surgery, either a tubal reconstructive procedure or a sterilization procedure. Other risk factors include one or more episodes of salpingitis, a previous ectopic gestation, current use of a progesterone-releasing IUD, use of a progestin-only oral contraceptive, use of pharmacologic methods of ovulation induction, or a history of infertility. In any woman with the symptoms of ectopic gestation, the diagnosis is facilitated by a quantitative assay for HCG and pelvic ultrasonography and can be established and treated by laparoscopy or laparotomy. Culdocentesis and measurement of serum progesterone levels may also be of assistance. Prior to the development of pelvic vaginal ultrasound, the finding of nonclotting blood at the time of culdocentesis, especially if the hematocrit was above 15%, was of great assistance in establishing the diagnosis of ruptured ectopic pregnancy. With the use of high-resolution pelvic ultrasound, the presence of intraperitoneal fluid can be easily visualized and culdocentesis is now not routinely done.

PROCEDURES USED FOR THE DIAGNOSTIC EVALUATION OF THE ASYMPTOMATIC OR MILDLY SYMPTOMATIC WOMAN WITH SUSPECTED ECTOPIC PREGNANCY

Human Chorionic Gonadotropin

About 85% of women with ectopic pregnancy have serum HCG levels lower than those seen in normal pregnancy at a similar gestational age. However, a single quantitative HCG assay cannot be used to diagnose ectopic pregnancy because the actual dates of ovulation and conception are often not known. Even if the date of ovulation is known, 2.5% of women with normal gestations will have HCG levels lower than the normal 95% confidence limits. Furthermore, low HCG levels are also found in women with various stages of spontaneous abortion, conditions that must be considered in the differential diagnosis. Intact HCG and free β-HCG levels were measured in a large group of women in early pregnancy who presented with symptoms of ectopic pregnancy. Although mean levels of intact HCG and free β-HCG were significantly lower in the group of women with ectopic pregnancy and those who aborted than in those with viable intrauterine pregnancies, the individual HCG levels among the three conditions overlapped too much to devise a cutoff level for diagnostic purposes (**Fig. 17-11**).

Figure 17-12, as constructed by Barnhart, shows the expected changes (increases) in HCG levels in women with an intrauterine pregnancy and in spontaneous abortion. Ninety-nine percent of normal intrauterine pregnancies have an increase of at least 53% in 2 days, which is less than the rise that was previously accepted (approximately 66%). This rate of increase should be similar in single or multiple gestations. Note in **Table 17-2** the expected decline in HCG levels in women who have an abnormal pregnancy destined for a spontaneous abortion. In women with an ectopic pregnancy, the rate of rise in HCG can mimic an intrauterine pregnancy 21% of the time and can mimic a spontaneous abortion 8% of the time. Note the overlap in this increase or decrease in HCG levels as depicted in **Figure 17-12**.

Today, the key to the diagnosis of ectopic pregnancy is vaginal ultrasound. The concept of a "discriminatory zone" has been advanced where if a level of HCG between 1500 and 2500 mIU/mL is reported, an intrauterine sac should be visible. Absent this observation, an abnormal pregnancy is present, and an ectopic pregnancy needs to be ruled out. It has been suggested further that as reliable as using the discriminatory zone is, the length of gestation is at least as important if accurate dating is available (as occurs with luteinizing hormone [LH] surge monitoring, etc.). Clearly by 5½ weeks from LMP (in a woman with normal ovulatory cycle length) an intrauterine sac should be visible in a normal intrauterine pregnancy. Important ultrasound findings include seeing a yolk sac at 5.5 weeks, a fetal pole by 6 weeks, and cardiac activity at 6.5 weeks. An abnormal pregnancy is likely if there is absence of a fetal pole with a gestational sac of 2 cm and if no cardiac activity is noted with a crown-rump length of >0.5 cm.

Thus, serial measurements of HCG are of great assistance in the early diagnosis of unruptured ectopic pregnancy. However, it must be realized that a differentiation between ectopic pregnancies and impending spontaneous abortion cannot be made with this technique because the rate of increase of HCG in women with an ectopic pregnancy is often similar to that found in women with an impending intrauterine abortion. An algorithm for possible treatment will be presented here.

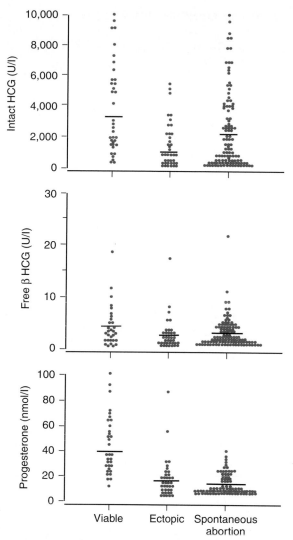

Figure 17-11 The distribution of serum concentrations of progesterone, intact human chorionic gonadotropin (HCG), and free β-HCG in viable and ectopic pregnancies and spontaneous abortions. Means are indicated by horizontal bars (—). (From Ledger WL, Sweeting VM, Chatterjee S: Rapid diagnosis of early ectopic pregnancy in an emergency gynaecology service—are measurements of progesterone, intact and free beta human chorionic gonadotrophin helpful? Hum Reprod 9:157, 1994.)

Table 17-2 Expected Change in Serum hCG Levels in First Week of Monitoring Women at Risk for Ectopic Pregnancy

Type of Pregnancy	Change in hCG	
	After 2 days	**After 7 days**
	percent	
Growing intrauterine pregnancy		
In 50% of women	124	500
In 85% of women	63	256
In 99% of women	53	133
Spontaneous abortion[†]		
Initial HCG, 50 mIU/mL	-12	-34
Initial HCG, 500 mIU/mL	-21	-60
Initial HCG, 2000 mIU/mL	-31	-79
Initial HCG, 5000 mIU/mL	-35	-84

[†]This change occurred in 90% of women with spontaneous abortion. Data from Barnhart KT, Sammel MD, Rinaudo PF, et al. Symptomatic patients with an early viable intrauterine pregnancy: HCG curves redefined, Obstet Gynecol 104:50-55, 2004. Data from N Engl J Med 361:4 2009.

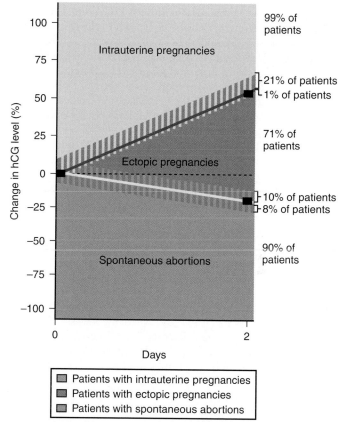

□ Patients with intrauterine pregnancies
□ Patients with ectopic pregnancies
□ Patients with spontaneous abortions

Figure 17-12 Change in the HCG level in intrauterine pregnancy, ectopic pregnancy, and spontaneous abortion. An increase or decrease in the serial human chorionic gonadotropin (HCG) level in a woman with an ectopic pregnancy is outside the range expected for that of a woman with a growing intrauterine pregnancy or a spontaneous abortion 71% of the time. However, the increase in the HCG level in a woman with an ectopic pregnancy can mimic that of a growing intrauterine pregnancy 21% of the time, and the decrease in the HCG level can mimic that of a spontaneous abortion 8% of the time. (Adapted from Barnhart K: Ectopic pregnancy. N Engl J Med 361[4]:384, 2009.)

Progesterone

Several investigators have shown that when an ectopic pregnancy is present, the corpus luteum does not secrete as much progesterone as occurs in normal pregnancies with similar levels of HCG. It has been found that in the women with ectopic pregnancies, mean serum progesterone levels were significantly lower at 4, 5, and 6 weeks gestational age than in the women with intrauterine gestations, whether or not these gestations subsequently aborted or continued to viability (see **Table 17-3**). It was also reported that at 4 weeks' gestation a threshold progesterone level of 5 ng/mL was able to differentiate ectopic from intrauterine gestations, with a sensitivity of 100% and a specificity of 97%. At 5 weeks' gestation, the threshold level of progesterone increased to 10 ng/mL and at 6 weeks to 20 ng/mL, but the sensitivity and specificity of the use of serum progesterone measurement to differentiate

ectopic from intrauterine gestations decreased as the gestational age increased. A significant difference in mean progesterone levels has been found between women in early pregnancy with a viable intrauterine gestation and those with an ectopic gestation or those

Table 17-3 Mean Progesterone Concentrations Obtained at Weeks 4, 5, and 6 of Gestation from Women Whose Pregnancies Subsequently Terminated in Live Births, Spontaneous Abortions, or Ectopic Pregnancies

| Pregnancy Outcome | n | Progesterone Concentrations at Different Gestational Ages (Weeks) (Mean ± SEM, ng/mL) | | | |
		4	5	6	Mean All Gestations
Live birth	242	35.5 ± 6.2	31.0 ± 6.0	27.5 ± 5.3	31.2 ± 5.9
Spontaneous abortion	81	32.9 ± 4.62	23.9 ± 2.8	23.3 ± 2.6	26.7 ± 3.0
Ectopic	15	*1.9 ± 0.9	*11.9 ± 1.4	*7.0 ± 3.3	*7.0 ± 2.9

*Significantly lower than other values in same column ($P = 0.0005$).
From Stern JJ, Voss, F, Coulam, CB: Early diagnosis of ectopic pregnancy using receiver-operator characteristic curves of serum progesterone concentrations. Hum Reprod 8:775, 1993.

who had a spontaneous abortion (see **Fig. 17-11**). It has also been found that in a group of women presenting with symptoms of ectopic pregnancy, no woman with a viable IUP had progesterone levels less than 10 ng/mL, whereas 88% of ectopic pregnancies and 83% of spontaneous abortions had progesterone values less than this amount.

Stovall and associates measured both HCG and serum progesterone levels in more than 1000 women in the first trimester of pregnancy. They found that all those women with a serum progesterone level less than 5 ng/mL had either an ectopic gestation or a nonviable intrauterine gestation, whereas 97% of women with a serum progesterone level above 25 ng/mL had a viable intrauterine gestation. They calculated that a single progesterone level of less than 15 ng/mL was as sensitive and more specific than lack of a rise of 66% of two HCG levels measured 48 hours apart for the detection of an abnormal pregnancy. This same group showed that the probability of an ectopic or abnormal IUP decreased with rising progesterone levels, with less than a 10% likelihood of an abnormal pregnancy occurring with the progesterone level above 17.6 ng/mL (**Fig. 17-13**).

Ultrasonography

Development of the transvaginal transducer probes with 7.0-MHz scanning frequency has enabled more precise imaging of the pelvic organs in early pregnancy than is possible with transabdominal ultrasonography. With these probes it is usually possible to identify an intrauterine gestational sac when the HCG level reaches 1500 mIU/mL and virtually always when the HCG level exceeds 2500 mIU/mL (First International Reference Preparation [1st IRP], now called the Third International Standard), about 5 to 6 weeks after the last menses. Kadar and colleagues reported that in both singleton and multiple gestations a gestational sac should always be seen sonographically beyond 24 days after conception, 38 days' gestational age. Because combined extrauterine and IUP is a rare event, the finding of an intrauterine gestational sac should nearly always exclude the presence of an ectopic pregnancy. When a gestational sac is not present and the HCG level is in the discriminatory zone, a pathologic pregnancy, either an ectopic or a nonviable intrauterine gestation, is most likely present and should be suspected. Usually an adnexal mass or a gestational saclike structure can be identified in the tube when an ectopic pregnancy is present that produces levels of HCG above 2500 mIU/mL.

Thus, diagnostic criteria for the ultrasonographic diagnosis of ectopic pregnancy with the use of a vaginal probe include the detection of a complex or cystic adnexal mass (often called an echogenic "bagel" sign) or visualization of an embryo fetal pole in the adnexa (**Fig. 17-14**). This is in the absence of an intrauterine

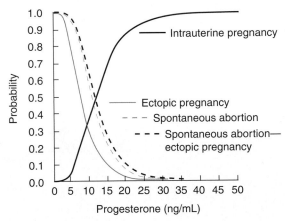

Figure 17-13 Predicted pregnancy outcome versus progesterone concentrations. The probability of ectopic pregnancy and spontaneous abortion decreases with rising progesterone levels, forming a negative-sloping sigmoid-shaped curve, a mirror image of the intrauterine pregnancy curve, with its slope decreasing sharply at approximately 5 ng/mL (15.9 nmol/L) and increasing sharply at approximately 17 ng/mL (54.1 nmol/L). (Reprinted from McCord ML, Arheart KL, Muram D, et al: Single serum progesterone as a screen for ectopic pregnancy: Exchanging specificity and sensitivity to obtain optimal test performance. Fertil Steril 66:513, 1996. Copyright 1996, with permission from The American Society for Reproductive Medicine.)

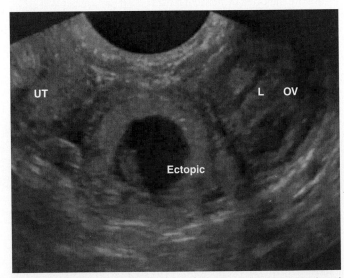

Figure 17-14 Ultrasound showing a left tubal ectopic. Note the bagel appearance of gestational sac, which here has a fetal pole. (Adapted from embryology.med.unsw.edu.au.)

gestational sac when the gestational age is known to be more than 38 days, or the HCG level is above a certain threshold, usually between 1500 and 2500 mIU/mL.

About two thirds of women presenting with symptoms of ectopic pregnancy have HCG levels above 2500 mIU/mL, and when this occurs, the diagnosis of ectopic pregnancy can usually be made by ultrasound. For the other one third with lower HCG levels, unless a gestational sac is evident on ultrasonography, other diagnostic techniques, such as measurement of a serum progesterone level and serial HCG determination, should be performed. Repeat ultrasonographic examinations at 3- to 5-day intervals are often helpful in establishing a correct diagnosis.

Several investigators have shown that with the use of endovaginal color Doppler flow imaging, it is possible to establish the diagnosis of ectopic pregnancy with greater sensitivity and specificity than with ordinary endovaginal sonography. With endovaginal color flow imaging of the pelvic structures in the presence of an ectopic pregnancy, about a 20% difference in

the degree of tubal blood flow between the adnexae has been found compared with less than an 8% difference with intrauterine gestations. Use of endovaginal color flow compared with routine transvaginal sonography increased the sensitivity of the diagnosis of ectopic pregnancy from 71% to 95%, with a specificity of 96% to 100% in various studies (**Fig. 17-15**).

Dilation and Curettage (D&C)

When serum HCG levels are more than 1500 mIU/mL, the gestational age exceeds 38 days, or the serum progesterone level is less than 5 ng/mL and no intrauterine gestational sac is seen with vaginal ultrasonography, a curettage of the endometrial cavity (by D&C) with histologic examination of the tissue removed, by frozen section if desired, can be undertaken to determine if any gestational tissue is present. This is a pragmatic approach reserved for those women who do not desire a pregnancy. Note that it has been shown that an endometrial biopsy (e.g., Pipelle) is inadequate in this scenario. Spandorfer and coworkers

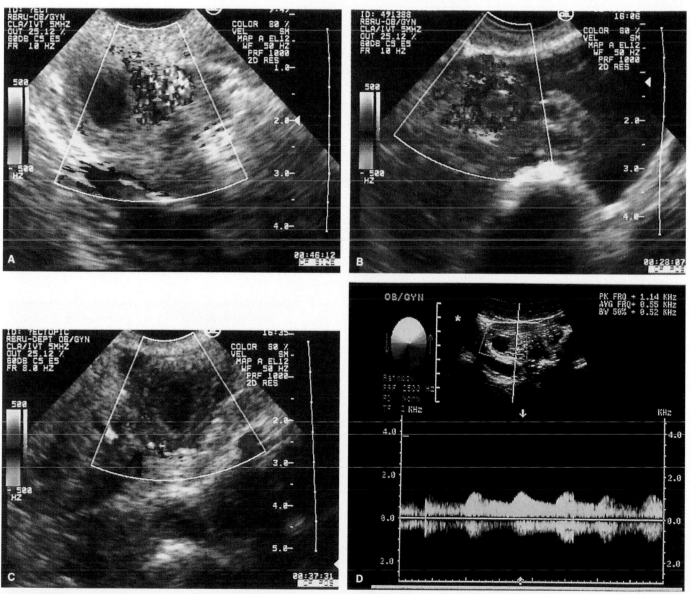

Figure 17-15 Ectopic pregnancy showing enhanced blood flow using color Doppler.

reported that frozen section was 93% accurate in identifying chorionic villi. If no chorionic villi are visualized in the removed tissue, a presumptive diagnosis of ectopic pregnancy can be made and treatment undertaken. A recent analysis by Ailawedi suggested that performing a dilatation and curettage in this setting results in fewer complications and is at least as cost effective as the empiric use of methotrexate.

Diagnostic Evaluation of Women with Suspected Ectopic Pregnancy

Several authors have developed flow sheets to aid the clinician in establishing the diagnosis of an asymptomatic or mildly symptomatic ectopic pregnancy. They involve the use of vaginal probe pelvic ultrasonography, measurements of serial quantitative HCG and single serum progesterone levels, and uterine curettage. One suggested algorithm is presented in **Figure 17-16**. Note that because of clinical variability, this is merely a guide to management. These diagnostic aids are of particular use when following an asymptomatic woman with risk factors for ectopic pregnancy, beginning shortly after conception. Performing a quantitative HCG assay twice weekly and calculating the rate of increase (measuring serum progesterone levels at 4, 5, and 6 weeks' gestational age) and performing serial ultrasonography beginning 3 weeks after ovulation will help to establish the diagnosis of ectopic pregnancy before tubal rupture. The combination of these two techniques is particularly applicable for stable women treated in institutions with adequate facilities for ultrasound and rapid serial quantitative β-HCG assays. If a woman with or without risk factors for ectopic pregnancy develops mild symptoms consistent with an ectopic gestation and is hemodynamically stable, vaginal sonography, measurement of serum progesterone and serial HCG levels, as well as uterine curettage, if indicated, will aid in establishing the diagnosis. The use of a quantitative serum HCG assay and transvaginal sonography enables the diagnosis of ectopic gestation in hemodynamically stable women to be

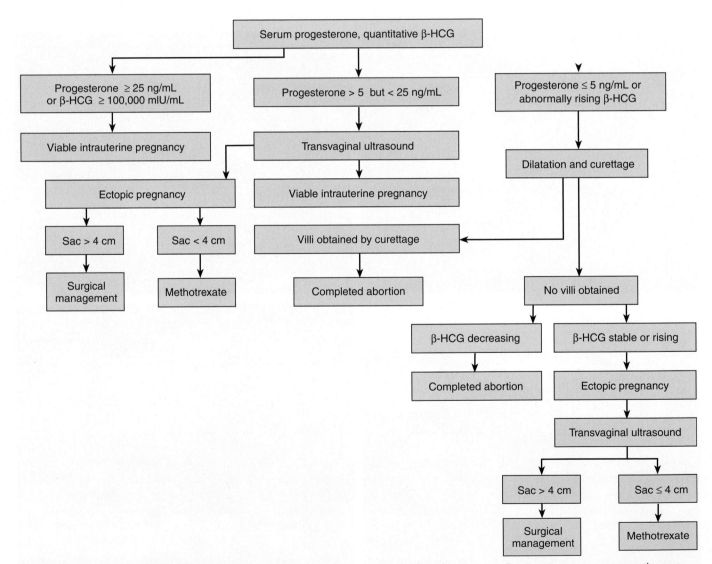

Figure 17-16 Algorithm for the diagnosis of an unruptured ectopic pregnancy without laparoscopy. Progesterone measurements increase the sensitivity of the algorithm by screening large numbers of patients inexpensively during the first trimester of pregnancy. A definitive diagnosis is made by transvaginal ultrasound or uterine curettage and does not depend on the serum progesterone concentrations obtained during screening. β-HCG, β-human chorionic gonadotropin. (From Buster JE, Carson SA: Ectopic pregnancy: New advances in diagnosis and treatment. Curr Opin Obstet Gynecol 7:168, 1995.)

made with a sensitivity of 97% to 100% and a specificity of 95% to 99% (**Fig. 17-17**).

Both suggested algorithms include the use of D&C. Although, as stated previously, this approach has been deemed to be cost effective, some women, particularly those who have been attempting pregnancy, are reluctant to have this treatment. In this setting it is reasonable to continue serial HCG and ultrasound monitoring. Unless HCG falls, it will be clear that with time, treatment of a nonviable pregnancy is needed. And this could be with either a D&C or use of methotrexate.

If a woman develops symptoms of a ruptured ectopic pregnancy that are of sufficient hemodynamic severity to require emergency care, a sensitive qualitative pregnancy test and vaginal sonography are usually all the diagnostic aids necessary to establish the diagnosis. If vaginal sonography is not immediately available, culdocentesis may be performed. If HCG is present and

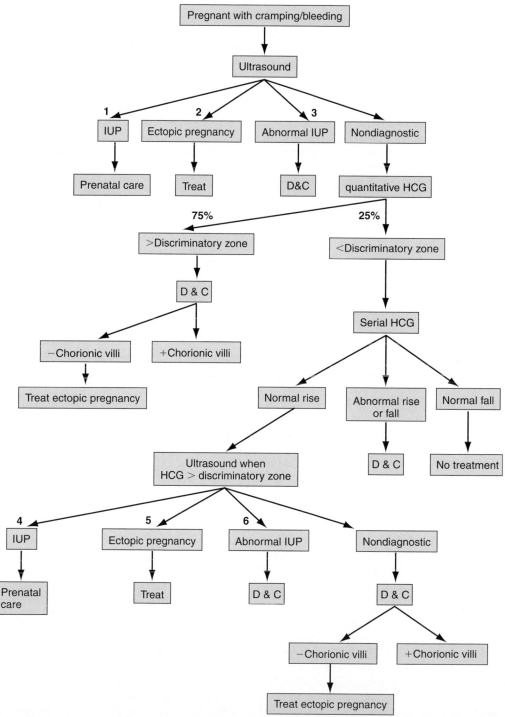

Figure 17-17 Sample schematic of strategy 1. Numbers refer to probabilities. D&C, dilatation and curettage; IUP, intrauterine pregnancy. (From Gracia C, Barnhart KT: Diagnosing ectopic pregnancy. Obstet Gynecol 97:465, 2001.)

peritoneal fluid is seen sonographically, it is most likely that an ectopic pregnancy is present, and laparoscopy should be performed.

MANAGEMENT

SURGICAL THERAPY

Laparoscopy is the procedure of choice for ruptured ectopic pregnancy as well as for cases when medical therapy (methotrexate) is contraindicated or refused. Laparoscopy is also useful at times when an accurate diagnosis cannot be made. Older studies have suggested that there is a false-positive and false-negative rate of approximately 2% with the use of laparoscopy for ectopics (i.e., either not being able to see the ectopic or confusing findings with hematosalpinx and other findings).

An **interstitial pregnancy** in the cornual area of the uterus can be treated laparoscopically; but it may require laparotomy with resection. A deep cornual resection is not deemed necessary and surprisingly does not decrease the risk of recurrent ectopic pregnancy. Subsequent intrauterine pregnancies should be delivered by C-section.

Rare ovarian pregnancies can be treated by laparoscopic surgical excision. With a routine tubal ectopic pregnancy, an oophorectomy should not be carried out, which had been advocated in the past. It does not improve the subsequent pregnancy rate or lower the risk of recurrence.

Conservative treatment (not performing a salpingectomy) for an unruptured ectopic pregnancy is considered to be the method of choice for women who desire future fertility. Although randomized trials have compared future fertility or the incidence of ectopic or intrauterine pregnancies after salpingostomy or salpingectomy, observational studies suggested that when conservative surgery is correctly performed, the repeat ectopic pregnancy rate is not increased compared with that occurring after salpingectomy, and the subsequent live birth rate is increased. In the large review by Yao and Tulandi of women with an ectopic pregnancy attempting to conceive after salpingostomy, 60% had an IUP and 15% an ectopic pregnancy. After salpingectomy, 38% had an IUP and 10% an ectopic pregnancy. Therefore, for hemodynamically stable women who wish to preserve fertility and have an unruptured tubal pregnancy, laparoscopic salpingostomy should be performed. The conservative surgical techniques used include **salpingotomy** (in which the tubal incision is closed primarily but is unnecessary and has worse subsequent pregnancy rates [discussed later]), salpingostomy (in which the tubal incision is allowed to close by secondary intention), fimbrial evacuation, and partial salpingectomy, also called segmental resection of the portion of the tube containing the ectopic pregnancy. Fimbrial evacuation usually traumatizes the endosalpinx and is associated with a high rate of recurrent ectopic pregnancy (24%), about twice as high as the rate after salpingectomy. In addition, this procedure may not remove the entire tubal gestation, and another procedure may be required a few days later. The best results of conservative management occur after salpingostomy (**Fig. 17-18**). Tulandi and Guralnick reported that the 2-year cumulative rates of IUP after salpingotomy and salpingostomy were similar, about 45%, but the 1-year rates were twice as great when salpingostomy was performed (45% versus 21%), indicating that there is a more rapid return of normal tubal function when the incision heals by secondary intention than when it is sutured (**Fig. 17-19**).

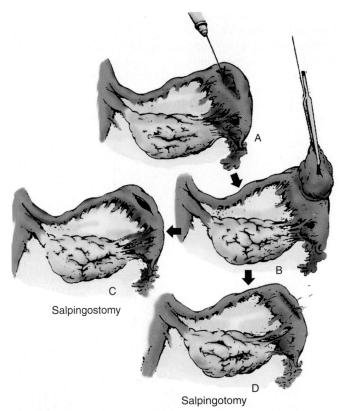

Salpingostomy

Salpingotomy

Figure 17-18 A, Incision is made into the antimesenteric border of the fallopian tube. **B,** Ectopic pregnancy is gently removed from within the fallopian tube. **C,** Salpingostomy site is allowed to heal by secondary intention. **D,** Salpingotomy is completed by primary closure. (From Leach RE, Ory SJ: Modern management of ectopic pregnancy. J Reprod Med 34:325, 1989.)

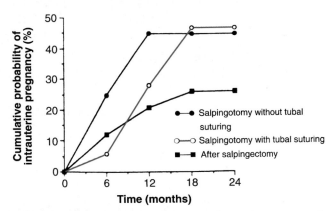

Figure 17-19 Cumulative probability of intrauterine pregnancy after conservative surgical treatment of tubal ectopic pregnancy by salpingotomy without tubal suturing, salpingotomy with tubal suturing, and after salpingectomy. (Reprinted from Tulandi T, Guralnick M: Treatment of tubal ectopic pregnancy by salpingotomy with or without tubal suturing and salpingectomy. Fertil Steril 55:53, 1991. Copyright 1991, with permission from The American Society for Reproductive Medicine.)

These techniques can be used to treat the majority of unruptured tubal pregnancies. When the unruptured pregnancy is small (<5 cm), it is preferable to perform the salpingostomy with a laparoscopic procedure, using delicate technique under the principals of microsurgery. A prospective trial has been carried out comparing laparoscopy or laparotomy for the treatment of unruptured ectopic gestation by linear salpingostomy. It was found both techniques are safe and effective, but the estimated blood loss, length of hospital stay, and cost were all significantly less in the group treated by laparoscopy and recovery was faster. However, the risk of **persistent ectopic pregnancy** (PEP) in several series has been found to be significantly greater if the salpingostomy is performed laparoscopically (a rate as high as 15 to 16%) rather than by laparotomy.

If a salpingostomy cannot be performed, an option short of salpingectomy is a segmental resection. This option is rarely used but may be considered if the opposite tube is absent or blocked, allowing for future tuboplasty if IVF-ET is not an option.

PERSISTENT ECTOPIC PREGNANCY (PEP)

With increasing use of conservative surgical treatment instead of salpingectomy for the treatment of ectopic pregnancy, the entity of PEP is becoming more common. The overall mean incidence of PEP after linear salpingostomy is about 5%, being higher when the procedure is performed laparoscopically and lower when performed by laparotomy. After fimbrial expression or tubal abortion, the incidence of persistence ranges from 12% to 15%.

PEP is uncommon when the preoperative HCG level is below 3000 mIU/mL. When preoperative HCG levels are greater than 3000 mIU/mL, the incidence of PEP has been reported to range from about 22% to 42%. If the HCG level is above 1000 mIU/mL 7 days after surgery or is more than 15% of the original level at this time, PEP is nearly always present. If the day 7 HCG level is under 1000 mIU/mL or less than 15% of the initial value, PEP is very unlikely. Vermesh and associates measured both HCG and progesterone levels preoperatively and every 3 days after conservative tubal surgery for an unruptured ectopic gestation in a group of 114 women. Of this group, 6 (5.3%) had PEP. All six had an initial sharp drop in HCG levels to 25% of the pretreatment levels 6 days after surgery, similar to the remainder of the group who did not have PEP. After 6 days, titers of the former group plateaued or rose slightly (**Fig. 17-20**). Progesterone levels showed the same type of pattern (**Fig. 17-21**).

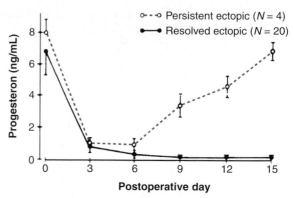

Figure 17-21 Serum progesterone patterns in persistent and resolved ectopic gestations after conservative surgery. (Reprinted from Vermesh M, Silva PD, Rosen GF, et al: Persistent tubal ectopic gestation: Patterns of circulating beta-human chorionic gonadotropin and progesterone, and management options. Fertil Steril 50:584, 1988. Copyright 1988, with permission from The American Society for Reproductive Medicine.)

Based on these data, PEP is presumed to be present if a day 9 serum HCG level is more than 10% of the initial level or a day 9 serum progesterone level is higher than 1.5 ng/mL. It is now recommended that after linear salpingostomy either HCG or progesterone levels be measured initially on day 6 postoperatively and at 3-day intervals thereafter. Increasing levels of either of these hormones beyond day 6 or a day 6 level of HCG more than 1000 mIU/mL or more than 15% of the original value are all indicators of persistent ectopic gestation. Because tubal rupture is likely to occur with PEP, it is best to treat the entity before this emergency situation occurs.

Methods used to treat PEP include salpingectomy, salpingostomy, methotrexate, or expectant management. Expectant management is usually reserved for the asymptomatic woman whose HCG titers plateau but do not rise. Surgical management should be utilized for those women who develop symptoms of persistent lower abdominal pain. The remaining women with PEP are best treated with methotrexate. A single dose of 50 mg/m^2 of methotrexate is usually sufficient to cause resolution of PEP. Graczykowski and Mishell performed a randomized trial in which a single dose of methotrexate or placebo was given within 24 hours after salpingostomy. The use of methotrexate reduced the risk of developing PEP by nearly 90%. The prophylactic use of a single dose of methotrexate may be considered in women with larger ectopics, higher initial levels of HCG, or when the surgery had been difficult.

Medical Treatment

Methotrexate (MTX) has become established as a reasonable primary treatment for ectopic pregnancy and is comparable with surgical therapy in observational studies. For medical and surgical therapy, rates of tubal pregnancy (62% to 90%) and recurrence rates (8% to 15%) are comparable.

MTX should be used in asymptomatic women who qualify for such treatment (see **Fig. 17-16**) and who have no contraindications (**Table 17-4**). Prior to treatment, several tests should be obtained, including a CBC, liver function test, BUN, and creatinine, blood type, and Rh.

There are two main protocols for MTX: single-dose and multidose regimens (see **Tables 17-5** and **17-6**). There is also an

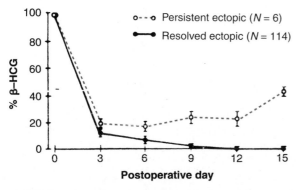

Figure 17-20 Serum β-human chorionic gonadotropin (β-HCG) patterns in persistent and resolved ectopic gestations after conservative surgery. (Reprinted from Vermesh M, Silva PD, Rosen GF, et al: Persistent tubal ectopic gestation: Patterns of circulating beta-human chorionic gonadotropin and progesterone, and management options. Fertil Steril 50:584, 1988. Copyright 1988, with permission from The American Society for Reproductive Medicine.)

Table 17-4 Contraindications to Medical Management of Ectopic Pregnancy with Systemic Methotrexate*

Contraindication	ACOG	ASRM
Absolute contraindications	Breast-feeding; laboratory evidence of immunodeficiency; preexisting blood dyscrasias (bone marrow hypoplasia, leukopenia, thrombocytopenia, or clinically significant anemia); known sensitivity to methotrexate; active pulmonary disease; peptic ulcer disease; hepatic, renal, or hematologic dysfunction; alcoholism; alcoholic or other chronic liver disease	Breast-feeding: evidence of immunodeficiency; moderate-to-severe anemia, leukopenia, or thrombocytopenia; sensitivity to methotremate; active pulmonary or peptic ulcer disease; clinically important hepatic or renal dysfunction; intrauterine pregnancy
Relative contraindications	Ectopic mass >3.5 cm; embryonic cardiac motion	Ectopic mass >4 cm detected by transvaginal ultrasonography; embryonic cardiac activity detected by transvaginal ultrasonography; patient declines blood transfusion; patient is not able to participate in follow-up; high initial HCG level (>5000 mIU/mL)
Choice of regimen based on HCG level	Multidose regimen of methotrexate may be appropriate if presenting HCG value > 5000 mIU/mL	Single-dose regimen of methotrexate better in patients with a low initial HCG level

*ACOG denotes American College of Obstetricians and Gynecologists, and ASRM American Society for Reproductive Medicine.
Data from American Society for Reproductive Medicine. The Practice Committee: Medical treatment of ectopic pregnancy, Fertil Steril 90:S206, 2008.

Table 17-5 Multiple-Dose MTX Treatment Protocol (28,29)

Treatment Day	Laboratory Evaluation	Intervention
Pretreatment	HCG, CBC with differential, liver function tests, creatinine, blood type and antibody screen	Rule out spontaneous Ab Rhogam if Rh negative
1	HCG	MTX 1.0 mg/kg IM
2		LEU 0.1 mg/kg IM
3	HCG	MTX 1.0 mg/kg IM if <15% decline day 1–day 3 If >15%, stop treatment and start surveillance
4		LEU 0.1 mg/kg IM
5	HCG	MTX 1.0 mg/kg IM if <15% decline day 3–day 5 If >15%, stop treatment and start surveillance
6		LEU 0.1 mg/kg IM
7	HCG	MTX 1.0 mg/kg IM if <15% decline day 5–day 7 If >15%, stop treatment and start surveillance
8		LEU 0.1 mg/kg IM

Note: Surveillance every 7 days (until HCG <5 mIU/mL).
Screening laboratory studies should be repeated 1 week after the last dose of MTX.
LEU = leucovorin; IM = intramuscularly.
American Society for Reproductive Medicine Practice Committee. Treatment of ectopic pregnancy, Fertil Steril, 90:S206, 2008.

Table 17-6 Single-Dose MTX Treatment Protocol (33)

Treatment Day	Laboratory Evaluation	Intervention
Pretreatment	HCG, CBC with differential, liver function tests, creatinine, blood type and antibody screen	Rule out spontaneous Ab Rhogam if Rh negative
1	HCG	MTX 50 mg/m² IM
4	HCG	
7	HCG	MTX 50 mg/m² IM if β-HCG decreased <15% between day 4 and day 7

Note: Surveillance every 7 days (until HCG <5 mIU/mL).
ASRM Practice Committee. Treatmens of ectopic pregnancy. Fertil Steril 2008.
Adapted from American Society for Reproductive Medicine Practice Committee: Treatment of ectopic pregnancy, Fertil Steril, 90:S208, 2008.

Table 17-7 Treatment and Side Effects Associated with MTX (25-27, 35, 42-44)

Treatment effects
  Increase in abdominal girth
  Increase in HCG during initial therapy
  Vaginal bleeding or spotting
  Abdominal pain

Drug side effects
  Gastric distress, nausea, and vomiting
  Stomatitis
  Dizziness
  Severe neutropenia (rare)
  Reversible alopecia (rare)
  Pneumonitis (rare)

ASRM Practice Committee. Treatmens of ectopic pregnancy. Fertil Steril 2008.
Adapted from American Society for Reproductive Medicine Practice Committee. Treatment of ectopic pregnancy, Fertil Steril, 90:S208, 2008.

intermediate two-dose regimen, which will be discussed later. The multidose regimen is more successful but involves more dosing, and therefore potentially has more side effects. It also includes the use of leukovorin (folinic acid), an antagonist to MTX, to reduce the risk of side effects. As shown in **Table 17-6**, the "multidose regimen" can be stopped if there is an appropriate decrease in HCG with treatment. The complications of MTX are listed in **Table 17-7**. In all regimens, the reduction in HCG is key to success, but complete resolution of HCG usually takes 2 to 3 weeks and can linger for up to 8 weeks after treatment.

Meta-analyses have confirmed the overall success of MTX to be 78% to 96%. The single-dose regimen has been reported to have a success of 88.1% (86 to 90) and the multiple-dose regimen was significantly more successful: 92 to 79 (89% to 96%). It is clear that there is a high failure rate with the single-dose

Table 17-8 Predictors of MTX Treatment Failure (38-41, 45)

Adnexal fetal cardiac activity
Size and volume of the gestational mass (>4 cm)
High initial HCG concentration (>5,000 mIU/mL)
Presence of free peritoneal blood
Rapidly increasing HCG concentrations (>50%/48 hours) before MTX
Continued rapid rise in HCG concentrations during MTX

ASRM Practice Committee. Treatmens of ectopic pregnancy. Fertil Steril 2008. Adapted from American Society for Reproductive Medicine Practice Committee: Treatment of ectopic pregnancy, Fertil Steril, 90:S209, 2008.

regimen, and this is clearly related to the viability of the ectopic, based on its size and level of HCG (**Table 17-8**). Seeing a yoke sac in the adnexa and a level of HCG >5000 mIU/mL affords a poorer prognosis of MTX single-dose therapy.

Figure 17-22 provides the correlation of failure rates with high levels of HCG. **Table 17-8** lists the predictions of failed responses. A two-dose regimen has been proposed as well, which is intermediate between the high and multiple-dose regiments. MTX (50 mg/m^2) is administered on days 1 and 4 without leukovorin. This regimen may be considered for patients who have HCG levels above 5000 mIU/mL.

About 85% of patients treated with methotrexate have a transient rise in HCG level between 1 and 4 days after treatment. Between 4 and 7 days after methotrexate is administered, the HCG levels should fall at least 15%. If this amount of decrease does not occur or there is less than a 15% decrease in HCG levels in each subsequent week, an additional dose of methotrexate should be given for a maximum of three doses. If after three doses of methotrexate HCG levels do not decline by 15% weekly, a surgical procedure should be performed. Serum progesterone levels fall more rapidly than HCG levels after methotrexate, and a progesterone level of less than 1.5 ng/mL has been found to be an excellent predictor of resolution of the ectopic pregnancy. Between 3 and 7 days after initiating therapy, severe pelvic pain lasting up to 12 hours frequently occurs. This symptom, probably caused by tubal abortion, needs to be differentiated from the symptoms of tubal rupture. Serial monitoring of vital signs and measurement of hematocrit levels are helpful. If the woman remains hemodynamically stable and the pain disappears, a tubal abortion has probably taken place and no further therapy is necessary.

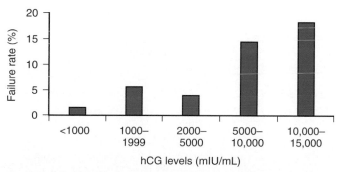

Figure 17-22 Single-dose MTX treatment failure based on HCG level. (American Society for Reproductive Medicine Practice Committee: Treatment of ectopic pregnancy, Fertil Steril, 90:S209, 2008.)

There have been two randomized trials comparing the results of systemic methotrexate with laparoscopic salpingostomy for the treatment of unruptured ectopic pregnancy. In a Dutch study, a similar degree of success was achieved with each treatment methodology. In the group treated medically, 14% required surgical intervention; in the group treated surgically, 20% required methotrexate treatment for persistent ectopic pregnancy.

In another study by Saraj and associates, 2 of 38 women treated with methotrexate required subsequent surgery, and 3 of 37 treated by salpingostomy required medical treatment for persistent ectopic pregnancy. Resolution following salpingostomy was more rapid than after methotrexate. The mean time to disappearance occurred about 20 days after salpingostomy and 27 days after methotrexate.

Observational data also support similar rates of tubal patency (62% to 90%) and recurrence rates of ectopic (8% to 15%) after medical and surgical therapy.

To avoid the toxicity of systemic methotrexate administration, a smaller dose of the drug has been administered directly into the tube with either laparoscopic or ultrasound visualization. In a summary of 11 series involving 295 women treated with tubal injection of methotrexate, 83% had successful resolution of the ectopic pregnancy, and subsequent tubal patency rates were 88% and fertility rates were 82%.

Because of the lower success rate and need for direct needle placement with local injection, most clinicians are now using systemic methotrexate. There have also been several reports of direct intratubal injection of other substances, including potassium chloride, hypertonic glucose, and prostaglandins, but use of these agents is generally less successful than the use of methotrexate.

Expectant Management

Although this is not a preferred plan of management, it is useful to know that certain ectopics may resolve without treatment. An overall success rate of 69% has been reported for expectant management. The lower the initial HCG level, the greater the success with spontaneous resolution.

Trio and coworkers, using multivariate analysis, reported that an initial HCG titer of less than 1000 mIU/mL and a decrease in HCG levels between the initial serum sample and one obtained a few days later were each independent predictors of successful spontaneous resolution, whereas sonographic visualization of an ectopic gestational sac was not an independent predictor of failure. In their series of 49 women managed expectantly, 88% of those with an initial HCG level of less than 1000 mIU/mL had successful resolution.

Korhonen and associates measured serial HCG levels before and during outpatient expectant management in a group of 118 women with ectopic pregnancies. This group comprised one fourth of all the women with the diagnosis of ectopic pregnancy seen at their institution during 3 years. When spontaneous resolution occurred, HCG levels declined to undetectable levels in 4 to 67 days, with a mean of 20 days. A distinct difference in the rate of decline of HCG levels in those who did and did not require surgery was not observed until 7 days after the initial examination (**Fig. 17-23**). If HCG levels had not fallen more than two thirds of the initial level in 7 days, two thirds of this group of women needed surgical treatment for rising HCG levels, clinical symptoms, or sonographic findings of

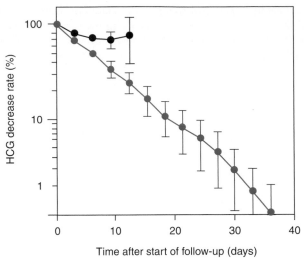

Figure 17-23 Mean value and 95% confidence limits for ratio of serum human chorionic gonadotropin (HCG) concentrations to starting value during expectant management in patients with a spontaneous resolution *(blue circles)* and in those later treated by laparoscopy *(black circles)*. The two groups diverged at 7 days. (Reprinted from Korhonen J, Stenman UH, Ylöstalo P: Serum human chorionic gonadotropin dynamics during spontaneous resolution of ectopic pregnancy. Fertil Steril 61:632, 1994. Copyright 1994, with permission from The American Society for Reproductive Medicine.)

intraperitoneal bleeding. It has been reported that when serial sonography is performed, some of the tubal pregnancies can increase in size and become more vascular as they resolve. Although knowledge of these facts is important, if an unruptured ectopic pregnancy is diagnosed by β-HCG and ultrasound, it is still preferable to treat with methotrexate or perform laparoscopy, depending on the clinical situation as discussed earlier.

TREATMENT OF NONTUBAL ECTOPICS

Less than 10% of ectopics do not arise exclusively from the tube. Heterotopic pregnancies (coexisting intrauterine and extrauterine pregnancies) are more common after ART (approximately 1% of pregnancies). Surgery for the extrauterine pregnancy is the only option.

Interstitial pregnancies (involving the cornua) are often large with high HCG levels and have a high associated morbidity. As discussed earlier, this is usually treated surgically, although potassium chloride injection into the embryo may be possible. Cervical pregnancy may also be injected directly if cardiac activity is witnessed. Systemic MTX and uterine artery embolization are also adjuncts for treatment.

THE DIAGNOSIS IN WOMEN WITH A HISTORY OF INFERTILITY

In women with a history of infertility, the diagnosis of ectopic pregnancy has been subjected to a risk-scoring assessment according to data by Coste (**Fig. 17-24**). In this scenario, methotrexate therapy is preferred unless the ectopic pregnancy involves a known hydrosalpinx, in which case salpingectomy should be preferred. The Cochrane database has shown that methotrexate therapy is equivalent to laparoscopic surgery; it has also been deemed more cost effective.

---

1. Calculate the score (number of points) for each risk factor:

Age (years)	Points		Smoking (cig/d)	Points		Other factors		Points	
								YES	NO
<35	0		0	0		EP history		10	0
35–39	3		1–20	2		Endometriosis		9	0
40	6		>20	4		History of infection [1]		8	0
						Clomiphene		7	0
						Tubal surgery		4	0

[1] Salpingitis history (confirmed or not), and/or positive serology for *Chlamydia trachomatis* (1/64)

2. Add the points and read the absolute risk of EP according to the number of points

0	2	4	6	8	10	12	14	16	18	20	22	24	26	28	30	32	34	36	38	40	42	44	46	48
1%	2%	2%	3%	5%	7%	11%	15%	21%	28%	37%	47%	57%	66%	74%	81%	87%	91%	93%	96%	97%	98%	99%	99%	99%

For example, a woman aged 36 years, smoking 25 cigarettes/day, with an EP history and a pregnancy induced by clomiphene would have a score of 3 + 4 + 10 + 7 = 24, for an EP risk of 57%.

Figure 17-24 Ectopic pregnancy (EP) risk scale. (From Coste J, Bouyer J, Fernandez H, Job-Spira N: Predicting the risk of extra-uterine pregnancy: Construction and validation of a French risk scale. Contacept Fertil Sex 26:643, 1998.)

PROGNOSIS FOR SUBSEQUENT FERTILITY

If a woman wishes to conceive after having an ectopic pregnancy, three possibilities exist: she may remain infertile, she may conceive and have an intrauterine gestation (with a viable birth or spontaneous abortion), or she may conceive and have an ectopic gestation. Overall the subsequent conception rate in women following all ectopic pregnancies is about 60%, with the other 40% remaining infertile. About one third of the pregnancies occurring after the initial ectopic pregnancy or another ectopic pregnancy, and one sixth are spontaneous abortions. Therefore, only about half the pregnancies are viable and only one third of all women with an ectopic pregnancy have a subsequent live birth. However, these overall figures are modified by several factors, particularly age, parity, history of infertility, evidence of contralateral tubal disease, whether the ectopic pregnancy is ruptured or intact, and use of an intrauterine device (IUD) at the time of the ectopic gestation. The subsequent fertility rate is significantly higher in parous women younger than age 30. However, if the ectopic pregnancy occurs in a woman's first pregnancy, her overall subsequent conception rate is only about 35%, being lower with a history of infertility and higher with no such history. On the other hand, women with high parity (more than three births) who develop an ectopic pregnancy have a relatively high rate, about 80%, of subsequent conception. The subsequent conception rate is lower in women who have a history of salpingitis, as well as those who have visual evidence of pathologic changes in the opposite oviduct as a result of previous salpingitis. Several studies have reported that women who were using an IUD at the time of ectopic pregnancy have normal rates of subsequent fertility and no increased risk of a subsequent ectopic pregnancy. Future fertility is significantly higher in women who have an unruptured tubal pregnancy than in those with tubal rupture, so early diagnosis is desirable. Only 65% of women with a ruptured ectopic pregnancy subsequently conceive, whereas the conception rate in women with an unruptured tubal pregnancy is approximately 82%.

In two large groups of women with unruptured ectopic pregnancy treated by conservative surgery, a high incidence of subsequent fertility (80% to 86%) and a low incidence of subsequent ectopic pregnancy (11% to 22%) have been reported.

The intrauterine pregnancy (IUP) rates were 64% to 70%. In both series, the IUP rates were highest (82% to 86%) in women with no history of infertility or gross evidence of prior salpingitis. The IUP rates were significantly lower (41% to 56%) in women with infertility. It has been shown that in women with evidence of prior tubal infection or a history of infertility, subsequent IUP rates were higher when they were treated with salpingostomy (73% to 76%) than when treated with salpingectomy (43% to 44%). Most studies in the literature indicate that the overall subsequent ectopic pregnancy rate is similar among women treated by salpingostomy or salpingectomy, and the data suggest that conservative surgery is most beneficial for women with evidence of contralateral tubal damage or a history of infertility.

When comparing salpingostomy outcomes after laparoscopy or laparotomy, the women treated by laparoscopy conceived sooner than those treated by laparotomy, and there were more ectopic pregnancies in the latter group. Overall, 68% and 71% of women in the two groups, respectively, had an IUP, and 5% and 19%, respectively, had an ectopic pregnancy.

In women with an unruptured ectopic a history of infertility (particularly resulting from tubal disease), previous salpingitis, a prior ectopic pregnancy, or the presence of only one tube were each independent factors that decreased the rate of subsequent fertility and also increased the risk of subsequent ectopic pregnancy (**Fig. 17-25**). It has been suggested therefore that if more than one of these factors were present it would be preferable to perform a salpingectomy than to perform a salpingostomy, as 80% of the recurrent ectopic pregnancies occurred in the same tube as the initial ectopic pregnancy.

The rate of repeat ectopic pregnancies after a single ectopic pregnancy ranges from 8% to 27%, with a mean of about 20%. Because the overall pregnancy rate is in the 60% to 80% range, about one of three to four conceptions after an ectopic pregnancy is a repeat ectopic pregnancy. Women with an ectopic pregnancy who become pregnant again should be monitored by ultrasound early in pregnancy. Only about one of three nulliparous women who have had an ectopic pregnancy ever conceives again (35%), and about one third of these conceptions are an ectopic pregnancy, for an overall rate of 13%. Risk factors for a repeat ectopic pregnancy were ectopic pregnancy as the first pregnancy, age younger than 25, evidence of tubal

Figure 17-25 Cumulative pregnancy rate according to the patients' history. IUP, intrauterine pregnancy.

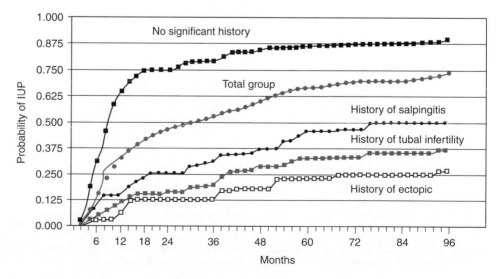

infection, and history of infertility (see **Table 17-1**). With two ectopic pregnancies, the subsequent fertility rate decreases even further. Of women who have had two consecutive ectopic pregnancies treated by salpingostomy, about half will subsequently conceive, but the majority of these will be a repeat ectopic pregnancy. There have been several reports on salpingostomy or salpingotomy in women with an unruptured tubal pregnancy in the only remaining tube. In the great majority of the subjects, the other tube had been removed because of another ectopic gestation. Of 90 women so treated in six different centers, the conception rate was 81%, with an IUP rate of 57%. About one fourth of the women who conceived had a subsequent ectopic pregnancy, which is similar to the rate among all ectopic pregnancies. Thus, conservative surgery or medical therapy may be considered when an unruptured ectopic pregnancy occurs in the only remaining tube.

KEY POINTS

- The rate of ectopic pregnancy in the United States has remained fairly constant since the early 2000s and is approximately 6.6/1000 pregnancies in women aged 15 to 24.
- The mortality rate has decreased over time and is approximately 0.5 deaths per 1000 per year.
- Risks of ectopic pregnancy include age, pelvic inflammatory disease, prior tubal surgery, smoking, and infertility.
- About 85% of women with an ectopic pregnancy have serum HCG levels lower than in normal pregnancy; the normal HCG doubling time is 1.4 to 3 days in early pregnancy. In 85% of pregnancies, there is a 66% increase every 48 hrs; a rise less than 53% in 48 hours is 99% sensitive for an abnormal pregnancy.
- An intrauterine sac should be seen in a normal pregnancy when HCG levels reach 1500 to 2500 mIU/mL. The so-called discriminatory zone is a gestational age over 38 days.
- Progesterone levels below 5 ng/mL indicate an abnormal pregnancy, and levels above 25 ng/mL indicate a normal pregnancy.
- When an unruptured ectopic pregnancy is present, the repeat ectopic pregnancy rate with salpingostomy does not increase compared with salpingectomy, whereas the subsequent live birth rate increases if the other tube is grossly abnormal or if there is a history of infertility.

- Overall, the subsequent conception rate in women with an ectopic pregnancy is about 60%. A little less than half of these pregnancies terminate in another ectopic pregnancy or spontaneous abortion; so only about one third of women with an ectopic pregnancy have a subsequent live birth.
- In women with one remaining tube, when an unruptured ectopic pregnancy is treated by salpingostomy, the conception rate is 81% with an IUP rate of 56% and a subsequent ectopic gestation rate of 24%.
- The overall risk of ectopic pregnancy after tubal sterilization failure is about 30%, reaching 50% if the sterilization technique was bilateral tubal fulguration.
- The incidence of heterotopic ectopic pregnancy is about 1% of all pregnancies and is more likely to occur after ART or in vitro fertilization.

Asymptomatic persistent ectopic pregnancy can be treated expectantly or with methotrexate (MTX). Several regimens are in use, and at least one third of women with ectopic pregnancies can be treated medically. The success of MTX depends on the size/age of the gestation and the initial HCG level. The HCG level should fall at least 15% between days 4 and 7 after the methotrexate injection (see **Fig. 17-11**) and at least 15% weekly thereafter.

REFERENCES CAN BE FOUND ON EXPERTCONSULT.com

SUGGESTED READING

Ailawad M, Lorch SA, Barnhart KT: Cost-effectiveness of presumptively medical treating women at risk for ectopic pregnancy compared with first performing a dilatation and curettage, *Fertil Steril* 83(2):376, 2005.

American Society for Reproductive Medicine, The Practice Committee: Medical treatment of ectopic pregnancy, *Fertil Steril* 90(3):S206–S212, 2008.

Barnhart K: Ectopic pregnancy, *N Engl J Med* 361 (4):379–387, 2009.

Barnhart K, Gosman G, Ashby R, et al: The medical management of ectopic pregnancy: A meta-analysis comparing "single dose" and "multidose" regimens, *Obstet Gynecol* 101(4):778, 2003.

Bixby S, Tello R, Kuligowska E: Presence of a yolk sac on transvaginal sonography is the most reliable predictor of single-dose methotrexate treatment failure in ectopic pregnancy, *J Ultrasound Med* 24(5):591–598.

Breen JL: A 21-year survey of 654 ectopic pregnancies, *Am J Obstet Gynecol* 106:1004, 1970.

Budowick M, Johnson TRB, Genadry R, et al: The histopathology of the developing tubal ectopic pregnancy, *Fertil Steril* 34:169, 1980.

Coste J, Bouyer J, Fernandez H, et al: Predicting the risk of extra-uterine pregnancy. Construction and validation of a French risk scale, *Contracept Fertil Sex* 26:643, 1998.

Fernandez H, Olivenes F, Pauthier S, et al: Ultrasound-guided injection of methotrexate versus laparoscopic salpingotomy in ectopic pregnancy, *Fertil Steril* 63:25, 1995.

Kadar N, Bohrer M, Kemmann E, et al: The discriminatory human chorionic gonadotropin zone for endovaginal sonography: A prospective, randomized study, *Fertil Steril* 61:1016, 1994.

Korhonen J, Stenman UH, Ylöstalo P: Serum human chorionic gonadotropin dynamics during spontaneous resolution of ectopic pregnancy, *Fertil Steril* 61:632, 1994.

Ledger WL, Sweeting VM, Chatterjee SP: Rapid diagnosis of early ectopic pregnancy in an emergency gynaecology service: Are measurements of progesterone, intact and free beta human chorionic gonadotrophin helpful? *Hum Reprod* 9:157, 1994.

O'Leary JL, O'Leary JA: Rudimentary horn pregnancy, *Obstet Gynecol* 22:371, 1963.

Peterson HB, for the US Collaborative Review of Sterilization Working Group: The risk of ectopic pregnancy after tubal sterilization, *N Engl J Med* 336:762, 1997.

Pouly JL, Canis M, Chapron C, et al: Multifactorial analysis of fertility after conservative laparoscopic treatment of ectopic pregnancy in a series of 223 patients, *Fertil Steril* 56:453, 1991.

Reece EA, Petrie RH, Sirmans MF, et al: Combined intrauterine and extrauterine gestations: A review, *Am J Obstet Gynecol* 146:323, 1983.

Rosman ER, Keegan DA, Krey L, et al: Ectopic pregnancy rates after in vitro fertilization: A look at the donor egg population, *Fertil Steril* 92 (5):1791–1793, 2009.

Saraj AJ, Wilcox JG, Najmabadi S, et al: Resolution of hormonal markers of ectopic gestation: A randomized trial comparing single-dose intramuscular methotrexate with salpingostomy, *Obstet Gynecol* 92:989, 1998.

Spandorfer SD, Menzin AW, Barnhart KT, et al: Efficacy of frozen-section evaluation of uterine curettings in the diagnosis of ectopic pregnancy, *Am J Obstet Gynecol* 175:603, 1996.

Stovall TG, Ling FW, Anderson RN, et al: Improved sensitivity and specificity of a single measurement of serum progesterone over serial quantitative beta-human chorionic gonadotrophin in screening for ectopic pregnancy, *Hum Reprod* 7:723, 1992.

Studdiford WE: Primary peritoneal pregnancy, *Am J Obstet Gynecol* 44:487, 1942.

Trio D, Lapinski RH, Strobelt N, et al: Prognostic factors for successful expectant management of ectopic pregnancy, *Fertil Steril* 63:469, 1995.

Tulandi T, Guralnick M: Treatment of tubal ectopic pregnancy by salpingotomy with or without tubal suturing and salpingectomy, *Fertil Steril* 55:53, 1991.

Vermesh M, Presser SC: Reproductive outcome after linear salpingostomy for ectopic gestation: A prospective 3-year follow-up, *Fertil Steril* 57:682, 1992.

Weström L, Bengtsson LPH, Mårdh PA: Incidence, trends and risks of ectopic pregnancy in a population of women, *Br Med J* 282:15, 1981.

Yao M, Tulandi T: Current status of surgical and nonsurgical management of ectopic pregnancy, *Fertil Steril* 67:421, 1997.

18

Benign Gynecologic Lesions
Vulva, Vagina, Cervix, Uterus, Oviduct, Ovary, Ultrasound Imaging of Pelvic Structures

Vern L. Katz

This book is divided primarily into chapters that deal with benign diseases and chapters that deal with malignant ones. For the clinician, however, the difference is not always clear. As in many areas of medicine, gynecologic problems do not fall into definitive categories, and those that include malignant disease often overlap with those that include benign disease. When the diagnosis from the history, physical examination, and laboratory tests is clear, management is usually self-evident. When a specific diagnosis is unclear, tissue biopsy is appropriate. This chapter deals primarily with benign lesions; however, the symptoms and differential diagnoses of these lesions have definite overlap with those of malignant disease. Thus, the clinical approach to many problems must be broad and not so focused as to prematurely exclude dangerous pathologies within the differential diagnosis, though they may be less common.

The discussions in this chapter are arranged anatomically, beginning with the vulva and subsequently covering the vagina, cervix, uterus, oviducts, and ovaries. This chapter does not attempt to be encyclopedic; rather, lesions have been selected based on their clinical importance and prevalence. Therefore, extremely rare lesions such as glomus tumors of the vulva or papillomas of the cervix have been omitted. Because several non-neoplastic abnormalities and lesions present in ways similar to those of benign tumors, this chapter also discusses entities that are not specifically abnormal growths. Clinical problems such as torsion of the ovary, lacerations of the vagina, and hematomas of the vulva are examples of common conditions included in this chapter.

The successful clinician must use both deductive and inductive reasoning in solving a problem. To have mastered both these techniques, he or she not only must be adept at history taking and physical examination but also must be able to form a complete list of possible lesions that may be involved in the patient's complaint. An understanding of the problems discussed in this chapter will be helpful in that endeavor.

The most common and least expensive of pelvic imaging techniques is diagnostic ultrasound. This topic is presented prior to the discussion of uterine abnormalities.

VULVA

URETHRAL CARUNCLE

A urethral caruncle is a small, fleshy outgrowth of the distal edge of the urethra. The tissue of the caruncle is soft, smooth, friable, and bright red and initially appears as an eversion of the urethra (Fig. 18-1). Urethral caruncles are generally small, single, and sessile, but they may be pedunculated and grow to be 1 to 2 cm in diameter. They occur most frequently in postmenopausal women and must be differentiated from urethral carcinomas. Urethral caruncles are believed to arise from an ectropion of the posterior urethral wall associated with retraction and atrophy of the postmenopausal vagina. The growth of the caruncle is secondary to chronic irritation or infection. Histologically, the caruncle is composed of transitional and stratified squamous epithelium with a loose connective tissue. Often the submucosal layer contains relatively large dilated veins. Caruncles are frequently subdivided by their histologic appearance into papillomatous, granulomatous, and angiomatous varieties. They are often secondarily infected, producing ulceration and bleeding. If the diagnosis of a urethral caruncle is entertained in a child, most likely the correct diagnosis is urethral prolapse (Fig. 18-2).

The symptoms associated with urethral caruncles are variable. Many women are asymptomatic, whereas others experience dysuria, frequency, and urgency. Sometimes the caruncle produces point tenderness after contact with undergarments or during intercourse. Ulcerative lesions usually produce spotting on contact more commonly than hematuria.

The differential diagnosis of urethral caruncles includes primary carcinoma of the urethra and prolapse of the urethral mucosa. Although urethral caruncles are not a precursor for urethral carcinoma, grossly the two are often confused. Marshall and colleagues reported a series of 394 urethral tumors. A clinical diagnosis of urethral caruncle was made in 376 of these women. Histologic examination of biopsy material demonstrated urethral carcinoma in nine patients in their series. Approximately 1 in 40 women with a clinical diagnosis of urethral caruncle has a malignant urethral neoplasm. Urethral carcinoma is primarily a disease of elderly women. The majority of urethral carcinomas are of squamous cell origin. Most of these rare carcinomas arise from the distal urethra. The symptoms of a urethral carcinoma include bleeding, urinary frequency, and dysuria, and the signs include a mass protruding from the urethra, with associated tenderness and induration of the urethra.

The diagnosis of a urethral caruncle is established by biopsy under local anesthesia. Initial therapy is oral or topical estrogen and avoidance of irritation. If the caruncle does not regress or is symptomatic, it may be destroyed by cryosurgery, laser therapy, fulguration, or operative excision. Following operative destruction, a Foley catheter should be left in place for 48 to

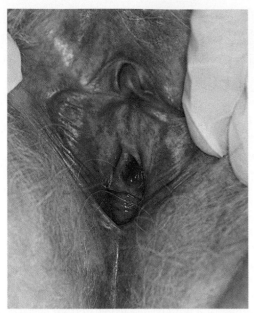

Figure 18-1 Urethral caruncle. Red popular lesion at the base of the meatus in a postmenopausal woman. (From Fisher BK, Margesson LJ: Genital Skin Disorders: Diagnosis and Treatment. St. Louis, Mosby, 1998.)

72 hours. Follow-up is necessary to ensure that the patient does not develop urethral stenosis. Often the caruncle may recur. Small, asymptomatic urethral caruncles do not need treatment.

Urethral prolapse is predominantly a disease of the premenarcheal female, although it does occur in postmenopausal women. Patients may have dysuria; however, most are asymptomatic. The annular rosette of friable, edematous, prolapsed mucosa does not have the bright red color of a caruncle and is not as circumscribed in gross configuration. It may be ulcerated

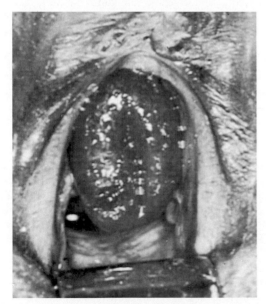

Figure 18-2 Prolapse of urethral mucosa in 7-year-old child. Edematous red collar of tissue surrounds urethral meatus. (From Kaufman RH: Solid tumors. In Kaufman RH, Faro S [eds]: Benign Diseases of the Vulva and Vagina, 4th ed. St. Louis, Mosby–Year Book, 1994.)

with necrosis or grossly edematous. Therapy of a prolapsed urethra is hot sitz baths and antibiotics to reduce inflammation and infection. Topical estrogen cream is sometimes an effective treatment. In rare cases it may be necessary to excise the redundant mucosa.

CYSTS

The most common large cyst of the vulva is a cystic dilation of an obstructed Bartholin's duct. Approximately 2% of new gynecologic patients present with an asymptomatic Bartholin's duct cyst. Treatment is not necessary in women younger than 40 unless the cyst becomes infected or enlarges enough to produce symptoms. A more complete discussion of Bartholin's duct cysts and abscesses is included in Chapter 22 (Infections of the Lower Genital Tract). Occasionally the ducts of mucous glands of the vestibule are occluded. The resulting cysts may be clear, yellow, or blue. Similar small mucous cysts occur in the periurethral region. Wolffian duct cysts or mesonephric cysts are rare, but when they do occur, they are found near the clitoris and lateral to the hymeneal ring. These cysts have thin walls and contain clear serous fluid.

Skene's duct cysts are rare, usually small, and may present with symptoms of discomfort or be found on routine examination. These cysts arise secondary to infection and scarring of the small ducts. The differential includes urethral diverticula. Clinically, physical compression of the cyst, unlike compression of a urethral diverticula, should not produce fluid from the urethral meatus. Imaging studies may also assist in establishing the diagnosis. Asymptomatic cysts in premenopausal women may be managed conservatively. Treatment is excision with careful dissection to avoid urethral injury.

The most common small vulvar cysts are epidermal inclusion cysts or sebaceous cysts. Because these cysts cannot be differentiated grossly and a continuing controversy exists with respect to their histogenesis, these two cysts are discussed together in this chapter. However, epithelial cysts are discovered much more frequently than sebaceous cysts. Epithelial cysts are located immediately beneath the epidermis. Most commonly they are discovered on the anterior half of the labia majora. These cysts are usually multiple, freely movable, round, slow growing, and nontender. They are firm to shotty in consistency, and their contents are usually under pressure. Grossly, they are white or yellow, and the contents are caseous, like a thick cheese. Local scarring of the adjacent skin sometimes occurs when rupture of the contents of the cyst produces an inflammatory reaction in the subcutaneous tissue.

An inclusion cyst may develop following trauma when an infolding of squamous epithelium has occurred beneath the epidermis in the site of an episiotomy or obstetric laceration. Most inclusion cysts of the vagina are directly related to previous trauma, whereas most inclusion cysts of the vulva are not related to trauma. Alternative theories of histogenesis include embryonic remnants and occlusion of pilosebaceous ducts of sweat glands. The histology of these cysts is characterized by an epithelial lining of keratinized, stratified squamous epithelium with a center of cellular debris that grossly resembles sebaceous material. Most vulvar epidermal cysts do not have sebaceous cells or sebaceous material identified on microscopic examination. Usually there are multiple cysts, with the majority being less than 1 cm in diameter. These cysts are asymptomatic unless they are

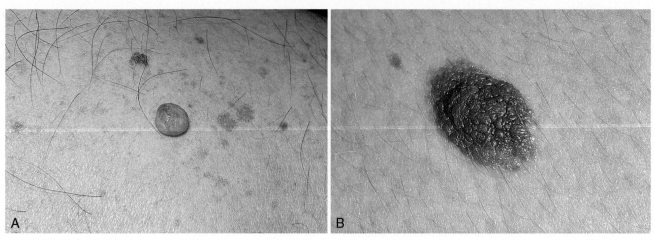

Figure 18-3 Vulvar nevi. **A,** Dome-shaped intradermal nevus. **B,** Compound nevus with irregular pigmentation. (From Fisher BK, Margesson LJ: Genital Skin Disorders: Diagnosis and Treatment. St. Louis, Mosby, 1998.)

secondarily infected. Large epidermal cysts may be confused with fibromas, lipomas, and **hidradenomas**.

Most of these cysts require no treatment. If the cyst becomes infected, treatment consists of heat applied locally and incision and drainage. Cysts that become recurrently infected or produce pain should be excised when the acute inflammation has subsided.

NEVUS

A nevus, commonly referred to as a *mole,* is a localized nest or cluster of melanocytes. These undifferentiated cells arise from the embryonic neural crest and are present from birth. Many nevi are not recognized until they become pigmented at the time of puberty. Vulvar nevi are one of the most common benign neoplasms in females. As with nevi in other parts of the body, they exhibit a wide range in depth of color, from blue to dark brown to black, and some may be amelanotic. The diameter of most nevi ranges from a few millimeters to 2 cm. Grossly, a benign nevus may be flat, elevated, or pedunculated. Other pigmented lesions in the differential diagnosis include hemangiomas, endometriosis, malignant melanoma, vulvar intraepithelial neoplasia, and seborrheic keratosis.

Vulvar nevi are generally asymptomatic. Most women do not closely inspect their vulvar skin and are unaware of biologic changes in gross appearance of these lesions. Histologically the lesions are subdivided into three major groups: junctional, compound, and intradermal nevi (**Fig. 18-3**).

Although the vulvar area contains approximately 1% of the skin surface of the body, 5% to 10% of all malignant melanomas in women arise from this region. The biologic reasons for this discrepancy are unknown. Speculation includes the hypothesis that junctional activity is common in vulvar nevi, and the many irritants to which vulvar skin is exposed may lead to malignancy. It is estimated that 50% of malignant melanomas arise from a preexisting nevus. The majority of women who develop melanomas are in their 50s. Family history of melanoma is one of the strongest risk factors for the disease.

Ideally, all vulvar nevi should be excised and examined histologically. Special emphasis should be directed toward the flat junctional nevus and the dysplastic nevus, for they have the greatest potential for malignant transformation (**Fig. 18-4**). The lifetime risk of a woman developing melanoma from a congenital junctional nevus that measures greater than 2 cm in diameter is estimated to be approximately 10%. The lifetime risk of a melanoma forming in women with dysplastic nevi is 15 times that of the general population. The dysplastic nevus is characterized by being more than 5 mm in diameter, with irregular borders and patches of variegated pigment. Removal may be accomplished with local anesthesia or coincidentally with obstetric delivery or gynecologic surgery. Proper excisional biopsy should be three-dimensional and adequate in width and depth. Approximately 5 to 10 mm of normal skin surrounding the nevus should be included, and the biopsy should include the underlying dermis as well. Some patients are reluctant to have a "normal" appearing

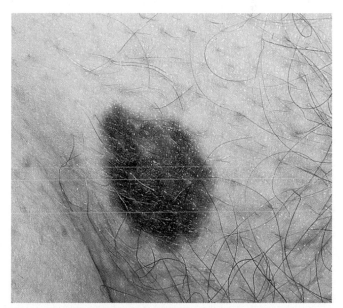

Figure 18-4 Suprapubic dysplastic nevus with an irregular shape, reddish hue to the edges, and indistinct margins. (From Fisher BK, Margesson LJ: Genital Skin Disorders: Diagnosis and Treatment. St. Louis, Mosby, 1998.)

nevus removed. Nevi that are raised or contain hair rarely undergo malignant change. However, if they are frequently irritated or bleed spontaneously, they should be removed. Recent changes in growth or color, ulceration, bleeding, pain, or the development of satellite lesions mandate biopsy. The characteristic clinical features of an early malignant melanoma may be remembered by thinking ABCD: *asymmetry, border* irregularity, *color* variegation, and a *diameter* usually greater than 6 mm.

HEMANGIOMA

Hemangiomas are rare malformations of blood vessels rather than true neoplasms. Vulvar hemangiomas frequently are discovered initially during childhood. They are usually single, 1 to 2 cm in diameter, flat, and soft, and they range in color from brown to red or purple. Histologically, the multiple channels of hemangiomas are predominantly thin-walled capillaries arranged randomly and separated by thin connective tissue septa. These tumors change in size with compression and are not encapsulated. Most hemangiomas are asymptomatic; occasionally they may become ulcerated and bleed.

There are at least five different types of vulvar hemangiomas. The strawberry and cavernous hemangiomas are congenital defects discovered in young children. The strawberry hemangioma is usually bright red to dark red, is elevated, and rarely increases in size after age 2. Approximately 60% of vulvar hemangiomas discovered during the first years of life spontaneously regress in size by the time the child goes to school. Cavernous hemangiomas are usually purple in color and vary in size, with the larger lesions extending deeply into the subcutaneous tissue. These hemangiomas initially appear during the first few months of life and may increase in size until age 2. Similar to strawberry hemangiomas, spontaneous resolution generally occurs before age 6. Senile or cherry angiomas are common small lesions that arise on the labia majora, usually in postmenopausal women. They are most often less than 3 mm in diameter, multiple, and red-brown to dark blue. Angiokeratomas are approximately twice the size of cherry angiomas, are purple or dark red, and occur in women between the ages of 30 and 50. They are noted for their rapid growth and tendency to bleed during strenuous exercise. In the differential diagnosis of an angiokeratoma is Kaposi's sarcoma and angiosarcoma. Pyogenic granulomas are an overgrowth of inflamed granulation tissue. These lesions grow under the hormonal influence of pregnancy, with similarities to lesions in the oral cavity. Pyogenic granulomas are usually approximately 1 cm in diameter and may be mistaken clinically for malignant melanomas, basal cell carcinomas, vulvar condylomas, or nevi. Treatment of pyogenic granulomas involves wide and deep excision to prevent recurrence.

The diagnosis is usually established by gross inspection of the vascular lesion. Asymptomatic hemangiomas and hemangiomas in children rarely require therapy. In adults, initial treatment of large symptomatic hemangiomas that are bleeding or infected may require subtotal resection. When the differential diagnosis is questionable, excisional biopsy should be performed. A hemangioma that is associated with troublesome bleeding may be destroyed by cryosurgery or use of an argon laser. Cryosurgical treatment usually involves a single freeze/thaw cycle repeated three times at monthly intervals. Obviously, if the histologic diagnosis is questionable, any bleeding vulvar mass should be treated by excisional biopsy so that the definitive pathologic

diagnosis can be established. Surgical removal of a large, cavernous hemangioma may be technically quite difficult. Lymphangiomas of the vulva do exist but are extremely rare.

Another rare malformation is the vulvar venous malformation. These lesions may become symptomatic at any age and are relatively prone to thrombosis. Venous malformations are different from vulvar varicosities, which are exacerbated with pregnancy and tend to regress postpartum. Marrocco-Trischitta and coworkers reported on the successful use of sclerotherapy for the malformations, after venography and Doppler ultrasound verified the diagnosis.

FIBROMA

Fibromas are the most common benign solid tumors of the vulva. They are more frequent than lipomas, the other common benign tumors of mesenchymal origin. Fibromas occur in all age groups and most commonly are found in the labia majora (**Fig. 18-5**). However, they actually arise from deeper connective tissue. Thus, they should be considered as dermatofibromas. They grow slowly and vary from a few centimeters to one gigantic vulvar fibroma reported to weigh more than 250 pounds. The majority are between 1 and 10 cm in diameter. The smaller fibromas are discovered as subcutaneous nodules. As they increase in size and weight, they become pedunculated. Smaller fibromas are firm; however, larger tumors often become cystic after undergoing myxomatous degeneration. Sometimes the vulvar skin over a fibroma is compromised by pressure and ulcerates.

Fibromas have a smooth surface and a distinct contour. On cut surface the tissue is gray-white. Fat or muscle cells microscopically may be associated with the interlacing fibroblasts. Fibromas have a low-grade potential for becoming malignant. Smaller fibromas are asymptomatic; larger ones may produce chronic pressure symptoms or acute pain when they degenerate. Treatment is operative removal if the fibromas are symptomatic or continue to grow. Occasionally they are removed for cosmetic reasons.

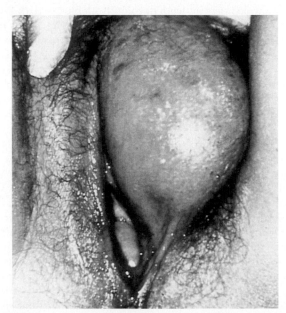

Figure 18-5 Vulvar fibroma, which is the most common benign solid tumor of the vulva. (From Friedrich EG [ed]: Vulvar Disease, 2nd ed. Philadelphia, WB Saunders, 1983.)

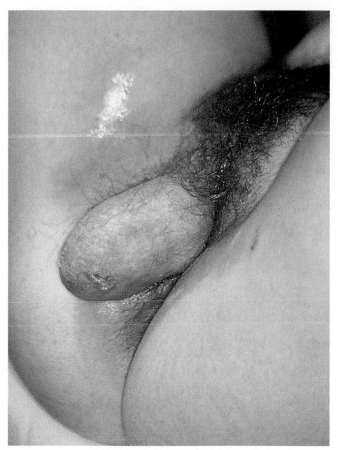

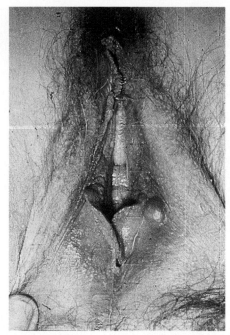

Figure 18-7 Hidradenoma. (From Shea CH, Stevens A, Dalziel KL, Robboy SJ: The vulva: Cysts, neoplasms, and related lesions. In Robboy SJ, Anderson MC, Russell P [eds]: Pathology of the Female Reproductive Tract. Edinburgh, Churchill Livingstone, 2002.)

Figure 18-6 Skin-colored pedunculated lipoma of labium major observed in a 15-year-old. (From Fisher BK, Margesson LJ: Genital Skin Disorders: Diagnosis and Treatment. St. Louis, Mosby, 1998.)

LIPOMA

Lipomas are benign, slow-growing, circumscribed tumors of fat cells arising from the subcutaneous tissue of the vulva (**Fig. 18-6**). Lipomas of the vulva are similar to lipomas of other parts of the body. When discovered they are softer and usually larger than fibromas. The majority of lipomas in the vulvar region are smaller than 3 cm in diameter. The largest vulvar lipoma reported in the literature weighed 44 pounds. Lipomas are the second most frequent benign vulvar mesenchymal tumor. Because of the fat distribution of the vulva, most lipomas are discovered in the labia majora and are superficial in location. They are slow growing, and their malignant potential is extremely low.

When a lipoma is cut, the substance is soft, yellow, and lobulated. Histologically, lipomas are usually more homogeneous than fibromas. Prominent areas of connective tissue occasionally are associated with the mature adipose cells of a true lipoma. Unless extremely large, lipomas do not produce symptoms. Excision is usually performed to establish the diagnosis, although smaller tumors may be followed conservatively.

HIDRADENOMA

The hidradenoma is a rare, small, benign vulvar tumor that originates from apocrine sweat glands of the inner surface of the labia majora and nearby perineum (**Fig. 18-7**). Occasionally, they may originate from eccrine sweat glands. For unknown reasons, they are discovered exclusively in white women between the ages of 30 and 70, most commonly in the fourth decade of life. These tumors have not been reported prior to puberty. Hidradenomas may be cystic or solid. In a review by Woodworth and colleagues 55% were cystic. Whereas 38% originated from the labia majora, 26% arose from the labia minora. Approximately 50% of hidradenomas are less than 1 cm in diameter.

These tumors are well defined and usually sessile, pinkish-gray nodules not larger than 2 cm in diameter. In most cases the surface epithelium is white, but occasionally necrosis of a central indented area occurs, with a protrusion of reddish-brown granulation tissue. These latter lesions may be confused with pyogenic granulomas.

These tumors have well-defined capsules. These papillary tumors arise deep in the dermis. Histologically, because of its hyperplastic, adenomatous pattern, a hidradenoma may be mistaken at first glance for an adenocarcinoma. On close inspection, however, although there is glandular hyperplasia with numerous tubular ducts, there is a paucity of mitotic figures and a lack of significant cellular and nuclear pleomorphism (**Fig. 18-8**). Hidradenomas are generally asymptomatic. However, they may cause **pruritus** or bleeding if the tumor undergoes necrosis. Excisional biopsy is the treatment of choice.

SYRINGOMA

The **syringoma** is a very rare, cystic, asymptomatic, benign tumor that is an adenoma of the eccrine sweat glands. It appears as small subcutaneous papules, less than 5 mm in diameter, that are either skin colored or yellow and that may coalesce to form cords of firm tissue. In the vulvar area, these asymptomatic papules are usually located in the labia majora. Identical tumors are often found in the eccrine glands of the eyelids. This tumor is usually

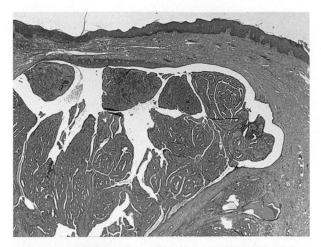

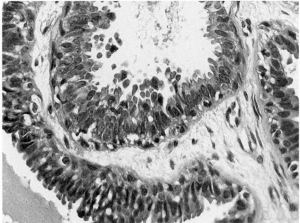

Figure 18-8 Histology, low-, and high-power micrographs of hidradenoma. (From Clement PB, Young RH: Atlas of Gynecologic Surgical Pathology. Philadelphia, WB Saunders, 2000.)

treated by excisional biopsy or cryosurgery. The most common differential diagnosis is Fox–Fordyce disease, a condition of multiple retention cysts of apocrine glands accompanied by inflammation of the skin. The latter disease often produces intense pruritus, while syringoma is generally asymptomatic. Fox–Fordyce disease is treated by oral or topical estrogens and topical retinoic acid.

ENDOMETRIOSIS

Endometriosis of the vulva is uncommon. Only 1 in 500 women with endometriosis will present with vulvar lesions. The firm, small nodule or nodules may be cystic or solid and vary from a few millimeters to several centimeters in diameter. The subcutaneous lesions are blue, red, or purple, depending on their size, activity, and closeness to the surface of the skin. The gross and microscopic pathologic picture of vulvar endometriosis is similar to endometriosis of the pelvis (see Chapter 19, Endometriosis). Vulvar adenosis may appear similar to endometriosis. The former condition occurs after laser therapy of condylomata acuminata.

Endometriosis of the vulva is usually found at the site of an old, healed obstetric laceration, episiotomy site, an area of operative removal of a Bartholin's duct cyst, or along the canal of Nuck. The pathophysiology of development of vulvar endometriosis may be secondary to metaplasia, retrograde lymphatic spread, or potential implantation of endometrial tissue during operation. Paull and Tedeschi documented 15 cases of vulvar endometriosis they believed were associated with prophylactic postpartum curettage of the uterus to prevent postpartum bleeding. In their series, there was not a single case of vulvar endometriosis in 13,800 deliveries without curettage, but 15 cases of vulvar endometriosis were associated with 2028 deliveries with prophylactic curettage. In general, symptoms do not appear for many months following implantation.

The most common symptoms of endometriosis of the vulva are pain and introital dyspareunia. The classic history is cyclic discomfort and an enlargement of the mass associated with menstrual periods. Treatment of vulvar endometriosis is by wide excision or laser vaporization depending on the size of the mass. Recurrences are common following inadequate operative removal of all the involved area.

GRANULAR CELL MYOBLASTOMA

Granular cell myoblastoma is a rare, slow-growing, solid vulvar tumor. The tumor originates from neural sheath (Schwann) cells and is sometimes called a *schwannoma*. These tumors are found in connective tissues throughout the body, most commonly in the tongue, and occur in any age group. Approximately 7% of solitary granular cell myoblastomas are found in the subcutaneous tissue of the vulva. Twenty percent of multiple granular cell myoblastomas are located in the vulva. The tumors are usually located in the labia majora but occasionally involve the clitoris.

These tumors are subcutaneous nodules, usually 1 to 5 cm in diameter. They are benign but characteristically infiltrate the surrounding local tissue. The tumors are slow growing, but as they grow, they may cause ulcerations in the skin. The overlying skin often has hyperplastic changes that may look similar to invasive squamous cell carcinoma. Grossly, these tumors are not encapsulated. The cut surface of the tumor is yellow. Histologically, there are irregularly arranged bundles of large, round cells with indistinct borders and pink-staining cytoplasm. Initially the cell of origin was believed to be striated muscle; however, electron microscopic studies have demonstrated that this tumor is from cells of the neural sheath.

The tumor nodules are painless. Treatment involves wide excision to remove the filamentous projections into the surrounding tissue. If the initial excisional biopsy is not adequate and aggressive enough, these benign tumors tend to recur. Recurrence occurs in approximately one in five of these vulvar tumors. The appropriate therapy is a second operation with wider margins, as these tumors are not radiosensitive.

VON RECKLINGHAUSEN'S DISEASE

The vulva is sometimes involved with the benign neural sheath tumors of von Recklinghausen's disease (generalized neurofibromatous and café-au-lait spots). The vulvar lesions of this disease are fleshy, brownish red, polypoid tumors. Approximately 18% of women with von Recklinghausen's disease have vulvar involvement. Excision is the treatment of choice for symptomatic tumors.

OTHER ABNORMAL TISSUES PRESENTING AS VULVAR MASSES

The differential diagnosis of vulvar masses includes a large array of rare lesions and aberrant tissues, including **leiomyomas**, squamous papillomas, sebaceous adenomas, **dermoids**, accessory breast tissue and Müllerian or Wolffian duct remnants, epidermal inclusion cysts, sebaceous cysts, mucous cysts, and skin diseases such as seborrheic keratosis, condylomata acuminata, and molluscum contagiosum. Some of these diseases are discussed in this chapter, others in Chapter 22.

HEMATOMAS

Hematomas of the vulva are usually secondary to blunt trauma such as a straddle injury from a fall, an automobile accident, or a physical assault. Traumatic injuries producing vulvar hematomas have been reported secondary to a wide range of recreational activities, including bicycle, motorcycle, and gocart riding; sledding; water skiing; cross-country skiing; and amusement park rides (**Fig. 18-9**). Spontaneous hematomas are rare and usually occur from rupture of a varicose vein during pregnancy or the postpartum period.

The management of nonobstetric vulvar hematomas is usually conservative unless the hematoma is greater than 10 cm in diameter or is rapidly expanding. The bleeding that produces a vulvar hematoma is usually venous in origin. Therefore, it may be controlled by direct pressure. Compression and application of an ice pack to the area are appropriate therapy. If the hematoma continues to expand, operative therapy is indicated in an attempt to identify and ligate the damaged vessel. Often identification of the "key responsible vein" is a futile operative procedure. However, obvious bleeding vessels are ligated, and a pack is placed to promote hemostasis. During the operation, careful inspection and, if needed, endoscopy is performed to rule out injury to the urinary bladder and rectosigmoid.

The majority of small hematomas regress with time. However, a "chronic expanding hematoma" may become particularly problematic. The most familiar clinical example of this type of problem is the chronic subdural hematoma, but a similar situation may accompany vulvar hematomas. The underlying pathophysiology is the repetitive episodes of bleeding from capillaries in the granulation tissue of the hematoma, which result in a chronic, slowly expanding vulvar mass. Treatment of a chronic expanding hematoma is drainage and débridement.

DERMATOLOGIC DISEASES

The skin of the vulva is similar to the skin over any surface of the body and is therefore susceptible to any generalized skin disease or involvement by systemic disease. The most common skin diseases involving the vulva include contact dermatitis, neurodermatitis, psoriasis, seborrheic dermatitis, cutaneous candidiasis, and lichen planus. The majority of vulvar skin problems are red, scalelike rashes, and the woman's primary complaint is of pruritus. The diagnosis and treatment of these lesions are often obscured or modified by the environment of the vulva. The combination of moisture and heat of the intertriginous areas may produce irritation; maceration; and a wet, weeping surface. Patients will commonly apply ointments and lotions, which may produce secondary irritation. Therefore, it is important that the gynecologist examine the skin of the entire body, because the patient may have more classic lesions of the dermatologic disease in another location. The skin of the vulva is susceptible to acute infections produced by *Streptococcus* or *Staphylococcus*, such as folliculitis, furunculitis, impetigo, and a special chronic infection, **hidradenitis suppurativa**.

The nonspecific symptom complex of vulvar pruritus and burning is presented next as an introduction to the discussion of dermatologic diseases of the vulva.

PRURITUS

Pruritus the single most common gynecologic problem; it is a symptom of intense itching with an associated desire to scratch and rub the affected area. Not uncommonly, secondary vulvar pain develops in association or subsequent to pruritus. In some women pruritus becomes an almost unrelenting symptom, with the development of repetitive "itch-scratch" cycles. The **itch-scratch cycle** is a complex of itching leading to scratching, producing excoriation and then healing. The healing skin itches, leading to further scratching. Pruritus is a nonspecific symptom. The differential diagnosis includes a wide range of vulvar diseases, including skin infections, sexually transmitted diseases, specific dermatosis, vulvar dystrophies, lichen sclerosus, premalignant and malignant disease, contact dermatitis, neurodermatitis, atrophy, diabetes, drug allergies, vitamin deficiencies, pediculosis, scabies, psychological causes, and systemic diseases such as leukemia and uremia.

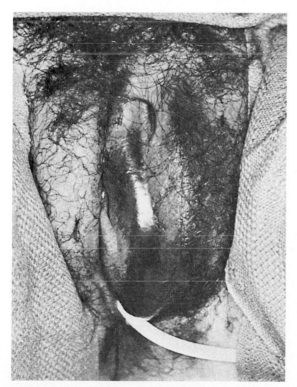

Figure 18-9 Vulva hematoma from straddle injury that produced urethral obstruction. (From Naumann RO, Droegemueller W: Unusual etiology of vulvar hematomas. Am J Obstet Gynecol 142:358, 1982.)

The management of pruritus involves establishing a diagnosis, treating the offending cause, and improving local hygiene. For successful treatment the itch-scratch cycle must be interrupted before the condition becomes chronic, resulting in **lichenification** of the skin, lichen simplex chronicus. During the latter process the skin becomes white, thickened, and "leathery." The resulting dry, scaly skin frequently cracks, forms fissures, and becomes secondarily infected, thus complicating the treatment. Chapter 30 (Neoplastic Diseases of the Vulva) discusses vulvar dystrophies.

VULVAR PAIN SYNDROMES: VULVAR VESTIBULITIS, VESTIBULODYNIA, AND DYSESTHETIC VULVODYNIA

Vulvar pain, **vulvodynia**, is one of the most common gynecologic problems. Studies have noted that up to 15% of women will develop an aspect of severe vulvar pain during their lifetimes. The disease has a wide spectrum of symptomatology. Large population based studies have noted that symptoms wax and wane, with many women having spontaneous remission. Reed et al. noted a 10% remission over a 2-year evaluation period. Interestingly, in the control group, approximately 2% of women developed symptoms.

The terminology for the syndrome of chronic vulvar pain is continually evolving. The terms *vulvar pain syndrome, vulvodynia,* and *vulvar vestibulitis* are often used interchangeably. Vulvar vestibulitis is somewhat of a misnomer, because it is not inflammation. Vulvar pain syndrome is described as the triad of severe pain to touch, localized to the vaginal vestibule and dyspareunia; pain and tenderness localized only to the vestibule; and mild to moderate erythema. Vulvar pain syndrome is further subdivided

into two categories: vestibulodynia and dysesthetic vulvodynia. The two conditions have a significant amount of overlap, although different etiologies and clinical course. In general, vestibulodynia is found in younger women, most commonly Caucasian, with onset shortly after puberty through the mid-20s. Dysesthetic vulvodynia is most common in peri- and postmenopausal women who have rarely if ever had previous vulvar pain.

The differential diagnosis of vulvar pain includes neurologic diseases, herpes simplex infection, chronic infections, abuse, pain syndromes, neoplasia, contact dermatitis, and psychogenic causes. Chronic pain is considered to be part of the vulvodynia spectrum, once the diagnoses of infection, invasive disease, and inflammation have been excluded. Severe chronic pain can be socially debilitating, and these patients have a wide spectrum of associated affective symptomatology as well. Women with vulvodynia, have greater psychologic distress than women who have other vulvar problems. Importantly, these psychologic concerns must be addressed as part of the therapeutic management.

Vestibulodynia involves the symptom of **allodynia**, which is hyperesthesia, a pain that is related to nonpainful stimuli. The pain is not present without stimulation. The diagnostic maneuver to establish the presence of allodynia is to lightly touch the vulvar vestibule with a cotton-tipped applicator. The vulvar areas most likely to be affected are from 4:00 to 8:00 along the vulvar-vaginal borders. Erythema is not always present, but when present it is confined to the vulvar vestibule (**Fig. 18-10**). Additionally, patients with vestibulodynia experience intolerance to pressure in the vulvar region. This pain is neurogenic in origin. The intolerance to pressure may be caused by tampon use, sexual activity, or tight clothing. The pain is described as raw and burning. It is not a spontaneous pain; it is invoked. However, it is severe in nature. Some authors have

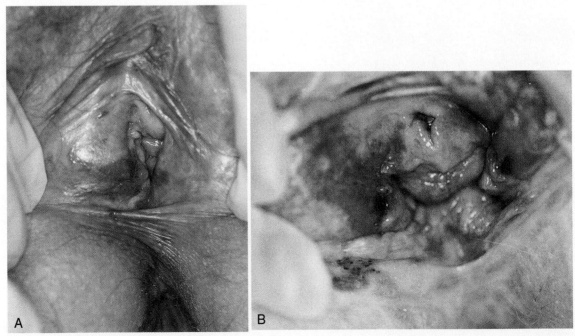

Figure 18-10 Vulvar vestibulitis. **A,** Redness localized to the right Bartholin's duct opening and, below it, vulvar vestibulitis. **B,** Discrete localized periglandular erythema in vulvar vestibulitis in a 60-year-old woman. (From Fisher BK, Margesson LJ: Genital Skin Disorders: Diagnosis and Treatment. St. Louis, Mosby, 1998.)

suggested that symptoms be present for at least 6 months prior to establishing the diagnosis. The symptoms may appear around the time of first intercourse, or within the next 5 to 15 years. Studies of women with vulvar vestibulodynia have found no increased incidence of sexual abuse compared with controls. However, many women are found to have erotophobia. Reports by Goetsch et al. note increased nerve density and normal estrogen receptors compared with controls. In contrast, other investigators have noted an increase in alpha-estrogen receptors. Theories of the etiology cite immunologic, and infectious factors, though no theory has been proved to date. Oral contraceptive use in younger women and hormone replacement in older women is not associated with incidence either.

Vulvar dysesthesia, vulvodynia, is a nonlocalized pain that is constant (not provoked by touch), mimicking a neuralgia. Allodynia is rarely noted, and erythema is also much less common than in vulvar vestibulodynia. Women with vulvodynia are more often perimenopausal or postmenopausal. Dyspareunia is currently present, but has usually not been present prior to the development of dysesthesia. Similar to women with vulvar vestibulodynia, there is *not* an increased history of sexual abuse compared with controls. Women with dysesthesia have been noted to have an increased incidence of chronic interstitial cystitis.

In general, both groups of women have an increased incidence of atopy. In some, a history of inflammation from topical agents may be elicited. These agents have usually either been self-prescribed or prescribed by a professional to treat initially what seems to be infection. Patients are often depressed and anxious, but this is thought to be a secondary reaction to the chronic pain. Edwards has presented an outline for evaluating these patients (**Table 18-1**). Prior to the diagnosis, she has suggested the exclusion of infection from atypical *Candida,* (which may not be obvious on inspection, and should be diagnosed by culture), as well as exclusion of infection by group B *Streptococcus.* Some authors have suggested that prior to extensive treatment a punch biopsy should be obtained to rule out dermatitis presenting atypically, including lichen sclerosis.

The therapeutic approach for these two conditions emphasizes a sensitivity to the debilitating social aspects of the problem. Similar to other chronic pain syndromes, tricyclic antidepressants or gabapentin have been, and found to be successful in several series. Doses of gabapentin range from 300 to 3600 mg, usually given with increasing doses every week. Most authors start at 300 mg daily, and then increase to 300 mg twice daily, then three times a day, then 600 mg t.i.d. to 900 t.i.d. and so on; the average affective dose is approximately 1800 mg a day.

Table 18-1 Evaluation of Patients with Vulvar Pain

Examination of vulva for abnormal redness, erosions, crusting, ulceration, hypopigmentation

Cotton swab test to identify areas of pain on pressure (e.g., vestibule)

Sensory neurologic examination for allodynia and symmetric sensation

Examination for vaginal redness, erosions, pallor, dryness

Biopsy of specific skin findings for evaluation by dermatopathologist

Microscopic evaluation of vaginal secretions for yeast, pH, increased white blood cells

Culture for *Candida* (exclusive of *C albicans*) and bacteria (especially group B *Streptococcus*)

Evaluation for depression and impact on quality of life

Classification of vulvar vestibulitis syndrome or dysesthetic vulvodynia

Approximately ⅔ to ¾ of women have a response to treatment with gabapentin. When the medication is discontinued, it should be tapered. Biofeedback and behavior modification therapy have also produced relief. Zoenoun and coworkers reported on 61 women treated successfully for vulvar vestibulitis with 5% lidocaine ointment nightly for a period of 6 to 8 weeks. In the past, women with refractory vulvar vestibulitis have been treated with surgical removal of the vulvar vestibule, and reapproximation of tissue. The surgery is difficult, with a significant complication rate, but results are generally good. Traas and colleagues reported on 126 women with vulvar vestibulitis. In their series, the complication rate was 39%; 89% of women felt that the surgery improved their condition enough to recommend it to other women. Importantly, 30% of women will have spontaneous relief of their symptoms without any treatment. Reports of multilevel nerve block given simultaneously for refractory cases have shown some response. Botulinium neurotoxin is also effective in some women, particularly for those with concurrent vaginismus and levator ani spasm. Series of treatments and combinations of treatments are often used.

For women with vestibulodynia unresponsive to other therapies, surgery is usually recommended. Vestibulectomy and modified vestibulectomy (partial or limited from 3 to 9:00) have shown resolution in 60% to 90% of women in multiple series. Bergerson et al. reviewed long-term results of women randomized to surgery for vestibulodynia and women treated with biofeedback and behavioral modification. At 6 months, all three therapies were effective, with surgery twice as effective as the other modalities. At two and a half years, all continued to be effective, with surgery having the greatest effects for pain. For dyspareunia, all treatments were equal. The authors, thus, recommended combination therapy when sexual issues were present. Treas et al. noted surgery to be most effective in younger women. Goetsch has advocated partial vestibulectomy, because most pain and painful skin occurs in the lower half of the vestibule. Complications from vestibulectomy include occlusion of Bartholin's gland leading to development of cysts. This problem requires surgical "unfoofing" of the duct.

CONTACT DERMATITIS

The vulvar skin, especially the intertriginous areas, is a frequent site of contact dermatitis. The vulvar skin is more reactive to exposure by irritants than other skin areas such as the extremities. Contact dermatitis may be one of two basic pathophysiologic processes: a primary irritant (nonimmunologic) or a definite allergic (immunologic) origin. Substances that are irritants produce immediate symptoms such as a stinging and burning sensation when applied to the vulvar skin. The symptoms and signs secondary to an irritant disappear within 12 hours of discontinuing the offending substance. In contrast, allergic contact dermatitis requires 36 to 48 hours to manifest its symptoms and signs. Often the signs of allergic contact, dermatitis persists for several days despite removal of the allergen. Commonly, biologic fluids such as urine and feces cause irritation of the vulvar skin. Rarely, some women will be allergic to latex or semen. The majority of chemicals that produce hypersensitivity of the vulvar skin are cosmetic or therapeutic agents, including vaginal contraceptives, lubricants, sprays, perfumes, douches, fabric dyes, fabric softeners, synthetic fibers, bleaches, soaps, chlorine, dyes in toilet tissues, and local anesthetic creams (**Fig. 18-11**).

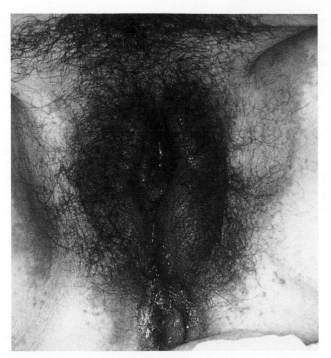

Figure 18-11 Acute contact dermatitis to chlorhexidine. Edema and erythema are present in areas where the antiseptic chlorhexidine solution was applied. (From Stevens A, Dalziel KL: Vulvar dermatoses. In Robboy SJ, Anderson MC, Russell P [eds]: Pathology of the Female Reproductive Tract. Edinburgh, Churchill Livingstone, 2002.)

External chemicals that trigger the disease process must be avoided. Some of the most severe cases of contact dermatitis involve lesions of the vulvar skin secondary to poison ivy or poison oak. Women with a history of atopy or eczema are more prone to contact dermatitis and tend to be more sensitive to skin irritations.

Acute contact dermatitis results in a red, edematous, inflamed skin. The skin may become weeping and eczematoid. The most severe skin reactions are from vesicles, and any stage may become secondarily infected. The common symptoms of contact dermatitis include superficial vulvar tenderness, burning, and pruritus. Chronic untreated contact dermatitis can evolve into a syndrome of lichenification, with the skin developing a leathery appearance and texture, *lichen simplex chronicus* (**Fig. 18-12**).

The foundation of treatment of contact dermatitis is to withdraw the offending substance. Sometimes the distribution of the vulvar erythema helps to delineate the irritant. For example, localized erythema of the introitus often results from vaginal medication, whereas generalized erythema of the vulva is secondary to an allergen in clothing. It is possible to use a vulvar chemical innocuously for many months or years before the topical vulvar "allergy" develops.

Initial treatment of severe lesions is with wet compresses of Burow's solution (diluted 1 to 20) for 30 minutes several times a day. This is followed by drying the vulva with cool air from a hair dryer. The vulvar skin should be kept clean and dry. Use of a lubricating agent such as petroleum jelly or Eucerin cream will reduce the pruritus by rehydrating the skin. Cotton undergarments that allow the vulvar skin to aerate should be worn, and

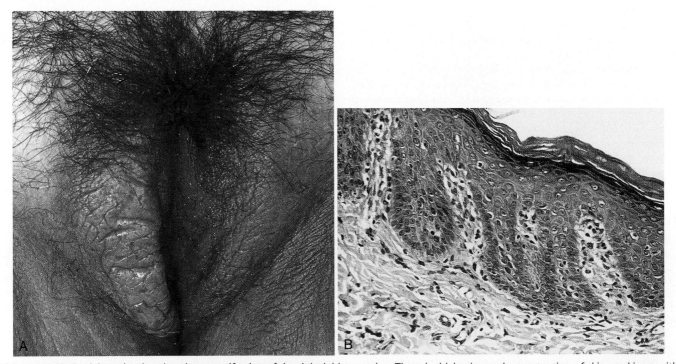

Figure 18-12 A, Lichen simplex chronicus manifesting of the right labium majus. There is thickening and accentuation of skin markings, with surface excoriation caused by recent scratching. **B,** Lichen simplex chronicus. The epidermis shows thickening of rete ridges, thickening of the granular layer, and overlying hyperkeratosis. (From Stevens A, Dalziel KL: Vulvar dermatoses. In Robboy SJ, Anderson MC, Russell P [eds]: Pathology of the Female Reproductive Tract. Edinburgh, Churchill Livingstone, 2002.)

constrictive, occlusive, or tight-fitting clothing such as pantyhose should be avoided. Vulvar dryness may be facilitated by using a nonmedicated cornstarch baby powder. Hydrocortisone (0.5% to 1%) and fluorinated corticosteroids (Valisone, 0.1%, or Synalar, 0.01%) as lotions or creams may be rubbed into the skin two to three times a day for a few days to control symptoms. Synthetic systemic corticosteroids (prednisone, starting with 50 mg/day for 7 to 10 days in a decreasing dose) are sometimes necessary for treatment of poison ivy and poison oak. Antipruritic medications, such as antihistamines, are not of great therapeutic benefit except as soporific agents. Women will often experience pruritus after steroid therapy for vulvar dermatitidis. This is not necessarily a recurrence but rather represents a type of withdrawal reaction. This rebound pruritus is seen most commonly with prolonged and higher doses of steroids. After examination, the optimal treatment is a step-down to a short course of a low-potency topical steroid such as 1% hydrocortisone.

PSORIASIS

Psoriasis is a common, generalized skin disease of unknown origin. Generally, women develop psoriasis during their teenage years, with approximately 3% of adult women being affected. Approximately 20% of these have involvement of vulvar skin. The disease is chronic and relapsing, with an extremely variable and unpredictable course marked by spontaneous remissions and exacerbations. Twenty-five percent of women have a family history of the disease. Genetic susceptibility to develop psoriasis is believed to be multifactorial. Common areas of involvement are the scalp and fingernails. When psoriasis involves the vulvar skin, it produces both anxiety and embarrassment. Similar to candidiasis, psoriasis may be the first clinical manifestation of HIV infection.

Vulvar psoriasis usually affects intertriginous areas and is manifested by red to red-yellow papules. These papules tend to enlarge, becoming well-circumscribed, dull-red plaques (**Fig. 18-13**). Though the presence of classic silver scales and bleeding on gentle scraping of the plaques may help to establish the diagnosis, the scales are less common in the vulva than on other areas of the body.

With psoriasis on the vulvar region, the number of scales is extremely variable and frequently they are absent. Under the influence of the moisture and heat of the vulva, vulvar psoriasis may resemble candidiasis. Importantly for the diagnosis, psoriasis does not involve the vagina. Sometimes dermatologists treat refractory cases of psoriasis with oral retinoids. The margins of psoriasis are more well defined than the common skin conditions in the differential diagnosis, including candidiasis, seborrheic dermatitis, and eczema. Initial treatment for mild disease is 1% hydrocortisone cream. If the patient has pain secondary to chronic fissures, more moderate disease, a 4-week course of a fluorinated corticosteroid cream should be given. If this treatment is not successful, a dermatologist should be consulted. Several newer antipsoriatic treatments may benefit this condition when it becomes moderate to severe. Systemic steroids often produce a rebound flare-up of the disease.

SEBORRHEIC DERMATITIS

Seborrheic dermatitis is a common chronic skin disease of unknown origin that classically affects the face, scalp, sternum, and the area behind the ears. Rarely, the mons pubis and vulvar

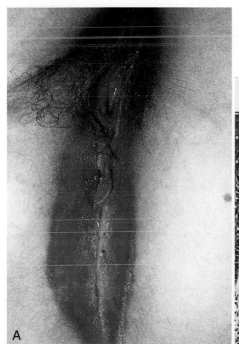 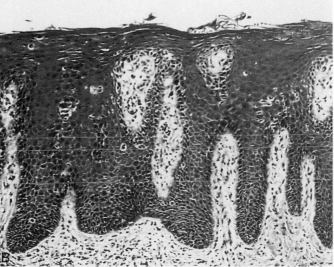

Figure 18-13 A, Psoriasis of perineum and vulva. Flexural psoriasis often lacks the typical parakeratotic scale of psoriasis on other body sites. Painful erosion of the natal cleft is common. **B,** Psoriasis. There is psoriasiform hyperplasia of rete ridges with papillary dermal edema and telangiectasia. The parakeratotic scale on the skin surface is not prominent in vulvar psoriasis. (From Stevens A, Dalziel KL: Vulvar dermatoses. In Robboy SJ, Anderson MC, Russell P [eds]: Pathology of the Female Reproductive Tract. Edinburgh, Churchill Livingstone, 2002.)

areas may be involved. Vulvar lesions are pale to yellow-red, erythematous, and edematous, and they are covered by a fine, nonadherent scale that is usually oily. Excessive sweating and emotional tension precipitate attacks. The cause of the condition is most likely a yeast, *Pityrosporum ovale*. Approximately 2% to 4% of women have some form of the disease. The pruritus associated with seborrheic dermatitis varies from mild to severe. Treatment is similar to that for contact dermatitis, with hydrocortisone cream being the most effective medication. Refractory cases sometimes respond to topical ketoconazole cream. The differential diagnosis of seborrheic dermatitis includes psoriasis, cutaneous candidiasis, and contact dermatitis. Often it is difficult to differentiate between the cutaneous manifestations of psoriasis and seborrheic dermatitis. Clinically and pragmatically, the exact diagnosis is only of academic interest because the treatment is similar.

LICHEN PLANUS

Lichen planus is an uncommon vulvovaginal dermatosis. Lichen planus is a unique, chronic eruption of shiny, violaceous papules. These tiny flat papules appear on flexor surfaces, mucous membranes, and vulvar skin in women older than 30 years of age. Most lesions are located on the inner aspects of the vulva, especially the labia minora and vestibule. Papules often develop in linear scratch marks. The lesions are intensely pruritic and usually painful. The initial onset usually follows a time of intense emotional stress. The disease presents most commonly as a

hypertrophic, coalesced plaque similar to lichen sclerosis. Lichen sclerosis, though, does not involve the vagina, whereas lichen planus can. Additionally, lichen planus may also present as a potentially severe and deforming erosive vaginitis, which is extremely painful and debilitating (**Fig. 18-14**). This ulcerative vaginitis may be mistakenly treated as atrophic vaginitis. If biopsy is necessary for diagnosis, punch biopsy is preferable.

The manifestation of symptoms include pruritus, and in the severe form, pain, burning, scarring, and eventually vaginal stenosis with loss of normal architecture. The cutaneous lesions of lichen planus tend to be self-limited. Often there is concomitant involvement of the oral mucous membranes, as well. The cause is thought to be an autoimmune phenomenon, which has been known to be initiated by certain drugs, including β-blockers, angiotensin-converting enzyme (ACE) inhibitors, and other medications. It may also arise spontaneously. Correct diagnosis is confirmed by a small punch biopsy of the vagina or vulva. Histologic findings (**Fig. 18-15**) include degeneration of the basal layers, a lymphocytic infiltrate of the dermis, as well as epidermal acanthosis.

This chronic disease tends to have spontaneous remissions and exacerbations that last for weeks to months. Treatment of local lesions is by use of a potent topical steroid cream such as clobetasol. If the patient is intensely symptomatic, oral steroids may be necessary. Dapsone for several months is sometimes effective in chronic resistant cases. Women with this condition should be monitored at periodic intervals because of an associated increased risk of developing vulvar carcinoma.

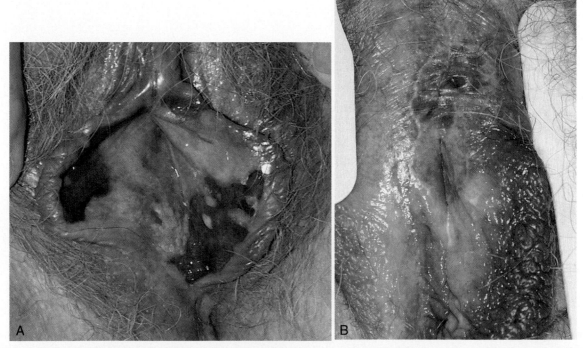

Figure 18-14 Lichen planus. **A,** Eroded ulcers in the vulva. **B,** Lacy reticulated pattern of lichen planus with periclitoral scarring in a 71-year-old woman who has had oral lichen planus for 10 to 15 years, cutaneous lichen planus of arms and legs for 18 months, and bouts of erosive vaginal lichen planus with scarring and partial vaginal stenosis. (From Fisher BK, Margesson LJ: Genital Skin Disorders: Diagnosis and Treatment. St. Louis, Mosby, 1998.)

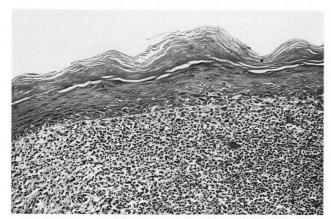

Figure 18-15 Lichen planus, histology. Note hyperkeratosis with extensive basal layer destruction and a dense lichenoid infiltrate at the dermoepidermal junction. (From Stevens A, Dalziel KL: Vulvar dermatoses. In Robboy SJ, Anderson MC, Russell P [eds]: Pathology of the Female Reproductive Tract. Edinburgh, Churchill Livingstone, 2002.)

BEHÇET SYNDROME

Behçet syndrome presents as recurrent, painful ulcers and papules on the vulva and oral mucosa, without other significant syndromes of inflammation. Women with eastern Mediterranean and Middle Eastern ancestry are the most susceptible to this autoimmune disease. The diagnosis is made after exclusion of herpetic lesions and other ulcerative diseases. The symptoms respond to topical anesthetics. Severe disease may require antineoplastic therapy including methotrexate, steroids, or other medications.

HIDRADENITIS SUPPURATIVA

Hidradenitis suppurativa is a chronic, unrelenting, refractory infection of skin and subcutaneous tissue that contains apocrine glands. The apocrine glands are found mainly in the axilla and the anogenital region. The disease is rare before puberty; 98% of cases are found in reproductive-age women, and most all disease regresses after menopause. As the infection progresses over time, deep scars and pits are formed (**Fig. 18-16**). The patient undergoes great emotional distress as this condition is both painful and is associated with a foul-smelling discharge. Current theories of the cause of this condition favor an inflammation beginning in the hair follicles (**Fig. 18-17**). Thus, the term sometimes used synonymously is acne inversa. The lesions involve the mons pubis, the genitocrural folds, and the buttocks. The differential diagnosis of hidradenitis suppurativa includes simple folliculitis, Crohn's disease of the vulva, pilonidal cysts, and granulomatous sexually transmitted diseases. The differentiation from Crohn's disease is usually made by history with an absence of gastrointestinal (GI) involvement. The early phase of the disease involves infection of the follicular epithelium, with what first appears as a boil. Erythema, involvement of multiple follicles, chronic infections that burrow and form cysts that break open and track through subcutaneous tissue creating odiferous and painful sinuses and fistula in the vulva. The chronic scarring, fibrosis, and hyperpigmentation with foul smelling discharge and soiling of underclothes leads to a socially debilitating condition. The diagnosis should be confirmed by biopsy.

With early disease during which there are small furuncles and folliculitis, topical and oral clindamycin is effective in the short term; 3-month courses of antibiotics should be given. Often, though, patients may relapse. If treatment is unsuccessful with long-term antibiotic therapy and topical steroids, other medical

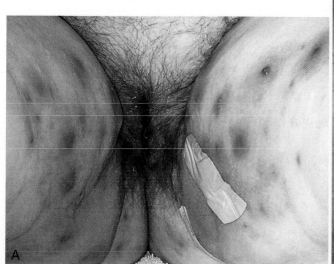

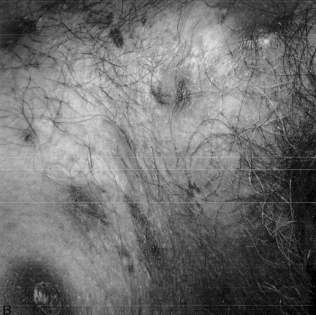

Figure 18-16 A, Multiple acneiform papules and nodules of hidradenitis suppurativa. **B,** Scars, nodules, and cysts in right inguinal area in hidradenitis suppurativa. (From Fisher BK, Margesson LJ: Genital Skin Disorders: Diagnosis and Treatment. St. Louis, Mosby, 1998.)

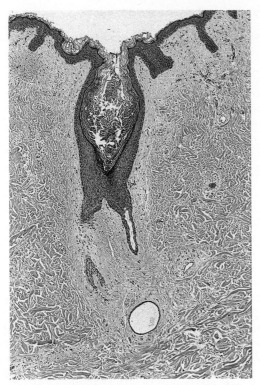

Figure 18-17 Hydradenitis suppurativa. Biopsy with follicular plugging and connection to dilated apocrine duct. (From Kelly P: Folliculitis and the follicular occlusion tetrad. In Bolognia JL, Jorizzo JL, Rapini RP [eds]: Dermatology. Edinburgh, Mosby, 2003.)

therapies have included antiandrogens, isotretinoin, and cyclosporine. The treatment of refractory cases is aggressive, wide operative excision of the infected skin.

EDEMA

Edema of the vulva may be a symptom of either local or generalized disease. Two of the most common causes of edema of the vulva are secondary reactions to inflammation or to lymphatic blockage. Vulvar edema is often recognized before edema in other areas of the female body is noted. The loose connective tissue of the vulva and its dependent position predispose to early development of pitting edema. Systemic causes of vulvar edema include circulatory and renal failure, ascites, and cirrhosis. Vulvar edema also may occur after intraperitoneal fluid is instilled to prevent adhesions or for dialysis. Local causes of vulvar edema include allergy, neurodermatitis, inflammation, trauma, and lymphatic obstruction caused by carcinoma or infection. Infectious diseases that are associated with vulvar edema include necrotizing fasciitis, tuberculosis, syphilis, filariasis, and lymphogranuloma venereum.

VAGINA

URETHRAL DIVERTICULUM

A urethral diverticulum is a permanent, epithelialized, saclike projection that arises from the posterior urethra. Often they present as a mass of the anterior vaginal wall. It is a common

Table 18-2 Location of the Ostium in 108 Female Patients with Diverticulum of the Urethra

Site	Number of Patients
Distal (external) third of the urethra	11
Middle third of the urethra	55
Proximal (inner) third of the urethra (including vesical neck)	18
Multiple sites	18
Unknown	6

From Lee RA: Diverticulum of the urethra: Clinical presentation, diagnosis, and management. Clin Obstet Gynecol 27:491, 1984.

problem, being discovered in approximately 1% to 3% of women. Blaivas and associates reported a series of 79 women referred to a urogynecology service because of periurethral masses (**Table 18-2**). Urethral diverticula accounted for 66/79 women (84%). Most urogynecologists have noted a decline in the prevalence of this condition since the early 1990s. The majority of cases are initially diagnosed in reproductive-age females, with the peak incidence in the fourth decade of life. The symptoms of a urethral diverticulum are nonspecific and are identical to the symptoms of a lower urinary tract infection. To diagnose this elusive condition, one should suspect urethral diverticulum in any woman with chronic or recurrent lower urinary tract symptoms. The urologic aspects of this condition are discussed in Chapter 21 (Urogynecology). Histologically the diverticulum is lined by epithelium; however, there is a lack of muscle in the saclike pocket.

Urethral diverticula may be congenital or acquired. Few urethral diverticula are present in children; therefore it is assumed that most diverticula are not congenital. Huffman made the analogy that anatomically the urethra is similar to a tree with many stunted branches that represent the periurethral ducts and glands. It is assumed that the majority of urethral diverticula result from repetitive or chronic infections of the periurethral glands. The suburethral infection may cause obstruction of the ducts and glands, with subsequent production of cystic enlargement and retention cysts. These cysts may rupture into the urethral lumen and produce a suburethral diverticulum. Occasionally a suburethral diverticulum has associated stone formation in the dilated retention cyst. Urethral diverticula are small, from 3 mm to 3 cm in diameter. The majority of urethral diverticula open into the midportion of the urethra (**Table 18-3**). Occasionally, multiple suburethral diverticula occur in the same woman.

Table 18-3 Final Diagnosis of Periurethral Mass and Frequency

Diagnosis	N (%)	95% Confidence Interval (%)
Urethral diverticulum	66 (84)	73, 91
Diverticulum with malignancy	4 (6)	2, 14.8
Vaginal cyst	6 (7)	3, 15
Leiomyoma	4 (5)	1, 12
Vaginal squamous cell carcinoma	2 (2.5)	0.03, 8.8
Etopic ureter	2 (2.5)	0.03, 8.8
Granuloma	1 (1)	0.03, 6.8

From Blaivas JG, Flisser AJ, Bleustein CB, Panagopoulos G: Periurethral masses: Diagnosis in a large series of women. Obstet Gynecol 103(5 Pt 1):842, 2004.

Classically, the symptoms associated with the urethral diverticulum are extremely chronic in nature and they have not resolved with multiple courses of oral antibiotic therapy. The most common symptoms associated with urethral diverticula are urinary urgency, frequency, and dysuria. Ginsburg and Genadry discovered that 90% of their patients had symptoms of chronic lower urinary tract infection as the presenting complaint. Approximately 15% of women with urethral diverticula experience hematuria. Other authors have stressed the three Ds associated with a diverticulum: *dysuria, dyspareunia,* and *dribbling* of the urine. Although for years, postvoiding dribbling has been termed a classic symptom of urethral diverticulum, it is reported by fewer than 10% of women with this condition. In Lee's series a palpable, tender mass was discovered in 56 of 108 patients. Ginsburg and Genadry found a palpable mass in 46 of 70 women with a urethral diverticulum. It is interesting that in most large series, approximately 20% of the women are asymptomatic. A classic sign of a suburethral diverticulum is the expression of purulent material from the urethra after compressing the suburethral area during a pelvic examination. Although the sign of producing a discharge by manual expression is specific, its sensitivity is poor.

The foundation of diagnosing urethral diverticulum is the physician's awareness of the possibility of this defect occurring in women with chronic symptoms of lower urinary tract infection. Subsequently, it is important to appreciate that a single diagnostic procedure may not identify the diverticulum. The two most common methods of diagnosing urethral diverticulum have been the voiding cystourethrography and cystourethroscopy. Approximately 70% of urethral diverticula will be filled by contrast material on a postvoiding radiograph with a lateral view. Cystourethroscopy will demonstrate the urethral opening of the urethral diverticulum in approximately 6 of 10 cases. Other diagnostic tests used to identify urethral diverticula include urethral pressure profile recordings, transvaginal ultrasound, computed tomography (CT) scans, magnetic resonance imaging (MRI), and positive-pressure urethrography. The latter test is done with a special double-balloon urethral catheter (Davis catheter) (**Fig. 18-18**). Classically, the recordings of the pressure profile of the urethra demonstrate a biphasic curve in a woman with a urethral diverticulum. No imaging modality has been shown to be superior to any other. If a woman has a urethral diverticulum and urinary incontinence, performing a stress urethral pressure profile will help to differentiate the etiology. The differential diagnosis includes **Gartner's duct cyst**, an ectopic ureter that empties into the urethra, and Skene's glands cysts.

Several different operations can correct urethral diverticula. Excisional surgery should be scheduled when the diverticulum is not acutely infected. Operative techniques can be divided into transurethral and transvaginal approaches, with most gynecologists preferring the transvaginal approach as described by Lee. The majority of diverticula enter into the posterior aspect of the urethra. Diverticula of the distal one third may be treated by simple marsupialization. Following operations, approximately 80% of patients obtain complete relief from symptoms. Some diverticula have multiple openings into the urethra. Complete excision of this network of fistulous connections is important. The recurrence rate varies between 10% and 20%, and many failures are due to incomplete surgical resection. The most serious consequences of surgical repair of urethral diverticula are urinary incontinence and urethrovaginal fistula. Postoperative

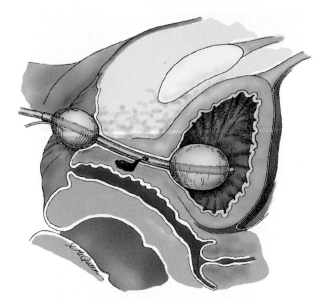

Figure 18-18 Double-balloon catheter in use for positive-pressure urethrography.

incontinence usually follows operative repairs of large diverticula that are near the bladder neck. This incontinence may be secondary to damage to the urethral sphincter. The incidence of each of these complications is approximately 1% to 2%.

INCLUSION CYSTS

Inclusion cysts are the most common cystic structures of the vagina. In Deppisch's series of 64 women with cystic masses of the vagina, 34 had inclusion cysts. The cysts are usually discovered in the posterior or lateral walls of the lower third of the vagina. Inclusion cysts vary from 1 mm to 3 cm in diameter. Deppisch reported a mean diameter of 1.6 cm. Similar to inclusion cysts of the vulva, inclusion cysts of the vagina are more common in parous women. Inclusion cysts usually result from birth trauma or gynecologic surgery. Often they are discovered in the site of a previous episiotomy or at the apex of the vagina following hysterectomy.

Histologically, inclusion cysts are lined by stratified squamous epithelium. These cysts contain a thick, pale yellow substance that is oily and formed by degenerating epithelial cells. Often these cysts are erroneously called sebaceous cysts in the misbelief that the central material is sebaceous. Similar to vulvar inclusion cysts, the cause is either a small tag of vaginal epithelium buried beneath the surface following a gynecologic or obstetric procedure or a misplaced island of embryonic remnant that was destined to form epithelium.

The majority of inclusion cysts are asymptomatic. If the cyst produces dyspareunia or pain, the treatment is excisional biopsy.

DYSONTOGENETIC CYSTS

Dysontogenetic cysts of the vagina are thin-walled, soft cysts of embryonic origin. Whether the cysts arise from the mesonephros (Gartner's duct cyst), the paramesonephricum (Müllerian cyst), or the urogenital sinus (vestibular cyst) is predominantly of academic rather than clinical importance. The cysts may be differentiated histologically by the epithelial lining (**Fig. 18-19**). Most mesonephric cysts have cuboidal, nonciliated epithelium.

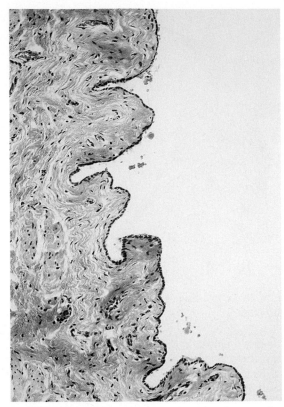

Figure 18-19 Histology of vaginal cyst. Gartner's duct cyst from the lateral vaginal wall. The cyst is lined by nonciliated cells. (From Clement PB, Young RH: Atlas of Gynecologic Surgical Pathology. Philadelphia, WB Saunders, 2000.)

Most perimesonephric cysts have columnar, endocervical-like epithelium. Occasionally pressure produced by the cystic fluid produces flattening of the epithelium, which makes histologic diagnosis less reliable. Although most commonly single, dysontogenetic cysts may be multiple. The cysts are usually 1 to 5 cm in diameter and are usually discovered in the upper half of the vagina (**Fig. 18-20**). Sometimes multiple small cysts may present like a string of large, soft beads. A large cyst presenting at the introitus may be mistaken for a cystocele, anterior enterocele, or obstructed aberrant ureter. Approximately 1 in 200 females develop these cysts.

Embryonic cysts of the vagina, especially those discovered on the anterior lateral wall, are usually Gartner's duct cysts. In the embryo the distal portion of the mesonephric duct runs parallel with the vagina. It is assumed that a segment of this embryonic structure fails to regress, and the obstructed vestigial remnant becomes cystic. These cysts are most commonly found in the lower one third of the vagina.

Most of these benign cysts are asymptomatic, sausage-shaped tumors that are discovered only incidentally during pelvic examination. Small asymptomatic Gartner's duct cysts may be followed conservatively. Deppisch, in a series of 25 women undergoing operations for symptomatic dysontogenetic cysts, reported a wide range of symptoms, including dyspareunia, vaginal pain, urinary symptoms, and a palpable mass. Sometimes large cysts interfere with the use of tampons.

Operative excision is indicated for chronic symptoms. Rarely, one of these cysts becomes infected, and if operated on during the acute phase, marsupialization of the cyst is preferred. Excision of the vaginal cyst may be a much more formidable operation than anticipated. The cystic structure may extend up into the broad ligament and anatomically be in proximity to the distal course of the ureter.

Rare tumors of the vagina include fibromas, angiomyxomas, and hemangiomas. All are usually found by the patient, and require surgical excision.

TAMPON PROBLEMS

The vaginal tampon has achieved immense popularity and ubiquitous use. It is not surprising that there are rare associated risks with tampon usage: vaginal ulcers, the "forgotten" tampon, and toxic shock syndrome. The latter, related to toxins elaborated by *Staphylococcus aureus,* is discussed in Chapter 22.

Wearing tampons for a few days has been associated with microscopic epithelial changes. The majority of women develop epithelial dehydration and epithelial layering, and some will develop microscopic ulcers. These minor changes take between 48 hours and 7 days to heal. In a study of colposcopic changes related to the tampon, Friedrich found serial changes of epithelial drying, peeling, layering, and ultimately microulceration. In his study, 15% of women wearing tampons only during the time of normal menstruation developed microulcerations. No clinical symptoms were associated with these microscopic changes. Theoretically, these microulcerations are a potential portal of entry for the HIV virus.

Barrett and colleagues were the first to describe large macroscopic ulcers of the vaginal fornix in four women who were tampon "abusers." Each of these young women wore vaginal tampons for prolonged lengths of time for persistent vaginal discharge or spotting, changing the individual tampon several times per day. The ulcers had a base of clean granulation tissue with smooth, rolled edges. Jimmerson and Becker found birefractal foreign body fragments in biopsy specimens (fibers from tampons) in the vaginal ulcers of 4 of 10 women. The pathophysiology of the ulcer is believed to be secondary to drying and pressure necrosis induced by the tampon. Obviously, many of these young women use tampons for the identical symptoms that are associated with a vaginal ulcer—that is, spotting and vaginal discharge. Often the intermenstrual spotting is believed to be breakthrough bleeding from oral contraceptives, and the possibility of a vaginal ulcer from chronic tampon usage is overlooked.

Vaginal ulcers are not uncommon secondary to several types of foreign objects, including diaphragms, pessaries, and medicated silicon rings. Management is conservative, because the ulcers heal spontaneously when the foreign object is removed. Any persistent ulcer should be biopsied to establish the cause.

A woman with a "lost" or "forgotten" tampon presents with a classic foul vaginal discharge and occasionally spotting. The tampon is usually found high in the vagina. The odor from a forgotten tampon is overwhelming. The woman should be treated with an antibiotic vaginal cream for the next 5 to 7 days.

LOCAL TRAUMA

The most frequent cause of trauma to the lower genital tract of adult females is coitus. Approximately 80% of vaginal lacerations occur secondary to sexual intercourse. Other causes of vaginal trauma are straddle injuries, penetration injuries by foreign objects, sexual assault, vaginismus, and waterskiing accidents.

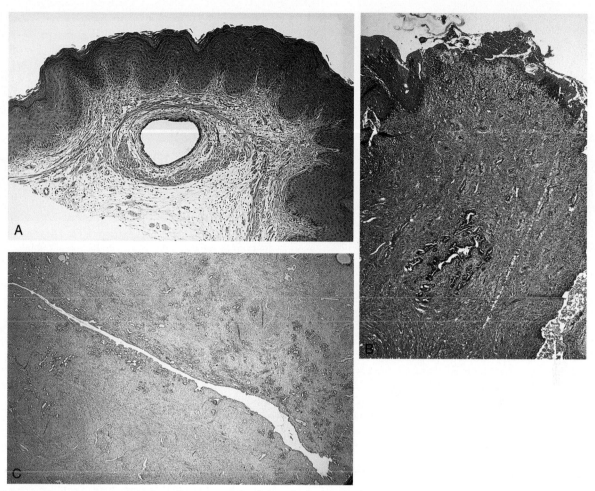

Figure 18-20 A, Normal mesonephric duct. On cross section it is a single duct in the submucosa surrounded by clusters of smooth muscle bands. **B,** Mesonephric duct. The mother duct, located deep in the wall of the vagina, is surrounded by smaller arborized offshoots. **C,** Elongated mesonephric duct. (From Robboy SJ, Anderson MC, Russell P, Morse A: The vagina. In Robboy SJ, Anderson MC, Russell P [eds]: Pathology of the Female Reproductive Tract. Edinburgh, Churchill Livingstone, 2002.)

The management of vulvar and vaginal trauma in children is discussed in Chapters 11 and 12.

The predisposing factors believed to be related to coital injury include virginity, the state of the postpartum and postmenopausal vaginal epithelium, pregnancy, intercourse after a prolonged period of abstinence, hysterectomy, and inebriation. Smith and colleagues reviewed 19 injuries from normal coitus; 12 of the women in his series were between the ages of 16 and 25 and 5 were older than 45. The most common injury is a transverse tear of the posterior fornix. Similar linear lacerations often occur in the right or left vaginal fornices. The location of the coital injury is believed to be related to the poor support of the upper vagina, which is supported only by a thin layer of connective tissue. The most prominent symptom of a coital vaginal laceration is profuse or prolonged vaginal bleeding. Many women experienced sharp pain during intercourse, and 25% noted persistent abdominal pain. The most troublesome but extremely rare complication of vaginal laceration is vaginal evisceration. Often the history of the coital injury is not obtained, and, for personal reasons, the woman may even give misleading information. However, coital injury to the vagina should be considered in any woman with profuse or prolonged abnormal vaginal bleeding. Sensitive but thorough history regarding abuse is always appropriate.

Management of coital lacerations involves prompt suturing under adequate anesthesia. Secondary injury to the urinary and gastrointestinal tracts should be ruled out.

CERVIX

ENDOCERVICAL AND CERVICAL POLYPS

Endocervical and cervical polyps are the most common benign neoplastic growths of the cervix. In an extensive series, Farrar and Nedoss reported an incidence of endocervical polyps in 4% of gynecologic patients. Endocervical polyps are most common in multiparous women in their 40s and 50s. Cervical polyps usually present as a single polyp, but multiple polyps do occur occasionally. The majority are smooth, soft, reddish purple to cherry red, and fragile. They readily bleed when touched. Endocervical polyps may be single or multiple and are a few millimeters to 4 cm in diameter. The stalk of the polyp is of variable

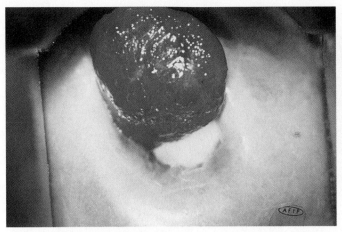

Figure 18-21 Cervical polyp. A large polyp protrudes from the external cervical os. The surface is red and rough, covered by endocervical epithelium. (From Anderson MC, Robboy SJ, Russell P, Morse A: The cervix—benign and non-neoplastic conditions. In Robboy SJ, Anderson MC, Russell P [eds]: Pathology of the Female Reproductive Tract. Edinburgh, Churchill Livingstone, 2002.)

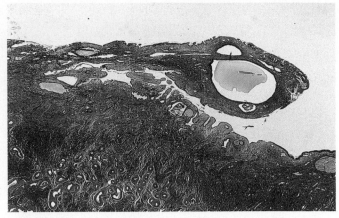

Figure 18-22 Cervical polyp. The stroma is fibromuscular and the base contains thick-walled blood vessels. Endocervical crypts, some dilated, are present within the polyp. (From Anderson MC, Robboy SJ, Russell P, Morse A: The cervix—benign and non-neoplastic conditions. In Robboy SJ, Anderson MC, Russell P [eds]: Pathology of the Female Reproductive Tract. Edinburgh, Churchill Livingstone, 2002.)

length and width (**Fig. 18-21**). Polyps may arise from either the endocervical canal (endocervical polyp) or ectocervix (cervical polyp). Endocervical polyps are more common than are cervical polyps. Often the terms *endocervical* and *cervical* polyps are used to describe the same abnormality. Polyps whose base is in the endocervix usually have a narrow, long pedicle and occur during the reproductive years, whereas polyps that arise from the ectocervix have a short, broad base and usually occur in postmenopausal women.

The hypothesis of the origin of endocervical polyps is that they are usually secondary to inflammation or abnormal focal responsiveness to hormonal stimulation. Focal hyperplasia and localized proliferation are the response of the cervix to local inflammation. The color of the polyp depends in part on its origin, with most endocervical polyps being cherry red and most cervical polyps grayish white.

The classic symptom of an endocervical polyp is intermenstrual bleeding, especially following contact such as coitus or a pelvic examination. Sometimes an associated leucorrhea emanates from the infected cervix. Many endocervical polyps are asymptomatic and recognized for the first time during a routine speculum examination. Often the polyp seen on inspection is difficult to palpate because of its soft consistency.

Histologically the surface epithelium of the polyp is columnar or squamous epithelium, depending on the site of origin and the degree of squamous metaplasia (**Fig. 18-22**). The stalk is composed of an edematous, inflamed, loose, and richly vascular connective tissue. Six different histologic subtypes have been described: adenomatous, cystic, fibrous, vascular, inflammatory, and fibromyomatous. Greater than 80% are of the adenomatous type. During pregnancy, focal areas of decidual changes may develop in the stroma. Often there is ulceration of the stalk's most dependent portion, which explains the symptom of contact bleeding. Malignant degeneration of an endocervical polyp is extremely rare. The reported incidence is less than 1 in 200. Considerations in the differential diagnosis include **endometrial polyps**, small prolapsed myomas, retained products of conception, squamous papilloma, sarcoma, and cervical malignancy. Microglandular endocervical hyperplasia sometimes presents

as a 1- to 2-cm polyp. This is an exaggerated histologic response, usually to oral contraceptives.

Most endocervical polyps may be managed in the office by grasping the base of the polyp with an appropriately sized clamp. The polyp is avulsed with a twisting motion and sent to the pathology laboratory for microscopic evaluation. The polyp is usually friable. If the base is broad or bleeding ensues, the base may be treated with chemical cautery, electrocautery, or cryocautery. After the polyp is removed, endometrium should be evaluated in women older than 40 who have presented with abnormal bleeding, to rule out coexisting pathology. In one study by Pradhan and coworkers, significant endometrial pathology was found in approximately 5% of asymptomatic women with endocervical polyps.

NABOTHIAN CYSTS

Nabothian cysts are retention cysts of endocervical columnar cells occurring where a tunnel or cleft has been covered by squamous metaplasia. These cysts are so common that they are considered a normal feature of the adult cervix. Many women have multiple cysts. Grossly, these cysts may be translucent or opaque whitish or yellow in color. Nabothian cysts vary from microscopic to macroscopic size, with the majority between 3 mm and 3 cm in diameter. Rarely, a woman with several large nabothian cysts may develop gross enlargement of the cervix. These mucous retention cysts are produced by the spontaneous healing process of the cervix. The area of the transformation zone of the cervix is in an almost constant process of repair, and squamous metaplasia and inflammation may block the cleft of a gland orifice. The endocervical columnar cells continue to secrete, and thus a mucous retention cyst is formed. Nabothian cysts are asymptomatic, and no treatment is necessary.

LACERATIONS

Cervical lacerations frequently occur with both normal and abnormal deliveries. Lacerations may occur in nonpregnant women with mechanical dilation of the cervix. Obstetric lacerations vary from minor superficial tears to extensive full-thickness lacerations at 3 and 9 o'clock, respectively, which may extend into the broad ligament. In gynecology the atrophic cervix of the postmenopausal woman predisposes to the complication of cervical laceration when the cervix is mechanically dilated for a diagnostic dilatation and curettage (D&C).

Acute cervical lacerations bleed and should be sutured. Cervical lacerations that are not repaired may give the external os of the cervix a fish-mouthed appearance; however, they are usually asymptomatic. The use of laminaria tents to slowly soften and dilate the cervix before mechanical instrumentation of the endometrial cavity has reduced the magnitude of iatrogenic cervical lacerations. Furthermore, the practice of routine inspection of the cervix, stabilized with one or more ring forceps, following every second- or third-trimester delivery has enabled physicians to discover and repair extensive cervical lacerations. Lacerations should be palpated to determine the extent of cephalad extension of the tear. Extensive cervical lacerations, especially those involving the endocervical stroma, may lead to incompetence of the cervix during a subsequent pregnancy.

CERVICAL MYOMAS

Cervical myomas are smooth, firm masses that are similar to myomas of the fundus (**Figs. 18-23** and **18-24**). A cervical myoma is usually a solitary growth in contrast to uterine myomas, which in general, are multiple. Depending on the series, 3% to 8% of myomas are categorized as cervical myomas. Because of the relative paucity of smooth muscle fibers in the cervical stroma, the majority of myomas that appear to be cervical actually arise from the isthmus of the uterus.

Most cervical myomas are small and asymptomatic. When symptoms do occur, they are dependent on the direction in which the enlarging myoma expands. The expanding myoma produces symptoms secondary to mechanical pressure on adjacent organs. Cervical myomas may produce dysuria, urgency, urethral or ureteral obstruction, dyspareunia, or obstruction of the cervix. Occasionally a cervical myoma may become pedunculated and protrude through the external os of the cervix. These prolapsed myomas are often ulcerated and infected. A very large

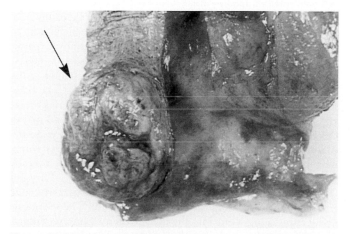

Figure 18-23 Leiomyoma (*arrow*), originating in cervix and dilating endocervical canal. It is soft, showing degenerative changes. (From Janovski NA [ed]: Color Atlas of Gross Gynecologic and Obstetric Pathology. New York, McGraw-Hill, 1969, p 71.)

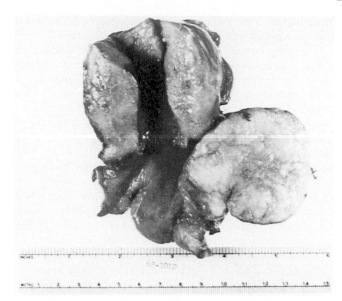

Figure 18-24 Leiomyoma of cervix most likely developing from lateral endocervix and protruding into broad ligament. Tumor is whitish, firm, and poorly encapsulated. (From Janovski NA [ed]: Color Atlas of Gross Gynecologic and Obstetric Pathology. New York, McGraw-Hill, 1969, p 69.)

cervical myoma may produce distortion of the cervical canal and upper vagina. Rarely, a cervical myoma causes dystocia during childbirth.

The diagnosis of a cervical myoma is by inspection and palpation. Grossly and histologically, cervical myomas are identical to and indistinguishable from myomas of the corpus of the uterus. Occasionally the histologic picture of cervical myomas will demonstrate many hyalinized, thick-walled blood vessels that are postulated to be the source of the neoplastic smooth muscle tumor. This latter subtype of cervical myoma is termed a *vascular leiomyoma*. Management is similar to that of uterine myomas in that asymptomatic, small myomas may be observed for rate of growth. The occurrence and persistence of symptoms from a cervical myoma are an indication for medical therapy with gonadotropin-releasing hormone (GnRH) agonists or myomectomy or hysterectomy, depending on the patient's age and future reproductive plans. Treatment of cervical myomas that grow laterally may become a challenge if myomectomy is the operation of choice, because of both a complex blood supply and involvement with the distal course of the ureter. Cervical myomas may be treated by radiologic catheter embolization. Prolapsed uterine myomas are discussed later in this chapter.

CERVICAL STENOSIS

Cervical stenosis most often occurs in the region of the internal os. Cervical stenosis may be divided into congenital or acquired types. The causes of acquired cervical stenosis are operative, radiation, infection, neoplasia, or atrophic changes. Cone biopsy and cautery of the cervix, either electrocautery or cryocoagulation, are the operations that most commonly cause cervical stenosis. Cervical stenosis may occur following loop electrocautery excision procedure (LEEP) procedures in women with low circulating estrogen levels such as secondary to periodic injections of medroxyprogesterone (Depo-Provera), postmenopausal women, and those who are breast-feeding. Peri- and postoperative treatment with vaginal or systemic estrogen may help prevent this complication.

The symptoms of cervical stenosis depend on whether the patient is premenopausal or postmenopausal and whether the obstruction is complete or partial. Common symptoms in premenopausal women include dysmenorrhea, pelvic pain, abnormal bleeding, amenorrhea, and infertility. The infertility is usually associated with endometriosis, which is commonly found in reproductive-age women with cervical stenosis. Post-menopausal women are usually asymptomatic for a long time. Slowly they develop a **hematometra** (blood), **hydrometra** (clear fluid), or **pyometra** (exudate).

The diagnosis is established by inability to introduce a 1- to 2-mm dilator into the uterine cavity. If the obstruction is complete, a soft, slightly tender, enlarged uterus is appreciated as a midline mass, and ultrasound examination demonstrating fluid within the uterine cavity. Management of cervical stenosis is dilation of the cervix with dilators under ultrasound guidance. If stenosis recurs, monthly laminaria tents may be used. Similarly, office follow-up and sounding of the cervix of women who have had a cone biopsy or cautery of the cervix is important to establish patency of the endocervical canal. Postmenopausal women with pyometra usually do not need antibiotics. After the acute infection has subsided, endometrial carcinoma and endocervical carcinoma should be ruled out by appropriate diagnostic biopsies. After cervical dilation, it is often useful to leave a T tube or latex nasopharyngeal airway as a stent in the cervical canal for a few days to maintain patency. Two small series from Birmingham, England, and Syracuse, New York, reported the use of the CO_2 laser for treatment of cervical stenosis. In these series approximately 70% of patients were relieved of their cervical stenosis. The success of treatment depends on the proper use of the laser and the quality and quantity of residual columnar epithelium remaining in the endocervix.

UTERUS

ULTRASOUND

Ultrasound, primarily endovaginal, is the most common and most efficient imaging technique for pelvic structures. For endovaginal ultrasound, transducers are configured on vaginal probes and placed in a sterile sheath, usually a glove or condom, prior to an examination. During the examination the woman is in a dorsal lithotomy position and has an empty bladder. Because the transducer is closer to the pelvic organs than when a transabdominal approach is employed, endovaginal resolution is usually superior. However, if the pelvic structures to be studied have expanded and extend into the patient's abdomen, the organs are difficult to visualize with an endovaginal probe. Most ultrasound machines are equipped with both types of transducers.

For transabdominal gynecologic examinations, a sector scanner is preferable. It provides greater resolution of the pelvis and an easier examination than the linear array. During abdominal pelvic ultrasound examination, it is helpful for the patient to have a full bladder. This serves as an acoustic window for the high-frequency sound waves. Ultrasound is more than 90% accurate in recognizing the presence of a pelvic mass, but it does not establish a tissue diagnosis.

Ultrasonography employs an acoustic pulse echo technique. The transducer of the ultrasound machine is made up of piezoelectric crystals that vibrate and emit acoustic pulses. Acoustic echoes return from the tissues being scanned and cause the crystals to vibrate again and release an electric charge. A computer within the ultrasound machine then integrates the electric charges to form the image. Present equipment provides resolution of less than 0.2 mm.

Doppler ultrasound techniques assess the frequency of returning echoes to determine the velocity of moving structures. Measurement of diastolic and systolic velocities provides indirect indices of vascular resistance. Muscular arteries have high resistance. Newly developed vessels, such as those arising in malignancies, have little vascular wall musculature and thus have low resistance. Three-dimensional ultrasound is a computer technique in which multiple two-dimensional images are compiled to render either a surface- or volume-based image that appears to occupy space, as opposed to being flat. Three-dimensional ultrasound has of yet not been shown to have a specific diagnostic advantage in gynecology compared with other modalities.

A disadvantage of ultrasound is its poor penetration of bone and air; thus, the pubic symphysis and air-filled intestines and rectum often inhibit visualization. Advantages of ultrasound include the real-time nature of the image, the absence of radiation, the ability to perform the procedure in the office before, during, or immediately after a pelvic examination, and the ability to describe the findings to the patient while she is watching. One of the most reassuring aspects of sonography is the absence of adverse clinical effects from the energy levels used in diagnostic studies.

Sonographic evaluation of endometrial pathology involves measurement of the endometrial thickness or stripe. The normal endometrial thickness is 4 mm or less in a postmenopausal woman not taking hormones. The thickness varies in premenopausal women at different times of the menstrual cycle and in women taking hormone replacement (**Fig. 18-25**). In this sense, a 5-mm cutoff cannot be applied to these women, other than postmenopausal women. The endometrial thickness is measured in the longitudinal plane, from outer margin to outer margin, at the widest part of the endometrium. Ultrasound is not a screening tool in asymptomatic women. However, several studies of postmenopausal women with vaginal bleeding have documented that malignancy is extremely rare in women with an endometrial thickness of 4 mm or less. Systematic reviews have noted that ultrasound may be reliably used to predict 96% to 99% of endometrial cancers in women with postmenopausal bleeding. The flip side of the coin is that 1% to 4% of malignancies will be missed using a cutoff of less than 4 mm. In addition, papillary-serous adenocarcinomas of the endometrium do not always develop endometrial stripe thickness. Two caveats for using ultrasound in screening of postmenopausal bleeding: (1) ultrasound does not provide a diagnosis—a tissue specimen is necessary for a diagnosis, and (2) all women with bleeding, no matter the endometrial thickness, need a tissue biopsy. If an endometrial biopsy obtains inadequate tissue and the endometrial thickness is 5 mm or greater, a repeat biopsy, hysteroscopically directed biopsy, or curettage should be performed.

Sonohysterography is an easily accomplished and validated technique for evaluating the endometrial cavity. The technique involves instilling saline into the uterine cavity. Sonohysterography is an alternative to office hysteroscopy. In this procedure, a thin balloon-tipped catheter or intrauterine insemination catheter is inserted through the cervical os, and 5 to 30 mL of warmed saline is slowly injected into the uterine cavity. Meta-analyses of

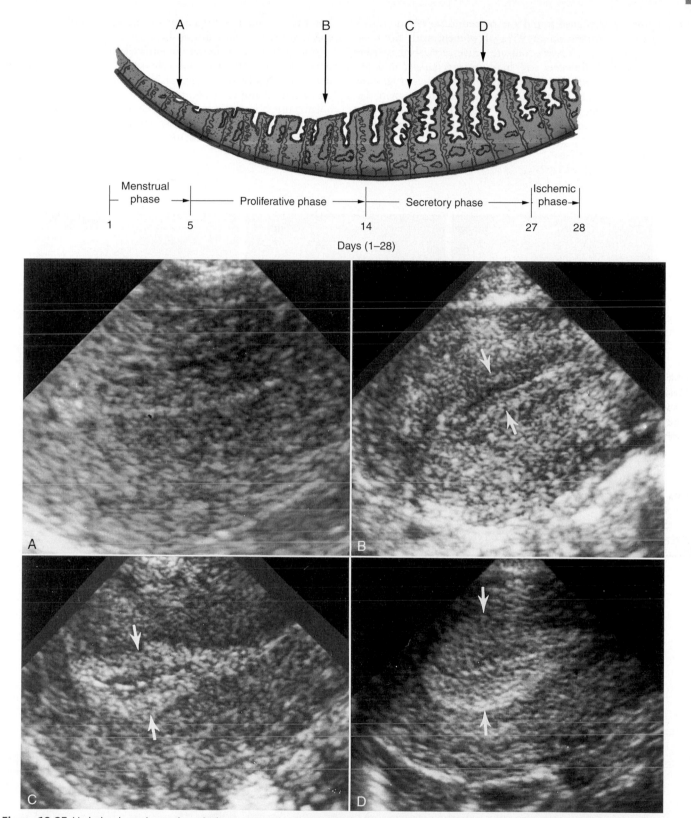

Figure 18-25 Variation in endometrium during menstrual cycle. **A,** Early proliferative phase. **B,** Late proliferative phase. **C,** Periovulatory phase. **D,** Late secretory phase. Note increase in endometrial thickness throughout the menstrual cycle. Also note multilayered appearance in the late proliferative phase. (From Fleischer AC, Kepple DM: Benign conditions of the uterus, cervix, and endometrium. In Nyberg DA, Hill LM, Bohm-Velez M, Mendelson EB [eds]: Transvaginal Ultrasound. St. Louis, Mosby–Year Book, 1992.)

sonohysterography have found the procedure to be successful in obtaining information in 95% of women, with minimal complications. Contraindications are active cervical or uterine infection. Some clinicians will have patients take a dose of ibuprofen prior to the procedure. Preferably, sonohysterography is performed in the proliferative phase of the cycle when the endometrial lining is at its lowest level. Sonohysterography has also been helpful in the evaluation of polyps, filling defects, submucous myomas, and uterine septae (**Fig. 18-26**).

Importantly, sonohysterography, as with all types of ultrasound, does not make a tissue diagnosis.

Sonography is the method of choice to locate a "missing" intrauterine device (IUD). It will help in diagnosing perforation of the uterus or unrecognized expulsion of the device. Endovaginal ultrasound transducers equipped with needle guides are frequently used for oocyte aspiration as part of in vitro fertilization.

In summary, ultrasound has become an extremely valuable adjunct to the bimanual examination. In many patients, particularly

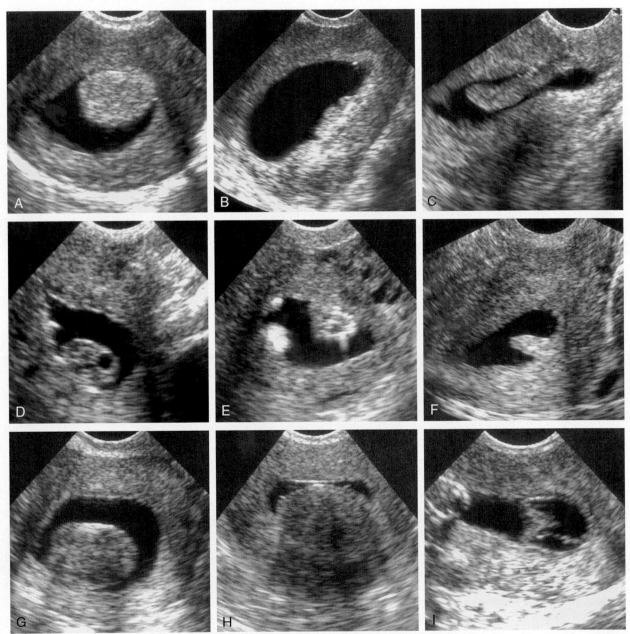

Figure 18-26 Sonohysterograms. **A,** Well-defined, round echogenic polyp. **B,** Carpet of small polyps. **C,** Polyp on a stalk. **D,** Polyp with cystic areas. **E,** Small polyp. **F,** Small polyp. **G,** Hypoechoic submucosal fibroid. **H,** Hypoechoic attenuating submucosal fibroid. **I,** Endometrial adhesions. Note bridging bands of tissue within fluid-filled endometrial canal. (From Salem S: The uterus and adnexa. In Rumack CM, Wilson SR, Charboneau JW [eds]: Diagnostic Ultrasound, 2nd ed. St. Louis, Mosby, 1998, p 538.)

obese patients, it is superior to perform bimanual examination alone. An endovaginal ultrasound of an early pregnancy has become a mainstay in the evaluation of the pregnant woman with first-trimester vaginal bleeding.

ENDOMETRIAL POLYPS

Endometrial polyps are localized overgrowths of endometrial glands and stroma that project beyond the surface of the endometrium. They are soft, pliable, and may be single or multiple. Most polyps arise from the fundus of the uterus. *Polypoid hyperplasia* is a benign condition in which numerous small polyps are discovered throughout the endometrial cavity. Endometrial polyps vary from a few millimeters to several centimeters in diameter, and it is possible for a single large polyp to fill the endometrial cavity. Endometrial polyps may have a broad base (sessile) or be attached by a slender pedicle (pedunculated). In Novak and Woodruff's review of 1100 women with polyps, the growths were discovered in all age groups, with a peak incidence between the ages of 40 and 49. The prevalence of endometrial polyps in reproductive-age women is 20% to 25%. Endometrial polyps are noted in approximately 10% of women when the uterus is examined at autopsy. The cause of endometrial polyps is unknown. Because polyps are often associated with endometrial hyperplasia, unopposed estrogen may be one cause.

The majority of endometrial polyps are asymptomatic. Those that are symptomatic are associated with a wide range of abnormal bleeding patterns. No single abnormal bleeding pattern is diagnostic for polyps; however, menorrhagia, premenstrual and postmenstrual staining, and scanty postmenstrual spotting are the most common. Occasionally a pedunculated endometrial polyp with a long pedicle may protrude from the external cervical os. Sometimes large endometrial polyps may contribute to infertility.

Polyps are succulent and velvety, with a large central vascular core. The color is usually gray or tan but may occasionally be red or brown. Histologically, an endometrial polyp has three components: endometrial glands, endometrial stroma, and central vascular channels (**Figs. 18-26** and **18-27**). Epithelium must be identified on three sides, like a peninsula. Approximately two of three polyps consist of an immature endometrium that does not respond to cyclic changes in circulating progesterone. This immature endometrium differs from surrounding endometrium and often appears as a "Swiss cheese" cystic hyperplasia during all phases of the menstrual cycle (**Fig. 18-28**). The other one third of endometrial polyps consist of functional endometria that will undergo cyclic histologic changes. The tip of a prolapsed polyp often undergoes squamous metaplasia, infection, or ulceration. The clinician cannot distinguish whether the abnormal bleeding originates from the polyp or is secondary to the frequently coexisting endometrial hyperplasia. Approximately one in four reproductive-age women with abnormal bleeding will have endometrial polyps discovered in her uterine cavity.

Malignancy in an endometrial polyp is related to patient's age and is most often of a low stage and grade. Bakour and colleagues from the U.K. reported on 67 women with polyps. The mean age was 54. Fifty-three of 62 (86%) of the polyps were benign, 7 of 62 (13%) were hyperplastic, and 2 of 62 (3%) were malignant. Another series from Goldstein and coworkers of 61 women with polyps found 54 of 61 (88%) to be benign and 3 of 61 (5%) to contain malignancy. A recent study of 1224 cases from Baiocchi et al. found that 3.5% contain malignant elements, and an additional 1.3% of polyps had premalignant changes. Overall the incidence of malignancy is 3% to 4%. The question of an association with endometrial polyps and endometrial carcinoma is still debated. A population-based, case-control study from Sweden by Pettersson and associates estimated that the increased risk of subsequent endometrial carcinoma in women with endometrial polyps is only twofold. It is interesting that benign polyps

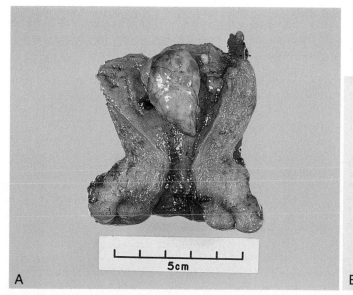
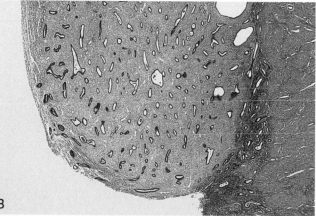

Figure 18-27 Endometrial polyp. **A,** Note cystic glands in the polyp. **B,** The fibrous stroma of the polyp contrasts with the cellular stroma of the adjacent endometrium. (From Anderson MC, Robboy SJ, Russell P, Morse A: Endometritis, metaplasias, polyps, and miscellaneous changes. In Robboy SJ, Anderson MC, Russell P [eds]: Pathology of the Female Reproductive Tract. Edinburgh, Churchill Livingstone, 2002.)

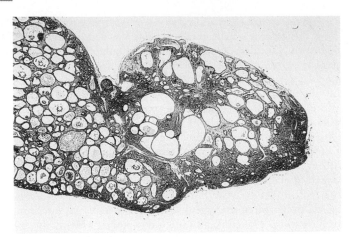

Figure 18-28 Endometrial polyp showing multiple cystic glands with flattened epithelial lining. (From Anderson MC, Robboy SJ, Russell P, Morse A: Endometritis, metaplasias, polyps and miscellaneous changes. In Robboy SJ, Anderson MC, Russell P [eds]: Pathology of the Female Reproductive Tract. Edinburgh, Churchill Livingstone, 2002.)

have been found in approximately 20% of uteri removed for endometrial carcinoma. In contrast, a large study from Montreal of 1467 women, by Perri et al. noted no increased incidence of associated malignancy.

Unusual polyps have been described in association with chronic administration of the nonsteroidal antiestrogen tamoxifen. The endometrial abnormalities associated with chronic tamoxifen therapy include polyps, 20% to 35%; endometrial hyperplasia, 2% to 4%; and endometrial carcinoma, 1% to 2%.

Most endometrial polyps are asymptomatic, and the diagnosis is not usually established until the uterus is opened following hysterectomy for other reasons. Endometrial polyps may be discovered by vaginal ultrasound, with or without hydrosonography, hysteroscopy, or hysterosalpingography during the diagnostic workup of a woman with a refractory case of abnormal uterine bleeding or pelvic mass (**Fig. 18-29**). A well-defined, uniformly hyperechoic mass that is less than 2 cm in diameter, identified by vaginal ultrasound within the endometrial cavity, is

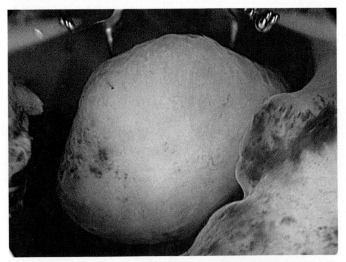

Figure 18-29 Endocervical polyp was seen at hysteroscopy. (From Goldberg JM, Falcone T: Atlas of Endoscopic Techniques in Gynecology. London, WB Saunders, 2000.)

usually a benign endometrial polyp (**Fig. 18-25A-C**). DeWaay and colleagues evaluated 64 asymptomatic women with polyps over a 2½-year period with hysterosonography. The polyps regressed in four of seven women. Interestingly, at the second ultrasound, seven women had developed new polyps.

The optimal management of endometrial polyps is removal by hysteroscopy with D&C. Because of the frequent association of endometrial polyps and other endometrial pathology, it is important to examine histologically both the polyp and the associated endometrial lining. Polyps, because of their mobility, often tend to elude the curette. Postcurettage hysteroscopic studies have demonstrated that routine use of a long, narrow polyp forceps at the time of curettage at best results in discovery and removal of only approximately one in four endometrial polyps. The differential diagnosis of endometrial polyps includes submucous leiomyomas, **adenomyomas**, retained products of conception, endometrial hyperplasia, carcinoma, and uterine sarcomas.

HEMATOMETRA

A hematometra is a uterus distended with blood and is secondary to gynatresia, which is partial or complete obstruction of any portion of the lower genital tract. Obstruction of the isthmus of the uterus, cervix, or vagina may be congenital or acquired. The two most common congenital causes of hematometra are an imperforate hymen and a transverse vaginal septum. Among the leading causes of acquired lower tract stenosis are senile atrophy of the endocervical canal and endometrium, scarring of the isthmus by synechiae, cervical stenosis associated with surgery, radiation therapy, cryocautery or electrocautery, endometrial ablation, and malignant disease of the endocervical canal.

The symptoms of hematometra depend on the age of the patient, her menstrual history and the rapidity of the accumulation of blood in the uterine cavity, and the possibility of secondary infection producing pyometra. Thus common symptoms of hematometra include primary or secondary amenorrhea and possibly cyclic lower abdominal pain. During the early teenage years, the combination of primary amenorrhea and cyclic, episodic cramping lower abdominal pains suggests the possibility of a developing hematometra. Occasionally the obstruction is incomplete, and there is associated spotting of dark brown blood. Hematometra in postmenopausal women may be entirely asymptomatic. On pelvic examination a mildly tender, globular uterus is usually palpated. Ultrasound may be used to confirm the diagnosis.

The diagnosis of hematometra is generally suspected by the history of amenorrhea and cyclic abdominal pain. The diagnosis is usually confirmed by vaginal ultrasound or probing the cervix with a narrow metal dilator, with release of dark brownish black blood from the endocervical canal. Sometimes the blood retained inside the uterus becomes secondarily infected and has a foul odor.

Management of hematometra depends on operative relief of the lower tract obstruction. Treatment of congenital obstruction is discussed in Chapter 11 (Congenital Abnormalities of the Female Reproductive Tract). Appropriate biopsy specimens of the endocervical canal and endometrium should be obtained to rule out malignancy when the cause of hematometra is not obvious. If the uterus is significantly enlarged or if there is any suspicion that the retained fluid is infected, drainage should be accomplished first. Biopsy should be postponed for approximately 2 weeks to diminish the chances of infection or uterine perforation. Hematometra following operations or cryocautery usually resolves with cervical dilation. Rarely, a hematometra may form following a first-trimester abortion. This is treated by repeat suction aspiration of the products of conception that are blocking the internal os.

LEIOMYOMAS

Leiomyomas, also called *myomas,* are benign tumors of muscle cell origin. These tumors are often referred to by their popular names, *fibroids* or *fibromyomas,* but such terms are semantic misnomers if one is referring to the cell of origin. Most leiomyomas contain varying amounts of fibrous tissue, which is believed to be secondary to degeneration of some of the smooth muscle cells.

Leiomyomas are the most frequent pelvic tumors and the most common tumor in women, with the highest prevalence occurring during the fifth decade of a woman's life. Estimates of the prevalence of myomas vary. A large population-based study from the Washington, D.C. area, using transvaginal ultrasound, found myomas in more than 80% of African-American women and greater than 70% of white women, by age 50. More conservative estimates have found myomas in 30% to 50% of perimenopausal women. In general, a third of myomas will become symptomatic. Myomas are more prone to grow and become symptomatic in nulliparous women. Why some women develop myomas while others do not is unknown. Symptomatic uterine leiomyomas are the primary indication for approximately 30% of all hysterectomies. Outside the United States, fibroids have been noted to be the most common indication for a hysterectomy in Malaysia, France, Nigeria, and Japan.

Risk factors associated with the development of myomata include increasing age, early menarche, low parity, tamoxifen use, obesity, and in some studies a high-fat diet. Smoking has been found to be associated with a decreased incidence of myomata. African-American women have the highest incidence, whereas Hispanic and Asian women have similar rates to white women. There appears to be a familial tendency to develop myoma. Studies of twins have noted than when identical and fraternal twins are compared, a significant proportion of myoma tend to have an inherited basis.

Although leiomyomas arise throughout the body in any structure containing smooth muscle, in the pelvis the majority are found in the corpus of the uterus. Occasionally, leiomyomas may be found in the fallopian tube or the round ligament, and approximately 5% of uterine myomas originate from the cervix. Rarely, myomas will arise in the retroperitoneum and produce symptoms secondary to "mass effects" on adjacent organs.

Myomas may be single but most often are multiple. They vary greatly in size from microscopic to multinodular uterine tumors that may weigh more than 50 pounds and literally fill the patient's abdomen. Initially most myomas develop from the myometrium, beginning as intramural myomas. As they grow, they remain attached to the myometrium with a pedicle of varying width and thickness. Small myomas are round, firm, solid tumors. With continued growth, the myometrium at the edge of the tumor is compressed and forms a pseudocapsule. Although myomas do not have a true capsule, this pseudocapsule is a valuable surgical plane during a myomectomy.

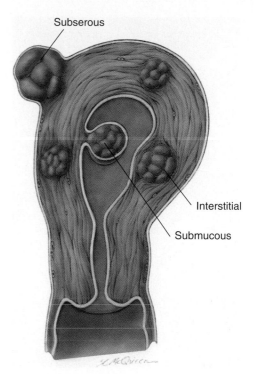

Figure 18-30 Drawing of cut surface of uterus showing characteristic whorl-like appearance and varying locations of leiomyomas. (From Novak ER, Woodruff JD [eds]: Novak's Gynecologic and Obstetric Pathology, 6th ed. Philadelphia, WB Saunders, 1967, p 215.)

Myomas are classed into subgroups by their relative anatomic relationship and position to the layers of the uterus (**Fig. 18-30**). The three most common types of myomas are intramural, subserous, and submucous, with special nomenclature for broad ligament and **parasitic myomas** (**Fig. 18-31**). Continued growth in one direction determines which myomas will be located just below the endometrium (submucosal) and which will be found just beneath the serosa (subserosal) (**Fig. 18-32**). Although only 5% to 10% of myomas become submucosal, they usually are the most troublesome clinically (**Fig. 18-33**). These submucosal tumors may be associated with abnormal vaginal bleeding or distortion of the uterine cavity that may produce infertility or abortion. Rarely, a **submucosal myoma** enlarges and becomes pedunculated. The uterus will try to expel it, and the prolapsed myoma may protrude through the external cervical os.

Subserosal myomas give the uterus its knobby contour during pelvic examination. Further growth of a subserosal myoma may lead to a pedunculated myoma wandering into the peritoneal cavity. This myoma may outgrow its uterine blood supply and obtain a secondary blood supply from another organ, such as the omentum, and become a parasitic myoma. Kho et al. in a recent series noted that laparoscopic morcellation of myomata led to occasional iatrogenic parasitic myomas that implanted and grew from fragments left after surgery. Growth of a myoma in a lateral direction from the uterus may result in a broad ligament myoma. The clinical significance of broad ligament myomas is that they are difficult to differentiate on pelvic examination from a solid ovarian tumor. Large, broad ligament myomas may produce a hydroureter as they enlarge.

Though the origin of uterine leiomyomas is incompletely understood, cytogenetic studies have yielded some clues to how and

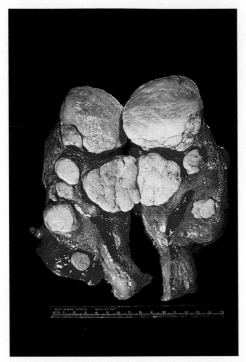

Figure 18-31 Multiple leiomyomas. These are predominantly intramural. The bulging cut surfaces are clearly shown. (From Anderson MC, Robboy SJ, Russell P: Uterine smooth muscle tumors. In Robboy SJ, Anderson MC, Russell P [eds]: Pathology of the Female Reproductive Tract. Edinburgh, Churchill Livingstone, 2002.)

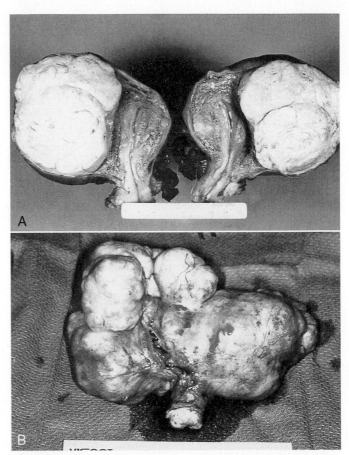

Figure 18-32 A, Large subserosal myoma. **B,** Hysterectomy specimen of myomatous uterus. (Courtesy of Vern L. Katz and William Droegemueller.)

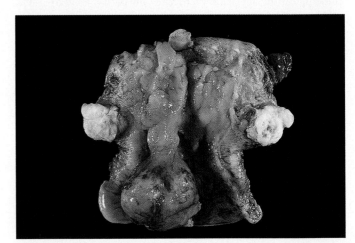

Figure 18-33 Uterus with multiple myomata. Note the large central submucosal myoma. (From Voet RL: Color Atlas of Obstetric and Gynecologic Pathology. St. Louis, Mosby-Wolfe, 1997.)

why myomas develop. Each tumor develops from a single muscle cell a progenitor myocyte, thus each myoma is monoclonal. Cytogenetic analysis has demonstrated that myomas have multiple chromosomal abnormalities. (Each myoma would have cells with the same abnormality.) Sixty percent are normal, 46XX. The larger the myoma, the more an abnormal karyotype will be detected. Interestingly, the chromosomal anomalies of myomata have a remarkable clustering of changes. Twenty percent of abnormalities involve translocations between chromosomes 12 and 14. Seventeen percent involve a deletion of chromosome 7. Twelve percent involve a deletion of chromosome 12, and some are trisomy 12. The affected regions on chromosome 12 are also abnormal in many other types of solid tumors. The regions of chromosome 12 and 7 involve genes that may regulate growth-inducing proteins and cytokines, including transforming growth factor β (TGF-β), epidermal growth factor (EGF), insulin-like growth factors (IGF) 1 and 2, and platelet-derived growth factor (PDGF) (**Fig. 18-34**). Many of these cytokines have been found in significantly higher concentrations in myomas than in the surrounding myometrium. Current theory holds that the neoplastic transformation from normal myometrium to leiomyomata is the result of a somatic mutation in the single progenitor cell. The mutation then affects cytokines that affect cell growth. Also, the growth may be influenced by relative levels of estrogen or progesterone. Both estrogen and progesterone receptors are found in higher concentrations in uterine myomas, as are other genomic changes that potentiate cellular proliferation. There also appear to be similarities between fibroids and keloid formation. Interestingly, Ishikawa et al. noted that myoma cells have increased expression of

aromatase. This potentiates more local estrogen. In their study, they found that African-American women had the highest levels of aromatase in myoma cells.

Myomas are rare before menarche, and most myomas diminish in size following menopause with the reduction of a significant amount of circulating estrogen. Myomas often enlarge during pregnancy and occasionally enlarge secondary to oral

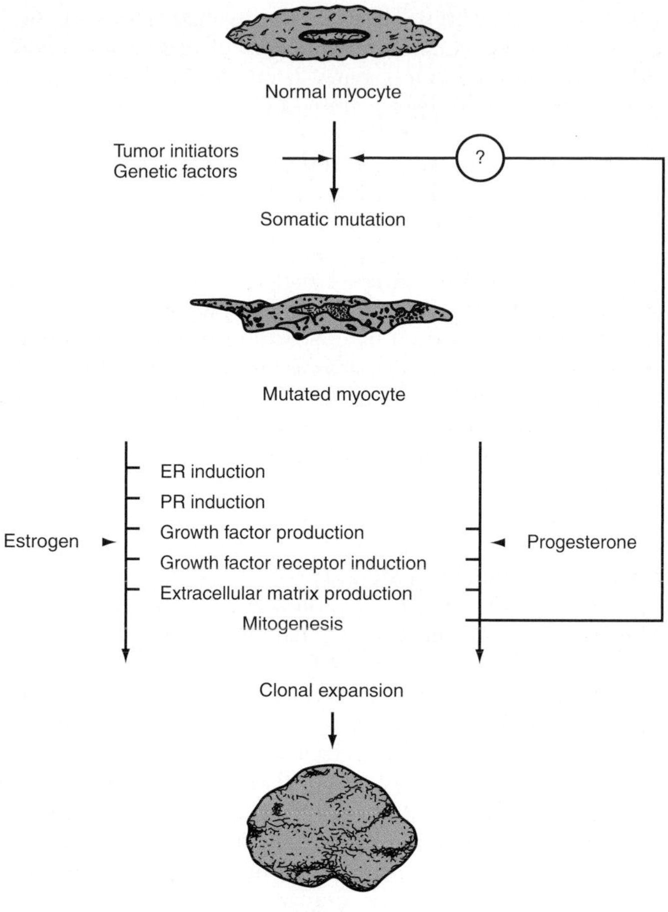

Normal myocyte

Tumor initiators
Genetic factors → ← ?

Somatic mutation

Mutated myocyte

Estrogen ►
- ER induction
- PR induction
- Growth factor production
- Growth factor receptor induction
- Extracellular matrix production
- Mitogenesis

◄ Progesterone

Clonal expansion

Myoma

Figure 18-34 The initiation and growth of myomas likely involves a multistep cascade of separate tumor initiators and promoters. The initial neoplastic transformation of the normal myocyte involves somatic mutations. Although the initiators of the somatic mutations remain unclear, the mitogenic effect of progesterone may enhance the propagation of somatic mutations. Myoma proliferation is the result of clonal expansion and likely involves the complex interactions of estrogen, progesterone, and local growth factors. Estrogen and progesterone appear equally important as promoters of myoma growth. ER, estrogen receptor; PR, progesterone receptor. (Modified from Rein MS, Barbieri RL, Friedman AJ: Progesterone: A critical role in the pathogenesis of uterine myomas. Am J Obstet Gynecol 172:14, 1995.)

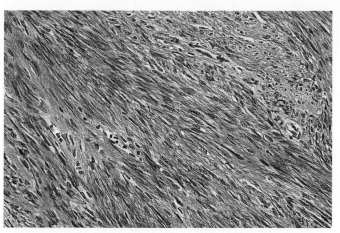

Figure 18-35 Leiomyoma. The smooth muscle cells are markedly elongated and have eosinophilic cytoplasm and elongated, cigar-shaped nuclei. The nuclei are uniform and mitotic figures absent or sparse. (From Anderson MC, Robboy SJ, Russell P: Uterine smooth muscle tumors. In Robboy SJ, Anderson MC, Russell P [eds]: Pathology of the Female Reproductive Tract. Edinburgh, Churchill Livingstone, 2002.)

contraceptive therapy. Medically induced hypoestrogenic states produce reductions in the size of myomas. Women who smoke cigarettes and are thus relatively estrogen-deficient have a lower incidence of myomas. Many women, though, have small myomas that do not grow under the influence of high circulating estrogen levels. Thus the relationship between estrogen and progesterone levels and myoma growth is complex.

Grossly, a myoma has a lighter color than the normal myometrium. On a cut surface, the tumor has a glistening, pearl-white appearance, with the smooth muscle arranged in a trabeculated or whorled configuration. Histologically there is a proliferation of mature smooth muscle cells. The nonstriated muscle fibers are arranged in interlacing bundles. Between bundles of smooth muscle cells are variable amounts of fibrous connective tissue, especially toward the center of any large tumor

(**Fig. 18-35**). The amount of fibrous tissue is proportional to the extent of atrophy and degeneration that has occurred over time. The intracellular structure of myoma cells is different from the surrounding normal myometrium. The abnormal cells contain more collagen and what Rogers et al. have described as a "stiffer" cytoskeleton secondary to the intracellular pressure generated by the densely packed surrounding myoma. Less than 5% of myomas exhibit hypercellularity, and these are termed "cellular leiomyomata" (**Fig. 18-35B**). Cellular leiomyoma tend to be larger in size and solitary. There is less accompanying **adenomyosis** or other uterine pathology. Turan et al. have noted that the clinical presentation of cellular leiomyoma is more similar to that of a sarcoma (leiomyosarcoma). Other authors have noted a genomic expression that is similar, as well, to leiomyosarcomas. However, cellular leiomyomata are not precursors to sarcoma and have a benign prognosis.

The eventual fate of some myomas is determined by their relatively poor vascular supply. This supply is found in one or two major arteries at the base or pedicle of the myoma. The arterial supply of myomas is significantly less than that of a similarly sized area of normal myometrium. Thus, with continued growth, degeneration occurs because the tumor outgrows its blood supply. The severity of the discrepancy between the myoma's growth and its blood supply determines the extent of degeneration: hyaline, myxomatous, calcific, cystic, fatty, or red degeneration and necrosis. The mildest form of **degeneration of a myoma** is hyaline degeneration (**Fig. 18-36**). Grossly, in this condition the surface of the myoma is homogeneous with loss of the whorled pattern. Histologically, with hyaline degeneration, cellular detail is lost as the smooth muscle cells are replaced by fibrous connective tissue. Huang and colleagues, using transvaginal color Doppler ultrasound, documented that the intratumoral blood flow correlated with reduced tumor size and tumor volume but did not correlate with angiogenesis or cell proliferation.

The most acute form of degeneration is red, or carneous, infarction (**Fig. 18-37**). This acute muscular infarction causes

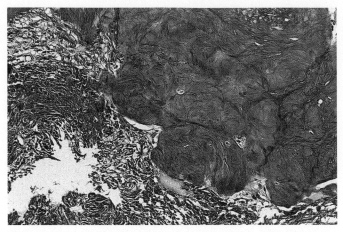

Figure 18-36 Hyaline degeneration is a leiomyoma. There is an eosinophilic ground-glass appearance. (From Anderson MC, Robboy SJ, Russell P: Uterine smooth muscle tumors. In Robboy SJ, Anderson MC, Russell P [eds]: Pathology of the Female Reproductive Tract. Edinburgh, Churchill Livingstone, 2002.)

severe pain and localized peritoneal irritation. The condition is best treated with nonsteroidal anti-inflammatory agents for 72 hours, as long as the woman is less than 32 weeks gestation. This form of degeneration occurs during pregnancy in approximately 5% to 10% of gravid women with myomas. The ultrasound appearance of painful myomas is one of mixed echodense and echolucent areas. Serial ultrasound examinations have also demonstrated that most (80%) myomas do not change size during pregnancy; if a change in size does occur, it is usually not associated with painful symptomatology. During pregnancy this complication should be treated medically, for attempts at operative removal may result in profuse blood loss. If the patient is not pregnant, acute degeneration is not a contraindication to myomectomy. The more advanced forms of degenerating myomas may become secondarily infected, especially when large necrotic areas exist. The histologic changes of degeneration

are found more commonly in larger myomas. However, two thirds of all myomas show some degree of degeneration, with the three most common types being hyaline degeneration (65%), myxomatous degeneration (15%), and calcific degeneration (10%).

The literature emphasizes that the incidence of malignant degeneration is estimated to be between 0.3% and 0.7%. The term *malignant degeneration* is incorrect. It is unknown as to whether myomas degenerate into sarcomas. Given the very high prevalence of myomas, most investigators believe that sarcomas arise spontaneously in myomatous uteri. In a series of 1429 hysterectomies, in patients with a preoperative diagnosis of symptoms related to myomas, leiomyosarcomas were found histologically in 0.49%. The incidence increases in each advancing decade of life. The possibility of a uterine tumor being a leiomyoma sarcoma is 10 times greater in a woman in her 60s than in a woman in her 40s.

The most common symptoms related to myomas are pressure from an enlarging pelvic mass, pain including dysmenorrhea, and abnormal uterine bleeding. The severity of symptoms is usually related to the number, location, and size of the myomas. However, over two thirds of women with uterine myomas are asymptomatic.

One of three women with myomas experiences pelvic pain or pressure. Acquired dysmenorrhea is one of the most frequent complaints. Various forms of vascular compromise, either acute degeneration or torsion of the pedicle, produce severe pelvic pain. Mild pelvic discomfort is described as pelvic heaviness or a dull, aching sensation that may be secondary to edematous swelling in the myoma. An enlarged myoma or myomas often produce pressure symptoms similar to those of an enlarging pregnant uterus. Sometimes a woman will notice that her abdominal girth is increasing without appreciable change in weight. Alternatively, an anterior myoma pressing on the bladder may produce urinary frequency and urgency. In general, urinary symptoms are more common than rectal symptoms. Extremely large myomas and broad ligament myomas may produce a unilateral or bilateral hydroureter.

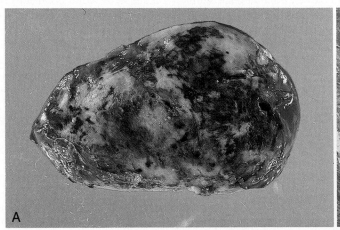
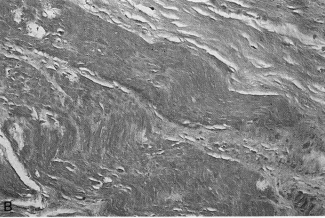

Figure 18-37 A, Gross view of an infracted leiomyoma. **B,** Red degeneration; the ghosts of the muscle cells and their nuclei remain. (**A,** From Anderson MC, Robboy SJ, Russell P: Uterine smooth muscle tumors. In Robboy SJ, Anderson MC, Russell P [eds]: Pathology of the Female Reproductive Tract. Edinburgh, Churchill Livingstone, 2002. **B,** From Voet RL: Color Atlas of Obstetric and Gynecologic Pathology. St. Louis, Mosby-Wolfe, 1997.)

Abnormal bleeding is experienced by 30% of women with myomas. The most common symptom is menorrhagia, but intermenstrual spotting and disruption of a normal pattern are other frequent complaints. Wegienka and colleagues evaluated the bleeding pattern of 596 women with myomas. Compared with a control group, bleeding was more frequently described as gushing. Menses were longer in duration and heavier. In this study, symptoms of bleeding were related to the size of myomas. Interestingly, location of the myomas, submucous versus intramural, was not related to bleeding symptoms. The exact cause-and-effect relationship between myomas and abnormal bleeding is difficult to determine and is poorly understood. The explanation is straightforward when there are areas of ulceration over submucous myomas. However, ulceration is a rare finding. The most popular theory is that myomas result in an abnormal microvascular growth pattern and function of the vessels in the adjacent endometrium. The older theory that the amount of menorrhagia is directly related to an increase of endometrial surface area has been disproved. One of three women with abnormal bleeding and submucous myomas also has endometrial hyperplasia, which may be the cause of the symptom.

Occasionally, myomas are the only identifiable abnormality after a detailed infertility investigation. Because the data relating myomas to infertility are weak, myomectomy is indicated only in long-standing infertility and recurrent abortion after all other potential factors have been investigated and treated. Studies suggest that submucous myomas that distort the uterine cavity are the myomas that may affect reproduction. Successful full-term pregnancy rates of 40% to 50% have been reported following a myomectomy. The success of an operation is most dependent on the age of the patient, the size of the myomas, and the number of compounding factors that affect the couple's fertility.

Rapid growth of a uterine myoma after menopause is a disturbing symptom. This is the classic symptom of a leiomyosarcoma, and thus the patient should have a total abdominal hysterectomy so that the tissue may be examined histologically.

Rarely, a secondary polycythemia is noted in women with uterine myomas. This syndrome is related to elevated levels of erythropoietin. The polycythemia diminishes following removal of the uterus.

Clinically, the diagnosis of uterine myomas is usually confirmed by physical examination. Upon palpation, an enlarged, firm, irregular uterus may be felt. The three conditions that commonly enter into the differential diagnosis include pregnancy, adenomyosis, and an ovarian neoplasm. The discrimination between large ovarian tumors and myomatous uteri may be difficult on physical examination, because the extension of myomas laterally may make palpation of normal ovaries impossible during the pelvic examination. The mobility of the pelvic mass and whether the mass moves independently or as part of the uterus may be helpful diagnostically. Ultrasound is diagnostic. Submucosal myomas may be diagnosed by vaginal ultrasound, hysteroscopy, or occasionally as a filling defect on hysterosalpingography. Occasionally, an abdominopelvic radiograph will note concentric calcifications. There are several reports promoting CT and MRI studies of uterine myomas. However, these imaging techniques are more expensive than ultrasound. Until CT and MRI can distinguish between benign and malignant myomas, they will rarely be ordered in routine clinical management of myomas. MRI is helpful in differentiating adenomyosis or an adenomyoma from a single, solitary myoma, especially in a woman desiring preservation of her fertility. Serial ultrasound examinations have been used to evaluate progression in size of myomas or response to therapy. However, in a recent study Cantuaria and coworkers compared bimanual pelvic exam and ultrasound imaging prior to hysterectomy for uterine myomas. They found a strong correlation in determining the size of myoma between bimanual and ultrasound exams.

The management of small, asymptomatic myomas is judicious observation. When the tumor is first discovered, it is appropriate to perform a pelvic examination at 6-month intervals to determine the rate of growth. The majority of women will not need an operation, especially those women in the perimenopausal period, where the condition usually improves with diminishing levels of circulating estrogens.

Cases of abnormal bleeding and leiomyomas should be investigated thoroughly for concurrent problems such as endometrial hyperplasia. If symptoms do not improve with conservative management, operative therapy may be considered. The choice between a myomectomy and hysterectomy is usually determined by the patient's age, parity, and most important, future reproductive plans. Myomectomy is associated with longer hospital stays and more pelvic adhesions than hysterectomy. Studies suggest that myomectomy results in approximately 80% resolution of symptoms. Hysterectomy is associated with a greater than 90% patient satisfaction rate. Though, hysterectomy has a higher rate of urinary tract injuries, particularly abdominal hysterectomy. When myomectomies are performed to preserve fertility, care must be taken to avoid adhesions, which may compromise the goal of the operation. In the past, full-thickness myomectomies (surgeries that entered the endometrial cavity) were considered an indication for cesarean delivery prior to labor. Currently, most clinicians recommend strong consideration for cesarean section for all degrees of myomectomy other than removal of a pedunculated leiomyomata, or small hysteroscopic resection.

Classic indications for a myomectomy include persistent abnormal bleeding, pain or pressure, or enlargement of an asymptomatic myoma to more than 8 cm in a woman who has not completed childbearing. The causal relationship of myomas and adverse reproductive outcomes is poorly understood. Long-standing infertility or repetitive abortion directly related to myomas is rare. Contraindications to a myomectomy include pregnancy, advanced adnexal disease, malignancy, and the situation in which enucleation of the myoma would severely reduce endometrial surface so that the uterus would not be functional. The choice between the two operations is not always an easy one. To quote Richard TeLinde, "All indications and contraindications in medicine are relative, a fact that is especially true when one considers hysterectomy versus myomectomy."

Within 20 years of the myomectomy operation, one in four women subsequently has a hysterectomy performed, the majority for recurrent leiomyomas. Myomectomy may be performed in selected women using laparoscopic techniques. Hurst and associates have emphasized careful, multilayer closure and the use of antiadhesive barriers. Some centers excise uterine myomas vaginally using an anterior or posterior colpotomy. They believe that vaginal myomectomy is an alternative surgical plan even in women with moderately enlarged tumors. Submucous myomas may be resected via the cervical canal using the hysteroscope. Although preliminary studies using laser surgery have been reported, most investigators advocate using an operative resectoscope. Three out of four women have long-term relief of their menorrhagia secondary to uterine myomas following hysteroscopic resection of the myomas.

The indications for hysterectomy for myomas are similar to indications for myomectomy, with a few additions. Some gynecologists selectively perform a hysterectomy for asymptomatic myomas when the uterus has reached the size of a 14- to 16-week gestation. The hypothesis is that most myomas of this size will eventually produce symptoms. However, it is impossible to predict which individual woman will develop symptoms. A previously mentioned indication for hysterectomy is rapid growth of a myoma after the menopause. Prolapse of a myoma through the cervix is optimally treated by vaginal removal and ligation of the base of the myoma, with antibiotic coverage. Hysteroscopic resection aids the transvaginal removal of a prolapsed myoma.

It is possible to treat leiomyomas medically by reducing the circulating level of estrogen and progesterone. GnRH agonists, medroxyprogesterone acetate (Depo-Provera), danazol, aromatase inhibitors, and the antiprogesterone RU 486 have undergone clinical trials. Randomized controlled trials of 5 and 10 mg of mifepristone (RU486) have shown significant reduction in size, bleeding, and improvement in quality of life. The use of GnRH agonists, sometimes with add-back hormonal therapy, has also been successful in treating myomas. Reductions in mean uterine volume and myoma size by 40% to 50% has been documented. However, individual responses vary greatly. With medical treatments, the majority of the reduction in size occurs within the first 3 months. After cessation of therapy, myomas gradually resume their pretreatment size. By 6 months after treatment, most myomas will have returned to their original size. During treatment, Doppler flow studies have demonstrated increased resistance in the uterine arteries and in the smaller arteries feeding the myoma. Also during treatment, the proliferative activity of the myoma and binding of epidermal growth factor is reduced. The use of medical suppressive therapies such as GnRH agonists for women with large myomas and those with anemia may reduce blood loss at the time of hysterectomy or myomectomy. However, one study found that tourniquets at the time of myomectomy were as effective as pretreatment with GnRH agonists in decreasing blood loss. Aromatase inhibitors are also successful for pretreatment and have fewer side effects.

Uterine myomas may also be treated with uterine artery embolization (UAE). Multiple embolic materials have been used including gelatin sponge (Gelfoam) silicone spheres, gelatin microspheres, metal coils, and most commonly polyvinyl alcohol (PVA) particles of various diameters. Postprocedural abdominal and pelvic pain is common for the first 24 hours and may last up to 2 weeks. Most patients remain overnight in the hospital for pain relief and observation; however, some women will go home a few hours after treatment. Large trials, including the EMMY trial (Uterine Artery Embolization for Treatment of Symptomatic Uterine Fibroid Tumors), have consistently documented shorter hospitalizations and shorter recoveries, with a similar complication rate to hysterectomy. Reviews of the large trials and reports find that the need for reoperation within the first few years after embolization is 20% to 30%, with an overall failure rate of 40%, failure rate being defined as a return of symptoms and decrement in quality of life measures. The 5-year failure rate from the EMMY trial as reported by van der Kooij et al. included a 28.4% subsequent hysterectomy rate. Risk factors for failure with UAE included younger age at embolization, bleeding as an indication for therapy, multiple myomas, and the finding at the time of imaging of collateral ovarian vessels feeding the myoma. Thus, the procedure itself, though a valuable alternative to hysterectomy, is not for all women, with such a significant proportion of women needing follow-up procedures.

Fertility after arterial embolization is difficult to quantify. Higher than expected rates of intrauterine growth restriction, preterm delivery, and miscarriage have been reported. In general, women choosing a conservative approach to preserve fertility should have a surgical myomectomy rather than UAE.

Complications of UAE affect about 5% of patients, and include postembolization fever; sepsis from infarction of the necrotic myometrium, which may occur several weeks to a few months post procedure; and ovarian failure, affecting up to 3% of cases in women younger than 45 and 15% in women older than 45. This is thought to occur from spread of emboli material into the ovarian circulation. There is, in general, a decreased ovarian reserve found in older women after embolization. Amenorrhea may occur secondary to an endometrial hypoxic injury, as well. Rarely, necrosis of surrounding tissues may present as a complication of embolization.

Another complication of UAE is shedding of necrotic myomata or portions of myomata into the intrauterine cavity. Shedding may lead to infection or abdominal pain as the uterus tries to pass the material. This may require either a uterine curettage or hysteroscopic removal, although some authors have reported removing the necrotic material in the office. Because shedding of necrotic material is a relatively common complication, several authors have recommended that submucous myomata be removed hysteroscopically rather than attempted through UAE because these types of myomata are more prone to be shed into the uterine cavity. Intra-abdominal adhesions, particularly after embolization of larger myomata, are also an uncommon but not rare complication.

Two associated but rare diseases should be noted: **intravenous leiomyomatosis** and **leiomyomatosis peritonealis disseminata**. *Intravenous leiomyomatosis* is a rare condition in which benign smooth muscle fibers invade and slowly grow into the venous channels of the pelvis (**Fig. 18-38**). The tumor grows by direct extension and grossly appears like a "spaghetti" tumor. Only 25% of tumors extend beyond the broad ligament. However, case series and reports document tumor growth into the vena cava and right heart. The tumors may present with cardiac symptomatology and usually require surgical resection. Series from Zhang et al. and Worley et al. noted good results with single staged surgeries. Most authors recommend antiestrogen therapy with aromatase inhibitors after resection of leiomyomatosis of any degree.

Leiomyomatosis peritonealis disseminata (LPD) is a benign disease with multiple small nodules over the surface of the pelvis and abdominal peritoneum. Grossly, LPD mimics disseminated carcinoma (**Fig. 18-39**). However, histologic examination demonstrates benign-appearing myomas (**Fig. 18-40**). This disorder is often associated with a recent pregnancy. Therapies with progestogens, SERMs, or aromatase inhibitors have all been used in management. A rare autosomal syndrome of uterine and cutaneous leiomyomata and renal cell carcinoma also exists. Consideration should be given to renal evaluation in families with this history and with cutaneous leiomyomas.

In summary, leiomyomas are the most common tumor in women, and certainly one of the most common problems facing

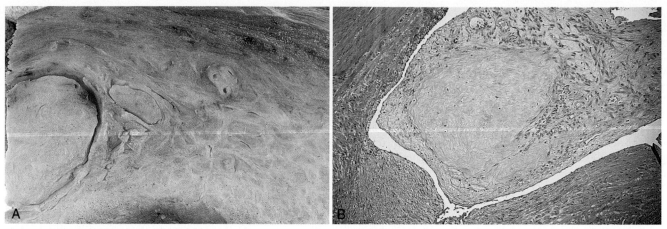

Figure 18-38 Intravenous leiomyomatosis. **A,** Tumor masses are present within distended blood vessels. **B,** This example shows hyaline degeneration of the intravascular element. (From Anderson MC, Robboy SJ, Russell P: Uterine smooth muscle tumors. In Robboy SJ, Anderson MC, Russell P [eds]: Pathology of the Female Reproductive Tract. Edinburgh, Churchill Livingstone, 2002.)

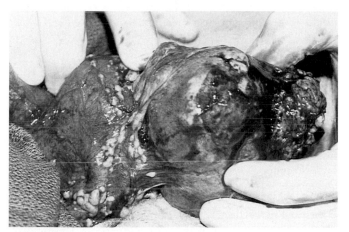

Figure 18-39 Photograph of leiomyomatosis peritonealis disseminate. (Courtesy of William Droegemueller and Vern L. Katz.)

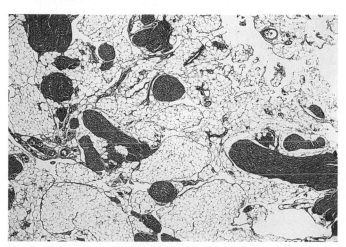

Figure 18-40 Peritoneal leiomyomatosis. Multiple tiny nodules of smooth muscle are scattered throughout the omentum. (From Anderson MC, Robboy SJ, Russell P: Uterine smooth muscle tumors. In Robboy SJ, Anderson MC, Russell P [eds]: Pathology of the Female Reproductive Tract. Edinburgh, Churchill Livingstone, 2002.)

the gynecologist. Symptoms will present in 30% to 50% of women with myomata. Management is individualized to fit the patient's symptoms and reproductive desires.

ADENOMYOSIS

Adenomyosis has often been referred to as *endometriosis interna.* This term is misleading because endometriosis and adenomyosis are discovered in the same patient in less than 20% of women. More important, endometriosis and adenomyosis are clinically different diseases. The only common feature is the presence of ectopic endometrial glands and stroma. Adenomyosis is derived from aberrant glands of the basalis layer of the endometrium. Therefore, these glands do not usually undergo the traditional proliferative and secretory changes that are associated with cyclic ovarian hormone production. The disease is common and may be found in up to 60% of hysterectomy specimens in women in the late reproductive years. Most studies have documented an incidence closer to 30%, with greater than 50% of these women being relatively asymptomatic. The symptoms of menorrhagia and dysmenorrhea form a spectrum and are subjective, thus delineating an incidence of associated symptomatology with adenomyosis is problematic.

Adenomyosis is usually diagnosed incidentally by the pathologist examining histologic sections of surgical specimens. The frequency of the histologic diagnosis is directly related to how meticulously the pathologist searches for the disease. Adenomyosis is also a common incidental finding during autopsy. Serial histologic slides confirm the continuity of benign growth of the basalis layer of the endometrium into the myometrium. Thus, the histogenesis of adenomyosis is direct extension from the endometrial lining.

The disease is associated with increased parity, particularly uterine surgeries and traumas. The pathogenesis of adenomyosis is unknown but is theorized to be associated with disruption of the barrier between the endometrium and myometrium as an initiating step. Parazzini and colleagues noted a 1.7 RR (1.1 to 2.6) of a dilation and curettage with an SAB in women with adenomyosis versus control subjects. Other studies have found a higher rate of induced abortion with presumed curettage in women with adenomyosis versus controls. Panganamamula and associates noted the history of any prior uterine surgery to be a significant risk factor in a set of 412 women with adenomyosis, RR 1.37 (1.05 to 1.79). These studies and experimental work in animals strongly support the theory that trauma to the endometrial-myometrial interface is a significant factor in the etiology of this condition. However, because adenomyosis was described well before uterine curettage and may occur (though uncommonly) in nulliparous women, the full pathogenesis is yet to be determined.

PATHOLOGY

There are two distinct pathologic presentations of adenomyosis. The most common is a diffuse involvement of both anterior and posterior walls of the uterus. The posterior wall is usually involved more than the anterior wall (**Fig. 18-41**). The individual areas of adenomyosis are not encapsulated. The second presentation is a focal area or adenomyoma. This results in an asymmetrical uterus, and this special area of adenomyosis may have a pseudocapsule. Diffuse adenomyosis is found in two thirds of cases.

In the more common, diffuse type of adenomyosis the uterus is uniformly enlarged, usually two to three times normal size. It is often difficult to distinguish on physical examination from uterine leiomyomas. However, the ultrasound appearance of leiomyomata helps to distinguish the two. Similarly on visual inspection the two entities are quite different. When a knife transects the myometrium, the cut surface protrudes convexly and has a spongy appearance. The cut surface of a uterus with adenomyosis is darker than the white surface of a myoma. Sometimes there are discrete areas of adenomyosis that are not densely encapsulated and contain small, dark cystic spaces. There is not a distinct cleavage plane around focal adenomyomas as there is with uterine myomas.

Histologic examination will note benign endometrial glands, and stromata are within the myometrium. These glands rarely undergo the same cyclic changes as the normal uterine endometrium. Studies have demonstrated both estrogen and progesterone receptors in tissue samples from adenomyosis.

The standard criterion used in diagnosis of adenomyosis is the finding of endometrial glands and stroma more than one low-powered field (2.5 mm) from the basalis layer of the endometrium. The small areas of adenomyosis have the same general appearance as the basalis layers of the endometrium. Histologically the glands exhibit an inactive or proliferative pattern. Rarely, one sees cystic hyperplasia or a pseudodecidual pattern. In general there is a lack of inflammatory cells surrounding the fossae of adenomyosis. Although the areas do not undergo full menstrual-type changes, bleeding may occur in these ectopic areas, as evidenced by both gross and microscopic findings. It is not unusual to see histologic variability in several different areas deep in the walls of the myometrium from the same uterus. Some fossae of adenomyosis undergo decidual changes either during pregnancy or during estrogen-progestin therapy for endometriosis. The reaction of the myometrium to the ectopic endometrium is hyperplasia and hypertrophy of individual muscle fibers (**Figs. 18-41** and **18-42**). Surrounding most foci of glands and stroma are localized areas of hyperplasia of the smooth muscle of the uterus. This change in the myometrium produces the globular enlargement of the uterus (see **Fig. 18-42**).

CLINICAL DIAGNOSIS

Over 50% of women with adenomyosis are asymptomatic or have minor symptoms that do not annoy them enough to seek medical care. They attribute the increase in dysmenorrhea or menstrual bleeding to the aging process and tolerate the symptoms. Symptomatic adenomyosis usually presents in women between the ages of 35 and 50. The severity of pelvic symptoms increases proportionally to the depth of penetration and the total volume of disease in the myometrium.

The classic symptoms of adenomyosis are secondary dysmenorrhea and menorrhagia. The acquired dysmenorrhea becomes increasingly more severe as the disease progresses. Occasionally the patient complains of dyspareunia, which is midline in location and deep in the pelvis. On pelvic examination the uterus is diffusely enlarged, usually two to three times normal size. It is most unusual for the uterine enlargement associated with adenomyosis to be greater than a 14-week-size gestation unless the patient also has uterine myomas. The uterus is globular and tender immediately before and during menstruation (**Fig. 18-43**). LevGur and colleagues evaluated the gynecologic histories of women with diffuse adenomyosis compared with women without such a history. In their series, the symptoms of dysmenorrhea and menorrhagia correlated with the amount of adenomyosis and the depth of myometrial invasion.

The diagnosis of adenomyosis is usually confirmed following histologic examination of the hysterectomy specimen. Frequently the clinical diagnosis is inaccurately assigned to the patient who has chronic pelvic pain. Traditionally the patient will have endometrial sampling to rule out other organic causes of abnormal bleeding. Many times adenomyosis is diagnosed retrospectively following a hysterectomy for other indications. Attempts have been made to establish the diagnosis preoperatively by transcervical needle biopsy of the myometrium. However, even with multiple needle biopsies, the sensitivity of the test is too low to be of practical clinical value. Adenomyosis may coexist with both endometrial hyperplasia and endometrial

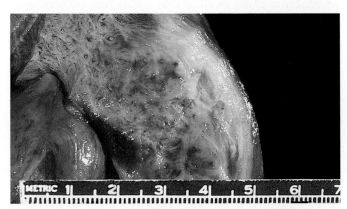

Figure 18-41 Adenomyosis. The myometrial wall is distorted and thickened by poorly circumscribed trabeculae that contain pinpoint hemorrhagic cysts. (From Anderson MC, Robboy SJ, Russell P: Uterine smooth muscle tumors. In Robboy SJ, Anderson MC, Russell P [eds]: Pathology of the Female Reproductive Tract. Edinburgh, Churchill Livingstone, 2002.)

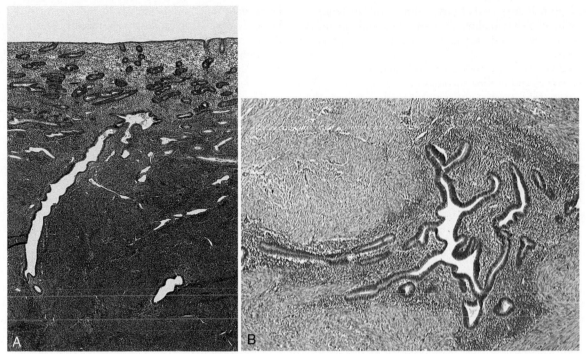

Figure 18-42 Adenomyosis, histologic appearance. **A,** Endometrial tissue infiltrates into the myometrium. **B,** The infiltrating islands of endometrium consist of both glands and stroma. The glands are inactive and of basal pattern. (From Anderson MC, Robboy SJ, Russell P: Uterine smooth muscle tumors. In Robboy SJ, Anderson MC, Russell P [eds]: Pathology of the Female Reproductive Tract. Edinburgh, Churchill Livingstone, 2002.)

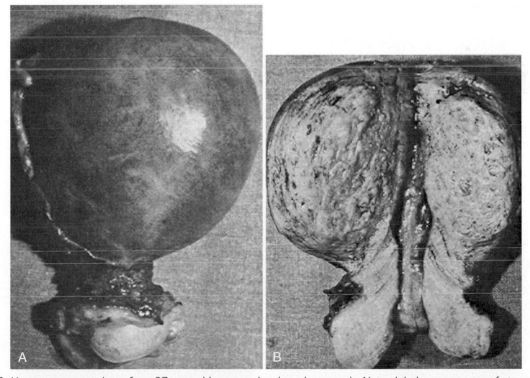

Figure 18-43 A, Hysterectomy specimen from 37-year-old woman showing adenomyosis. Note globular appearance of uterus. **B,** Bisection of posterior wall of uterus. (From Emge LA: The elusive adenomyosis of the uterus: Its historical past and its present state of recognition. Am J Obstet Gynecol 83:1551, 1962.)

carcinoma. Approximately two of three women with adenomyosis have coexistent pelvic pathology, most commonly myomas but also endometriosis, endometrial hyperplasia, and salpingitis isthmica nodosa.

Ultrasound and MRI are both useful to help differentiate between adenomyosis and uterine myomas in a young woman desiring future childbearing. Diagnosing adenomyosis by transvaginal ultrasonography has a reported sensitivity between 53% and 89% and a specificity of 50% to 89%. In some series, MRI is more sensitive, ranging between 88% and 93%, and has a higher specificity (66% to 91%) than ultrasonography in the diagnosis of adenomyosis. Recently, Verma et al. have reported the addition of sonohysterography with vaginal ultrasound, with an increase in sensitivity and specificity comparable with MRI. T2-weighted images are superior in making the diagnosis and documenting widened junctional zones. Findings of poorly defined junctional zone markings in the endometrial-myometrial interface help confirm the diagnosis. Ascher and coworkers describe high signal intensity striations emanating from the endometrium and trailing into the myometrium as helpful findings. These bands most likely represent the glands and hypertrophied muscle of adenomyosis. MRI is clinically useful in differentiating adenomyosis from uterine leiomyoma, especially preoperatively in women who desire future fertility or who may choose uterine artery embolization for treatment of myomata. The success of uterine artery embolization for adenomyosis is unproved.

MANAGEMENT

There is no satisfactory proved medical treatment for adenomyosis. Patients with adenomyosis have been treated with GnRH agonists, progestogens, and progesterone-containing IUDs, cyclic hormones, or prostaglandin synthetase inhibitors for their abnormal bleeding and pain. Hysterectomy is the definitive treatment if this therapy is appropriate for the woman's age, parity, and plans for future reproduction. Size of the uterus, degree of prolapse, and presence of associated pelvic pathology determine the choice of surgical approach. For the woman in her late 40s, the ovaries are often removed as a risk-reducing measure against ovarian carcinoma. Women who become pregnant with adenomyosis are at increased risks of pregnancy complications. Juang et al. noted an increase in premature labor and delivery, low birthweight, and preterm premature rupture of membranes in a large case-control series of women with adenomyosis.

OVIDUCT

LEIOMYOMAS

Both benign and malignant tumors of the oviduct are uncommon compared with other gynecologic neoplasms. Although these tumors are underreported, fewer than 100 women with myomas or leiomyomas of the oviduct are described in the literature. Tubal leiomyomas may be single or multiple and usually are discovered in the interstitial portion of the tubes. They usually coexist with the more common uterine leiomyomas. Myomas may originate from muscle cells in the walls of the tube or blood vessels or from smooth muscle in the broad ligament.

Leiomyomas of the tube present as smooth, firm, mobile, usually nontender masses that may be palpated during the bimanual examination. Similar to uterine myomas, they may be subserosal, interstitial, or submucosal. During laparoscopy the myomas appear as a spherical mass that protrudes from beneath the peritoneal surface. They vary from a few millimeters to 15 cm in diameter. Histologically they are identical to uterine leiomyomas.

The majority of the myomas of the oviduct are asymptomatic. Rarely, they may undergo acute degeneration or be associated with unilateral tubal obstruction or torsion. Treatment of a symptomatic tubal leiomyoma is excision.

ADENOMATOID TUMORS

The most prevalent benign tumor of the oviduct is the *angiomyoma* or *adenomatoid tumor* (**Fig. 18-44**). They are small, gray-white, circumscribed nodules, 1 to 2 cm in diameter. These tumors are usually unilateral and present as small nodules just under the tubal serosa. These small nodules do not produce pelvic symptoms or signs. These benign tumors also are found below the serosa of the fundus of the uterus and the broad ligament. Microscopically, they are composed of small tubules lined by a low cuboidal or flat epithelium. Histologic studies have established that the thin-walled channels that comprise these tumors are of mesothelial origin (**Fig. 18-45**). These tumors do not become malignant; however, they may be mistaken for a low-grade neoplasm when initially viewed during a frozen-section evaluation.

PARATUBAL CYSTS

Paratubal cysts are frequently incidental discoveries during gynecologic operations for other abnormalities. They are often multiple and may vary from 0.5 cm to more than 20 cm in diameter. Most cysts are small, asymptomatic, and slow growing and are discovered during the third and fourth decades of life. When paratubal cysts are *pedunculated* and near the fimbrial end of the oviduct, they are called **hydatid cysts of Morgagni** (**Figs. 18-46** and **18-47**). Cysts near the oviduct may be of mesonephric,

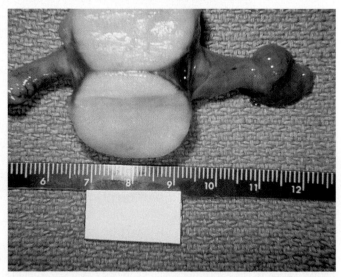

Figure 18-44 Adenomatoid tumor. (From Anderson MC, Robboy SJ, Russell P: The fallopian tube. In Robboy SJ, Anderson MC, Russell P [eds]: Pathology of the Female Reproductive Tract. Edinburgh, Churchill Livingstone, 2002.)

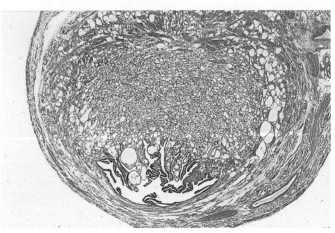

Figure 18-45 Adenomatoid tumor arising in the fallopian tube. (From Voet RL: Color Atlas of Obstetric and Gynecologic Pathology. St. Louis, Mosby-Wolfe, 1997.)

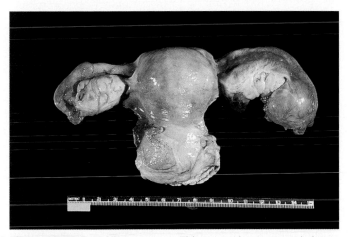

Figure 18-46 Broad ligament cyst. This parovarian, or paratubal cyst, is thin walled and contains clear watery fluid. (From Anderson MC, Robboy SJ, Russell P: The fallopian tube. In Robboy SJ, Anderson MC, Russell P [eds]: Pathology of the Female Reproductive Tract. Edinburgh, Churchill Livingstone, 2002.)

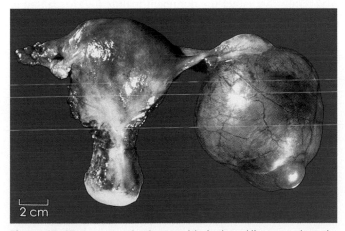

Figure 18-47 A nonneoplastic cyst with the broad ligament abuts the normal ovary. (From Clement PB, Young RH: Atlas of Gynecologic Surgical Pathology. Philadelphia, Saunders, 2000.)

mesothelial, or paramesonephric origin. Sometimes the histologic differentiation is difficult because of mechanically produced changes in the cells that line the cyst. These cysts are translucent and contain a clear or pale yellow fluid.

The histogenesis of the majority of paratubal cysts had been believed to be from the mesonephric duct, with the cysts arising from the main duct or accessory tubules. These latter cysts often develop between the leaves of the broad ligament in the mesosalpinx, with the ovary being separate. However, a histologic study of 79 paratubal cysts by Samaha and Woodruff has documented that 60 of the cysts were of tubal origin. Thus, the majority of grossly identified "paratubal cysts" are in reality accessory lumina of the fallopian tubes. The remaining 19 cysts in Samaha and Woodruff's series were of mesothelial origin. Paratubal cysts are thin walled and smooth and contain clear fluid. Often there are multiple small cysts. Occasionally there is a papillomatous proliferation on the internal wall of these cysts. Inflammatory cysts of the peritoneum may be found anywhere in the pelvis.

The majority of paratubal cysts are asymptomatic and are usually discovered incidentally during ultrasound or during gynecologic operations. When paratubal cysts are symptomatic, they generally produce a dull pain. During a pelvic examination it is difficult to distinguish a paratubal cyst from an ovarian mass. At operation the oviduct is often found stretched over a large paratubal cyst. The oviduct should not be removed in these cases because it will return to normal size after the paratubal cyst is excised. Stein and associates recently reported a retrospective 10-year review of 168 women with parovarian tumors. Three low-grade malignant neoplasms were found in this series. These malignancies were in women of reproductive age who had cysts greater than 5 cm in diameter with internal papillary projections. The authors cautioned that the differentiation between benign and malignant parovarian masses cannot be made by external examination of the cyst. The practice of aspirating cysts via the laparoscope should be limited to cysts that are completely simple and associated with normal cancer antigen-125 (CA-125) levels.

Paratubal cysts may grow rapidly during pregnancy, and most of the cases of torsion of these cysts have been reported during pregnancy or the puerperium. Treatment is simple excision.

TORSION

Acute torsion of the oviduct is a rare event; however, it has been reported with both normal and pathologic fallopian tubes. Pregnancy predisposes to this problem. Tubal torsion usually accompanies torsion of the ovary, as they have a common vascular pedicle. (See the discussion of ovarian torsion later in this chapter.) Torsion of the fallopian tube is secondary to an ovarian mass in approximately 50% to 60% of patients. The right tube is involved more frequently than is the left (**Fig. 18-48**). The degree of tubal torsion varies from less than one turn to four complete rotations. Torsion of the oviduct is usually seen in women of reproductive age. However, it occurs also in preadolescent children, especially when part of the tube is enclosed in the sac of a femoral or inguinal hernia.

Tubal torsion may be divided into intrinsic and extrinsic causes. Prominent intrinsic causes include congenital abnormalities, such as increased tortuosity caused by excessive length of the tube, and pathologic processes, such as hydrosalpinx, hematosalpinx, tubal neoplasms, and previous operation, especially

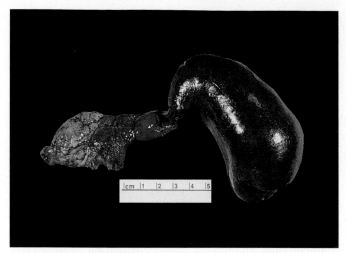

Figure 18-48 Hematosalpinx with torsion. (From Voet RL: Color Atlas of Obstetric and Gynecologic Pathology. St. Louis, Mosby-Wolfe, 1997.)

tubal ligation. Torsion of the fallopian tube following tubal ligation is usually of the distal end. Extrinsic causes of tubal torsion are ovarian and peritubal tumors, adhesions, trauma, and pregnancy.

The most important symptom of tubal torsion is acute lower abdominal and pelvic pain. The onset of this pain may be gradual or sudden, and the pain is usually located in the iliac fossa, with radiation to the thigh and flank. The duration of pain is generally less than 48 hours, and it is associated with nausea and vomiting in two thirds of the cases. Usually, the pelvic pain, secondary to hypoxia, is so intense that it is difficult to perform an adequate pelvic exam. Unless there is associated torsion of the ovary, a specific mass is usually not palpable on pelvic examination.

The preoperative diagnosis of tubal torsion is made in less than 20% of reported cases. However, the number of cases diagnosed preoperatively has increased dramatically with the use of vaginal ultrasonography. Because of the severity of the pain, a wide differential diagnosis of abdominal and pelvic pathology must be considered. The differential diagnosis includes acute appendicitis, ectopic pregnancy, pelvic inflammatory disease, and rupture or torsion of an ovarian cyst.

Exploratory operation determines the extent of hypoxia and the choice of operative techniques. With tubal torsion, usually the tubes are gangrenous and must be excised. The twisted tube is usually filled with a bloody or serous fluid. It may be possible to restore normal circulation to the tube by manually untwisting it. The tube is usually sutured into a secure position to prevent recurrence.

OVARY

Ovarian masses are a frequent finding on pelvic examination and pelvic imaging. The task of the clinician is to determine whether the mass should be removed or may be managed expectantly. The very general factors used to consider removal include the symptoms produces by the mass, the chances that the mass is malignant, and the likelihood of spontaneous resolution.

FUNCTIONAL CYSTS

Follicular Cysts

Follicular cysts are by far the most frequent cystic structures in normal ovaries. They may be found as early as 20 weeks gestation in female fetuses and throughout a woman's reproductive life. Follicular cysts are frequently multiple and may vary from a few millimeters to as large as 15 cm in diameter. A normal follicle may develop into a physiologic cyst. A minimum diameter to be considered as a cyst is generally considered to be between 2.5 and 3 cm. Follicular cysts are not neoplastic and are believed to be dependent on gonadotropins for growth. They arise from a temporary variation of a normal physiologic process. Clinically they may present with the signs and symptoms of ovarian enlargement and therefore must be differentiated from a true ovarian neoplasm. Functional cysts may be solitary or multiple. These cysts are found most commonly in young, menstruating women. Solitary cysts may occur during the fetal and neonatal periods and rarely during childhood, but there is an increase in frequency during the perimenarcheal period. Wolf and coworkers studied 149 postmenopausal women and found simple cysts ranging in size from 0.4 to 4.7 cm in 15% of them. Large solitary follicular cysts in which the lining is luteinized are occasionally discovered during pregnancy and the puerperium. CA-125 may be used to evaluate such cysts in pregnancy. The values for CA-125 should be within the normal range past 12 weeks' gestation. Multiple follicular cysts in which the lining is luteinized are associated with either intrinsic or extrinsic elevated levels of gonadotropins. Interestingly, reproductive-age women with cystic fibrosis appear to have an increased propensity for developing individual follicular cysts.

Follicular cysts are translucent, thin-walled, and are filled with a watery, clear to straw-colored fluid. If a small opening in the capsule of the cyst suddenly develops, the cyst fluid under pressure will squirt out. These cysts are situated in the ovarian cortex, and sometimes they appear as translucent domes on the surface of the ovary. Histologically the lining of the cyst is usually composed of a closely packed layer of round, plump granulosa cells, with the spindle-shaped cells of the theca interna deeper in the stroma. In many cysts the lining of granulosa cells is difficult to distinguish, having undergone pressure atrophy. All that remains is a hyalinized connective tissue lining. The temporary disturbance in follicular function that produces the clinical picture of a follicular cyst is poorly understood. Follicular cysts may result from either the dominant mature follicle's failing to rupture (persistent follicle) or an immature follicle's failing to undergo the normal process of atresia. In the latter circumstance, the incompletely developed follicle fails to reabsorb follicular fluid. Some follicular cysts lose their ability to produce estrogen, and in others the granulosa cells remain productive, with prolonged secretion of estrogens. Occasionally, follicular cysts are better termed **follicular hematomas**, because blood from the vascular theca zone fills the cavity of the cyst.

Most follicular cysts are asymptomatic and are discovered during ultrasound imaging of the pelvis or a routine pelvic examination. Ultrasound cannot differentiate absolutely a benign from a malignant process. However, several characteristics of ovarian masses correlate with malignancy, including septations, internal papillations (echogenic structures protruding into the mass), loculations, solid lesions or cystic lesions with solid components, and smaller cysts adjacent to or part of the wall of the larger cyst–daughter cysts (**Fig. 18-49**).

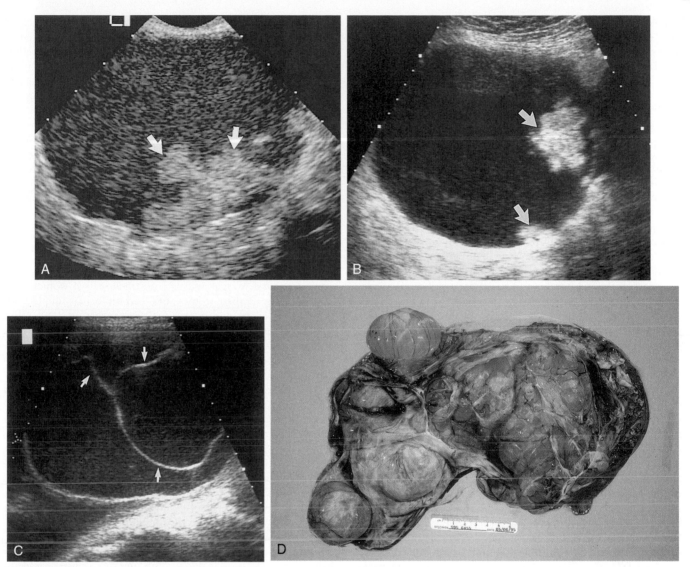

Figure 18-49 Serous cystadenocarcinoma, varying appearances. **A,** Transvaginal scan shows large cystic mass containing multiple low-level internal echoes and solid echogenic components (*arrows*). **B,** Transabdominal scan shows large cystic mass with irregular solid echogenic mural nodules (*arrows*) and low-level internal echoes. **C,** Mucinous cystadenoma. Transabdominal scan shows large cystic mass with multiple thin septations (*arrows*) and fine low-level internal echoes. **D,** Gross pathologic specimen shows multiple cystic loculations. (From Salem S: The uterus and adnexa. In Rumack CM, Wilson SR, Charboneau JW [eds]: Diagnostic Ultrasound. St. Louis, Mosby, 1998, pp 555-556.)

These cysts may rupture during examination, because of their thin walls. The patient may experience tenesmus, a transient pelvic tenderness, deep dyspareunia, or no pain whatsoever. Rarely is significant intraperitoneal bleeding associated with the rupture of a follicular cyst. However, women who are chronically anticoagulated or those with von Willebrand's disease may bleed. Occasionally, menstrual irregularities and abnormal uterine bleeding may be associated with follicular cysts, which produce elevated blood estrogen levels. The syndrome associated with such follicular cysts consists of a regular cycle with a prolonged intermenstrual interval, followed by episodes of menorrhagia. Some women with larger follicular cysts notice a vague, dull sensation or heaviness in the pelvis.

The initial management of a suspected follicular cyst is conservative observation. The majority of follicular cysts disappear spontaneously by either reabsorption of the cyst fluid or silent rupture within 4 to 8 weeks of initial diagnosis. However, a persistent ovarian mass necessitates operative intervention to differentiate a physiologic cyst from a true neoplasm of the ovary. There is no way to make the differentiation on the basis of signs, symptoms, or the initial growth pattern during early development of either process. Endovaginal ultrasound examination is helpful in differentiating simple from complex cysts and is also helpful during conservative management by providing dimensions to determine if the cyst is increasing in size. When the diameter of the cyst remains stable for greater than 10 weeks or enlarges, a neoplasia should be ruled out. Oral contraceptives may be prescribed for 4 to 6 weeks for young women with adnexal masses. This therapy removes any influence that pituitary gonadotropins may have on the persistence of the ovarian cyst. It also allows for several weeks of observation. In Spanos's series, 80% of cystic masses 4 to 6 cm in size disappeared during the time the patient was taking oral contraceptives. Steinkampf and colleagues performed a randomized prospective study of the effect of oral contraceptives on functional ovarian masses in women of reproductive age. Their study group consisted of women with infertility who had recently been treated by ovulation induction. In their series there was no difference in the rate of disappearance of functional ovarian cysts between the group that received oral contraceptives and the control group, perhaps because so many cysts will resolve spontaneously.

The evaluation of an asymptomatic cyst, found incidentally, is based on the principle that the cyst should be removed if there is any suspicion of malignancy. Suspicion may develop because of history, including family history, patient age, and other nongynecologic signs and symptoms. The size and physical characteristics of the cyst are as important as are other laboratory parameters. CA-125 is helpful in evaluating the adenexal mass in postmenopausal women. In premenopausal women, CA-125 is rarely helpful unless the mass is extremely suggestive of malignancy. Ultrasound cannot differentiate absolutely a benign from a malignant process. However, several characteristics of ovarian masses correlate with malignancy, including septations; thickness of septations, internal papillations (echogenic structures protruding into the mass), loculations, solid lesions or cystic lesions with solid components, smaller cysts adjacent to or part of the wall of the larger cyst–daughter cysts, bilaterality, and free fluid in the cul de sac (see **Fig. 18-49A-D**). As discussed earlier, measurement of diastolic and systolic velocities provide indirect indices of vascular resistance. Muscular arteries have high resistance. Newly developed vessels, such as those arising in malignancies, have little vascular wall musculature and thus have low resistance. Color flow Doppler is a technique that usually displays shades of red and blue delineating blood flow within a neoplasm. For example, benign ovarian lesions have little color flow. When a color flow Doppler scan does demonstrate vascularity, the vascular resistance can be calculated. Low resistance is associated with malignancy, and high resistance usually is associated with normal tissue or benign disease. Color flow Doppler has been shown to be sensitive in evaluating ovarian malignancy.

The appearance of the other ovary should be noted. Color Doppler indicating vascular resistance is advocated by some authors, but it is neither sensitive nor specific enough to be used as a determining study. In most cases, simple small cysts may be observed. In general, complex cysts or persistent simple cysts larger than 10 cm should be evaluated. In women with cysts in pregnancy, if the cyst is simple with a normal CA-125, conservative management is acceptable. (CA-125 is generally not obtained in pregnant women with cysts less than 5 cm if they are simple.)

A cyst in a perimenopausal or postmenopausal woman should be removed if it is anything other than a simple cyst, if the CA-125 is abnormal (>35), or if the cyst is persistent or large (>10 cm). A small simple cyst in a perimenopausal or postmenopausal woman (<5 cm) with a normal CA-125 may be observed with regular reevaluation including ultrasound. Several studies, including the large prospective series from Greenlee et al., examined the issue of simple cysts in postmenopausal women with simple cysts. These studies have noted that expectant management is safe and reasonable. In the series by Greenlee, The Prostate, Lung, Colorectal, and Ovarian cancer Screening Trial, women were followed for 4 years with transvaginal ultrasound. Of 15,735 women, 2217 (14%) had at least one simple cyst. Cysts were more common in women in the 50- to 59-year-old age group and women with hysterectomies prior to age 40. Cysts were less common among smokers and older women. In all, 54% of cysts were present on scans 1 year later; 8% of women had more than one cyst. Only 0.4% of the entire population developed ovarian cancer, and half of the women who developed cancer did not have cysts. The 14% incidence of cysts in postmenopausal women is similar to rates of simple cysts in other large series. Thus, women with simple cysts who are asymptomatic and with negative CA-125 may be reassured and if desired, followed expectantly. Management of cysts between 5 and 10 cm that are otherwise not suggestive should be individualized. Ekerhovd and coworkers reported on 927 premenopausal women and 377 postmenopausal women with ovarian cysts. Of these women, 660 had unilocular simple cysts, 3 were borderline, and 4 were malignant (total of 1%). All of the borderline and malignant tumors were found in cysts greater than 7.5 cm. In women with cysts that had echodensity and papulations (644 women), 24 (3.7%) turned out to be borderline or malignant. Cysts that were multiseptate were not included in the study. All cysts with internal structures were excised and had a much higher rate of malignancy. The authors, as well as others, have confirmed the recommendation that unilocular cysts less than 5 cm may be followed if there is no family history, a normal CA-125, or other significant findings.

In premenopausal women, operative management of nonmalignant cysts is cystectomy, not oophorectomy. Many clinicians will manage simple cysts with the laparoscope. Because this procedure has an accompanying risk of spilling malignant cells into the peritoneal cavity if the cyst is an early carcinoma, strict preoperative criteria should be fulfilled before laparoscopy is attempted. These include the woman's age; size of the mass; and ultrasound characteristics, such as nonadherent, smooth, and thin-walled cysts, without papillae or internal echoes (simple). DeWilde and associates, reporting on a series of follicular cysts averaging 6 cm in diameter, found that the recurrence rate following laparoscopic fenestration was approximately 2%. Higher rates of recurrence, up to 40%, have been reported for simple drainage of multiple types of benign cysts, the point being that drainage or fenestration is effective for follicular cysts and poorly effective for other cysts. When cysts are drained, it is essential to remember that cytologic examination of cyst fluid has poor predictive value and poor sensitivity in differentiating benign from malignant cysts. One recent report of fine-needle aspiration of ovarian cysts found sensitivity of 25%, specificity of 90%, a false-positive rate of 73%, and a false-negative rate of 12%. If there is any suspicion of malignancy, the cyst should be removed and a histopathologic evaluation obtained. Several investigators have noted that intraoperative spillage is associated with a greater than expected rate of recurrence. The size of the cyst is not a necessary reason to avoid laparoscopy. Most all simple cysts, even those >10 cm, can be managed through the laparoscope.

Corpus Luteum Cysts

Corpus luteum cysts are less common than follicular cysts, but clinically they are more important. This discussion collectively combines corpus luteum cysts and persistently functioning

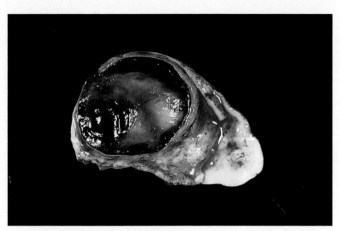

Figure 18-50 Hemorrhagic corpus luteum with an outer yellow rim and central hemorrhage. (From Voet RL: Color Atlas of Obstetric and Gynecologic Pathology. St. Louis, Mosby-Wolfe, 1997.)

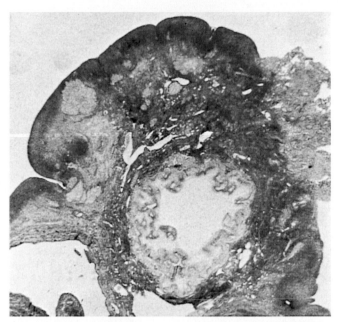

Figure 18-51 Corpus albicans cyst. Lining of cyst is composed of hyalinized connective tissue. (From Blaustein A: Nonneoplastic cysts of the ovary. In Blaustein A [ed]: Pathology of the Female Genital Tract. New York, Springer-Verlag, 1977, p 396.)

mature corpora lutea (**Fig. 18-50**). Pathologists are sometimes able to distinguish between a hemorrhagic cystic corpus luteum and a corpus luteum cyst, but at other times this difference cannot be established. All corpora lutea are cystic with gradual reabsorption of a limited amount of hemorrhage, which may form a cavity. Clinically, corpora lutea are not termed *corpus luteum cysts* unless they are a minimum of 3 cm in diameter. Corpus luteum cysts may be associated with either normal endocrine function or prolonged secretion of progesterone. The associated menstrual pattern may be normal, delayed menstruation, or amenorrhea.

Corpora lutea develop from mature graafian follicles. Intrafollicular bleeding does not occur during ovulation. However, 2 to 4 days later, during the stage of vascularization, thin-walled capillaries invade the granulosa cells from the theca interna. Spontaneous but limited bleeding fills the central cavity of the maturing corpus luteum with blood. Subsequently this blood is absorbed, forming a small cystic space. When the hemorrhage is excessive, the cystic space enlarges. If the hemorrhage into the central cavity is brisk, intracystic pressure increases and rupture of the corpus luteum is a possibility. If rupture does not occur, the size of the resulting corpus luteum cyst usually varies between 3 and 10 cm. Occasionally a cyst may be 11 to 15 cm in diameter. If a cystic central cavity persists, blood is replaced by clear fluid, and the result is a hormonally inactive corpus albicans cyst (**Fig. 18-51**). A corpus luteum of pregnancy is normally 3 to 5 cm in diameter with a central cystic structure, occupying at least 50% of the ovarian mass.

Most corpus luteum cysts are small, the average diameter being 4 cm. Grossly, they have a smooth surface and, depending on whether the cyst represents acute or chronic hemorrhage, are purplish red to brown. When a corpus luteum is cut, the convoluted lining is yellowish orange, and the center contains an organizing blood clot. Both the granulosa and the theca cells undergo luteinization. In chronic corpus luteum cysts, the wall becomes gray-white, and the polygonal luteinized cells usually undergo pressure atrophy. Hallatt and colleagues reviewed 173 ruptured corpora lutea with hemoperitoneum. In their institution the frequency of serious bleeding from a corpus luteum cyst compared with ectopic pregnancy was one in four.

Corpus luteum cysts vary from being asymptomatic masses to those causing catastrophic and massive intraperitoneal bleeding associated with rupture. Many corpus luteum cysts produce dull, unilateral, lower abdominal and pelvic pain. The enlarged ovary is moderately tender on pelvic examination. Depending on the amount of progesterone secretion associated with cysts, the menstrual bleeding may be normal or delayed several days to weeks with subsequent menorrhagia. Halban in 1915 described a syndrome of a persistently functioning corpus luteum cyst that has clinical features similar to an unruptured ectopic pregnancy. Halban's classic triad was a delay in a normal period followed by spotting; unilateral pelvic pain; and a small, tender, adnexal mass. This triad of symptomatology is similar to the triad of an anomalous period or delay in a normal period, spotting, and unilateral pelvic pain that are exhibited by the classic ectopic pregnancy. The differential diagnosis between these two conditions without a sensitive pregnancy test is difficult.

Corpus luteum cysts may cause intraperitoneal bleeding. The amount of bleeding varies from slight to clinically significant hemorrhage, necessitating blood transfusion. Internal bleeding often follows coitus, exercise, trauma, or a pelvic examination. However, episodes of bleeding usually do not recur, which differs from an ectopic pregnancy. Women with a bleeding diathesis or those undergoing chronic warfarin (Coumadin) therapy are especially prone to developing ovarian hemorrhage from a corpus luteum cyst. Bleeding occurs usually between days 20 and 26 of their cycle, and these women have a 31% chance for subsequent hemorrhage from a recurrent corpus luteum cyst. Oral contraceptives are sometimes used to suppress ovulation and avoid recurrent hemorrhage.

Hallatt and colleagues reported that sudden, severe, lower abdominal pain was a prominent symptom in women with hemoperitoneum caused by a ruptured corpus luteum cyst (**Table 18-4**). One of three women also noted unilateral cramping and lower abdominal pain for 1 to 2 weeks before overt rupture. The right ovary was the source of hemorrhage in

Table 18-4 Symptoms of 173 Women with Ruptured Corpus Luteum

Location	Number	Percentage
Right ovary	114	66
Left ovary	56	32
Unknown	3	2
Abdominal pain	173	100
Right ovary	21	72
Left ovary	8	28
Duration		
Less than 24 hours	94	54
1 to 7 days	40	23
Over 7 days	14	8
Unknown	25	15
Nausea or vomiting or diarrhea	60	35

From Hallatt JG, Steele CH Jr, Snyder M: Ruptured corpus luteum with hemoperitoneum: A study of 173 surgical cases. Am J Obstet Gynecol 149:6, 1984.

66% of their series. Tang and coworkers have also reported a right-sided predominance in the incidence of hemorrhage from corpus luteum cysts. They postulated that the difference is related to a higher intraluminal pressure on the right side because of the differences in ovarian vein architecture. Most ruptures occur between days 20 and 26 of the cycle, although in the series of Hallatt and colleagues, 28% of the women had a delay in menses not explained by pregnancy (**Table 18-5**).

The differential diagnosis of a woman with acute pain and suspected ruptured corpus luteum cyst includes ectopic pregnancy, a ruptured endometrioma, and adnexal torsion. A sensitive serum or urinary assay for human chorionic gonadotropin (HCG) will help to differentiate a bleeding corpus luteum from ectopic pregnancy (see Chapter 17). Vaginal ultrasound is useful in establishing a preoperative diagnosis. Culdocentesis has been used in the past to establish the severity of the hemorrhage, but it is rarely necessary today. If the hematocrit of the fluid obtained from the posterior cul-de-sac is greater than 15%, operative therapy becomes a necessity. Cystectomy is the operative treatment of choice, with preservation of the remaining portion of the ovary. In the series by DeWilde and associates reporting on

Table 18-5 Menstrual History in 173 Women with Ruptured Corpus Luteum

Last Menstrual Period to Operation	
Under 14 days	5
14 to 31 days (pregnant = 2)	77
31 to 60 days (pregnant = 15)	56
Over 60 days (pregnant = 10)	18
No menstrual period	14
Hysterectomy	5
Amenorrhea after oral contraceptives	5
Secondary amenorrhea	2
Menarche	1
Menopause	1
History of irregular menses	14
Unknown	3

From Hallatt JG, Steele CH Jr, Snyder M: Ruptured corpus luteum with hemoperitoneum: A study of 173 surgical cases. Am J Obstet Gynecol 149:6, 1984.

persistent corpus luteum cysts treated by fenestration via the laparoscope, 6 of 44 (14%) recurred. Obviously, it was impossible for the authors to distinguish between a recurrent corpus luteum cyst and the development of a new corpus luteum. Unruptured corpus luteum cysts may be followed conservatively. Raziel and coworkers reported on a series of 70 women with ruptured corpora lutea. Ultrasonic evidence of large amounts of peritoneal fluid and severe pain were indications for operative intervention. In 12 of 70 patients with small amounts of intraperitoneal fluid and mild to moderate pain, observation alone was associated with resolution of symptoms.

Theca Lutein Cysts

Theca lutein cysts are by far the least common of the three types of physiologic ovarian cysts (**Fig. 18-52**). Unlike corpus luteum cysts, theca lutein cysts are almost always bilateral and produce moderate to massive enlargement of the ovaries. The individual cysts vary in size from 1 cm to 10 cm or more in diameter. These cysts arise from either prolonged or excessive stimulation of the ovaries by endogenous or exogenous gonadotropins or increased ovarian sensitivity to gonadotropins. The condition of ovarian enlargement secondary to the development of multiple luteinized follicular cysts is termed **hyperreactio luteinalis**. Approximately 50% of molar pregnancies and 10% of choriocarcinomas have associated bilateral theca lutein cysts (Chapter 35, Gestational Trophoblastic Disease). In these patients the HCG from the trophoblast produces luteinization of the cells in immature, mature, and atretic follicles. The cysts are also discovered in the latter months of pregnancies, often with conditions that produce a large placenta, such as twins, diabetes, and Rh sensitization. It is not uncommon to iatrogenically produce theca lutein cysts in women receiving medications to induce ovulation. Theca lutein cysts are occasionally discovered in association with normal pregnancy, as well as in newborn infants secondary to transplacental effects of maternal gonadotropins. Rarely, these cysts are found in young girls with juvenile hypothyroidism.

Grossly the total ovarian size may be voluminous, 20 to 30 cm in diameter, with multiple theca lutein cysts. Bilateral ovarian enlargement is produced by multiple gray to bluish-tinged cysts.

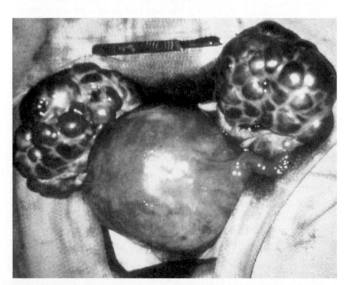

Figure 18-52 Bilateral theca lutein cysts. (Courtesy of Daniel R. Mishell, Jr., MD)

The bilateral enlargement is secondary to hundreds of thin-walled locules or cysts, producing a honeycombed appearance. Grossly the external surface of the ovary appears lobulated. The small cysts contain a clear to straw-colored or hemorrhagic fluid. Histologically the lining of the cyst is composed of theca lutein cells (paralutein cells), believed to originate from ovarian connective tissue. Occasionally there is also luteinization of granulosa cells. These voluminous and congested ovaries are slow growing. The majority of women with smaller cysts are asymptomatic. Generally only the larger cysts produce vague symptoms, such as a sense of pressure in the pelvis. Ascites and increasing abdominal girth have been reported with hyperstimulation from exogenous gonadotropins. Rarely, associated adnexal torsion may occur. Montz and colleagues, in reviewing the natural history of 102 women with theca lutein cysts, found that approximately 1% of patients experienced acute complications of either torsion or intraperitoneal bleeding. They also discovered that theca lutein cysts persisted in some women for weeks after HCG levels were nondetectable.

The presence of theca lutein cysts is established by palpation and often confirmed by ultrasound examination. Treatment is conservative because these cysts gradually regress. If these cysts are discovered incidentally at cesarean delivery, they should be handled delicately. No attempt should be made to drain or puncture the multiple cysts because of the possibility of hemorrhage. Bleeding is difficult to control in these cases because of the thin walls that constitute the cysts.

A condition related to theca lutein cysts is the **luteoma of pregnancy**. The condition is rare and not a true neoplasm but rather a specific, benign, hyperplastic reaction of ovarian theca lutein cells (**Figs. 18-53** and **18-54**). These nodules do not arise from the corpus luteum of pregnancy. Fifty percent of luteomas are multiple, and approximately 30% of those reported have bilateral nodules. In appearance they are discrete and brown to reddish brown and may be solid or cystic.

The majority of patients with luteomas are asymptomatic. The solid, fleshy, often hemorrhagic nodules are discovered incidentally at cesarean delivery or postpartum tubal ligation. Most cases have been reported in multiparous African-American women. Masculinization of the mother occurs in 30% of cases, and masculinization of the external genitalia of the female fetus

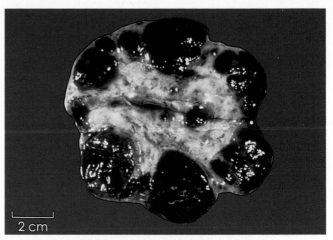

Figure 18-54 Luteoma with multiple reddish nodules. (From Clement PB, Young RH: Atlas of Gynecologic Surgical Pathology. Philadelphia, WB Saunders, 2000.)

may sometimes occur. These tumors regress spontaneously following completion of the pregnancy.

BENIGN NEOPLASMS OF THE OVARY

Benign Cystic Teratoma (Dermoid Cyst, Mature Teratoma)

Benign ovarian teratomas are usually cystic structures that on histologic examination contain elements from all three germ cell layers. The word *teratoma* was first advanced by Virchow and translated literally means "monstrous growth." Teratomas of the ovary may be benign or malignant. Although *dermoid* is a misnomer, it is the most common term used to describe the benign cystic tumor, composed of mature cells, whereas the malignant variety is composed of immature cells (immature teratoma). *Dermoid* is a descriptive term in that it emphasizes the preponderance of ectodermal tissue with some mesodermal and rare endodermal derivatives. Malignant teratomas that are immature are usually solid with some cystic areas and histologically contain immature or embryonic-appearing tissue. (See Chapter 33 [Neoplastic Diseases of the Ovary] for further discussion of malignant teratomas.) Benign teratomas may contain a malignant component, usually in women older than 40. The malignant component is generally a squamous carcinoma and is found in less than 1% of cases. A series of malignancy found in mature teratomas, from Hurwitz et al., noted the mean age of patients to be 48, ranging from 27 to 69. Nonovarian teratomas may arise in any midline structure of the body where the germ cell has resided during embryonic life.

Benign teratomas are among the most common ovarian neoplasms. They account for more than 90% of germ cell tumors of the ovary. These slow-growing tumors occur from infancy to the postmenopausal years. Depending on the series, dermoids represent 20% to 25% of all ovarian neoplasms and approximately 33% of all benign tumors, if follicular and corpus luteum cysts are excluded. Dermoids are the most common ovarian neoplasm in prepubertal females and are also common in teenagers. More than 50% of benign teratomas are discovered in women between the ages of 25 and 50 years. In the series by Lakkis and coworkers of 118 women with dermoids, 86% of the women were younger than 40 years of age, and 3.4% had recurrences (**Fig. 18-55**).

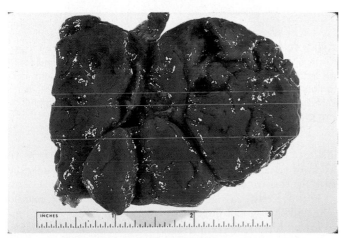

Figure 18-53 Luteoma of pregnancy with numerous solid brown nodules. (From Voet RL: Color Atlas of Obstetric and Gynecologic Pathology. St. Louis, Mosby-Wolfe, 1997.)

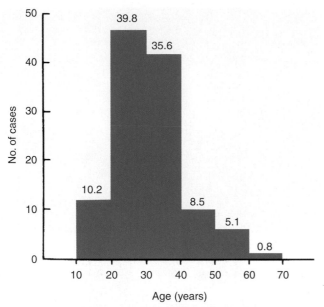

Figure 18-55 Age distribution of cystic teratomas. (From Lakkis WG, Martin MC, Gelfand MM: Benign cystic teratoma of the ovary: A 6-year review. Originally published in Canadian Journal of Surgery 28:444, 1985.)

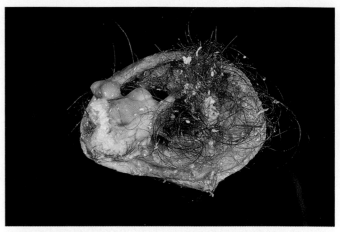

Figure 18-56 Mature cystic teratoma (dermoid cyst) filled with hair and keratinous debris with one solid nodular area (Rokitansky protuberance). (From Voet RL: Color Atlas of Obstetric and Gynecologic Pathology. St. Louis, Mosby-Wolfe, 1997.)

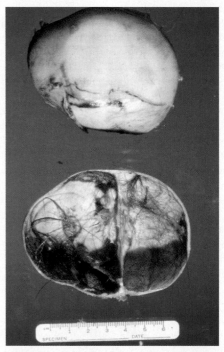

Figure 18-57 Bilateral mature cystic teratomas in pregnancy. The cyst is bilocular. Dermal papillae are noted. Teeth are also present in the left lobule. (From Russell P, Robboy SJ, Anderson MC: Germ cell tumors of the ovaries. In Robboy SJ, Anderson MC, Russell P [eds]: Pathology of the Female Reproductive Tract. Edinburgh, Churchill Livingstone, 2002.)

Similarly, in the series by Comerci and colleagues of 573 tumors in 517 women, the mean age was 32 years and 86% were younger than 43 years of age. With routine obstetric ultrasound, the mean age at diagnosis is expected to fall. In most large series of benign tumors in postmenopausal women, dermoids account for approximately 20% of the neoplasms.

Dermoids vary from a few millimeters to 25 cm in diameter. Comerci and colleagues reported a large tumor weighing 7657 g in a woman who was asymptomatic. However, 80% are less than 10 cm. These tumors may be single or multiple, with as many as nine individual dermoids having been reported in the same ovary. Benign teratomas occur bilaterally 10% to 15% of the time. Often, dermoid cysts are pedunculated. These cysts make the ovary heavier than normal, and thus they are usually discovered either in the cul-de-sac or anterior to the broad ligament. On palpation these tumors, which have both cystic and solid components, have a doughy consistency.

The cysts are usually unilocular. The walls of the cyst are a smooth, shiny, opaque white color. When they are opened, thick sebaceous fluid pours from the cyst, often with tangled masses of hair and firm areas of cartilage and teeth (**Figs. 18-56** and **18-57**). The sebaceous material is a thick fluid at body temperature but solidifies when it cools in room air.

Benign teratomas are believed to arise from a single germ cell after the first meiotic division. Therefore, they develop from totipotential stem cells, and they are neoplastic sequelae from a transformed germ cell. Dermoids have a chromosomal makeup of 46,XX. Linder and coworkers, in a series of experiments using chromosome banding techniques and electrophoretic variance, discovered that the chromosomes of dermoids were different from the chromosomes of the host. They postulated that dermoids began by parthenogenesis from secondary oocytes. An alternative hypothesis was that the dermoid resulted from fusion of the second polar body with the oocyte. The studies by Linder and coworkers ruled out the possibility that dermoids arise from somatic cells or from an oogonium before the first stage of meiosis. The first meiotic division occurs at approximately 13 weeks of gestation. Thus, dermoids begin in fetal life sometime after the first trimester.

Histologically, benign teratomas are composed of mature cells, usually from all three germ layers (**Fig. 18-58**). A combination of skin and skin appendages, including sebaceous glands, sweat glands, hair follicles, muscle fibers, cartilage, bone, teeth, glial cells, and epithelium of the respiratory and gastrointestinal tracts, may be visualized. Teeth are predominantly premolar and molar forms. The fluid in dermoid cysts is usually sebaceous.

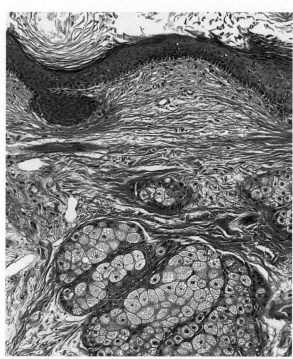

Figure 18-58 Mature cystic teratoma. This cyst is lined by mature epidermis and is subtended by connective tissue containing exuberant dermal appendages (pilosebaceous follicles). (From Russell P, Robboy SJ, Anderson MC: Germ cell tumors of the ovaries. In Robboy SJ, Anderson MC, Russell P [eds]: Pathology of the Female Reproductive Tract. Edinburgh, Churchill Livingstone, 2002.)

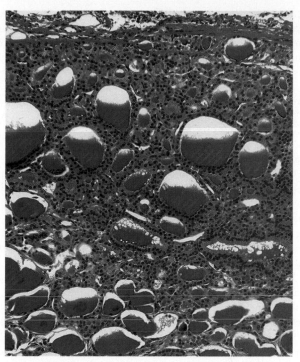

Figure 18-59 Struma ovarii. Variably sized banal thyroid follicles. (From Russell P, Robboy SJ, Anderson MC: Germ cell tumors of the ovaries. In Robboy SJ, Anderson MC, Russell P [eds]: Pathology of the Female Reproductive Tract. Edinburgh, Churchill Livingstone, 2002.)

Most solid elements arise and are contained in a protrusion or nipple (mamilla) in the cyst wall, termed the **prominence or tubercle of Rokitansky**. This prominence may be visualized by ultrasound as an echodense region, thus aiding in the sonographic diagnosis. If malignancy occurs, it is most always found in this nest of cells. The wall of the cyst will often contain granulation tissue, giant cells, and pseudoxanthoma cells.

From 50% to 60% of dermoids are asymptomatic and are discovered during a routine pelvic examination, coincidentally visualized during pelvic imaging, or found incidentally at laparotomy. Presenting symptoms of dermoids include pain and the sensation of pelvic pressure. Specific complications of dermoid cysts include torsion, rupture, infection, hemorrhage, and malignant degeneration. Three medical diseases also may be associated with dermoid cysts: thyrotoxicosis, carcinoid syndrome, and autoimmune hemolytic anemia, the latter two being quite rare.

Adult thyroid tissue is discovered microscopically in approximately 12% of benign teratomas. **Struma ovarii** is a teratoma in which the thyroid tissue has overgrown other elements and is the predominant tissue (**Fig. 18-59**). Strumae ovarii constitute 2% to 3% of ovarian teratomas. These tumors are usually unilateral and measure less than 10 cm in diameter. Less than 5% of women with strumae ovarii develop thyrotoxicosis, which may be secondary to the production of increased thyroid hormone by either the ovarian or the thyroid gland.

Another rare finding with dermoids is the presence of a primary carcinoid tumor from the gastrointestinal or respiratory tract epithelium contained in the dermoid. One of three of these tumors is associated with the typical carcinoid syndrome even without metastatic spread. If the carcinoid is functioning, it may be diagnosed by measuring serum serotonin levels or

urinary levels of 5-hydroxyindoleacetic acid. The autoimmune hemolytic anemia associated with dermoids is the rarest of the three medical complications.

Rupture or perforation of the contents of a dermoid into the peritoneal cavity or an adjacent organ is a potentially serious complication. The incidence varies between 0.7% and 4.6%. However, most series report less than 1%. Rupture is more common in pregnancy. If a rupture occurs during surgery, the abdomen should be copiously irrigated with saline, with careful removal of any particulate matter. Chemical peritonitis is reported in less than 1% of ruptured dermoids. Rupture may occur either catastrophically, which produces an acute abdomen, or by a slow leak of the sebaceous material. The latter is clinically more common, with the sebaceous material producing a severe chemical granulomatous peritonitis. Waxman and Boyce warn that this possibility should be considered and a frozen section obtained so that the true diagnosis is established. Thus, a young woman will not be mistakenly treated for suspected ovarian carcinoma with metastasis because of the identical gross appearance of a slow-leaking dermoid cyst. Infection, hemorrhage, and malignant degeneration are all unusual complications of dermoids, occurring in less than 1% of patients.

Torsion of a dermoid is the most frequent complication, occurring in 11% of the series by Pantoja and associates and 3.5% of the time in Comerci and colleagues' series. Because of its weight, the benign teratoma is often pedunculated, which may predispose to torsion. Torsion is more common in younger women. Small dermoid cysts, less than 6 cm in diameter, grow slowly at an approximate rate of 2 mm per year.

The diagnosis of a dermoid cyst is often established when a semisolid mass is palpated anterior to the broad ligament. Approximately 50% of dermoids have pelvic calcifications on radiographic examination. Often an ovarian teratoma is an incidental finding during radiologic investigation of the genitourinary or gastrointestinal tract. Most dermoids have a characteristic ultrasound picture. These characteristics include a dense echogenic area within a larger cystic area, a cyst filled with bands of mixed echoes, and an echoic dense cyst. Laing and coworkers have found that only one of three dermoids has this "typical picture." In their series of 45 patients with 51 biopsy-proved dermoid cysts, 24% of the dermoid cysts were predominantly solid, 20% were almost entirely cystic, and 24% were not visible. Ultrasound has a more than 95% positive predictive value and a less than 5% false positive rate.

Operative treatment of benign cystic teratomas is cystectomy with preservation of as much normal ovarian tissue as possible. Laparoscopic cystectomy is an accepted approach. Rates of spillage are comparable with that from open laparotomy. However, adequate irrigation in such cases is essential and often more time consuming. Many authors use a 10-cm diameter cutoff as the upper limit for a laparoscopic approach.

When a teratoma is diagnosed incidentally during pregnancy, conservative management is acceptable. Though dermoids have a higher incidence of torsion and potential for rupture during pregnancy, most large series have not shown that an aggressive approach to asymptomatic teratomas, less than 10 cm confers any advantage for the mother or pregnancy. Though laparoscopy is safe during pregnancy, a small periumbilical minilaparotomy may be a faster, less traumatic approach. The treatment is cystectomy, and with the recommendation for reduced intraoperative time this approach may be preferable during pregnancy.

Endometriomas

Endometriosis of the ovary is usually associated with endometriosis in other areas of the pelvic cavity. Approximately two out of three women with endometriosis have ovarian involvement. Interestingly, only 5% of these women have enlargement of the ovaries that is detectable by pelvic examination. However, because of the prevalence of the disease, endometriosis is one of the most common causes of enlargement of the ovary. Because most authors do not classify endometriosis as a neoplastic disease, the diagnosis of endometriosis may not be given due consideration in the differential diagnosis of an adnexal mass. Ovarian endometriosis is similar to endometriosis elsewhere and is described in greater detail in Chapter 19.

The size of ovarian endometriomas varies from small, superficial, blue-black implants that are 1 to 5 mm in diameter to large, multiloculated, hemorrhagic cysts that may be 5 to 10 cm in diameter (**Fig. 18-60**). Clinically, large ovarian endometriomas, greater than 20 cm in diameter, are extremely rare. Areas of ovarian endometriosis that become cystic are termed *endometriomas*. Rarely, large chocolate cysts of the ovary may reach 15 to 20 cm (**Fig. 18-61**). Larger cysts are frequently bilateral. The surface of an ovary with endometriosis is often irregular, puckered, and scarred. Depending on their size, endometriomas replace a portion of the normal ovarian tissue.

Although most women with endometriomas are asymptomatic, the most common symptoms associated with ovarian endometriosis are pelvic pain, dyspareunia, and infertility. Approximately 10% of the operations for endometriosis are for acute symptoms, usually related to a ruptured ovarian endometrioma that was previously asymptomatic. Smaller cysts generally have thin walls, and perforation occurs commonly secondary to cyclic hemorrhage into the cystic cavity.

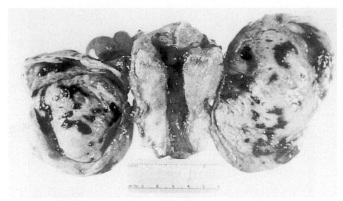

Figure 18-60 Endometriosis of ovaries. Wall of endometriotic cyst is thickened and fibrotic. Inner surface shows areas of dark brown discoloration. (From Janovski NA [ed]: Color Atlas of Gross Gynecologic and Obstetric Pathology. New York, McGraw-Hill, 1969, p 159.)

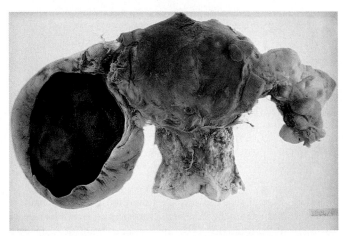

Figure 18-61 "Chocolate cyst" of ovary. The endometrioma is large, but it has not yet completely replaced the ovary. (From Robboy SJ: Endometriosis. In Robboy SJ, Anderson MC, Russell P [eds]: Pathology of the Female Reproductive Tract. Edinburgh, Churchill Livingstone, 2002.)

On pelvic examination, the ovaries are often tender and immobile, secondary to associated inflammation and adhesions. Most commonly the ovaries are densely adherent to surrounding structures, including the peritoneum of the pelvic sidewall, the oviduct, the broad ligament, and sometimes the small or large bowel. Endometrial glands, endometrial stroma, and large phagocytic cells containing hemosiderin may be identified histologically (see Fig. 19-10). Pressure atrophy may lead to the loss of architecture of the endometrial glands. The ultrasound characteristics include a thick-walled cyst with a relatively homogeneous echo pattern that is somewhat echolucent. This appearance confers a greater than 95% positive predictive value in some studies.

The choice between medical and operative management depends on several factors, including the patient's age, future reproductive plans, and severity of symptoms. Medical therapy is rarely successful in treating ovarian endometriosis if the disease has produced ovarian enlargement. Often surgical therapy is complicated by formation of de novo and recurrent adhesions.

On pathologic examination, it is important to distinguish endometriosis from benign endometrial tumors, which are usually adenofibromas. The latter tumor is a true neoplasm, and there is a malignant counterpart.

Fibroma

Fibromas are the most common benign, solid neoplasms of the ovary. Their malignant potential is low, less than 1%. These tumors make up approximately 5% of benign ovarian neoplasms and approximately 20% of all solid tumors of the ovary.

Fibromas vary in size from small nodules to huge pelvic tumors weighing 50 pounds. One of the predominant characteristics of fibromas is that they are extremely slow-growing tumors. The average diameter of a fibroma is approximately 6 cm; however, some tumors have reached 30 cm in diameter. In most series, less than 5% of fibromas are greater than 20 cm in diameter. The diameter of a fibroma is important clinically, because the incidence of associated ascites is directly proportional to the size of the tumor. Many ovarian fibromas are misdiagnosed and are believed to be leiomyomas prior to operation. Ninety percent of fibromas are unilateral; however, multiple fibromas are found in the same ovary in 10% to 15% of cases. The average age of a woman with an ovarian fibroma is 48. Thus, this tumor often presents in postmenopausal women. The tumor arises from the undifferentiated fibrous stroma of the ovary. Bilateral ovarian fibromas are commonly found in women with the rare genetic transmitted basal cell nevus syndrome.

The pelvic symptoms that develop with growth of fibromas include pressure and abdominal enlargement, which may be secondary to both the size of the tumor and ascites. Smaller tumors are asymptomatic because these tumors do not elaborate hormones. Thus, there is no change in the pattern of menstrual flow. Fibromas may be pedunculated and therefore easily palpable during one examination yet difficult to palpate during a subsequent pelvic examination. Sometimes on pelvic examination the fibromas appear to be softer than a solid ovarian tumor because of the edema or occasional cystic degeneration.

Meigs' syndrome is the association of an ovarian fibroma, ascites, and hydrothorax. Both the ascites and the hydrothorax resolve after removal of the ovarian tumor. The ascites is caused by transudation of fluid from the ovarian fibroma. Samanth and Black reported that the incidence of ascites was directly related to the size of the fibroma. Fifty percent of patients have ascites if the tumor is greater than 6 cm. However, true Meigs' syndrome is rare, occurring in less than 2% of ovarian fibromas.

The hydrothorax develops secondary to a flow of ascitic fluid into the pleural space via the lymphatics of the diaphragm. Statistically the right pleural space is involved in 75% of reported cases, the left in 10%, and both sides in 15%. The clinical features of Meigs' syndrome are not unique to fibromas, and a similar clinical picture is found with many other ovarian tumors.

Grossly, fibromas are heavy, solid, well encapsulated, and grayish white. The cut surface usually demonstrates a homogeneous white or yellowish white solid tissue with a trabeculated or whorled appearance similar to that of myomas. The majority of fibromas are grossly edematous (**Fig. 18-62**). Less than 10% of fibromas have calcifications or small areas of hyaline or cystic degeneration. Histologically, fibromas are composed of connective tissue, stromal cells, and varying amounts of collagen interposed between the cells. The connective tissue cells are spindle-shaped, mature fibroblasts. They are arranged in an imperfect pattern. A few smooth muscle fibers may be occasionally identified. It is sometimes difficult to distinguish fibromas from nonneoplastic thecomas. Histologically the pathologist must differentiate fibromas from stromal hyperplasia, fibrosarcomas, and also look for epithelial elements of an associated **Brenner tumor**.

The management of fibromas is straightforward because any woman with a solid ovarian neoplasm should have an exploratory operation soon after the tumor is discovered. Simple excision of the tumor is all that is necessary. Following excision of the tumor, there is resolution of all symptoms, including ascites. Because these tumors are frequently discovered in postmenopausal women, often a bilateral salpingo-oophorectomy and total abdominal hysterectomy are performed. Conversely, it is important to note that most women who preoperatively have the combination of a solid ovarian tumor and ascites are found to have ovarian carcinoma.

Transitional Cell Tumors-Brenner Tumors

Brenner tumors are rare, small, smooth, solid, fibroepithelial ovarian tumors that are generally asymptomatic. The semantic classification of neoplasms changes, and the current preferred term for benign Brenner tumor is *transitional cell tumor*. The benign, proliferative (low malignant potential), and malignant forms together constitute approximately 2% of ovarian tumors.

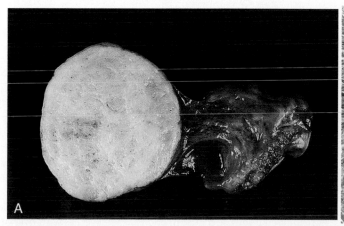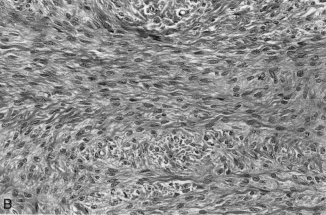

Figure 18-62 A, Fibroma of the ovary with a well-circumscribed light tan mass. **B,** Histology of fibroma of the ovary, demonstrating bland fibrous differentiation. (From Voet RL: Color Atlas of Obstetric and Gynecologic Pathology. St. Louis, Mosby-Wolfe, 1997.)

These tumors usually occur in women ages 40 to 60 years. Approximately 30% of transitional cell tumors are discovered as small, solid tumors in association with a concurrent serous cystic neoplasia, such as serous or mucinous cystadenomas of the ipsilateral ovary. Some are microscopic, with the entire tumor contained in a single low-powered microscopic field, and others may reach a diameter of 20 cm; the majority are less than 5 cm in diameter. The tumor is unilateral 85% to 95% of the time.

The Brenner tumor was first described in 1898. In 1932, Robert Meyer postulated that it was a distinct, independent neoplasm from granulosa cell tumors. Since that time there has been a controversy in the gynecologic pathology literature as to the histogenesis of the neoplasm. Presently, most authorities accept the theory that most of these tumors result from metaplasia of coelomic epithelium into uroepithelium. Detailed three-dimensional histologic studies have demonstrated a downward growth in a cordlike fashion of epithelium from the surface of the ovary to deeper areas in the ovarian cortex. Others have postulated that sometimes the solid nests of epithelial cells of the tumor originate from the rete ovarii or Walthard rests. Shevchuk and coworkers, in an electron microscopy study, confirmed the histologic and ultrastructural similarity between epithelium in Brenner tumors and transitional epithelium. These authors argue that because of the histogenesis from coelomic inclusion cysts and also the mixture of Müllerian-type epithelium in 30% of Brenner tumors, it might be appropriate to classify Brenner tumors in the epithelial group of ovarian neoplasms.

Approximately 90% of these small neoplasms are discovered incidentally during a gynecologic operation, although large tumors may produce unilateral pelvic discomfort. Postmenopausal bleeding is sometimes associated with Brenner tumors, as endometrial hyperplasia is a coexisting abnormality in 10% to 16% of cases. It is postulated that luteinization of the stroma produces estrogen with resulting hyperplasia. Recent reports by Moon and associates and Outwater and colleagues describe the CT and MRI characteristics of Brenner tumors of the ovary. The extensive fibrous content of these tumors results in lower signal intensity in T2-weighted images. During CT scanning, Brenner tumors characteristically demonstrate a finding of extensive amorphous calcification within the solid components of the ovarian mass.

Grossly, Brenner tumors are smooth, firm, gray-white, solid tumors that grossly resemble fibromas. Similar to fibromas, transitional cell tumors are slow growing. On sectioning, the tumor usually appears gray; however, occasionally there is a yellowish tinge with small cystic spaces (**Fig. 18-63**). Approximately 1% to 2% of these tumors undergo malignant change (Chapter 33, Neoplastic Diseases of the Ovary). Histologically, Brenner tumors have two principal components: solid masses or nests of epithelial cells and a surrounding fibrous stroma. The epithelial cells are uniform and do not appear anaplastic (**Fig. 18-64**). The histology and ultrastructure of the epithelial cells of a Brenner tumor are similar to transitional epithelium of the urinary bladder. The pale epithelial cells have a coffee bean–appearing nucleus, which is also described as a longitudinal groove in the cell's nucleus.

Electron microscopy has demonstrated that the longitudinal groove during routine microscopy is produced by prominent indentation of the nuclear membrane. An additional ovarian neoplasm is frequently found associated with Brenner tumors. Balasa and colleagues, in a review of 302 tumors, reported

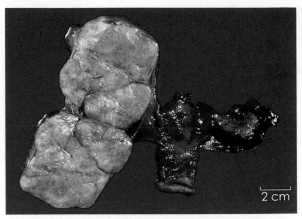

Figure 18-63 Brenner tumor. (From Clement PB, Young RH: Atlas of Gynecologic Surgical Pathology. Philadelphia, WB Saunders, 2000.)

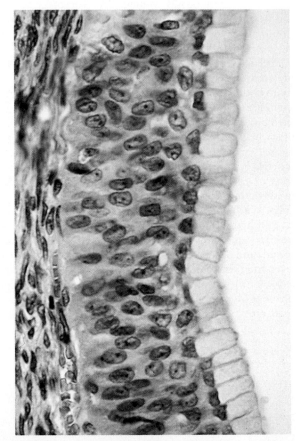

Figure 18-64 Benign Brenner tumor. A cyst in the Brenner tumor is lined by an inner layer of endocervical-type mucinous cells and an outer layer of stratified transitional cells, a few of which have grooved nuclei. (From Clement PB, Young RH: Atlas of Gynecologic Surgical Pathology. Philadelphia, WB Saunders, 2000.)

100 other concurrent neoplasms, with the majority being serous and mucinous cystadenomas or teratomas.

Management of Brenner tumors is operative, with simple excision being the procedure of choice. However, as with ovarian fibromas, the patient's age often is the principal factor in deciding the extent of the operation.

Adenofibroma and Cystadenofibroma

Adenofibromas and cystadenofibromas are closely related. Both of these benign firm tumors consist of fibrous and epithelial components. The epithelial element is most commonly serous, but histologically may be mucinous and endometrioid or clear cell. They differ from benign epithelial cystadenomas in that there is a preponderance of connective tissue. Most pathologists emphasize that at least 25% of the tumor consists of fibrous connective tissue. Obviously, cystadenofibromas have microscopic or occasional macroscopic areas that are cystic. The varying degree of fibrous stroma and epithelial elements produces a spectrum of tumors, which have resulted in a confusing nomenclature with terms such as *papillomas, fibropapillomas,* and *fibroadenomas.*

Adenofibromas are usually small fibrous tumors that arise from the surface of the ovary. They are bilateral in 20% to 25% of women. They usually occur in postmenopausal women and are 1 to 15 cm in diameter. Grossly, they are gray or white tumors, and it is difficult to distinguish them from fibromas. Papillary adenofibromas, which project from the surface of the ovary, at first glance may appear to be external excrescences of a malignant tumor. Histologically, small precursors of adenofibromas are identified in many normal ovaries. Under the microscope, true cystic gland spaces lined by cuboidal epithelium are characteristic. However, differing from serous cystadenomas, the fibrous connective tissue surrounding the cystic spaces is abundant and is the predominant tissue of the tumor.

Smaller tumors are asymptomatic and are only discovered incidentally during abdominal or pelvic operations. Large tumors may cause pressure symptoms or, rarely, undergo adnexal torsion. Recently a small series of the MRI features of these tumors has been reported. Similar to Brenner tumors, the fibrous component produces a very low signal intensity on T2-weighted images. This interest in imaging results from an attempt to distinguish, prior to operation, whether a predominantly solid ovarian mass is benign or malignant. Because adenofibromas are usually discovered in postmenopausal women, the treatment of choice is bilateral salpingo-oophorectomy and total abdominal hysterectomy. Because these tumors are benign and because malignant transformation is rare, simple excision of the tumor and inspection of the contralateral ovary is appropriate in younger women.

Torsion

Torsion of the ovary or both the oviduct and the ovary (adnexal torsion) is uncommon but an important cause of acute lower abdominal and pelvic pain. Recent series have noted that torsion may cause up to 3% of all acute abdomens presenting to emergency departments. Torsion of the ovary may occur separately from torsion of the fallopian tube, but most commonly the two adnexal structures are affected together.

Adnexal torsion occurs most commonly during the reproductive years, with the average patient being in her mid-20s. However, adnexal torsion is also a complication of benign ovarian tumors in the postmenopausal woman. Pregnancy appears to predispose women to adnexal torsion, with approximately one in five women being pregnant when the condition is diagnosed. Most susceptible are ovaries that are enlarged secondary to ovulation induction during early pregnancy. One series reported four cases of adnexal torsion in 648 pregnancies resulting from ovulation induction. The most common cause of adnexal torsion is ovarian enlargement by an 8- to 12-cm benign mass of the ovary. However, smaller ovaries may also undergo torsion.

Ovarian tumors are discovered in 50% to 60% of women with adnexal torsion. Torsion of a normal ovary or adnexum is also possible and occurs more frequently in children. Hibbard reports that because of their relative prevalence, dermoids are the tumor most frequently reported in a series of women with adnexal torsion. However, the relative risk of adnexal torsion is higher with parovarian cysts, solid benign tumors, and serous cysts of the ovary. The right ovary has a greater tendency to twist (3 to 2) than does the left ovary. Torsion of a malignant ovarian tumor is comparatively rare.

Patients with adnexal torsion present with acute, severe, unilateral, lower abdominal and pelvic pain. Often the patient relates the onset of the severe pain to an abrupt change of position. A unilateral, extremely tender adnexal mass is found in more than 90% of patients. Approximately two thirds of patients have associated nausea and vomiting. These associated gastrointestinal symptoms sometimes lead to a preoperative diagnosis of acute appendicitis or small intestinal obstruction. Many patients have noted intermittent previous episodes of similar pain for several days to several weeks. The hypothesis is that previous episodes of pain were secondary to partial torsion, with spontaneous reversal without significant vascular compromise. With progressive torsion, initially venous and lymphatic obstruction occurs. This produces a cyanotic, edematous ovary, which on pelvic examination presents as a unilateral, extremely tender adnexal mass. Further progression of the torsion interrupts the major arterial supply to the ovary, resulting in hypoxia, adnexal necrosis, and a concomitant low-grade fever and leukocytosis. Fever is more common in women who have developed necrosis of the adnexa. Approximately 10% of women with adnexal torsion have a repetitive episode affecting the contralateral adnexum.

Most patients with adnexal torsion present with symptoms and signs severe enough to demand operative intervention (**Fig. 18-65**). Some authors have reported the successful use of Doppler ultrasound to evaluate ovarian arterial blood flow to help diagnose torsion. Abnormal color Doppler flow is highly predictive of torsion of the ovary. However, approximately 50% of women with surgically confirmed adnexal torsion will have a normal Doppler flow study. The false negative rate is high enough that normal Doppler studies should never trump clinical suspicion. Women with ovarian torsion may be treated via

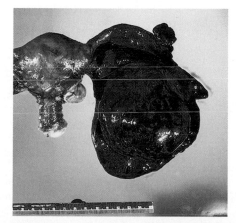

Figure 18-65 Adnexal torsion with hemorrhagic infarction. A benign cyst was found in the ovary. (From Clement PB, Young RH: Atlas of Gynecologic Surgical Pathology. Philadelphia, WB Saunders, 2000.)

laparoscopic surgery. The most common gynecologic conditions that may be confused with adnexal torsion are a ruptured corpus luteum or an adnexal abscess. In recent series emphasizing the early diagnosis of adnexal torsion, conservative operative management has been possible in 75% of cases.

Because the majority of cases of adnexal torsion occur in young women, a conservative operation is ideal. The clinician should maintain a high index of suspicion for adnexal torsion so that early and conservative surgery is possible. With severe vascular compromise, the appropriate operation is unilateral salpingo-oophorectomy. The vascular pedicle should be clamped with care so as not to injure the ureter, which may be tented up by the torsion.

Although salpingo-oophorectomy has been the routine treatment for ovarian torsion, large series of conservative management have been reported. Conservative surgery either through the laparoscope or via laparotomy entails gentle untwisting of the pedicle, possibly cystectomy, and stabilization of the ovary with sutures. The risk of recurrence of torsion in women without cystectomy and or stabilization of the ovary is problematic. A series by Pausky et al. noted a rate of recurrence of 64% in older women. Other series note similar rates in both gravid and nongravid patients and in younger women as well.

The risk of pulmonary embolus (PE) with adnexal torsion is small, approximately 0.2%. One series noted the risk of PE to be similar when torsion was managed by conservative surgery with untwisting or adnexal removal without untwisting.

Ovarian Remnant Syndrome

Chronic pelvic pain secondary to a small area of functioning ovarian tissue following intended total removal of both ovaries is termed *ovarian remnant syndrome.* Most of the women who develop this condition had endometriosis or chronic pelvic inflammatory disease and extensive pelvic adhesions discovered during previous surgical procedures. A more recently described risk factor is laparoscopic oophorectomy.

The chronic pelvic pain is usually cyclic and exacerbated following coitus. Approximately half of women present with pain, and half with a pelvic mass. Usually the masses are small, approximately 3 cm in diameter, and most commonly located in the retroperitoneal space immediately adjacent to either ureter. Histologically, the mass contains both ovarian follicles and

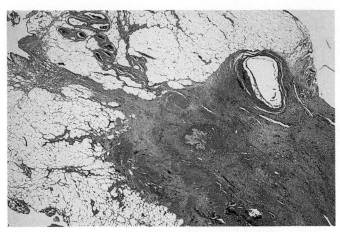

Figure 18-66 Ovarian remnant syndrome. Ovarian tissue that was left behind at the time of oophorectomy has regrown and is functional. (From Robboy SJ, Bentley RC, Russell P, Anderson MC: The peritoneum. In Robboy SJ, Anderson MC, Russell P [eds]: Pathology of the Female Reproductive Tract. Edinburgh, Churchill Livingstone, 2002.)

stroma (**Fig. 18-66**). If the mass cannot be palpated during pelvic examination, imaging studies such as vaginal ultrasound or MRI are often helpful. Premenopausal levels of follicle-simulating hormone or estradiol help to establish the diagnosis in a woman who has a history of a bilateral salpingo-oophorectomy. However, sometimes a small area of ovarian tissue does not produce enough circulating estrogen to suppress gonadotropins. Difficult cases have been diagnosed by challenging and stimulating the suspected ovarian remnant with either clomiphene citrate or a GnRH agonist.

Once the diagnosis is suspected, the most effective treatment is surgical removal of the ovarian remnant. The tissue should be removed by laparoscopy or laparotomy with wide excision of the mass using meticulous techniques so as to protect the integrity of the ureter. The recurrence rate is approximately 10%. A series by Magtibay et al. noted a 10% rate of intraoperative complications, illustrating that removal is a difficult procedure secondary to the associated pathologies that had necessitated the original surgery.

KEY POINTS

- The vulva contains 1% of the skin surface of the body, but 5% to 10% of all malignant melanomas in women arise from this region. Ideally, all vulvar nevi should be excised and examined histologically. Special emphasis should be directed toward the flat junctional nevus and the dysplastic nevus, for they have the greatest potential for malignant transformation. The dysplastic nevus is characterized by being more than 5 mm in diameter, with irregular borders and patches of variegated pigment.
- The management of nonobstetric vulvar hematomas is usually conservative unless the hematoma is greater than 10 cm in diameter or rapidly increasing.
- The most common causes of vulvar contact dermatitis are cosmetic and local therapeutic agents. External chemicals that trigger the disease process must be avoided.

- Women usually develop psoriasis during their teenage years, with approximately 3% of adult women being affected. Approximately 20% of these have involvement of the vulvar skin.
- The margins of psoriasis are better defined than the common skin conditions in the differential diagnosis, including candidiasis, seborrheic dermatitis, and eczema. Psoriasis does not involve the vagina, only the vulva.
- Lichen sclerosus does not involve the vagina, whereas lichen planus may involve the vagina.
- Classically, the symptoms associated with the urethral diverticulum are extremely chronic in nature and they have not resolved with multiple courses of oral antibiotic therapy.
- Cervical stenosis may occur following loop electrocautery excision procedures (LEEPs) in women with low circulating

KEY POINTS—CONTINUED

- estrogen levels such as secondary to periodic injections of medroxyprogesterone (Depo-Provera), postmenopausal women, and those who are breast-feeding. Peri- and postoperative treatment with vaginal or systemic estrogen may help prevent this complication.
- Endocervical polyps are smooth, soft, red, fragile masses. They are found most commonly in multiparous women in their 40s and 50s. After the endocervical polyp is removed, endometrial sampling should be performed to diagnose a coexisting endometrial hyperplasia or carcinoma.
- Endometrial polyps are noted in approximately 10% of women when the uterus is examined at autopsy. Approximately one in four women with abnormal bleeding will have an endometrial polyp.
- Leiomyomas are the most frequent pelvic tumors, with the highest prevalence occurring during the fifth decade of a woman's life.
- The cause of uterine leiomyomas is incompletely understood. It is known that each tumor results from an original single muscle cell. Each individual uterine myoma is monoclonal. All the cells are derived from one progenitor myocyte.
- Abnormal bleeding is experienced by a third of women with myomas, the most common pattern being intermenstrual spotting. Women with myomas and abnormal bleeding should be thoroughly evaluated for concurrent causes of bleeding.
- Adenomyosis is frequently asymptomatic. If multiple serial sections of the uterus are obtained, the incidence may exceed 60% in women 40 to 50 years of age.
- Adenomyosis rarely causes uterine enlargement greater than a size at 14 weeks' gestation unless there is concomitant uterine pathology.
- The initial management of a suspected follicular cyst is conservative observation. The majority of follicular cysts disappear spontaneously by either reabsorption of the cyst fluid or silent rupture within 4 to 8 weeks of initial diagnosis.
- The practice of aspirating cysts via the laparoscope should be limited to cysts that are completely simple and associated with normal CA-125 levels. Several investigators have noted that intraoperative spillage of malignant cystic tumors is associated with greater than expected recurrence.
- The differential diagnosis of a woman with acute pain and a suspected ruptured corpus luteum cyst includes ectopic pregnancy, a ruptured endometrioma, and adnexal torsion.

- The treatment of unruptured corpus luteum cysts is conservative. However, if the cyst persists or intraperitoneal bleeding occurs, necessitating operation, the treatment is cystectomy.
- Drainage or fenestration is effective for follicular cysts and poorly effective for cystadenomas. They will tend to recur. When cysts are drained, it is essential to remember that the cytologic examination of cyst fluid has poor predictive value and poor sensitivity in differentiating benign from malignant cysts.
- Theca lutein cysts arise from either prolonged or excessive stimulation of the ovaries by endogenous or exogenous gonadotropins or increased ovarian sensitivity to gonadotropins. The condition of ovarian enlargement secondary to the development of multiple luteinized follicular cysts is termed *hyperreactio luteinalis.* Approximately 50% of molar pregnancies and 10% of choriocarcinomas have associated bilateral theca lutein cysts.
- Benign ovarian teratomas vary from a few millimeters to 25 cm, may be single or multiple, and are bilateral 10% to 15% of the time. Dermoids are believed to arise during fetal life from a single germ cell. They are 46,XX in karyotype.
- Operative treatment of benign cystic teratomas is cystectomy with preservation of as much normal ovarian tissue as possible.
- Fifty percent of patients with an ovarian fibroma will have ascites if the tumor is greater than 6 cm. The incidence of associated ascites is directly proportional to the size of the tumor.
- Transitional cell tumors (Brenner tumors) are small, smooth, solid, fibroepithelial tumors of the ovary. They usually occur in women between the ages of 40 and 60 and are predominantly unilateral.
- Adnexal torsion occurs most commonly in the reproductive years, with the average age of patients being in the mid-20s. Pregnancy predisposes to adnexal torsion.
- Ovarian tumors are discovered in 50% to 60% of women with adnexal torsion.
- Abnormal color Doppler flow is highly predictive of torsion of the ovary. However, approximately 50% of women with surgically confirmed adnexal torsion will have a normal Doppler flow study.
- The risk of pulmonary embolus with adnexal torsion is approximately 0.2%. The risk is similar regardless of whether the condition is managed by conservative surgery with untwisting or adnexal removal without untwisting.

ACKNOWLEDGMENTS

We wish to acknowledge Martha Goetsch for her advice with portions of this chapter.

REFERENCES CAN BE FOUND ON
EXPERTCONSULT.com

SUGGESTED READING

Baiocchi G, Manci N, Pazzaglia M, et al: Malignancy in endometrial polyps: A 12-year experience, *AJOG* 201:462, 2009.

Baird DD, Dunson DB, Hill MC, et al: High cumulative incidence of uterine leiomyoma in black and white women: Ultrasound evidence, *Am J Obstet Gynecol* 188:100, 2003.

Bergeron S, Khalife S, Glazer HI, et al: Surgical and behavioral treatments for vestibulodynia, two and one half year follow up and predictors of outcome, *American College of Obstetrics and Gynecologists* 111:159, 2008.

Boardman LA, Cooper AS, Blais LR, et al: Topical Gabapentin in the Treatment of localized and Generalized Vulvodynia, *AJOG* 112:579, 2008.

Ghezzi F, Cromi A, Bergamini V, et al: Should adnexal mass size influence surgical approach? A series of 186 laparoscopically managed large adnexal masses, *BJOG* 1020, 2008.

Goetsch MF: Incidence of Bartholin's duct occlusion after superficial localized vestibulectomy, *AJOG* 200:688, 2009.

Gonzalez AB, Stafford I, Mancuso P, et al: Delivery of a polyp, *American College of Obstetrics and Gynecologists* 488, 2008.

Greenlee RT, Kessel B, Williams CR, et al: Prevalence, incidence, and natural history of simple ovarian cysts among women >55 years old in a large cancer screening trial, *AJOG* 202:373, 2010.

Guthrie BD, Adler MD, Powell EC: *Incidence and Trends of Pediatric Ovarian Torsion Hospitalizations in the United States, 2000-2006,* 2010.

Kho KA, Nezhat C: Parasitic Myomas, *American College of Obstetricians and Gynecology* 114:611, 2009.

Magtibay PM, Nyholm JL, Hernandez JL, et al: Ovarian remnant syndrome, *AJOG* 193, 2005.

Pansky M, Smorgick N, Herman A, et al: Torsion of normal adnexa in postmenarchal women and risk of recurrence, *American College of Obstetricians and Gynecology* 109:355, 2007.

Perri T: Are endometrial polyps true cancer precursors? *AJOG* 203:232, 2010.

van der Kooij SM, Hehenkamp WJK, Volkers NA, et al: Uterine artery embolization vs hysterectomy in the treatment of symptomatic uterine fibroids: 5-year outcome from the randomized EMMY trial, *AJOG* 203:105, 2010.

19

Endometriosis
Etiology, Pathology, Diagnosis, Management

Roger A. Lobo

ENDOMETRIOSIS

Endometriosis is a benign but, in many women, a progressive and aggressive disease. The wide spectrum of clinical problems that occur with endometriosis has frustrated gynecologists, fascinated pathologists, and burdened patients for years. Although endometriosis was first described in 1860, the classic studies by Sampson in the 1920s were the first to emphasize the clinical and pathologic correlations of endometriosis. Even today, many aspects of the disease remain enigmatic.

By definition, endometriosis is the presence and growth of the glands and stroma of the lining of the uterus in an aberrant or heterotopic location. **Adenomyosis** is the growth of endometrial glands and stroma into the uterine myometrium to a depth of at least 2.5 mm from the basalis layer of the endometrium. Adenomyosis is sometimes termed *internal endometriosis*; however, this is a semantic misnomer because most likely they are separate diseases.

It is usually stated that the incidence of endometriosis has been increasing since the 1980s. This "opinion" is secondary to an enlightened awareness of mild endometriosis as diagnosed by the increasing use of laparoscopy. Since the early 2000s, diagnostic delay, the average time to the first diagnosis of the disease, has decreased dramatically. However, it has been estimated to take an average time of 11.7 years in the United States and 8 years in the United Kingdom to make the diagnosis. Evers has advanced a provocative hypothesis that endometrial implants in the peritoneal cavity are a physiologic finding secondary to **retrograde menstruation**, and their presence does not confirm a disease process. The prevalence of pelvic endometriosis in the general female population has been suggested to be 6% to 10%. The age-specific incidence or prevalence of endometriosis is not known and has only been estimated. Many patients are diagnosed incidentally during surgery performed for a variety of other indications. Conservative estimates find that endometriosis is present in 5% to 15% of laparotomies performed on reproductive-age females. The prevalence of active endometriosis is approximately 33% in women with chronic pelvic pain. The incidence of endometriosis is 30% to 45% in women with infertility. Over one year of observation, it has been found that 17% to 29% of lesions may resolve spontaneously, whereas 24% to 64% progress, and 9% to 59% do not change.

The cause of endometriosis is uncertain and involves many mechanisms including retrograde menstruation, vascular dissemination, metaplasia, genetic predisposition, immunologic changes, and hormonal influences, as discussed later. In addition, there is increasing evidence that environmental factors may also play a role, including exposure to dioxin and other endocrine disruptors. Clinically, it is most difficult to predict the natural course of endometriosis in any one individual. For example, the clinician cannot know which woman with mild disease in her 20s will progress to severe disease at a later age.

The typical patient with endometriosis is in her mid-30s, is nulliparous and involuntarily infertile, and has symptoms of secondary dysmenorrhea and pelvic pain, but it must be stressed that symptoms and signs may be extremely variable. The classic symptom of endometriosis is pelvic pain. However, in clinical practice the majority of cases are not "classic." The diagnosis and treatment of infertility associated with endometriosis is discussed in Chapter 41 (Infertility). Aberrant endometrial tissue grows under the cyclic influence of ovarian hormones and is particularly estrogen dependent; therefore, the disease is most commonly found during the reproductive years. However, 5% of women with endometriosis are diagnosed following menopause. Postmenopausal endometriosis is usually stimulated by exogenous estrogen. Endometriosis in teenagers should be investigated for obstructive reproductive tract abnormalities that increase the amount of retrograde menstruation. Although previously thought to be rare in adolescents, in teens with pelvic pain, endometriosis has been found in approximately half the cases.

Endometriosis is a disease not only of great individual variability but also of contrasting pathophysiologic processes. It is a benign disease, yet it has the characteristics of a malignancy—that is, it is locally infiltrative, invasive, and widely disseminating. Although the growth of ectopic endometrium is stimulated by physiologic levels of estrogen, the use of contraceptive steroids of various doses is usually beneficial for treatment. Another contrast often noted is the inverse relationship between the extent of pelvic endometriosis and the severity of pelvic pain. Women with extensive endometriosis may be asymptomatic, whereas other patients with minimal implants may have incapacitating chronic pelvic pain. However, as would be expected, women with deep infiltrating endometriosis, especially in retroperitoneal spaces, often experience severe episodes of pain. Recently, pelvic lesions of endometriosis have been found to have positive immunostaining for smooth muscle as well as nerve cells.

The clinical variability in responses among women with endometriosis may relate to differences in immunologic function and variations in cytokine production.

ETIOLOGY

There are several theories to explain the pathogenesis of endometriosis. However, no single theory adequately explains all the manifestations of the disease. Most important, there is only speculation as to why some women develop endometriosis and others do not. One popular theory is that there is a complex interplay between a dose-response curve of the amount of retrograde menstruation and an individual woman's immunologic response.

Retrograde Menstruation

The most popular theory is that endometriosis results from retrograde menstruation. Sampson suggested that pelvic endometriosis was secondary to implantation of endometrial cells shed during menstruation. These cells attach to the pelvic peritoneum and under hormonal influence grow as homologous grafts. Indeed, reflux of menstrual blood and viable endometrial cells in the pelvis of ovulating women has been documented. Endometriosis is discovered most frequently in areas immediately adjacent to the tubal ostia or in the dependent areas of the pelvis.

Endometriosis is frequently found in women with outflow obstruction of the genital tract. The attachment of the shed endometrial cells involves the expression of adhesion molecules and their receptors. This is thought to be an extremely rapid process as demonstrated in vitro. **Figures 19-1** and **19-2** depict the process of implants from retrograde menstruation and early invasion.

Metaplasia

In contrast to the theory of seeding from retrograde menstruation is the theory that endometriosis arises from metaplasia of the coelomic epithelium or proliferation of embryonic rests.

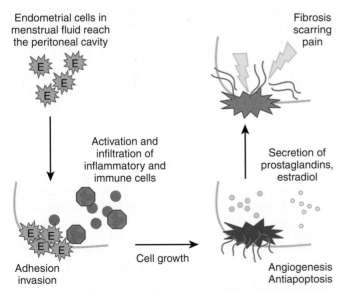

Figure 19-1 Proposed establishment of peritoneal endometriotic implants via retrograde menstruation, attachment, proliferation, migration, neovascularization, inflammation, and fibrosis. E, endometrial cell. (From Flores I, Rivera E, Ruiz LA, et al: Molecular profiling of experimental endometriosis identified gene expression patterns in common with human disease. Fertil Steril 87(5):1180-1199, 2007.)

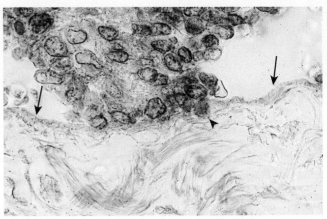

Figure 19-2 Early invasion of an endometrial implant through the mesothelium. The mesothelium is labeled with monoclonal antibody to cytokeratin and stained with diaminobenzidine (arrows). An endometrial stromal cell (arrowhead) passing through the mesothelium is thought to represent the initial step of invasion into the stroma of the peritoneum. Original magnification, ×31,000. Counterstained with hematoxylin. (From Witz CA, Monotoya-Rodrigueez I, Schenken RS: Whole explants of peritoneum and endometrium: A novel model of the early endometriosis lesion. Fertil Steril 71[1]:56-60, 1999.)

The Müllerian ducts and nearby mesenchymal tissue form the majority of the female reproductive tract. The Müllerian duct is derived from the coelomic epithelium during fetal development. The metaplasia hypothesis postulates that the coelomic epithelium retains the ability for multipotential development. The decidual reaction of isolated areas of peritoneum during pregnancy is an example of this process. It is well known that the surface epithelium of the ovary can differentiate into several different histologic cell types. Endometriosis has been discovered in prepubertal girls, women with congenital absence of the uterus, and very rarely in men. These examples support the **coelomic metaplasia** theory.

Metaplasia occurs after an "induction phenomenon" has stimulated the multipotential cell. The induction substance may be a combination of menstrual debris and the influence of estrogen and progesterone. Batt and Smith have hypothesized that the histogenesis of endometriosis in peritoneal pockets of the posterior pelvis results from a congenital anomaly involving rudimentary duplication of the Müllerian system. The peritoneal pockets that they describe are found in the posterior pelvis, the posterior aspects of the broad ligament, and the cul-de-sac (**Fig. 19-3**). Similarly, Nisolle and Donnez have postulated that metaplasia of the coelomic epithelium that invaginates into the ovarian cortex is the pathogenesis for the development of ovarian endometriosis.

Lymphatic and Vascular Metastasis

The theory of endometrium being transplanted via lymphatic channels and the vascular system helps to explain rare and remote sites of endometriosis, such as the spinal column and nose. Endometriosis has been observed in the pelvic lymph nodes of approximately 30% of women with the disease. Hematogenous dissemination of endometrium is the best theory to explain endometriosis of the forearm and thigh, as well as multiple lesions in the lung.

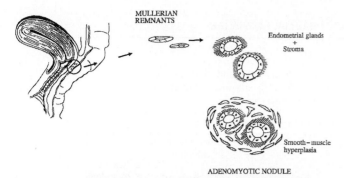

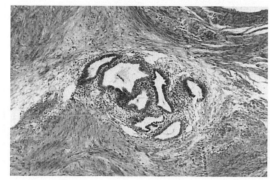

Figure 19-3 Proposed derivation of endometriotic lesion in the rectovaginal septum. (From Strauss JF, Barbieri R: Yen & Jaffe's Reproductive Endocrinology, 5th ed. Philadelphia, Saunders, 2004, pp 692-693.)

Table 19-1 Cytokines and Growth Factors in Peritoneal Fluid

Concentrations Increased in Endometriosis
Complement
Eotaxin
Glycodelin
IL-1
IL-6
IL-8
MCP-1
PDGF
RANTES
Soluble ICAM-1
TGF-β
VEGF
Concentrations Unchanged in Endometriosis
EGF
Basic FGF
Interferon-γ
IL-2
IL-4
IL-12
Concentrations Decreased in Endometriosis
IL-13

EGF, epidermal growth factor; FGF, fibroblast growth factor; ICAM, intercellular adhesion molecule; IL, interleukin; MCP, membrane cofactor protein; PDGF, platelet-derived growth factor; RANTES, regulated upon activation, normal T cell expressed and secreted; TGF, transforming growth factor; VEGF, vascular endothelial growth factor.
References are from the original source.
From McLaren J, Deatry G, Prentice A, et al: Decreased levels of the potent regulator of monocyte/macrophage activation, interleukin-13, in the peritoneal fluid of patients with endometriosis. Hum Reprod 12:1307, 1997.

Iatrogenic Dissemination

Endometriosis of the anterior abdominal wall is sometimes discovered in women after a cesarean delivery. The hypothesis is that endometrial glands and stroma are implanted during the procedure. The aberrant tissue is found subcutaneously at the abdominal incision. Rarely, iatrogenic endometriosis may be discovered in an episiotomy scar.

Immunologic Changes

One of the most perplexing, unanswered questions concerning the pathophysiology of endometriosis is that some women with retrograde menstruation develop endometriosis, but most do not. Multiple investigations have suggested that changes in the immune system, especially altered function of immune-related cells, are directly related to the pathogenesis of endometriosis. Whether endometriosis is an autoimmune disease has been intensely debated for many years. Studies have demonstrated abnormalities in cell-mediated and humoral components of the immune system in both peripheral blood and peritoneal fluid. **Table 19-1** depicts various cytokines and growth factors that have been implicated in the pathogenesis of endometriosis.

Most likely the primary immunologic change involves an alteration in the function of the peritoneal macrophages so prevalent in the peritoneal fluid of patients with endometriosis. It has been hypothesized that women who do not develop endometriosis have monocytic-type macrophages in their peritoneal fluid that have a short life span and limited function. Conversely, women who develop endometriosis have more peritoneal macrophages that are larger. These hyperactive cells secrete multiple growth factors and cytokines that enhance the development of endometriosis. The attraction of leukocytes to specific areas is controlled by chemokines, which are chemotactic cytokines (**Fig. 19-4**). Changes in the expression of integrins also may be an important local factor. Following the theory of different macrophage populations in endometriosis is the finding that the destroying of normally extruded endometrial cells in endometriosis may be deficient. It has been shown that natural killer (NK) cells have decreased cytotoxicity against endometrial and hematopoietic cells in women with endometriosis. Also, peritoneal fluid of women with endometriosis has less influence of NK activity than is found in fertile women without endometriosis.

Another attractive theory is the recent finding of a protein similar to haptoglobin in endometriosis epithelial cells called Endo 1. This chemoattractant protein-enhanced local production of interleukin-6 (IL-6) self-perpetuates lesion/cytokine interactions. Further compounding the proliferative activity of endometriosis lesions are angiogenic factors that are increased in lesions. Here the expression of basic fibroblast factor, IL-6, IL-8, platelet-derived growth factor (PDGF), and vascular endothelial growth factor (VEGF) are all increased.

Steroid interactions also enhance the progression of disease. Estrogen production is enhanced locally, and there is evidence for upregulation of aromatase activity, increased Cox-2 expression, and dysregulation of 17β-dehydrogenase activity, where there is a deficiency in 17β-dehydrogenase II activity and possibly an enhancement of type II activity favoring local estradiol production. **Figure 19-5** shows abnormalities of Cox-2, aromatase, and HSD 17β2 in disease free women, and endometrium and ectopic lesions in women with endometriosis where high local concentrations of estrogen and prostaglandin E_2

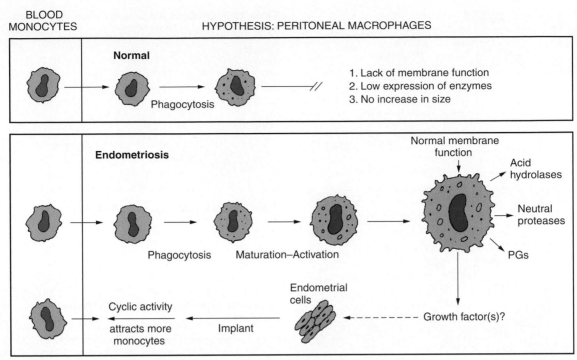

Figure 19-4 Hypothesis regarding pathophysiologic characteristics of human peritoneal macrophages in endometriosis. PG, prostaglandins. (Redrawn from Halme J, Becker S, Haskill S, et al: Altered maturation and function of peritoneal macrophages: Possible role in pathogenesis of endometriosis. Am J Obstet Gynecol 156:787, 1987.)

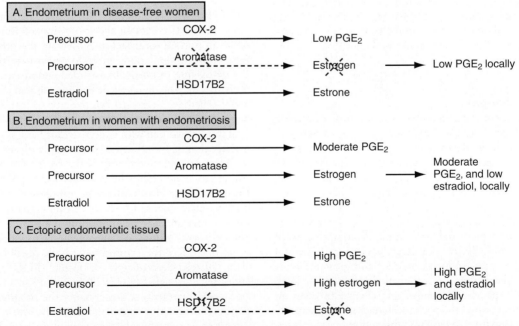

Figure 19-5 Normal endometrium and endometriosis. In normal endometrial tissue (panel A), activity of the enzyme cyclooxygenase-2 (CO-2), and thus production of prostaglandin E_2 (PGE_2), is low. Estrogen is not produced locally, owing to the absence of aromatase. During the luteal phase, the progesterone-dependent 17β-hydroxysteroid dehydrogenase 2(HSD17B2) enzyme catalyzes the conversion of the biologically active estradiol to estrone that is less estrogenic. In the endometrium of women with endometriosis (panel B), there is a subtle increase in COX-2 activity. In ectopic endometriotic tissue (panel C), full-blown molecular abnormalities include high COX-2 and aromatase levels. Increased PGE_2 formation in endometrial and endometriotic tissues can cause severe menstrual cramps and chronic pelvic pain. Tissue estradiol levels should be high, because estradiol is overproduced by aromatase and is not metabolized owing to deficient HSD17B2 activity. Increasing enzyme activity is denoted by the increasing thickness of arrows. (Modified from Bulun SE, Lin Z, Imir G, et al: Mechanisms of disease. N Engl J Med 360:270, 2009, Figure 1.)

predominate. Enhanced aromatase activity appears to be the result of overexpression of the orphan nuclear receptor steroidogenic factor-1 (SF-1) in lesions. The local production of estrogen through aromatase activity explains why progression of lesions may occur even with ovarian suppression. Further, there is evidence for progesterone "resistance" (**Fig. 19-6**). This is occasioned by a dysregulation of the isoform B of the progesterone receptor in most endometriotic lesions where levels may be undetectable. The latter propensity may be on a genetic basis, as discussed later on.

Autoimmunity may well exist in women with endometriosis, and although the finding of abnormalities of the histocompatibility locus antigen (HLA) system have not been consistent, there are reports of increased B and T cells, and serum immunoglobulin (IgG, IgA, and IgM) autoantibodies in endometriosis. A survey of the U.S. Endometriosis Association has provided suggestive evidence of the higher prevalence of other autoimmune diseases. The association of all these immune processes in the symptoms and signs of endometriosis is depicted in **Figure 19-7**.

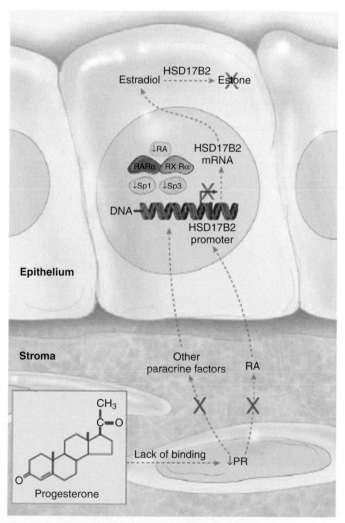

Figure 19-6 Disrupted paracrine action of progesterone in endometriotic tissue. (Modified from Bulun SE, Lin Z, Imir G, et al: Mechanisms of disease. N Engl J Med 360:270, 2009, Figure 3.)

Genetic Predisposition

Several studies have documented a familial predisposition to endometriosis with grouping of cases of endometriosis in mothers and their daughters. An investigation by Simpson and coworkers demonstrated a sevenfold increase in the incidence of endometriosis in relatives of women with the disease compared with controls. One of 10 women with severe endometriosis will have a sister or mother with clinical manifestations of the disease. The incidence of endometriosis in first-degree relatives, women with severe endometriosis, has been thought to be 7%. Women who have a family history of endometriosis are likely to develop the disease earlier in life and to have more advanced disease than women whose first-degree relatives are free of the disease. Recent studies have identified deletions of genes, most specifically increased heterogenicity of chromosome 17 and aneuploidy, in women with endometriosis compared with controls. Loci on 9q and 10q have also been found to increase the susceptibility for endometriosis. The expression of this genetic liability most likely depends on an interaction with environmental and epigenetic factors. Preliminary data suggest some bilateral ovarian endometrial cysts may arise independently from different clones. Although no consistent abnormality has been found in women with endometriosis, there are several candidate genes. **Table 19-2** provides a list of genes and gene products aberrantly expressed in endometriosis.

Several of these aberrantly expressed gene products, for example, the matrix metalloproteinases (MMPs) and integrins, have important implications for endometrial lesion attachment and for implantation defects, which may exist in infertile women with endometriosis. Reflux of MMPs into the peritoneal cavity at menstruation may contribute to peritoneal attachment in susceptible women.

Finally, Bulun and others have suggested that genetic predisposition, or exposure to environmental factors (toxics), may program fetal progenitor cells in an epigenetic way to overexpress SP1 and estrogen receptor β, which increase the risk of developing endometriosis.

Pathology

The majority of endometrial implants are located in the dependent portions of the female pelvis (**Fig. 19-8**). The ovaries are the most common site, being involved in two of three women with endometriosis. In most of these women the involvement is bilateral. The pelvic peritoneum over the uterus; the anterior and posterior cul-de-sac; and the uterosacral, round, and broad ligaments are also common sites where endometriosis develops. Pelvic lymph nodes have been found to be involved in up to 30% of cases.

The cervix, vagina, and vulva are other possible pelvic locations. Brosens has emphasized the importance of distinguishing between superficial and deep lesions of endometriosis. Deep lesions, penetrations of greater than 5 mm, represent a more progressive form of the disease. Distinguishing superficial implant lesions on peritoneal surfaces, including the ovary, from deep endometriotic ovarian cysts and cul-de-sac modules is important for therapy (discussed later on) in that these latter abnormalities may suggest different causes of the disease (e.g., metaplasia), which require a surgical approach.

Approximately 10% to 15% of women with advanced disease have lesions involving the rectosigmoid. Depending on the amount of associated scarring, endometriosis of the bowel

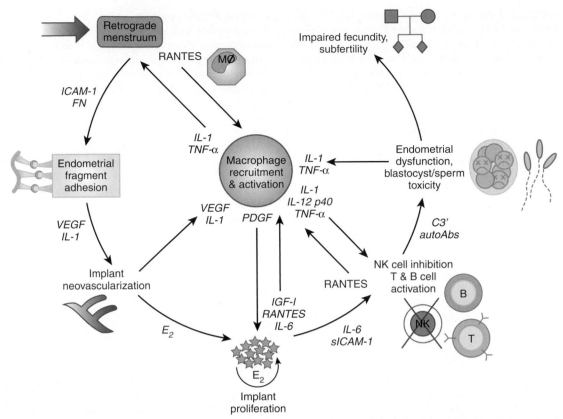

Figure 19-7 Schematogram depicting the network of chemokines, cytokines, and growth factors in the pathophysiology of endometriosis, autoAbs, autoantibodies; C3; complement 3; E$_2$, estradiol; FN, fibronectin; sICAM, soluble intercellular adhesion molecule; IGF-1, insulin-like growth factor-1;IL, interleukin; MØ, macrophage; NK cell, natural killer cell; PDGF, platelet-derived growth factor; RANTES, regulated on activation, normal IT cell expressed and secreted; TNF, tumor necrosis factor; VEGF, vascular endothelial growth factor.

Table 19-2 Genes and Gene Products Aberrantly Expressed in Endometrium from Women with Endometriosis

Aromatase
Endometrial bleeding factor
Hepatocyte growth factor
17β-hydroxysteroid dehydrogenase
HOX A10
HOX A11
Leukemia inhibitory factor
Matrix metalloproteinases 3, 7, and 11
Tissue inhibitors of metalloproteinases
Progesterone-receptor isoforms
Complement 3
Glutathione peroxidase
Catalase
Thrombospondin 1
Vascular endothelial growth factor
Integrin α$_v$β$_3$
Glycodelin

may be difficult to differentiate grossly from a primary neoplasm of the large intestine. Endometriosis may be found in a wide variety of sites, including the umbilicus, areas of previous surgical incisions of the anterior abdominal wall or perineum, the bladder, ureter, kidney, lung, arms, legs, and even the male urinary tract (**Table 19-3**).

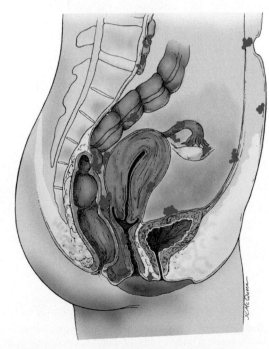

Figure 19-8 Common pelvic sites of endometriosis.

Table 19-3 Anatomic Distribution of Endometriosis

Common Sites	Rare Sites
Ovaries	Umbilicus
Pelvic peritoneum	Episiotomy scar
Ligaments of the uterus	Bladder
Sigmoid colon	Kidney
Appendix	Lungs
Pelvic lymph nodes	Arms
Cervix	Legs
Vagina	Nasal mucosa
Fallopian tubes	Spinal column

Gross pathologic changes of endometriosis exhibit wide variability in color, shape, size, and associated inflammatory and fibrotic changes. The visual manifestations of endometriosis in the female pelvis are protean and have many appearances. Increased awareness and anticipation have focused on the subtle lesions of endometriosis. Recently, clinicians closely inspect the pelvic peritoneum to identify abnormal areas and small, non-hemorrhagic lesions. More emphasis has been placed on biopsy confirmation of endometriosis because of increasing awareness of subtle lesions. The gross appearance of the implant depends on the site, activity, relationship to the day of the menstrual cycle, and chronicity of the area involved. The color of the lesion varies widely and may be red, brown, black, white, yellow, pink, clear, or a red vesicle. The predominant color depends on the blood supply and the amount of hemorrhage and fibrosis. The color also appears related to the size of the lesion, degree of edema, and the amount of inspissated material (**Table 19-4**). **Figure 19-9** depicts the spectrum of lesions with black and white lesions reflecting older lesions with inflammatory and fibrotic changes. Other peritoneal lesions that grossly appear similar to endometriosis, but on histologic examination are not, include necrotic areas of an ectopic pregnancy, fibrotic reactions to suture, hemangiomas, adrenal rest, Walthard's rest, breast cancer, ovarian cancer, epithelial inclusions, residual carbon from laser surgery, peritoneal inflammation, psammoma bodies, peritoneal reactions to oil-based hysterosalpingogram dye, and splenosis.

New lesions are small, bleblike implants that are less than 1 cm in diameter. Initially these areas are raised above the surrounding tissues. Red, blood-filled lesions have been shown, by histologic and biochemical studies, to be the most active phase of the disease (see **Fig. 19-9**). With time the areas of endometriosis become larger and assume a light or dark brown color, and they may be described as "powder burn" areas or "**chocolate cysts**." The older

Table 19-4 Preoperative Symptoms in 130 Patients Undergoing Colorectal Resection for Endometriosis

Symptom	No. of Patients	(%)
Pelvic pain	111	(85)
Rectal pain	68	(52)
Cyclic rectal bleeding	24	(18)
Diarrhea	55	(42)
Constipation	53	(41)
Diarrhea and constipation	18	(14)
Dyspareunia	83	(64)

From Bailey HR, Ott MT, Hartendorp P: Aggressive surgical management for advanced colorectal endometriosis. Dis Colon Rectum 37:747, 1994.

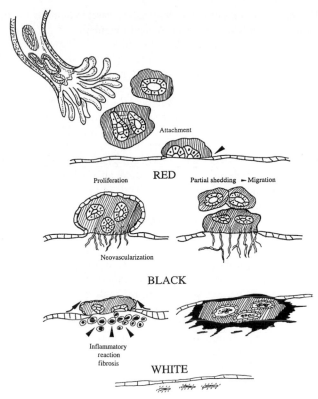

Figure 19-9 Proposed establishment of peritoneal endometriotic implants via retrograde menstruation and the like. (From Strauss JF, Barbieri R: Yen & Jaffe's Reproductive Endocrinology, 5th ed. Philadelphia Saunders, 2004, pp 692-693.)

lesions are white, have more intense scarring, and are usually puckered or retracted from the surrounding tissue. White or mixed colored lesions are more likely to provide histologic confirmation of endometriosis. Also, the progression from red to white lesions also seems to correlate with age.

The pattern of ovarian endometriosis is also variable. Individual areas range from 1 mm to large chocolate cysts greater than 8 cm in diameter (**Fig. 19-10**). The associated adhesions may be

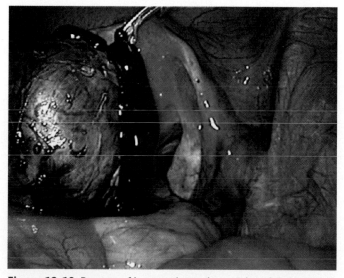

Figure 19-10 Rupture of large endometrioma "chocolate cyst." (From www.pathologystudent.com.)

filmy or dense. Larger cysts are usually densely adherent to the surrounding pelvic sidewalls or broad ligament.

The three cardinal histologic features of endometriosis are ectopic endometrial glands, ectopic endometrial stroma, and hemorrhage into the adjacent tissue (**Fig. 19-11**). Previous hemorrhage can be discovered by identifying large macrophages filled with hemosiderin near the periphery of the lesion. In the majority of cases, the aberrant endometrial glands and stroma respond in cyclic fashion to estrogen and progesterone. These changes may or may not be in synchrony with the endometrial lining of the uterus. The ectopic endometrial stroma will undergo classic decidual changes similar to pregnancy when exposed to high physiologic or pharmacologic levels of progesterone.

In approximately 25% of the cases of endometriosis, viable endometrial glands and stroma cannot be identified. Repetitive episodes of hemorrhage may lead to severe inflammatory changes and result in the glands and stroma undergoing necrobiosis secondary to pressure atrophy or lack of blood supply. In these cases, a presumptive diagnosis of endometriosis is made by visualizing the intense inflammatory reaction and the large macrophages filled with blood pigment.

The natural history of endometriosis is a subject of intense speculation. Spontaneous regression or disappearance of active disease may occur and lesions may regress in approximately one quarter of cases. The pathophysiology of progression from subtle endometriosis to severe disease may be expected from the multiple mechanisms of potential disease acceleration discussed earlier, but in reality is not known, although it is likely that immune mechanisms are involved.

CLINICAL DIAGNOSIS

Symptoms

It is important to reemphasize that endometriosis has many different clinical presentations, with one in three women being asymptomatic. Most important, the disease has an extremely unpredictable course. The classic symptoms of endometriosis are cyclic pelvic pain and infertility. The chronic pelvic pain usually presents as secondary dysmenorrhea or dyspareunia (or both). Secondary dysmenorrhea usually begins 36 to 48 hours

prior to the onset of menses. However, approximately one third of patients with endometriosis are asymptomatic, with the disease being discovered incidentally during an abdominal operation or visualized at laparoscopy for an unrelated problem. Conversely, endometriosis is discovered in approximately one of three women whose primary symptom is chronic pelvic pain.

Clinicians have appreciated the paradox that the extent of pelvic pain is often inversely related to the amount of endometriosis in the female pelvis. Women with large, fixed adnexal masses sometimes have minor symptoms, whereas other patients with only a few small foci with deep infiltration may experience moderate to severe chronic pain. The cyclic pelvic pain is related to the sequential swelling and the extravasation of blood and menstrual debris into the surrounding tissue. The chemical mediators of this intense sterile inflammation and pain are believed to be prostaglandins and cytokines. Infiltrative endometriosis, which involves extensive areas of the retroperitoneal space, often is associated with moderate to severe pelvic pain. Studies of pain mapping by laparoscopy under minimal sedation have found that the pelvic pain arises from areas of normal peritoneum adjacent to areas of endometriosis.

Secondary dysmenorrhea is a common component of pain that varies from a dull ache to severe pelvic pain. It may be unilateral or bilateral and may radiate to the lower back, legs, and groin. Patients often complain of pelvic heaviness or a perception of their internal organs being swollen. Unlike primary dysmenorrhea, the pain may last for many days, including several days before and after the menstrual flow.

The dyspareunia associated with endometriosis is described as pain deep in the pelvis. The cause of this symptom seems to be immobility of the pelvic organs during coital activity or direct pressure on areas of endometriosis in the uterosacral ligaments or the cul-de-sac. Sometimes patients describe areas of point tenderness. The acute pain, experienced during deep penetration, may continue for several hours following intercourse.

Abnormal bleeding is a symptom noted by 15% to 20% of women with endometriosis. The most frequent complaints are premenstrual spotting and menorrhagia. Usually this abnormal bleeding is not associated with anovulation and may be related to abnormalities of the endometrium. On the other hand, patients with endometriosis frequently have ovulatory dysfunction. Approximately 15% of women with endometriosis have coincidental anovulation or luteal dysfunction.

An increased incidence of first-trimester abortion in women with untreated endometriosis has been reported, although this notion has been challenged and remains an unproven association. Less common, yet troublesome, are the symptoms resulting from endometriosis influencing the gastrointestinal and urinary tracts. Cyclic abdominal pain, intermittent constipation, diarrhea, **dyschezia**, urinary frequency, dysuria, and hematuria are all possible symptoms. Bowel obstruction and hydronephrosis may occur. One rare clinical manifestation of endometriosis is catamenial hemothorax, bloody pleural fluid occurring during menses. Massive ascites is a rare symptom of endometriosis, but it is important because the disease process initially masquerades as ovarian carcinoma.

Signs

The classic pelvic finding of endometriosis is a fixed retroverted uterus, with scarring and tenderness posterior to the uterus. The characteristic nodularity of the uterosacral ligaments and

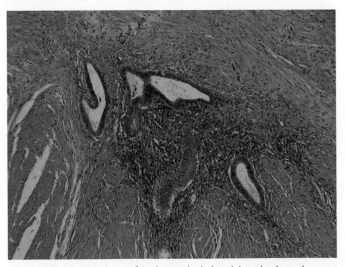

Figure 19-11 Histology of endometriosis involving the bowel. (From www.ispub.com/journal, 2007.)

cul-de-sac may be palpated on rectovaginal examination in women with this distribution of the disease. Advanced cases have extensive scarring and narrowing of the posterior vaginal fornix. The ovaries may be enlarged and tender and are often fixed to the broad ligament or lateral pelvic sidewall. The adnexal enlargement is rarely symmetrical, as one might expect in some benign pelvic conditions. In one study of 561 women with ovarian **endometriomas**, bilateral cysts were observed in 158 (28%). In women with unilateral endometriomas, 63% were found in the left ovary.

Speculum examination may demonstrate small areas of endometriosis on the cervix or upper vagina. Lateral displacement or deviation of the cervix is visualized or palpated by digital exam of the vagina and cervix in approximately 15% of women with moderate or severe endometriosis. An experienced clinician may instruct the patient to return for a pelvic examination during the first or second day of her menstrual flow when the diagnosis of endometriosis is in doubt. This is the time of maximum swelling and tenderness in the areas of endometriosis. The diagnosis can be confirmed in most cases by direct laparoscopic visualization of endometriosis with its associated scarring and adhesion formation. In many patients it is discovered for the first time during an infertility investigation. Biopsy of selected implants confirms the diagnosis.

When laparoscopy is undertaken to establish the diagnosis of endometriosis, it is important to describe systematically the extent of the pathology. The American Society for Reproductive Medicine developed a point-scoring system in 1996, designed primarily to record the progress of the disease in fertility patients. The focus here was intended to provide characterization of disease extent for fertility and not for pain assessment. Nevertheless, there are no data supporting this correlation of scoring with pregnancy rates. More recently, a proposed scoring system by Adamson focuses on the fertility potential of patients with endometriosis, the Endometriosis Fertility Index (EFI), and it has been shown in prospective evaluation to correlate with pregnancy rates. For example, a low score of 0.3 was shown to have a 3-year cumulative pregnancy rate of only 10% to 11% (**Figs. 19-12** and **19-13**).

Ultrasound examination shows no specific pattern to screen for pelvic endometriosis but may be helpful in differentiating solid from cystic lesions and may help distinguish an endometrioma from other adnexal abnormalities. Because the lesions are vascular, increased Doppler flow may be demonstrated in endometriosis (**Fig. 19-14**).

Magnetic resonance imaging (MRI) provides the best diagnostic tool for endometriosis but is not always a practical modality for its diagnosis. With a detection ratio and specificity of around 78% for implants, MRI for endometriosis has a reported sensitivity and specificity of approximately 91% to 95%. There is a characteristic hyperintensity on T1-weighted images and a hypointensity on T2-weighted images.

Although a benign disease, endometriosis exhibits characteristics of both malignancy and sterile inflammation. Therefore, the common considerations in the differential diagnosis include chronic pelvic inflammatory disease, ovarian malignancy, degeneration of myomas, hemorrhage or torsion of ovarian cysts, adenomyosis, primary dysmenorrhea, and functional bowel disease.

Occasionally a large endometrioma of the ovary may rupture into the peritoneal cavity. This results in an acute surgical abdomen and brings into the differential diagnosis conditions such as ectopic pregnancy, appendicitis, diverticulitis, and a bleeding corpus luteum cyst.

COURSE OF DISEASE

The rate of progression of the disease varies widely from one patient to another. Serial pelvic examinations are a poor indicator of progression of the disease. Serum levels of cancer antigen-125 (CA-125) have been used as a marker for endometriosis. CA-125 levels are elevated in most patients with endometriosis and increases incrementally with advanced stages. However, assays for serum levels of CA-125 have a low specificity because they also increase with other pelvic conditions such as leiomyomas, acute pelvic inflammatory disease, and the first trimester of pregnancy. Similarly, serum CA-125 levels have a low sensitivity for the diagnosis of early or minimal endometriosis.

Glycodelin, previously known as placental protein 14, has been shown to be elevated in endometriosis and is produced in endometriotic lesions. Levels also fall with removal of the disease. However, because of great variability in levels, glycodelin has not proved to be useful clinically.

Although it is generally thought that endometriosis improves during pregnancy, this is not always the case and an increase in lesions has been documented, although primarily in the first trimester. Ovarian endometriomas, which may have a different pathogenetic origin, from surface implants of endometriosis on the ovary may persist during pregnancy. Also, ovarian endometriosis rupture during pregnancy may occur.

Endometriosis may be associated with ovarian cancer. Not only are lesions found at the time of diagnosis of ovarian cancer, but the risk of developing ovarian cancer may increase fourfold in women with endometriosis. Loss of heterozygosity and mutations in suppressor genes, for example, *p53,* may explain this association. These findings warrant caution in the long-term follow-up of women who have extensive disease and ovarian endometriomas.

The association of other cancers with endometriosis, although suggested, has not been substantiated. However, cervical endometriosis is a particular condition that can produce abnormalities in cervical cytology.

Endometriosis is dependent on ovarian hormones to stimulate growth. With natural menopause, there is a gradual relief of symptoms. Following surgical menopause, areas of endometriosis rapidly disappear. However, it is important to note that 5% of symptomatic cases of endometriosis present after menopause. The majority of cases in women in their late 50s or early 60s are related to the use of exogenous estrogen.

TREATMENT

The two primary short-term goals in treating endometriosis are the relief of pain and promotion of fertility. The primary long-term goal in the management of endometriosis is attempting to prevent progression or recurrence of the disease process. Presently, there is a paucity of definitive, evidence-based literature to select the most appropriate method of treatment. The appropriate treatment for endometriosis varies widely because of the vast differences in the spectrum of clinical symptoms and in

ENDOMETRIOSIS FERTILITY INDEX (EFI)
SURGERY FORM

LEAST FUNCTION (LF) SCORE AT <u>CONCLUSION</u> OF SURGERY

Score		Description		Left	Right
4	=	Normal	Fallopian tube	☐	☐
3	=	Mild dysfunction			
2	=	Moderate dysfunction	Fimbria	☐	☐
1	=	Severe dysfunction			
0	=	Absent or nonfunctional	Ovary	☐	☐

Lowest score ☐ + ☐ = ☐
　　　　　　　Left　　Right

To calculate the LF score, add together the lowest score for
the left side and the lowest score for the right sides. If an ovary
is xxxxxxx xxx the sides, the LF score is xxxxx xxx by xxxxxxx the
lowest scores on the side with the ovary.

ENDOMETRIOSIS FERTILITY INDEX (EFI)

Historical factors

Factors	Description	Points(?)
Age		
	If age is 35 years	2
	If age is 35 to 39(?) years	1
	If age is 40 years	0
XXXXX XXXX		
	If years xxxx is 3	2
	If years xxxx is > 3	0
False Pregnancy		
	If there is a liability of a prior pregnancy	1
	If there is no liability of a prior pregnancy	0

Total historical factors ☐

Surgical factors

Factors	Description	Points(?)
Lf Scores(?)		
	If LF Score = X to X (high score)	3
	If LF Score = X to X (moderate score)	2
	If LF Score = X to X (low score)	0
Aps(?) Endometriosis(?) Score		
	If APS endometriosis lesion score is < 15	1
	If APS endometriosis lesion score is 15	0
Aps Total Score(?)		
	If APS total score is < 35	1
	If APS total score is 35	0

Total surgical factors ☐

EFI + total historical factos + total surgical factors

☐ + ☐ = ☐
Historical　Surgical　EFI Score

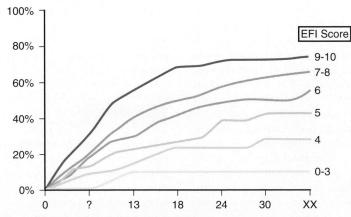

ESTIMATED PERCENT PREGNANT BY EFI SCORE

Figure 19-12 Endometriosis Fertility Index (EFI) surgery form. (From Adamson GD, Pasta DJ: Endometriosis fertility index: The new, validated endometriosis staging system. Fertil Steril, 2009. E pub available.)

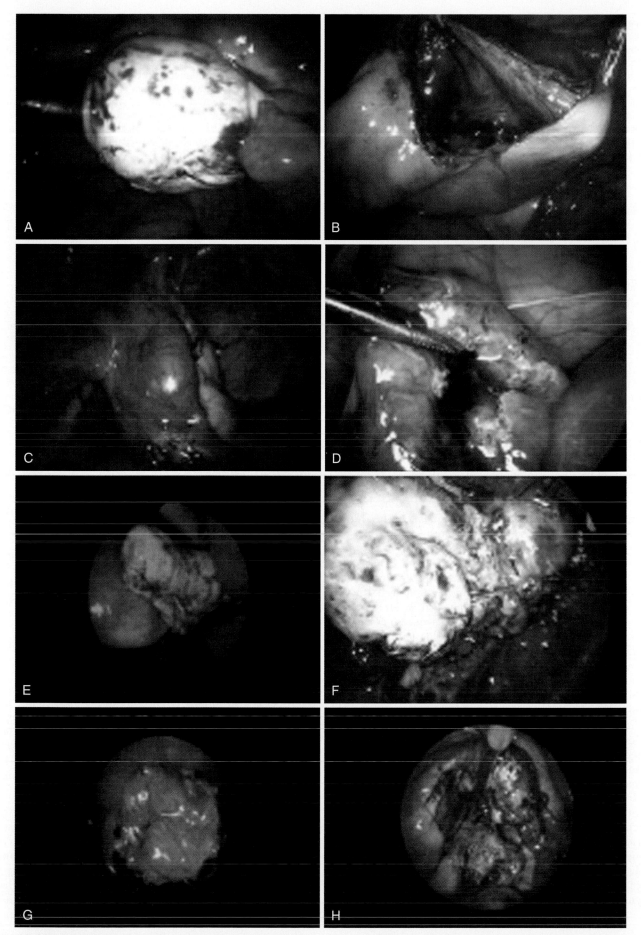

Figure 19-13 See legend to next page

Figure 19-13 Least function scores. **A,** Ovary=3: not normal, but only minor trauma to the surface. Fimbria = 3: slight blunting. **B,** Ovary = 2 (high): large endometrioma cleanly resected, good volume of ovary remaining, but more than minor damage. **C,** Tube = 2 (high): distal tubal endometriosis moderately significant, cleanly vaporized by CO_2 laser. Could be associated with postoperative adhesions and loss of function. **D,** Fimbria = 2 (high): clear intrafimbrial adhesions, treated with some damage to fimbria, still some reasonable architecture and function, but more than minor damage. **E,** Ovary = 2 (low): large endometrioma has been removed, suture required for ovarian reconstruction, some damage to ovarian surface, and relatively small ovarian volume. **F,** Tube = 2 (low): extensive resection and vaporization of tubal endometriosis seen in tube at 12 o'clock with resultant reduction in tubal function. Ovary = 2 (low): small endometrioma removed with loss of ovarian volume, and extensive invasive ovarian surface endometriosis vaporized, with postoperative high risk of adhesions. **G,** Fimbria = 2 (low): fimbrioplasty has been performed in obviously damaged tube, but with good patency expected. Very close to a score of 1. **H,** tube = 1: both tubes have extensive salpingitis isthmica nodosa. (From Adamson GD, Pasta DJ: Endometriosis fertility index: The new, validated endometriosis staging system. Fertil Steril 94:1609-15, 2010, Figure 3.)

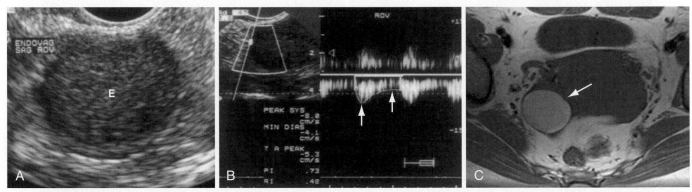

Figure 19-14 Ultrasound of endometriosis. **A,** Endovaginal ultrasound showing an endometrioma. Note low-level echoes. **B,** Doppler showing increased flow (RI = 0.48), which is suggestive of a malignancy. **C,** T1–weighted MRI showing an endometrioma *(arrow)* with a high-intensity similar to fat. (Adapted from Web MD, img.medscape.com.)

the extent of the disease from one woman to another. Therefore, the treatment plan must be individualized. Choice of therapy, for women whose primary symptom is pelvic pain, depends on multiple variables, including the patient's age, her future reproductive plans, the location and extent of her disease, the severity of her symptoms, and associated pelvic pathology. Most patients should undergo a diagnostic evaluation, which may necessitate a diagnostic laparoscopy to establish the nature and extent of endometriosis before embarking on prolonged therapy. However, if other gynecologic conditions such as chronic pelvic inflammatory disease or neoplasia have been ruled out, empiric medical therapy for 3 months is a reasonable option. Various suppressive treatments and where they act in the pathophysiology of endometriosis may be found in **Figure 19-15.**

Treatment of endometriosis can be medical, surgical, or a combination of both. Most of the sex steroids, alone or in combination, have been tried in clinical studies to suppress the growth of endometriosis. Optimal regression secondary to medical treatment is observed in small endometriomas that are less than 1 to 2 cm in diameter. Response in larger areas of endometriosis may be minimal with medical therapy. A poor therapeutic result may be governed by the reduction of blood supply to the mass caused by surrounding scar tissue.

Surgical therapy is divided into conservative and definitive operations. Conservative surgery involves the resection or destruction of endometrial implants, lysis of adhesions, and attempts to restore normal pelvic anatomy. Definitive surgery involves the removal of both ovaries, the uterus, and all visible ectopic foci of endometriosis. This type of surgery is analogous to cytoreductive surgery in ovarian carcinoma.

MEDICAL THERAPY

Medical therapy is aimed at suppression of lesions and associated symptoms, particularly pain. This is best achieved by menstrual suppression, ideally without inducing hypoestrogenism. Unfortunately, once suppressive therapy is stopped, symptoms tend to recur at variable rates. The choice of medical therapy should be individualized, weighing in potential adverse effects, side effects, cost of therapy, and expected patient compliance. The clinical effectiveness, as measured by relief of symptoms and recurrence rates of current medical therapies, are largely similar. The recurrence rate following medical therapy is 5% to 15% in the first year and increases to 40% to 50% in 5 years. Obviously the chance of recurrence is directly related to the extent of initial disease. In summary, medical therapy usually suppresses symptomatology and prevents progression of endometriosis, but it does not provide a long-lasting cure of the disease. The recurrence rate in women who initially had minimal disease is approximately 35%, whereas in those women whose initial disease was severe the rate is approximately 75%. Although there are several medical therapies for endometriosis, the Food and Drug Administration (FDA) has approved only **danazol** and gonadotropin-releasing hormone (GnRH) agonists.

Danazol

The FDA approved danazol in the mid-1970s for the treatment of endometriosis. In recent years, clinicians are less likely to prescribe danazol and most frequently select **GnRH agonists,** progestogens, or oral contraceptives danazol also may be prescribed for women with benign cystic mastitis, menorrhagia, and hereditary angioneurotic edema. Danazol is an attenuated

A. Sources of estradiol in endometriotic tissue

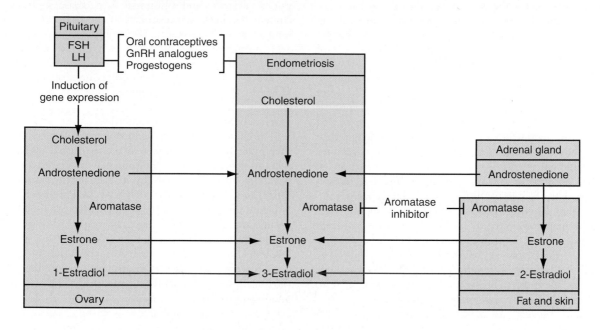

B. Survival and inflammation of endometriotic tissue

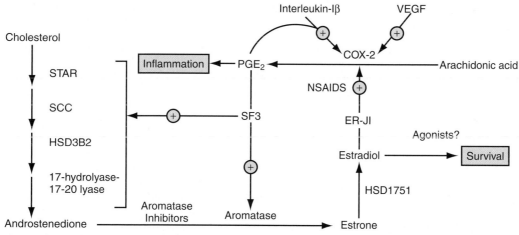

Figure 19-15 Molecular distinctions between endometriotic tissue and endometrium. **A** shows the three sources of estradiol, biologically active estrogen, in endometriotic tissue. The first sources are follicle-stimulating hormone (FSH) and luteinizing hormone (LH), which induce the expression of ovarian steroidogenic genes, including aromatase, for biosynthesis of estradiol. Ovarian secretion of estradiol can be reduced through suppression of FSH and LH by gonadotropin-releasing hormone (GnRH) analogues, combination oral contraceptives, or progestins. The second source of estrogen is the estradiol that arises from aromatase activity in fat or skin. The third source of estradiol is local production in endometriotic tissue. Aromatase inhibition in peripheral tissue (fat and skin) and endometriotic tissue stops estradiol biosynthesis and is therapeutic in endometriosis. As shown in **B,** high levels of local estradiol and prostaglandin E_2 (PGE_2) are maintained in endometriotic tissue by autoregulatory positive-feedback mechanisms (indicated by plus signs) that involve nuclear receptors (steroidogenic factor 1 [SF1] and estrogen receptor β [ER-β]), enzymatic pathways, cytokines, and growth factors. COX-2 denotes cyclooxygenase-2, HSD17B1 17β-hydroxysteroid dehydrogenase 1, HSD3B2 3β-hydroxysteroid dehydrogenase 2, side-chain cleavage (SCC) enzyme, steroidogenic acute regulatory (STAR) protein, and vascular endothelial growth factor (VEGF). (Adapted from Bulun SE, Lin Z, Imir G, et al: Mechanisms of disease. N Engl J Med 360:271, 2009, Figure 2.)

androgen that is active when given orally. Chemically it is a synthetic steroid that is the isoxazole derivative of ethisterone (17-α-ethinyltestosterone). Many years ago, oral androgens such as methyl testosterone were also used, as they induce endometrial atrophy. Danazol produces a hypoestrogenic and hyperandrogenic effect on steroid-sensitive end organs. The drug is mildly androgenic and anabolic. Many of danazol's side effects

are directly related to these two properties, which has limited its modern-day use.

Danazol induces atrophic changes in the endometrium of the uterus and similar changes in endometrial implants. It may also modulate immunologic function. Although doses of 400 to 800 mg of danazol have been prescribed, many clinicians reduce the total daily dosage of the drug down to 200, and even 100 mg of danazol daily. Danazol is usually begun during menses (days 1 to 5). Because the relief of the symptoms is directly related to the incidence of amenorrhea, the lower dosages of danazol are not as effective but may be tried. Side effects of the hormonal changes are encountered by 80%, and approximately 10% to 20% of women discontinue danazol because of side effects. Virtually all of the symptoms disappear on cessation of drug therapy. However, there are scattered reports of deepening of the voice that did not resolve after discontinuation. Mild elevation in serum liver enzyme levels has been reported in women treated for endometriosis, and women who take danazol for longer than 6 months should have serum liver enzyme determinations. An androgenic effect on lipids occurs, with reduction in high-density lipoprotein (HDL) cholesterol and triglycerides and an increase in low-density lipoprotein (LDL) cholesterol.

The standard length of treatment with danazol is 6 to 9 months. Approximately three of four patients note significant improvement in their symptoms, and about 90% have objective improvement discovered at second-look laparoscopy. The uncorrected fertility rate following danazol therapy is approximately 40%. Unfortunately, symptoms will recur in 15% to 30% of women within 2 years following therapy.

Several randomized, double-blind clinical studies have compared the therapeutic effectiveness of danazol with GnRH agonists. The results do not show significant differences between the efficacies of these two drugs.

GnRH AGONISTS

Several GnRH agonists have been developed and approved for the treatment of endometriosis. Representative agonists are leuprolide acetate (Lupron, injectable), nafarelin acetate (Synarel, intranasal), and goserelin acetate (Zoladex, subcutaneous implant). The usual dose of leuprolide acetate is 3.75 mg intramuscularly once per month or a 11.25-mg depot injection every 3 months. Nafarelin acetate nasal spray is given in a dose of one spray (200 μg) in one nostril in the morning and one spray (200 μg) in the other nostril in the evening up to a maximum of 800 μg daily. Goserelin acetate is given in a dosage of 3.6 mg every 28 days in a biodegradable subcutaneous implant.

Studies have determined the dose-response curve of the GnRH agonists, establishing the optimal dose to produce sufficient downregulation and desensitization of the pituitary to produce extremely low levels of circulating estrogen and amenorrhea. Chronic use of GnRH agonists produces a "medical oophorectomy." A dramatic reduction occurs in serum estrone, E_2, testosterone, and androstenedione to levels similar to the hormonal levels in oophorectomized women. The total serum estrone and estradiol levels and the free serum E_2 concentration are 25% to 50% of those measured in women taking danazol chronically for endometriosis.

GnRH agonists have no effect on sex hormone-binding globulin. Thus, the androgenic side effects from danazol caused by the increase in free serum testosterone are not observed. Similarly, no significant changes occur in total serum cholesterol, HDL, or LDL levels during therapeutic periods of as long as 6 months. Endometrial samples obtained after several months of chronic agonist therapy demonstrated either atrophic or early proliferative endometrium.

The side effects associated with GnRH agonist therapy are primarily those associated with estrogen deprivation, similar to menopause. The three most common symptoms are hot flushes, vaginal dryness, and insomnia. A decrease in bone mineral content has been demonstrated in the trabecular bone of the lumbar spine by quantitative computer tomography. This decrease in bone density is not seen in the compact bone of the distal radius. There is a decrease in measured bone mass of 2% to 7% during a 6-month course of agonist therapy. However, it has been established that the decrease in bone density associated with 6 months of therapy agonist completely recovers between 12 and 24 months.

The clinical response to agonist therapy depends on when the therapy is initiated in regard to the menstrual cycle. If agonist therapy is begun during the follicular phase, an agonist phase results in an initial rapid rise in follicle-stimulating hormone (FSH) and E_2, for approximately 3 weeks. FSH levels fall to basal levels by the third to fourth week of therapy. E_2 levels rapidly decline after 21 days of therapy. The expected surge in luteinizing hormone (LH) does not occur, and serum progesterone levels do not become elevated. Amenorrhea is induced within 6 to 8 weeks. In contrast, beginning agonist therapy during the luteal phase, or if artificially manipulated by the concurrent administration of oral progestogen, serum E_2 levels are suppressed to those postoophorectomy within 2 weeks. Amenorrhea is induced in 4 to 5 weeks. It is important to ensure that the patient is not pregnant when beginning GnRH agonist therapy during the luteal phase.

GnRH agonist therapy ameliorates symptomatology in 75% to 90% of patients with endometriosis, depending on the extent of the disease in the study group. Growth of endometriosis is arrested, diminished, or eliminated. The greatest therapeutic effects are seen in patients whose areas of endometriosis are less than 1 cm in diameter. Ovarian function usually returns to normal in 6 to 12 weeks after 6 months of GnRH agonist therapy. Large ovarian endometriomas and severe adhesive disease have not responded to hormonal therapy. The primary advantage of GnRH agonists over danazol is better patient compliance. Most patients find the side effects of GnRH agonists more tolerable. Currently, many clinicians "add back" hormone replacement therapy with dosages similar to menopausal therapy in combination with chronic GnRH agonist regimens. The clinical hypothesis is that the add-back medication will reduce or eliminate the vasomotor symptoms and vaginal atrophy and also diminish or overcome the demineralization of bone. Barbieri has suggested that there is a therapeutic window that he estimates is a circulating level of approximately 30 pg/mL of E_2. He postulated that this level of E_2 is enough to protect the body from substantial bone loss and is not high enough to interfere with the inhibition of growth of endometriosis (see **Fig. 19-15**). Multiple randomized trials have demonstrated that add-back therapy does not interfere with the effectiveness of agonists to relieve the pelvic pain from endometriosis. The majority of studies have also demonstrated no diminished therapeutic efficacy when add-back therapy is initiated simultaneously with the GnRH agonist. Some clinicians additionally give bisphosphonates and calcium with the low-dose progestins and estrogen, but bisphosphonates are not recommended in younger women who may wish to become pregnant. Add-back regimens not only reduce or eliminate adverse clinical and metabolic side effects associated with hypoestrogenism but also facilitate safe and effective prolongation of GnRH agonist therapy for up to 12 months. Additional agents that have been used for add back therapy are tibolone and raloxifene.

GnRH antagonists have also been considered an attractive option in that they have no "flare" effect. A direct effect on lesions has also been hypothesized. Novel oral agents are also in early development.

For women not wishing to conceive, who predominantly have pain and no indication for surgery (which may include failed medical therapy), stopping and starting various treatments and interchanging them is a reasonable approach to control symptoms.

ORAL CONTRACEPTIVES

In the late 1950s, very large doses of norethynodrel with mestranol daily were given to produce amenorrhea and a "pseudopregnancy." Most of the published studies involved the first-generation, high-estrogen–content oral contraceptives. However, more recent reports have established that the present low-estrogen monophasic combination pills, specifically the ones with a relatively high progestin potency, are equally effective when used in a continuous fashion. It has been accepted that the most economical regimen for the treatment of women with mild or moderate symptoms of endometriosis has been continuous daily oral contraceptives for 6 to 12 months. Continuous dose regimens are aimed at more complete suppression and the only concern is with breakthrough bleeding, which can be dealt with in a variety of ways as with contraceptive therapy (see Chapter 13).

One potential risk of using oral contraceptives or progestogens is that there is some risk of rupture if a large endometrioma is present. Rupture of large endometriomas may result in an acute surgical abdomen during the first 6 weeks of oral contraceptive therapy. During prolonged therapy the endometrial glands atrophy and the stroma undergoes a marked decidual reaction. Some smaller endometriomas (3 cm) can undergo necrobiosis and resorption.

The most common side effects of inducing amenorrhea with oral contraceptives include weight gain and breast tenderness. Approximately one in three women discontinue this therapy because of side effects.

The results of continuous oral contraceptive therapy include a decrease in symptomatology in approximately 80% of patients during therapy.

NSAIDs

Nonsteroidal anti-inflammatory drugs (NSAIDs) are beneficial for pain relief and as concomitant therapy may improve the bleeding control of patients on oral contraceptives. There may also be a direct therapeutic value in endometriosis. Although cyclooxygenase-2 (Cox-2) inhibitors are now infrequently used because of cardiovascular concerns in older individuals, this therapy for endometriosis has a rationale in that lesions of endometriosis have been found to express high levels of Cox-2 (see **Fig. 19-15**). In summary, anti-inflammatory agents may be beneficial for pain relief as well as potentially for the treatment of endometriosis, particularly when other suppressive therapy cannot be used.

Other Hormonal Treatments

For women who cannot tolerate the high dosage of estrogen in an oral contraceptive or who have a contraindication to estrogen therapy, treatment with progestogens only has been successful.

Medroxyprogesterone acetate (Provera) in a dosage of 20 to 30 mg orally per day or depomedroxyprogesterone acetate (Depo-Provera) in a dosage of 150 mg intramuscularly every 3 months to a maximum of 200 mg every month will produce a prolonged amenorrhea. The medication is most appropriate for the older woman who has completed childbearing. The time of resumption of ovulation following discontinuation of injectable medroxyprogesterone is prolonged and extremely variable. Some women will not ovulate for more than a year after their last injection. Therefore, this form of therapy should not be prescribed for a young woman who is contemplating pregnancy in the near future. Oral medroxyprogesterone in a dosage of 30 mg/day is an alternative mode of therapy, as is norethindrone acetate (10 to 40 mg) daily. This more androgenic progestogen, although quite effective, has a similar symptom profile to that for continuous medroxyprogesterone.

Gestrinone is a progestogen originally developed as a once-a-week oral contraceptive. Recently, this drug has undergone clinical trials for endometriosis with dosages ranging from 2.5 to 7.5 mg/week. Gestrinone acts as an agonist–antagonist of progesterone receptors and an agonist of androgen receptors and also binds weakly to estrogen receptors. At completion of therapy in a randomized trial, a tendency for prolonged pain relief was observed for gestrinone when compared with GnRH agonist.

Dienogest is a selective progestogen that causes anovulation, has an antiproliferative effect on endometrial cells, and may inhibit cytokine secretion. In clinical trials at 2 mg/day orally, it has been found to be as effective as GnRH agonists.

OTHER POSSIBLE MEDICAL THERAPIES

There are several other less well-proved therapies. These include the peroxisome proliferator-activated receptor (PPAR) ligands, which have been shown to inhibit macrophage action in animal models; targeting haptoglobin because of structural similarity to Endo-1; targeting MMPs; and tumor necrosis factor α and VEGF. Also, antiprogestogens like mifepristone have shown efficacy in small clinical trials, and several compounds are being studied further. ERβ agonists may also play some role in the future trials in that some of the estrogen action involved in increasing VEGF and angiogenetic factors are mediated through ERβ (**Fig. 19-15**). ERβ may also modulate immune function. It should be noted that SERMS, specifically tamoxifen and raloxifene, have not been shown to be beneficial. Another anti-inflammatory immunomodulator, pentoxifylline, has also shown promise.

Aromatase inhibitors show promise in that endometriotic lesions specifically make estrogen. Both anastrozole 1 mg and letrozole 2.5 and 5 mg have been shown to be beneficial. They often need to be combined with oral contraceptives, progestogens, or GnRH agonists because of their tendency to stimulate the ovaries in premenopausal women. Preliminary trials have shown efficacy with the addition of aromatase inhibitors, although the side effect profile (including bone loss) may be worse because of the profound hypoestrogenism unless an oral contraceptive is used.

Various medicinal herbs have been suggested for use based on their antiproliferative and anti-inflammatory and pain-relieving properties as reviewed by Weiser. However, no rigorous clinical trial data are available at present.

ROUTE OF ADMINISTRATION

Delivering progestogens or danazol locally (intrauterine or vaginally) may also enhance effectiveness. Small clinical trials have suggested the benefit of using suppositories and local agents, particularly in those women with cul-de-sac disease.

SURGICAL THERAPY

Surgery has been the foundation of treatment for women with moderate or severe endometriosis, especially those with adhesions and when the disease involves nonreproductive organs. However, consideration is often given to beginning with medical therapy and reserving surgery for those patients with suboptimal results. A surgical approach is mandatory in cases involving acute rupture of large endometriomas, ureteral obstruction, compromises in intestinal function, or for large ovarian endometriomas.

Laparoscopy is employed frequently for both diagnostic and therapeutic reasons. The major advantage of treating endometriosis with the laparoscope, using surgical instruments, the laser, or electrocautery is that patients may be treated at the time of diagnosis. Depending on the operative technique chosen, endometriosis is coagulated, vaporized, or resected. Surgical treatment for endometriosis should mainly be carried out via laparoscopy rather than by laparotomy because of a shorter recovery period and reduction in the extent of subsequent adhesions.

Adhesions in the pelvis have varying characteristics. They may be minimal or extensive, filmy or dense, and avascular or vascular. If the laser is used, the surgeon must adjust spot size, power setting (watts), and time of application to control depth of penetration. The laser or bipolar electrocautery should be used, but with caution when endometriosis is adjacent to the ureter, bladder, or bowel. Follow-up studies have documented pain improvement in 70% to 80% of patients treated via the laparoscope.

In a prospective randomized trial, Sutton demonstrated the efficiency of laser laparoscopy over expectant management after diagnostic laparoscopy. Pain decreased by 62.5% compared with 22.6% with expectant management, and pain relief continued in 55% of women over 72 months. The median time to pain recurrence after surgery has been estimated to be 20 months. It has been suggested that photosensitization of lesions in endometriosis may also add some therapeutic value in terms of infertility, although this approach is still considered experimental.

The surgical difficulties in treating invasive carcinoma and endometriosis are similar. The infiltrative nature of both disease processes and the associated scarring result in a loss of cleavage planes and result in difficult dissections. Technically it is easier to palpate rather than visualize the extent of the infiltrative process of endometriosis.

Conservative surgery has as its goal the removal of all macroscopic, visible areas of endometriosis with the preservation of ovarian function and restoration of normal pelvic anatomy. Conservative operations include removal or destruction of implants, removal of endometriomas, lysis of adhesions, appendectomy, and sometimes presacral neurectomy. Throughout these procedures, the surgeon observes the principles of microsurgery and plastic surgery, including minimal and gentle handling of tissues, avoiding hypoxia of the peritoneum, and attempting to restore the pelvic anatomy to normal. Approximately one in four women will have a second operation for a recurrence of endometriosis. Laparoscopy has proven to be as effective and reliable as laparotomy in the treatment of ovarian endometriomas.

The rate of recurrence is directly dependent on the duration of follow-up and is highest in women with extensive disease and a history of previous surgery for endometriosis. Recent studies have documented that excision of an ovarian endometrioma is associated with a lower reoperation rate than using a fenestration technique, and both are superior to cyst aspiration alone.

If the patient has midline pain, such as dysmenorrhea or dyspareunia, occasionally a presacral neurectomy or resection of the uterosacral ligaments may be performed. Ablation of the uterosacral nerves when performed via the laparoscope is called laser uterosacral nerve ablation (LUNA). This procedure is less frequently performed today because of questionable efficacy and concerns of surgical complications. A successful presacral neurectomy relieves only midline pain and does not diminish pain in other areas of the pelvis.

Somewhere between conservative and definitive surgery for endometriosis, there is a place for total abdominal hysterectomy with ovarian preservation of one or both ovaries. This operation is selected for women who have completed childbearing and are in their late 20s or 30s. Without repetitive episodes of retrograde menstruation, the endometriosis remains quiescent in the majority of these women. Approximately one out of three women develop recurrent symptoms, and they subsequently have a second operation involving oophorectomy. Definitive surgical treatment is reserved for patients with far-advanced disease and for whom future fertility is no longer a consideration. Patients with pain that continues after medical and conservative surgery are treated by definitive surgery. Definitive surgery involves total abdominal hysterectomy, bilateral salpingo-oophorectomy, and the removal of all visible endometriosis. If a fair amount of disease was left and was resectable, then consideration should be given to treating a premenopausal woman with progestogens or continuous oral contraceptives for approximately 6 months before beginning estrogen alone.

Medical therapy and surgical therapy are often performed in combination for advanced stages of the disease. Clinicians debate the advantages of either preoperative or postoperative medical therapy. Presently many surgeons favor preoperative medical treatment followed by surgery in women with extensive disease. It is postulated that preoperative therapy facilitates the subsequent operative procedure, although this perception is not evidence based. Depending on the extensiveness of the disease and the success of surgery, medical therapy postoperatively may also be considered, although not usually in women actively trying to conceive.

Photodynamic therapy for endometriosis is undergoing preliminary trials as noted earlier. This procedure involves intravenous injection of a special dye that is concentrated in areas of endometriosis. A laser light produces a photochemical reaction to destroy the areas.

Most surgeons routinely remove the appendix when performing surgery for endometriosis not related to infertility. In a series of more than 100 consecutive patients with endometriosis, 13% had histologic evidence of endometriosis in the appendix. This involvement could be discovered by gross examination in only 60% of patients.

THERAPY FOR FERTILITY

Medical therapy cannot be first-line treatment for endometriosis because suppression of ovulation interferes with the ability to conceive. Occasionally as an adjunct, more prolonged (than usual) GnRH agonist therapy may be used before in vitro fertilization (IVF). In this section, surgical options are considered.

It is clear that for symptomatic women with ovarian endometriomas, laparoscopic surgical excision should be undertaken. However, in cases of extensive pelvic disease where in vitro fertilization/embryo transfer (IVF-ET) is a necessary approach, and when pelvic pain is not a significant issue, the removal of endometriomas is of no benefit and may be harmful in that it may compromise ovarian reserve. The size of an endometrioma also comes into play in cases of IVF-ET; if all visible normal ovarian tissue is replaced by endometriomas, surgical excision may be necessary. Otherwise for small lesions (>2 cm), follicle aspiration can be accomplished avoiding the endometriomas. In general, the presence of endometriomas tends to decrease the number of oocytes aspirated but may not impair oocyte or embryo quality.

There has long been a debate as to whether treating mild endometriotic lesions or implants would improve fertility. Two prospective randomized trials have provided some guidance. Data from the Canadian and Italian studies, taken together, both suggest that the pregnancy rates are improved with implant ablation (**Figs. 19-16** and **19-17**). Thus, one additional pregnancy may be expected for eight surgical procedures. The way these data should be extrapolated into practice is that if

a laparoscopy is being performed in a woman wishing to conceive, visible lesions should be ablated if technically possible rather than ignoring them.

Apart from the mechanical factors (endometriomas, adhesions, fibrosis) affecting pregnancy rates, in endometriosis, macrophage and cytokine abnormalities are thought to play a significant role in inhibiting fertility (see **Fig. 19-9**). These factors may affect oocyte quality, fertilization, and embryo quality as well as endometrial receptivity. Therefore, in addition to ablating lesions when present, several strategies have been devised to enhance fecundity. Controlled ovarian stimulation and intrauterine insemination, an approach to enhance fecundity in women with unexplained infertility, has been found to be beneficial in women with endometriosis. Finally, if IVF-ET is undertaken (because of mechanical factors or with other failed approaches), although pregnancy rates are generally favorable, one meta-analysis has suggested that the pregnancy rates are lower than for women with tubal disease alone (odds ratio: 0.81) (**Fig. 19-18**). Indeed, a Cochrane systematic review of three RCTs found that prior suppression of endometriosis with a GnRH agonist for 3 to 6 months prior to IVF-ET improves outcomes with an odds ratio of 9.19. This reemphasizes the pathophysiologic consequences involved with having endometriosis (described earlier).

Figure 19-16 Estradiol therapeutic window. The concentration of estradiol required to cause the growth of endometriosis lesions may be greater than the concentration required to stabilize bone mineral density. (From Barbieri RL: Hormone treatment of endometriosis: The estrogen threshold hypothesis. Am J Obstet Gynecol 166:740, 1992.)

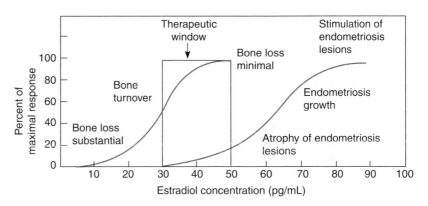

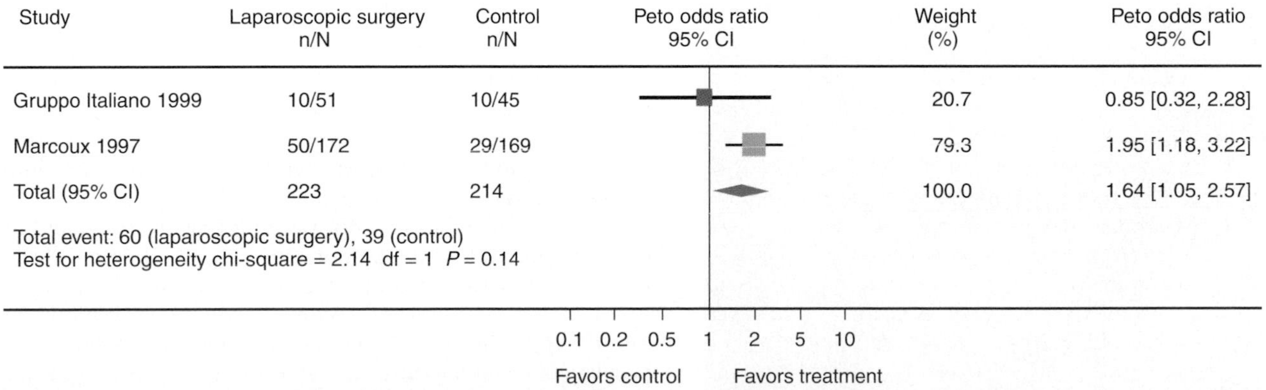

Study	Laparoscopic surgery n/N	Control n/N	Peto odds ratio 95% CI	Weight (%)	Peto odds ratio 95% CI
Gruppo Italiano 1999	10/51	10/45		20.7	0.85 [0.32, 2.28]
Marcoux 1997	50/172	29/169		79.3	1.95 [1.18, 3.22]
Total (95% CI)	223	214		100.0	1.64 [1.05, 2.57]

Total event: 60 (laparoscopic surgery), 39 (control)
Test for heterogeneity chi-square = 2.14 df = 1 *P* = 0.14

0.1 0.2 0.5 1 2 5 10

Favors control   Favors treatment

Figure 19-17 Meta-analysis of the two randomized trials assessing the efficacy of laparoscopic surgery in the treatment of subfertility associated with minimal-to-mind endometriosis. Combing live birth and ongoing pregnancy data from the two studies shows an improvement with laparoscopic surgical treatment (OR 1.64, 95%; C1 1.05-2.57). (From Jacobson TZ, Barlow DH, Koninckx PR, et al: Laparoscopic surgery for subfertility associated with endometriosis: Df, degrees of freedom. Cochrane Database Syst Rev 4: CD001 398, 2002.)

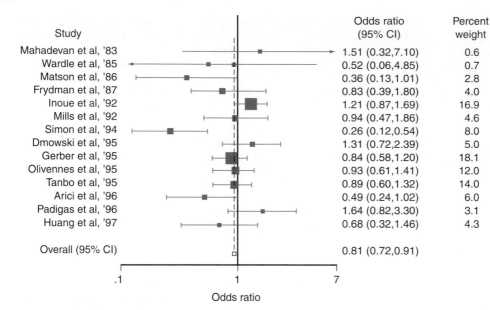

Study		Odds ratio (95% CI)	Percent weight
Mahadevan et al, '83		1.51 (0.32,7.10)	0.6
Wardle et al, '85		0.52 (0.06,4.85)	0.7
Matson et al, '86		0.36 (0.13,1.01)	2.8
Frydman et al, '87		0.83 (0.39,1.80)	4.0
Inoue et al, '92		1.21 (0.87,1.69)	16.9
Mills et al, '92		0.94 (0.47,1.86)	4.6
Simon et al, '94		0.26 (0.12,0.54)	8.0
Dmowski et al, '95		1.31 (0.72,2.39)	5.0
Gerber et al, '95		0.84 (0.58,1.20)	18.1
Olivennes et al, '95		0.93 (0.61,1.41)	12.0
Tanbo et al, '95		0.89 (0.60,1.32)	14.0
Arici et al, '96		0.49 (0.24,1.02)	6.0
Padigas et al, '96		1.64 (0.82,3.30)	3.1
Huang et al, '97		0.68 (0.32,1.46)	4.3
Overall (95% CI)		0.81 (0.72,0.91)	

Odds ratio

Figure 19-18 Unadjusted meta-analysis of 14 studies comparing pregnancy by in vitro fertilization in endometriosis patients versus tubal factor infertility controls. Horizontal bars depict study-specific 95% confidence intervals, and solid squares indicate weighting in the meta-analysis. References are from the original source. (Modified from Barnhart K, Dunsmoor-Su R, Coutifaris C: Effect of endometriosis on in vitro fertilization, Fertil Steril 77:1148. Copyright 2002, with permission from The American Society for Reproductive Medicine.)

ENDOMETRIOSIS AT OTHER SITES

GASTROINTESTINAL TRACT ENDOMETRIOSIS

The frequency of gastrointestinal tract involvement in series of women with histologically proven endometriosis varies from 3% to 34%. Most large series document a frequency of approximately 5%. Implants that involve the gastrointestinal tract are the most common site of extrapelvic endometriosis. The severity and extent of involvement of the bowel by ectopic endometrium varies from the incidental finding of a spot on the serosa of the bowel to obstruction of the rectosigmoid. In most cases, the implants do not produce clinical symptoms. In the majority of cases, endometriosis of the gastrointestinal tract involves the sigmoid colon and the anterior wall of the rectum. An important clinical marker is the finding that women with endometriosis of the ovaries have an increased frequency of extensive, invasive disease of the large intestine (**Fig. 19-19**).

Endometriosis of the appendix is fairly common with an incidence reported to be between 1% and 13%. Endometriosis

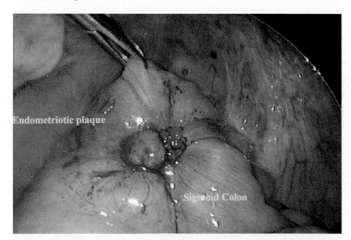

Figure 19-19 Endometriosis involving the sigmoid colon. (From Hemmings R, Falcone T, Clinical Reproductive Medicine and Surgery, Mosby, 2007.)

of the small bowel is rare. Approximately 200 cases of endometriosis of the ileum have been reported in the literature. This is a troublesome process because of the high incidence of associated small bowel obstruction.

Classic symptoms of endometriosis of the large bowel include cyclic pelvic cramping and lower abdominal pain and rectal pain with defecation, especially during the menstrual period. Associated with the abdominal and pelvic pain is a change in bowel function, diarrhea or constipation (or both). A distinct dysfunction of the enteric nervous system has been suggested to be the primary cause of the abnormalities of bowel function in women with endometriosis. It is difficult to differentiate the symptoms associated with endometriosis from the constellation of symptoms associated with inflammatory disease of the colon or malignancy. Women with a gastrointestinal malignancy usually experience intermittent rather than cyclic intestinal bleeding. Early diagnosis of gastrointestinal endometriosis demands a high index of suspicion by the physician. The initial clue to the diagnosis of the patient with multiple symptoms is the cyclic nature of these symptoms. Bowel resection is indicated for obstruction of the bowel or with extensive lesions in which malignancy may not be ruled out. On pathologic examination, the aberrant endometrial glands and stroma penetrate the serosa of the bowel and muscularis. It is unusual for endometriosis to involve the submucosa of the bowel. However, studies have demonstrated that 25% to 35% of women with advanced endometriosis of the large bowel experience episodic rectal bleeding from endometriosis extending into the submucosa.

Diagnosis of endometriosis invading the rectosigmoid is usually suspected by palpation of a pelvic mass or "rectal shelf" on rectovaginal examination. Sigmoidoscopy usually demonstrates absence of a mucosal lesion in addition to fixation and immobility of the anterior rectal wall. Donnez and coworkers speculate that endometriosis of the rectovaginal septum is a disease process more closely related to foci of adenomyosis than endometriosis. They postulate that the nodules originate from Müllerian rests in the rectovaginal space. Such lesions are usually unresponsive to medical therapy and require surgical resection.

URINARY TRACT ENDOMETRIOSIS

Endometriosis in the female pelvis occasionally produces dysfunction in adjacent pelvic organs. Approximately 10% of women with endometriosis have involvement of the urinary tract by implants of endometriosis and associated retroperitoneal fibrosis. In most cases an incidental finding of aberrant endometrial glands and stroma is discovered on the bladder peritoneum and anterior cul-de-sac. The most serious consequence of urinary tract involvement is ureteral obstruction, which occurs in about 1% of women with moderate or severe pelvic endometriosis. The pathogenesis of endometriosis of the bladder is controversial. Interestingly, approximately 50% of women with endometriosis of the urinary tract have a history of previous pelvic surgery. The lesions may develop from implanted endometrium during cesarean delivery or may be an extension from adenomyosis of the anterior uterine wall.

Patients with endometriosis involving the urinary tract have nonspecific clinical presentations. Hematuria and flank pain are experienced by less than 25% of women. One of three women with documented complete ureteral obstruction secondary to endometriosis has no pelvic symptoms whatsoever. The clinical challenge is to diagnose minimal ureteral obstruction at an early stage, before loss of renal function. The obstruction is almost always in the distal one third of the course of the ureter. The importance of an imaging study to diagnose ureteral compromise in all women with retroperitoneal endometriosis cannot be overemphasized.

Endometriosis of the bladder is discovered most often in the region of the trigone or the anterior wall of the bladder. Bladder endometriosis produces midline, lower abdominal, and suprapubic pain, dysuria, and, occasionally, cyclic hematuria. Treatment of endometriosis of the peritoneum over the bladder can be accomplished by medical or surgical means. Ureteral obstruction may be intrinsic, from active endometriosis, or extrinsic, from long-standing fibrotic reactions to retroperitoneal inflammation. Extrinsic endometriosis is three to five times more common than the intrinsic form. There are few reports of endometriosis of the ureter responding to danazol or GnRH agonists. However, long-term follow-up with serial ultrasound imaging or intravenous pyelograms must be undertaken to ensure that the disease process does not recur.

Surgical therapy is preferred for ureteral obstruction secondary to endometriosis. The operations are rare and should be individualized. However, operative removal of the uterus and both ovaries and the relief of urinary obstruction by ureterolysis or by ureteroneocystostomy are the most common choices. If ureterolysis is the operation chosen, peristalsis in the involved segment of the ureter should be observed, along with adequate resection of the endometriosis and surrounding inflammation in the retroperitoneal space. Ureteroneocystostomy has the

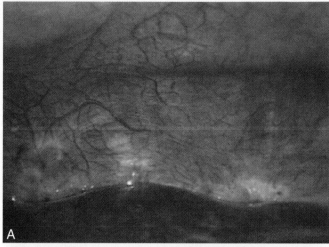

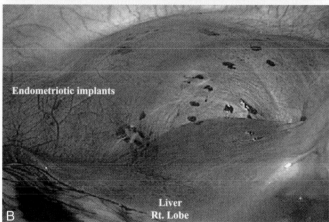

Figure 19-20 A, Fibrotic-type endometriosis involving the right hemidiaphragm. The lesions are seen above the liver. Most are obscured by the liver. **B,** Hemorrhagic-type endometriosis lesions of the right hemidiaphragm. (From Hemmings RR, Falcone T: Endometriosis. In Falcone T, Hurd WW: Clinical Reproductive Medicine and Surgery, Mosby/Elsevier, 2007, p 741, Figure 49-8.)

advantage of bypassing the urinary obstruction and making it technically easier to resect the area of endometriosis and associated retroperitoneal fibrosis.

EXTRA PELVIC ENDOMETRIOSIS

Endometriosis can also involve the diaphragm (**Fig. 19-20**). This may be an incidental finding at laparoscopy but may cause abdominal pain or even hemothorax and hemoptysis. Medical suppressive therapy is the first approach, although surgery including pleurodesis may be required.

KEY POINTS

- Endometriosis is a benign, usually progressive, and sometimes recurrent disease that invades locally and disseminates widely.
- Possible causal factors of endometriosis include retrograde menstruation, coelomic metaplasia, vascular metastasis, immunologic changes, iatrogenic dissemination, and a genetic predisposition.

- Endometriosis lesions produce estrogen locally and have increased secretion of prostaglandins and inflammatory cytokines, which cause pain and contribute to infertility. There is also a relative resistance to progesterone in endometriosis lesions.
- Grossly, endometriosis appears in many forms, including red, brown, black, white, yellow, pink, or clear vesicles and

lesions. Red, blood-filled lesions are in the most active phase of endometriosis.

- Approximately 10% of teenagers who develop endometriosis have associated congenital outflow obstruction.
- The two primary short-term goals in treating endometriosis are the relief of pain and the promotion of fertility. The primary long-term goal in the management of a woman with endometriosis is attempting to prevent progression or recurrence of the disease process.
- The recurrence rate following medical therapy is 5% to 15% in the first year and increases to 40% to 50% in 5 years.
- The side effects associated with GnRH agonist therapy are primarily those associated with estrogen deprivation, similar to menopause. The three most common symptoms are hot flushes, vaginal dryness, and insomnia. A decrease in bone mineral content of trabecular bone has been demonstrated in the cortical bone on the lumbar spine by quantitative computed tomography.

- Many clinicians "add back" very low doses of estrogen, low doses of progestins, or both in combination with chronic GnRH agonist therapy.
- The incidence of endometriosis is 30% to 45% in women with infertility. There is probably some benefit to abrading endometriosis lesions when seen at laparoscopy. In patients with endometriosis, the success of IVF-ET may decrease by 20%.
- Classic symptoms of endometriosis of the large bowel include cyclic pelvic cramping and lower abdominal pain and rectal pain with defecation, especially during the menstrual period.
- Endometriosis of the bladder is discovered most often in the region of the trigone or the anterior wall of the bladder. Bladder endometriosis produces midline, lower abdominal, and suprapubic pain, dysuria, and, occasionally, cyclic hematuria.

REFERENCES CAN BE FOUND ON EXPERTCONSULT.com

SUGGESTED READING

Adamson GD, Pasta DJ: Endometriosis fertility index: The new, validated endometriosis staging system, *Fertil Steril* 94:1609–1615, 2010.

American College of Obstetricians and Gynecologists (ACOG) Committee on Adolescent Health Care: Endometriosis in Adolescents, Committee Opinion 310:1–9, 2005.

Barbieri RL: Hormone treatment of endometriosis: The estrogen threshold hypothesis, *Am J Obstet Gynecol* 166:740, 1992.

Barnhart K, Dunsmoor-Su R, Courtifaris C: Effect of endometriosis on in vitro fertilization, *Fertil Steril* 77:1148, 2002.

Batt RE, Smith RA: Embryologic theory of histogenesis of endometriosis in peritoneal pockets, *Obstet Gynecol Clin North Am* 16:15, 1989.

Brosens IA, Brosens JJ: Redefining endometriosis: Is deep endometriosis a progressive disease? *Hum Reprod* 15:1, 2000.

Bulun SE: Mechanisms of Disease: Endometriosis, *N Engl J Med* 360(3):268–279, 2009 (Review).

Evers JLH: Endometriosis does not exist; all women have endometriosis, *Hum Reprod* 9:2206, 1994.

Gestrinone Italian Study Group: Gestrinone versus a gonadotropin-releasing hormone agonist for the treatment of pelvic pain associated with endometriosis: A multicenter, randomized, double-blind study, *Fertil Steril* 66:911, 1996.

Giudice LC: Endometriosis, *N Engl J Med* 362 (24):2389–2398, 2010.

Hornstein MD, Surrey ES, Weisberg GW, et al: Leuprolide acetate depot and hormonal add-back in endometriosis: A 12-month study, *Obstet Gynecol* 91:16, 1998.

Kettel L, Murphy A, Morales A, et al: Preliminary report on the treatment of endometriosis with low-dose mifepristone (RU 486), *Am J Obstet Gynecol* 178:1151, 1998.

Nisolle M, Donnez J: Peritoneal endometriosis, ovarian endometriosis, and adenomyotic nodules of the rectovaginal septum are three different entities, *Fertil Steril* 68:585, 1997.

Odagiri K, Konno R, Fujiwara H, et al: Smooth muscle metaplasia and innervation in interstitium of endometriotic lesions related to pain, *Fertil Steril* 92(5):1525–1531, 2009.

Sallam HN, Garcia-Velasco JA, Dias S, et al: Long-term pituitary down-regulation before in vitro fertilization (IVF) for women with endometriosis, *Cochrane Database Syst Rev* (1): CD004635, 2006 (Review).

Strauss JF III, Barbieri RL: Yen and Jaffe's Reproductive Endocrinology, ed 6, 2009, Saunders/Elsevier.

Strowitzki T, Marr J, Gerlinger C, et al: Dienogest is as effective as leuprolide acetate in treating the painful symptoms of endometriosis: A 24-week, randomized, multicentre, open-label trial, *Hum Reprod* 25(3):633–641, 2010.

Sutton ES, Whitelaw N, et al: Prospective randomized double-blind, controlled trial of laser laparoscopy in the treatment of pelvic pain associated with minimal, mild, and moderate endometriosis, *Fertil Steril* 62:696, 1994.

Yang J, Van Dijk-Smith JP, Van Vugt DA, et al: Fluorescence and photosensitization of experimental endometriosis in the rat after systemic 5-aminolevulinic acid administration: A potential new approach to the diagnosis and treatment of endometriosis, *Am J Obstet Gynecol* 174:154, 1996.

20

Anatomic Defects of the Abdominal Wall and Pelvic Floor

Abdominal and Inguinal Hernias, Cystocele, Urethrocele, Enterocele, Rectocele, Uterine and Vaginal Prolapse: Diagnosis and Management

Gretchen M. Lentz

The structural supports of the abdomen and pelvis are susceptible to a number of stresses. In the female these supports are affected by congenital anatomic weaknesses, the stresses of childbearing, injury, surgical damage, and straining. In addition, a combination of chronic stresses, such as lifting heavy objects, chronic cough, straining at stool, or activities that require frequent stretching, plus the aging process, may make older women more susceptible to such abnormalities. This chapter considers hernias of the abdominal wall and pelvic region, as well as conditions that are a result of the loss of pelvic supports.

ABDOMINAL WALL HERNIAS

The abdominal wall is made up of the following structures beginning externally: skin; subcutaneous connective tissue; external oblique, internal oblique, and transversus abdominis muscles with their investing fascia; and parietal peritoneum. The rectus abdominis muscles run longitudinally in the midline from the xiphoid to the pubic symphysis. The investing fasciae of the external oblique, internal oblique, and transversus abdominis muscles completely encase the rectus abdominis muscles cephalad to the semilunar line. Caudally from the semilunar line the muscle is completely behind the aponeurosis of the fasciae of these muscles and lies directly on the peritoneum (**Fig. 20-1**). Normally the investing fasciae join in the midline after surrounding the rectus abdominis muscles.

In the male, the descent of the testes from their original retroperitoneal site to the scrotum necessitates passing through the abdominal wall to the inguinal region. At the level of the transversalis fascia where the descent begins, the internal inguinal ring is formed. The inferior epigastric artery defines the medial margin of this ring as it courses from the external iliac artery medially and superiorly into the rectus sheath. The inguinal canal runs from the internal inguinal ring obliquely downward, emerging through the external inguinal ring and opening in the external oblique aponeurosis just above the pubic spine and then continuing into the scrotum. This allows for passage of the testes and for the presence of part of the spermatic cord.

In the female, the round ligament courses in the same direction but ends short of the labia. An **inguinal hernia**—that is, a bulge of peritoneum through the internal inguinal ring and into the inguinal canal—is less common in the female than in the male and is frequently identified after stretching of the abdominal wall during or after pregnancy. It may be related to a congenital weakness of this area. Occasionally a femoral-type groin hernia may develop. In this case the defect in the transversalis fascia occurs in Hesselbach's triangle, which is an area bounded laterally by the inferior epigastric artery, inferiorly by the inguinal ligament, and medially by the lateral margin of the rectus sheath (**Fig. 20-2**). The hernia sac passes under the inguinal ligament into the femoral triangle rather than coursing through the inguinal canal. **Femoral hernias** are more common in females than in males.

With a **reducible hernia**, the contents can be returned to the abdominal cavity. If the contents cannot be reduced, the hernia is said to be incarcerated. An **incarcerated hernia** may be acute, accompanied by pain, or may be long-standing and asymptomatic. If the blood supply to the incarcerated structure is compromised, the hernia is said to be *strangulated*. Because the hernia sac is primarily prolapsed peritoneum, the hernia itself is not strangulated but only its contents.

On rare occasions a portion of the wall of the hernia sac is composed of an organ such as the sigmoid colon or the cecum. In these instances, the hernia is called a **sliding hernia**.

A **ventral hernia** occurs in the abdominal wall away from the groin. Examples include **umbilical hernias**, which are caused by congenital relaxation of the umbilical ring, and **incisional hernias**, which are herniations through separation of fascial planes after operative incision. Two special ventral hernias include the epigastric hernia, which occurs in a defect of the linea alba above the umbilicus, and the rare **spigelian hernia**, which is a herniation at a point where the vertical linea semilunaris joins the lateral border of the rectus muscle. Spigelian hernia is a congenital or acquired defect. These are rather rare hernias (1% to 2% of all hernias), so they are not mentioned any further.

Incisional hernias generally involve the separation of the fascia of the abdominal wall with the hernia sac palpated beneath

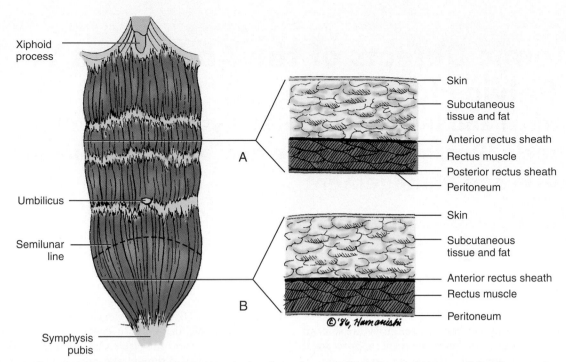

Figure 20-1 Graphic representation of layers of the abdominal wall. **A,** Above semilunar line. **B,** Below semilunar line.

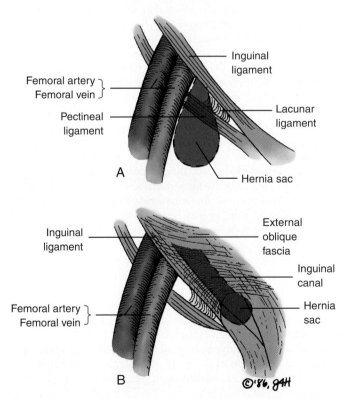

Figure 20-2 Graphic representation of right femoral **(A)** and right inguinal **(B)** hernias in the female.

the skin and subcutaneous tissue. The sac wall is composed of peritoneum.

Because the umbilicus consists of a fusion of skin, fascia, and peritoneum, an umbilical hernia generally occurs because the

fascial ring is grossly separated, allowing the hernia sac to protrude. This occurs most frequently in obese women. The hernia sac itself is made up of peritoneum and subcutaneous tissue beneath the skin (**Fig. 20-3**).

Rectus diastasis is an acquired abdominal wall defect in which the rectus muscles on either side of the midline separate. This is not a true hernia as there is no fascial defect, but it is mentioned here for differential diagnosis purposes. Also, pregnancy is a common risk factor.

ETIOLOGY

Hernias may be the result of a congenital malformation. The umbilical hernia is the best example. Before 10 weeks' gestation, the abdominal contents are partially herniated through the umbilicus into the extra embryonic coelomic cavity. However, after 10 weeks the viscera normally return to the abdominal cavity, and the defect in the abdominal wall closes during subsequent fetal growth. Generally at birth only the space occupied by the umbilical cord remains patent. After the cutting of the cord, the area heals so that the skin in the area of the umbilicus fuses above the closed fascial layer. Some infants at birth will show a

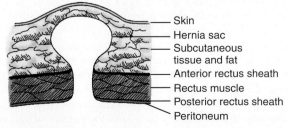

Figure 20-3 Graphic representation of umbilical hernia.

small umbilical hernia, but in most instances the fascial defect closes during the first 3 years of life. If it does not close, an umbilical hernia will form. In rare cases the abdominal wall closure process is less complete, leading to an omphalocele, which is a hernia sac at the umbilicus covered only by peritoneum and including bowel and other abdominal contents. Omphaloceles are usually seen in infants with other malformations and possibly chromosome anomalies, such as trisomy 13.

Black infants have umbilical hernias more often than do white infants. Occasionally, umbilical hernias occur in adults after the distention of the abdominal cavity with pregnancy or with ascites.

Inguinal hernias are more common in males than in females. Femoral hernias occur primarily in females. Hernias that occur in adults are often associated with trauma or injury. In many instances, the hernia bulge develops slowly after years of heavy labor. It is likely that a congenital anatomic defect was always present but became exaggerated over time, leading to the development of a hernia. Zimmerman and Anson thought that such lesions resulted from inadequate muscle support at the lower area of the inguinal canal, primarily caused by a defect in the internal oblique muscle. Stretching of this area in pregnancy may initiate a hernia, but other factors, such as chronic cough caused by smoking or chronic respiratory disease, may be responsible.

Incisional hernias generally occur because of poor healing of the fascia. This may be secondary to poor nutrition, infection, or necrosis of the fascia secondary to suturing. It may also occur because absorbable suture loses its tensile strength before healing is complete or excessive wound tension. Stress and strain secondary to chronic cough or retching in the postoperative period may contribute to the process. Emergency surgery increases the risk of incisional hernia. Other conditions that inhibit wound healing include obesity, smoking, connective tissue disorders, and immunosuppressant medications. Incisional hernias may develop 10% to 15% of the time after an abdominal laparotomy incision.

SYMPTOMS AND SIGNS

Bulges in the abdominal wall lead to the discovery of most ventral or groin hernias in women, either by a physician at the time of physical examination or by the patient. These hernias are generally symptom free. Occasionally, excessive straining or trauma will be implicated, and the patient may experience a feeling of tearing of tissue. Frequently the bulges are noted during an increase in intraabdominal pressure such as with coughing, pregnancy or ascites. Most hernias are asymptomatic, but in some cases, particularly with larger ones, there may be aching or discomfort. Should intraabdominal organs move into the sac, the patient may experience some discomfort. Organs that strangulate within the sac cause acute pain and discomfort. Incarcerated organs may give nonspecific visceral pain, which is most likely the result of mesenteric stretching. An incisional hernia with incarceration may present with a bowel obstruction.

In cases where a hernia exists but no contents are within the sac, physical examination reveals a weakening at the site of the hernia. It is often possible to feel the "ring" of the hernia as one palpates the defect through the skin and subcutaneous tissue. The patient's straining will generally accentuate the hernia, making it more palpable and visible. In the case of inguinal and femoral hernias, it may be necessary for the patient to be standing for one to palpate the hernia.

When there are intraabdominal contents within the hernia sac, the hernia is more easily palpated. The physician should then decide, based on his or her attempts to gently milk the contents from the sac back through the defect ring, whether the contents are reducible. For a hernia that does not reduce easily but in which there is no evidence of vascular compromise, it is sometimes useful to apply ice packs to the abdomen in the area of the incarcerated hernia before additional attempts are made to reduce it. In cases of **strangulated hernia**, evidence of devitalization of an organ, such as fever, leukocytosis, and evidence for an acute abdomen, may be noted.

MANAGEMENT

Nonoperative management of hernias of the ventral wall and groin in women is often feasible. Umbilical hernias in little girls will generally close by age 3 or 4 years and rarely become incarcerated. An incisional hernia, if not too large, can frequently be managed by a corset, which prevents it from becoming incarcerated. Unincarcerated groin hernias are often small and become uncomfortable only with an increase in intraabdominal pressure, such as occurs with pregnancy. Many authors advocate repair, however, because the small neck of these hernias may make incarceration more likely. With pregnancy the opportunity for incarceration is reduced because the increasing size of the uterus pushes bowel contents away from the area of the herniation. Trusses and other supports are generally difficult to fit and are of little value in women.

Larger hernias, hernias that continuously contain intraabdominal contents, hernias that cause continuing discomfort, and those that have been incarcerated should be repaired. Most incisional hernias should be repaired, but asymptomatic groin hernias can be safely managed conservatively. Some general principles of operative repair can be stated. The first principle involves the anatomy of the hernia. The hernia almost always consists of a sac of peritoneum with a narrow neck and a fascial defect of some sort. In rare instances, if a peritoneal sac is broad based, it may be possible to simply reduce the sac through the fascial defect without opening it and then to repair the fascial defect. However, if a narrow-necked sac exists, it must be dissected free of the fascial defect, emptied of its contents, and then excised and sutured at the neck (base). The fascial defect is then mobilized completely to remove stress and scarring, and it is closed with permanent suture. In many cases the fascial defect may be large and the degree of mobilization that is required may be impossible. In such instances, patching with inert material, such as polypropylene (Marlex, Prolene) or expanded Polytetrafluoroethylene (ePTFE, Gortex) mesh, may be necessary. Mesh repairs have become the preferred technique for incisional hernias because the recurrence rate is lowered. Recent studies are conclusive regarding lower recurrence risk for hernia using permanent mesh. However, the infection risk is higher. Sutured repair without mesh is still acceptable for small hernias (<2 to 3 centimeters).

The second principle involves management of the contents of the hernia sac. Usually the hernia sac reduces with ease, but if intraabdominal contents are fixed to the sac wall by adhesions, the sac must be opened and the adhesions carefully separated.

Care must be taken not to damage the organs or their blood supply. When these organs are reduced from the sac, the sac may be handled in the usual fashion. When incarceration has occurred, the organs must be inspected for viability before replacement.

Umbilical Hernia

A curved incision is made at the inferior margin of the umbilicus (**Fig. 20-4**). The umbilicus is dissected free of the sac and reflected upward. The sac is then dissected free of the fascial defect and either reduced or excised, depending on the

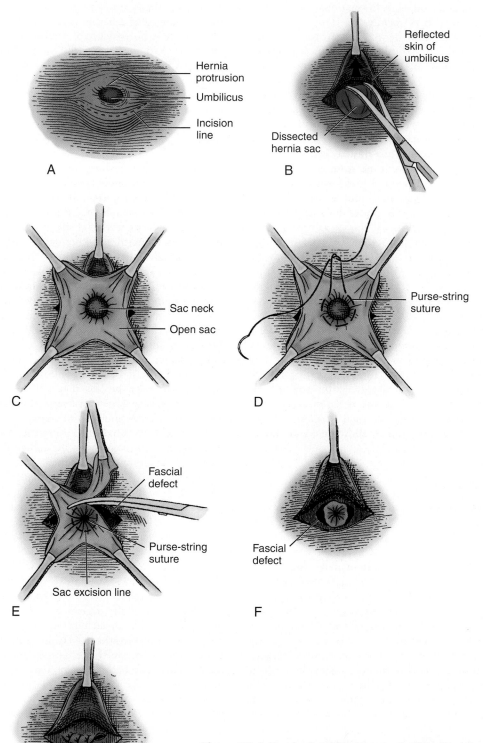

Figure 20-4 Repair of umbilical hernia. **A,** Site of incision. **B,** Umbilicus dissected free of sac and reflected upward. **C,** Appearance of sac that is cut open. **D,** Placement of purse-string suture at neck of sac. **E,** Sac dissected free of fascial defect after suture is tied. **F,** Appearance of fascial defect after sac has been excised. **G,** Fascial defect closed; umbilicus will be tacked to it.

circumstances. The fascial edges are freshened and either closed by direct approximation anterior to posterior using nonabsorbable sutures or mobilized and closed in a "vest over pants" manner, suturing the anterior edge to the posterior edge in an overlapping fashion. Studies have not shown that either of these closures is superior to the other, and the approach taken generally is the one that best fits the circumstances. The umbilicus is then tacked to the fascial defect and the skin margin approximated. Large defects may require mesh placement to avoid tension on the closure. Laparoscopic repair is also possible.

Incisional Hernia

Repair of an incisional hernia can be accomplished by incising the skin through the old scar or via a parallel incision and dissecting through the subcutaneous tissue to identify both margins of the separated fascial defect. The peritoneum of the hernia sac is then isolated, dissected free of the margins, and reduced in the most appropriate fashion, with the surgeon exercising care not to damage any organs that may be fixed in the sac by adhesions. The fascial edges are then mobilized completely and closed with a mass suture technique. Outcome studies show a sutured repair is more likely to result in a recurrence than a mesh repair. Sutured repair may be adequate for small hernias (<2 to 3 centimeters) and when the risk of using a mesh prosthesis is unacceptable. Laparoscopic repairs appear to reduce perioperative complications of wound and mesh infections, lower the recurrence risk, and shorten hospital stays, although larger randomized trials are needed to confirm this.

Prevention of incisional hernias bears mention because 10% to 15% of abdominal incisions will develop a hernia. Preventing wound infection with appropriate antibiotic prophylaxis if indicated and careful surgical technique is worthwhile because the hernia rate increases to 23% with postoperative wound infection. A meta-analysis of abdominal fascial closure concluded a continuous nonabsorbable suture closure resulted in significantly lower rates of incisional hernia. Weight loss and smoking cessation should be discussed, as these are risk factors for hernia development.

Groin Hernia

To repair an inguinal or femoral hernia, an incision is made above the inguinal ligament, usually parallel to its medial portion. Subcutaneous tissue is separated, and the aponeurosis of the external oblique muscle is exposed. The external oblique is then incised from above, down through the external inguinal ring, with the surgeon taking care to avoid the ilioinguinal nerve, which is frequently adherent to the external ring. The sac is identified and, by careful dissection, excised down to its emergence through the transversalis fascia. The sac is opened, and the intraperitoneal contents are reduced. The surgeon should place his or her finger through the sac neck into the peritoneal cavity and palpate the structures immediately within to be sure that there are no other hernia sacs protruding, particularly into the femoral canal. The sac neck is then ligated and transfixed away from the ring, often to Cooper's ligament. The transversalis fascia is approximated with nonabsorbable suture. The external oblique aponeurosis is then closed with nonabsorbable suture, and the skin and subcutaneous tissue are closed. Occasionally on opening the external oblique aponeurosis, only a mass of fat is found. In such instances the diagnosis of a hernia was made in error and no sac is present. Often, however, there is both fat and a sac, and the surgeon must be careful to determine the contents of the inguinal canal.

Femoral Hernia

When the sac is protruding beneath the inguinal ligament and through the femoral canal, an attempt may be made to reduce it from above. Frequently it is necessary to incise the inguinal ligament to free up the sac neck. In either case the sac should be ligated at its base, with the surgeon making sure that its contents are not damaged and that they are reduced. The sac, as in all cases, is generally handled by excising excess peritoneum and placing a purse-string suture of absorbable material about the base. Although it is probably not necessary to repair the inguinal ligament, most surgeons will do so. To prevent recurrent hernia in the transversalis fascia, the sac neck is sutured to Cooper's ligament beneath the inguinal ligament. To support the transversalis fascia repair, the external oblique aponeurosis is sutured over the transversalis fascia for extra support, all with interrupted, nonabsorbable suture material. Recurrence rates are reported to be less than 2% in a randomized trial of open mesh repairs.

Recently, many groin hernias have been repaired laparoscopically. This may be carried out both in the preperitoneal space and intraperitoneally. In most instances, a mesh patch is placed across the defect and fixed with either staples or sutures. Intraperitoneal exploration by laparoscopy often makes it possible to see a small hernia developing on the opposite side, which can also be fixed. In a study of 79 patients undergoing a repair of inguinal hernia, Panton and Panton determined that 25% were found to have a hernia on the contralateral side. Operative complications occur in 5% 10% of patients and include lateral thigh paresthesia, inferior epigastric artery injury, enterotomy from adhesiolysis, bowel obstruction secondary to herniation through trocar sites, and bladder injury. A 2010 meta-analysis by Dedemadi reported that laparoscopic or open mesh repair for recurrent inguinal hernia is equivalent in outcomes. Similarly, a 2010 Cochrane Collaboration reviewed 41 laparoscopic versus open groin hernia repairs involving 7161 patients, and hernia recurrence risk was similar as long as mesh was utilized. However, the laparoscopic repair takes longer (15 minutes) and has a more serious complication rate including visceral injury to the bladder or bowel and vascular injury. This needs to be weighed against the shorter recovery time with less persisting pain and numbness. Mesh reduced the risk of recurrent hernia by 30% to 50%.

DISORDERS OF PELVIC SUPPORT

Pelvic organ prolapse (POP) is a condition characterized by the failure of various anatomic structures to support the pelvic viscera. POP is common in parous women, with a lifetime prevalence of 30% to 50%, although many are asymptomatic. Prevalence of symptomatic POP ranges from 4% to 8% in recent studies. Racial prevalence data from a Kaiser population-based study finds significant difference in the symptoms of POP with African-American women having less symptomatic POP than white women (OR 0.4, confidence interval [CI] 0.2 to 0.8). The Women's Health Initiative found Hispanic women had the highest risk of POP and similarly, and African-American women had the lowest risk compared with white women. Pelvic support structure defects are often associated with vaginal childbirth–related injury (either neuropathy or muscular injury), other pelvic trauma, stress and strain from heavy lifting, and the aging process. Abnormalities that result from these relaxation problems include **urethrocele**, **cystocele**, **rectocele**, **enterocele**, and **uterine prolapse** (**descensus of the cervix and uterus**). If a hysterectomy has been performed, prolapse of the vaginal vault may also be a problem. It is unusual to have only one of these conditions. In most cases the relaxation affects all the support structures of the pelvis. More than 200,000 surgical repairs are performed each year for POP. Frequently, relaxation of the urethra, the bladder neck, and the bladder (urethrocele, cystocele) is associated with urinary incontinence, which is discussed in Chapter 21 (Urogynecology).

PATHOPHYSIOLOGY

The pelvic organs are supported by several key anatomic structures including the pelvic floor muscles, the fascial attachments, and the nervous system. Increasing parity, age and weight are commonly reported risk factors. The risk for symptomatic POP rises threefold with one vaginal delivery and fivefold for three or more vaginal deliveries. Interestingly, age and body mass index (BMI) have been inconsistently reported as risk factors in newer studies. Higher weight of the largest infant delivered vaginally, lower education, and vaginal trauma or episiotomies during labor are reported risk factors in some studies. Recent research finds irritable bowel syndrome and constipation as independent risk factors for POP, but other studies have not found an association with constipation. Genetic predisposition, estrogen deficiency, and pelvic floor damage from prior surgery might also be risk factors (**Box 20-1**).

The pathophysiology of POP is probably multifactorial. Bump and Norton outlined a useful concept in looking at risk

factors as predisposing, inciting, promoting, or decompensation events (**Fig. 20-5**). A study from Hove et al in the Netherlands surveyed 1869 women with validated questionnaires on risk factors for POP and used the four categories Bump and Norton outlined. The three greatest risk factors for developing POP in reproductive-age women were POP during pregnancy (OR 2.06; CI 1.42 to 3.00), maternal history of POP (OR 1.67; CI 1.10 to 2.54), and current heavy physical work (OR 1.48; CI 0.98 to 2.23). Forty-six percent of all POP in this population was attributed to these three factors. For this reproductive age group, only one risk factor can be modified: heavy lifting.

Box 20-1 Risk Factors for Development of Pelvic Organ Prolapse
Vaginal childbirth
Aging
Obesity
Prior pelvic surgery
Hysterectomy
Constipation
Irritable bowel syndrome
Genetic conditions
Neurologic injury
Controversial Risk Factors for Development of Pelvic Organ Prolapse
Episiotomy
Higher weight of the largest infant delivered vaginally
Chronic cough and respiratory diseases
Exercise
Heavy lifting
Lower education

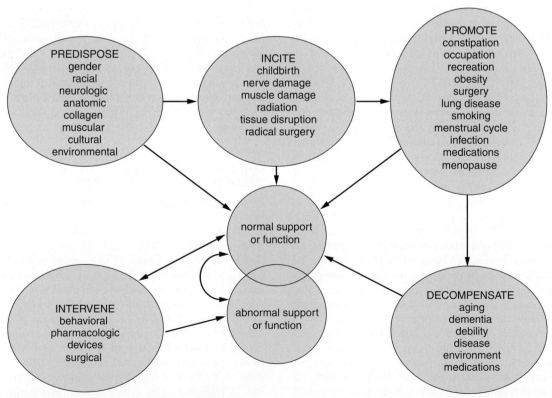

Figure 20-5 Model for the development of pelvic floor dysfunction in women. (From Bump RC, Norton PA: Epidemiology and natural history of pelvic floor dysfunction. Obstet Gynecol CINA 25[4]:723, 1998.)

The Women's Health Initiative studied postmenopausal women and reported that a history of at least one delivery was associated with twice the risk of POP compared to nulliparous controls. Other epidemiologic studies estimate that 75% of POP can be attributed to pregnancy and childbirth. For the general population, obesity and smoking may be modifiable risk factors. Besides environmental factors, there also appears to be genetic factors that contribute to POP. Twin studies support this as well as an early report of significant genome-wide association analysis, which is used in looking for genetic contributions to complex diseases.

Much research has been reported recently on the use of magnetic resonance imaging (MRI) for evaluating healthy female pelvic anatomy and anatomic variations to compare to women with pelvic floor dysfunction. Hoyte and colleagues used three-dimensional color thickness mapping to compare the levator ani of 30 women: 10 asymptomatic, 10 with urodynamic stress incontinence, and 10 with POP. Thicker, bulkier levator ani muscles were found in the asymptomatic women. Loss of levator muscle bulk was found in women with POP and stress incontinence. Theoretic explanations for these findings include muscle atrophy from denervation from childbirth injuries or muscle wasting from muscle insertion detachment also from childbirth, and possibly age and hormonal status (**Fig. 20-6**). More women with POP show levator muscle defects and increased size of the levator hiatus on MRI compared to women with stress urinary incontinence and controls. Imaging is not usually necessary in women with prolapse, but current research with MRI, defecography, and 3-D and 4-D ultrasound is furthering our understanding of support defects.

GENERAL SYMPTOM ASSESSMENT

Symptoms of POP are often not specific to the area that is prolapsing, and many women have no symptoms. In general, four categories of symptoms should be reviewed with the patient for complete clinical evaluation (**Box 20-2**). First, urinary symptoms might include urinary incontinence, difficulty voiding, slow urinary stream, or a sensation of incomplete bladder emptying. Second, bowel symptoms of constipation, straining, incomplete evacuation, anal incontinence, or splinting to achieve bowel movement might be present. Third, sexual symptoms should be discussed to assess for discomfort, irritation, and decreased sexual desire. Fourth, other local symptoms can occur, such as the classic symptoms of vaginal heaviness and bulge, a vaginal mass or low back pain, pelvic pain, or vaginal bleeding. Questions about how these symptoms are affecting the woman's quality of life address role and social limitations such as the ability to do usual daily chores, exercise and social event participation, as well as emotional health limitations. Validated, self-administered questionnaires are available such as the Pelvic Organ Prolapse Quality of Life (P-QOL) scale and the Urinary Distress Inventory, which cover these categories. Understanding the woman's goals for treatment is important, because often there are multiple symptoms in each area discussed earlier.

QUANTIFICATION OF PELVIC ORGAN PROLAPSE

A prolapse into the upper barrel of the vagina is called **first degree**. If the prolapse is through the vaginal barrel to the region of the introitus, it is **second degree**. If the cervix and uterus prolapse out through the introitus, it is called **third degree**. Some staging systems incorporate a **fourth degree** prolapse, which refers

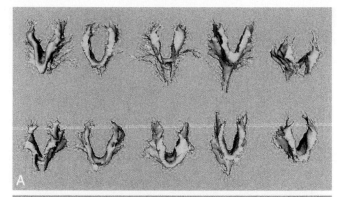

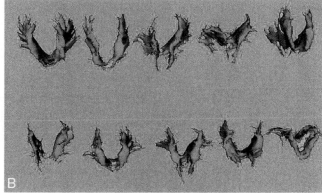

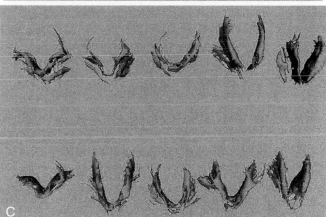

Figure 20-6 Color images of reconstructed levator ani muscles from three subject groups: Asymptomatic group **(A)**, GSI group **(B)**, prolapse group **(C)**. (From Hoyte L, Jakab M, Warfield SK: Levator ani thickness variations in symptomatic and asymptomatic women using magnetic resonance-based 3-dimensional color mapping. Am J Obstet Gynecol 191:856, 2004.)

to complete eversion of the uterus and cervix (procidentia) or vaginal apex. These terms are still widely used clinically but are imprecise. In 1996, the International Continence Society, the American Urogynecologic Society, and the Society of Gynecologic Surgeons adapted a standardized terminology for the description of female pelvic organ prolapse and pelvic floor dysfunction. This is an objective, site-specific system for describing, quantifying, and staging pelvic support and was developed to enhance both clinical and academic communication with respect to individual patients and populations of patients. The terminology replaces such terms as *cystocele, rectocele, enterocele,* and *urethrovesical junctions* with precise descriptions relating to specific anatomic landmarks. The first points are on the anterior vaginal

Box 20-2 Pelvic Organ Prolapse Symptom Categories for Clinical Evaluation

Lower urinary tract symptoms
  Urinary incontinence
  Frequency, urgency, nocturia
  Voiding difficulty: slow stream, incomplete emptying, obstruction
  Urinary splinting
Bowel symptoms
  Constipation
  Straining
  Incomplete evacuation
  Bowel splinting
  Anal incontinence
Sexual symptoms
  Interference with sexual activity
  Dyspareunia
  Decreased sexual desire
Other symptoms
  Pelvic pressure, heaviness, pain
  Presence of vaginal bulge/mass
  Low back pain
  Tampon not retained
  Quality of life impacts

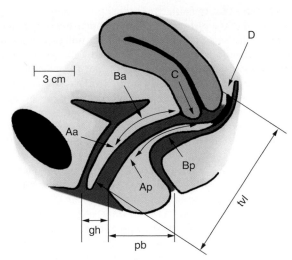

Figure 20-7 Quantitative description of pelvic organ prolapse six sites (points Aa, Ba, C, D, Bp, and Ap), genital hiatus (gh), perineal body (pb), and total vaginal length (tvl) used for pelvic organ support quantitation. (From Bump RC, Mattiasson A, Bo K: The standardization of terminology of female pelvic organ prolapse and pelvic floor dysfunction. Am J Obstet Gynecol 175:10, 1996.)

wall and categorize anterior vaginal wall prolapse accordingly. Point Aa is a point located in the midline of the anterior wall 3 cm proximal to the urethral meatus and is roughly the location of the urethrovesical crease. Point Ba represents the most distal position of any part of the anterior vaginal wall. Point C represents either the most distal edge of the cervix or the leading edge of the vagina if a hysterectomy has been performed. Point D represents the location of the posterior fornix (pouch of Douglas) in a woman with a cervix. Point Bp is a point most distal of any part of the upper posterior vaginal wall, and point Ap is a point located in the midline of the posterior vaginal wall 3 cm proximal to the hymen. To record measurements, these points should be expressed in centimeters above or below the hymen. It is important for the examining individual to express the position and other circumstances of the examination (i.e., straining or not, patient flat on table or in examining chair, etc.). **Figure 20-7** shows a diagram of the points and sites described earlier.

When the examination is recorded according to the anatomic points just cited, staging may be performed (listed in **Table 20-1**). These organizations hope that by using this system, a clearer understanding of a patient's prolapse will be achieved and the transmittal of this information to others will be made more accurate. They also expect that this system will make it possible to standardize research information. Because the old terminology remains commonly used outside academic centers, both will be referred to in this chapter.

URETHROCELE AND CYSTOCELE

Loss of anterior vaginal wall support is the most common site of primary POP. A cystocele is the protrusion of the bladder into the vagina, signifying the relaxation of fascial supports of the anterior vaginal wall.

Anterior compartment defects may allow the descent of the urethra (urethrocele), bladder neck, or bladder (cystocele) into the vaginal canal. Pelvic supports likely depend on interplay

Table 20-1 Staging of Pelvic Floor Prolapse Using International Continence Society Terminology

Stage 0
No prolapse is demonstrated. Points Aa, Ap, Ba, and Bp are all at −3 cm and either point C or D is between total vaginal length −2 cm.

Stage I
Criteria for stage 0 are not met, but the most distal portion of the prolapse is >1 cm above the level of the hymen.

Stage II
The most distal portion of the prolapse is less or equal to 1 cm proximal or distal to the plane of the hymen.

Stage III
The most distal portion of the prolapse is >1 cm below the plane of the hymen but protrudes no farther than 2 cm less than the total vaginal length in centimeters.

Stage IV
Essentially complete eversion of the total length of the lower genital tract.

between the endopelvic fascia and its attachments to the bony pelvis, the supporting pelvic musculature, and its innervation. Specifically, the trapezoidal anterior vaginal wall has distal and medial attachments near the pubic symphysis, lateral attachments to the arcus tendineus fascia pelvis and proximal, and lateral attachments near the ischial spine. Anatomic studies have identified fascial breaks in these facial attachments. Lateral breaks correspond to paravaginal defects; apical detachments from the pubocervical fascia of the cervix or vaginal apex are transverse cystoceles, and distal detachments from near the pubic symphysis appear as urethroceles or urethral hypermobility. Often only a cystocele is present, and generally in these cases the patient is continent. Although the patient may have stress urinary incontinence in this situation, the cystocele could also lead to voiding dysfunction from urethral kinking or compression. When a urethrocele is present as well, the woman usually often suffers from stress incontinence.

Symptoms and Signs

Symptoms and signs of urethrocele and cystocele consist of a sensation of fullness, pelvic pressure or vaginal bulge and at times a feeling that organs are falling out, occasional urgency, and often a feeling of incomplete emptying with voiding or slow urinary stream. The patient and the physician note a soft, bulging mass of the anterior vaginal wall. In some patients this mass must be replaced manually before the patient can void. Strain, cough, or prolonged standing accentuates the bulge. Often POP symptoms are less bothersome in the morning and worsen later in the day after upright activities. The mass may descend to or beyond the introitus. Although urethroceles and cystoceles almost always occur in parous women, they have been noted in nulliparous women who have poor structural supports. This is particularly true in women who have congenital malformations or weaknesses of the endopelvic connective tissue and musculature of the pelvic floor. Most parous women demonstrate some degree of cystocele, and when asymptomatic, they do not require therapy.

Women with prolapse often have other urinary symptoms. Some women have stress incontinence caused by urethral hypermobility, and others are continent despite lack of urethral support. Besides urethral hypermobility, probably urethral closure pressure and intrinsic urethral factors are more important than support for continence, which may explain these findings. Another group of women may have occult or latent stress incontinence because their continence depends on urethral kinking or obstruction from severe prolapse.

Sexual function symptoms should be considered. Dyspareunia, vaginal dryness or irritation, and other difficulty with intercourse may occur with POP in any compartment.

Diagnosis

The urethrocele and the cystocele are best demonstrated with a patient in the lithotomy position. A retractor or posterior wall blade of a Graves speculum is used to depress the posterior vaginal wall. The patient is then asked to strain, and the degree of the cystocele or urethrocele is noted. The physician should palpate the bladder neck and note whether it is well supported. Generally, if the supports of the bladder neck are adequate, the urethra is adequately supported. If a cystocele and a urethrocele are present, it invariably follows that the bladder neck is not supported. For determining the type of cystocele present, a ring forceps can be used with the split speculum. If supporting the lateral anterior vaginal walls to the arcus tendineus fascia pelvis causes the cystocele to disappear with straining, a paravaginal defect is present. If apical support with the ring forceps causes the cystocele to resolve with straining, a transverse detachment is present. The examination for cystocele and urethrocele is best performed with the bladder at least partially filled (100 to 250 mL). A standing exam with Valsalva often allows the physician to see the maximal descent of the POP.

At the time of all POP exams, it is useful to determine the maximal descent of the most severe portion of the prolapse, as often more than one compartment is affected. Pelvic floor muscle bulk, symmetry, and function can easily be assessed during the bimanual exam and by asking the woman to tighten her muscles like she is trying to inhibit voiding. Checking the vaginal tissues for ulceration and bleeding should be done.

Urethroceles must be differentiated from inflamed and enlarged Skene's glands and urethral diverticula. Cystoceles must be differentiated from bladder tumors and bladder diverticula, both of which are rare but may occur. Urethroceles and cystoceles are generally soft, pliable, and nontender. Although diverticula may be reducible, a sensation of a mass is usually present. Inflamed Skene's glands are generally tender, and it may be possible to express pus from the urethra when they are palpated. Pus may be expressed also in the presence of a diverticulum of the urethra. In such cases, gonococcal and chlamydial infections should be considered.

Management

Treatment of urethroceles and cystoceles may be nonoperative or operative and depends on patient preferences and goals. Nonoperative treatment consists of supporting the herniation of the anterior vaginal wall with the use of the Smith-Hodge, ring, cube, or inflatable **pessary** (Fig. 20-8), or even with the intermittent use of a large tampon. Kegel exercises (see Chapter 21, Urogynecology) help to strengthen the pelvic floor musculature and thereby may relieve some of the pressure symptoms produced by the cystocele. Although there is little direct evidence that pelvic floor muscle training prevents or treats POP, it may be beneficial for mild POP and it is effective for concomitant symptoms of urinary and fecal incontinence. Braekken's 2010 randomized controlled trial investigated morphologic and functional changes after pelvic floor muscle training in 109 women with stage 1-III POP. This supervised training led to a 44% increase in muscle strength, a 15% increase in muscle thickness, a decreased levator hiatus area, shortened muscle length, and elevation of the bladder and rectum position. It took 6 months of muscle hypertrophy training to achieve these results, so this option requires motivated patients. A follow-up study by the same group reported that 11 (19%) of women in the exercise group improved one stage on the Pelvic Organ Prolapse Quantification system compared with 4 (8%) of controls. This did correlate with reduced frequency and bother of vaginal bulging

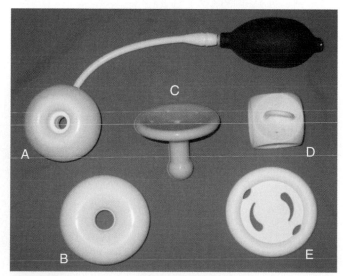

Figure 20-8 Examples of pessaries. **A,** inflatable; **B,** donut; **C,** Gellhorn; **D,** cube; **E,** ring with support.

and heaviness by 74% and 67%, respectively. It is reasonable to offer pelvic floor muscle training for POP symptoms because it is without adverse effects. Women who have performed Kegel exercises on their own and have not improved may still benefit from working with a physical therapist. In an older woman, the use of a vaginal estrogen product may improve vaginal atrophy and patient comfort if the prolapsed vaginal mucosa is irritated or ulcerated. There is no evidence that estrogen therapy will prevent or treat POP. Behavioral modification may help urinary symptoms such as urgency and will be discussed in Chapter 21.

A younger woman with a large cystocele should be encouraged to avoid operative repair until she has completed her family. Occasionally the abnormality is so uncomfortable that repair must be performed before childbearing is complete. If this is the case, cesarean delivery should be considered for subsequent pregnancies.

Operative repair of a cystocele is generally performed in conjunction with the repair of all other pelvic support defects. It is unusual for anterior supports of the vagina to relax without an accompanying relaxation of the apical compartment. Repair therefore usually consists of an anterior colporrhaphy, correction of uterine descensus or apical defect posthysterectomy if noted, and possibly posterior colporrhaphy for rectocele. Frequently an enterocele accompanies a cystocele and apical defect and where present must be repaired. These problems are discussed later in this chapter.

Anterior wall repair (colporrhaphy) is performed by incising the vaginal epithelium transversally just above the anterior lip of the cervix in the region of the bladder reflection (**Fig. 20-9**). The midline vaginal cuff is grasped with Allis clamps if a hysterectomy has just been performed. If the woman has undergone a hysterectomy in the past, the incision may be made approximately 1 to 1.5 cm anterior to the vaginal scar. The vagina is then incised longitudinally from the transverse incision

to the level of the bladder neck. If no urethrocele is present, this incision is sufficient. If a urethrocele is present, the incision must be continued under the urethra as well. The longitudinal incision is made by separating the vaginal wall from the underlying fibromuscular layer progressively, using Metzenbaum scissors. When the longitudinal incision is complete, the cut edge of the vagina is held under tension, and the pubocervical fascia that is attached is separated from it by blunt and sharp dissection. This is repeated on each side. At this point the bladder is free of the pubocervical fascia, which is itself free of the vaginal wall. The surgeon then places a suture over the bladder neck (Kelly stitch), bringing together the pubocervical fascia on either side. The stitch should be placed in such a fashion that the pubocervical fascia is sutured as far away from the cut edge as possible and parallel to the previous incision. A similar stitch is taken on the opposite side and the suture tied. Most appropriate for this closure is 0 or 2-0 polyglycol suture. With the bladder neck well identified and supported, the pubocervical fascia is then closed with progressive similar stitches to completely imbricate the fascia over the bladder. For larger cystoceles, a two-layer plication may be needed. If the urethrocele is present, similar sutures are also placed over the urethra. (Additional procedures to correct stress incontinence are discussed in Chapter 21, Urogynecology.) After the plication of the pubocervical fascia is completed, the vaginal edges are trimmed and the vagina closed with a row of interrupted 2-0 polyglycol sutures. Addition of graft materials to the anterior vaginal wall has been studied in several small trials. In 2008, the Society of Gynecologic Surgeons convened a group to review vaginal graft use. A systematic review of the literature was published, suggesting permanent mesh grafts placed in the anterior vaginal wall may improve anatomic support in the short term, but long-term outcome studies are lacking. Mesh exposure, pelvic pain, dyspareunia, and increased risk of stress incontinence have all

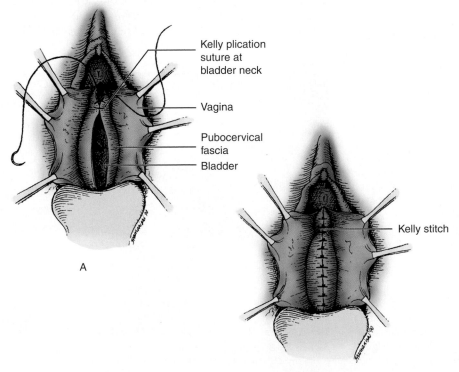

Figure 20-9 Cystourethrocele repair. **A,** The placement of Kelly stitch in the pubocervical fascia at the junction of the urethra with the bladder neck. **B,** The repair of the cystocele as the pubocervical fascia is sutured. Thus, the cystocele is plicated. (Redrawn from Symmonds RE: Relaxation of pelvic supports. In Benson RC [ed]: Current Obstetric and Gynecologic Diagnosis and Treatment, 5th ed. Los Altos, CA, Lange Medical, 1984.)

Kelly plication suture at bladder neck

Vagina

Pubocervical fascia

Bladder

Kelly stitch

A

B

been reported significantly more often with mesh inlays than with traditional anterior colporrhaphy. In 2008, an FDA public health notification summarized more than 1000 reports of surgical complications. A 2010 Cochrane Database systematic review concluded that the risk of recurrent cystocele may be reduced with synthetic graft placement, but there is still insufficient evidence to make firm recommendations. Although vaginal mesh kits are widely available, long-term outcome studies are still lacking. Certainly careful patient selection, detailed patient counseling, and a skilled surgeon with proper training is needed for these procedures and to manage the complications.

Postoperatively, the bladder should be drained for about 1 to 2 days. There are several ways to accomplish this. The first is to leave a No. 16 Foley catheter in place for 1 to 2 days, remove the catheter when the woman is ambulatory, and allow the patient to try to void with spontaneous bladder filling. After voiding at least 200 mL, the patient should be catheterized for the presence of residual urine or, alternatively, a bladder ultrasound can estimate residual volume. If residual urine is found in a quantity of more than 150 mL on two successive voidings or if the amount voided is less than 200 mL, the physician should consider replacing the catheter for 24 to 48 hours. If residual urine amounts are less than 150 mL on two consecutive voidings, no further steps are necessary. Another method for assessing postoperative voiding dysfunction is to retrograde fill the bladder via the Foley catheter with 300 mL of saline. The catheter is removed, the woman's voided volume is recorded, and the postvoid residual is calculated by subtracting the voided volume from 300 mL. One randomized trial of 50 subjects found retrograde and spontaneous fill were equivalent methods of evaluating postoperative voiding after surgery for POP or urinary incontinence. Two thirds of subjects failed the voiding trial on postoperative day 1. This is helpful information in counseling women on the chance going home with a Foley catheter given short hospital stays for these procedures.

After an anterior repair if voiding does not occur prior to hospital discharge, the woman may be treated with a Foley catheter for continuous drainage for a week and rechecked for voiding and residual urine as an outpatient. Prophylactic antibiotics are rarely recommended; however, symptomatic lower urinary tract infections are common and should be treated as they occur.

Alternatives to the above-mentioned regimen include suprapubic catheter drainage or teaching the patient clean intermittent self-catheterization (CISC). With a suprapubic catheter, the drainage tube can be clamped, allowing the patient to void when she can and allowing residual urine measurements to be taken. The suprapubic technique is simple to use and seems to have a lower incidence of infection than does transurethral catheterization, but patients may complain of extravasation of urine around the site and occasionally of hematoma formation. CISC can be threatening for patients to learn, but once learned, many patients prefer not having an indwelling catheter and can measure their own postvoid residual urine volumes. CISC is generally not necessary if short periods of catheterization are anticipated. The surgeon should decide which method is best suited to the patient's needs and develop a system that the surgeon and nursing team understand and can follow.

Postoperatively it is important to emphasize to the patient that heavy lifting, straining, or prolonged periods of standing should be avoided for 3 months. The healing process is slow, and the tissue is generally weak initially. Complete healing should be ensured before the tissue is stressed by normal activities.

Certainly, recurrent anterior vaginal wall prolapse remains as the most frustrating problem for the gynecologic surgeon and patients. In fact, George R. White was quoted in 1909 saying, "Ahlfet states that the only problem in plastic gynecology left unsolved by the gynecologist is that of permanent cure of cystocele." It is still the problem of the current century with reported failure rates of 30% to 40% for anterior colporrhaphy. The reintroduction of the paravaginal repair by Richardson brought hopes of reducing the recurrence of cystoceles. However, studies show failure rates of 3% to 14%, and controlled studies reporting long-term outcomes are lacking. So when POP repair is planned vaginally, anterior colporrhaphy is still indicated for cystocele correction with careful attention to the likely need for apical vaginal vault support. Synthetic mesh to augment the anterior vaginal wall repair seems to improve the short-term anatomic success rate, but at the price of increased complications, many of which require further operation. Abdominal sacral **colpopexy** will be discussed later in this chapter and offers another surgical option for women with anterior vaginal wall prolapse associated with uterine or apical prolapse. If stress incontinence is also present, a specific repair such as a midurethral sling is indicated along with the anterior colporrhaphy.

RECTOCELE

Symptoms and Signs

The patient with a rectocele often complains of heavy pelvic pressure or "falling out" feeling in the vagina. She may complain of constipation and occasionally may need to splint the vagina with her fingers to affect a bowel movement. She may also have a feeling of incomplete emptying of the rectum at the time of the bowel movement. Protrusion of the prolapse may worsen later in the day and be aggravated by prolonged standing or exertion. Any impairment of sexual activity should be discussed.

In general 24% to 67% of women with POP have defecation symptoms. Although reported symptoms might be related to the rectocele, there are many other potential causes of evacuation problems that are not (sigmoidocele, rectal prolapse, rectal intussusception).

Diagnosis

A rectocele is a protrusion of the rectum into the vagina, signifying a relaxation of the posterior vaginal wall. It may be identified by retracting the anterior vaginal wall upward with one half of a Graves or Pederson speculum and having the patient strain. The rectum will bulge into the vagina, and this bulge may protrude through the introitus (**Fig. 20-10**). The physician should then place one finger in the rectum and one in the vagina and palpate the defect. Often the rectovaginal septum is paper thin, and the rectocele can be palpated to its upper margin. If an enterocele is present, it may be possible to differentiate it from the rectocele by having the patient strain. Frequently, however, the diagnosis of a small enterocele is established only at the time of operation.

Management

Nonoperative management of a rectocele is similar to that mentioned for a cystocele. Pessaries, Kegel exercises, and estrogen may be useful in the appropriate situations. Gastrointestinal symptoms

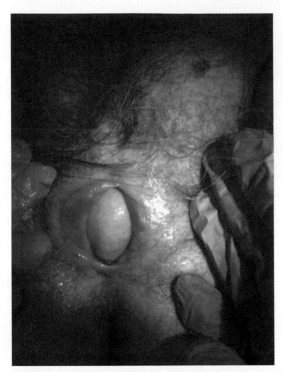

Figure 20-10 Rectocele. Although this may appear to be a cystocele, split speculum exam revealed a rectocele.

must be thoroughly evaluated, including screening for colorectal cancer if appropriate. If constipation and straining are issues, a dietary fiber and fluid intake review should be obtained. At least 25 g of fiber, six to eight glasses of fluid, regular exercise, and allowing time for defecation after meals can be recommended to regulate bowel habits as first-line therapy. Evacuation symptoms suggestive of an obstructive process or seeming out of proportion to the degree of rectocele bear further investigation by an expert such as defecography or dynamic MRI.

Operative management of a rectocele (posterior colporrhaphy) is often performed at the time of an anterior colporrhaphy with or without enterocele repair or operation for uterine descensus or **vaginal vault prolapse** after hysterectomy. Most women with rectoceles also have a gaping genital hiatus and a defect in their perineal body. Therefore, as part of a rectocele repair, a **perineorrhaphy** is performed as well. The surgeon should estimate at the time of starting the posterior repair what degree of perineorrhaphy he or she wishes to perform. The margins of the perineum to be narrowed are generally marked by placing Allis clamps at their extreme at the introital opening (**Fig. 20-11**). The tissue of the introitus is then incised between these clamps, and the vaginal wall is separated from the underlying tissue and rectum in a progressive manner longitudinally in the midline, beginning at the introital incision and being carried forward to the apex of the vagina above the limit of the rectocele. This is done by progressive separation and incision using the Metzenbaum scissors in a fashion similar to that described for cystocele repair.

When the vaginal wall is completely incised, the edges are grasped and placed under tension, and the perirectal connective tissue is separated from the vaginal mucosa by blunt and sharp (if necessary) dissection. This is carried out bilaterally until it is possible for the operator to palpate the perirectal space on each side. The operator then places a finger of his or her nondominant hand into the rectum using a double-gloved technique while

an assistant picks up perirectal (fibro muscularis) tissue on either side. The operator then places a delayed absorbable suture into the perirectal tissue on either side. Approximately three to five of these stitches are placed, and these are held without tying. The operator should use his or her finger in the rectum to ensure that no suture is placed into the rectum. The perirectal tissue usually includes portions of the connective tissue over the levator ani muscles. When the sutures are tied, these tissues are interposed between rectum and vagina, thereby reducing the rectocele. These sutures also serve to tack the vagina to the levator ani area, thereby, it is hoped, avoiding future vaginal prolapse if a hysterectomy has also been performed. Care must be taken to avoid creating a "shelf" in the posterior vaginal wall, which may narrow the vagina too much and lead to dyspareunia. Therefore, levator ani plication may best be indicated in nonsexually active women. If vaginal vault prolapse is also present, a separate repair is indicated for support of the vaginal apex, and this is discussed later. The vaginal edges are then trimmed and the vagina closed with a row of either continuous or interrupted absorbable suture.

Attention is then turned to the perineorrhaphy when there is perineal muscle separation and a perineal body defect. It is closed in the following fashion. Polyglycol sutures are placed in the lateral margins of the transverse incision, essentially bringing bulbocavernosal and superficial perineal muscles together from either side to the midline. The operator should be sure that the bulbocavernosal muscle insertions are included in the sutures by pulling on the suture and noting whether the tension identifies the muscle bundles. Over tightening the introitus might cause dyspareunia. The remainder of the perineal incision is then closed with a row of 2-0 polyglycol sutures to the deep tissue, and the skin of the perineum is closed with either interrupted or continuous subcuticular suture of 3-0 absorbable suture.

Although anatomic position is often corrected by a posterior colporrhaphy, function may not be corrected. Defecatory problems may remain, so patients should be forewarned. The 2008 systematic review covering vaginal graft materials also studied the posterior compartment. The meta-analysis concluded there was insufficient data to make any recommendations.

ENTEROCELE

An enterocele is a herniation of the pouch of Douglas (cul-de-sac) between the uterosacral ligaments into the rectovaginal septum and usually contains small bowel. It frequently occurs after an abdominal or vaginal hysterectomy and generally is the result of a weakened support for the pouch of Douglas and the loss of vaginal apical support by the uterosacral ligaments. In the prevention of an enterocele, the uterosacral and cardinal ligaments are the most important support structures and should be incorporated into the vault repair at the time of a hysterectomy and the ligaments from each side joined together.

Diagnosis

An enterocele is not always easy to diagnose. It is a true hernia of the peritoneal cavity emanating from the pouch of Douglas between the uterosacral ligaments and into the rectovaginal septum (**Fig. 20-12**). It may be noticed as a separate bulge above the rectocele, and at times it may be large enough to prolapse through the vagina (**Figs. 20-13** and **20-14**). If such is the case, it may be possible to make the specific diagnosis of enterocele by transilluminating the bulge and seeing small bowel shadows within the sac. It may also be possible to differentiate the enterocele from

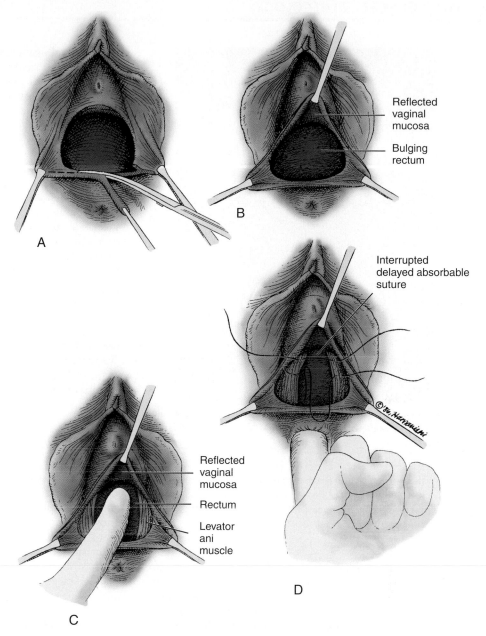

Figure 20-11 Repair of rectocele. **A,** Placement of Allis clamps at margins of perineal incision; perineal incision is being made. **B,** Reflected vaginal mucosa with rectum bulging. **C,** Depression of rectum identifying margins of levator ani muscle. **D,** Placement of sutures in perirectal tissue and levator ani bundles.

Reflected vaginal mucosa

Bulging rectum

Interrupted delayed absorbable suture

Reflected vaginal mucosa

Rectum

Levator ani muscle

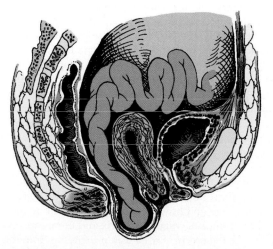

Figure 20-12 Enterocele and uterine prolapse. (Reproduced with permission from Symmonds RE: Relaxation of pelvic supports. In Benson RC [ed]: Current Obstetric and Gynecologic Diagnosis and Treatment, 5th ed. Los Altos, CA, Lange Medical, 1984.)

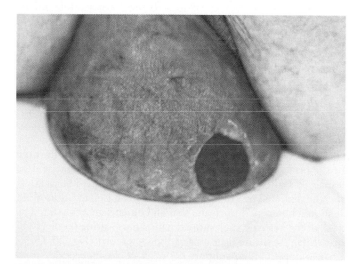

Figure 20-13 Elderly patient with vaginal prolapse who proved to have stage IV apical eversion and enterocele with ulcers on the vagina.

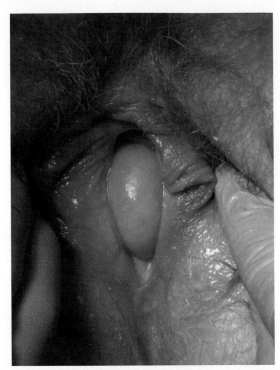

Figure 20-14 Enterocele with vaginal apical prolapse. Split speculum exam and digital exam with palpation of bowel in the sac helped define this defect.

a rectocele by rectovaginal examination. The contents of an enterocele are always small bowel and may also include omentum. The contents may be easily reducible or may be fixed to the peritoneum of the sac by adhesions.

Management

Enteroceles may be reduced transabdominally as a primary procedure or at the time of other abdominal procedures. In the primary procedure the sac should be reduced upward if possible and dissected free from the bladder and rectum. If the uterosacral ligaments are present, these may be brought together in the midline and attached to the vaginal cuff after closing the anterior and posterior fascia of the vaginal apex. If the uterosacral ligaments cannot be identified, as with large enteroceles after previously performed hysterectomy, concentric purse-string sutures in the endopelvic fascia may obliterate the cul-de-sac. Care must be taken to avoid damaging the ureters, rectum, and sigmoid colon. It is best to perform this procedure with permanent sutures. The enterocele has probably occurred because of weakening of the apical supports (uterosacral ligaments), so an abdominal sacrocolpopexy is usually necessary for resuspension and closure of the enterocele defect.

Repair of the enterocele can be carried out vaginally at the time of the posterior colporrhaphy and apical repair. The sac will be visualized as the vagina is separated from the rectum. The sac must then be dissected free of underlying tissue and isolated at its neck. It should be opened to ensure that all contents are replaced. The neck of the hernia is then sutured with a purse-string 0 polyglycol or permanent suture ligature and the sac excised (**Fig. 20-15**).

It is important to support the neck of the enterocele sac as much as possible. Approximating the anterior and posterior vaginal connective tissue is important to close the defect. Usually with an enterocele, support of the vaginal apex is indicated.

If uterosacral ligaments can be identified or if they are present when a vaginal hysterectomy has been performed in association with an enterocele repair, they can be used in the repair. This can be accomplished by fixing the uterosacral ligaments to the peritoneum of the sac and the vaginal vault connective tissue using a suture of 0 polyglycol, beginning on one side of the vagina and continuing through the uterosacral ligament of that side, the peritoneum of the sac, and the uterosacral ligament and vagina of the opposite side. Multiple sutures can be placed if space allows. This technique was described by McCall and is often called the *McCall stitch*. It effectively shortens the cul-de-sac and supports the enterocele neck. If uterosacral ligaments cannot be identified, as is often the case if the uterus has been previously removed, the rectocele repair should be continued to the area of the enterocele sac neck to reinforce this area and support the cul-de-sac as high as possible. This usually involves the joining of the levator ani muscles up to the area of the enterocele sac. Often a vaginal sacrospinous ligament suspension is needed for optimal apical repair.

Correctly repaired enteroceles usually will not recur. Enteroceles repaired without proper attention to ligation of the neck of the sac, closure of the anterior and posterior vaginal connective tissue of the vaginal cuff, and without appropriate rectocele repair may recur. In such cases, a subsequent operation with special attention to these surgical principles is indicated.

UTERINE PROLAPSE (DESCENSUS, PROCIDENTIA)

Descensus of the uterus and cervix into or through the barrel of the vagina is associated with injuries of the endopelvic fascia, including the cardinal and uterosacral ligaments, as well as injury to the neuromuscular unit with relaxation of the pelvic floor muscles, particularly the levator ani muscles (**Fig. 20-16**). Occasionally, prolapse is the result of increased intraabdominal pressure, such as with ascites or large pelvic or intraabdominal tumors superimposed on poor pelvic supports. In some instances, sacral nerve disorders, especially injuries to S1 to S4, or diabetic neuropathy may be responsible. Using computed tomography, Sze and associates demonstrated that women with advanced genital prolapse had larger transverse inlet diameters, but not anterior-posterior diameters, than do women without prolapse, suggesting an anatomic predisposition. Associated factors that increase tension on pelvic floor musculature, such as chronic respiratory disease including chronic bronchitis, asthma, and bronchiectasis, or severe obesity, may be associated. Congenitally damaged or relaxed pelvic floor supports may cause prolapse in young, nulliparous women. Most of the time, however, the patients are multiparous, with the prolapse being at least in part a result of childbirth trauma. Descensus is almost always associated with rectocele and cystocele and, at times, enterocele, supporting the concept of overall damage to the pelvic support structures.

Symptoms and Signs

Major symptoms noted by patients with descensus are a feeling of pelvic pressure and heaviness, fullness, or "falling out" in the perineal area. In cases where the cervix and uterus are low in the vaginal canal, the cervix may be seen protruding from the introitus, giving the patient the impression that a tumor is bulging out of her vagina. Where stage IV prolapse has occurred, the patient is aware that a mass has actually prolapsed out of the introitus. Because prolapse almost always is related to anterior and

Figure 20-15 Repair of enterocele.
A, Appearance of enterocele sac with vaginal wall reflected. **B,** Appearance of open enterocele sac with sac neck identified. **C,** Placing of purse-string suture at the neck of the enterocele sac. **D,** Excision of enterocele sac.

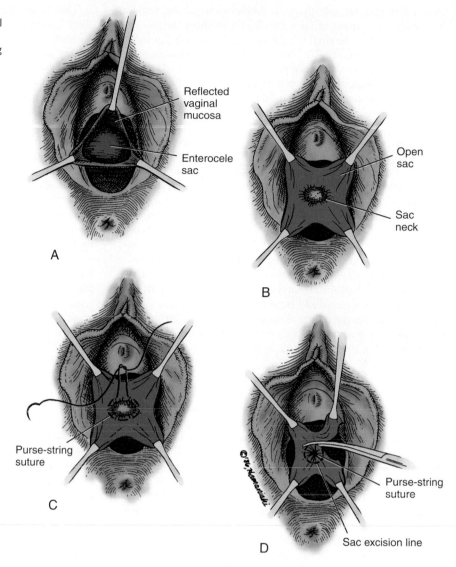

Reflected vaginal mucosa

Enterocele sac

A

Open sac

Sac neck

B

Purse-string suture

C

Purse-string suture

Sac excision line

D

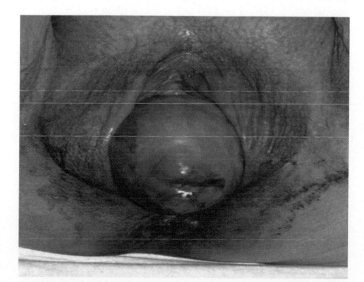

Figure 20-16 Uterine prolapse.

posterior vaginal wall relaxation, symptoms that were reported earlier for cystocele and rectocele may be present as well.

In stage IV prolapse, the vagina is everted around the uterus and cervix and completely exteriorized. When this occurs, the patient is in danger of developing dryness, thickening, and chronic inflammation of the vaginal epithelium and cervix if present. It is not uncommon for the cervix or vaginal epithelium to cause pain or vaginal bleeding. There is often discharge, and secondary infection can occur. Stasis ulcers may result as edema and interference with blood supply to the vaginal wall occur. These ulcers rarely become cancerous, but biopsies should be considered to ensure that they are not. Evisceration of abdominal contents is a rare complication, but a surgical emergency. In almost every case of acquired prolapse, the perineal supports are poor and the perineal body is damaged.

Management

Stage I uterine prolapse does not require therapy unless the patient is very uncomfortable. Degrees of prolapse that place the cervix at or through the introitus probably cause greater discomfort and are usually more bothersome to the patient. Medical management of such conditions involves the use of a pessary, usually of the ring, Smith-Hodge, donut, cube, or inflatable variety (see **Fig. 20-8**). These require the replacement of the uterus and cervix to their usual position in the pelvis and then the institution of support using one of these devices. Pessaries are available in varying sizes and should be properly fitted to the patient. In general, the perineum must be capable of holding the pessary in place, or the pessary will frequently fall out. Women who choose a pessary are often poor surgical candidates, have had a prior failed POP surgery, wish to delay surgery because of future childbearing desires, or simply prefer a nonsurgical option. There is currently no evidence from randomized controlled trials on pessary use to direct the selection of the device or to compare pessaries with other treatments or surgery. Surveys of physicians fitting pessaries reported that a ring pessary was the most commonly selected shape. Usually a support pessary is tried first, such as a ring or Gehrung because they are easier for the patient to use. Space occupying pessaries such as the cube, Gellhorn, donut, and inflato-ball are a second option. Gellhorn is reported in one study to be successfully fit with stage IV POP more often than rings. A prospective trial found that 75% of 203 women fitted with a pessary successfully retained the device at 2 weeks. Failure to retain the pessary was significantly associated with increasing parity, prior POP surgery, and past hysterectomy. Forty-eight percent of the women completed a questionnaire at 4 months. The pessary reduced symptoms of POP, including general symptoms of a vaginal bulge. It also relieved urinary symptoms such as voiding problems in 40% of women, urinary urgency in 38%, and urge incontinence in 29%. There was no improvement in stress urinary incontinence. Bowel symptoms improved as well.

Complications from vaginal pessaries are rare with proper use. This includes regular removal, cleaning, and replacement, as well as use of vaginal cream for postmenopausal women with vaginal atrophy. Complications include vaginal infections, bleeding, discomfort, vaginal erosion and ulceration, and pessary incarceration. More serious complications have been rarely reported, usually from neglect.

If the patient is a young woman and pregnant, it is important to replace the uterus before it enlarges and becomes trapped in the lower pelvis or vagina. If this happens, edema may cause incarceration and even loss of blood supply to the uterus. In a postmenopausal woman, estrogen replacement for at least 30 days with vaginal estrogen cream may help improve the vitality of the vaginal epithelium, the cervix, and the vasculature of these organs, making fitting of a pessary or the operative procedure and the healing process more efficient. The patient should not undergo operation until all ulcers of the vagina and cervix are healed, because to do otherwise is to risk infection and breakdown of the repair.

Operative repair for prolapse of the uterus and cervix generally involves a vaginal hysterectomy with a vaginal vault suspension. The hysterectomy is performed carefully, isolating the uterosacral and cardinal ligaments so that they may be used in the support of the vaginal vault. The uterosacral ligaments should be sutured together so that the cul-de-sac is shortened or obliterated; the anterior and posterior fascia of the vaginal apex should be closed together and, thus, the risk of a subsequent enterocele is lessened. Other vaginal vault suspension procedures can be used instead of the McCall type.

The American College of Obstetricians and Gynecologists' 2009 committee opinion and a Cochrane systematic review the same year state evidence demonstrating that vaginal hysterectomy is associated with better outcomes and fewer complications than laparoscopic or abdominal hysterectomy. This is a general recommendation and with POP, often there are many other considerations including concomitant procedures needed, concern about failure rates, and restoration of bowel, bladder, and sexual function. In some cases, a vaginal hysterectomy is not advisable. These circumstances include a previous intraabdominal operation for an inflammatory process, such as endometriosis or pelvic inflammatory disease. Where such is the case, an abdominal, laparoscopically assisted vaginal, or total laparoscopic hysterectomy may be performed. This can be followed by a vaginal anterior and posterior colporrhaphy, if needed. Under these circumstances, the cardinal and uterosacral ligaments should be treated as noted earlier.

In some women the cervix is hypertrophied and elongated to the area of the introitus, but the supports of the uterus itself are intact. A cystocele and rectocele may be present, and operative repair can consist of a Manchester (Donald or Fothergill) operation. This operation combines an anterior and posterior colporrhaphy with the amputation of the cervix and the use of the cardinal ligaments to support the anterior vaginal wall and bladder. Although it was suggested for repair in young women who wish to maintain their reproductive abilities, the loss of the cervix may interfere with fertility or lead to incompetence of the internal cervical os. The operation has value in elderly women with comorbid medical conditions who have an elongated cervix and well-supported uterus because it is technically easier and has a shorter operative time than the vaginal hysterectomy in such cases and the entering of the peritoneal cavity is avoided.

In elderly women who are no longer sexually active, a simple procedure for reducing prolapse is an obliterative procedure called a **colpocleisis**. The classic partial colpocleisis procedure was described by Le Fort in 1877 (**Fig. 20-17**) and involves the removal of a strip of anterior and posterior vaginal wall, with closure of the margins of the anterior and posterior wall to each other. This procedure may be performed with or without the presence of a uterus and cervix, and when it is completed, a small vaginal canal exists on either side of the septum, which is produced by the suturing of the lateral margins of the excision. The line of dissection of the vaginal wall is carried to the level of the bladder neck anteriorly and to the reflection of bladder onto the cervix at the upper margin of the vagina. Posteriorly the dissection is carried from just inside the introitus to a position just posterior to the cervix. If a hysterectomy has been previously performed, the dissection may begin approximately 1 cm on either side of the vaginal scar. When the procedure is completed, the bladder neck is spared from any scarring, and urinary incontinence is generally avoided. An operation such as a midurethral synthetic sling may be carried out if the patient has stress urinary incontinence. After healing, a small introital area is noted; this has cosmetic benefits in older women. In addition, narrow canals are noted on each lateral vaginal wall. If the cervix and uterus are still present and intrauterine pathology occurs, bleeding along these canals could take place, alerting the physician to a potential problem.

The Goodall–Power modification of the Le Fort operation (**Fig. 20-18**) allows for the removal of a triangular piece of vaginal wall beginning at the cervical reflection or 1 cm above the vaginal scar at the base of the triangle, with the apex of the

Figure 20-17 Le Fort procedure. **A,** Incision of anterior vaginal wall strip. **B,** Incision of posterior wall strip. **C,** Removal of vaginal strip. **D** and **E,** Placement of sutures. **F,** Appearance of vagina after procedure is completed but before perineorrhaphy is performed.

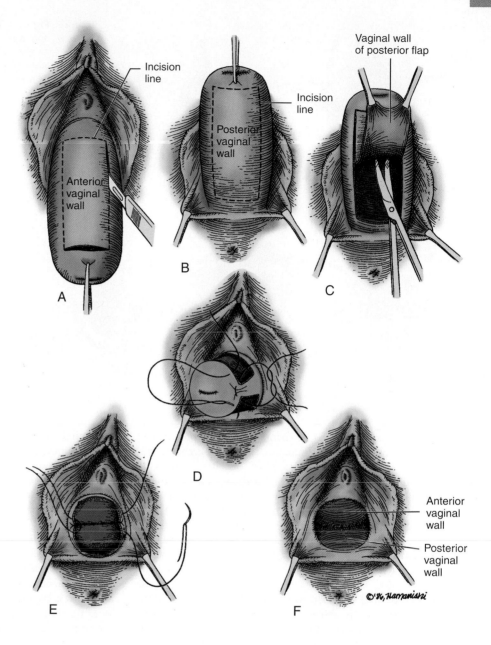

triangle just beneath the bladder neck anteriorly and just at the introitus posteriorly. The cut edge of vaginal wall making up the base of the triangle anteriorly is sutured to the similar wall posteriorly, and the vaginal incision is then closed with a row of interrupted sutures beginning beneath the bladder neck and carried side to side to the area of the introitus. This procedure works well for relatively small prolapses, whereas the Le Fort is best for larger ones.

When a colpocleisis is performed, if an enterocele is found when the vaginal wall is stripped away, the sac must be identified, its neck ligated, and the peritoneum of the sac excised to prevent recurrence of the enterocele behind the colpocleisis. In most cases a perineorrhaphy is performed with a colpocleisis to reduce the size of the genital hiatus and restore the perineal body.

Prognosis for a colpocleisis procedure to reduce the prolapse and prevent recurrence is generally excellent. Case series report 91% to 100% success rates. Overall, patient satisfaction is over 90%. Careful counseling must be done preoperatively to be sure

the woman will never desire coital activity because occasional regret over closure of the vagina has been reported.

Denehy and coworkers compared 25 elderly women (average age 82 years) in poor health and with an uterovaginal prolapse treated by colpocleisis with 42 women who also had a similar prolapse but were treated with vaginal hysterectomy, anterior colporrhaphy, and posterior colporrhaphy. Members of the vaginal hysterectomy group were considerably younger, with an average age of 66 (range 39 to 80). Average operating time for the Le Fort procedure was 75 minutes compared with 150 minutes for the vaginal hysterectomy. There was one postoperative death in the Le Fort group, but 19 of the 20 remaining Le Fort patients had excellent results for a follow-up of an average of 25 months (range 4 to 40 months). These authors performed Kelly urethral plication and posterior colpoperineoplasty in all patients.

A special circumstance involves the treatment of women who wish to maintain their fertility despite the fact that they have symptomatic uterine prolapse. Kovac and Cruikshank have

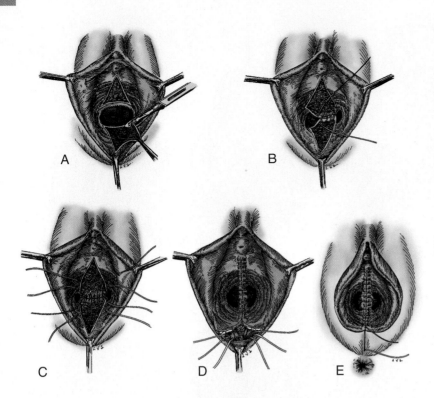

Figure 20-18 Goodall–Power modification of Le Fort operation. **A**, Representation of vaginal incision on anterior and posterior wall. **B**, Early placement of sutures. **C**, Later placement of sutures. **D**, Vaginal incision completely closed; perineorrhaphy being performed. **E**, Appearance at completion of procedure. (Reprinted with permission from Symmonds RE: Relaxation of pelvic supports. In Benson RC [ed]: Current Obstetric and Gynecologic Diagnosis and Treatment, 5th ed. Los Altos, CA, Lange Medical, 1984.)

demonstrated that uterosacral ligaments bilaterally could be sutured to the sacrospinous ligaments, thereby reversing the prolapse. In 19 such patients treated, 5 delivered a total of 6 babies (1 delivered twice). In 2005, Diwan, in an uncontrolled trial, compared laparoscopic uterosacral ligament uterine suspension with vaginal hysterectomy and vault suspension. Using the pelvic organ prolapse quantification system, both groups had excellent support and no laparoscopic uterine suspension patient had reoperation for recurrence. Laparoscopic sacrocervicopexy for treatment of uterine prolapse has been described. In 2008, Rosenblatt retrospectively reported a case series of 40 women who desired retention of fertility. At 1 year, the cervix was −4.84 centimeters above the hymenal ring. It is unclear what the role of uterine suspension should be in current practice and the longevity of such repairs. Young women with POP who desire further childbearing should be encouraged to try a pessary first.

APICAL VAGINAL WALL PROLAPSE

Prolapse of the vaginal apex at some time remote to the performance of either abdominal or vaginal hysterectomy has been reported as occurring in 0.1% to 18.2% of patients. Apical prolapse may be accompanied by a cystocele, a rectocele, an enterocele, or some combination thereof. Occasionally the prolapse involves only one of those entities and not the entire vaginal apex. In a study in Munich, Richter reported that of 97 vaginal stump prolapses, 6.2% were cystocele only, 5.1% rectocele only, 9.3% primarily an enterocele type, and 72.2% of mixed type. Specific classification was not given for 7.2%. A 2006 study by Rooney confirmed it is rare to find isolated support defects of the anterior or posterior vaginal walls or an isolated apical defect.

Vaginal apex prolapse is probably the result of continuing pelvic support defects in the connective tissues, namely, the cardinal and uterosacral ligaments attachments to the vaginal cuff. Multiple vaginal wall defects are usually found because the connective tissue defects, the pelvic floor muscles, and innervation are globally affected and usually not isolated damage to one site.

Symptoms and Signs

Symptoms and signs of vaginal apex prolapse are similar to those delineated for descensus of the uterus. They include pelvic heaviness, backache, and a mass protruding through the introitus. At times, stress incontinence, urgency, frequency, dribbling, vaginal bleeding or discharge (if there is an ulcer), and, depending on the size of the mass, difficulty with sitting or walking may occur.

Diagnosis

Examination may help determine the contents of the herniation depending on where the vaginal scar is located in relation to the protruding mass and the extent to which the supports of the pelvis are lost. Rectovaginal examination is often helpful in delineating an enterocele from a rectocele.

Management

Although the management of descensus with the uterus present is uniformly agreed to be vaginal hysterectomy with vaginal vault suspension and, if indicated, anterior and posterior colporrhaphy, there is much controversy over the appropriate procedure for apical vaginal wall prolapse. Nevertheless, certain principles and facts are important. The first is that the normal position of the vagina in the standing position is against the rectum and no more than 30 degrees from the horizontal (**Fig. 20-19**). The second principle is that pelvic relaxation is a part of the problem and dictates that an existing cystocele, rectocele, or enterocele must

Figure 20-19 Pelvis of a dissected cadaver in supine position demonstrating vaginal canal orientation in the pelvis. (Courtesy of Richard Hebertson, MD.)

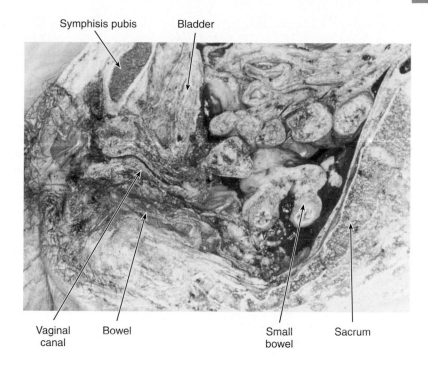

Symphisis pubis   Bladder

Vaginal canal   Bowel   Small bowel   Sacrum

be repaired as part of the procedure. The third principle acknowledges that the perineal body is almost always severely weakened in such patients and must therefore be reconstructed as well. Nonsurgical management, such as the use of pessaries, vaginal estrogen, and the healing of ulcers, should be used as appropriate. Pessaries, however, are rarely retained in such patients, and attempts to treat these patients nonsurgically are generally met with frustration.

The choices of operative procedures are many. These include those that use the abdominal route, the vaginal route, laparoscopic or robotic route, or some combination thereof. Randomized, controlled trials are few, but Maher reported in a 2010 Cochrane Collaboration that abdominal sacral colpopexy has significantly lower vault failure rate (RR 0.23, CI 0.07 to 0.77) and dyspareunia rate (RR 0.39, CI 0.18 to 0.86) compared with vaginal sacrospinous colpopexy, although there was no significant difference in reoperation rates (RR 0.46, CI 0.19 to 1.11). However, the benefits of vaginal surgery with shorter operative times, fewer complications, and quicker return to daily activities must be weighed against the improved durability with the abdominal approach.

Because apical vaginal wall suspensions still have a role in the pelvic surgeon's armamentarium, several will be discussed. A variety of other vaginal procedures have been designed. The best success, however, occurs in procedures in which adequate vaginal length is maintained and the vagina is positioned against the rectum nearly parallel to the horizontal. Fixation to various aspects of the pelvis like the uterosacral ligaments, iliococcygeus ligaments, or to the sacrospinous ligament have had encouraging degrees of success, the latter being the most successful. Using the sacrospinous ligament can frequently be accomplished vaginally. Randall and Nichols reported excellent success with both abdominal and vaginal approaches. In 18 patients treated with fixation of the vaginal vault to the sacrospinous ligament via the vaginal route, all had successful outcomes.

Morley and DeLancey reported the results of 100 patients treated at the University of Michigan for vaginal vault prolapse

or posthysterectomy enterocele with sacrospinous ligament suspension of the vaginal vault. Of 71 patients who were followed for 1 year or more, 64 (90%) had complete symptomatic relief, 10 had some asymptomatic relaxation of the vaginal walls, and 9 had either vaginal stenosis or stress incontinence. In addition, 4 patients developed cystoceles, and 3 had recurrent prolapse of the vagina. Other authors have reported equally encouraging results using this procedure.

Sze and Karram reviewed the literature on transvaginal vault prolapse repair in 1997. They compared the cumulative results for sacrospinous ligament fixation ($n = 1062$) and endopelvic fascia vault fixation ($n = 322$). Of the sacrospinous ligament fixation group, 193 (18%) developed recurrent relaxation, including 32 vault eversions, 81 anterior wall and 24 posterior wall prolapses, and 56 with other or multiple defects. Of the endopelvic fascia fixation groups, 34 (11%) developed recurrent relaxation, including 9 vault prolapses, 2 anterior and 11 posterior wall prolapses, and 12 developed other defects. Follow-up was from 1 to 12 years, and these authors concluded that the true efficacy of these procedures remains inconclusive.

Figure 20-20 depicts the fixation of the vaginal vault to the sacrospinous ligament and the direction of the vagina after the procedure. Miyazaki reported the use of an instrument, the Miya hook ligature carrier, to lessen the difficulty of placing a suture into the sacrospinous ligament. This is depicted in **Figure 20-21**. Some surgeons favor the use of this instrument in the performance of this procedure. Sharp has reported equally good results using an orthopedic instrument, the Shutt suture punch system, as an alternative to the Miya hook ligature carrier. Several special ligature carriers and auto suturing devices (Endostitch, Capio device) have also been found useful. It is likely that other instruments will be developed for this purpose.

Operative risks of sacrospinous colpopexy include injury to the pudendal and inferior gluteal arteries and the pudendal and sciatic nerves. Rectal injury is rare, although care must be taken when dissecting the rectal pillars to reach the ligament and to retract the bowel away when placing the sutures.

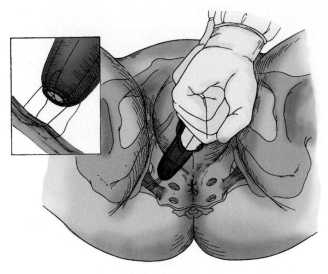

Figure 20-20 Sutures tied to bring the new vaginal apex into contact with the ligament and overlying muscle. Vaginal wall is advanced toward the sacrospinous ligament while tying sutures. A "suture bridge" is to be avoided. (Redrawn from Morley GW, DeLancey JOL: Sacrospinous ligament fixation for eversion of the vagina. Am J Obstet Gynecol 158:872, 1988.)

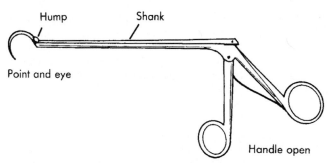

Figure 20-21 The Miya hook ligature carrier. (From Miyazaki FS: Miya hook ligature carrier for sacrospinous ligament suspension. Obstet Gynecol 70:286, 1987.)

Thornton and Peters reported on 41 women who underwent repair of vaginal apex, in which the vaginal approach was used with good, lasting success. Of these patients, 20 required a repair of an enterocele and a posterior repair, which especially detailed the attachment of the posterior wall of the vagina to the perirectal fascia and levator ani muscles. In addition, 21 patients underwent a repair of an enterocele with both an anterior and a posterior repair because a cystocele was believed to be a major part of their prolapse problem. Long-term follow-ups were affected, and the success rate was said to be excellent.

Maher published a case control study in 2001 comparing 50 women who had iliococcygeus and 78 women who had sacrospinous fixation for vaginal vault prolapse. Subjective success rates were 91% and 94%, respectively, but objective success rates were substantially lower at 53% and 67%. Neither of these findings was significantly different. Patient satisfaction was statistically different on a visual analogue scale with 78 of 100 reported for iliococcygeus and 91 of 100 for sacrospinous. Follow-up times were similar at 21 months and 19 months, respectively. The complication rates for postoperative cystocele, buttock pain, and hemorrhage were similar.

Using the uterosacral ligaments to suspend an apical vaginal wall prolapse is not a new idea in vaginal reconstructive surgery. It lost favor to the sacrospinous ligament for a time, but has had a resurgence of popularity although no randomized trials have been published. Because these ligaments are thought to be key in supporting the vaginal apex, and because suspension here replaces the vagina in the normal anatomic position, the procedure has advantages. Shull described opening the anterior and posterior vaginal walls in the midline and opening the enterocele sac. With packing the bowel out of the field, the uterosacral ligaments can be identified and grasped with a long Allis clamp taking care to avoid the ureter. A series of three sutures are placed in each uterosacral ligament, which are then used to reconstruct the vaginal apex with the anterior vaginal endopelvic fascia and the posterior vaginal rectovaginal septum closed together. Any enterocele defect is also closed with this technique.

A 2010 systematic review of 10 observation studies reported on 930 women undergoing uterosacral ligament suspension. A successful anatomic outcome was considered present when women had "optimal" or "satisfactory" (pelvic organ prolapse quantification system stage 0 or 1) outcomes. In the anterior, apical, and posterior compartments, the pooled rates for a successful outcome were 81.2% (95% confidence interval [CI], 67.5 to 94.5%), 98.3% (95% CI, 95.7 to 100%), and 87.4% (95% CI, 67.5 to 94.5%). In the anterior compartment, women with preoperative stage 2 prolapse were more likely than those with preoperative stage 3 prolapse to have a successful anatomic outcome (92.4% versus 66.8%; P = 0.06). Subjective symptom outcomes could not be reported because of the differing study designs.

This technique can also be used for vaginal apical suspension at the time of initial hysterectomy. The major risks are kinking or obstruction of the ureters, and cystoscopy is advised at the end of the procedure. Injury to the sacral nerves from sutures that are placed too deeply in the side wall has also been reported and usually presents as pain.

For the abdominal approach, a variety of procedures have been tried. These include fixation of the vaginal vault to the anterior abdominal wall, to the lumbar spine, to the sacral promontory, to various tendinous lines in the musculature of the true pelvis, and to the sacrospinous ligament. The anterior abdominal wall fixation increases the diameters of the pouch of Douglas and frequently adds to the risk of subsequent enterocele development, often creating a recurrence in short order. Fixation to the lumbar spine or the sacral promontory is often difficult to achieve directly and requires the interposition of a different material. In the past, ox fascia lata, fascial aponeurosis from the patient, or inert materials such as polypropylene graft have been used. In randomized trials, cadaveric fascia was associated with a higher rate of recurrent prolapse than synthetic mesh. Currently, a wide pore, monofilament mesh is widely used for abdominal sacral colpopexy. The mesh graft is sutured to the anterior and posterior upper vaginal vault and the opposite end to the ligamentum flavum of the sacral promontory or the anterior longitudinal ligament of the sacrum. Care must be taken to avoid the middle sacral artery and the plexus of veins in its vicinity. The mesh graft should be made retroperitoneal by closing the peritoneum in front of it. This renders the graft retroperitoneal to avoid troublesome adhesions and internal hernias at a future date. After such procedures, the pouch of Douglas may still be large enough to allow an enterocele to develop. Therefore, the procedure might also require obliteration of the cul-de-sac.

Benson and associates performed a randomized trial of bilateral sacrospinous vault suspensions and paravaginal repair ($n = 48$) and colposacral suspension and paravaginal repair ($n = 40$). Surgical effectiveness as judged by recurrent prolapse was optimal in 29% of the vaginal and 58% of the abdominal group and was unsatisfactory, leading to reoperation in 33% of the vaginal and 16% of the abdominal group. Only a few other randomized trials have reported since this study, but as mentioned earlier, the abdominal sacral colpopexy has a higher success rate than vaginal apex support procedures. Anatomic success rates range in studies from 76% to 100%. In addition, information from the CARE randomized trial of abdominal sacral colpopexy with or without Burch colposuspension showed that women reported significant improvement in urinary, bowel, prolapse, and sexual function using validated pelvic floor scales.

Operative complications from abdominal sacral colpopexy include cystotomy (3.1%), enterotomy (1.6%), incisional problems (4.6%), ileus (3.6%), thromboembolic event (3.3%), transfusion (4.4%), and small bowel obstruction or ileus (1% to 5%). Abdominal sacral colpopexy has downsides with longer operating time and longer return to normal activities of daily living compared with vaginal vault suspensions. Also, synthetic mesh complications occur 3% to 5% of the time with most being vaginal erosions. Some of these problems can be offset by laparoscopic or robotic approaches to this surgery. Short-term outcome studies show similar success rates with shorter hospital stays and less blood loss. One of the most dreaded operative complications is presacral hemorrhage when dissecting or placing sutures on the sacral promontory. Care must be taken to visualize the blood vessels and be prepared in the event of hemorrhage.

If an abdominal sacrocolpopexy (ASC) is to be performed for treatment of POP, urinary continence must be considered. A multicenter 2006 trial by Brubaker and colleagues randomized 322 women with no stress incontinence symptoms to have a concomitant Burch colposuspension or not (controls). Three months after surgery, 24% of women in the Burch group and 44% of controls had stress incontinence, even though none reported stress incontinence preoperatively. Burch colposuspension significantly reduced postoperative stress incontinence when performed at the time of ASC, without an increase in other urinary problems.

In elderly women who are no longer sexually active, and particularly in those who have medical reasons to avoid a longer procedure, a Le Fort–type colpocleisis operation may be performed with an excellent result, which was discussed earlier in the uterine prolapse section. Perineorrhaphy almost always needs to be performed as part of any procedure to repair a vaginal apex prolapse.

The question of continuing sexual activity after vaginal vault repairs is obviously an important one. With an adequate vaginal operation (with the exception of colpocleisis), intercourse is achievable in most patients who wish to maintain this activity.

Weber and coworkers studied sexual function in 81 women who were sexually active before undergoing surgery for pelvic prolapse or urinary incontinence or both. All remained sexually active after surgery, but dyspareunia was likely to occur if a combination of the Burch procedure and posterior colporrhaphy was performed.

RECTAL PROLAPSE

Rectal prolapse will be covered in Chapter 22 on anal incontinence.

CONCLUSIONS

In all women with symptomatic pelvic organ prolapse, several areas of function need to be discussed including urinary, bowel, sexual, and other pelvic complaints. Nonsurgical treatments are limited, but many women can be observed with mild symptoms. Motivated, symptomatic women can benefit from a pessary trial.

If surgical treatment is desired, there are many factors to consider including patient characteristics and desires as well as the surgeon's skills. Recurrent pelvic organ prolapse is a substantial problem and little is known about prevention of pelvic organ prolapse, so much research is still needed in this field.

KEY POINTS

- Femoral hernias are more common in females than in males, whereas inguinal hernias are more common in males.
- In the female, large hernias, hernias that continuously have intraabdominal contents, hernias that cause continuing discomfort, and hernias that have been incarcerated should be operatively repaired.
- Women have a lifetime risk of 11% of undergoing a single operation for pelvic organ prolapse or urinary incontinence by age 80.
- Pelvic organ prolapse is defined as the downward descent of the pelvic organs resulting in protrusion of the vaginal walls or uterus and cervix.
- Vaginal delivery is a major risk factor for the development of pelvic organ prolapse.
- The cardinal and uterosacral ligaments hold the uterus and upper vagina in the proper location over the levator plate.

- The major goals of surgery for pelvic organ prolapse are to correct the woman's urinary and bowel symptoms and to restore sexual function if desired when repairing the anatomic defects. It is important for the woman to articulate her goals before surgery.
- Prolapse of the vaginal apex at some time after hysterectomy has been reported in 0.1% to 18.2% of patients, and hysterectomy may be a risk factor for later prolapse.
- Vaginal prolapse after hysterectomy includes a mixture of cystocele, rectocele, and enterocele in 72% of cases, and an isolated prolapse of one compartment is rare.
- Vaginal vault prolapse can be repaired abdominally or vaginally. An abdominal sacral colpopexy with synthetic mesh appears to have a higher long-term success rate for the vaginal apex, but at the risk of more surgical complications.

REFERENCES CAN BE FOUND ON EXPERTCONSULT.com

SUGGESTED READING

Braekken IH, Majida M, Engh ME, et al: Can pelvic floor muscle training reverse pelvic organ prolapse and reduce prolapse symptoms? An assessor-blinded, randomized, controlled trial, *Am J Obstet Gynecol* 203(2):170.e1–170.e7, 2010.

Bump RC, Mattiasson A, Bo K: The standardization of terminology of female pelvic organ prolapse and pelvic floor dysfunction, *Am J Obstet Gynecol* 175:10, 1996.

Hoyte L, Jakab M, Warfield SK: Levator ani thickness variations in symptomatic and asymptomatic women using magnetic resonance-based 3-dimensional color mapping, *Am J Obstet Gynecol* 191:856, 2004.

Maher CF, Qatawneh AM, Dwyer PL, et al: Abdominal sacral colpopexy or vaginal sacrospinous colpopexy for vaginal vault prolapse: A prospective randomized study, *Am J Obstet Gynecol* 190:20, 2004.

McCall ML: Posterior culdoplasty-surgical correction of enterocele during vaginal hysterectomy: A preliminary report, *Obstet Gynecol* 10:595, 1957.

Olson AL, Smith VJ, Bergstrom JO, et al: Epidemiology of surgically managed pelvic organ prolapse and urinary incontinence, *Obstet Gynecol* 89:501, 1997.

Sung VW, Rogers RG, Schaffer JI, et al: Graft use in transvaginal pelvic organ prolapse repair: A systematic review, *Obstet Gynecol* 112 (5):1131–1142, 2008.

21

Urogynecology
Physiology of Micturition, Voiding Dysfunction, Urinary Incontinence, Urinary Tract Infections, and Painful Bladder Syndrome

Gretchen M. Lentz

The gynecologist frequently consults on and treats urologic problems in the female patient. Perhaps the most commonly seen of these problems involves infection and inflammation of the lower tract. Urinary tract infections (UTIs) occur in up to 50% of women over their lifetime. **Painful bladder syndrome** affects fewer women, but they often have chronic pain and may make frequent visits to the gynecologist's office before a diagnosis is made. Furthermore, there is considerable overlap of symptoms with other gynecologic problems such as UTIs, endometriosis, and dyspareunia. Gynecologists are frequently involved in the care of women with pelvic pain and need to understand this syndrome.

Many women suffer from some degree of urinary **incontinence**. Various prevalence studies have reported that approximately 30% of women noted some degree of incontinence during the preceding 12 months. Ten percent of women suffer from weekly incontinence and 5% have daily incontinence. Urinary incontinence problems increase in incidence with age and, because the number of older women in our population is increasing, it is likely that this problem will grow in magnitude. A 2008 survey of pelvic floor disorders by Nygaard and colleagues found at least one pelvic floor disorder in 24% of women. At least weekly or monthly urine leakage was reported by 7% of women ages 20 to 39, 17% ages 40 to 59, 23% ages 60 to 79, and 32% 80 years of age and older. This study may actually underpredict the prevalence of these disorders because women in the survey may have been successfully treated and not counted. Overweight and obese women were more likely to report urinary incontinence than women of normal weight. Among older adults, only about 38% of women actually discuss incontinence with a physician.

Continence depends on a number of factors, including the neurologic control of micturition, the anatomic relationships of the urinary tract, and the specific effects of a number of systemic, infectious, and neoplastic conditions. Older women have additional challenges to the urinary system with comorbid medical conditions, ambulatory difficulties, and cognitive impairments. Not only the prevalence but the severity of urinary incontinence increases with age. Incontinence has been associated with depression, increased social isolation, falls, hip fractures, and admission to nursing homes, which has additional morbidity. Furthermore, incontinence decreases quality of life and increases costs to society. This chapter discusses the physiology of micturition and diagnosis and evaluation of pathologic entities that affect the female urologic system, and offers suggestions on treatment.

PHYSIOLOGY OF MICTURITION

A number of factors are involved in maintaining continence. The central nervous system (CNS) and peripheral ganglia coordinate function of the lower urinary system through complex neural pathways—those that maintain a urethral closure mechanism and those that affect detrusor function. It is a balance between bladder storage, which is organized primarily in the spinal cord and coordinates urethral closure and detrusor relaxation, and micturition, which is controlled by reflex mechanisms mediated by the brain. Voluntary voiding is a learned function and is not automatic, like heart rate control.

Bladder detrusor contractility is stimulated by the activity of the parasympathetic nervous system, mediated primarily through the neurotransmitter acetylcholine. This stimulates muscarinic (primarily M_3) receptors in the bladder wall, which then activate detrusor contraction. Sympathetic nervous system β receptors within the bladder cause bladder relaxation when stimulated. Bladder contraction may also be affected by irritation and inflammation of the bladder wall lining, causing uninhibited contractions. Inhibitory input to the urethral smooth muscle is conveyed by nitric oxide via parasympathetic nerves. Somatic cholinergic motor nerves supply the striated muscles of the external urethral sphincter from the sacral spinal cord.

The act of voiding is under the control of four basic autonomic and somatic nervous system feedback loops. The first loop (loop I) involves a circuit from the cerebral cortex to the brain stem, which inhibits micturition by modifying sensory stimuli emanating from loop II. Loop II, which originates in the sacral micturition center (S2 through S4) and the detrusor muscle wall itself, represents sensory fibers to the brain stem, where modulation of the stimuli by loop I takes place. If cerebral inhibition is not imposed (loop I), the stimuli are returned to the sacral micturition center as a response to the bladder filling,

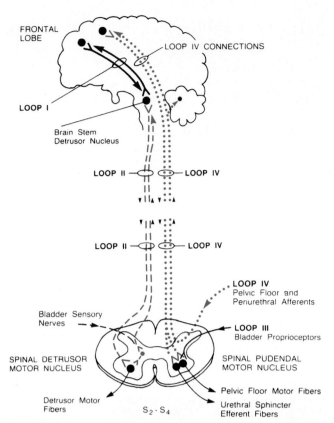

FRONTAL LOBE

LOOP IV CONNECTIONS

LOOP I

Brain Stem
Detrusor Nucleus

LOOP II — LOOP IV

LOOP II — LOOP IV

LOOP IV
Pelvic Floor and
Periurethral Afferents

Bladder Sensory
Nerves

LOOP III
Bladder Proprioceptors

SPINAL DETRUSOR
MOTOR NUCLEUS

SPINAL PUDENDAL
MOTOR NUCLEUS

Detrusor Motor
Fibers

Pelvic Floor Motor Fibers

Urethral Sphincter
Efferent Fibers

S_2-S_4

Figure 21-1 Central nervous system feedback loops. (From Williams ME, Pannill FC 3 rd: Urinary incontinence in the elderly: Physiology, pathophysiology, diagnosis, and treatment. Ann Intern Med 97:895, 1982.)

allowing activation of loop III. Loop III involves sensory flow from the bladder wall to the sacral micturition center with returning motor fibers to the urethral sphincter striated muscle, which allows the voluntary relaxation of the urethral sphincter as the detrusor contracts. Loop IV originates in the frontal lobe of the cerebral cortex and runs to the sacral micturition center and then to the urethral striated muscle, allowing urethral voluntary muscles to relax, thus leading to the initiation of voiding. **Figure 21-1** demonstrates these four loops, as visualized by Williams and Pannill. **Table 21-1** summarizes the important aspects of each loop as reviewed by Ostergard.

Both the parasympathetic and sympathetic nervous systems function with the CNS in these feedback loops via the pontine micturition center. The parasympathetic system is involved in the act of voiding via nuclei in S2 through S4 (micturition center) and mediates its activity through the neurotransmitter acetylcholine, directly stimulating muscarinic receptors in the bladder wall. This signal is transmitted via the pelvic nerve and causes the detrusor to contract. At the same time, the pontine micturition center (PMC) in the brain inhibits the sympathetic pathway as well as the somatic pathway to the urethra. This allows the urethra to relax so that coordinated voiding can occur. Functional brain imaging studies (e.g., positron emission tomography [PET]) during voiding show activation of the cortex, insula, and PMC. The sympathetic system, on the other hand, acts to prevent micturition. Norepinephrine is secreted via this system, stimulating both α- and β-adrenergic receptors. The bladder contains primarily β receptors, stimulation of which causes relaxation of the detrusor muscle. The urethra contains primarily α receptors. Stimulation of these α receptors causes contraction of the urethral sphincter. Thus, the overall effect is to prevent micturition (**Fig. 21-2**). Estrogen and progesterone receptors are present in the bladder and urethra, although their role in affecting continence has not been fully elucidated. Many other neurotransmitters, neuropeptides, and receptors have been identified in the lower urinary tract, including dopamine, serotonin, nitric oxide, γ-aminobutyric acid (GABA), glutamine, neurokinin A, nerve growth factor, and adenosine triphosphate (ATP).

Because the neurogenic control of micturition is so complex and depends on the interaction of so many factors, it is understandable that a host of general systemic diseases or diseases involving the nervous system may affect bladder control. These include, but are not limited to, demyelinating diseases (e.g., multiple sclerosis), diabetes mellitus, vascular diseases, and CNS trauma and tumors. In addition, medications that have an effect on the CNS or autonomic nervous system may affect bladder control. Compounds with atropine-like effects may interfere with the initiation of micturition, whereas those with cholinergic effects may cause bladder overactivity (**Table 21-2**).

In summary, bladder control depends on the ability of the bladder to store urine under low pressure, which involves inhibition of the detrusor muscle and contraction of the smooth and striated urethral sphincters. Emptying the bladder requires coordination with pelvic floor and urethral sphincter relaxation and detrusor contraction. There are local reflexes and central

Table 21-1 Neurologic Control of Micturition: Clinical Considerations on Central Nervous System Reflex Loops

Loop	Origin	Termination	Function	Associated Conditions
I	Frontal lobe	Brain stem	Coordinates volitional control of micturition	Parkinson's disease, brain tumors, trauma, micturition
II	Brain stem Bladder wall	Brain stem	Detrusor muscle contraction to empty bladder	Spinal cord trauma, multiple sclerosis (MS), spinal cord tumors, neuropathy, local urinary tract disease
III	Sensory afferents of tumors, diabetic detrusor muscle disease	Striated muscle of urethral sphincter via pudendal motor neurons and sacral micturition center	Allows relaxation of urethral sphincter in synchrony with detrusor contraction	MS, spinal cord trauma or neuropathy, local urinary tract
IV	Frontal lobe	Pudendal nucleus	Volitional control of striated external urethral sphincter	Cerebral or spinal trauma or tumor, MS, cerebrovascular disease, lower urinary tract disease

Adapted from Ostergard DR: The neurological control of micturition and integral voiding reflexes. Obstet Gynecol Surv 34:417, 1979.

CONTINENCE   MICTURITION

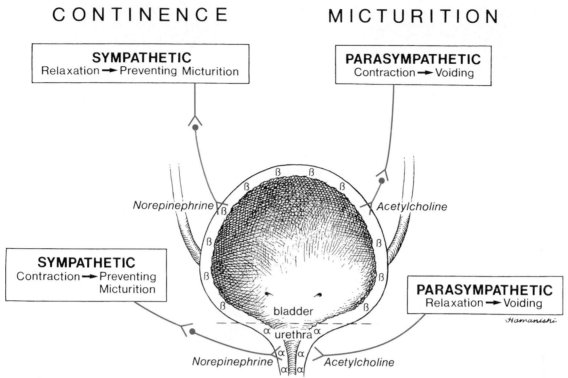

Figure 21-2 Innervation of the bladder and urethra. Parasympathetic fibers arising in S2-S4 have long preganglionic fibers and pelvic ganglia close to the bladder and urethra. These parasympathetic fibers excrete acetylcholine. Sympathetic fibers that have long postganglionic fibers discharge norepinephrine to β receptors, primarily in the bladder, and α receptors, primarily in the urethra. (Adapted from Raz S: Pharmacological treatment of lower urinary tract dysfunction. Urol Clin North Am 5:323, 1978.)

inhibitory influences involved. The system can be disrupted by a stroke, which is a suprapontine lesions leading to loss of central inhibition, resulting in detrusor overactivity and reemergence of reflex micturition. A spinal cord injury above the lumbosacral level eliminates voluntary control of voiding, leading to acute urinary retention. Later, neurogenic detrusor overactivity occurs from spinal reflex pathways, which are uncoordinated, so the urethral sphincter may not relax simultaneously, leading to detrusor-sphincter dyssynergia. A lumbosacral burst fracture can result in detrusor overactivity with urethral sphincter hyporeflexia or sphincter hyperreflexia. A radical hysterectomy or subsacral cauda equine lesion might disrupt the local reflexes and lead to overflow incontinence because of detrusor and sphincter hyporeflexia. If the pudendal nerve is intact, the sphincter function will be normal.

BLADDER AND URETHRAL ANATOMY AND FUNCTION

With the neurologic principles of micturition in mind, it is appropriate to assess other factors that may influence continence. Asmussen and Ulmsten noted that the bladder and urethra are essentially a functional unit, with the bladder's subfunction being to store urine and the urethra's to allow it to pass. For urine to pass through the urethra, the maximum urethral pressure must be lower than the **intravesical pressure**. Intravesical pressure depends on the following: (1) the volume of fluid in the bladder; (2) the part of the intraabdominal pressure transmitted to the bladder; and (3) the tension in the bladder wall related to

muscular and nervous system activity and elastic properties. The resting pressure in the bladder is between 20 and 30 cm H_2O although, on urodynamic testing, the resting pressure if often calibrated to 0 cm H_2O.

The intraurethral pressure depends on the following: (1) striated muscle fibers of the urethral wall; (2) smooth muscle fibers of the urethral wall (a circular and longitudinal layer); (3) vascular content of the urethral submucosal cavernous plexus; (4) passive elasticity of the urethral wall; and (5) the part of the intraabdominal pressure transmitted to the urethra. The urethra has primarily receptors from the sympathetic nervous system, which, when stimulated, cause contraction of the urethral sphincter. The urethral smooth and striated (skeletal) muscles add to the resting urethral tone, whereas the skeletal fibers react when **intraabdominal pressure** rises, such as with a cough.

Anatomically, the exact border between the bladder and urethra is difficult to determine. The functional length of the urethra, however, is that part in which the urethral pressure exceeds the bladder pressure. Asmussen and Ulmsten have noted that the **urethral closure pressure** (UCP) is defined as the maximum **urethral pressure** minus the bladder pressure. For continence to be present, the UCP must be higher than the bladder pressure. Urethral pressure varies with age, increasing up to the age of 20 years and then gradually decreasing until menopause. However, after menopause, the fall of this pressure is more rapid. Asmussen and Ulmsten have demonstrated that the highest pressure zone in the urethra is approximately at the midpoint of the functional urethral length. The anatomic urethral length is approximately 3 to 4 cm. Westby and coworkers have located this high-pressure zone at approximately 0.5 cm proximal to the

Table 21-2 Drugs That Affect Continence and Micturition

Drug	Action
Sympathetic (relaxes bladder; controls urethral sphincter)	
Dopamine	α-Adrenergic stimulator
Methamphetamine	α-Adrenergic stimulator
Norepinephrine	α-Adrenergic stimulator
Phenylephrine	α-Adrenergic stimulator
Albuterol	β-Adrenergic stimulator
Isoproterenol	β-Adrenergic stimulator
Terbutaline	β-Adrenergic stimulator
Parasympathetic (stimulates bladder contraction; relaxes urethral sphincter)	
Pilocarpine	Stimulates acetylcholine, incontinence
Pyridostigmine	Stimulates acetylcholine, incontinence
Sympathetic Blockers	
Hydralazine	Adrenergic blocker, stress incontinence
Methyldopa	Adrenergic blocker, stress incontinence
Reserpine	Adrenergic blocker, stress incontinence
Parasympathetic Blockers	
Atropine	Parasympathetic inhibitor, impaired emptying
Papaverine	Parasympathetic inhibitor, impaired emptying
Scopolamine	Parasympathetic inhibitor, impaired emptying

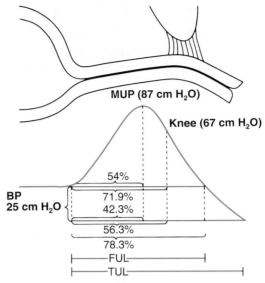

Figure 21-3 Location of maximum urethral pressure in relation to the urogenital diaphragm (average value of 25 normal women). Knee indicates the location of the urogenital diaphragm seen on X-ray film and transformed to the pressure curve. BP, Blood pressure; MUP, maximal urethral pressure. (From Asmussen M, Ulmsten U: On the physiology of continence and pathophysiology of stress incontinence in the female. Contrib Gynecol Obstet 10:32, 1983.)

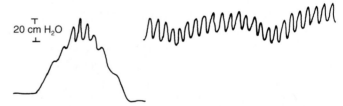

Figure 21-4 Maximum urethral pressure shows great variation synchronously with the heartbeat. Variations of 20 cm H_2O as shown in the curve are not uncommon. (From Asmussen M, Ulmsten U: On the physiology of continence and pathophysiology of stress incontinence in the female. Contrib Gynecol Obstet 10:32, 1983.)

Table 21-3 Topography of Urethral and Paraurethral Structures*

Approximate Location†	Region of the Urethra	Paraurethral Structures
0-20	Intramural urethra	Urethral lumen traverses bladder wall
20-60	Midurethra	Striated urethral sphincter muscle Pubourethral ligament Vaginolevator attachment
60-80	Urogenital diaphragm	Compressor urethrae muscle Urethrovaginal sphincter muscle
80-100	Distal urethra	Bulbocavernosus muscle

*Smooth muscle of the urethra was not considered.
†Expressed as a percentile of total urethral length.
From DeLancey JOL: Correlative study of paraurethral anatomy. Obstet Gynecol 68:91, 1986.

urogenital diaphragm. Most of the functional urethral length is actually above the urogenital diaphragm (**Fig. 21-3**). Asmussen and Ulmsten, and Gosling and associates, have pointed out that the submucosal cavernous plexus of vessels, the bulk of the smooth and striated muscle, and the bulk of the autonomic nerve supply are most prominent in the area in which they record the maximum urethral pressure. Because the urethral pressure displays high-pressure zone oscillations that are synchronous with the heartbeat, the submucosal cavernous plexus is probably important in helping to maintain continence (**Fig. 21-4**). Estrogen receptors are found in the bladder and urethra. Enhorning and Asmussen and Ulmsten have demonstrated that urethral pressure can oscillate as much as 25 cm H_2O in young women but seldom more than 5 cm H_2O in postmenopausal women. The cavernous plexus is thicker walled and less elastic in older women. Thus, not only is the epithelium of the bladder and bladder neck dependent on hormone stimulation, but probably so is the vascular system of these areas.

DeLancey made some interesting observations on functioning periurethral anatomy by studying serial histologic sections of intact pelvic viscera and surrounding tissue, and by dissecting 22 fresh and embalmed cadavers. Because the length of the urethra varies among women, the topography of urethral and paraurethral structures was expressed in terms of the location along the urethra as a percentage of the total urethra. DeLancey considered the zero location as that point at which the urethra leaves the bladder lumen and the 100th percentile as that point at which the urethra terminates on the perineum. From the standpoint of functional anatomy, there is excellent agreement among the measurements made from each of his specimens when

percentiles are used; **Table 21-3** depicts these anatomic relationships. It can be seen that the intramural urethra represents approximately 20% of the length of the urethra. The portion of the urethra encircled by striated urethral sphincter muscle

URETHRAL LANDMARKS

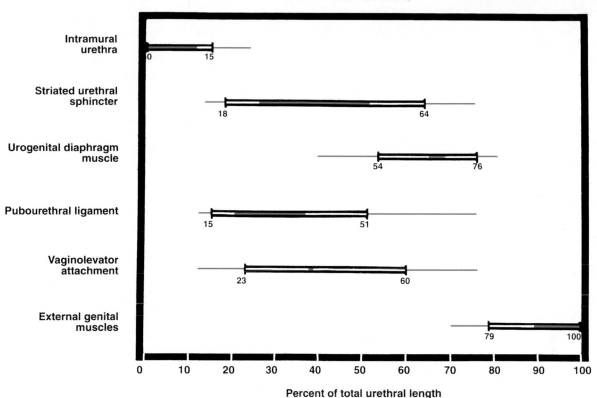

Figure 21-5 Average spatial distribution of paraurethral structures, as well as the range of values found. Urogenital diaphragm muscles are the compressor urethrae and urethrovaginal sphincter. (From DeLancey JOL: Correlative study of paraurethral anatomy. Obstet Gynecol 68:91, 1986.)

and associated with the pubourethral ligament and vaginal levator attachment concerns the midurethra—that is, that portion from the 20th to 60th percentile along the total length. The 60th to 80th percentile of the urethral length passes through the urogenital diaphragm and is under the influence of the urethrovaginal sphincter muscles. Finally, the last 20%, or distal urethra, traverses the bulbocavernosus muscles. These urethral landmarks are depicted in **Figure 21-5**, which highlights the actual ranges and values found in DeLancey's study. The actual anatomic relationships are depicted in **Figure 21-6**. DeLancey's observations help correlate the anatomic relationships with the physiologic observations that others have made.

In a subsequent paper, DeLancey noted that additional anatomic factors might influence continence. Using serial histologic sections from eight female cadavers and the dissections of 34 other cadavers, he noted that the proximal urethra gets added support because the anterior vagina is attached to the muscles of the pelvic diaphragm and to the arcus tendineus fasciae pelvis. Contraction of the pelvic diaphragm thus pulls the vagina against the posterior surface of the urethra, helping to close it. At rest, the urethra is supported by its attachment to the arcus tendineus fasciae pelvis and the tone of the pelvic diaphragm muscles. Two striated muscle arches, the compressor urethrae and urethrovaginal sphincter, support the distal urethra in the region of the urogenital diaphragm. These muscles help compress the distal urethra, helping to maintain continence during a cough.

In summary, continence depends on the bladder, urethra, pelvic muscles, and surrounding connective tissue supports.

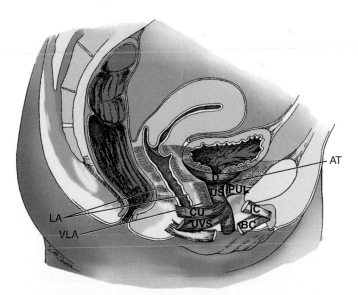

Figure 21-6 Interrelationships of approximate location of paraurethral structures. Levator ani muscles are shown as light lines running deep to the pelvic viscera. The vaginal levator attachment is shown as a darker area. AT, Arcus tendineus fasciae pelvis; BC, bulbocavernosus muscle; CU, compressor urethrae; D, detrusor muscle; IC, ischiocavernosus muscle; LA, levator ani muscles; PUL, pubourethral ligament; US, urethral sphincter; UVS, urethrovaginal sphincter; VLA, vaginal levator attachment. (Adapted from DeLancey JOL: Correlative study of paraurethral anatomy. Obstet Gynecol 68:91, 1986.)

DIAGNOSTIC PROCEDURES

The clinical history is useful in the diagnosis of urinary incontinence. Several validated scales are available, such as the Urogenital Distress Inventory (UDI), Incontinence Impact Questionnaire (IIQ), Bristol Female Lower Urinary Tract Questionnaire, and King's Health Questionnaire, although one has not become the preferred instrument. Useful testing can be done in the gynecologist's office without the need for sophisticated equipment. These procedures are described and their benefits noted. The description is followed by a discussion of more sophisticated diagnostic techniques requiring specialized equipment.

URINALYSIS AND CULTURE

A simple urinalysis and urine culture may provide much information. The presence of white or red blood cells (RBCs) and bacteria in a catheterized or clean voided sample, in which the perineum around the urethra has been appropriately prepared with an antiseptic solution, may suggest a UTI, urethral diverticulum, or even urinary tract malignancy in rare cases. UTI may be associated with **urgency**, frequency, dysuria, and even incontinence. In such cases, the urinalysis and urine culture may be diagnostic. Several dipstick methods are available to detect bacteriuria and pyuria. The accuracy of these methods is variable, but they do have some use in screening patients who are incontinent or have symptoms suggestive of infection. In some cases, a culture should be obtained to identify the specific organism involved and verify the presence of an infection. Urinalysis is also useful to screen for microscopic hematuria (RBCs) in women with new-onset urgency and frequency because underlying urinary tract pathology may be present. A formal microscopic urinalysis should be carried out to confirm screening results because urine dipstick tests can often yield a false-positive result and actual RBCs need to be identified. A catheterized specimen should be obtained if abnormal results are questioned because of vaginal contamination. This is common in women with pelvic organ prolapse, obesity, postmenopausal bleeding, or menses, or in older women with arthritis and poor hand function.

TEST FOR RESIDUAL URINE

This simple procedure can be extremely helpful in the evaluation of a woman with incontinence with pelvic organ prolapse, voiding symptoms such as frequency or incomplete bladder emptying, or recurrent UTIs. It is not necessary in the initial evaluation in a woman without complicating factors. The woman is asked to void and a catheter is inserted into the bladder no more than 10 to 15 minutes later. The urine remaining in the bladder is measured and may be sent for urinalysis and culture. Under normal circumstances, the amount of **residual urine** should be less than 50 mL after the woman has voided at least 250 mL. The measurement is most accurate if done with a full bladder. Large amounts of residual urine suggest urinary retention resulting from inadequate bladder emptying. A reasonable accuracy of measuring residual urine volume can also be obtained noninvasively by ultrasound. Bladder scan ultrasound units are available and patients prefer to avoid urethral catheterization. Postvoid residual urine volume by ultrasound may be falsely elevated in women with large uterine fibroids or a large adnexal mass. Confirmation is necessary with catheterization if this is suspected.

BLADDER DIARY

Asking the woman to complete a bladder diary is a simple, inexpensive way to obtain information about her fluid intake, voiding habits, voided volumes, and incontinent episodes. An example diary form is shown in **Figure 21-7**. A 2006 systematic review concluded that a large proportion of cases of **urodynamic stress incontinence** could be correctly diagnosed in a primary care setting from the clinical history alone. The bladder diary appears to be the most cost-effective tool and is useful for diagnosing detrusor overactivity with reasonable sensitivity and specificity when used with the clinical history.

OFFICE CYSTOMETRICS

It is possible to gain a great deal of information about bladder capacity and bladder function with relatively simple tools. Once a catheter is inserted to check for residual urine, the catheter is left in place and attached to a graduated Asepto syringe without a bulb. It is possible to pour sterile saline (or sterile water) into the syringe and measure the amount of saline that first causes the woman to have the urge to void. This first urge should normally occur after 150 to 200 mL of saline has been infused. Women with normal bladder function should be able to continue to maintain continence at that level. Similarly, a strong, normally controllable urge to void usually occurs when 400 to 500 mL has been instilled. Thus, a normal bladder first transmits an urge to void at 150 to 200 mL and functional capacity is reached at 400 to 600 mL. Larger volumes can be reached without incontinence, but this is usually accomplished with a great deal of conscious effort. If, during filling, the women reports urgency and the column of fluid in the Asepto syringe rises, leakage may be seen around the catheter and detrusor overactivity confirmed.

COUGH STRESS TEST AND PAD WEIGHT TEST

If a bladder has been previously filled to measure capacity, it should then be emptied to approximately 250 mL of saline, or if the bladder is empty, 250 mL of saline should be instilled. The catheter is then removed and the woman is asked to cough while in the recumbent position. If urine spurts from the urethral meatus, stress incontinence may be present and a positive cough stress test (CST) is noted. After the stress test is performed in a recumbent woman, it should be repeated with the woman standing if no leakage is seen. Frequently, she will appear to be continent with stress while lying down but may demonstrate incontinence when the influence of gravity on the pelvic organs is brought into play in the standing position. For research studies, 250 mL of saline is instilled, the woman is asked to cough 10 times, and any leakage is considered a positive CST. The clinical stress test is effective in diagnosing stress incontinence.

Because urine loss with cough should be immediate if stress incontinence is the problem, it may be possible to detect evidence of detrusor instability by observing the time of the spurt of urine in the stress test. Typically, the detrusor reacts a few seconds after the stimulus; therefore, a spurt that occurs after a delay after a cough suggests the presence of a cough-induced involuntary detrusor contraction.

If no leakage is seen and anterior vaginal wall prolapse is present, occult stress incontinence is possible. Currently, it can be challenging to determine whether a woman with anterior vaginal

Your Daily Bladder Diary

This diary will help you and your health care team. Bladder diaries help show the causes of bladder control trouble. The "Example" line (below) will show you how to use the diary.

Time	Drinks		Urine		ACCIDENTS			
	What kind?	How many?	How many times?	How much? sm med lg	Accidental leaks sm med lg	Did you feel a strong urge to go?	What were you doing at the time? Sneezing, exercising, driving, lifting, etc.
Example	*coffee*	*2 cups*	//	☐ ☒ ☐	☐ ☒ ☐	☒ Yes ☐ No	*Running*
6–7 am				☐ ☐ ☐	☐ ☐ ☐	☐ Yes ☐ No	
7–8 am				☐ ☐ ☐	☐ ☐ ☐	☐ Yes ☐ No	
8–9 am				☐ ☐ ☐	☐ ☐ ☐	☐ Yes ☐ No	
9–10 am				☐ ☐ ☐	☐ ☐ ☐	☐ Yes ☐ No	
10–11 am				☐ ☐ ☐	☐ ☐ ☐	☐ Yes ☐ No	
11–12 noon				☐ ☐ ☐	☐ ☐ ☐	☐ Yes ☐ No	
12–1 pm				☐ ☐ ☐	☐ ☐ ☐	☐ Yes ☐ No	
1–2 pm				☐ ☐ ☐	☐ ☐ ☐	☐ Yes ☐ No	
2–3 pm				☐ ☐ ☐	☐ ☐ ☐	☐ Yes ☐ No	
3–4 pm				☐ ☐ ☐	☐ ☐ ☐	☐ Yes ☐ No	
4–5 pm				☐ ☐ ☐	☐ ☐ ☐	☐ Yes ☐ No	
5–6 pm				☐ ☐ ☐	☐ ☐ ☐	☐ Yes ☐ No	
6–7 pm				☐ ☐ ☐	☐ ☐ ☐	☐ Yes ☐ No	

Your name: _____   Date: _____

Figure 21-7 Daily bladder diary. (From Vasavada SP, Appell R, Sand PK, et al [eds]: Female Urology, Urogynecology, and Voiding Dysfunction. New York, Marcel Dekker, 2005, p 127.)

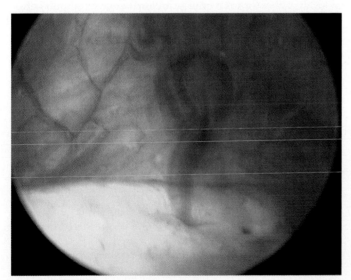

Figure 21-8 Cystoscopy after indigo carmine was infused IV to confirm the duplicated ureters on the left side and that both were functioning.

wall relaxation is likely to develop overt stress incontinence after a pelvic organ prolapse repair. Urodynamic testing is often performed with and without a pessary to reduce the cystocele and to see whether stress incontinence occurs.

A 1-hour pad weight test is another research tool for documenting pre- and postintervention urinary leakage volumes. Again, with a 250-mL bladder volume, a pad is given to the woman and she is asked to complete a series of activities over the hour, including walking, climbing stairs, coughing, and other events. If the pad weighs more than 2 to 3 g, the test is considered positive. Both this test and the CST are commonly used as objective measures of outcome for surgical incontinence trials.

Thus, with urinalysis, urine culture, measuring postvoid residual urine, bladder diary, documented first urge to void, bladder capacity, and the cough stress test, the physician will have a great deal of information concerning the cause of the woman's urinary complaint. More sophisticated urodynamic evaluations using specific and often costly equipment should be performed by those who are trained and experienced in these tests. A short discussion of these procedures and the equipment involved follows.

URODYNAMICS

Urodynamic investigation attempts to measure bladder and urethral function and voiding function. **Cystometry**, part of the urodynamic test, measures bladder pressure during the filling phase of the micturition cycle. First urge to void, normal desire to void, and bladder capacity are noted. The woman can cough and/or perform the Valsalva maneuver to detect stress incontinence in the absence of a detrusor contraction. Detrusor overactivity may be noted with the symptom of urgency, with or without leakage in association with a **detrusor pressure** rise. Poor compliance from a nonelastic bladder is noted with a gradual pressure rise to more than 15 cm H_2O rather than phasic contractions of detrusor overactivity. In attempting to understand the basis of urinary stress incontinence, the practitioner must realize that what must be determined is the relationship between the simultaneous intraurethral and intravesical pressures (**Fig. 21-9**). For greatest accuracy, these should be measured with the woman in the sitting position as well as standing, at rest, and with straining. The ideal means of evaluating a woman for incontinence is to use a multichannel recorder that permits pressure determinations at two points within the urethra (proximal and midpoint to distal), one within the bladder, and one intraabdominally as recorded by an intrarectal sensor or by a sensor within the vagina if the vagina is in a relatively normal position (not prolapsed). Pressure flow studies measure voiding in terms of detrusor and urethral function. **Figure 21-10** (NEW) shows a multichannel urodynamic study during the pressure/flow or voiding phase and highlights a woman with a voiding disorder which was the main reason the study was ordered.

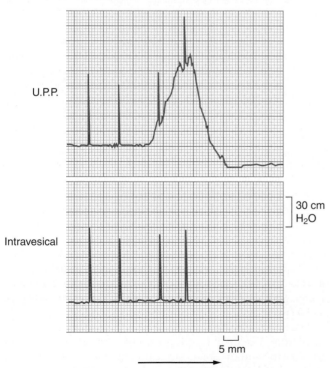

Figure 21-9 Simultaneous recordings of urethra and intravesical pressures during coughing. Stress produces a parallel increase of bladder and urethral pressure because the intraabdominal position of the bladder and proximal two thirds of the urethra are displayed. U.P.P, urethral pressure profile (From Raz S: Pharmacological treatment of lower urinary tract dysfunction. Urol Clin North Am 5:323, 1978.)

Several authors have described the concept of leak point pressure tests for evaluating urethral function in stress incontinence. Instead of measuring the intravesical pressure needed to overcome passive urethral resistance, this test measures the intravesical pressure necessary to overcome urethral resistance under stress (cough or strain). Studies have reported many variations in techniques to measure leak point pressures. The International Continence Society defines an **abdominal leak point pressure** (ALPP) as the lowest of the intentional or actively increased intravesical pressure that provokes urinary leakage in the absence of a detrusor contraction. This increased pressure can result from a Valsalva maneuver (VLPP) or coughing. The ALPP has been used to separate urinary stress incontinence as either related to an anatomic defect (hypermobility of the urethra) or **intrinsic sphincter deficiency**. However, is has become clear there is significant overlap in these conditions and using a simple cut off of less than 60 cm H_2O to define intrinsic sphincter deficiency is too simplistic. The woman's history and clinical picture must be considered carefully and not just an arbitrary cut off point.

Maximal urethral closure pressure is another measure of urethral function in stress incontinence. Below 20 cm H_2O is the criteria used to define intrinsic sphincter deficiency. Using the MUCP for choosing therapy in subtypes of stress incontinence or for outcome results in surgical trials has been criticized because unlike the VLPP, the test is not performed during stress. A 2010 randomized, controlled trial by Nager and colleagues studied the relationship between various measurements of urethral function and subjective scores of urinary incontinence. They actually found VLPP and MUCP have moderate correlation with each other, but each had little or no correlation with the woman's subjective scores of incontinence severity or objective tests like the supine empty bladder stress test. These data call into question the use of urodynamic measures of urethral function when they do not correlate with urinary incontinence severity. However, many stress incontinence surgical trials use the MUCP and leak point pressures to categorize incontinence and to predict risk of surgical failure so being familiar with the tests is useful.

Other recent studies have called into question the usefulness of urodynamics for stress or **urge incontinence** symptoms in uncomplicated cases. The test correlates poorly with symptoms and often does not affect the outcome of treatment, even with stress incontinence surgery. When urodynamic testing is done, it must be correlated with the woman's symptoms and exam as those factors may be more revealing than the test.

Multichannel devices involve more expensive equipment and require continuous maintenance. It is possible to add a video urodynamic system to the multichannel recorders, making it possible via fluoroscopy to identify reflux into the ureters under pressure situations. The video system also makes it possible to actually observe the act of micturition, any anatomic changes, and the effect of stress. The data obtained by multi-channel pressure recordings with the ability to actually visualize micturate makes urodynamics the most accurate diagnostic information the clinician can obtain. This technique is considered the standard against which other tests are measured.

Urodynamic testing is not necessary for beginning a conservative treatment program for stress, urge, or mixed incontinence symptoms or for routine evaluation. However, if the diagnosis is unclear, the woman has failed conservative therapy, has had prior incontinence surgery, has voiding complaints, had pelvic organ

Figure 21-10 Multichannel urodynamic study of a 44-year-old woman, G5 P1, with complaints of mixed incontinence and difficulty emptying her bladder. She had some minor neurologic symptoms suggestive of multiple sclerosis but her evaluation had not proved a definite diagnosis. Her voiding study revealed an acontractile bladder and abdominal straining to void, with poor urine flow.

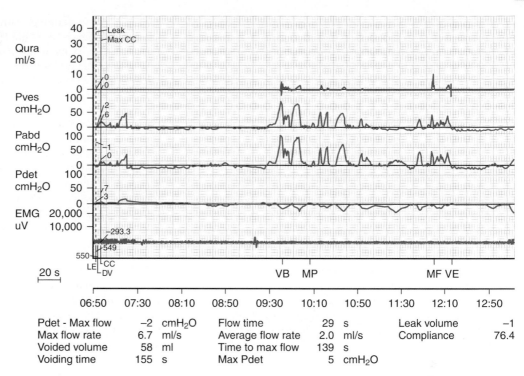

Pdet - Max flow	−2	cmH$_2$O	Flow time	29	s	
Max flow rate	6.7	ml/s	Average flow rate	2.0	ml/s	
Voided volume	58	ml	Time to max flow	139	s	
Voiding time	155	s	Max Pdet	5	cmH$_2$O	
			Leak volume	−1		
			Compliance	76.4		

prolapse beyond the hymen, or has a complicated medical history (such as neurologic disease), then urodynamic testing may provide useful information.

CYSTOURETHROSCOPY

Cystourethroscopy, or simply cystoscopy, may be performed with a flexible or rigid telescope that allows visualization of the urethra, bladder, and ureteral orifices in an office setting (**Box 21-1**). Generally, saline or sterile water is used for the

---

Box 21-1 Common Findings on Urethrocystoscopy

Normal urothelium—pale, fine blood vessels
- Normal—squamous metaplasia in trigone (benign overgrowth)
- Abnormal—hypervascularity
- Abnormal—cystic lesions in the trigone; could be benign cystitis (UTI)
- Abnormal—stitch or mesh from incontinence surgery
- Abnormal—bladder stone or kidney stone that has passed
- Abnormal—lesion growing from wall; biopsy, could be carcinoma
- Abnormal—grapelike clusters; biopsy, could be transitional cell carcinoma
- Abnormal—trabeculations (hypertrophied detrusor muscle), benign; seen in OAB or outlet obstruction
- Abnormal—Hunner's ulcer; pathognomonic for interstitial cystitis

Normal urethra—collapsed in absence of fluid flow
- Abnormal—fronds or pseudopolyps, benign response to inflammation
- Abnormal—stricture; prior surgery, especially urethral diverticulum excision

Ureteral orifices with bilateral jets of urine flow
- Abnormal—sluggish flow, could mean partial obstruction
- Abnormal—no flow, could mean obstruction from current or past surgery, stone, or stricture

---

infusion fluid to expand the bladder. Local lidocaine jelly is inserted into the urethra for analgesia in the office. A small 17 Fr sheath is commonly used for routine inspection and a larger sheath for operative procedures. Examination of the bladder is best accomplished using a 30- or 70-degree lens, which offers the angles needed to examine the bladder in its entirety. A 0- or 12-degree lens is best for examining the urethra. The bladder may need to be flushed for optimal viewing if blood obscures the view; this can easily be done by filling, emptying, and refilling the bladder. A systematic survey should be done inspecting the bladder base and **trigone**, ureteral orifices, dome, and all other surfaces all the way back to the bladder neck. The bladder may be visualized and the presence of inflammation, foreign bodies, urinary tract stones, anatomic abnormalities such as a duplicated ureter (see **Fig. 21-8**) or benign or malignant lesions noted. Urethroscopy, using the same cystoscopy equipment, is excellent for visualizing the urethra and provides information about inflammatory processes within the urethra, urethral diverticula, other anatomic defects such as a urethral stricture or foreign body (e.g., mesh from an midurethral tape sling) and permits some estimate of urethral tone.

INFECTIONS OF THE LOWER URINARY TRACT

CYSTITIS

A UTI (cystitis) is the most common bacterial infection seen in an outpatient setting. Infections of the urethra and bladder are almost always associated with some combination of the following: frequency, urgency, dysuria, pyuria, hematuria, acute or chronic pelvic pain, backache, and at times fever. As many as 50% of all women develop UTIs at some time during their life and, by age 70, as many as 10% of women will have recurrent UTIs. At times, incontinence is associated with acute and recurrent infections. Although *Escherichia coli* is the cause of most UTIs (80% to 85%), a myriad of organisms, including *Enterobacter, Klebsiella, Pseudomonas, Proteus, Streptococcus faecalis, Staphylococcus saprophyticus, Enterococcus,* and *Chlamydia* can be found. The presence of bacteria in the urine (bacteriuria) does not necessarily prove clinical infection. Bacteriuria is fairly common in women, especially older women. For example, cumulative data from several studies have suggested that 20% of women older than 65 years will demonstrate bacteriuria, but the percentage increases from approximately 15% in the 65- to 70-year group to 20% to 50% for women older than 80 years. Bacteriuria is present in women who are on chronic catheterization and common in women in nursing homes who are chronically incontinent. Asymptomatic bacteriuria is not treated, even in older women or diabetics, with no change in their morbidity or mortality. Exceptions exist to this recommendation if the woman is undergoing an invasive procedure, is pregnant, has had a renal transplant, or is incontinent and her incontinence resolves with treatment. If a woman with asymptomatic bacteriuria becomes symptomatic, treatment is appropriate.

Many explanations have been offered as to why the female urinary tract is vulnerable to infection. These include the following: short female urethra, thereby allowing easier access of bacteria to the bladder; proximity of the vulva, vagina, and rectum to the opening of the urethra; effects of sexual intercourse on the entrance of bacteria into the urethra and lower urinary tract; and effect of loss of estrogen on the reproductive tract of older women. After menopause, the vaginal pH rises and may alter the vaginal flora, allowing for colonization of uropathogenic species, especially *E. coli*. It is probably appropriate to add personal immunologic and genetic variations to this list, which may make one woman more susceptible than another to certain bacteria. Nonsecretors of certain blood group antigens are at increased risk.

The definition of a symptomatic UTI is a woman with dysuria, frequency, urgency, and/or suprapubic pain with pyuria. Uncomplicated UTIs occur in healthy women with normal urinary function. UTIs are classified as complicated when there are comorbid conditions that require longer treatment courses, such as underlying urologic abnormalities, presence of a foreign body (e.g., catheter), urinary calculi, obstruction of urine flow, diabetes mellitus, spinal cord injury, pregnancy, renal transplantation, or other illnesses. Acute uncomplicated UTIs can often be diagnosed successfully with symptom assessment and clean-catch midstream urine for dipstick testing for leukocyte esterase, or microscopic unspun urine evaluation for white blood cells (pyuria), because the pathogens are predictable. Pyuria should always be seen in the urine when UTI occurs and is the most valuable and fastest laboratory test. RBCs may be present in microscopic or macroscopic numbers. Hematuria is common in acute infections, and infection is the most common cause of hematuria. Gross hematuria may occur as a result of the extravasation of blood across dilated and inflamed capillaries. If microscopic or macroscopic hematuria persists after UTI treatment, it must be evaluated.

If a culture is done, it usually grows a single organism. The number of organisms per milliliter is not important. In cases of urethritis and trigonitis, the presence of as few as 100 organisms/mL may indicate an infection because of the dilution of the urine. Complicated UTIs often require urine culture. The Infectious Diseases Society of America (IDSA) and Council for Appropriate and Rational Antibiotic Therapy (CARAT) have developed evidence-based guidelines for the treatment of UTIs. If local *E. coli* bacterial resistance rates are less than 20%, trimethoprim-sulfamethoxazole (TMP-SMX) is recommended. If resistance is greater than 20%, a fluoroquinolone is advised. Three-day therapy is adequate for acute uncomplicated UTIs. The resistance of *E. coli* to TMP-SMX has recently increased dramatically, so fluoroquinolone use has increased. Unfortunately, resistance to ciprofloxacin has been reported at 9.5% and is rising. Short course (3-day) therapy improves patient tolerability and compliance and reduces cost. This treatment strategy results in more than a 90% cure rate. If nitrofurantoin is used for mild to moderate symptoms of an uncomplicated UTI, at least 5 to 7 days of drug treatment is recommended. Resistance rates of *E. coli* to nitrofurantoin have remained low. Other alternatives include fosfomycin and cefpodoxime. With uncomplicated UTIs, progression to pyelonephritis is extremely rare. For complicated UTIs, a 7- to 10-day course of a fluoroquinolone is recommended. If a culture is obtained and results are reported, the antibiotic may be changed if the organisms noted are not sensitive to the antibiotic in use. The woman should remain well hydrated and be encouraged to continue treatment, even though symptoms generally disappear within 48 hours. Infections frequently recur because they are not adequately eradicated. This may result from physician error (treating with too low a dose of antibiotic, the wrong antibiotic, or for too short a period of time) or patient error (not taking the medication as prescribed).

Persistent or recurrent cystitis following the initial infection presents in approximately 20% of women (**Fig. 21-11**). Frequent infections with the same organism (relapse) suggest the possibility that a nidus of infection exists. Recurrent infections of different organisms (reinfection) should alert the physician to the need for a more complete evaluation. However, radiographic imaging—seeking structural abnormalities of the bladder, kidney, or ureters—is rarely useful in otherwise healthy women. More than 90% of recurrences in young women are exogenous reinfection with new isolates arising from local flora. Behavioral modification has become popular for preventing recurrent acute cystitis. Possible modifications in lifestyle include discontinuing use of a diaphragm and spermicide for contraception.

Occasionally, continuous antibiotic therapy at a lower dose for a more prolonged period is necessary to ensure that the woman is no longer infected. Approximately 75% of episodes of acute bacterial infection in women with recurrent cystitis occur within 24 hours of coitus. These women are excellent candidates to be treated with prophylactic antibiotics. The type of prophylaxis depends on the individual woman's history to determine whether broad-spectrum antibiotics should be prescribed continuously, postcoitally, or when the woman believes she is developing an infection. The broad-spectrum antibiotics most commonly chosen for low-dose antibiotic prophylaxis include trimethoprim, TMP-SMX, nitrofurantoin, and a cephalosporin. Prophylaxis may be given for months without significant emergence of antibiotic-resistant bacteria. Postmenopausal women with recurrent UTIs often benefit from vaginal estrogen therapy because this restores the acidic environment of the vagina and restores normal bacteria and lactobacilli. Raz and Stamm have shown significant reduction in recurrent UTIs in postmenopausal women using vaginal estrogen cream. Their review suggested that cranberries can reduce the risk of recurrent UTIs

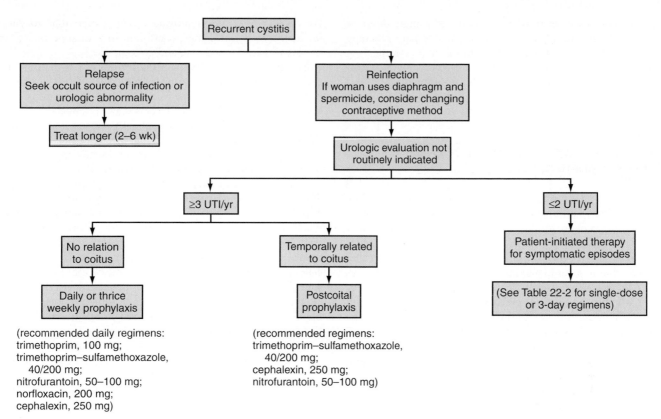

Figure 21-11 Strategies for managing recurrent cystitis in women. (From Stamm WE, Hooton TM: Management of urinary tract infections in adults. N Engl J Med 329:1328, 1993.)

but the correct dosage or formulation is unknown; some studies used cranberry juice and others used concentrates or pills. D-Mannose also has limited evidence of benefit in this situation.

Frequent catheterizations or manipulation of the lower urinary tract often cause UTIs. An indwelling catheter for 24 hours leads to bacteriuria in as many as 50% of patients. When left in place for 96 hours, an indwelling catheter causes bacteriuria in almost 100% of patients. There is no good evidence supporting the use of prophylactic antibiotics in patients who must continue catheter use. A woman with an indwelling catheter should be monitored for the possibility of a symptomatic UTI, be kept well hydrated, have a urine culture if symptoms occur, and be treated with the appropriate antibiotic. However, it is difficult to eradicate infection in the presence of an indwelling catheter. Removing the catheter or switching to clean intermittent self-catheterization would be optimal. Postoperative and debilitated patients are at greatest risk.

Although physicians commonly recommend measures to their patients for preventing UTIs, studies do not support these practices. These include wiping the rectum away from the urethra, voiding after intercourse, and drinking more fluid.

Additional circumstances that may be responsible for infections in women include the dilation of the urinary tract in pregnancy, urinary tract obstruction, urinary stones, diverticulum, foreign bodies (e.g., mesh placed for a midurethral sling for incontinence), ureteral reflux, and pelvic organ prolapse. Other causes of UTIs in men and women include the need for frequent catheterization, instrumentation, and overdistention of the bladder in neurogenic conditions in which stasis becomes a problem.

URETHRITIS

Patients with acute urethritis generally have the typical findings of lower tract UTIs, which include dysuria, frequency, and urgency. They often have a urethra that is tender to palpation. Under certain circumstances, it may be possible to express pus from the urethra; this is particularly common in acute infections with gonococcal or *Chlamydia* organisms. In these situations, the infection involves not only the urethra but also the periurethral glands. Frequently, significant pyuria is noted in a clean-catch urine sample, particularly when taken early in the voiding. The urine should be inspected, because *Trichomonas* infestation is occasionally noted in such cases. Herpes simplex virus has also been associated with urethritis.

Pus expressed from the urethra should be submitted for culture and for smear with Gram stain. Intracellular diplococci are suggestive of gonorrhea. *Neisseria gonorrhoeae* or *Chlamydia* is usually cultured in such situations. Nucleic acid amplification tests enable detection of both organisms. In particular, this is the preferred test for *C. trachomatis*. It should be kept in mind that these are reportable diseases to the state health department. Urine obtained by the clean-catch method should also be cultured.

If no specific organism is identified on smear, a broad-spectrum coverage such as a sulfa preparation for 3 days or nitrofurantoin, 50 or 100 mg three or four times daily, should be prescribed for 10 days. If *Chlamydia* is suspected or cultured, doxycycline, 100 mg twice daily, should be prescribed for at least 7 days, or azithromycin, 1 g orally, in a single dose, should be given. If gonorrhea is diagnosed, the current recommended treatment consists of ceftriaxone 125 mg IM (single dose) or cefixime, 400 mg orally, in a single dose. An alternative therapy is oral ofloxacin or levofloxacin. Penicillin is no longer the drug of choice because of the many penicillin-resistant gonococcal strains now present. Resistance to fluoroquinolones is also spreading. Coinfections with *N. gonorrhoeae* and *C. trachomatis* are common, so dual therapy is often indicated.

PAINFUL BLADDER SYNDROME AND INTERSTITIAL CYSTITIS

Painful bladder syndrome is a more global definition adopted by the International Continence Society to deal with patients with pain syndromes of the lower urinary tract without evidence of bladder pathology or infection. By definition, painful bladder syndrome (PBS) is the complaint of suprapubic pain related to bladder filling accompanied by other symptoms, such as daytime frequency and nocturia, in the absence of proven UTIs or other pathology. **Interstitial cystitis** (IC) is a complex, painful bladder condition that may be the same entity as PBS or may be at the far end on the severity spectrum. There is no consensus on how to define this condition. They will be referred to together as PBS-IC or individually, according to research study definition. The cause and pathophysiology are poorly understood but are most likely multifactorial. Theories regarding cause include an altered bladder epithelial permeability, mast cell activation, and an upregulation of sensory afferent nerves. Studies have found that C fiber bladder afferent neurons have changes in their electrical and chemical properties affecting bladder sensitivity. It is a common syndrome, seen in women more often than men, but the actual incidence is unknown, although it has been estimated to be as high as 500/100,000 women.

The most common symptoms of PBS-IC are bladder-pelvic pain, urgency, daytime frequency, and nocturia, without evidence for infection or other causes. Dyspareunia is also a common complaint in sexually active women. It is often confused with other bladder conditions such as UTIs, **overactive bladder**, and urethral syndrome (an outdated term, but it may be part of the spectrum of the syndrome). The differential diagnosis includes several gynecologic conditions including pelvic inflammatory disease, vulvodynia, and endometriosis. A voiding diary will often demonstrate frequent small voids of less than 150 mL each and as many as 20 or more voids daily. Sleep can be disrupted by a frequent need to void. On examination, suprapubic and anterior vaginal wall tenderness may be found.

On cystoscopy, the bladder frequently appears normal during filling but, with distention under anesthesia, characteristic petechial hemorrhages resembling glomeruli usually appear. Oozing of blood is often seen. However, glomerulations may be a nonspecific finding because they can be seen in asymptomatic women. This cystoscopic finding is not diagnostic of IC, although it is used to differentiate IC from PBS in some studies. Hunner's ulcers are diagnostic of IC but are infrequently seen in women with bladder pain. If a biopsy under anesthesia is taken, ulcers with granulation tissue, mucosal hemorrhage, monocytic infiltration, and mast cells in the lamina propria and detrusor muscle are often seen. Parsons has proposed that these changes are related to a defective or altered glycosaminoglycan mucus layer, which results in altered bladder permeability. However, investigations to date have not shown whether this alteration is cause or effect. Some authors believe that these changes are the result of an autoimmune disease. The presence of immunoglobulins and complement in the bladder wall and the increase in interleukin-6 level in patients' urine may support this. Naturally occurring feline interstitial cystitis (FIC) shows changes in electrical currents that control neuronal excitability in sensory neurons.

Several symptom indices are useful for evaluating women with painful bladder complaints, although they were not developed for screening. The pain, urgency, frequency (PUF) scale (**Table 21-4**) and O'Leary-Sant scale are helpful in characterizing a woman's complaints, especially in light of the lack of definitive diagnostic testing. PBS-IC should be considered in the differential diagnosis of any woman with chronic pelvic pain.

To date, there is no laboratory test or urine test that is diagnostic of IC. Although urodynamic testing may reveal that these patients have early first sensation to void and low bladder capacities, there is no range in volume that is specific for IC. Parsons

Table 21-4 Pelvic Pain, Urgency, Frequency (PUF) Patient Symptom Scale (PUF)

Question	Points 0	1	2	3	4	Score
1. How many times do you go to the bathroom during the day?	3-6	7-10	11-14	15-19	20 +	
2. a. How many times do you go to the bathroom at night?	0	1	2	3	4 +	
b. If you get up at night to go to the bathroom, does it bother you?	Never	Occasionally	Moderate	Severe		
3. Are you currently sexually active? Yes/No						
4. a. If you are sexually active, do you now or have you ever had pain or symptoms during or after sexual intercourse?	Never	Occasionally	Usually	Always		
b. If you have pain, does it make you avoid sexual intercourse?	Never	Occasionally	Usually	Always		
5. Do you have pain associated with your bladder or in your pelvis (vagina, labia, lower abdomen, urethra, perineum)?	Never	Occasionally	Usually	Always		
6. Do you still have urgency after you go to the bathroom?	Never	Occasionally	Usually	Always		
7. a. If you have pain, is it usually mild, moderate, or severe?		Mild	Moderate	Severe		
b. Does your pain bother you?	Never	Occasionally	Usually	Always		
8. a. If you have urgency, is it usually mild, moderate, or severe?		Mild	Moderate	Severe		
b. Does your urgency bother you?	Never	Occasionally	Usually	Always		
					Total Score:	

and associates have developed the potassium sensitivity test (PST). The PST involves inserting a catheter into the bladder and instilling a saline solution, followed by a potassium chloride solution. A positive PST test result is noted if increased pain occurs with the potassium solution. In Parsons and associates' study in gynecologic offices, 244 women with pelvic pain, vulvodynia, or urgency-frequency syndrome diagnoses underwent the PST. Of these women ($N=206$), 84% had genitourinary symptoms and 88% had a positive PST compared with 76% without urinary symptoms. The International Consultation on Incontinence (ICI) stated in 2005 that these are "inadequate data to recommend using the PST for diagnosis" of IC.

Many treatments are available, but few have been uniformly helpful. Women are encouraged to see this as a chronic problem that is not malignant and to try to reduce stress, encourage family support, and avail themselves of the writings and support of the Interstitial Cystitis Association. A multipronged treatment strategy is often necessary. These women should be instructed to avoid acidic, alcoholic, and carbonated beverages, spicy foods, coffee, tea, chocolate, tomatoes, vinegar, and artificial sweeteners, all of which have been associated with increased pain in patients with PBS-IC. Tobacco should also be avoided. Bladder retraining to increase the interval between voiding may help. Pelvic floor muscle exercises also might be of benefit in women with increased pelvic floor muscle tone and tenderness.

Standard medical therapy has included dimethyl sulfoxide (DMSO) bladder instillation often accompanied by heparin, steroids, or local anesthetics. DMSO is an anti-inflammatory agent that acts as a bladder anesthetic, relaxes muscles, causes mast cell inhibition, and may dissolve collagen. Often, DMSO is given as a single treatment followed by heparin therapy for up to 1 year. Many other drugs have been instilled, including heparin, lidocaine, and oxybutynin, but trials are insufficient to show a benefit. A heparin analogue, pentosan polysulfate sodium (PPS, Elmiron), has been given orally 100 mg three times daily, with some reported improvement. PPS is the only U.S. Food and Drug Administration (FDA)–approved oral drug for IC and may help repair the glycosaminoglycan layer of the bladder epithelium. It can take 6 months to be effective and improvements are modest; 38% of patients have a more than 50% improvement at 12 weeks. Tricyclic antidepressants may also be helpful because they can inhibit the neural activation that leads to pain. Amitriptyline is not FDA-approved for IC but doses of 10 to 75 mg nightly have produced pain relief in two thirds of women and decreases in urgency and frequency. Unfortunately, in another trial, when reviewing all randomized subjects, amitriptyline with education and behavioral modification did not significantly improve symptoms. However, in this study, it was found that amitriptyline may be beneficial in those who can tolerate a daily dose of 50 mg or more, although this subgroup comparison was not specified in advance. The side effects of sedation, dry mouth, and constipation are often bothersome. Antihistamines such as hydroxyzine may be of benefit for patients with concurrent allergies and for decreasing mast cell degranulation, but most studies have not shown benefit. Antidepressants may be useful in depressed women.

Hydrodistention of the bladder under anesthesia is therapeutic in 20% to 30% of patients and is sometimes done at the initial evaluation when performing cystoscopy to rule out other pathology. However, most experts do not use hydrodistention as a diagnostic criterion any longer because the findings of glomerulations are nondiagnostic. Three to 6 months of symptom improvement occurs with distention in responders.

Because PBS-IC is a complex disease, it is best treated by an experienced physician with the expertise and patience to deal with the woman and her needs over a prolonged period. Usually, multiple interventions are necessary, with a combination of behavioral changes, pelvic floor physical therapy, counseling, oral medications, and bladder instillation. Hormonal manipulation in premenopausal women with menstrual flares may provide benefit.

URETHRAL SYNDROME (URETHRAL PAIN SYNDROME)

The so-called **urethral syndrome** is poorly characterized but most reports suggest the same symptoms of dysuria, frequency, urgency, and pain that are seen with urethritis or UTIs. In the case of urethral syndrome, however, the symptoms are generally of long standing, and no specific organism can be identified. The International Continence Society standardization report in 2002 added a new genitourinary pain syndrome category. It defined urethral pain syndrome as the "occurrence of recurrent episodic urethral pain usually on voiding, with daytime frequency and nocturia, in the absence of proven infection or other obvious pathology." This problem may be part of the PBS-IC group. Typically, urethroscopy has revealed a reddened, chronically inflamed urethra, with spasm at the bladder neck. The prevalence of this condition is unknown but may affect as many as 20% to 30% of all women at one time or another. The cause is unknown but there are many theories, including allergic, immunologic, infectious, neurologic, atrophic, and psychogenic causes. Some think that the problem resides in the paraurethral glands (analogous to the prostate in men) and that infection with organisms such as *Mycoplasma, Ureaplasma,* or *Chlamydia* might be responsible. The incidence of these infections, however, has been approximately the same as in populations of women without the syndrome. Nevertheless, these organisms should be sought and eradicated with appropriate antibiotic therapy when they are found, because this may alleviate symptoms. Baerheim and colleagues have compared the success of treatment with antibacterial therapy in 51 patients with acute lower UTIs and 58 patients with acute urethral syndrome and found improvement by 3 days in approximately 50% of each group.

Because the cause in most cases is unknown, various therapies have been devised, with varying success. These include dilation of the urethra with progressive dilators (of historic interest only), antispasmodics, estrogen (in postmenopausal women), and cryosurgery. Patients diagnosed as having the urethral syndrome deserve a careful evaluation before specific therapy is initiated. Most of the studies on urethral syndrome were published before 1990. Many reports have indicated that suprapubic pain is a feature, with relief after voiding. Chronic urethral syndrome may be a subset of PBS-IC.

URETHRAL DIVERTICULUM

Causes

Urethral diverticula occur in perhaps as many as 1% to 6% of all women at some time during their lifetime. Age distribution in published reports ranges from 19 to 76 years, but most diverticula seem to occur between the ages of 30 and 50 years. Andersen has suggested that the disease occurs more frequently in blacks, with a ratio perhaps as high as 6:1.

A variety of causes have been suggested, including congenital, acute and chronic inflammatory, and traumatic. The congenital theory stems from the fact that rare cases have been reported in children and neonates. Evidence for acute and chronic infection comes from observations noting infection and obstruction of the periurethral glands, which result in the formation of retention cysts that when repeatedly infected, may rupture into the lumen of the urethra and remain as an outpouching, giving rise to the diverticulum. Several authors have suggested that the gonococcus is the cause of this, but *E. coli* and other organisms have been found in such processes. Urethral trauma from multiple catheterizations or from childbirth has also been suggested as a causative factor. However, many women with diverticula have neither been catheterized nor given birth. The infectious origin is probably the most commonly espoused and the prevalence in women with recurrent UTIs may be as high as 40%.

Symptoms and Signs

The classic description of symptoms in a woman with urethral diverticula includes the three Ds—postvoid dribbling, dysuria, and dyspareunia. More common are complaints of frequency and urgency, dysuria, history of recurrent UTIs, dribbling, and incontinence. Occasionally, hematuria occurs. In a series reported from the Mayo Clinic, Lee noted that a palpable, tender, suburethral mass was present in 51 of 85 patients (60%) and that protrusion of the diverticulum from the vaginal introitus occurred in 4 patients. More recent reports have suggested that a tender mass is only found 35% of the time. Occasionally, patients have urinary stones in the diverticula or discharge or pus from the urethra. Malignancy is rarely found.

Diagnosis

Diagnosis is generally suggested by physical examination. The distal anterior vaginal wall overlying the urethra or bladder neck may be tender or a cystic mass may be found about the midurethra. Pus or cloudy urine may be expressed as the urethra and mass are massaged. A normal examination and nonclassic symptoms are often typical of how a woman presents, which is why the diagnosis is often delayed. Historically, the double-catheter balloon technique, which essentially closes the urethra at each end and forces contrast medium into the diverticulum under pressure during cystography, has been the gold standard. Now, magnetic resonance imaging (MRI) with cross-sectional imaging offers the most detailed anatomic study; it can also image diverticula that do not communicate with the urethra, as well as multiple outpouchings. Other tests are used, such as urethroscopy, voiding cystourethrography, urodynamics (because 35% to 50% will have incontinence), transvaginal ultrasound, and virtual computed tomography (CT) urethroscopy.

Treatment

No treatment is indicated for asymptomatic urethral diverticula. Mild symptoms of frequency and urgency can be treated with anticholinergics and infections with antibiotics. Carcinoma has been reported in diverticula so caution is needed if no surgical therapy is planned. A variety of procedures have been suggested for the management of urethral diverticula. Lapides has suggested a technique for transurethral marsupialization that involves the resection of the roof of the diverticulum using transurethral electrocautery. Essentially, this technique enlarges the orifice of the diverticulum by incising its roof; however, the orifice can be challenging to identify or not found at all. Spence and Duckett reported a marsupialization technique in which the diverticulum was opened and sutured to the vaginal epithelial surface. Generally, this leads to a fistula and requires secondary closure, making this technique useful in only rare circumstances. Diverticulectomy is the more common procedure done today.

Urethroscopy occasionally identifies the location of the diverticulum and careful inspection might show multiple diverticula. In Lee's report from the Mayo Clinic, the diverticulum was noted coming from the distal third of the urethra in only 10 of 85 patients, whereas 38 patients demonstrated an origin from the middle third and 13 from the proximal third, including the bladder neck. Lee noted multiple diverticula in 18 of 85 patients.

After the diverticulum is identified and evaluated, an incision is made in the anterior vaginal wall and the diverticulum is dissected free of the pubocervical fascia. The diverticulum's neck is noted and excised by sharp dissection, and the urethral wall is closed with a row of interrupted 4-0 polyglycol sutures. The closure line is generally in the longitudinal axis. Occasionally, however, a transverse closure is necessary because of the nature of the attachment. The pubocervical fascia is then reinforced with a row of 3-0 polyglycol reabsorbable interrupted sutures. Hemostasis is scrupulously secured with electrocautery and the vaginal incision is closed with polyglycol sutures (**Fig. 21-12**).

Most diverticula emanate from the ventral wall of the urethra. Occasionally, however, the diverticulum is noted to be arising from the lateral wall of the urethra or even from the anterior wall. In these cases, the dissection must be carefully carried to the base of the diverticulum and the procedure carried out as stated. In all cases, a no. 16 or 18 Foley or suprapubic catheter is left in place for 7 to 14 days. Postoperative videocystourethrography can be performed to ensure that there are no urethrovesical fistulas before discontinuing use of the catheter.

Several nuances have been offered to make dissection and subsequent repair easier. One involves placing a ureteral catheter into the diverticulum and allowing it to coil so that the diverticulum is more easily observable during dissection. Some surgeons have attempted to dilate the neck of the diverticulum before beginning the excision and, occasionally, have even tried to pack foreign substances such as gauze through the neck to make the dissection easier. Often, a Martius flap is brought into the field between the periurethral fascial closure and vaginal wall. This is thought to prevent fistula formation.

Complications

Major complications of this procedure include urethrovaginal fistula formation, development of stress urinary incontinence, recurrence of the diverticulum, missing diverticula when multiple diverticula are present, and stricture of the urethra. Reported urethrovaginal fistula rates are 5% to 8.3%. If the diverticulum recurs within the first few months after operation, it may represent a second diverticulum that was overlooked or an inappropriate repair of the diagnosed diverticulum. If the diverticulum occurs after 1 year, it is probably a new lesion. Stricture of the urethra has rarely been reported in any of the operative series but it is a theoretical possibility.

A 2010 study reported the largest series of 122 women undergoing urethral diverticulectomy. Recurrence of diverticula that required repeat excision occurred in 10.7%, which is higher than

Figure 21-12 Resection of urethral diverticulum. **A,** Diverticulum exposed with vaginal lining and endopelvic fascia retracted. **B,** Fingers hold diverticulum on traction, which aids in dissection and identification of ostium. **C,** After complete resection of diverticulum, urethra is closed with fine, interrupted extramucosal sutures. (Adapted from Lee RA: Diverticulum of the female urethra: Postoperative complications and results. Obstet Gynecol 61:52, 1983.)

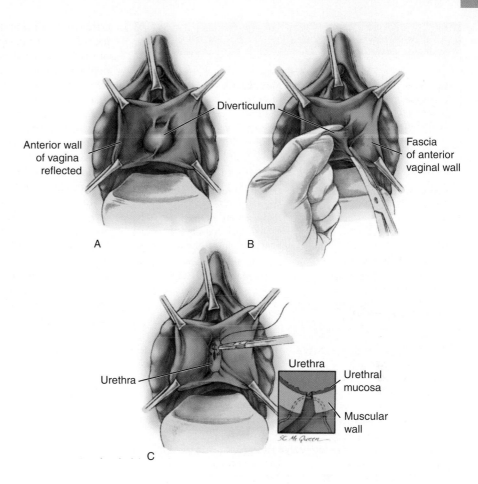

that in earlier reported studies. Risk factors for recurrence included proximal diverticulum, multiple diverticula, and previous pelvic or vaginal surgery, excluding previous diverticulectomy. Of the patients in this study, 26% had persistent pain or discomfort with urination. Other studies have also reported the development of the urethral syndrome, probably caused by continuing inflammation and irritation.

Other complications involve stress incontinence, which may be related to the dissection of the bladder neck away from its usual location and injury to the urethral sphincter mechanism. If intrinsic sphincter deficiency results, the incontinence can be difficult to treat because of tissue compromise from repair.

UROLITHIASIS

Urinary tract stones, renal or ureteral, may occur in patients of both genders and at any age. Approximately 5% of women will develop a symptomatic stone by the age of 70 years. These may be related to metabolic abnormalities, such as gout or errors of calcium metabolism, but usually relate to chronic infection and stasis of urine. The leading risk factor for stones is genetic. Other risk factors for calculi in women include pregnancy, during which time the urinary tract becomes dilated and stasis is more common, a history of kidney stones or family history, certain medications, excessive vitamin C intake, low calcium intake, chronic diarrhea, and dehydration.

Symptoms occur most often when a stone passes from the kidney to the ureter. Pain occurs on the side of the stone and varies from a dull ache to severe paroxysms of pain, called renal colic. Flank pain, lower abdominal pain, and groin pain can occur; the location can vary as the stone moves down the ureter with radiation of pain to the groin. Gross or microscopic hematuria is usually present. Noncontrast CT scanning has become the gold standard for diagnosis, particularly if the abdominal radiograph is normal. Ultrasound misses small stones but is recommended for pregnant women.

Various treatment modalities are available, including observation with pain medications and fluids awaiting spontaneous passage, endoscopic removal, surgical removal, and destruction of the stone with laser or shockwave lithotripsy. Although not FDA-approved, alpha blockers may aid in passage of the stone. The principal consideration, however, should be correction of the basic problem that caused the stone. Urgent intervention is necessary if the woman has fever, chills, nausea and vomiting, and pain uncontrolled by narcotics. An obstructing stone in the presence of infection can be life-threatening.

URINARY INCONTINENCE

RISK FACTORS

Box 21-2 lists the currently known risk factors associated with incontinence, summarizing the work of several authors. Some of the factors will be highlighted in this section. The prevalence of urinary incontinence increases until approximately 50 years of age and then stabilizes before increasing again after age 65.

Box 21-2 Factors Independently Associated with Urinary Incontinence in Women

Modifiable Factors

Gynecologic
Cystocele
Uterine prolapse
Nonnormal gynecologic examination
Poor pelvic floor muscle contraction

Medications
Diuretics
Estrogen
Benzodiazepines
Tranquilizers
Antidepressants
Hypnotics
Laxatives

Urologic and Gastrointestinal
Antibiotics
Recurrent urinary tract infections
Dysuria
Fecal incontinence
Constipation
Bowel problems

Other Factors
Smoking
High caffeine intake
Higher body mass index
Functional impairment

Comorbid Diseases
Diabetes
Stroke
Elevated systolic blood pressure
Cognitive impairment
Parkinsonism
Arthritis
Back problems
Hearing and visual impairment

Nonmodifiable Factors

Gynecologic Factors
Hysterectomy in older women
Prolapse surgery

Pregnancy-Related Factors
Vaginal delivery
Forceps delivery
Cesarean section
Increased parity
Fetal birth weight

Other Factors
Age
White race
Higher education
Childhood enuresis
Presence of two or more comorbid diseases

From Holroyd-Leduc JM, Straus SE: Management of urinary incontinence in women. Clinical applications. JAMA 291: 996, 2004.

Prevalence estimates were presented earlier in this chapter. Bump and McClish compared risk factors and determinants of urodynamic stress incontinence between smokers and nonsmokers using a case-control method. In this study, 71 smokers and 118 nonsmokers were compared following a complete urogynecologic evaluation. Smokers were found to have stronger urethral sphincters and generated a greater increase in bladder pressure with coughing, but similar findings with respect to urethral mobility and pressure transmission ratios were found when compared with nonsmokers. Urodynamic stress incontinence developed in smokers despite their stronger urethral sphincter findings, probably because of more violent coughing leading to earlier development of anatomic defects.

Another area of interest involves racial and ethnic differences with respect to the presence of urinary incontinence. Bump noted that black women with urinary incontinence have a different distribution of symptoms and different reasons for their incontinence than white women. Black women had a significantly lower prevalence of pure urodynamic stress incontinence than white women. These conclusions were based on a study of 200 consecutive women, 54 of whom were black, referred for evaluation of urinary stress incontinence or pelvic organ prolapse. The findings may possibly relate to differences in collagen and connective tissue in these individuals. Several other studies have found a higher prevalence of urinary incontinence in non-Hispanic white woman and Mexican-American women compared with rates in Asian and black women, although at least two studies have found no difference between racial or ethnic groups.

Obesity has a strong association with incontinence and, for every five-unit increase in body mass index, the risk increases. Depression and anxiety are associated with incontinence. This has been further evaluated in overweight and obese women. These women reported a higher number of weekly incontinence episodes than women without depressive symptoms, as well as more bothersome symptoms and poorer quality of life.

Epidemiologic studies have suggested increased risk with hysterectomy but short-term clinical studies have not, so more research is needed to clarify this issue. Vaginal childbirth and higher fetal weight are risk factors in younger women but the effect diminishes in older women, possibly because the neuromuscular decline with aging becomes a more important factor. The prevalence of incontinence is significantly higher for women in nursing homes and women with cognitive impairment and poor mobility.

STRESS URINARY INCONTINENCE

Stress urinary incontinence occurs when bladder pressure exceeds urethral pressure, with increases in intraabdominal pressure. Urethral hypermobility and urethral closure are factors to consider in issues of continence. In 1971, the saline-moistened or lubricated cotton swab test (Q-tip test) was introduced to differentiate the defects in the posterior urethrovesical angle, which we now relate to loss of bladder neck support or urethral hypermobility. The concept of the posterior urethrovesical angle is no longer applicable, but the test and its association with urethral hypermobility is still useful and has been reported in stress incontinence surgery research studies. This test involves placing a cotton swab into the urethra to the bladder neck and observing the angle that the urethra makes with the horizontal with a Valsalva maneuver. The cotton swab test suggests defects in the anterior vaginal wall supports of the bladder neck, but not a specific urologic diagnosis. The test quantifies the mobility of the bladder neck and proximal urethra in continent and incontinent women, with and without pelvic support relaxation, but offers no additional information about incontinence.

Bladder neck funneling, position, and hypermobility can be evaluated by perineal ultrasound, and this test may have many useful applications in the future. Ultrasound examination of the urethral sphincter may also be helpful in measuring length, thickness, and striated muscle volume. Athanasiou and associates, using three-dimensional ultrasound, have shown that women with stress urinary incontinence have significantly shorter, thinner, and smaller volumes of striated muscle in their urethras than continent women of comparable ages and parity. Urethral closure is affected by the mucosa and vasculature,

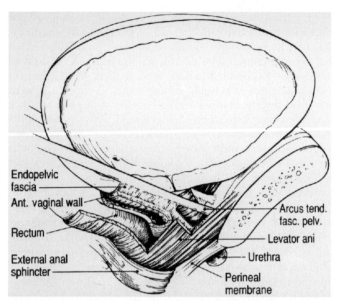

Figure 21-13 Lateral view of the components of the urethral support system. Note how the levator ani muscles support the rectum, vagina, and urethrovesical neck. Also note how the endopelvic fascia next to the urethra attaches to the levator ani muscle; contraction of the levator muscle leads to elevation of the urethrovesical neck. (From DeLancey JOL, Ashton-Miller JA: Pathophysiology of adult urinary incontinence. Gastroenterolgy 126(Suppl 1):S23, 2004.)

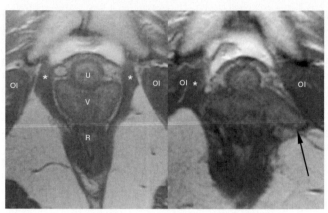

Figure 21-14 Axial MRI scan at the level of the midurethra in a normal nullipara (*left*) and a woman 9 months after vaginal birth (*right*) in whom the pubovisceral portion of the levator ani muscle has been lost. The pubovisceral muscle (*) is seen between the urethra (U) and obturator internus (OI) muscle in the normal woman but is missing in the woman on the right. R, Rectum; V, vagina. (From DeLancey JOL, Ashton-Miller JA: Pathophysiology of adult urinary incontinence. Gastroenterolgy 126(Suppl 1):S23, 2004.)

adjacent connective tissue structures, striated and smooth muscles, and involuntary and voluntary muscle contractions that prevent incontinence in response to stress.

In addition to the importance of the urethral sphincteric system to continence, the support system has been studied further. DeLancey's hammock theory explains that the urethra sits on the endopelvic fascia and anterior vaginal wall. Because that support layer is attached to the pelvic wall via the arcus tendineus fascia pelvis and levator ani, the urethra is actually compressed with increased abdominal pressure. This maintains urethral closure pressures above increases in abdominal and bladder pressure and prevents urinary leakage (**Fig. 21-13**). Anatomically, if hypermobility is present, this corresponds to the loss of the backstop support at the bladder neck. This is a likely explanation for the success of midurethral slings for relieving stress incontinence.

Stress incontinence may occur with injury or degeneration to the urethral support women or urethral sphincter mechanism; it is more likely that most women have elements of both problems. Although we try to classify women with stress incontinence as having urethral hypermobility or the more severe leakage associated with urethral musculature damage, termed *low-pressure urethra* or *intrinsic sphincter deficiency* (ISD), there is actually great overlap. Women with a cystourethrocele or anterior vaginal wall relaxation have urethral hypermobility but not necessarily stress incontinence. If they have stress incontinence, they must have some urethral sphincter compromise along with the hypermobility.

The possibility of trauma from obstetric delivery or another traumatic experience has been implicated in the cause of stress incontinence. Meyer and colleagues studied 149 patients during pregnancy and 9 weeks postpartum. They found that 36% of women who were delivered by forceps and 21% who delivered spontaneously suffered from urinary incontinence. Bladder neck mobility was significantly increased after all vaginal births, but bladder neck position at rest was only lowered in the forceps group. Women who underwent cesarean delivery were unaffected. DeLancey and coworkers have reported MRI images showing levator ani injuries in 10% to 15% of primiparous women. These injuries may lead to later pelvic floor dysfunction and incontinence, although long-term follow-up studies are needed (**Fig. 21-14**). Considering other forms of pelvic floor trauma, Nygaard studied female American Olympic athletes and could not find a difference between the low-impact (swimmers) and high-impact (gymnasts, track and field performers) athletes with respect to the development of stress incontinence later in life.

Treatment
Conservative Management

Inquiring about a woman's goals for treatment of stress incontinence is useful, as is identifying the most bothersome aspects of her complaints. Conservative measures should be discussed and offered to the woman (**Box 21-3**). The first-line treatment is pelvic floor muscle training directed toward the strengthening of the levator ani and pubococcygeal muscles, which affect the urethral closure mechanism. This can be affected by isometric exercises, as described by Kegel. Although there are a number of modifications of these exercises, one useful application is to teach the woman to contract these muscles slowly, 8 to 12 times, for a count of 6 to 8 seconds each, and to repeat this series for three sets. Interestingly, Kegel, in 1956, suggested that the woman contract her pubococcygeal muscles five times on waking, five times on rising, and five times every half-hour throughout the day. According to modern physiology principles, this is not optimal and might be a reason for a woman stating that her trial of

Box 21-3 Methods of Pelvic Muscle Strengthening
Kegel exercises
Biofeedback
Isometric with vaginal cones (weights)
Electrical stimulation of pelvic floor

Kegel exercises failed. For general strength training, three or four times weekly may be adequate. The woman can be instructed on how to contract these muscles by being told to attempt to stop the urinary stream while she is voiding. After she learns which muscles to contract, she should perform the exercises at other times without any relationship to voiding. Pelvic muscle exercise success is improved with specific training by a health professional or physical therapist. Improvement in the muscular supports may be enough to overcome the anatomic weakness that originally led to the stress incontinence.

The 2006 Cochrane Database review of pelvic floor muscle training analyzed 12 trials involving 836 women. There was variation in study design, study populations, and outcome measures, making comparisons challenging. Women who did pelvic floor muscle training were more likely to be cured or improved than the control group and experienced fewer daily incontinence episodes. A supervise training program for at least 3 months was supported by the review. Interestingly, these exercises helped women with all types of incontinence, although the women with stress incontinence enjoyed more benefit. Better efficacy was noted in younger women.

Many patients enjoy prolonged relief, even after stopping pelvic floor muscle exercises. Bø and Talseth studied 23 women who participated in a 6-month intensive pelvic floor muscle exercise routine and noted that 5 years later, 75% demonstrated no leakage during a stress test and 70% were satisfied with their continence. Of these patients, 70% were still exercising their pelvic muscles at least once weekly and demonstrated pelvic floor muscle strength. Nygaard noted similar findings. These authors noted improvement of incontinence, not only in patients with stress incontinence but also in those with urge and **mixed urinary incontinence**.

It is important to ensure that the woman is aware of how to perform the exercises correctly. In a study by Bump and co-workers in which 47 women were given simple verbal or written instructions, 23 (49%) had an ideal Kegel effort signified by an increase in force of the urethral closure. However, 12 subjects (25%) were performing the technique poorly and in such a way that incontinence might be promoted. The authors recommended a demonstration approach rather than a written or verbal approach.

A variation in pelvic muscle training is the use of weighted vaginal cones. This involves a set of cones of increasing weight that require pelvic muscle contraction to hold them within the vagina. Peattie and associates demonstrated an improvement in 70% of 30 premenopausal women with stress incontinence after only 1 month of exercise. A correlation was noted between decreased urine loss and the ability to retain cones of increased weight. A 2007 Cochrane review found evidence that vaginal cones were better than no active treatment for stress incontinence and may be of similar efficacy to pelvic muscle exercises and electrical stimulation, although this was based on less than optimal study designs in the trials.

Pelvic floor electrical stimulation has also been studied for improving pelvic floor muscle strength and decreasing symptoms of stress incontinence. A small, removable vaginal probe is placed in the vagina or anus and the electrical stimulation activates a pelvic muscle contraction. A 2003 randomized controlled trial by Goode and colleagues studied 200 women with stress incontinence and found that pelvic floor electrical stimulation did not increase effectiveness in a comprehensive behavioral training program.

An incontinence pessary is a silicone ring device with a knob placed in the vagina, with the goal of stabilizing the urethra to eliminate hypermobility or raise urethral pressure. This is a safe and effective conservative treatment. The FemSoft urethral insert device (Rochester Medical, Stewartville, MN) is basically a urethral plug. Although women with stress incontinence may have greatly reduced leakage when wearing the insert, it is not popular as self-catheterization is needed to insert the device and a new one needs to be placed after each void. The occasional woman who leaks only with vigorous exercise might choose to use this insert during her workout. **Figure 21-15** shows each of these devices.

Weight loss in overweight and obese women significantly reduces urinary leakage, as shown in a 2009 randomized controlled trial of 338 women. A 6-month behavioral intervention for weight loss included diet, exercise, and behavioral modification and was compared with a control group that received structured education not related to weight loss. The women in the intervention group lost 8% of their body weight (7.8 kg) compared with 1.6% (1.5 kg) in the control group. Incontinence episodes declined by 47% and 28%, respectively ($P = .01$), but this was only for stress incontinence, not urge incontinence.

In postmenopausal women, estrogen therapy was thought to increase the vasculature and mucosal seal of the urethra, thereby increasing urethral closing pressure and overcoming the effects that might have led to mild degrees of stress incontinence. However, randomized studies have called into question these effects and, in fact, the opposite effect has been shown. The Heart and Estrogen/Progestin Replacement Study (HERS) found that women taking combined hormone replacement actually reported worsened incontinence. Both the Women's Health Initiative (WHI) and Nurses' Health Study also found increased risk of incontinence; the WHI found that the risk was greatest

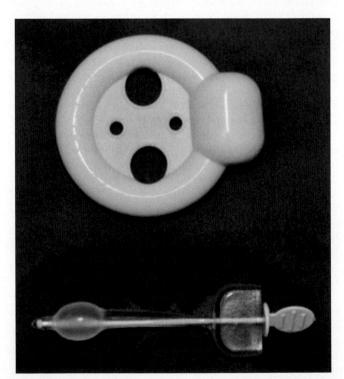

Figure 21-15 Incontinence ring pessary and FemSoft urethral insert.

for stress incontinence. Oral estrogen is no longer advised for stress incontinence. (See later, Estrogen and the Lower Urinary Tract.)

Other non-FDA approved drugs and combinations of drugs have been studied to determine whether pharmacologic therapy can aid stress-incontinent women. Although imipramine is a tricyclic antidepressant, it has α-adrenergic enhancement characteristics. Its action on the alpha receptors in the bladder neck and urethra may cause muscle contraction and could theoretically lessen stress incontinence. Imipramine has limited benefit for treating stress incontinence and weak evidence to suggest that any other adrenergic drug is better than placebo treatment.

Duloxetine is not FDA-approved for treating stress incontinence in the United States but has been approved in Europe. Duloxetine is a serotonin and norepinephrine reuptake inhibitor that stimulates pudendal motor neuron activity in Onuf's nucleus in the spinal cord and causes rhabdosphincter contraction in the urethra. Several large randomized trials have compared duloxetine to placebo, but reduction in incontinence is modest and cure rates are no different than placebo. Nausea is a frequent side effect. For a woman considering treatment for depression, who also has bothersome stress incontinence, duloxetine is a reasonable medication to consider. **Table 21-5** summarizes classes of other agents that may affect urinary function or therapy.

Surgical Treatment

Hundreds of surgical procedures have been developed to treat stress incontinence. Before the 1950s, the operative approach to treat stress incontinence primarily involved vaginal procedures, which included plication of the bladder neck (Kelly procedure) with anterior colporrhaphy to reduce a cystocele. Bergman and Giovanni, and Harris and coworkers, have published studies demonstrating that retropubic urethropexy operations have a higher cure rate than anterior colporrhaphies for stress incontinence when the patients are followed long term. Anterior colporrhaphy has been largely abandoned as a surgical procedure for treating stress incontinence.

For historic reasons, several surgical procedures no longer in use will be mentioned here; familiarity with them is necessary because these women often present with recurrent stress incontinence. Further surgery can be complicated by scarring in the vagina and retropubic space and increase the risk of bladder injury. Transvaginal needle suspensions (TVNSs) were introduced in the late 1950s as a less invasive alternative to retropubic operations. Special needles were developed by Pereyra that could be used to guide sutures from the paravaginal tissue through the space of Retzius, suspended from the rectus fascia. The suture was tied over the rectus fascia, just above the bladder neck. This was carried out through a small suprapubic and vaginal incision. Stamey's 1973 modification of the Pereyra procedure used a small tube of Dacron material to buttress the suture, thereby keeping it from pulling through. Many other modifications of TVNS have been described and popularized.

Several national and international organizations convened and reviewed the long-term success rates of incontinence operations when it became apparent that TVNS held up poorly after 2 to 3 years. Consensus statements suggested slings and retropubic suspensions have more durable results than TVNS or anterior repair for stress incontinence. TVNS have rapidly declined as a primary treatment option for stress incontinence, as have anterior repairs.

Before midurethral synthetic slings for women with stress incontinence were popularized, the surgery of choice was a suprapubic approach or a pubovaginal bladder neck sling. The Marshall-Marchetti-Krantz suprapubic urethrovesical suspension operation was first reported in 1949 and was the mainstay of many surgeons attempting to alleviate stress incontinence in these patients. The space of Retzius is entered, the bladder neck is identified, generally with a 30-mL bulb Foley catheter in the bladder, and the paravaginal tissue adjacent to the bladder neck is identified and sutured to the pubic symphysis using two or three interrupted sutures on each side of the bladder neck. The surgeon must be careful not to place undue stress on the bladder neck (**Fig. 21-16**). A rare (1% to 2%) but painful complication of the Marshall-Marchetti-Krantz procedure is **osteitis**

Table 21-5 Drugs with Possible Effects on the Lower Urinary Tract

Class	Possible Side Effects	Drug and Usual Indication	Action
Antihypertensives	Incontinence	Reserpine, hypertension	Pharmacologic sympathectomy by depleting catecholamines
		Methyldopa, hypertension	
		Angiotensin-converting enzyme inhibitors	Side effect of cough—may worsen stress incontinence
Dopaminergic agonists	Bladder neck obstruction	Bromocriptine, galactorrhea	Increased urethral resistance, decreased detrusor contractions
		Levodopa, Parkinson's disease	
Cholinergic agonists	Decreased bladder capacity and increased intravesical pressure	Digitalis, cardiotropic	Increased bladder wall tension
Neuroleptics	Incontinence	Major tranquilizers—prochlorperazine, promethazine, trifluoperazine, chlorpromazine, haloperidol	Dopamine receptor blockade, with internal sphincter relaxation
β-Adrenergic agents	Urinary retention	Isoxsuprine, vasodilator	Inhibited bladder muscle contractility
		Terbutaline, bronchodilator	
Estrogen	Incontinence		Worsens stress and mixed UI
Xanthines	Incontinence	Caffeine	Decreased urethral closure pressure
Alcohol	Frequency, urgency		Sedation and immobility may inhibit ability to recognize urgency

UI, Urinary incontinence.

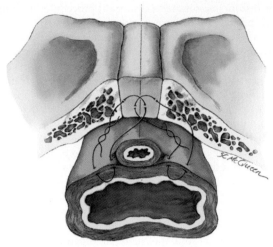

Figure 21-16 Demonstration of the relative position of a pair of sutures adjacent to the urethra, securely placed into the pubic symphysis. (Adapted from Buchsbaum HJ, Schmidt JD [eds]: Gynecologic and Obstetric Urology. Philadelphia, WB Saunders, 1982.)

pubis. This condition is an inflammatory reaction in the periosteum of the pubic bone that is more often associated with permanent suture material

In 1961, Burch advocated a modification of the suprapubic bladder neck suspension by suspending the vaginal wall to Cooper's ligament (**Fig. 21-17**). Polyglycol or nonabsorbable sutures are appropriate. At times, patients have difficulty voiding for prolonged periods, and the occasional woman may report that she needs to rise off the commode to a semistanding position to void.

Colombo and coworkers performed a prospective randomized clinical trial using the Burch and Marshall–Marchetti–Krantz procedures. The follow-up was 2 to 7 years. They reported subjective and objective cure rates of 92% and 80%, respectively, for the

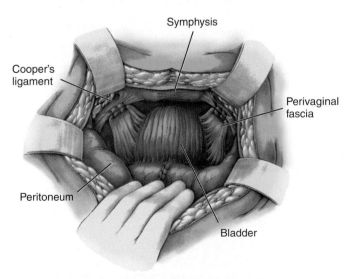

Figure 21-17 Burch procedure. The lateral edges of the vagina have been sutured to Cooper's ligament. (Adapted from Burch JC: Urethrovaginal fixation to Cooper's ligament for correction of stress incontinence, cystocele, and prolapse. Am J Obstet Gynecol 81:281, 1961.)

Burch procedure and 85% and 65%, respectively, for the Marshall-Marchetti-Krantz procedure. These differences were not statistically significant. In a 2005 Cochrane Database review of 39 trials of the Burch procedure, Lapitan and associates noted that the success rate reported ranged from 85% to 90% at 1 year, and 70% were dry at 5 years. Other studies have shown a 69% success rate at 10 to 20 years. Follow-up urodynamic studies performed 10 years later in one study reported a surgical cure rate of 90.3%, but five of the seven patients who were considered failures though that their symptoms had improved.

A 2007 multicenter randomized trial compared 655 women assigned to have an autologous fascial sling or Burch procedure. At 24 months, the success rates were higher for women who had the fascial sling than the Burch procedure, 44% versus 38% ($P = .01$), using the strictest outcome criteria and 66% versus 49% ($P < .001$), respectively, if specifically considering stress incontinence outcomes. However, the fascial sling group had more complications with UTIs, voiding difficulty, and postoperative urge incontinence. This well-done trial was overshadowed by the rapid popularity and simplicity of the midurethral slings.

The Burch procedure can also be performed laparoscopically. Saidi and colleagues have reported comparable 12-month cure rates in 70 patients undergoing laparoscopic procedures (91.4%) and 87 patients undergoing open procedures (92%). The laparoscopic procedures had a somewhat shorter operative time and a much shorter hospital stay. Ross followed 48 consecutive patients who underwent laparoscopic Burch procedures and found a cure rate of 93% and 89% at 1 and 2 years, respectively, using multichannel urodynamic studies. Further studies have not been large enough to clarify the proposed benefits; one randomized study found a higher 3-year failure rate compared with an open technique. With the introduction of minimally invasive vaginal midurethral slings, the use of laparoscopic Burch procedures has declined.

Shull and Baden reported on 149 consecutive patients who were assessed anatomically and found to have a paravaginal defect causing stress urinary incontinence. In these patients, they performed an abdominal repair in which the anterior vaginal wall was sutured with permanent suture to the white line bilaterally. In follow-up for as long as 48 months, 97% of patients remained continent. However, 6% suffered vaginal cuff prolapse, 5% developed an enterocele in addition to cuff prolapse, and 5% redeveloped the cystocele after the operation. When the paravaginal fascial defect is noted on anatomic examination, this operation has a good application as an alternative to other described procedures. It may also be used in conjunction with other procedures when multiple anatomic defects are identified, and can be performed abdominally or vaginally. Most surgeons do not perform a paravaginal defect repair as the sole operation for stress incontinence because of the paucity of studies. However, it may be useful for anatomic correction of a paravaginal support defect.

Midurethral vaginal tape slings using permanent mesh have become the most commonly used surgical procedures for stress incontinence. The first to be introduced was the retropubic tension-free vaginal tape sling (TVT). This was developed based on the theory that the tension on the pubourethral ligaments interacts with muscles of the pelvic floor and suburethral vaginal support structure. Ulmsten and coworkers published a 1996 article on 75 women treated with a midurethral sling made of permanent mesh (**Fig. 21-18**). The sling was placed under local

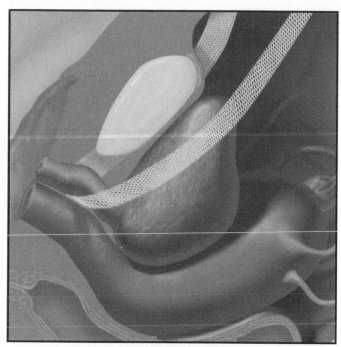

Figure 21-18 Tension-free vaginal tape (TVT) sling with Prolene mesh placed midurethrally, without the need for fixation. (Courtesy of Gynecare, Ethicon, Somerville, NJ.)

anesthesia with sedation. A small vaginal incision was made under the midurethra. Small tunnels were made bilaterally to aid in passage of the trocar from the vaginal area through the retropubic space against the pubic bone, and exiting through abdominal skin punctures suprapubically. Cystoscopy was performed to evaluate for bladder perforation before the sling was brought into place. The sling was a monofilament polypropylene synthetic mesh, 1 cm wide and 40 cm long. An 84% cure rate was reported, an additional 8% were improved, and 8% failed. At 3 years after surgery, Ulmsten and colleagues reported an 86% cure rate.

Many other researchers worldwide have published similar success rates. Studies in older and obese populations also have similar success. Complications have included retropubic hematoma, bladder perforation, intraoperative bleeding, urinary retention, mesh exposure and, rarely, bowel and urethral injuries and vascular injury. Ward, Hilton, and the UK and Ireland TVT trial group have published a prospective randomized study comparing TVT with Burch colposuspension for primary urodynamic stress incontinence. With strict outcome data, the TVT procedure appears to be as effective as the Burch procedure at 2 years, with 63% and 51% cured by objective outcome data, respectively. The lower cure rates in this trial are likely because of the strict outcome criteria. Although the Burch procedure is often successful, the 2- to 3-day hospital stay, 4- to 6- week recovery, and additional risks are much less attractive than a short outpatient procedure (usually less than 30 minutes) with three small incisions and a 2-week recovery time. However, the placement of a permanent mesh has additional risks of mesh erosion and infection not seen with the Burch procedure.

Delorme introduced the transobturator (TOT) tape sling approach in 2001 with the hope of avoiding vascular, bladder, and bowel injuries. TOT sling trocars traverse the obturator canal instead of the retropubic space via small groin incisions at the level of the clitoris bilaterally. Delorme described an out-to-in passage through the obturator membrane along the inferior pubic ramus. Two years later, an in-to-out passage was described and touted to reduce urethral injury. Complications include bleeding, groin or leg pain, and urethral injuries. Objective and subjective cure rates have been similar in a randomized trial comparing a TOT tape sling with a Burch colposuspension. A 2010 multicenter randomized trial compared retropubic TVT with TOT sling. In this study, 597 women were randomized and 95% completed 12-month follow-up for treatment success analysis. Objective treatment success required a negative cough stress test, pad test, and no retreatment. Objective success was 80.8% for the retropubic sling and 77.7% for a TOT sling; subjective success rates were 62.2% and 55.8%, respectively. Voiding dysfunction was significantly more common in the retropubic sling group (2.7% versus 0%; $P=.004$). Neurologic symptoms of thigh and groin pain were higher in the TOT group (9.4% versus 4%; $P=.01$). Although this is the single best trial to date, many randomized trials have shown similar success rates of the TOT sling compared with the retropubic TVT sling in women with normal pressure urethras (except in ISD; see later). Although in single trials they have equivalent outcomes, the complication profile is different. Either procedure can also lead to de novo development of urge incontinence, mesh erosion, mesh infection, or dyspareunia.

A 2010 systematic review of 39 randomized controlled trials studied midurethral mesh slings, Burch colposuspension, and fascial pubovaginal slings. The results were similar to the studies detailed earlier, although the large number of trials reported allowed enough patients to find differences that were not found in individual studies. However, the study was limited by the wide variation in study design, outcome reporting, and length of follow-up. The retropubic midurethral tape sling women had a slightly higher objective cure rate (odds ratio [OR], 0.8; $P=.04$) than women treated with the transobturator sling, although the subjective cure rates were similar. The transobturator sling group had a significantly lower risk of bladder and vaginal perforation, lower urinary tract symptoms, and hematoma. The in-to-out versus out-to-in style of transobturator sling was not significantly different. Compared with the Burch colposuspension, the retropubic midurethral sling group had significantly higher continence success overall (OR, 0.61; $P=.00009$), but more intraoperative complications of bladder perforation. The fascial pubovaginal bladder neck sling and retropubic midurethral sling had similar cure rates, but the pubovaginal sling group had significantly more storage lower urinary tract symptoms (OR, 0.3; $P=.04$).

It is usual postoperatively to check a woman for residual urine after she voids; residuals of less than 100 to 150 mL, after the woman voids at least 200 mL, and double the residual volume, are considered acceptable. Larger residuals should indicate the use of continuing catheterization for 48 to 72 hours or intermittent self-catheterization.

A note on the use of preoperative urodynamic studies is warranted here. Urodynamics are often done before surgery for stress incontinence to confirm the diagnosis and evaluate for any voiding abnormality that might increase the postoperative risk of urinary retention. Recent studies have questioned the role of urodynamics, particularly in women with only stress incontinence symptoms, no urge incontinence, no voiding complaints, and no prior incontinence surgery. One study of a carefully selected group of women at low risk of voiding problems found that preoperative urodynamic studies did not predict postoperative voiding dysfunction or the risk of surgical revision in the pubovaginal sling group. Another study reported that the level of Valsalva leak point pressure (VLPP) and presence of detrusor overactivity did not predict the success of a Burch colposuspension or an autologous fascial sling in women with pure stress incontinence. Clearly, more research is needed to clarify the benefits and role of urodynamics in the evaluation of incontinence.

INTRINSIC SPHINCTER DEFICIENCY

Sand and associates offered some insight into why at least some retropubic urethropexy procedures fail. In a study of 86 patients evaluated preoperatively and postoperatively with urodynamic studies, they noted that in women younger than 50 years, there was a significant risk of failure if the preoperative urethral closure pressure was less than 20 cm H_2O. Although low urethral closure pressure was found to be an independent risk factor in women younger than 50 years, it was not found to be the case in women older than 50.

In 1981, McGuire noted the loss of intrinsic urethral tone in a number of women, particularly those with a history of pelvic trauma, radiation, underlying neurologic conditions, or scarring of the urethral sphincter. This has been termed *intrinsic sphincter deficiency* (ISD). Currently, the two types of stress incontinence, hypermobility and ISD, are thought to be interdependent and not separate entities. However, it is still useful to discuss severe stress incontinence in women with a fixed and poorly functioning urethra.

Horbach and Ostergard retrospectively evaluated 263 consecutive patients undergoing a complete urodynamic evaluation because of urinary leakage. Intrinsic sphincter dysfunction was defined as maximum urethral closure of 20 cm H_2O or less in the sitting position at maximum cystometric capacity; 132 women (50.2%) were found to have intrinsic sphincter dysfunction. Women in this group tended to be older and more likely to have undergone a hysterectomy and at least one anti-incontinence procedure compared with women with continence problems who had normal urethral pressure. By multivariate analysis, it was noted that age older than 50 years was the only independent variable that could predict the presence of intrinsic sphincter dysfunction in women with stress urinary incontinence.

At present, treatment for urinary stress incontinence caused by ISD consists of one of the following: periurethral bulking substance injections; urethral bladder neck sling procedures in select women retropubic midurethral synthetic sling; or use of an artificial sphincter device. A number of substances have been used for periurethral bulking injections. These include the individual's blood or fat, polytetrafluoroethylene (Teflon), bovine collagen, silicone microspheres, and pyrolytic zirconium oxide. Injection of blood or fat has provided only transient relief and the use of Teflon has resulted in several complications, primarily caused by wandering of the Teflon to distant sites. Glutaraldehyde cross-linked (GAX) collagen has been used as a urethral bulking agent. This is a bovine dermal collagen first used by Appell and colleagues, who reported a high success rate. It has a relatively high incidence of hypersensitivity reaction and therefore women should be skin-tested before its use. Without hypersensitivity, it appears to be a relatively safe and minimally invasive means of closing the urethra, and centers have been

using it for this purpose. It seems to have a positive effect for at least 2 years and it is possible to reinject patients. Long-term follow-up has been disappointing, with a 26% success rate at 5 years. Part of the failure may be because collagen is biodegradable and not necessarily durable. Permanent materials of silicone microimplants and pyrolytic zirconium oxide beads have been studied. Short-term success rates have ranged widely from 33% to 60% for cure or improvement. No material has proved better than another. Nonetheless, for older unfit women and women who have failed other incontinence surgeries, an injectable material for stress incontinence might be an attractive option.

Midurethral synthetic slings have been studied for ISD. The differing definitions of ISD with urethral hypermobility versus a fixed nonmobile urethra have made comparisons difficult. In published trials of a retropubic midurethral sling with hypermobility and a low maximum urethral closure pressure (MUCP), the low MUCP did not seem to affect the outcome. Reported cure rates range from 73% to 86%. One study with a 5-year follow-up found that 57% of the women were very satisfied and another 17% had improved continence. In contrast, using a TOT approach in this circumstance resulted in more failures. In the setting of a fixed urethra, only 33% of women reported being cured of incontinence.

A variety of traditional sling procedures, including the use of fascia lata, anterior rectus fascia tissue, cadaveric fascia lata, and inert materials such as polyethylene terephthalate (Mersilene) mesh, can be used. These procedures mobilize the bladder neck, often by a vaginal or vaginal and abdominal approach, and allow the interposition of a strip of material under the proximal urethra surrounding the bladder neck, which is attached to the anterior rectus sheath. This creates support and compression to the urethra and prevents urethral movement during increased abdominal pressure. This procedure is generally effective in creating continence.

The surgeon must exercise care in determining the tension to be applied on the bladder neck when the sling is fixed. Making it too tight may interfere with voiding and may actually damage the bladder neck and/or lead to de novo development of urge incontinence; making it too loose will abrogate its effectiveness. Generally, with a no. 16 or 18 Foley catheter in the urethra, it should be possible for the surgeon to judge the tension so that the sling fits comfortably against the urethra without compressing it. Concomitant cystoscopy may also be used.

Many other reports using other sling materials have shown success rates (cure or improvement) of 86% to 92%, with complications of UTIs, urinary retention, and de novo development of urgency.

An anterior rectus sheath fascial sling procedure is now generally reserved for patients with intrinsic sphincter deficiency or women whose previous anti-incontinence procedure failed and have a fixed urethra, because midurethral slings do not work well with a fixed urethra. Fascia lata slings have been used by many surgeons and can be performed mostly vaginally in a relatively short operative time. However, the woman then has a leg incision to harvest the fascia lata, which can be painful. Autologous fascia lata is more effective than irradiated and freeze-dried donor fascia lata, with the use of the latter type leading to a concern about graft degeneration and, thus, procedure failure.

The use of the artificial urinary sphincter may be a viable option for some women and will generally produce continence.

Artificial urinary sphincters are generally placed by abdominal and vaginal surgical approaches. Erosion and mechanical problems with these devices are potential side effects. The artificial sphincter consists of a cuff surrounding the urethra. The device is controlled by a pressure balloon placed in the space of Retzius. The woman controls the device by releasing pressure via a pump in the labia when she wishes to void and reestablishing pressure when she wishes to be continent. Diokno and coworkers reported a 91% success rate in 32 patients in whom they implanted the device. Others have reported similar results.

OVERACTIVE BLADDER

Overactive bladder (OAB) is defined as the symptom of urgency, with or without urge incontinence, usually with frequency and nocturia. Urgency is the complaint of a sudden compelling desire to pass urine, which is difficult to defer. Urge incontinence is the complaint of involuntary leakage of urine accompanied by or immediately preceded by urgency. This condition is generally chronic and may wax and wane, but is slowly progressive and associated with an urgency-frequency problem that is often accompanied by painless, involuntary urine loss. Generally, a large volume of urine is lost; leakage may occur in any position and often with a change in position. Rarely, an event usually associated with stress incontinence, such as coughing, will trigger this urge incontinence, but it is generally delayed until seconds after the stress has occurred. Large-volume urine loss is more characteristic of urge incontinence compared with stress incontinence. Stress incontinence frequently disappears when recumbent but urge incontinence continues, often with nocturia. **Table 21-6** summarizes the differences in symptoms. OAB occurs in approximately 17% of the population and the incidence increases with age. OAB patients have a lower quality of life than women with stress incontinence.

Detrusor overactivity is a urodynamic observation; it is the result of sudden, spontaneous detrusor contraction. It has previously been termed *detrusor dyssynergia, unstable bladder,* or *detrusor overactivity*. The term *idiopathic detrusor overactivity* is used as

Table 21-6 Typical Symptom Differences in Stress and Urge Incontinence

Symptom	Stress Incontinence	Urge Incontinence
Leakage with exertion, cough, sneeze, activity	Yes	No
Leakage with sensation or urgency	No	Yes
Frequency, nocturia	No	Yes
Large volume urine loss	No	Yes
Leakage with running water, key in the door	No	Yes
Leakage with position change from sitting to standing	Possible	Yes
Leakage while recumbent	No	Possible
History of childhood bedwetting	No	Yes

a urodynamic definition when there is no defined cause of the condition. If a neurologic disorder, such as stroke, Parkinson's disease, multiple sclerosis, spinal cord injury, or other CNS pathology is present, the term *neurogenic detrusor overactivity* is appropriate. In older women, both urge incontinence and urgency can coexist, with an elevated residual urine volume. Dribbling often results. This condition is termed *detrusor hyperactivity with impaired contractile function* (DHIC) and these two conditions may have different causative factors.

The loss of urine in OAB is probably triggered by sudden uninhibited stimulation of receptors in the bladder wall. The problem may be caused by the breakdown of normal neurologic and inhibitory reflexes. A postal survey of 6000 women in a Washington State health maintenance organization estimated the prevalence of urinary incontinence to be 42% and major depression 3.7%. However, the depression rate was significantly higher in women with incontinence and, in particular, women with moderate and severe incontinence (5.7% and 8.3%, respectively). It also differed by incontinence type (4.7% stress, 6.6% in urge or mixed). The study did not indicate that one condition caused the other; however, there is an increased risk of major depression in women with urinary incontinence, so it is worth screening for depression in this population. It is possible that altered neurotransmitter function, such as serotonin or norepinephrine, could alter bladder function, contributing to uninhibited detrusor contractions and urge incontinence.

Sands and colleagues reported a study of 86 women with urodynamic stress incontinence. Of these, 20 (23.3%) also had detrusor overactivity preoperatively and, of these 20, 11 (55%) had stable detrusor function after retropubic urethropexy, whereas 5 of 66 patients (7.6%) who had stable detrusor function preoperatively developed unstable detrusors postoperatively. Overall, women with both stress incontinence and OAB experienced a cure rate of only 30% with surgery. No relationship could be found among preoperative symptoms, age, history of previous procedures, and cystometric parameters between those who were cured and those who were not. In addition, none of these criteria could predict which woman who was detrusor-stable before surgery would develop overactivity after surgery. Risks of developing detrusor overactivity or having persistent detrusor overactivity after surgery must be recognized and incorporated into the preoperative counseling because it may require further medical therapy.

Diagnosis

A bladder diary such as that shown in **Figure 21-7** can be useful in diagnosing OAB because it can document frequency (more than eight daytime voids), nocturia (more than one nighttime void), and episodes of incontinence preceded by urgency. Additional information can be obtained about incontinence related to activity (stress incontinence), fluid intake, pad usage, and voided volumes (a measure of bladder capacity). The ideal diary duration has yet to be established, but 2 to 3 days is generally recommended. **Filling cystometry**, which evaluates the pressure-volume relationship of the bladder, allows the detection of spontaneous involuntary detrusor contractions in the bladder, which are noted as the bladder fills. These techniques are also useful for detecting urodynamic stress incontinence in patients who have an urgency component to their incontinence. It is important that both problems be treated in these patients, or it is unlikely that incontinence will be cured.

TREATMENT

Behavioral therapy is first-line treatment. In women who have stress and urge incontinence, a surgical procedure may have a place in the specific therapy. However, if the major part of the problem seems to be urge incontinence, this should be treated first, because an operative procedure may not be necessary. Similarly, patients who have undergone an operation for stress urinary incontinence and continue to be incontinent should be evaluated for detrusor overactivity. Bates and coworkers have demonstrated that a high percentage of such failures would be found to have detrusor overactivity on urodynamic studies.

Behavioral management includes fluid management and bladder training. Because most patients with detrusor overactivity have abnormal voiding habits, bladder retraining or bladder drills are useful. This involves a programmed progressive lengthening of the period between voiding, with or without the addition of **biofeedback** techniques. Women need to be taught urge suppression using distraction or relaxation techniques. The goal is to increase the voiding interval to 2 to 3 hours with normal fluid intake. In their study, Millard and Oldenburg demonstrated improvement in 74% of women with detrusor instability using these techniques. Cystometric studies performed on these patients revealed a reversion to stable bladder function. However, compliance with bladder retraining by patients is often a problem. Visco and associates studied 123 women who were offered bladder retraining and found that 55% never started treatment or were noncompliant. They noted that women who were given concurrent pharmacologic therapy had an 87% compliance rate, compared with 53% for those who started training, did not complete it, and were not given medication. Other behavioral treatments such as scheduled voiding, fluid management, and a bedside commode may be particularly helpful for older women with OAB.

In a 2006 Cochrane Database review, it was concluded that women with incontinence who performed pelvic floor muscle training were more likely to report cure or improvement, although only approximately one less incontinence episode daily. Although women with urge incontinence may experience less benefit than women with stress incontinence, there did appear to be improvement and few adverse effects. Women also need a strategy for urge suppression to prevent leakage and a few quick Kegel exercises followed by deep breathing and relaxation may help reduce urge. Given the noninvasive nature of muscle training, it makes sense as initial therapy for all urinary incontinence problems over a 3-month period.

Anticholinergic (antimuscarinic) drugs may be useful; **Table 21-7** shows currently available drugs. At times, these medications, in conjunction with bladder retraining, have greater efficacy than either alone. In one trial, combination therapy yielded better outcomes over time on the Urogenital Distress Inventory and Overactive Bladder Questionnaire ($P < .001$) at both time points studied for patient satisfaction and perceived improvement but not health-related quality of life.

Overall, in clinical studies, anticholinergic or antimuscarinic drugs reduce incontinence episodes by 60% to 75%, but only 20% to 40% of patients have no incontinent episodes. Although efficacy has been proven in many randomized trials, poor patient compliance is often found with these medications because of continued incontinence, expense without cure, and anticholinergic side effects. The most common side effect is dry mouth.

Table 21-7 Medications for Overactive Bladder

Drug	Dosage
Oxybutynin (Ditropan IR)*	5 mg b.i.d. t.i.d. q.i.d.
Oxybutynin (Ditropan XL)†	5 or 10 mg qd
Tolterodine (Detrol IR)*	1 or 2 mg b.i.d
Tolterodine (Detrol LA)‡	4 mg qd
Oxybutynin transdermal (Oxytrol)	3.9-mg patch (twice weekly)
Darifenacin (Enablex)	7.5 or 15 mg qd
Solifenacin (VESIcare)	5 or 10 mg qd
Trospium (Sanctura)	20 mg b.i.d or 60 mg qd (ER)†
Fesoterodine (Toviaz)	4 mg to 8 mg qd

*Intermediate-release (IR).
†Extended release (XL, ER).
‡Long acting (LA).

Flexible-dosing schedules of several drugs, changing to a different drug, or using a drug patch delivery system are options for finding a tolerable drug for this chronic condition. However, one report by Salvatore and colleagues found that two thirds of women discontinued therapy within 4 months, likely because they do not provide long-lasting symptom relief. A randomized trial of adding behavioral training to medication therapy reduced incontinence frequency but did not allow the woman to stop the drug and maintain improvement. Intravesical instillation of anticholinergic medication can provide an alternative delivery mechanism for women who fail or cannot tolerate oral therapy.

Pelvic floor electrical stimulation has been studied for improving a woman's ability to inhibit involuntary detrusor contractions and decreasing symptoms of urge incontinence. A small removable vaginal probe is placed in the vagina or anus; electrical stimulation activates a pelvic muscle contraction. This transvaginal neuromodulation appears to be of benefit compared with placebo. Peripheral nerve stimulation is being studied via the tibial nerve with neuromodulation to the sacral nerve plexus at the S2-S4 junction for treating OAB. A 2010 study by Fnazzi and associates recruited 35 female patients presenting with **detrusor overactivity incontinence** that did not respond to antimuscarinic therapy. They were randomly assigned to percutaneous tibial nerve stimulation or a control group. The percutaneous tibial nerve stimulation group (18 patients) was treated with 12 percutaneous tibial nerve stimulation sessions. The control group (17 patients) received a placebo treatment using a 34-gauge needle placed into the medial part of the gastrocnemius muscle. The sessions lasted for 30 minutes and were performed three times weekly. Patients showing a reduction in urge incontinence episodes more than 50% were considered responders; 71% of the intervention group and 0% in the placebo group responded ($P < .001$). A randomized controlled trial with 1-year follow-up showed significant and lasting improvement, although larger studies are needed.

Women with intractable detrusor overactivity who have failed conservative treatment and medications have surgical options. **Figure 21-19** shows a therapeutic pathway that leads to more invasive options for treatment. Botulinum toxin A theoretically blocks presynaptic acetylcholine from parasympathetic nerves, causing paralysis of the detrusor smooth muscle, although it may also affect bladder afferent and/or urothelial cell neurotransmitters. Botulinum toxin A is injected into the bladder wall via cystoscopy. It is FDA-approved, for neurogenic detrusor overactive which includes women with multiple sclerosis and spinal cord injuries, and many studies have been published showing 60% to 70% cure or improvement rates.

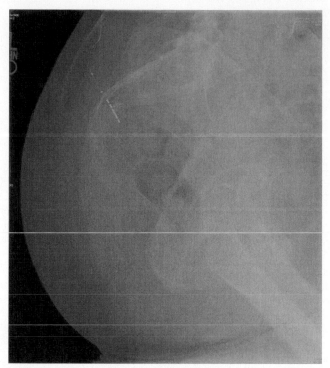

Figure 21-21 Lateral x-ray showing the lead wire in the final implantation site at S3. (Courtesy of Dr. Jane L. Miller, Department of Urology, School of Medicine, University of Washington, Seattle.)

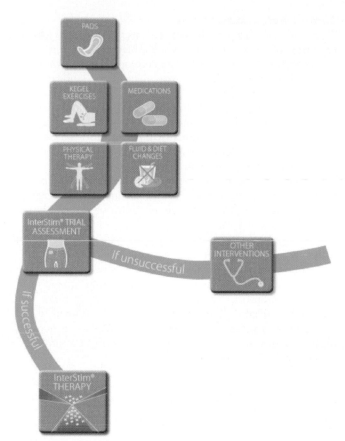

Figure 21-19 Treatment algorithim for urge incontinence. (Courtesy of Medtronics, Minneapolis.)

Temporary urinary retention is reported as high as 40%, which caused one randomized trial to be halted early. Long-term efficacy data show that reinjection is necessary, but just as effective. Benefit is maintained for 9 to 12 months. The optimal injection dose and location of injection need to be determined and long-term outcome studies are needed.

Sacral neuromodulation involves an implantable device, which chronically stimulates the sacral nerves and reduces symptoms. The FDA approved InterStim (Medtronic, Minneapolis) in 1997 for urgency, urge incontinence, and later for urinary retention (**Fig. 21-20**). A 2006 retrospective study of 41 patients used a stimulation test. If the results showed a 50% improvement in urge incontinence symptoms, the permanent stimulator was implanted. Of these patients, 90% had a greater than 50% reduction in symptoms when assessed at 12 months. However, 29% of patients had some complication. This complication rate has decreased with improvement in the wire lead that is placed (**Fig. 21-21**) and other improvements in standardizing the implantation procedure. Multiple long-term outcome studies have been published confirming that this is a feasible option for many women with refractory urge incontinence.

Table 21-8 summarizes the treatment options for the two most common types of urinary incontinence. **Figure 21-22** shows an evaluation and treatment algorithm for stress, urge, and mixed incontinence.

Figure 21-20 InterStimtest generator and permanent implantable generator, along with spinal cord model. (Courtesy of Medtronics, Minneapolis.)

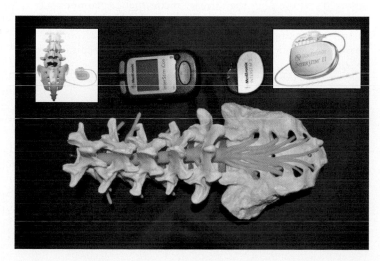

Table 21-8 Effective Treatment Options for Women with Urinary Incontinence by Type of Incontinence

Treatment Option	Stress Incontinence	Urge Incontinence
Nonpharmacologic	Pelvic floor muscle training	Pelvic floor muscle training
	Bladder training	Bladder training
	Prompted voiding	Prompted voiding
	Incontinence pessary	Pelvic floor electrical stimulation or tibial nerve
Pharmacologic		Anticholinergic drugs (antimuscarinic)
Surgical	Midurethral synthetic sling	Botulinum toxin A injection*
	Retropubic colposuspension	Neuromodulation, InterStim
	Suburethral fascial sling	

*Not FDA-approved.
Adapted from Holroyd-Leduc JM, Straus SE: Management of urinary incontinence in women. Clinical applications. JAMA 291:996, 2004.

MIXED URINARY INCONTINENCE

As the term implies, mixed urinary incontinence means that a woman complains of both stress and urge incontinence. Walter and Olesen studied 303 patients complaining of urinary incontinence and discovered that 43% had stress incontinence, 21% urge incontinence, and 36% both urge and stress incontinence. The pathophysiology and treatment of mixed incontinence have not been well studied despite the fact that it accounts for one third of incontinence complaints. Asking a woman about the stress or urge component can be unrevealing because it is only just urine leakage to the woman. Sometimes, the woman can articulate which problem is worse and treatment can begin for the more bothersome condition. Pelvic floor muscle exercises and behavioral training are appropriate first-line therapies (see earlier, stress and urge incontinence sections). The literature supports trying antimuscarinic drugs, which in one trial significantly reduced incontinence episodes. Of five published studies of surgical trials for mixed incontinence, varied cure rates have been reported. Although the stress incontinence component of the leakage may decrease, the woman is often disappointed to still be leaking because the urge component has not improved. The condition often responds poorly to medications or surgery.

OTHER FACTORS RELATED TO INCONTINENCE

Nocturnal enuresis is the complaint of loss of urine during sleep. The term *continuous urinary incontinence* has been defined by the International Continence Society as the continuous leakage of urine where the woman does not describe urgency or activity associated with the leakage. **Extraurethral incontinence** is defined as the observation of urine leakage through channels other than the urethra, including urinary fistulas and an ectopic ureter.

Chronic Retention of Urine

Overflow incontinence is the old term used to describe **chronic retention of urine**. It occurs when a bladder does not empty. The problem may be caused by a neurologic disorder that interferes with normal bladder reflexes, neuropathy, and myogenic failure or by obstruction of the urethra. Typically, the woman complains of voiding small amounts and still feeling that there is urine in the bladder, or she may only complain of incontinence and lose small amounts of urine without any control. Typically, the bladder is nonpainful and may be palpable after the woman has voided. The diagnosis is made when there is persistence of a significant amount of urine left in the bladder after voiding, as confirmed with ultrasound bladder scanning or catheterization. Typically, the retention of urine volume is more than 300 mL.

This condition is commonly seen in patients after incontinence surgery, with multiple sclerosis, diabetic neuropathy, and trauma or tumors of the central nervous system. A complete general medical and urologic workup is necessary to clarify the patient's condition. Therapy directed at the primary cause may be beneficial. Often, the woman must be trained in techniques of intermittent self-catheterization. Alpha blockers used for men with prostatic hypertrophy are not FDA-approved for women and rarely work.

Estrogen and the Lower Urinary Tract

Estrogen has long been known to play a role in lower urinary tract function because estrogen and progesterone receptors are found throughout the vagina, bladder, and urethra. Estrogens had been prescribed for years for the treatment of stress incontinence, until controlled trials (HERS, WHI, Nurses' Health Study) and the Hormones and Urogenital Therapy (HUT) Committee reported that estrogen was not an efficacious treatment for stress incontinence and actually increased the risk of incontinence. In postmenopausal women with vaginal atrophy, there may also be urethral mucosal epithelium atrophy because there are estrogen receptors in the urethra, which may lead to irritative symptoms. Estrogen does appear to be superior to placebo for recurrent cystitis and vaginal and urethral atrophy in the postmenopausal woman. Urethral atrophy and inflammation might contribute to irritate the bladder and lead to symptoms of urgency and frequency. A systematic review of the effects of vaginally administered estrogen has reported significant improvement in frequency, nocturia, urgency, incontinence episodes, and bladder capacity in postmenopausal women. In doses used for the treatment of genital atrophy (0.5 g of unconjugated estrogen cream three times weekly), serum levels were low and endometrial thickness unchanged. An intravaginal estrogen ring that releases very low levels of estrogen over a 3-month period is a convenient method of administration for many women. The estrogen benefit may be caused by the treatment of vaginal atrophy rather than a specific bladder and urethral effect. Possible confounding effects of progestogens and the multitudes of different estrogen preparations, oral and vaginal, hamper most studies. Progestogens have been associated with increased bladder irritability. Low-dose vaginal estrogens relieve urogenital atrophy symptoms and likely reduce recurrent UTI symptoms, but have no proven role in continence.

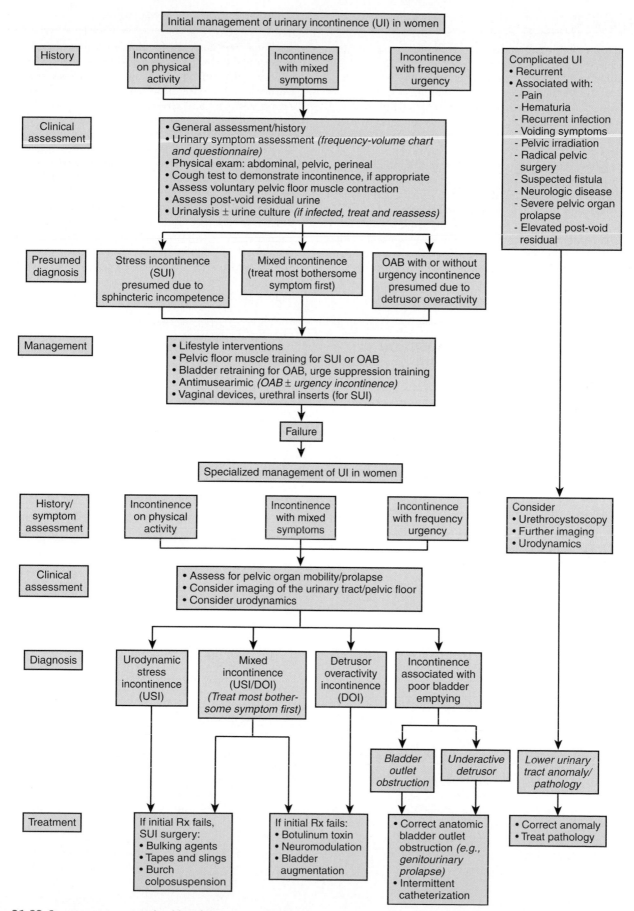

Figure 21-22 Summary treatment algorithm for stress, urge, and mixed incontinence.

- As many as 30% of all women may suffer from some degree of urinary incontinence during their lifetime.
- Continence is determined by the balance between forces that maintain urethral closure and those that affect detrusor function. Parasympathetic nervous system activity via the neurotransmitter acetylcholine stimulates receptors in the bladder wall to activate detrusor contraction. Sympathetic nervous system
- The highest pressure zone in the urethra is approximately midpoint in the functional urethra, which is roughly 0.5 cm proximal to the urogenital diaphragm.
- Approximately 50% of all women will develop urinary infections at some point in their lifetime and, by age 70 years, as many as 10% of women will have recurrent UTIs.
- Painful bladder syndrome–interstitial cystitis is a painful, chronic bladder condition that is not related to infection and is associated with symptoms of bladder and pelvic pain, urinary frequency, urgency, and/or nocturia, and often dyspareunia.

- The long-term cure rate for the Burch procedure is usually greater than 80% in properly selected women. The midurethral synthetic tape slings appear to have similar efficacy for the surgical treatment of stress incontinence, with a shorter surgery and recovery time.
- Retropubic and transobturator midurethral slings have similar success rates for stress incontinence, although with different risk profiles. The retropubic approach has a significantly higher risk of voiding dysfunction and the obturator approach has a higher risk for groin and leg pain.
- Approximately 20% of women with urinary incontinence suffer from detrusor overactivity. Behavioral changes and antimuscarinic medications are first-line treatment for this condition, although often have disappointing cure rates. Surgical procedures are available and effective.
- Being obese or overweight increase the risk of incontinence and weight loss can reduce stress incontinence significantly.

REFERENCES CAN BE FOUND ON EXPERTCONSULT.com

22

Anal Incontinence
Diagnosis and Management

Gretchen M. Lentz

Anorectal disorders are common in women and anal incontinence is particularly distressing. Women may be reluctant to discuss this with their physician because of embarrassment. In the woman, these supports are affected by the stresses of childbearing, so the obstetrician-gynecologist will often be the first to assess the problem. However, anal incontinence prevalence increases with age, so the physician must be ready to address these problems in the postmenopausal woman and be aware of the significant effects that these disorders can have on a woman's quality of life. **Anal incontinence** is a general term that refers to loss of gas or fecal material via the anus. **Fecal incontinence** is the inability to prevent loss of stool from the anus until desired. This chapter considers the causes, diagnosis, and treatment of anal incontinence.

ANAL INCONTINENCE

Fecal incontinence (FI) is one of the most devastating of all physical disabilities but, because of the social embarrassment and psychological effects, most patients fail to report their symptoms and many physicians do not ask. Therefore, the exact prevalence of this condition is unknown. Estimates range from 11% to 15% of community-dwelling women older than 64 years, although in reviewing many studies, it can range from 1% to 24%. Part of this variability relates to study definition differences for fecal incontinence. Occasional fecal soiling will not be as devastating as gross fecal incontinence, but both may be reported as part of the same study definition. Approximately 10% of women will report some change in bowel habits after one vaginal delivery. Prevalence increases with age. Little is known about racial differences in fecal incontinence, but a 2010 study found a prevalence of 6.1% in noninstitutionalized African Americans aged 52 to 68 years. Over 30% of women reporting urinary incontinence also report fecal incontinence, known as dual incontinence. Fecal incontinence is the second leading cause of nursing home placement. **Box 22-1** lists common risk factors for this condition. Late-onset fecal incontinence may have a different set of risk factors and, in one nested case-control study, bowel disturbances rather than obstetric events were more important.

Anal incontinence is the inability to defer the elimination of stool or gas until there is a socially acceptable time and place to do so. Fecal incontinence is the inability to defer the elimination of stool. Because maintaining continence is a complex physiologic process that requires a person's ability to perceive the type of fecal bolus, store or retain when necessary, and excrete when desirable, the loss of that ability is equally complex.

In the evaluation of anal incontinence, it is important for the physician to understand the woman's symptoms, type of loss (i.e., flatus or stool), frequency of incontinence, and effect on the quality of her life. Fecal incontinence affects each woman's life in a different manner. What may be acceptable for one woman may be intolerable to another. Evaluation and treatment should be directed by the severity of the woman's symptoms and the expected goals of therapy.

PHYSIOLOGY OF FECAL CONTINENCE

Fecal continence requires normal stool consistency and volume, normal colonic transit time, a compliant rectum, innervation of the pelvic floor and anal sphincter, and interplay among the puborectalis muscle, rectum, and anal sphincters. Loss of one or more of these functions can lead to fecal incontinence.

As a bolus of stool or gas passes from the sigmoid colon to the rectal canal, receptors in the wall of the puborectalis sense the distention of the rectum. As long as the pressure in the anal canal is maintained at a higher level than the rectal pressure, continence is maintained. Anal canal pressure depends on a functional internal anal sphincter (IAS) and external anal sphincter (EAS). The IAS is a thickened continuation of the circular muscle of the colon and provides 75% to 85% of the resting tone of the anal canal, but there is a lower rectal sphincter pressure when the anal canal is distended with stool. The IAS, under autonomic control, maintains the high-pressure zone or continence zone and, along with the EAS, keeps the anal canal closed. The shape of the combined IAS and EAS is almost cylindrical as it encircles the anal canal. Recent magnetic resonance imaging (MRI) scans from nulliparous women have shown that the EAS does not appear as a cylinder, but rather has lateral winged projections. The function of this component is not known. The sphincter complex averages 18.3 mm in thickness and 2.8 cm in length in the midline anteriorly; 54% of the anterior thickness is attributable to the IAS and the remainder to the EAS. The EAS provides the voluntary squeeze pressure that prevents incontinence with increasing rectal or abdominal pressure. The EAS is innervated by the hemorrhoidal branch of the pudendal nerve from the S2-S4 nerve roots. Contraction of the EAS, voluntarily or through a spinal reflex, increases the anal canal pressure by 25% but this tone cannot be maintained indefinitely because these are fatigable, fast twitch muscles.

The third muscular component of the sphincter complex is the puborectalis muscle (**Fig. 22-1**). The puborectalis, part of the levator ani muscle complex, originates from the pubic bone on either side of the midline, passes beside the vagina and rectum, and fuses posteriorly behind the anorectal junction to form the U-shaped sling that cradles the rectum while sending some fibers onto the walls of the anal canal. Unlike most other striated muscles, the puborectalis, like the IAS, maintains a constant muscle tone that is directly proportional to the volume of the rectal content and pressure, and relaxes at the time of defecation. Both the puborectalis and EAS contain a majority of type I, or slow twitch, muscle fibers, which are ideally suited to maintaining a constant contraction or tone. Each muscle group also contains a small proportion of type II, or fast twitch, fibers that allow for quick responses to rapid increases in intraabdominal pressure. The puborectalis is innervated by direct branches from S3 and S4 and, to a lesser degree, from the pudendal nerve.

The constant contraction of the puborectalis creates a 90-degree angle between the rectum and anal canal. This angle, known as the anorectal angle, has been the source of much discussion and evaluation in determining its role in the maintenance of continence. Parks has postulated that this angle creates a flap valve effect that presses the anterior rectal wall down onto the upper anal canal and thereby prevents the rectal contents from entering the anal canal when intraabdominal pressure is applied. The anterior rectal wall therefore acts as a plug. However, Bartolo has found that when the anal sphincter is maximally stressed and the rectum is visualized radiographically, there is no contact between the rectal wall and anal canal. In addition, surgical procedures that try to re-create this angle in an attempt to restore continence have not proved effective.

When a bolus of stool or gas is sensed in the rectum, the IAS has a reflex relaxation that allows for colonic contents to be sampled by the anal canal to distinguish solid, liquid, and gas forms of fecal material. After the sampling, the IAS contracts and the fecal material is pushed back into the rectum. This reflex, known as the rectoanal inhibitory reflex, or RAIR, is absent in patients with Hirschsprung's disease. This reflex can also be inhibited by chronic dilation of the anus with fecal impaction and lead to incontinence. If the impaction is cured, the reflex and anal tone can return to normal.

If the rectum has normal compliance and the person chooses to defer defecation, the IAS and EAS sphincters and puborectalis remain contracted until the appropriate time to eliminate. As seen in **Table 22-1**, loss of any of these important components can lead to incontinence of flatus, liquid, or solid stool.

CAUSES AND PATHOPHYSIOLOGY

There are many causes of fecal incontinence (**Table 22-2**). One way to categorize the reasons for fecal incontinence is to separate the initial cause into those that start outside the pelvis with a normal pelvic floor from those that start with an abnormal pelvic

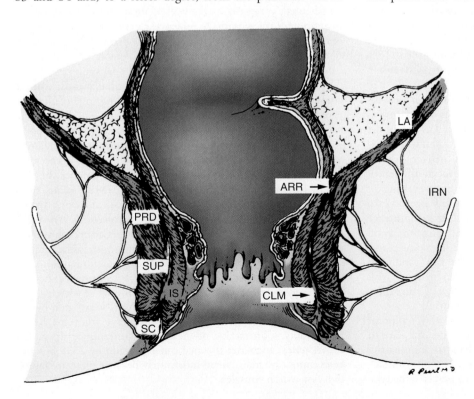

Figure 22-1 Coronal section of the anal canal and lower rectum. ARR, Level of anorectal ring; CLM, conjoined longitudinal muscle; IRN, inferior rectal nerve; LA, levator ani muscles; PRD, puborectalis/deep external sphincter complex; SC, subcutaneous external sphincter. (From Pearl RK: In Smith L [ed]: Practical Guide to Anorectal Testing. New York, Igaku-Shoin, 1995.)

Table 22-1 Anal Incontinence: Components of the Continence Mechanism

Component	Function	Symptoms of Deficit
External anal sphincter	Provides emergency control for liquid stool and flatus	Fecal urgency; urge-related incontinence of liquid stool and flatus
Puborectalis	Maintains continence of solid stool	Incontinence of solid stool
Internal anal sphincter	Keeps anal canal closed at rest; allows sampling of stool content and enhances continence of liquid stool and flatus	Fecal soiling Incontinence of liquid stool and flatus
Anal sensation	Allows discrimination of gas, liquid, and solid stool; provides warning of impending incontinence	Fecal soiling; fecal leakage that is promptly halted by voluntary contraction on conscious detection
Colonic motility	Controls stool volume, consistency, and delivery rate to the rectum	Incontinence of liquid or loose stools during prolonged or severe diarrheal states
Rectal reservoir	Maintains adequate reservoir under low pressure	Incontinence of solid stool associated with sudden rectal distention; fecal urgency and urge-related incontinence

From Toglia M: Anal incontinence: An underrecognized, undertreated problem. Female Patient 21:27, 1996.

Table 22-2 Common Causes of Fecal Incontinence

Obstetric injury
    Disruption of internal anal sphincter
    Disruption of external anal sphincter
    Pelvic floor denervation
Trauma
    Pelvic fracture
    Accidental injury
    Anal intercourse
    Anorectal surgery
    Rectovaginal fistula
Diarrheal states
    Irritable bowel syndrome
    Infectious diarrhea
    Inflammatory bowel disease
    Short gut syndrome
    Laxative abuse
    Radiation enteritis
Malabsorption
Rectal neoplasia
Rectal prolapse
Rectocele
Hemorrhoids
Overflow
    Impaction
    Encopresis
Neurologic disease
    Congenital anomalies (e.g., myelomeningocele)
    Multiple sclerosis
    Diabetic neuropathy
    Neoplasms or injury of brain, spinal cord, cauda equina
    Pudendal neuropathy (e.g., from childbirth, chronic straining, perineal descent)
Congenital anomalies of the anorectum or pelvis

floor. Causes that start outside the pelvis include all the pathologies that cause diarrhea or increased intestinal motility, overflow incontinence from fecal impaction, and rectal neoplasms. Known or diagnosable neurologic conditions such as multiple sclerosis, diabetic neuropathy, trauma, or neoplasms in the spinal cord or cauda equina initially begin as pathologies outside the pelvis, and the pelvic floor is presumed to be normal. As these neuropathies progress, there is damage to the pelvic floor musculature or rectal sensation, resulting in fecal incontinence.

Fecal incontinence secondary to an abnormal pelvic floor is caused by congenital anorectal malformations, surgery, obstetric injury, aging, or pelvic floor denervation without a known neurologic disease. Historically, incontinence secondary to denervation has been designated as idiopathic and represents 80% of patients with fecal incontinence. Pelvic floor denervation has been studied extensively in the last 15 years in women with urinary and fecal incontinence, as well as pelvic organ prolapse. Denervation may be secondary to vaginal delivery, chronic straining with constipation, rectal prolapse, or descending perineal syndrome. Histologic studies of the EAS and puborectalis show fibrosis, scarring, and fiber-type grouping consistent with nerve damage and reinnervation in women with idiopathic fecal incontinence. Electromyography (EMG) studies have demonstrated reinnervation of the pelvic floor with increased fiber density and prolongation of nerve conduction on **pudendal nerve terminal motor latency** (PNTML) studies.

In healthy women, the most common cause of fecal incontinence is damage to the anal sphincters at the time of vaginal delivery, with or without neuronal injury. This type of incontinence is often referred to as anal incontinence. Damage can occur by mechanical disruption or separation of the IAS, EAS, or both, or by damage to the muscle innervation by stretching or crushing the pudendal and pelvic nerves. Sultan and coworkers 1993 landmark study showed that 13% of primiparas and 23% of multiparas developed fecal incontinence or fecal urgency 6 weeks postpartum. By **endoanal ultrasound**, all but one of the women had evidence of anal sphincter disruption. The incidence of occult external anal sphincter disruption after vaginal delivery determined by endoanal ultrasound ranged from 11% to 35%. Most of the women showed pudendal nerve conduction prolongation, but recovered by 6 months postpartum. Because anal sphincter injury correlated with the development of symptoms, reducing anal sphincter injury and understanding risk factors are critical to prevention. The chance of anatomic sphincter injury is increased with midline episiotomy, instrumented delivery, vaginal delivery of larger infants, and persistent occiput posterior presenting head position. Other risk factors include increasing maternal age, prolonged second stage (longer than 2 hours), epidural anesthesia, and clinically diagnosed sphincter laceration at the time of delivery. The first vaginal delivery appears to have the greatest effect on pelvic floor function and risk of EAS disruption, but subsequent deliveries can increase the risk of permanent damage, especially in women with transient symptoms of fecal incontinence after their first delivery. Not all risk factors are known, and not all women are susceptible to pelvic floor and sphincter damage with vaginal delivery.

Diabetes mellitus deserves mention because of its rising prevalence. Diabetics can develop autonomic neuropathy and can have decreased IAS resting pressure. Either of these might contribute to fecal incontinence.

DIAGNOSIS AND ASSESSMENT

For fecal incontinence, even more than urinary incontinence, if the physician does not ask, the woman will not volunteer the information. Ideally, a question such as, "How often do you leak gas, liquid, or solid stool?" should be placed on the standard office intake questionnaire. Several reports have shown that twice as many patients complain of fecal or flatal incontinence when given a written questionnaire rather than answering verbal questioning.

Because approximately 1 in 10 women will develop some fecal incontinence or fecal urgency after one vaginal delivery, it is especially important to incorporate open-ended questions concerning flatal or fecal incontinence as part of the 6-week postpartum visit. In addition, as women age, the chance of developing fecal incontinence increases, so it is also important to target older women for questioning.

Evaluation

Assessment of the woman with fecal incontinence must include a thorough history because the origin of the problem may be the single most important criterion of therapy. **Table 22-3** lists some questions to be asked when taking a history regarding fecal incontinence.

The history should include onset, duration, severity of the condition, effect on the woman's daily activities, pad use, frequency of bowel movements, and consistency of bowel movements, use of laxatives, fiber intake, and dietary habits. Specific questions

Table 22-3 History in a Patient with Suspected Fecal Incontinence

Onset and precipitating event(s)
Duration, severity, and timing
Stool consistency and urgency
Coexisting problems, surgery, urinary incontinence, back injury
Obstetric history—forceps, tears, presentation, repair
Drugs, caffeine, diet
Clinical subtypes—passive or urge incontinence or fecal seepage
Clinical grading of severity
History of fecal impaction

concerning diarrhea, amount of flatus, average number of stools per day, passage of mucus, and bloating should be asked. Physicians and patients define normal bowel function differently. Diarrhea may mean frequent bowel movements to one person but loose and watery bowel movements to another. It is best to have the woman quantitate the number of bowel movements and incontinent episodes and describe the stool consistency. A diary of bowel habits and incontinent episodes can be useful, and several standardized classification systems are available. **Table 22-4** gives a frequently used scoring system developed by Jorge and Wexner. The woman circles the appropriate number on each line of the scale. The numbers are then added. A perfect score, or 0, indicates no incontinence and a score of 20 indicates complete incontinence. The value of this continence grading scale is that it can be used before and after treatment to determine the efficacy of the intervention. A standardized questionnaire should be used whenever possible to direct diagnosis and treatment and assess treatment success.

The history should also identify specific complaints such as feelings of incomplete emptying, straining with bowel movements, fecal urgency, pain with defecation, and insensible loss of stool. It is important to determine whether the woman senses the need to have a bowel movement or if she is unaware that she needs to defecate, but finds stool in her undergarments. A sensory impairment or hygiene problem is implied when stool leakage occurs without warning. If the woman is aware of impending incontinence, but cannot prevent the passage of stool, a motor impairment is suggested. Patients may have pseudoincontinence secondary to soiling from prolapsing hemorrhoids or rectovaginal or anovaginal fistulas.

The review of systems should include abdominal pain or cramping, lower back or pelvic pain, any changes in pelvic or lower extremity sensation, and changes in sexual response. Changes in the neurologic function of the pelvis or lower extremities or a history of an acute onset of fecal incontinence should direct the physician to rule out a neurologic disease, such as multiple sclerosis or a neoplasm of the brain or lumbosacral spinal cord.

The past medical history should include detailed history of vaginal deliveries, including birth weights, length of second stage, episiotomies or lacerations, and use of forceps. Any breakdown or complications of episiotomy healing should be noted. The past history of abdominal and pelvic surgeries or trauma to the back or pelvis should be reviewed. Details and operative reports of any anal dilatations, anal sphincterotomy, hemorrhoidectomy, rectovaginal fistula repairs, or posterior colporrhaphy should be obtained. Patients should also be questioned about previous evaluations and results of flexible sigmoidoscopy, colonoscopy,

Table 22-4 Continence Grading Scale*

Type of Incontinence	Frequency				
	Never	**Rarely**	**Sometimes**	**Usually**	**Always**
Solid	0	1	2	3	4
Liquid	0	1	2	3	4
Gas	0	1	2	3	4
Wears pad	0	1	2	3	4
Lifestyle alteration	0	1	2	3	4

*The continence score is determined by adding points from this table, which takes into account the type and frequency of incontinence and the extent to which it alters the patient's life.
0 = perfect, 20 = complete incontinence; never = 0 (never); rarely = <1/month; sometimes = <1/week, ≥1/month; usually = <1/day, ≥1/week; always = ≥1/day.
From Jorge JM, Wexner SD: Etiology and management of fecal incontinence. Dis Colon Rectum 36:77, 1993.

Stool Diary								
PLEASE RECORD YOUR STOOL HABITS FOR ONE WEEK:							Name: Hosp #:	
Date	Time of bowel movement	Incontinence	Stool seepage or straining	Stool consistency (Type 1–7) See below	Urgency – unable to postpone BM for more than 15 minutes	Use of pads	Medications	Comments
		Yes / No	Yes / No		Yes / No	Yes / No		

Use the following descriptors for describing stool consistency:

Type 1: **Separate hard lumps.** Type 2: **Sausage shaped but lumpy.** Type 3: **Like a sausage but with cracks on its surface.**
Type 4: **Like a sausage or snake, smooth and soft.** Type 5: **Soft blobs with clear-cut edges (passed easily).**
Type 6: **Fluffy pieces with ragged edges, a mushy stool.** Type 7: **Watery.**

Figure 22-2 Stool diary. This is a sample stool diary for assessing patients with fecal incontinence. (From Rao SS: American College of Gastroenterology Practice Parameters Committee. Diagnosis and management of fecal incontinence. American College of Gastroenterology Practice Parameters Committee. Am J Gastroenterol 99:1585, 2004.)

and barium enemas. Any family history of colon cancer, inflammatory bowel disease, or familial polyposis should be elicited.

Many medications also affect bowel function. The woman should not only be asked about laxatives and bowel stimulants, but a complete list of all prescription and over-the-counter medications, as well as any dietary or herbal supplements, should be reviewed. Many drugs, including anticholinergics, antidepressants, iron, narcotics, nonsteroidal anti-inflammatory drugs (NSAIDs), and pseudoephedrine, can cause chronic constipation that may contribute to overflow incontinence or pelvic floor neuropathy secondary to straining.

Women can be instructed on how to keep a daily stool diary (**Fig. 22-2**). This is a good baseline evaluation tool and can later be used to assess conservative treatment with dietary changes and fiber intake.

Physical Examination

Undergarments or pads should be inspected for stool, mucus, blood, or pus. If material is found, the woman should be asked if this is her normal leakage. Physical examination begins with inspection of the perineum and anal region. Pruritus ani, or discoloration and irritation of the perianal skin, is commonly seen with fecal incontinence of liquid stool and chronic diarrhea. Perianal skin creases or folds should completely encircle the anus. Note the presence of protruding tissue around or from the anus and determine whether there are external hemorrhoids or mucosal or full-thickness rectal mucosal prolapse (**Fig. 22-3**). The **dovetail sign**, or loss of anterior perineal folds, indicates a

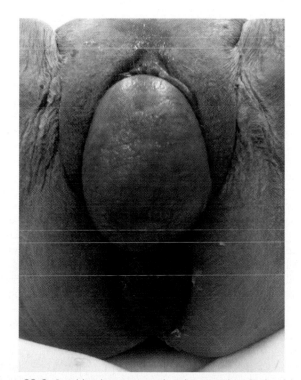

Figure 22-3 Combined severe rectal prolapse and vaginal pelvic organ prolapse. Note the protrusion of the rectal mucosa from the anus.

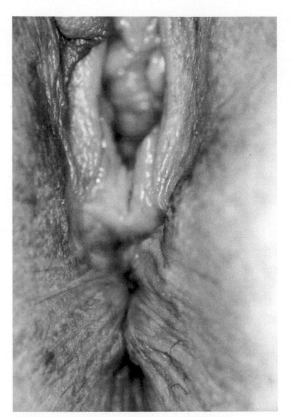

Figure 22-4 Perineum with chronic laceration of external anal sphincter (EAS). Inspection of the perineum shows the classic dovetail sign with loss of the anal skin creases anteriorly because of a chronic third-degree laceration of the EAS. Normally, with an intact sphincter, the skin creases are arranged radially around the anus. (From Stenchever MA, Benson JT [eds]: Atlas of Clinical Gynecology. New York, McGraw-Hill, 2000.)

defect in the EAS or chronic third-degree laceration (**Fig. 22-4**). Previous episiotomy, laceration, or surgical scars should be noted. The size of the genital hiatus and presence of genital prolapse should be assessed as an indicator of pelvic floor neuromuscular function. The innervation of the EAS can be grossly tested by eliciting the clitoral-anal or bulbocavernosus reflex. Using a cotton swab, a gentle quick touch beside the clitoris or over the bulbocavernosus muscle should elicit a contraction of the EAS. If intact, the reflex implies that the pudendal nerve afferents and rectal or external hemorrhoidal branch of the pudendal efferent nerves are functional. Unlike men, who should always exhibit this reflex, approximately 10% of women lack this reflex naturally. However, if absent, and in the presence of fecal incontinence, further neurologic testing is indicated. Sensation in the S2-S4 dermatomes should be screened by dull and pinprick discrimination when touching the perineum. The same wooden cotton swab used to elicit bulbocavernosus reflexes can be broken and then used for pinprick (broken end) and dull (cotton end) sensation testing. Loss of sensation should direct the clinician to further neurologic or radiologic assessment of the nervous system.

Next, the woman should be asked to squeeze as if trying not to pass gas. Inspection of the perianal folds should be evaluated for a concentric contraction and some upward movement of the perineal body as she contracts the EAS and levator ani. Substitution with contraction of the buttocks, upper thighs, or abdomen should be noted. The woman should then be asked to bear down as if trying to have a bowel movement. She should be reassured that it is expected that she might pass flatus during this part of the examination. The degree of perineal descent and any prolapse of the vagina, pelvic viscera, or rectum should be noted. If there appears to be any pelvic organ prolapse, the examination should be performed with the woman in the standing position or after straining on a commode to maximize the prolapse.

Rectal examination is used to assess resting and squeeze tones of the anal canal. The resting tone of the anal canal is an indicator of IAS function. When asked to squeeze, a circumferential contraction and tightening should be felt. An upward movement of the rectum and posterior compartment of the pelvis should be seen as the levator ani muscles contract. Because these muscles also play an important role in anal continence, palpation of the levators for strength and symmetry should be performed by palpating the muscles on each side of the vagina at the introitus.

In addition to assessing rectal tone, the anal canal and rectum should be palpated for masses and a dilated rectum or the presence of stool in the rectal vault. A chronically distended rectum, with stool, a tumor, or an intussuscepting bowel, will disrupt the normal **rectoanal inhibitory reflex** that allows the highly sensitive anal canal to sample the stool contents by relaxing the IAS while time-contracting the EAS to prevent incontinence. If this reflex is suppressed, the anal canal remains dilated, the EAS fatigues, and incontinence will occur.

While doing the rectal examination, the woman is also asked to strain to diagnose the presence of a **rectocele**, enterocele, rectal prolapse, or bowel intussusception. With the examiner's finger in the rectum, the integrity of the rectovaginal septum, posterior vaginal wall, and perineal body can be assessed by palpating through the vagina via bimanual examination.

Testing

Clinical diagnosis based on physical examination and history alone will be accurate in most patients. However, further evaluation, including radiologic and physiologic tests, have been shown in a prospective study at a tertiary colorectal referral clinic to alter the final diagnosis of the cause of fecal incontinence in 19% of cases. Which tests to consider should be based on history and physical examination, prior treatment, and proposed therapy. The algorithm outlined in **Figure 22-5** recommends further evaluation based on history and the rectal tone. Normal rectal tone directs the clinician away from anal incontinence and toward a metabolic or colonic origin. Metabolic tests, including determination of thyroid-stimulating hormone and glucose levels, should be carried out. If chronic diarrhea is present with normal rectal sphincter tone, stool cultures, colonoscopy, and diarrhea evaluation are indicated. Differential diagnosis for a diarrhea workup will include lactose intolerance, celiac sprue, inflammatory bowel disease, irritable bowel syndrome, and bacterial overgrowth from diabetic gastroparesis. In cases of fecal incontinence with normal rectal sphincter tone without diarrhea, **anal manometry** to evaluate rectal sensation is useful and can help in the consideration of peripheral neuropathy causes.

Poor resting tone on rectal examination directs the clinician to a neuromuscular cause. A normal resting tone, but with poor squeeze, suggests an anterior sphincter defect and chronic third-degree laceration of the EAS. If poor rectal squeeze is detected, endoanal ultrasonography is the best first-line test.

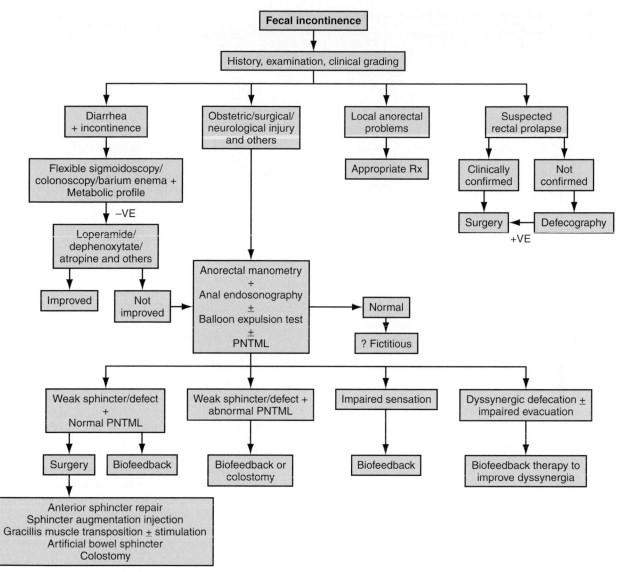

Figure 22-5 Algorithmic approach to the evaluation and management of fecal incontinence. A detailed history differentiates incontinence of gas, liquid, or solid stool, along with frequency, onset, and effect on the patient's quality of life. The history should assess the possibility of Crohn's disease, ulcerative colitis, irritable bowel syndrome, radiation to the pelvis, neurologic diseases such as multiple sclerosis, and prior anorectal surgeries. A detailed obstetric history should include type of delivery, weight of largest infant, length of second stage, episiotomy or lacerations, and use of forceps or vacuum extraction. Rectal examination should assess resting and squeeze tone, presence of a rectocele or rectal mass, and fecal impaction. Inspection of the rectum and vagina should evaluate for a rectovaginal fistula, prolapsing hemorrhoids, or rectal prolapse. Further evaluation, including radiologic and physiologic tests, have been shown in a prospective study at a tertiary colorectal referral clinic to alter the final diagnosis of the cause of fecal incontinence in 19% of cases. (From Rao SS: American College of Gastroenterology Practice Parameters Committee. Diagnosis and management of fecal incontinence. American College of Gastroenterology Practice Parameters Committee. Am J Gastroenterol 99:1585, 2004.)

Evaluation or further testing is not only performed for diagnostic purposes, but also to determine which nonsurgical and surgical therapies are most likely to benefit the woman. In addition, certain tests, such as anal manometry or an anal sphincter ultrasound, can be used for baseline assessment to which post-treatment assessment or function can be compared. Whenever the woman's history does not match her physical examination findings, further testing should be considered. In addition, if the woman has had prior surgery or has other pelvic floor dysfunction, testing before treatment, especially surgical, may help direct care. It is important to remember that the woman may have more than one cause or pathology contributing to her fecal incontinence, such as pudendal neuropathy and an anal sphincter defect or irritable bowel in combination with a weakened pelvic floor (**Table 22-5**).

Diagnostic Procedures
Colonoscopy
A colonoscopy is indicated for any woman with chronic diarrhea to evaluate for inflammatory bowel disease and infectious diarrhea. Endoscopic evaluation detects mucosal disease or neoplasia effectively. This is also acceptable bowel screening for any woman older than 50 years, particularly if an acute change in bowel habits is reported.

Table 22-5 Tests of Anorectal Function for Patients with Fecal Incontinence

Test	Measures	Indication
Anal manometry	Resting anal pressures	Low resting and squeeze pressure on rectal examination
	Maximum squeeze pressure	Prior radiation treatment
	Rectoanal inhibitory reflex	Fecal urgency
	Rectal sensation	Fecal impaction
Single-fiber EMG	Fiber density	Denervation
	Muscle activity	Reinnervation injury
		Map EAS defect
Pudendal nerve motor latency	Speed of signal along pudendal nerve	Pudendal nerve damage from childbirth or straining
Endoscopic ultrasound	IAS and EAS defect	Obstetric or traumatic sphincter injuries
Defecating proctography	Movement of pelvic floor	Perineal descent
	Pelvic floor defects	Posterior compartment deficits

EAS, External anal sphincter; EMG, electromyography; IAS, internal anal sphincter.

Endoanal Ultrasound

Endoanal ultrasound has significantly enhanced the ability to delineate defects of the IAS and EAS. This is one of the simplest and least expensive tests for imaging sphincter defects. The integrity, thickness, and length of the IAS and EAS can be determined. The IAS is visible as a hypoechoic circle and the EAS is seen as a hyperechoic circle (**Fig. 22-6**). Endoanal ultrasound is most useful in evaluation of patients for chronic third-degree lacerations or occult sphincter tears. Breaks in the EAS can be readily noted. Knowing the boundaries of the sphincter defect and whether both the EAS and IAS are disrupted can direct the surgeon at the time of anal sphincteroplasty. Similar information can be obtained from EMG of the EAS when used to map the sphincter defect. In general, transanal ultrasound is less painful and better tolerated by the woman.

Anal Manometry

Anal manometry was a commonly used test that objectively assesses the resistance to spontaneous defecation provided by the anorectal sphincter mechanism and the sensory capabilities of the rectum to provide a feeling of imminent defecation. Anal manometry is helpful for patients who have had prior surgery to the anorectal canal or radiation therapy that could have altered the rectal storage function. In patients who, by history, report a normal sensation to defecate, anal manometry has been largely replaced by endoanal ultrasound.

Anal manometry uses a rectal balloon to assess rectal sensation, rectal compliance, the RAIR, and maximal tolerable rectal volume (**Fig. 22-7**). The RAIR is a reflex response to increased pressure in the rectum from gas or stool. Normally, the IAS relaxes to allow a sampling of the rectal contents by the anal canal to determine whether the contents are gas or stool and whether it is an appropriate time to defecate or pass flatus. At the same time, the EAS squeezes to prevent incontinence.

In addition to rectal function, resting and squeeze pressures in the anal canal are obtained by pulling a perfusion catheter with radial ports (four or eight) through the anal canal. The IAS contributes 80% of the resting pressure. Voluntary contraction of the EAS should double the resting pressure (**Fig. 22-8**). Both resting and anal squeeze pressures are reduced in woman with anorectal incontinence. Although objective documentation is useful for diagnosis or preoperative baseline, normal resting and squeeze pressures can be accurately assessed on rectal examination by most experienced clinicians. Rectal sensation evaluation is the most useful information obtained from anal manometry testing.

Electromyography

EMG is used for mapping the EAS defect and for determining the presence and degree of neuropathy, denervation, and reinnervation. EMG evaluates the bioelectrical action potentials generated by the depolarization of skeletal striated muscle. This evaluation consists of systematic examination of spontaneous activity, recruitment patterns, and the waveform of the motor unit action potentials (MUAPs).

Performance and interpretation of EMG of the EAS requires special training and experience. A needle electrode is inserted into the skeletal muscle of the EAS. First, spontaneous activity is heard and seen. Next, the woman voluntarily squeezes her pelvic floor and recruitment activity is recorded. Straining should decrease activity and coughing should increase recruitment. The final step in analysis is evaluation of the MUAP waveform. Following nerve damage, as seen with a vaginal delivery, reinnervation of the muscle fibers leads to a single motor unit innervating multiple muscle fibers. On single-fiber EMG, the MUAPs have larger amplitudes, longer duration, and more phases or crossings of the baseline. Because discomfort and pain can occur with needle electrodes, endoanal ultrasound has replaced EMG for assessing the anatomy of the anal sphincter.

Pudendal Nerve Terminal Motor Latency

Nerve conduction studies measure the time from stimulation of a nerve to a response in the muscle it innervates. The PNTML is determined by using a glove-mounted electrode known as a St. Mark's pudendal electrode, connected to a pulsed stimulus generator; with the examiner's index finger in the vagina or anus, the pudendal nerve is stimulated at the ischial spine.

The latent period between the pudendal nerve stimulation and the electromechanical response of the muscle is measured. Normal PNTML is 2.0 ± 0.2 milliseconds. A normal PNTML is the measurement of the fastest response of the pudendal nerve and does not necessarily mean that the entire nerve is normal (**Fig. 22-9**). Prolonged PNTMLs have been found in patients with idiopathic fecal incontinence and in patients with rectal prolapse and may be predictive of continence following surgical repair. Gilliland's 1998 study suggested that PNTML was the most sensitive predictor of functional outcome of overlapping EAS repairs. However, these tests are rarely performed now because newer research shows poor correlation of prolonged pudendal terminal latencies with clinical symptoms and PNTML does not seem to directly reflect nerve function in the way that quantitative EMG can.

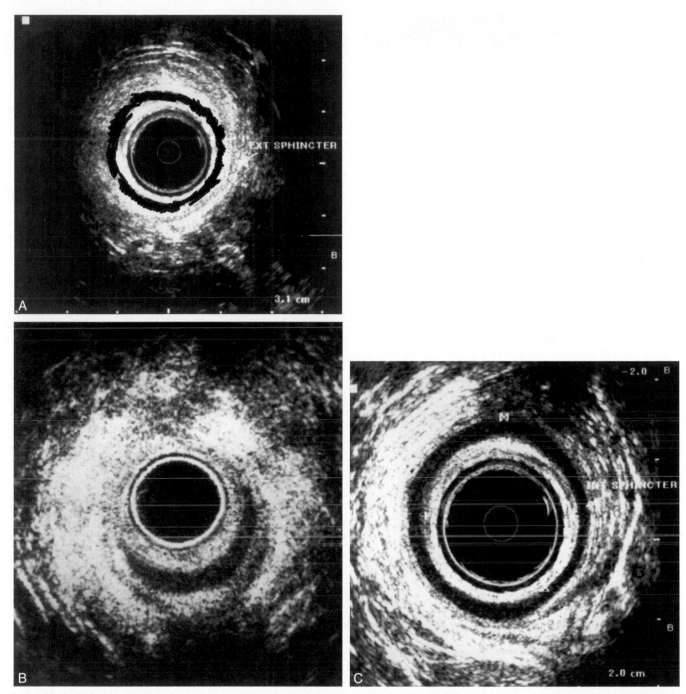

Figure 22-6 Anal ultrasound. **A,** Anal ultrasound has significantly enhanced the ability to delineate defects of the internal and external anal sphincters. The internal anal sphincter (IAS) is visible as a hypoechoic circle and the external anal sphincter (EAS) is seen as a hyperechoic circle. Scarred areas have a homogeneous gray appearance. Both the IAS and EAS are intact. **B,** With the patient supine, a defect in the IAS from 3 to 9 o'clock and a defect at 12 o'clock in the EAS is shown. **C,** Again, with the vagina at the 12 o'clock position, there is an intact IAS and defect in the EAS. (From Stenchever MA, Benson JT [eds]: Atlas of Clinical Gynecology. New York, McGraw-Hill, 2000.)

Defecography

Dynamic cystoproctography, or defecography, is an imaging technique that has been widely used in the evaluation of anorectal function and anatomy, dating back to the mid-1960s. Defecography may be used as an adjunct to physical examination in patients with chronic constipation and pelvic floor defects or hernias that may be contributing to their fecal incontinence. Rectal intussusceptions, rectal prolapse, and sigmoidocele can be seen on defecography, along with rectoceles that do not empty at the time of defecation. Stool retained in the rectocele can cause chronic distention of the rectum and loss of rectal sensation. The loss of rectal sensation leads to chronic constipation or impaction, causing further neuromuscular damage to the pelvic floor and ultimately fecal incontinence. Perineal descent and the anorectal angle can be objectively measured using defecography.

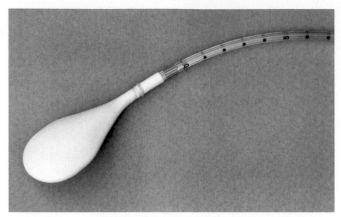

Figure 22-7 Anal manometer, a four-channel perfusion catheter with balloon tip. There are many different types and methods for performing anal manometry. A balloon or probe is inserted into the rectum, and a pressure transducer relays information to a recorder or computer. Important manometric parameters include sphincter length, resting and squeeze pressures, rectal sensation, and presence of the anorectal inhibitory reflex (RAIR). The balloon is placed in the rectum and inflated by 10-cm^3 increments to determine rectal sensation and compliance. The presence of the RAIR is determined with balloon inflation and observing the IAS relax and the EAS contract to allow for the sampling of rectal contents. The four radical ports are perfused with sterile water, and resting and squeeze pressures around the anal canal are measured at 1-cm intervals along the anal canal. The catheter can be pulled at a constant rate to determine the length of the sphincter and high-pressure or continence zone.

Magnetic Resonance Imaging of the Anal Sphincters

MRI of the anal sphincters can evaluate muscular and connective tissue supports of the pelvis. Recent advances in MRI technologies using the endoanal coil, rapid sequencing, and cinematic display have replaced defecography for the evaluation of the pelvic floor and defecation disorders in a few centers. Muscular defects, along with pelvic organ prolapse and perineal descent, can be assessed. Specialized dynamic MRI may replace defecography and endoanal ultrasound in the future, but limited availability of these MRI scanners and their expense limit its use.

Transit Study

A colonic transit study is used to evaluate colonic motility and is most often used for the evaluation of chronic constipation. For patients for whom fecal impaction or overflow incontinence is high on the differential, a transit study may be indicated. There are numerous variations of the study. The woman ingests a Sitzmark capsule containing 20 or 25 radiopaque rings. She does not take any laxatives or bowel stimulants. Five days after taking the capsule, an abdominal flat radiographic plate is obtained. Normally, 80% of the capsules should have been passed. Diffuse or global colon dysfunction is indicated if the rings are dispersed throughout the colon or segmental abnormalities can be seen if the rings are clustered in one area or trapped in a rectocele.

TREATMENT

Treatment of fecal incontinence includes lifestyle changes, dietary management, biofeedback, electrical stimulation, medications, sacral nerve stimulation, and surgery (**Box 22-2**). Obstructive devices, including transanal plugs, have been marketed but are not widely used. Obviously, fecal incontinence should be treated based on the diagnosis as in medications or surgery for inflammatory bowel disease or surgery for a neoplasm of the cauda equina. For all women with fecal incontinence, maintaining normal stool consistency and frequency is essential first-line treatment. For women with associated liquid or watery stools, dietary modifications and medications are first-line therapy.

Education, Diet, and Lifestyle Interventions

Education regarding good bowel function makes sense, but little research exists to support this strategy. Having a predictable, regular bowel evacuation program and optimizing stool consistency to avoid the loose stool or frank diarrhea that taxes the system seems to improve fecal incontinence. Having a larger and more well-formed stool, rather than liquid stool, allows for rectal distention and sensation that may provide earlier warning and better emptying.

Increasing dietary fiber with diet changes or bulking agents or fiber supplements such as methyl cellulose or psyllium helps increase stool size. Eating high-fiber cereals and drinking hot coffee or tea at breakfast are encouraged to stimulate the gastrocolic reflex and elimination before leaving home. There is reasonable evidence that adding soluble dietary fiber compared with placebo in women with loose stools reduces the rate of FI. However women must be warned that fiber supplements can worsen diarrhea in some people. Increases in fiber also had benefit for women with mild FI, without loose stools. By keeping a food diary, women may identify offending foods (e.g., lactose, fructose) that aggravate their FI and learn to avoid those foods. Nicotine can

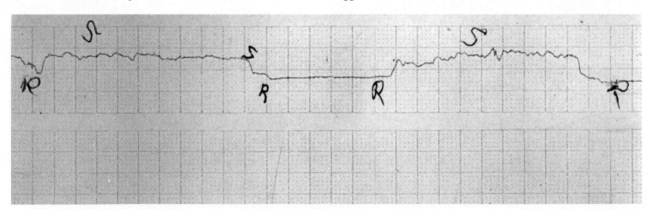

Figure 22-8 A single-channel recording of the resting pressure of the anal canal (R) and the squeeze pressure (S). The IAS contributes 80% of the resting pressure. Voluntary contraction or squeezing of the EAS should double the resting pressure.

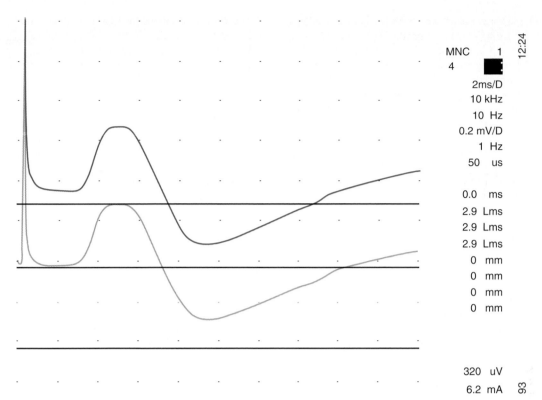

Figure 22-9 Pudendal nerve terminal motor latencies (PNTML). Normal bilateral PNTML have been shown to be 2.0 ± 0.2 milliseconds. The latency response is measured from the onset of the stimulus to the onset of the response in the EAS. A normal PNTML is the measurement of the fastest response of the pudendal nerve and does not necessarily mean that the entire nerve is normal, and neither does an abnormal latency indicate abnormal muscle function. A damaged nerve can heal and reinnervate the muscle and, although the PNTML may be slightly prolonged, the muscle functions normally. (From Stenchever MA, Benson JT [eds]: Atlas of Clinical Gynecology. New York, McGraw-Hill, 2000.)

Box 22-2	Treatment of Fecal Incontinence	
Management	**Option**
Education and lifestyle interventions	Regular bowel evacuation, optimization of stool consistency, unclear role for caffeine restriction, weight reduction, smoking cessation, gastrointestinal medication review and change, treatment of reversible causes of diarrhea
Diet	Dietary manipulation with soluble fiber for avoiding loose stools and for mild FI
Anal sphincter exercises and/or biofeedback training	Weak evidence suggesting efficacy for exercises, but safe, noninvasive treatment; biofeedback has insufficient evidence to recommend because of inadequate trials, but is noninvasive.
Electrical stimulation	Insufficient evidence to recommend but small trials show some benefit
Medications	Loperamide, diphenoxylate plus atropine (concern of central nervous system side effects) for diarrhea; enemas, laxatives, suppositories for complete bowel emptying
Sacral nerve stimulation	FDA-approved in 2011 and multiple studies show benefit up to 5 years.
Surgery	Anal sphincteroplasty indicated for postobstetric laceration or highly symptomatic women who have failed conservative measures with defined sphincter defect.

FDA, U.S. Food and Drug Administration.

hasten rectosigmoid transit time and stimulate distal colonic motility, so it might exacerbate fecal urgency. In a nursing home study, a daily exercise program with education around toileting opportunities improved FI. Brisk exercise, particularly after meals, may precipitate FI because of increased colonic activity.

Biofeedback

For fecal incontinence, like urinary incontinence, biofeedback requires a motivated woman, feedback device, and planned exercise program. Although the woman may not perceive normal sensation or be able to contract her pelvic floor voluntarily,

she must be neurologically intact to benefit from biofeedback. No correlation has been seen with premanometry testing as long as some neuromuscular function is present.

One trial has reported 60% to 70% of patients with fecal incontinence secondary to an abnormal pelvic floor will have a 90% reduction in incontinence with biofeedback. Further studies have shown varying success rates of 38% to 100%. A National Institutes of Health (NIH) consensus statement has concluded that biofeedback is effective in the first year postpartum for reversing some pregnancy-related fecal incontinence. The largest prospective study, by Norton and others, compared standard care with biofeedback. The improvement was 54% in the biofeedback group and 53% in the standard care group. Although this questions the effectiveness of biofeedback, it is important to consider that the standard group received nine 40- to 60-minute sessions with a nurse specialist on diet, fluid management, bowel evacuation techniques, bowel training, and use of antidiarrheal medications. Also, biofeedback helped over 50% of patients with this difficult problem. The other lesson from this trial is that more than 50% of patients improved with conservative measures.

Biofeedback of any type is based on the woman hearing, seeing, or sensing a response from a planned exercise. A measuring device, electrode or pressure transducer, is used transvaginally or transanally to record and provide feedback to the woman on how she is squeezing the pelvic floor. She then uses this feedback to increase or lengthen the pelvic floor contraction. If the woman has incontinence secondary to a sensory deficit in the rectum, rectal balloons can be used to "retrain" the woman to perceive rectal distention while squeezing her external sphincter in response to rectal distention. The woman can be taught by a physical therapist, who not only provides encouragement but also instructs on proper technique. Although initially laborintensive, biofeedback has no side effects or morbidity and can be used in conjunction with other treatment modalities, including surgery. The American College of Gastroenterology recommends biofeedback therapy despite imperfect evidence to support its use. In addition, for patients with urinary and fecal incontinence, a single therapy may improve both conditions.

Electrical Stimulation Therapy

Functional electrical stimulation therapy has been shown to improve fecal incontinence in patients with a weakened pelvic floor who are unable to contract their EAS or puborectalis on command. Because of the expense, electrical stimulation is generally reserved for patients who are unable to respond to traditional biofeedback protocols. Both transvaginal and transrectal probes are available. Most protocols recommend high-frequency stimulation at a maximum tolerable stimulation of 50 Hz for 15 to 20 minutes twice daily. Response to therapy is usually seen in 6 weeks, with maximum improvement by 12 weeks, but reported benefits are slight. New stimulation protocols with both biofeedback and electrical stimulation in a 2010 randomized trial of 158 patients was promising at 3 months, with 50% continence rate.

Medications

No specific medication is approved for fecal incontinence except for antidiarrheal medications. To slow intestinal transit and allow for increased water absorption, several medications (**Table 22-6**) are available. Loperamide appears more effective than diphenoxylate for fecal urgency related incontinence and also increases IAS tone. Hyoscyamine is recommended for women with fecal incontinence after meals. Taking this before meals is recommended. For some patients, a daily cleansing of the rectum with an enema allows for several hours of freedom from their incontinence.

Sacral Nerve Stimulation

In 2011, a sacral nerve stimulation device was FDA-approved for treating chronic fecal incontinence. One randomized controlled trial, 54 of 120 patients with severe fecal incontinence improved with the test stimulation and had the permanent generator placed, and 22 (47%) were continent. Observational studies

Table 22-6 Medications for Treatment of Diarrhea

Drug	Dosage	Mechanism of Action
Loperamide	2 mg tid or 4 mg followed by 2 mg after loose bowel movement Maximum, 8 mg/day	Inhibits circular and longitudinal muscle contraction
Diphenoxylate with atropine	5 mg qid initial dose	Direct action of circular smooth muscle to decrease peristalsis
Hyoscyamine sulfate	0.375 mg bid timecaps	Anticholinergic
Cholestyramine	4-mg pack qd or bid	Binds bile acids after cholecystectomy

have reported similar improvements. A 2010 study reported on long-term outcomes in a cohort analysis of consecutive patients. Treatment success was defined as a more than 50% reduction in episodes of fecal incontinence compared with baseline. Temporary sacral nerve stimulation was performed in 118 patients and 91 (77%) were considered suitable for permanent implantation. The median follow-up period was 22 months (range, 1 to 138 months); 70 patients were followed for 1 year, with success in 63 (90%). Of 18 patients followed for 5 years, 15 (83%) reported continued success—1 (61%) maintained full efficacy, 4 (22%) reported some loss, and 3 (17%) reported complete loss. Three patients with a 10-year follow up had no loss in efficacy. This is a less invasive treatment than other surgical alternatives and has few complications, so it is a promising option. In several studies, the long-term success rate appeared higher than that for anal sphincteroplasty, although no randomized comparative trials have been carried out.

Surgery

Surgical management of fecal incontinence includes repair of rectal prolapse, anal sphincteroplasty, radiofrequency treatment of the anal canal, injectable perianal bulking materials, anal sphincter neomuscular flaps, and implantation of artificial sphincters. Unfortunately, postanal repair or posterior levatorplasty has not been shown to be effective for the treatment of fecal incontinence in most patients and will not be discussed here. Perianal injection of bulking agents for fecal incontinence has been done with several materials, including silicone, collagen, and carbon-coated microbeads. The largest trial included 82 patients; it involved injecting silicone biomaterial to augment the IAS, with significant improvement at 1 year. Better and longer outcome studies are needed. Radiofrequency waves delivered to the anal canal denature collagen and change tissue compliance. One small trial with a 12-month follow-up showed modest improvement, but only limited data are available for this study.

Repair of rectal prolapse, transrectally or transabdominally, restores continence in 50% of patients. Success depends on the neuromuscular function of the pelvic floor. Laparoscopic rectopexy is associated with fewer postoperative complications and a shorter hospital stay than open rectopexy. Bowel resection during rectopexy was associated with lower rates of constipation in a systematic review. Rectal prolapse is commonly associated

Table 22-7 Outcomes after Sphincteroplasty

Study, Year[*]	Institution	No. of Patients	Follow-Up Period (mean [range]; mo)	Outcome Success (%)	Outcome Improved (%)
Fang et al, 1984	Minnesota	76	35 (2-62)	82	89
Browning and Motson, 1988	St. Marks	83	39.2 (4-116)	78	91
Ctercteko et al, 1988	Cleveland Clinic, Ohio	44	50	75	
Laurberg et al, 1988	St. Marks	19	18 (median, 9-36)	47	79
Yoshioka and Keighley, 1989	Birmingham	27	48 (median, 16-108)		74.1
Wexner et al, 1991	Cleveland Clinic, Florida	16	10 (3-16)	76	87.5
Fleshman et al, 1991	Washington University	55	0 (12-24)	72	87
Simmang et al, 1994	Washington University	14	0 (6-12)	71	93
Engel et al, 1994	St. Marks	55	15 (6-36)	60.4	
Engel et al, 1994	Amsterdam	28	46 (median, 15-116)	75	
Londono-Schimmer et al, 1994	St. Marks	94	58.5 (median, 12-98)	50	75
Sitzler and Thompson, 1996	St. Marks	31	0 (1-36)	74	
Felt-Bersma et al, 1996	Vrije University	18	14 (3-39)		72
Oliveira et al, 1996	Cleveland Clinic, Florida	55	29 (3-61)	70.1	80
Nikiteas et al, 1996	Birmingham	42	38 (median, 12-66)	60	
Gilliland et al, 1998	Cleveland Clinic, Florida	100	24 (median, 2-96)	55	69
Malouf et al, 2000[†]	St. Marks	474	77(60-96)		50
Grey et al, 2007[‡]	Manchester	47	>60		60

*All references from the original source (Gilliand et al, 1998), except the last two.
[†]Malouf AJ, Norton CS, Engel AF, et al: Long-term results of overlapping anterior anal-sphincter repair for obstetric trauma. Lancet 355:260, 2000.
[‡]Grey BR, Sheldon RR, Telford KJ, Kiff ES: Anterior anal sphincter repair can be of long-term benefit: A 12-year case cohort from a single surgeon. BMC Surg 7:1, 2007.
From Gilliand R, Altomare DF, Moreira H, et al: Pudendal neuropathy is predictive of failure following anterior overlapping sphincteroplasty. Dis Colon Rectum 41:1516, 1998.

with severe pelvic organ prolapse, especially after colpectomy and colpocleisis.

Overlapping anterior anal sphincteroplasty provides symptomatic control of incontinence in 60% to 80% of patients with anatomic EAS defects in the short term. Long-term outcome studies show a more modest success rate, and few women are completely continent. Overlapping sphincteroplasty cure rates 5 to 10 years after surgery may be as low as 1% to 28% (**Table 22-7**). Patients who have an anal sphincter defect and prolonged PNTML should be counseled that their chance of continence following surgery may be decreased, but unless there is absolutely no nerve function, surgical repair should be considered. Repair of an anal sphincter laceration includes not only repair of the EAS but identification and repair of any IAS defects. Because the IAS maintains the resting tone of the anus, it is important to restore sphincter integrity, especially for control of flatus.

The surgery is performed through a transperineal incision from the 11 to 2 o'clock position over the EAS defect. With the examiner's gloved hand in the rectum, the internal sphincter is identified and plicated in the midline with 3-0 prolonged absorbable sutures. Next, the ends of the EAS are identified. The use of a nerve stimulator can facilitate identification of the sphincter ends. The fibrous scar tissue at the ends of the sphincter is kept for added strength. The sphincter ends are dissected free to allow overlap in the midline without tension. The sphincter is then closed with 2-0 or 3-0 prolonged absorbable sutures by overlapping the sphincter ends (**Fig. 22-10**). The advantage of the overlapping sphincteroplasty over the traditional end-to-end repair is decreased tension to prevent separation of the suture line once anesthesia no longer prevents sphincter contraction.

When anal sphincter injury occurs during vaginal delivery, the type of repair needed has been debated. To date, according to only a few studies, there is no significant difference between end-to-end and overlapping anal sphincteroplasties. The outcome of anal sphincteroplasties after delivery is unacceptably poor, with 47% to 67% of women complaining of defecatory symptoms such as flatus incontinence, fecal urgency, and fecal incontinence. Although frank fecal incontinence is reported at a much lower rate, 2% to 9%, the other defecatory symptoms are nonetheless bothersome to women. Furthermore, endoanal ultrasound examinations after sphincteroplasty show persistent anatomic defects in 40% to 85% of repairs.

Because the outcome after anal sphincteroplasty is suboptimal, prevention emerges as an even more important consideration. Vaginal childbirth injury to the anal sphincter is such a common cause of fecal incontinence that prevention should start here. Midline episiotomy has been shown repeatedly in various studies to be strongly associated with anal sphincter damage. Avoidance of routine episiotomy and consideration of a mediolateral episiotomy when absolutely necessary could be beneficial in prevention efforts.

Neosphincters

There are basically two types of neosphincters, one using the woman's own skeletal muscle, usually the gracilis, and the other using an artificial Silastic cuff connected to a fluid reservoir to occlude the anal canal. The gracilis muscle wrap has been shown to have inconsistent results. Initially described by Pickrell and colleagues in 1952, the entire muscle is mobilized and its distal portion wrapped snugly around the anus, anchored to the contralateral ischial tuberosity. The addition of chronic, low-frequency electrical stimulation of the nerve or muscle has been used to convert fatigue-prone type II to fatigue-resistant type I muscle fibers. Once converted, the muscle may be continuously stimulated, resulting in prolonged closure of the anal canal. A report by Baeten and colleagues for the Dynamic Gracioplasty Therapy Study Group reported on 123 adults treated at 20 institutions with dynamic gracioplasty and found that 63% of

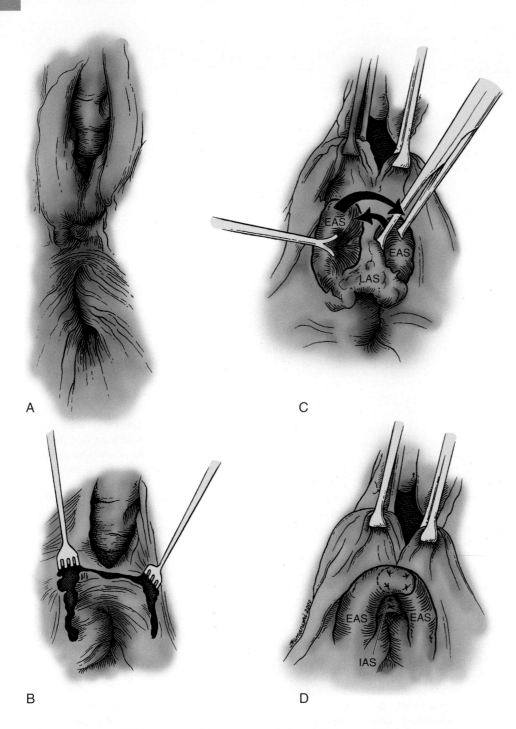

A

B

C

D

Figure 22-10 Sphincter drawing. **A,** Dovetail sign with loss of anal skin creases anteriorly. **B,** Transperineal incision. **C,** EAS identified. **D,** Overlapping sphincteroplasty and IAS repaired.

patients reported a 50% or greater improvement in incontinent events 1 year after surgery. Another 11% noted some improvement and 26% reported no improvement or worsened incontinence. There was one surgery-related death; 74% of patients experienced an adverse event related to the treatment, with 40% of patients requiring additional surgery. Despite these frequent complications, most patients showed a significant improvement in quality of life postsurgery.

Artificial sphincters are indicated for patients with anal incontinence caused by neuromuscular disease or trauma. These use a Silastic cuff connected to a fluid reservoir that encircles the anal canal to cause closure. The cuff is deflated before defecation. Complications include infection and mechanical breakdown; 75% success rates and 33% complication rates, similar to those for the muscle transpositions have been reported. Colostomy can be offered if all other acceptable treatments have failed. Although this sounds extreme, it can greatly improve the quality of life for woman with severe fecal incontinence.

RECTOVAGINAL FISTULAS

Although not a true source of fecal incontinence by definition, rectovaginal fistulas (RVFs) are common enough complications of vaginal birth and gynecologic surgeries to be addressed under this heading. A RVF is an abnormal connection between the

Table 22-8 Origin of Rectovaginal Fistula

Category	Condition	Mechanism
Traumatic		
Obstetric	Prolonged second stage of labor	Pressure necrosis of rectovaginal septum
	Midline episiotomy Perineal lacerations	Extension directed into rectum
Foreign body	Vaginal pessaries	Pressure necrosis
	Violent coitus	Mechanical perforation
	Sexual abuse	Mechanical perforation
Iatrogenic	Hysterectomy	Injury to anterior rectal wall
	Stapled colorectal anastomosis	Staple line includes vagina
	Transanal excision of anterior rectal tumor	Deep margin of resection into vagina
	Enemas	Mechanical perforation
	Anorectal (e.g., incision and drainage of intramural abscesses)	Mechanical perforation
Inflammatory	Crohn's disease	Transmural inflammation-perforation
	Pelvic radiation	Early tumor necrosis
	Pelvic abscess	Late transmural inflammation
	Perirectal abscess	
Neoplastic	Rectal	Local tumor growth into neighboring structure
	Cervical	
	Uterine	
	Vaginal	
	Primary or recurrent tumors	

From Stenchever MA, Benson JT (eds): Atlas of Clinical Gynecology. New York, McGraw-Hill, 2000.

vagina and rectum. Whenever a woman presents with complaints of fecal or flatal incontinence, an RVF should be included in the differential diagnosis.

The causes of RVF, as seen in **Table 22-8**, include traumatic, inflammatory, and neoplastic origins, but obstetric injuries are the most common cause. It is estimated that 0.1% of vaginal births will result in an RVF.

A fistula occurring caudad or adjacent to the EAS is termed an *anovaginal fistula* and is managed differently from an RVF. Fistulas that occur more than 3 cm above the anal verge are true RVFs. Most RVFs secondary to obstetric injury occur in the lower third of the vagina and may be associated with a sphincter defect in the EAS. It is important to evaluate the EAS (see earlier) with transanal ultrasound or EMG to map any defects prior to surgical treatment.

Fistulas secondary to surgical trauma, malignancy, or an inflammatory process may occur at any point along the vaginal wall, including the apex. If a fistula develops after a difficult surgery, such as after pelvic inflammatory disease, or radiotherapy, it is important to check for more than one fistula prior to repair. If the woman has a history of malignancy, examination with biopsy specimens should be performed to rule out cancer as the cause of the fistula.

Depending on the size and location of the fistula, the woman may be almost asymptomatic or complain of a small amount of flatus passing into her vagina with a low small fistula. With a large fistula, she may have formed stool coming through the

vagina with every bowel movement, causing significant distress and hygiene problems. Rectal bleeding is more likely to be reported with a neoplastic process or post–pelvic radiation.

Evaluation of a woman includes a history and physical examination to determine cause. If there is suspicion of inflammatory bowel disease, a colonoscopy is warranted. Perineal skin and rectal examinations are important to visualize the fistula tract and determine the integrity of the anal sphincters and quality of the tissues surrounding the fistula, and to palpate for abscesses and other masses. Most obstetric-related RVFs show the fistula along the scar line. Methylene blue mixed in lubricant and placed in the rectum can help identify the fistula. If still not identified, a dilute methylene blue enema with a tampon in the vagina may help in isolating the fistula. If the vaginal orifice is found, but not the rectal opening, insertion of an angiocatheter with a squirting of hydrogen peroxide can show bubbling on the rectal side. A small lacrimal duct probe might allow passage through the vaginal tract to identify the rectal exit site.

An office anoscopy or proctoscopy may also help evaluate the surrounding tissues. In general, a mature epithelialized fistula that is not infected is not painful on digital examination. If the examination in the office is not successful in locating the fistula or is too painful for the woman, she should be taken to the operating room for examination under anesthesia. If the fistula has still not been identified, filling the vagina with water and insufflating the rectum should produce bubbling in the vagina that can be traced to the opening. A barium enema may also be helpful for identifying high fistulas. Vaginography using dilute barium solution may also help identify a fistula.

Surgical management of an anovaginal or anoperineal fistula is accomplished by opening the fistula tract, curetting the tract, and leaving the tract open to heal secondarily. Excision of the tract and primary closure will result in recurrent fistula formation in most cases.

Many surgical procedures have been described for the treatment of RVF. Regardless of the procedure chosen, basic surgical principles must be followed. The tissue must be healthy, well vascularized, and free of infection and induration. This may require waiting for up to 3 months following the original trauma or surgery for complete healing. If there is significant fecal contamination, prior radiation, or persistent abscess, a diverting colostomy should be considered. After a colostomy, a delay of 8 to 12 weeks is generally required for the inflammation and cellulites around the fistula to heal. At the time of repair, a Martius fat pad graft can be used to increase the vascular supply to the area. Preoperatively, the woman should have a complete mechanical bowel preparation starting several days before the surgery to prevent liquid stool from contaminating the field. Some surgeons may place the woman on a liquid diet several days before surgery with no mechanical bowel preparation except enemas until clear the night before surgery. The goal is to have no liquid stool in the rectum and to have the woman's first postoperative bowel movement, several days after surgery, be soft but formed. Antibiotic bowel prophylaxis is warranted.

Other surgical principles include excision of the entire fistulous tract, wide mobilization of the rectal tissue, and broad tissue to tissue closure without tension. The rectal side is the high-pressure side and requires attention to repair. The vaginal side may be closed or left open to drain, if indicated, and should close spontaneously. A delayed absorbable suture, such as 3-0 Polysorb (glycolide-lactide copolymer), is used on all layers. Alternatively, a monofilament delayed absorbable suture such as Maxon (monofilament polyglyconate) or PDS (polydioxanone) might lower the risk of infection over a braided suture. Permanent sutures are not used.

Transvaginal and transrectal repairs have been described, but gynecologists generally prefer the transvaginal approach. Depending on the location and need to repair the anal sphincters, an uncomplicated fistula can be repaired as for a fourth-degree laceration as a perineoproctotomy with layered closure. After cutting from the perineal body, through the sphincters and to the fistulous tract, care must be taken to excise the tract and any surrounding scar tissue. A two-layered closure of the rectum and anal canal is then performed, as in a fourth-degree closure. Care should be given to closing the EAS.

To preserve an intact sphincter, the RVF can be cored out by placing a pediatric Foley transvaginally, filling the balloon on the rectal side, and then using the Foley for traction by pulling upward. After excision, depending on the size, a small fistula can be closed with two-layer purse-string sutures or with an interrupted two-layer closure.

Transrectal repairs, preferred by many colorectal surgeons, generally involve the development of rectal mucosal flaps, mobilized and brought down or lateral to cover the excised fistula site. In 23 patients treated at the Cleveland Clinic with rectal advancement flaps, fistulas were successfully cured in 77% of patients with obstetric or surgical injury and 60% of patients with Crohn's disease.

Postoperatively, the woman's diet and medications should be managed to keep her bowel movements soft, but formed. In most cases, a clear liquid diet is continued for the first 3 days after surgery, followed by a low-residue diet. Broad-spectrum antibiotics should be continued for 2 weeks. Sitz baths, two or three times daily, followed by the use of a blow dryer or heat lamp, keep the area clean and dry.

KEY POINTS

- Estimates of fecal incontinence range from 11% to 15% of community-dwelling women older than 64 years.
- Over 30% of women reporting urinary incontinence also report fecal incontinence, known as dual incontinence.
- The IAS, under autonomic control, maintains the high-pressure zone or continence zone and, along with the EAS, keeps the anal canal closed.
- The EAS provides the voluntary squeeze pressure that prevents incontinence with increasing rectal or abdominal pressure. The EAS is innervated by the hemorrhoidal branch of the pudendal nerve from the S2-S4 nerve roots.
- A common cause of fecal incontinence is damage to the anal sphincter at the time of vaginal delivery, with or without neuronal injury. Prevention of these injuries is critical.
- The incidence of occult external anal sphincter disruption after vaginal delivery determined by endoanal ultrasound ranges from 11% to 35%. The chance of muscular injury is increased with midline episiotomy, instrumented delivery, and vaginal delivery of larger infants.
- Approximately 1 in 10 women will develop some fecal incontinence or fecal urgency after one vaginal delivery.
- At a tertiary colorectal referral clinic, a prospective study showed that further evaluation, including radiologic and physiologic tests, altered the final diagnosis or the cause of fecal incontinence in 19% of cases.
- Biofeedback for patients with fecal incontinence shows a similar reduction in incontinence episodes as intense education on bowel care, medications, and dietary and fluid management by a nurse specialist. This highlights the importance of conservative management techniques.
- Overlapping anterior anal sphincteroplasty provides symptomatic control of incontinence in 60% to 80% of patients initially, but long-term outcomes are not nearly as successful.

REFERENCES CAN BE FOUND ON
EXPERTCONSULT.com

23

Infections of the Lower and Upper Genital Tracts
Vulva, Vagina, Cervix, Toxic Shock Syndrome, Endometritis, and Salpingitis

Linda O. Eckert and Gretchen M. Lentz

The Centers for Disease Control and Prevention (CDC) regularly revises its treatment protocols for sexually transmitted diseases. The recommendations and medications in this edition are based on the 2010 CDC guidelines. Readers are urged to consult any updates in the CDC guidelines, because bacterial sensitivities and epidemiologic concerns may lead to changes in treatment protocols. The latest information may be found on the CDC website (http://www.cdc.gov).

The discussion of infectious diseases of the female genital tract is divided into those of the lower genital tract, the vulva, vagina, and cervix; and those of the upper genital tract, endometritis and salpingitis. These separations are made for clarity of presentation. The female genital tract has anatomic and physiologic continuity. Thus, infectious agents that colonize and involve one organ often infect adjacent organs. To understand the pathophysiology and natural history of infectious diseases of the genital tract, one must keep this continuity in mind.

The symptoms caused by infections of the lower genital tract produce the most common conditions seen by gynecologists. Therefore, the initial focus of this chapter is on clinical presentation and the differential diagnosis of vulvitis, vaginitis, and cervicitis.

Toxic shock syndrome (TSS) and syphilis are also discussed in this chapter. Although the most devastating pathologic processes from these diseases occur in sites other than the genital tract, they often obtain entry into the body through the vulvar, rectal, vaginal, or cervical epithelium.

Many of the infections discussed in this chapter may be acquired through sexual contact and are termed *sexually transmitted infections* (STIs). STIs often coexist—for example, vulvar herpes and condyloma acuminatum or infections of *Chlamydia trachomatis* and *Neisseria gonorrhoeae*. When one disease is suspected, appropriate diagnostic methods must be used to detect other infections. This principle cannot be overemphasized.

INFECTIONS OF THE VULVA

The skin of the vulva is composed of a stratified squamous epithelium containing hair follicles and sebaceous, sweat, and apocrine glands. The subcutaneous tissue of the vulva also contains specialized structures such as the Bartholin glands. Similar to skin elsewhere on the body, the vulvar area is subject to primary and secondary infections. The three most prevalent primary viral infections of the vulva are herpes genitalis, condyloma acuminatum, and molluscum contagiosum. However, symptoms from secondary infections of the vulva caused by organisms that produce vulvovaginitis are among the most common of all gynecologic conditions. To understand the differential diagnosis of vulvar infections, one must consider that vulvar skin is also sensitive to hormonal, metabolic, and allergic influences.

Vulvar itching or burning of acute onset and short duration suggests infection or contact dermatitis. Approximately 10% of outpatient visits to gynecologists are for vulvar pruritus. The signs of erythema, edema, and superficial skin ulcers of the vulva also suggest infection. Skin fissures and excoriation may be signs of primary infection, may be caused by the woman's scratching as a result of irritation from a vaginal discharge, or may be the manifestation of a primary dermatologic disease.

INFECTIONS OF BARTHOLIN'S GLANDS

Bartholin's glands normally are two rounded, pea-sized glands deep in the perineum that are nonpalpable unless enlarged. They are located at the entrance of the vagina at 5 and 7 o'clock. Mucinous secretions from Bartholin's glands provide moisture for the epithelium of the vestibule but are not important for vaginal lubrication. The Bartholin's ducts are approximately 2 cm in length; they open in a groove between the hymen and labia minora in the posterior lateral wall of the vagina. Approximately 2% of adult women develop enlargements of one or both glands. The most common cause is cystic dilation of Bartholin's duct (**Fig. 23-1**).

The cause of a Bartholin's duct cyst is obstruction of the duct secondary to nonspecific inflammation or trauma. Histologically, Bartholin's ducts are lined by transitional epithelium. These ducts are easily obstructed, usually near the distal orifice. Following obstruction, there is continued secretion of glandular fluid, which results in the cystic dilation. Years ago, bilateral enlargement of Bartholin's glands was believed to be a pathognomonic sign of gonococcal infection. This is no longer true. Unilateral or bilateral Bartholin's gland infection in most cases

The treatment of infections or enlargement of Bartholin's glands depends on their symptomatology. Asymptomatic cysts in women younger than 40 years do not need treatment. The therapy for acute adenitis without abscess formation is broad-spectrum antibiotics and frequent hot sitz baths. The treatment of choice for a symptomatic cyst or abscess is the development of a fistulous tract from the dilated duct to the vestibule. Simple incision and drainage of a Bartholin gland abscess are complicated by a tendency for the abscess to recur. The classic surgical treatment is to develop a fistulous tract to marsupialize the duct. After an elliptical wedge of tissue has been removed, the remaining edges of the duct or abscess are everted and sutured to the surrounding skin with interrupted sutures. This forms an epithelialized pouch that provides drainage for the gland. The recurrence rate following marsupialization is approximately 5% to 10%. An alternative surgical approach is to insert a Word catheter, a short catheter with an inflatable Foley balloon, through a stab incision into the abscess and leave it in place for 4 to 6 weeks (**Fig. 23-2**). During this period, a tract of epithelium will form. All the procedures mentioned may be performed with local anesthesia. Antibiotics are not necessary unless there is an associated cellulitis surrounding the Bartholin gland abscess.

Women older than 40 years with gland enlargement require a biopsy to exclude adenocarcinoma of Bartholin's gland. Excision of a Bartholin duct and gland is indicated for persistent deep infection, multiple recurrences of abscesses, or recurrent enlargement of the gland in women older than 40 years. Removal of a Bartholin gland for recurrent infection should be performed when the infection is quiescent. Excision can be challenging because of the rich vascular supply to the region and may be accompanied by morbidity, including intraoperative hemorrhage, hematoma formation, fenestration of the labia, postoperative scarring, and associated dyspareunia. It is best to use regional block or general anesthesia for excision.

PEDICULOSIS PUBIS AND SCABIES

The skin of the vulva is a frequent site of infestation by animal parasites, the two most common being the crab louse and the itch mite. Ideally, early diagnosis and treatment are of the utmost importance in controlling parasitic infection.

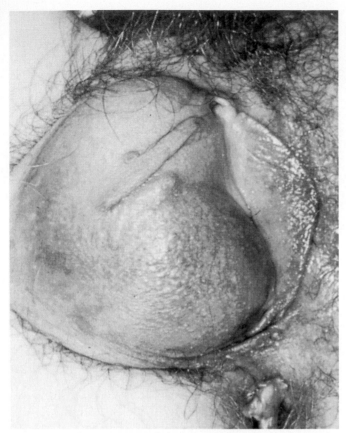

Figure 23-1 Bartholin's abscess. The mass is tender and fluctuant and is situated on the lower lateral aspect of labium minus at 5 o'clock. (From Kaufman RH: Cystic tumors. In Kaufman RH, Faro S [eds]: Benign Diseases of the Vulva and Vagina, 4th ed. St. Louis, Mosby–Year Book, 1994.)

is not caused by a sexually transmitted infection. Positive cultures from Bartholin's gland abscesses are often polymicrobial and contain a wide range of bacteria similar to the normal flora of the vagina.

The differential diagnosis of Bartholin's gland cysts includes mesonephric cysts of the vagina and epithelial inclusion cysts. Mesonephric cysts are generally more anterior and cephalad in the vagina, whereas epithelial inclusion cysts are more superficial. Rarely, a lipoma, fibroma, hernia, vulvar varicosity, or hydrocele may be confused with a Bartholin's duct cyst. Bartholin's duct cysts are found in the labia majora and the duct orifices are at the base of the labia minora, just distal to the hymen.

Most women with Bartholin's duct cysts are asymptomatic. The cysts may vary from 1 to 8 cm in diameter and are usually unilateral, tense, and nonpainful. Most cysts are unilocular. However, in chronic or recurrent cysts there occasionally are multiple compartments.

In contrast, an abscess of a Bartholin's gland tends to develop rapidly over 2 to 4 days with significant symptoms, including difficulty in ambulation. Acute pain and tenderness can be severe and are secondary to rapid enlargement, hemorrhage, or secondary infection. The signs are those of a classic abscess—erythema, acute tenderness, edema and, occasionally, cellulitis of the surrounding subcutaneous tissue. Without therapy, most abscesses tend to rupture spontaneously by the third or fourth day.

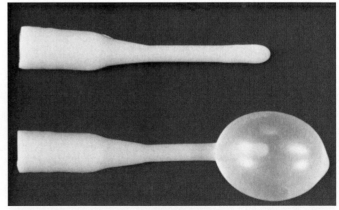

Figure 23-2 Word catheters before and after inflation. They are used to develop a fistula from Bartholin's cyst or abscess to the vestibule. (From Friedrich EG: Vulvar Disease, 2nd ed. Philadelphia, WB Saunders, 1983.)

Pediculosis pubis is an infestation by the crab louse, *Phthirus pubis*. The crab louse is also called the pubic louse and is a different species from the body or head louse. Lice in the pubic hair are the most contagious of all STIs, with over 90% of sexual partners becoming infected following a single exposure. The louse is usually transmitted by close contact, although nonsexual transmission of pubic lice has been documented from towels or bedding. *P. pubis* is generally confined to the hairy areas of the vulva. It may occasionally be found in other areas, such as the eyelids. The major nourishment of the louse is human blood.

The louse's life cycle has three stages, egg (**nit**), nymph, and adult. The entire life cycle is spent on the host. Eggs are deposited at the base of hair follicles. The adult parasite is approximately 1 mm long and dark gray when its alimentary tract is not filled with blood (**Fig. 23-3**). Of clinical importance for diagnosis is the fact that the louse moves slowly. The incubation period for pediculosis is approximately 30 days.

The predominant clinical symptom of louse infestation is constant pubic pruritis caused by allergic sensitization. Usually, initial sensitization takes several weeks to develop but may be as rapid as 5 days following initial infection. Following a reinfection, pruritus may occur within 24 hours. Examination of the vulvar area without magnification demonstrates eggs and adult lice and pepper grain feces adjacent to the hair shafts (**Fig. 23-4**). The tiny rough spots visualized with the naked eye are the alimentary tracts of lice filled with human blood. The vulvar skin may become secondarily irritated or infected by constant scratching. For definitive diagnosis, one can make a microscopic slide by scratching the skin papule with a needle and placing the crust under a drop of mineral oil. The louse's body looks like that of a miniature crab, with six legs that have claws on them.

Scabies is a parasitic infection of the itch mite, *Sarcoptes scabiei*. Similar to the crab louse, it is transmitted by close contact. Unlike louse infestation, scabies is an infection that is widespread over the body, without a predilection for hairy areas. The adult female itch mite digs a burrow just beneath the skin. She lays eggs in this home during her life span of approximately 1 month. The adult itch mite is usually less than 0.5 mm long, approximately the size of a grain of sand. Unlike the crab louse, an itch mite travels rapidly over skin and may move up to 2.5 cm in 1

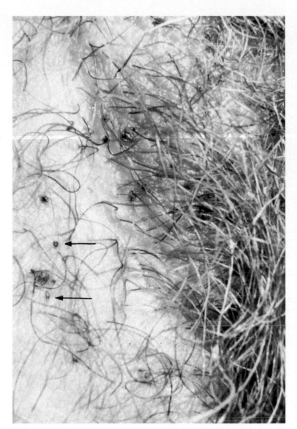

Figure 23-4 Crab lice and nits of pediculosis pubis *(arrows)*. (From Kaufman RH: Miscellaneous vulvar disorders. In Kaufman RH, Faro S [eds]: Benign Diseases of the Vulva and Vagina, 4th ed. St. Louis, Mosby-Year Book, 1994.)

minute. Mites are able to survive for only a few hours away from the warmth of skin.

The predominant clinical symptom of scabies is severe but intermittent itching. Generally, more intense pruritus occurs at night when the skin is warmer and the mites are more active. Initial symptoms usually present approximately 3 weeks after primary infestation. Scabies may present as papules, vesicles, or burrows. However, the pathognomonic sign of scabies infection is the burrow in the skin. The burrow usually has the appearance of a twisted line on the skin surface, with a small vesicle at one end. Any area of the skin may be infected, with the hands, wrists, breasts, vulva, and buttocks being most commonly involved. A handheld magnifying lens is helpful for examining suspicious areas. Microscopic slides may be made using mineral oil and a scratch technique (**Fig. 23-5**). Mites lack lateral claw legs but have two anterior triangular hairy buds. Scabies has been termed the *great dermatologic imitator,* and the differential diagnosis includes almost all dermatologic diseases that cause pruritus. The treatment of pediculosis pubis or scabies involves an agent that kills both the adult parasite and the eggs. The therapy currently recommended by the CDC 2010 guidelines for pediculosis pubis involves the use of permethrin, 1% cream rinse, applied to affected areas and washed off after 10 minutes, or pyrethrins, with piperonyl butoxide applied to the affected area and washed off after 10 minutes. Alternative regimens include malathion, 0.5% lotion, applied for 8 to 12 hours and washed off, or ivermectin, 250 µg/kg, repeated in 2 weeks. None of these

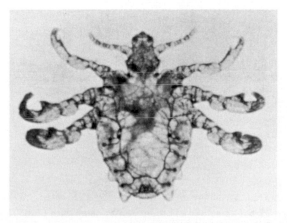

Figure 23-3 Pubic louse, *Phthirus pubis*, after blood meal. (From Billstein S: Human lice. In Holmes KK, Mårdh PA, Sparling PF, et al [eds]: Sexually Transmitted Diseases. New York, McGraw-Hill, 1984.)

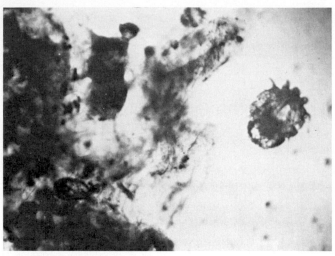

Figure 23-5 Skin scrapings of unexcoriated papules fortuitously disclose adults, larvae, eggs, and fecal pellets, any of which would be diagnostic of scabies. (From Orkin M, Howard IM: Scabies. In Holmes KK, Mårdh PA, Sparling PF, et al [eds]: Sexually Transmitted Diseases. New York, McGraw-Hill, 1984.)

should be applied to the eyelids. Retreatment may be necessary if lice are found or if eggs are observed at the hair-skin junction. Patients with pediculosis pubis should be evaluated for other STIs and evaluated after 1 week if symptoms persist. Those who do not respond to one of the recommended regimens should be retreated with an alternative regimen.

The CDC recommendation for scabies is permethrin cream, 5%, applied to all areas of the body from the neck down and washed off after 8 to 14 hours or ivermectin, 200 µg/kg orally, repeated in 2 weeks, if necessary. Alternative regimens include lindane, 1%, 1 oz of lotion or 30 g of cream applied thinly to all areas of the body from the neck down and thoroughly washed off after 8 hours. Resistance to lindane has been reported in some parts of the United States. Lindane is not recommended as first-line therapy because of toxicity. It should only be used as an alternative if the woman cannot tolerate other therapies or if they have failed. Lindane should not be used immediately after a bath or shower and should not be used by persons who have extensive dermatitis, women who are pregnant or lactating, or children younger than 2 years. Patients with scabies have intense pruritus that may persist for many days following effective therapy. An antihistamine will help alleviate this symptom. Similar to pediculosis pubis, women should be examined 1 week following initial therapy and retreated with an alternative regimen if live mites are observed.

To avoid reinfection by pediculosis pubis or scabies, treatment should be prescribed for sexual contacts within the previous 6 weeks and other close household contacts. Those with close physical contact should be treated at the same time as the infected woman, regardless of whether they have symptoms. Bedding and clothing should be decontaminated (i.e., machine-washed, machine-dried using the heat cycle, or dry-cleaned) or removed from body contact for at least 72 hours. Fumigation of living areas is not necessary. Importantly, women and physicians should not confuse the 1% cream rinse of permethrin dosage recommended for pubic lice with the permethrin cream, 5%, that is recommended for scabies.

MOLLUSCUM CONTAGIOSUM

Molluscum contagiosum is a pox virus that replicates in the cytoplasm of cells and causes a chronic localized infection consisting of flesh-colored, dome-shaped papules with an umbilicated center. Like many viruses in the pox family, molluscum is spread by direct skin to skin contact. The incubation period is 2 to 7 weeks. In children, molluscum contagiosum may present over the entire body. In adults, it is primarily an asymptomatic disease of the vulvar skin and, unlike most STIs, it is only mildly contagious. However, lesions can be spread by autoinoculation, during contact sports, or by fomites on bath sponges or towels. Widespread infection in adults is most closely related to underlying cellular immunodeficiency, such as during an HIV infection. It can also occur in the setting of chemotherapy or corticosteroid administration.

Diagnosis is made by the characteristic appearance of the lesions. The small nodules or domed papules of molluscum contagiosum are usually 1 to 5 mm in diameter (**Fig. 23-6**). Close inspection reveals that many of the more mature nodules have an umbilicated center. An infected woman will typically have 1 to 20 solitary lesions randomly distributed over the vulvar skin. A crop of new nodules will persist from several months to years. If the diagnosis cannot be made by simple inspection, the white waxy material from inside the nodule should be expressed on a microscopic slide. The finding of intracytoplasmic molluscum bodies with Wright or Giemsa stain confirms the diagnosis. The major complication of molluscum contagiosum is bacterial superinfection. The umbilicated papules may resemble furuncles when secondarily infected.

Molluscum contagiosum is usually a self-limiting infection and spontaneously reduces after a few months in immunocompetent individuals. However, treatment of individual papules will decrease sexual transmission and autoinoculation of the virus. After injection of local anesthesia, the caseous material is then evacuated and the nodule excised with a sharp dermal curette. The base of the papule is subsequently chemically treated with ferric subsulfate (Monsel solution) or 85% trichloroacetic

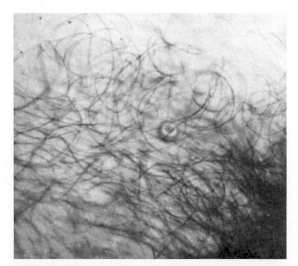

Figure 23-6 Papule of molluscum contagiosum with umbilicated center. (From Brown ST: Molluscum contagiosum. In Holmes KK, Mårdh PA, Sparling PF, et al [eds]: Sexually Transmitted Diseases. New York, McGraw-Hill, 1984.)

acid. An alternative method is cantharidin, a chemical blistering agent.

In one retrospective study, 90% of 300 children had clearance of lesions with an average of two visits. In immunocompromised individuals, treatment is more difficult. In the HIV-infected woman, there have been multiple reports of recalcitrant molluscum lesions resolving only after initiating highly active antiretroviral therapy (HAART).

GENITAL ULCERS

Herpes, granuloma inguinale (donovanosis), lymphogranuloma venereum, chancroid, and syphilis may all present as ulcerations in the genital area. However, their causes, disease courses, and treatments are different. **Table 23-1** lists some of their major characteristics. Physicians must always consider the possibility of more than one STI concurrently infecting an individual.

Genital Herpes

Genital herpes is a recurrent infection that is incurable and highly contagious, with 75% of sexual partners of infected individuals contracting the disease. It is among the most frequently encountered STIs; a study of 5452 asymptomatic adults in private community-based clinics in six geographic regions in the United States found that the seroprevalence of herpes simplex virus type 2 (HSV-2) was 25.5%. Approximately 80% of individuals are unaware that they are infected. Frequently, herpes is transmitted by asymptomatic shedding, which may occur as frequently as 1 in 5 days. It is important that the woman understand the natural history of disease with emphasis on probability of recurrent attacks, effect of antiviral agents, and risks of neonatal infection. Although recurrent genital herpes is not a debilitating physical disease, it may present an overwhelming psychological burden.

There are two distinct types of HSV, type 1 (HSV-1) and type 2 (HSV-2). In the past, a broad generalization was that

HSV-I tends to infect epithelium above the waist and HSV-2 tends to cause ulceration below the waist. However, HSV-1 is the most commonly acquired genital herpes in women younger than 25 years and, in some series, HSV-1 may cause lower genital tract infection in 13% to 40% of patients. HSV-1 does not protect against HSV-2, but HSV-2 does offer some protection against HSV-1. Most initial genital infections occur in women between the ages of 15 and 35 years.

In primary herpes, the incubation period is between 3 and 7 days (average, 6 days). Although subclinical primary herpes infection is common, both local and systemic disease manifestations occur when the primary infection is symptomatic. The woman typically experiences paresthesias of the vulvar skin followed by the eruption of multiple vesicles, which progress to shallow, superficial ulcers over a large area of the vulva. Patients experience multiple crops of ulcers for 2 to 6 weeks. The ulcers usually heal spontaneously without scarring (**Fig. 23-7**). Viral shedding may occur for 2 to 3 weeks after vulvar lesions appear and, during primary infections, positive cultures for herpesvirus may be obtained from lesions in 80% of women. Most symptomatic women have severe vulvar pain, tenderness, and inguinal adenopathy and simultaneous involvement of the vagina and cervix is common (**Fig. 23-8**).

Systemic symptoms, including general malaise and fever, are experienced by 70% of women during the primary infection. Rarely, there is central nervous system (CNS) infection, with the reported mortality rate from herpes encephalitis being approximately 50%. Primary infections of the urethra and bladder may result in acute urinary retention, necessitating catheterization. The symptoms of vulvar pain, pruritus, and discharge peak between days 7 and 11 of the primary infection. The average woman experiences severe symptoms for approximately 14 days.

Recurrent genital herpes is a local disease with less severe symptoms. On average, a woman will have four recurrences during the first year and, in 50% of women, the first recurrence occurs within 6 months of the initial infection. The probability

Table 23-1 Clinical Features of Genital Ulcers

	Type				
Parameter	**Syphilis**	**Herpes**	**Chancroid**	**Lymphogranuloma Venereum**	**Donovanosis**
Incubation period	2-4 wk (1-12 wk)	2-7 days	1-14 days	3 days-6 wk	1-4 wk (up to 6 mo)
Primary lesion	Papule	Vesicle	Papule or pustule	Papule, pustule, or vesicle	Papule
Number of lesions	Usually one	Multiple, may coalesce	Usually multiple, may coalesce	Usually one	Variable
Diameter (mm)	5-15	1-2	2-20	2-10	Variable
Edges	Sharply demarcated Elevated, round or oval	Erythematous	Undermined, ragged, irregular	Elevated, round or oval	Elevated, irregular
Depth	Superficial or deep	Superficial	Excavated	Superficial or deep	Elevated
Base	Smooth, nonpurulent	Serous, erythematous	Purulent	Variable	Red and rough (beefy)
Induration	Firm	None	Soft	Occasionally firm	Firm
Pain	Unusual	Common	Usually very tender	Variable	Uncommon
Lymphadenopathy	Firm, nontender Pseudoadenopathy bilateral	Firm, tender, often bilateral	Tender, may suppurate, usually unilateral	Tender, may suppurate, loculated, usually unilateral	

From Holmes KK, Mårdh PA, Sparling PF, et al (eds): Sexually Transmitted Diseases, 2nd ed. New York, McGraw-Hill, 1990.

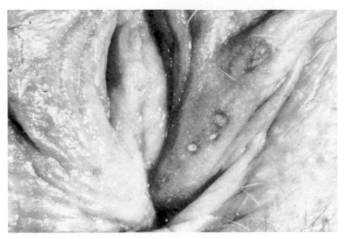

Figure 23-7 Recurrent herpes genitalis. Superficial ulcers are noted following rupture of vesicles. (From Kaufman RH, Faro S: Herpes genitalis: Clinical features and treatment. Clin Obstet Gynecol 28:156, 1985.)

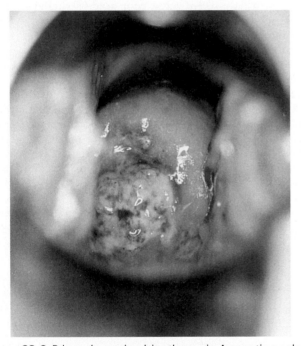

Figure 23-8 Primary herpes involving the cervix. A necrotic exophytic mass is seen on posterior lip. This was clinically thought to be invasive carcinoma. Herpes simplex virus culture was positive. The lesion spontaneously disappeared. (From Kaufman RH, Faro S: Herpes genitalis: Clinical features and treatment. Clin Obstet Gynecol 28:154, 1985.)

and frequency of recurrence of herpes are related to the HSV serotype. Approximately 80% of women with an initial genital HSV-2 infection will experience a recurrence within 12 months. If her primary HSV-2 infection was severe, she will have recurrences approximately twice as often, with a shorter time to recurrence intervals compared with women with milder initial episodes of the disease. In contrast, if the initial pelvic infection was HSV-1, there is a 55% chance of a recurrence within 1 year, with the average rate of recurrence slightly less than one episode.

For recurrences, vulvar involvement is usually unilateral, recurrent attacks last an average of 7 days, and viral shedding

occurs for approximately 5 days. The ability to culture herpesvirus successfully from recurrent herpetic ulcers is 40%. A common feature of recurrence is a prodromal phase of sacroneuralgia, vulvar burning, tenderness, and pruritus for a few hours to 5 days before vesicle formation. Extragenital sites of recurrent infection are common. The herpesvirus resides in a latent phase in the dorsal root ganglia of S2, S3, and S4.

The clinical diagnosis of genital herpes is often made by simple clinical inspection. Women come to their physician when they develop symptoms from vulvar ulcers. Herpetic ulcers are painful when touched with a cotton-tipped applicator, whereas the ulcers of syphilis are painless. Viral cultures are useful in confirming the diagnosis in primary episodes when culture sensitivity is 80%, but less useful in recurrent episodes. Most herpesvirus cultures will become positive within 2 to 4 days of inoculation. The most accurate and sensitive technique for identifying herpesvirus is the polymerase chain reaction (PCR) assay. Serologic tests are helpful in determining whether a woman has been infected in the past with herpesvirus. The Western blot assay for antibodies to herpes is the most specific method for diagnosing recurrent herpes, as well as unrecognized or subclinical infection. However, Western blot tests are not widely available and are difficult to perform. Type-specific HSV serologic assays might be useful in the following situations: (1) recurrent genital symptoms or atypical symptoms, with negative HSV cultures; (2) clinical diagnosis of genital herpes without laboratory confirmation; or (3) partner with genital herpes. HSV serologic testing should be considered for persons presenting for an STI evaluation, especially for those with multiple sex partners or HIV infection and at increased risk for HIV acquisition. Screening for HSV-1 or HSV-2 in the general population is not indicated.

Enzyme-linked immunoassay (ELISA) and immunoblot tests are available for HSV-1 and HSV-2. Rapid serologic point of care tests are now available for HSV-2 antibodies. Appropriate screening tests for other STIs should be obtained, because they may coexist with herpes.

Treatment of HSV-1 or HSV-2 may be used for three different clinical scenarios:

1. Primary episode
2. Recurrent episode
3. Daily suppression

In primary episodes, the duration and severity of symptoms are lessened and shedding is shortened with antiviral therapy. Antiviral therapy is recommended for in all patients with primary episodes.

Episodic therapy for recurrences can shorten the duration of the outbreak if started within 24 hours of prodromal symptoms or lesion appearance. Because of the necessity of starting antiviral therapy immediately after recognizing symptoms, it is important that the woman with HSV be given a prescription for antiviral therapy to have at home.

Patient-initiated therapy has been found to be superior to therapy ordered by a physician because patients initiate therapy earlier in the course of a recurrence. The antiviral medication should be started as early as possible during the prodrome, and definitely within 24 hours of the appearance of lesions. Daily suppressive therapy is recommended when the woman has six or more episodes annually or for psychological distress. It is important for patients to be aware that asymptomatic viral shedding can occur even when on daily suppressive therapy.

Box 23-1 Antiviral Treatment for Herpes Simplex Virus in the Nonpregnant Patient

	Antiviral Agent		
Indication	Valacyclovir	Acyclovir	Famciclovir
First clinical episode	1000 mg bid, 7-10 days	200 mg five times/day; or 400 mg tid, 7-10 days	250 mg tid, 7-10 days
Recurrent episodes	1000 mg daily, 5 days; or 500 mg bid, 3 days	400 mg tid, 5 days; 800 mg bid, 5 days; or 800 mg tid, 2 days	125 mg bid, 5 days; 500 mg once then 250 mg bid, 2 days; 100 mg bid, 1 day
Daily suppressive	1000 mg daily (≥10 recurrences/year) or 500 mg daily (≤9 recurrences/year)	400 mg bid or 1000 mg/day	250 mg bid

Workowski KA, Berman S; Centers for Disease Control and Prevention (CDC): Sexually transmitted diseases treatment guidelines, 2010. MMWR 59(RR-12):20-22.

In serodiscordant couples a prospective placebo-controlled randomized trial has demonstrated that daily use of valacyclovir for suppression in the seropositive partner results in significantly fewer cases of HSV acquisition in the seronegative partner. Regular use of condoms in serodiscordant couples also decreases transmission, but is not 100% protective. HSV-seronegative women are three times as likely to acquire HSV infection from seropositive male partners compared with seronegative males acquiring HSV from infected female partners. A summary of CDC-recommended treatment regimens is presented in **Box 23-1**.

Acyclovir is a drug with relatively minimal toxicity and recent reports have documented its safety in patients receiving daily therapy with acyclovir for as long as 6 years and with valacyclovir or famciclovir for 1 year. However, the CDC recommends that acyclovir or other suppressive drugs be discontinued after 12 months of suppressive therapy to determine the subsequent rate of recurrence for each individual woman. Even if herpes is not treated over time, clinical recurrences tend to dramatically decrease in number.

A vaccine would be the logical approach for optimum prevention of herpes. Research is ongoing.

Granuloma Inguinale (Donovanosis)

Granuloma inguinale, also known as donovanosis, is a chronic, ulcerative, bacterial infection of the skin and subcutaneous tissue of the vulva. Rarely, the vagina and cervix are involved in advanced untreated cases. Granuloma inguinale is common in tropical climates such as New Guinea and the Caribbean Islands, but fewer than 20 cases are reported each year in the United States. This disease can be spread sexually and through close nonsexual contact. However, it is not highly contagious, and chronic exposure is usually necessary to contract the disease. The incubation period is extremely variable, from 1 to 12 weeks. It is caused by an intracellular, gram-negative, nonmotile, encapsulated rod, **Klebsiella granulomatis,** which is very difficult to culture on standard media. There are no U.S. Food and Drug Administration (FDA)–approved molecular tests for the detection of *K. granulomatis* DNA. Serologic tests are nonspecific.

The initial growth of granuloma inguinale is a nodule that gradually progresses into a painless, slowly progressing ulcer surrounded by highly vascular granulation tissue. This gives the ulcer a beefy red appearance and it bleeds easily when touched. Unless secondarily infected, the ulcers are painless and without regional adenopathy. Typically, multiple nodules are present, resulting in ulcers that grow and coalesce and, if untreated, will eventually destroy the normal vulvar architecture. If untreated, the chronic form of the disease is characterized by scarring and lymphatic obstruction, which produces marked enlargement of the vulva. In endemic areas, the disease is usually diagnosed by its clinical manifestations. The diagnosis may also be established by identifying **Donovan bodies** in smears and specimens taken from the ulcers (**Fig. 23-9**). Donovan bodies appear as clusters of dark-staining bacteria with a bipolar (safety pin) appearance found in the cytoplasm of large mononuclear cells. The differential diagnosis includes lymphogranuloma venereum, vulvar carcinoma, syphilis, chancroid, genital herpes, amebiasis, and other granulomatous diseases.

Granuloma inguinale may be managed by a wide range of oral broad-spectrum antibiotics. The CDC recommends doxycycline, 100 mg orally, twice daily for a minimum of 3 weeks. Alternative antibiotic regimens include the following: a minimum 3-week course of azithromycin, 1 g orally/week; ciprofloxacin, 750 mg orally twice daily; erythromycin base, 500 mg orally four times daily; or trimethoprim-sulfamethoxazole (TMP-SMZ), one double-strength tablet orally twice daily. Therapy should be continued until the lesions have healed completely. Alternative antibiotic therapy such as an aminoglycoside has been used

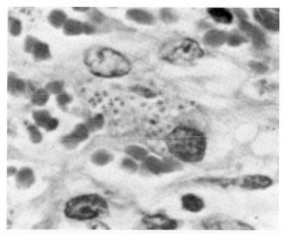

Figure 23-9 Donovanosis. Biopsy specimen shows intracytoplasmic Donovan bodies (H&E stain). (From Hart G: Donovanosis. In Holmes KK, Mårdh PA, Sparling PF, et al [eds]: Sexually Transmitted Diseases. New York, McGraw-Hill, 1984.)

in refractory cases. Rarely, medical therapy fails and surgical excision is required. Co-infection with another sexually transmitted pathogen is a distinct possibility. Sex partners of women who have granuloma inguinale should be examined if they have had sexual contact during the 60 days preceding the onset of symptoms.

Lymphogranuloma Venereum

Lymphogranuloma venereum (LGV) is a chronic infection of lymphatic tissue produced by *Chlamydia trachomatis*. It is found most commonly in the tropics. Cases occur infrequently in the United States, with fewer than 150 new cases being reported each year, most of which occur in men. In women, the vulva is the most frequent site of infection, but the urethra, rectum, and cervix may also be involved. This sexually transmitted infection is caused by serotypes L1, L2, and L3 of *C. trachomatis*. Serologic studies in high-risk populations have found that subclinical infection is common. The incubation period is between 3 and 30 days.

There are three distinct phases of vulvar and perirectal LGV. The primary infection is a shallow painless ulcer that heals rapidly without therapy. It is typically located on the vestibule or labia but occasionally in the periurethral or perirectal region. One to 4 weeks after the primary infection, a secondary phase marked by painful adenopathy develops in the inguinal and perirectal areas. Two thirds of women have unilateral adenopathy and 50% have systemic symptoms, including general malaise and fever. When the disease is untreated, the infected nodes become increasingly tender, enlarged, matted together, and adherent to overlying skin, forming a **bubo** (tender lymph nodes). A classic clinical sign of LGV is the double genitocrural fold, or **groove sign** (**Fig. 23-10**), a depression between groups of inflamed nodes. Within 7 to 15 days, the bubo will rupture

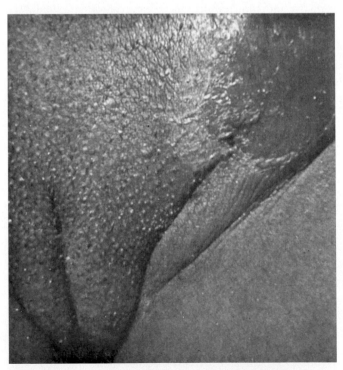

Figure 23-10 Lymphogranuloma venereum bubo with groove sign. (From Friedrich EG: Vulvar Disease, 2nd ed. Philadelphia, WB Saunders, 1983.)

spontaneously and form multiple draining sinuses and fistulas. These are classic signs of the tertiary phase of the infection. Extensive tissue destruction of the external genitalia and anorectal region may occur during the tertiary phase. This tissue destruction and secondary extensive scarring and fibrosis may result in elephantiasis, multiple fistulas, and stricture formation of the anal canal and rectum.

Diagnosis is established by detecting *C. trachomatis* by culture, direct immunofluorescence, or nucleic acid detection from the pus or aspirate from a tender lymph node. *Chlamydia* serology (complement fixation titers >1:64) can support the diagnosis in the appropriate clinical context. However, the diagnostic usefulness of serologic methods other than complement fixation and some microimmunofluorescence procedures remains unclear. In the absence of specific LGV diagnostic testing, patients should be treated based on the clinical presentation, including proctocolitis or genital ulcer disease with lymphadenopathy. The differential diagnosis of LGV includes syphilis, chancroid, granuloma inguinale, bacterial lymphadenitis, vulvar carcinoma, genital herpes, and Hodgkin's disease.

The CDC recommends doxycycline, 100 mg twice daily for at least 21 days, as the preferred treatment. An alternative therapy choice is erythromycin base, 500 mg four times daily orally for 21 days. Azithromycin, 1 g orally once weekly for 3 weeks, is probably effective, but clinical data are lacking. Fluoroquinolone-based treatments may also be effective, but extended treatment intervals are likely required.

Antibiotic therapy cures the bacterial infection and prevents further tissue destruction. However, fluctuant nodes should be aspirated to prevent sinus formation. Rarely, incision and drainage of infected nodes is necessary to alleviate inguinal pain. The late sequelae of the destructive tertiary phase of LGV often require extensive surgical reconstruction. It is important to administer antibiotics during the perioperative period.

Chancroid

Chancroid is a sexually transmitted, acute, ulcerative disease of the vulva caused by *Haemophilus ducreyi*, a highly contagious, small, nonmotile, gram-negative rod. Chancroid is a common disease in developing countries, but infrequent in the United States. Epidemiologic studies have suggested that chancroid tends to occur in clusters and may account for a substantial portion of genital ulcer cases when present. However, difficulty in making the diagnosis may cause underreporting. The clinical importance of chancroid has been enhanced by recent reports that the genital ulcers of chancroid facilitate the transmission of HIV infection.

The soft chancre of chancroid is always painful and tender. In comparison, the hard chancre of syphilis is usually asymptomatic. On Gram stain, this facultative anaerobic bacterium exhibits a classic appearance of streptobacillary chains, or what has been described as an extracellular school of fish. The incubation period is short, usually 3 to 6 days. Tissue trauma and excoriation of the skin must precede initial infection because *H. ducreyi* is unable to penetrate and invade normal skin.

The initial lesion is a small papule. Within 48 to 72 hours, the papule evolves into a pustule and subsequently ulcerates. The extremely painful ulcers are shallow, with a characteristic ragged edge, and usually occur in the vulvar vestibule and rarely in the vagina or cervix. The ulcers have a dirty, gray, necrotic, foul-smelling exudate and lack induration at the base (the soft chancre). Multiple papules and ulcers may be in different phases of maturation secondary to autoinoculation. Within 2 weeks of an untreated infection, approximately 50% of women develop acutely tender inguinal adenopathy, a bubo, which is typically unilateral. Fluctuant nodes should be treated by needle aspiration to prevent rupture or by incision and drainage if larger than 5 cm.

A definitive diagnosis of chancroid requires the identification of *H. ducreyi* on special culture media that are not widely available from commercial sources; even when these media are used, sensitivity is less than 80%. No FDA-approved PCR test for *H. ducreyi* is available in the United States, but this testing can be performed by clinical laboratories that have developed their own PCR test and conducted a Clinical Laboratory Improvement Amendments (CLIA) verification study. Sometimes, the clinical diagnosis is made in a woman with painful vulvar ulcers after excluding other common STIs that produce vulvar ulcers, including genital herpes, syphilis, LGV, and donovanosis.

Because of antibiotic resistance to tetracyclines and sulfonamides, the CDC recommends the following: azithromycin, 1 g orally in a single dose; ceftriaxone, 250 mg IM in a single dose; ciprofloxacin, 500 mg orally twice daily for 3 days; or erythromycin base, 500 mg orally three times daily for 7 days. Sexual partners should be treated in a similar fashion. Successful antibiotic therapy results in symptomatic and objective improvement within 5 to 7 days of initiating therapy. Large ulcers may require 2 to 3 weeks to heal, with clinical resolution of lymphadenopathy slower than that of ulcers. Bubos respond at a slower rate than skin ulcers. Approximately 10% of women whose ulcers initially heal have a recurrence at the same site. Women with HIV infection have an increased rate of failure to the standard treatments for chancroid and therefore often require more prolonged therapy. Co-infection with another ulcer causing an STI should be considered, especially in women lacking an appropriate response to treatment.

Syphilis

Syphilis is a chronic, complex systemic disease produced by the spirochete *Treponema pallidum*. The infection initially involves mucous membranes. Syphilis remains one of the important STIs in the United States, and epidemiologists speculate that only one of four new cases of syphilis is reported. Early syphilis is a cofactor in the transmission and acquisition of HIV and, currently, 25% of new syphilis cases occur in persons coinfected with HIV. Even with mandatory screening, congenital syphilis continues to be a public health problem. Mothers who experience the tragedy of stillbirth or neonatal death from syphilis usually have not received prenatal care. Syphilis should be included in the differential diagnosis of all genital ulcers and cutaneous rashes of unknown origin, and all women diagnosed with syphilis should be screened for HIV.

T. pallidum is an anaerobic, elongated, tightly wound spirochete. Because of its extreme thinness, it is difficult to detect by light microscopy. Therefore, the presence of spirochetes is diagnosed by use of specially adapted techniques, **dark-field microscopy** or direct fluorescent antibody tests (**Fig. 23-11**). These organisms have the ability to penetrate skin or mucous membranes. The incubation period is from 10 to 90 days, with an average of 3 weeks. They replicate every 30 to 36 hours, which accounts for the comparatively long incubation period.

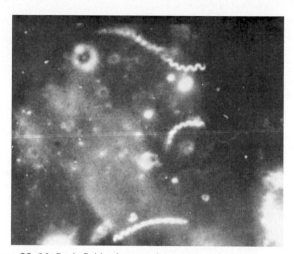

Figure 23-11 Dark-field microscopic appearance of *Treponema pallidum*. (From Larsen SA, McGrew BE, Hunter EF, et al: Syphilis serology and dark field microscopy. In Holmes KK, Mårdh PA, Sparling PF, et al [eds]: Sexually Transmitted Diseases. New York, McGraw-Hill, 1984.)

Syphilis is a moderately contagious disease. Approximately 3% to 10% of patients contract the disease from a single sexual encounter with an infected partner. Similar studies have documented that 30% of individuals become infected during a 1-month exposure to a sexual partner with primary or secondary syphilis. Patients are contagious during primary, secondary, and probably the first year of latent syphilis. Syphilis can be spread by kissing or touching a person who has an active lesion on the lips, oral cavity, breast, or genitals. Case transmission can occur with oral-genital contact.

The diagnosis of syphilis is complicated by the fact that the organism cannot be cultivated in vitro. Hence, serologic tests have been the foundation of screening programs to detect early syphilis. There are two types of serologic tests, the nonspecific nontreponemal and the specific antitreponemal antibody tests. The nonspecific tests, such as the VDRL (Venereal Disease Research Laboratory) slide test and the RPR (rapid plasma reagin) card test are inexpensive and easy to perform. They are used as screening tests for the disease, typically become positive 4 to 6 weeks after exposure, and are also a useful index of treatment response. These tests evaluate the woman's serum for the presence of reagin IgG and IgM antibodies as they react with an antigen from beef heart. Quantitative nontreponemal antibody titers usually correlate with the activity of the disease. Serologic testing is an indirect method of diagnosis because it relies on a humoral immune response to infection. As such, it has some inherent limitations. Approximately 1% of patients have technical or biologic false-positive results with the nonspecific tests. Many conditions produce biologic false-positive results, including a recent febrile illness, pregnancy, immunization, chronic active hepatitis, malaria, sarcoidosis, IV drug use, HIV infection, advancing age, acute herpes simplex, and autoimmune diseases such as lupus erythematosus or rheumatoid arthritis. Biologic false-positive serum tests usually are associated with extremely low titers (< 1:8). A false-negative result is a possibility, occurring in approximately 1% to 2% of tests. This negative reaction occurs in women in whom there is an excess of anticardiolipin antibody in the serum, termed the ***prozone phenomenon***.

Table 23-2 Potential Causes of Biologic False-Positive Results in Syphilis Serology

Cause	Acute	Chronic
		BFP Reaction
Physiologic	Pregnancy	Advanced age, multiple blood transfusions
Infectious	Varicella, vaccinia, measles, mumps, infectious mononucleosis, herpes simplex, viral hepatitis, HIV seroconversion illness, cytomegalovirus, pneumococcal pneumonia, *Mycoplasma* pneumonia, chancroid, lymphogranuloma venereum, psittacosis, bacterial endocarditis, scarlet fever, rickettsial infections, toxoplasmosis, Lyme disease, leptospirosis, relapsing fever, rat bite fever	HIV, tropical spastic paraparesis, leprosy,* tuberculosis, malaria,* lymphogranuloma venereum, trypanosomiasis,* kala-azar*
Vaccinations	Smallpox, typhoid, yellow fever	
Autoimmune disease		Systemic lupus erythematosus, discoid lupus, drug-induced lupus, autoimmune hemolytic anemia, polyarteritis nodosa, rheumatoid arthritis, Sjögren's syndrome, Hashimoto's thyroiditis, mixed connective tissue disease, primary biliary cirrhosis, chronic liver disease, idiopathic thrombocytopenic purpura
Other		IV drug use, advanced malignancy hypergammaglobulinemia, lymphoproliferative disease

*BFP reaction resolves with resolution of infection.
BFP, Biologic false-positive; HIV, human immunodeficiency virus.
Data from Nandwani R, Evans DTP: Are you sure it's syphilis? A review of false-positive serology. Int J STD AIDS 1995; 6:241; and Hook EW III, Marra CM: Acquired syphilis in adults. N Engl J Med 1992; 326:1062.

Women with immunocompromise also may have false-negative tests because of their inability to produce the antibodies detected by these screening tests.

If a nonspecific test result is positive, the significance of this result must be confirmed by a specific antitreponemal test. Specific tests are more sensitive; however, occasionally, they may produce false-positive results. Most false-positive results occur in women with lupus erythematosus (**Table 23-2**). The standard for specific tests had been the TPI (*Treponema* immobilization) test. It has largely been replaced by the FTA-ABS (fluorescent-labeled *Treponema* antibody absorption) test and the MHA-TP (microhemagglutination assay for antibodies to *T. pallidum*). The MHA-TP does not have as high a rate of false-positive results as the FTA-ABS. A woman with a positive reactive treponemal test usually will have this positive reaction for her lifetime, regardless of treatment or activity of the disease.

Clinically, syphilis is divided into primary, secondary, and tertiary stages. In primary syphilis, a papule, which is usually painless, appears at the site of inoculation 2 to 3 weeks after exposure. This soon ulcerates to produce the classic finding of primary syphilis, a chancre that is a painless ulcer, 1 to 2 cm, with a raised indurated margin and a nonexudative base (**Fig. 23-12**). Usually, the chancre is solitary, painless, and found on the vulva, vagina, or cervix, although extragenital primary lesions, including lesions of the mouth, anal canal, and breast nipple, have been reported in approximately 5% of patients. Nontender and firm regional adenopathy is present during the first week of clinical disease. Within 2 to 6 weeks, the painless ulcer heals spontaneously. Hence, many women do not seek treatment, a feature that enhances the likelihood of transmission. Confirmation that the ulcer is primary or secondary syphilis depends on the identification of *T. pallidum* by dark-field microscopy from wet smears of the ulcer. Special preparations must be made to obtain suitable smears. It is important to clean and abrade the ulcer with gauze before obtaining the serum for the slides. At the time of dark-field identification of *T. pallidum* from a primary chancre,

approximately 70% of women will have a positive serologic test. If the serologic test result remains negative for 3 months, it is unlikely that the ulcer was syphilis. Syphilis is not frequently diagnosed in the primary stage in women.

If primary syphilis is untreated, approximately 25% of individuals develop secondary syphilis, which is the result of hematogenous dissemination of the spirochetes. Secondary syphilis is a systemic disease that develops between 6 weeks and 6 months (average, 9 weeks) after the primary chancre. The stages are not exclusive. Approximately 25% of women still have a primary chancre when the secondary lesions appear. An untreated attack of secondary syphilis will last 2 to 6 weeks and a multitude of systemic symptoms may occur, depending on the major organs involved, such as rash, fever, headache, malaise, lymphadenopathy, and anorexia. The classic rash of secondary syphilis is red macules and papules over the palms of the hands and the soles of the feet (**Fig. 23-13**). Vulvar lesions of **condyloma latum** are large, raised, flattened, grayish-white areas (**Fig. 23-14**). On wet surfaces of the vulva, soft papules often coalesce to form ulcers. These ulcers are larger than herpetic ulcers and are not tender unless secondarily infected. A woman with syphilis is most infectious during the first 1 to 2 years of disease, with decreasing infectivity thereafter.

The latent stage of syphilis follows the secondary stage and varies in duration from 2 to 20 years; it is characterized as positive serology without symptoms or signs of disease. Women with syphilis in the primary or secondary stages and during the first year of latent syphilis are believed to be infectious. Most women diagnosed with syphilis are detected via positive blood tests during the latent stage of the disease. Early latent syphilis is an infection of 1 year or less. All other cases are referred to as late latent or latent syphilis of unknown duration. Women who have been sexually active with latent syphilis should have a pelvic examination to discover potential lesions involving the vagina or cervix.

The tertiary phase of syphilis is devastating in its potentially destructive effects on the central nervous, cardiovascular, and musculoskeletal systems. Tertiary syphilis develops in

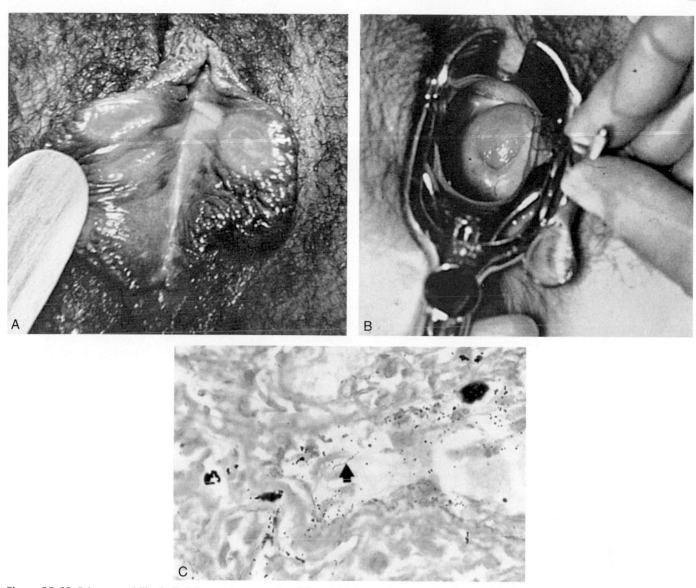

Figure 23-12 Primary syphilis. **A, B,** Primary chancres of syphilis, which began as a papule, erode, and develop into painless ulcers with raised, firm, indurated borders and a clean smooth base. **C,** silver staining reveals a spirochete 6 to 15 μm in length with regularly spaced spiral coils (*arrow*). (**A, B** from U.S. Public Health Service: Syphilis: A Synopsis. Washington, DC, U.S. Government Printing Office, 1967, pp 47, 50; **C** from Wong TY, Mihm MC Jr: Images in clinical medicine. Primary syphilis. N Engl J Med 331:1492, 1994.)

approximately 33% of patients who are not appropriately treated during the primary, secondary, or latent phases of the disease (**Fig. 23-15**). The manifestations of late syphilis include optic atrophy, tabes dorsalis, generalized paresis, aortic aneurysm, and **gummas** of the skin and bones. A gumma is similar to a cold abscess, with a necrotic center and the obliteration of small vessels by endarteritis.

Parenteral penicillin G is the drug of choice for syphilis. *T. pallidum* is exquisitely sensitive to penicillin. However, because of the slow replication time of the spirochete, blood levels must be maintained for 7 to 14 days. The CDC recommends 2.4 million units of benzathine penicillin G IM in one dose for early syphilis (primary and early latent secondary syphilis). Patients who are allergic to penicillin should receive oral tetracycline, 500 mg every 6 hours for 14 days, or doxycycline, 100 mg orally twice a day for 2 weeks. Standard treatment protocols for syphilis are detailed in **Box 23-2**. Approximately 60% of women

develop an acute febrile reaction associated with flulike symptoms such as headache and myalgia within the first 24 hours after parenteral penicillin therapy for early syphilis. This response is known as the Jarisch-Herxheimer reaction.

All women with early syphilis should be reexamined clinically and serologically at 6 and 12 months following therapy. With successful therapy in early syphilis, the titer should decline fourfold in 6 months and become negative within 12 months. Women with latent syphilis should have quantitative nontreponemal serologic tests 6, 12, and 24 months following therapy. During the first 3 to 4 years of the latent phase, a woman may experience relapses of secondary syphilis. Women who have a sustained fourfold increase in nontreponemal test titers have failed treatment or become reinfected. They should be retreated and evaluated for concurrent HIV infection. When women are retreated, the recommendation is three weekly injections of benzathine penicillin G, 2.4 million units IM. For long-term

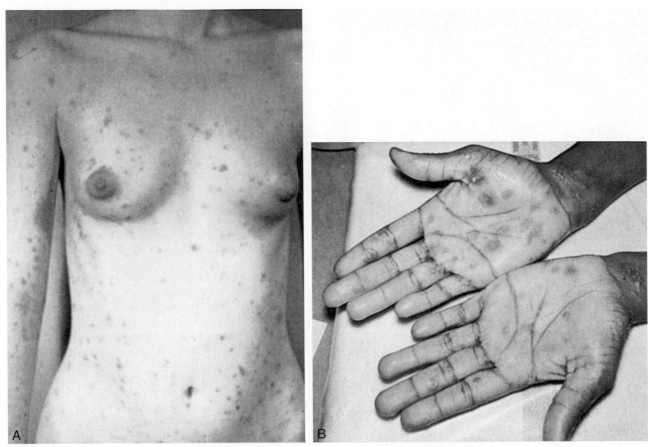

Figure 23-13 Rash of secondary syphilis. **A,** Common presentation on the trunk and arms. **B,** Red maculopapular lesions involve palms and soles. From Kissane JM: Bacterial diseases. In Kissane JM [ed]: Anderson's Pathology. St. Louis, Mosby–Year Book, 1985.)

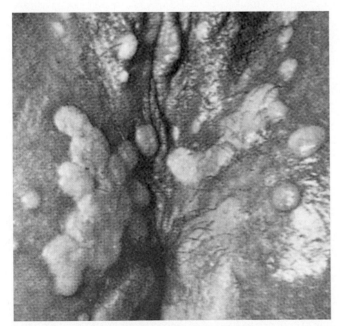

Figure 23-14 Multiple lesions of condylomata lata on vulva and perineum. Dark-field microscopic findings were positive.
(From Faro S: Sexually transmitted diseases. In Kaufman RH, Faro S [eds]: Benign Diseases of the Vulva and Vagina, 4th ed. St. Louis, Mosby–Year Book, 1994.)

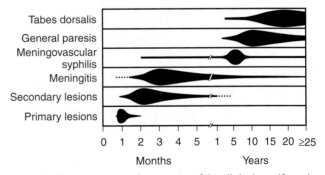

Figure 23-15 Approximate time course of the clinical manifestations of early syphilis and neurosyphilis. *Shaded areas* corresponding to each syndrome represent the approximate proportion of patients with the syndrome specified and do not indicate the proportion of all patients with syphilis who have that syndrome. (From Hook EW III, Marra CM: Acquired syphilis in adults. N Engl J Med 326:1060, 1992.)

follow-up, the same serologic tests should be ordered. Optimally, the test should be obtained from the same laboratory. The VDRL and RPR tests are equally valid, but RPR titers tend to be slightly higher than VDRL titers. With successful treatment, the VDRL titer will become nonreactive or, at most, be reactive, with a lower titer within 1 year. There is a 1% to 2% chance that the woman will not exhibit a fourfold titer decline and these cases are considered therapeutic failures. They should

Box 23-2 CDC Recommended Treatment of Syphilis (2010)

Early Syphilis (primary, secondary, and early latent syphilis of less than 1 year's duration)

Recommended regimen: Benzathine penicillin G, 2.4 million U IM, one dose

Alternative regimen (penicillin-allergic nonpregnant patients): Doxycycline, 100 mg orally bid for 2 wk *or* tetracycline, 500 mg orally qid for 2 wk

Late Latent Syphilis (>1 year's duration, gummas, and cardiovascular syphilis)

Recommended regimen: Benzathine penicillin G, 7.2 million U total, administered as three doses of 2.4 million U IM at 1-wk intervals

Alternative regimen (penicillin-allergic nonpregnant patients): Doxycycline 100 mg orally 2 times a day for 2 wk if < 1 year, otherwise, for 4 wk; *or* tetracycline, 500 mg orally qid for 2 wk if < 1 year; otherwise, for 4 wk

Neurosyphilis

Recommended regimen: Aqueous crystalline penicillin G, 18-24 million U daily, administered as 3-4 million U IV every 4 hr, for 10-14 days

Alternative regimen: Procaine penicillin, 2.4 million U IM daily, for 10-14 days plus probenecid, 500 mg PO qid for 10-14 days

Syphilis in Pregnancy

Recommended regimen: Penicillin regimen appropriate for stage of syphilis. Some experts recommend additional therapy (e.g., second dose of benzathine penicillin, 2.4 million U IM) 1 wk after the initial dose for those who have primary, secondary, or early latent syphilis.

Alternative regimen (penicillin allergy): Pregnant women with a history of penicillin allergy should be skin-tested and desensitized.

Syphilis in HIV-Infected Patients

Primary and secondary syphilis: Benzathine penicillin G, 2.4 million U IM. Some experts recommend additional treatments, such as three weekly doses of benzathine penicillin G, as in late syphilis. Penicillin-allergic patients should be desensitized and treated with penicillin.

Latent syphilis (normal CSF examination): Benzathine penicillin G, 7.2 million U as three weekly doses of 2.4 million U each

CSF, Cerebrospinal fluid.

Workowski KA, Berman S; Centers for Disease Control and Prevention (CDC): Sexually transmitted diseases treatment guidelines, MMWR 59(RR-12):26-36, 2010.

be retreated. Patients with syphilis lasting longer than 1 year should have quantitative VDRL titers for 2 years following therapy because their titers will decline more slowly. A specific test for syphilis, such as the FTA-ABS, remains reactive indefinitely. In summary, all women with a first attack of primary syphilis should have a negative nonspecific serology within 1 year, and women treated for secondary syphilis should have a negative serology within 2 years. If they are not, treatment failure, reinfection, and concurrent HIV infection should be investigated.

Syphilis often involves the CNS. The diagnosis is complicated and there is no established diagnostic test that is a gold standard for neurosyphilis. All women with suspected neurosyphilis should be tested for HIV infection. The diagnosis of neurosyphilis is based on a combination of clinical findings, reactive serologic tests, and abnormalities of cerebrospinal fluid, serology, cell count, or protein. Infection of the CNS by spirochetes may occur during any stage of syphilis. Women should undergo a cerebrospinal fluid examination if they develop neurologic or ophthalmologic signs or symptoms, evidence of active tertiary syphilis, treatment failures, and HIV infection with late latent syphilis or syphilis of an unknown duration. To treat neurosyphilis, the CDC recommends aqueous crystalline penicillin G, 18 to 24 million units daily, administered as 3 to 4 million units IV every 4 hours for 10 to 14 days. An alternative regimen is procaine penicillin, 2.4 million units IM daily, plus probenecid, 500 mg orally four times daily for 10 to 14 days. The duration of both these regimens for neurosyphilis is shorter than that of the regimen used for late syphilis in the absence of neurosyphilis. Therefore, some experts administer benzathine penicillin, 2.4 million units IM, after completion of either regimen to provide a comparable total duration of therapy.

It is important for all women with syphilis to be tested for HIV infection. Simultaneous syphilis and HIV infections alter the natural history of syphilis, with earlier involvement of the CNS. Women with HIV infection may have a slightly increased rate of treatment failure with currently recommended regimens. Similarly, they may exhibit unusual serologic responses. Usually, serologic titers are higher than expected. However, false-negative serologic tests or delayed appearance of seroreactivity has been reported. Nevertheless, the CDC's recommendation for treating early syphilis in women is the same whether or not they are concurrently infected with HIV. Following penicillin treatment for syphilis, women with HIV should be followed with quantitative titers at more frequent intervals—for example, at 3, 6, 9, 12, and 24 months following therapy.

Sexual partners of women with syphilis in any stage should be evaluated clinically and serologically. The time intervals used to identify an at-risk sex partner are 3 months plus duration of symptoms for primary syphilis, 3 months plus duration of symptoms for secondary syphilis, and 1 year for early latent syphilis. Those who are exposed within the 90 days preceding the diagnosis of primary, secondary, or early latent syphilis in their sexual partners should be treated presumptively because they may be infected, even if seronegative.

VULVAR IRRITATION CAUSED BY VAGINITIS

Anatomic distribution of symptoms occasionally creates a semantic misinterpretation of the clinical reality. This is true for vulvar disease. The sensory nerve endings are more numerous in the vulvar skin than in the vagina. Hence, the presence of excessive vaginal fluid is not appreciated until the fluid flows from the vagina onto the vulva. Also, women whose chief complaint is vaginal itching or burning may have symptoms caused by irritation of the vestibule and adjacent vulvar epithelium. Thus, the first symptom of vaginal infection is often vulvar pruritus and the first sign of vaginal infection may be secondary erythema and edema of the vulvar skin.

A semantic compromise is to refer to most vaginal infections as vulvovaginitis. This is especially true with candidiasis. There is a separate clinical entity of primary cutaneous candidiasis, but it is rare and is most often found in women with diabetes mellitus. The skin involvement of primary candidiasis is most prominent on the labia and genitocrural folds. In this condition, the vulva appears beefy red, the labia are edematous, and the skin of the vulva has fissures and often small vesicles and pustules.

The differential diagnosis for women with symptoms of vulvovaginitis is complex. Discharge, burning, and pruritus are the common symptoms, and signs of vulvar irritation include erythema and excoriation of the vulvar skin. Discharge may be caused by a cervical or vaginal infection. Vulvar irritation may be produced by primary or secondary infections, primary skin irritant, or contact dermatitis. Vaginal spermicides, soaps, perfumes, and feminine hygiene sprays can cause skin irritation, as can self-medication for a vaginal infection. Physiologic fluids such as urine and normal cervical secretions and vaginal fluid may cause maceration of the vulvar skin when the epithelium remains constantly moist. Hence, emphasis on keeping the vulvar skin dry can help alleviate the symptoms of vulvovaginitis. The woman should be encouraged to wear loose-fitting cotton undergarments.

The clinical symptoms of vulvovaginitis are usually not helpful in establishing the cause. Physical examination, including vulvar skin inspection and microscopic examination of cervical and vaginal secretions, is necessary.

VAGINITIS

Vaginal discharge is the most common symptom in gynecology. Other symptoms associated with vaginal infection include superficial dyspareunia, dysuria, odor, and vulvar burning and pruritus. The three common infections of the vagina are produced by the following: (1) a fungus (candidiasis); (2) a protozoon (*Trichomonas*); and (3) a disruption of the vaginal bacterial ecosystem leading to bacterial vaginosis. Relative prevalence differs depending on the population studied; in a group of middle-class women in the reproductive range, bacterial vaginosis represents approximately 50% of cases, whereas candidiasis and *Trichomonas* infection each constitute approximately 25% of cases. Vaginal discharge resulting from viral infections such as herpes was discussed earlier in this chapter. Vaginitis in prepubertal and postmenopausal women is discussed elsewhere in the text in Chapter 12 (Pediatric and Adolescent Gynecology) and Chapter 14 (Menopause and Care of the Mature Woman).

Accurate diagnosis of vaginitis is critical. HIV acquisition is increased in women with *Trichomonas* vaginitis or bacterial vaginosis. Hence, timely diagnosis with appropriate treatment is paramount.

The vaginal environment has been described as a dynamic and delicate ecosystem. The normal vaginal pH is approximately 4.0 in premenopausal women. The maintenance of an optimum pH balance involves a complex interplay of hormonal, microbiologic, and other unknown factors. In women of reproductive age, estrogen stimulates the glycogen content of vaginal epithelial cells. The glycogen is metabolized to lactic acid and other short-chain organic acids, principally by the lactobacilli but also by other vaginal bacteria and enzymes. *Lactobacillus,* an aerobic, gram-positive rod, is found in 62% to 88% of asymptomatic women and is the regulator of normal vaginal flora. Lactobacilli make lactic acid, which maintains the normal vaginal pH of 3.8 to 4.5 and inhibits the adherence of bacteria to vaginal epithelial cells. Approximately 60% of vaginal lactobacilli strains make hydrogen peroxide, which inhibits the growth of bacteria and destroys HIV in vitro. Estrogen improves lactobacilli concentration by enhancing the vaginal epithelial cell production of glycogen, which breaks down into glucose and acts as a substrate for the bacteria.

One of the most helpful diagnostic aids in the differential diagnosis of vaginitis is the measurement of vaginal acidity with pH indicator paper. A vaginal pH higher than 5.0 indicates bacterial vaginosis or *Trichomonas* infection, or possibly an atrophic vaginal discharge. A vaginal pH less than 4.5 represents a physiologic discharge or fungal infection, although fungal infection can occur concurrently with bacterial vaginosis or *Trichomonas*. Cervical mucus, vaginal fluids produced during sexual excitement, and semen all have a neutral or basic pH and may temporarily change the normal acidity. Semen has been found to buffer vaginal acidity for 6 to 8 hours following intercourse. The vaginal pH is slightly higher in postmenopausal than in premenopausal women.

Normal physiologic vaginal discharge consists of cervical and vaginal epithelial cells, normal bacterial flora, water, electrolytes, and other chemicals. The quantitative concentration of bacterial organisms is 10^8 to 10^9 colonies/mL of vaginal fluid. The concentrations of anaerobic and aerobic bacteria vary considerably during the menstrual cycle. Qualitatively, the number of bacterial species may vary from 17 to 29. Anaerobic bacteria are quantitatively the most prevalent, five times more common than aerobic bacteria.

In addition to lactobacilli, other common aerobic bacteria found in the vagina are diphtheroids, streptococci, *Staphylococcus epidermidis,* and *Gardnerella vaginalis.* The most common gram-negative bacillus is *Escherichia coli.* Anaerobic bacteria have been detected in approximately 80% of women, with the most prevalent being *Peptococcus, Peptostreptococcus,* and *Bacteroides* spp. (**Table 23-3**). *Candida* spp. and mycoplasmas are also common inhabitants of asymptomatic women. Our knowledge of vaginal flora has traditionally relied on classic microbiology. Newer molecular techniques are demonstrating even greater complexity in vaginal flora.

The clinical diagnosis of vaginitis depends on the examination of the vaginal secretions under the microscope and measurement of the vaginal pH. Nevertheless, it is helpful to generalize about the classic characteristics of normal secretions and the three common vaginal infections (**Table 23-4**).

Table 23-3 Bacterial Vaginal Flora in Asymptomatic Women without Vaginitis

Organism	Range of Recovery (%)
Facultative Organisms	
Gram-positive rods	
Lactobacilli	50-75
Diphtheroids	40
Gram-Positive Cocci	
Staphylococcus epidemidis	40-55
Staphylococcus aureus	0-5
Beta-hemolytic streptococci	20
Group D streptococci	35-55
Gram-Negative Organisms	
Escherichia coli	10-30
Klebsiella spp.	10
Other organisms	2-10
Anaerobic Organisms	
Peptococcus spp.	5-65
Peptostreptococcus spp.	25-35
Bacteroides spp.	20-40
Bacteroides fragilis	5-15
Fusobacterium spp.	5-25
Clostridium spp.	5-20
Eubacterium spp.	5-35
Veillonella spp.	10-30

From Eschenbach DA: Vaginal infection. Clin Obstet Gynecol 26:187, 1983.

Table 23-4 Typical Features of Vaginitis

Condition	Symptoms and Signs*	Findings on Examination*	pH	Wet Mount	Comment
Bacterial vaginosis†	Increased discharge (white, thin), Increased odor	Thin, whitish gray, homogeneous discharge, cocci, sometimes frothy	>4.5	Clue cells (>20%) shift in flora Amine odor after adding potassium hydroxide to wet mount	Greatly decreased lactobacilli Greatly increased cocci Small curved rods
Candidiasis	Increased discharge (white, thick)‡ Dysuria Pruritus Burning	Thick, curdy discharge Vaginal erythema	<4.5	Hyphae or spores	Can be mixed infection with bacterial vaginosis, *T. vaginalis*, or both, and have higher pH
Trichomoniasis§	Increased discharge (yellow, frothy) Increased odor Dysuria Pruritus	Yellow, frothy discharge, with or without vaginal or cervical erythema	>4.5	Motile trichomonads Increased white cells	More symptoms at higher vaginal pH

*Although these features are typical, their sensitivity and specificity are generally inadequate for diagnosis.
†For a diagnosis of bacterial vaginosis, a report of increased discharge has a sensitivity of 50% and a specificity of 49%; odor, a sensitivity of 49% and a specificity of 20%; and pH > 4.7, a sensitivity of 97% and a specificity of 65%, compared with the use of a Gram stain.
‡Of patients presenting with symptoms of vaginitis, 40% report increased (white) discharge, but this discharge is not related to *Candida albicans* in many studies.
§A report of a yellow discharge has a sensitivity of 42% and a specificity of 80%; a frothy discharge on examination has a sensitivity of 8% and a specificity of 99%.
From Eckert LO: Clinical practice: Acute vulvovaginitis. N Engl J Med 355:1246, 2006.

Normal vaginal secretions are white, floccular or curdy, and odorless. In a woman with a normal or physiologic discharge, it is important to note that the vaginal discharge is present only in the dependent portions of the vagina. Pathologic discharges usually involve the anterior and lateral walls of the vagina. It should be emphasized that vaginal discharge characteristics, especially the amount of discharge, are insensitive and nonspecific diagnostic criteria for vaginitis. However, thick, white, curdy, patchy discharge, when present, is highly associated with fungal infections. Gray-white discharges that are thin and usually profuse suggest a differential diagnosis of *Trichomonas* or bacterial vaginosis, as do vaginal discharges that have a foul odor. The odor secondary to necrotic gynecologic tumors of the lower genital tract may be minimized by treating the woman topically for bacterial vaginosis.

BACTERIAL VAGINOSIS

Bacterial vaginosis reflects a shift in vaginal flora from lactobacilli-dominant to mixed flora, including genital mycoplasmas, *G. vaginalis*, and anaerobes, such as peptostreptococci, and *Prevotella* and *Mobiluncus* spp. Although *Gardnerella* and anaerobic organisms can be found in women with normal vaginal flora, their concentration increases several-fold in women with bacterial vaginosis concurrent with a marked decrease in lactobacilli.

The origin of bacterial vaginosis remains elusive. No causative agent has been identified. Because of the inability to find a transmissible agent, bacterial vaginosis has not been classified as an STI. However, risk factors for bacterial vaginosis include new or multiple sexual partners. It is also prevalent in women who have sex with women; genotyping has revealed identical bacterial strains between monogamous lesbian partners. Also, bacterial vaginosis is more common in lesbian couples who share sex toys with each other without cleaning the toys between use. Recently, molecular techniques have identified a cluster of noncultivable bacteria related to *Clostridium* in women with bacterial vaginosis. As newer techniques analyzing vaginal flora evolve, it may be

possible to determine a causal agent. Currently, bacterial vaginosis is described as a "sexually associated" infection rather than a true sexually transmitted infection.

Other risk factors include douching as least monthly or within the prior 7 days, and social stressors (e.g., homelessness, threats to personal safety, insufficient financial resources) have been reported to increase risk. A lack of hydrogen peroxide–producing lactobacilli is also a recognized risk factor for bacterial vaginosis and may explain, in part, the higher prevalence of bacterial vaginosis in black women independent of other risk factors. Bacterial vaginosis is the most prevalent cause of symptomatic vaginitis, with a prevalence of approximately 15% to 50%.

Histologically, there is an absence of inflammation in biopsies of the vagina—thus, the term *vaginosis* rather than vaginitis. Bacterial vaginosis has been associated with upper tract infections, including endometritis, pelvic inflammatory disease, postoperative vaginal cuff cellulitis, and multiple complications of infection during pregnancy, such as preterm rupture of the membranes, endomyometritis, decreased success with in vitro fertilization, and increased pregnancy loss of less than 20 weeks' gestation.

In women with bacterial vaginosis, the most frequent symptom is an unpleasant vaginal odor, which patients describe as musty or fishy (**Table 23-5**). The odor is often sensed following intercourse, when the alkaline semen results in a release of aromatic amines.

The vaginal discharge associated with bacterial vaginosis is thin and gray-white. The consistency of the discharge is similar to a thin paste made from flour. Speculum examination reveals that the discharge is mildly adherent to the vaginal walls, in contrast to a physiologic discharge, which is discovered in the most dependent areas of the vagina. The vaginal discharge is frothy in approximately 10% of women and it is rare to have associated pruritus or vulvar irritation.

Bacterial vaginosis is clinically diagnosed. The classic findings on wet smear are clumps of bacteria and clue cells, which are

Table 23-5 Diagnostic Tests Available for Vaginitis

Test	Sensitivity (%)	Specificity (%)	Comments
Bacterial Vaginosis			
pH > 4.5	97	64	
Amsel's criteria	92	77	Must meet three of four clinical criteria (pH > 4.5, thin watery discharge, >20% clue cells, positive whiff test), but similar results achieved if two of four criteria meet Nugent criteria. Gram stain morphology score (1-10) based on lactobacilli and other morphotypes; score of 1-3 indicates normal flora, score of 7-10 bacterial vaginosis; high interobserver reproducibility
Pap smear	49	93	
Point-of-care tests			
QuickVue Advance, pH + amines	89	96	Positive if pH > 4.7
QuickVue Advance, *G. vaginalis**	91	>95	Tests for proline iminopeptidase activity in vaginal fluid; if used when pH > 4.5, sensitivity is 95% and specificity is 99%
OSOM BV blue*	90	<95	Tests for vaginal sialidase activity
Candida			
Wet mount			
Overall	50	97	
Growth of 3-4+ on culture	85		*C. albicans* a commensal agent in 15%-20% of women
Growth of 1+ on culture	23		
pH ≤ 4.5	Usual		If symptoms present, pH may be elevated if mixed infection with bacterial vaginosis or *T. vaginalis* present
Pap smear	25	72	
Trichomonas vaginalis			
Wet mount	45-60	95	Increased visibility of microorganisms with a higher burden of infection
Culture	85-90	>95	
pH > 4.5	56	50	
Pap smear	92	61	False-positive rate of 8% for standard Pap test and 4% for liquid-based cytologic test
Point-of-care test: OSOM	83	98.8	10 min required to perform tests for *T. vaginalis* antigens

From Eckert LO: Clinical practice: Acute vulvovaginitis. N Engl J Med 355:1246, 2006.

vaginal epithelial cells with clusters of bacteria adherent to their external surfaces (**Fig. 23-16**). Leukocytes are not nearly as frequent as epithelial cells underneath the microscope.

The four criteria for the diagnosis of bacterial vaginosis are as follows: (1) a homogeneous vaginal discharge is present; (2) the vaginal discharge has a pH of 4.5 or higher; (3) the vaginal discharge has an amine-like odor when mixed with potassium

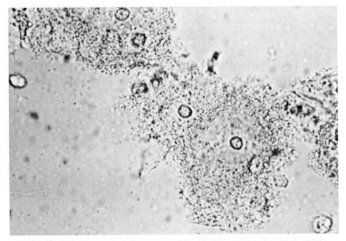

Figure 23-16 Vaginal epithelial cells from woman with bacterial vaginosis. These are typical clue cells, heavily covered by coccobacilli, with loss of distinct cell margins (×400). (From Holmes KK: Lower genital tract infections in women: Cystitis/urethritis, vulvovaginitis, and cervicitis. In Holmes KK, Mårdh PA, Sparling PF, et al [eds]: Sexually Transmitted Diseases. New York, McGraw-Hill, 1984.)

hydroxide, the **whiff test**; and (4) a wet smear of the vaginal discharge demonstrates clue cells more than 20% of the number of the vaginal epithelial cells. For the clinician, three of these four criteria are sufficient for a presumptive diagnosis. Ironically, 50% of women who have three of the four clinical criteria for bacterial vaginosis are asymptomatic. If readily available, Gram staining of vaginal secretion is an excellent diagnostic method. A colorimetric test that detects proline iminopeptidase has been developed for office use. Enzyme levels in vaginal fluid are elevated in women with bacterial vaginosis.

A positive whiff test may be obtained with bacterial vaginosis or *Trichomonas* infection. It is usually more prominent with bacterial infections because of the degree of anaerobic metabolism. The common aromatic amines are cadaverine and putrescine, both of which result from anaerobic metabolism. It should be stressed that vaginal bacterial culture has no role in the evaluation of bacterial vaginosis.

Because there are no effective means of replacing lactobacilli, the treatment for bacterial vaginosis is to decrease anaerobes with antibiotic therapy and hope the woman will then regenerate her own lactobacilli. **Table 23-6** provides treatment options. Cure rates are comparable; the agent used should depend on the woman's preference and cost factors. Treatment results in an 80% symptomatic and 70% microbiologic cure at 1 month. Single-dose oral therapy of 2 g of metronidazole is no longer recommended because of high failure rates. alternative regimens include the following: tinidazole, 2 g orally for 3 days or 1 g orally for 5 days; clindamycin, 300 mg orally, twice daily for 7 days; and clindamycin ovules, 100 mg intravaginally, once at bedtime for 3 days.

Table 23-6 CDC Recommendations for Treatment of Acute Vaginitis (2010)

Disease	Drug	Dose	Cost[†]
Bacterial vaginosis[*]	Metronidazole (Flagyl)	500 mg PO, bid for 7 days[†]	$
	Tinidazole	2-g dose PO daily for 2 days	$$$
	Tinidazole	1-g dose PO daily for 5 days	$$$
	0.75% metronidazole gel (Metrogel)	One 5-g application intravaginally daily for 5 days[‡]	$$$
	2% clindamycin cream (Cleocin vaginal)	One 5-g application intravaginally every night for 7 days	$$$
Vulvovaginal candidiasis, uncomplicated			
Intravaginal therapy[‡ §]	Azoles		
	2% butoconazole cream (Mycelex-3)	5 g/day for 4 days[§]	$$
	2% sustained-release butoconazole cream (Gynazole)	One 5-g dose	$$$
	1% clotrimazole cream (Mycelex-7)	5 g for 7-14 days[§]	$
	Clotrimazole (Gyne-Lotrimin 3)	Two 100-mg vaginal tablets/day for 3 days; one 500-mg vaginal tablet	$ $
	2% miconazole cream	5 g/day for 7 days[§]	$$
	Miconazole (Monistat-7)	One 100-mg vaginal suppository/day for 7 days[§]	$$
	Miconazole (Monistat-3)	One 200-mg vaginal suppository/day for 3 days	$$
	Miconazole (Monistat-1)	One 1200-mg vaginal suppository[§]	
	6.5% tioconazole ointment (Monistat 1-day)	One 5-g dose[§]	$
	0.4% terconazole cream (Terazol 7)	5 g/day for 7 days	$$$
	0.8% terconazole cream (Terazol 3)	5 g/day for 3 days	$$
	Terconazole vaginal	One 80-mg vaginal suppository/day for 3 days	$$$
	Nystatin vaginal	One 100,000-U vaginal tablet/day for 14 days	$$$
Oral therapy	Fluconazole (Diflucan)	One 150-mg dose PO	$
Vulvovaginal candidiasis, complicated[†,‖]			
Intravaginal therapy[‡]	Azole	7-14 days	$$
Oral therapy[¶]	Fluconazole (Diflucan)	Two 150-mg doses PO, 72 hr apart	$$$
Trichomoniasis	Metronidazole (Flagyl)	One 2-g dose PO, 500 mg orally bid for 7 days	$
	Tinidazole (Tindamax)	One 2-g dose PO**	$$

[*†]Oral therapy is recommended for pregnant women.
[††]Drug may cause gastrointestinal upset in 5% to 10% of patients; a disulfuram reaction is possible; alcohol should be avoided for 24 hr after ingestion.
[‡§]Vaginal treatments cause local vaginal irritation in 2% to 5% of patients.
[§]This agent is available over the counter.
[‖]Complicated vulvovaginitis refers to disease in women who are pregnant, women who have uncontrolled diabetes, women who are immunocompromised, or women who have severe symptoms, non-*Candida albicans* candidiasis, or recurrent episodes (four or more/year).
[¶]Oral therapy is not recommended for pregnant women.
[**]Drug may cause gastrointestinal upset in 2% to 5% of patients; disulfuram reaction is possible; alcohol should be avoided 72 hr after ingestion.
Adapted from Eckert LO: Clinical practice: Acute vulvovaginitis. N Engl J Med 355:1250, 2006.

Recurrent bacterial vaginosis (three or more episodes in the previous year) is a common clinical problem. One double-blind, randomized, placebo-controlled trial has demonstrated that after 10 days of daily induction therapy with vaginal metronidazole, the twice-weekly use of 0.75% metronidazole gel for 16 weeks maintains a clinical cure in 75% of patients at 16 weeks and 50% by 28 weeks.

Concurrent treatment of the male partner is not recommended at this time. Alternative therapies such as the use of oral or vaginal *Lactobacillus* are not efficacious.

TRICHOMONAS *VAGINAL INFECTION*

Trichomonas vaginalis is a unicellular intracellular parasite that is sexually transmitted and inhabits the vagina and lower urinary tract, especially Skene's ducts in the female. It is estimated that there are 5 million new cases of trichomoniasis annually in the

United States. The prevalence of the disease remains high, despite the availability of effective treatments since the early 1960s. *Trichomonas* vaginal infection is the cause of acute vaginitis in 5% to 50% of cases, depending on the population studied, and is the most prevalent nonviral, nonchlamydial STI of women.

Many women with *Trichomonas* in their vaginal secretions are symptom-free. In one study of women with positive cultures, only one out of two women had symptoms of abnormal vaginal discharge and only one out of six women complained of vulvar pruritus. Positive wet smears or cultures for *Trichomonas* are reported in 3% to 10% of asymptomatic gynecology patients, with a much higher percentage being found in women attending an STI clinic.

This infection is a highly contagious STI; following a single sexual contact, at least two thirds of male and female sexual partners become infected. The protozoa is isolated from 30% to 40%

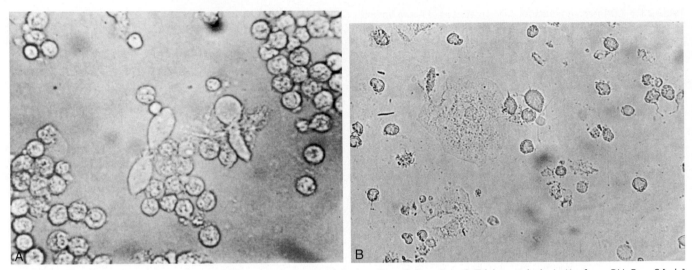

Figure 23-17 A, B, Trichomonads in wet mount prepared with physiologic saline. (**A** from Faro S: Trichomoniasis. In Kaufman RH, Faro S [eds]: Benign Diseases of the Vulva and Vagina, 4th ed. St. Louis, Mosby-Year Book, 1994. **B** from Friedrich EG: Vulvar Disease, 2nd ed. Philadelphia, WB Saunders, 1983.)

of male partners of women with a positive culture and approximately 85% of female partners of a male with a positive culture. The incubation period is 4 to 28 days. *Trichomonas* is a hardy organism and will survive for up to 24 hours on a wet towel and up to 6 hours on a moist surface. However, experimental studies have established that successful vaginal infection depends on the deposition of an inoculum of several thousand organisms. Hence, it is unlikely that infection may be related to exposure from infected towels or swimming pools.

Trichomoniasis is caused by the anaerobic flagellated protozoon, *T. vaginalis* (**Fig. 23-17**), a unicellular organism that is normally fusiform in shape. It exists only in the trophozoite form or vegetative cell, and is slightly larger than a white blood cell. Three to five flagella extend from one end of the organism and provide active movement of the protozoon.

Vaginitis from *Trichomonas* is a disease primarily of women in their reproductive years. The normal highly acidic vaginal environment is resistant to *Trichomonas* infection. In such an environment, the *Trichomonas* organism assumes a spherical shape. Motion is then restricted to waves of the undulating membrane of the protozoon. When lactobacilli predominate in the vaginal fluid, a woman will not develop symptoms. However, menstrual blood, semen, or other vaginal pathogens that alter the vaginal pH to a more basic level favor the growth of *Trichomonas* organisms.

Trichomonas produces a wide variety of patterns of vaginal infection. The primary symptom of *Trichomonas* vaginal infection is profuse vaginal discharge. Patients often complain that the copious discharge makes them feel "wet." Approximately 50% of symptomatic women also detect an abnormal vaginal odor and experience vulvar pruritus; dysuria is a symptom in approximately one of five women with symptomatic *Trichomonas* infection. Women with chronic infection may have a malodorous discharge as their only complaint.

On physical examination, a woman with *T. vaginalis* may have erythema and edema of the vulva and vagina. Vulvar skin involvement is limited to the vestibule and labia minora, which helps distinguish it from the more extensive vulvar involvement of *Candida* vulvovaginitis. The discharge color may be white, gray, yellow, or green, and the classic discharge of *Trichomonas* infection is termed *frothy* (with bubbles) and often has an unpleasant odor. A frothy discharge is only noted in 10% to 25% of women with proven *Trichomonas* infection, but is nondiagnostic because it may be seen also with bacterial vaginosis. The classic sign of a strawberry appearance of the upper vagina and cervix is rare and is noted in less than 10% of women.

The diagnosis of *Trichomonas* vaginal infection is confirmed by examination of vaginal fluid mixed with physiologic saline under the microscope (see **Table 23-6**). To visualize *Trichomonas* organisms optimally, it is best to use high power and dampen the condenser to produce the greatest contrast. If the wet smear is fresh and warm, the organisms will exhibit forward motion. If the slide is cold, the organisms are surrounded by white blood cells, or the saline is too hypertonic, the *Trichomonas* organisms will assume an ovoid configuration and exhibit minimal motion. The wet smear usually contains a large number of inflammatory cells and many vaginal epithelial cells. The only other vaginitis with an abundance of white blood cells is atrophic vaginitis, in which the epithelial cells are normal in appearance and have distinct edges.

The accuracy of diagnosis by wet smear varies widely throughout the literature. If the woman is symptomatic, the sensitivity of a saline wet preparation is 80% to 90%. Because the elevated vaginal pH associated with *T. vaginalis* is from 5.0 to 7.0, measurement of vaginal fluid pH with colorimetric paper can be useful. Vaginal culture for *T. vaginalis* has an 85% to 90% sensitivity and 75% specificity. A point of care enzymatic test, OSOM (Genzyme, Cambridge, MA), has 83% sensitivity and 98% specificity and requires only 10 minutes to perform. This test may be particularly useful when a microscope is unavailable. Attempts to diagnose *T. vaginalis* infection by Papanicolaou (Pap) smear results in an error rate of at least 50%. There have been a large number of false-positive and false-negative reports.

Nitroimidazoles are the only class of drugs recommended for treatment of *Trichomonas* vaginitis. A single oral dose (2 g) of metronidazole or tinidazole is recommended. An alternate regimen is metronidazole, 500 mg orally, twice daily for 7 days.

Tinidazole is a second-generation nitroimidazole and has a longer half-life of 24 hours. Metronidazole is safe in all trimesters of pregnancy. Tinidazole is categorized as a category C drug in pregnancy. Nausea is the most frequent complication and is experienced by 5% of women. Patients should be warned that nitroimidazoles inhibit ethanol metabolism. Women should avoid alcohol for 24 hours after metronidazole and 72 hours after tinidazole therapy to avoid a disulfiram-like reaction. Topical therapy for *Trichomonas* vaginitis is not recommended because it does not eliminate disease reservoirs in Bartholin's and Skene's glands. Recent data have shown that metronidazole, 2-g single oral dose, was not as effective as 500 mg twice daily for 7 days for trichomoniasis in HIV-infected women. Therefore, a multi-dose treatment regimen for *T vaginalis* may be considered for HIV-infected women.

In most cases, women who have a recurrence have been reinfected or complied poorly with therapy. The prevalence of low-level metronidazole resistance in *T. vaginalis* is 2% to 5%; in case series, prolonged treatment with higher doses of metronidazole and tinidazole has been successful. Because *T. vaginalis* is sexually transmitted, treatment of the woman's partner is important and increases cure rates. If reexposure is not an issue, and the infection is not cleared after adequate therapy, one should consult the CDC treatment guidelines for further therapeutic options or for assistance in performing susceptibility testing.

The asymptomatic woman who has *Trichomonas* identified in the lower genital urinary tract definitely should be treated. Extended follow-up studies have shown that one of three asymptomatic women will become symptomatic within 3 months. Furthermore, HIV acquisition is increased in women with *Trichomonas* infection. Similar to bacterial vaginosis, *T. vaginalis* is associated with upper genital tract infections, including infections after delivery, surgery, abortion, pelvic inflammatory disease, preterm delivery, infertility, and cervical dysplasia treatment. Because all STIs have common epidemiologic backgrounds, finding one dictates carrying out appropriate studies to rule out colonization or infection with another STI.

CANDIDA *VAGINITIS*

Candida vaginitis (**Fig. 23-18**) is produced by a ubiquitous, airborne, gram-positive fungus. In most populations, more than 90% of cases are caused by *Candida albicans,* with 5% to 10% of vaginal fungal infections produced by *Candida glabrata* or *Candida tropicalis. Candida* spp. are part of the normal flora of approximately 25% of women, being a commensal saprophytic organism on the mucosal surface of the vagina. Its prevalence in the rectum is three to four times greater and in the mouth two times greater than in the vagina. *Candida* organisms develop filamentous (hyphae and pseudohyphae) and ovoid forms, termed *conidia, buds,* or *spores.* The filamentous forms of *C. albicans* have the ability to penetrate the mucosal surface and become intertwined with the host cells (**Fig. 23-19**). This results in secondary hyperemia and limited lysis of tissue near the site of infection. In contrast, *C. glabrata* does not produce filamentous forms.

When the ecosystem of the vagina is disturbed, *C. albicans* can become an opportunistic pathogen. Hormonal factors, depressed cell-mediated immunity, and antibiotic use are the three most important factors that alter the vaginal ecosystem. The hormonal changes associated with pregnancy and

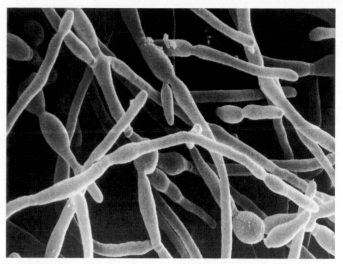

Figure 23-18 Scanning electron micrograph shows a pure culture of *Candida albicans* (× 6030). (From Phillips DM: Images in clinical medicine. N Engl J Med 328:1322, 1993.)

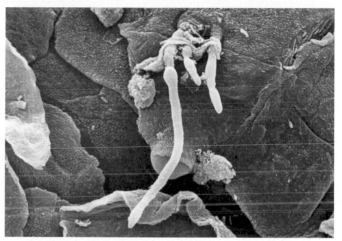

Figure 23-19 Scanning electron micrograph of intraluminal debris of specimen of vaginal wall taken from patient with vaginal candidiasis (× 3500). The hyphae of *C. albicans* penetrate the epithelial layers of vaginal surface. (From Merkus JM, Bisschop MP, Stolte LA: The proper nature of vaginal candidosis and the problem of recurrence. Obstet Gynecol Surv 40:499, 1985.)

menstruation favor growth of the fungus. The prevalence of *Candida* vaginitis increases throughout pregnancy, probably as a result of the high estrogen levels. The literature was initially mixed with respect to the relationship between oral contraceptives and candidiasis. However, with the currently used low-dose estrogen oral contraceptives, there is no increase in the incidence of fungal vaginitis. Women tend to report recurrent episodes of vaginitis immediately preceding and immediately following their menstrual periods.

Lactobacilli inhibit the growth of fungi in the vagina. Therefore, when the relative concentration of lactobacilli declines, rapid overgrowth of *Candida* spp. occurs. Broad-spectrum antibiotics, especially those that destroy lactobacilli (e.g., penicillin, tetracycline, cephalosporins), are notorious for precipitating acute episodes of *C. albicans* vaginitis. Women with diabetes mellitus, or even a low renal threshold for sugar, have a higher incidence of vaginal and vulvar candidiasis. Obesity and debilitating disease are other predisposing factors.

Probably the most important host factor is depressed cell-mediated immunity. Women who take exogenous corticosteroids and women with AIDS often experience recurrent *Candida* vulvovaginitis. Altered local immune responses, such as hyper–IgE-mediated response to a small amount of *Candida* antigen, may occur in women with recurrent vulvovaginal candidiasis. Also, some women with recurrent vulvovaginal candidiasis have tissue infiltration with polymorphonuclear (PMN) leukocytes. This high density of PMNs correlates with symptomatology but does not result in clearance of *Candida.*

Vaginitis caused by fungal infection is primarily a disease of the childbearing years. It is estimated that three of four women will have at least one episode of vulvovaginal candidiasis during their lifetime. The greatest enigma of this condition is the recurrence rate after an apparent cure, varying from 20% to 80%. Approximately 3% to 5% of these women experience recurrent vulvovaginal candidiasis (RVVC), which is defined as four or more documented episodes in 1 year.

Fungal vaginitis usually presents as a vulvovaginitis. Pruritis is the predominant symptom. Depending on the degree of vulvar skin involvement, pruritus may be accompanied by vulvar burning, external dysuria, and dyspareunia. The vaginal discharge is white or whitish gray, highly viscous, and described as granular or floccular, with no have an odor. The amount of discharge is highly variable. The vulvar signs include erythema, edema, and excoriation. With extensive skin involvement, pustules may extend beyond the line of erythema. During speculum examination, a cottage cheese–type discharge is often visualized, with adherent clumps and plaques (thrush patches) attached to the vaginal walls. These clumps, or raised plaques, are usually white or yellow. The vaginal pH associated with this infection is below 4.5, in contrast to bacterial vaginosis and *Trichomonas* vaginitis, which are associated with an elevated pH.

The diagnosis is established by obtaining a wet smear of vaginal secretion and mixing this with 10% to 20% potassium hydroxide (Fig. 23-20). The alkali rapidly lyses red blood cells and inflammatory cells. Active disease is associated with filamentous forms, mycelia, or pseudohyphae, rather than spores. However, it may be necessary to search the slide and scan many different microscopic fields to identify hyphae or pseudohyphae. The average concentration of organisms is 10^3 to 10^4/mL. Although symptoms can be present at a low colony count, the ability to detect *C. albicans* on a wet mount is 80% when semiquantitative culture growth is 3 to 4+, but only 20% when culture growth is 2+. Hence, a negative smear does not exclude *Candida* vulvovaginitis. The diagnosis can be established by culture with Nickerson or Sabouraud medium. These cultures will become positive in 24 to 72 hours. Vaginal culture for *Candida* is particularly useful when a wet mount is negative for hyphae but the patients have symptoms and discharge or other signs suggestive of vulvovaginal candidiasis on examination. Fungal culture may also be useful for women who have recently treated themselves with an antifungal agent; up to 90% have a negative culture within 1 week after treatment. It should be stressed that obtaining a vaginal culture for bacteria is not useful because anaerobes, coliforms, and *G. vaginalis* all are part of normal vaginal flora. The differential diagnosis includes other common causes of vaginitis, such as bacterial vaginosis, *Trichomonas* vaginitis, and atrophic vaginitis. Also, one should consider noninfectious conditions such as allergic reactions, contact dermatitis, chemical irritants, and rare diseases such as lichen planus.

The over-the-counter (OTC) availability of vaginal antifungal therapy makes self-treatment an option for many women. However, it must be recognized that symptoms suggestive of uncomplicated vulvovaginal candidiasis may reflect an alternative diagnosis. One study of women seen at a clinic for STIs found that self-treatment of the symptoms listed on the package insert of an OTC medication for candidiasis would correctly treat only 28% of patients; 53% had bacterial vaginosis, infection with *T. vaginalis,* gonorrhea, or chlamydia. In another study involving women purchasing OTC antifungal therapy, only 34% had vulvovaginal candidiasis and no other vaginal infection. If a woman chooses self-treatment, she should be advised to come in for examination if the symptoms are not eliminated with a single course of OTC therapy.

For treatment of vulvovaginal candidiasis, the CDC recommends placing the woman into an uncomplicated or complicated category to guide treatment (Box 23-3). A number of

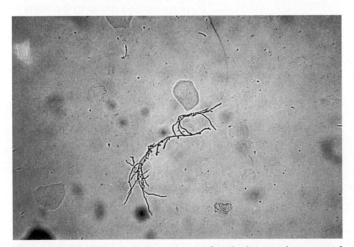

Figure 23-20 Microscopic appearance of vaginal smear in a case of vaginal candidiasis (potassium hydroxide preparation, yeast cells and pseudomycelia; × 320). (From Merkus JM, Bisschop MP, Stolte LA: The proper nature of vaginal candidosis and the problem of recurrence. Obstet Gynecol Surv 40:495, 1985.)

Box 23-3 Classification of Vulvovaginal Candidiasis (VVC)	
Uncomplicated VVC	**Complicated VVC**
■ Sporadic or infrequent vulvovaginal candidiasis *and*	■ Recurrent vulvovaginal candidiasis *or*
■ Mild to moderate vulvovaginal candidiasis *and*	■ Severe vulvovaginal candidiasis *or*
■ Likely to be *C. albicans and*	■ Non-*albicans* candidiasis *or*
■ Nonimmunocompromised women	■ Women with uncontrolled diabetes, debilitation, or immunosuppression

Workowski KA, Berman S; Centers for Disease Control and Prevention (CDC): Sexually transmitted diseases treatment guidelines, MMWR 59(RR-12):62, 2010.

azole vaginal preparations and a single oral agent, fluconazole, are approved for treatment. In patients with uncomplicated vulvovaginal candidiasis, topical antifungal agents are typically used for 1 to 3 days, or a single oral dose of fluconazole. Patient preference, response to prior therapy, and cost should guide the choice of therapy.

For patients with complicated vaginitis, topical azoles are recommended for 7 to 14 days. If using oral therapy, a second dose of fluconazole (150 mg) given 72 hours after the first dose is recommended.

In women with RVVC, the resolution of symptoms typically requires longer duration of therapy. Seven to 14 days of topical therapy or three doses of oral fluconazole 3 days apart (e.g., days 1, 4, and 7) are options. After this initial treatment, maintenance therapy will help prevent recurrence of symptoms. Oral fluconazole (e.g., 100-, 150-, or 200-mg dose) weekly for 6 months is typically first-line treatment. However, topical treatments used intermittently as a maintenance regimen may be considered. Women with recurrent vulvovaginitis should receive a vaginal fungal culture to determine species and sensitivities.

Infections with *Candida* spp. other than *C. albicans* are often azole-resistant. However, one study of terconazole for non–*C. albicans* fungal vaginitis resulted in a mycologic cure in 56% of patients and a symptomatic cure in 44% of women. Vaginal boric acid capsules (600 mg in O gelatin capsules) are another option. In one study, treatment for a minimum of 14 days resulted in a symptomatic cure rate of 70% for women with non–*C. albicans* infection. Boric acid inhibits fungal cell wall growth. It may also be used for suppression in women with recurrent vulvovaginal candidiasis. Following 10 days of therapy, one 600-mg capsule intravaginally twice weekly for 4 to 6 months decreases symptomatic recurrences. Boric acid is toxic if ingested, so it should be stored in a safe manner.

Studies of alternative therapies for vulvovaginal candidiasis (such as oral or vaginal *Lactobacillus,* garlic, or diet alterations such as yogurt ingestion) do not show efficacy. A summary of diagnostic tools for determining the cause of vaginitis and of treatment options are provided in **Tables 23-5** and **23-6**.

TOXIC SHOCK SYNDROME

TSS is an acute febrile illness produced by a bacterial exotoxin, with a fulminating downhill course involving dysfunction of multiple organ systems. The cardinal features of the disease are its abrupt onset and rapidity with which the clinical signs and symptoms may present and progress. It is not unusual for the syndrome to develop from a site of bacterial colonization rather than from an infection.

A woman with TSS may develop a rapid onset of hypotension associated with multiorgan system failure. TSS was first described in 1978 by Todd as a sometimes fatal sequela of *Staphylococcus aureus* infection in children. In the early 1980s, more than 95% of the reported cases of TSS were diagnosed in previously healthy, young (<30 years), menstruating females. *S. aureus* was isolated from the vagina in more than 90% of these cases.

Between 1979 and 1996, 5,296 TSS cases were reported. Menstrual cases accounted for 74% of total cases, although the proportion has decreased over time (91% from 1979 to 1980, 71% from 1981 to 1986, and 59% from 1986 to 1996). The number of cases of menstrual TSS has declined from 9 of 100,000 women in 1980 to 1 of 100,000 women since 1986. The case-fatality rate has also declined; it was 1.8% from 1987 to 1996 after a high of 5.5% in 1979 to 1980. Most likely, the withdrawal of highly absorbent tampons and polyacrylate rayon–containing products from the market partially explains the decrease. However, tampon use remains a risk factor for TSS. Women who develop TSS are more likely to have used higher absorbency tampons, several cycle days of tampons, and kept a single tampon in for a longer period of time.

Presently, approximately 50% of cases of TSS are not related to menses. Nonmenstrual TSS may be a sequelae of focal staphylococcal infection of the skin and subcutaneous tissue, often following a surgical procedure. In the past few years, it has been recognized that occasionally severe postoperative infections by *Streptococcus pyogenes* produce a similar "streptococcal toxic shocklike syndrome." TSS related to a surgical wound occurs early in the postoperative course, usually within the first 48 hours. The proportion of cases following surgical procedures increased from 14% in 1979 to 1986 to 27% in 1987 to 1996.

There are three requirements for the development of classic TSS: (1) the woman must be colonized or infected with *S. aureus*; (2) the bacteria must produce TSS **toxin 1** (TSST-1) or related toxins; and (3) the toxins must have a route of entry into the systemic circulation. Most strains of *S. aureus* are unable to produce TSS toxin 1. Interestingly, approximately 85% of women have antibodies against TSST-1.

If an individual woman continues to use tampons when the vagina is colonized with *S. aureus,* there is a significant chance of recurrence. It has been reported that one woman experienced five episodes of the disease. There appears to be no pattern to these recurrent episodes. Interestingly, women with menstrual-related TSS do not respond immunologically to TSST-1 as do women with nonmenstrual-related TSS. It is rare for a woman with nonmenstrual TSS to have a recurrence.

The signs and symptoms of TSS are produced by the exotoxin named toxin 1. Toxin 1 is a simple protein with a molecular weight of 22,000 kDa and is accepted as the underlying cause of the disease. Thus, toxins act as superantigens, molecules that activate up to 20% of T cells at once, resulting in massive cytokine production. Pathophysiologically, superantigens do not require processing by antigen-presenting cells. The primary effects of toxin 1 are to produce increased vascular permeability, thus resulting in profuse leaking of fluid (capillary leak) from the intravascular compartment into the interstitial space and an associated profound loss of vasomotor tone, causing decreased peripheral resistance.

Studies of the bacteriology of the vagina of normal menstruating females have documented that 5% to 17% of women are colonized with *S. aureus*. Approximately 5% test positive when the culture is obtained at midcycle and the percentage increases to 10% to 17% during menses. Rarely are blood cultures positive for *S. aureus* in a woman with TSS. Thus, the exotoxin is believed to be absorbed directly from the vagina. It is possible that microulcerations produced by use of tampons facilitate the toxin's entry into the systemic circulation. The risk of nonmenstrual TSS is definitely increased in women who use barrier contraceptives such as a diaphragm, cervical cap, or a sponge containing nonoxynol 9.

Because of the severity of the disease, gynecologists should have a high index of suspicion for TSS in a woman who has an unexplained fever and a rash during or immediately following her menstrual period. The syndrome has a wide range of symptoms. The varying degree of severity of symptoms and signs depends on the magnitude of involvement of individual organs. Most women experience a prodromal flulike illness for the first 24 hours. Between days 2 and 4 of the menstrual period, the patient experiences an abrupt onset of a high temperature associated with headache, myalgia, sore throat, vomiting, diarrhea, generalized skin rash, and often hypotension. It is important to consider that not all women with TSS experience the full-blown manifestations of the disease. The rigid criteria developed by the CDC are used for epidemiologic studies. Clinically, many women present with a forme fruste of TSS, with low-grade fever and dizziness rather than hypotension.

The most characteristic manifestations of TSS are the skin changes. During the first 48 hours, the skin rash appears similar to intense sunburn. During the next few days, the erythema will become more macular and resemble a drug-related rash. From days 12 to 15 of the illness, there is a fine flaky desquamation of skin over the face and trunk, with sloughing of the entire skin thickness of the palms and soles. The vaginal mucosa is hyperemic during the initial phase of the syndrome. During pelvic examination, patients complain of tenderness of the external genitalia and vagina. Myalgia, vomiting, and diarrhea are experienced by more than 90% of women with TSS (**Box 23-4**). Many abnormal laboratory findings are associated with the

---

Box 23-4 Case Definition of Toxic Shock Syndrome

1. Fever (temperature 38.9° C [102° F])
2. Rash characterized by diffuse macular erythroderma
3. Desquamation occurring 1-2 wk after onset of illness (in survivors)
4. Hypotension (systolic blood pressure ≤ 90 mm Hg in adults) or orthostatic syncope
5. Involvement of three or more of the following organ systems:
   a. Gastrointestinal (vomiting or diarrhea at onset of illness)
   b. Muscular (myalgia or creatine phosphokinase level twice normal)
   c. Mucous membrane (vaginal, oropharyngeal, or conjunctival hyperemia)
   d. Renal (BUN or creatinine level ≥ twice normal or ≥ 5 WBCs/HPF in absence of UTI)
   e. Hepatic (total bilirubin, SGOT, or SGPT twice normal level)
   f. Hematologic (platelets ≤ 100,000/mm^3)
   g. Central nervous system (disorientation or alteration in consciousness without focal neurologic signs when fever and hypotension are absent)
   h. Cardiopulmonary (adult respiratory distress syndrome, pulmonary edema, new onset of second- or third-degree heart block, myocarditis)
6. Negative throat and cerebrospinal fluid cultures (a positive blood culture for *Staphylococcus aureus* does not exclude a case)
7. Negative serologic test results for Rocky Mountain spotted fever, leptospirosis, rubeola

BUN, Blood urea nitrogen; HPF, high-powered field; SGOT, serum glutamic-oxaloacetic transaminase; SGPT, serum glutamic-pyruvic transaminase; UTI, urinary tract infection; WBC, white blood cell count.
From Centers for Disease Control (CDC): Toxic-shock syndrome, United States, 1970-1982. MMWR Morb Mortal Wkly Rep 31:201, 1982.

Box 23-5 Laboratory Abnormalities in Early Toxic Shock Syndrome

Present in > 85% of patients
Coagulase-positive staphylococci in cervix or vagina
Immature and mature polymorphonuclear cells > 90% of WBCs
Total lymphocyte count < 650/mm^3
Total serum protein level < 5.6 mg/dL
Serum albumin level < 3.1 g/dL
Serum calcium level < 7.8 mg/dL
Serum creatinine clearance > 1.0 mg/dL
Serum bilirubin level > 1.5 mg/dL
Serum cholesterol level ≤ 120 mg/dL
Prothrombin time > 12 seconds
Present in > 70% of patients
Platelet count < 150,000/mm^3
Pyuria > 5 WBCs/HPF
Proteinuria ≥ 2+
BUN > 20 mg/dL
Aspartate aminotransferase (formerly SGOT) > 41 U/liter
BUN, Blood urea nitrogen; HPF, high-powered field; SGOT, serum glutamic-oxaloacetic transaminase; WBCs, white blood cells.

*Results were available for at least 18 patients per category with the following exceptions: cervicovaginal cultures (12 patients), cholesterol level (15 patients), and prothrombin time (14 patients).
From Chesney PJ, Davis JP, Purdy WK, et al: Clinical manifestations of toxic shock syndrome. JAMA 246:746, 1981.

---

disease and, again, they reflect the severity of involvement of individual organ systems (**Box 23-5**). The differential diagnosis of toxic shock syndrome includes Rocky Mountain spotted fever, streptococcal scarlet fever, and leptospirosis.

The management of a classic case of severe TSS demands an intensive care unit and the skills of an expert in critical care medicine. The first priority is to eliminate the hypotension produced by the exotoxin. Copious amounts of IV fluids are given while pressure and volume dynamics are centrally monitored. Mechanical ventilation is required for women who develop adult respiratory distress syndrome.

When the woman is initially admitted to the hospital, it is important to obtain cervical, vaginal, and blood cultures for *S. aureus*. Although there have been no controlled series documenting its efficacy, it is prudent to wash out the vagina with saline or dilute iodine solution to diminish the amount of exotoxin that may be absorbed into the systemic circulation.

Women with TSS caused by methicillin-susceptible *S. aureus* should be treated with clindamycin, 600 mg IV every 8 hours, plus nafcillin or oxacillin, 2 g IV every 4 hours. Most experts recommend a 1- to 2-week course of therapy with an antistaphylococcal agent such as clindamycin or dicloxacillin, even in the absence of a positive *S. aureus* culture. In patients with TSS caused by methicillin-resistant *S. aureus* (MRSA), clindamycin plus vancomycin (30 mg/kg/day IV in two divided doses) or linezolid (600 mg oral or IV every 12 hours) is used. If the diagnosis is questionable, it is best to include an aminoglycoside to obtain coverage for possible gram-negative sepsis. Antibiotic therapy probably has little effect on the course of an individual episode of TSS. However, if the underlying cause of toxic shock syndrome is a skin infection, the infected site should be drained and débrided. Treatment with mupirocin to decrease colonization is recommended, applying half of the ointment from a single-use tube into one nostril and the other half into the other nostril twice daily for 5 days.

In summary, the treatment of TSS depends on the severity of involvement of individual organ systems. Not all patients develop a temperature higher than 38.9° C and hypotension. Thus, clinicians should be aware of the forme fruste manifestations of the syndrome. The foundation of treatment of the disease is prompt and aggressive management because of the rapidity with which the disease may progress.

It is possible to decrease the incidence of TSS by a change in the use of catamenial products. Women should be encouraged to change tampons every 4 to 6 hours. The intermittent use of external pads is also good preventive medicine. Women will usually accept the recommendation to wear external pads during sleep. The incidence of TSS has decreased dramatically with the removal of super-absorbing tampons from the market. A study by Tierno and Hanna reported that all-cotton tampons are the safest choice to avoid menstrual TSS.

Finally, there are cases of streptococcal toxic shock–like syndrome that are secondary to life-threatening infections with group A streptococcus (*Streptococcus pyogenes*). Several different exotoxins have been identified and M types 1 and 3 are the two most common serotypes. In gynecology, most of these cases involve massive subcutaneous postoperative infections. One of the most distinguishing characteristics of a necrotizing skin infection is the intense localized pain in the involved area. Older women and women who are diabetic or immunocompromised are at much greater risk to develop invasive streptococcal infection and streptococcal toxic shock–like syndrome. The mortality rate is approximately 30% when TSS is secondary to group A streptococcal infections.

CERVICITIS

Cervicitis, an inflammatory process in the cervical epithelium and stroma, can be associated with trauma, inflammatory systemic disease, neoplasia, and infection. Although it is clinically important to consider all causes of inflammation, this section will focus on infectious origins.

The cervix acts as a barrier between the abundant bacterial flora of the vagina and the bacteriologically sterile endometrial cavity and oviducts. Cervical mucus is much more than a simple physical barrier; it exerts a definite bacteriostatic effect. Mucus may also act as a competitive inhibitor with bacteria for receptors on the endocervical epithelial cells. Cervical mucus also contains antibodies and inflammatory cells that are active against various sexually transmitted organisms.

Often, the woman is asymptomatic, even though the cervix is colonized with organisms. The cervix is a potential reservoir for *Neisseria gonorrhoeae, Chlamydia trachomatis,* HSV, human papillomavirus, and *Mycoplasma* spp. Cervical infection can be ectocervicitis or endocervicitis. Ectocervicitis can be viral (HSV) or from a severe vaginitis (e.g., strawberry cervix associated with *T. vaginalis* infection) or *C. albicans.* Endocervicitis may be secondary to infection with *C. trachomatis* or *N. gonorrhoeae.* Bacterial vaginosis and *Mycoplasma genitalium* have also been associated with endocervicitis. Infection of the endocervix becomes a major reservoir for sexual and perinatal transmission of pathogenic microorganisms. Primary endocervical infection may result in secondary ascending infections, including pelvic inflammatory disease and perinatal infections of the membranes, amniotic fluid, and parametria.

The histologic diagnosis of chronic cervicitis is so prevalent that it should be considered the norm for parous women of reproductive age. The histopathology of endocervicitis is characterized by a severe inflammatory reaction in the mucosa and submucosa. The tissues are infiltrated with a large number of PMNs and monocytes and, occasionally, there is associated epithelial necrosis. Physiologically, there is a resident population of a small number of leukocytes in the normal cervix. Thus, the emphasis is on a severe inflammatory reaction by a large number of PMNs. This section will focus on mucopurulent cervicitis and techniques to diagnose common cervical infections.

MUCOPURULENT CERVICITIS

The diagnosis of cervicitis continues to rely on symptoms, examination, and microscopic evaluation. Two simple, definitive, objective criteria have been developed to establish mucopurulent cervicitis—gross visualization of yellow mucopurulent material on a white cotton swab (**Fig. 23-21**) and the presence of 10 or more PMN leukocytes per microscopic field (magnification, × 1000) on Gram-stained smears obtained from the endocervix. Alternative clinical criteria that may be used are erythema and edema in an area of cervical ectopy or associated with bleeding secondary to endocervical ulceration or friability when the endocervical smear is obtained. Women may also report increased vaginal discharge and intermenstrual vaginal bleeding. In their original study, the Seattle group discovered that 40% of patients with STIs had mucopurulent cervicitis (24% diagnosed by grossly visualized purulent material, 16% without mucopus but positive Gram stains of cervical mucus). However, the sensitivity, specificity, and positive predictive value of objective criteria have varied markedly in follow-up studies.

The prevalence of mucopurulent cervicitis depends on the population being studied. Approximately 30% to 40% of women attending clinics for STIs and 8% to 10% of women

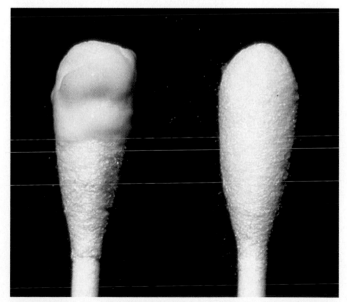

Figure 23-21 Mucopurulent cervicitis demonstrated by cotton swab test.

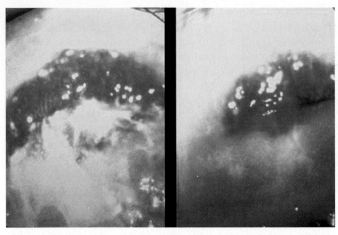

Figure 23-22 Patient with *C. trachomatis* mucopurulent cervicitis with resolution post-treatment.

in university student health clinics have the condition. More than 60% of women with this disease are asymptomatic. Symptoms that suggest cervical infection include vaginal discharge, deep dyspareunia, and postcoital bleeding. The physical signs of a cervical infection are a cervix that is hypertrophic and edematous.

C. trachomatis is the cause of cervical infection in many women with mucopurulent cervicitis (**Fig. 23-22**). Depending on the geographic region, gonorrhea is also an important cause of mucopurulent cervicitis. However, most women who have lower reproductive tract infections caused by *C. trachomatis* or *N. gonorrhoeae* do not have mucopurulent cervicitis. The corollary is that most women who have mucopurulent cervicitis are not infected by *C. trachomatis* or *N. gonorrhoeae*. Mucopurulent cervicitis is present in approximately 40% to 60% of women in whom no cervical pathogen can be identified. Thus, this condition often persists following adequate broad-spectrum antibiotic therapy. The presence of active herpes infection is correlated with ulceration of the ectocervix but not with mucopus.

When mucopurulent cervicitis is clinically diagnosed, empirical therapy for *C. trachomatis* is recommended for women at increased risk of this common STI (age < 25 years, new or multiple sex partners, unprotected sex). If the prevalence of *N. gonorrhoeae* is more than 5%, concurrent therapy for *N. gonorrhoeae* is indicated. Concomitant trichomoniasis should also be treated if detected, as should bacterial vaginosis. If presumptive treatment is deferred, the use of a sensitive nucleic acid test for *C. trachomatis* and *N. gonorrhoeae* is needed.

Recommended regimens for presumptive cervicitis therapy include azithromycin, 1 g orally in a single dose, or doxycycline, 100 mg orally twice daily for 7 days, adding gonococcal treatment if the prevalence is over 5% in the population assessed. Women treated for chlamydia should be instructed to abstain from sexual intercourse for 7 days after single-dose therapy or until completion of the 7-day regimen.

Mycoplasma genitalium, which is noncultivable, has been associated in women with mucopurulent cervicitis by DNA testing. Bacterial vaginosis has also been associated with mucopurulent cervicitis; cervicitis resolved with bacterial vaginosis treatment.

The key teaching point is that many women harboring sexually transmitted pathogens in the cervix are asymptomatic.

DETECTION OF PATHOGENIC CERVICAL BACTERIA

Neisseria gonorrhoeae

Nucleic acid amplification testing (NAAT) of the urine or cervix is the most sensitive and specific diagnostic tool for identifying gonorrheal infections. Urine tests should be first void (either the first void in morning, or at least 1 hour since last void). This technique allows for the sensitive detection of DNA particles originating from the urethra or endocervix, which fall into the vaginal pool and vestibule.

Most women who are colonized with *N. gonorrhoeae* are asymptomatic. Therefore, it is important to screen women at high risk for gonorrheal infection routinely. Screening of high-risk individuals is the primary modality to control the disease. Gonorrheal NAAT results are over 95% sensitive and specific.

As of April 2007, quinolones are no longer recommended in the United States for the treatment of gonorrhea and associated conditions. Consequently, only one class of antimicrobials, the cephalosporins, is still recommended and available for the treatment of gonorrhea in the United States. Two other considerations are given high priority when choosing an antibiotic, single-dose efficacy and simultaneously treating coexisting chlamydial infection. *C. trachomatis* has frequently been found to simultaneously colonize women with gonorrhea. The present recommended parenteral regimen is ceftriaxone, 250 mg IM, once. Alternatively, cefixime may be given in a single oral dose, although parenteral ceftriaxone has a higher efficacy for pharyngeal gonococcal disease. These regimens have documented cure rates higher than 95% in uncomplicated anogenital gonorrhea. Single-dose, injectable, cephalosporin regimens, other than ceftriaxone, 250 mg IM, that are safe and highly effective against uncomplicated urogenital and anorectal gonococcal infections include ceftizoxime (500 mg IM), cefoxitin (2 g IM, with probenecid 1 g orally), and cefotaxime (500 mg IM). None of the injectable cephalosporins offer any advantage over ceftriaxone for urogenital infection, and efficacy at the pharynx is less certain. For patients who are allergic or intolerant to cephalosporins, spectinomycin, 2 g IM in a single dose, is effective, but is no longer available in the United States. Azithromycin, 2 g, may be used in cephalosporin-allergic patients. Treatment regimens for gonorrhea and chlamydial infection are given in **Boxes 23-6 and 23-7**). In addition to the antibiotics for gonorrhea, the CDC recommends treating with azithromycin, 1 g orally in a single dose, or oral doxycycline, 100 mg twice daily for 7 days, if chlamydia has not been ruled out.

If the woman is asymptomatic, follow-up testing is no longer recommended by the CDC as a test of cure for lower tract

---

Box 23-6 CDC Recommended Treatment of Uncomplicated Gonococcal Infections of the Cervix, Urethra, and Rectum in Adults (2010)

Ceftriaxone, 250 mg IM, single dose
  or, if not an option
Cefixime, 400 mg PO, single dose
  or
Single-dose injectable cephalosporin regimen
  plus treatment for chlamydia

Workowski KA, Berman S; Centers for Disease Control and Prevention (CDC): Sexually transmitted diseases treatment guidelines, MMWR 59(RR-12):50, 2010.

Box 23-7 Recommended Regimens for Treatment of Chlamydial Infection

Azithromycin, 1 g PO, single dose*
  or
Doxycycline, 100 mg PO bid for 7 days

Alternative Regimens
Erythromycin base, 500 mg PO qid for 7 days,
  or
Erythromycin ethylsuccinate, 800 mg PO qid for 7 days,
  or
Ofloxacin, 300 mg PO bid for 7 days
  or
Levofloxacin, 500 mg PO once daily for 7 days

*Consider concurrent treatment for gonococcal infection if prevalence of gonorrhea is high in the patient population under assessment. Workowski KA, Berman S; Centers for Disease Control and Prevention (CDC): Sexually transmitted diseases treatment guidelines, MMWR 59(RR-12):45, 2010.

infections (uncomplicated gonorrhea). However, studies have shown a high rate of reinfection, so rescreening patients is prudent. Women with positive cultures for gonorrhea should have a serologic test for syphilis in 4 to 6 weeks, even though patients with incubating syphilis are usually cured by antibiotic combinations of ceftriaxone and tetracycline. Similarly, patients should be offered informed consent and testing for HIV infection.

It is important to remember that *N. gonorrhoeae* attaches to the columnar epithelium, so a vaginal cuff swab in women with prior hysterectomies is not recommended.

Chlamydia trachomatis

As with gonorrhea, the gold standard of techniques used to identify *C. trachomatis* infection is NAAT. *C. trachomatis* also attaches to the columnar epithelium. Hence, vaginal specimens should not be collected from women who have had a hysterectomy. When a culture is used for diagnosis, *C. trachomatis* is an obligatory intracellular organism; hence, it is mandatory to obtain epithelial cells to maximize the percentage of positive cultures. A Dacron, rayon, or calcium alginate swab is placed in the endocervical canal. It is rotated for 15 to 20 seconds to abrade the columnar epithelium gently. The cytobrush, which was developed primarily to enhance sampling of endocervical cells for cytology, has been found to be the optimal instrument for appropriate sampling for *Chlamydia* culture as well. Chlamydial antigen detection is insensitive and nonspecific compared with NAAT and is no longer recommended.

C. trachomatis infection is frequently asymptomatic. Chlamydial screening programs have been successful at decreasing the prevalence of the disease. The CDC recommends annual screening of all sexually active women 25 years of age or younger, and screening of older women with risk factors (e.g., those who have a new sex partner or multiple partners).

For all women with a chlamydial or gonorrheal infection, partners should be treated. Patients should be instructed to refer all sex partners of the last 60 days for evaluation and treatment and to avoid sexual intercourse until therapy is completed and they and their partner have resolution of symptoms.

If a woman is unsure whether her partner will be treated, delivery of antibiotic therapy (by prescription or medication) is an option. Studies have demonstrated that patient-delivered partner

therapy result in lower rates of chlamydial persistence or recurrence. All women with *C. trachomatis, N. gonorrhoeae,* or mucopurulent cervicitis of unknown origin need evaluation to rule out pelvic inflammatory disease.

ENDOMETRITIS

Once an infection ascends through the cervix into the endometrium or into the salpinx, it is an upper genital tract infection. Nonpuerperal endometritis is infection of the uterine lining. Although endometritis commonly coexists with salpingitis, several studies have supported endometritis as a distinct clinical syndrome. In one large study of 152 women with suspected pelvic inflammatory disease (PID), all of whom underwent laparoscopy and endometrial biopsy, 43 (28%) had neither endometritis nor salpingitis, 26 (17%) had isolated endometritis, and 83 (55%) had acute salpingitis. Those with endometritis alone had distinct risk factors (douching in last 30 days, current intrauterine device [IUD] in place, and douching in days 1 to 7 of menstrual cycle). Also, among those women with suspected PID, endometritis was associated with clinical manifestations (e.g., cervical motion tenderness, rebound, fever) and infection with *N. gonorrhoeae, C. trachomatis,* or both intermediate in frequency between women with salpingitis and those with neither salpingitis nor endometritis.

The gold standard diagnosis of endometritis is based on endometrial biopsy. At least one plasma cell/$\times 120$ field of endometrial stroma combined with five or more neutrophils in the superficial endometrial epithelium/$\times 400$ field is the histopathologic criteria for endometritis. In severe cases, diffuse lymphocytes and plasma cells in the endometrial stroma or stromal necrosis may be present.

The concept of subclinical endometritis has evolved, in part, because many women with tubal infertility have no history of clinical symptoms consistent with prior PID. Several large cross-sectional studies in various geographic regions have studied women with no symptoms or signs of acute salpingitis (no cervical motion or adnexal or uterine tenderness) to define subclinical endometritis further. Most of these studies were conducted in STI clinics or emergency rooms in women at risk for PID; endometritis is associated with young age (20 to 22 years old in most studies), abnormal uterine bleeding (menorrhagia or metrorrhagia), menstrual cycle day less than 14, douching in last 30 days, and history of prior PID.

Lower genital tract infections with *C. trachomatis, N. gonorrhoeae,* bacterial vaginosis, *M. genitalium,* and *T. vaginalis* and mucopurulent cervicitis are associated with histologic endometritis with an odds ratio (OR) of 1.5 to 3.0, depending on the study. One study demonstrated that in women with current *N. gonorrhoeae* or *C. trachomatis* infection, endometritis was apparent in 43% of those with a history of prior PID and 23% of those without prior PID. This is suggestive of possible immunologic memory. Some women with endometritis do not have an isolated pathogen.

Because many of the symptoms and signs associated with endometritis are subtle, a clinician needs to have a low threshold for performing an endometrial biopsy to aid in the diagnosis. Treatment for endometritis is the same as outpatient salpingitis treatment (**Table 23-7**). Treatment should last 14 days. The addition of metronidazole should be strongly considered, especially if the woman has bacterial vaginosis.

Table 23-7 Endometritis Treatment Regimens: 2010 CDC Guidelines

Ceftriaxone, 250 mg IM, single dose
or
Cefoxitin, 2 g IM, single dose, and probenecid, 1 g PO administered concurrently in a single dose
or
Other parenteral third-generation cephalosporin (e.g., ceftizoxime, cefotaxime)
plus
Doxycycline, 100 mg PO bid for 14 days
with or without
Metronidazole, 500 mg PO bid for 14 days

Workowski KA, Berman S; Centers for Disease Control and Prevention (CDC): Sexually transmitted diseases treatment guidelines, MMWR 59(RR-2):66, 2010.

Antimicrobial therapy for endometritis is effective. One study has demonstrated significant reduction in abnormal bleeding, cervicitis, uterine tenderness, and histologic endometritis following treatment with cefixime, 400 mg orally, azithromycin, 1000 mg, with or without metronidazole, 500 mg orally twice daily for 7 days. Endometritis in HIV-seropositive women has not been well characterized. One series of 42 seropositive women, none of whom had *C. trachomatis* or *N. gonorrhoeae,* has demonstrated a 38% prevalence of endometritis. Compared with the seropositive women without endometritis, the seropositive women with endometritis did not have increased uterine tenderness, lower counts of CD4$^+$ lymphocytes, or other findings. A small subset of those with endometritis had a repeat endometrial biopsy following antimicrobial therapy and 50% of the endometritis had resolved histologically. The authors concluded that endometritis in HIV-infected women might be related to pathogens that were not evaluated, to prior infection, or to reduced immunity from HIV.

The sequelae of endometritis distinct from salpingitis are difficult to determine. In a series of 614 women in the PID evaluation and clinical health (PEACH) study, women with endometritis, upper genital tract infection with *N. gonorrhoeae* or *C. trachomatis,* or both were compared with women without endometritis or upper genital tract infection for outcomes of pregnancy, infertility, recurrent PID, and chronic pelvic pain. The women with endometritis or upper genital tract infection had higher age- and race-specific pregnancy rates than the national average after adjusting for age, race, education, PID history, and baseline infertility. In the group with clinically suspected mild PID treated with standard antimicrobial therapy, endometritis or upper genital tract infection was not associated with reproductive morbidity.

PELVIC INFLAMMATORY DISEASE

PID is an infection in the upper genital tract not associated with pregnancy or intraperitoneal pelvic operations. Thus, it may include infection of any or all of the following anatomic locations: endometrium (endometritis; see previous section), oviducts (salpingitis), ovary (oophoritis), uterine wall (myometritis), uterine serosa and broad ligaments (parametritis), and pelvic peritoneum. Many authors prefer the term *salpingitis* because infection of the oviducts is the most characteristic and common

component of PID. Importantly, most long-term sequelae of PID result from destruction of the tubal architecture by the infection. In most clinical situations, the terms acute *salpingitis* and *pelvic inflammatory disease* are used synonymously to describe an acute infection.

The incidence of PID in the United States is decreasing. However, the prevalence of STIs and corresponding PID is a major public health concern. The estimated number of cases in women 15 to 44 years of age was 189,662 in 2002 and 168,837 in 2003 (National Ambulatory Medical Care Survey [NAMCS]). The number of hospitalizations for acute PID steadily declined in the 1980s and 1990s, increased somewhat in the period from 2001 to 2004 but, by 2006, had dropped back to 50,000/year, levels consistent with those in 2000. Outpatient visits have also declined. From 2001 to 2008, the number of visits to physician's offices for PID declined from 244,000 to 104,000. Reduction of the medical impact of acute PID requires aggressive therapy for lower genital tract infection and early diagnosis and treatment of upper genital tract infection. Public health emphasis also must be placed on primary prevention involving attempts to prevent exposure and acquisition of STIs. This includes teaching adolescents safe sex practices and promoting the use of condoms and chemical barrier methods. Secondary prevention of PID involves the universal screening of women at high risk for chlamydia and gonorrhea, screening for active cervicitis, increasing use of sensitive tests to diagnose lower genital infection, treatment of sexual partners, and education to prevent recurrent infection.

Acute PID results from ascending infection from the bacterial flora of the vagina and cervix in more than 99% of cases. This ascending infection occurs along the mucosal surface, resulting in bacterial colonization and infection of the endometrium and fallopian tubes. The process sometimes extends to the surface of the ovaries and nearby peritoneum, and rarely into the adjacent soft tissues, such as the broad ligament and pelvic blood vessels. Acute PID is rare in the woman without menstrual periods, such as the pregnant, premenarcheal, or postmenopausal woman. In less than 1% of cases, acute PID results from transperitoneal spread of infectious material from a perforated appendix or intraabdominal abscess. Hematogenous and lymphatic spread to the tubes or ovaries is another remote possibility. Unlike an infection in many other areas of the body that may be caused predominantly by one species of microorganism, acute PID is usually a polymicrobial infection that is a mixture of aerobic and anaerobic bacteria, clinically appearing as a complex infection. More than 20 species of microorganisms have been cultured from direct tubal aspiration of purulent material. Therapeutic strategies and regimens are of a broad range, seeking to suppress aerobic and anaerobic organisms.

Annually, acute PID occurs in 1% to 2% of all young, sexually active women. It is the most common serious infection of women ages 16 to 25 years. Approximately 85% of infections are spontaneous in sexually active females. The other 15% of infections develop following procedures that break the cervical mucus barrier, allowing the vaginal flora the opportunity to colonize the upper genital tract. These procedures include endometrial biopsy, curettage, IUD insertion, hysterosalpingography, and hysteroscopy. For emphasis, PID is extremely rare in women who are amenorrheic or not sexually active. When PID is found in the postmenopausal woman, associated conditions such as genital malignancies, diabetes, or concurrent intestinal diseases, such as diverticulitis, appendicitis, or carcinoma, are usually discovered.

One in four women with acute PID experiences medical sequelae. Following acute PID, the rate of ectopic pregnancy increases 6- to 10-fold, and the chance of developing chronic pelvic pain increases fourfold. In the United States, each year, 26,100 ectopic pregnancies and 90,000 new cases of chronic abdominal pain are directly related to PID. The incidence of infertility following acute PID varies widely (6% to 60%), depending on the severity of the infection, number of episodes of infection, and age of the woman. Weström has reported that hospitalized patients have an incidence of infertility caused by tubal obstruction of 11.4% after one episode of PID, 23.1% after two episodes, and 54.3% after three or more episodes. Women with one episode of acute PID are also more susceptible to developing a subsequent infection. It is difficult to distinguish whether this tendency is related primarily to mucosal damage or to reinfection by a potentially infected mate.

The clinical symptoms and signs of acute PID vary considerably and are usually nonspecific. Importantly, some patients may have very little symptomatology, a condition called **silent,** or **asymptomatic pelvic inflammatory disease**. These women may have tubal infertility without a prior history of symptoms or signs consistent with an acute infection (see earlier, Endometritis).

Ideally, laparoscopy with direct visualization of the internal female organs not only improves the diagnostic accuracy but also affords the opportunity for direct culture of purulent material, which might help establish optimum therapy. However, most women do not undergo this procedure because of the expense and risk.

In summary, the CDC has emphasized that physicians should treat women aggressively if there is any suspicion of the disease because the sequelae are so devastating and the clinical diagnosis made from symptoms, signs, and laboratory data is often incorrect.

ETIOLOGY

As noted, acute PID is usually a polymicrobial infection caused by organisms ascending from the vagina and cervix along the mucosa of the endometrium to infect the mucosa of the oviduct. In many cases, no causative organism is found. The two classic sexually transmitted organisms associated with PID, *N. gonorrhoeae* and *C. trachomatis,* cause acute PID in many cases. These two organisms may frequently coexist in the same individual. Endogenous aerobic and anaerobic bacteria that originate from the normal vaginal flora are cultured from tubal fluid in approximately 50% of cases. In women with bacterial vaginosis (BV) and PID, BV-associated microorganisms have been isolated laparoscopically from the fallopian tubes, demonstrating ascension of these organisms. Direct cultures have shown that tubal infections are usually polymicrobial throughout the active infectious process. One investigator found an average of seven different species in intraabdominal cultures obtained via the laparoscope. Laparoscopic studies have demonstrated a correlation of no more than 50% between endocervical and tubal cultures. Thus, endocervical cultures are, at best, a crude index of the specific cause of upper genital tract infection.

Approximately 15% of women with cervical infection by *N. gonorrhoeae* subsequently develop acute PID. The virulence of the strain or colony type of *N. gonorrhoeae* helps predict the incidence of upper genital tract infection. Transparent colonies of *N. gonorrhoeae* on culture medium attach more readily to epithelial cells and thus produce tubal infection more frequently than opaque-appearing colonies. Immunologic studies have demonstrated that an antibody against the outer membrane protein of the gonococcus develops in approximately 70% of women following severe pelvic infection. The lack of significant antibody titers may help explain why teenagers are more likely to develop upper genital tract disease than women in their late 20s.

There is an extremely wide variation in the recovery rates of *N. gonorrhoeae,* depending on the geographic location of the study (**Table 23-8**). However, the prevalence of *N. gonorrhoeae* cervicitis in young women is significantly increased in the South and southeastern regions of the United States. Therefore, the proportion of patients with salpingitis from *N. gonorrhoeae* in these regions is likely much higher than in the Pacific Northwest or other geographic regions with a low gonorrhea prevalence.

Once the gonococcus ascends to the fallopian tube, it selectively adheres to nonciliated mucus-secreting cells. However, most damage occurs to the ciliated cells, most likely because of an acute complement-mediated inflammatory response with the migration of polymorphonuclear leukocytes, vasodilation, and transudation of plasma into the tissues (**Figs. 23-23 and 23-24**). This robust inflammatory response causes cell death and tissue damage. The process of repair with removal of dead cells and fibroblast presence results in scarring and tubal adhesions.

C. trachomatis is an intracellular, sexually transmitted bacterial pathogen. A report from Edinburgh has found a ratio of chlamydial-to-gonococcal PID diagnosed by laparoscopy of 4:1. However, there is a widespread difference in isolation rates (**Table 23-9**). Chlamydia has become more prevalent than gonorrhea. From 20% to 40% of sexually active women have antibodies against *C. trachomatis.* From 10% to 30% of women with acute PID who do not have cultures positive for *Chlamydia* have evidence of acute chlamydial infection by serial antibody titer testing. Approximately 30% of women with documented acute cervicitis secondary to chlamydia subsequently develop acute PID. Studies have shown that upper tract chlamydial infection increases the risk of an ectopic pregnancy by three to six times compared with women without chlamydial infection.

Whereas *N. gonorrhoeae* remains in the fallopian tubes for at most a few days in untreated patients, *Chlamydia* may remain in the fallopian tubes for months after initial colonization of the upper genital tract. Sophisticated PCR assays, in situ hybridization, and electron microscopy studies have demonstrated the persistence of the *C. trachomatis* in the fallopian tubes for years. Whether this represents persistent or recurrent infection of the upper genital tract is unknown.

Cell-mediated immune mechanisms appear to be important in tissue destruction associated with *C. trachomatis* infection. Primary infection appears to be self-limited, with mild symptoms and little permanent damage. In animals, repeat genital exposures to *C. trachomatis* can induce a chronic hypersensitivity response to chlamydial antigens. Because chlamydial 57-kDa protein and human 60-kDa heat shock protein have homologous regions, repeat exposures to *Chlamydia,* such as may occur in asymptomatic untreated *C. trachomatis* cervical infection, may lead to an autoimmune response that causes severe tubal damage, even if *C. trachomatis* is no longer present. Immunologically

Table 23-8 Comparison of *C. trachomatis* and *N. gonorrhoeae* Cervical Isolation and *N. gonorrhoeae* Tubal Isolation in Women with Acute Pelvic Inflammatory Disease

| First Author of Study[†] | No. of Patients | Cervical Infection | | Tubal or Peritoneal Infection* |
		C. trachomatis	*N. gonorrhoeae*	*N. gonorrhoeae*
Henry-Suchet	17	6/16 (38%)	0/4	1/4 (25%)
Møller	166	37 (22%)	9 (5%)	
Mårdh	60	23 (38%)	4 (5%)	
Gjønnaess	65	26/56 (46%)	5 (8%)	0/65
Mårdh	63	19/53 (36%)	11 (17%)	1/14 (7%)
Adler	78	4 (5%)	14 (18%)	
Ripa	206	52/156 (33%)	39 (19%)	
Osser	209	52/111 (47%)	41 (20%)	
Paavonen	106	27 (25%)	27 (25%)	
Paavonen	101	32 (32%)	25 (25%)	
Paavonen	228	69 (30%)	60 (26%)	
Eilard	22	6 (27%)	7 (32%)	1/22 (5%)
Bowi	43	22 (51%)	15 (35%)	
Eschenbach	204	20/100 (20%)	90 (44%)	7/54 (13%)
Sweet	39	2 (5%)	18 (46%)	8/35 (23%)
Cunningham	104		56 (54%)	30/104 (29%)
Thompson	30	3 (10%)	24 (80%)	10/30 (33%)
Total	1741	400/1365 (29%)	445/1728 (26%)	58/328 (18%)

*Isolation of *N. gonorrhoeae* from the peritoneum of the total number of women studied.
[†]Reference to studies appear in original source.
From Eschenbach DA: Acute pelvic inflammatory disease, vol 1. In Gynecology and Obstetrics, Philadelphia, Harper & Row, 1985, p 8.

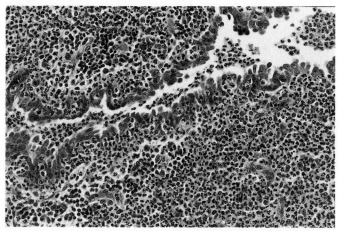

Figure 23-23 Acute salpingitis with a mixture of neutrophils, lymphocytes, and plasma cells in the fallopian tube destroying some of the epithelial lining. (From Voet RL: Color Atlas of Obstetric and Gynecologic Pathology. St. Louis, Mosby, 1997, p 107.)

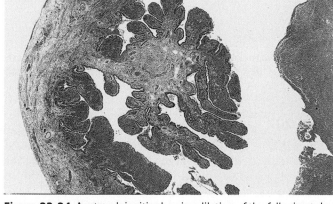

Figure 23-24 Acute salpingitis showing dilation of the fallopian tube and blunting of the papillary fronds. (From Voet RL: Color Atlas of Obstetric and Gynecologic Pathology. St. Louis, Mosby, 1997, p 102.)

sensitized studies have demonstrated that women with antibodies to chlamydial heat shock protein are more likely to have severe tubal scarring and **Fitz-Hugh–Curtis syndrome** (adhesions between the liver and diaphragm indicating prior peritonitis) than women who do not mount this antibody response. Recent basic research has demonstrated a genetic modulation of the immune response to *C. trachomatis* infection, with an increased risk in women with HLA-1. Preliminary evidence has suggested that the specific chlamydial strain also may be an important variable.

The past decade has produced a clinical awareness of a syndrome known as atypical, or silent, PID. This is an asymptomatic, or relatively asymptomatic, inflammation of the upper genital tract often associated with chlamydial infection. The

sequelae of repeated asymptomatic chlamydial infections are tubal infertility and ectopic pregnancy. Some investigators believe that atypical PID may be the more common form of upper tract infection, and symptomatic PID may just be the tip of the iceberg. As many as 40% of women with cervicitis without upper tract symptoms will also have endometritis noted on endometrial biopsy. Studies of women with tubal infertility have found that many women, although not diagnosed as having had overt PID, have had symptoms of acute pelvic pain (see earlier, Endometritis).

The role of genital mycoplasmas as the cause of acute PID is unclear. Cervical cultures positive for *Mycoplasma hominis* and *Ureaplasma urealyticum* may be obtained from most young, sexually active women; the rate of isolation of genital mycoplasmas

Table 23-9 *Chlamydia trachomatis* in Acute Pelvic Inflammatory Disease

Upper Genital and Study*	Fourfold Rise in Number of Patients	Isolation Rate of C. trachomatis		
		Endocervix (%)	Peritoneal Cavity (%)	Serum Antibodies (%)
Eilard et al	22 (23)	6 (27)	2 (9)[†]	5
Mårdh et al	53	19 (37)	6/20 (30)[†]	
Treharne et al	143 (62)[‡]			88
Paavonen et al	106 (26)	27 (26)		19/72
Paavonen	228 (19)	68 (30)		32/167
Mårdh et al	60 (40)	23 (38)		24/60
Ripa et al	206 (57)[§]	52/156 (33)		118
Gjønnaess et al	56 (46)	26 (46)	5/42 (12)[†]	26/52
Møller et al	166 (21)	37 (22)		34
Osser and Persson	111 (51)	52 (47)		37/72
Eschenbach et al	100 (20)	20 (20)	1/54 (2)[‖]	15/74
Sweet et al	37 (23)	2 (5)	0[†]	5/22
Thompson et al	30	3 (10)	3 (10)[¶]	
Sweet et al	71	10 (14)	17 (24) **	
Wasserheit et al	22	10 (45)	8 (36) **	
Kiviat et al	55	12 (22)	12 (22) **	
Brunham et al	50 (40)	7 (14)	4 (8)[¶]	20
Landers et al	148	41 (28)	32 (22) **	
Soper et al	84	13 (15)	1 (1)[¶], 6 (7) **	
Kiviat et al	69		16 (23)	

*References appear in the original source.
[†]Fallopian tube.
[‡]Chlamydial immunoglobulin G (IgG) ≥ 1:64; 23% had IgM = 1:8.
[§]Chlamydial IgG ≥ 1:64; fourfold rise in 28/80 (35%).
[‖]Culdocentesis.
[¶]Exudate from fallopian tube.
**Fallopian tube and/or endometrial cavity
From Sweet RL, Gibbs RS: Infectious Diseases of the Female Genital Tract, 3 rd ed. Baltimore, Williams & Wilkins, 1995.

from the cervix is approximately 75% and similar in populations of women who are sexually active, with and without PID. Direct tubal cultures have demonstrated *M. hominis* in 4% to 17% and *U. urealyticum* in 2% to 20% of women with acute PID. However, serologic studies in women with acute PID have demonstrated that only one woman in four develops a significant rise in antibody titers to these organisms. Experimental inoculation of the cervix of the grivet monkey has demonstrated that the route of spread of mycoplasmas is via the parametria rather than the mucosa. Thus, the primary upper genital tract infection is in the parametria and the tissue surrounding the tubes, not in the tubal lumen. This may help explain the low success rate of direct tubal cultures. Histologically, *Mycoplasma* does not appear to produce damage to the tubal mucosa. These organisms are not highly pathogenic. In summary, in vitro and in vivo studies have suggested that *Mycoplasma* may be a commensal bacterium rather than a pathogen in the oviducts.

However, *M. genitalium*, which is noncultivable and identified by PCR, has recently been associated with cervicitis, endometritis, and tubal factor infertility. In one study of 123 women with laparoscopically determined acute salpingitis, *M. genitalium* was detected in 9 (7%), including 1 woman with a positive fallopian tube specimen. In a different study, *M. genitalium* was detected in the cervix, endometrium, or both of 58 women with histologically confirmed endometritis.

The endogenous aerobic and anaerobic flora of the vagina frequently ascend to colonize and infect the upper reproductive tract. Direct cultures of purulent material (**Fig. 23-25**) from the tubal lumen or posterior cul-de-sac have demonstrated a

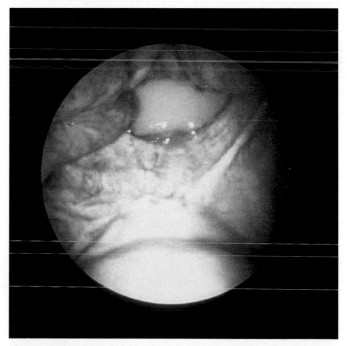

Figure 23-25 Laparoscopic view of the pouch of Douglas with pus from acute PID.

wide range of organisms. The most common aerobic organisms are nonhemolytic *Streptococcus, E. coli,* group B *Streptococcus,* and coagulase-negative *Staphylococcus.* Anaerobic organisms tend to predominate over aerobes, and the most common anaerobic organisms are *Bacteroides* spp., *Peptostreptococcus,* and *Peptococcus.* Anaerobic organisms are almost ubiquitous in pelvic abscesses associated with acute PID. A **tubo-ovarian complex** and abscess are more common in women with concurrent bacterial vaginosis or HIV infection. The findings of concurrent bacterial vaginosis and PID, as well as the association of bacterial vaginosis with endometritis, serve to emphasize the contributory role of these organisms in the pathogenesis of PID. Regardless of the initiating event, the microbiology of PID should be treated as mixed.

RISK FACTORS

Risk factors are important considerations in the clinical management and prevention of upper genital tract infections. There is a strong correlation between the incidence of STIs and acute PID in any given population. In epidemiologic studies, age at first intercourse, marital status, and number of sexual partners are all gross indicators of the frequency of exposure to STIs and PID. Having multiple sexual partners increases the chance of acquiring acute PID by approximately fivefold. Social factors such as involvement with a child protective agency, prior suicide attempt, and alcohol use before intercourse have also been identified in case-control studies as risk factors for PID. The frequency of intercourse with a monogamous partner is not a risk factor.

The age distribution of uncomplicated STI is usually the same as that for acute PID. It is a condition of young women, with 75% of cases occurring in women younger than 25 years. The sexual behavior of teenagers, including lack of contraception, predisposes them to STIs and, correspondingly, acute PID. The incidence decreases with advancing age. The risk that a sexually active adolescent female will develop acute PID is 1 in 8, which decreases to 1 in 80 for women older than 25 years. For unknown reasons, young women with colonization of the cervix by *Chlamydia* have a higher incidence of upper genital tract infection than older women. A hypothesis to explain the increased infection rate in teenagers includes the comparative lack of antibody protection and the wider area of cervical columnar epithelium, which allows colonization by *C. trachomatis* and *N. gonorrhoeae.*

Stone and associates have tabulated proven and hypothetical methods of preventing STIs and acute PID (**Table 23-10**). Clinical and laboratory studies have documented that the use of contraceptives changes the relative risk of developing acute PID. Barrier methods (e.g., condoms, diaphragms, spermicidal preparations) are effective as mechanical obstructive devices and as chemical barriers. Nonoxynol 9, the material ubiquitous in spermicidal preparations, is bactericidal and viricidal. Laboratory tests have demonstrated that nonoxynol 9 kills *N. gonorrhoeae,* genital *Mycoplasma* spp., *T. vaginalis, T. pallidum,* HSV, and HIV. However, doses of 100-mg gel, alone or in a contraceptive sponge, are associated with increased epithelial abrasions and ulcers. The porosity of latex in condoms is more than 1000 times smaller than viral particles. Thus, routine condom use prevents the deposition and transmission of infected organisms from the semen to the endocervix. Many studies have found that women who frequently use a vaginal douche have a threefold to fourfold increased relative risk of PID over women who douche less frequently than once a month.

Multiple case-control studies carried out 20 to 30 years ago reported an increased risk of acute PID in women who were using an IUD. There has been just criticism of these early epidemiologic studies for their selection of control groups and the bias of including women with Dalkon shield IUDs in their statistics. The increase in risk for PID occurs only at the time of insertion of the IUD and in the first 3 weeks after placement. An analysis from the World Health Organization (WHO) has found the rate of PID to be 9.7/1000 woman-year for the first 20 days after insertion compared with 1.4/1000 woman-year for the next 8 years of follow-up. Studies evaluating the newer progesterone-containing IUD have not shown an increased risk of intrauterine infection. Many experts believe that IUDs may be considered in carefully selected nulliparous patients.

Acute salpingitis occurring in a woman with a previous tubal ligation is extremely rare and, when it does occur, the symptoms of the infection are less severe. Phillips and D'Ablaing have reported the incidence of acute PID developing in the proximal stump of previously ligated fallopian tubes as 1 in 450 women hospitalized for acute salpingitis.

Epidemiologic studies have documented that previous acute PID is a definite risk factor for future attacks of the disease. Approximately 25% of women with acute PID subsequently develop another acute tubal infection. Direct cultures have proven that the disease is another primary infection. The microscopic tubal damage produced by the initial upper genital tract infection may facilitate repeat infection. It is possible that prior infection causes an immunologic priming effect, making upper genital tract infection more likely with repeated cervical exposure (see earlier previous discussion of *C. trachomatis* pathology). The increased risk may also be related to an untreated male partner.

Transcervical penetration of the cervical mucus barrier with instrumentation of the uterus is a risk factor because it may initiate iatrogenic acute PID. The incidence of upper genital tract infection associated with first-trimester terminations is approximately 1 in 200 cases. Recent practice has emphasized the use of prophylactic antibiotics to decrease the incidence of associated acute PID. Women with concurrent bacterial vaginosis have a higher risk for postabortal infection and thus should be treated with oral antibiotics with anaerobic coverage.

A growing area of research involves the identification of changes in the virulence of organisms and the host's response to the organisms. Virulence factors of an organism may explain why some lower tract infections progress to upper tract disease but others do not. The gonococcus has characteristics that may become activated in certain environments to increase the virulence of the organism. Similarly, other organisms that are usually of low virulence may have features that affect their virulence and pathogenicity. Both bacterial virulence factors, such as hemolysin enzymes and proteases, and bacterial defense mechanisms that inhibit host responses may become activated in varying microenvironments. Genetic variation may be another risk factor. Some women may be genetically predisposed to mount a robust inflammatory process that may lead to tubal scarring (e.g., chlamydial heat shock protein).

SYMPTOMS AND SIGNS

Patients with acute PID present with a wide range of nonspecific clinical symptoms and signs. The severity of the clinical presentation of acute PID varies from lack of discernible symptoms to diffuse peritonitis and a life-threatening illness. Because the diagnosis is usually based on clinical criteria, there are high false-positive and high false-negative rates. The diagnosis of acute PID, even by experienced clinicians, is imprecise. The differential diagnosis of

Table 23-10 Methods of Preventing STDs, Mechanisms of Action, and Efficacy

Method	Mechanism	Efficacy in Prevention of STDs
Behavioral		
Monogamy	Decreases likelihood of exposure to infected persons	Not well studied; theoretic efficacy
Reducing number of partners	Decreases likelihood of contact with infectious agents	
Avoiding certain sexual practices		
Inspecting and questioning partners		
Barriers		
Condom	Protects partner from direct contact with semen, urethral discharge, or penile lesion	Effective in vitro barrier to chlamydiae, CMV, and HIV, partial protection HSV
	Protects wearer from direct contact with partner's mucosal secretions	Appears to decrease risk of acquiring urethral/cervical GC, PID, and male urethral *Ureaplasma* colonization; partial HPV protection
		Effect on risk of acquiring NGU not established
Spermicide	Chemically inactivates infectious agents	Nonvaginal use has not been studied
		Inactivates gonococci, syphilis spirochetes, trichomonads, HSC, ureaplasmas, and HIV in vitro. In vivo studies disappointing.
		100 mg gel dose and contraceptive sponge associated with epithelial ulcers and abrasiors
Diaphragm/spermicide	Mechanical barrier covers cervix	Diaphragm alone has not been studies
	Used with spermicides	Appears to decrease risk of acquiring cervical GC and PID
Vaccines	Induce antibody response that renders host immune to disease	Commercially available hepatitis B vaccine is safe and effective
		Results of clinical trials of gonococcal and herpes simplex vaccines ongoing
		Gonococcal, HIV, and HSV vaccines research in progress
		Effective guardravalent HPV vaccine safe and effective
Oral Antibiotics		
Penicillin	Kill infectious agent on or shortly after exposure before infection is established	No studies among women or civilian men
Sulfathioazole		Appears to decrease risk of acquiring GC and hard and soft chancres, but use not recommended
Tetracycline analogues		
Local		
Postcoital urination		
Postcoital washing	Flushes infectious agents out of urethra and washes infectious agents of genital skin and mucous membrane	Poorly studied
Postcoital antiseptic douching	Inactivates and washes infectious agents out of vagina	Poorly studied. Not recommended. Increases risk of endometritis

CMV, cytomegalovirus; GC, gonorrhea; HIV, human immunodeficiency virus; HPV, human pappilomavirus; HSV, herpes simplex virus; NGU, nongonococcal urethritis. PID, pelvic inflammatory disease.

From Stone KM, Grimes DA, Magder LS: Primary prevention of sexually transmitted diseases. A primer for clinicians. JAMA 255:1763, 1986. Copyright 1986, American Medical Association.

acute PID includes lower genital tract pelvic infection, ectopic pregnancy, torsion or rupture of an adnexal mass, acute appendicitis, gastroenteritis, and endometriosis.

Laparoscopic studies of women with a clinical diagnosis of acute PID have established the inadequacy of diagnosis by the usual criteria of history, and physical examination, and laboratory studies. In these studies, approximately 20% to 25% of women had no identifiable intraabdominal or pelvic disease. Another 10% to 15% of patients were found to have other pathologic conditions, such as ectopic pregnancy, acute appendicitis, or torsion of the adnexa (**Tables 23-11** and **23-12**). In one study of women in whom laparoscopy was performed because of clinically suspected acute PID, the clinical diagnosis was confirmed at laparoscopy in 532 women (65%). Laparoscopic studies also demonstrate a lack of correlation among the number and intensity of symptoms, signs, and degree of abnormality of laboratory values and the severity of tubal inflammation. Women with

C. trachomatis infections may exhibit minor symptoms but have a severe inflammatory process visualized by laparoscopic examination. Criteria for establishing the severity of acute PID by laparoscopic examination are listed in **Table 23-13**.

Historically, the diagnosis of acute PID was not established unless the woman had the triad of fever, elevated erythrocyte sedimentation rate (ESR), and adnexal tenderness or a mass. Only 17% of laparoscopically identified cases have this classic triad. Thus, reliance on these stringent clinical criteria generally results in most cases being overlooked and untreated. In practice, most women with acute PID do not undergo laparoscopy because of the expense of this invasive technique. Endometrial biopsy is more readily available as a diagnostic tool.

More recently, the PEACH trial found that for women with endometritis diagnosed on endometrial biopsy, the requirement of all three clinical criteria—lower abdominal tenderness, adnexal tenderness, and cervical motion tenderness—resulted in decreased

Table 23-11 Laparoscopic Findings in Patients with False Positive Clinical Diagnosis of Acute PID but with Pelvic Disorders Other Than PID

Laparoscopic Finding	Number
Acute appendicitis	24
Endometriosis	16
Corpus luteum bleeding	12
Ectopic pregnancy	11
Pelvic adhesions only	7
Benign ovarian tumor	7
Chronic salpingitis	6
Miscellaneous	15
Total	98

From Jacobson LJ: Differential diagnosis of acute pelvic inflammatory disease. Am J Obstet Gynecol 138: 1006, 1980.

Table 23-12 Preoperative Diagnoses in Patients with False-Negative Clinical Diagnosis of Acute PID Prior to Laparoscopy/Laparotomy

Clinical Diagnosis	Visual Diagnosis: Acute PID (Number)
Ovarian tumor	20
Acute appendicitis	18
Ectopic pregnancy	16
Chronic salpingitis	10
Acute peritonitis	6
Endmetriosis	5
Uterine myoma	5
Uncharacteristic pelvic pain	5
Miscellaneous	6
Total	91

From Jacobson LJ: Differential diagnosis of acute pelvic inflammatory disease. Am J Obstet Gynecol 138: 1006, 1980.

Table 23-13 Severity of Disease by Laparoscopic Examination

Severity	Findings
Mild	Erythema, edema, no spontaneous purulent exudates*; tubes freely movable
Moderate	Gross purulent material evident; erythema and edema, marked; tubes may not be freely movable, and fimbria stoma may not be patent
Severe	Pyosalpinx or inflammatory complex abscess†

*The tubes may require manipulation to produce purulent exudate.
†The size of any pelvic abscess should be measured.
From Hager WD, Eschenbach DA, Spence MR, et al: Criteria for diagnosis and grading of salpingitis. Obstet Gynecol 61:114, 1983.

Box 23-8 CDC Guidelines for Diagnosis of Acute Pelvic Inflammatory Disease: Clinical Criteria for Initiating Therapy

Minimum Criteria
Empirical treatment of PID should be initiated in sexually active young women and others at risk for STIs if the following minimum criteria are present and no other causes(s) for the illness can be identified:
Lower abdominal tenderness *or*
Adnexal tenderness *or*
Cervical motion tenderness

Additional Criteria for Diagnosing PID
Oral temperature > 38°C
Abnormal cervical or vaginal discharge (mucopurulent)
Presence of abundant WBCs on microscopy of vaginal secretions
Elevated erythrocyte sedimentation rate
Elevated C-reactive protein
Laboratory documentation of cervical infection with *N. gonorrhoeae* or *C. trachomatis*

Definitive Criteria for Diagnosing PID
Histopathologic evidence of endometritis on endometrial biopsy
Transvaginal sonography or MRI showing thickened fluid-filled tubes, with or without free pelvic fluid or tubo-ovarian complex
Laparoscopic abnormalities consistent with PID
Although initial treatment can be made before bacteriologic diagnosis of *C. trachomatis* or *N. gonorrhoeae* infection, such a diagnosis emphasizes the need to treat sex partners.

PID, Pelvic inflammatory disease; STI, sexually transmitted infection; WBC, white blood cells.
Workowski KA, Berman S; Centers for Disease Control and Prevention (CDC): Sexually transmitted diseases treatment guidelines, MMWR 59(RR-12):64, 2010.

unlikely that the woman has acute PID. Approximately 75% of patients with acute PID have an associated endocervical infection or coexistent purulent vaginal discharge. Abnormal uterine bleeding, especially spotting or menorrhagia, is noted in approximately 40% of patients. Nausea and vomiting are relatively late symptoms in the course of the disease.

The symptoms of acute pelvic infection secondary to *N. gonorrhoeae* are of rapid onset, and the pelvic pain usually begins a few days after the start of a menstrual period. Acute pelvic infection caused by *C. trachomatis* alone often may have an indolent course with slow onset, less pain, and less fever. It is important to remember that up to 50% of women with tubal damage never experience any symptoms consistent with PID.

Five percent to 10% of women with acute PID develop symptoms of perihepatic inflammation, the Fitz-Hugh–Curtis syndrome (**Fig. 23-26**). Persistent symptoms and signs include right upper quadrant pain, pleuritic pain, and tenderness in the right upper quadrant when the liver is palpated. The pain may radiate to the shoulder or into the back. Liver transaminase levels may be elevated. The condition is often mistakenly diagnosed as pneumonia or acute cholecystitis. Fitz-Hugh–Curtis syndrome develops from transperitoneal or vascular dissemination of the gonococcal or *Chlamydia* organism to produce the perihepatic inflammation. Other organisms, including anaerobic streptococci and coxsackievirus, have also been associated with this syndrome. When laparoscopy is performed, the liver capsule will appear inflamed, with classic violin string adhesions to the parietal peritoneum beneath the diaphragm. Women with

sensitivity. Hence, in 2006, the CDC treatment guidelines were changed to state that empirical therapy for PID should be initiated in sexually active young women and other women at risk for STIs with pelvic or lower abdominal pain if cervical motion tenderness, uterine tenderness, or adnexal tenderness is present. The CDC 2010 diagnostic criteria are summarized in **Box 23-8**.

The most frequent symptom of acute PID is new-onset lower abdominal and pelvic pain. Typically, the pain is diffuse, bilateral, and usually described as constant and dull. It may be exacerbated by motion or sexual activity and, on occasion, the pain may become cramping. The duration of pain is usually less than 7 days. If the pain has been present for longer than 3 weeks, it is

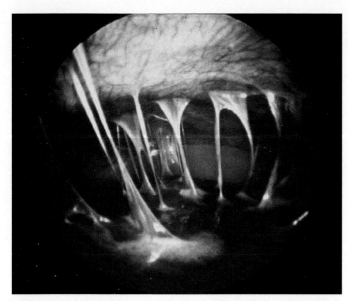

Figure 23-26 Classic violin string sign of Fitz-Hugh–Curtis syndrome in PID.

perihepatitis have a higher prevalence of moderate to severe pelvic adhesions and a higher prevalence and titers of antibodies to chlamydial heat shock protein 60. Treatment is the same as the treatment for acute salpingitis.

Lower abdominal and pelvic tenderness during examination is the hallmark of acute PID. On abdominal examination, patients have tenderness to direct palpation in the lower abdomen, and occasionally rebound tenderness. On pelvic examination, bilateral tenderness of the parametria and adnexa is present and may be exacerbated with movement of the uterus or cervix during the pelvic examination. An ill-defined adnexal fullness is frequently noted, which may represent edema, inflammatory adhesions to the small or large intestine, or an adnexal complex or abscess. The incidence of true adnexal abscess is approximately 10% in women with acute PID.

DIAGNOSIS

Direct visualization via the laparoscope is the most accurate method of diagnosing acute PID. If the woman has impending septic shock, acute surgical abdomen, or a complicated differential diagnosis in a postmenopausal woman, laparoscopy or laparotomy is strongly indicated. The laparoscopy is diagnostic but also offers the additional advantage of concurrent operative procedures such as lysis of adhesions, potential drainage of an abscess, and irrigation of the pelvic cavity. To date, operative laparoscopy during acute infection has not been proved to reduce the prevalence of long-term sequelae. With the change in management toward outpatient therapy, laparoscopy is used less frequently. Acute PID should be included in the differential diagnosis of any sexually active young woman with pelvic pain.

Elevated temperature is an unreliable diagnostic sign because only one of three women with acute PID present with a temperature higher than 38° C. Laboratory tests may be ordered but are also insensitive and nonspecific. Less than 50% of women with acute PID have a white blood cell count higher than 10,000 cells/mL. Leukocytosis does not correlate with the need for hospitalization or the severity of tubal inflammation. The ESR is elevated (>15 mm/hr) in approximately 75% of women with laparoscopically confirmed acute pelvic infection. However, 53% of women with pelvic pain and visually normal pelvic organs have an elevated ESR. C-reactive protein levels have been used, but are not reliable enough to guide clinical management. Combinations of positive test results improve diagnostic specificity and positive predictive value. However, this results in a diminution of sensitivity and negative predictive value (**Table 23-14**). Women with acute PID should have a sensitive test for human chorionic gonadotropin to help in the differential diagnosis of ectopic pregnancy. Approximately 3 to 4 of every 100 women who are admitted to a hospital with a diagnosis of acute pelvic infection have an ectopic pregnancy.

Because most cases of upper genital tract infection are preceded by lower genital tract infection, it is important to examine the endocervical mucus for inflammatory cells and perform the

Table 23-14 Diagnostic Test Characteristics of Laboratory Tests for the Diagnosis of Acute Upper Genital Tract Infection

Test	Sensitivity (%)	Specificity (%)	30% NPV	30% PPV	60% NPV	60% PPV
Entire Cohort (N = 120)						
ESR	70	52	80	38	54	69
CRP	71	66	84	47	60	76
WBC	57	88	83	67	58	88
Vaginal WBC	78	39	80	35	54	66
Classical PID (N = 70)						
ESR	72	53	82	40	56	70
CRP	76	59	85	44	62	74
WBC	66	80	85	59	61	83
Vaginal WBC	87	38	87	38	66	68
Nonclassical PID (N = 50)						
ESR	64	51	77	36	49	66
CRP	58	73	80	48	54	76
WBC	38	97	78	84	51	95
Vaginal WBC	62	41	72	31	42	6

CRP, C-reactive protein; ESR, erythrocyte sedimentation rate; NPV, negative predictive value; PPV, positive predictive value; WBC, white blood cell count.
From Peipert JF, Boardman L, Hogan JW, et al: Laboratory evaluation of acute upper genital tract infection. Obstet Gynecol 87:733, 1996. Reprinted with permission from the American College of Obstetricians and Gynecologists.

NAAT for *N. gonorrhoeae* and *C. trachomatis.* The presence of an increased number of vaginal white blood cells is the most sensitive laboratory indicator of acute PID. If the cervical discharge appears normal and no white blood cells are found on the wet preparation of vaginal fluid, the diagnosis of PID is unlikely and alternative causes of pain should be considered.

Because clinical symptoms and signs are nonspecific for the disease, the rates of false-positives and false-negatives are high when the diagnosis is based on clinical criteria. However, because of the long-term sequelae of the disease, most clinicians maintain a low threshold in entertaining a diagnosis of acute PID, readily accepting that they are treating many women who actually do not have pelvic infection so as not to omit treating those with early or mild disease. For the CDC guidelines for the diagnosis of acute PID, see **Box 23-8**.

An endometrial biopsy for evidence of endometritis can be a useful tool. This test is primarily used to help confirm clinical suspicion because of the time required to obtain the result. Although most women with acute salpingitis have coexisting endometritis, the converse—that most women with endometritis have salpingitis—has not been established. In one study of women with biopsy-proven endometritis, the accuracy of coexistent acute PID confirmed by laparoscopy had a sensitivity of 89% and a specificity of 87%.

Ultrasonography is of limited value for patients with mild or moderate PID because of its low sensitivity, but vaginal ultrasonography is helpful in documenting an adnexal mass. It is also a noninvasive diagnostic aid for patients who are so tender during pelvic examination that the physician cannot determine the presence or absence of a pelvic mass. Although ultrasonography is neither specific nor sensitive in distinguishing the cause of a pelvic mass, findings of dilated and fluid-filled tubes, free peritoneal fluid, and adnexal masses may be confirmatory of symptoms and physical signs (**Figs. 23-27 to 23-30**). Thus, vaginal ultrasound has a high positive predictive value when used in a high-risk population. Magnetic resonance imaging (MRI) is sensitive, but its expense and limited acute availability in some locations have restricted its role in PID diagnosis.

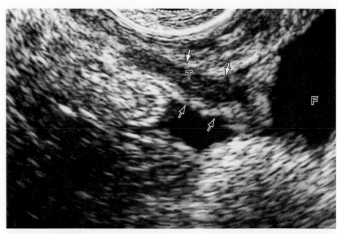

Figure 23-28 Longitudinal section of a slightly dilated and fluid-filled tube (T). Its walls are slightly thickened *(arrows)*. Endometrial biopsy showed plasma cell endometritis. F, Free fluid. (From Cacciatore B, Leminen A, Ingman-Friberg S, et al: Transvaginal sonographic findings in ambulatory patients with suspected pelvic inflammatory disease. Obstet Gynecol 80:912, 1992.)

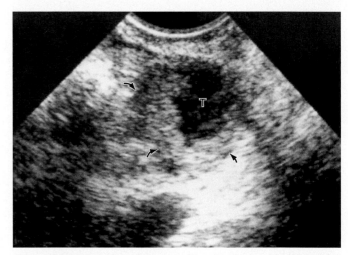

Figure 23-29 Sonographic image of a cross section of a dilated and fluid-filled fallopian tube (T). The wall is thickened and irregular in shape *(arrows)*. Endometrial biopsy revealed plasma endometritis. (From Cacciatore B, Leminen A, Ingman-Friberg S, et al: Transvaginal sonographic findings in ambulatory patients with suspected pelvic inflammatory disease. Obstet Gynecol 80:912, 1992.)

The percentage of American women with acute PID who also are infected with HIV has been estimated to be 6% to 22%. Women with acute PID and HIV infection have a higher incidence of adnexal masses. However, an acute pelvic infection responds to antibiotic therapy in a similar fashion to that in women who are not infected with HIV. The CDC continues to emphasize the importance of treating partners of women with STIs.

TREATMENT

Treatment of the woman with PID encompasses more than just prescribing the appropriate antimicrobial regimen. Determining the need for hospitalization, patient education, treatment of

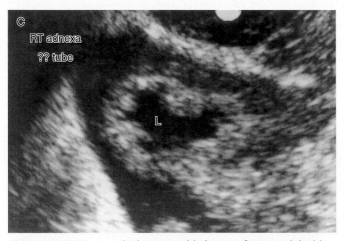

Figure 23-27 Transvaginal sonographic image of acute salpingitis. The central sonolucent fluid in the lumen (L) and the thickened endosalpingeal folds give this a cogwheel appearance. (From Timor-Tritsch IE, Lerner JP, Monteagudo A, et al: Transvaginal sonographic markers of tubal inflammatory disease. Ultrasound Obstet Gynecol 12:56, 1998.)

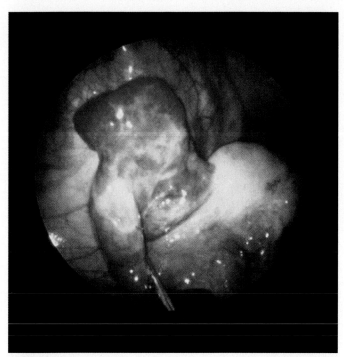

Figure 23-30 Laparoscopic view of acute PID and a tubo-ovarian abscess.

Table 23-15 Microorganisms Isolated from Fallopian Tubes of Patients with Acute Pelvic Inflammatory Disease

Type of Agent	Organism
Sexually transmitted disease	Chlamydia trachomatis
	Neisseria gonorrhoeae
	Mycoplasma hominis
Endogenous agent aerobic or facultative	Streptococcus species
	Staphylococcus speciesHaemophilus
	Escherichia coli
Anaerobic	Bacteroides species
	Peptococcus species
	Peptostreptocccus species
	Clostridium species
	Actinomyces species

From Weström L: Introductory address: Treatment of pelvic inflammatory disease in view of etiology and risk factors. Sex Transm Dis 11:439, 1984.

sexual partners, and careful follow-up are key issues. The two most important goals of the medical therapy of acute PID are the resolution of symptoms and preservation of tubal function. Antibiotic therapy should be started as soon STI screening results have been obtained and the diagnosis has been suggested. Early diagnosis and early treatment will help reduce the number of women who suffer from the long-term sequelae of the disease. Women who are not treated in the first 72 hours following the onset of symptoms are three times as likely to develop tubal infertility or ectopic pregnancy as those who are treated early in the disease process. Animal and human studies have suggested that early antibiotic treatment improves long-term fertility. In the management of acute PID, one should not forget the treatment and education of the male partner for the prevention of the disease, including the use of proper contraceptives, which help reduce the rate of upper genital tract infection.

Although the choice of antibiotic therapy for most infectious diseases is usually based on cultures and sensitivity of bacteria obtained directly from the site of the infection in PID, direct tubal cultures are not practical. Because most cases of PID are polymicrobial, broad-spectrum antibiotic coverage is indicated. Empirical antibiotic protocols should cover a wide range of bacteria, including *N. gonorrhoeae, C. trachomatis,* anaerobic rods and cocci, gram-negative aerobic rods, and gram-positive aerobes (**Table 23-15**). Selection of one antibiotic protocol over another may be influenced by the clinical history. For example, acute PID following an operative procedure is usually caused by endogenous flora of the vagina, whereas acute PID in a 19-year-old college student is likely secondary to *C. trachomatis.*

A failure of outpatient oral therapy may be related to non-compliance, reinfection, or inadequate antibiotic coverage for **penicillinase-producing gonorrhea,** chromosomally mediated resistant *N. gonorrhoeae,* or facultative or anaerobic organisms involved in upper genital tract infection that are resistant to

the drug prescribed. It is important to know resistance profiles in your geographic region. Inpatient failure rates for resolution of acute symptoms with IV antibiotics are approximately 5% to 10%.

A variety of oral and parenteral antibiotic regimens have been effective in achieving short-term clinical and microbiologic cures in randomized clinical trials. However, there are a paucity of data comparing the effect of various protocols on the incidence of long-term complications and elimination of bacterial infection in the endometrium and fallopian tubes. The CDC has published recommendations for the outpatient treatment of PID (**Box 23-9**). Ceftriaxone, 250 mg IM once, or cefoxitin, 2 g IM, plus probenecid, 1 g orally in a single dose, concurrently once, or another parenteral third-generation cephalosporin such as ceftizoxime or cefotaxime together with doxycycline, 100 mg orally twice daily for 14 days, is the recommended outpatient regimen. The optimal cephalosporin choice is not known. Ceftizoxime has unparalleled coverage against *N. gonorrhoeae;* cefotaxime has better anaerobic coverage. The clinician should individualize the choice of regimens depending on his or her estimate of the need for anaerobic coverage. Importantly, if the woman has bacterial vaginosis, adding prolonged coverage with metronidazole, 500 mg orally twice daily for 14 days, is preferable.

Box 23-9 CDC Recommendations for Ambulatory Management of Acute Pelvic Inflammatory Disease

Ceftriaxone, 250 mg IM, single dose
  or
Cefoxitin, 2 g IM, single dose, and probenecid, 1 g PO administered concurrently in a single dose
  or
Other parenteral third-generation cephalosporin (e.g., ceftizoxime, cefotaxime)
  plus
Doxycycline, 100 mg PO bid for 14 days
  with or without
Metronidazole, 500 mg PO bid for 14 days

Workowski KA, Berman S; Centers for Disease Control and Prevention (CDC): Sexually transmitted diseases treatment guidelines, MMWR 59(RR-2):66, 2010.

Other regimens with at least one trial include amoxicillin–clavulanic acid and doxycycline. However, this regimen may be difficult to tolerate because of adverse gastrointestinal symptoms. Azithromycin has demonstrated short-term effectiveness in one randomized trial; another trial used azithromycin combined with ceftriaxone, 250 mg IM single dose, with azithromycin, 1 g orally once weekly for 2 weeks. Also, with these regimens, consider the addition of metronidazole, because anaerobic organisms are suspected in the cause of PID and metronidazole will also treat BV, which is frequently associated with PID. Quinolone-containing regimens are no longer routinely recommended because of gonorrhea resistance. However, if parenteral cephalosporin therapy is not feasible, the use of fluoroquinolones (levofloxacin, 500 mg orally once daily, or ofloxacin, 400 mg twice daily for 14 days), with or without metronidazole, may be considered if the community prevalence and individual risk of gonorrhea are low, or if the diagnostic test result for gonorrhea performed prior to instituting therapy is negative.

It is important to reexamine women within 48 to 72 hours of initiating outpatient therapy to evaluate the response of the disease to oral antibiotics. The woman should be hospitalized when the therapeutic response is not optimal. If the disease is responding well, approximately 4 to 6 weeks after therapy the woman should be reexamined to assess the resolution of clinical symptoms and establish a post-treatment baseline.

In the past, many practitioners preferred to hospitalize nulliparous women for the treatment of PID, but this is no longer recommended. A multicenter trial of 831 women has found no advantage to inpatient treatment of mild to moderate PID randomized to inpatient versus outpatient treatment. In over 84 months of follow-up, there were an equivalent number of pregnancies, live births, time to pregnancy, infertility, recurrent PID, chronic pelvic pain, and ectopic pregnancy in the inpatient and outpatient treatment groups. This was true even in teenagers and women without a previous live birth.

The CDC has established criteria for hospitalization (**Box 23-10**). These include unsure diagnosis, being too ill to tolerate oral therapy, no improvement with oral therapy, and presence of a tubo-ovarian abscess or pregnancy. Acute PID associated with the presence of an IUD may be more advanced at the time of diagnosis than infection without a foreign body. Patient and physician delays in diagnosis are not unusual. Often, women misinterpret the early signs and symptoms of an infection as being related to the IUD. Pelvic infections with an IUD in place and pelvic infections following operative or diagnostic procedures often are caused by anaerobic bacteria. Outpatient therapy leaving the IUD in situ may be attempted if close

---

Box 23-10 Indications for Hospitalizing Patients with Acute Pelvic Inflammatory Disease

Surgical emergencies (e.g., appendicitis) cannot be excluded.
The patient is pregnant.
The patient does not respond clinically to oral antimicrobial therapy.
The patient is unable to follow or tolerate an outpatient oral regimen.
The patient has severe illness, nausea and vomiting, or high fever.
The patient has a tubo-ovarian abscess.

Adapted from Workowski KA, Berman S; Centers for Disease Control and Prevention (CDC): Sexually transmitted diseases treatment guidelines, MMWR 59 (RR-12):65, 2010.

Box 23-11 Inpatient Management of Acute Pelvic Inflammatory Disease

Parenteral Regimen A
Cefotetan, 2 g IV every 12 hr
or
Cefoxitin, 2 g IV every 6 hr
plus
Doxycycline, 100 mg PO or IV every 12 hr
NOTE: Because of pain associated with infusion, doxycycline should be administered orally when possible, even when the patient is hospitalized. PO and IV administration of doxycycline provide similar bioavailability.

Parenteral Regimen B
Clindamycin, 900 mg IV every 8 hr
plus
Gentamicin, loading dose IV or IM (2 mg/kg of body weight) followed by a maintenance dose (1.5 mg/kd) every 8 hr. Single daily dosing may be substituted.

Alternative Parenteral Regimens
Limited data support the use of other parenteral regimens. The following regimen has been investigated in a least one clinical trial, and has broad-spectrum coverage:
Ampicillin-sulbactam, 3 g IV every 6 hr
plus
Doxycycline, 100 mg PO or IV every 12 hr
One trial has demonstrated high short-term clinical cure rates with azithromycin, either as monotherapy for 1 wk (500 mg IV × one or two doses followed by 250 mg PO, 5-6 days) or combined with a 12-day course of metronidazole.

Adapted from Workowski KA, Berman S; Centers for Disease Control and Prevention (CDC): Sexually transmitted diseases treatment guidelines, MMWR 59 (RR-12):65, 2010.

---

follow-up of the woman is possible. If the pelvic infection worsens or does not improve, the IUD should be removed. Concurrent immunodeficiency, especially HIV infection with a low $CD4^+$ count, is another reason to consider hospitalization. If a therapeutic response or compliance with oral medications has not been optimal or is questionable, or if follow-up in 72 hours is not possible, the woman should be admitted for IV antibiotic therapy.

The 2010 CDC guidelines for inpatient treatment of acute PID with parenteral therapy are listed in **Box 23-11**. The protocols stress the polymicrobial origin of acute pelvic infection, increasing importance of *C. trachomatis,* and emergence of penicillin-resistant *N. gonorrhoeae.* With IV protocols, the CDC recommends that IV antibiotics be continued for at least 24 hours after substantial improvement in the patient. When the woman has a mass, we add ampicillin to clindamycin and gentamicin. However, for patients without a mass, we switch to oral antibiotics when the symptoms have diminished and the woman has been afebrile for 24 hours. In both regimens, doxycycline is continued for a total of 14 days.

Regimen A is a combination of doxycycline and IV cefoxitin. It is excellent for community-acquired infection. Doxycycline and cefoxitin provide excellent coverage for *N. gonorrhoeae,* *C. trachomatis,* and penicillinase-producing *N. gonorrhoeae.* Cefoxitin is an excellent antibiotic against *Peptococcus* and *Peptostreptococcus* spp. and *E. coli.* The disadvantage of this combination is that the two drugs are less than ideal for a pelvic abscess or anaerobic infections. To date, cefotetan has been found to be as effective as cefoxitin. There is no clinically significant difference in the bioavailability of doxycycline whether it is given by the oral or IV route. Thus, doxycycline should be administered orally whenever possible because of the marked superficial phlebitis produced by IV infusion.

Doxycycline should be included in the regimen of follow-up oral therapy. Sweet and associates have observed 17 women with PID who initially had endometrial cultures positive for *Chlamydia*. Clinically, 16 of 17 women responded to treatment with cephalosporins alone. However, posttreatment endometrial cultures remained positive for *Chlamydia* in 12 of 13 women. Therefore, without tetracycline or erythromycin, a woman may appear free of symptoms but may still be harboring *Chlamydia*. Antibiotics active against *C. trachomatis* must be present in effective dosages for at least 7 days for clinical and microbiologic cures to occur. *C. trachomatis* has a 48- to 72-hour life cycle inside the mucosal cell. Thus, prolonged therapeutic levels of the antichlamydial antibiotic are imperative.

Regimen B is a combination of clindamycin and an aminoglycoside (gentamicin). It has the advantage of providing excellent coverage for anaerobic infections and facultative gram-negative rods. Therefore, it is preferred for patients with an abscess, IUD-related infection, and pelvic infection after a diagnostic or operative procedure. Studies have demonstrated that high IV levels of clindamycin, such as 900 mg every 8 hours, provide activity against 90% of bacterial strains of *Chlamydia*. Most infectious disease experts recommend the use of a single daily dose of gentamicin rather than a dose given every 8 hours. The initial once-daily aminoglycoside dosage is based on nomograms that take body weight into consideration. The advantages of a once-daily aminoglycoside program are decreased toxicity, increased efficacy, and decreased cost. Also, no serum drug levels need to be measured. Aztreonam, a monobactam, has an antibiotic spectrum similar to that of the aminoglycosides but without renal toxicity but is much more expensive. It may be given in a dose of 2 g IV every 8 hours. Also, a third-generation cephalosporin may be used instead of an aminoglycoside in a woman with renal disease. Parenteral antibiotic therapy may be discontinued when the woman has been afebrile for 24 hours, and oral therapy with doxycycline (100 mg twice daily) should continue to complete 14 days of therapy.

Alternative inpatient regimens include ampicillin-sulbactam plus doxycycline because they have excellent anaerobic coverage and would be a good choice for women with a tubo-ovarian complex. The alternative regimen has less extensive clinical trials.

In summary, no regimen is uniformly effective for all patients. To date, there are insufficient clinical data to suggest the superiority of one regimen over another with respect to initial response or subsequent fertility.

Operative treatment of acute PID has decreased markedly in the past 15 years. Operations are restricted to life-threatening infections, ruptured tubo-ovarian abscesses, laparoscopic drainage of a pelvic abscess, persistent masses in some older women for whom future childbearing is not a consideration, and removal of a persistent symptomatic mass. Because of the techniques of in vitro fertilization, every effort is made to perform conservative surgery and preserve ovarian and uterine function in women who are not done with childbearing. Unilateral removal of a tubo-ovarian complex or an abscess is a frequent conservative procedure for acute PID. Similarly, drainage of a cul-de-sac

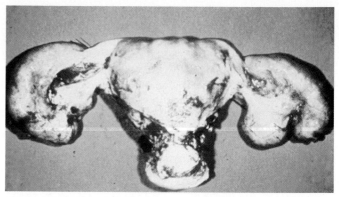

Figure 23-31 Hysterectomy specimen from a 23-year-old woman with bilateral tubo-ovarian abscesses.

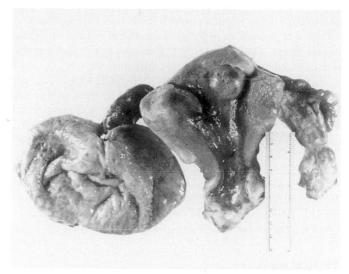

Figure 23-32 Pyosalpinx. The right tube is markedly enlarged and contains 50 mL of creamy pus. The tubal wall is thickened. (From Janovski NA [ed]: Color Atlas of Gross Gynecologic and Obstetric Pathology. New York, McGraw-Hill, 1969, p 131.)

abscess via percutaneous drainage or a colpotomy incision results in preservation of the reproductive organs.

Rigorously defined, an abscess is a collection of pus within a newly created space. In contrast, a tubo-ovarian complex is a collection of pus within an anatomic space created by the adherence of adjacent organs. Abscesses caused by acute PID contain a mixture of anaerobes and facultative or aerobic organisms (**Figs. 23-31** and **23-32**). The environment of an abscess cavity results in a low level of oxygen tension. Therefore, anaerobic organisms predominate and have been cultured from 60% to 100% of reported cases. Basic studies have discovered that clindamycin penetrates the human neutrophil, and it is possible that this property facilitates the level of clindamycin within the abscess. Clindamycin is also stable in the abscess environment, which is not true of many other antibiotics. Thus, a combination of clindamycin and an aminoglycoside is considered the standard for treatment of a tubo-ovarian abscess. This combination does not treat *Enterococcus*, and ampicillin should be added if there is suspicion that this organism is involved. Metronidazole alone is an effective alternative to clindamycin for anaerobic infections but does not provide gram-negative coverage. If abscesses do not respond to parenteral broad-spectrum antibiotics, drainage is imperative.

Transvaginal or transabdominal percutaneous aspiration or drainage of pelvic abscesses may be accomplished under ultrasonic or computed tomography (CT) guidance. This technique has shown excellent results. In one small randomized trial, early transvaginal drainage and intensive antibiotic therapy were compared with intensive antibiotic therapy alone. A favorable short-term outcome occurred in 90% of those who underwent ultrasound-guided transvaginal drainage in contrast to 65% of the control group. However, fertility and ectopic pregnancy rates after percutaneous drainage are unknown at this time. Long-term recurrence and sequelae need to be evaluated before this technique is accepted as a therapeutic standard. A strong contraindication to percutaneous aspiration is any suspicion of an infected carcinoma in the differential diagnosis. Laparoscopic aspiration of tubo-ovarian complexes is another alternative. This procedure has shown good results but does not have greater benefit than percutaneous ultrasound-guided aspiration of abscess cavities. Laparoscopic aspiration obviously carries more operative risks than ultrasound-guided aspiration.

Postmenopausal women with suspected PID should have appropriate imaging studies to rule out other concurrent diseases, especially malignancies. The bacterial cause in postmenopausal women does not usually include a sexually transmitted microorganism, but rather bacteria from the intestinal tract or normal vaginal flora. The disease process involves tubo-ovarian complexes and abscesses. Medical treatment should emphasize broad-spectrum antibiotic regimens with adequate anaerobic coverage. Operative intervention in a postmenopausal woman should be considered early in the disease, especially if the condition does not improve rapidly with medical treatment.

SEQUELAE

Before antibiotic therapy, the mortality rate associated with acute PID was 1%. Grimes has estimated that there is presently one death every other day in the United States directly related to PID. Most of these deaths result from rupture of tubo-ovarian abscesses. The current mortality rate is 5% to 10% for ruptured tubo-ovarian abscesses, even with modern medical and operative treatment.

Recurrent acute PID is experienced by approximately 25% of women. Younger women become reinfected twice as often as older women. A great challenge to health care providers is to educate women with PID to reduce their chances of a second episode of infection. It is essential and imperative that preventive medicine include treatment and education of the male partner. Liberal prescriptions for treatment of lower genital tract disease and selection of contraceptives that will reduce the chance of upper genital tract infections are also important for these women. Because sequelae to PID, overt and silent, are related to the number of infections, prevention cannot be overemphasized. Because most PID in the United States is related to STIs, increased attention to partner treatment and education is appropriate.

The morbidity, suffering, and cost of PID arise from the scarring and adhesion formation that accompany healing of damaged tissues after the infection itself is eradicated. These effects result in ectopic pregnancy, chronic pain, and infertility. Approximately 10% to 15% of pregnancies will be ectopic after laparoscopically mild to moderate PID, and almost 50% after severe PID. The number of hospitalizations for ectopic

Table 23-16 Summary of Reproductive Events after Index Laparoscopy in the Total Sample of 1732 Patients and 601 Control Subjects

Category	No. of Patients (%)	No. of Control Subjects (%)
Total no. followed	1732	601
Avoiding pregnancy	370 (21.4)	144 (24.0)
Not pregnant for unknown reasons*	53 (3.1)	6 (1.0)
Attempting pregnancy	1309	451
Pregnant	1100 (80.8)	439 (96.1)
First pregnancy ectopic	100 (9.1)	6 (1.4)
Not pregnant	209 (16.0)	12 (2.7)
Completely examined	162	3
With proved TFI	141	0
With nTFI (other cause of infertility)	21	3
Incompletely examined	47	9

*Reporting no use of contraceptive and not consulting for infertility.
nTFI, nontubular factor infertility. TFI, tubal factor infertility.
From Weström L, Joeseof R, Reynolds G, et al: Pelvic inflammatory disease and fertility. A cohort study of 1,844 women with laparoscopically verified disease and 657 control women with normal laparoscopic results. Sex Transm Dis 19:185, 1992.

pregnancies peaked around 1989 at 90,000 and declined to 20,000 in 2009. This decline is partially a result of outpatient management of ectopic pregnancies, but is mostly a result of successful chlamydia screening and prevention programs. One case-control study has suggested that chlamydia-associated PID alone causes almost half of all ectopic pregnancies (**Table 23-16**).

Studies have found that chronic pain is a common sequela of a symptomatic pelvic infection. In one study, the chance that a woman will develop chronic pelvic pain following acute salpingitis was four times greater than the risk for control subjects. Approximately 20% of women with acute pelvic infections subsequently developed chronic pelvic pain versus approximately 5% in controls without pelvic infection. Other studies have found similar results (**Table 23-17**). Among women with chronic pelvic pain, approximately two of three are involuntarily infertile, and a similar percentage have deep dyspareunia. In a study from Oxford of 1355 women with PID and 10,507 controls, chronic abdominal pain developed 10 times more commonly in those who had PID (**Table 23-18**). Chronic pelvic pain may be caused by a **hydrosalpinx**, a collection of sterile watery fluid in the fallopian tube. A hydrosalpinx (**Fig. 23-33**) is the end-stage development of a pyosalpinx. Chronic pain often develops in a woman, even though she may have had a normal pelvic examination when examined 4 to 8 weeks following her acute infection. The pain may result from adhesions and the resultant fixation or tethering of organs intended to have freedom of movement during physical activity, coitus, and ovulation (**Table 23-19**). Women with chronic pelvic pain and a history of acute PID may benefit from laparoscopy to establish the diagnosis and rule out other diseases, such as endometriosis. Often, conservative surgery for this sequelae via laparoscopy or celiotomy is successful.

Acute pelvic infection is one of the major causes of female infertility. Epidemiologic studies have estimated that between 4% and 13% of women are infertile or undergo an operative procedure secondary to acute PID.

The sequelae of infections include a damaged yet patent oviduct, peritubular and periovarian adhesions that may hinder

Table 23-17 Frequency and Predictors of Long-Term Sequelae of Acute Pelvic Inflammatory Disease

Sequela	Frequency (No. and %)	Risk Factor	*Univariate Analysis*		Multivariate Analysis *P* Value
			P	Relative Risk and 95% Confidence Interval	
Involuntary infertility	17/42 (40%)	History of pelvic inflammatory disease (PID)	0.05	1.8 (1.0-3.3)	0.05
		Age at time of first sex	0.04	0.39	0.07
		≥2 days of pain before therapy	0.02	2.0 (1.1-3.6)	
Chronic pelvic pain	12/51 (24%)	History of PID	0.03	1.5 (1.0-2.2)	
PID after index episode	22/51 (43%)	History of PID	0.06	1.7 (0.9-3.1)	0.02
		Mean no. of days of pain before therapy	0.04	—	0.04
		Age at time of first sex	0.0008	—	0.01
Ectopic pregnancy	2/51 (2.4%)	*			

*Risk analysis not performed because of small numbers involved.
From Safrin S Schacter J, Dahrouge D, Sweet RL: Long-term sequelae of acute inflammatory disease. A retrospective cohort study. Am J Obstet Gynccol 166:1300, 1992.

Table 23-18 Standardized (Indirect Standardization) First Event Rates Per 1000 Woman-Years for Specified Outcomes*

Outcome Condition	Women with PID (*N* = 1,200)	Women with Control Conditions (*N* = 10,507)	Relative Risk
Nonspecific abdominal pain	16.7 (155)	1.7 (158)	9.8
Gynecologic pain	3.6 (38)	0.8 (70)	4.5
Endometriosis	2.2 (18)	0.4 (34)	5.5
Hysterectomy	18.2 (152)	2.3 (204)	7.9
Ectopic pregnancy	1.9 (19)	0.2 (14)	9.5

*After admission with acute pelvic inflammatory disease or a control event in cohorts of women in the Oxford Record Linkage Study followed from 1970 to 1985. Number of women shown in parentheses.
From Buchan H, Vessey M, Goldacre M, Fairweather J: Morbidity following pelvic inflammatory disease. Br J Obstet Gynaecol 100:558, 1993.

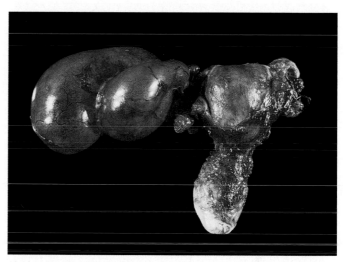

Figure 23-33 Hydrosalpinx with marked dilation of the fallopian tube and blunting of the fimbriated end. (From Voet RL: Color Atlas of Obstetric and Gynecologic Pathology. St. Louis, Mosby, 1997, p 107.)

Table 23-19 Associations among History of Acute Pelvic Inflammatory Disease and Adnexal Adhesions, Distal Tubal Occlusion, and/or Perihepatic Adhesions

Laparoscopic Findings	Pelvic Inflammatory Disease		OR	95% CI	*P*
	Yes (*N* = 22)	No (*N* = 90)			
Distal tubal occlusion	4 (18.2%)	7 (7.8%)	2.6	0.7-10.0	0.14
Tubal adhesions	8 (36.4%)	21 (23.3%)	1.9	0.7-5.1	0.16
Ovarian adhesions	9 (40.9%)	21 (23.3%)	2.3	0.9-6.5	0.08
Perihepatic adhesions	3/21 (14.3%)	2/84 (2.4%)	6.8	1.1-43.9	0.05
Any adhesions	11 (50.0%)	25 (27.8%)	2.6	1.0-6.8	0.04

CI, Confidence interval; OR, odds ratio.
From Wølner-Hanssen P: Silent pelvic inflammatory disease: Is it overstated? Obstet Gynecol 86:321, 1995.

ovum pickup, and finally complete tubal obstruction. Tubal obstructions secondary to infection are commonly found at the fimbrial end or cornual region of the oviduct. An alarming factor that has been documented with chlamydial infection is the tubal damage from subacute PID. Patton and colleagues found almost equally severe tubal damage, adhesion, degeneration of endosalpingeal structures, and cilia dysfunction in women with acute chlamydial PID and women with silent chlamydial infection.

Weström followed a large cohort of women with PID in southern Sweden from 1960 through 1984. He discovered that the infertility rate was significantly lower in younger women than in older women following a single episode of infection (**Table 23-20**). The milder the episode of acute PID, the less likely a woman was to suffer tubal obstruction and infertility. The infertility rate also increased directly with the number of episodes of acute pelvic infection. These data are not surprising because the prevalence of

Table 23-20 Percentage and Number of Patients Attempting to Conceive*

No. of Episodes of PID	Age (Years)		
	<25 % (n/N)	≥25 % (n/N)	Total % (n/N)
One	7.7 (59/771)	9.1 (20/220)	8.0 (79/991)
Mild	0.8 (2/241)	0.0 (0/71)	0.6 (2/312)
Moderate	6.4 (23/361)	5.6 (5/89)	6.2 (28/452)
Severe	20.1 (34/169)	25.0 (15/60)	21.4 (49/229)
Two	18.4 (29/158)	25.9 (7/27)	19.5 (36/185)
Three or more	37.7 (23/61)	75.0 (3/4)	40.0 (26/65)
Total	11.2 (111/990)	12.0 (30/251)	11.4 (141/1241)

*Women had tubal factor infertility by age, number of acute PID episodes, and severity of PID, excluding those with nontubal factor infertility and with incomplete infertility examinations.

n, Total number of cases followed; N, total number of evaluable cases; PID, pelvic inflammatory disease.

From Weström L, Joeseof R, Reynolds G, et al: Pelvic inflammatory disease and fertility. A cohort study of 1,844 women with laparoscopically verified disease and 657 control women with normal laparoscopic results. Sex Transm Dis 19:185, 1992.

long-term sequelae is directly proportional to the number and severity of the episodes of acute PID. Lepine and coworkers reported additional data from the largest and longest prospective cohort study of women with acute PID. They found that increasing severity of the initial episode of acute pelvic infection correlates with a longer low-term probability of live birth. The cumulative proportion of women achieving a live birth after 12 years was 90% for women whose initial infection was mild, 82% for women with moderate disease, and 57% for women with severe PID. Subsequent episodes of pelvic infection had a greater effect on women whose initial episode was judged as severe as for those with milder disease.

ACTINOMYCES INFECTION

Actinomyces is a rare cause of upper genital tract infection. *Actinomyces israelii*, the most common species found, is a gram-positive anaerobic bacterium that is difficult to culture. To culture this organism successfully, an anaerobic environment must be maintained for 2 to 3 weeks.

A. israelii is discovered by histologic examination or culture from women with tubo-ovarian abscesses. There are many large series of tubo-ovarian abscesses without a single case of *A. israelii* described. Most cases described have been in women chronically wearing an IUD for an average of 8 years. Usually, *A. israelii* is part of a polymicrobial infection, and whether its role is primary or secondary in the infectious process is unknown.

There is controversy about the significance of discovering actinomycetes on a Pap smear of women wearing an IUD. The contrasting, relatively high detection rate of actinomycetes observed on Pap smears from IUD users, and extreme rarity of subsequent development of pelvic actinomycosis, has led most experts to conclude that progression to upper tract infection is highly unlikely to be related. The decision to remove the IUD to treat a woman is influenced by the presence or absence of clinical symptoms. Unless there are associated symptoms, such as fever, abdominal pain, or abnormal uterine bleeding, the identification of the organism in any cervical smear should not prompt antibiotic therapy or IUD removal.

Actinomycetes may produce a chronic endometritis, with an associated foul-smelling discharge. The clinical infection may be manifest by widespread adhesions, induration, and fibrosis. The diagnosis of *Actinomyces* infection is usually not made until a tubo-ovarian abscess is examined by the pathologist. Then, the classic sulfur granules are observed histologically, along with gram-positive filaments.

Although much has been written about chronic draining sinuses with *Actinomyces* infection, this complication is unusual in gynecology. However, when this organism is present in a tubo-ovarian abscess, the woman should receive oral penicillin, doxycycline, or a fluoroquinolone for 12 weeks following an operative procedure.

TUBERCULOSIS

Tuberculosis of the upper genital tract, primarily chronic salpingitis and chronic endometritis, is a rare disease in the United States. Most gynecologists may never encounter a single case. However, pulmonary tuberculosis has been steadily increasing in the United States and it is likely that the incidence of pelvic tuberculosis also may rise. Tuberculosis is a frequent cause of chronic PID and infertility in other parts of the world. Thus, it should be suspected in immigrants, especially those from Asia, the Middle East, and Latin America. Although the disease is usually found in premenopausal women, it occurs in postmenopausal women 10% of the time.

Pelvic tuberculosis may be produced by *Mycobacterium tuberculosis* or *Mycobacterium bovis*. The primary site of infection for tuberculosis is usually the lung. Early in the course of pulmonary infection, the bacteria spread hematogenously and the infection becomes located in the oviducts, which are the primary and predominant site of pelvic tuberculosis. Subsequently, the bacilli usually spread to the endometrium and, less commonly, to the ovaries. In developing countries without pasteurization of milk, bovine tuberculosis produces primary infections in the human gastrointestinal tract. Subsequent lymphatic or hematogenous dissemination results in pelvic tuberculosis. Autopsy studies published 25 years ago demonstrated that 4% to 12% of women who died of pulmonary tuberculosis concurrently had evidence of upper genital tract infection. In a large study from India, 117 women had tubal blockage secondary to tuberculosis. When these women underwent laparoscopy, the findings were 50% simple tubal blockage, 15% tubo-ovarian masses, and 24% a frozen pelvis.

In general, extrapulmonary tuberculosis may present as an insidious or rapidly progressing disease. The clinical symptoms and signs of pelvic tuberculosis are similar to the chronic sequelae of nontuberculous acute PID. The predominant presentations of this chronic infection are infertility and abnormal uterine bleeding. Mild to moderate chronic abdominal and pelvic pain occur in 35% of women with the disease. Advanced cases are often accompanied by ascites. Some women may be asymptomatic. The findings at pelvic examination are normal in approximately 50% of cases. The remaining patients have mild adnexal tenderness and bilateral adnexal masses, with an inability to manipulate the adnexa because of scarring and fixation.

Tuberculous salpingitis may be suspected when a woman is not responding to conventional antibiotic therapy for acute bacterial PID. Results of a tuberculin skin test will be positive. However, approximately one in three women does not have evidence of pulmonary tuberculosis on chest radiographic films.

The diagnosis may be established by performing an endometrial biopsy late in the secretory phase of the cycle. A portion of the endometrial biopsy should be sent for culture and animal inoculation and the remaining portion should be examined histologically. The findings of classic giant cells, granulomas, and caseous necrosis confirm the diagnosis (**Fig. 23-34**). Approximately two of three women with tuberculous salpingitis will have concomitant tuberculous endometritis. Pelvic tuberculosis may not be diagnosed until laparotomy or celiotomy, when the characteristic changes may be visualized. The distal ends of the oviduct remain everted, producing a tobacco pouch appearance. When the diagnosis has been established, the woman should have a chest radiographic examination, IV pyelography, serial gastric washings, and urine cultures for tuberculosis. Approximately 10% of women with pelvic tuberculosis have concomitant urinary tract tuberculosis.

The treatment of pelvic tuberculosis is medical. Not uncommonly, patients will be admitted to the hospital for initiation of therapy, for observation, and to ensure appropriate compliance. Initial therapy in a woman with newly diagnosed tuberculosis usually will include five drugs because of the emergence of multidrug-resistant organisms. **Multidrug-resistant** (MDR) **tuberculosis** is defined as infection from a strain of *M. tuberculosis* that is resistant to two or more agents, including isoniazid. The mortality rate in HIV-negative patients who develop MDR infection may be as high as 80%. Often, health care workers become infected during outbreaks of MDR tuberculosis. The CDC has recommended starting a woman on a multidrug regimen until the culture results yield specific sensitivity. At that time, medications may be decreasedto two or three agents. Patients who have infection from MDR strains are

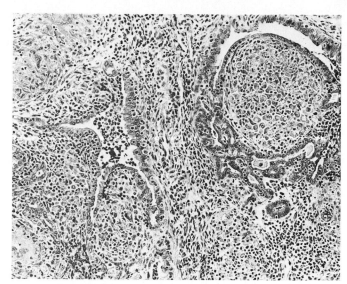

Figure 23-34 Tuberculous salpingitis—Langerhans' giant cell granuloma. (From Gompel C, Silverberg SG (eds): Pathology in Gynecology and Obstetrics, 2nd ed. Philadelphia, JB Lippincott, 1977, p 258.)

usually kept on a five-drug regimen. Operative therapy for pelvic tuberculosis is reserved for women with persistent pelvic masses, some women with resistant organisms, women older than 40 years, and women whose endometrial cultures remain positive. Although the major sequela of pelvic tuberculosis is infertility, occasionally a woman will become pregnant after medical therapy.

KEY POINTS

- The CDC regularly revises its treatment protocols for STIs. This information may be accessed online at www.cdc.gov/publications.
- Pediculosis pubis, an infestation by the crab louse *Phthirus pubis,* is characterized by constant itching, predominantly vulvar involvement, and the finding of eggs and lice by visual inspection. It may be treated by topical application of 1% permethrin cream rinse (Nix) or 1% lindane shampoo (Kwell).
- Scabies, an infection by the itch mite *Sarcoptes scabiei,* is characterized by intermittent pruritus, most commonly in the hands, wrists, breasts, vulva, and buttocks. It may be treated by topical application of 5% permethrin cream (Nix) or 1% lindane lotion or 30 g of cream.
- Genital herpes is a recurrent incurable STI. Approximately 80% of individuals are unaware that they are infected. It is usually transmitted by individuals who are asymptomatic and unaware that they have the infection at the time of transmission.
- Nonspecific tests for syphilis, the VDRL and RPR, have a 1% false-positive rate. Therefore, specific tests such as the TPI, FTA-ABS, and MHA-TP must be used when a positive nonspecific test result is encountered.
- In women in the reproductive age range, bacterial vaginosis represents approximately 50% of vaginitis cases and

candidiasis and *Trichomonas* infection represent approximately 25% each. HIV acquisition is increased in women with bacterial vaginosis and *T. vaginalis* infection.
- *T. vaginalis* infection is a highly contagious STI. It is the most prevalent nonviral, nonchlamydial STI of women. An asymptomatic female who has *Trichomonas* identified in the lower female genital urinary tract should definitely be treated.
- Symptoms that suggest cervical infection include vaginal discharge, deep dyspareunia, and postcoital bleeding. Most women who have lower reproductive tract infections caused by *C. trachomatis* or *N. gonorrhoeae* do not have **mucopurulent cervicitis**. The corollary is that most women who have mucopurulent cervicitis are not infected by *C. trachomatis* or *N. gonorrhoeae.*
- Acute PID is usually caused by a polymicrobial infection of organisms ascending from the vagina and cervix, traveling along the mucosa of the endometrium to infect the mucosa of the oviduct. It should be diagnosed with a minimum of suspicion with the knowledge that overtreatment is preferable to missed diagnosis.
- Approximately one in four women with acute PID experiences further medical sequelae, including recurrent acute PID, ectopic pregnancy, and chronic pelvic pain.

REFERENCES CAN BE FOUND ON
EXPERTCONSULT.com

24

Preoperative Counseling and Management
Woman Evaluation, Informed Consent, Infection Prophylaxis, and Avoidance of Complications

Vern L. Katz

Preoperative evaluation is a challenge to the gynecologist, because it involves both the art and science of clinical medicine. Excellent preparation for the operation facilitates a successful end result. Optimum preparation involves two personality traits, compulsive attention to detailed planning and a deep empathy for the woman. For the gynecologist, preoperative planning can be divided into three basic aspects—obtaining preoperative information, reducing the woman's anxieties and fears, and obtaining **informed consent**. Moore has stated that the first aphorism of preoperative preparation is to avoid surprises. This dictum should be applied to protect the woman and physician.

In regard to the task of obtaining preoperative information, there are two goals. The first is to ensure that the procedure is appropriate for the woman's problem. This decision is made initially, prior to the preoperative workup, but must be confirmed again. The content of this part of the clinician's task is covered elsewhere in this text; the process of the task involves the physician-patient relationship. Just as crucial is the second goal, making sure that the woman is safe for the procedure and has no comorbidities that might need special attention. The physician must work through all the major organ systems—cardiac, pulmonary, gastrointestinal, renal, musculoskeletal, and endocrine—to assess for comorbidities. This will be apparent primarily from the history. Some comorbidities will require further consultation with other specialists, such as a cardiologist for cardiac problems, or an anesthesiologist for spinal impairment.

The gynecologist, as leader of the surgical team, has an obligation to prepare the woman, her family, and the hospital personnel, including nurses, anesthesiologists, and operating room team, about the details of the surgical procedure. Most gynecologic operations are elective and thus allow sufficient time to prepare. However, even in emergency situations, preoperative preparation should be as detailed as possible because shortcuts during an emergency can result in further compromise to the woman.

For the woman, there are no small, insignificant, or minor operations. Almost any surgical procedure is a major event in her life. Associated with an elective operation are the anxiety and apprehension of the anticipated surgical procedure coupled with the ambivalence of deciding whether to have the operation. To help her decide, it is important for the physician to outline the natural history of the gynecologic disease so that the woman can understand the benefits of surgery. Most women have questions concerning the return of normal body functions and the cosmetic changes produced by the operation; these must be answered. Questions about the woman's perception of the operation's impact on her sexuality must be discussed. Prospective studies have documented that sexual function is most likely to remain the same or improve following gynecologic surgery for benign disease. As always, the physician is an educator. His or her goal should be to outline the reason and approximate time frame for each preoperative step and procedure for the woman. If the woman is ambivalent concerning the need for a surgical procedure, this often may be resolved by suggesting that she seek another professional opinion. Many third-party payer programs insist that patients obtain a second opinion before elective gynecologic operations.

Few events assault human dignity and challenge the emotional defenses as much as the events surrounding an elective operation. The woman is stripped of her clothing, bombarded with questions, and sometimes clipped of her pubic hair, all when she is feeling the most vulnerable because of the impending surgery. It is important for the physician to protect the woman's privacy and human dignity during the preoperative period. The gynecologist must appreciate that the preoperative period is one of great psychological stress for the woman. The time of the anticipated surgical procedure is a catalyst for emotional responses, ranging from vulnerability and helplessness to the grief produced by possible anticipated loss of a reproductive organ. The physician-patient relationship is far more than the legally described contractual one. An important aspect of the relationship is the physician's encouragement of the woman to be a partner in the mutual goal of a return to normal function. The understanding and trust built between the woman and physician during the preoperative period will help her build confidence and cope with the stress of the postoperative period.

One of the most important aspects of the preoperative preparation is a discussion with the physician before the procedure. Ideally the physician, the woman, and her family have a private meeting. During this time, it is important for the physician to answer all the woman's questions, as well as those of her family. It is acceptable to answer a question with the statement, "I don't know." Patients admire the honesty that this response expresses.

The gynecologist must remember that just as he or she studies the woman for verbal and nonverbal information, so does the woman watch the gynecologist. It is essential for the gynecologist to display gentleness and patience at this time. Sincere interest may be reinforced by eye contact and a gentle touch of the hands.

A thorough and detailed history and physical examination, considering the entire woman, not just the pelvis, detect approximately 90% of the facts pertinent to the surgical procedure. A number of studies have demonstrated that the most significant risk factors for postoperative morbidity are preoperative conditions. Preoperative laboratory screening tests discover fewer than 10% of significant surgical risk factors. It is an established surgical axiom that operative morbidity and mortality are directly proportional to preexisting conditions. Known or unsuspected medical illnesses may affect the operation, anesthesia, and postoperative course and, in rare cases, may preclude the procedure altogether. Also, it is important to evaluate the influence of gynecologic disease on other organ systems. For example, is a pelvic mass producing obstruction of the ureters?

This chapter outlines the preoperative preparations for gynecologic operations for benign disease. The preparations and plans for surgery extend into the postoperative period in a continuous spectrum. Thus, several topics will be started here and discussed further in Chapter 25 (Postoperative Counseling and Management). Emphasis is placed on obtaining a standard complete history, performing an adequate physical examination, and educating the woman and family, including obtaining informed consent. Special considerations for a woman with a concurrent common medical disease are also included. Two recurrent themes are stressed here—avoiding surprises during each step in the preoperative period and alleviating the woman's fears and anxiety. This chapter is not intended to be an exhaustive discussion of all medical and surgical conditions that may have some effect on preoperative planning. Rather, the focus is on common preoperative problems encountered in benign gynecologic surgery. Cost containment strategies have placed increasing emphasis on same-day admission for almost all major gynecologic operations, regardless of the woman's age. This practice has abruptly changed the timing of many preoperative events. Laboratory tests, electrocardiography, and radiographic examinations are performed on an outpatient basis before surgery.

Two considerations are helpful for women who must run the preoperative hospital gauntlet. It is helpful to give the woman a specific list of instructions for the 24 hours prior to surgery. Second, the woman may need a drug that will help relieve anxiety, such as diazepam, lorazepam, or alprazolam to be taken the evening before surgery.

PREOPERATIVE HISTORY

A detailed complete history not only obtains information but also helps relieve the woman's fears and anxieties. When the history is obtained in an unhurried manner, the process is reassuring. The woman should perceive the gynecologist as a gentle and reassuring clinician rather than as a detective trying to solve a crime rapidly. The extent and depth of the general history may be modified to a minor degree by the age and general health of the woman and the surgical procedure that is contemplated.

However, even minor operations may have major complications, so it is best to be overprepared. The possibility of degenerative multiple organ disease necessitates a meticulous review before any surgical procedure in geriatric patients. A detailed history is important, even for an emergency operation.

For elective operations, the preoperative history usually is taken on two separate occasions. Studies have documented that women often omit important medical information, particularly when under stress. Repetitive history taking provides additional information and helps decrease the risk of omission of significant information. The interview occurs initially in the physician's office several weeks before the operation and is repeated 1 to 7 days before the procedure. The second interval is valuable because it gives the woman an opportunity to reconsider her decision. Similarly, the physician uses the time to collect necessary information, such as records of previous surgical procedures. An important question to include in the history is whether the woman or anyone in her family has had problems with surgery, including bleeding or anesthesia. This question may provide information about potential medical issues and alert the surgeon to sources of anxiety for the woman that are better addressed prior to the procedure. In reviewing the history the second time, the woman often recalls important information that she may have omitted during the initial history. For example, she may have recently talked to a sister who has had a history of excessive bleeding during an operation.

There are two purposes in obtaining a detailed and comprehensive history from the woman. The first is to put the woman at ease; the second is to cover a formalized and extremely thorough set of questions. These two processes demand time and gentle consideration of the woman's anxiety. It is best to let the woman offer her perspective first. Subsequently, the physician may direct the questions to a standard format. Obviously, the format must be covered in a systematic manner so that essential areas are not omitted. Many gynecologists have the woman complete a standardized historical questionnaire prior to the outpatient appointment.

Although this chapter does not review all the components of a complete history, which are discussed further in Chapter 7 (History, Physical Examination, and Preventive Health Care), it is advantageous to group questions under the specific organ systems—pulmonary, cardiovascular, renal, hepatic, metabolic, endocrine, neurologic, hematologic, and immunologic. Several specific questions should be included to fill any holes and to cross-check the review of symptoms. These questions cover problems with surgery, anesthesia, or bleeding in the woman or her family.

The next general category is drug allergy and current medications. Questions must be constructed to include prescribed and over-the-counter (OTC) medications, as well as herbals and supplements. Approximately 0.5% of the general population and 1.5% of women older than 55 years are receiving continuous glucocorticoids. Thus, a specific question about glucocorticoid therapy for chronic medical problems is essential. It is important to inquire regarding OTC vitamins, nutritional, and herbal supplements. Many of these have the potential to affect surgery through coagulation, healing, and cross-reactivity with other medications. In general, herbal treatments should be stopped 7 days prior to surgery.

Many women do not consider aspirin or oral contraceptives as medication; therefore, specific questions regarding these substances are needed. General questions regarding smoking, alcohol, exercise tolerance, and recent upper respiratory infections are often grouped together. Specific questions should be directed toward sensitivity to iodine or latex. Latex allergy is directly responsible for 12% of the perioperative anaphylactic reactions in adult women and for 70% in children. Health care workers are particularly prone to latex allergy. Women with spinal cord injuries, or those who have had to perform self-catheterization, are at higher risk for latex allergy.

The woman's contraceptive history, including any recent change, must be known. Over the years, there has been no greater embarrassment in the operating room than the realization that a recent contraceptive practice has been abandoned and the woman is pregnant. Included with the contraceptive history are key questions concerning possible exposure to the human immunodeficiency virus (HIV). Also, the physician should estimate the probability of blood transfusion and, together with the woman, decide whether autologous blood should be donated for possible transfusion. Many women and their families are deeply concerned about the potential risk of acquiring HIV via allogeneic blood. Presently, the risk of an HIV-contaminated unit of donated blood passing through screening tests and infecting the woman is approximately 1/1,000,000 U of blood. Using a decision analysis model to assess the cost-effectiveness of autologous blood donation, Etchason and colleagues have found considerable additional cost ($68 to $4783) per unit of blood. Managed care programs struggle with this ethical dilemma. Finally, there is no evidence that blood from directed donors, selected by the woman, is safer than blood from volunteer donors.

PHYSICAL EXAMINATION

The preoperative physical examination should answer three basic questions:

1. Has the primary gynecologic disease process changed since the initial diagnosis?
2. What is the effect of the primary gynecologic disease on other organ systems?
3. What deficiencies in other organ systems may affect the proposed surgery and hospitalization?

A pelvic examination performed the day before surgery may demonstrate that a myoma has undergone acute degeneration or an ovarian cyst may have ruptured and disappeared. Pelvic masses adherent to the large intestine suggest the potential need for mechanical cleansing of the bowel before surgery. A woman with cardiac murmurs secondary to valvular heart disease needs antibiotic prophylaxis against subacute bacterial endocarditis. Often, the morbidly obese woman has impairments in the function of the circulatory and respiratory systems. Observations and findings in the physical examination may prompt further laboratory and diagnostic tests.

The most important feature of the preoperative physical is that it should be performed in a thorough and compulsive manner. The gynecologist should use the same sequence every time to help focus attention on the evaluation of each organ system.

The physical examination is best performed in the physician's office. To diminish the woman's anxiety, the physical examination should not be performed in silence. Conversation with the woman may involve further history taking or questions and answers about the proposed operation. Gentle palpation is important. A gentle touch helps to build the trust and confidence that are the foundation of the physician-patient relationship.

Two important axioms should be stressed. First, in emergency situations, it is imperative to perform a complete physical examination. This should include an evaluation of blood pressure and pulse in the recumbent and sitting positions; orthostatic hypotension and tachycardia are crude indices of a decrease in circulating intravascular volume. Second, it is important to perform a pelvic and rectal examination the day before the operation and again in the operating room immediately before the surgical incision. Pelvic masses sometimes change in size when the bladder and gastrointestinal tracts are empty. These measures help avoid surprises and may alter the surgical plan.

LABORATORY AND DIAGNOSTIC PROCEDURES

The general purpose of preoperative laboratory procedures is to identify conditions that will alter or aid in perioperative management. Specifically, screening tests are used to find unsuspected asymptomatic diseases that may affect, alter, or postpone the anticipated surgical procedure. Preoperative laboratory tests also help establish the extent of known disease that may influence the scheduling of elective surgery. Gynecologists should individualize their preoperative approach to patients and select specific tests for each woman. The downside of multiple routine preoperative tests is that they increase the likelihood of false-positive results, especially if the disease has a low prevalence in the population being tested. A false-positive test has many negative features, including anxiety for the woman, additional testing, and financial cost, and often delays scheduling the operation. Sometimes, special imaging procedures are used to determine the effects of pelvic disease on other organ systems.

Age-appropriate screening tests should be reviewed with women prior to elective surgery. For example, Papanicolaou (Pap) smears and mammograms should be up to date prior to an elective gynecologic procedure. A workup of a potential breast cancer would take precedence over elective surgery for benign pelvic disease. Screening colonoscopy should be discussed with women older than 50 years. Few women will avail themselves of this test if they are asymptomatic but testing the stool for occult blood in women older than 50 detects bleeding from a colon cancer in approximately 2 of 1000 asymptomatic women.

Presently, there is debate over which preoperative laboratory procedures should be standard. Attention has been drawn to the cost-benefit ratio of preoperative screening. Although the cost of each individual test is usually low, the aggregate costs are substantial. Often, the cost argument is overcome by the individual gynecologist's concern to practice defensive medicine in the present medicolegal climate. Many preoperative laboratory tests are ordered simply by convention, for years being standard orders in an individual's or hospital's practice.

In a classic study, Kaplan and coworkers retrospectively studied the usefulness of preoperative laboratory procedures. They estimated that 60% of routinely ordered tests, such as differential cell count, platelet count, and 12-factor automated body chemistry analyses, would not have been performed if tests had been ordered only for an indication discovered by history or physical examination. Most important, only 0.22% of these tests

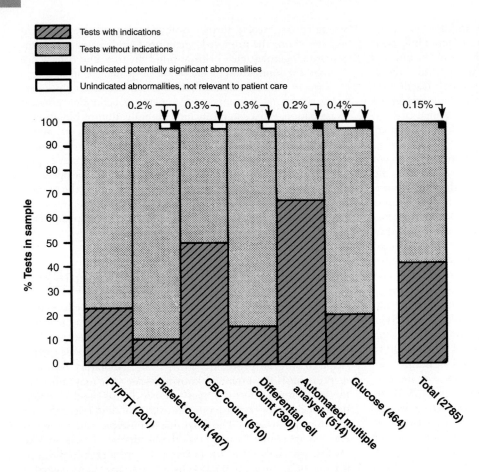

Figure 24-1 Proportions of indicated and unindicated preoperative tests, drawn to scale. Numbers in parentheses represent sample sizes used. CBC, Complete blood count; PT/PTT, prothrombin time/partial thromboplastin time;. Automated multiple analysis is sixth factor. (From Kaplan EB, Scheiner LB, Boeckmann AJ, et al: The usefulness of preoperative laboratory screening. JAMA 253:3578, 1985.)

demonstrated an abnormality that might influence perioperative management (**Fig. 24-1**). The final conclusion in their assessment of 2000 women undergoing elective operations was that in the absence of specific indications, routine preoperative laboratory tests do not significantly contribute to patient care and could be eliminated. Many authorities perform no routine preoperative clinic screening test on healthy women younger than 40 years.

Two of the most important considerations in the choice of preoperative tests are the age of the woman and extent of the surgical procedure. Preoperative laboratory procedures should be determined in each woman based on the findings of the complete history and a physical examination. Women who benefit from preoperative testing have significant risk factors or positive findings discovered during the complete history and physical examination. Most important, abnormal results from any laboratory test should result in some change in perioperative treatment. Regretfully, unexpected abnormalities in many standard preoperative laboratory tests are frequently overlooked or ignored. Studies have found that between 30% and 60% of unexpected abnormalities detected by preoperative laboratory tests are not actually noted or investigated prior to surgery.

The preoperative complete blood count and urinalysis are required by almost all hospitals. For gynecologists, the most important is the test for anemia. A woman should not be admitted for elective gynecologic surgery with a low hematocrit level that will necessitate transfusion during the perioperative period, unless a delay in surgery is contraindicated or medical therapy to improve the hematocrit level has been unsuccessful. The results

of the urinalysis, white blood cell count, and differential count rarely alter management. Before major gynecologic surgery, with an anticipated potential blood loss of more than 750 mL, a blood sample should be sent to the blood bank for typing and screening for unusual antibodies. This should replace the expensive routine typing and cross-matching. However, it is important that the blood bank have the capability of providing cross-matched blood within a reasonable period if serious intraoperative bleeding does occur. Routine preoperative typing and screening for uncomplicated abdominal or vaginal hysterectomy are not cost-effective. Also, routine clotting studies are not cost-effective and rarely provide useful clinical information unless indicated by history and physical examination (**Table 24-1**).

It is beneficial to order limited blood screening tests for women older than 40 years or who have positive family histories or questionable past histories of hepatic or renal disease. Determining the preoperative creatinine or blood urea nitrogen (BUN) level is especially important if the woman is going to be treated with antibiotics excreted by the kidneys. A test for human chorionic gonadotropin may be appropriate, depending on contraceptive and sexual history. A pregnancy test should almost always be performed if the patient is a teenager. Menstrual history is at best an imperfect indication of an early pregnancy. Serum electrolyte levels are ordered for women taking diuretics or those with a history of renal disease or heart disease. Also, serum electrolyte levels should be evaluated for women with vomiting, diarrhea, ileus, bowel obstruction, or any condition that affects water or electrolyte balance.

Table 24-1 Platelet and Clotting Factor Disorders

Parameter	Platelet Disorder	Clotting Factor Disorder
Site of bleeding	Skin; mucous membrane (e.g., nasal, oral, vaginal, gastrointestinal)	Deep or soft tissue (e.g., muscles, joints)
Bleeding after cuts and scratches	Yes	No
Petechiae	Yes	No
Ecchymoses	Small, superficial	Large, deep (often palpable)
Hemarthroses	Rare	Common
Bleeding after surgery	Immediate, usually mild	Delayed (several hours or 1-2 days), then severe

From Clarke-Pearson DL: Obstet Gynecol Forum 6:2, 1992.

The tradition of ordering chest radiographs on all patients has been abandoned. A history and physical examination are sufficient for screening and chest radiographs only need to be ordered for patients with positive findings. A meta-analysis of studies of routine preoperative chest radiographs has demonstrated that false-positive results leading to invasive procedures and associated morbidity are more frequent than the discovery of new findings leading to a change in management. Currently, chest films should be ordered for women who are 20-pack/year smokers, women with cardiac or pulmonary symptoms, immigrants who have not had a recent chest film, and women older than 70 years, although this age varies at different hospitals.

A baseline preoperative electrocardiogram (ECG) has been found to be cost-effective in asymptomatic patients only after age 60 years in women without a history of cardiac disease or significant risk factors. Electrocardiography may be indicated for women with a history of smoking and those with diabetes or renal disease, depending on the severity.

At the conclusion of the complete history, physical examination, and screening laboratory procedures, the gynecologist should determine whether consultation with other specialists is necessary. This decision should be based on the seriousness of the concurrent disease and the complexity of the proposed operation.

PATIENT-FAMILY EDUCATION AND INFORMED CONSENT

One of the primary responsibilities of the gynecologic surgeon is to educate the woman and her family about the anticipated surgical procedure, hospitalization, and recovery. Providing this information is an ethical and legal responsibility. Informed consent is an important principle to ensure that the woman's right to self-determination is respected. The ethical concept of the process of informed consent includes two important components, comprehension and free consent. Most important, in almost all circumstances, the woman and her family want to know about the operation. Similar to the history and physical examination, educational discussions should take place on at least two occasions. Throughout the educational process, questions from the woman or family should be welcomed. The woman and family should be informed about the potential use of IV fluids, urinary catheters, and monitoring equipment. Often, physicians take these devices for granted, not realizing that such equipment may cause anxiety and fears in laypersons not familiar with modern postoperative care.

Educating the woman is a great step in relieving anxiety. If the woman is aware of the sequence of events, the stress during this period becomes more tolerable. It is difficult to overeducate the woman on details of the preoperative area, operating room, and recovery room routines. Written information, when available, is also helpful. Psychological preparation of the family is equally important, and arrangements should be made for a specific location for a meeting with family members immediately following the operation. An informed family is one of the surgeon's greatest assistants. An uninformed family may harass the entire health care delivery team.

Few concepts bring more ambivalence and concern to the physician than the doctrine of informed consent. In the present medicolegal climate, the absence of informed consent is cited as a major problem in many lawsuits. Some critics have pointed out that true informed consent would involve sending the woman to medical school and then through several hours of intensive discussion. Some of these issues are discussed further in Chapter 6 (Medical-Legal Risk Management).

It is important to differentiate between the concepts of consent and informed consent. Consent involves a simple yes-no decision, but informed consent is an educational process. If a gynecologist were to operate without consent, he or she would be vulnerable to charges of assault and battery. The right of an adult woman to have final authority to consent to an operation has more than 200 years of legal precedent. The preoperative consent form that is standard in most hospitals simply documents that consent, hopefully informed consent, has been obtained.

To obtain informed consent, the surgeon must explain the following to the woman in understandable terms: the nature and extent of the disease process; the nature and extent of the contemplated operation; the anticipated benefits and results of the surgery, including a conservative estimate of successful outcome; the risks and potential complications of the operative procedure; alternative methods of therapy; and any potential changes in sexual, reproductive, and other functions. The gynecologist should also discuss with the woman what the operation will not accomplish. Many patients expect surgery to cure a large constellation of symptoms magically. Questions from the woman should be encouraged and welcomed. After being educated and considering the information, the woman acquires an understanding of the risks and benefits of the proposed procedures, and may make a fully informed decision and give informed consent for the operation to be performed. In the physician's note, the mnemonic PARQ is often used, which indicates that the **p**rocedure, **a**lternatives, **r**isks, and **q**uestions have been addressed. Any details specific to the situation should be clarified in that note in addition to stating the mnemonic.

The possibility of unanticipated pathologic conditions should be discussed with the woman and permission obtained on the written consent form for the most extensive operative procedure that may be necessary. Patients readily accept the necessity of freedom of judgment by the gynecologist during the operation about the extent of the operative procedure, depending on what is discovered during surgery. For example, permission to remove both fallopian tubes and ovaries along with the uterus should be obtained in the event that extensive adnexal disease is an unanticipated finding.

One of the greatest dilemmas in the doctrine of informed consent is the extent and depth of discussions concerning potential complications of an operation. Attorneys who specialize in defending gynecologists in medical malpractice litigation strongly advise discussing all major complications, including death from surgery and rare, serious complications, such as urinary tract fistulas following hysterectomy. Studies have documented that approximately 70% of patients do not read the consent form before signing it. Ideally, to protect the gynecologist, the final discussion of the informed consent process should be witnessed by a family member and another member of the health care delivery team. Highlights of this discussion should be documented by a paragraph written by the gynecologist in the progress notes of the chart.

Regretfully, some patients may become overwhelmed by multiple caregivers' perceived obligation to provide information. The excessive and conflicting information provided by physicians, nurses, and other caring individuals in the typical tertiary care hospital may confuse and increase the fears of the woman and her family. Adding to this problem is the abundance of conflicting, non–peer-reviewed information available in the lay press and the Internet. In summary, a caring gynecologist must not only educate the woman, but be prepared to discuss other information that the woman has received. During a woman's educational process, so much information may be given that it causes confusion. Studies have noted that the more information given, the less information is actually retained, much less correctly retained. A study by Sandberg and colleagues has noted that during the preoperative evaluation, information given by anesthesiologists and other health care providers vastly exceeds the short-term capacity of patients. Thus, it is extremely helpful to provide written lists of preoperative instructions and important information.

PREOPERATIVE PREPARATION

Rarely, a woman is admitted to the hospital prior to the operation. The preoperative orders should communicate the gynecologist's preoperative preparation for the woman. To avoid omissions, it is important to develop a systematic method of writing preoperative orders. The orders should be individualized, depending on the previous history and physical examination obtained as an outpatient, the woman's age, and the extent of the proposed surgical procedure. Unusual or infrequent orders should be written in specific detail to avoid confusion by nursing and other hospital personnel. Because of the increasing emphasis on same-day admission to the hospital, most procedures and orders are accomplished on an outpatient basis. Therefore, it is important to give the woman a specific list of instructions for the 24 hours before surgery.

The first two or three lines of the order sheet should include the proposed operation and a list of the woman's diseases. Further orders are subdivided into four broad categories—general measures, medication, laboratory tests, and preventive therapies.

General measures include orders for activity, diet, ordinary medication usage, and vital signs. The woman should have nothing more than sips of water with essential medications for the 2 to 4 hours prior to elective surgery. If the operation is not scheduled until the middle of the afternoon, it is acceptable for the woman to have an early liquid breakfast. Interestingly the extent of preoperative anxiety does not influence gastric fluid volume or acidity.

The second category of orders is for medications. When prophylactic antibiotics are ordered, the time of injection should ensure that significant blood and tissue levels will have been attained at the time of bacterial contamination during the surgical procedure. An additional subgroup is special medications for specific medical illnesses. It is presumed that the anesthesiologist will write orders for preoperative medication to alleviate anxiety and reduce tracheobronchial secretions.

The third major group of orders involves preoperative laboratory tests. This includes standard laboratory tests and specifically indicated laboratory tests.

The fourth and last group of orders involves preventive therapies. Thrombophlebitis remains a major complication of gynecologic surgery. Prophylactic subcutaneous heparin, intermittent pneumatic leg compression devices, or both are indicated for women at moderate and high risk for thromboembolic disease. Patients who have been NPO for a prolonged period or who have lost fluid from cleansing of the gastrointestinal tract should be given IV fluids before induction of anesthesia to ensure proper hydration. If removal of hair is necessary, it should be clipped immediately before the operation.

CONSULTATION WITH THE ANESTHESIOLOGIST

The preoperative interaction between the woman and anesthesiologist in a preoperative screening clinic is most important. For the woman, the reassurance of meeting the anesthesiologist and of exchanging information greatly alleviate anxiety. For the anesthesiologist, it is an opportunity to obtain necessary medical information, evaluate the woman, determine the risk of the perioperative period, and write preoperative medication orders. This meeting had traditionally occurred the afternoon or evening before surgery. However, with emphasis on cost containment and greater use of outpatient facilities, and with admission to the hospital the morning of the operation, this meeting frequently occurs in an out patient clinic several days before surgery. Anesthesiologists have now assumed more responsibility for postoperative pain management, primarily using epidural narcotics. This subject should be discussed with the woman. Recovery is more rapid when a woman's concerns are addressed and when she knows what to expect regarding postoperative therapy for pain.

Anesthesiologists classify surgical procedures according to the woman's risk of mortality. In 1961, Dripps first published guidelines to determine the risk of death related to major operative procedures. This physical status scale (**Table 24-2**) has been adopted by the American Society of Anesthesiologists (ASA).

Table 24-2 American Society of Anesthesiologists (ASA) Physical Status Classification

ASA Physical Status Class	Description
1	A normal healthy patient
2	A patient with mild systemic disease
3	A patient with severe systemic disease
4	A patient with severe systemic disease that is a constant threat to life
5	A moribund patient who is not expected to survive without the operation
6	A declared brain-dead patient whose organs are being removed for donor purposes

Adapted from American Society of Anesthesiologists:ASA Physical Status Classification System, 2011 (http://www.asahq.org/clinical/physicalstatus.htm).

The scale has been revalidated many times over the years. With minor modifications, these anesthetic risk classes are still widely used. An emergency operation doubles the mortality risks for classes 1, 2, and 3, produces a slightly increased risk in class 4, and does not change the risk in class 5. Class 6 has been added more recently; it includes patients who have been declared brain-dead and whose organs are being removed for donor purposes.

Most deaths caused by anesthesia are ascribable to human error. The most common serious morbidity associated with elective surgery is cardiovascular complications. Evaluations by anesthesiologists in a preoperative clinic have provided information leading to changes in treatment for more than 15% of healthy patients. In this report, the most common medical conditions of concern that tend to be changed by anesthesia are gastric reflux, insulin-dependent diabetes mellitus, asthma, and anticipated difficulties in intubation.

A problem frequently encountered by gynecologists and anesthesiologists is whether to continue or interrupt medications that the woman is taking. If the drug is prescribed for a medical illness, it is best to continue the drug throughout the perioperative period. The physician must determine whether the drug will adversely affect the course of the anesthesia or surgery and whether it will interact with other drugs to be given during the procedure. It is acceptable to have the woman take oral medications the morning of surgery. The 30 to 60 mL of water needed to swallow the oral medication is negligible compared with gastric fluid volumes.

The primary goals of preoperative medication are to relieve anxiety and produce sedation. Many patients desire amnesia. This may not be a reasonable goal for early discharge following the operation. Sedation is easy to accomplish; however, relief of anxiety does not invariably accompany sedation. Narcotics and sedatives should be used with caution in women with chronic respiratory or liver disease. A task force of the ASA has recommended against the routine prophylactic use of anticholinergics, antihistamines, and histamine-2 (H2) receptor antagonists to reduce the risks of pulmonary aspiration.

PROPHYLACTIC ANTIBIOTICS

The use of prophylactic antibiotics in gynecologic surgical procedures has become standard. Wound infections and pelvic cellulitis, although infrequent, are important causes of postoperative morbidity. Gynecologic operations may result in the production of hypoxic tissue and collections of bloody and serous fluids, both of which are excellent culture media. Rigidly defined, prophylactic antibiotic use involves the administration of antibiotics to women without evidence of pelvic infection to prevent postoperative morbidity related to infection. The major use of prophylactic antibiotics is in operations such as vaginal hysterectomy, following which there is the potential for a high incidence of postoperative pelvic cellulitis. The goal of antibiotic therapy is to prevent infection by the endogenous flora of the lower female reproductive tract. Prophylactic antibiotics are given occasionally when the incidence of postoperative infection is low, but the results of the surgical procedure would be severely compromised if an infection did occur, such as with reconstructive operations on the fallopian tubes.

In general, the use of prophylactic antibiotics results in fewer operative site infections (e.g., abdominal wound and pelvic cellulitis), reduced febrile morbidity, and shorter hospital stays. The major risk of allergic or toxic reactions is small, especially with a short course of prophylactic antibiotics. The increased cost of the antibiotics is justified by a lower total cost from a shorter hospitalization. Certainly, the economic costs of prolonged hospitalization for even a minor postoperative infection are substantial.

The foundation of our understanding of prophylactic antibiotics is the classic research of John Burke, published in 1961. He stressed the fact that maximum antibacterial activity in subcutaneous wounds results from a combination of host resistance and antibiotics. His experimental studies proved that the antibiotic must be present in damaged tissue at the time of contamination with bacteria or shortly thereafter. Burke termed the first 3 hours of decreased tissue resistance following a surgical insult as the *effective period.* He found that there was no protective effect in preventing the development of subcutaneous wound infections if the antibiotics were given later than 3 hours following bacterial contamination.

Subsequent studies have documented two other important facts concerning prophylactic antibiotics in gynecology. First, the goal of prophylactic antibiotics is to reduce the total number of bacteria present in the operative site. It is not necessary to kill all the bacteria. Second, for prophylaxis to be successful, adequate tissue levels of antibiotics need to be maintained only for the duration of the operation. The normal endogenous vaginal flora has 1×10^8 bacteria/mL of vaginal secretions, consisting of a wide spectrum of aerobic and anaerobic organisms. Thus, theoretically, the choice of a single antibiotic for prophylaxis in gynecology is most difficult. Ideally, the drug chosen as a prophylactic antibiotic should be nontoxic, inexpensive, and effective against most organisms encountered in the endogenous flora. Multiple reports have documented a linear relationship between the incidence of bacterial vaginosis and incidence of postoperative pelvic infection. Therefore, a woman should not have an elective hysterectomy if bacterial vaginosis is discovered during the 2 weeks prior to surgery. It is important for the gynecologist to identify women with bacterial vaginosis. Following treatment, the vaginal ecosystem should return to normal prior to the operation.

There is abundant literature supporting the use of prophylactic antibiotics in gynecology. The incidence of febrile morbidity may be reduced from 40% to 15% and the incidence of pelvic infection decreased from 25% to 5%. Presently, first- or second-generation cephalosporins are the most popular choice for prophylactic antibiotics in gynecology (e.g., a single dose of a cephalosporin, first or second generation, 1 to 2 g IV no more than 30 minutes before the skin incision. Often, nursing personnel give prophylactic antibiotics prematurely by optimistically anticipating when the woman will go to the operating room. This practice may result in lower than desirable antibiotic levels during the time of bacterial contamination.

With the wide spectrum of bacteria involved in the constantly changing ecologic system of the vagina, a single antibiotic does not have the spectrum to be bactericidal or bacteriostatic against all the bacteria present. The important feature sought in a prophylactic antibiotic is its ability to reduce the total number of bacteria present in the bacterial inoculum; it does not have to affect all organisms. A reduction in overall number allows the woman's natural defense mechanisms to eradicate the remaining bacteria.

Emphasis has focused on an extremely short duration of therapy for prophylactic antibiotics. Comparative studies have documented that single-dose therapy is as effective as 24 hours of antibiotics. No advantage exists to continuing prophylactic antibiotics beyond the immediate operative period. This short duration of administration also reduces cost and complications. The incidence of serious complications, such as drug allergy and resistant bacteria, is directly related to the length of administration of the antibiotic. With **prophylactic antibiotics**, the major concern is the potential threat of increasing bacterial resistance. This results in two problems, more **nosocomial infections** with resistant organisms and alterations of the normal vaginal flora. If infection develops following prolonged use of prophylactic antibiotics, cultures must be obtained and antibiotic coverage selected that is different from the antibiotic used for prophylaxis. Other potential complications from prophylactic antibiotics include antibiotic-associated diarrhea or colitis and the more serious pseudomembranous enterocolitis often secondary to *Clostridium difficile* infection. This complication usually follows chronic use of antibiotics but, rarely, may occur after a short exposure to antibiotics. Antibiotic therapy at any time in the previous 6 weeks may be responsible for precipitating the onset of this disease.

Many factors affect the risk of postoperative infection. The most important include the length of the operation, whether the woman is premenopausal or postmenopausal, obesity, low socioeconomic status, malnutrition, immunosuppression, use of prophylactic antibiotics, and operative approach. A randomized clinical trial reported by Greif and coworkers studied supplemental perioperative oxygen in 500 patients undergoing operations involving the large bowel. They found that the administration of supplemental oxygen during the operation and in the first 2 hours of the perioperative period results in a 50% reduction in the incidence of wound infection. In one study, it was found that keeping a woman warm is also helpful to reduce perioperative infection.

In summary, prophylactic antibiotics are routinely ordered for gynecologic operations. The most popular choice is a single dose of a cephalosporin given close enough to surgery so that tissue levels will be adequate when the operation begins. Whatever broad-spectrum antibiotic is selected, the gynecologist must know the pharmacokinetics of the drug. The half-life of the antibiotic is important for selecting the proper timing and route of preoperative administration and the possible necessity of an intraoperative dose for longer operations. The antibiotic selected should be active against most endogenous vaginal flora. The drug should be present at the time of surgical insult and should be used only during the operative procedure. Obviously, prophylactic antibiotics are helpful, but they should not be exchanged or substituted for meticulous surgical technique. Approximately 25% of all surgical infections are caused by *Staphyloccus aureus*. Recent studies have suggested that women at high risk for infection—those with previous *S. aureus* infection or colonization, obese women, and women with diabetes—would benefit from preoperative *S. aureus* screening by nasal culture. If positive cultures are documented, eradication of colonization with chlorhexidine baths and twice-daily intranasal mupirocin is indicated. A study by Bode and associates has noted a decrease in surgical site infection from 7.7% (32 of 413 patients with placebo) to 3.4% (17 of 504) in the decolonization group (relative risk [RR], 4.2; 95% confidence interval [CI], 0.23 to 0.75).

ASSOCIATED RISK FACTORS AND COMPLICATIONS

BLEEDING DISORDERS AND THROMBOEMBOLIC DISEASE

Thrombophlebitis of the pelvic or the leg veins is a frequent complication of gynecologic surgery. Studies using sophisticated ^{125}I-fibrinogen scanning techniques have documented that approximately 15% of women having gynecologic surgery for a benign disease and approximately 22% of women having surgery for malignant disease develop thrombophlebitis (**Table 24-3**). Many, if not most, of these women will be asymptomatic. In one study, almost 40% of patients with deep vein thrombophlebitis who had no symptoms of pulmonary embolus had documented evidence of a pulmonary embolus by ventilation perfusion studies of the lung. The two potentially serious outcomes associated with thrombosis are pulmonary embolus early

Table 24-3 Incidence of Venous Thrombosis after Gynecologic Operations with ^{125}I-Fibrinogen Scanning

Reference*	No. of Patients	Type of Operation	Incidence of Leg Vein Thrombosis
Adolf et al	75	Major	29
Ballard et al	55	Major benign disease	29
Clyton et al	231	Major	16
Endl and Auinger	43	Major	37
Walsh et al	100	Vaginal hysterectomy	7
	117	Abdominal hysterectomy	13
	23	Wertheim's operation	25
	22	Other malignant disease	45

*References are from the original source.
From Bonnar J: Venous thromboembolism and gynecologic surgery. Clin Obstet Gynecol 28:433, 1985.

in the course of the disease and the chronic complication of post-thrombotic venous insufficiency, which may greatly impair a woman's quality of life. Many aspects of pelvic surgery predispose the woman to develop thrombophlebitis, including venous stasis, surgical injury to the walls of large veins, associated anaerobic infection, and hormonal status. Typically, the three major pathophysiologic changes that facilitate the development of thrombophlebitis and pulmonary embolus are venous injury, circulatory stasis, and hypercoagulable conditions (Virchow's triad).

Approximately 40% of deaths following gynecologic surgery are related to pulmonary emboli. Although the initial venous injury most often occurs at the time of the operation, approximately 15% of symptomatic emboli do not present until the first week following discharge from the hospital. Because of the significant morbidity and mortality associated with a postoperative pulmonary embolus, every effort should be made to reduce the incidence of thrombophlebitis.

Thromboprophylaxis includes treatments and protocols that are given to a woman to prevent a thrombosis. To prescribe the optimum thromboprophylaxis protocol, a risk assessment of every woman undergoing surgery is undertaken. The first step is to determine during the history which factors place the woman at increased risk for thromboembolic disease. One category of these factors includes a tendency, either inherited or acquired, to form a thrombosis, a thrombophilia. A history of previous thrombophlebitis or embolus or family or personal history of

hypercoagulability should prompt a laboratory evaluation for a thrombophilia. The thrombophilia screen should include assessment of factor V Leiden with an activated protein C resistance or a genetic analysis, prothrombin G20210A mutation, proteins C, S, and antithrombin III levels, genotype of the methylenetetrahydrofolate reductase (MTHFR) enzyme for homocysteinemia and, in the case of a personal history, assessment for anticardiolipin antibody, beta-2 glycoprotein, and lupus anticoagulant (**Fig. 24-2**). With a strong history and a negative thrombophilia workup, consideration is given to a more extensive screen for less common thrombophilias, including plasminogen activator inhibitor levels and factors VIII, IX, XI, and VII. The thrombophilias are discussed further in Chapter 16 (Spontaneous and Recurrent Abortion). The presence of a thrombophilia places the woman at an increased risk for thrombotic disease during the perioperative period. If there is a potent thrombophilia, such as antithrombin III deficiency or high levels of anticardiolipin, the woman is considered at the highest risk. Women with two thrombophilias are also at the highest risk for thrombosis; for example, women who are homozygous for factor V Leiden or who have both the prothrombin mutation and protein C deficiency. A review by Donahue and coworkers has noted that if thromboprophylaxis is given, there is no increased risk of a thrombosis from factor V Leiden.

Other risk factors for thrombosis include malignant disease, previous radiation therapy, congestive heart failure, chronic pulmonary disease, nephrotic syndrome, morbid obesity, venous

Figure 24-2 Mechanisms in the control of coagulation and inherited thrombophilias. (From Seligsohn U, Lubetsky A: Genetic susceptibility to venous thrombosis. N Engl J Med 344:1223, 2001.)

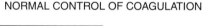

NORMAL CONTROL OF COAGULATION

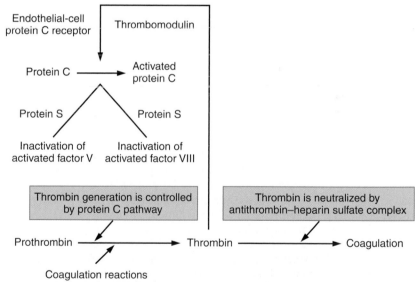

MECHANISMS OF INHERITED THROMBOPHILIAS

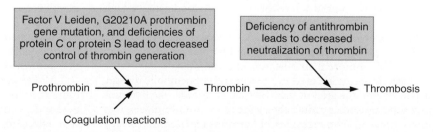

Table 24-4 Risk Assessment Profile for Thromboembolism in Gynecologic Surgery

Low Risk
Minor surgery (<30 min) with no other risk factors
Major surgery (<30 min) but with age <40 yr and no other risk factors
Age <40 yr, no other risk factors

Moderate Risk
Minor surgery (<30 min) in patients with personal or family history or DVT, pulmonary embolism, or thrombophilia
Major surgery (>30 min)
Laparoscopic extended surgery
Obesity (>80 kg [176 lb])
Moderate to severe varicose veins
Current infection
Immobility before operation (>3 days)
Major current illness (e.g., cardiovascular disease, cancer, inflammatory bowel disease, nephritic syndrome, malignancies other than gynecologic, chronic pulmonary disease)
Heart failure or recent myocardial infarction
Single thrombophilia other than antithrombin III deficiency, anticardiolipin antibody, or lupus anticoagulant
Recent pregnancy
Hormonal therapy within 4 weeks, including OCP, HRT, or SERM
Recent surgery or trauma
Long-distance travel within 3 weeks
IV drug use

High Risk
Presence of three moderate risk factors from moderate risk list
Major pelvic or abdominal surgery for gynecologic cancer
Major surgery (>30 min) in patients with personal or family history of previous DVT, pulmonary embolism, or thrombophilia; paralysis or immobilization of lower limbs
Age >60 yr
Active malignancy
Thrombosis within 1 mo
Two thrombophilias, or antithrombin III deficiency, lupus anticoagulant, oranticardiolipin

DVT, Deep vein thrombosis; HRT, hormone replacement therapy; OCP, oral contraceptive pills; SERM, selective estrogen receptor modulator.
Adapted from Bonnar J: Can more be done in obstetric and gynecologic practice to reduce morbidity and mortality associated with venous thromboembolism? Am J Obstet Gynecol 180:784, 1999.

Box 24-1 Thrombophrophylaxis

1. In the low-risk group, provide early mobilization and support stockings.
2. In the moderate-risk group, administer 60 mg enoxaparin or 5000 U dalteparin 6-12 hr after surgery and then give daily as long as patient is hospitalized, or intermittent pneumatic compression stockings intraoperatively and throughout hospitalization.
3. In the high-risk group, intermittent pneumatic compression and LMWH, 30 mg enoxaparin or equivalent half-dose of other LMWH 1-2 hr before surgery, repeated 12 hr after surgery, and then 60 mg enoxaparin/day or equivalent. Alternatively, heparin may be given as 60 mg enoxaparin or 5000 U dalteparin given 6-12 hr postoperatively and then daily.

Note: Dosing may be altered in mobidly obese patients or very thin patients.

disease, edema of the legs, active pelvic infection, age older than 40 years, current use of oral contraceptives or hormone replacement therapy up to the time of the operation, and length of immobilization or preoperative hospitalization. Not uncommonly, the clinician is asked to consult for a hospitalized woman who is subsequently taken to surgery. Three or more days of limited ambulation confer a greater risk for thromboembolism. The length of the procedure is also a risk factor. In general, surgeries longer than 30 minutes put the woman at an increased risk. Laparoscopy is not less of a risk than a laparotomy if the laparoscopy lasts longer than 30 minutes. All these factors are evaluated and the woman is assigned a level of risk—low, moderate, or high (**Table 24-4**). Women in the lowest risk group have less than a 3% risk of thrombosis, women in the moderate group have a 10% to 30% risk of thrombosis, and women in the high-risk groups have a more than 30% risk of a thrombosis.

Various means are used to prevent thromboembolic disease, depending on the level of risk (**Box 24-1**). Ideally, the first prophylactic measure to reduce the incidence of embolic disease is to discontinue oral contraceptives or hormone replacement therapy

(HRT) 4 weeks before major elective surgery. The increase in absolute risk from oral contraceptives is low so, pragmatically, the risk avoided by stopping oral contraceptives must be weighed against the possible risk of an unwanted pregnancy. The level of risk from HRT is also small. Several large cohort studies have shown no significant increase in incidence of deep vein thrombosis (DVT) in women using hormonal therapies as long as thromboprophylaxis is used. Thus, women who are taking HRT or oral contraceptives should receive thromboprophylaxis, even if they are younger. Other simple prophylactic measures include elastic stockings, early ambulation, and leg exercises in bed. Support hose should be thigh-high to avoid venous stasis at the knee. The appearance of the support hose also serves a teaching function to remind women and nursing personnel of the importance of ambulation and exercise to prevent venous stasis. The preventive effect from support hose in themselves is low; however, the added effects and risk-benefit ratio are large.

The key decision for the prophylaxis of thromboembolic diseases is whether to order prophylactic heparin, pneumatic inflated sleeve devices, or a combination of both. A meta-analysis reviewing more than 70 randomized trials of more than 16,000 general surgery, orthopedic, and urologic patients has demonstrated that perioperative subcutaneous heparin prevents approximately two thirds of DVT and 50% of all deaths from pulmonary emboli. The most striking data in this study related the reduction in death directly to pulmonary emboli, with 19 deaths in the patients given perioperative heparin and 55 deaths in the control group. Randomized clinical trials have demonstrated that pharmacologic agents, such as heparin, or mechanical methods, such as intermittent pneumatic compression of the legs, are equally effective in preventing thrombophlebitis. The complication from heparin prophylaxis is bleeding. Some women are transiently anticoagulated by the heparin and may experience excessive bleeding during or following the operative procedure. This complication is experienced by approximately 2% of women. The risk of bleeding is significantly lower with low-molecular-weight heparin (LMWH). Obese or extremely thin women should have their dosage of heparin adjusted.

LMWH are superior to standard unfractionated heparin because they have a longer half-life, almost 100% bioavailability, dose-independent clearance, and a more consistent anticoagulation effect from dose to dose. Most studies have reported significantly fewer hemorrhagic complications with LMWH than with unfractionated heparin. Also, the incidence of heparin-induced thrombocytopenia is significantly lower in women given LMWH than in those receiving unfractionated heparin. There are two major protocols for heparin prophylaxis. One uses a reduced dose prior to the procedure, with a half-dose 1 to 2 hours before surgery (30 mg enoxaparin or 2500 U dalteparin). A second dose is given 12 hours after surgery. A full dose (60 mg enoxaparin or 5000 U dalteparin) is given every 24 hours. The second protocol uses a full dose 6 to 12 hours after surgery and every 24 hours thereafter. A meta-analysis of studies summarizing 1600 surgeries for elective hip repair, as high risk as gynecologic procedures, has found perioperative and postoperative LMWH administration to be equally effective. The rates of DVT were 12.4% and 14.4%, respectively. The risks of bleeding were higher in the perioperative protocol groups, 6.3% versus 2.5% for postoperative dosing. It was concluded that dosing may begin 12 hours after the procedure in most cases, and no less than 6 hours after the procedure. Trials comparing administration 6 and 12 hours postprocedure will help elucidate optimum timing.

The primary alternative to anticoagulation is intermittent pneumatic compression modalities, which include foot pumps and calf- and thigh-level stockings. Together, these not only prevent stasis and the endothelial injury that may occur with extreme venous distention, but also stimulate the fibrinolytic system. Thus, the effect is more than just physical. In one meta-analysis of 11 randomized clinical trials, there was an almost 70% reduction in the incidence of DVT in patients using intermittent pneumatic calf compression. One study in trauma patients found full-length compression stockings to be superior to foot pumps. Compression stockings are relatively inexpensive; their only disadvantage is poorly fitting stockings that produce a tourniquet effect at the knee. They should be used intraoperatively and for the entire hospitalization because the fibrinolytic effect is maintained only while they are in use. Complications or side effects are extremely rare, but injuries to the common peroneal nerve and compartment syndrome have been reported. Contraindications to the use of pneumatic stockings include known DVT, severe atherosclerotic disease, congestive heart failure, and open wounds on the legs. Nursing personnel, patients, and their families must be educated about the benefits of the devices or their compliance with this mechanical method is poor. The decision of which method to use is primarily based on the differences in bleeding complications between the two regimens. Maxwell and colleagues randomized 211 gynecologic oncology patients to LMWH or compression stockings. The rates of DVT were similar and were low in both groups.

In women who are currently taking oral anticoagulants for thromboprophylaxis because of previous DVT, oral anticoagulants should be stopped 5 days prior to surgery. Heparin and oral medications should be restarted shortly after surgery. The operation should be delayed if the previous event was within 3 months. Women who must be operated on within 6 months of a previous DVT should be converted from oral agents to IV heparin and given perioperative thromboprophylaxis until oral agents can be restarted postoperatively. This is termed *bridging therapy*; oral anticoagulants, when discontinued, need about 5 days to lose their effects, and for laboratory clotting studies to reach normal levels. IV heparin is used perioperatively. In older patients, it may take longer for the international normalized ratio

(INR) to become normal. The timing of bridging therapy thus needs to be adjusted. If the risk for thrombosis is high, and the surgery cannot be postponed, a temporary vena cava filter may be placed transcutaneously. These patients should also have mechanical prophylaxis. Each woman should have her therapy individualized after assessment of risk. Patients should discontinue aspirin and aspirin-containing medications 2 to 3 weeks prior to surgery.

In contrast to thrombophilias, bleeding disorders usually cause symptomatic issues in most patients earlier in their lives. Thus, most bleeding problems have come to patients' awareness earlier. It is estimated that approximately 1% to 2% of patients have some type of bleeding diathesis in the United States; the most common is von Willebrand disease. Patients who have had symptoms of easy bruising, frequent nosebleeds, anemia, menorrhagia, and excessive bleeding with surgical procedures should be considered for a hematologic assessment. This should include a complete blood count (CBC), prothrombin time (PT), partial thromboplastin time (PTT), and von Willebrand factor assay. Any positive test result should be followed by consultation with a hematologist. Women with already confirmed bleeding problems should have a consultation for appropriate prophylaxis.

GASTROINTESTINAL TRACT SYMPTOMS

Gastrointestinal symptoms are rare in women being evaluated for elective operations for benign gynecologic conditions. However, if the woman has these symptoms, the gynecologist should consider preoperative endoscopy or imaging studies of the gastrointestinal tract. The effect of nausea, vomiting, or diarrhea on serum electrolyte levels and on the nutritional status of the woman needs to be evaluated.

Colonoscopy may be indicated for benign disease if there is a left-sided adnexal mass in a woman older than 40 years, a positive stool guaiac test, or bowel symptoms. Again, the evaluation of each woman must be individualized in an attempt to determine whether a primary gynecologic process is pressing on the bowel or directly invading the large intestine.

The woman should not eat solid food for 6 to 8 hours before surgery. Clear liquids are emptied from the stomach within minutes; however, fatty foods greatly delay gastric emptying. Obviously, incomplete preparation of the upper gastrointestinal tract increases the risk of aspiration, which is a serious complication of anesthesia and operations. Studies have documented the safety of allowing inpatients and outpatients to ingest clear liquids up until 2 hours before elective surgery.

If there is a suspicion that the operation will necessitate entry into the lumen of the large intestine, mechanical cleansing of the colon should be considered. Mechanical cleansing is also desirable for obese women and those in whom the intestines will need to be packed. Mechanical cleansing is helpful in women undergoing laparoscopic or robotic surgery. Almost all gynecologists use a single day of an oral solution. Magnesium citrate, sodium phosphate (Fleet enema), and polyethylene glycol (PEG; GoLYTELY) are the three most commonly used agents. Oliveria and associates reported a large randomized trial comparing sodium phosphate and PEG-based oral lavage solutions. The efficacy of the two preparations was similar. However, there was superior subjective patient tolerance to the 90-mL dose of sodium phosphate. Care must be taken in selecting patients who are to receive oral sodium phosphate because it produces hypokalemia and is contraindicated in women with hepatic, renal, or heart disease. In older patients, the bowel preparation is often omitted or given on an inpatient basis with an IV solution to prevent dehydration. Women taking medications need also to be watched to ensure that the cleansing does not interfere with drug absorptions.

URINARY TRACT DISEASE

The lower urinary tract is in close anatomic proximity to the pelvic organs. Benign and malignant gynecologic diseases frequently produce anatomic distortion of the urethra, urinary bladder, or ureters. Similarly, gynecologic neoplasias may produce partial or complete obstruction of one or both ureters, resulting in hydroureter or hydronephrosis. Preoperative evaluation may include blood chemistry studies (e.g., BUN, creatinine), imaging studies (e.g., computed tomography [CT] scan), and function studies (e.g., glomerular filtration rate).

Preoperative imaging may help diagnose congenital abnormalities of the urinary tract. Congenital urinary anomalies are rare but are more common in women with congenital anomalies of the reproductive tract. The presence of a pelvic kidney is important information in the differential diagnosis of a large, fixed adnexal mass. The presence of a double ureter is another anomaly discovered by preoperative imaging studies. Preoperative knowledge of a double ureter is advantageous for the anatomic identification of structures in the retroperitoneal spaces.

Imaging also helps confirm the patency of the lower urinary tract. It is important to establish whether the enlargement, inflammation, or displacement of the gynecologic organs has produced distortion, obstruction, and possibly associated chronic infection of the urinary tract. For example, when a uterus is enlarged to the pelvic brim with myomas, hydronephrosis is noted in approximately one third of women. Common indications for enhanced CT scanning with benign gynecologic disease include cervical myomas, lateral projection of uterine myomas, adnexal masses that are fixed and adherent, endometriosis, and large pelvic masses that produce urinary symptoms. Using these conservative indications, approximately 25% of studies will demonstrate an abnormal finding. However, a preoperative IV pyelogram (IVP) will not give the gynecologist information that necessarily reduces the incidence of operative injury to the ureters. During the operation, the ureters must be identified along their entire course. The exact incidence of ureteral injury associated with benign surgery is unknown because many injuries do not produce symptoms.

One serious problem with contrast media used for imaging is an allergic reaction triggered by immunoglobulin E antibodies to the radiologic contrast medium. An imaging study of the kidneys using conventional ionic contrast media has an adverse reaction rate of approximately 8%, and life-threatening reactions occur following 1 in every 1000 injections. Pretreating patients with oral corticosteroids, giving methylprednisolone (32 mg) 12 and 2 hours before the injection of IV contrast material, significantly reduces the incidence of allergic reaction. This treatment is an alternative to using monomeric, nonionic, iodinated compounds as contrast media, with a lower incidence of allergic reactions. Studies have demonstrated a decrease in severe allergic reactions of five- to 30-fold with nonionic compared with ionic contrast media.

Another serious concern when ordering an enhanced imaging study is the rare possibility of clinically significant nephrotoxicity being caused by the contrast material. Nephropathy has been a common cause of iatrogenic acute renal failure. Patients with diabetes, existing renal impairment, chronic hypertension, moderate to severe congestive heart failure, or reduced effective arterial volume, and those receiving drugs that impair renal function, are at high risk for contrast nephrotoxicity. A normal serum creatinine level should be verified prior to ordering these scans. For example, up to 15% of women with diabetic nephropathy will develop renal failure requiring dialysis, despite adequate hydration and the use of low-osmolar agents. The pathogenesis of contrast nephrotoxicity is believed to be direct tubular insult and ischemic injury. Low-osmolar nonionic contrast media are less nephrotoxic than high-osmolar ionic media in high-risk patients. One study of 83 patients with chronic renal insufficiency has demonstrated that a combination of prophylactic oral administration of the antioxidant acetylcysteine, along with hydration, was an effective means of preventing further renal damage produced by a nonionic, low-osmolar contrast agent. A randomized trial by Aspelin and colleagues using an iso-osmolar contrast medium found an almost ninefold reduction in renal toxicity when compared with a low-osmolar contrast medium.

As many as 5% of women have some form of renal disease. Insufficient renal function is a major risk factor in elective operations because of the woman's decreased ability to excrete medications. Women with insufficient renal function do poorly if they develop perioperative infections. Women with azotemia have a threefold greater risk of adverse drug reactions than women with normal renal function. However, renal insufficiency is infrequent in an asymptomatic woman younger than 40 years, especially compared with the incidence of unsuspected respiratory disease. The frequency of abnormal serum BUN or creatinine levels is directly dependent on the woman's age. Most authorities recommend that serum creatinine and BUN levels be determined in all women with a history of renal disease and in those older than 45 years. Baseline and interval tests of renal function in women who are to be treated with aminoglycosides are necessary and valuable studies. Women with chronic renal disease usually have platelet dysfunction that should be evaluated preoperatively.

Women with chronic renal insufficiency, diabetes, jaundice, and congestive heart failure, as well as older women, are at high risk of developing acute renal failure during the perioperative period. Prior to surgery, they should be evaluated to ensure that they have normal blood volume and osmolar status. They should be carefully monitored to avoid hypotension and nephrotoxins. Perioperative ketorolac (Toradol) should be avoided in women with elevated serum creatinine levels. Assessment of volume status is particularly important if these women have received a mechanical bowel preparation. Because women with chronic renal insufficiency have a decreased reserve, small insults to the kidney, such as a relative hypovolemia, may push these women into renal failure. A not uncommon scenario occurs when a women with marginal renal function begins to develop a movement of intracellular volume into her third space after surgery. If IV hydration is inadequate, the woman will have normal vital signs but decreased urine output. The oliguria is a response to the relative hypovolemia. At the same time, nonsteroidal anti-inflammatory drugs (NSAIDs) may be prescribed. The combination of chronic renal insufficiency with decreased reserve, hypovolemia, and exposure to an NSAID leads to a transient tubular necrosis, with a worsening oliguria and azotemia.

RESPIRATORY DISEASE

Pulmonary complications are the most frequent form of postoperative morbidity experienced by women following gynecologic operative procedures, occurring in more than 1 in 20 postoperative patients. The goals of the preoperative assessment of the respiratory system are to identify women at risk for developing postoperative pulmonary complications and prescribe appropriate preoperative therapy to reduce these risks. Common pulmonary complications include bronchospasm, atelectasis, pneumonia, and exacerbation of underlying chronic lung disease. A rare but most serious problem is respiratory failure with prolonged mechanical ventilation usually seen in women with severely diminished pulmonary reserve. Predicting and preventing postoperative cardiac problems will dramatically reduce postoperative pulmonary morbidity. Arozullah and coworkers, in a study of 161,000 operations, was able to derive a model for predicting the likelihood of developing postoperative pneumonia (**Table 24-5**). Only rarely, a woman cannot be anesthetized and well oxygenated intraoperatively. The primary goal should be to avoid postoperative pulmonary complications. Similar to the evaluation of other organ systems, the history and physical examination are the most important parts of the pulmonary evaluation. Pulmonary function tests of lung volumes and flow rates are indicated only to evaluate women with a history or physical findings suggestive of restrictive or obstructive pulmonary disease.

Preoperative assessment must determine whether the woman has the pulmonary reserve to overcome the normal postoperative decrease in pulmonary function. Women who have compromised preoperative pulmonary function are especially susceptible to develop clinically significant postoperative atelectasis, which occurs following approximately 10% of gynecologic operations. Predisposing factors that increase the incidence of atelectasis include morbid obesity, smoking, pulmonary disease, and advanced age. Increased pain, the supine position, abdominal distention, impaired function of the diaphragm, and sedation also contribute to decreased lung volumes and reduced dynamic measurements of pulmonary function for the postoperative woman. The sequence of events that predispose a woman to postoperative pulmonary complications are depicted in **Figure 24-3**.

Important questions in the history relate to smoking, recent upper respiratory infection, cough, amount of sputum production, degree of dyspnea, wheezing and, most important, exercise tolerance. In women with known respiratory disease, a complete medication history should be obtained, including antibiotics, bronchodilators, mucolytic agents, and corticosteroids. Some women exhibit suppression of their hypothalamic pituitary axis function if they have received low daily doses of oral or inhaled corticosteroids. Thus, if low daily doses of oral or inhalation corticosteroids have been taken during the past year for longer than 2 weeks, the woman should receive parenteral hydrocortisone to cover potential adrenal insufficiency during the perioperative period. The history should also include questions about exposure to industrial air pollution. With the increase in obesity in the population, there has been a concomitant increase in the incidence of sleep apnea. Several apnea screens have been validated to identify patients who should be referred for further evaluation. The easiest screen is the STOP mnemonic: *s*noring, *t*iredness, *o*bserved stopping of breathing, blood *p*ressure. Women in whom there is a potential for sleep apnea such as those who are morbidly obese and those with a large neck circumference should be questioned and referred when appropriate.

If the woman is currently a smoker, the risk of postoperative pulmonary complications increases approximately fourfold. The basic defense mechanisms of the lungs, such as the ciliary action of the epithelial cells that line the respiratory tract, are significantly impaired by smoking. Even young women with normal lungs who smoke a half-pack of cigarettes daily are at increased risk. Ideally, women should stop smoking 8 weeks preoperatively. However, abstinence from cigarettes for 2 to 4 weeks preoperatively is a more practical goal. Providing transdermal nicotine replacement is helpful in alleviating the symptoms of acute nicotine withdrawal. Smoking is most detrimental in women with chronic bronchitis or chronic obstructive pulmonary disease (COPD). Several studies have found that referral to preoperative smoking cessation programs not only decreases the percentage of women who smoke around the time of surgery, but also leads to an increased incidence of long-term cessation of smoking. In one multicenter study, Lindstrom and associates noted that the patients in a smoking cessation program had perioperative complication rates of 21% versus 41% in controls. The number needed to treat (NNT) in this study was five patients to prevent perioperative complications.

Table 24-5 Postoperative Pneumonia Risk Index

Preoperative Risk Factor	Point Value
Type of Surgery	
Abdominal aortic aneurysm repair	15
Thoracic	14
Upper abdominal	10
Neck	8
Neurosurgery	8
Vascular	3
Age	
≥80 yr	17
70–79 yr	13
60–69 yr	9
50–59 yr	4
Functional Status	
Totally dependent	10
Partially dependent	6
Weight loss >10% in past 6 mo	7
History of chronic obstructive pulmonary disease	5
General anesthesia	4
Impaired sensorium	4
History of cerebrovascular accident	4
Blood Urea Nitrogen Level	
<2.86 mmol/L (<8 mg/dL)	4
7.85–10.7 mmol/L (22–30 mg/dL)	2
≥10.7 mmol/L (≥30 mg/dL)	4
Transfusion >4 units	3
Emergency surgery	3
Steroid use for chronic condition	3
Current smoker within 1 year	3

Class I, <15 points, probability of pneumonia, 0.24; class II, 16-25 points, 1.20 probability; class III, 26-40 points, probability 4.0: class IV, 41-55 points, probability 9.4; class V, >55 points, probability of pneumonia 15.4.
From Arozullah AMJ, Khuri SF, Henderson WG: Development and validation of a multifactorial risk index for predicting postoperative pneumonia after major noncardiac surgery. Ann Intern Med 135:847, 2001.

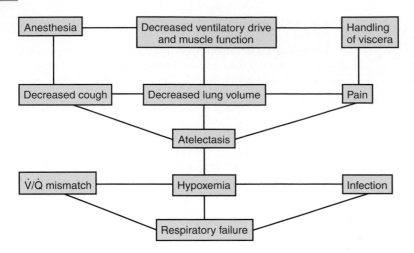

Figure 24-3 The administration of anesthesia and handling of viscera precipitate a series of changes that may lead to postoperative pulmonary complications. $\dot{V}/\dot{Q}$, ventilation-perfusion. (From Celli BR: What is the value of preoperative pulmonary function testing? Med Clin North Am 2:309, 1993.)

During the physical examination, special attention should be given to findings of tachypnea, wheezing, rhonchi, rales, decreased breath sounds, and prolonged expiration. Direct observation of exercise tolerance, such as climbing a flight of stairs, is helpful in evaluating the extent of pulmonary reserve. This is a crude index of pulmonary function. Women with any positive findings on history or physical examination should have a chest radiographic examination and, in select cases, arterial blood gas values should be obtained and pulmonary function tests performed. Preoperative pulmonary function tests should be carried out on women with productive sputum (more than 2 ounces/day), 20 pack-years or longer smoking history, morbid obesity, asthma, and COPD. Women with chronic lung disease often have shunting of blood in the lungs and arterial hypoxemia. Thus, preoperative arterial blood gas levels should be measured. When arterial blood gases are evaluated, the oxygen tension should exceed 65 mm Hg and the carbon dioxide tension should be less than 45 mm Hg. An elevated arterial CO_2 is an important warning sign because the respiratory drive has become refractory to hypercarbia. In a study of 272 patients referred for preoperative pulmonary assessment, 8% eventually developed postoperative pulmonary complications. Age older than 65 years, a 40 pack-year history, and short laryngeal height (<4 cm) were independently associated with pulmonary morbidity. Preoperative hypercarbia and poor forced expiratory volumes and times were related to the independent variables.

Pulmonary function tests help assess the pulmonary reserve and identify the extent to which the dysfunction is reversible. These tests help to identify women at increased risk for pulmonary problems during the postoperative period. Pulmonary function tests that measure lung volumes and flow rates help distinguish restrictive defects or a decrease in the amount of lung tissue from obstructive defects in which there is a reduction and prolongation of airflow during expiration. The two most common pulmonary function tests used for screening are forced vital capacity (FVC) and forced expiratory volume in 1 second (FEV_1). A woman with a FVC volume less than 50% of the predicted normal for her age and body size should have more extensive testing for significant lung disease. Similarly, the FEV_1 should be more than 75% of the predicted normal volume. When pulmonary function test results are lower than predicted, or the history uncovers notable issues, a pulmonary consult

should be obtained. Pulmonologists may prescribe bronchodilators or steroids to maximize pulmonary function in women with obstructive disease. A systematic review by Smith found level I evidence that chest physiotherapy, intermittent positive pressure breathing, and epidural anesthesia are three modalities that reduce postoperative pulmonary morbidity, in addition to smoking cessation.

Postoperative pulmonary morbidity is strongly associated with a low serum albumin level, less than 3.5 g/dL. Women with chronic disease, malnutrition, or malabsorption should have their albumin level checked in a preoperative blood screen, usually part of a metabolic panel. Age is an additional risk factor for pulmonary complications. Women older than 60 to 69 years have a twofold risk over younger women and those 70 to 79 years have a threefold risk. Age alone, without other respiratory symptoms, is not an indication for spirometry. However, many clinicians obtain chest x-rays in women older than 70 years as part of the preoperative evaluation. The guidelines for what age (if any) to order a preoperative chest x-ray in an asymptomatic woman are not firmly established, and vary from institution to institution.

Women who are morbidly obese or with symptoms of sleep apnea—or a suspicious history obtained from the woman's spouse or partner—should have a pulmonary consultation. They may benefit from the use of a continuous positive airway pressure (CPAP) device. Women with sleep apnea should not be placed on low levels of oxygen and narcotics without CPAP because they have lost their respiratory stimulus from chronically higher levels of CO_2. Thus, if they are given inspired oxygen, there will be nothing to stimulate breathing, thereby leading to apnea and acidosis. Women with sleep apnea also have a higher incidence of hypertension and cardiac disease secondary to sympathetic nervous system activation during periods of apnea. These women should have an ECG and anesthesia consultation as well.

Over 25 million Americans have asthma, so this condition is frequently encountered during the preoperative evaluation. Asthma increases the incidence of perioperative respiratory problems approximately fourfold. Asthmatic women are susceptible to perioperative respiratory complications secondary to bronchial hyperresponsiveness, airflow obstruction, and hypersecretion of mucus. Ideally, an asthmatic woman should have elective surgery when she is free of wheezing and has optimal

Table 24-6 Risk Reduction Strategies

Preoperative
Encourage cessation of cigarette smoking for at least 8 wk.
Treat airflow obstruction in patients with chronic obstructive pulmonary disease or asthma.
Administer antibiotics and delay surgery if respiratory infection is present.
Begin patient education regarding lung expansion maneuvers.

Intraoperative
Limit duration of surgery to less than 3 hr.
Use spinal or epidural anesthesia.*
Avoid use of pancuronium.
Use laparoscopic procedures when possible.
Substitute less ambitious procedure for upper abdominal or thoracic surgery when possible.

Postoperative
Use deep-breathing exercises or incentive spirometry.
Use continuous positive airway pressure.
Use epidural analgesia.*

*This strategy is recommended, although variable efficacy has been reported in the literature.
Adapted from Smetana GW: Preoperative pulmonary evaluation. N Engl J Med 340:937, 1999.

Table 24-7 Mechanisms Causing Adverse Outcomes from Poorly Controlled Diabetes

Hyperglycemia
Dehydration
Academia from keto acids and lactate
Nonenzymatic glycosylation of proteins central to immune function: complement, impaired IgG, inhibited neutrophil activity
Fatigue and muscle wasting from lipolysis and protein catabolism
Increased circulating fatty acids
Increased skeletal muscle breakdown
Cell membrane instability
Decline in myocardial contractility and increased cardiac arrhythmias
Inhibited endothelial function
Insulin resistance
Increased lipolysis
Presence of insulin inhibits inflammatory factors
Decreased endothelial-derived relaxing factor—nitric oxide
Insulin and glucose inhibit proinflammatory cytokines

Adapted from the American College of Endocrinology: Position Statement on Inpatient Diabetes and Metabolic Control. Endocr Pract 10:77, 2004.

pulmonary status, as measured by pulmonary function tests (peak flow >80% of predicted or her personal best value).

Preoperative preparation of women with asthma or other COPD includes cessation of smoking, instruction in incentive spirometry, combination of inhaled ipratropium and inhaled β-adrenergic receptor agonist, chest physiotherapy, and postural drainage, adequate hydration, sometimes high-dose oral corticosteroids, and antibiotics for purulent sputum for several days before the anticipated surgery. Most authorities advise combining multiple therapeutic regimens to try to reduce the risk of postoperative pulmonary complications.

In summary, the major factors in postoperative respiratory morbidity are underlying pulmonary disease, smoking, advanced age, obesity, low serum albumin level, and the associated decrease in functional respiratory capacity normally produced by the events surrounding an operation. Prophylactic lung expansion programs are the foundation of effective plans to decrease the risk of postoperative atelectasis in high-risk individuals. A meta-analysis of studies of incentive spirometer or deep-breathing exercises has found a decrease in relative risk of pulmonary complications by approximately 50%. Effective pain control by epidural analgesia also reduces the risk of pulmonary complications (**Table 24-6**).

ENDOCRINE SYSTEM: DIABETES MELLITUS

The prevalence of diabetes in adult women is approximately 10% in women younger than 65 years, and the incidence increases rapidly as women get older. The rule of thumb for diabetes management is that elective operations should be scheduled for the diabetic woman only if she is in nutritional balance and under good diabetic control. Associated electrolyte problems must be recognized and corrected before the operation. The stress of an operation and of anesthesia often produces changes in glucose tolerance and insulin resistance. Because pancreatic reserve is a continuum, even women who are not diabetic by standard blood glucose criteria may develop detrimental hyperglycemia secondary to the physiologic stresses of surgery.

During the perioperative period, the physiologic stress response involves the release of catecholamines, cortisol, growth hormone, and glucagon, all of which may produce hyperglycemia. The combined effects of these three hormones tend to elevate the blood sugar level by 20 to 40 mg/dL; physiologically, they act synergistically to amplify the proglycemic response at the cellular level. In 2004, the American College of Endocrinology published a position paper, "Inpatient Diabetes and Metabolic Control," emphasizing not only the effects of elevated blood glucose levels but the beneficial effects of adequate insulin (**Table 24-7**). Insulin decreases lipolysis. Elevated free fatty acid levels are associated with arrhythmias. Insulin inhibits several inflammatory mediators, especially the proinflammatory cytokines. Adequate insulin also leads to an increase in nitric oxide levels in the endovasculature, inducing vasodilation.

The principal postoperative complications in diabetic women are increased operative site infections, cardiac morbidity, and wound disruptions. The increase in infection rate is believed to be secondary to a decrease in cellular and humoral responses to bacteria. Women with diabetes have approximately a fivefold increase in incidence of wound infection compared with age-matched controls. The increased incidence of wound disruptions is caused by a decreased tensile strength during healing associated with insulin resistance and an elevated blood sugar level.

Preoperative evaluation requires meticulous attention to the details of the woman's disease during the history and physical examination. Important questions center on the severity of the diabetes, types of medications, and recent diabetic control, including blood glucose levels. Specific inquiries should be made about the complications of chronic diabetes, especially those affecting the cardiovascular and renal systems. During the physical examination, attention should be directed toward the diagnosis of peripheral neuropathy. Diabetic neuropathy may be the explanation of persistent pain during the perioperative period. Autonomic neuropathy may cause postoperative gastrointestinal or genitourinary dysfunction. Autonomic dysfunction also predisposes the diabetic woman to postural hypotension, cardiac arrhythmias, and cardiac arrest. Preoperative blood studies should include some measurement of recent diabetic control, such as a glycosylated hemoglobin, hemoglobin A1c (HbA1c), and electrolyte and renal profiles. An ECG should be obtained regardless of the woman's age. Special emphasis should be directed to screening for asymptomatic infection, especially in the urinary tract.

The medical sequelae of diabetes mellitus, such as renal and cardiac insufficiency, peripheral neuropathy, and peripheral vascular disease, are related to the severity and chronicity of the disease. The woman's history will help differentiate mild insulin-dependent diabetes from severe insulin-dependent diabetes. When diabetes is treated with oral agents, consideration should be directed to preoperative dosage. Longer acting sulfonylureas may be discontinued 24 hours before surgery. Short-acting sulfonylureas should be discontinued 12 hours before the operation.

Metformin is associated with lactic acidosis in the setting of renal compromise. Many fatalities have occurred in the perioperative and postoperative periods. Decreased renal function may occur even in women who have otherwise seemingly normal renal activity. Women who take metformin for treatment of polycystic ovary syndrome should stop their medication 4 days prior to surgery. Women who take metformin for glucose control should be changed to subcutaneous insulin if necessary 3 to 4 days prior to surgery.

Perioperative and postoperative treatment of women with glucose intolerance or overt diabetes is based on glucose control, with the general goal of management being to avoid hyperglycemia and hypoglycemia. Regional anesthesia has less of an effect on blood glucose than general anesthesia and, when appropriate, is a better option for diabetic women. Current evidence has shown clearly that the closer the blood sugar level is maintained toward normal, the greater the improvement in patient outcomes. Populations of patients undergoing surgery for cardiac, vascular, neurosurgical, and bariatric indications, as well as those having general surgery or experiencing trauma and those in intensive care, have all been studied. All have been shown to have a decreased incidence of morbidity and mortality with glucose regulation of a serum levels less than 140 mg/dL, compared with control groups, with sliding scales starting at 200 mg/dL or higher. Fasting blood glucose levels higher than 126 mg/dL and random levels higher than 200 mg/dL in general surgery patients were noted to correlate with mortality rates 18 times higher and twice longer lengths of stay compared with patients with tight control and glucose levels less than 120 mg/dL.

In a landmark trial by Van Den Berghe and colleagues, 1548 intensive care unit (ICU) patients were randomized into tight control, glucose levels 80 to 110 mg/dL, versus controls for whom insulin was given for glucose levels above 215 mg/dL. The mortality rate was 4.6% versus 8% in controls. The increase in mortality was related primarily to sepsis. Tight control was associated with a significant reduction in septicemia by 46%, reduction in renal failure by 41%, reduction in transfusion by 50%, and reduction in neuropathy by 44%. Importantly, this study evaluated blood glucose levels in all patients, not just diabetics, which emphasizes that the stresses of surgery can produce detrimental hyperglycemia in any patient. The greater the perioperative stress, the greater the insulin resistance. Studies from the Mayo Clinic of 1026 patients showed that the increased morbidity could be directly related to increasing glucose levels; thus, threshold glucose levels to start treatment should occur as close to the physiologic range as possible. In contrast, patients undergoing short and simple surgeries with short

hospitalizations do not show as much benefit from tight control and sometimes risk hypoglycemia, with dangerous consequences. The risk-benefit ratio for these women favors maintaining glucose levels lower than 180 to 200 mg/dL.

Patients with laparotomies, those at higher risk with comorbid medical conditions, those with long hospital stays, and the morbidly obese should be considered for close glucose control. The preprandial glucose level should be less than 110 mg/dL and maximum glucose levels at any time should not exceed 180 mg/dL. ICU patients should have insulin infusions to maintain glucose levels under 110 mg/dL. For patients with minor surgeries who will be resuming regular oral intake shortly after surgery, glucose levels may be controlled with hourly glucose measurements and subcutaneous insulin. For patients who have mild diabetes and who may resume oral intake, checking hourly glucose levels is appropriate. If these patients are taking oral agents for their diabetes, the oral agent should be discontinued the evening prior to surgery and restarted when the diet is restarted. For patients with more complex surgeries, in whom oral intake will not be resumed soon, insulin infusions beginning preoperatively or intraoperatively should be considered (Table 24-8). An insulin infusion should be begun when the blood sugar level reaches 180 mg/dL. Patients should have glucose levels checked in the preoperative screening area and then at regular intervals until surgery and recovery are concluded and a steady state is reached. Postoperative glucose management is discussed further in Chapter 25 (Postoperative Counseling and Management).

With the increase in undiagnosed type 2 diabetes, some preliminary studies have evaluated office finger stick glucose measurements in the preoperative assessment. This cost-effective

Table 24-8 Perioperative Insulin Protocol

1. Test woman in preoperative holding area. If woman is on oral medications, and procedure is <1 hr in duration with anticipated return to regular diet, check glucose regularly. If blood glucose level is >180 mg/dL, begin insulin infusion.
2. If blood glucose level is <110 mg/dL check every 2 hr; IV D$_5$W solution should be used.
3. If blood glucose level is 110-179 mg/dL, check hourly and begin insulin when glucose level surpasses 180 mg/dL.
4. If blood glucose level is >200 mg/dL, check every 30 min.
5. If woman is type 1 diabetic, begin insulin infusion in holding area when blood glucose level is > 100 mg/dL.
6. Begin infusion with solution run through line and on a pump piggybacked into main line.

Sample Infusion Protocol		
Blood Glucose (mg/dL)	**Insulin Bolus (U)**	**Insulin Rate (U/hr)**
100-120	0	0.5
121-150	0	1
151-180	0	1.5
181-200	1	2
201-220	2	2.5
221-220	3	4
251-280	4	5
281-300	6	6
301-330	8	7

Note: Infusion rates should be adjusted for complexity of surgery, blood loss, emergent nature, and woman's degree of control.

technique will highlight patients who will benefit from closer perioperative glucose evaluation.

Continuous IV infusion of regular insulin should be mixed in normal saline with 10 mEq of potassium or 5% dextrose in half-normal saline with 10 mEq of potassium. Lactate induces gluconeogenesis. Thus, one should be cautious in giving large volumes of lactated Ringer's solution because it may produce hyperglycemia. One last caveat should be stated here. For obvious reasons, elective operations on women with diabetes mellitus should be scheduled early in the morning.

THYROID DISEASE

Women with thyroid disease should take their regular dose of thyroxine with a sip of water the morning of surgery. If their thyroid has not been checked for several months prior, it is helpful to determine the thyroid-stimulating hormone (TSH) or free thyroxine (T_4) level during the preoperative evaluation. Also, women with thyroid disease should have an ECG and their electrolyte levels should be determined.

Women with poorly controlled hyperthyroidism may be vulnerable to thyroid storm in response to the stress of surgery. Symptoms of storm may include tachycardia and hyperthermia. Initial treatment is beta blockade, iodine, and antithyroid medication. Women with poorly controlled hypothyroidism may have hypertension, myocardial dysfunction, and hypoglycemia. Thyroid hormone enhances the cellular response to catecholamines, and women with hypothyroid disease respond poorly to stress.

ADRENAL DISEASE

Glucocorticoids are prescribed for a variety of illnesses. Exogenous glucocorticoids will blunt the natural response of the hypothalamic-pituitary-adrenal axis in the necessary response to stress. Steroid use for longer than a 2- to 3-week period within the year prior to surgery necessitates augmented steroid administration during the perioperative period. Even if the dosing was small (as little as 5 to 7.5 mg of daily prednisone), adrenal insufficiency may occur. Supplemental cortisone should be given, 100 mg every 12 hours for most women. Minor surgery will only need one dose; major surgeries entail dosing for the surgery and up to 24 hours postoperatively.

CARDIOVASCULAR DISEASE

The greatest single cause of surgical mortality, including postoperative mortality, is cardiovascular disease. It has been estimated that over 1 million postoperative cardiac complications, including fatal myocardial infarctions, will occur each year in the United States. Many of these deaths occur with emergency surgeries and are unavoidable. However, for elective procedures, it is the responsibility of the gynecologist to assess the risks and, if possible, take steps to improve the woman's cardiac status or decide whether the benefits of the surgery are appropriate for the risks involved.

The goals of cardiovascular assessment are twofold—to determine the risks for women with cardiac symptomatology and to assess risk levels in women without cardiac disease. Surgery presents a significant challenge to the cardiovascular system. Cardiac output must increase in proportion to the complexity of the operation. Intravascular volume may increase and at times fall into a hypovolemic or relative hypovolemic state. Both these states would be challenges to cardiac and vascular status. One of the greatest challenges comes from the catecholamine surges that accompany an operation and that produce a rise in myocardial oxygen demand. If the woman has limited reserves, she may not be able to respond adequately to these challenges. The surge in activity of the sympathetic nervous system can sometimes be ameliorated by the use of beta blockers, but at other times may present specific and significant challenges to the gynecologic surgeon. Also, several physiologic responses to surgery and medications, including anesthesia, antidiuretic hormones, angiotensin, and other hormonal secretions may depress myocardial function.

The American College of Cardiology (ACC) and American Heart Association (AHA) have developed a four-part assessment for evaluating cardiac risk associated with surgery. The first group of risk factors arises from the history, physical examination, laboratory evaluation, and diagnostic tests. The second assessment is the woman's preoperative functional status. The next is the complexity and nature of the anticipated surgery. Fourth is an evaluation of a woman's cardiac disease, which may be low to nonexistent in many women.

For all patients, the assessment of cardiac risk begins with a history and physical examination. In this step, asymptomatic cardiac disease may be uncovered. A history of cardiac symptoms, previous cardiac disease, hypertensive disease, vascular disease, comorbidities, including renal disease, hepatic disease, pulmonary disease, and diabetes, a history of hyperlipidemia, obesity, and smoking all need to be taken into account. The physical examination should focus not only on the examination of the heart, but also on the lungs and peripheral vasculature, including the extremities. Laboratory assessment in many patients should include assessment of renal status, including BUN and creatinine levels, metabolic state with serum albumin level, and consideration of blood gases in those with chronic pulmonary disease.

An ECG should be obtained in patients older than 55 years, those with diabetes, those with a previous cardiac history or symptoms, and those with other comorbidities. A routine ECG obtained on postmenopausal women may diagnose asymptomatic myocardial infarction or serious arrhythmias. Although no study has shown that routine preoperative electrocardiography in asymptomatic women who are at low risk changes management or outcome, most hospitals require an ECG in all older women, which varies from 55 to 70 years old, depending on the hospital. This may necessitate postponing elective surgery. It should be noted, though, that electrocardiography is a fairly nonsensitive test. Two weeks following a documented myocardial infarction, a normal ECG is found in approximately one of four patients. The potential observation for arrhythmias is valuable at this time. The dangers of an operation in a woman with multiple premature ventricular contractions (PVCs) are most significant if the PVCs are associated with a decrease in left ventricular function. Women with previously uncategorized arrhythmias need to be evaluated by a specialist prior to surgery.

An assessment of the woman's functional capacity is the next step in the preoperative assessment. This evaluates what the woman can normally do in her daily life (**Table 24-9**). The question, "Can you climb a flight of stairs?," which is the ability to perform an exercise of 4 metabolic equivalents (METs), is an important separation point. Patients who cannot climb a flight of

Table 24-9 Energy Used for Assessing Functional Capacity Levels

Energy Used (MET)	Activity
1-3	Daily household activities—eating, dressing using the bathroom without help, walking around the house, walking on level ground around the block at a slow pace.
4-6	Light housework, climbing a flight of stairs, walking at about 4 mph, jogging a short distance, extensive work around the house (e.g., moving furniture, scrubbing floors).
7-10	Tennis, jogging, moderate recreational activities.
≥10	Strenuous exercises—running, basketball, skiing, aerobics

MET, Metabolic equivalent.

Table 24-10 American College of Physicians Modified Cardiac Risk Index*

Variable	Points, n
Coronary Artery Disease	
Myocardial infarction <6 mo earlier	10
Myocardial infarction >6 mo earlier	5
Canadian Cardiovascular Society Angina Classification[†]	
Class III	10
Class IV	20
Alveolar Pulmonary Edema	
Within 1 wk	10
Ever	5
Suspected critical aortic stenosis	20
High-grade atrioventricular (AV) block	10
Arrhythmias	
Rhythm other than sinus or sinus plus atrial premature beats on electrocardiogram	5
More than five premature ventricular contractions on ECG	5
Poor general medical status, defined as any of the following:	5
Po_2 <60 mm Hg; Pco_2 >50 mm Hg; K^+ level <3 mmol/liter; blood urea nitrogen level >50 mmol/liter; creatinine level >260 μmol/liter; bedridden; diabetes mellitus	
Age >70 yr	5
Emergency surgery	10
Low functional capacity	5
Hypertension	5
History of stroke	5

*Class I = 0-15 points; class II = 20-30 points; class III = more than 30 points.
[†]Canadian Cardiovascular Society classification of angina: 0 = asymptomatic; I = angina with strenuous exercise; II = angina with moderate exertion; III = angina with walking 1 or 2 level blocks or climbing one flight of stairs or less at a normal pace; IV = inability to perform any physical activity without development of angina. Adapted from American College of Physicians: Guidelines for assessing and managing the perioperative risk from coronary artery disease associated with major noncardiac surgery. Ann Intern Med 127:309, 1997.

stairs without difficulty, whose functional capacity is less than 4 METs, will usually have more difficulty with surgery, whereas those whose functional capacity is more than 4 METs usually do well. Tasks such as dressing oneself and moving about the house are the equivalent of 1 to 2 METs; activities such as tennis or jogging are closer to 10 METs.

In grading risk, the complexity of the operation may be divided into associated high, intermediate, and low cardiac risk. High cardiac risk has more than a 5% risk of cardiac complications, intermediate less than 5%, and low risk less than 1%. Elective major gynecologic procedures usually present an intermediate risk and endoscopic and minor procedures are usually of low risk; however, extensive gynecologic resections that are lengthy and involve significant fluid shifts pose a high risk. Emergency surgery will increase the risk of cardiovascular complications two- to fivefold over the baseline risk.

When the composite risks are pulled together, the risk to the woman can be estimated (**Tables 24-10** and **24-11**). If the risks of cardiac complications are high or the cardiac history is worrisome, more intensive evaluation is indicated. Stress or exercise electrocardiography and invasive cardiac angiography may be considered. The ACC, in association with AHA guidelines, has published an algorithm for assessing risk and guiding clinicians about further investigations of the woman's cardiac status prior to surgery. If a clinician is unsure about safety for a woman undergoing surgery, referral is indicated. Also, many signs and symptoms may be ambiguous, such as inability to sleep well at night, atypical chest pain, and questions about functional capacity, which may be caused by physical problems other than cardiovascular ones. When such a history is unclear, testing is indicated, such as exercise stress tests in conjunction with cardiac consultation.

If surgery is necessary, but the woman is at increased risk, several treatment measures may be given to decrease cardiac risk. One of the more commonly used interventions is perioperative beta blockade, which is preferable begun approximately 1 to 4 weeks prior to surgery. Beta blockade should be titrated to a resting heart rate of approximately 60 beats/min. In one study, the mortality rate was reduced by more than 55% with the use of beta blockade. It is important to note that the mortality rate in this study was decreased for up to 24 months after surgery compared with that for controls. Longer acting agents are preferred to shorter acting agents. Several studies have looked at the use of beta blockade preoperatively, and there is a general consensus about who should receive preoperative medication.

Most physicians believe that any high-risk woman, based on the algorithms explained earlier, should receive perioperative beta blockade. However, some physicians think that patients at intermediate risk should be considered for beta blockers as well, depending on what puts them at risk, such as personal characteristics versus type of surgery. In contrast, patients at low risk and most patients at moderate risk have an increased complication rate, with an increase in morbidity from prophylactic beta blockers. Several studies have also investigated the use of prophylactic calcium channel blockers and prophylactic statins in high-risk patients.

The preoperative hematocrit level is inversely associated with cardiac complications. The lower the hematocrit, the higher the risk for an adverse outcome. If surgery is elective, it is desirable to give oral (or parenteral) iron to obtain a hematocrit more than 38%. Wu and coworkers have noted that in patients older than 65 years, perioperative mortality increases 1.6% for every percentage point less than a 39% hematocrit value in noncardiac surgery. When surgery is not elective, consideration for transfusion should be given to high-risk patients with anemia.

Other mechanisms to decrease cardiac risk include perioperative continuous monitoring for ST-segment changes. The development of ST-segment changes intraoperatively may

Table 24-11 Cardiac Risk Classes for Patients Going to Surgery

Risk Class	Point Score	No or Minor Complications (%)	Life-Threatening Complications* (%)	Cardiac Death (%)
I	0-5	99	0.7	0.2
II	6-12	93	5.7	2.7
III	13-25	86	11.7	2.7
IV	>26	22	22.7	56.7

*Myocardial infarction, ventricular tachycardia, pulmonary edema.
Adapted from Goldman L, Caldera DL, Southwick FS, et al: Cardiac risk factors and complications in non-cardiac surgery. Medicine 57:357, 1978; Salem DN, Homans D, McNally JW, et al: Cardiology. In Molitch ME (ed): Management of Medical Problems in Surgical Patients. Philadelphia, FA Davis, 1982, p 76.

potentially signify myocardial ischemia. Biochemical markers should then be checked (levels of creatinine kinase, MB fraction), which if positive may lead to the need for coronary revascularization. Certainly, all women at high risk should be strongly considered for intensive monitoring. Routine intraoperative transesophageal echocardiography has not been shown to be helpful, nor has prophylactic placement of a pulmonary artery catheter. Other medications, such as angiotensin-converting enzyme (ACE) inhibitors, aspirin, and statins should be continued throughout the perioperative period in women who are at intermediate or high risk for morbidity.

HYPERTENSIVE DISEASE

Women with controlled essential hypertension in the absence of cardiac or renal complications are not at an increased risk for major problems with elective surgery. However, women with poorly controlled hypertension and a diastolic pressure higher than 110 mm Hg should have more intense medical management of their hypertension before elective surgery. No increased risk of cardiovascular complications from surgery occurs in women with uncomplicated mild to moderate hypertension when the diastolic blood pressure is less than 110 mm Hg. If mild or moderate hypertension is complicated by angina, congestive heart failure, abnormal ECG, left ventricular hypertrophy, or renal insufficiency, the surgery should be postponed until the woman is completely evaluated by a cardiologist.

During the induction of anesthesia, there is a potential abrupt rise of blood pressure of 20 to 50 mm Hg. This transient hypertension is experienced during intubation in 6% of normotensive patients and 17% of women with hypertension. Rapid hemodynamic fluctuations are directly related to morbidity in hypertensive women. Major differences between preoperative and intraoperative blood pressures correlate directly with episodes of myocardial ischemia. Perioperative hypotension or hypertension will occur in 20% to 30% of hypertensive women in whom the blood pressure is controlled prior to surgery.

Antihypertensive medication should be continued throughout the perioperative period. The only exception is monoamine oxidase inhibitors, primarily used to treat depression, which should be discontinued for at least 2 weeks before surgery. Discontinuing some antihypertensive agents is potentially harmful. For example, if beta blockers are withdrawn, patients may develop a hypersensitivity to adrenergic stimulation and exacerbation of ischemic heart disease. Myocardial infarction, ventricular tachycardia, and abrupt cardiac arrest have all been documented in women in whom beta blockers have been abruptly discontinued prior to surgery. Similarly, patients taking clonidine develop abrupt hypertensive rebound if the drug is withdrawn. Diuretic

therapy need not be discontinued before surgery. Potential hazards of diuretics include a relative hypovolemia and hypokalemia. Although diuretics often produce hypokalemia, and associated arrhythmias are a concern in women with organic heart disease, they are rarely seen in women without significant heart disease.

CORONARY ARTERY DISEASE

Medically significant coronary artery disease is a problem of older women. It is unusual for a premenopausal woman to have ischemic heart disease unless she has diabetes, hyperlipidemia, severe hypertension, or a strong family history of coronary disease. Nevertheless, women older than 50 years often have elective gynecologic surgery. Thus considerations of angina and previous myocardial infarctions are essential when planning elective surgery.

Unstable angina of less than 3 months' duration is a strong contraindication to an elective operation. Conversely, most women with stable angina without a previous history of myocardial infarction do not have an increased risk of infarction during operations. Regardless of the duration of angina, the woman should be evaluated by a cardiologist prior to elective surgery. When a woman has had a myocardial infarction, it is important to delay an elective operation for approximately 6 months. The excessive mortality rate associated with a noncardiac operative procedure within 3 months of an acute myocardial infarct is 27% to 37%. Following a 6-month interval, the chance of a reinfarction is 4% to 6% with elective operations. Randomized controlled studies of preoperative percutaneous transluminal coronary stent placement or coronary angioplasty have not been published. It is difficult to prove that revascularization operations on the heart reduce the short-term likelihood of mortality in patients subsequently undergoing noncardiac surgery within 6 months of an acute myocardial infarction. No advantage exists in delaying surgery longer than 6 months, because the woman's risk remains constant for the rest of her life.

The induction of anesthesia is an especially vulnerable time for myocardial ischemia. Myocardial ischemia occurs when the heart has to increase its rate and respond to an increase in systemic blood pressure. Approximately 60% of postoperative myocardial infarctions are not accompanied by chest pain. The woman develops congestive heart failure, arrhythmia and, in the older woman, confusion. Most postoperative myocardial infarcts occur during the first 48 hours following surgery. However, it is not unusual for the heart attack to present on the third or fourth postoperative day. Thus, women with coronary artery disease should be closely monitored, hemodynamically and electrocardiographically, for at least 3 to 4 days postoperatively.

VALVULAR HEART DISEASE

Women with valvular heart disease who are at significant risk during surgery are those with aortic and mitral stenosis. Physiologically, these lesions are similar in that the fixed cardiac output may lead to decompensation secondary to the need for changes in cardiac output during surgical procedures.

The major perioperative consideration in women with valvular heart disease is the use of prophylactic antibiotics to reduce the incidence of subacute bacterial endocarditis developing from a bacteremia associated with the surgical procedure. Even without antibiotic coverage, this is a rare complication. However, because of the substantial morbidity and mortality associated with bacterial endocarditis, antibiotic prophylaxis is the standard of care.

Mitral valve prolapse is presently the leading indication for endocarditis prophylaxis. Mitral valve prolapse is a common finding; it is diagnosed in 4% to 8% of women having gynecologic surgery. A report by Fried has documented that the prevalence of mitral valve prolapse is considerably lower than previously reported. The prevalence of mitral valve prolapse is highest in young thin women. The incidence of bacterial endocarditis is threefold to eightfold higher in women with mitral valve prolapse than in the general population. An ad hoc group of the AHA has developed an algorithm to define when prophylaxis is recommended for patients with mitral valve prolapse (**Fig. 24-4**). Women with a history of mitral valve prolapse should have an echocardiogram after diagnosis to document whether they are at risk for endocarditis and thus may need antibiotics.

Women who are in the high-risk category for endocarditis include those with prosthetic cardiac valves, previous endocarditis, complex cyanotic congenital heart disease, and surgically constructed systemic pulmonary shunts or conduits. Women who are in the moderate-risk category include those with most other congenital cardiac malformations, acquired valvular dysfunction such as that associated with rheumatic heart disease, hypertrophic cardiomyopathy, and mitral valve prolapse with valvular regurgitation or thickened leaflets. Women in the high-risk and moderate-risk categories definitely should receive antibiotics prophylactically to prevent endocarditis. Women in the negligible-risk category for whom endocarditis prophylaxis is not recommended include those with an isolated secundum atrial septal defect, previous coronary artery bypass graft surgery, cardiac pacemakers, and previous surgical repair of atrial septal, ventricular septal, or patent ductus arteriosis. Appropriate antibiotic coverage for moderate-risk women undergoing gynecologic surgery is ampicillin (2 g IV); for high-risk women, gentamicin (1.5 mg/kg body weight, not to exceed 120 mg) should be added within 30 minutes of starting the procedure. Depending on the time of expected bacteremia, the same dosage of both drugs is often repeated 6 hours later, or amoxicillin, 1.0 g orally 6 hours following the parenteral antibiotics. If the woman is allergic to ampicillin, vancomycin (1 g) may be substituted; this should be given slowly IV, over a 2-hour period, to avoid systemic flushing, known as so-called red man syndrome.

Special consideration should be given to women with valvular heart disease who are receiving chronic oral anticoagulation. It is preferable to discontinue the oral medication 3 to 4 days before surgery. The INR should be less than 1.5 prior to beginning the operation. There has been a recent change in clinical opinion concerning the need for IV heparin in these patients. Kearon and Hirsh have postulated that the absolute risk of thromboembolism associated with a few days of perioperative subtherapeutic anticoagulation is generally low. In contrast, the risk of bleeding associated with perioperative IV heparin is often relatively high. Therefore, they believe that the risk-benefit ratio does not favor the use of perioperative heparin. Oral anticoagulants are usually resumed postoperatively with heparin. Exceptions include patients with caged ball valves and women with recent thromboemboli. These women should be converted to perioperative heparin prior to the procedure.

SURGERY IN OLDER WOMEN

Performing surgery in the older woman requires careful preoperative preparation. Physical changes of aging affect comorbidities, functional reserve, tissue healing and frailty of tissue, and a delayed return to baseline function after the procedure. The number of older women is increasing. By 2030, 20% of the American population will be older than 65 years. The definition

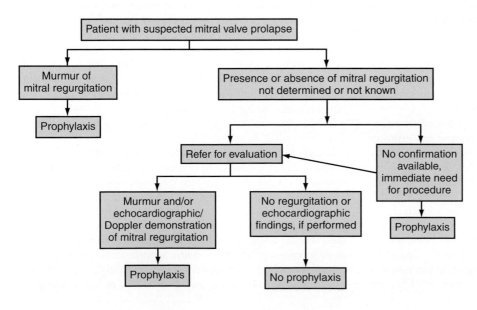

Figure 24-4 Clinical approach to determination of the need for prophylaxis in patients with suspected mitral valve prolapse. (From Dajani AS, Taubert KA, Wilson W, et al: Prevention of bacterial endocarditis. Recommendations by the American Heart Association. JAMA 277:1796, 1997.)

of "elderly" is also changing; it has been said that the older the surgeon, the older the definition of elderly. Although risks factors for surgery begin to increase at age 40, and then increase steadily, the general set point for elderly is age 70 years.

Cardiac morbidity is the single greatest source of morbidity and mortality in the older surgical population. Women older than 70 years experience a 7% to 10% risk of cardiac morbidity with major surgery. Important physiologic changes that must be accounted for include alterations in the cardiac musculature, with connective tissue and fat replacing myocardial tissue. Rosenthal and Zenilman have summarized those changes. Alterations occur in the heart's conduction system, with connective tissue replacing electrical conduction cells. An increased incidence of arrhythmias results. Aging leads to weakening in the valve with dilation of the valve rings and decreased distensibility, thus leading to impaired functional reserve. A decreased response to sympathetic stimulation leads to poorer diastolic filling and a reduced compensation to hypovolemic changes. Thus, failure occurs at a lower cardiac threshold. Symptoms of cardiac failure may be less specific in the geriatric population. The first sign may be confusion, which is common in the older population. Because the older woman has less cardiac reserve, anemia is particularly problematic. Preoperative hematocrit should be obtained. A study by Wu and coworkers of older patients with myocardial infarction has noted that a hematocrit more than 33% is associated with a significantly increased rate of survival. Similarly, hypovolemia must be avoided. Older patients who need a bowel preparation should be admitted and given IV fluids to maintain normal volume and electrolyte levels. If there is a less stringent need for mechanical bowel preparation, a Fleet's enema may be sufficient. All women older than 70 are candidates for perioperative beta blockade.

The pulmonary reserve also decreases with advancing age. Chest wall compliance, inspiratory effort, and pulmonary elasticity all decline, leading to a drop in vital capacity. As women age, their response to hypoxia decreases. Older women are more susceptible to sepsis if they develop pneumonia. The biliary, renal, neurologic, and immune systems all steadily deteriorate with age. All are important components for the necessary response to surgery. Thus, careful preoperative attention to electrolyte levels, pulmonary reserve, liver function, and preexisting functional capacity are also part of the preoperative assessment. Weighing the risks and benefits of the operation must take into account the complication rate, particularly in women with comorbidities. Toglia and Nolan have published a series of 54 major gynecologic surgeries in women between the ages of 70 and 85 years (mean, 77 years). Of these women, 10% developed cardiac complication, including three myocardial infarctions in the perioperative period and two more within 1 week. Two patients developed significant arrhythmias and one patient had a stroke. Parker and colleagues reported on 62 women between the ages of 80 and 94 years (mean, 84 years), who underwent 77 procedures (49 major), with a 14% complication rate. Friedman and associates reported on 120 women in their 80s and 90s. Compared with a cohort of women 50 to 79 years of age, the length of stay was increased but mortality and major complications were similar.

When obtaining consent from an older woman, the American College of Surgery has emphasized several issues. If the woman has a hearing impairment, consent should be obtained in a quiet room, with the surgeon speaking slowly. Family members should be present. A discussion of postoperative recovery and any changes in the woman's level of independence need to be discussed. Not all older women judge risks and long-term problems similar to younger women; their perspective is different.

THE MORNING OF THE OPERATION

PREOPERATIVE NOTE

A brief preoperative note helps to serve as a final summary of preoperative preparation. This abbreviated checklist should summarize important findings in the preoperative history, physical examination, and laboratory screening tests. It is designed to ensure that no step has been forgotten and to summarize in a few words pertinent details for others who subsequently attend the woman. The surgeon should make a brief notation that all the woman's questions have been answered and that both woman and physician are in agreement over the proposed operative procedure.

HAIR REMOVAL

Multiple studies have documented a twofold to threefold increase in infection rate directly related to perioperative shaving. Cruse and Ford studied approximately 63,000 operations over a 10-year period and found a 0.9% incidence of infection when patients were not shaved as opposed to 2.5% when they were shaved. Razors produce macroscopic and microscopic nicks and cuts that allow a protective environment for colonization by skin bacteria. Depilatory agents often produce intense burning if used on the perineum. A systematic review by Kjonniksen and associates has concluded that if the hair is mechanically in the way, it should be clipped just before the operation. Patients should be advised not to shave themselves prior to surgery for this reason.

REASSURANCE

Many women are extremely anxious on the morning of their operation, and admission to the hospital the morning of surgery usually intensifies their anxiety. In many hospitals, this process offers little emotional support to the individual woman but rather gives her the idea that she is being treated in an impersonal fashion. The physical presence of her gynecologist, when she enters the operating room, provides great reassurance. The kindness of touching the woman's hand or standing by her side as the induction of anesthesia begins is greatly appreciated.

PELVIC EXAMINATION

After the woman is asleep or the conduction anesthesia has taken effect, the gynecologic surgeon has two important responsibilities—performing the preoperative pelvic examination and supervising the positioning of the woman. A pelvic examination following catheterization and just before surgical incision should be standard practice, regardless of the type or extent of the proposed gynecologic operation. The relaxation of the abdominal wall produced by anesthesia and the advantage of an empty bladder and lower intestinal tract afford the surgeon the optimum environment for performing a pelvic examination. The findings may change the choice of incision or operative approach. Before draping the woman, the gynecologist should make sure that the woman is properly positioned on the operating room table.

This is especially true for obtaining good exposure in the lithotomy position. Pressure points should be avoided to protect against neuromuscular and skin injury, especially over bony prominences.

KEY POINTS

- For the woman, there are no small, insignificant, or minor operations. Almost any operation is a major event in her life.
- The goals of preoperative planning are to obtain appropriate information, reduce the woman's anxieties and fears, and obtain informed consent.
- Highlights of the discussion regarding informed consent should be documented by a paragraph written by the gynecologist in the progress notes of the chart.
- A detailed history and physical examination will detect approximately 90% of the information pertinent to the surgical procedure.
- Studies have documented that patients often omit important medical information, particularly when under stress. Repetitive history taking provides additional information and helps decrease the risk of omission of significant history information.
- Specific questions should be directed toward sensitivity to iodine or latex. Latex allergy is directly responsible for 12% of the perioperative anaphylactic reactions in adult patients and for 70% in children.
- The preoperative physical examination should answer three basic questions. Has the primary gynecologic disease process changed since the initial diagnosis? What is the impact of the primary gynecologic disease on other organ systems? What deficiencies in other organ systems may affect the proposed surgery and hospitalization?
- A pregnancy test should almost always be performed if the woman is in her childbearing years.
- Serum electrolyte levels should be evaluated for patients with vomiting, diarrhea, ileus, bowel obstruction, or any condition that affects water or electrolyte balance.
- Routine chest radiographic films are not cost-effective unless the woman is older than 75 years or has findings in the history or physical examination suggestive of cardiac or respiratory disease.
- A baseline preoperative ECG is appropriate and cost-effective for women older than 60 years and in women with preexisting comorbidities.

- Oral medications that a woman may be taking for a specific condition or illness may be taken the morning before surgery with 30 to 60 mL of water.
- Antibiotic prophylaxis is effective by reducing the number of bacteria present, not by killing all bacteria. To be effective, the antibiotic must be present at the time of tissue injury or shortly thereafter.
- Approximately 40% of deaths following gynecologic surgery are directly or indirectly related to pulmonary emboli.
- There is a threefold increase in morbidity and a twofold increase in mortality if surgery is performed on diabetic patients who are in a state of poor glucose control.
- Women with diabetes have approximately a fivefold increase in incidence of wound infection compared with age-matched controls.
- The perioperative blood glucose levels in diabetic women should be maintained at less than 180 mg/dL. It is preferable to be as close to normoglycemia as possible.
- The use of insulin lispro (Humalog) has facilitated the perioperative management of diabetes. The advantages of this medication are its extremely short onset, peak levels and duration of action, and more predictable subcutaneous absorption.
- Elective surgical procedures on diabetic women should be scheduled early in the morning.
- The presence of congestive failure is the single most important predictive factor of cardiovascular complications during the perioperative period.
- No increased risk of cardiovascular complications from surgery occurs in women with uncomplicated mild to moderate hypertension when the diastolic blood pressure is less than 110 mm Hg.
- The excessive mortality associated with noncardiac surgery within 3 months of an acute myocardial infarction is 27% to 37%.
- If the older woman has a hearing impairment, consent should be obtained in a quiet room, with the surgeon speaking slowly; family members should be present.

REFERENCES CAN BE FOUND ON
EXPERTCONSULT.com

25

Postoperative Counseling and Management
Fever, Respiratory, Cardiovascular, Thromboembolic, Urinary Tract, Gastrointestinal, Wound, and Operative Site Complications; Neurologic Injury; Psychological Sequelae

Vern L. Katz

The goal of postoperative care is the restoration of a woman's normal physiologic and psychological health. The postoperative period encompasses the time from the end of the procedure in the operating room until the woman has resumed her normal routine and lifestyle. Classically, this continuum may be divided into three overlapping phases based on the woman's functional status. The role and concerns of the gynecologist gradually evolve as the woman moves from one phase to another. The first phase, perioperative stabilization, draws the surgeon's attention to the resumption of normal physiologic functions, particularly respiratory, cardiovascular, and neurologic. The older the woman, the more comorbidities she has and, the more complex the procedure, the longer this period lasts. This period encompasses recovery from anesthesia and the stabilization of homeostasis, with resumption of oral intake. Usually, the time period is 24 to 48 hours. The second phase, postoperative recovery, usually lasts 1 to 4 days. This phase may occur in the hospital and at home. During this period, patients will resume regular diet, ambulation, and move from parenteral to oral medications for treatment of pain. Most traditional postoperative complications become apparent in this time. The last phase is termed the *return to normalcy*, which lasts 1 to 6 weeks. Care during this time occurs primarily in the outpatient setting. During this phase, the woman gradually increases strength and transitions from a sick role back to full and normal activity.

As the woman moves through these phases, physically and psychologically, her needs will change and the interaction with staff and her physician also change. She will gradually leave the patient role and resume a nondependent role. The communication among physicians, patients, and family varies over the course of recovery. For example, in the immediate postoperative period, the primary psychological task of dealing with pain and nausea is the immediate concern. Later, however, the return of dignity and dealing with changes in body image will dominate a woman's attention. It is common for the main questions on the first postoperative day to be "When can I get these tubes out?" and "When can I shower?" Information or bad news about surgical findings must be tailored and given honestly but appropriately for the woman's physical and psychological status. In the first phase of recovery, discussion regarding surgical results is usually concrete and simple as the woman drifts in and out of an awake state. Later, in the postoperative recovery, details can be discussed. As the woman enters the third phase of returning to normalcy, the implications, perspectives, and treatments become much more of an issue and are reviewed in detail.

Postoperative complications may occur at any time; however, early recognition and management will often preclude larger problems from developing. Thus, attention to postoperative details cannot be overemphasized. Often, the woman and her family judge the competence of the gynecologist by the compassion displayed and attention to detail during this postoperative period. Complications increase the duration of the postoperative stay in the hospital. In a study of women readmitted for postoperative complications, approximately 40% had been discharged earlier than the mean length of stay for the corresponding operative procedure. Because many procedures are now laparoscopic, patients will usually leave less than or close to 24 hours after surgery. When complications begin to develop, the woman is at home. Particularly close attention to a postoperative woman's or family's questions is necessary to detect problems before they reach severe levels. The office receptionist or triage nurse must have special training and sensitivity to this very important issue.

General caveats of postoperative management emphasize attention to the particular needs of each woman. Flexibility and individual considerations should take precedence over standard orders, but guidelines can help the physician develop his or her own preferences. Individualization is especially important in the postoperative care of geriatric women. Special nursing attention and minimal doses of narcotics help prevent confusion and disorientation. Ongoing verbal communications with the nursing staff help eliminate misunderstandings that might result in less than ideal postoperative care.

Surgical stress invokes several physiologic responses meant as the body's defenses. Many of these responses may be more problematic than the actual surgery. For example, some women will respond to the insulin resistance of surgical trauma with severe hyperglycemia, which is detrimental to healing. Peri- and postoperative management strategies are aimed at minimizing or preventing these adverse effects, such as prevention of thromboembolism, or beta blockade in older patients to prevent cardiac complications (**Fig. 25-1**). The clinician must be aware of the physiologic stressors.

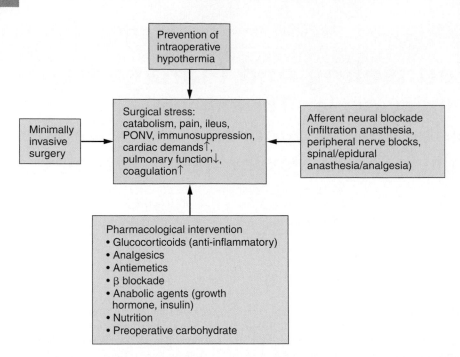

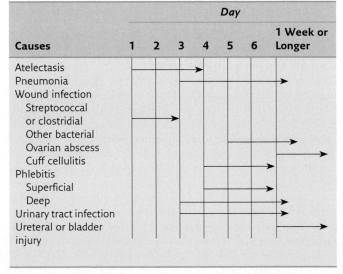

Figure 25-1 Stresses of surgery and interventions to counteract adverse responses. (Adapted from Kehlet H, Dahl JB: Anaesthesia, surgery, and challenges in postoperative recovery. Lancet 362:1922, 2003.)

This chapter discusses major issues of management during the period from the end of surgery until the return to normal physiologic and psychological function. Problems and complications arise over the whole spectrum of the postoperative time frame and are interrelated. Thus, the clinician must be aware at all times of a woman's changing status during recovery. For simplicity, this chapter is organized around organ systems and their potential complications. However, few problems arise in a single organ system.

POSTOPERATIVE FEVER

The exact definition of postoperative febrile morbidity varies greatly among authors. Diurnal fluctuations are characteristic of the normal daily body temperature patterns of humans. Most definitions use a temperature greater than 38° C 24 hours after surgery as the indicator of febrile morbidity. It is not unusual for gynecologic patients to have a mild temperature elevation during the first 72 hours of the postoperative period, especially during the late afternoon or evening. Up to 75% of patients develop a temperature greater than 37° C, which is usually not associated with an infectious process. In a study of 686 women with hysterectomy for benign indications, Peipert and colleagues documented a febrile morbidity rate of 14%.

Fever is the most common diagnostic problem in the postoperative patient. Common causes of a fever include **atelectasis**, pneumonia, urinary tract infection (UTI), nonseptic phlebitis, wound infection, and operative site infection. Two intraoperative factors that dramatically increase the risk of postoperative fever are an operative time longer than 2 hours and the necessity for intraoperative transfusion. In Peipert and associates' study, increased intraoperative blood loss was associated with a 3.5 relative risk (RR; 95% confidence interval [CI], 1.8 to 6.8) of developing fever postoperatively.

The physician's primary goal in examining the postoperative febrile patient is to determine whether the fever is caused by an infection. Approximately 20% of postoperative fevers are directly related to infection and 80% are related to noninfectious causes. Some conditions necessitate active intervention, whereas others are self-limiting. Thus, it is imperative not to treat a postoperatively febrile patient empirically with broad-spectrum antibiotics. The pathophysiology of postoperative fever is primarily related to the release of cytokines. The cause of a postoperative fever may be simple and common, such as atelectasis or dehydration, or unusual, such as malignant hyperthermia or septicemia. The temporal relationship of the onset of a woman's febrile response to common postoperative complications is depicted in **Table 25-1**.

WORKUP FOR FEVER

The initial workup for a postoperative fever should emphasize the most common problems. Medical students memorize the five Ws in the differential diagnosis: **w**ind (atelectasis), **w**ater

Table 25-1 Onset of Fever for Various Postoperative Complications

	Day						
Causes	1	2	3	4	5	6	1 Week or Longer
Atelectasis							
Pneumonia							
Wound infection							
Streptococcal or clostridial							
Other bacterial							
Ovarian abscess							
Cuff cellulitis							
Phlebitis							
Superficial							
Deep							
Urinary tract infection							
Ureteral or bladder injury							

(UTI), *w*ound (infection or hematoma), *w*alk (superficial or deep vein phlebitis), and *w*onder drugs (drug-induced fever).

The proper workup of a postoperative fever, similar to that of any problem in gynecology, involves the three classic steps of history, physical examination, and laboratory evaluations, with major emphasis placed on the physical examination. The physical examination emphasizes the following: examination of the lungs for atelectasis and pneumonia; the wound and operative site for infection or hematoma formation; the costovertebral angles for tenderness, which might suggest pyelonephritis; and superficial veins in the arms for superficial phlebitis and deep veins in the legs for deep vein phlebitis.

The findings of the history and especially the physical examination and considerations of cost containment all influence the extent of laboratory tests ordered. Ordering a specific list of laboratory tests is unrewarding. The three most commonly ordered laboratory tests are complete blood count, chest roentgenography, and urinalysis. A study by Schwandt and coworkers has emphasized that chest radiography and urine cultures are best ordered only for specific clinical signs not as reflex orders. Other common tests include culture and Gram stains of body fluids, including sputum, urine, and blood. One study of over 300 women who were febrile following hysterectomy did not identify a single positive blood culture. Women with persistent and undiagnosed fevers may need liver function tests or special imaging studies, such as pelvic ultrasound or computed tomography (CT) to detect problems such as compromised ureters, abscesses, or foreign bodies.

Each major complication will be discussed in detail later in the chapter. However, several specific generalizations concerning the type and characteristics of fever patterns should be emphasized. Fever is a common postoperative finding, occurring in approximately 75% of women. Rarely is the cause of the fever a serious infection. Microatelectasis is thought to be the cause of approximately 90% of fevers occurring in the first 48 hours after operation. Patients who develop fever as a result of an indwelling catheter, such as plastic intravenous (IV) lines or Foley catheters, are afebrile for several days and then experience an abrupt temperature spike. In contrast, wound or pelvic infections, which are usually clinically diagnosed from the fourth to seventh postoperative days, usually are associated with a low-grade fever that begins early in the postoperative period. An empiric trial of IV heparin for 72 hours is often a diagnostic and therapeutic trial for pelvic thrombophlebitis in refractory cases of postoperative fever of unknown origin.

Importantly, infection in the older woman will not always present with classic findings. The amount of temperature elevation may not reflect the severity of the infection. Not uncommonly, the first signs of infection in older adults will be mental status changes. Additionally, the degree of leukocytosis, being blunted or absent, may not reflect infection.

A woman with a drug-induced fever feels better and does not look as ill as her temperature course indicates. The tachycardia associated with the elevated temperature is usually much less than usually anticipated with a similar temperature elevation secondary to inflammation or infection. The presence of eosinophilia suggests a drug-induced fever. However, drug fever is rare and is usually a diagnosis of exclusion. Presumptive evidence of a drug-induced fever is established when the fever disappears after discontinuation of the drug.

Superficial thrombophlebitis often produces an enigmatic fever. Often, there is tenderness at the IV site. Thus, it is important to change any IV lines empirically that have been in place for longer than 48 to 72 hours. This is particularly true for central venous catheters and epidural catheters, in which an infection may not show clinical signs of localized tenderness or erythema. The cause of febrile transfusion reactions is a concern. However, usually the reactions are caused by leukocyte or platelet antibodies. As long as a major blood type incompatibility is not found, treatment may be conservative.

The basic fever workup should be repeated at intervals until the diagnosis is established. The woman should be reexamined and selective laboratory tests reordered. Rare causes of postoperative fever include pulmonary embolism (PE), thyroid storm, and malignant neoplasms. These diagnoses usually present with other signs and symptoms as well as temperature elevation. It is important to consider that fever is a potentially beneficial physiologic response to the patient. Therefore, unless the woman is markedly symptomatic secondary to the elevated temperature, it is not necessary to order an **antipyretic** medication. Cellular damage only occurs when the core temperature exceeds 41° C. Active cutaneous cooling does not reduce core temperature and may have undesirable effects, such as increasing the metabolic rate and activating the autonomic nervous system.

MANAGEMENT OF A FALLING HEMATOCRIT

Bleeding is one of the most feared postoperative complications. Significant arterial bleeding in the first 24 hours often necessitates reoperation. This complication is discussed later in the chapter, along with the management of shock and pelvic hematomas.

Vital signs should be ordered at frequent intervals during the first 24 hours to detect hypovolemia. Most women will have sufficient intravascular volume to compensate (during the early phases of hemorrhage) through the redistribution of blood flow from less vital to more vital organs. Low urine output may be the earliest sign of a decrease in intravascular volume. Thus, following an operation, sizable amounts of unrecognized intraperitoneal or retroperitoneal bleeding are sometimes present without the woman having subjective symptoms or appreciable changes in her vital signs or urine output. Minimum urine output should be 0.5 mL/kg/hr. Women of medium and larger size should produce more urine, just as petite patients will produce less. A consistent orthostatic decrease in blood pressure of more than 10 mm Hg may indicate a possible decrease of 20% of the blood volume. Thus, a hematocrit may be helpful at two intervals during the postoperative course. I prefer a hematocrit at 24 and 72 hours following the operative procedure. A hematocrit drawn 24 hours following an operation may not truly reflect postoperative blood loss.

The normal physiologic response to the stress of the operation and tissue destruction is a release of increased levels of aldosterone, cortisol, and antidiuretic hormone (ADH). The higher levels of aldosterone produce an increase in sodium and water retention, whereas increased levels of ADH promote free water retention. This has been called the **ebb phase** of postoperative physiology. It is common for women to have notable lower extremity edema for the first few postoperative days, because they are often given significant amounts of IV fluids. Depending on the type and amount of intraoperative and postoperative IV fluids, the hematocrit on the first postoperative day may be misleading and reflect fluid changes rather than intraoperative or postoperative hemorrhage. The hematocrit from the third postoperative day is a more accurate measurement of postoperative change. If the woman is doing well, stress hormone levels decline and water retention stops. The woman will begin to experience a brisk diuresis, sometimes termed the *flow phase*, beginning around the third postoperative day. Hematocrits should be obtained in a standard fashion to eliminate sampling errors. For example, hematocrit samples drawn from central lines or during blood gas determinations often give false values because of the heparin or saline flush solutions.

After the effects of the operative blood loss are subtracted from the preoperative hematocrit, each further reduction in hematocrit of 3 to 5 points reflects a postoperative hemorrhage of approximately 500 mL. The safe level of postoperative anemia is a controversial issue. Most young healthy women without complicating medical illness will tolerate a hematocrit value of 20% to 22% without transfusion. These patients should be observed for orthostatic changes in their vital signs. Importantly, and in stark contrast, women with cardiac and pulmonary disease and women older than 60 years should be transfused to maintain a hematocrit above 30%. The morbidity and mortality associated with a surgical procedure are directly related to the amount of intraoperative and postoperative blood loss and not the corresponding level of preoperative anemia.

RESPIRATORY COMPLICATIONS

Alterations of pulmonary function are an expected physiologic change in women having general anesthesia and operations that open the peritoneal cavity. Of importance, respiratory complications directly cause 25% of deaths in women who die during the first 7 postoperative days. Many respiratory problems are secondary to inadequate ventilation by women as they try to minimize acute pain from the operative incision.

ATELECTASIS

The term *atelectasis* is derived from two Greek words that mean "imperfect expansion." The severity of atelectasis ranges from lack of expansion of a small group of terminal bronchioles and alveoli to complete collapse of a lung. In most patients, atelectasis is the failure to maintain patency of the small pulmonary airways and alveoli. Atelectasis is the most common cause of postoperative temperature elevations. Studies have demonstrated that there is no association between fever and the amount of atelectasis diagnosed radiologically. The incidence of atelectasis depends on the number of predisposing risk factors and the vigor with which the clinical diagnosis is established.

Of all postoperative respiratory complications, 90% are related to atelectasis. The immediate postoperative period is characterized by a decrease in functional residual capacity and lung compliance (**Fig. 25-2**). Thus, the work of breathing is increased. Microatelectasis is most common when small airways (<1 mm in diameter) become blocked by secretions. When small airways remain closed by a combination of mucous plugs and bronchospasm, the gas distal to the obstruction is absorbed. This process results in atelectasis. These changes occur during the first 72 hours following an operation. When atelectasis becomes progressive and involves a large area of lung tissue, there is an associated decrease in oxygen saturation and a decrease in arterial oxygen pressure (Po_2). This is associated with a normal to low arterial carbon dioxide pressure (Pco_2).

Pulmonary and nonpulmonary factors that favor premature airway closure and development of atelectasis are listed in **Box 25-1**. The supine position decreases the functional residual capacity by approximately 20% compared with the erect position. Obesity, smoking, age older than 60 years, prolonged operative time, presence of a nasogastric tube, and coexisting

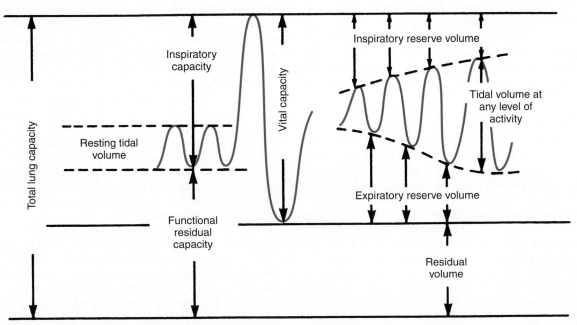

Figure 25-2 Graphic illustration of lung volumes and capacities. (From Wellman JJ: Respiratory care in the surgical patient. In Lubin MF, Walker HD, Smith RB [eds]: Medical Management of the Surgical Patient. Stoneham, MA, Butterworth, 1982.)

Nonpulmonary Factors
  Supine position
  Obesity
  Increased abdominal girth (ileus, pneumoperitoneum)
  Breathing at low lung volumes
    Bindings around the chest and abdomen
    Incisional pain
    Sedative narcotic drugs
    Prolonged effect of paralyzing drugs
    Immobility
    Excessively high concentrations of oxygen for prolonged periods

Pulmonary Factors
  Interstitial edema
  Loss of surfactant with air space instability
  Airway obstruction
    Inflammatory with swelling of bronchial and interbronchial tissue
    Constriction of bronchial smooth muscle
    Retained secretions

From Wellman JJ: Respiratory care in the surgical patient. In Lubin MF, Walker HK, Smith RB (eds): Medical Management of the Surgical Patient. Stoneham, MA, Butterworth, 1982.

medical conditions, such as cardiac or lung disease and pulmonary infection, all predispose women to atelectasis.

In normal breathing periodic, involuntary deep inspirations help expand all areas of the lung. Pain, the supine position, narcotics, and abdominal distention contribute to a pattern of monotonous shallow breathing without spontaneous deep sighs in the postoperative period. Because of the pain of an abdominal incision, chest wall breathing dominates over abdominal breathing. The resultant decrease in the movement of the diaphragm contributes to the development of atelectasis. A further decrease in functional residual capacity, a decrease in surfactant, and a depression of mucociliary transport all contribute to ventilation-perfusion ($\dot{V}/\dot{Q}$) mismatches and reduced $\dot{V}/\dot{Q}$ ratios. The end results are gas trapping, atelectasis, and vascular shunting. In most individuals, microatelectasis is patchy and localized to small areas. However, the severity of atelectasis varies and may involve a complete lung. Distribution of pulmonary blood flow is influenced by gravity. A greater proportion of pulmonary blood flows to dependent areas of the lungs in the supine patient. This increased blood flow, combined with the atelectasis in dependent areas, results in an increased impairment of oxygenation, as well as a decrease in the elimination of carbon dioxide. Obese patients, in general, should be kept slightly upright, not prone, for the first 24 hours to improve vital capacity and ventilation, thus decreasing atelectasis.

The endotracheal tube may contribute to the development of atelectasis. Even correctly placed endotracheal tubes are associated with destruction of cilia in the respiratory tract epithelium. Women with nasogastric tubes have a higher incidence of atelectasis, more commonly related to a decrease in deep breathing than to aspiration of stomach contents. Atelectasis may present as the classic triad of fever, tachypnea, and tachycardia developing within the first 72 hours following an operation. On physical examination, tubular breathing, decreased breath sounds, and moist inspiratory rales may be heard. These findings are most prominent over the bases of the lung. If the condition progresses, an increase in productive cough and leukocytosis result. Chest radiographic films may demonstrate a patchy infiltrate with elevations of the diaphragm. There may be a corresponding shift of the trachea and mediastinum when atelectasis involves a large segment of the lung.

Atelectasis usually resolves spontaneously by the third to fifth postoperative day. Nevertheless, major efforts are made to prevent atelectasis, especially in high-risk individuals. The foundations of prevention of atelectasis are the encouragement of uneven ventilation and the production of episodes of prolonged inspiration to increase functional residual capacity. Thus, the patient is encouraged to walk, take deep breaths, cough, turn from side to side, and remain semierect rather than supine. Early mobilization and ambulation have been documented to be as effective as chest physical therapy in the prevention of pulmonary complications. Keeping pain relief to a level at which the woman will be able to cooperate and not have monotonous shallow breathing is also helpful. The most important aid to prevent and treat atelectasis is a simple bedside incentive spirometry device. Many women need encouragement by the hospital staff to use these devices effectively. The primary risk of atelectasis is progression to pneumonia. Randomized clinical trials and systematic reviews have noted that preventive measures significantly reduce problematic atelectasis and pneumonia. Thus, these simple measures should be ordered for all patients.

In summary, basilar atelectasis is the most common postoperative pulmonary problem experienced by gynecologic patients. If atelectasis does not clear, the woman should be treated with chest physical therapy, intermittent positive pressure breathing, aerosol therapy, or intermittent continuous positive airway pressure by mask. Rarely, bronchoscopy may be indicated to remove large mucus plugs.

PNEUMONIA

Postoperative pneumonia is commonly associated with atelectasis because bacterial infections often begin in collapsed areas of the lungs. Predisposing factors to the development of pneumonia include chronic pulmonary disease, heavy cigarette smoking, alcohol abuse, obesity, advanced age, nasogastric tubes, long operative procedures, gram-negative bacterial infections, postoperative peritonitis, and debilitating illnesses.

The symptoms and signs of pneumonia are fever, cough, dyspnea, tachypnea, and purulent sputum. When pain occurs, it may be felt in the back or chest. The classic physical finding of pneumonia is coarse rales over the infected area. The patient usually has a higher temperature and more systemic toxicity than a woman with atelectasis. Leukocytosis is pronounced in most patients, although it may be delayed or attenuated in older women. Chest roentgenograms often demonstrate diffuse patchy infiltrates of the lung. Radiographic diagnoses are approximately 60% accurate for bacterial or viral pneumonia in women with laboratory-proven pneumonia. Gram staining of the sputum helps differentiate between bacterial colonization and infection. In cases of pneumonia, the smear contains a large number of inflammatory cells with both intracellular and extracellular bacteria.

The management of pneumonia is similar to the management of atelectasis, with the addition of parenteral antibiotics. The initial choice of parenteral antibiotics is usually based on the Gram stain and subsequently on sputum cultures. Most lung infections result when the contents of the mouth (mucus and bacteria that have a physiologic pH) are inhaled and subsequently produce bacterial pneumonia.

One in 3000 procedures may be complicated by pneumonitis produced by the aspiration of gastric fluid (sterile and highly acidic). The aspiration produces a severe chemical pneumonitis. Aspiration and its complications are a cause of approximately 30% of anesthetic mortalities. Women at high risk for aspiration pneumonia include older women, obese women, and those with a hiatal hernia or emergency surgery associated with a full stomach. The morbidity from aspiration is secondary to particulate matter entering into the lungs and the caustic nature of gastric acid. The combination of these insults leads to a destructive inflammatory response. When aspiration is significant and severe, adult respiratory distress syndrome often develops. Secondary infection usually complicates aspiration pneumonitis, and broad-spectrum antibiotics should be given when this diagnosis is entertained. Preventive measures include early removal of nasogastric suction, antacid ingestion, and H2 blockers in the perioperative period, as well as careful use of narcotics and sedatives.

SLEEP APNEA

Sleep apnea has become a significant concern because the incidence of obese and morbidly obese patients has risen. Increased fatty tissue in the neck may produce compression and narrowing of the airway, leading to intermittent apnea while a woman sleeps. In addition, the chronic airway narrowing in obese patients may also lead to hypoventilation. Increased chest wall thickness and adipose tissue in the abdominal wall and neck lead to a decrease in pulmonary compliance. The lowered Po_2 may induce systemic as well as pulmonary hypertension. Patients will also develop a chronically increased Pco_2. Respiratory drive shifts from a CO_2-driven response to a response to low levels of oxygen. When morbidly obese patients are given higher levels of oxygen, as well as narcotics, they are at increased risk for apnea. These patients develop an increased sensitivity to narcotics that shuts down the respiratory drive. Patients with chronic hypoxia from any cause will often have an increased sensitivity to narcotics, but it is particularly problematic in the obese patient who is dependent on low levels of oxygen for respiratory stimulation. These patients should be given oxygen as needed. However, during the postoperative period, when narcotics are given, continuous pulse oxymetry should be used to keep the oxygen saturation in the 94% range. At saturation levels of 96% to 99% these patients may lose respiratory drive and become hypercarbic and acidotic.

CARDIOVASCULAR PROBLEMS

HEMORRHAGIC SHOCK

Shock is defined as a condition in which circulatory insufficiency prevents adequate vascular perfusion of vital organs. Systemic hypotension results in poor tissue perfusion and reduced capillary filling. If this pathophysiologic state is neglected, prolonged hypotension results in oliguria, progressive metabolic acidosis, and multiple organ failure. Shock may be produced by hemorrhage, cardiac failure, sepsis, and anaphylactic reactions. Hypovolemic shock is the most common cause of acute circulatory failure in gynecologic patients. Cardiogenic shock and septic shock are rare. Shock from postoperative hemorrhage is usually seen in the first several hours following surgery. In the perioperative period, hypovolemia may be secondary to several factors, including preoperative volume deficiency, unreplaced blood loss during surgery, extracellular fluid loss during surgery, inadequate fluid replacement and, most commonly, continued blood loss following the surgical procedure. Tachycardia is the classic cardiovascular physiologic response to hypotension. Progressive hypovolemia results in diminished urine output.

The vast majority of perioperative cases of shock are related to hemorrhage secondary to inadequate hemostasis. The development of shock from acute blood loss depends on the rate of bleeding; for example, a slow venous ooze may produce a large amount of blood loss but not produce shock. Rapid loss of 20% of a woman's blood volume produces mild shock, whereas a loss of greater than 40% of blood volume results in severe shock. Actual measurement of intraoperative blood loss is imprecise, even with the extensive use of suction equipment. Studies have demonstrated that 15% to 45% of surgical blood loss is absorbed on the drapes, laparotomy pads, and other areas. Thus, the level of blood in the suction bottle does not accurately represent the true loss from the procedure. Massive blood loss has been defined as hemorrhage that results in replacement of 50% of the circulating blood volume in less than 3 hours.

Hypotension in the immediate postoperative period may be secondary to the residual effects of anesthesia or oversedation. For example, older patients often experience prolonged vasodilation secondary to the sympathetic blockade produced by epidural or spinal anesthesia. The most common cause of postoperative bleeding is a less than ideal ligature or hemorrhage from a vessel that has retracted during the operation. Bleeding may come from an isolated artery or vein or may be more generalized when the bleeding is secondary to a clotting diathesis. The differential diagnosis of postoperative hemorrhagic shock includes conditions such as pneumothorax, PE, massive pulmonary aspiration, myocardial infarction, and acute gastric dilation.

The differential diagnosis of ineffective coagulation includes sepsis, fibrinolysis, diffuse intravascular coagulation, and a previously unrecognized coagulation defect, such as von Willebrand's disease. Inadequate hemostasis sometimes develops from excessive transfusion. The progressive acidosis associated with shock increases hemostatic problems. Hypothermia further complicates hemostasis because it produces platelet dysfunction and coagulopathy secondary to decreased activity of thromboxanes. Thrombocytopenia, impaired platelet function, and a decrease in factors V, VIII, and XI occur with massive transfusions. Coagulopathy begins with the transfusion of more than 5 units of blood. Hypofibrinogenemia is the first to develop, followed by deficiencies of other coagulation factors. Thrombocytopenia is the last recognized defect in the coagulopathy cascade. However, the timing of its development varies among individuals. Thus, transfusion of platelets should be determined by serial platelet counts (**Box 25-2**). Similarly, preset formulas for the transfusion of fresh-frozen plasma, such as 2 units of plasma for every 5 units of packed cells, should be replaced by selective transfusion of plasma as needed to match a clotting deficiency.

Tachycardia and decreased urine output are two early signs of hypovolemia caused by hidden internal bleeding. The body's adrenergic response to hemorrhage includes perspiration, tachycardia, and peripheral vasoconstriction. Urine output decreases

Box 25-2 Suggested Transfusion Guidelines for Platelets

Recent (within 24 hr) platelet count < 10,000/mm^3 (for prophylaxis)

Recent (within 24 hr) platelet count < 50,000/mm^3 with demonstrated microvascular bleeding (oozing) or a planned surgical/invasive procedure

Demonstrated microvascular bleeding and a precipitous fall in platelet count

Adult patients in the operating room who have had complicated procedures or have required more than 10 units of blood *and* have microvascular bleeding. Giving platelets assumes that adequate surgical hemotasis has been achieved.

Documented platelet dysfunction (e.g., prolonged bleeding time > 15 min, abnormal platelet function tests) with petechiae, purpura, microvascular bleeding (oozing), or surgical or invasive procedure

Unwarranted indications:

    Empirical use with massive transfusion when patient is not having clinically evident microvascular bleeding (oozing)

    Prophylaxis in thrombotic thrombocytopenic purpura, hemolytic-uremic syndrome, or idiopathic thrombocytopenic purpura

    Extrinsic platelet dysfunction (e.g., renal failure, von Willebrand's disease)

From Rutherford EJ, Skeet DA, Schooler WG: Hematologic principles in surgery. In Townsend CM, Beauchamp RD, Evers BM (eds): Sabiston Textbook of Surgery, 17th ed. Philadelphia, Saunders, 2004.

Box 25-3 Management Priorities in Massive Transfusion*

Restore circulating blood volume.
Maintain oxygenation.
Correct coagulopathy.
Maintain body temperature.
Correct biochemical abnormalities.
Prevent pulmonary and other organ dysfunction.
Treat underlying cause of hemorrhage.

*The exact priority depends on the circumstances. From Donaldson MDJ, Seaman MJ, Park GR: Massive blood transfusion. Br J Anaesth 69:621, 1992.

to less than 0.5 mL/kg/hr (20 to 25 mL/hr) as a result of poor perfusion of the kidneys. With further loss of blood, the woman becomes agitated, appears weak, and develops skin pallor, with cold and clammy extremities. The systolic blood pressure drops below 80 mm Hg. Again, because of adaptive cardiovascular changes, it takes a rapid loss of approximately one third of the blood volume to produce significant hypotension.

After an operation, occult intraperitoneal and retroperitoneal bleeding often occur without significant local symptoms. Extraperitoneal bleeding may present as bleeding from the vaginal vault if the vaginal cuff was left open. Abdominal distention, muscle rigidity, and shoulder pain are late signs of intraperitoneal hemorrhage. The diagnosis of clinically significant postoperative bleeding may be confirmed by serial changes in hematocrit levels or by paracentesis. However, it is important to caution that marked changes in hematocrit and hemoglobin levels require time to develop. Imaging studies may demonstrate obliteration of the psoas shadow and deviation of the ureter by a large retroperitoneal hematoma. Ultrasound may demonstrate significant intraperitoneal fluid collections.

The goals of management of postoperative shock are to replace, restore, and maintain the effective circulating blood volume and establish normal cellular perfusion and oxygenation (see **Box 25-3**). To accomplish this, an adequate cardiac output and appropriate peripheral vascular resistance must be maintained. The first priority is to provide adequate ventilation because poor respiratory gas exchange is the most frequent cause of death in these patients. The second, almost simultaneous, priority is rapid fluid replacement with adequate amounts of blood and crystalloid solution (normal saline or lactated Ringer's solution). The 3:1 rule suggests a ratio of 3 mL of crystalloid solution for every 1 mL of blood loss. The optimal fluid replacement is a fluid evenly distributed throughout multiple body compartments. Optimal replacement includes packed red blood cells

and a balanced electrolyte solution, such as lactated Ringer's solution. In February 1995, the University Hospital Consortium developed guidelines for the use of albumin, nonprotein colloid, and crystalloid solutions. They recommended that crystalloids should be considered the initial resuscitation fluid of choice in hemorrhagic shock; colloids are appropriate for resuscitation in conjunction with crystalloids when blood products are not immediately available. A meta-analysis of patients with hypovolemia found an excess mortality of approximately 6% (1 excess death per 17 treated patients) in those who received albumin instead of or in addition to crystalloid solutions. Guidelines for transfusion of red blood cells are listed in **Box 25-4**.

The goals of fluid replacement are to obtain and maintain a systolic blood pressure that is similar to preoperative readings, maintain urine output greater than 0.5 mL/kg/hr (usually, >30 mL/hr), and maintain a pulmonary wedge pressure between 10 and 15 mm Hg. **Table 25-2** lists types of blood components used for replacement therapy. To monitor the rapid replacement of large volumes of IV fluid, central venous

Box 25-4 Suggested Transfusion Guidelines for Red Blood Cells

Hemoglobin < 8 g/dL or acute blood loss in an otherwise healthy patient with signs and symptoms of decreased oxygen delivery with two or more of the following:

    Estimated or anticipated acute blood loss of > 15% of total blood volume (750 mL in 70- kg man)

    Diastolic blood pressure < 60 mm Hg

    Systolic blood pressure drop > 30 mm Hg from baseline

    Tachycardia (>100 beats/min)

    Oliguria, anuria

    Mental status changes

Hemoglobin < 10 g/dL in patients with known increased risk of coronary artery disease or pulmonary insufficiency who have sustained or are expected to sustain significant blood loss

Symptomatic anemia with any of the following:

    Tachycardia (>100 beats/min)

    Mental status changes

    Evidence of myocardial ischemia, including angina

    Shortness of breath or dizziness with mild exertion

    Orthostatic hypotension

Unfounded or questionable indications:

    To increase wound healing

    To improve the patient's sense of well-being

    7 g/dL < hemoglobin < 10 g/dL (or 21% < hematocrit < 30%) in otherwise stable, asymptomatic patient

Mere availability of predonated autologous blood without medical indication

From Rutherford EJ, Skeet DA, Schooler WG: Hematologic principles in surgery. In Townsend CM, Beauchamp RD, Evers BM (eds): Sabiston Textbook of Surgery, 17th ed. Philadelphia, Saunders, 2004.

Table 25-2 Indications for Administration of Various Blood Products

Product	Content	Acceptable	Unacceptable
		Indication	
Red blood cells	Red cells	To increase oxygen-carrying capacity in anemic women; for orthostatic hypotension secondary to blood loss	For volume expansion; to enhance wound healing; to improve general well-being
Platelet concentrates	Platelets	To control or prevent bleeding associated with deficiencies in platelet number or function	In patients with immune thrombocytopenic purpura (unless bleeding is life-threatening)
Fresh-frozen plasma	Plasma, clotting factors	To increase the level of clotting factors in patients with demonstrated deficiency	For volume expansion; as a nutritional supplement; prophylactically with massive blood transfusion
Cryoprecipitate	Factors I, V, VIII, XIII, von Willebrand factor, fibronectin	To increase the level of clotting factors in patients with demonstrated deficiency of fibrinogen, factor VIII, factor XIII, fibronectin, or von Willebrand factor	Prophylactically with massive blood transfusion

From American Congress of Obstetricians and Gynecologists: ACOG Tech Bull 199:1, 1994.

catheters may be necessary. It is important to measure the pressure with the woman at a 45-degree angle. Studies have demonstrated that a central venous pressure measurement in the supine position will severely underestimate the volume of intravascular depletion. A Foley catheter, with urometer, facilitates measurement of hourly urine outputs.

Returning a patient to the operating room to control hemorrhage is often a difficult decision. However, this decision should not be postponed. The woman should have an exploratory operation as soon as possible after volume replacement. During this second operation, excellent anesthesia, a full selection of surgical instruments, and the value of good assistance cannot be overemphasized. Proper exposure is paramount for the success of this operation. Initially the old clots are removed and further bleeding is reduced by direct pressure over the pelvic vessels. A systematic search is conducted in an effort to identify the individual vessels that are bleeding. Often, the offending artery or vein cannot be identified, or friability of the tissues results in further bleeding.

In situations requiring reoperation, there is usually a need for transfusion. There is a proven, time-honored surgical axiom: "The greater the blood loss, the more the surgeon underestimates." Many clinicians will add 25% to 35% to their estimated blood loss when hemorrhage occurs to be on the safe side when calculating replacement. The ratio of 2 units of packed red blood cells to 1 unit of fresh-frozen plasma is desirable. For every 6 units of packed red blood cells, a six-pack of platelets should be given. Each unit or pack of platelets will raise the platelet level by 15,000/mm^3. The platelet count should be maintained above 50,000/mm^3 in a woman who is bleeding. The importance of adequate transfusion is not only support of intravascular volume, but supply of oxygen. The greater a woman's comorbidities, the greater the risks from perioperative anemia.

Coagulation studies, prothrombin time, and activated prothrombin time should be obtained regularly during the bleeding episode. The term *washout* is used to describe the loss of clotting factors as a woman uses up her blood volume and is replaced with packed cells and crystalloid. DIC (disseminated intravascular coagulation) is an intravascular consumption and is different than washout. However, both conditions require replacement and ongoing evaluation. Importantly, with continued severe bleeding, the use of recombinant factor VIIa (70 to 90 μg/kg) should be considered. Although expensive, factor VIIa initiates

a rapid burst of thrombin production and stimulates the entire clotting cascade. Many studies have shown it to be very effective in situations of continued bleeding from small vessels in the face of reoperation with washout.

Bilateral ligation of the anterior divisions of the hypogastric arteries distal to the posterior parietal branch is an effective operation to control persistent postoperative pelvic hemorrhage. This procedure results in a reduction of pulse pressure, which allows a stable clot to form at the site where the pelvic vessels are injured. Classically, two ligatures are placed and tied around each hypogastric artery (**Fig. 25-3**). The major potential complication of this procedure is injury to the hypogastric vein. If there is generalized oozing, thrombocytopenia, DIC, or factor VIII deficiency should be suspected. If these conditions are excluded, venous oozing from small vessels in the pelvis may be controlled by the local application of microfibrillar collagen compounds (e.g., Avitene, Gelfoam, Floseal).

Intraoperative rapid autologous blood transfusion is a technique that is used extensively in cardiovascular and trauma surgery. Regretfully, it is underused or rarely performed by gynecologists. Grimes has described a simple device that can

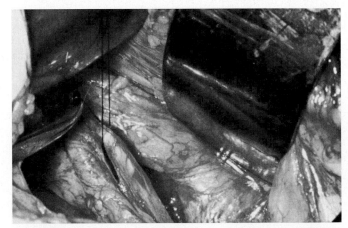

Figure 25-3 Ligation of internal iliac artery. Double loop is being directed toward bifurcation of common iliac artery. (From Breen JL, Gregori CA, Kindzierski JA: Hemorrhage in gynecologic surgery. In Shaefer G, Graber EA [eds]: Complications in Obstetric and Gynecologic Surgery. Hagerstown, physician, Harper & Row, 1981.)

adapt this technique for use in any operating room. The major complication of rapid autologous transfusion is a 10% hemolysis rate. The risks of air embolism or infusion of particulate matter are minimal. Obviously, autologous blood does not contain platelets or clotting factors, so platelets and fresh-frozen plasma will have to be given concurrently for severe hemorrhage. Rapid autologous transfusion is contraindicated in advanced pelvic infection or malignancy.

In many cases, angiographic embolization instead of exploratory laparotomy is preferable (**Fig. 25-4**). Introduction of digital road mapping technology has improved the rapid identification of bleeding vessels. Similarly, treatment of recurrent postoperative hemorrhage or hemorrhage late in the postoperative course (7 to 14 days) may be performed with angiographic arterial embolization. Absorbable gelatin sponges, which produce vascular occlusion for 10 to 30 days, or metal coils with Dacron fibers, which produce permanent occlusion, may be used.

HEMATOMAS

This section will describe the management of wounds or pelvic hematomas that develop slowly and are diagnosed after the first postoperative day. Proper management of postoperative hematomas is one of the most challenging and controversial subjects in operative gynecology. The incidence of hematomas is inversely related to the extent to which meticulous hemostasis is obtained intraoperatively. Women who are given low-dose heparin or who take aspirin chronically are at a slightly higher risk of hematoma formation. Hematomas result from intermittent or slow, continuous venous bleeding and are almost always self-limiting. Eventually, the pressure of the expanding hematoma will exceed the venous pressure and a stable clot will form.

The extent of the hematoma is determined partially by the potential size of the compartment into which the bleeding occurs. Retroperitoneal or broad ligament hematomas may contain several units of blood. The diagnosis of a wound or pelvic hematoma is usually suspected on the morning of the third postoperative day when the laboratory reports an unexpectedly low hematocrit. The woman may have mild to moderate tenderness over the affected area. By the fifth postoperative day, the hematoma liquefies and is easier to outline during bimanual examination. Distinguishing between an uninfected hematoma and a hematoma that has become secondarily infected is difficult before incision and drainage. Both clinical situations produce tenderness and fever secondary to the inflammation surrounding the hematoma. The diagnosis of most retroperitoneal hematomas may be made by physical examination. Most important is a careful rectovaginal examination. Radiologic imaging studies are indicated when the hematoma cannot be palpated.

Hematomas smaller than 5 cm in diameter may be treated conservatively. Larger hematomas may be drained transcutaneously with CT or ultrasound direction as soon as they liquefy. If not treated, most large hematomas will become secondarily infected, even when the woman is treated with parenteral antibiotics. Effective drainage of most pelvic and broad ligament hematomas usually can be accomplished vaginally or radiographically. Small subcutaneous hematomas or fascial hematomas usually resolve. However, they are associated with an increased incidence of wound infection.

Any operation is accompanied by the potential risk of an unrecognized retained sponge or laparotomy pad. The exact

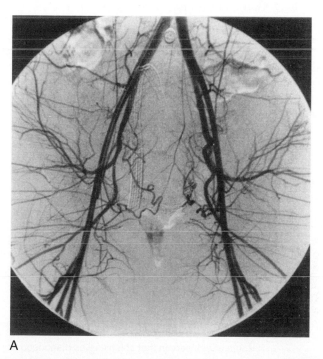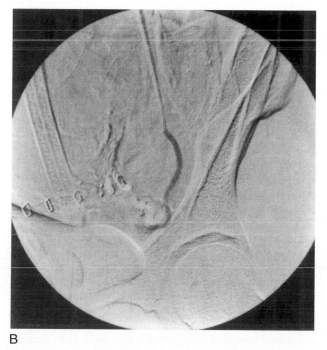

A   B

Figure 25-4 A, Anteroposterior digital subtraction pelvic angiogram in 37-year-old woman with persistent pelvic bleeding after surgical myomectomy for uterine leiomyomas demonstrates contrast pooling (*arrows*) from branches of left uterine artery, consistent with active hemorrhage. **B,** Postembolization left uterine arteriogram shows occluded left uterine artery (*long arrows*) with no evidence of active bleeding. (From Vedantham S, Goodwin SC, McLucas B, Mohr G: Uterine artery embolization: An underused method of controlling pelvic hemorrhage. Am J Obstet Gynecol 176:938, 1997.)

incidence of this worrisome complication is difficult to establish but is estimated to be from 1 in 1200 to 1500 laparotomies. Usually, the sponge counts at surgery have been correct. When this complication is discovered during the first postoperative week, the woman usually has a tender pelvic mass that is infected. When this mass is discovered after the immediate postoperative course, patients are often asymptomatic or exhibit minimal tenderness. The possibility of a retained foreign body should be considered in the differential diagnosis of pelvic hematomas and abscesses. A retrospective study of retained sponges by Gawande and associates has noted that retained foreign bodies are more commonly associated with a higher body mass index (BMI), emergency surgeries, and an intraoperative change in the type of procedure to be performed.

THROMBOPHLEBITIS AND PULMONARY EMBOLUS

Surgery is a time of hypercoagulability secondary to the stress response. As such, the surgeon must be aware of the potential complications of thromboembolism throughout the postoperative course. Prophylaxis against deep vein thrombosis (DVT) is discussed in Chapter 24 (Preoperative Counseling and Management). However, prophylaxis needs to be continued throughout the hospital stay and, in certain high-risk cases, even after discharge. For example, patients with both a malignancy and a thrombophilia, or previous DVT and thrombophilia, and those who will have decreased ambulation may benefit from 1 to 3 weeks of low-molecular-weight (LMW) heparin after leaving the hospital. Studies in patients with hip replacements and with abdominal pelvic malignancies have shown significant reductions (50% to 66%) in the incidence of DVT with prolonged anticoagulation. Currently, there is insufficient evidence to make recommendations for prolonged thromboprophylaxis for gynecology patients, except in high-risk situations. Without specific guidelines, the length of time for thromboprophylaxis should be individualized. Prophylaxis will not prevent all DVTs; thus, part of daily rounds includes assessments for this complication.

Superficial Thrombophlebitis

Superficial thrombophlebitis is one of the most frequently occurring postoperative complications and is most commonly associated with IV catheters. Superficial thrombophlebitis is a benign disease. However, it is associated with deep vein thrombophlebitis in approximately 5% of cases. Superficial thrombophlebitis is frequently overlooked or disregarded as a cause of postoperative fever. Superficial tenderness and erythema outline the course of the veins. Women with established superficial varicosities in the lower extremities are especially susceptible because of localized stasis or pressure during the operative procedure and inactivity during the first 24 hours after operation. Patients with superficial thrombophlebitis of the legs also may have concomitant deep venous disease. Thus, the finding of superficial thrombophlebitis does not eliminate the necessity to consider DVT as well. Recurrent superficial phlebitis, in varying anatomic sites, may be a sign of occult malignant disease. Detailed basic investigations have identified fibrin sheaths surrounding IV catheters in 60% to 100% of patients studied. The exact fate of the several inches of clot and fibrin sheath after the removal of the IV catheter is uncertain. Venography studies have found that these clots and fibrin sheaths do not break up on catheter removal but initially remain in situ. IV catheters are an important source of

nosocomial infections. Approximately 30% of all hospital-acquired bacteremias are secondary to IV lines. The most serious complication of IV catheter use is infection of the thrombus, producing suppurative phlebitis or catheter sepsis.

The natural history of IV catheter-associated phlebitis was documented by Hershey and colleagues. The classic symptom of phlebitis is inflammation of the subcutaneous tissue along the course of a vein or over the area of merging varicosities. The woman develops a painful, tender, erythematous induration (nodule or core). In most severe cases, there is associated fever. The duration of phlebitis is prolonged if the catheter is not immediately removed when the diagnosis of superficial phlebitis is made. I have recommended that all IV catheters be removed and replaced at 48-hour intervals, regardless of whether signs or symptoms of superficial phlebitis are present. In addition, the use of an IV team decreased the incidence of catheter-associated phlebitis from 32% to 15% in one series. Strict aseptic techniques should be used during catheter insertion. Catheters inserted into the hand or forearm, through which antibiotics are infused, should be changed at least every 36 hours. Although not all studies have affirmed that recommendation, most authors have suggested all IV lines be changed every 48 to 72 hours. The longer the catheter is left in place, the greater the risk of catheter related phlebitis (see **Fig. 25-5**). In one study, heparin flushes of IV catheters decreased the risks of phlebitis by an RR of 6 (95% CI, 4 to 8) over saline flushes. Recent series have documented the association of inherited thrombophilias with superficial phlebitis, increasing the risk by 4- to 13-fold. The more potent the thrombophilia, the higher the risk.

In summary, venous catheters should be removed at the first sign of induration, erythema, or edema. Superficial phlebitis is the leading cause of an enigmatic postoperative fever during the third, fourth, or fifth postoperative day.

The clinical management of mild superficial thrombophlebitis includes rest, elevation, and local heat. Moderate to severe superficial thrombophlebitis may be treated with a nonsteroidal anti-inflammatory drug (NSAID) such as ibuprofen or low-dose heparin. The rare case of proximal progression of the inflammatory process should be treated with therapeutic doses of IV heparin and antibiotics.

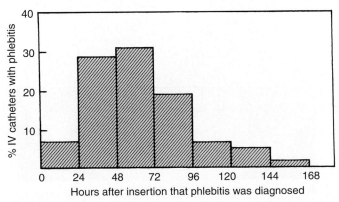

Figure 25-5 Intravenous catheters and development of infection. Phlebitis was diagnosed hours after insertion of catheter. (From Hershey CO, Tomford JW, Mclaren CE, et al: The natural history of intravenous catheter-associated phlebitis. Arch Intern Med 144:1374, 1984.)

Deep Vein Thrombophlebitis

Thromboembolic complications generally occur early in the postoperative course, 50% within the first 24 hours and 75% within 72 hours. Approximately 15% occur after the seventh postoperative day. Diagnosis of deep vein thrombophlebitis by physical examination is insensitive. Thus, imaging studies are essential for establishing the correct diagnosis. Venous thrombosis and PE are the direct causes of approximately 40% of deaths in gynecologic cases. The incidence of fatal pulmonary emboli following gynecologic operations is approximately 0.2%. Because women often die within a few hours of the appearance of initial symptoms, emphasis must be placed on prevention rather than treatment of this complication. PE is not the only major consequence of deep venous thrombophlebitis. Many women develop chronic venous insufficiency or postphlebitic syndrome of the legs as a major sequela following thrombophlebitis. The resulting damage to valves of the deep veins produces shunting of blood to superficial veins, chronic edema, pain on exercise, and skin ulceration.

The reported incidence of DVT with gynecologic operations without prophylaxis varies from 7% to 45%, with an average of approximately 15%. Walsh and associates have found the incidence of DVT to be 7% after vaginal hysterectomy, 13% after abdominal hysterectomy for benign disease, 25% after a Wertheim hysterectomy, and 45% after extensive gynecologic cancer surgery. The incidence of thrombophlebitis is directly dependent on risk factors such as the type and duration of operation, age of the woman, thrombophilias, history of deep vein thrombophlebitis, peripheral edema, amount of blood lost at operation, restrictions in preoperative ambulation, obesity, immobility, malignancy, sepsis, diabetes, current oral contraceptive or hormone use, and conditions that produce venous stasis, such as ascites and heart failure (**Table 25-3**). Older and obese women have an increased incidence of thrombophlebitis because of dilation of their deep venous system. There is a two- to fourfold increased risk for venous thrombophlebitis in women taking postmenopausal estrogen therapy. The length of the surgical procedure also has an important influence on the development of thrombophlebitis. If the operation is 1 to 2 hours in duration, approximately 15% of women develop the disease; if the surgery is longer than 3 hours, the risk is greater (**Table 25-4**).

Table 25-3 Conditions Associated with Increased Risk for Deep Vein Thrombosis

Active cancer
Acute medical illness (e.g., acute myocardial infarction, heart failure, respiratory failure, infection)
Advancing age
Antiphospholipid syndrome
Behçet's syndrome
Central venous catheter
Chronic care facility stay
Congenital venous malformation
Dyslipoproteinemia
Heparin-induced thrombocytopenia
Hormone replacement therapy
Immobilization
Inflammatory bowel disease
Intravenous drug abuse
Limb paresis
Long-distance travel
Myeloproliferative diseases
Nephrotic syndrome
Obesity
Oral contraceptives
Other drugs
   Antipsychotics
   Chemotherapeutic agents
   Tamoxifen
   Thalidomide
Paroxysmal nocturnal hemoglobinuria
Pregnancy, puerperium
Previous venous thromboembolism
Prolonged bed rest
Superficial vein thrombosis
Surgery
Trauma
Varicose veins
Vena cava filter

From Kyrle PA, Eichinger S: Deep vein thrombosis. Lancet 365:1164, 2005.

Table 25-4 Risk Categories of Thromboembolism in Gynecologic Operations

Risk Category	Risk Level		
	Low	Medium	High
Age (yr)	40	40	50
Contributing factors			
Operation	Uncomplicated or minor	Major abdominal or pelvic	Major, extensive
Weight		Moderately obese—75 to 90 kg or >20% above ideal weight	Morbidly obese—>115 kg or >30% above ideal weight
			Previous venous thrombosis
			Varicose veins
			Cardiac disease
			Diabetes (insulin-dependent)
Calf vein thrombosis (%)	2	10-35	30-60
Iliofemoral vein thrombosis (%)	0.4	2-8	5-10
Fatal pulmonary emboli (%)	0.2	0.1-0.5	1
Recommended prophylaxis	Early ambulation	Low-dose heparin or intermittent pneumatic compression	Low-dose heparin or intermittent pneumatic compression

From Mattingly RF, Thompson JD (eds): Te Linde's Operative Gynecology, 6th ed. Philadelphia, JB Lippincott, 1985.

The process of thrombosis most often begins in the deep veins of the calf. It is estimated that 75% of pulmonary emboli originate from a thrombus that began in the leg veins. If one leg is involved, the other leg has thrombophlebitis in approximately 33% of women. Usually, the thrombophlebitis remains localized, the clot lyses spontaneously, and the woman is free of symptoms. In approximately 1 in 20 cases the process extends centrally to the veins of the upper leg and pelvis. Involvement of the femoral vein often results in swelling caused by obstruction of this large vein. Pulmonary emboli from calf veins alone are rare, with only 4% to 10% of pulmonary emboli originating from this area. In contrast, there is a 50% risk of a PE if thrombophlebitis of the femoral vein is not treated.

In 1854, Virchow described the three key predisposing or precipitating factors in the production of thrombi: an increase in coagulation factors, damage to the vessel wall, and venous stasis. Subsequent studies have documented that all three events occur with gynecologic operations. Blood flow in the iliac vein decreases by approximately 55% during an operation. During an operation, there are several normal physiologic changes that produce hypercoagulability, including increases in factors VIII, IX, and X, number of platelets, platelet aggregation and adherence, fibrinogen, and lastly, thromboplastin-like substance from tissue necrosis.

Kakkar has described the cascade of events leading to the development of thrombophlebitis. The initial event in the cascade is stasis. Stasis leads to localized anoxia with subsequent generation of thrombi at the anoxic site. This produces changes in the lining of the vessel, with exposure of the basement membrane, platelet adhesion, and local coagulation. Thus, the most important event in thrombophlebitis is the generation of thrombi in the presence of venous stasis. A thrombus may generate in an area of stasis or it may generate wherever a vessel wall is damaged, with resultant exposure of the subendothelial collagen, to which platelets will adhere.

The site of initial formation of the thrombus is most often near the base of a valve cusp in the calf of the leg (**Fig. 25-6**). The thrombus propagates and grows by repetitive layers of platelet aggregation and deposition of fibrin from fibrinogen. The most recently formed portion of the propagating thrombi are free-floating (not attached to the vein) and are most likely to become pulmonary emboli. The body attempts to repair the area of thrombosis through an invasion of fibroblasts from the vein wall to encompass the base of the thrombus. Eventually, the thrombus is attached to the vein wall, the area is reepithelialized, organization occurs, and symptoms resolve.

The signs and symptoms of deep vein thrombophlebitis depend directly on the severity and extent of the process. Many localized cases of deep vein thrombophlebitis in the calf are asymptomatic and are only recognized by a screening procedure such as duplex ultrasonography. However, even extensive areas of deep vein thrombophlebitis may be asymptomatic; the first sign may be the development of a PE. In a woman who is asymptomatic, the pathophysiologic process may not totally obstruct the individual vein and drainage is obtained via associated competent collateral circulation.

Studies using ^{125}I-labeled fibrinogen to screen the legs have documented that approximately one of two women who develop deep vein thrombophlebitis following gynecologic surgery is totally free of symptoms. Among women who develop signs and symptoms, approximately 68% have induration of the calf

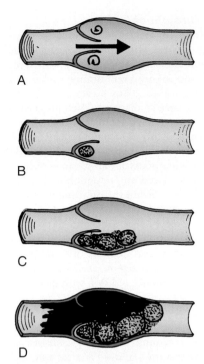

Figure 25-6 Stages in development of thrombus in valve pocket of deep veins of leg. **A**, Stasis in valve pocket results in thrombin generation. **B**, Platelet aggregation and fibrin formation. **C**, Propagation of platelet-fibrin nidus. **D**, Blockage of venous flow with resultant retrograde extension. (From Bloom AL, Thomas DP [eds]: Haemostases and Thrombosis. Edinburgh, Churchill Livingstone, 1981, p 684.)

muscles, 52% have minimum edema, 25% have calf tenderness, and 11% develop a difference of more than 1 cm in diameter of the leg. **Homans' sign** is present in 10% and differential pain over the calf with a blood pressure cuff is present in approximately 40%. The clinical diagnosis of iliofemoral thrombosis is much easier—the woman usually develops severe symptoms caused by obstruction of venous return. Usually, there is an acute onset of severe pain, swelling, and a sensation that the leg will burst.

The clinician must maintain a high degree of suspicion to begin the diagnostic workup for deep vein thrombophlebitis. The clinical symptoms and signs of DVT are nonspecific. A clinical clue is the persistence of a low-grade fever with unexplained tachycardia. The tachycardia is often more rapid than one would expect with a low-grade fever. The finding of a definite difference in leg circumference is supportive evidence of DVT. Physical examination of the legs produces false-positive findings in approximately 50% of cases. At the time of the initial bedside examination, the physician will develop a level of suspicion for DVT based on physical findings and clinical characteristics. If the likelihood is low, the next step would, in nonsurgical patients, be a D-dimer level; however in the postoperative patient, D-dimer is not reliable. D-Dimer is a protein from cross-linked fibrin after it has been degraded by plasmin in the fibrinolytic process. Thus, D-dimer may be elevated because of trauma, surgery, intravascular hemolysis, pregnancy, and other inflammatory states. If the signs and symptoms are suggestive, or the woman is at high risk, the next step should be imaging. Interestingly, the more symptomatic the disease, the more adherent the thrombus. The greater the symptoms, the less likely the development of a PE.

Ascending contrast venography (phlebography) is the most accurate method for detecting deep vein thrombophlebitis, but is rarely if ever used. **Duplex ultrasound**, the combination of Doppler and real-time B-mode ultrasound, and color Doppler are the preferred methods for diagnosing deep vein thrombophlebitis. The diagnostic accuracy of venography is more than 95% for peripheral disease and more than 90% for iliofemoral thrombophlebitis. Contrast venography is more expensive, painful, and time-consuming. Duplex ultrasonography has remarkably high sensitivity and specificity in symptomatic women. Real-time ultrasound imaging provides visualization of the larger veins and sensitive Doppler ultrasound is focused simultaneously on the suspicious vessel. The technology depends on changes in venous flow for a positive diagnosis. A meta-analysis from White and coworkers has documented that the sensitivity of duplex ultrasonography in detecting proximal thrombi is 95% (95% CI, 92% to 98%) and the specificity is 99% (95% CI, 98% to 100%). The advantages of this method are that it is noninvasive, easy to use, highly accurate, objective, simple, and reproducible. Color Doppler ultrasonography may improve the diagnostic accuracy in larger veins. The main disadvantage of duplex ultrasound is its limited accuracy when investigating small vessels in the calf. The inability to compress the deep vein by moderate pressure with the ultrasound probe is the most widely used criterion for the positive diagnosis of DVT.

Lensing and colleagues, in a prospective study of 220 patients, used compressibility of the vein as the sole criterion for diagnosis of DVT. For all patients in their study, including both proximal vein and calf vein thrombosis, the sensitivity was 91% and the specificity was 99%.

The objectives of the clinical management of deep vein thrombophlebitis associated with gynecologic surgery are early detection and early therapy. In reality, antithrombotic therapy is preventive medicine, because the therapeutic agent interrupts progression of the disease (thrombus formation) but does not actively resolve the disease process. Anticoagulation with heparin (unfractionated or LMW heparin) is the treatment of choice for the initial diagnosis of DVT (**Table 25-5**). LMW heparin is as effective and is safer than unfractionated heparin. LMW heparin, although more expensive than unfractionated heparin, has several advantages and has effectively replaced unfractionated heparin as the gold standard for treatment of DVT. LMW heparin may be given subcutaneously once or twice daily. It does not require monitoring in women with normal and stable renal function. It induces significantly less heparin-induced thrombocytopenia and has a lower risk of inducing bleeding. Because blood levels are more reproducible, there is actually a lower incidence of complications noted in some studies in terms of progression from DVT to pulmonary emboli. Additionally, studies comparing LMW heparin with unfractionated heparin have shown a greater effect with thrombus regression within the veins themselves. Testing of levels of LMW heparin is based not on the activated partial thromboplastin time (aPTT), but on the antifactor Xa activity level. Levels are calculated specifically for each LMW heparin. An aPTT of 1.5 times normal corresponds approximately to an antifactor Xa activity level of 0.2. Therapeutic levels are found between 0.4 and 0.8. Bleeding usually occurs when levels of the antifactor Xa activity level rise more than 1.0 to 1.2. If needed in patients with unstable renal status, levels may be checked approximately 4 hours after dosing.

If unfractionated heparin is desired as an IV infusion, the initial loading dose is 5,000 to 10,000 IU, followed by a continuous infusion of 1000 to 1500 IU/hr. The dosage of unfractionated IV heparin should be adjusted to prolong an aPTT to 2.5 times control values. Continuous heparin infusion is preferred over periodic bolus injections because there are fewer hemorrhagic complications (6% versus 14%). The average half-life of heparin is 1 to 2 hours after IV injection. Failure to achieve adequate anticoagulation in the first 24 hours of therapy increases the risk of recurrent venous thromboembolism 15-fold. Heparin should be continued for 5 to 7 days. Oral warfarin (Coumadin), 15 mg daily, should be initiated within the first 48 hours of heparin therapy. Following 2 to 3 days of 10 to 15 mg of warfarin daily, the international normalized ratio

Table 25-5 Options for Initial Anticoagulant Treatment of Deep Vein Thrombosis

| Drug | Method of Administration | Dosage* | Reported Risks (no./total no. [%]) | |
			Heparin-Induced Thrombocytopenia†	Major Bleeding
Unfractionated heparin	IV	Loading dose, 5000 U or 80 U/kg of body weight with infusion adjusted to maintain aPTT within therapeutic range	9/332 (2.7)	35/1853 (1.9)
LMW heparin			0/333 (0)	20/1821 (1.1)
Dalteparin	Subcutaneous	100 U/kg every 12 hr or 200 U/kg daily; maximum, 18,000 U/day		
Enoxaparin	Subcutaneous	1 mg/kg every 12 hr or 1.5 mg/kg daily; maximum, 180 mg/day		
Tinzaparin	Subcutaneous	175 U/kg daily; maximum, 18,000 U/day		
Nadroparin	Subcutaneous	86 U/kg every 12 hr or 171 U/kg daily; maximum, 17,100 U/day		

*Doses vary in patients who are obese or who have renal dysfunction. Monitoring of antifactor Xa levels has been suggested for these patients, with dose adjustment to a target range of 0.6-1.0 U/mL 4 hr after injection for twice-daily administration or 1.0-2.0 U/mL for once-daily administration. Even though there are few supporting data, most manufacturers recommend capping the dose for obese patients at that for a 90-kg patient.

†The therapeutic range of activated partial thromboplastin time corresponds to heparin levels of 0.3-0.7 U/mL, as determined by antifactor Xa assay. High levels of heparin-binding proteins and factor VIII may result in so-called heparin resistance. In patients requiring more than 40,000 U/day to attain a therapeutic aPTT, the dosage can be adjusted on the basis of plasma heparin levels.

From Bates SM, Ginsberg JS: Treatment of deep-vein thrombosis. N Engl J Med 351:271, 2004.

(INR) will usually be 1.5 to 2. This therapeutic level—an INR of 2—should be maintained by appropriate adjustment of the warfarin dosage. The biologic half-life of warfarin is 2 to 3 days. Anticoagulation with warfarin should be continued for 6 to 9 months for adequate secondary prophylaxis. A meta-analysis from Ost and colleagues has evaluated the duration of anticoagulation following venous thromboembolism. Studies of 3 months of therapy were compared with studies of 6 months or longer. The risks of bleeding (the major complication) were similar between short- and long-term therapy. However, the relative risk of recurrent thromboembolism was 0.21 (95% CI, 0.14 to 0.31) comparing long-term with short-term heparin use. Some patients with large DVT, antiphospholipid antibody syndrome, or malignancies may require extended therapy beyond 6 to 9 months because of increased risks of recurrence (**Table 25-6**).

The primary risk of chronic anticoagulation therapy is the potential for major bleeding complications. Major bleeding occurs in approximately 4% woman-years of therapy. Thus, it is important to follow these women carefully with serial coagulation studies. Approximately 1% of patients on full-dose heparin develop thrombocytopenia (platelet count $< 100,000/mm^3$). If thrombocytopenia develops, heparin should be discontinued because of the potential risk of paradoxic thrombosis.

Rarely, patients will not be candidates for anticoagulation. In these patients, inferior vena caval filters may be used to protect against pulmonary emboli. Temporary vena caval filters may be placed with fluoroscopic guidance. In some patients with large DVT and other risk factors, such as compound thrombophilias and malignancy, consideration may be given to both anticoagulation and filter placement.

Many clinicians will obtain laboratory studies to identify thrombophilic states when a DVT occurs. These tests should be obtained with any idiopathic DVT. However, there is less support for the cost-benefit ratio in obtaining this information for a surgically related DVT. If management decisions, including the duration of therapy or the use of estrogens in the future, might be changed, thrombophilia studies should be obtained. Additionally, in a woman with a family history of thrombosis, it would be reasonable to obtain these studies.

There is no evidence that bed rest is helpful for patients with DVT or that immobilization will prevent pulmonary embolism. Patients with confirmed DVT may receive NSAIDs, because coagulation factors will be monitored. Patients should also be prescribed support stockings, which should be worn for several months to 2 years. The use of support stockings decreases the risks of post-thrombotic syndrome. In their systematic review, Segal and associates summarized trials that noted that women who used stockings up to 2 years after DVT had reductions in the incidence of post-thrombotic syndrome of more than 50%.

Pulmonary Embolism

The accurate diagnosis of PE is essential for the prevention of morbidity from lack of treatment or unnecessary anticoagulation therapy. Autopsy studies have documented that pulmonary emboli are undiagnosed clinically in approximately 50% of women who experience this complication. Approximately 10% of women with a PE die within the first hour. The mortality of women with correctly diagnosed and treated pulmonary emboli is 8%, in contrast to approximately 30% if the disease is not treated. Most pulmonary emboli in gynecologic patients originate from thrombi in the pelvic and femoral veins. Predisposing risk factors are found in most women with PE. Anticoagulation therapy is also dangerous, because heparin is one of the leading causes of drug-related deaths in hospitalized patients.

No combination of symptoms or signs is pathognomonic for PE. The signs and symptoms of PE are nonspecific, and similar symptoms are caused by many other forms of cardiorespiratory disease. Many patients with PE will be asymptomatic. Common conditions considered in the differential diagnosis of pulmonary embolism include pneumonia, cardiac failure, atelectasis, aspiration, acute respiratory distress syndrome, and sepsis. Although the differential diagnosis is broad in scope, the symptoms should alert the physician to the possibility of a PE, thus allowing a proper diagnostic workup to establish or rule out the disease. A national study of 327 patients with angiographically proven PE found that chest pain, dyspnea, and apprehension are the most common symptoms. The dyspnea is often of abrupt onset. The classic triad of shortness of breath, chest pain, and hemoptysis is seen in less than 20% of women with proven PE. Tachycardia, tachypnea, rales, and an increase in the second heart sound over the pulmonic area are the most frequently found signs of pulmonary emboli (**Table 25-7**). Approximately 15% of women with pulmonary emboli have an unexplained low-grade fever associated with a PE. A high fever is rarely associated with a PE but definitely may occur. The clinical manifestations of PE are produced primarily by occlusion of the large branches of the pulmonary arteries by embolic material.

Table 25-6 Recommendations for Duration of Anticoagulant Therapy for Patients with Deep Vein Thrombosis

Characteristics of Patient*	Risk of Recurrence in Year after Discontinuation (%)	Duration of Therapy
Major transient risk factor	3	3 mo
Minor risk factor, no thrombophilia	<10 if risk factor avoided	6 mo
	>10 if risk factor persistent	Until factor resolves
Idiopathic event; no thrombophilia or low-risk thrombophilia	<10	6 mo†
Idiopathic event; high-risk thrombophilia	>10	Indefinite
More than one idiopathic event	>10	Indefinite
Cancer; other ongoing risk factor	>10	Indefinite

*Examples of major transient risk factors are major surgery, major medical illness, and leg casting. Examples of minor transient risk factors are the use of an oral contraceptive and hormone replacement therapy. Examples of low-risk thrombophilias are heterozygosity for factor V Leiden and G20210A prothrombin gene mutations. Examples of high-risk thrombophilia are antithrombin, protein C, and protein S deficiencies, homozygosity for factor V Leiden or prothrombin gene mutation or heterozygosity for both, and presence of antiphospholipid antibodies.
†Therapy may be prolonged if the patient prefers to prolong it or if the risk of bleeding is low.
From Bates SM, Ginsberg JS: Treatment of deep-vein thrombosis. N Engl J Med 351:273, 2004.

Table 25-7 Symptoms and Signs of Pulmonary Embolism

Symptoms	Patients with Finding (%)
Predisposing factors*	94
Dyspnea	84
Pleuritic chest pain	74
Apprehension	59
Cough	53
Hemoptysis	30
Syncope	14
Signs	
Tachypnea	92
Rales	58
Accentuation of pulmonic valve closure	53
Tachycardia	44
Cyanosis	20

*Prolonged immobilization, postoperative state, congestive heart failure, carcinomatosis, and so on.
From Blinder RA, Coleman RE: Evaluation of pulmonary embolism. Radiol Clin North Am 23:392, 1985.

Pathophysiologically, associated reflex bronchial constriction and vasoconstriction intensify the symptomatology. More than 50% of clinically recognized pulmonary emboli are multiple. The most frequent location of pulmonary emboli is in the lower lobes of the right lung. Shock and syncope are associated with massive pulmonary emboli.

Although imaging techniques are the gold standard for establishing the diagnosis of pulmonary emboli, several studies have found that clinical assessment is almost as accurate. Chunilal and coworkers have referred to the so-called clinical gestalt and noted a similar accuracy of diagnosis to imaging. Clinical assessment of signs and symptoms by an experienced clinician may approximate a low, medium, and high probability of PE.

Laboratory studies that may help in diagnosis and management include electrocardiograms (ECGs), chest radiographs, blood gas analyses, assessment of troponin, and brain natriuretic peptide (BNP). Less than 15% of ECGs demonstrate significant changes of right ventricular strain, with T wave inversion in V_1 to V_4 with a PE. Most women with pulmonary emboli demonstrate hypoxemia on blood gas determinations but, as with other routine tests, these findings do not occur invariably. Diminished pulmonary vascular markings may be a suggestive finding on a chest film, but are fairly nonspecific. The chest radiograph may be helpful in the differential diagnosis by demonstrating other pulmonary processes. The most common findings on chest film examination with a PE are infiltrate, pleural effusion, atelectasis, and enlargement of the heart or descending pulmonary artery, although these findings are nonspecific. The rapid measurement of plasma D-dimer levels may sometimes be useful for screening women with a suspected PE, but is not reliable in the postoperative patient.

In women who are in mild to moderate distress, IV heparin should be started while imaging studies are being ordered. If there is any question of severe distress or hemodynamic instability, thrombolytic therapy may be indicated. In stable patients, a stepwise approach is useful. Many clinicians will order Doppler studies of the lower extremities. No radiation is involved and the tests are simple. If the Doppler studies are positive, the woman will be anticoagulated and no further workup is necessary. If the tests are negative, further imaging is still necessary, because in the postoperative patient, pelvic clots may be the origin of the pulmonary embolus, not lower extremity clots. The next two options are a $\dot{V}/\dot{Q}$ **scan** or helical CT.

Helical CT increases the risk of breast cancer by a little less than 1%; thus, in a young woman, a $\dot{V}/\dot{Q}$ scan is preferable. Prior to $\dot{V}/\dot{Q}$ scanning, a chest x-ray should be obtained. If the chest x-ray shows other findings, such as atelectasis, the $\dot{V}/\dot{Q}$ scan has a much higher chance of being nondiagnostic and CT should be ordered instead. Helical CT has replaced $\dot{V}/\dot{Q}$ scanning as the most common imaging technique to establish or exclude the diagnosis of PE (**Fig. 25-7**). Helical CT, sometimes called spiral CT, uses imaging of the pulmonary vessels. Imaging of the pulmonary vessels is facilitated by the use of IV contrast media. The procedure is minimally invasive and provides a volumetric image of the lung by rotating the detector at a constant rate around the woman. A cost-effective analysis from Doyle and colleagues has found that helical CT is the most cost-effective first-line test to diagnose pulmonary embolus. In addition to radiation, the other problem with CT is the overdiagnosis of small peripheral emboli, which are probably not of clinical significance.

The alternative to helical CT is $\dot{V}/\dot{Q}$ scanning. This test is safe and relatively easy to perform. The scan involves the injection of small radiocolloid particles into the circulation. They are trapped in small vessels; their distribution depends on regional pulmonary blood flow. Ventilation scintigraphy uses radionuclides of technetium aerosol or xenon gas. The combination of lack of symmetry and a mismatch in the ventilation scan is the abnormality that leads to the diagnosis. However, the clinician should not rely too much on the ability of the $\dot{V}/\dot{Q}$ scan as a single test to diagnose a PE. In patients with a suspected PE, 40% will have a normal scan. A normal result effectively rules out the diagnosis of PE. The multicenter Prospective Investigation of Pulmonary Embolism Diagnosis (PIOPED) found that 4% of patients with normal or near-normal perfusion lung scans subsequently were discovered to have pulmonary emboli. This study emphasized a high sensitivity of 98% but a low specificity of 10% for $\dot{V}/\dot{Q}$ scans in the diagnosis of PE. The authors noted that almost all patients with acute PE had abnormal scans, but so did most patients without emboli. $\dot{V}/\dot{Q}$ scans have a high sensitivity but a variable specificity for the diagnosis of PE. For example, other cardiorespiratory diseases such as asthma may result in regional areas of decreased perfusion. If the scan documents multiple segments or lobar perfusion defects with a ventilation mismatch, the probability of pulmonary emboli is more than 85%. $\dot{V}/\dot{Q}$ scans with less extensive perfusion abnormalities or matching ventilation defects do not reliably exclude the diagnosis of PE.

The management of the vast majority of pulmonary emboli is with anticoagulation with IV unfractionated heparin or full-dose LMW heparin, similar to the management of deep vein thrombophlebitis (**Fig. 25-8**). Prompt and early therapy with heparin provides anticoagulation and inhibits the release of serotonin from platelets. Potentially, this results in a decrease in the associated bronchoconstriction. Some women are candidates for thrombolytic therapy (streptokinase-urokinase). The time window for effective use of thrombolysis is up to 14 days following the initial symptoms or signs of a PE, although it is rarely used beyond 48 to 72 hours. Thrombolytic therapy works by transforming plasminogen to plasmin. Use of thrombolytic therapy during the early postoperative period is a subject of great debate because of the increased risk of serious hemorrhage. Goldhaber and associates completed a randomized controlled study

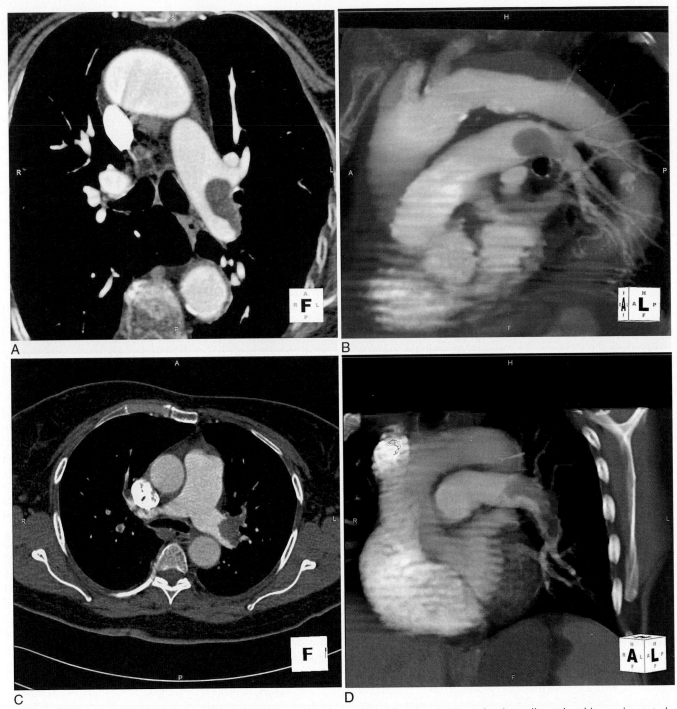

Figure 25-7 Helical CT of pulmonary embolism. The letters on the cube help orient the viewer as the three-dimensional image is rotated. A, Anterior; F, foot; H, head; L, left. (Courtesy of Dr. Charles McGlade, Sacred Heart Medical Center, Eugene, OR.)

comparing urokinase and recombinant human tissue-type plasminogen activator. The latter was found to act more rapidly and to be safer than urokinase. Thrombolytic therapy is the method of choice in patients with massive pulmonary emboli (angiographically, >50% obstruction of the pulmonary arterial bed) with associated moderate to severe hemodynamic embarrassment, lobular obstruction, or multiple segmental profusion defects. Random trials of heparin versus thrombolytic therapy have shown that emboli clear more rapidly with initial thrombolytic therapy.

The MAPPET-3 trial (Management Strategies and Prognosis of Pulmonary Embolus-3) found that in severely affected patients (but not those in shock), thrombolytic therapy was superior to heparin. However, for all patients, particularly those with small emboli, the increased risks of intracranial bleeding may outweigh the benefits (1% to 3% of patients). Trials have evaluated thrombolytic therapy with heparin and found the combination superior to heparin alone. A thrombolytic agent is infused IV for the first 12 to 24 hours and heparin therapy is continued for 7 to 10 days. The clinical assumption is that approximately

Figure 25-8 Algorithm for treatment of pulmonary embolism. (From Taj MR, Atwal AS, Hamilton G: Modern management of pulmonary embolism. Br J Surg 86:853, 1999.)

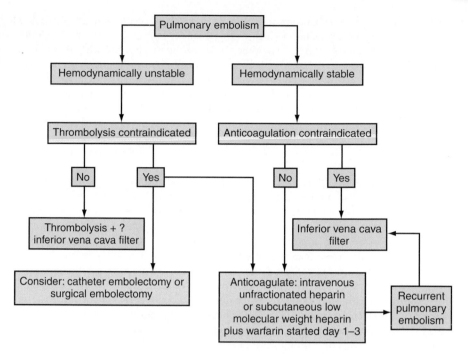

7 days are needed for the intravascular venous thrombus to become firmly attached to the vein's side wall. In patients who have heparin allergies, or develop heparin-induced thrombocytopenia (HIT), thrombin inhibitors are an alternative therapy.

An adjunct for treatment is vena caval filters. The most widely accepted indication for vena cava filters is failure of medical management or a contraindication to heparin therapy. Approximately 35% of vena cava filters are placed for prophylactic indications. A randomized trial reported by Decousos and co-workers compared vena cava filters with LMW or unfractionated heparin. They concluded that the initial beneficial effect of vena cava filters for the prevention of PE is counterbalanced by an excess of recurrent DVT, without any difference in mortality rates. Treatment of a massive PE in an unstable woman involves a choice of thrombolytic therapy, pulmonary artery embolectomy, transvenous catheter embolectomy, or filter placement in the inferior vena cava.

All patients with pulmonary emboli should have warfarin therapy after heparin treatment for 3 to 9 months. The risk of a woman developing a subsequent fatal PE during the 3 months of anticoagulation therapy is approximately 1 in 70 to 100. Trials from Canada and from Sweden have found better long-term survival with extended anticoagulation, 18 months to 2 years. Some authors believe that if there are additional risk factors, such as very potent thrombophilias, indefinite anticoagulation is indicated.

URINARY TRACT PROBLEMS

INABILITY TO VOID

Many women experience an inability to void or an incomplete emptying of the bladder during the postoperative period. The cause is complex, but the inability to void is more frequent and lasts longer after an operation that involves the urethra or bladder neck. The major pathophysiologic change is the direct trauma and edema produced by the surgical procedure to the perivesical tissues. Other factors that contribute include the potential of overdistention from excessive hydration and dyssynchronous contractions from the bladder neck. The differential diagnosis includes anxiety, mechanical interference, obstruction by swelling and edema, neurologic imbalance, and drug-associated detrusor hypotonia.

The woman's initial attempts at voiding should be made in a sitting position. Obviously, privacy is important to minimize performance anxiety. It is best not to remove the Foley catheter until the woman is ambulatory. Most women have difficulty in emptying their bladder completely on a bedpan or in a semirecumbent position during the first 24 hours after abdominal hysterectomy. Catheter drainage keeps the bladder at rest and avoids acute bladder distention with resulting detrusor dysfunction and possibly retrograde reflux of urine. The age-old tradition of intermittent clamping and releasing of the Foley catheter to regain bladder tone is counterproductive and is not based on sound physiologic principles.

Most problems with voiding resolve without medication and with time. If mechanical obstruction is not suspected to be a major factor, intermittent straight catheterization is indicated. This will result in a lower incidence of UTI and a more rapid return to normal function than periodic replacement and removal of a Foley catheter for the evaluation of residual urine volume. Although bacteriuria occurs secondary to intermittent catheterization, development of pyelonephritis is rare unless the woman has concomitant vesicoureteral reflux. Bacteriuria may occur more frequently with indwelling catheters. Most women prefer self-catheterization. They especially appreciate intermittent self-catheterization because it gives them control over part of their postoperative care. Routine culture of the urine with removal of a catheter in an asymptomatic woman is not necessary. Rarely, medications may be given to patients who experience prolonged periods of inability to void. Reflex urethral spasm is common after plastic surgery to repair an enterocele or rectocele. Urethral spasm may be diminished by an α-adrenergic receptor blocking agent such as phenoxybenzamine (Dibenzyline). However, hypotension may be associated with this drug. Bladder hypotonia may occur as a result of overdistention, prolonged inactivity, or use of medications such as beta blockers. Bladder hypotonia may be treated with bethanechol (Urecholine), 25 to 50 mg every 8 hours. Urecholine effectively produces detrusor contractions. However, this is rarely prescribed in the postoperative setting.

INFECTION

The most commonly acquired infection in the hospital and the most frequent cause of gram-negative bacteremia in hospitalized patients is catheter-associated UTI. Approximately 40% of nosocomial infections are UTIs, and 60% of these are directly related to an indwelling urethral catheter. Of patients with infections from bladder catheters, 1% will develop bacteremia. However, patients without catheters may develop overdistention and bladder atony as a result of postoperative pain. Overdistention produces a temporary paralysis of the detrusor activity that may take several days to resolve. The atonic bladder is also prone to UTI. Thus, after a gynecologic operation, the woman is susceptible to UTI, with or without a catheter in place.

The normal uroepithelium inhibits adherence of surface bacteria to the walls of the urethra and bladder. A bladder catheter disrupts this property and surface bacteria are able to colonize the lower urinary tract. Additionally, bacteria form a sheet or **biofilm** of microorganisms and bacterial bioproducts that adheres to the catheter. These biofilms protect bacteria from antibiotics. This characteristic of biofilms explains why antibiotic suppression is ineffective for patients with chronic catheterization and why replacement of a catheter is necessary in the treatment of systemic infection secondary to a colonized urinary tract. The incidence of a positive culture increases dramatically with time. After a Foley catheter has been in place for 36 hours, approximately 20% of women have bacterial colonization and, after 72 hours, more than 75% have positive cultures. If the catheter drains into an open system for longer than 96 hours, 100% develop bacteriuria. Women with an indwelling catheter in place with a closed drainage system develop UTIs at the rate of approximately 5%/24 hours; this increases to 50% of women after 7 days of continuous catheterization.

Catheter-related UTIs are related to the patient's age. In one study, 30% of women older than 50 years developed an infection, compared with 16% of postoperative women younger than age 50. Diabetes increased the incidence of catheter-related UTIs threefold. The incidence of infection is directly related to how long the catheter is in place. The incidence of a positive urine culture after a single in-and-out catheterization is approximately 1%.

Sterile technique used during insertion, strict aseptic catheter care, and maintenance of a closed drainage system are all important steps for reducing the incidence of infection through reduced colonization. Bacteria ascend from the exterior to the bladder via the lumen of the catheter or around the outside of the catheter. A meta-analysis by Saint and colleagues has noted that silver alloy–coated urinary catheters are significantly more effective in preventing UTIs than silver oxide catheters. The silver alloy–coated catheters are more expensive than standard Foley catheters. However, they reduce nosocomial UTIs by approximately 50%. A sterile, closed drainage system is another prophylactic measure to reduce the incidence of UTIs. In one study,

strict closed drainage reduced the rate of infection from 80% to 23%. Studies have documented a lower risk of infection with a suprapubic, transabdominal urinary catheter. The latter technique also decreases patient discomfort and permits earlier spontaneous voiding. Systemic prophylactic antibiotics exert a short-term effect, decreasing the initial incidence of infection. However, the negative effect of prophylactic antibiotics has been an increased emergence of antibiotic-resistant bacteria. Therefore, prophylactic antibiotics are not used to cover a catheter, except in immunocompromised patients. With catheterization for longer than 3 weeks, all patients have bacterial colonization, regardless of the use of prophylactic antibiotics and a closed system.

The symptoms of UTI usually develop 24 to 48 hours after the Foley catheter is removed. Of interest, the signs and symptoms associated with a catheter-acquired lower UTI are not nearly as pronounced or as specific as those associated with cystitis unrelated to catheter use. Patients with lower UTIs usually do not have fever but experience urinary frequency and mild dysuria, which are difficult to distinguish from normal postoperative discomfort. As noted, older women may manifest mental status changes as the first sign of problems. Women with upper UTIs usually have a high fever, chills, and flank pain. If urinary tract symptoms persist after appropriate antibiotic therapy, one should obtain imaging studies to evaluate the possibility of obstruction in the urinary tract. Obstruction of the ureter without associated infection may be asymptomatic or produce only mild flank tenderness. No appreciable change will be noted in urinary output with an isolated unilateral ureteral obstruction.

The diagnosis of UTI is established by urinalysis and urine culture. Women with high-volume urine outputs may demonstrate minimal findings on urinalysis but have a positive urine culture. Stark and Maki have emphasized that a bacterial concentration of 10^2 organisms/mL in a catheterized specimen is significant. In their studies, more than 95% of patients with 10^2 colony-forming units (CFU)/mL subsequently developed the standard criterion of infection, which is 100,000 CFU/mL for a midstream culture.

A minimum of 3 days of antibiotic therapy for a woman who has developed cystitis after catheter use is the recommended treatment. One-day, single-dose antibiotic treatment is not an effective treatment for UTI.

To reduce the incidence of UTI, the Foley catheter should be used judiciously. When possible, use of a suprapubic catheter or intermittent in-and-out catheterization is preferable to continuous drainage with a Foley catheter. If a Foley catheter is used, retrograde flow of urine from the bag to the bladder during ambulation should be avoided. Preventive measures, such as aseptic care of the catheter and a closed, sterile drainage system, are also important. It is not necessary to treat catheter-associated urinary tract colonization unless the patient becomes febrile (develops infection). If signs and symptoms of infection occur with a Foley in place, the woman should be treated with systemic antibiotic therapy for 10 days. Prophylactic antibiotics are not used unless the patient is immunosuppressed, because they often result in a UTI with a *Proteus* or *Pseudomonas* sp. rather than the more common *Escherichia coli.*

URETERAL INJURY AND URINARY FISTULA

Vesicovaginal and ureterovaginal fistulas are infrequent yet significant complications of operations for benign gynecologic conditions. In the United States, gynecologic operations are found to be the cause of approximately 75% of urinary tract fistulas. Surprisingly, it is not the difficult cancer operation but rather the simple total abdominal hysterectomy for benign disease, such as myomas or abnormal bleeding, that is most frequently associated with this complication. Fistulas following gynecologic surgery are secondary to abdominal hysterectomy in 75% of cases and to vaginal surgery in the remaining 25%. The exact incidence of injury to the ureter associated with gynecologic surgery is unknown because many patients do not exhibit symptoms. However, it has been estimated that ureteral injury occurs as frequently as 1/200 abdominal hysterectomies. The ratio of injuries to the urinary bladder to ureteral injuries in nonlaparascopic surgeries is approximately between 3:1 and 5:1. Ibeanu and associates have performed concomitant cystoscopy on 839 women undergoing hysterectomies for benign disease (few laparoscopic procedures). They noted that 2.9% of patients had bladder injuries and 1.8% had ureteral injuries. Other studies have reported similar results. The site of ureteral injury is usually near the uterine artery. Injuries may include transection, close sutures that constrict or devascularize the ureter, and thermal injuries from cautery. Stanhope and coworkers have noted a mean increase of only 0.8 mg/dL in the serum creatinine level following unilateral ureteral obstruction secondary to gynecologic surgery.

The classic clinical symptom of a urinary tract fistula is the painless and almost continuous loss of urine, usually from the vagina. On occasion, the uncontrolled loss of urine may be related to change in position or posture. When urine loss is intermittent and related to position, one should suspect a ureterovaginal rather than a vesicovaginal fistula. Urinary incontinence that presents within a few hours of the operative procedure is usually secondary to a direct surgical injury to the bladder or ureter that was not appreciated during the surgery. Most fistulas become symptomatic in 8 to 12 days and occasionally as late as 25 to 30 days after the operation. Damage to the blood supply from clamping, cautery, or figure-of-eight sutures produces avascular necrosis and subsequent sloughing of the urogenital tissue. Pelvic examination often reveals a small reddened area of granulation tissue at the site of the fistula.

A small fistula may be clinically identified by placing a tampon in the vagina and instilling a dilute solution of methylene blue dye into the urinary bladder. This will also help differentiate between a vesicovaginal fistula and ureterovaginal fistula. If the blue coloring is discovered on the tampon, the defect is most likely in the bladder. If the tampon is not colored, 3 to 5 mL of indigo carmine should be injected IV. The subsequent finding of blue coloring on the tampon is presumptive evidence of an ureterovaginal fistula. An IV pyelogram or enhanced CT scan should be obtained in either case to detect obstruction of the ureter and diagnose compound (ureter and bladder) fistulas.

As with most other postoperative complications, preventive medicine is paramount. Optimum operative technique should emphasize the standard axioms in the prevention of urinary tract injury. The woman should have an empty bladder and the physician should obtain adequate exposure of the site. Sharp dissection should be made along tissue planes with proper traction and countertraction. When operating near the bladder or ureter, bleeding vessels should be ligated individually rather than with random clamping of tissue. If possible, the ureter should not be completely detached from the overlying peritoneum. With extensive dissection of the periureteral tissue, care should be taken to avoid interference with the longitudinal vascular supply of the ureter. In the most difficult cases, in which anatomic landmarks are obscure, opening of the dome of the bladder and palpation with the index finger and thumb may help identify the proper surgical plane. The urinary system, especially the bladder, is very forgiving if given a short period of rest to recover. If trauma to the bladder is suspected, continuous catheter drainage for 3 to 5 days usually results in spontaneous healing. Selective cystoscopy following complicated or difficult operative procedures—when the gynecologist wonders whether the integrity of the lower urinary tract has been compromised—should be a strong consideration.

When leakage from the urinary tract is first discovered, the bladder should be drained with a large-bore Foley catheter. Ureteral injuries should be treated with retrograde ureteral catheters. Approximately 20% of bladder injuries and 30% of ureteral injuries that are drained and stented will heal spontaneously without further surgery. Ureteral injuries that occur secondary to cauterization or coagulation may present several days to a few weeks after surgery. Symptoms may vary from pain, bloating, ileus, leukocytosis, and urinary ascites. Serum creatinine levels may be normal or elevated with intra-abdominal leaking of urine. If levels are elevated in the presence of fever or ileus, imaging studies should be considered. With the increase in laparoscopic and robotic surgery, the incidence of thermal injury to the urinary tract has significantly increased. A recent report from Harmanli and coworkers has noted a fourfold increase in urinary injury in laparoscopic hysterectomies compared with supracervical cases. Many injuries go unrecognized at the time, resulting in readmission. In cases in which the injury is seen at or around the time of surgery, splinting of the urinary tract facilitates healing of the defect before epithelialization of the aberrant tract occurs. Spontaneous healing usually occurs within the first 4 weeks. With a ureteral fistula, follow-up imaging should be ordered at 3, 6, and 12 months to detect delayed ureteral strictures.

Operative repair of a vesicovaginal fistula is usually accomplished via a multilayered closure performed by the vaginal route. The principles for a successful operation include the following: adequate exposure, dissection, and mobilization of each tissue layer; excision of the fistulous tract; closure of each layer without tension on the suture line; and excellent hemostasis with closure of the dead space. Reliable bladder drainage is provided to avoid tension on the suture line for approximately 10 days. The Latzko operation is the simplest means of repairing a fistula at the vaginal apex. This technique of partial colpocleisis involves denudation of the vaginal mucosa surrounding the fistula and subsequent multilayer closure, without entering the bladder. The primary disadvantage of the procedure is postoperative shortening of the vagina.

Many ureteral injuries discovered during the immediate postoperative period will heal when treated by percutaneous nephrostomy and ureteral catheters. Ureterovaginal fistulas that do not heal spontaneously are usually repaired 2 to 3 months after the original operation. Most persistent ureterovaginal fistulas involving the lower third of the ureter are repaired by reimplanting the ureter into the bladder.

GASTROINTESTINAL COMPLICATIONS

POSTOPERATIVE DIET

Most patients may be put on a regular diet as soon as tolerated. This section discusses nausea and postoperative gastrointestinal (GI) complications. Relevant to postoperative nutrition is glucose control. Part of the physiologic stress response to surgery is a drive for gluconeogenesis. This process is enhanced by a hormonally mediated insulin resistance. The resultant hyperglycemia is advantageous in the teleologic sense of the fight-or-flight response, but is detrimental for wound healing, cardiovascular function, and inflammatory processes. Several studies have correlated clinical outcomes with glucose levels. The American Association of Endocrinology has noted an 18-fold increase in hospital mortality in general medicine and general surgery patients with glucose levels above 200 mg/dL.

Glucose control begins preoperatively and is discussed in detail in Chapter 24 (Preoperative Counseling and Management). Women who are given insulin infusions during surgery, should have their infusions continued until they are taking regular meals. At this point, they may be given subcutaneous insulin, if necessary. Metformin (Glucophage) should not be used in the perioperative setting because of the potential risks of metabolic acidosis associated with this agent. In women with a history of insulin resistance, women who are morbidly obese, and those older than 60 years, glucose levels should be checked at the bedside every 4 to 6 hours during the first postoperative day. If a woman's glucose rises above 160 to 180 mg/dL, she should be treated.

American Diabetic Association recommendations suggest that critically ill patients have better outcomes with tighter glucose control—fasting levels less than 110 mg/dL and postprandial levels less than 140 mg/dL. Non–critically ill patients should have fasting levels less than 120 mg/dL and postprandial levels less than 180 mg/dL. However, a recent large study of 6100 critically ill patients (NICE-SUGAR) has suggested that tight control of 80- to 108-mg/dL fasting levels may actually be associated with worse outcomes because of complications from iatrogenic hypoglycemia. Studies of non–critically ill patients, in contrast, have found that hyperglycemia is associated with more wound infections. Ramos and associates have noted an increased incidence of infection by 30% for every increase in glucose of 40 mg/dL over the recommended 110 mg/dL.

Sliding scale insulin treatments are less effective in the first 24 hours but are easier than infusions. Sliding scale regular insulin is most appropriate for women without a previous history of diabetes and without risk factors, and those with short surgeries who will resume normal activity and diet within 24 hours. Infusions are preferable if glucose levels are elevated significantly and early in the postoperative course and for women with longer surgeries who will not resume regular eating and activity for a few days. Insulin infusions are begun with concomitant infusions of D_5 half-normal saline (5% dextrose in half-strength normal saline) with 10 mEq of KCl. The Portland Insulin Protocol allows for control of glucose levels and, with nursing support, can be effective (see **Appendix A** online).

When transitioning off insulin infusions, it is reasonable to use the rule of thumb of 80% of the previous 24-hour total insulin dose. This amount may be divided into split doses of NPH insulin or longer acting glargine. Glargine is associated with less hypoglycemia. Initially, a bolus of fast-acting insulin, lispro, may be added with meals. The bedside glucose level is measured every 4 hours. In patients who go home at 24 hours, oral medications or insulin may be restarted at the time of discharge with the same dose as that which was used before the operative period.

POSTOPERATIVE NAUSEA AND GASTROINTESTINAL FUNCTION

Minor disturbances in GI function are a normal consequence of anesthesia, perioperative medications, and surgical manipulation. Most women experience some nausea for approximately 12 hours, pass flatus some time during the first 48 hours, and have a spontaneous bowel movement by the third or fourth postoperative day. Current best practice for women without bowel resections and those younger than 70 years is clear liquids within 6 hours of surgery and a regular diet with cessation of nausea. Traditionally, patients were to have nothing by mouth until the passage of flatus and then given a gradual resumption of diet from clear liquid to full liquid to soft to regular diet, terned *step-up diets*. Several studies have shown that delayed feeding and step-up diets are unnecessary and, in some ways detrimental. Steed and colleagues, in a study of major gynecologic surgeries, including oncologic cases, have compared restricted oral intake with step-up diets to early full diet and found no adverse effects, as well as a shorter length of stay in the early feeding group. McMillan and associates, in a study of major gynecologic surgeries, compared low-residue diet at 6 hours followed by a regular diet with a traditional delayed feeding and a step-up diet after bowel function had returned. They found more nausea and emesis in the delayed feeding group, with a shorter length of stay in the early feeding group. Cutillo and Pearl and their coworkers have found similar results in their studies of gynecologic oncology patients (**Table 25-8**).

Approximately one third of adult women experience postoperative nausea and vomiting (PONV). Several factors affect the likelihood and severity of postoperative nausea, including preoperative anxiety, decreased threshold for nausea and vomiting, previous history of PONV, duration of surgery, drugs used for anesthesia, obesity, and postoperative pain medications. Certain preventive measures may be used to minimize PONV, including adequate hydration, minimizing use of narcotics and inhalation agents, avoiding nitrous oxide, choice of regional

Table 25-8 Gastrointestinal Information

Category	Clear Liquid (N = 107)	Regular Diet (N = 138)
Morbidity		
Nausea	21 (19.6)	26 (18.8)
Vomiting	10 (9.3)	19 (13.8)
Abdominal distention	10 (9.3)	18 (13.0)
Nasogastric tube use	1 (0.9)	8 (5.8)
Tolerance		
Diet on first attempt	101 (94.4)	121 (87.7)
Regular diet on first attempt	103 (96.3)	
If intolerant, time to tolerance (days)	5.3 ± 1.5	3.6 ± 1.5
Flatus before discharge	55 (51.4)	69 (50.0)
Intervals (days)		
Bowel sounds	1.2 ± 0.5	1.2 ± 0.5
Flatus	2.8 ± 1.4	2.8 ± 1.0
Regular diet*	2.4 ± 2.5	1.1 ± 0.3
Hospital stay	3.6 ± 3.0	3.4 ± 1.7

*$P < .05$; no other significant differences between groups.
Data presented as mean ± standard deviation or N (%).
From Pearl MI, Frandina M, Mahler L, et al: A randomized controlled trial of a regular diet as the first meal in gynecologic oncology patients undergoing intraabdominal surgery. Obstet Gynecol 100:232, 2002.

anesthesia, and avoiding excessive movement in the immediate postoperative period. Many physicians prescribe medications prophylactically for women to prevent PONV (see **Appendix B** online). Serotonin is the most important neurotransmitter and intestinal hormone affecting nausea. Serotonin affects the GI nerves and also central nevous system (CNS) receptors, specifically through the 5-HT3 receptors. Specific serotonin antagonists, such as ondansetron (Zofran), and dolasetron (Anzemet), are particularly effective as agents for treating PONV.

A large randomized clinical trial of 5199 patients by Apfel and colleagues has examined several regimens for the prophylaxis of PONV. This large multicenter trial documented several important principles for postoperative management. The antiemetic interventions of dexamethasone, the 5-HT3 antagonist ondansetron, and droperidol were found to be equally effective for treating nausea. Droperidol is associated with a rare but problematic side effect of prolonged QT intervals and has subsequently led to most pharmacies removing this medication from their formularies. Dexamethasone, 2.5 to 5 mg, should be given at the beginning of surgery to be most effective The repeat use of medications for rescue effects are less efficacious if an agent has been given previously. Previous studies have found that agents such as metoclopramide are ineffective for prophylaxis. Antiemetics in the phenothiazine class, such as promethazine and prochlorperazine, are effective but have some limitations because of side effects of sedation, dry mouth, and extrapyramidal effects, which may be worse for older women. Acupressure, or electrical stimulation to acupressure points, has also been found to be effective. The stimulation point is at point 6, on the dorsal wrist above the ulna. Some hospitals use adjunctive **acustimulation** in addition to pharmacologic agents, with good results.

Apfel and associates' study also looked at risk factors for PONV. Female gender is one of the strongest risk factors for PONV (RR, 3.13; 95% CI, 2.33 to 4.20). Thus, all women should be considered for prophylactic measures. Other factors include 1.78 RR (95% CI, 1.35 to 2.95) for patients with hysterectomies, 1.57 RR (95% CI, 1.32 to 1.07) for nonsmokers, and 2.14 (95% CI, 1.75 to 2.61) for use of postoperative opioids. With patients going home within 24 hours of surgery, the term *postdischarge nausea and vomiting* (PDNV) is used. Treatments for this problem are by nature nonparenteral. General treatments include oral 5-HT3 antagonists combined with antihistamines such as promethazine, or scopolamine patches for patients without contraindications.

ILEUS

Ileus is an inhibition of the normal propulsive reflexes of the bowel regulated by the autonomic nervous system. Adynamic (paralytic) ileus is a normal event defined as an ileus of minor to moderate degree. It may be expected to follow any intraperitoneal or pelvic operation. Brief declines in the motility of the GI tract are normal responses after surgery. The stomach returns to full motility in 24 to 72 hours after surgery. However, some gastric secretions will continually pass into the duodenum. The stomach secretes 500 to 1000 mL of fluid/day. The pancreas secretes an additional liter. The small intestine resumes peristalsis within 6 hours after surgery. The colon resumes full motility in 18 to 48 hours. Most women will have a bowel movement within 72 hours of surgery. The incidence and duration of **adynamic ileus** are lower following vaginal hysterectomy than abdominal

hysterectomy and even less following laparoscopic surgery. If adynamic ileus persists longer than 5 days, a diagnosis of mechanical bowel obstruction should be strongly considered.

Adynamic ileus is believed to result from a lack of coordinated motor activity of the intestine, which results in disorganized propulsive activity. Electrical activity is present, but the pathophysiologic problem is continuous activity of the intrinsic inhibitor neurons in the wall of the small intestine. Usually, the process is generalized, but occasionally may be localized, involving only an isolated loop of small intestine. The cause of prolonged postoperative ileus is a subject of continued debate. Generally, the mechanisms include an increased neurologic inhibition of intestinal motility caused by sympathetic nerve activity, as well as an inflammation within the intestinal wall. Bauer and Boeckxstaens have describe leukocytic infiltration secondary to cytokine production from manipulation of the bowel during surgery. The inflammation inhibits the appropriate neuromuscular reactions, which then decrease motility. Opioid receptors become stimulated with abdominal surgery, further decreasing motility.

Early carbohydrate intake as well as postoperative gum chewing have improved rates for return of bowel function and decreased rates of postoperative ileus. Importantly, early feeding, as noted, decreases the incidence of postoperative ileus, most likely through stimulation of intestinal reflexes. The workup of postoperative ileus should include dtermination of serum electrolyte and magnesium levels, because hypokalemia and abnormal magnesium levels may cause ileus. Narcotics, intraabdominal infection, urinary ascites, and retroperitoneal hematomas may all affect GI motility. Overall, a multifactorial peri- and postoperative approach to postoperative ileus is indicated (**Table 25-9**).

The classic symptoms of a prolonged ileus include absence of flatus, abdominal distention, and obstipation. Often, these symptoms are associated with nausea and effortless vomiting. Bowel sounds may be hypoactive or absent. This condition may be associated with abdominal tenderness and the abdomen is usually tympanic to percussion. Nausea and vomiting that persist more than 24 hours after surgery are a cause for concern.

Diagnostic films of the abdomen (supine, erect, lateral) help establish the correct diagnosis (**Table 25-10**). In a woman with adynamic ileus, the intestinal gas is scattered throughout the GI tract, including the small intestine and colon. Air-fluid levels, if present, tend to be at the same level. In some studies, CT has been found to be sensitive and specific for differentiating adynamic ileus from complete obstruction and helpful for differentiating ileus from partial obstruction.

Oral administration of radiocontrast material may be a therapeutic and diagnostic test. The osmolality of the radiocontrast material is approximately six times greater than that of normal saline. Thus, a large amount of fluid enters the small bowel and acts as a direct stimulant of peristalsis. In one study, after preliminary abdominal films were obtained, 120 mL of 66% diatrizoate meglumine, 10% diatrizoate sodium (Gastrografin), was administered orally or via nasogastric tube. Passage of liquid stool occurred within a few hours in patients with adynamic ileus. Gastrografin, unlike barium, is nontoxic if it accidentally contaminates the peritoneal cavity during an operation for bowel obstruction.

Severe adynamic ileus is a self-limiting condition that responds to GI rest, IV fluids, and time. During the period of watchful expectancy, adequate fluid and electrolyte replacement

Table 25-9 Treatment Options for Postoperative Ileus

Treatment	Potential Mechanism	Comments
Nonpharmacologic Options		
Nasogastric tube	Gastric, small bowel decompression	No evidence NG tubes reduce duration of POI. May increase pulmonary postoperative complications pulmonary postoperative complications
Early enteral nutrition	Stimulates GI motility by eliciting reflex response and stimulating release of several hormonal factors	Appears safe, well tolerated. Some, but not all, studies suggest decrease in POI
Sham feeding	Cephalic-vagal reflex	Small clinical trials suggest some benefit
Early mobilization	Possible mechanical stimulation	No significant change in duration of POI, but may decrease other postoperative complications
Laparoscopic surgery	Decreased opiate requirements, decreased pain, less abdominal wall trauma	Most studies find decreased duration of POI with laparoscopy
Psychological preoperative preparation	Improves bowel motility through visceral learning	One study found positive benefit in decreasing time to flatus and hospital discharge
Pharmacologic Treatment Options		
Metoclopramide	Dopamine antagonist, cholinergic agent	
Cisapride	Dopamine antagonist, cholinergic agonist, serotonin receptor agonist	Possibly effective, withdrawn from U.S. market due to cardiovascular side effects
Erythromycin	Motilin agonist	2 RCTs suggest no benefit
Opiate antagonists	Block peripheral opiate receptors	One RCT shows ADL8-2698 decreases time to flatus, bowel movement, and hospital discharge, but not currently available outside of clinical trials. Other agents have not been evaluated in POI movement, and hospital discharge, but not currently available outside of clinical trials. Other agents have not been evaluated in POI
Epidural anesthesia	Inhibits sympathetic reflex at cord level, opioid-sparing analgesia	Several RCTs suggest benefit in decreasing POI, most effective when inserted at thoracic level
NSAIDs	Opiate-sparing analgesia, inhibits COX-mediated prostaglandin synthesis	Probable benefit. COX-2 selective medications need further evaluation
Laxatives	Stimulant, prokinetic effects	No RCTs. One nonrandomized, unblinded study suggests possible benefit
Antiadrenergic agents	Blocks sympathetic neural reflex	Little practical benefit in POI drugs often limited by cardiovascular side effects
Cholinergic agents	Acetylcholine modulation	Frequent systemic side effects. Neostigmine has possible benefit
Multimodality Therapy	Combination therapy may work via multiple mechanisms	Possible benefit in reducing POI. No RCTs have been reported

COX, Cyclooygenase; NSAIDs, nonsteroidal anti-inflammatory drugs; POI, postoperative ileus; RCTs, randomized controlled trials.
From Behm B, Stollman N: Postoperative ileus: Etiologies and interventions. Clin Gastroenterol Hepatol 1:74, 2003.

Table 25-10 Differential Radiographic Findings in Ileus and Mechanical Obstruction

Adynamic Ileus	Mechanical Obstruction
Small and large bowel distended in proportion to each other	In small bowel obstruction, there is dilated small bowel proximal to site of obstruction; in colonic obstruction, the colon is distended and small bowel distention is present with an incompetent ileocecal valve.
Air-fluid levels in small bowel infrequent; when present, they at the same levels	Air-fluid levels are common and at different levels in the bowel.
Quantitative difference in small bowel distention	Greater small bowel distention than with ileus
Small bowel distention in central part of abdomen with colon in periphery	Small bowel distention present in central part of abdomen; no peripheral large bowel distention

From Buchsbaum HJ, Mazer J: The gastrointestinal tract. In Buchsbaum HJ, Walton LA (eds): Strategies in Gynecologic Surgery. New York, Springer-Verlag, 1986.

is necessary. Patients experience mild cramping and passage of flatus and regain their appetite with the return of normal peristalsis. If adequate bowel sounds are present, a rectal tube, Fleet's enema, or rectal suppository may facilitate the initial passage of flatus. Some advocate the routine postoperative administration of a wetting agent, such as simethicone (Mylicon), to reduce surface tension of intestinal mucus and liberate entrapped gas. Opinions are mixed as to whether such an agent reduces the incidence or intensity of adynamic ileus. Randomized trials of the

prokinetic agents erythromycin and metoclopramide have shown these agents to be ineffective in relieving ileus. Importantly, prophylactic nasogastric suctioning will not prevent ileus. In many studies, prophylactic nasogastric suctioning is associated with an increased risk of aspiration as well as an increased rate of ileus—the very symptom the treatment is supposed to prevent. However, if a severe ileus does not resolve, nasogastric suctioning will be necessary. Nasogastric suction prevents progression of the intestinal distention. During periods when

Table 25-11 Average Daily Volume and Electrolyte Concentrations of Gastrointestinal Secretions

Secretion	Volume (mL/day)	Electrolyte Concentration (mEq/L)		
		Na⁺	K⁺	Cl⁻
Saliva	1000-1500	10-40	10-20	6-30
Gastric juice	2000-2500	60-120	10-20	10-30
Hepatic bile	600-800	130-155	2-12	80-100
Pancreatic juice	700-1000	150-155	5-10	30-50
Duodenal secretions	300-800	90-140	2-10	70-120
Jejunal and ileal secretions	2000-3000	125-140	5-10	100-130
Colonic mucosal secretions	200-500	140-148	5-10	60-90
Total:	8000-10,000			

Table 25-12 Composition of Intravenous Solutions

Solution	Glucose (g/liter)	Component (mEq/liter)							
		Na⁺	Cl⁻	HCO₃⁻	K⁺	Ca²⁺	Mg²⁺	HPO₄⁻	NH₄⁻
Extracellular fluid	1000	140	102	27	4.2	5	3	0.3	
5% dextrose and water	50								
10% dextrose and water	100								
0.9% sodium chloride (normal saline)		154	154						
0.45% sodium chloride (half-normal saline)		77	77						
0.21% sodium chloride (¼ normal saline)		34	34						
3% sodium chloride (hypertonic saline)		513	513						
Lactated Ringer's solution		130	109	28*	4		2.7		
0.9% ammonium chloride		168							168

*Present in solution as lactate but is metabolized to bicarbonate.
From Miller TA, Duke JH: Fluid and electrolyte management. In Dudrick SJ, Baue AE, Eiseman B, et al (eds): Manual of Preoperative and Postoperative Care, 3rd ed. Philadelphia, WB Saunders, 1983.

nasogastric suctioning is used, special attention should be given to correct replacement of fluid and electrolytes (**Tables 25-11** and **25-12**). A rare but worrisome complication of prolonged ileus is massive dilation of the cecum. Massive dilation of the colon related to a pseudo-obstruction produced by severe adynamic ileus in the absence of mechanical obstruction is known as Ogilvie's syndrome. This condition may be treated medically by evacuating the air with colonoscopy or, in severe cases, cecostomy may be necessary. An alternative method of treating this condition is IV neostigmine.

INTESTINAL OBSTRUCTION AND ADHESIONS

Adhesions are the most common cause of intestinal obstruction postoperatively. During subsequent operations, up to 90% of women are found to have some adhesions following abdominal laparotomy, although most are filmy. In a large retrospective cohort study covering a 10-year period following laparotomy for gynecologic conditions, approximately one in three women had adhesion-related readmissions to the hospital. Less common causes of intestinal obstruction are hernias, mesenteric defects, intussusception, volvulus, and neoplasm. Large raw areas of the pelvis with hypoxic tissue facilitate the attachment of small intestine following pelvic surgery. Previous gynecologic surgeries are the most common cause of small bowel obstruction in women. The incidence of operation for obstruction of the small intestine after an abdominal hysterectomy is estimated to be approximately 2%. Interestingly, in one series, adhesions involving the pelvic peritoneum were responsible for the intestinal obstruction in 85% of cases, and adhesions to the closure of the anterior

abdominal wall accounted for the other 15%. Fortunately, the fibrous adhesions that form during the first 2 to 3 weeks after an operation are soft and filmy. Thus, intestinal strangulation during the postoperative period is extremely rare. Dense adhesions may develop several months after surgery. Adhesion formation after surgical procedures appears to be related to irritation of the peritoneum. The reaction of injured peritoneum involves a reepithelialization by peritoneal cells to cover raw intra-abdominal surfaces. The process begins within 24 hours of surgery. Fibrin-rich exudates cover areas of denuded viscera and abdominal wall. Factors that increase adhesion formation include inflammation, infection, and trauma. Thus, suturing of peritoneum should be kept to a minimum. The greatest risk, as noted by Dubisson and coworkers in a recent series of 1000 consecutive laparoscopies, was in previous midline incisions, with more than 50% having adhesions, compared with less than 3% after a previous laparoscopy. The incidence of intestinal obstruction depends on the type of gynecologic surgery performed. Approximately 2 in 1000 women develop an obstruction after a benign gynecologic operation, whereas approximately 8% develop intestinal obstruction after radical cancer surgery. Intestinal obstruction occurs in the small intestine in approximately 80% of cases and in the colon in the remaining 20%. As noted, the differential diagnosis between bowel obstruction and ileus is difficult (**Table 25-13**).

The acute symptoms of intestinal obstruction usually present between the fifth and seventh postoperative days. Most patients have a short period of normal intestinal function before the onset of symptoms. Women with bowel obstruction appear to have more toxicity and more acute distress than women with ileus.

Table 25-13 Differential Diagnosis Between Postoperative Ileus and Postoperative Obstruction

Clinical Features	Postoperative Ileus	Postoperative Obstruction
Abdominal pain	Discomfort from distention but not cramping pains	Cramping, progressively severe
Relationship to previous operation	Usually within 48-72 hr of operation	Usually delayed; may be 5-7 days for remote onset
Nausea and vomiting	Present	Present
Distention	Present	Present
Bowel sounds	Absent or hypoactive	Borborygmi with peristaltic rushes and high-pitched tinkles
Fever	Only if related to associated peritonitis	Rarely present unless bowel becomes gangrenous
Abdominal radiograph	Distended loops of small and large bowels; gas usually present in colon	Single or multiple loops of distended bowel, usually small bowel with air-fluid levels
Treatment	Conservative with nasogastric suction, enemas, cholinergic stimulation	Partial—conservative with nasogastric decompression, *or* Complete—surgical

The abdominal pain is intermittent, colicky, and sharp in nature. Episodes of colicky pain usually last from 1 to 3 min. Associated symptoms include vomiting, abdominal distention, and constipation. Bowel sounds are loud, high-pitched, and metallic. Occasionally, they may be heard without a stethoscope. Nasogastric drainage is more profuse than in patients with severe adynamic ileus. A patient with a complete small bowel obstruction may have a bowel movement, eliminating fecal material that already existed in the colon.

Abdominal radiographs demonstrate a stepladder appearance—multiple air-fluid levels throughout the small intestine, with an absence of gas in the colon and rectum. Pneumoperitoneum from an exploratory celiotomy usually persists for 7 to 10 days. Thus, in the early postoperative period, free air under the diaphragm is not diagnostic of perforation of a hollow viscus. Obstruction of the colon may be diagnosed by retrograde infusion of contrast material or by flexible endoscopy.

The foundation of early treatment of postoperative intestinal obstruction is decompression of the small intestine and adequate replacement of fluids and electrolytes. Decompression may be accomplished by means of a nasogastric tube. Serial monitoring of white blood cell counts with differentials should be performed. Repeat abdominal radiographic examinations at regular intervals are used to assess the degree of intestinal distention. Expectant management is successful in many patients. In an older series by Wolfson and colleagues, less than 40% of 112 patients with small bowel obstruction caused by adhesions required surgery. A small series from Gowen has also noted more than 70% success with long tube decompression. Conservative therapy was most successful in patients in whom the long intestinal drainage tube was successfully advanced from the stomach into the small intestine.

The major cause of morbidity and death with bowel obstruction is delay in diagnosis, with resultant strangulation and secondary sepsis. Women who develop strangulation experience a dramatic increase in the intensity of abdominal pain, and the pain becomes continuous. Strangulation of the small bowel is associated with localized peritoneal irritation, increase in temperature, and marked leukocytosis. Bowel obstruction may also lead to translocation of intestinal bacteria across the bowel wall, promoting sepsis. A series by Sagar and associates has found that the more distal the obstruction, the greater the incidence of anaerobic septicemia.

Fecal impaction is most often seen in older patients. It results from loss of peristalsis in the colon, with an impaired perception of rectal fullness. Fecal impaction is a humiliating experience for

the woman. She may have diarrhea around the impaction or obstipation. Treatment involves obtaining partial analgesia with lidocaine jelly and, subsequently, manually fragmenting and extracting the fecal mass.

RECTOVAGINAL FISTULA

Rectovaginal fistulas and fecal incontinence secondary to perineal tears are usually obstetric complications and are only rarely associated with gynecologic surgery. In general, rectovaginal fistulas following hysterectomy or repair of an enterocele are usually located in the upper third of the vagina, whereas those secondary to a posterior colporrhaphy are in the lower third of the vagina. Other causes of rectovaginal fistula are carcinoma, radiation therapy, perirectal abscess, inflammatory bowel disease, lymphogranuloma venereum, and trauma.

The initial signs and symptoms associated with potential fistulous tracts between the rectum and vagina usually present 7 to 14 days after an operation. The first warning may be the rectal passage of several blood clots, indicating that a hematoma has ruptured into the rectum. Distressing symptoms include passage of gas from the vagina and, depending on the size of the opening, the passage of fecal material from the vagina. Associated with these classic symptoms and signs are a chronic, foul-smelling vaginal discharge and subsequent dyspareunia. Aside from the physical symptoms of the anatomic defect, fistulas cause severe emotional distress because they affect almost every aspect of the woman's daily life.

The diagnosis is not difficult to establish and only very small openings present a diagnostic problem. What appears to be granulation tissue in the posterior aspect of the vagina is the dark red rectal mucosa, which stands out in contrast to the lighter vaginal mucosa. Usually, the defect may be successfully defined with a small, malleable metal probe. If this is not successful, a Foley catheter should be placed in the rectum. Methylene blue dye or milk may then be instilled into the rectum with a tampon in the vagina, similar to the procedure for establishing the diagnosis of a vesicovaginal fistula.

For initial treatment the woman should be obstipated with a low-residue diet and diphenoxylate hydrochloride (Lomotil). Approximately one in four anatomic defects heals spontaneously before epithelialization of the tract. A low-residue diet or hyperalimentation may be helpful in facilitating spontaneous closure of some anatomic defects.

Timing of the operative repair is important. The gynecologist should inspect the area surrounding the fistula to ensure that the tissues are free of edema, induration, and infection. Preoperative evaluation includes visualization of the entire vagina and sigmoidoscopy of the rectal mucosa in an attempt to discover more than one opening. Imaging studies and endoscopy are important diagnostic tools if there is any suspicion of coexistence of Crohn's disease.

The operative technique used depends on the size and location of the fistula. Standard operative principles include removal of the entire fistulous tract and closure of tissue layers without tension on the suture line. In the repair of large rectovaginal fistulas in the lower part of the vagina, it is usually easier to convert the rectovaginal fistula into a fourth-degree laceration. Diverting colostomy should be used for all radiation-induced fistulas, most fistulas associated with inflammatory bowel disease, and some large postoperative fistulas at the apex of the vagina. The woman may be discharged from the hospital after the first bowel movement. The stool should be kept soft with low-residue diets and stool softeners such as mineral oil for the first 2 weeks after the operation.

ANTIBIOTIC-ASSOCIATED DIARRHEA

Patients may develop diarrhea in the postoperative period after exposure to antibiotics. Oral and parenteral antibiotics produce similar rates of diarrhea, with some studies noting that up to one third of patients receiving antibiotics will develop diarrhea. Antibiotic therapy, for prophylaxis or treatment, can disrupt the normal intestinal flora. The result is a disturbed breakdown of bile acids and carbohydrates that induce loose stools. Diarrhea may develop secondary to medications other than antibiotics, including oral contrast media, diabetic foods that contain artificial sweeteners, and many cardiac medications. If the woman is afebrile, the diarrhea is mild, and the abdominal examination is unremarkable, stopping or changing antibiotics and providing supportive care are all that is necessary. If the woman has a temperature higher than 38° C, a leukocytosis, abdominal tenderness, severe abdominal distention, bloody diarrhea, or persistent diarrhea, evaluation for *Clostridium difficile* infection is indicated (**Table 25-14**).

C. difficile is a species of spore-forming, gram-positive anaerobic bacteria found normally in 5% of healthy adults. However, after antibiotic treatment and disruption of normal enteric flora, up to 25% of hospitalized adults will become colonized with *C. difficile*. The organism is spread by nosocomial oral-fecal contamination. Persistence of the spores of *C. difficile* and contamination of the environment are primary factors in cross infection. After colonizing the intestine, the organism may secrete toxins, which produce a spectrum of clinical disease. Symptoms from the infection are varied and range from a mild diarrhea to colitis to a pseudomembranous colitis that in rare cases may be fatal. Almost all antibiotics have been associated with the development of *C. difficile* diarrhea (**Table 25-15**). Second- and third-generation cephalosporins (e.g., clindamycin, ampicillin, amoxicillin) are the antibiotics associated with the highest risk of developing *C. difficile* diarrhea. Symptoms usually appear 5 to 10 days after the initiation of antibiotic therapy. However, they may appear from a few days to a few weeks after antibiotic exposure. Diagnostic tests include the following: culture for the organism; *C. difficile* cell cytotoxin B assay; enzyme-linked immunosorbent assay (ELISA) kits for the *C. difficile* toxins A and B; stool leukocyte assay, which is nonspecific; colonoscopy for direct evaluation of pseudomembranes; abdominal radiography; and CT. The test for *C. difficile* cell cytotoxin B in the stool is the gold standard for diagnosis because it is the most sensitive and specific and is also relatively inexpensive. The results are usually available within 24 hours.

Discontinuing antibiotic therapy is the only treatment required in approximately one in four women. Use of drugs that

Table 25-14 Differences between Antibiotic-Associated Diarrhea from *Clostridium difficile* and Diarrhea from Other Causes

Characteristic	*Cause*	
	C. difficile **Infection**	**Other Causes**
Most commonly implicated antibiotics	Clindamycin, cephalosporins, penicillins	Clindamycin, cephalosporins, or amoxicillin-clavulanate
History	Usually no relevant history of antibiotic intolerance	History of diarrhea with antibiotic therapy common
Clinical features		
Diarrhea	May be florid; evidence of colitis with cramps, fever, and fecal leukocytes common	Usually moderate in severity (i.e., nuisance diarrhea) without evidence of colitis
Findings on CT or endoscopy	Evidence of colitis (not enteritis) common	Usually normal
Complications	Hypoalbuminemia, anasarca, toxic megacolon, relapses with treatment with metronidazole or vancomycin	Usually none except occasional cases of dehydration
Results of assay for *C. difficile* toxin	Positive	Negative
Epidemiologic pattern	May be epidemic for endemic in hospitals or long-term care facilities	Sporadic
Treatment		
Withdrawal of implicated antibiotic	May resolve but often persists or progresses	Usually resolves
Antiperistaltic agents	Contraindicated	Often useful
Oral metronidazole or vancomycin	Prompt response	Not indicated

CT, computed tomography

From Bartlett JG: Antibiotic-associated diarrhea. N Engl J Med 346:335, 2002.

Table 25-15 Antimicrobial Agents That Induce *Clostridium difficile*-Associated Diarrhea and Colitis

Frequent Induction	Infrequent Induction	Rare or No Induction
Ampicillin and amoxicillin	Tetracyclines	Parenteral aminoglycosides
Cephalosporins	Sulfonamides	Bacitracin
Clindamycin	Erythromycin	Metronidazole
	Chloramphenicol	Vancomycin
	Trimethoprim	
	Quinolones	

From Kelly CP, Pothoulakis C, LaMont JT: *Clostridium difficile* colitis. N Engl J Med 330:257, 1994.

slow intestinal transit time, such as diphenoxylate atropine (Lomotil) or narcotics, are definitely contraindicated because the toxins of *C. difficile* remain in the GI tract for a longer period. Therapy for the infection is metronidazole, 250 mg PO, four times daily, or vancomycin PO, 125 mg four times daily. Gastrointestinal symptoms usually improve within the first 72 hours of therapy and complete resolution of symptoms occurs within 10 days. Host factors are involved in the pathogenesis of the disease; older and more chronically ill patients usually develop more severe symptoms. Patients with ileus may receive high-dose vancomycin through a long tube. Up to 25% of women may develop a recurrence or relapse. Studies have confirmed that more than 50% of recurrences of symptoms after initial response to treatment are caused by reinfection rather by a relapse. Recurrences usually can be successfully treated in the same manner as the initial therapy.

Probiotic agents have been studied for the prevention of antibiotic-associated diarrhea as well as for treatment of *C. difficile* disease. Probiotics are live microbes that may act in the intestinal tract to colonize with less problematic organisms. Other actions include the secretion of compounds that may inhibit *C. difficile* or inactivate the toxin. To be most effective, probiotics should be given at the same time as the antibiotic. Several trials in the United States and Europe have found that the probiotic yeast *Saccharomyces boulardii* significantly decreases the incidence of antibiotic-associated diarrhea. Trials of *Lactobacillus* have not found significant efficacy. Although the complete mechanism of action is theoretical at this point, *S. boulardii* does seem to inactivate the *C. difficile* toxin. The yeast also appears to stimulate immunoglobulin A (IgA) production in the intestinal mucosa against *C. difficile*.

WOUND COMPLICATIONS

INFECTION

A major wound infection prolongs the hospital stay approximately 2 to 6 days. In their extensive review of 23,649 operations, Cruse and Foord determined that the incidence of abdominal wound infection varied depending on risk factors; however, for abdominal hysterectomy, the incidence was approximately 5%. In a population of women not at high risk, the incidence of infection should be 1% to 2%. Abdominal hysterectomy is classified as a clean-contaminated operative procedure because the bacterial flora of the vagina is in continuity

with the operative site during the surgery. The Centers for Disease Control and Prevention has revised their nomenclature describing incisional infection. They subdivide incisional infections into superficial infections that involve only the skin and subcutaneous tissue and deep infections that involve the deep soft tissues, including fascia and muscles. Although some infections are generally associated with specific organisms such as streptococcus or clostridia, most gynecologic infections are polymicrobial. Thus, antibiotic treatments are aimed at providing broad-spectrum coverage for aerobic, anaerobic, and gram-negative organisms. A list of common antibiotics is found in **Appendix C** online.

The pathophysiology of wound infection depends on an interaction between the number and virulence of bacterial contamination and the resistance of the woman. Inoculation of bacteria into the wound occurs in the operating room during the surgical procedure. A wide spectrum of common endogenous bacteria produce wound infections, including most gram-positive cocci and aerobic and anaerobic rods. Small numbers of bacteria are present in all surgical wounds; however, bacterial growth is facilitated by decreased tissue oxygen and excessive amounts of necrotic tissue. It takes from 100,000 to 1,000,000 bacteria/g of tissue to produce infection in a surgical wound of the skin and subcutaneous tissue. The incidence of superficial skin infection is directly related to the length of the operative procedure. Each additional hour of surgery results in a doubling of the incidence of superficial skin infections. The primary source of bacterial contamination of an abdominal wound may be exogenous to the woman (e.g., a break in sterile technique) or endogenous (e.g., purulent material from a pelvic abscess).

Local and systemic factors contribute to the level of host resistance and thus to the incidence of wound infections. Local factors are more significant and include the presence of hematomas, necrotic tissue, foreign bodies, dead space, use of cauterization, and decreased local tissue perfusion. Systemic factors include obesity, diabetes, liver disease, malnutrition, immunosuppression, defects in the reticuloendothelial system, age, and duration of preoperative hospitalization (**Box 25-5**). The incidence of postoperative wound infection is increased eightfold when the

---

Box 25-5 Factors Associated with Wound Infections

Preexisting skin and operative site infection
Tissue with poor oxygenation
Hematoma
Necrotic tissue
Foreign bodies
Cauterized tissue
Poor circulation from vascular disease
Dead space within the wound
Anemia
Decreased perfusion from tension
Obesity
Long preoperative hospitalization
Poor nutrition
    Vitamin deficiencies
    Mineral deficiencies (e.g., zinc)
Glucocorticoids, other immunosuppressive medications
Diabetes
Liver disease
Ionizing radiation
Advanced age

woman's preoperative weight exceeds 200 pounds. Soper and colleagues have noted that the thickness of subcutaneous tissue is the greatest risk factor for wound infection in a series of women undergoing abdominal hysterectomy. If an abdominal incision is more than 4 cm in depth, the risk of a superficial skin infection is increased approximately threefold. Multiple regimens and protocols have been studied to decrease rates of wound infection. Skin warming to improve circulation, supplemental oxygen, and antibiotics to be given well before incision time have all been emphasized as techniques for infection prevention.

The first symptom of most wound infections appears between the fifth and tenth postoperative days. Wound infection may occur as late as several months following surgery, but more than 90% of cases present within the first 2 weeks of the postoperative period. The first sign is usually fever, followed by tachycardia and varying degrees of increased tenderness and pain. As the infection progresses, many wounds develop areas that are fluctuant or firm, and some develop crepitus. The incision is swollen, erythematous, edematous, and tender. Occasionally, subcutaneous gas may be seen on radiographic examination. There may be associated spontaneous purulent drainage from the wound later in the course of the infection.

Fever during the first 24 to 48 hours is usually secondary to atelectasis. However, two rare types of wound infections are so virulent that they produce toxicity within the first 48 hours. Typically, these early infections are those produced by *Clostridium* spp. and acute β-hemolytic streptococcal infection. Clinically, wound infections secondary to β-hemolytic streptococci appear swollen and red and have an odorless discharge. In contrast, infections secondary to *Clostridium* are boggy and edematous and the discharge has a sweet odor.

Initial treatment of any wound infection consists of opening and draining the wound. The wound opens easily following removal of the skin sutures or clips. Purulent material exhibits a wide range of consistency from the thin watery discharge typical of a streptococcal infection to the thick pus associated with staphylococcal subcutaneous infections. Gram staining and aerobic and anaerobic cultures of the wound should be carried out at this point. These initial cultures are most valuable if the woman does not respond to initial management. In such cases, the differential diagnosis would be between infections involving deeper tissue planes and infection for which host resistance has failed, even after drainage of the wound.

Once a wound infection has been opened and drained, care is directed toward initial packing of the wound with gauze to effect débridement and periodic irrigation. If necrotic tissue is seen, the tissue should be resected back to the point where vital tissue can be identified. If there is a distinct zone of diffuse erythema surrounding a wound infection, the most likely organism is a streptococcal infection, and IV antibiotics are indicated. If methicillin-resistant *Staphylococcus aureus* (MRSA) is cultured, the great majority of women will respond solely to débridement. If the woman does not respond or responds slowly, antibiotics specific for MRSA should be used, such as clindamycin or sulfamethoxazole-trimethoprim. Systemic antibiotics are always indicated for women with immunosuppression or concomitant disease with impaired defense mechanisms.

Most women with a wound infection will become afebrile within 48 to 72 hours after the wound has been opened and débrided. When the woman becomes afebrile and granulation tissue begins to form, consideration may be given to delayed secondary

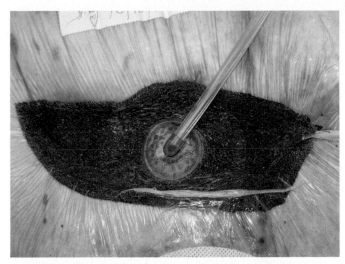

Figure 25-9 Wound-Vac device on an abdominal wound. The *black area* is the sponge within the incision. (From Heridge RT, Leong M, Phillips L: Wound healing. In Townsend CM, Beauchamp RD, Evers BM, Mattox KL [eds]: Sabiston Textbook of Surgery, 18th ed. Philadelphia, Saunders, 2008, pp 191-216.)

closure. If the incision is large and débridement has been extensive, closure may be facilitated with the use of vacuum-assisted devices. The wound is cleaned daily and, between cleaning, topical negative pressure is maintained with the vacuum-assisted device. The vacuum promotes granulation, reduces edema in the subcutaneous tissue, and greatly speeds healing. It may be used on an outpatient basis (**Fig. 25-9**).

Prevention is the foundation of any approach to the treatment of wound infections. Prevention involves consideration of local and systemic factors, which, if unattended, predispose to infection. Prophylactic antibiotics decrease the incidence of wound infection. These antibiotics are discussed in Chapter 24 (Preoperative Counseling and Management).

If the wound is grossly contaminated, it should be left open. Delayed primary closure on the third or fourth postoperative day may be appropriate. Women who should be considered as candidates for delayed primary closure include those who are immunosuppressed or malnourished, who have far-advanced malignancies, or who are markedly obese. Women having operative procedures that involve a simultaneous abdominal and vaginal approach and those with a surgical opening of unprepared large intestine are also candidates for delayed primary closure. In a small series, Brown and associates have reported that the latter technique reduces the incidence of wound infection from 23% in a control group to 2% in the group having delayed closure. When delayed primary closure is planned, sutures may be placed at the time of surgery and secured, but not tied. The incision should be packed loosely with gauze. If the wound is dry and without evidence of infection on postoperative day 3, the edges may be approximated with the preplaced sutures.

Delayed secondary closure may be accomplished in previously infected wounds after several days of drainage and débridement. Delayed secondary closure markedly reduces the time necessary for eventual closure of the skin defect by secondary intention. The woman's satisfaction is dramatically increased with delayed secondary closure. If delayed closure does not appear to be a likely option, such as in women who have more than 3 cm of subcutaneous tissue, application of a closed vacuum system is initiated.

A virulent, rapidly progressing form of soft tissue wound infection is **necrotizing fasciitis**. Often, the diagnosis is not suspected during the early part of the infection because of the relative minor changes in the skin overlying the deeper infection. The early symptoms are local pain with systemic symptoms of tachycardia and fever, which are higher than would be expected with an uncomplicated wound infection. The woman may experience marked tenderness when the infected area is palpated. Conversely, necrotic tissue may become hypoesthetic, or completely numb. An appearance of an area that appears infected but is anesthetic should heighten the suspicion for the diagnosis of necrotizing fasciitis. As the disease progresses, the wound edges usually darken, with crepitance and bullae formation and anesthetic areas developing. Necrotizing fasciitis involves the subcutaneous tissue and superficial fascia. In a series of gynecologic and obstetric patients, Gallup and coworkers have found that 35% displayed radiographic evidence of subcutaneous gas. Obesity and diabetes were common comorbidities in this series. They treated many patients with hyperbaric oxygen after débridement. Others have also emphasized this management option for necrotizing fasciitis.

The infection rapidly expands in the subcutaneous spaces and often tracks far beyond the superficial margins of the involved skin. If the diagnosis is questionable, a full-thickness core biopsy and frozen section of the tissue should be performed. This condition is a life-threatening surgical emergency and patients should have débridement as soon as possible. It is most important for the gynecologist to have a high degree of suspicion for this condition because even with adequate surgical débridement, the mortality rate is 30% to 50%. This rare but potentially fatal condition necessitates wide débridement of all necrotic tissue, high levels of broad-spectrum antibiotics, and sometimes hyperbaric oxygen. Débridement to freely bleeding tissue helps determine the surgical margin. It is not unusual for the woman to need repetitive débridements. Women with diabetes, malnutrition, immunosuppression, malignancy, obesity, and poor tissue perfusion are most susceptible to this complication.

DEHISCENCE AND EVISCERATION

Dehiscence is a failure of normal healing and literally means disruption of any of the layers of a surgical incision. The physiologic, biochemical, and structural changes that characterize normal wound healing are complex and, at best, imperfectly understood. However, clinically, the most important fact to the clinician is that the strength of the wound increases over time (**Fig. 25-10**). The strength of a skin incision increases at a rapid and almost constant rate for the first 4 months and at a much slower rate for the first year. Clinically, dehiscence usually means that the previous incision of the skin, subcutaneous tissue, and fascia has separated, but not the peritoneum. This complication usually occurs during the first several days. Often, dehiscence is recognized immediately or within the first 24 hours following the removal of skin clips. **Wound evisceration** is a complete breakdown of the healing process through all levels of the abdominal incision, with omentum or bowel presenting through the incision.

The incidence of **wound dehiscence** is approximately 1 in 200 gynecologic operations. The major short-term result of

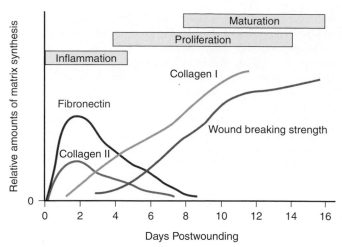

Figure 25-10 Wound healing over time. (From Heridge RT, Leong M, Phillips L: Wound healing. In Townsend CM, Beauchamp RD, Evers BM, Mattox KL [eds]: Sabiston Textbook of Surgery, 18th ed. Philadelphia, Saunders, 2008, pp 191-216.)

wound dehiscence is the prolongation of hospital stay. Over the long term, dehiscence predisposes to incisional hernias. Wound dehiscence is a rare cause of surgical mortality, especially in debilitated patients. Wound infection is present in approximately 50% of women with wound disruption. As with wound infections, preventive management is the most important therapeutic consideration. The incidence of dehiscence has decreased with the use of longer lasting and stronger sutures. Many clinicians prefer to use polydioxanone suture (PDS), a treated Vicryl, or a permanent suture such as polypropylene (Prolene) for greater strength and prolonged presence in the tissue. The rule of thumb is that the suture should remain strong in the tissue until the tissue can resume its original strength. In patients with a propensity for poor or prolonged healing, such as women with malignancy, diabetes, or immune suppression, the use of a permanent suture should be strongly considered. When infection is present, a monofilament suture is preferable to a braided or polyfilament suture (**Tables 25-16** and **25-17**).

The consensus regarding fascial disruption is that local factors are much more important in the pathophysiology of wound disruption than systemic factors, although both should be considered in preventive management. Important mechanical factors predisposing to disruption are conditions that increase the tension on the incision line, such as abdominal distention and chronic lung disease, or a technically inadequate closure of the wound. Other factors include obesity, advanced age, malignancy, uremia, liver failure, diabetes, hypoproteinemia, hematoma formation, sepsis, corticosteroids or chemotherapy, prior radiation therapy, and whether the incision is made through an area of a previous incision. Whether an incision is horizontal or vertical has little effect on the incidence of wound disruption. The pathophysiology of fascial dehiscence involves exaggerated collagen lysis in the wound. Clinically, the sutures tear through the fascia rather than dissolving or becoming untied. For example, approximating and tying sutures too vigorously, especially with a figure-of-eight suture, may lead to strangulation and necrosis of the tissue and subsequent wound dehiscence. Primary mass closure with a continuous monofilament, delayed absorbable suture helps avoid this problem in high-risk patients.

Table 25-16 Comparison of Absorbable Sutures

Suture Reaction	Types	Raw Material	Tensile Strength Retention In Vivo	Tissue
Surgical gut suture	Chromic	Collagen derived from healthy beef and sheep	Individual patient characteristics can affect rate of tensile strength loss.	Moderate reaction
Monocryl suture (poliglecaprone 25)	Monofilament	Copolymer of glycolide and epsilon-caprolactone	~50%-60% (violet, 60%-70%) remains at 1 wk; ~20%-30% (violet, 30%-40%) remains at 2 wk; lost within 3 wk (violet, 4 wk)	Minimal acute inflammatory reaction
Coated vicryl (polyglactin 910)	Braided	Copolymer of lactide and glycolide coated with 370 and calcium stearate	~75% remains at 2 wk	Minimal acute inflammatory reaction
Suture	Monofilament		~50% remains at 3 wk, 25% at 4 wk	
PDS II suture (polydioxanone)	Monofilament	Polyester polymer	~70% remains at 2 wk; ~50% remains at 4 wk; ~25% remains at 6 wk	Slight

Adapted from Neumayer L, Vargo D.: Principles of perioperative and operative surgery. In Townsend CM, Beauchamp RD, Evers BM, Mattox KL (eds): Sabiston Textbook of Surgery, 18th ed. Philadelphia, Saunders, 2008, pp 251-279.

Table 25-17 Comparison of Nonabsorbable Sutures

Suture	Types	Raw Material	Tensile Strength Retention in vivo	Tissue Reaction
Perma-Hand—silk suture	Braided	Organic protein called fibroin	Progressive degradation of fiber may result in gradual loss of tensile strength over time.	Acute inflammatory reaction
Ethilon—nylon suture	Monofilament	Long-chain aliphatic polymers nylon 6 or nylon 6,6	Progressive hydrolysis may result in gradual loss of tensile strength over time.	Minimal acute inflammatory reaction
Nurolon—nylon suture	Braided	Long-chain aliphatic polymers nylon 6 or nylon 6,6	Progressive hydrolysis may result in gradual loss of tensile strength over time.	Minimal acute inflammatory reaction
Mersilene—polyester fiber suture	Braided Monofilament	Poly(ethylene terephthalate)	No significant change known to occur in vivo.	Minimal acute inflammatory reaction
Ethibond *Excel*—polyester fiber suture	Braided	Poly (ethylene terephthalate) coated with polybutilate	No significant change known to occur in vivo.	Minimal acute inflammatory reaction
Prolene—polypropylene suture	Monofilament	Isotactic crystalline stereoisomer of polypropylene	Not subject to degradation or weakening by action of tissue enzymes.	Minimal acute inflammatory reaction
Pronova—poly (hexafluoropropylene-VDF suture)	Monofilament	Polymer blend of poly(vinylidene fluoride) and poly(vinylidene fluoride-cohexafluoropropylene)	Not subject to degradation or weakening by action of tissue enzymes	Minimal acute inflammatory reaction

Adapted from Neumayer L, Vargo D.: Principles of perioperative and operative surgery. In Townsend CM, Beauchamp RD, Evers BM, Mattox KL (eds): Sabiston Textbook of Surgery, 18th ed. Philadelphia, Saunders, 2008, pp 251-279.

The classic symptom and sign of wound disruption is the spontaneous passage of copious serosanguineous fluid from the abdominal incision. This usually occurs between the fifth and eighth postoperative days. Patients with uninfected wounds generally have been asymptomatic, but often report a "pop" after an episode of coughing or emesis. Patients who develop wound defects often lack the normal healing ridge of tissue that can be palpated in normal healing wounds.

Imperative for prevention of wound dehiscence is proper closure of the incision in a woman at high risk for less than optimum healing. Although there are many regional preferences for the choice of suture and method of closure, the most popular technique is some modification of the Smead-Jones closure with permanent suture (**Fig. 25-11**). Closure with the Smead-Jones technique results in a dehiscence rate of approximately 1 in 1000 operations. With this technique, it is important to place individual sutures at least 1 to 1.5 cm away from the adjacent sutures and include at least 2 cm of fascia on either side of the incision. The alternative technique is a mass closure using a monofilament permanent suture material such as nylon or Prolene.

Rarely, the vaginal cuff may rupture, producing dehiscence and vaginal evisceration of abdominal contents. This complication often presents with sudden vaginal bleeding and pain. In their series, Croak and colleagues have noted that prior pelvic surgery and postmenopausal surgery for enterocele are common predisposing factors (**Table 25-18**). If there is no evidence of infection, the vaginal cuff may be closed primarily without opening the abdomen. If secondary issues are present that may inhibit healing (e.g., immunosuppression) or if infection is suspected, an abdominal approach should be considered. Antibiotic treatment with broad-spectrum coverage should be strongly considered. Vaginal evisceration is uncommon but, when it occurs, it is usually several weeks after surgery, and may follow intercourse. Recent reports have noted an increase in vaginal cuff disruption and evisceration with robotic surgery. This is postulated to be secondary to increased use of cauterization, leading to poor wound healing. This complication may present up to 8 weeks

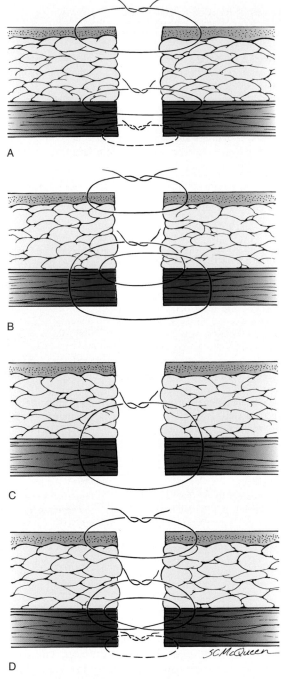

Figure 25-11 Types of abdominal incision closures. **A,** Layered. **B,** Smead-Jones. **C,**Through-and-through. **D,** Far-near. (From Braun TE: Wound dehiscence. In Schaefer G, Graber EA [eds]: Complications in Obstetric and Gynecological Surgery. Hagerstown, physician, Harper & Row, 1981.)

after surgery. Many gynecologists ask patients to refrain from intercourse for 12 weeks to give time for the sutures to dissolve completely and for the tissue to heal.

The treatment of wound disruption is prompt reclosure in the operating room. On the hospital ward, once the diagnosis is recognized, the wound and viscera should be covered with sterile gauze and broad-spectrum antibiotics begun. Once the woman is anesthetized, the wound may be completely reopened

Table 25-18 Predisposing Factors to Evisceration*

Predisposition	Clinical No./No. with Data Reported (%)
Postmenopausal (age > 51 yr)	9/12 (75)
Prior pelvic surgery	10/12 (83)
Postmenopausal with surgery	9/12 (75)
Enterocele and vaginal vault	10/12 (83)
Posterior enterocele	6/12 (50)
Vaginal cuff defect	4/12 (33)
Coital trauma	1/12 (8)
Spontaneous	7/12 (58)
Trauma	1/12 (8)

*Total numbers reported for each predisposition were limited by availability of data. Some patients had more than one predisposition.
From Croak AJ, Gelshart JB, Kingele CJ, et al: Characteristics of patients with vaginal vault rupture and evisceration. Obstet Gynecol 103:573, 2004.

and evaluated, depending on the size and depth of the defect. Similar to the management of wound infections, digital examination of the defect is important so that the full extent of the problem will be recognized. With larger defects, the wound edges must be débrided and the wound closed with a modified Smead-Jones or mass closure technique.

When a closure of a hernia is indicated during surgery, either as part of the primary surgery or after débridement, two principles are emphasized. The closure should be sterile, with all signs of infection resolved. Secondly, mesh should be used to close the defect. Studies have noted a significantly lower disruption rate with mesh closure than with suture.

WOUND CARE FOR OBESE PATIENTS

Obesity is one of the most significant risk factors for wound infection and disruption. As noted, hyperglycemia is an associated risk factor in this population of patients. Optimal healing, collagen synthesis, and reepithelialization require good oxygenation. Adipose tissue is poorly vascularized and thus has suboptimal oxygenation. Poor ventilation after surgery in the obese woman further exacerbates this problem. Techniques to improve wound healing in obese patients have ben summarized by Walsh and associates; these include maintaining normothermia in the operating suite, which decreases vasoconstriction, and closure of the subcutaneous space if it is larger than 2 cm. Subcutaneous drains do not decrease the infection or wound disruption rate. When patients have a BMI more than 35, many clinicians will double the prophylactic antibiotic dose (e.g., from 1 g of cefazolin to 2 g). However, extending the dosing beyond surgery is not helpful. See **Box 25-6.**

Box 25-6 Techniques to Decrease Wound DIsruption and Infection in Obese Surgical Patients

1. Chlorhexidine bath or shower the night before surgery
2. Women with BMI > 35—double the dosage of prophylactic antibiotics
3. Maintain core normothermia during the operation.
4. Close subcutaneous tissue if >2 cm in depth
5. Sterile dressing for 24-48 hr
6. Maintain euglycemia.
7. Excess oxygen during surgery and subcutaneous drains do not improve outcomes.

OPERATIVE SITE COMPLICATIONS

PELVIC CELLULITIS AND ABSCESS

Infections of the contiguous retroperitoneal space immediately above the vaginal apex are common complications following abdominal or vaginal hysterectomy. However, the frequency of this postoperative complication has dramatically decreased in direct relation to the use of prophylactic antibiotics. These soft tissue infections range in severity from localized minor cellulitis to large pelvic abscesses and have many names, from **cuff cellulitis** to infected hematoma. Nevertheless, they are similar to soft tissue infections in other parts of the body and are a cellulitis or an abscess. These infections prolong hospital stay and increase the cost of patient care. The bacterial spectrum that produces these infections includes aerobic and anaerobic bacteria from exogenous and endogenous sources. Most postoperative pelvic infections are polymicrobial, usually from endogenous vaginal flora, and approximately 60% to 80% involve anaerobic organisms.

The pathophysiology of the development of retroperitoneal infection is straightforward. The classic "clamp, crush, cut and tie technique" used in pelvic surgery produces an abundance of hypoxic and anoxic tissue that helps establish an optimal environment for infection. This environment is further enhanced by the normal retroperitoneal hysterectomy site, producing an average of 40 mL of serosanguineous fluid daily during the first 72 postoperative hours. The endogenous flora of the upper vagina colonize and multiply in this retroperitoneal serosanguineous fluid and in pelvic hematomas after the surgery.

The major symptoms of an operative site infection are fever associated with lower quadrant abdominal and pelvic pain. The fever usually becomes prominent between the third and fifth postoperative days. As the infection becomes more severe, the fever becomes spiking in character, the pain intensifies, and the patient develops moderate leukocytosis.

The diagnosis of cuff cellulitis is confirmed by pelvic examination. Pelvic tenderness and induration are prominent during the bimanual examination. A subtle difference exists between normal postoperative pelvic tenderness and induration and the tenderness and induration produced by infection. Postoperative infection is accompanied by an increase in suprapubic pain and lateral parametrial tenderness. Cuff cellulitis sometimes responds to drainage by opening the vaginal cuff. Appropriate cultures of the site are difficult with cellulitis because of vaginal contamination. Persistent cellulitis, one encompassing a large area, or a pelvic abscess necessitates parenteral antibiotic therapy. Often, the diagnosis of a retroperitoneal abscess is confirmed when the patient has ongoing fever and pelvic tenderness after 2 to 3 days of parenteral antibiotics for a suspected cuff cellulitis. Eason and colleagues have reported that the volume of pelvic fluid 3 to 5 days postoperatively after a hysterectomy is a nonspecific finding and does not predict febrile morbidity or the need for drainage. They further commented that large or complex fluid collections may be present without adverse clinical consequences. CT-directed biopsy may aid in diagnosis.

Because of their polymicrobial origin, infections are usually treated with an aminoglycoside (gentamicin) and an antibiotic specific for anaerobic infection (clindamycin). Metronidazole (Flagyl) may be substituted for clindamycin. An alternative therapy is substitution of a third-generation cephalosporin or the monobactam agent aztreonam (Azactam) for the aminoglycoside.

Aztreonam has a similar spectrum of antibiotic coverage, with much less renal toxicity; however, it is much more expensive. IV antibiotics should be continued until the patient is afebrile for 24 hours. Studies have documented that oral antibiotic therapy is unnecessary following successful parenteral therapy. Alternatives to the aminoglycoside-clindamycin regimen include broad-spectrum antibiotics combined with β-lactamase inhibitors such as ampicillin-sulbactam, amoxicillin-clavulanate, piperacillin-tazobactam, or ticarcillin-clavulanate. These drugs have better coverage of *Enterobacteriaceae* spp. and *Enterococcus*. Although many pelvic abscesses drain spontaneously, patients should have serial pelvic examinations and endovaginal ultrasound or CT imaging to determine the most appropriate time and modality to effect drainage. Appropriate cultures should be obtained from the center of an abscess cavity when the abscess is operatively incised. If a woman does not become afebrile within 48 hours of adequate drainage of a retroperitoneal abscess, a concomitant complication of pelvic thrombophlebitis should be suspected. If pelvic thrombophlebitis is suspected, a 72-hour trial of IV heparin therapy with concurrent antibiotics should be instituted.

GRANULATION TISSUE

Granulation tissue at the apex of the vaginal vault is a frequent complication following hysterectomy. Small areas of friable, red granulation tissue are seen at the 6-week postoperative pelvic examination in more than 50% of women. Granulation tissue is more common following abdominal than vaginal hysterectomy. Colombo and associates have found that the incidence of cuff cellulitis and formation of granulation tissue is no different between women with the vaginal cuff left open and those in whom it is closed after abdominal hysterectomy. Manyonda and coworkers have conducted a prospective randomized trial of women with total abdominal hysterectomies comparing polyglactin (Vicryl) and chromic catgut for closure of the cuff. In this study, 32% of women had developed vault granulation tissue by their 6-week postoperative checkup. Of women who developed granulation tissue, chromic catgut was implicated twice as frequently as polyglactin suture, 68% versus 32%, respectively.

Excessive granulation tissue is the result of an exaggerated healing response of the vascular-rich pelvic tissues. One of the causes is believed to be inversion of the vaginal epithelium between the margins of the edges of the incision at the apex of the vaginal vault.

Some patients are asymptomatic, but many women experience spotting or a bloody discharge after intercourse. A rare woman may have mild pelvic discomfort. On speculum examination, the granulation tissue appears as a polypoid projection hanging from the vaginal suture line. The differential diagnosis includes a prolapsed fallopian tube and recurrent carcinoma in a woman with a pelvic malignancy. The polypoid mass is easily avulsed from the vaginal apex. The remaining areas of granulation tissue should be treated with a chemical cautery (e.g., silver nitrate, Monsel's solution) or by cryocauterization or electrocauterization.

INCISIONAL HERNIA

Vertical midline incisions produce the highest rate of abdominal wall hernias, 10% to 15%. Most will present within 1 year of surgery. Diabetes, poor nutrition, and obesity are all predisposing factors for postoperative hernia. Transverse and Pfannenstiel incisions have a low rate, followed by laparoscopic incisions, with the lowest rate of hernia. In obese and diabetic patients, it is prudent to close the fascia if the laparoscopic incision extends beyond 1 cm. Studies have noted a 2% to 3% hernia rate in laparoscopic sites of 12 mm or larger. More recent studies with modern trocars have noted that 1% of patients will develop hernias.

PROLAPSED FALLOPIAN TUBE

Prolapse of the distal end of the fallopian tube is a rare complication of abdominal or vaginal hysterectomy. It is usually discovered during a routine visit during the first few months (up to 6 months) following surgery. Factors that may predispose a woman to develop prolapse of the fallopian tube include hematoma formation and postoperative pelvic infection.

Many women with this complication are free of symptoms, but others experience a watery discharge, postcoital spotting and pain, or moderate lower abdominal and pelvic pain. Differing from granulation tissue, the fallopian tube is not friable and is firmly attached. Grasping the fallopian tube with an instrument and applying traction produces much more pain than traction on granulation tissue. Treatment is the destruction of the segment of the fallopian tube protruding through the vaginal vault with cryocauterization or laser. Because the fallopian tube is well innervated, any destructive procedure must be performed with anesthesia. The fallopian tube may be removed during a subsequent outpatient procedure with adequate anesthesia. Most clinicians opt for a vaginal approach, with ligation of the fallopian tube as high as possible. The stump of the tube is buried retroperitoneally and the vaginal epithelium is closed. Some difficult cases must be performed transabdominally via laparoscope or minilaparotomy. An alternative treatment is coagulation of the segment of fallopian tube protruding through the vaginal apex with cryocauterization. Because of the tube's innervation, this must be done with anesthesia. Often, the vaginal wall reepithelializes over the area, thereby excluding the tube from any connection with the vaginal cavity.

LYMPHOCYST

A **lymphocyst** is a local collection of lymphatic fluid within the retroperitoneal spaces of the pelvis resulting from retrograde drainage of lymph. It is a rare complication, discovered most frequently after pelvic node dissections. In the past, this complication occurred in approximately 20% of patients having undergone radical surgery. However, with meticulous attention to ligation of distal lymphatic channels and abandonment of the practice of reperitonealization, this complication is reported in less than 5% of these cases. A peritoneal opening, or peritoneal window, allows flow of the lymphatic fluid into the peritoneal cavity, with subsequent peritoneal resorption. The incidence is lower in series in which palpation alone is used to identify the cysts. If ultrasound examination is used postoperatively to screen for lymphocysts, the incidence is 10-fold greater. Conditions that predispose the woman to formation of a lymphocyst are previous radiation and anticoagulation.

Lymphocysts usually present during the first 6 postoperative weeks. They vary greatly in size and seldom become infected. The cyst usually begins anteriorly and medially to the iliac vessels. As it expands, it may produce pelvic pain, leg pain, fever, obstruction or angulation of the ureter, pressure symptoms on the bladder, or partial venous obstruction. Small lymphocysts (< 4 cm in diameter) are usually asymptomatic and regress spontaneously within 8 weeks. Larger cysts may necessitate treatment by intermittent aspiration or marsupialization performed laparoscopically, or placement of an omental flap.

OVARIAN ABSCESS

Ovarian abscess is a rare but serious postoperative complication. This condition is potentially fatal because of intraperitoneal rupture of the abscess. Ovarian abscesses arise from bacterial colonization of the ovarian cortex without primary involvement of the fallopian tube. This may occur via disruption of the ovarian capsule by the presence of a recently ruptured corpus luteum or via an operative disruption, such as cystectomy performed during vaginal hysterectomy.

The disease may follow a slow indolent course or a rapidly progressive one. Some patients with this complication present during the first postoperative week with high fever and severe pain, which are continuous until rupture occurs. Other patients will be afebrile, but return at some time during the first few months with a persistent low-grade fever and mild pain. Chronologically, most ovarian abscesses appear later in the postoperative course compared with other retroperitoneal abscesses. Ovarian abscesses usually appear 2 to 3 weeks postoperatively, but cases have been reported as late as 3 to 4 months later. Willson and Black, in a classic work describing 28 patients with ovarian abscess, noted that the predominant symptom was abdominal pain associated with persistent tachycardia and high fever. This abscess is found higher in the pelvis than a retroperitoneal abscess at the apex of the vagina.

Initial treatment is medical therapy with IV antibiotics. However, most patients do not respond to medical therapy and drainage of the abscess becomes a necessity, either percutaneously with imaging-directed aspiration or surgically. If surgical drainage is required, the abdominal approach is preferable. This rare problem should be considered in any woman having a gynecologic operation in which the integrity of the ovarian capsule is disrupted physiologically or operatively.

POSTOPERATIVE NEUROPATHY

Postoperative neuropathy is an uncommon but significant and sometimes debilitating problem. A review of gynecologic injuries by Irvin and associates has found the three most common causes of neuropathy to be related to self-retaining retractors, overly flexed thighs when women are placed in the dorsal lithotomy position, and surgical resection.

The femoral nerve is the largest branch of the lumbar plexus and arises from the primary dorsal rami of L2, L3, and L4. It provides motor function to several leg muscles, including the quadriceps, and sensory fibers that innervate the anterior and medial surfaces of the thigh and leg. The vascular supply to the femoral nerve may be compromised during an abdominal or vaginal hysterectomy. The cause of this complication is usually related to continuous pressure, usually by a self-retaining retractor producing ischemic necrosis of the nerve. The vascular circulation of the nerve itself is compromised by diminished blood flow in the vasa nervorum. The most common site of nerve compression is 4 to 6 cm above the inguinal ligament where the nerve pierces the psoas muscle.

Factors that contribute to the development of this complication are thinness of the woman, long retractor blades, prolonged operative times, and systemic diseases such as diabetes mellitus, gout, alcoholism, and malnutrition. The classic woman who develops this complication is a short, thin, athletic woman who has a transverse incision in which a self-retaining retractor is used. A similar problem may develop after vaginal operations or laparoscopy in thin women who are placed into exaggerated hip flexion or abduction in the dorsal lithotomy position. Dunnihoo and colleagues have reported on 33 cases of femoral neuropathy after vaginal hysterectomy. Femoral neuropathy following vaginal surgery is believed to be secondary to compromise of the nerve by severe angulation of the woman, not secondary to pressure injury from retractors. In a recent series, Bohrer and associates found peripheral nerve injury in 1.8% of 616 patients with elective gynecologic procedures, with almost all related to positioning. Most of these could be related to exaggerated flexion for laparoscopic and vaginal surgeries. Two patients had motor and sensory losses. in this series, all but one woman had resolution of neuropathy with medical treatment.

Patients with this complication may experience numbness, paresthesias, and difficulty with their gait. Patients may have difficulty lifting the affected knee because of the involvement of the quadriceps. Symptoms may present with a spectrum of severity. Usually, the neurologic symptoms develop within the first 24 to 72 hours following surgery. These symptoms are causes of great anxiety to the woman. Because of the inability to lift the leg, climbing stairs is a particular problem. Muscle and sensory function recover spontaneously over several weeks to several months. The woman should be seen by a physical therapist to facilitate ambulation and prevent muscle atrophy.

To prevent this complication, it is important to palpate the lateral pelvic wall and femoral artery after placement of a self-retaining retractor. With the woman in the lithotomy position, one should check for pulsations in the popliteal or posterior tibial vessels. In a thin woman, placing folded towels between the skin surface and self-retaining retractor helps prevent this complication by decreasing the depth of penetration of the lateral retractor blades.

The ilioinguinal and iliohypogastric nerves pass in a transverse and diagonal course through the anterior lower abdominal musculature medial to the inguinal ligament and through the inguinal canal. The nerves supply sensory fibers to the labia, mons pubis, and medial thigh. The nerves may become injured during surgery with a Pfannenstiel incision or during a urinary incontinence procedure (**Fig. 25-12**). Pathophysiologically, the nerve may be transected or entrapped by suture or scar formation. Sharp or burning pain may develop immediately postoperatively or usually within a few days. The pain may radiate to the groin or vulva. Most symptoms will resolve spontaneously. Severe pain may necessitate nerve block, suture removal, or segmented removal of the involved nerve. Several specific postoperative neuropathies are related to specific procedures. Uterosacral ligament suspension may affect the sacral plexus (S2 to S4) and produce pain and numbness in the posterior thigh and buttocks. Pudendal neuropathy has been reported with cystocele repairs and graft placement producing pain and numbness in the vulva and perineum. If symptoms are not relieved with analgesics and other medications, such as gabapentin, surgical removal of the sutures may be necessary.

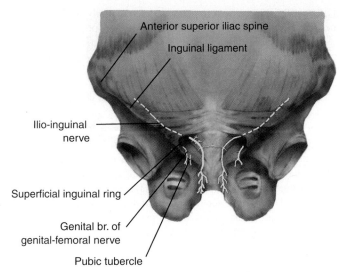

Figure 25-12 Ilioinguinal nerve entrapment during needle suspension for stress incontinence. (From Miyazaki F, Shook G: Ilioinguinal nerve entrapment during needle suspension for stress incontinence. Obstet Gynecol 80:246, 1992.)

When pain does not resolve and becomes chronic, it develops a CNS component. Thus, many patients with long-standing pain will respond to CNS-directed therapies. Mendell and Sahenk have reviewed sensory neuropathies. Tricyclic antidepressants, selective serotonin reuptake inhibitors (SSRIs), and anticonvulsants such as carbamazepine, gabapentin, and lamotrigine, have been found to be effective adjunctive agents for this complication, although gabapentin is the most studied. Long-term pain in the incision may also be related to small neuromas.

ESTROGEN REPLACEMENT

Bilateral salpingo-oophorectomy is sometimes performed on young women for conditions such as pelvic inflammatory disease. National surveys have documented that bilateral salpingo-oophorectomy concomitant with hysterectomy is performed in approximately 25% of premenopausal women. Removal of the ovaries in a premenopausal woman reduces the serum estradiol concentration by approximately 80% and serum testosterone concentration by approximately 50%. The possible consequences of estrogen deprivation include vasomotor symptoms, urogenital tissue atrophy (e.g., atrophic vaginitis, dyspareunia, urethral syndrome), and osteoporosis. Removal of the ovaries in premenopausal women may lead to clinically significant sexual dysfunction.

Estrogen replacement is indicated for the vast majority of premenopausal women having bilateral oophorectomy. The increase in hypercoagulability produced by the doses of estrogen used for postmenopausal symptoms is negligible. Nevertheless, because of the physiologic hypercoagulability and injury to the intima of vessels associated with the operative procedure, oral estrogen therapy should not be started immediately after the procedure. Estradiol given via a cutaneous patch or vaginal ring is more acceptable in the immediate postoperative period than oral estrogen because of the difference in effect of the associated relative decrease in the liver's production of clotting factors. An oral tablet of 0.625 mg of conjugated estrogens daily is sufficient to protect from bone demineralization and osteoporosis. A higher dose may be required to alleviate hot flushes. Most women in the perimenopausal age range who undergo oophorectomy will also develop symptomatic hot flushes. In general, women may be given estrogen replacement when they become symptomatic. This may occur within a few days to 1 week after surgery. Transdermal estrogen produces significantly fewer changes in coagulation factors than oral estrogen. A 0.05- to 0.1-mg estradiol patch to premenopausal women without risk factors to use estrogen, starting 2 days after surgery, is also effective. In women older than 45 years, many clinicians await symptoms. If estrogen is contraindicated, SSRIs may be helpful alternatives. The small amount of evidence regarding estrogen replacement in this setting indicates that quality of life improves after hysterectomy and that sexual function is not adversely affected. Estrogen replacement is usually limited to 5 years.

PSYCHOLOGICAL SEQUELAE

PAIN RELIEF

The proper management of pain during the postoperative period should be an essential task and goal of all gynecologists. Most women experience moderate to severe pain during the first 36 to 48 hours following a gynecologic operation. However, pain and suffering are personal internal events, the extent and presence of which may best be measured by direct communication with the woman. Pain is initiated at the local level through the trauma of the surgery. Systemic and neurologic pathways are then activated (**Fig. 25-13**). The most effective pain management strategies involve inhibiting the initiation and activation of these broader pain reflexes. Such inhibition is also associated with the fewest side effects. A systematic review from Virian and coworkers has considered factors that might predict postoperative pain and the use of pain medications. Preoperative pain, mental state (e.g., high levels of anxiety, depression, negative

affect), and type of surgery were directly correlated with analgesic use. Age was inversely correlated with pain and pain medication usage. Gender did not correlate with pain. Studies comparing types of hysterectomy, abdominal, vaginal, and laparoscopic have found a descending order of postoperative pain, as might be anticipated. However, selection bias in these studies is a significant confounder.

The current literature documents that pain relief is often treated inadequately in postoperative patients. For many women who undergo gynecologic surgery, dosages of analgesics are prescribed that are less than adequate to relieve pain, and many nurses further reduce the amount of medication. The many misconceptions concerning postoperative pain include the dangers of addiction and the fear of respiratory depression. Kuhn and colleagues have emphasized that it is not only physicians and nurses who contribute to ineffective treatment, but patients also contribute by having a lower level of pain relief expectation. They believe that pain relief is poor because of inadequate education of patients about what to expect from pain relief. Inadequate pain relief prolongs hospital stay and has adverse psychological consequences. Also, several investigators have noted that inadequately treated pain increases secondary morbidities, including atelectasis from decreased mobility, increased inflammatory response, and elevated glucose levels, with higher catecholamine levels. Studies have shown that epidural anesthesia (presumably by inhibiting the spinal pain reflexes) has a significantly diminished effect on the immune response in patients undergoing laparotomy. Syndromes of chronic pain are presumed to begin with inadequate pain relief in the postoperative period.

More than 3 decades ago, White presented a schematic representation of the pain cycle and the potential delays in pain relief with traditional PRN analgesic regimens (**Fig. 25-14**). Many studies have confirmed that regular-interval preventive pain relief is superior to conventional on demand analgesic medication during the first 36 to 48 hours after surgery. However, there is great variability in absorption. In addition, the therapeutic window—the range of effective blood concentration before undesired side effects occur—is narrow. In White's study, peak concentrations varied as much as fivefold among the 10 different individuals and the time to reach peak blood level varied as much as sevenfold. Thus, patient-controlled analgesia (PCA) systems have become one of the preferred methods of pain relief during

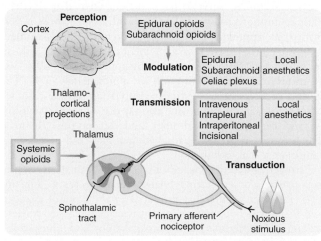

Figure 25-13 Schematic drawing of the pathways for transmission of painful stimuli. (From Sherwood E, Williams CG, Prough DS: Anaesthesiology principles, pain management, and conscious sedation. In Townsend CM, Beauchamp RD, Evers BM, et al [eds]: Sabiston Textbook of Surgery, 17th ed. Philadelphia, Saunders, 2004.)

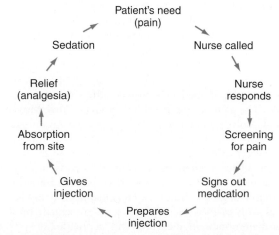

Figure 25-14 Pain cycle. (From White PF: Pain management (special report). Postgrad Med 80:8, 1986.)

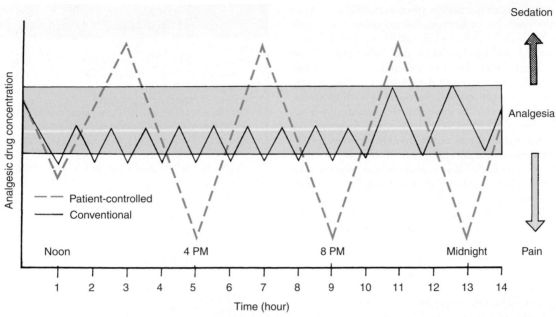

Figure 25-15 Theoretical relationships among dosing interval, analgesic drug concentration, and clinical effects when comparing patient-controlled analgesia (PCA) system *(solid lines)* with conventional intramuscular therapy *(dashed lines)*. (Adapted from White PF: Semin Anesthesiol 4:255, 1985.)

the immediate postoperative period (**Fig. 25-15**). PCA systems dramatically decrease patients' anxiety because they are in control, rather than the hospital staff. These systems are safe and effective as long as there is a lockout period, and they help minimize individual differences in pharmacokinetics. Modern PCA systems minimize the risk of drug overdose and allow the patient to titrate and therefore maximize analgesic effectiveness. In general, patients use the PCA for approximately 12 to 36 hours until they are completely tolerating oral feeding. A meta-analysis from Remy and associates has found that the addition of acetaminophen with an opioid PCA reduces the amount of opioid needed. Sample dosing for PCA is listed in **Appendix D** (online). Women should be given instructions concerning PCA to help alleviate inherent fears of addiction. Their families need instruction in not pushing the medication for the patient to help alleviate pain. PCA is less effective in older patients, who are more affected by confusion and disorientation.

Perioperative intrathecal or epidural injections of opioids effectively relieve postoperative pelvic pain in most situations. Side effects are primarily itching and a small risk of hypotension.

Continuous PCA epidurals may also be used. The advantages and disadvantages of PCA and epidural anesthesia are presented in **Table 25-19**.

In addition to narcotics, NSAIDs are valuable as adjunctive agents. NSAIDs are most effective when given as scheduled medications and as early as possible in the postoperative period. Their mechanism of action is the inhibition of prostaglandin production. Through inhibition of prostaglandins, pain is prevented rather than blocked centrally. NSAID have three potential side effects. The first is increased gastric acid, best treated by H2 blockers or proton pump inhibitors. Second, renal toxicity which may be prevented by using set doses and prescribing only for women with normal renal function with adequate intravascular volume. Third is inhibition of platelet function with higher doses of NSAIDs. Some clinicians will wait 1 to 2 hours after surgery before giving these agents to avoid excessive bleeding. Advantages of prostaglandin synthetase inhibitors are a lack of effect on gastrointestinal motility and a much smaller effect on sensorium than narcotic agents. Commonly used NSAIDs for postoperative pain include ibuprofen, naproxen, and

Table 25-19 Advantages and Disadvantages of Epidural Analgesia and Patient-Controlled Analgesia

Epidural Analgesia	Patient-Controlled Analgesia	Comments
Advantages	Immediate pain relief	Requires no special nursing or anesthesia support postoperatively
	May improve colon motility	Gives the patient personal control over administration of pain medication
	May improve postoperative pulmonary function after lower abdominal and pelvic surgery	
	Less sedating than patient-controlled analgesia	
Disadvantages	Requires a skilled anesthesiologist for correct placement	Patient may experience pain in the recovery room until an adequate serum level of medication is achieved
	May interfere with ambulation	
	May delay removal of Foley catheter	

From Baker VV: Principles of postoperative care. In Baker VV, Deppe G (eds): Management of Perioperative Complications in Gynecology. Philadelphia, WB Saunders, 1997.

ketorolac (Toradol). Ketorolac may be given as an IM or IV injection during the operative procedure. IM injections reach peak plasma levels in 40 to 50 min, with a half-life of 4 to 6 hours. The dose is an IM loading dose of 30 mg, followed by 15 to 30 mg every 6 hours during the first 24 to 36 hours. More commonly, ketorolac is given IV every 4 to 6 hours, 15 to 30 mg. The drug works well when given concomitantly with narcotics. Ketorolac should not be used for more than 4 consecutive days because of GI side effects. In older adults, changes in GI function may limit the usefulness of these agents. Stomach colonization with *Helicobacter pylori* increases with increasing age. Of women older than 80 years, 80% are colonized. These bacteria increase sensitivity to GI irritation. Prophylactic H2 blockers or proton pump inhibitors should be considered when administering NSAID to older patients.

Many of the side effects of the NSAIDs are caused by cyclooxygenase-1 (COX-1) inhibition. The development of selective COX-2 inhibitors has promise, although warnings regarding cardiovascular side effects have limited their acceptance at this time. Sample protocols for pain orders are listed in **Appendix D** (online).

Many surgeons and anesthesiologists believe that giving analgesics in the perioperative period prior to the patient's sensation of pain (giving them preemptively) leads to better pain control. Many studies have noted that the beneficial effects are significant when infiltration is given prior to the surgical incision. Because much pain arises from peritoneal irritation and fascial trauma, incisional infiltration is most effective with minimally invasive procedures such as laparoscopy. Infiltration is most commonly used with a local anesthetic, lidocaine 1%, or bupivacaine, 0.25%. Temporary indwelling infusion catheters that use local anesthetics have been shown in multiple studies and systematic reviews to benefit patients through decreased opioid use, earlier ambulation, and decreased PONV. Catheters are placed above and below the fascia and removed on day 3. In patients who are expected to require large amounts of opioid, such as those already on chronic narcotics for pain, the addition of gabapentin decreases narcotic use, perceived pain levels, and PONV. A meta-analysis has found a 35% reduction in pain (95% CI, 0.59 to 0.72). Most studies used 1200 mg/day.

Patients with persistent incisional pain, longer than 4 to 6 months, should be evaluated for incisional neuromas. Neuromas are thought to arise from damaged and transected peripheral nerves that the develop a fibrous capsule. If a superficial small trigger area can be identified, an injection of 1% hydrocortisone with 2 to 3 mL of 0.25% bupivacaine may be attempted. If this is unsuccessful, referral to a surgeon with expertise in peripheral nerves should be considered.

POSTOPERATIVE CONCERNS IN OLDER SURGICAL PATIENTS

Patients older than 70 years, particularly those 80 years and older, need special consideration in the perioperative period. Studies of older women undergoing gynecologic surgery have found that for elective procedures, the complication rates are no different from those of younger women after adjusting for comorbidities. **Box 25-7** summarizes physical changes that should be kept in mind when caring for older surgical patients. The cardiovascular system is affected with increased systemic vascular resistance and a poorer response to systemic catecholamines. Many anesthetic agents decrease cardiac contractility.

Box 25-7 Physiologic Changes in Older Adults That Might Affect Surgery

Cardiovascular
- Approximate 1% decrease in cardiac output/yr after age 30 yr
- Decreased vascular compliance and increased systemic vascular resistance (SVR)
- Increased cardiovascular disease
- Decreased cardiac output in response to stress
- Increased susceptibiity to conduction abnormalities

Pulmonary
- Decreased pulmonary reserve
- Dectreased mucus-producing cells, with increased susceptibility to infection
- Decreased elasticity in the lungs
- Decreased forced expiratory volume in 1 second (FEV_1)
- Decreased functional residual capacity (FRC), exacerbated with postoperative pain and atelectasis

Renal
- Decreased glomerular filtration rate (GFR), $\approx$1% decrease/yr after age 20
- Serum creatinine level not effective measure of renal function in this situation

Skeletal
- Increased osteoporosis, with increase in injury from falls
- Decreased rib expansion, so poorer response to need for postoperative lung expansion

Nutritional
- Poorer nutrition
- Greater incidence of vitamin deficiencies, including vitamin B_{12}

The hematocrit level, as noted, should be maintained above 30%. Atrial fibrillation and cardiac failure are the two most common cardiac complications and attention to intravascular volume is important to maintain cardiac output. Many older women have decreased appetites and poor nutrition; this should be addressed prior to elective surgery. The nursing staff often is hesitant to give enough pain medications for fear of oversedation. However, inadequate pain relief is a worse sequela. Epidural PCA is a desirable postoperative tool for pain relief.

Postoperative delirium and postoperative cognitive dysfunction (POCD) are altered levels of mental function occurring after surgery. These conditions are more common in the older adults. Prolonged and delayed mental status changes may be caused by decreased oxygen, decreased cardiac output, medications, and drug-drug interactions. In general, postoperative delirium occurs 24 to 72 hours after surgery. Disorientation, sleep deprivation, and pain may all be contributing factors. The condition occurs in 5% to 15% of older patients and increases the risk of patient falls. Postoperative cognitive dysfunction may occur for a few months after surgery and has been noted to some degree in up to 5% of older surgical patients.

Postoperative disorientation and agitation are related to patient falls. Patients will try to get out of bed on their own. The nursing staff needs to be attentive to bowel and bladder needs and to help patients get out of bed in a timely routine.

PSYCHOSEXUAL PROBLEMS AND DEPRESSION

The time immediately before and after a surgical procedure is a stressful period for all women and their families. Anxiety and fear are normal responses and should be anticipated by health care providers. Any surgery on the female reproductive organs stimulates questions and conflicts concerning body image, feminine identity, sexuality, and possibly future childbearing. The period after a gynecologic operation is one of transition and is a unique psychological challenge to the woman. The reader should review Chapter 9 (Emotional Aspects of Gynecology) for a more detailed discussion of the problems of loss and grief. After gynecologic surgery, every woman needs support to deal with this challenge, and it is important to emphasize that it may take many months to complete the process.

Personal issues that relate to a woman's body image and sexuality are particularly affected by hysterectomy. In premenopausal women who have undergone bilateral salpingo-oophorectomy, physiologic dosages of transdermal testosterone have been demonstrated to improve sexual function. The exogenous androgens also resulted in a beneficial effect on well-being and depression. Open discussions with the woman that allow her to discuss issues regarding sexuality are important during preoperative and postoperative visits. Psychological studies have confirmed that sexual function after a hysterectomy is related to a number of factors. Poor knowledge of reproductive anatomy, a negative expectation of sexual recovery after the operation, preoperative psychiatric morbidity, and a history of unsatisfactory sexual relationships are all associated with a poor outcome. A review by Farrell and Kieser has noted that although many studies have been done, their methodology is vastly different and does not allow definitive conclusions. Individual factors are more important determinants of sexual function than the particular surgery. In summary, the effect of hysterectomy on sexual function is an exceedingly complex topic, with both physical and psychological factors known to have varying and almost unquantifiable influences.

MENTAL STATUS CHANGES

Anxiety and mental status changes are not uncommon in the postoperative period. Medications, hemodynamic changes, fever, and altered sleep patterns contribute to changes in sensorium. These changes are most pronounced in older adults. Multivariate analyses have correlated pain levels, hematocrit under 30%, smoking, and a history of psychiatric disorders with postoperative mental status changes. Other than hematocrit levels, these factors are difficult to control. Mental status change does require evaluation (**Box 25-8**). Changes in oxygenation,

---

Box 25-8 Causes of Acute Delirium

Drug intoxication (alcohol, antihistamines, sedatives)
Drug withdrawal (alcohol, narcotics, anxiolytics)
Acute cerebral disorders (edema, transient ischemic attack stroke, neoplasm)
Metabolic disturbances (electrolyte, imbalance, hypoglycemia)
Hemodynamic disturbances (hypovolemia, myocardial infarction, congestive heart failure)
Infections (septicemia, urinary tract infection, pneumonia)
Respiratory disorders (respiratory failure, pulmonary embolism)
Trauma (head injury, burns)

From Dayton MT: Surgical complications. In Townsend CM, Beauchamp RD, Evers BM, et al (eds): Sabiston Textbook of Surgery, 17th ed. Philadelphia, Saunders, 2004.

---

electrolyte imbalance, sepsis, medication interactions, and acute anemia need to be excluded.

A syndrome of nausea, sweating, tachycardia, tremors, delirium, and even grand mal seizures postoperatively is often misdiagnosed as a drug or anesthetic reaction. This constellation of signs and symptoms is usually caused by alcohol withdrawal. The presence of a tremor should alert health care providers to the correct diagnosis. In the treatment of postalcohol withdrawal symptoms, benzodiazepines are the drug of choice. In older women, especially after emergency surgery, postoperative confusion, anxiety, changes in personality, and memory impairment are frequent findings, and a large differential diagnosis must be considered.

DISCHARGE INSTRUCTIONS AND POSTOPERATIVE VISITS

Simple but complete discharge instructions are an important component of postoperative care. The physician should anticipate the most common questions and give the woman explicit instructions. Particular attention should be given to limitations in physical activity, such as heavy lifting and resumption of sexual relations. Information should be given about vaginal spotting as sutures dissolve. Appropriate contact information should be provided in case of unanticipated complications and to schedule return appointments. An accomplished clinician, Eugene A. Stead, Jr., has taught that discharge instructions should not be given on the morning of discharge. Rather, patients should receive these instructions the day before discharge; then, a post-test is given on the morning of discharge to ensure that the patient understands the instructions. Instructions should be given in verbal and written forms. Because an increasing number of procedures are performed as outpatient surgery or short stays, the physician must modify instructions to accommodate the gradual resumption of activity. The 24- to 48-hour postdischarge phone call to the recovering woman provides an excellent forum for answering questions and providing reassurance. Studies of outpatient surgeries have found this contact to be most important. Additionally, it is difficult for the woman and her significant others to remember instructions received during the first 24 hours after surgery. Written guidelines are extremely valuable for outpatient procedures. Careful training of nursing and triage staff in regard to postoperative questions cannot be overemphasized. Patients will usually be home when the first signs of complications occur. These signs and symptoms may in themselves be minor, but may presage a more serious complication that could evolve. Thus, a much higher index of suspicion should be used with these patients.

Most clinicians will see patients from 1 to 3 weeks and again at 5 to 6 weeks after surgery. The first visit is an important time to review and answer questions about surgical findings and hospital interactions. Many patients and their families will hold off on expressing concerns until after discharge for fear of creating problems. An open-ended question, such as, "Did things go as you expected?" will help clear up any problems before they become deeper sources of anxiety or mistrust. From 1 to 3 weeks, patients are transitioning back to routine activities. Questions about appropriate levels of activity can be answered at the first postoperative visit. Discussions of reestablishing sexual relations and physical activity are important to review at this time.

Physical examination of the incision, IV sites, and extremities are indicated at the first visit. Unless there is a problem or a specific issue, a pelvic examination may be deferred until the second visit at 5 to 6 weeks after the procedure. If vaginal surgery or vaginal pain or pressure is present, then a vaginal examination may be indicated.

The discussion of surgical findings occurs at several points during the postoperative period. Initially, patients are drowsy after waking up from anesthesia or IV analgesics. Families may want to know the results prior to the patient hearing them. Preoperatively, it is important to clarify with the woman who in the family can know what information. During the early postoperative period, the gynecologist must judge how much information to provide. This should be tailored to what the patient can understand, depending on her level of wakefulness. Honesty at all times is the basic ethical principle; however, if the woman is waking up from anesthesia, she obviously will not be able to understand a detailed description of operative findings. The art of medicine is called into play at this point in knowing how much to explain. By the end of the first few days, the discussion may move to details of surgical findings as well as treatment options, sequelae, and prognosis if a long-term problem has been found.

KEY POINTS

- Often, the woman and her family judge the competence of the gynecologist by the compassion displayed during the immediate postoperative period.
- Postoperative febrile morbidity is related to infection in approximately 20% of cases and noninfectious causes in 80% of cases.
- Infection in older adults will not always present with classic findings. The amount of temperature elevation may not reflect the severity of the infection. Not uncommonly, the first signs of infection in older adults will be mental status changes. Also, the degree of leukocytosis may not reflect infection, being blunted or absent.
- Minimum urine output should be 0.5 mL/kg/hr. The use of a 20-mL/hr benchmark for all women is only an approximation and should be adjusted for the patient's weight.
- Because of the shifts in water balance, the postoperative hematocrit at 72 hours is a more accurate measurement of operative and postoperative blood loss than a hematocrit at 24 hours.
- The normal physiologic response to the stress of an operation and tissue destruction is release of increased levels of antidiuretic hormone and aldosterone, causing sodium and water retention.
- After subtracting the effects of the operative blood loss from the preoperative hematocrit, a further reduction in hematocrit of 3 to 5 points reflects a postoperative hemorrhage of approximately 500 mL.
- Women older than 60 years, and those with significant cardiac and pulmonary comorbidity, should be transfused if their hematocrit falls below 30%.
- Microatelectasis is a common occurrence developing during almost all pelvic surgery and is persistent 24 hours postoperatively in approximately 50% of women. Current studies have demonstrated that there is no association between fever and the amount of atelectasis diagnosed radiologically.
- Radiographic diagnoses are approximately 60% accurate for bacterial or viral pneumonia in women with laboratory-proven pneumonia.
- Rapid loss of 20% of a woman's blood volume produces mild shock, whereas a loss of greater than 40% of blood volume results in severe shock.
- From 15% to 45% of surgical blood loss is absorbed onto drapes, pads, and other areas. Thus, blood levels in the suction bottle are inaccurate markers of total operative blood loss.
- Massive blood loss has been defined as hemorrhage that results in replacement of 50% of circulating blood volume in less than 3 hours.
- Returning a patient to the operating room to control hemorrhage is often a difficult decision. However, this decision should not be postponed, and the patient should have an exploratory operation as soon as possible after volume replacement.
- The extent of wound or pelvic hematomas is determined by the potential size of the compartment into which the bleeding occurs. Retroperitoneal or broad ligament hematomas may contain several units of blood.
- Superficial phlebitis is the leading cause of an enigmatic postoperative fever during the third, fourth, or fifth postoperative day.
- The clinical management of mild superficial thrombophlebitis includes rest, elevation, and local heat. Moderate to severe superficial thrombophlebitis may be treated with nonsteroidal antiinflammatory agents.
- Venous thrombosis and PE are the direct causes of approximately 40% of deaths in gynecologic cases once the diagnosis is confirmed.
- Signs and symptoms of pulmonary emboli are nonspecific; however, the most common symptoms are chest pain, dyspnea, apprehension, tachypnea, rales, and an increase in the second heart sound over the pulmonic area.
- Intermittent in-and-out catheterization is preferable to continuous drainage with a Foley catheter for women with intermediate-term voiding dysfunction. Women especially appreciate intermittent self-catheterization because it gives them control over part of their postoperative care.
- Although symptoms of urinary incontinence may present within a few hours of the operative procedure, most fistulas usually present 8 to 12 days after operation, and occasionally as late as 25 to 30 days after the operation.
- If there is a suspicion that trauma to the bladder has occurred during an operative procedure, continuous catheter drainage for 3 to 5 days usually results in spontaneous healing.
- Approximately 25% of adult women experience postoperative nausea and vomiting.
- An uncomplicated ileus may last 24 to 48 hours in the stomach, only a few hours in the small intestines, and 48 to 72 hours in the colon.

KEY POINTS—CONTINUED

- If adynamic ileus persists for longer than 5 days, a diagnosis of mechanical bowel obstruction should be strongly considered.
- Postoperative oral feeding is safe and efficacious. This practice is preferred by women because it facilitates their recovery and shortens hospital stay.
- The difference between small bowel obstruction and adynamic ileus is subtle, because adynamic ileus is normally associated with partial obstruction of the small intestine.
- Second- and third-generation cephalosporins—clindamycin, ampicillin, and amoxicillin—are the antibiotics associated with the highest risk of developing *C. difficile* diarrhea.
- The incidence of postoperative wound infection is increased eightfold when the woman's preoperative weight exceeds 200 pounds. The thickness of subcutaneous tissue is the greatest risk factor for wound infection in women undergoing abdominal hysterectomy.
- Necrotizing fasciitis involves the subcutaneous tissue and superficial fascia. It rapidly expands in the subcutaneous spaces. If the diagnosis is questionable, a full-thickness core biopsy and frozen section of the tissue should be performed.
- This condition is a surgical emergency and patients should have operative débridement as soon as possible.
- The incidence of wound dehiscence is approximately 1 in 200 gynecologic operations. Wound infection is found in approximately 50% of women with wound disruption.
- The classic feature of an impending wound disruption is the spontaneous passage of copious serosanguineous fluid from the abdominal incision.
- Most postoperative pelvic infections are polymicrobial, usually from endogenous vaginal flora, and approximately 60% to 80% involve anaerobic organisms.
- The volume of pelvic fluid 3 to 5 days postoperatively after a hysterectomy is a nonspecific finding and does not predict febrile morbidity or the need for drainage.
- Common causes of femoral neuropathy are continuous pressure from self-retaining retractors or exaggerated hip flexion or abduction in the dorsal lithotomy position in thin women.
- Discharge instructions should be given in verbal and written forms, and the gynecologist should anticipate the most common questions. Office personnel should be particularly attuned to patients with minor complaints that might presage significant postoperative issues.

REFERENCES CAN BE FOUND ON
EXPERTCONSULT.com

26

Molecular Oncology in Gynecologic Cancer
Immunologic Response, Cytokines, Oncogenes, and Tumor Suppressor Genes

Premal H. Thaker and Anil K. Sood

Cancer develops because of the accumulation of successive and multiple molecular lesions that result in an altered cellular phenotype that is self-sufficient in growth signaling, insensitive to anti-growth signals and capable of tissue invasion and metastasis, limitless replicative potential, sustained **angiogenesis**, and evading **apoptosis**. These molecular changes can include **overexpression**, **amplification**, or **mutation** of **oncogenes**, the failure of **tumor suppressor gene** function because of a mutation, deletion, or viral infection, and the inappropriate expression of **cytokines**, growth factors, or cellular receptors. Also, natural or induced immune responses may play a role in the modulation of cancer growth because immune cells such as tumor-associated **macrophages** may actually cause tumors to grow. Based on a growing understanding of the immune response, biologic pathways, and cancer development, new immunotherapy and targeted therapies to gynecologic malignancies are being developed, and are reviewed and summarized in this chapter.

THE IMMUNOLOGIC RESPONSE

The immune system has adapted to fight off bacterial or viral infections, but it also plays a role in the surveillance and control of cancer cell growth. The immune system has two types of responses, innate and adaptive. Innate responses are non–antigen-specific, rapid, and do not increase with repetitive exposure to a given **antigen**. Components of the innate immune system include physical barriers such as epithelial surfaces, macrophages, **natural killer** (NK) cells, neutrophils, dendritic cells, and components of the **complement** system. Dendritic cells and macrophages are phagocytic cells that act as **antigen-presenting cells** (APCs). Macrophages also play an important role in the production of cytokines. Innate immune responses form the initial immune response to invading pathogens and contribute to adaptive immunity, which is comprised of **T lymphocytes** (T cells) and **B lymphocytes** (B cells) that are involved in cell-mediated immunity and **humoral immunity**, respectively.

INNATE IMMUNITY

In contrast to the adaptive immune system, which can recognize a variety of foreign substances, including tumor antigens, the innate immune system can only recognize microbial substances. For the most part, neutrophils, macrophages, NK cells, and dendritic cells are involved in the innate immune response and depend on the recognition of pattern recognition receptors (PRRs), which are encoded in the germline and identically expressed by effector cells. These receptors recognize pathogen-associated molecular patterns (PAMPs), which are expressed by microbes and trigger intracellular signaling cascades that result in inflammation and microbial death. PRRs are expressed constitutively in the host, and are not dependent on immunologic memory (**Fig. 26-1**). Toll-like receptors (TLRs) are PRRs that stimulate type 1 **interferon** (IFN) production, which has antimicrobial, antiviral, and anticancer activity. TLR agonists are being evaluated for use as vaccine adjuvants in immunotherapy trials for ovarian cancer. NK cells are a subset of the lymphocyte population, can directly kill infected cells, and recognize cells that lack **major histocompatibility complex** (MHC) class I molecules, such as bacteria. Moretta and colleagues have reported that NK cells are cytotoxic to tumor cells, probably because of a similar lack of MHC class I molecules.

The complement system plays an important role in the innate immune system and is a complex system, consisting of a large group of interacting plasma proteins. Activation by binding to antigen-complexed **antibody** molecules activates what is termed the *classical pathway*. In contrast, the alternative pathway is activated by recognition of microbial surface structures in the absence of antibody. Activation of these pathways leads to cleavage of C3 protein into a larger C3b fragment that is deposited on the microbial surface, leading to complement activation of C3a, which serves as a chemoattractant for neutrophils. Complexing of downstream complement proteins C6, C7, C8, and C9 produces a membrane pore in tagged cells that ultimately results in cell lysis. Unfortunately, tumor cells are often resistant to complement-dependent cytotoxicity. The innate immune system is intricately linked to the adaptive immune system by

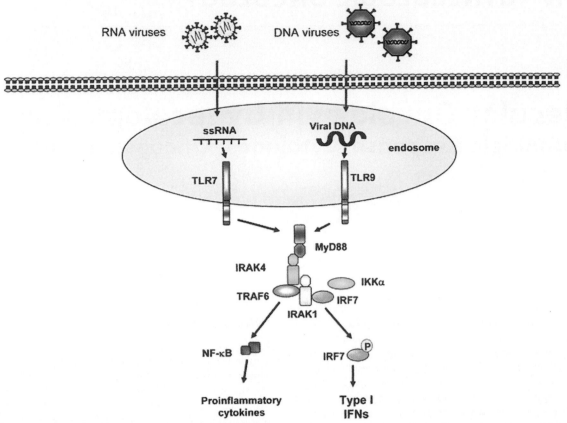

Figure 26-1 Toll-like receptors (TLRs). TLRs are pattern recognition receptors that recognize microbes, viruses, and cancer cells. TLRs recruit MyD88, which is an adaptor protein that ultimately activates interferon and proinflammatory cytokines. IKK, Inhibitor of nuclear factor-κB (IκB) kinase; IRAK-4, interleukin-1R-associated kinase-4; IRF-3, interferon regulatory factor-3; pDCs, plasmacytoid dendritic cells; TNF, tumor necrosis factor; TRAF6, TNF receptor–associated factor 6. (From Takeuchi O, Akira S: Recognition of viruses by innate immunity. Immunol Rev 220:214-224, 2007.)

activated macrophages that enhance T cell activation and complement fragments that can activate B cells and antibody production.

ADAPTIVE IMMUNITY

Humoral Immunity: B Cells and Immunoglobulins

In humans, B cells are derived from hematopoietic stem cells and aggregate in the lymph nodes, gastrointestinal tract, or spleen. B lymphocytes synthesize antibodies in response to an activated $CD8^+$ cell or **helper T cell** (Th2). Then, the B lymphocytes differentiate into **plasma cells** that secrete large quantities of antibody (**immunoglobulin**) in response to an antigen. Unlike T cells, B cells recognize antigens in an unprocessed state. Each B cell is programmed to secrete a specific type of antibody, and it is estimated that more than 10^7 different antibodies are capable of being produced in response to the presence of foreign antigens (**Fig. 26-2**).

Overall, antibodies have the same basic structure, except for extensive variability in the portion of the structure binding to the specific antigen. Two identical heavy and light chains comprise the basic immunoglobulin (Ig) structure. Each pair is connected by a disulfide bond. Both the heavy and light chains have a variable (V) region at the amino terminus and a constant region (C) at the carboxy terminus. The V region participates in antigen recognition and confers specificity and the C region enables

the antibody to bind to the phagocyte. Five immunoglobulin molecules (IgG, IgM, IgA, IgD, and IgE) exist and serve different effector functions. Early in the antibody response, IgM and IgD production occurs and the membrane-bound form of IgM and IgD binds antigen and activates naïve B cells, leading to B cell proliferation and clonal selection. Also, IgM is involved in the activation of the classical pathway of the complement system. Later in the antibody response the IgG response develops, which has a higher specificity for particular antigens. IgG is also responsible for neonatal immunity in the transfer of maternal antibodies across the placenta and gut. Also, IgG causes **opsonization** of the antigen for phagocytosis by macrophages and neutrophils, as well as activation of the classical pathway of the complement system. NK cells and other leukocytes can bind to IgG- and IgE-coated cells to facilitate antibody-dependent cytotoxicity. IgE mediates hypersensitivity reactions and IgA is responsible for mucosal immunity.

Cellular Immunity: T Cells

T cells originate in the bone marrow, differentiate in the thymus, and then circulate in the blood or are harbored in the lymph nodes, spleen, or Peyer's patches of the intestine. In contrast to the humoral response, the cellular immune response **cellular immunity**) depends on direct cell-cell contact. Although antibodies and B cell receptors may recognize multiple types of antigens, T cells are restricted to peptide antigens and only

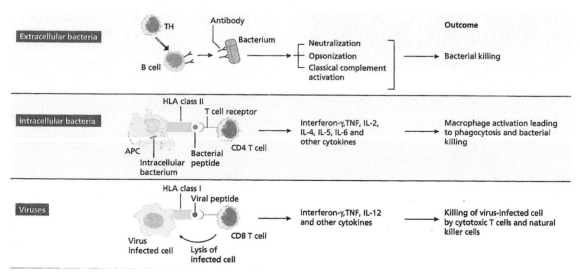

Figure 26-2 Overview of specific immune responses. *Top row,* Humoral immunity. B lymphocytes eliminate microbes by secreting antibodies. *Middle and lower rows,* Cell-mediated immunity. Helper T lymphocytes activate macrophages or dendritic cells that kill phagocytosed molecules or cytotoxic T lymphocytes that eliminate infected cells. (From Chapel H, Haeney M, Misbah S, Snowden N: Essentials of Clinical Immunology, 5th ed. Malden, Mass, Blackwell, 2006, p 35.)

recognize peptide sequences in the context of membrane-bound host proteins called MHC molecules (**Fig. 26-3**). There are two classes of MHC molecules. Each class presents antigens to different populations of T cells and is responsible for various functions in the cellular immune response. Th cells (which are CD4$^+$) respond to antigens bound to class II MHC molecules to secrete cytokines that stimulate the proliferation and differentiation of T cells as well as other B cells and macrophages. Class II MHC molecules are expressed primarily by professional APCs, which present phagocytosed and processed extracellular peptides to Th cells. There are two subsets of Th cells, which differ in their cytokine profiles and elicit different responses. Th1 cells secrete **interleukin** (IL)-2 and interferon-gamma (IFN-γ) to elicit a cell-mediated inflammatory response. Th2 cells secrete IL-4, IL-5, IL-6, and IL-10 to promote antibody secretion and the humoral response. Although both types are involved in most immune responses, they regulate the magnitude of each through mutual inhibition of cytokine production such that Th2 cell cytokines suppress production of Th1 cell cytokines and vice versa.

Unlike class II MHC molecules, class I MHC molecules are expressed by all nucleated cells in the body and are used to present intracellular peptides for surveillance to circulating **cytotoxic T lymphocytes** (CTLs). CTLs are also known as CD8$^+$ T cells and directly destroy cells that express foreign antigens that arise after a viral infection or are expressed as a result of tumorigenesis. Therefore, CTLs are considered to be primarily responsible for the antitumor immune response. Zhang and colleagues have reported that the presence of intratumoral T cells results in improved progression-free and overall survival in ovarian cancer patients. This effect was confirmed by Sato and colleagues, who documented a survival advantage in patients with a higher CD8$^+$/CD4$^+$ ratio of intratumoral cells in ovarian cancer patients. Han and associates have found that antigen-processing machinery component downregulation and subsequent lack of intratumoral T cells are independent prognostic factors for decreased survival in ovarian cancer patients.

A third class of T cells, regulatory T cells (Tregs), is CD4$^+$ T cells that are present in the peripheral circulation, inhibit immune responses and prevent autoimmunity. Because most tumor-associated antigens are self-antigens, recognition by immune effector cells is regulated by Tregs through peripheral tolerance. High numbers of Tregs have been found in the peripheral blood of patients with epithelial ovarian cancer and Tregs preferentially accumulate in the tumor environment, such as ascites and ovarian tumor islets. Curiel and associatess have shown that high levels of Tregs are found to be predictive of poor overall survival in a cohort of 70 patients with ovarian cancer. Based on these data, a goal of immunotherapy is to eliminate Tregs in the hope of enhancing innate antitumor immunity. Denileukin diftitox, a drug that selectively eliminates Tregs, has been investigated in ovarian cancer patients and preliminary results indicate that it induces tumor regression or stabilization, with low toxicity.

CYTOKINES

Cytokines are proteins secreted by immune cells that are produced in different phases of the immune response to control its duration and extent. During the activation phase of the immune response system, cytokines stimulate growth and differentiation of lymphocytes, whereas in the effector phase of the immune response, they activate other effector cells to help eliminate antigens and microbes. The major classes of cytokines include those that regulate innate immunity, regulate adaptive immunity, and stimulate hematopoiesis.

Cytokines That Mediate Innate Immunity
Interleukins
Interleukins are potent cytokines produced by some leukocytes to affect other leukocytes. IL-1 is released in response to cell damage by macrophages, endothelial cells, and some epithelial cells. Although IL-1 has actions similar to those of **tumor necrosis factor** (TNF), it lacks the ability to cause septic shock

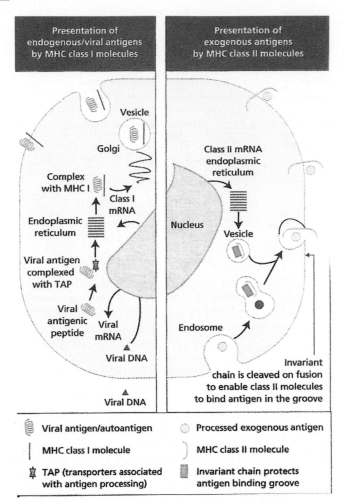

Presentation of endogenous/viral antigens by MHC class I molecules	Presentation of exogenous antigens by MHC class II molecules

Figure 26-3 Different routes of antigen presentation. After the antigen is processed into smaller fragments, the major histocompatability complex class (I or II) and these fragments interact with the receptor on the surface of the T cell to activate cytotoxic or helper T cells. (From Chapel H, Haeney M, Misbah S, Snowden N: Essentials of Clinical Immunology, 5th ed. Malden, Mass, Blackwell, 2006, p 7.)

symptoms. Macrophages can secrete a variety of ILs. M1 macrophages secrete IL-12, IL-18, IL-23, IFN-γ, and TNF-α and promote immune responses against tumors and intracellular microbes. IL-12 plays an important role in the transition between cell-mediated immunity and adaptive immunity. IL-12 stimulates NK cells and T cells to produce IFN-γ, which activates macrophages to kill phagocytosed foreign substances. Also, IL-12 increases cytolytic activity by stimulating CD8$^+$ cells. M2 macrophages produce vascular endothelial growth factor (VEGF), IL-6, IL-10, and prostaglandin E2, all of which have immunosuppressive functions and are found selectively in established tumors. The other ILs stimulate NK and T cell activation and proliferation, as well as IFN-γ synthesis.

Chemokines
Chemokines are small secreted proteins that are part of the largest known cytokine family. There are approximately 53 peptides and 23 G protein–coupled receptors in humans. Functionally, chemokines released in response to inflammatory stimuli that cause leukocyte recruitment are considered to be inflammatory whereas chemokines that cause migration of leukocytes to lymphoid organs are considered to be homeostatic. Chemokines affect tumor establishment in the following ways: determining the extent and type of leukocyte infiltration, promoting angiogenesis, controlling site-specific metastasis, and affecting tumor cell proliferation. The CXC chemokines (CXCL9, CXCL10, and CXCL11) are induced by IFN-γ and are typical chemoattractants of NK cells. In ovarian cancer patients, the expression of CXCR4/CXCL12 correlates with decreased progression-free and overall survival. Because of the importance of chemokines in gynecologic and other malignancies, CXCR4 inhibitors such as peptide antagonists and neutralizing antibodies are being developed.

Interferons
Type 1 IFN, IFN-α and IFN-β, are stimulated by intracellular TLRs and mediate the early innate immune response to viral infections. These cytokines inhibit viral replication, increase expression of class I MHC molecules, and promote a Th1 cell-mediated immune response by promoting T cell proliferation and NK cell cytolytic activity. IFN-γ, a type II IFN, is principally responsible for macrophage activation and the effector functions of innate and adaptive immune responses.

Cytokines That Mediate Adaptive Immunity
In addition to IFN-γ and transforming growth factor beta (TGF-β), IL-2, IL-4, IL-5, and IL-13 are all involved in the regulation of adaptive immunity. After T cells recognize the antigen, the T cells produce IL-2, which causes clonal expansion of activated T cells and additional production of cytokines such as IFN-γ and IL-4. IL-2 stimulates antibody synthesis and B cells by acting as a growth factor. IL-4 not only promotes IgE production from B cells, but also stimulates the development of Th2 cells from naïve T cells. IFN-γ is produced by T cells in response to antigen recognition or by NK cells in response to microbes or IL-12. IFN-γ activates the microbicidal function of macrophages, stimulates the expression of class I and II MHC and costimulatory molecules by antigen-presenting cells (APC), promotes the maturation of cells expressing CD4 into Th1 cells, and inhibits the Th2 cell pathway, thereby effectively promoting a cellular immune response. Currently, intraperitoneal and intrapleural administration of IFN-γ using gene therapy vectors to avoid the toxic effects of systemic IFN administration is being tested in clinical trials of ovarian cancer. TGF-β inhibits the proliferation of and differentiation of T cells and contributes to immune evasion of tumor cells by inhibiting antitumor host immune responses.

Cytokines That Mediate Hematopoiesis
Colony-Stimulating Factors
IL-3 is a multi-lineage **colony-stimulating factor** that allows for the differentiation of cells into myeloid progenitor cells, granulocytes, monocytes, and dendritic cells. Granulocyte colony-stimulating factor (G-CSF) is a cytokine produced by macrophages, fibroblasts, and endothelial cells and promotes the mobilization of neutrophils from the bone marrow. Granulocyte-macrophage colony-stimulating factor (GM-CSF) is produced by T cells, macrophages, endothelial cells, and fibroblasts. GM-CSF stimulates the maturation of bone marrow cells

into dendritic cells and monocytes. G-CSF and GM-CSF are available pharmacologically and are used in patients undergoing chemotherapy and bone marrow transplantation.

TUMOR CELL KILLING AND IMMUNOTHERAPY

Immunotherapy has been developed to recognize and destroy tumor cells. Immune modulation, passive therapy, and active therapy are the three major classes of immunotherapy. Immune modulation relies on nonspecific means such as the administration of IL-2, IFNs, or bacille Calmette-Guerin to elicit an immune response. Passive therapy transfers components of the acquired immune system to the cancer patient (**passive immunity**). An example of passive therapy is the use of monoclonal antibodies directed toward **tumor-specific antigens**. Active therapy uses the woman's immune system to elicit a response; an example would be vaccines comprised of peptides, proteins, DNA, or RNA.

Immune modulation has been used in ovarian cancer in the form of adjuvant IFN treatment after surgery and as consolidation therapy after surgery and standard chemotherapy. A phase III trial in advanced ovarian cancer patients randomized patients to IV cisplatin and cyclophosphamide chemotherapy versus the same regimen with intraperitoneal IFN-γ. Windbichler and colleagues have shown an improvement in progression-free but not overall survival in the IFN arm, with acceptable toxicity. Possible explanations for the improvement in the chemotherapy plus IFN include induction of cytotoxic T lymphocytes, stimulation of NK cells and macrophages, an anti-angiogenic effect on tumor vasculature, and the direct inhibition of oncogene expression by high IFN-γ levels in the tumor microenvironment. This study was redone with the standard chemotherapy of carboplatin and paclitaxel with IFN-γ versus chemotherapy alone and showed a survival disadvantage in patients receiving IFN-γ, but no difference in progression-free survival. Because of the mixed results, further trials investigating the potential synergistic effect of IFN administration and cytotoxic chemotherapy are needed to rigorously evaluate this approach for treatment rigorously.

Tumor cells have specific tumor-associated antigens or receptors on their surface that may distinguish them from normal cells. The antigen most often targeted in ovarian cancer is cancer antigen 125 (CA-125), a glycoprotein present at elevated levels in the serum of more than 80% of patients with epithelial ovarian cancer. A murine monoclonal antibody (MAb) to CA-125 (oregovomab) was investigated for its therapeutic usefulness as a consolidation treatment in ovarian cancer patients but did not demonstrate overall survival advantage over control. However, a subset of patients who had evidence of a robust antiantibody immune response in the form of anti-murine antibodies had evidence of tumor protection after treatment. Trials of oregovomab, with or without chemotherapy, have also been conducted in patients with recurrent disease, and induction of anti–CA-125 T cell responses may correlate with improved survival times. Bevacizumab (Avastin) is a monoclonal antibody directed against VEGF. In a phase II study of persistent or recurrent ovarian cancer patients, it showed an unprecedented 21% response rate and 40% of patients did not have progression at 6 months. Therefore, bevacizumab is currently being investigated in phase III trials (GOG218 and ICON 7) .

Adoptive T cell immunotherapy uses the transfer of T cells expanded *ex vivo* in large numbers because of their ability to kill tumor cells specifically and to proliferate and persist for long periods after transfer. A strong rationale exists for the development of adoptive T cell therapies in the treatment of ovarian cancer. First, tumor-specific T cells can be found in the peripheral circulation or in tumors in up to 50% of ovarian cancer patients. Second, the presence of intratumoral T cells being associated with improved survival suggests that administering adoptive immunotherapy could produce clinical results. Currently, adoptive immunotherapy is being investigated in ovarian cancer patients expressing Wilms' tumor gene product (WT-1) as a phase I study at Memorial Sloan-Kettering Cancer Center.

Another promising immunotherapy in gynecology has been the human papillomavirus vaccine (HPV) for the prevention of vulvar, vaginal, or cervical dysplasia and the corresponding cancers. A study conducted by Garland and workers has shown that the quadrivalent vaccine against HPV 6, 11, 16, and 18 decreases the incidence of dysplasia or cancer significantly; the vaccine was 100% effective. Currently, *Listeria monocytogenes*, which secretes the antigen HPV-16 E7 and is fused to a non-hemolytic listeriolysin O protein, has been used as a therapeutic vaccine for patients with advanced cervical cancer. The use of HPV vaccine therapy is efficacious and has tremendous implications for the treatment of gynecologic HPV-related dysplasias and cancers.

MOLECULAR ONCOLOGY

Cancer development can be sporadic if it is caused by an acquired mutations or can be hereditary if caused by inheritance of a mutated gene followed by acquisition of an acquired mutation in the other **allele**. Genetic alterations occur in three major categories of genes—oncogenes, tumor suppressor genes, and DNA **mismatch repair genes** (MMRs). Knowledge of how these genes function is a rapidly expanding field and well beyond the scope of this text, but a general overview is provided here.

ONCOGENES

An oncogene refers to a set of genes that when altered are associated with the development of a malignant cell. Functionally, oncogenes are involved in cell proliferation, signal transduction, and transcriptional alteration. Mechanisms of alteration in oncogene function include gene amplification (increase in the number of copies of the genes in the cell), **translocation**, or overexpression, which refers to excessive and abnormal protein production. Several classes of oncogenes such as peptide growth factors, cytoplasmic factors, and nuclear factors exist. Examples are described in the following section (**Table 26-1**).

Peptide Growth Factors
Epidermal Growth Factor Receptor (EGFR) Family
There are four type of *Erb*B receptors—*Erb*B1 (commonly known as EGFR, human epidermal growth factor receptor [HER]1), *Erb*B2 (also known as HER2/neu), *Erb*B3 (also known as HER3), and *Erb*B4 (also known as HER4). All *Erb*B receptors share an extracellular domain that binds ligand, a transmembrane domain, and an intracellular tyrosine kinase domain. In the *Erb*B pathway, homodimers and heterodimers are formed from the various classes of receptors, resulting in activation of the Ras-Raf-MAPK pathway and the phosphoinositide 3-kinase

Table 26-1 Classes of Genes Involved in Growth Stimulatory Pathways

Peptide Growth Factors	Corresponding Receptors
Epidermal growth factor (EGF) and transforming growth factor-α (TGF-α) Heregulin	EGF receptor (*erb*-B1), *erb*-B2 (Her-2/Neu), *erb*-B3, *erb*-B4
Vascular endothelial growth factor (VEGF) A, VEGF-B, VEGF-C, VEGF-D, VEGF-E, placental growth factor (PlGF) 1, PlGF2	VEGFR-1, VEGFR-2, VEGFR-3, neuropilins
Insulin-like growth factors (IGF-I, IGF-II)	IGF-I and IGF-II receptors
Platelet-derived growth factor (PDGF)	PDGF receptor
Fibroblast growth factor (FGF)	FGF receptors
Macrophage colony-stimulating factor (M-CSF)	M-CSF receptor (FMS)
Cytoplasmic Factors	**Examples**
Tyrosine kinases	Eph family
G proteins	K-Ras, H-Ras, N-Ras
Serine-threonine kinases	AKT
Nonreceptor tyrosine kinases	Focal Adhesion Kinase (FAK), Src
Nuclear Factors	**Examples**
Transcription factors	C-myc, C-jun, C-fos
Cell cycle progression factors	Cyclins, E2F

Adapted from Boyd J, Berchuck A: Oncogenes and tumor suppressor genes. In Hoskins WJ, Young RC, Markman M, et al (eds): Principles and Practice of Gynecologic Oncology. Philadelphia, Lippincott Williams & Wilkins, 2005, p 93-122.

(PI3K)–activated AKT pathway. Although the *Erb*B3 lacks intrinsic kinase activity and *Erb*B2 has no specific ligand, the formation of heterodimers leads to activation of these classes of receptors.

The Ras-Raf-MAPK pathway is a major downstream target of the *Erb*B family of receptors and leads to the activation of Ras, causing the activation of MAPKs to regulate transcription of molecules linked to cell proliferation, survival, and transformation. Also, the PI3K-activated AKT pathway serves as another downstream target of the *Erb*B pathway; it drives tumor progression via cell growth, proliferation, survival, and motility. A number of mechanisms such as receptor gene amplification and overexpression, receptor mutations, and autocrine ligand production cause *Erb*B pathway disruption, leading to tumor formation. EGFR gene mutations have been found in glioblastomas, non–small cell lung cancer, and ovarian cancer. Slamon and colleagues have reported that Her2/neu amplification is found in 20% to 30% of breast cancers and 10% of ovarian cancers. Because of the multitude of cancers with genetic alterations or changes in the ErbB family, several potential strategies exist for targeting EGFR, including monoclonal antibodies, low-molecular-weight tyrosine kinase inhibitors (TKIs, many of which are in advanced clinical development), antisense oligonucleotides, and intracellular single-chain Fv fragments of antibodies. Currently, monoclonal antibodies such as cetuximab have been approved by the U.S. Food and Drug Administration (FDA) for the treatment of metastatic colorectal cancer along with chemotherapy, as well as for the treatment of locally or regionally advanced head and neck cancer with radiation therapy.

Angiogenesis and Vascular Endothelial Growth Factor

Cancer growth requires a sufficient blood supply to extend beyond 1 mm^3 in size. Angiogenesis occurs by sprouting (branching of new blood vessels from preexisting blood vessels) or by nonsprouting (requires the enlargement and splitting of preexisting blood vessels). The tumor vascular environment is characterized by vessels that are irregular in shape, dilated, tortuous, and disorganized. Angiogenesis is dependent on the relative increase of proangiogenic factors such as VEGF, platelet derived-growth

factor (PDGF), and ephrins and their receptors. Also, endothelial cells are genetically stable, unlike tumor cells, thereby increasing the therapeutic value of targeting angiogenesis for cancer therapy.

VEGF is critical to endothelial cell survival, vascular permeability, cell fenestration, and vasodilation. There are seven proteins in this family—VEGF-A, VEGF-B, VEGF-C, VEGF-D, VEGF-E, placental growth factor (PlGF) 1, and PlGF2. Most human tumors, including those of the lung, thyroid, breast, gastrointestinal, female reproductive tract, and urinary tract, have marked expression of VEGF. There are three vascular endothelial growth factor receptors, VEGFR-1, VEGFR-2, and VEGFR-3. VEGFR-3 is expressed on the vascular and lymphatic endothelium, unlike the other two receptors, which are expressed only on the vascular endothelium. Also, there is a second class of VEGFRs known as the neuropilins (NRPs), which potentiate VEGF-A– and VEGFR-2–mediated actions. Similar to the EGFR family, there are many ligands to receptors in the VEGF family. Ultimately, activation of the VEGF receptors can lead to downstream effects on the mitogen-activated protein kinase (MAPK) pathway, v-src sarcoma viral oncogene homologue (SRC), PI3K-AKT, focal adhesion kinase (FAK), and Ras-Raf-MAPK (Ras-Raf-MAPK) superfamily. Because of the clinical significance of the VEGF pathway in many cancers, anti-VEGF antibodies such as bevacizumab, VEGFR tyrosine kinase inhibitors, and vascular targeting agents have been developed to target this critical pathway. Thaker and associates have shown in an orthotopic mouse model of ovarian cancer that dual inhibition of EGFR and VEGFR by the tyrosine kinase inhibitor AEE788, along with paclitaxel, inhibits the progression of cancer by causing apoptosis of tumor cells and tumor-associated endothelial cells. In ovarian cancer, bevacizumab is being evaluated in conjunction with standard carboplatin and paclitaxel for first-line treatment, as well as for consolidation therapy.

Ephrin Family of Ligands and Receptors

Tyrosine kinases provide a transfer of a phosphate from adenosine triphosphate (ATP) to tyrosine residues on specific cellular proteins; however, they can also play a role in the development of cancer and tumor progression. Recently, attention has been given to elucidating the role of the ephrin receptor A2 (EphA2) in tumorigenesis and therapeutic targeting. EphA2 belongs to the largest known family of protein tyrosine kinase receptors, the Eph family, and there are two Eph receptors, A and B that have corresponding ligands. The normal cellular function of EphA2 in epithelial tissue is not completely understood, but in cancer, EphA2 modulates cell growth, survival, migration, and angiogenesis. EphA2 overexpression has been correlated with disease severity and is predictive of a poor outcome in ovarian cancer patients. There are several therapeutic approaches for targeting EphA2, including agonist monoclonal antibody, immunotherapy, soluble EphA receptors, and neutral liposomal **small interfering RNA** (siRNA), some of which are already in clinical trials.

Phosphoinositide 3-Kinase Pathway

The PI3K family is comprised of lipid and serine-threonine kinases that control second messengers through phosphorylation. AKT is the predominant downstream target of PI3K and has many targets, including mammalian target of rapamycin (mTOR), signal transducer and activation of transcription (STAT), MAPK, nuclear factor-κB, and protein kinase C. The activation of the PI3K-AKT pathway controls cell survival with inhibition of apoptosis, cell growth, cell metabolism, RNA translation, and cell proliferation. Also, this pathway has been implicated in chemotherapy resistance.

RAS is another cytoplasmic factor. It is a G protein involved in the transmission of growth stimulatory signals from the cell membrane to the nucleus. The RAS family of G proteins is positioned downstream of cell surface receptor tyrosine kinases and upstream of the cytoplasmic cascade of kinases, such as mitogen-activated protein (MAP) kinases. MAP kinases in turn activate nuclear transcription factors such as c-myc, c-jun, and c-fos. Currently, it is estimated that about one third of cancers have point mutations in RAS genes, such as *KRAS, HRAS,* and *NRAS*. Because RAS requires the post-translational modification of the addition of a farnesyl group to the C-terminus to move from the cytoplasm to the inner plasma membrane, inhibitors to farnesylation have been developed and are in clinical trials.

Tumor Suppressor Genes

Tumor suppressor genes control cell growth cellular proliferation and aberrations in tumor suppressor genes can cause malignancy. The retinoblastoma (*Rb*) gene was the first tumor suppressor gene to be identified and encodes a nuclear protein that regulates G1 phase cell cycle arrest. Knudson and colleagues have proposed the "two-hit" theory to explain the action of tumor suppressor genes. The first hit is the inheritance of the *Rb* mutated gene and the second hit is the somatic mutation that occurs later and leads to cancer.

In gynecologic malignancies, the most common tumor suppressor gene is *p53*, which is located on the short arm of chromosome 17. *p53* has key roles as a transcription factor and regulator of the cell cycle and apoptosis. Normal *p53* binds to transcriptional regulatory elements in the DNA and acts as a gatekeeper of the genome by responding to DNA damage with the activation of apoptotic effectors such as BAX, FAS, and bcl-2. Missense mutations that change a single amino acid in the encoded protein in exons 5 to 8 are the most common mutations of *p53*. The resultant mutant proteins can no longer bind to

DNA, but can bind to and inactivate any normal *p53* in a cell. Cells with mutant *p53* do not experience cell cycle arrest at the G_1-S checkpoint before DNA replication and at the G_2-M checkpoint prior to mitosis, nor do they undergo apoptosis.

Tumor suppressor genes such as *p53* are found in approximately 10% to 20% of endometrioid cancers, predominantly grade 3, and in many late and sporadic ovarian cancers. In cervical carcinogenesis, the E6 oncoprotein of HPV types 16 and 18 associates with *p53* and targets it for degradation, and the E7 oncoprotein of HPV type 16 binds to *Rb* in infected cells to upregulate proliferation. Although *p53* mutations are one of the most common mutations in cancer, therapeutic targeting of *p53* has met with less than optimal results in several disease sites.

Phosphatase and tensin homologue (PTEN) is the regulatory counterpart of PI3K by dephosphorylating proteins phosphorylated by PI3K. *PTEN* is a tumor suppressor gene and is found in approximately 20% of endometrial hyperplasia and 50% of endometrioid cancers. Mutations of *PTEN* occur in exons 3, 4, 5, 7, and 8 targeting the phosphatase domain and regions that control protein stability and localization. Decreased or absent expression of *PTEN* result in many of the mutations found in endometrioid cancers. Also, **epigenetic** mechanisms such as promoter hypermethylation and subcellular localization can affect *PTEN* function in the absence of intragenic mutations.

BRCA1 and BRCA2

Approximately 5% to 10% of breast and ovarian cancers arise in the setting of a genetic predisposition. The vast majority of these cases are associated with germline mutations in the **BRCA1** gene located on chromosome 17q21 and the **BRCA2** gene located on chromosome 13q12.3. The pattern of inheritance is autosomal dominant, and the prevalence of the mutated gene occurs more frequently in Ashkenazi Jewish and certain French Canadian women. The following women should be tested for a BRCA mutation:

- A woman with a family history of two or more women with breast cancer before the age of 50 years or ovarian cancer at any age

or

- A woman with breast cancer before the age of 50 years or ovarian cancer at any age plus Ashkenazi Jewish ancestry

or

- A woman with bilateral breast cancer and/or a history of both breast and ovarian cancers

The cumulative risk of developing ovarian cancer by the age of 70 years is 40% to 50% for *BRCA1* mutation and 20% to 25% for *BRCA2* mutation carriers, but there is equal breast cancer penetrance in *BRCA1* or *BRCA2* mutation carriers. The *BRCA2* mutation is also associated with male breast cancer and pancreatic, urinary tract, and biliary tract cancers. Unfortunately, a woman with this mutation develops breast or ovarian cancer at a younger age than sporadic cancers.

BRCA1 and *BRCA2* are tumor suppressor genes that encode for large proteins. Similar to other hereditary cancer syndromes, inheritance of a *BRCA* mutation confers an increased susceptibility to cancer, but not an absolute guarantee of developing cancer unless a second inactivation of the allele occurs.

Both *BRCA1* and *BRCA 2* encode proteins that are involved in the repair of DNA strand breaks. Most detected mutations are nonsense or frameshift alterations that lead to truncated proteins. BRCA1 and BRCA2 proteins are involved in the pathway mediated by RAD51, which is a protein important in repairing double DNA strand breaks. BRCA1 is also involved in tumor suppression by transcriptional regulation of gene expression, such as being a *p53* independent transactivator of cyclin kinase inhibitor p-21. *BRCA2* has been identified as a FANCD1 gene, a member of the Fanconi anemia complex. Cells with deficient *BRCA1* or *BRCA2* are incapable of repairing DNA strand breaks, which leads to genetic instability and tumorigenesis. In *BRCA*-deficient cells, the defective maintenance of genomic integrity may not only accelerate cancer initiation and progression, but may also render the cancer more susceptible to therapeutic agents whose cytotoxic potential is mediated through the induction of a specific type of DNA damage that *BRCA* normally functions to repair. For example, cisplatin and radiation cause DNA interstrand cross-links. Recently, in a phase I study, poly(adenosine diphosphate [ADP]-ribose polymerase (PARP) inhibitors such as olaparib have been used in the treatment of *BRCA1* and *BRCA2* mutation carriers with predominantly breast and ovarian cancer and were found to have an acceptable toxicity profile. PARPs are a family of multifunctional enzymes that repair DNA single-strand breaks through the repair of base excisions. The inhibition of PARPs leads to the accumulation of DNA double-strand breaks, which are normally repaired by BRCA proteins and thereby provide selectivity of treatment in this *BRCA* mutation population. Currently, clinical trials combining PARP inhibitors and chemotherapy are ongoing in a *BRCA* mutation positive cancer population, but the use of PARP inhibitors for therapy is a good example of how molecular oncology can be exploited for therapeutic value. Cass and colleagues, as well as others, have demonstrated that women with *BRCA* mutations survive longer than their sporadic cancer counterparts.

DNA Mismatch Repair Genes

Hereditary nonpolyposis colorectal cancer (HNPCC), also known as Lynch syndrome, is an autosomal dominant cancer syndrome that predisposes an individual to colorectal, endometrial, gastric, biliary tract, urinary tract, or ovarian cancer. This syndrome is thought to account for all cases of hereditary endometrial cancer and up to 5% of hereditary ovarian cancers. The estimated lifetime risk for endometrial cancer in HNPCC gene carriers is 40% to 60%, corresponding to a relative risk of 13 to 20, whereas that of ovarian cancer is 6% to 20%, corresponding to a relative risk of 4 to 8. Linkage analysis of high-risk families led to the discovery of Lynch syndrome. It was found to be caused by germline mutations in genes responsible for recognizing and fixing errors in the DNA helix, resulting from incorrect pairings of nucleotides during replication or the formation of abnormal loops of DNA. *MSH2* (MutS homologue 2) and *MLH1* (Mut L homologue 1) are the most commonly mutated mismatch repair genes and are located on chromosomes 2p16 and 3p21, respectively. Other mismatch repair genes are *MSH6*, *PMS1*, and *PMS2*, but these occur at a lower frequency. Cells with a defective mismatch repair system exhibit **microsatellite instability** (MSI). MSI occurs as DNA mismatches cause a shortening or lengthening of repetitive DNA sequences and

---

Box 26-1 Bethesda and Amsterdam II Criteria for Hereditary Nonpolyposis Colorectal Cancer

Any one of the following meet Bethesda Criteria:
- Colorectal cancer less than 50 years
- Presence of synchronous or metachronous HNPCC-related carcinomas regardless of age (colorectal, endometrial, stomach, ovarian, pancreas, ureter, renal pelvis, biliary tract, sebaceous gland, and small bowel)
- Colorectal cancer with specific histologic features in individuals less than 60 years of age
- Colorectal cancer diagnosed in one or more first-colorectal degree relatives with colorectal cancer or other HNPCC-related tumors. One of the cancers must have been diagnosed before the age of 50 years (this includes adenomas, which must have been diagnosed before the age of 40 years)
- Colorectal cancer in two or more first- or second-degree relatives with a HNPCC-related tumor, regardless of age

or

All of the following meet Amsterdam II Criteria:
- Colorectal and/or endometrial cancer or transitional cancer of the ureter or renal pelvis or cancer of the small bowel in at least three individuals in the same family
- One of the patients is a first-degree relative of the other patients
- Disease occurs in at least two other family members
- At least one of the diagnoses was made before the age of 50
- The diagnoses must be histologically confirmed
- Familial adenomatous polyposis is excluded.

Adapted from Karlan BY, Berchuck A, Mutch D: The role of genetic testing for cancer susceptibility in gynecologic practice. Obstet Gynecol 110:155-167, 2007.

---

these mismatches go unchecked. This results in the cancer containing a greater or lesser number of repeats than are present in the normal cells of the individual. There is a consensus panel of five microsatellite markers (D2S123, D5S346, D17S250, Bat 25, and Bat 26) that can be used to identify HNPCC-related cancers compared with sporadic ones. In endometrial cancer, MSI can occur from promoter methylation and must be distinguished from MSI caused by an inherited mismatch repair defect.

Taking a family history is the first step in identifying patients with HNPCC. The Bethesda criteria (**Box 26-1**) seem to be the most sensitive for predicting mismatch repair mutations, but the Amsterdam II criteria are more specific. Amsterdam II criteria include the following: colorectal carcinoma and/or endometrial cancer or transitional cell of the ureter or renal pelvis or carcinoma of the small bowel in at least three individuals; one of the patients is a first-degree relative of two other patients; disease occurs in at least two other family members; one of the diagnoses should be made before the age of 50 years; histologic confirmation of the diagnosis; and familial adenomatous polyposis has been excluded.

FUTURE DIRECTIONS

With the continued improved understanding of molecular oncogenesis and tumor progression, promising biologically targeted therapies will emerge. One such therapy is siRNA, which can be designed to target and silence oncogenes involved in all steps of cancer initiation, proliferation, and metastasis. Unlike small molecule inhibitors or fully humanized antibodies, siRNAs can target multiple downstream pathways or targets specifically and effectively based on direct, homologydependent, post-transcriptional gene silencing. The major challenges to the development of siRNA as a therapeutic tool have been its degradation by serum nucleases, poor cellular uptake, and rapid renal clearance following administration. However, the development of nuclease-resistant chemically modified siRNAs and neutral nanoliposomes such as 1,2-dioleoyl-*sn*-glycero-3-phosphatidylcholine (DOPC) for improved delivery should overcome these obstacles. Preclinically, neutral nanoliposomal EphA2 siRNA injection every 4 days decreased tumor growth in two ovarian cancer cell lines compared with control siRNA and, when EphA2-targeted siRNA was combined with paclitaxel, there was a statistically significant decrease in tumor growth in both cell lines. Clinical development will follow completion of safety studies.

Another potential therapeutic target is noncoding RNA (ncRNA). This includes a broad range of regulatory RNA molecules, such as ribozymes, antisense, siRNA, micro-RNA, and aptamers. Small ncRNAs elicit at least four types of responses that trigger specific gene inactivation, which are important in a variety of cancers—destruction of homologous messenger RNA, inhibition of translation, de novo methylation of genomic regions that block transcription of target genes, and chromosomal rearrangement. These flexible molecules have proven to have enormous potential as diagnostic and therapeutic tools in cancer medicine.

GYNECOLOGIC MALIGNANCIES

Cancer is a complex multistep process that requires self-sufficient growth signals, insensitivity to anti-growth signals, tissue invasion and metastasis, limitless replicative potential, sustained angiogenesis, and evasion of apoptosis. The clinical diversity of gynecologic cancers such as histologic type, stage, and outcome is probably attributable to molecular differences among cancers. The role of oncogenes and tumor suppressor genes vary not only among cancers but also within a given type of cancer. To date, an understanding of the molecular pathogenesis of gynecologic cancers is in its infancy but, with new molecular profiling technologies, this understanding is expanding rapidly. With this improved characterization, new insights into the origin, prevention, and treatment of gynecologic cancers should follow. In the following sections, we describe the role of oncogenes and tumor suppressor genes that lead to the development of gynecologic cancers.

ENDOMETRIAL CANCER

Endometrial Cancer and Tumor Suppressor Genes

Endometrial cancer is divided into two types—type I, which is thought to be unopposed estrogen and develops in a background of endometrial hyperplasia, and type II, which is comprised of nonendometrioid and more aggressive cancers. Inactivation of tumor suppressor gene *p53* is among the most frequent genetic events in endometrial cancer. Also, overexpression of *p53* occurs more frequently in advanced stage endometrial cancer and has

been associated with worse survival after controlling for stage, suggesting that loss of *p53* tumor suppressor function leads to a more aggressive phenotype. Recently, endometrial glandular dysplasia has been proposed as a precursor for type 2 serous carcinomas, and both the precursor and serous carcinoma have demonstrated overexpression of *p53*. In uterine sarcomas, overexpression of mutant *p53* occurs in malignant mixed mesodermal tumors (MMMTs), leiomyosarcomas, and undifferentiated endometrial sarcomas.

The *PTEN* gene is on chromosome 10q and encodes a phosphatase that functions by opposing the activity of PI3K. Mutations in this gene are usually deletions, insertions, or nonsense mutations that lead to truncated protein products and are associated with endometrioid histology, early stage, and favorable clinical behavior. Dellas and workers have recently found that loss of *PTEN* and p27 protein expression in obese endometrial cancer patients is associated with a significantly better prognosis. Sometimes, *PTEN* mutation status can be used to differentiate an ovarian metastasis from an endometrial cancer versus a synchronous primary cancers.

Germline mutations in DNA mismatch repair genes are essential to HNPCC. Endometrial cancer is the second most common malignancy observed in women with HNPCC after colon cancer. Unlike in colon cancer, loss of mismatch repair function in endometrial cancer has not been consistently associated with improved survival (see earlier section on HNPCC for further details).

Endometrial Cancer and Oncogenes

Unlike inactivation of tumor suppressor genes, fewer alterations in oncogenes have been found in endometrial cancer. *Her2/neu* has been found to be expressed in approximately 20% of endometrioid and serous carcinomas and was associated with aggressive phenotype and poor survival in a recent population-based series. Racial differences in the expression of *Her2/neu* have been found as well. Regardless, the levels of *Her2/neu* overexpression are much lower than in breast cancer, but nonetheless there have been reports of using trastuzumab (anti-*Her2/neu* antibody) for the treatment of endometrial cancer.

KRAS mutations occur most often in type I endometrial cancers as well as in hyperplasias, suggesting that *KRAS* mutation is an early event in the development of type I endometrial cancers. The *BRAF* mutations were found in endometrial cancers with mismatch repair deficiency and have different frequencies in various populations.

The beta-catenin (β-catenin) gene maps to chromosome 3p21 and is important for cell differentiation, maintenance of normal tissue architecture, and signal transduction. Mutations in exon 3 of β-catenin result in stabilization of the protein, cytoplasmic and nuclear accumulation, and participation in signal transduction and transcriptional activation through the formation of complexes with DNA binding proteins. These mutations occur in approximately 14% to 44% of endometrial cancers and are independent of the presence of microsatellite instability and the mutational status of *PTEN* and *KRAS*. Data regarding the prognostic significance of these mutations are unclear, but are thought to be associated with good prognosis.

The fibroblast growth factor receptor 2 (*FGFR2*) gene encodes one of a family of tyrosine kinase growth factor receptors that receive signals from a large family of ligands. Pollack and colleagues have recently evaluated the *FGFR2* gene for activating mutations in a series of endometrial cancers and found them in approximately 10% of endometrioid cancers. Currently, the Gynecologic Oncology Group has a phase II trial evaluating an anti-*FGFR2* tyrosine kinase inhibitor in recurrent endometrial cancer.

Immunotherapy and Endometrial Cancer

Although endometrial cancer is the most frequent gynecologic cancer and the fourth most common cancer in women, immunotherapy has not been investigated as a viable option for the treatment of endometrial cancer. Recent investigations have revealed that endometrial cancer is immunogenic and could be a reasonable target for immunotherapy. Santin and coworkers found that a strong *in vitro* tumor-specific response could be generated by tumor lysate–pulsed autologous dendritic cells in uterine papillary serous carcinoma. Although limited by few patients, a strong cytotoxic T cell and Th1 response was characterized by enhanced IFN-γ and low IL-4 expression. However, therapeutic immunotherapy trials for endometrial cancer have not been completed.

OVARIAN CANCER

Ovarian Cancer and Tumor Suppressor Genes

To date, alteration of the *p53* tumor suppressor gene is the most frequent genetic event in ovarian cancers. Advanced stage and serous cancers have a higher frequency of *p53* mutations than early stage and non-serous cancers. Overall, 70% of advanced stage ovarian cancers have missense or truncation mutations in *p53*. Evidence suggests that inactivation of *Rb* greatly enhances tumor formation in ovarian cells with *p53* mutations.

Cyclin-dependent kinase inhibitors (CDKIs) also act as tumor suppressors because they inhibit cell cycle progression from the G1 to S phase. The *p16* gene (CDKN2A) undergoes homozygous deletion in approximately 15% of ovarian cancers. *BRCA1* and *p16* may be inactivated by transcriptional silencing because of promoter methylation rather than mutation and/or deletion.

Oncogenes and Ovarian Cancer

Unlike in breast cancer, in which 30% express increased levels of *Her2/neu*, a minority of ovarian cancers have increased *Her2/neu* expression. The Gynecologic Oncology Group has conducted a trial to evaluate the response rate of ovarian cancer patients to single-agent anti-*Her2/neu* antibody therapy and found the rate of response to be approximately 7%. *KRAS* mutations are commonly found in borderline tumors of the ovary and mucinous ovarian cancers, but not in serous ovarian tumors. PI3K and β-catenin are rarer mutations, but are more likely to be found in endometrioid and clear cell tumors of the ovary.

Immunotherapy and Ovarian Cancer

Since the clinical history of ovarian cancer entails periods of remission and relapse of sequentially shortened duration as chemotherapy resistance develops, immune-based strategies should be contemplated in women with minimal disease burden. The immune system protects the host against the development of cancer, but also creates tumor immunogenicity. Currently, immunotherapy trials are now generally focused on the effector phase of the immune response to elicit primarily an antibody response, produce humoral and cellular responses, or cause the activation and/or generation of antigen-specific CTLs and Th cells. The cancer-testis antigen NY-ESO-1 vaccines have been developed and used in a clinical trial of high-risk ovarian cancer patients in first clinical remission. Overall, these vaccines were found to have a low side effect profile and induced specific T cell immunity, but did not delay progression-free survival. Also, anti-idiotype vaccines, which try to increase the immunogenicity of tumor-associated antigens by presenting the desired **epitope** to the host in a different molecular environment, have been used to increase antibody production. Abagovomab vaccination is safe, and an ongoing phase III investigation is being conducted through the Arbeitsgemeinschaft Gynakologische Oncologie group. Radionuclides conjugated with antibodies such as yttrium conjugated to the *MUC1* gene have been shown to have no difference in overall survival in ovarian cancer patients. Although, to date, numerous nonrandomized phase II immune targeted trials have shown benefit in terms of survival and presence of respective effectors, these have not been confirmed in phase III trials, but further investigation is warranted in ovarian cancer.

CERVICAL CANCER: ONCOGENES, TUMOR SUPPRESSOR GENES, AND IMMUNOTHERAPY

Because only a small proportion of women with HPV develop cervical cancer, additional genetic alterations must occur. However compared with other gynecologic cancers, the roles of oncogenes and tumor suppressor genes are not as well elucidated. The allelic loss of possible tumor suppressor genes at loci on chromosomes 3p, 11p, and others has been noted, but specific tumor suppressor genes remain unidentified. Also, Mammas and colleagues have found that the oncogenes *Hi* and *NRAS* are upregulated in cervical cancer independently of HPV infection. Similar to endometrial and ovarian cancers, gene silencing caused by promoter hypermethylation may also be involved in cervical cancer development. The methylation status of the oncogene human telomerase reverse transcriptase and the tumor suppressor genes death-associated protein kinase and O6-methylguanine DNA methyltransferase could be used to distinguish the progression from normal to cervical dysplasia to invasive cancer. In terms of immunotherapy for the treatment of cervical cancer, many resources are being used in developing therapeutic HPV vaccines. Fortunately, because cell pellets from liquid-based Pap smears can be obtained, molecular studies can be easily performed to characterize the molecular pathogenesis of cervical cancer better.

CONCLUSION

Cancer pathogenesis is a complex process, but with the advent of high-throughput molecular technologies, a new understanding is rapidly advancing. This understanding of the biology and immunology of the disease offers hope for better means for prevention, early detection, and treatment.

KEY POINTS

- The immune system consists of the innate and adaptive immune systems. The innate system is present at birth and consists of natural barriers, NK cells, macrophages, and the complement system. The adaptive immune system adapts to infection and consists of T and B cells.
- The cellular immune response occurs as a result of T lymphocytes reacting via a surface **T cell receptor** (TCR) that processes antigens presented to it by an APC in conjunction with HLA (MHC) molecules.
- T cell activation can result in activation of helper or inducer (Th) cells, cytotoxic or **suppressor T cells**, or cytokine production.
- Helper or inducer T (Th) cells recruit macrophages and cytotoxic or suppressor cells.
- Cytotoxic T cells have the ability to lyse infected cells or signal B cells to produce antibody.
- Humoral immunity results from antigenic stimulation of a B lymphocyte, which differentiates into a plasma cell and secretes antibody (immunoglobulin).
- The complement cascade provides a basis for the inflammatory response and can also mediate cytotoxicity.
- Cytokines (**lymphokines**) are regulatory substances of the immune system produced as a result of T cell activation, cell damage by a virus or other cells, such as macrophages and monocytes, involved in the immune response.
- Passive therapy transfers components of the acquired immune system to the recipient with cancer (e.g., monoclonal antibodies directed toward tumor-specific antigens).
- Active immunotherapy uses a patient's own immune system for protection against infection (e.g., vaccines).

- There are three types of genes associated with malignant development—oncogenes, tumor suppressor genes, and DNA mismatch repair genes.
- Malignant change is seen with point mutations, chromosomal aberration, gene amplification (increase in number of copies), or chromosomal translocation.
- *Ras* oncogenes are part of a group of signal transducer oncogenes that relay messages from the membrane to the cell nucleus. They are activated generally by point mutations.
- Growth factor genes include *C-erb-B2 (Her-2/neu),* which can be overexpressed and act as a tumor-specific target for monoclonal antibody therapy; these are especially useful in breast cancer therapy.
- Nuclear oncogenes include *myc* and *fos* and can activate other genes as well as stimulate DNA replication.
- Angiogenesis is the formation of new blood vessels in order for tumors to grow.
- Tumor suppressor genes such as *Rb* and *p53* restrain cell growth. They have two copies and, in general, alteration of both copies leads to a mutant expression, which allows tumorigenesis to occur.
- *BRCA1* and *BRCA2* mutations confer a high lifetime risk of breast and/or ovarian cancer. Mutation screening may be appropriate for women with family histories suggesting a hereditary predisposition to breast or ovarian cancer.
- DNA mismatch repair genes act by recognizing and fixing errors in the DNA helix resulting from incorrect pairings of nucleotides. They prevent the accumulation of genetically damaged material in the cell.

REFERENCES CAN BE FOUND ON EXPERTCONSULT.com

ACKNOWLEDGMENTS

Portions of this chapter were supported by grants from the National Institutes of Health (CA110793, CA109298, P50CA083639, CA104825, P50 CA098258, AND U54 CA151668, CA128797, RC2GM092599, P50CA134254), Ovarian Cancer Research Fund (Program Project Development Grant), Department of Defense (OC073399, W84XWH-10-0158, BC085265), Meyer and Ida Gordon Foundation 2, Zarrow Foundation, Marcus Foundation, Gynecologic Cancer Foundation, and Betty Anne Asche Murray Distinguished Professorship.

27

Principles of Radiation Therapy and Chemotherapy in Gynecologic Cancer
Basic Principles, Uses, and Complications

Judith A. Smith and Anuja Jhingran

In this chapter, the general principles of **radiation** therapy and chemotherapy are discussed with the intent of describing the underlying concepts and principles of therapy that pertain to the treatment of gynecologic malignancies. The rationale and logistics of individual cancer treatments are detailed separately in other chapters specifically dedicated to each gynecologic malignancy.

Included with the basic concepts of radiation physics are discussions of atomic and nuclear structure, particles, and nomenclature, radiation production, interactions of radiation with bodily tissues, biologic effects of radiation on cells, and the factors that modify these effects. Common radiation sources and their properties are illustrated as they relate to the treatment of specific gynecologic malignancies. Basic principles of normal tissue tolerance and the complication risks of radiation therapy as they relate to gynecologic malignancies are also presented.

Cell growth, division, and metabolism are modified by cancer-related changes in gene expression and protein regulation and by chemotherapeutic alteration of cellular metabolism. Treating physicians must recognize the various classes of chemotherapeutic agents, their actions in gynecologic malignancies, and their treatment-related toxicities. General approaches are to be followed in administering chemotherapy, specifically including the monitoring of patients receiving these agents. These are reviewed in this chapter.

RADIATION THERAPY

RADIATION THERAPY PRINCIPLES

Radiation therapy is the safe clinical application of radiation for the local treatment of abnormally proliferating benign or malignant tumors. The principles of radiation physics and radiobiology underlying treatment are discussed, but several key therapeutic goals deserve mentioning first. The dose response of tumor cells after radiation treatment follows a sigmoid curve, with increasingly effective tumor cell kill or arrest of division associated with increasing dose (**Fig. 27-1**). A similar treatment response exists for normal tissues, and the ability of radiation therapy to control malignancy depends on the greater tolerance of normal tissues to radiation exposure and a diminished

capacity of cancer cells to recover from radiation-induced damage. Thus, if one were to treat up to the total radiation dose that causes no normal tissue damage, only a small proportion of a tumor would be controlled by radiation-induced damage. Conversely, if one were to treat to a total dose that could eradicate almost the entire tumor, irreparable damage to normal tissue would often occur. This would lead to an unacceptable series of complications or even patient death after radiation treatment. The therapeutic goal of radiation therapy is to balance attempts at maximum local tumor control while minimizing adverse symptoms of treatment and normal tissue damage. Basic radiation therapy principles are detailed throughout the chapter, but briefly include the following:

- *Fractional cell kill:* Each radiation dose kills a constant fraction of the tumor cell population. Tumor cell kill follows a linear-quadratic relationship with the potential for cell-mediated repair of radiation-induced damage between radiation dose fractions.
- *Radiation dose rate:* Large radiation doses per fraction produce the greatest number of tumor cell kills; these same large radiation doses also produce the greatest damage burden on normal tissues, leading to early and late adverse complications.
- *Radiation resistance:* Although all tumor cells are sensitive to the effects of radiation, select malignant tumor cells show reduced **radiosensitivity**, resulting in slow tumor regression or renewed tumor repopulation during or after radiation treatment. Radiation resistance is associated with (1) enhanced cell-mediated repair of radiation-induced damage, (2) active concentration of chemical **radioprotectors**, or (3) cellular hypoxia or nutritional deficiency.
- *Cell cycle dependency of cell kill:* Actively proliferating tumor cells are most often killed by radiation therapy. Ionizing radiation imparts its greatest cell kill effect during the mitotic phase (M phase) and, to a lesser extent, during the late Gap1 phase and early DNA synthesis phase (G1/S). Radiation has little effect during the late synthetic phase (S phase). Before each phase of the cell cycle, genomic integrity is monitored and, if found intact, a cell then progresses through the next phase. If, however, genomic damage is detected, a cell arrests the cell cycle so that the damage may be repaired. If the normal monitors of genomic integrity are faulty, as in the case of most

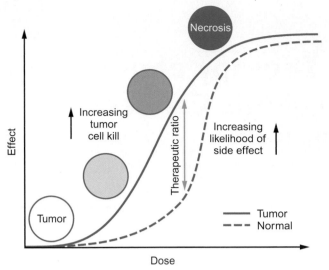

Figure 27-1 Therapeutic ratio. The concept of the therapeutic ratio for radiation therapy compares the radiation dose-response curves for tumor control and normal tissue side effect rate. Optimally, the tumor control curve lies to the left of the normal tissue curve. For every incremental increase in total dose needed to control tumor, there is a corresponding increase in the likelihood of normal tissue side effects from treatment. The magnitude of the difference between effective tumor cell kill and the likelihood of treatment-related side effects corresponds to the therapeutic ratio *(gray arrow)*. Improved tumor-directed, image-guided radiotherapy planning, use of radiation sensitizers, and use of chemotherapeutic agents (which push the tumor control curve to the left) or the use of radioprotectors (which push the normal tissue curve to the right) can widen the therapeutic ratio.

cancers, then a cell traverses the cell cycle with radiation-induced damage, leading to mitotic cell death or loss of critical genomic information vital to future cell survival.

With these basic fundamental principles of radiation therapy discussed, it is important to examine in depth the effects of electromagnetic radiation on biologic systems as they pertain to the treatment of gynecologic malignancies.

BASIC RADIATION PHYSICS

Matter is made up of subatomic particles bound together by energy to form atoms. The simplest representation of the atom consists of a central core of one or more positively charged protons (+1; 933 MeV [mega **electron volt**]) and zero or more uncharged neutrons (±0; 933 MeV) surrounded by a cloud of negatively charged orbital electrons (−1; 0.511 MeV). As described by Bowland, four fundamental forces hold these subatomic particles together: the strong force (10^1 N), electromagnetic or coulomb force (10^{-2} N), weak force (10^{-13} N), and gravitational force (10^{-42} N). The strong nuclear force acts over a short range (10^{-14} m), keeping an atom's protons from repelling one another because of the similar electrostatic charge. The coulomb force of attraction binds orbital electrons to the nucleus so that the closer an electron is to the nucleus, the higher the binding energy of the electron. As described later, the strength of the binding energy of orbital electrons relates to the interaction of radiation on matter and its subsequent biologic effects. The chemical identity of an atom relates to its number of

protons, and this number identifies the atom's **atomic number** (Z). The neutron number (N) varies among atoms and increases as the atomic number increases to stabilize the nucleus. An atom's **atomic mass number** (A) is approximately the sum of the proton number and the neutron number (A = Z + N). Radionuclides are represented by the following notation: $^A X$.

When an atom is neutral, it has no electric charge, meaning that the number of protons equals the number of electrons. If incident energy is transferred to an atom, an ionization event can occur whereby the atom acquires a positive or negative charge. When a charge is acquired, an atom is said to be ionized. Removal of an orbital electron results in an atom with a positive charge; the energy required to strip an electron off an atom must exceed the binding energy of that particular electron. Addition of an orbital electron results in an atom with a negative charge. This can occur when an electron passes close enough to an atom to experience a strong attractive force from the nucleus. Atoms can also undergo excitation, a process whereby an incident particle's energy is not sufficient to eject an atom's orbital electron but rather raises one or more electrons to a higher orbital energy state. It is through these types of interactions in atoms that radiation therapy elicits biologic consequences within tissues.

Radiation itself can be defined as the emission and propagation of energy through space or a physical medium. Radiation can be particulate, meaning that units of matter with discrete mass and momentum propagate energy (e.g., **alpha particles**, protons, neutrons, electrons) or can be electromagnetic (**photons**), meaning that energy travels in oscillating electric and magnetic fields that have no mass and no charge, with a velocity of the speed of light ($c = 3.8 \times 10^8$ m/sec). Both particulate radiation and electromagnetic radiation can ionize atoms, events that occur randomly throughout the medium.

In the treatment of gynecologic malignancies, the most common source of radiation is electromagnetic (photon) radiation. Photons are generally referred to as **x-rays** (extranuclear or from the atom) or **gamma rays** (from the nucleus) based on their origin. Important properties of a photon include its wavelength (λ), frequency (ν), speed c = (λν), and energy E = (hν), where h is **Planck's constant**. A photon's energy (E) is proportional to its frequency; that is, higher energies are transmitted at a higher frequency. Because the frequency of a photon is inversely proportional to the wavelength, electromagnetic radiation with a shorter wavelength has a higher frequency and thus a higher energy. As described by Kahn in his textbook on the physics of radiation therapy, the energy that is produced is measured in electron volts; 1 eV = 1.6×10^{-19} J, and it takes approximately 34 eV to generate one ion pair in water. The photons used to treat gynecologic malignancies can be generated externally at a distance from the woman's tumor (**teletherapy**) or internally, close to the woman's tumor (**brachytherapy**). Teletherapy x-ray radiotherapy units can deliver a range of photon energies from 50,000 eV (50 keV) to more than 30 MeV, depending on their radiation source or **linear accelerator** design. Nuclear decay of radioactive isotopes generates the gamma ray photons used in brachytherapy; such decay or disintegration was measured historically in a unit called a **curie** (Ci). One Ci is defined as 3.7×10^{10} disintegrations/sec, which is equivalent to the rate of disintegration of 1 g of radium. The modern standard unit for activity is the becquerel (Bq), which is one disintegration/sec, or 2.7×10^{-11} Ci.

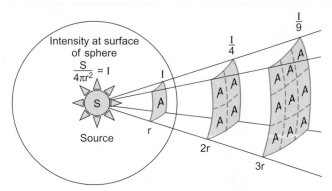

Figure 27-2 Inverse square law. Radiation intensity decreases with the square of the distance away from a point source of radiation. The intensity (I) of radiation at any given radius (r) is the source strength (S) divided by the area (A) of the sphere. For example, the energy intensity three times as far from a point source is spread over nine times the area—hence, one ninth the intensity.

Regardless of the source of electromagnetic or photon radiation, the transmitted energy diverges as the distance it travels from the source increases. This divergence causes a decrease in energy, a relationship described by the inverse square law. The inverse square law states that the energy dose of radiation per unit area decreases proportionately to the square of the distance from the site to the source $(1/r^2)$. For example, the dose of radiation 3 cm from a point source is only one ninth of the value of the dose at 1 cm (**Fig. 27-2**).

THERAPEUTIC RADIATION PRODUCTION

In general, two techniques are used in radiation therapy treatment, teletherapy (external) and brachytherapy (internal). Teletherapy in the form of external beam radiation treatment produces ionizing radiation through radioactive decay of unstable radionuclides such as cobalt (^{60}Co) or, more commonly, through acceleration of electrons. In a typical ^{60}Co teletherapy unit, the shielded ^{60}Co source resides in a treatment head mounted to a gantry that has a 360-degree rotation around the patient. Collimators consisting of interleaved bars or custom-made blocks of high Z materials can shape the treatment beam to conform the dose to the target volume. With the decay of each ^{60}Co atom, two gamma ray photons are emitted at 1.17 and 1.33 MeV (average,1.25 MeV). Over a specified time limit of exposure, these gamma ray photons deliver a specific radiation dose. Absorbed radiation dose is measured in a unit called a **gray** (1 Gy = 1 J/kg). Typical dose rates are 3 Gy/min at 80 cm from the source. The ^{60}Co source decays with a half-life of 5.263 years; thus, the source must be replaced every 5 to 7 years.

In a typical linear accelerator teletherapy unit, electrons are "boiled" off a filament and accelerated under vacuum along an accelerating wave guide using alternating microwave fields. These accelerated electrons can be used to treat the patients themselves or can hit a high Z material transmission target to produce photons of various energies by a interaction known as *bremsstrahlung,* which means braking radiation. Currently, most treatment machines generate photon energies of 4 to 20 MeV and, similar to ^{60}Co teletherapy units, have 360-degree gantry rotation around a patient. Typical linear accelerator dose rates are 3 Gy/min at 100 cm from the source. It is important to

realize key differences between these two types of treatment machines: (1) a ^{60}Co unit is always "on" when the source is not shielded because radioactive decay always occurs, whereas a linear accelerator is "on" only when energized because there is no radionuclide source; (2) the photon spectra are different in that ^{60}Co has a discrete average monoenergetic energy, whereas linear accelerators produce photons of variable energies and an average energy of one third the maximum generated energy; and (3) ^{60}Co produces treatment beams using only gamma ray photons, whereas a linear accelerator produces treatment beams of electrons or x-ray photons, depending on its treatment mode.

Alternate forms of teletherapy treatment are available, but are rarely used to treat gynecologic malignancies. A teletherapy radiation dose can be delivered using alpha particles (helium nucleus), neutrons, or protons. Alpha particles produce a large number of ionizations over a short distance, but have limited use as a mode of therapy because of their short range in tissue. Neutrons are highly penetrating into tissue because of their lack of charge; they cause high-energy collisions with atomic nuclei, principally of hydrogen, to produce recoil protons that then lose energy in surrounding tissues by ionization. Accelerated protons, as positively charged particles, used as therapy deposit a radiation dose sparingly along their path until near the end of their range, where the peak dose is delivered, the so-called Bragg peak. Neutron and proton therapies are used to treat cancer, but are not used routinely in the treatment of gynecologic malignancies.

To produce a consequential radiobiologic effect in tissues or tumor, incident photons or other forms of radiation must interact with matter. Kahn has noted that there are five possible electromagnetic (photon) interactions with matter:

1. *Coherent scattering* ($<$10 keV) occurs when an incident photon scatters off an atom's outer orbital electron without losing energy. This produces no radiobiologic effect.
2. *Photoelectric effect* (10 to 60 keV) occurs when an incident photon interacts with an inner orbital electron and the photon's energy is completely absorbed by that electron. If enough energy is transferred to the orbital electron to exceed the binding energy of the inner orbital electron, it is ejected, leaving a vacancy that an outer orbital electron fills. When an outer orbital electron fills the vacancy, a characteristic x-ray is produced with energy equal to the difference in binding energy between the two electron orbitals. The probability of a photoelectric effect event happening is proportional to Z^3/E^3. Diagnostic radiographic or computed tomography (CT) images that are acquired at relatively low photon energies have high tissue–bone contrast detail because the Z^3/E^3 ratio is maximized.
3. *Compton effect* (60 keV to 10 MeV) occurs when an incident photon (Eγ) loses some or all of its energy to an outer orbital electron. The photon, if it remains, is scattered at some angle away from the atom. An electron that has acquired energy exceeding its binding energy (E$_{BE}$) leaves the atom with sufficient kinetic energy (E$_{KE}$ = Eγ $-$ E$_{BE}$) to penetrate tissue and produce molecular damage through downstream ionizations. For simplicity, at common therapeutic photon energies (4 to 18 MeV), the Compton effect is biologically most important in that incident photons interact predominantly with cellular water. Human and mammalian tissues are principally composed of water ($\approx$90%) and functional biomolecules such as proteins and DNA (**Fig. 27-3**). Incident photons ionize

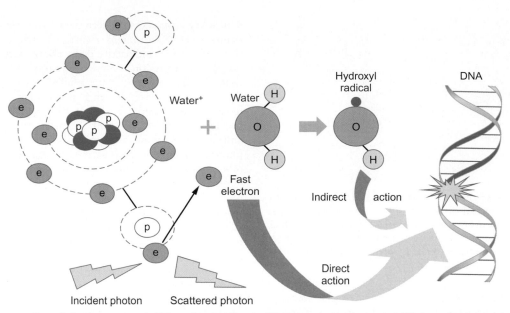

Figure 27-3 Compton effect. Cells are composed of biomolecules dissolved in an aqueous solution (≈90% water by weight). Incident photons (p) randomly ionize (*left*) cellular water to produce an ion radical (water$^+$) and a free fast electron (e$^-$) that can damage biomolecules such as DNA. The water ion radical interacts with another molecule of water to form a hydroxyl radical (·OH). Most often (≈66%), formed hydroxyl radicals diffuse throughout the cell, breaking chemical bonds in target molecules such as proteins and DNA (R, *right*). Breaks in the chemical bonds of DNA can lead to DNA base damage, DNA cross-links, DNA single-strand breaks, and DNA double-strand breaks, contributing to the loss of vital genomic material during subsequent cell divisions and possibly mitotic death of the damaged cell.

water to produce an ion radical (H_2O^+) and a free electron (e$^-$). The ion radical is highly reactive (half-life of 10^{-10} second) and can interact with another molecule of water to form a hydroxyl radical (·OH). Hydroxyl radicals are also highly reactive (half-life of 10^{-9} second) and can break chemical bonds in target molecules such as proteins and DNA (·R). Breaks in the chemical bonds of DNA can lead to DNA base damage, DNA cross-links, DNA single-strand breaks, and DNA double-strand breaks. As discussed later, DNA strand breaks can result in the loss of vital genomic material during subsequent cell divisions, potentially leading to mitotic death of the damaged cell. In this way, therapeutic radiation leads to significant radiobiologic effects by functionally modifying cellular proteins and damaging DNA.

4. *Pair production* (>10 MeV) occurs when an incident photon has an energy greater than 1.022 MeV. This threshold is required because the photon disappears to form an electron-positron pair, with each particle having an energy of 0.511 MeV. Once formed, free electrons slow by nuclear attraction and are quickly stopped in tissue. However, the formed positron is highly reactive and short-lived in that it is annihilated with surrounding electrons to create two photons of 0.511 MeV, each traveling 180 degrees apart from one another. Positron emission tomography (PET) scanners build images based on the coincident detection of photons formed by this process.

5. *Photodisintegration* (>10 MeV) occurs when an energetic photon penetrates the nucleus of an atom and dislodges a neutron. Emitted neutrons cannot ionize tissue themselves because they have no charge, but rather collide with surrounding atomic nuclei to produce recoil, positively charged protons that elicit radiobiologic effects through subsequent ionizations.

Radiation Biology

Munro has shown that nuclear DNA is unquestionably one essential target of therapeutic radiation. In his textbook on radiobiology, Hall reported that one third of radiation-induced DNA damage is from the direct interaction of incident photons ionizing atoms within DNA itself. Two thirds of radiation-induced DNA damage is a consequence of the indirect damage done by freely diffusing hydroxyl radicals (·OH). However, Hall and Hei have described a bystander effect whereby lethal damage to cellular proteins, organelles, or the cell membrane in an irradiated cell can lead to neighboring cell death in cells that would not have died on their own. The bystander effect suggests that damage to cellular proteins or organelles in one cell may also result in cell lethality. Note that not all radiation damage is lethal to the cell; some damage to DNA can undergo repair—namely, sublethal DNA damage repair. Sublethal DNA damage repair occurs in normal cells and malignant cells, but much less so in malignant cells because these often have abnormal DNA repair mechanisms. A variety of complex and redundant repair mechanisms have been identified, including base excision repair and nucleotide excision repair for damage to the DNA base and deoxyribose backbone, homologous recombination repair for DNA single-strand breaks, and nonhomologous end-joining repair for DNA double-strand breaks. As the time interval between radiation doses lengthens, cell survival increases because of the prompt repair of radiation-induced damage. The repair process is usually complete within 1 to 2 hours, although this period may be longer in some slowly renewing cellular tissues. Before discussing the consequences of DNA damage, it is important to understand key factors that can modify the rate at which DNA damage accumulates.

Intracellular molecular oxygen importantly modifies radiation-induced DNA damage as it fixes damage done by free hydroxyl radicals. Palcic and Skarsgard have reported that molecular oxygen, when present during or within microseconds of photon-induced ionization events, reacts with the altered chemical bonds of ionized molecules ($\cdot$R) to produce organic peroxides (RO_2), a nonreparable form of the target molecule. Molecules fixed in this manner are permanently altered and may function abnormally. Thus, tumor and tissue oxygenation have practical implications in radiation therapy insofar as a rapidly proliferating gynecologic malignancy may have a poor blood supply, which decreases tumor cell oxygenation, particularly at the center of large tumors. Tumor tissue hypoxia leads to radiation resistance, as reflected by increased cell survival after radiation treatment. Laboratory experiments have shown that the radiation dose necessary to kill the same proportion of hypoxic cells as compared with aerated cells approaches 3:1. This ratio is commonly referred to the oxygen enhancement ratio. For oxygen to have its maximal effect, the dissolved oxygen concentration in a tumor must be approximately 3 mm Hg (venous blood is 30 to 40 mm Hg), according to Hall. In the treatment of gynecologic malignancies, Dunst and coworkers have found that cervical cancer patients undergoing radiation therapy with a serum hemoglobin level greater than 10 mg/dL have improved tumor oxygenation, resulting in superior local control and superior clinical outcomes compared with patients whose hemoglobin level is less than 10 mg/dL. Also, hypoxic cell sensitizers such as the nitroimidazoles, as studied by Adams and colleagues, and the bioreductive drug tirapazamine, as reported by Goldberg and coworkers, improve he radiosensitivity of hypoxic cells within tumors. The potential benefit of these agents in the treatment of gynecologic cancers has been explored in clinical trials.

The rate at which energy is lost per unit path length of medium, or **linear energy transfer** (LET), also has an effect on the accumulation of radiation-induced DNA damage. For photons, energy loss is infrequent along its path length, typical of low-LET radiation. Sparsely ionizing, low-LET radiation produces one or more sublethal events and thus multiple hits are needed to kill the cell. Heavy particulate radiation from alpha particles or protons is densely ionizing because energy is deposited more diffusely along its path length. This is typical of high-LET radiation. Because the probability of producing a lethal event in a cell is much higher with high- LET radiation, cell death in this case is independent of tumor oxygenation. Thus, research efforts have been directed toward the development of heavy particle generators that can overcome the limitation of poor oxygenation of cancer cells.

Within the cell, molecules that have sulfhydryl moieties at one end and a strong base such as an amine at the other end are capable of scavenging free radicals produced by radiation-induced ionization events. These molecules can also donate hydrogen atoms to ionized molecules before molecular oxygen can fix the damage done by radiation-induced hydroxyl radicals. As reported by Utley and associates, amifostine is a nonreactive phosphorothioate that accumulates (1) readily in normal tissues by active transport to be metabolized into an active compound to scavenge free radicals and (2) slowly in tumors by passive diffusion, with limited or no conversion to the active compound. It is reasonable to conclude that the presence of a radioprotector such as amifostine would decrease radiation-induced DNA damage and limit normal tissue radiation-related side effects. Clinical trials have been investigating the radioprotective effect of amifostine in gynecologic malignancies but, at present, amifostine has

shown the most promise as a chemoprotectant and has been approved to reduce the renal toxicity associated with repeated administration of cisplatin chemotherapy in women with advanced ovarian cancer.

What constitutes cell death in the traditional sense—cessation of cellular respiration and vital function—is not the same in radiation biology. Death in radiation biology is the loss of reproductive integrity or the inability to maintain uninterrupted cellular proliferation with high fidelity. Thus, radiation kills without the actual physical disappearance of malignant cells, although body macrophages often remove the dead cells, causing tumors to shrink in size. Malignant cells may remain a part of a tumor, but have discontinued cellular metabolism and proliferation. Most cells, when exposed to radiation, die a mitotic death, meaning that cells die at the next or a subsequent cell division, with all progeny also dying. Inflammation can accompany mitotic cell death, potentially resulting in local adverse side effects. Jonathan and associates have noted that alternative forms of loss in reproductive capacity caused by radiation include terminal differentiation, senescence, and apoptosis. In apoptosis, cells undergo a complex process of programmed cellular involution and phagocytosis by neighboring cells. There is no inflammatory response resulting from apoptosis. One remarkable example of apoptosis is the formation of the spaces between the digits of the hand during human fetal development.

Returning to radiation-induced DNA damage, electromagnetic radiation (x-ray or gamma) deposits energy in cells, which may damage DNA directly or indirectly through hydroxyl radicals ($\cdot$OH). In relative terms, more than 1000 DNA base-damaging events, 1000 DNA single-strand breaks, and 40 DNA double-strand breaks occur with each typical radiation dose fraction. Although base and DNA single-strand breaks need to be repaired so that mutations are not propagated, DNA double-strand breaks are believed to be the most crucial radiobiologic effect of radiation therapy. There is an increased statistical probability that a cell will be unable to repair a DNA double-strand break, resulting in the loss of genetic material at cell division. Also, attempts by cells to repair the DNA double-strand breaks often result in bizarre chromosome arrangements that interfere with the normal division of the cell. Cell death ensues through loss of critical genes or impaired cell division.

Cell death following radiation therapy is modeled by a linear-quadratic relationship (**Fig. 27-4**). The initial slope of the cell survival curve is shallow and curvilinear, whereas the terminal slope is more linear. In the low-dose region of the survival curve typical of daily-dose fractions used in radiation therapy, the fraction of cells surviving is high because of the repair of single-event sublethal damage (e.g., multiple base damage or DNA single-strand breaks). In the high-dose region of the survival curve, the fraction of cells surviving is low because of multiple event damage in the form of DNA double-strand breaks or the accumulation of too many sublethal events that can be repaired before the next cell division. Capacity to repair sublethal damage depends on radiation quality (LET), tissue oxygenation, and cell cycle time.

As shown in **Figure 27-5**, and as described by Deshpande and associates and Pawlik and Keyomarsi, there are four highly regulated phases of the cell cycle. After completing mitosis, cells enter a gap phase (G1), variable in time span, in which the cell performs protein synthesis and other functional metabolic and biologic processes. Under the influence of complex, finely

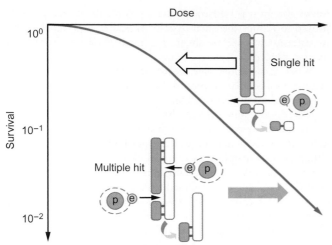

Figure 27-4 Cell survival curves. A radiation survival curve plots cell survival on a logarithmic scale against radiation dose on a linear scale. Survival represents the number of cells retaining reproductive capacity to form approximately 50 cell colonies (i.e., approximately five to six cell divisions) after a specified radiation dose. The initial slope is shallow, forming a shoulder in the low-dose region (1 to 3 Gy/fraction) caused by repair of sublethal damage. Occasionally, a single hit will produce a DNA double-strand break, resulting in the loss of genetic material (*open arrow*). In the high-dose region (>3 Gy/fraction), the slope steepens caused by multiple damaging events leading to DNA double-strand breaks. If not repaired, significant vital genetic material may be lost at a subsequent cell division and the cell may die. e, Electron; p, photon.

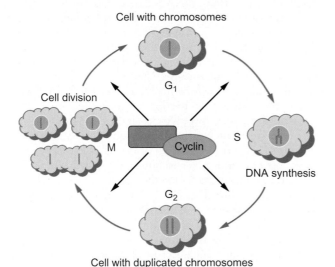

Figure 27-5 Phases of the cell. After mitosis (M), there is an interval of variable duration during which there is RNA and protein synthesis and a diploid DNA content (G1 [Gap1]). The cell may also enter a prolonged or resting phase (G0) and then reenter the cycle during DNA synthesis, the S phase, in which DNA is duplicated. During the G2 (Gap2) phase, there again is protein and RNA synthesis. During the M phase, the cell divides into two cells, each of which receives diploid DNA content. CDK, Cyclin-dependent kinase.

regulated intercellular and intracellular signaling, cells then enter the DNA replication phase (S phase) in which the cell must exactly replicate its DNA to produce an identical set of chromosomes. Entry into the S phase is controlled by sequentially activated, highly regulated cyclin-dependent kinases (CDKs)

responsible for differentially recruiting and amplifying specific gene products necessary for DNA replication. Moreover, there are corresponding cell cycle inhibitory proteins (CDKIs) that negatively regulate cell cycle **progression**. After DNA replication, the cell enters a second gap phase (G2), in part to ensure high DNA replication fidelity in the newly formed chromosomes. At the completion of the G_2 phase, cells undergo mitosis, whereby two identical daughter cells are produced.

To maintain genetic integrity through the cell cycle, the cell has multiple checkpoints through which it must pass, notably at the G1/S and G2/M transitions, as described by Pawlik and Keyomarsi. The G1/S checkpoint prevents the replication of damaged DNA, as in the case of radiation therapy. Malumbres and Barbacid have reported that proteins critical to the G1/S checkpoint include p53, p21, and the retinoblastoma protein (Rb), all of which modulate the activity of CDKs responsible for the transition to S phase. Briefly, Rb lacks phosphorylated subunits in its active form, binding to the E2F transcription factors and preventing E2F translocation to the nucleus to recruit genes needed for the S phase. Sequential phosphorylation of RB by CDK 4/6-cyclin D and CDK2-cyclin E complexes releases the E2F transcription factors. Radiation-induced DNA damage results in the accumulation of the G1 checkpoint regulatory protein p53, which in turn activates the CDKI p21; p21 inhibits the phosphorylation of RB, delaying the G1/S transition. The G2/M checkpoint prevents the segregation of aberrant chromosomes at mitosis. Two molecularly distinct checkpoints have been identified, one that is regulated by the ataxia-telangiectasia mutated gene product (ATM) and one that is ATM-independent. ATM has multiple phosphorylation products that modulate CDKs at the G2/M transition (Chk1 and Chk2) as well as p53 expression through modification of its degradation pathway. According to Xu and associates, phosphorylation of Chk1 and Chk2 inhibits the cdc2 protein kinase, blocking cells at the G2/M transition. ATM's essential role in DNA damage recognition is highlighted by the extreme radiosensitivity of patients with mutated ATM. Malignant cells that often have mutated cell cycle checkpoint proteins have an impaired ability to repair damage done to nuclear DNA, and thus accumulate lethal DNA-damaging events that lead to cell kill in a few cell cycles.

Cells show different radiosensitivities during the cell cycle. M-phase cells are particularly radiosensitive because the DNA is packaged tightly into chromosomes, so that ionization events have a high likelihood of causing lethal DNA double-strand breaks. S-phase cells are particularly radioresistant because enzymes responsible for ensuring high-fidelity DNA replication are relatively overexpressed and recognize altered DNA bases or inappropriate strand breaks. Cells in the G1 or G2 phase of the cell cycle are relatively radiosensitive compared with the S phase. Chemotherapies that inhibit cell cycle–dependent pathways or impede DNA repair enhance the radiobiologic effect of radiation.

RADIATION TREATMENT: BRACHYTHERAPY AND TELETHERAPY THERAPY

In general, two techniques are used in radiation treatment, brachytherapy (internal) and teletherapy (external). Brachytherapy involves the placement of radioactive sources within an existing body cavity (e.g., the vagina) in close proximity to the tumor. In the treatment of gynecologic malignant tumors, radioactive sources can be placed within hollow needles that are implanted directly into the tissue to be irradiated (interstitial implant) or within a hollow cylinder, or inserted in tandem into the vagina or through the cervical os, respectively. For the treatment of cervical cancer, two vaginal ovoids, one on each side of the tandem, are positioned in the vaginal fornices (intracavitary therapy). In clinical practice, interstitial or intracavitary brachytherapy needles or applicators without radioactive sources are placed first in the operating room with the patient under anesthesia. After postanesthesia patient recovery, the position of the needles or applicators is confirmed by radiographic imaging. These radiographic images help guide radiotherapy planning. Radioactive sources are afterloaded some time later to reduce radiation exposure to medical personnel treating the woman. The most widely used intracavitary applicator is the Fletcher-Suit applicator, which is useful for the treatment of a cervical tumor or a tumor located near the cervix (**Fig. 27-6**). For interstitial and intracavitary brachytherapy, the radiation dose delivery to the tumor and surrounding tissues follows the inverse square law as modified by source and tissue photon attenuation and scattering.

Several radioisotopes with various photon energies and half-lives are used in gynecologic brachytherapy. Although

uncommon, radioisotopes with a short half-life (e.g., ^{198}Au [gold]) may be placed within the woman and left permanently. Radioisotopes with a long half-life (e.g., ^{137}Cs [cesium]) are placed temporarily within interstitial or intracavitary needles or applicators and are removed after a prescribed radiation dose has been administered. Historically, brachytherapy for most gynecologic malignancies consisted of temporary low-dose rate (40 to 70 **centigray** [cGy]/hr) sources in place for 1 to 3 days. A low-dose rate requires that the woman be in a shielded hospital room with medical personnel supervision, on bed rest, with prolonged analgesia and prophylactic anticoagulation, and limited family contact during radiation dose administration. Recently, high-dose rate, catheter-based brachytherapy has become popular because the procedure can be performed in 1 day on an outpatient basis. The high-dose rate uses a thin wire tipped with iridium (^{192}Ir) to deliver radiation doses at rates exceeding 200 cGy/min. Unlike low-dose rate therapy, high-dose rate therapy is performed in a shielded treatment room requiring patient immobilization for a short period and minimal patient analgesia and anesthesia. **Table 27-1** indicates the half-lives of some of the isotopes commonly used in treating gynecologic cancers. It is also important that a uniform distribution of radiation be achieved in the adjacent tissues to avoid hot spots, which can damage normal tissue, as well as cold spots, which can lead to reduced dose delivery to the tumor.

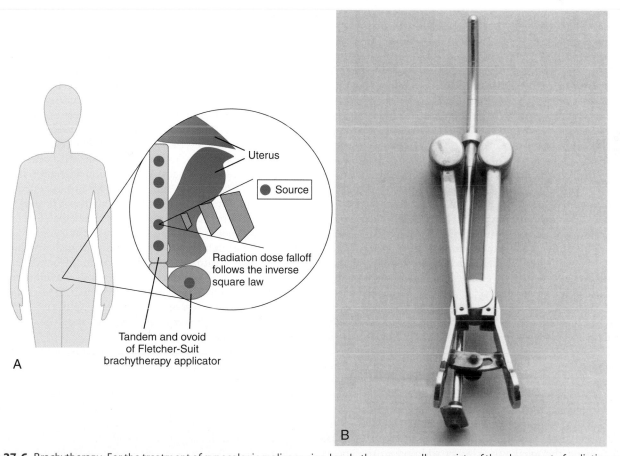

Figure 27-6 Brachytherapy. For the treatment of gynecologic malignancies, brachytherapy usually consists of the placement of radiation sources (*dark circles*) in close proximity to the tumor. This can be accomplished by the intracavitary placement of hollow applicators such as the Fletcher-Suit applicator (*inset*) placed within the uterine cavity and vaginal vault or by the interstitial placement of hollow needles through the tissues themselves. The radiation dose decreases as the square of the distance away from the radiation source.

Table 27-1 Half-Lives of Commonly Used Radioisotopes for Gynecologic Malignancies

Radionuclide	Half-Life
Gold (^{198}Au)	2.7 days
Phosphorus (^{32}P)	14.3 days
Iridium (^{192}Ir)	73.8 days
Cobalt (^{60}Co)	5.26 yr
Cesium (^{137}Cs)	30 yr
Radium (^{226}Ra)	1620 yr

Teletherapy in the form of external beam radiotherapy means that the source of radiation is at a distance from the woman, sometimes located at a distance 5 to 10 times more than the depth of the tumor being irradiated. This distance is referred to as the **source-to-surface distance** (SSD) and is used to calculate dose using the inverse square law. When using an SSD patient treatment setup, the SSD is used along with tumor depth, radiation beam energy, depth of the point of maximum dose, and output parameters for a given treatment field size to determine the daily radiation dose. Alternatively, with the use of different angles and ports of treatment, the concept of source-axis distance has been introduced; it denotes the distance from the radiation source to the central axis of machine rotation. The woman is positioned so that this axis passes through the center of the tumor, and treatment ports are arranged around this axis to optimize tumor dose. When using a source-axis distance patient treatment setup, the daily radiation dose is calculated using machine output and beam attenuation at the depth for a given treatment field size.

Conventional external beam radiation is delivered with beams of uniform intensity. Advances in computer-guided planning and treatment have made the use of beams of varying intensity more commonplace. This approach of planned dose intensification allows the high-dose region to be conformed precisely to the shape of the planned treatment volume, a technique called intensity-modulated radiotherapy. Recent advances in radiotherapy delivery systems have allowed linear accelerators to be coupled with helical CT scanners. Image-guided radiation therapy using this type of device is called helical tomotherapy. In conventional therapy, and in intensity-modulated radiotherapy and helical tomotherapy, beams from the external radiation source can be sculpted using high electron-dense material collimators. Collimators limit scatter radiation and block portions of the treatment beam from delivering an intolerant radiation dose to critical tissues (**Fig. 27-7**). In general, the higher the energy source of the radiation, the deeper the beam can penetrate into tissue. Thus, high-energy radiation has its predominant effect in deeper tissues and spares the surface of the skin of a radiation effect.

An **isodose curve** is a line that connects points in the tissue that receive equivalent doses of irradiation. **Figure** 27-7 contrasts the isodose curves for 6- and 22-MeV machines. For the 6-MeV machine, the maximum dose is near the surface, with a more rapid falloff in the deeper tissues. For the 22-MeV machine, the maximum dose is deep to the surface, sparing the effects of radiation on the overlying skin. In addition to the energy of the beam, the energy of radiation absorbed at various depths is affected by the size of the field being treated. Larger fields contain more scattered radiation, which leads to a greater dose at a given depth. **Figure** 27-7 shows the effect of increasing the size of the field with an increasing dose at a given depth for three different types of energy sources.

Thus, the radiation dose delivered to the tumor is affected by the energy of the source, depth of the tumor beneath the surface, and size of the field undergoing irradiation. With external therapy, usually 180 to 200 cGy/day is given five times per week. There has been experimental work evaluating hyperfractionation, which involves smaller multiple doses given more frequently (e.g., 120 cGy three times daily or 160 cGy twice daily, with 6 hours between doses to allow sublethal damage repair in normal tissues). Hyperthermia, or the use of high-temperature heat to denature cellular proteins, has also been explored to enhance the therapeutic effectiveness of radiation because malignant cells are particularly vulnerable to heat-induced killing during the S-phase portion of the cell cycle. It appears to offer the most promise for tumors localized in an area that can effectively and safely tolerate increased temperatures (42° to 43° C [107.6° to 109.4° F]).

TISSUE TOLERANCE AND RADIATION COMPLICATIONS

Adverse radiation effects are commonly divided into two broad categories, early and late, which demonstrate markedly different patterns of response to radiation dose **fractionation**. It is important for the treating physician to understand critical tissues and organ systems at risk of radiation damage. **Table 27-2** presents the approximate tolerance of tissues to radiation therapy.

Early or acute effects manifest as the result of death in a large population of cells and can occur within days to weeks after the initiation of radiation therapy. For early effects, the total dose of radiation and, to a lesser extent, the dose per fraction determine the severity of the side effect. Radiation acutely affects tissues undergoing rapid cell division to replace lost normal functioning cells. This is most pronounced in areas such as the skin, intestinal mucosa, mucosa of the vagina and bladder, and hematopoietic system, in which precursor stem cells are renewing functional mature cells. The radiation dose given in multiple small fractions reduces the untoward adverse effects of cell damage on normal tissue and allows normal healing to occur between treatment fractions through sublethal DNA damage repair (the shallow curvilinear portion of the cell survival curve). During the treatment of gynecologic malignancies, most adverse early treatment-related toxicities can be managed with medication. It is preferred practice that radiation treatment not be interrupted for treatment-related toxicities caused by radiation-induced tumor accelerated repopulation. Only rarely does a treatment program need to be temporarily discontinued for treatment-related toxicities.

Late effects occur after a delay of months or years after radiation therapy. Late effects are often the product of parenchymal connective tissue cell loss and vascular damage. Late effects may be seen in slowly renewing tissues such as the lung, kidney, heart, and liver and in the central nervous system. In the treatment of gynecologic malignancies, late adverse effects include tissue necrosis and fibrosis, as well as fistula formation and ulceration. In contrast to early effects, late effects depend primarily on the dose per fraction. Fractionated radiation therapy using a daily radiation dose of 180 to 200 cGy minimizes the risk of late effects. Second cancers (mostly sarcomas) induced after radiation are

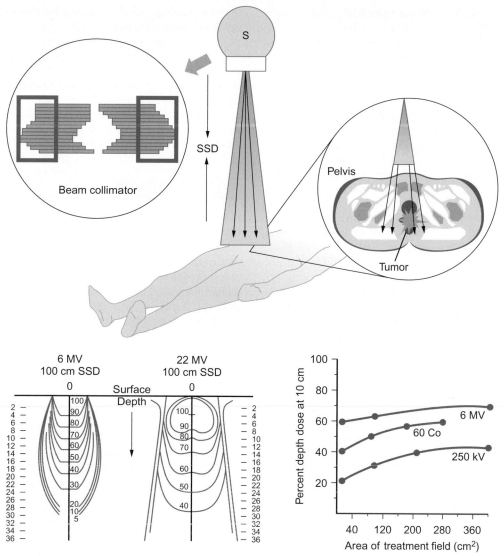

Figure 27-7 Teletherapy. Conventional external beam radiotherapy is the delivery of radiation dose to tissues at a distance (SSD) away from the radiation source (S). As the beam emerges from the treatment machine, the beam diverges and can be shaped by high-Z material leaflets of a beam collimator *(top)* or custom blocks. As the treatment beam hits the patient, photon interactions occur, producing ionization events *(inset)*. Energy deposition within tissue creates isodose curves. Isodose curves and depth-dose distributions for 6- and 22-MV photons are shown *(bottom left)*. Note that the higher energy machine delivers radiation to a greater depth for the same surface dose, resulting in skin sparing. As treatment field size varies, the dose delivered at a specified depth varies *(bottom right)*.

Table 27-2 Normal Tissue Tolerance to Radiation Therapy

Tissue	Tolerance (Gy)
Kidney	20-23
Liver	25-35
Small bowel	45-50
Rectum	60-70
Bladder	60-70
Vaginal mucosa	70-75
Cervix	>120

rare (1 in 500 to 1000 cases) and do not usually appear until 15 to 20 years after radiation exposure. Arai and associates have noted an excess of rectal cancer, bladder cancer, and leukemia in women with carcinoma of the cervix treated by radiation in comparison with those treated by surgery.

The skin overlying the tumor being treated visibly reveals the effects of radiation-induced normal tissue damage. Skin effects are manifest by reddening of the skin and loss of hair where the radiation treatment beam enters the body. Erythema may progress to dry or moist skin breakdown or desquamation caused by loss of the actively proliferating basal layer of the epidermis that renews the overlying epithelium. This is less common now than in prior years because higher energy radiation beams, which spare the surface dose, are used. However, during the treatment of vulvar malignancies, the skin surface and superficial groin nodes are the radiotherapeutic target, so desquamation is more commonly observed. Medical treatment consisting of non–metal-containing creams and emollients during therapy reduce discomfort and allows healing within 2 to 4 weeks after completion of radiation therapy. Late skin fibrosis may produce a rough leathery texture to the skin in the irradiated field. Chiao and Lee, and Gothard and coworkers, have reported on the use of pentoxifylline and vitamin E to promote healing of late subcutaneous and deep tissue fibrosis after radiation.

In the treatment of gynecologic malignancies, other sites at risk of radiation-induced normal tissue damage are the bladder, rectum, and large and small bowel. The bladder epithelium consists of a basal layer of small diploid cells covered by large transitional cells. Radiation damage to the diploid cells results in slow renewal of the overlying transitional cells that are periodically sloughed off during urination. Radiation cystitis manifested as dysuria and urinary frequency results in bladder irritation. Treatment with analgesics such as phenazopyridine (Pyridium) can alleviate symptoms. Hematuria may also occur. Therapy with sclerosing solutions or fulguration through a cystoscope may be necessary. McIntyre and colleagues have noted that ureteral stricture after radiation for stage I carcinoma of the cervix is 1% at 5 years and 2.5% at 20 years, a rare but important complication. In rare cases, urinary diversion may be required. Bladder fibrosis and reduced bladder capacity are late effects of pelvic radiation therapy.

In the intestine, the renewing stem cells are found at the bottom of the crypts of Lieberkuhn. Within 2 to 4 days after the start of radiation, these cells can become depleted, leading to atrophy of intestinal mucosa. Damage to the bowel usually occurs in the form of inflammation (sigmoiditis or enteritis), which commonly results in increased bowel motility or diarrhea but also, rarely, may be associated with severe bleeding and cramping pain. Less severe cases can often be controlled with a low-roughage diet and antispasmodic medications. Although uncommon, severe cases may require bowel resection or permanent bowel diversion through a colostomy. Covens and coworkers have noted that those who require operation for radiation damage to the bowel have an approximately 25% risk of dying in 2 years, with ileal damage being the most risky. Those with complications not requiring surgery frequently have decreased vitamin B_{12} and bile acid absorption. Late bowel toxicities include radiation proctitis caused by small vessel vascular damage in the epithelium, which may progress to intermittent rectal bleeding. Bowel stenosis or obstructions resulting from fibrosis and adhesion formation may occur, especially in patients who have had previous pelvic or abdominal surgery. Occasionally, enteric fistulas can develop, and bowel perforation may occur. In the latter case, surgical therapy is required, usually to bypass the affected area of the intestine. As a rule, extensive dissection of irradiated tissue is avoided. Montana and Fowler have shown that the risks of proctitis and cystitis are dose-related. For example, they found severe proctitis and cystitis at doses of 6750 and 6900 cGy, respectively, whereas such complications were not observed in patients whose median dose was 6300 and 6500 cGy.

A lowering of circulating lymphocytes, granulocytes, platelets, and red blood cells can be seen with pelvic radiation therapy for gynecologic malignancies. The stem cells of the bone marrow in an adult reside in the axial skeleton (vertebrae, ribs, and pelvis). Usual external beam radiation therapy treatment fields for gynecologic malignancies encompass the sacrum and lower vertebrae and pelvis, thereby reducing precursor stem cells for circulating blood cells. This is an important consideration if the woman is to receive concurrent radiosensitizing chemotherapy or subsequent cytotoxic chemotherapy. Growth factor support with synthetic **erythropoietin** and/or granulocyte colony-stimulating factor (G-CSF) is often required for patients receiving multiagent chemotherapy following treatment with pelvic radiation therapy.

Finally, fistulas between the vagina and bladder or between the vagina and rectum may develop when there has been extensive radiation damage to the intervening tissues. This usually takes place during therapy for large carcinomas of the cervix. As a rule, such complications will occur 6 to 24 months after treatment, although they may occur many years after primary therapy. Diverting surgery or resection of the fistulas is often needed to correct these serious complications.

CHEMOTHERAPY

Although many patients with gynecologic cancers present initially with a clinically appreciable mass or tumor, only a minority of patients have localized disease, curable with surgery or radiation treatment alone. More often, the cancer has spread to regional lymph nodes or disseminated to other organs, even though these sites may not be clinically appreciated at the time of initial diagnosis.

Chemotherapy regimens for gynecologic cancers have evolved over the past 7 decades. Initially, Li and colleagues demonstrated the first successful effort in gynecologic cancer using the **antimetabolite** methotrexate, which could cause permanent remission of metastatic trophoblastic disease. Shortly thereafter, treatment regimens emerged with single-agent melphalan followed by single-agent cyclophosphamide. When cisplatin was introduced into clinical practice, it added significant improved activity to cyclophosphamide; this combination then became the standard of care. In the 1980s, clinical studies to evaluate paclitaxel for treatment of ovarian cancer were undertaken. Paclitaxel soon replaced cyclophosphamide and paclitaxel plus cisplatin became the standard of care for ovarian cancer and, since then, has become a popular treatment option for all gynecologic malignancies. Because of toxicity associated with cisplatin, numerous studies were conducted to justify substitution with carboplatin for cisplatin because of its improved toxicity profile, but controversy still remains over which **taxane** or platinum agent is preferred. Overall, the consensus is that primary chemotherapy should include a taxane and a platinum agent.

Historically, there has been no clear difference or advantage in regard to which taxane or platinum agent was used or which dose intensity was selected until the recent clinical trial by Katsumata and colleagues. This study suggested that there is an advantage with a weekly schedule or dose density compared with the standard platinum-taxane, every 3-week regimen. However, there are concerns about the toxicity associated with the dose-dense regimen; questions about the feasibility of this regimen have arisen with the typical older women seen in clinical practice, so a confirmatory Gynecologic Oncology Group (GOG) phase III study is ongoing.

In addition to dosing schedule, the route of chemotherapy administration has also been an area of research interest. For decades, many researchers have conducted numerous clinical trials of intraperitoneal (IP) chemotherapy. Recently, in 2006, Armstrong and colleagues published the first IP therapy clinical trial to demonstrate a survival advantage over the standard IV regimen (**Box 27-1**). However, these advances in chemotherapy for the treatment of ovarian cancer have not translated into major changes in overall 5-year survival, which remains less than 20%.

A number of general principles have been developed during the study of chemotherapeutic agents. These provide guidelines for their recommended use and administration (see **Box 27-1**).

CHEMOTHERAPY PRINCIPLES AND GUIDELINES

Some of the concepts used in antibiotic therapy for infections have been applied to the chemotherapeutic approach to cancer management. However, major differences exist. Infections are frequently caused by a single virus or even multiple types of bacteria with specific growth patterns and sensitivities to antibiotics. Although it is believed that a cancer can originate from a single cell, clinically evident disease is composed of a heterogeneous population of cells with different cell cycle durations, varying **growth fractions**, and diverse expression of genes, potential mutations, and proteins responsible for cell proliferation and metastasis. Intrinsic and acquired drug resistance remains one of the daunting challenges in the treatment of gynecologic cancers.

Basic principles for cancer chemotherapy arose from experiments in murine tumor models, notably mice leukemias, conducted by Skipper and colleagues at the Southern Research Institute. These principles include the following:

- *Fractional cell kill:* Each dose of chemotherapy kills a constant fraction of the tumor cell population. Tumor cell kill usually correlates in a linear relationship with the pharmacokinetic parameter of the area under the drug concentration curve (AUC).
- *Dose intensity:* High chemotherapy doses interspersed with short rest periods produce the greatest tumor cell kill in rapidly proliferating malignancies.
- *Drug resistance:* Single-agent chemotherapy administration selectively isolates drug-resistant tumor cells, leading to an outgrowth of hardy, resistant malignant cells. Chemotherapy drug resistance has been associated with the following: (1) cell-mediated modification of drug targets; (2) active drug transport out of the cell; and (3) alteration of drug activation or targeting.
- *Cell cycle dependency of cell kill:* Actively proliferating tumor cells are most often killed by chemotherapy agents; drugs inhibiting DNA processing act during the S phase and those impairing cell division act during the M phase. If the normal monitors of genomic integrity are intact, a cell may suspend the cell cycle to repair any detected damage. If, however, these monitors are abnormal, a cell may continue progression through the cell cycle, which may lead to unrecoverable cell cycle arrest or irreparable damage to critical genes vital for future cell survival. Malignant cancer cells often demonstrate abnormal monitors of genomic integrity, in part permitting their rapid proliferation but also increasing their sensitivity to chemotherapies.

APPROACHES TO TREATMENT

The dose of an anticancer chemotherapy agent is usually calculated as a function of body surface area (square meters), which provides a better measure of potential toxicity than body weight. This is partly because of the observation that body surface area more closely reflects cardiac output and blood flow than body weight alone. Chemotherapeutic agents have varying toxicities (see later). A major problem with most agents is bone marrow toxicity, requiring careful monitoring of mature and stem cell turnover in the hematopoietic system. Most gynecologic cancer chemotherapy agents are administered IV in cycles varying from weekly to 3- or 4-week intervals between each cycle. If mature white blood cells (i.e., absolute neutrophil count) and platelets have not recovered adequately by the time the next cycle is due, treatment delay and/or a dose reductions is often considered. In patients with a history of prolonged myelosuppression and/or with regimens associated with significant myelosuppression, the proactive use of growth factor support is often helpful in allowing chemotherapy treatments to continue at full dose and on time, as scheduled.

Additional considerations about the toxicity of chemotherapeutic agents relate to hepatic metabolism and/or renal excretion. It may be necessary to modify the dose of the drug administered when renal or hepatic function is compromised. For example, consider the following:

- Doxorubicin (Adriamycin) and paclitaxel are metabolized in the liver, and dose reductions must be made if the drug is administered to a woman with hepatic dysfunction.
- Methotrexate and cisplatin effects are increased in patients with renal damage, necessitating dose reduction in these patients.
- Cisplatin not only has its effects intensified in patients with renal damage but also is toxic to the kidney, requiring particular caution if administered to those with compromised renal function or those undergoing therapy with other renal toxic medications.

Plasma protein binding (PPB) can also alter toxicity profile. For example, paclitaxel and topotecan both are associated with PPB greater than 80%. When PPB drugs are displaced, the unbound or free fraction of drug will increase, which may increase toxicity and/or effects of the chemotherapy. Furthermore, a low serum albumin level leads to an increase in the free fraction of the chemotherapeutic agent, which is one reason why malnourished patients have a heightened toxicity to chemotherapy.

Various chemotherapeutic agents can be differentially toxic to other organ systems of the body, including the gastrointestinal, nervous, pulmonary, and reproductive systems. The primary toxicities affecting gynecologic cancer patients are nausea and vomiting, prolonged myelosuppression, and neuropathies. Acute nausea and vomiting can usually be prevented with the combination of a serotonin antagonist with a steroid. Despite the introduction of newer agents such as aprepitant and palonosetron, delayed nausea and vomiting remains a therapeutic challenge. Unfortunately there are limited options for the prevention and management of chemotherapy-induced neuropathy other than dose reduction or switching chemotherapy agents. Myelosuppression is a manageable toxicity with most chemotherapy regimens. Prevention of myelosuppression with the use of a myeloid growth factor (e.g., G-CSF) has better efficacy than waiting until prolonged neutropenia develops. Although not often relevant for patients with gynecologic cancer, loss of ovarian function and fertility is often an important consideration when selecting adjuvant treatments for younger women with other cancers. The goal of treatment is to provide as high a dose of the chemotherapeutic agent at a planned frequency, as defined by clinical trial data to produce maximum chemotherapeutic effectiveness without causing unacceptable toxicity or side effects.

There are four ways in which chemotherapy is generally used for the treatment of gynecologic cancers: (1) as an induction treatment for advanced disease (neoadjuvant therapy) in gynecologic setting, it is used to shrink tumor prior to surgery to improve the potential for optimal tumor debulking, which is followed by additional chemotherapy; (2) as an adjunct to radiation therapy; (3) as primary treatment for cancer in the gynecologic cancer setting, it is often administered after completion of tumor debulking surgery; or (4) as consolidation after a **complete response** is achieved to target undetectable microscopic disease.

In assessment of the effect of chemotherapeutic agents, a number of definitions are used to describe the response of the tumor being treated. Clinical response should be assessed on an individual basis, with tumors in some patients monitored by physical examination and in some patients through imaging, typically with CT or magnetic resonance imaging (MRI). Other means of assessing response to therapy include serial assessment of specific tumor markers (e.g., CA-125 for ovarian cancer or β-human chorionic gonadotropin for gestational trophoblastic disease) or identification of changes in hypermetabolic foci by PET.

In 2000, an international committee endorsed a technique for measuring tumors by CT and MRI that is easy and highly reproducible. This is known as RECIST (*r*esponse *e*valuation *c*riteria in *s*olid *t*umors) and is applicable for subjects with at least one measurable target lesion. The greatest diameters of all target lesions are summed and changes in this sum during treatment are used to assign response (**Table 27-3**).

CHEMOTHERAPEUTIC AGENTS

A large number of chemotherapeutic drugs have been used in the treatment of gynecologic cancers (**Fig. 27-8**). In general, these agents can be classified into platinum compounds, taxanes, **antitumor antibiotics**, topoisomerase I inhibitors, **alkylating agents**, antimetabolites, **vinca alkaloids**, biologic and **targeted**

Table 27-3 RECIST (Response Evaluation Criteria in Solid Tumors) Criteria to Assess Clinical Response to Therapy

Criterion	Features
CR (complete response)	Disappearance of all target lesions
PR (**partial response**)	30% decrease in sum of greatest diameters of target lesions
PD (progressive disease)	20% increase in sum of greatest diameters of target lesions
SD (stable disease)	Small changes that do not meet the above criteria

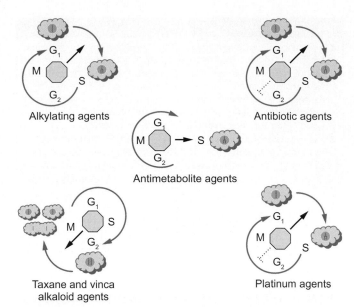

Figure 27-8 Chemotherapy cell cycle activity. Chemotherapeutic agents demonstrate variable antitumor cytotoxic and radiosensitizing activities, depending on their mechanism of action during the cell cycle. Alkylating agents facilitate the transfer of alkyl groups to DNA, disrupting the G1/S transition (*top left*). Agents derived from bacteria deregulate normal DNA and RNA processing, slowing progression through the G1/S and G2/M transitions (*top right*). Antimetabolites result in faulty base insertion into replicated DNA or specifically inhibit rate-limiting enzymes such as ribonucleotide reductase that are needed to produce deoxyribonucleotides for DNA replication during the S phase (*center*). Taxane and vinca alkaloid agents alter the mitotic spindle during mitosis, preventing cell division (*bottom left*). Platinum agents show activity throughout the cell cycle and form DNA structural adducts, limiting progression at various cell cycle checkpoints. Chemotherapeutic agents themselves are cytotoxic, but also increase tumor cell sensitivity to ionizing radiation during critical periods of the cell cycle in which radiation has a maximal effect. The safe combination of these various classes of chemotherapeutic agents and radiation is an area of active clinical research.

therapy, and anticancer hormones. Agents currently used alone or in combination for the treatment of gynecologic cancer are discussed here.

Platinum Analogues

Cisplatin and carboplatin are two of the most active and widely used chemotherapeutic agents in the treatment of gynecologic malignancies and are used in the primary treatment of ovarian, tubal, peritoneal, endometrial, cervical, and vulvar cancers, as well as some cases of metastatic gestational trophoblastic disease.

Platinum (PLT) analogues form PLT-DNA adducts that intercalate the DNA, interrupting DNA synthesis. Although its cell cycle specificity has not been clearly defined, cisplatin's radiosensitizing mechanisms include the formation of toxic intermediates in the presence of radiation-induced free radicals, radiation-induced increased cellular platinum uptake, inhibition of radiation-induced DNA repair, and cell cycle arrest at the G2-M transition. For the treatment of most gynecologic malignancies, cisplatin is given by an IV or IP infusion. Cisplatin is emetogenic but can be appropriately managed with serotonin antagonists. Hypomagnesemia is a problem in patients receiving cisplatin, often requiring frequent magnesium replacement.

Because cisplatin is nephrotoxic, copious hydration and mannitol infusion usually accompany cisplatin administration to prevent renal tubular necrosis because the drug is excreted in the urine in its active form. Cisplatin also induces myelosuppression and high-frequency ototoxicity. Audiograms may be obtained before and during treatment to assess ototoxicity. Cisplatin induces severe peripheral neuropathy, which may improve somewhat after cessation of therapy but tends to be long-lasting.

Carboplatin is an analogue of cisplatin; a study conducted by Ozols and colleagues has reported that it has activity in ovarian epithelial carcinoma comparable with that of cisplatin. Its mechanism of action and antitumor activity throughout the cell cycle are similar to those of cisplatin, but carboplatin is less potent in producing DNA interstrand cross-links compared with cisplatin. Yang and coworkers have found that the cellular uptake of carboplatin increases after ionizing radiation treatment with a concomitant increase in drug-DNA binding.

Carboplatin is dosed based on the woman's specific renal function. Often, the calculated creatinine clearance is used in place of the measured glomerular filtration rate (GFR) to estimate renal function. Carboplatin is dosed based on a target area under the curve (AUC) from 5 to 7 mg/mL; the dose is calculated using the Calvert formula:

$$\text{Dose (mg)} = \text{target AUC} \times (\text{GFR} + 25)$$

Although carboplatin is renally eliminated because of this dose algorithm, it is not associated with the degree of nephrotoxicity as cisplatin; thus, rigorous prehydration is not required, allowing for it to be administered on an outpatient basis. The adverse drug effects associated with carboplatin include neurotoxicity, nausea, and vomiting, but to a lesser extent compared with cisplatin. Myelosuppression, primarily thrombocytopenia, is the dose-limiting toxicity (DLT) associated with carboplatin.

The DLT of carboplatin is myelosuppression, primarily thrombocytopenia, although neutropenia and anemia also occur. Typically, after dosing single-agent carboplatin, the nadir occurs between 15 and 20 days. Because carboplatin's typical dose is individualized based on the woman's specific renal function, it appears to have an improved toxicity profile. It is important to keep in mind that appropriate parameters need to be used to estimate renal function to minimize toxicity. Less common toxicities include alopecia, hepatotoxicity, neurotoxicity, and ototoxicity.

Both platinum analogues can be associated with delayed hypersensitivity reactions. Because carboplatin is used more often in a recurrent setting, there are more hypersensitivity reactions reported with carboplatin. There is a high cross-sensitivity, so patients who react to one platinum agent will be at significant risk for another reaction if exposed to another platinum analogue. Desensitization protocols with complete histamine blockade (H1 and H2) and steroids have been successful and allow continuation of treatment with the platinum agent.

Taxanes

Paclitaxel is a taxane that is naturally derived from the bark of the Pacific or Western yew (*Taxus brevifolia*). Docetaxel are derived from the bark of the English yew (*Taxus baccata*). Both chemotherapeutic agents promote microtubule assembly, stabilizing microtubules to prevent and inhibit depolymerization of tubulin during mitosis (M phase). By arresting cell division through a functional block of the M phase, paclitaxel and docetaxel are potent chemotherapeutic agents, with activity in most solid tumors. Although administration of both taxanes can be accompanied by severe hypersensitivity reactions and hypotension, it is more commonly observed with paclitaxel because of its diluent, polyethoxylated castor oil (Cremophor EL) and ethanol. Thus, premedication with antihistamines and steroids are recommended to minimize infusion-related hypersensitivity reactions. Neutropenia is the major toxic side effect, but sensory peripheral neuropathy is also a serious problem. Bradycardia and severe cardiac problems have been reported with the administration of paclitaxel, but they are rare. A rare complication has been the report of bowel perforation in a few individuals while on paclitaxel therapy, as noted by Rose and Piver. In addition to its use in the treatment of ovarian cancer, paclitaxel and/or docetaxel are being used in the treatment of other cervical cancers, endometrial cancer, and uterine sarcomas.

Antitumor Antibiotics

Antitumor antibiotics are derived from products of bacterial or fungal cultures. The chemotherapeutic agents generally used for gynecologic malignancies are actinomycin D (Dactinomycin), doxorubicin, and bleomycin (Blenoxane).

Actinomycin D is derived from the bacteria *Streptomyces parvulus* and is used primarily in the treatment of gestational trophoblastic disease. It lodges between adjacent purine-pyrimidine (guanine-cytosine) base pairs, blocking DNA-dependent ribosomal RNA synthesis by RNA polymerase. Actinomycin D is maximally effective in the G1 phase of the cell cycle, but data suggest that this drug may act throughout the entire cell cycle. Because bound actinomycin D dissociates slowly from DNA, cells actively progressing through the cell cycle are stopped from doing so at the G1/S checkpoint for genomic integrity, leading to cell death. If radiation is delivered in the presence of the drug, treated cells show a radiosensitizing effect. The drug causes severe myelosuppression, often leading to leukopenia and thrombocytopenia (nadir, 7 to 10 days). Toxicity to the gastrointestinal mucosa is associated with vomiting within 20 hours, stomatitis, and nonbloody diarrhea. Reversible alopecia may also occur. Dermatitis resulting from radiation recall has also been noted, meaning that skin erythema and inflammation arise in skin areas previously irradiated.

Doxorubicin and its newer liposomal formulation (Doxil) are anthracyclines derived from the bacteria *Streptomyces peucetius*, var. *caesius*. Within the cell nucleus, doxorubicin wedges between stacked nucleotide pairs in the DNA helix and, because of its bulk, inhibits binding of enzymes needed for DNA-directed RNA and DNA transcription, as well as DNA replication. Doxorubicin therefore has maximal activity in the G1 and S phases of the cell cycle. A second mechanism of action noted for doxorubicin includes the inhibition of topoisomerase II in the G2 phase of the cell cycle. Topoisomerase II assists in the coiling and supercoiling of DNA prior to mitosis by facilitating enzymatic DNA double-strand breaks. Doxorubicin has been shown to stabilize the double-strand break generated by topoisomerase II, thereby promoting loss of genetic material during mitotic division. Doxorubicin must be administered carefully by IV injection because extravasation leads to soft tissue and skin necrosis and ulceration. Doxorubicin is metabolized by the liver, and dosages must be reduced in patients with compromised hepatic function. Myelosuppression occurs regularly with

Table 27-4 Side Effects of Drugs Often Used or Being Tested in Gynecologic Oncology

Agent	Common Toxicities
Altretamine	Nausea and vomiting, diarrhea, abdominal cramping, myelosuppression
Bevacizumab	Hypertension (DLT), proteinuria, congestive heart failure, increase risk of bleeding, thromboembolism, GI perforation
Bleomycin	Interstitial pneumonitis, pulmonary fibrosis (DLT), mucocutaneous toxicity, fever
Capecitabine	Diarrhea (DLT), paresthesias, palmar-plantar erythrodyesthesia (PPE), dermatitis, hyperbilibinemia, fatigue, anorexia
Carboplatin	Nausea and vomiting, myelosuppression (DLT), nephrotoxicity, electrolyte wasting, diarrhea, stomatitis, hypersensitivity reactions
Cyclophosphamide	Hemorrhagic cystitis, SIADH, alopecia, myelosuppression (DLT)
Dactinomycin	Myelosuppression (DLT), hepatotoxicity, alopecia, fatigue, myalgia, pneumonitis, malaise, lethargy
Docetaxel	Myelosuppression, fluid retention, hyperlacrimation, nail disorders
Etoposide	Myelosuppression, nausea and vomiting, hypotension, anorexia, alopecia, headache, fever
5-Flurouracil	Nausea and vomiting, diarrhea, anorexia, myelosuppression, PPE, cardiotoxicity
Gemcitabine	Myelosuppression (DLT), flulike symptoms, headache, somnolence, nausea and vomiting, stomatitis, diarrhea, constipation, rash
Letrozole	Nausea and vomiting, bone pain, arthralgias, hot flashes
Leuprolide acetate	Peripheral edema, gynecomastia, hot flashes, hyperphosphatemia, nausea and vomiting, weight gain
Liposomal Doxorubicin	Myelosuppression, stomatitis, mucositis, alopecia, flushing, shortness of breath, hypotension, headaches, cardiotoxicity, hand-foot syndrome
Methotrexate	Stomatitis, nausea and vomiting, myelosuppression, nephrotoxicity, elevation in hepatic enzymes, Interstitial pneumonitis
Paclitaxel	hypersensitivity reactions, peripheral neuropathy (DLT), nausea and vomiting, alopecia
Tamoxifen	Thromboembolism, hot flashes, decreased libido, nausea and vomiting, thrombocytopenia, anemia
Topotecan	Myelosuppression (DLT), nausea and vomiting, diarrhea, stomatitis, abdominal pain, alopecia, SGOT and SGPT elevation
Vincristine	Neurotoxicity, constipation (DLT), alopecia,
Vinorelbine	Myelosuppression (DLT), neurotoxicity, constipation, asthenia, fatigue

DLT, Dose-limiting toxicity, GI, gastrointestinal; SGOT, serum glutamic pyruvic transaminase; SGPT, serum glutamic pyruvic transaminase; SIADH, syndrome of inappropriate antidiuretic hormone secretion.

therapeutic doses. Complete but reversible alopecia is a side effect (**Table 27-4**). Because the doxorubicin metabolism creates free radicals that bind to cardiac myocytes, it can cause significant cardiac toxicity, leading to irreversible congestive heart failure. Therefore, cardiac function is assessed routinely before administration and cumulative doses are kept to less than 450 mg/m^2. Liposomal doxorubicin has a synthetic lipid-like membrane around the doxorubicin molecule that is proposed to promote tumor uptake and protect against cardiotoxicity. Cardiomyopathy is less common with liposome-encapsulated doxorubicin, but skin toxicity, notably palmar plantar erythrodysesthesia (PPE), is more common.

Bleomycin is derived from the bacteria *Streptomyces verticillus* and, when complexed with ferrous iron, is a potent oxidase, producing single-strand DNA breaks by hydroxyl radical formation. Bleomycin may be administered IV, IM, or SC. It is excreted via the kidney, and some dose reduction is made if renal function is compromised. The drug does not produce significant myelosuppression, in contrast to most of the other cytotoxic agents. It is, however, highly toxic to the lungs in that pneumonitis and pulmonary fibrosis occurs in 10% of patients. Thus, particular care must be used in persons with compromised lung function. To prevent this complication, cumulative doses of less than 400 units are given. If pneumonitis develops, as evidenced by symptoms of low-grade fever and nonproductive cough, treatment is a tapered course of oral corticosteroid therapy. Bleomycin is also toxic to skin and can produce erythema, peeling, and pigmentation. It has been used as part of combination therapy, with particular effectiveness against ovarian germ cell tumors, and has been tried for a variety of other gynecologic malignancies, particularly carcinoma of the cervix.

Topoisomerase I and II Inhibitors

As noted, topoisomerases are DNA enzymes that control the topology of DNA double-helix cellular functions during transcription and replication of genetic material. There are two classes of topoisomerases, I and II. Drugs that prevent these functions are referred to as topoisomerase inhibitors.

Topotecan

Topotecan is in the class of camptothecins and is used for the treatment of cervical and epithelial ovarian cancers. Camptothecins inhibit topoisomerase I, causing stabilization of the cleavable complex and resulting in an accumulation of single-strand and double-strand DNA breaks, and ultimately cell death. It has recently been approved by the U.S. Food and Drug Administration (FDA) to be used in combination with cisplatin for the treatment of platinum-sensitive recurrent cervical cancer.

Topotecan is a semisynthetic analogue of camptothecin, a chemical derived from the *Camptotheca accuminata* tree native to China. This drug stabilizes single-strand breaks made by topoisomerase I, an enzyme that relaxes DNA structural tension by facilitating single-strand breaks and subsequent religation. Topotecan has the greatest activity during the G1/S phases of the cell cycle. Toxicities include bone marrow suppression, nausea and vomiting, alopecia, mucositis, and diarrhea.

Etoposide

Etoposide is an epipodophyllotoxin derived from the root of the Mayapple or mandrake plant that stabilizes DNA strand breaks made by topoisomerase II during coiling and supercoiling of DNA during mitosis. The primary toxicity of etoposide is myelosuppression, leading to depression of leukocytes and platelets.

Other common toxicities include anorexia, nausea and vomiting, stomatitis, and severe hypotension if infused in less than 30 minutes. Uncommon toxicities include cardiotoxicity, bronchospasm, and somnolence. It is important to recognize that oral etoposide has an erratic absorption, with significant interpatient variability, from 0% to 100% bioavailability. Oral etoposide is typically used in the recurrent setting after failure of other second-line agents. Oral etoposide should never be used in place of the IV formulation when there is a curative intent—that is, a BEP regimen (**b**leomycin sulfate, **e**toposide phosphate, and cisplatin for germ cell tumors.

Alkylating Agents

Alkylating agents are chemical compounds that facilitate the replacement of hydrogen for an alkyl group, potentially disrupting normal function of the altered molecule. As chemotherapeutic agents, alkylating agents interact directly with DNA by transferring positively charged alkyl groups to negatively charged chemical groups intrinsic to the DNA molecule. Examples of this class include cyclophosphamide and ifosfamide. In general, the effectiveness of these agents appears to be similar, but there are some variations in toxicity. As a drug class, alkylating agents affect rapidly dividing cells and are particularly toxic to bone marrow, leading to severe myelosuppression.

Cyclophosphamide and its structural analogue ifosfamide are bifunctional cyclic phosphamide esters of nitrogen mustard. Both drugs interact with the N7 position of guanine in the DNA helix to form cross-link bridges between the same strand of DNA (intrastrand), opposite strands of DNA (interstrand), and DNA and cellular proteins. By forming intrastrand and interstrand DNA bridges, cyclophosphamide and ifosfamide impair the functional binding of enzymes used to process and replicate DNA, disrupting the G1/S phase transition of the cell cycle. These drugs are inactivated in the liver and exclusively excreted by the kidney. Their urinary metabolite acrolein may accumulate within the urinary system, causing severe urothelial damage that may result in hemorrhagic cystitis within 24 hours or weeks after administration. Prophylactic hydration (3 liters/day) to increase dilute urinary output and administration of 2-mercaptoethane sulfonate (mesna), a compound that binds to acrolein and prevents urotoxicity, can be used to prevent this complication. Administration of these agents also leads to leukopenia (nadir, 8 to 14 days) and thrombocytopenia (nadir, 18 to 21 days), alopecia, nausea and vomiting, and amenorrhea. Therapy with alkylating agents has been associated with a subsequent risk of developing acute leukemia. This risk may range from 2% to 10% and appears to be related to the dose of and duration of alkylating agent treatment. They may be administered IV or orally but are only rarely used in the primary treatment of gynecologic malignancies.

Antimetabolites

Antimetabolites interfere with cell metabolism by competing with naturally occurring purines or pyrimidines, whose chemical structure they resemble. In this way, they interfere or prevent vital biochemical reactions.

5-Fluorouracil (5-FU) is a fluorinated pyrimidine analogue resembling the DNA nucleoside thymine; it differs from the RNA nucleoside uracil by a fluorinated carbon in the fifth position in the nucleoside ring, as described by Grem. Conversion of 5-FU into fluorodeoxyuridine monophosphate blocks DNA synthesis by covalently binding to thymidylate synthase. This inhibits the formation of de novo thymidylate, a necessary precursor of thymidine triphosphate essential for DNA synthesis and cell division. The conversion of 5-FU into fluorouridine triphosphate results in the erroneous incorporation of fluorouridine triphosphate into RNA strands, which interferes with RNA processing and protein synthesis. By these actions, 5-FU perturbs normal progression through the G1/S transition, bringing about impaired cell division caused by altered nucleotide pools and DNA repair. As such, 5-FU is a potent **radiosensitizer**. One advantage of the drug is that 5-FU can be administered as a bolus or continuous IV infusion or orally as a prodrug (e.g., capecitabine) that is metabolized to 5-FU. Common toxicities associated with 5-FU include myelosuppression, stomatitis, diarrhea, alopecia, nail changes, dermatitis, acute cerebellar syndrome, cardiac toxicity, hyperpigmentation over the vein used for infusion, and PPE have been reported (**Table 27-4**). The 5-FU given IV is normally used in conjunction with cisplatin as a radiation sensitizer in the treatment of advanced cervical and vulvar cancers. Oral 5-FU (capecitabine) is often used in the treatment of recurrent ovarian and endometrial cancers.

Methotrexate is a folic acid analogue that binds tightly to dihydrofolate reductase, which plays a critical role in intracellular folate metabolism. This prevents the metabolic transfer of one carbon unit within the cell and thereby arrests DNA, RNA, and protein synthesis. Cells exhibit sensitivity to this drug predominantly in the S phase portion of the cell cycle. The effects of methotrexate can be overcome by the administration of folinic acid (citrovorum factor) 24 hours after methotrexate, which replenishes the tetrahydrofolate. Some chemotherapeutic protocols have used very high doses of methotrexate to treat the tumor, followed by citrovorum rescue to avoid severe toxic side effects (see **Table 27-4**). Methotrexate is administered IV, IM, or orally using a variety of dose regimens. It is excreted in the urine and dose adjustments must be made if there is decreased renal function. Methotrexate results in severe myelosuppression (nadir, 6 to 13 days). Stomatitis, nausea, and vomiting are reported. Hepatotoxicity resulting in liver enzyme elevation may be seen within 12 hours after high-dose treatment. Therapeutic serum methotrexate levels are evident long after treatment in patients with ascites or pleural effusion because these act as a reservoir for the drug. The predominant use of the drug for gynecologic malignancies has resulted in the effective treatment of trophoblastic disease.

Gemcitabine, a synthetic deoxycytidine nucleoside analogue, targets ribonucleotide reductase (RR), the rate-limiting enzyme in deoxyribonucleotide metabolism during the S phase. Gemcitabine is triphosphorylated in tumor cells by the enzyme deoxycytidine kinase, inhibiting DNA polymerase activity and interrupting DNA replication. As a nucleoside analogue, gemcitabine is incorporated as a fraudulent base pair in DNA; as a diphosphate, it inhibits the regulatory subunit of the RR enzyme, which leads to the depletion of deoxyribonucleotide pools needed for DNA synthesis in the S phase of the cell cycle. Reported treatment toxicities include myelosuppression, transient elevation of liver enzyme levels, nausea, vomiting, flulike symptoms, and fatigue (see **Table 27-4**). Gemcitabine is used in the treatment of recurrent ovarian cancer, endometrial cancer, and uterine sarcomas.

Vinca Alkaloids

The vinca alkaloids bind to the β-tubulin subunits of the mitotic spindles, blocking polymerization of the microtubules in mitosis. For gynecologic malignancies, the vinca alkaloids used most often include vinorelbine and vincristine. Vincristine is derived from the periwinkle plant (*Vinca rosea*) and acts in a cell cycle–dependent manner, blocking the assembly of tubulin and causing toxic destruction of the mitotic spindle, which arrests cellular mitosis. Vinorelbine is a semisynthetic vinca alkaloid derived from vinblastine. By affecting the late G2 and M phases of the cell cycle, these drugs are potent cytotoxins and increase cell radiosensitivity by slowing the G2/M transition in which radiation effects are maximal. Vincristine is severely neurotoxic and can produce numbness, motor weakness, and constipation as a result of its autonomic effects. The DLT of vinorelbine is myelosuppression (see **Table 27-4**).

Altretamine

Altretamine has been used for a number of years, but in recent years has been replaced with more active agents. The exact mechanism of action of altretamine is not known. It does not act as an alkylating agent in vitro, but is possibly activated to one in vivo. Altretamine is metabolized by cytochrome P450 (CYP450) and the reduced form of nicotinamide adenine dinucleotide phosphate (NADPH) to N-hydroxymethyl pentamethylmelamine, which has been shown to bind covalently to DNA. Additional N-methylmelamines formed may also mediate some of the cytotoxicity of this agent.

It is an oral agent that is usually given in four divided doses. Altretamine therapy may be associated with some nausea, vomiting, diarrhea, abdominal cramping, and myelosuppression (see **Table 27-4**). In addition, a pharmacist should monitor for potential CYP450-drug interactions in patients on multiple prescriptions and alternative medications.

Biologic and Targeted Agents

Over the past 5 years, there have been major efforts toward the incorporation of monoclonal antibodies such as bevacizumab and cetuximab and small-molecule tyrosine inhibitors such as sunitinib, gefitinib, and sorafenib into first-line and recurrent treatment regimens for gynecologic cancers. Although as single-agent therapy the biologic agents have not demonstrated significant activity against gynecologic cancers, there are mounting clinical data to support the implementation of agents such as bevacizumab into first-line and maintenance regimens to improve progression-free survival, specifically for ovarian cancer.

Bevacizumab

Bevacizumab is a recombinant humanized monoclonal antibody that targets and inactivates vascular endothelial growth factor (VEGF) to inhibit the angiogenesis pathway. As a single agent in the recurrent ovarian cancer setting, bevacizumab has had only a moderate response. However, in combination with chemotherapy, bevacizumab has had promising response rates, ranging from 15% to 80%. There are significant limitations to incorporating bevacizumab with chemotherapy regimens because of the high risk of bowel perforation in ovarian cancer patients that was first observed in phase II studies. Hence, the current recommendation is that patients should not have had recent bowel surgery or a history of significant bowel resections.

Bevacizumab has been evaluated in combination with oral cyclophosphamide, paclitaxel, and gemcitabine for the treatment of recurrent ovarian cancer. The integration of bevacizumab into a first-line treatment regimen has focused on the benefits with paclitaxel plus carboplatin followed by maintenance with bevacizumab alone. However, the duration of maintenance bevacizumab remains an area of therapeutic and pharmacoeconomic controversy. Although there is some improvement in response rates to chemotherapy and in progression-free survival, it is premature to determine the overall benefit of bevacizumab in the treatment of ovarian cancer.

Targeted Agents

Tyrosine kinase inhibitors (TKIs) such as sorafenib, sunitinib, pazopanib, and cediranib also target the VEGF angiogenesis pathway via inhibition of the VEGF receptor (VEGFR). Current research efforts have been focused on combination regimens of these TKIs with cytotoxic agents for first-line treatment and also for the treatment of recurrent ovarian cancer. Another agent of interest is aflibercept (VEGF Trap), which is a fusion protein that targets VEGF-A. Initial studies have demonstrated that it is beneficial in the treatment of malignant ascites. Unfortunately, the popular epidermal growth factor receptor (EGFR) agents such as erlotinib, which have had so much benefit in the treatment of other cancers, have not demonstrated activity alone or in combination with chemotherapy or with bevacizumab for the treatment of gynecologic cancers. Finally, the newer classes of targeted therapies, such as platelet-derived growth factor (PDGF) inhibitors and poly (ADP-ribose) polymerase (PARP) inhibitors, are being incorporated into numerous clinical studies in an attempt to improve progression-free and overall survival.

Anticancer Hormone Therapy

Hormone therapy has been effectively developed for the treatment of breast cancer. Estrogen and progesterone receptors have been clearly identified in endometrial carcinomas and have been found in other types of gynecologic cancers, particularly ovarian epithelial carcinomas. Progestins such as megestrol (Megace), depot medroxyprogesterone acetate (Depo-Provera), and 17-hydroxyprogesterone caproate (Delalutin), as well as antiestrogens such as tamoxifen and raloxifene, have been used in the treatment of endometrial carcinomas and seem to have their best effects against well-differentiated tumors.

DRUG RESISTANCE

A daunting challenge is overcoming drug resistance, which occurs fairly often in the recurrent setting of all gynecologic malignancies. Platinum sensitivity is defined by a disease-free interval longer than 6 months after treatment with a platinum agent. If platinum-sensitive, patients can be retreated with a platinum agent, which usually will be single-agent carboplatin because it is tolerated better. Platinum resistance is present when there is tumor progression while receiving a platinum agent or disease relapse within less than 6 months after the completion of chemotherapy, and alternative agents need to be considered. Taxane resistance follows the same parameters.

The optimal chemotherapeutic agent or regimen in the treatment of platinum-resistant disease is currently unknown. Ideally, the agent should be active in gynecologic cancer and should be non–cross-resistant with taxanes or platinum agents. Overall, regardless of the agent, the response rate is low for all the agents in platinum-refractory (resistant) cancer. Typically, it is recommended to give three cycles prior to evaluation for response to the new agent unless there is a more than 50% doubling of CA-125. Because tumor regression is so rare in the recurrent setting, even achieving **stable disease** is considered a treatment success. If no response is observed after three cycles, an alternative chemotherapy regimen may be selected.

EVALUATION OF NEW AGENTS

In the development of new oncology drugs, serial evaluations are necessary to assess the effectiveness of the drug and ascertain its toxicity. A number of trials are necessary to move a new agent from the point of evaluation to allow it to be used in regular medical practice. Unlike other areas of drug development, clinical trials for cytotoxic agents can only be conducted in those with active cancer, often those who have already failed current standard therapy treatment options.

A standard method frequently used to measure a patient's general functional condition before enrollment in clinical chemotherapy trials of new agents is the Karnofsky Performance Status Scale (**Table 27-5**). In general, patients are poor candidates from clinical trials if their score is 50 or less. Cooperative research groups, such as the GOG, have modified the Karnofsky scoring system to reflect a five-point graded classification.

After extensive preclinical evaluation, investigational new drug (IND) applications are filed to move new drugs into human studies. The human clinical trial process is a fairly rigorous and costly process to determine not only safety and efficacy but also improvement over the current standard of care for each new agent proposed, sometimes alone or in various combination regimens. A general outline of phase trials is outlined as follows:

- *Phase I trial:* A phase I trial tests new drugs at various doses to evaluate toxicity and determine tolerance to the drug. At the various doses tested, some therapeutic effects may be observed, although this is not the primary aim of the trial.
- *Phase II trial:* A phase II trial tests the therapeutic effectiveness and extent of toxicity of the drug at doses expected to be effective against a specific tumor type.
- *Phase III trial:* A phase III trial compares new treatment therapies against the current treatment standard of care. For example, this trial design assesses whether a new drug therapy is superior, equivalent, or inferior to the chemotherapeutic agent currently used.

There have been numerous programs implemented to help facilitate drug approval and access to investigational drugs, such as the Fast Track Drug Approval Program and Orphan Drug Approval. Special consideration for either program requires preapplication and approval by the FDA. Often, in the gynecologic oncology setting, FDA approval for new gynecologic indications is not sought because of small patient populations and the inability to conduct phase III studies in a timely fashion. Compendia listings are often granted based on

Table 27-5 Assessment of Performance Status

Score	Karnofsky Performance Status Scale
100	Normal, no complaints; no evidence of disease
90	Able to carry on normal activity; minor signs or symptoms of disease
80	Normal activity with effort; some signs or symptoms of disease
70	Cares for self but unable to carry on normal activity or do active work
60	Requires occasional assistance but is able to care for most personal needs
50	Requires considerable assistance and frequent medical care
40	Disabled; requires special care and assistance
30	Severely disabled; hospitalization indicated, although death not imminent
20	Very sick; hospitalization necessary; active support treatment necessary
10	Moribund; fatal process progressing rapidly
0	Dead

Grade	Gynecologic Oncology Group Performance Status Scale
1	Fully active, able to carry on all predisease performance without restriction
2	Restricted in physically strenuous activity but ambulatory and able to carry out work of a light or sedentary nature (e.g., light housework, office work)
3	Capable of only limited self-care, confined to bed or chair >50% of waking hours
4	Completely disabled; cannot carry on any self-care; totally confined to bed or chair
5	Dead

peer-reviewed published literature, which expands reimbursement for treatment recommendations.

Progress has been slow and unsuccessful in finding a cure for ovarian cancer and recurrent endometrial or cervical cancers. In the absence of a curative treatment for recurrent disease, selecting an investigational trial treatment still remains the best option for ovarian cancer patients. Research is needed to identify and develop new approaches for the prevention of recurrence and new options for the treatment of advanced primary and recurrent disease. Efforts should especially focus on agents to modulate or overcome drug resistance or new molecular targets to optimize chemotherapy outcomes.

KEY POINTS

- Electromagnetic radiation is a form of energy that has no mass or charge and travels at the speed of light.
- The inverse square law states that the energy measured from a radiation source is inversely proportional to the square of the distance from the radiation source.
- Each delivered radiation dose kills a constant fraction of tumor cells irradiated. Oxygen can render radiation-induced DNA damage permanent.
- The effect of photon radiation (low LET) on tissues is altered by tissue oxygenation, whereas neutron radiation (high LET) is independent of oxygenation.
- The cell replication cycle consists of M (mitosis), G1 (Gap1 = RNA and protein synthesis), S (DNA synthesis), and G2 (Gap2 = RNA and protein synthesis). When the cell is not in the replication cycle, it is in the G0 phase.
- The dose of radiation delivered to a tumor depends on the energy of the source, the size of the treatment field, and the depth of the tumor beneath the surface. Increasing the dose increases the depth of maximum dose beneath the skin surface.
- Radiation acts on cells primarily in the M phase, making rapidly proliferating cells the most radiosensitive.

KEY POINTS—CONTINUED

- Normal tissues repair the radiobiologic effects of radiation more effectively than tumor tissue.
- Radiation side effects usually involve erythema of the skin, without desquamation and mild fatigue.
- Uncommon side effects include lowering of the circulating blood cells, dysuria and urinary frequency, diarrhea, bowel injury, and fistula formation:
  - Cytotoxic chemotherapeutic agents act on various phases of the cell cycle, primarily affecting rapidly proliferating cells, and at a given dose destroy a constant fraction of tumor cells.
  - Growth factors or G-CSF are used to limit the hematologic toxicity of chemotherapy.
- After the completion of the staging and primary surgical treatment, the current standard of care is six cycles of a taxane–platinum-containing chemotherapy regimen.
- If recurrence is less than 6 months after completion of chemotherapy, the tumor is defined to be platinum- and/or taxane-resistant.
- The antitumor activity of second-line chemotherapy regimens is similar; the choice of treatment for recurrent disease depends on residual toxicities, physician preference, and patient convenience. Participation in a clinical trial is also a reasonable option for these patients.

REFERENCES CAN BE FOUND ON
EXPERTCONSULT.com

28

Intraepithelial Neoplasia of the Lower Genital Tract (Cervix, Vulva):
Etiology, Screening, Diagnostic Techniques, Management

Kenneth L. Noller

Carcinoma of the cervix is one of the most common malignancies in women, estimated to be the second or third most common cause of cancer death in women worldwide, despite the fact that a screening test, the Pap smear, is available that has been demonstrated to reduce the incidence of the disease by at least 70%. Unfortunately, many developing countries lack the ability to carry out widespread Pap screening.

HISTORY, EPIDEMIOLOGY, AND INFECTION

It is likely that carcinoma of the cervix has been a major cause of cancer death for centuries, although histologic confirmation has only been available more recently. For example, in Paris in the 19th century, cervical cancer was reported to be the most common malignancy in women.

In the early part of the 20th century, epidemiologic studies demonstrated that the cancer was closely linked to sexual activity. Early age at first intercourse and multiple sexual partners were the most consistent risk factors. This suggested that there might be an infectious agent passed through sexual activity that "causes" cervical carcinoma. Although some studies found associations with herpes simplex virus, *Chlamydia*, and gonorrheal infections, all these were ultimately discarded. It was only when it became possible to identify **human papillomavirus** (HPV) infection that the true cause of cervical cancer was discovered. In 2008, Professor Harald zur Hausen received the Nobel Prize in Medicine for his discovery that HPV was the causative organism.

The papillomaviruses are found in almost all mammalian species and are generally species-specific. They are double-stranded DNA viruses that replicate within epithelial cells, as described in a 2005 ACOG Practice Bulletin. The group that infects humans includes more than 120 types. Within these types, there is further grouping, so that the types that commonly are found on one anatomic part of the body are not the same as found on other parts. For example, plantar warts on the feet are not caused by the same HPV types as warts on the hands. In several locations, infection with HPV is associated with a clinically evident lesion, the wart. Unfortunately, this has led to HPV being labeled as the wart virus despite the fact that many infections, indeed most in the genital tract, do not form warts.

Approximately 40 types of HPV are known to infect the genital tracts of men and women. Of these, at least 13 are associated with cancer. The other types are associated with genital warts or are unimportant infections with no clinical symptoms. Because it is not possible to grow the virus in the laboratory, it has taken many years and much indirect evidence to determine that an infection with one of the cancer-associated types is a necessary precursor to squamous cell carcinoma and most cases of adenocarcinoma of the uterine cervix. However, the virus is an incomplete cause because the vast majority of genital HPV infections do not result in cancer.

Epidemiologic evidence is conclusive that the virus can be passed from one individual to another through sexual activity. However, HPV DNA can be found on clothing and other surfaces and, thus, fomite transmission might be possible. However, according to Winer and colleagues, it is unlikely. It will not be possible to determine whether such material is infective until a method of culturing HPV is developed.

Studies of college students and other groups performed by Wheeler and colleagues in 1996, and Moscicki and associates in 1998, 2004, and 2008 have confirmed that most men and women acquire a genital HPV infection within a few years of the onset of sexual activity. The most common type identified in the general U.S. population is type 16, which is also the type most highly associated with cancer. Studies by Ho and associates in 1998 tested participants for evidence of the virus at regular intervals several months apart; most of the detected infections cleared within a few months, although some persisted for as long as 36 months. Recently, it has been found that many infections last only a few weeks, suggesting that the previous studies underestimated the cumulative incidence of the disease. Many investigators now believe that in sexually active individuals, infection with HPV at some time is almost universal.

Despite almost uniform infection with HPV, the vast majority of women do not develop cervical cancer. That is, of the millions and millions of women who are infected with HPV, only a few will ever develop cervical cancer, even if they are never screened and/or treated for preinvasive lesions. Longitudinal studies have now confirmed this (**Fig. 28-1**). The search for a predictive measure that will distinguish between those women who are infected and will clear the disease and those in whom the infection will persist and lead eventually to carcinoma has

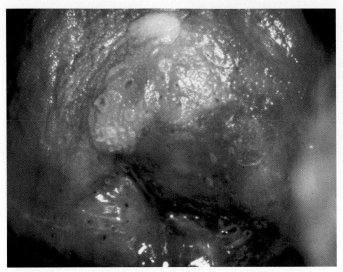

Figure 28-1 Colpophotograph of a cervix with an active human papillomavirus infection. The patient had a cytology sample reported as a low-grade squamous intraepithelial lesion. She was followed without treatment, and the lesions regressed over the next year.

been frustrating. Although it is clear that women who have a compromised immune system from any cause (e.g., genetic, iatrogenic, infectious) have a greater risk of developing a persistent HPV infection, there is as yet no way to predict which healthy women will be unable to clear the disease spontaneously. The only other independent risk factor that has been identified is smoking, which increases the risk of **cervical intraepithelial neoplasia** (CIN) 3 by as much as a factor of 3, according to McIntyre-Seltman and associates.

A cancer-associated HPV type causes neoplastic cellular changes when its DNA becomes integrated into the host cell genome. When this happens, certain repressor areas of the viral genome are lost. Consistently, the loss of these control mechanisms allows for the expression of the viral E6 and E7 genes. As described by Munger and colleagues, the production of oncoproteins results in the inactivation of the p53 and retinoblastoma tumor repressors. These changes theoretically lead to cell immortalization and rapid cell proliferation. However, in most cases, the transformed cells are managed by the individual's immune system and the infection or intraepithelial neoplasia is defeated. In some women, for reasons that are still not clear, the transformed cells begin to replicate and, if the lesion is not treated, a cancer can develop after a period of several years.

Testing for the presence of HPV DNA is useful in a few specific clinical settings. These are described in the sections on cytology screening and management of abnormal cytology reports.

Recently, two vaccines that protect against the acquisition of HPV types 16 and 18, the two most common cancer-associated HPV types, have become available commercially. A number of studies, in particular one by Mao and colleagues, have confirmed that they protect against the development of significant preinvasive neoplasia and that the protection remains effective for many years. A comprehensive review of these vaccines was published by Saslow and associates in 2007. These vaccines have the potential to prevent approximately 70% of all cases of squamous cancer of the cervix. However, to be most effective, they must be given before exposure—that is, at the onset of sexual activity. Noller and

coworkers, in 1987, reported the age of onset of sexual activity for a large group of U.S. women. Ideally, all girls (and boys) would receive the series of three injections at approximately 11 or 12 years of age. It is not yet known whether vaccination protection is lifelong or whether a booster dose will be needed later. The vaccine is derived from virus-like particles that do not contain any viral DNA.

Because the vaccines currently available do not provide protection against all cancer-associated HPV types, screening with the **Pap** (Papanicolaou) **test** will need to be continued indefinitely. Vaccines that protect against more than two cancer-associated HPV types are currently being studied, but are not yet available.

CERVICAL CYTOLOGY TESTING

Cervical cytology testing (the Pap test) became available in many developed countries in the 1950s after the studies of Papanicolaou had shown that by examining a properly prepared and stained cellular sample scraped from the uterine cervix, the presence of cancer and its precursors could be identified. The 1941 monograph by Papanicolaou and Traut remains one of the sentinel breakthroughs in the history of preventive medicine. Their work led to the demonstration that when cancer precursors are identified, local therapy prevents the development of cancer. Despite the fact that Pap testing has a low sensitivity (many false-negatives), the incidence of cervical cancer has been reduced by 50% to 70% in almost all countries that use it. The success of the technique relies on the facts that it takes many years for invasive cancer to develop following an HPV infection and that most women are tested repeatedly. Most women who develop invasive cervical cancer in the United States have never been tested or have not been tested for many years.

The technique requires that the cervix be visualized after placement of a speculum into the vagina. The portio of the cervix is then scraped using a "broom" or the combination of a plastic spatula and endocervical brush (**Figs. 28-2** and **28-3**). Noller and colleagues' 2003 survey of the Fellows of the American College of Obstetricians and Gynecologists showed great uniformity in the use of Pap testing.

Originally, the clinician would place the collected sample on a glass slide and fix it with alcohol. In recent years, that method has been replaced almost entirely by a liquid-based approach. The sample is now placed in a liquid medium for transport to the laboratory where the slide is prepared. The transport medium also can be used for HPV DNA testing and for the detection of some sexually transmitted diseases. A 2009 American College of Obstetricians and Gynecologists (ACOG) Practice Bulletin has recommended Pap testing for all women beginning at age 21. This change to an older age of onset of testing was based on the fact that the risk of invasive cervical cancer occurring in a woman younger than 21 years is approximately 1 in a million.

The frequency of Pap testing remains controversial. Although annual testing was the norm in the United States for many years, other developed countries have seen similar in the incidence of cervical cancer with less frequent testing. It is likely that biennial or triennial testing will become more common in the future. It is also likely that testing for high risk HPV DNA will be accepted as an alternative to cytology for women over age 30. Perhaps the

Figure 28-2 A plastic spatula is often used to obtain a specimen from the exocervix. It must be used with an instrument that samples the endocervix. **A,** Cervix as seen through a speculum, with the spatula being used to obtain a cell sample. **B,** Longitudinal view at the same point in the procedure.

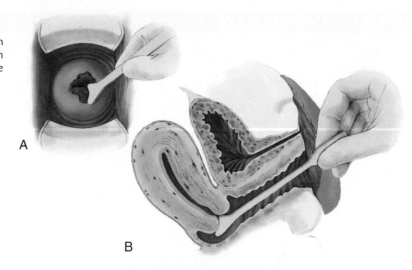

Figure 28-3 Both these instruments can be used to obtain a cytologic sample from the endocervix: cervical broom (Unimar) (*top*); cytobrush (Medscand, Cooper Surgical, Trumbull, CT) (*bottom*).

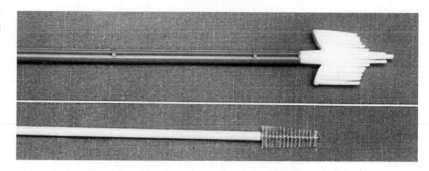

most effective testing after age 30 is the use of the combination of the Pap test and HPV DNA testing, according to studies by Bellinson, Schiffman, Naucler, and their associates. If both tests are negative, the risk of HSIL during the next 3 to 5 years is extremely low. Annual testing with cytology alone is acceptable although not necessary for most women.

The combination of two tests for screening will occasionally result in disparate results—that is, when one test is positive and the other is negative. A group of experts in this area met under the leadership of the National Cancer Institute to develop interim guidelines for patient management in these situations. Results were published by Wright and colleagues in 2004. Consensus guidelines published in 2007 by Wright and associates further specified how to follow women with disparate results. In general, if one test is positive and one negative, the clinician should repeat both tests in 6 to 12 months.

In the past, many women were advised to continue to have Pap testing after hysterectomy, despite the fact that vaginal carcinoma is exceedingly rare. Pearce and colleagues have shown that most abnormal Pap tests after hysterectomy result in false-positives. Therefore, the current recommendation is that women cease to have Pap testing after a total hysterectomy (i.e., the cervix has been removed completely). The only exceptions are women who have a history of an HSIL, are immunocompromised, or were exposed in utero to diethylstilbestrol.

Testing may also be discontinued in women who have no history of HSIL, have no new sexual partner, and have reached an advanced age, according to a study by Sawaya and associates. Unfortunately, the various guideline organizations do not agree

on the age at which testing can be stopped, but the age range of 65 to 70 is most commonly cited.

Several investigators have examined the cost benefits of various cytology methods, intervals, and techniques. In most cases, according to studies by Kim, Goldie, and their colleagues, following the current guidelines is the most efficient method to care for a patient and maximize the expense of screening.

CERVICAL CYTOLOGY REPORTING: THE BETHESDA SYSTEM

In 1988, the National Cancer Institute convened a conference to develop a uniform terminology for the reporting of Pap test reports. The **Bethesda System** (TBS) has been modified twice, with the most recent modification occurring in 2001 and reported by Solomon and associates. **Box 28-1** shows the currently used classification. Almost all laboratories in the United States (and many countries throughout the world) use this terminology. Unfortunately, this cytology nomenclature is often confused with the terms used to describe histologic diagnoses. **Figure 28-4** shows how TBS, CIN, and **dysplasia** categories correspond to tissue changes.

The first part of any TBS report states whether the sample is satisfactory or unsatisfactory. Reasons for an unsatisfactory report include such items as lack of a label, loss of transport medium, scant cellularity, and contamination by foreign material. Few samples are reported as unsatisfactory if a liquid-based technique is used.

Box 28-1 Bethesda System for Reporting Cervical Cytology

Adequacy of sample
  Satisfactory
  Unsatisfactory
Squamous cell abnormalities
  Atypical squamous cells (ASC)
    ASC of undetermined significance
    ASC cannot exclude high-grade lesion
  Low-grade squamous intraepithelial lesion

High-grade squamous intraepithelial lesion
Squamous cell carcinoma
Glandular cell abnormalities
  Atypical glandular cells, specify site of origin, if possible
  Atypical glandular cells, favor neoplastic
  Adenocarcinoma in situ
  Adenocarcinoma
Other cancers (e.g., lymphoma, metastatic, sarcoma)

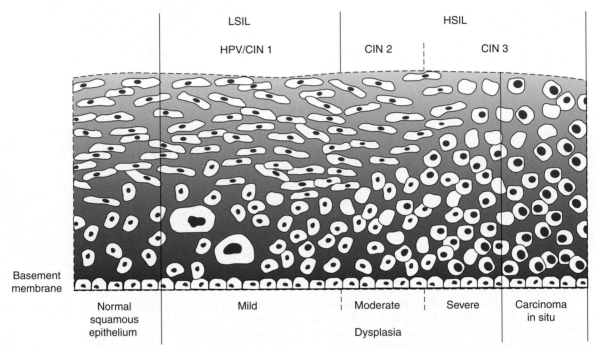

Figure 28-4 Diagram of cervical epithelium showing various terminologies used to characterize progressive degrees of cervical neoplasia. CIN, Cervical intraepithelial neoplasia; HSIL, high-grade squamous intraepithelial lesion; HPV, human papillomavirus; LSIL, low-grade squamous intraepithelial lesion.

The report next indicates whether the cellular material was normal. If other than normal, the abnormalities are further divided into squamous and glandular. The cytologist may also comment on the presence of evidence of infections such as yeast and changes consistent with a diagnosis of bacterial vaginosis.

Squamous abnormalities are found in approximately 5% to 6% of all cytology samples. The most common is **atypical squamous cells** (ASC) of undetermined significance (ASC-US). This indicates that there are cells on the slide that show some of the features associated with squamous lesions, but there are few of these cells present or the changes are not consistent with a more precise report. In most laboratories, ASC-US changes are reported in 3% to 5% of all samples.

ASC-US reports require a management plan. Kinney and associates have demonstrated that although an ASC-US report is usually not indicative of HSIL, because ASC-US reports are common, the absolute number of women with HSIL and ASC-US is high. The National Cancer Institute sponsored a prospective randomized study, the ASCUS LSIL Transmission Study (ALTS), to determine the most efficacious method of further evaluation of women with this report. One third of the women had immediate colposcopy, one third had repeat cytology in 4 to 6 months, and one third had HPV DNA testing, followed by colposcopy if the test was positive for high-risk HPV types. Although the HPV DNA arm performed slightly better than the others, all three approaches were found to be acceptable.

The second abnormality is ASC-H (atypical squamous cells, cannot exclude a higher grade lesion). This report indicates that there are cells present that are worrisome for a significant lesion, but are few in number. All women with this report should be evaluated with a colposcopic examination because there is a high likelihood that a significant lesion is present, as reported by Sherman and coworkers in 1999.

A low-grade squamous intraepithelial lesion (LSIL) is the next category. In the ALTS trial, it was shown that almost all of the women with this report were HPV DNA–positive. This report is most often found to be consistent with histology reports of

CIN 1, HPV, and/or mild dysplasia. With the light microscope, it is not possible to determine which of these lesions represents a transient viral infection and which has the potential to progress to a higher grade lesion.

Colposcopy is not appropriate for some women with LSIL lesions. While Pap testing is no longer recommended for women under age 21, if a sample is taken and reported as LSIL, the patient should be followed with cytology in 12 months. The second exception is in menopausal women. If LSIL is reported in these women, HPV DNA testing or repeat cytology in 6 and 12 months is preferred to colposcopy, according to the Consensus Guidelines published by Wright and coworkers.

HSIL is the next category. Women with this report often have a CIN 2 or 3 lesion and, very occasionally, cancer. All should be evaluated with colposcopy, according to the ACOG Practice Bulletin 99. This is the most straightforward of all the categories in TBS.

If solid evidence of carcinoma is present in the cytology specimen, it will be reported as such. In countries in which cytology screening has been in place for many years, this is a rare finding. Other malignancies can also rarely be identified on cytology (e.g., lymphoma, sarcoma, metastatic cancer).

As discussed in Zweitig and colleagues' study, a cytology sample will contain **abnormal glandular cells** approximately three times in 1000 samples. Sometimes, these can be classified by the site of origin (e.g., endometrium, ovary), but often they cannot. The classification of these glandular lesions is long and complicated (see **Box 28-1**), but they are managed similarly. All these women should have colposcopy and, if no lesion is identified, additional tests are needed. **Conization** of the cervix, scalpel excision, is preferred to **loop electrosurgical excision** (LEEP) in this case and should be performed unless there are other explanations for the abnormal glandular cells. For example, in pregnancy and with certain cervical infections such as *Chlamydia*, abnormal glandular cells are occasionally seen. If colposcopy is negative, these women can be followed until after the condition is resolved. However, if the abnormal glandular cells persist, conization is necessary. If the woman is older than 35 years, an endometrial biopsy should be performed. When atypical glandular cells are present, there is approximately a 7% to 10% risk of invasive cancer, making this a very worrisome report.

The first step in the management of women with the various abnormal cytology reports is shown in the **Box 28-2**. Because colposcopy is the predominant method of evaluation of women with abnormal reports, the technique is discussed in detail below.

ALTERNATIVE TO CYTOLOGY SCREENING FOR CERVICAL CANCER

Although the Pap test is the only screening procedure for cervical cancer that has been shown to reduce the incidence of that disease, there is increasing evidence that screening with HPV tests might be superior. A number of studies, including those of Mayrand, Ronco, and their coworkers have demonstrated that HPV testing is more sensitive than Pap testing, with only a small loss in positive predictive value (PPV). Dillner and colleagues have reported a study from Sweden that showed that after 6 years, significantly more CIN 3+ was detected in a group of women who were HPV-positive than among those who were cytology-positive. Although the Pap test is still the only approved screening test for the detection of cervical cytology in the United States, it is possible that HPV testing may also be approved within the next few years.

In many areas of the world, Pap testing is not available because of the lack of enough cytotechnicians and cytopathologists. In those settings, HPV testing would be beneficial at the present time.

NATURAL HISTORY OF CERVICAL INTRAEPITHELIAL NEOPLASIA

CIN is graded as 1, 2, or 3 depending on the percentage of the thickness of the epithelium that demonstrates cells with nuclear atypia. There is now general agreement that the histologic changes known as CIN 1, or mild dysplasia, result from an infection with HPV (**Fig. 28-5**). In most cases, these lesions disappear spontaneously, often within weeks to months although, according to Moscicki and associates, it may take up to 36 months in some cases. In a few women, for reasons that have not as yet been discovered, these infections persist and the virus becomes integrated into the host genome, allowing for the development of malignant transformation. Fortunately, this process is slow and requires several years from first infection to the development of cancer.

When the process of cell transformation involves one half to two thirds of the thickness of the epithelium, it is designated as CIN 2 (**Fig. 28-6**). The process still remains reversible at this stage, with approximately 40% disappearing spontaneously without treatment, according to Castle and colleagues.

When the neoplastic process involves the full or almost full thickness of the epithelium, it is designated as CIN 3 (**Fig. 28-7**). This term encompasses what was once called severe dysplasia and **carcinoma in situ**. Because CIN 3 is believed to be the precursor to invasive cancer, treatment is recommended (see later). However, approximately one third of these lesions may spontaneously disappear.

Fortunately, it takes several to many years for CIN to progress to invasive cancer. Treatment at any time during the intraepithelial stage will halt further progression. There is even an early stage of invasive cancer called microinvasive carcinoma. These lesions are not visible to the naked eye, but may be identified by colposcopic examination (**Fig. 28-8**). Management of theses lesions is covered in Chapter 29.

Box 28-2   First Step in Evaluation of a Woman with an Abnormal Cervical Cytology Report

Squamous lesions
  ASC-US: HPV DNA testing for HR types; repeat Pap test in 6 months; colposcopy (all three options acceptable)
  ASC-H: Colposcopy
  LSIL: Colposcopy or HPV DNA testing
  HSIL: Colposcopy
  Glandular lesions: All reports require colposcopy and further evaluation if negative.

ASC-H, Atypical squamous cells, cannot exclude a higher grade lesion; ASC-US, atypical squamous cells of undetermined significance; HR, high risk; HSIL, high-grade intraepithelial lesion; HPV DNA, human papillomavirus DNA; LSIL, low-grade squamous intraepithelial lesion.

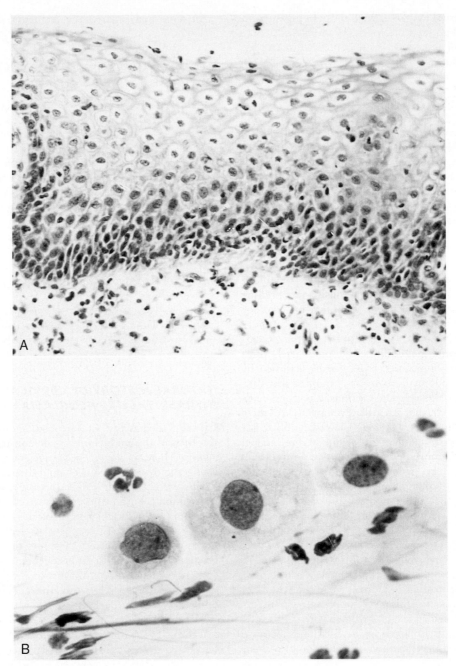

Figure 28-5 A, Cervical intraepithelial neoplasia 1 (mild dysplasia). Atypical cells are present in the lower one third of the epithelium (H&E stain, ×250). **B, Low-grade squamous intraepithelial lesion** cytology. These cells show an altered nuclear-to-cytoplasmic ratio with enlargement and have granular chromatin (Pap stain, ×800).

EVALUATION OF ABNORMAL CYTOLOGY: COLPOSCOPY

As noted, the technique of colposcopy is often the first step in the evaluation of women with abnormal cytology results.

The **colposcope** is a low-power binocular microscope with a powerful light source that is focused 30 cm beyond the front objective. Its useful magnification is from approximately 3× to 15×. The instrument is placed just outside the vagina after a speculum has been inserted and the cervix brought into view.

After any obscuring mucus is removed with a swab, the cervix is carefully examined for the presence of lesions. Dilute acetic acid, 3% to 5%, is then applied to the cervix and, after approximately 30 seconds, the cervix is again examined. Although the exact mechanism of action has never been determined, the acetic acid causes areas of increased nuclear density to be seen. With experience, a colposcopist can distinguish those tissue patterns associated with CIN from normal epithelium.

A good colposcopist becomes facile in the recognition of tissue patterns, much as a pathologist relies on that ability to make

Figure 28-6 Cervical intraepithelial neoplasia 2 (moderate dysplasia). The atypical cells extend approximately halfway through to the epithelium (H&E, ×300).

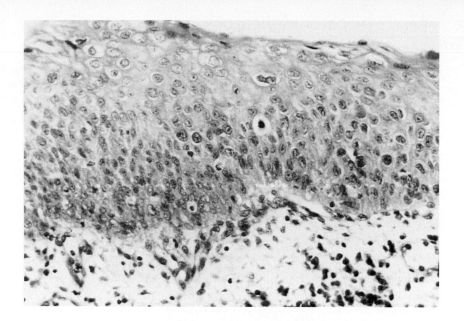

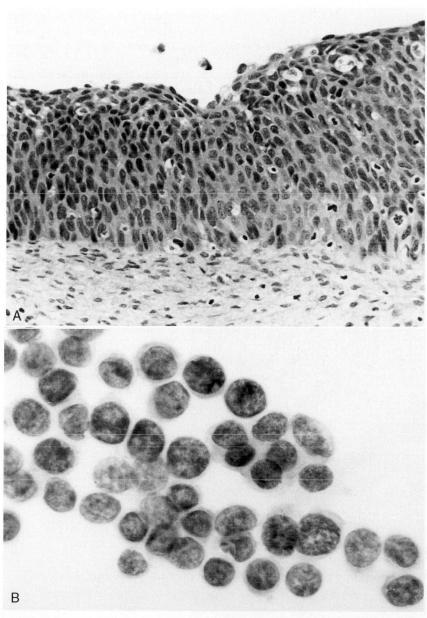

Figure 28-7 A, Cervical intraepithelial neoplasia 3 (severe dysplasia, carcinoma in situ). There is a lack of squamous maturation throughout the thickness of the epithelium. Almost all the cells have enlarged nuclei with granular chromatin. Note that the basement membrane is intact, showing that this process is confined to the epithelial layer only. **B,** High-grade squamous intraepithelial lesion. These cells exhibit large nuclei with granular chromatin. Very little cytoplasm can be seen (Pap stain, ×800).

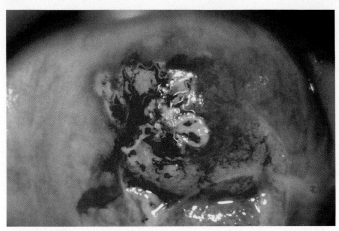

Figure 28-8 Colpophotograph of a microinvasive carcinoma of the anterior lip of the cervix at 6× magnification. Abnormal vessels can be seen, and one of these is bleeding because of the application of acetic acid.

histologic diagnoses. However, recent publications have shown that colposcopy is not as accurate as once believed. Although published several decades ago, there are no better descriptions and illustrations of the technique and findings of colposcopy than in the textbooks of Coppleson and coworkers and Kolstad and Stafl.

The colposcopist must also determine whether the **transformation zone** (TZ) can be seen in its entirety (**Fig. 28-9**). The TZ is the area that lies between normal columnar epithelium and mature squamous epithelium. The TZ is important because most cases of squamous neoplasia of the cervix begin in this anatomic area, probably because it is an area of rapid cell turnover. Almost all women are born with an area of columnar epithelium on the portio (face) of the cervix. When the vagina becomes acidic at the time of menarche, this single columnar cell layer is gradually replaced by squamous epithelium through the process of squamous **metaplasia**. Squamous epithelium is much more resistant to the low pH of the mature vagina.

It is important to be able to assess the entire TZ. If some portions extend into the endocervical canal beyond visibility, the examiner will not be able to determine whether there is more significant disease above. In these cases, the lesion should not be treated with ablative methods (see later), but rather by one of the techniques that provides a tissue sample for histologic examination. If the entire TZ is visible, and the patient has not previously been treated for CIN, any of the common methods of treatment of CIN can be used. However, if there is any finding that suggests that the lesion might extend into the canal or if it is not possible to see the TZ, it is wise to evaluate the endocervix with a cytologic specimen from the canal or an endocervical curettage.

If a lesion is seen, one or more biopsy specimens should be taken to confirm the diagnosis (**Fig. 28-10**), and increasing the number of biopsies also increases detection. Because the cervix has few if any pain fibers that respond to a cutting action, the samples can be taken with minimal or no pain. However, it is

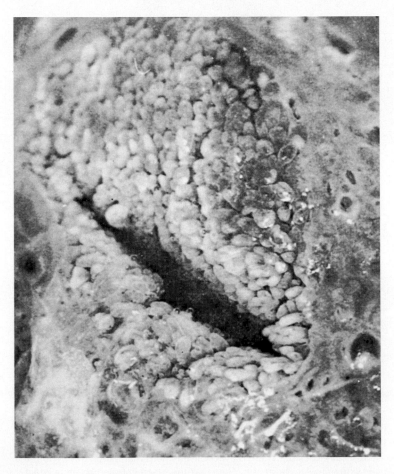

Figure 28-9 Normal cervix as seen through a colposcope at approximately 6× magnification. The central grapelike structures are covered with columnar epithelium. The tissue outside this area represents squamous metaplasia. There are multiple gland openings in this area, indicating that columnar epithelium is being replaced by squamous epithelium. This area between the columnar and squamous epithelia is known as the transformation zone. (From Coppleson M, Pixley E, Reid B: Colposcopy—A Scientific and Practical Approach to the Cervix in Health and Disease. Springfield, IL, Charles C Thomas, 1971.)

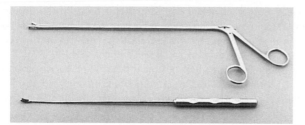

Figure 28-10 Cervical biopsy instruments: punch biopsy (*top*); endocervical curette (*bottom*).

important to maintain a sharp cutting edge on the biopsy instruments because the cervix has pain fibers that respond to stretch. If bleeding occurs, the base of the biopsy site can be touched with Monsel's solution or a silver nitrate stick. Cervical biopsy specimens are very small, usually only approximately 4 × 5 mm. Therefore, no restrictions are needed and the sites heal within a few days (**Fig. 28-11**). The exception is if a biopsy is performed during pregnancy. In that case, the patient should be advised to place nothing in the vagina for 3 weeks.

Colposcopy during pregnancy is difficult. The cervix becomes larger, the vaginal side walls tend to obstruct the view of the cervix, the blood supply to the cervix is increased, and decidual changes in the epithelium can be confused with CIN. Nonetheless, colposcopy plays a key role in a pregnant woman with an abnormal Pap test result. Invasive cancer must be ruled out, a determination that can be made by a careful colposcopic examination of the cervix. If there is no evidence of invasion, further evaluation can be postponed until 6 to 12 weeks after delivery. Biopsies during pregnancy can be performed safely in the physician's office. However, the examiner must be ready to respond with prolonged local pressure and, on rare occasions, with suture ligation should brisk bleeding occur.

The only indication for an excisional procedure in pregnancy is the possible presence of invasive disease. In those cases, a conization procedure under anesthesia is recommended.

If CIN was identified during pregnancy, a follow-up colposcopic examination should be scheduled postpartum. However, it should not be attempted until at least 6 weeks have passed. Often, the lesion will have disappeared, even if it was CIN 3.

TREATMENT

There has been a great change in the approach to treatment of CIN lesions over the past 4 decades. Now that it is known that most early lesions disappear spontaneously, treatment is indicated only for those lesions that have demonstrated a potential for further progression.

CERVICAL INTRAEPITHELIAL NEOPLASIA

CIN 1

Treatment of CIN 1 is no longer the preferred method of management of these lesions at any age. Exceptions should be made on a patient by patient basis and only if the lesion has persisted for at least 12 months. Treatment of CIN 1 in women younger than 21 years is not recommended, unless the lesion persists for more than 24 months. Almost all CIN 1 is a manifestation of a transient HPV. Because the lesion is so far removed from cancer, it should not be regarded as a serious finding. Patients with CIN 1 require follow-up to ensure that the lesion regresses, but clinicians should not present the finding in a way that alarms the patient.

Some small fraction of CIN 1 lesions progress to CIN 2 or 3 but, at present, it is not possible to determine which ones have that potential. However, because the treatment of CIN 2 and 3 is easy and office-based, there is no penalty for waiting to determine whether spontaneous resolution of a CIN 1 lesion will occur. In addition, all the treatments are associated with a risk of long-term complications, such as cervical stenosis and premature delivery, according to Kyrgiou and colleagues (**Fig. 28-12**).

CIN 2

Approximately 40% of CIN 2 lesions also regress spontaneously. For many years, almost all CIN 2 lesions were treated. It slowly became more common not to treat women younger than 21 years. As the transient nature of these lesions has become more evident, many clinicians now follow patients beyond age 21, particularly if they are not through with childbearing. If a lesion progresses to CIN 3, it should be treated.

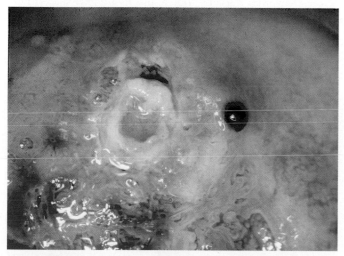

Figure 28-11 Colpophotograph (≈ ×12) of a cervical biopsy site 72 hours after the procedure. The eschar is already beginning to separate from the cervix.

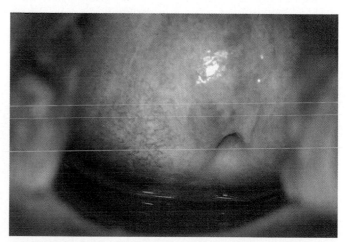

Figure 28-12 Mild cervical stenosis following **cryocautery** for cervical intraepithelial neoplasia 2. The colposcopic examination is unsatisfactory because the transformation zone cannot be seen (colpophotograph, ≈ ×6).

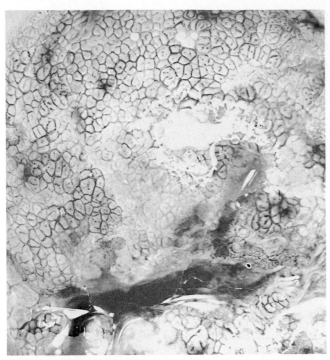

Figure 28-13 Extensive cervical intraepithelial neoplasia 3 (CIN 3) lesion covering most of the epithelium visible in this colpophotograph. The predominant feature is a **mosaic** pattern. There is umbilication of many of the tiles with a punctate vessel, a common feature of CIN 3. Although this large lesion needs to be examined carefully for evidence of atypical vessels, a hallmark of invasive cancer, none are seen in this view (colpophotograph, ×8). (From Kolstad P, Stafl A: Atlas of Colposcopy. Baltimore, University Park Press, 1972.)

CIN 3

Although some of these lesions regress, most persist or, in some cases, progress to invasive cancer (**Fig. 28-13**). Therefore, according to ACOG Practice Bulletin 99, they should be treated. If the involved area is removed in its entirety, the disease is cured. Several methods have similar treatment success (see later).

Women who have had one CIN 3 lesion are slightly more likely to develop another lesion in the future. Therefore, long-term follow-up is necessary.

TREATMENT METHODS

The goal of treatment of CIN is to remove the lesion, and any technique that accomplishes that goal can be used. Currently, most treatment is office-based. It is hard to justify the expense and increased risk of treatment under general anesthesia, except in rare cases with specific indications.

Treatment can be accomplished by ablation (e.g., cryotherapy, thermoablation, CO_2 laser ablation) or excision (e.g., LEEP [also known as large loop excision of the transformation zone, LLETZ], cold knife conizacion, CO_2 laser conization). All these methods have first-treatment success rates of approximately 95%; the choice of method depends on the availability of equipment and experience and expertise of the clinician. Hysterectomy is not recommended for treatment of CIN, even if cervical biopsy specimens have been reported carcinoma in situ.

As early as 1976, Kolstad and Klem demonstrated that hysterectomy for carcinoma in situ was no better than an excisional cone. In addition, hysterectomy carries risks that are much more common and serious than office-based therapy of CIN 3.

When a first treatment fails, it is because of incomplete excision of the entire lesion. Involved tissue can be left behind in the endocervix or on the exocervix. The latter does not represent a difficult treatment problem because colposcopy can easily identify the area and office excision is easy and curative.

When the endocervical margin of an excised specimen is positive for CIN, the patient should be followed with **endocervical sampling** and colposcopy in 3 to 6 months. Many of these women will not have persistent disease, according to Lopes and colleagues, probably because very little of the lesion remains and the normal healing process destroys the remainder. However, when there is evidence that CIN remains in the endocervical canal 4 to 6 months after the procedure, repeated excision of the canal is indicated. An endocervical margin that is positive is not an indication for hysterectomy or immediate repeat excision.

Ablative Methods
Cryotherapy
This outpatient method was the most commonly used treatment for CIN lesions in the 1970s and 1980s, but has largely been supplanted by LEEP. If patients are carefully selected, the success rate is approximately 95%. Larger CIN lesions have higher failure rates, most likely because the whole lesion is not covered by the cryoprobe. It is not appropriate to use cryotherapy if the lesion extends into the endocervix.

The procedure is simple. After colposcopy and sampling have shown that the lesion is confined to the exocervix, a probe is selected that will cover the entire lesion (**Fig. 28-14**). In most systems, N_2O is used as the refrigerant. The probe is applied to the cervix and the system is activated. The cervix will freeze quickly, but the probe must remain in place until the ice ball that forms extends to at least 5 mm beyond the edge of the instrument. In most cases, this takes 3 to 4 minutes. The refrigerant is then turned off and the probe is allowed to thaw and separate from the cervix. Several studies have suggested that repeating the freeze–thaw cycle a second time results in a higher success rate, whereas others have shown equal success with a single freeze.

Most patients experience almost no discomfort during the procedure, although some complain of menstrual-type cramping.

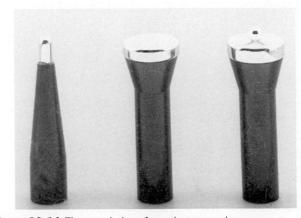

Figure 28-14 Three varieties of cryotherapy probes.

Because the tissue that was destroyed remains on the cervix, the patient will begin to experience vaginal discharge within a few hours to a day. As the tissue sloughs, the amount of discharge increases and malodor is common. It may take as long as 3 weeks for the discharge to stop. The patient should be cautioned to place nothing in the vagina for at least 3 weeks after the procedure to avoid dislodgment of the eschar.

The first follow-up should occur in approximately 4 to 6 months and include cytology and colposcopy. The cytology sample should include the endocervix.

Short-term complications from the procedure include the nuisance of the discharge and occasional bleeding. Long-term complications include cervical stenosis and a small increase in preterm labor. Unfortunately, the instrument is sometimes used by inexperienced individuals, and cases of invasive cancer following treatment have been reported.

Thermoablation

This technique is rarely used in the United States at present. Various loops, needles, and paddles are used to destroy CIN lesions. Although the success rate is similar to other techniques, it often requires general anesthesia and perhaps results in more cervical stenosis than other methods.

CO_2 Laser Ablation

This technique became available to clinicians in the 1980s. When a focused CO_2 laser beam is directed at the cervical epithelium, the laser energy is absorbed by the water in the cells. The water turns to steam and the cell wall disrupts, killing the cell. The cell protein is largely exploded in a plume of smoke that is drawn out of the vagina by suction. Because little dead tissue is left after the procedure, there is no prolonged vaginal discharge as there is with cryotherapy. The success rate is similar to other techniques.

The technique became popular because the area of tissue destruction could be minimized and there was no prolonged discharge as with cryotherapy. In addition, because the instrument is attached to a colposcope, usually those who used the technique were familiar with CIN. However, additional training is required because treatment success depends on the correct choice of laser energy delivered (calculated as power density) and proper depth and extent of treatment.

For several years, CO_2 laser ablation was the method of choice for treatment of CIN. It can be performed in the office with no anesthesia. (I have personally treated several hundred patients in the office with this technique.) However, the equipment is expensive. When LEEP became available, use of the laser treatment began to wane. Currently, it is used almost exclusively when the lesion extends far out onto the exocervix. In these cases, the CO_2 laser can remove less tissue than other methods.

Excisional Methods

Loop Electrosurgical Excision

LEEP is currently the most common method for the treatment of CIN 2 and 3. It involves the removal of the TZ of the cervix under local anesthesia and can be performed safely and without discomfort in the office.

Typically, 3 or 4 mL of lidocaine with epinephrine is injected into the cervix in a circumferential manner, making five to eight injections at the distal edge of the resection margin. The lidocaine is injected just under the epithelium rather than deep

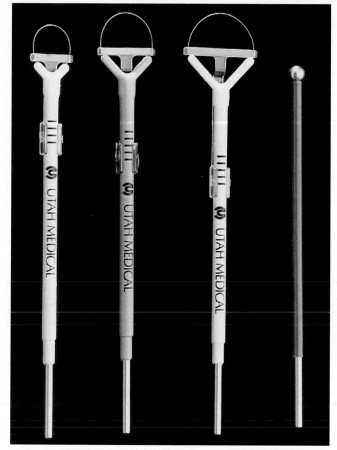

Figure 28-15 Electrodes (Utah Medical, Midvale, UT) used for a loop electroexcision procedure. The width of the excised tissue specimens can range from 1.0 to 2.0 cm, and the specimen depth can be adjusted by sliding the guard attached to the electrode shaft. Following excision, the base of the cervix is often gently cauterized with a ball electrode. (Courtesy of Dr. Steven E. Waggoner, University of Chicago, Chicago.)

into the cervix. One to 2 minutes should be allowed for the epinephrine to cause vasoconstriction. A wire loop attached to a cautery instrument that can provide a cutting current is then used to remove the tissue. Various sizes of loops are available (**Fig. 28-15**). If there is any bleeding, the edge of the defect can be cauterized with a ball electrode attached to the current generator set to cautery. In most cases, there is less than 5 mL of blood loss. There is no reason to perform curettage of the endocervical canal above the resected margin because the management of the patient is the same whether the sample is positive or negative, and curettage can cause additional scarring.

The LEEP specimen is sent to the laboratory for histologic evaluation. In most cases, the whole lesion will have been excised and the margins of the specimen will be free of CIN. If either margin is positive for CIN, a colposcopic examination should be performed, with the first follow-up cytology in 4 to 6 months. If the exocervical margin was positive, that area should be evaluated carefully. If a small bit of the original lesion was left behind, treatment is usually easy.

If the endocervical margin showed signs of CIN, there is no urgency to perform a repeat procedure. Many of these women will have no residual disease at the time of follow-up in 4 to 6 months. At that time, the endocervix should be evaluated by cytology or endocervical curettage. A repeat LEEP should be performed only if persistent CIN is demonstrated in the canal. A positive endocervical margin or evidence of persistent disease in the canal is not an indication for hysterectomy. Hysterectomy is almost never indicated for the treatment of CIN. Only if CIN 3 persists despite multiple local treatment attempts should it be considered, and evaluation by an expert colposcopist is strongly recommended. There is recent evidence that HPV testing can be used to predict the persistence and recurrence of CIN after LEEP.

Cold Knife Conization

This term is used to describe removal of the CIN lesion with a scalpel (the cold knife). Before colposcopy was widely used in the evaluation of women with abnormal Pap tests, cold knife conization was the standard diagnostic procedure. Under general anesthesia, the cervix would be stained with an iodine-containing solution and all the epithelium that did not stain would be removed. The knife would be angled toward the endocervical canal, thus removing a cone-shaped piece of tissue that could be evaluated by a pathologist. Often, extensive suturing of the defect bed would be performed.

With the advent of colposcopy and office-based therapy, cold knife conization is used less and less often. For the evaluation of squamous lesions, it offers no advantage over LEEP, which does not require the use of general anesthesia. Its sole unique indication at present is for the diagnostic evaluation of patients with glandular lesions in which the absence of the thermal artifact introduced at the endocervical margin by LEEP is problematic. In addition, some clinicians still use the technique when a LEEP has failed, although there are few data to support this approach.

The technique has evolved over time. Because colposcopy should always be performed before cold knife conization, the exocervical extent of the lesion will be known. There is no reason to excise more tissue than necessary, so the excision should be tailored to the lesion. In many cases, a small cylinder of tissue can be removed instead of the larger cone. In most cases, bleeding can be controlled with the application of Monsel's solution (ferrous subsulfate) to the defect, especially if a vasoconstrictive solution is injected into the cervix before the excision. Sutures are only rarely necessary. If a bleeding site is encountered, a simple or figure-of-eight ligature of the bleeder suffices. There is no indication for the Sturmdorf sutures that were often used in the past. This technique rolled the exocervical epithelium into the canal, making subsequent evaluation almost impossible. In addition, it is not necessary to control bleeding.

FOLLOW-UP

All the treatment methods described have a first-time success rate of approximately 95%. According to ACOG Practice Bulletin Number 99, because women who have been treated for CIN 2 and 3 have a somewhat higher risk of developing a new lesion, they should be followed closely. A first Pap test should be performed 6 to 12 months after the treatment and repeated at that interval until three negative cytology results have been reported. At that time, the woman can be returned to routine annual screening examinations.

If a Pap test is reported as showing a squamous abnormality, colposcopy should be performed. The examination should include an evaluation of the endocervix, with cytology or endocervical curettage. If a lesion is seen on the distal exocervix, it most likely represents an edge that was not included in the initial treatment. However, if a lesion is seen to be involving the endocervical canal or if the endocervical specimen is positive, an excisional procedure that includes the endocervix should be performed.

VAGINAL INTRAEPITHELIAL NEOPLASIA

The least common malignancy of the lower female genital tract is vaginal cancer. The lesions are almost all squamous carcinomas, and it is believed that most are preceded by an intraepithelial lesion. However, cancer is so rare that it is no longer advised to screen for the malignancy in women who have had a total hysterectomy unless they have a recent history of CIN 2 or 3. Because most abnormal vaginal cytology specimens are false-positives, women who have undergone hysterectomy should be actively discouraged from having cytology samples taken. The exceptions, according to Kalogirou and colleagues, are women who have been treated for HSIL, women exposed in utero to diethylstilbestrol, and women who are immunocompromised.

VULVAR INTRAEPITHELIAL NEOPLASIA

Vulvar cancer occurs primarily in postmenopausal women who have had an untreated preinvasive lesion for many years. Unfortunately, cytologic screening of the vulva is not useful because it is unreliable. Most cases are identified when a patient complains of a sore or an area that itches. Some asymptomatic cases are identified when a clinician performs a vulvar examination and identifies an abnormal-appearing area.

NATURAL HISTORY

The natural history of vulvar intraepithelial neoplasia (VIN) lesions is not as well worked out as for CIN lesions. Most cases of invasive squamous cancer of the vulva go through an intraepithelial stage similar to cervical lesions. It is known that most invasive squamous cancers of the vulva contain HPV DNA, but the percentage of positive cases is lower than those of the cervix, for which it is almost 100%. When vulvar cancer occurs in a reproductive-age woman (a rather rare event), HPV DNA can almost always be identified. In postmenopausal women, the percentage of cancers with HPV DNA is lower.

Vulvar histology is much less helpful than cervical histology. For example, it is known that some CIN 3 lesions will progress to cancer if not treated. However, a much larger fraction of VIN 3 lesions disappear spontaneously, particularly when they occur in women younger than 35 years. Currently, VIN 1 lesions are not treated, as are fewer and fewer VIN 2 lesions as both represent transient manifestations of active HPV infection.

Invasive vulvar cancer is probably preceded by VIN 3 in most cases. Because there is no way to distinguish between those lesions that will and will not regress, treatment of VIN 3 is still recommended for all ages.

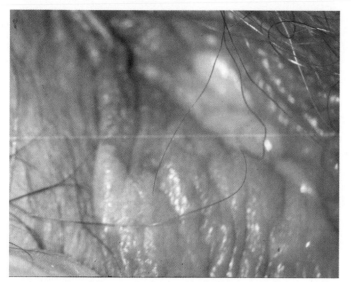

Figure 28-16 Vulvar intraepithelial neoplasia (VIN) 3 lesion as seen through a colposcope after the application of acetic acid. A second lesion is out of focus, but can be seen in the background. VIN is often multifocal.

TREATMENT

Before a decision to treat is made, according to Wright and Chapman, it is important to have histologic confirmation of the lesion to be certain that it is truly VIN 3 and to rule out invasion (**Fig. 28-16**). For some reason, many clinicians are reluctant to perform vulvar biopsies in the office. These can be performed with a minimal of discomfort by using a small (30-gauge) needle and lidocaine.

If a decision is made to treat a VIN lesion, there are several techniques that can be used. The goal is to destroy the lesion, and any method that removes the epithelium can accomplish that. Unlike the cervix, there are no crypts (commonly called glands) in the vulvar epithelium, so excisions can be superficial.

In the past, excision with a scalpel was used almost universally to treat VIN. Fortunately, many of these lesions are small and require only a small excision, especially in younger women. Because of the multiple folds of skin on the vulva, it is almost always possible to close the incision primarily. If lesions recur, a relatively common event, there may not be sufficient skin remaining for primary closure without relaxing incisions. It is not necessary to remove more than the lesion. In the past, a skinning vulvectomy, in which all the skin of the vulva was removed and a skin graft placed on the defect, was commonly used to treat vulvar carcinoma in situ (VIN 3). That procedure is no longer indicated, because simple local excision of the individual lesion(s) has a similar cure rate.

The CO_2 laser can be used to ablate areas of VIN. It is especially useful in the area surrounding the clitoris, where it is possible to remove the minimum amount of tissue consistent with removal of the entire lesion. However, the skill of the operator is important with this technique because the ablation should not be carried through the dermis. The raw edges, actually burns, left after laser surgery are much more painful than excision and primary closure.

Cryosurgery has been used, but there is poor control of the depth of the tissue destruction and healing is slow and painful. LEEP is used by some. There is better control of depth with LEEP than with cryosurgery, but it is still rarely used.

A novel approach in young women with VIN 3 lesions, particularly in the periclitoral area, is the application of imiquimod. Although no large studies have been reported, small case series, such as that reported by van Seters and colleagues, have shown a reasonable rate of clearance for those who can tolerate the irritation that always accompanies its use. Long-term data are not available.

KEY POINTS

- The Pap test is the most effective cancer screening procedure ever developed.
- When Pap testing is used widely, it decreases the incidence of cervical cancer by approximately 70%.
- TBS terminology is used for the reporting of cervical cytology specimens.
- Cervical cancer is caused by HPV.
- Almost all HPV infections regress spontaneously.
- Smoking increases the likelihood that an HPV infection will persist or progress.
- A vaccine is available that prevents HPV infection if given before exposure to the HPV types in the vaccine.
- In some cases, an HPV infection can lead to a precancer of the cervix, called CIN. CIN is graded as 1, 2, or 3 depending on the percentage of the epithelial thickness involved in the process.

- CIN 1 should be observed rather than treated because it usually regresses spontaneously.
- Treatment of CIN 2 and 3 can be performed in the office with any one of several techniques.
- CIN 2 and 3 occur more commonly in women who are immunocompromised.
- An HPV DNA test can be used to triage women with ASC-US cytology reports. It can also be combined with cervical cytology for screening for CIN in women older than 30.
- The colposcope is used to evaluate women with abnormal Pat tests.
- The LEEP procedure is the most common method used to treat CIN 2 and 3.
- Cervical stenosis, infertility, and premature birth are increased slightly in women who have been treated for CIN, regardless of the treatment method used.

**REFERENCES CAN BE FOUND ON
EXPERTCONSULT.com**

29

Malignant Diseases of the Cervix
Microinvasive and Invasive Carcinoma: Diagnosis and Management

Anuja Jhingran and Charles Levenback

Malignancies of the cervix are almost always carcinomas; a summary of the more common histologic types are shown in **Box 29-1**. Approximately 80% to 85% of these tumors are squamous cell carcinomas and from 15% to 20% are adenocarcinomas. The incidence of adenocarcinomas has increased in most developing countries, particularly among younger women. Carcinoma of the cervix is closely associated with early and frequent sexual contact and cervical viral infection, particularly human papillomavirus (HPV), as detailed in Chapter 28 (Intraepithelial Neoplasia of the Lower Genital Tract). According to the American Cancer Society, the frequency of cervical cancer has been steadily decreasing, in part because of the effect of widespread screening for premalignant cervical changes by cervical cytology (Pap smear). An estimated 12,200 new cases of invasive cervical cancer are expected to be diagnosed in 2010 and 4,210 patients were estimated to die of cervical cancer in 2010. The incidence of cervical carcinoma in the United States is higher among the Hispanic population (12.7%) compared with whites (8.0%) and African Americans (11.0%). However, the mortality rate from cervical cancer is the highest among African Americans compared with other races, partly because African Americans tend to have their cancers diagnosed at a later stage. Invasive cervical cancers are diagnosed at a localized stage in 51% of white women and 43% of African American women. This chapter details the various types of cervical carcinomas and considers their natural history, methods of diagnosis and evaluation, and details of therapy. Primary sarcomas and melanomas of the cervix are extremely rare and are not considered separately (**Fig. 29-1**).

HISTOLOGIC TYPES

Varieties of squamous cell carcinoma of the cervix are illustrated in **Figure 29-2**. An early form, **microinvasive carcinoma**, is considered separately in the next section. Most squamous cell carcinomas of the cervix are reported to be of the large cell, nonkeratinizing type, but many are keratinized, and squamous pearls may be seen. The degree of differentiation of tumors is usually designated by three grades: G1, well differentiated; G2, intermediate; and G3, undifferentiated. However, there is no consensus on the value of tumor grade as a major prognostic factor for squamous cell carcinoma of the cervix.

A rare variety of squamous cell carcinoma is the so-called **verrucous carcinoma**, which is morphologically similar to those found in the vulva (see Chapter 30). These warty tumors appear as large bulbous masses (**Fig. 29-3**). They rarely metastasize but unfortunately may be admixed with the more virulent, typical squamous cell carcinomas, in which case metastatic spread is more likely.

Adenocarcinomas may have a number of histologic varieties. As noted by Brinton and colleagues, adenocarcinomas do not appear to be affected by the usual sexual factors associated with squamous carcinomas. However, HPV DNA, oral contraceptive use, and lack of cervical cytologic screening have heightened the risk of developing these tumors. The typical variant often contains intracytoplasmic mucin and is related to the mucinous cells of the endocervix (endocervical pattern; **Fig. 29-4**). However, on occasion, the cells contain little or no mucin, and then the tumor may resemble an endometrial carcinoma (endometrioid pattern). It may be difficult histologically to ascertain whether these carcinomas arise in the cervix or endometrium. Endocervical tumors more frequently stain positive for carcinoembryonic antigen than endometrial tumors, and this histochemical observation has been used to try to distinguish the tumors microscopically by an immunoperoxidase reaction.

A rare but important virulent variety of adenocarcinoma is the **adenoma malignum**. These microscopically innocuous-appearing tumors consist of well-differentiated mucinous glands (**Fig. 29-5**) that vary in size and shape and infiltrate the stroma. Despite their bland histologic appearance, they tend to be deeply invasive and metastasize early. The term *minimal deviation adenocarcinoma* is applied to these tumors. According to McGowan and associates, patients with Peutz-Jeghers syndrome are at increased risk of the development of these tumors.

Clear cell adenocarcinomas of the cervix are histologically identical to those of the ovary (see Chapter 33) and vagina (see Chapter 31). They are uncommon in the cervix and can also be associated with intrauterine diethylstilbestrol exposure, although they also often develop spontaneously in the absence of diethylstilbestrol exposure.

Adenoid cystic carcinomas are rare. Berchuk and Mullin have summarized 88 cases reported in the literature. These tumors

Box 29-1 Summary of Major Categories of Cervical Carcinoma

Squamous Cell Carcinomas
Large cell (keratinizing or nonkeratinizing)
Small cell
Verrucous

Adenocarcinomas
Typical (endocervical)
Endometrioid
Clear cell
Adenoid cystic (basaloid cylindroma)
Adenoma malignum (minimal deviation adenocarcinoma)

Mixed Carcinomas
Adenosquamous
Glassy cell carcinoma

are aggressive and may resemble cylindromas of salivary gland or breast origin and histologically may resemble basal cell carcinomas of the skin (adenoid basal, or basaloid, carcinomas). Most patients with these tumors are older than 60 years. The basaloid variety appears to be less aggressive. King and coworkers have reported four unusual cases in women younger than 40 years. One woman was noted to survive longer than 5 years.

Adenosquamous carcinomas, as the name implies, consist of squamous carcinoma and adenocarcinoma elements in varying proportions (**Fig. 29-6**). They occur frequently in pregnant women. A particularly virulent variety is termed *glassy cell carcinoma* (**Fig. 29-7**). This is an undifferentiated tumor consisting of large cells containing cytoplasm, with a ground-glass appearance. Glassy cell carcinomas tend to metastasize early to lymph nodes as well as to distant sites and usually have a fatal outcome.

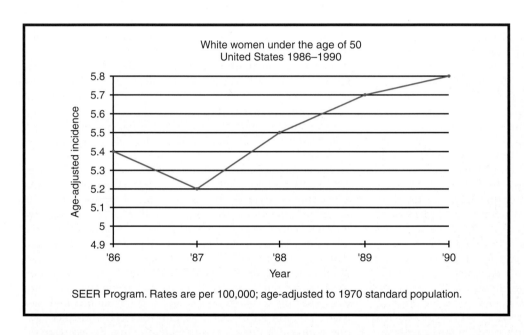

White women under the age of 50
United States 1986–1990

SEER Program. Rates are per 100,000; age-adjusted to 1970 standard population.

Figure 29-1 Incidence rates of invasive carcinoma. (From Ries ALG, Miller BA, Hankey BF, et al: SEER Cancer Statistics Review, 1973-1991 [NIH Publ. No. 94-2789]. Bethesda, MD, National Institutes of Health, 1994, pp 136-144.)

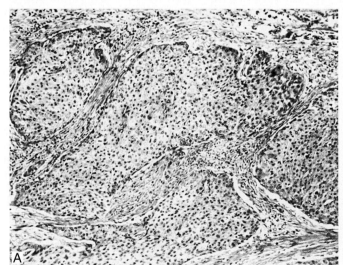

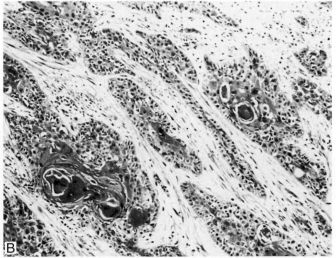

Figure 29-2 A, Large cell, nonkeratinizing squamous cell carcinoma. Discrete islands of uniform, large cells with abundant cytoplasm are separated by fibrous stroma (×160). **B,** Keratinizing squamous cell carcinoma. Irregular nests of squamous cells forming several pearls are separated by fibrous stroma. The nests have pointed projections (×160).

Continued

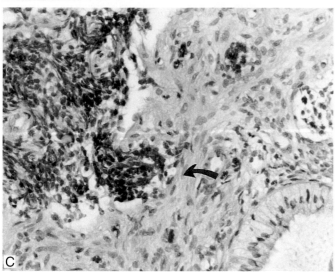

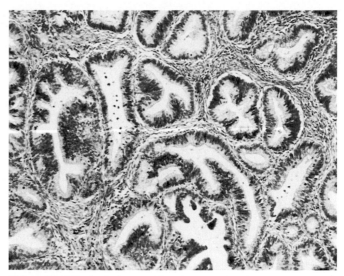

Figure 29.2—cont'd C, Small cell neuroendocrine carcinoma of the cervix (*arrow*) infiltrating between normal endocervical glands (H&E, × 240.) (**A, B** from Clement PB, Scully RE: Carcinoma of the cervix: Histologic types. Semin Oncol 9:251, 1982; **C** courtesy of Dr. Anthony Montag, Department of Pathology, University of Chicago, Chicago.)

Figure 29-4 Typical adenocarcinoma. Irregular glands are lined by stratified mucin-containing epithelium. Mitotic figures are numerous (× 160). (From Clement PB, Scully RE: Carcinoma of the cervix: Histologic types. Semin Oncol 9:251, 1982.)

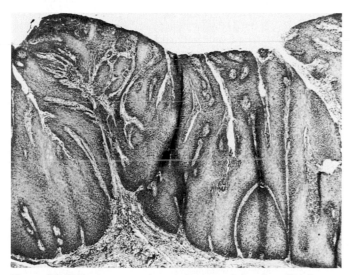

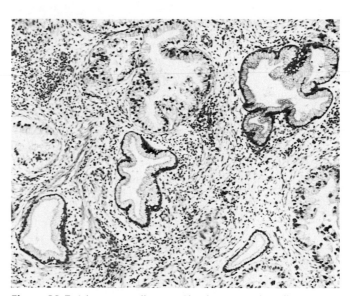

Figure 29-3 Verrucous carcinoma. Downgrowths of papillae have broad bases. Tumor cells are well differentiated (× 34). (From Clement PB, Scully RE: Carcinoma of the cervix: Histologic types. Semin Oncol 9:251, 1982.)

Figure 29-5 Adenoma malignum. Glands are mostly well differentiated, appearing normal except for their irregular shapes. A few obviously malignant glands are also present (× 160). (From Clement PB, Scully RE: Carcinoma of the cervix: Histologic types. Semin Oncol 9:251, 1982.)

Small cell carcinoma of the cervix is rare, comprising less than 5% of all carcinomas of the cervix. Women with small cell carcinoma are likely to be 10 years younger than those with squamous cell carcinoma. The cells are small anaplastic cells with scant cytoplasm. They behave aggressively and are frequently associated with widespread metastasis to multiple sites, including bone, liver, skin, and brain. Efforts to treat these cancers with approaches typically used for small cell carcinoma of the lung have had mixed results.

Another variant that is not in the World Health Organization (WHO) classification is non–small cell neuroendocrine tumors. These tumors contain intermediate to large cells, high-grade

nuclei, and eosinophilic cytoplasmic granules of the type seen in neuroendocrine cells. Reported survival rates for patients with these aggressive carcinomas are similar to those of patients with small cell tumors, and optimal therapy has yet to be established.

CARCINOMA OF THE CERVIX

CLINICAL CONSIDERATIONS

Patients with carcinoma of the cervix characteristically present with abnormal bleeding or brownish discharge, frequently noted following douching or intercourse and also occurring spontaneously

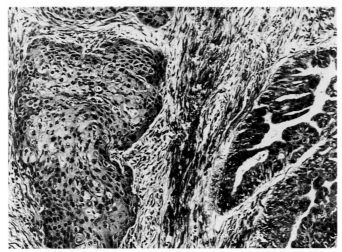

Figure 29-6 Well-differentiated adenosquamous carcinoma. Glandular structure lies adjacent to a nest of nonkeratinizing large squamous cells (×400). (From Clement PB, Scully RE: Carcinoma of the cervix: Histologic types. Semin Oncol 9:251, 1982.)

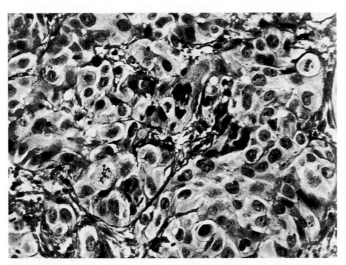

Figure 29-7 Glassy cell carcinoma. Cells have sharp borders, ground-glass–type cytoplasm, and nuclei containing prominent nucleoli (×1000). (From Clement PB, Scully RE: Carcinoma of the cervix: Histologic types. Semin Oncol 9:251, 1982.)

between menstrual periods. These patients often have a history of not having had a cytologic (Pap) smear for many years. Other symptoms, such as back pain, loss of appetite, and weight loss, are late manifestations and occur when there is extensive spread of cervical carcinoma. The patients tend to be in their 40s to 60s, with a median age of 52 years, as noted worldwide by Pecorelli and colleagues. Preinvasive intraepithelial carcinoma of the cervix (see Chapter 28) occurs primarily in women in their 20s and 30s and has become more common in those in their 20s, leading to a gradual increase in the incidence of invasive carcinoma in younger patients.

The diagnosis is established by biopsy of the tumor; a specimen can easily be obtained at office examination. A Kevorkian, Eppendorf, Tishler, or similar punch biopsy instrument is convenient to use. Occasionally, it is necessary to biopsy nodularity or induration in the vagina near the cervix to ascertain the limit

of tumor spread and define a correct tumor stage. If the woman's cytologic smear is suggestive of invasive carcinoma, with no gross lesion visible, and endocervical curettage does not demonstrate carcinoma, or if an adequate biopsy specimen to establish carcinoma cannot be obtained, cervical conization should be performed.

STAGING

The staging of carcinoma of the cervix depends primarily on the pelvic examination; the designation may be modified by general physical examination, chest radiographic examination, intravenous pyelography (IVP), or computed tomography (CT) and is not changed based on operative findings. **Table 29-1** shows the definitions of the four stages of cervical carcinoma according to the International Federation of Gynecology and Obstetrics

Table 29-1 Clinical Stages of Carcinoma of the Cervix Uteri

Stage	Characteristics
I	Carcinoma is strictly confined to the cervix (extension to the corpus should be disregarded)
IA	Invasive cancer which can be diagnosed only by microscopy, with deepest invasion ≤ 5 mm and largest extension ≥ 7 mm (Fig. 29-8)
IA1	Measured stromal invasion ≤ 3.0 mm in depth and extension of ≤7 mm (Fig. 29-9)
IA2	Measured stromal invasion of >3 mm and not >5.0 mm, with an extension of not >7.0 mm
IB	Clinically visible lesions limited to the cervix uteri or preclinical cancers greater than IA*
IB1	Clinically visible lesion ≤ 4 cm in greatest dimension
IB2	Clinically visible lesion > 4 cm in greatest dimension
II	Cervical carcinoma invades beyond the uterus, but not to the pelvic wall or lower third of vagina
IIA	No obvious parametrial involvement
IIA1	Clinically visible lesion ≤ 4.0 cm in greatest dimension
IIA2	Clinically visible lesion > 4.0 cm in greatest dimension
IIB	Obvious parametrial involvement
III	The tumor extends to the pelvic wall and/or involves lower third of the vagina and/or causes hydronephrosis or nonfunctioning kidney†
IIIA	Tumor involves lower third of the vagina, with no extension to the pelvic wall
IIIB	Extension to the pelvic wall and/or hydronephrosis or a nonfunctioning kidney
IV	The carcinoma has extended beyond the true pelvis or has involved (biopsy-proven) mucosa of the bladder or rectum. A bullous edema, as such, does not permit a case to be allotted to stage IV.
IVA	Spread of growth to adjacent pelvic organs
IVB	Spread to distant organs

*All macroscopiclly visible lesions, even with superficial invasion, are allotted to stage IB carcinomas. Invasion is limited to a measured stromal invasion, with a maximum depth of 5.0 mm and a horizontal extension of not >7.0 mm. Depth of invasion should not be >5.0 mm taken from the base of the epithelium of the original tissue, superficial or glandular. The depth of invasion should always be reported in millimeters, even in those cases with early (minimal) stromal invasion (minus 1.0 mm). The involvement of vascular or lymphatic spaces should not change the stage allotment.
†On rectal examination, there is no cancer-free space between the tumor and the pelvic wall.
All cases with hydronephrosis or nonfunctioning kidney are included, unless they are known to be from another cause.
Adapted from Pecorelli S: Revised FIGO staging for carcinoma of the vulva, cervix, and endometrium. Int J Gynaecol Obstet 105:103, 2009.

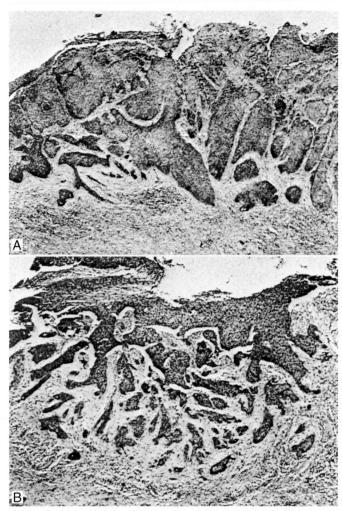

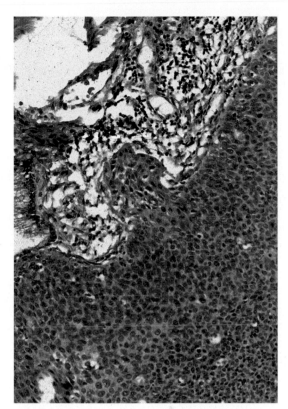

Figure 29-9 Photomicrograph showing early stromal invasion. (Courtesy of Dr. Anthony Montag, Department of Pathology, University of Chicago, Chicago.)

Figure 29-8 A, Tumor with only 0.5 mm of invasion (×40). **B,** Example of so-called spray pattern with multiple invasive nodules in stroma. Invasion is only 1 mm (×50). (From Creasman WT, Fetter BF, Clarke-Pearson DL, et al: Management of stage IA carcinoma of the cervix. Am J Obstet Gynecol 153:164, 1985.)

(FIGO; revised in 2009). The various types of tumor distribution that may be observed in the various stages are illustrated in **Figure 29-10.**

NATURAL HISTORY AND SPREAD

Carcinoma of the cervix is initially a locally infiltrating cancer that spreads from the cervix to the vagina and paracervical and parametrial areas. Grossly, the tumors may be ulcerated (**Fig. 29-11**), similar to carcinomas occurring elsewhere in the female genital tract, and may have an **exophytic** growth pattern or cauliflower-like appearance extruding from the cervix, usually producing abnormal bleeding and staining. Alternatively, they may be **endophytic,** in which case they are asymptomatic, particularly in the early stage of development, and tend to be deeply invasive when diagnosed. These usually start initially from an endocervical location and often fill the cervix and lower uterine segment, resulting in a **barrel-shaped cervix**. The latter tumors tend to metastasize to regional pelvic nodes and, because of the tendency of late diagnosis, are often more advanced than the exophytic variety. The primary path for distant spread is through lymphatics to the regional pelvic nodes. Bloodborne metastases from cervical carcinomas do occur, but are less frequent and are usually seen late in the course of the disease.

Initially, cervical carcinoma spreads to the primary pelvic nodes, which include the pericervical node, presacral, hypogastric (internal iliac) and external iliac nodes, and nodes in the obturator fossa near the vessels and nerve. From this primary group, tumor spread proceeds secondarily to the common iliac and para-aortic nodes. Rarely, the inguinal nodes are involved; however, if the lower third of the vagina is involved, the median inguinal nodes should be considered a primary node. The distribution of lymph node involvement was studied in detail in 26 cases of untreated carcinoma of the cervix by Henriksen (**Fig. 29-12**). A series studying the incidence and distribution pattern of retroperitoneal lymph node metastases in 208 patients with stages IB, IIA, and IIB cervical carcinomas who underwent radical hysterectomy and systemic pelvic node dissection reported that 53 patients (25%) had node metastasis. The obturator lymph nodes were the most frequently involved, with a rate of 19% (39 of 208), and the authors proposed them as sentinel nodes for cervical cancers. An important distal node that becomes involved after the para-aortic group is the left scalene node—that is, the left supraclavicular node. A clinical correlation is that biopsy of this node is frequently performed in the assessment of advanced cervical carcinoma to clarify whether the tumor has spread outside the abdomen. In addition to nodal spread, hematogenous spread of cervical carcinoma occurs primarily to the lung, liver and, less frequently, bone (see later, Recurrence).

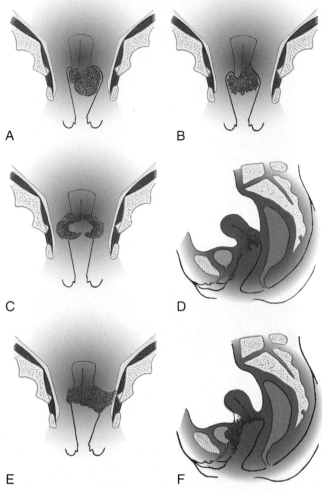

A

B

C

D

E

F

Figure 29-10 Staging of cervical carcinoma. **A,** Stage IB, nodular cervix. **B,** Stage IIA, carcinoma extending into left vault. **C,** Stage IIB, parametrium involved on both sides, but carcinoma has not invaded pelvic wall; endocervical crater. **D,** Stage IIIA, submucosal involvement of anterior vaginal wall and small papillomatous nodule in its lower third. **E,** Stage IIIB, parametrium involved on both sides; at left, carcinoma has invaded pelvic wall. **F,** Stage IVA, involvement of bladder. (From Pettersson F, Bjorkholm E: Staging and reporting of cervical carcinoma. Semin Oncol 9:289, 1982.)

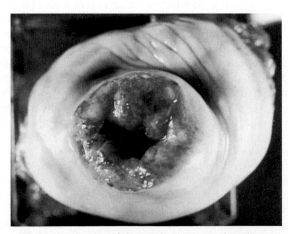

Figure 29-11 Carcinoma of the cervix (gross specimen).

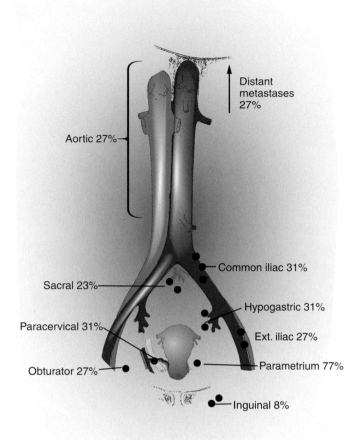

Figure 29-12 Frequency of lymph node metastases in cervical carcinoma. Shown is the incidence of node group involvement in 26 nontreated cases of cervical carcinoma. (From Henriksen E: The lymphatic spread of carcinoma of the cervix and of the body of the uterus. Am J Obstet Gynecol 58:924, 1949.)

PROGNOSTIC FACTORS

FIGO stage is the most important determinant of prognosis for carcinoma of the cervix (**Table 29-2**); however, there are other factors, including tumor and patient characteristics, that are prognostic and are not included in the FIGO staging system. One of the most important predictors is tumor size for local recurrence and death for patients treated with surgery or radiation

Table 29-2 Carcinoma of the Uterine Cervix: Distribution by Stage and 5-Year Survival Rates for Patients Treated in 1990–1992 (N = 11,945)

Stage	No. of Patients (n)	5-Year Survival
Ia	902	95.01%
Ib	4657	80.1%
II	3364	64.2%
III	2530	38.31%
IV	492	14%

Modified from Pecorelli S, Creasman WT, Pettersson F, et al: FIGO Annual Report on the Results of Treatment in Gynaecological Cancer, vol 23. Milan, Italy, International Federation of Gynecology and Obstetrics, 1998.

therapy. The FIGO staging classification for stage I disease has been modified to include tumor diameter (i.e., ≤ 4 cm, stage IB1; >4 cm, stage IB2). Another important prognostic factor is involvement of lymph nodes, which also is not part of the clinical staging system. In several surgical series, after a radical hysterectomy, patients with positive pelvic lymph nodes had a 35% to 40% lower 5-year survival rate than patients with negative nodes. Patients with positive para-aortic nodes have a survival rate that is approximately 50% that of patients with similar stage disease and negative para-aortic nodes. With extended-field radiation therapy, patients with positive para-aortic nodes have approximately a 40% to 50% 5-year survival rate. There is a strong correlation between positive nodes and positive lymph–vascular space invasion (LVSI) in the tumor specimen in patients with cervical carcinoma. However, LVSI may be an independent predictor of prognosis as shown in a number of larger surgical series.

In patients who have had a radical hysterectomy, histologic evidence of extracervical spread (≥ 10 mm), deep stromal invasion ($>70\%$ invasion), and LVSI are associated with a poorer prognosis. A randomized trial from the Gynecologic Oncology Group (GOG) compared observation versus adjuvant radiation therapy in patients after radical hysterectomy with a combination of two of the factors mentioned earlier; patients who received radiation therapy had better local control as well as improved overall survival. Involvement of the parametrium in the hysterectomy specimen has been correlated with higher rates of lymph node involvement, local recurrence, and death from cancer. Uterine body involvement is associated with an increased rate of distant metastases in patients treated with radiation or surgery.

Patients with adenocarcinomas of the cervix have a poorer prognosis than patients with squamous cell carcinomas of the cervix. Investigators have found that among patients treated surgically, patients with adenocarcinomas have high relapse rates compared with rates in patients with squamous cell carcinomas. In an analysis of 1767 patients treated with radiation for FIGO stage IB disease, Eifel and associates found that independent of age, tumor size, and tumor morphology, patients with adenocarcinomas had the same pelvic control rate but twice as high a rate of distant metastasis as patients with squamous cell carcinomas of the cervix. Although the prognostic significance of histologic grade for squamous carcinomas has been disputed, there is a clear correlation between the degree of differentiation and clinical behavior of adenocarcinomas.

There has been a great interest in molecular markers regarding prognosis and treatment in carcinoma of the cervix. One of the most studied markers is the serum squamous cell carcinoma antigen. Studies have shown that pretreatment levels of this antigen correlate well with stage of disease, tumor histology, grade, type of tumor (exophytic versus infiltrative), microscopic depth of invasion, and risk of lymph node metastases in patients with early-stage disease. However, the most important properties of this antigen may be its ability to predict clinical outcome as well as a marker for monitoring the course of disease and response to treatment in patients with cervical cancer. Several investigators have reported significantly lower survival rates in patients with elevated values compared with patients with normal baseline levels, independent of stage. For detection of tumor recurrence, serial squamous cell carcinoma antigen testing has been proven to be more specific than sensitive, with specificities ranging from 90% to 100% and sensitivities ranging from 60% to 90%.

Further investigation is needed in these areas. Some investigators have found a higher rate of recurrence in patients with HPV-positive nodes (although negative for malignancies) and poor prognosis with the presence of HPV mRNA in the peripheral blood of cervical cancer patients. Other markers that have been investigated include epidermal growth factor receptor, cyclooxygenase-2, DNA-ploidy, tumor vascularity, and S-phase fraction.

TREATMENT

Pretherapy Evaluation

Once a woman has been diagnosed as having an invasive carcinoma, pretreatment evaluation is conducted to determine the extent of disease, arrive at an accurate clinical staging, and plan the program of therapy. The usual evaluation consists of a thorough history and physical examination, routine blood studies, IVP or CT, and chest radiography. Demonstration of an obstructed ureter or nonfunctioning kidney caused by tumor automatically assigns the case at least to stage III (see **Table 29-1**). A barium enema test or flexible sigmoidoscopy, as well as a cystoscopy, is sometimes performed in the case of large tumors or for patients who will be receiving radiation treatment.

CT and magnetic resonance imaging (MRI) is more expensive than IVP, but has the advantage of being able to provide greater information concerning tumor spread to lymph nodes, particularly in cases of higher stage disease. CT, MRI, and IVP provide approximately equivalent information for most cases of stages I and IIA, but CT and MRI allow detection of enlarged pelvic and para-aortic nodes that were suspicious for involvement of tumor. However, CT is not particularly useful to detect the parametrial extent of cervical carcinoma, which is evaluated more reliably by pelvic examination. MRI has also been used to evaluate local spread, but the test is not used routinely. The suggestion of tumor in retroperitoneal nodes by CT does not affect stage, which relies primarily on clinical examination and the status of the ureters.

The best radiographic imaging technique for detecting lymph node metastases is unclear. CT and MRI are good for identifying enlarged nodes; however, the accuracy of these techniques in the detection of positive nodes is compromised by their failure to detect small metastases, and many enlarged nodes are caused not by metastases but by inflammation associated with advanced disease. The accuracy of MRI in the detection of lymph node metastases (72% to 93%) is similar to that of CT, but is better than CT and physical examination for the evaluation of tumor location, tumor size, depth of stromal invasion, vaginal extension, and parametrial extension of cervical cancer. However, with regard to detecting lymph node metastases or other distant disease, positron emission tomography (PET) shows promise. Several studies from a single institution have shown that ^{18}F-fluorodeoxyglucose PET (FDG-PET) detects abnormal lymph nodes more often than CT and that findings with PET are a better predictor of survival than those with CT or MRI in patients with carcinoma of the cervix. Recently, Medicare has approved PET-CT as part of the initial staging evaluation for patients with cervical carcinoma.

Surgical staging is probably the most sensitive method of evaluating whether regional lymph nodes contain metastases; however, it is invasive, expensive, and delays treatment to the primary lesions. Laparoscopic lymph node dissection may decrease the time between surgery and the start of treatment and may be associated with less late radiation-related morbidity than the old standard of open transperitoneal staging. Several studies are exploring the role of intraoperative lymphatic mapping for patients with cervical cancer and other gynecologic malignancies.

Treatment for Stage I
Stage IA
The term *microinvasion* has been used for years to describe patients with minimally invasive cervical cancer, but this term is not part of the FIGO staging system. Microinvasion was used to describe patients with 3-mm invasion or less and essentially no risk of metastatic spread. Several investigators went a step further to measure not only the depth of invasion but also tumor volume by measuring lateral spread. Volumetric measurements are generally more difficult and have not been embraced by pathologists (at least not in North America). Nevertheless, volumetric measurements are used in the FIGO staging scheme. There is ample evidence that patients with small-volume tumors measured only by depth of invasion or by two-dimensional measurement have a low risk of relapse and death with radical surgery or more conservative surgical approaches.

The diagnosis of microinvasive tumor cannot be made based on a biopsy specimen alone; a cervical conization must be performed. If the margin of the cervical cone specimen contains neoplastic epithelium, the risk of invasive tumor in the remaining uterus is increased. Decisions on treatment should be based on an adequate cone biopsy specimen. If a woman has positive margins, the cone can be repeated. Sometimes, deeper invasion will be uncovered and more radical treatment will be required. In some patients, conization alone is adequate.

Stage IA1 tumors measured stromal invasion is 3 mm or less, with lateral extension of 7 mm or less. These measurements are determined on a cone biopsy, which also determines other prognostic factors (e.g., lymph vascular space involvement, histologic subtype, grade). These factors do not alter the stage assignment, in spite of their adverse prognostic significance. In the absence of LVSI or high-risk histologic subtypes, the risk of lymph node metastases is remote and nonradical surgery is adequate. This may include cone biopsy, simple trachelectomy, or simple hysterectomy, depending on the circumstances.

Patients with Stage 1A2 tumors have a measured stromal invasion of 5 mm or less. Patients in this category, even without LVSI, are at a low risk of nodal involvement. Thus, radical or modified radical approaches are usually recommended, which includes modified radical hysterectomy or trachelectomy and pelvic lymph adenectomy. Stage IA1 patients who have LVSI are treated in the same manner as stage IA2 patients.

There continues to be interest in determining the necessity of treating the parametrium in patients with low-stage cervical cancer. Several investigators have noted that the risk of parametrial involvement is 1% or less in patients undergoing radical hysterectomy in low-risk situations. Parametrial resection contributes significant short-term and long-term morbidity to surgery. Lymphatic mapping techniques suggest that parametrial sentinel lymph nodes can be identified and resected without a radical dissection. In the future, we expect that the indications for surgery that omits the parametrial resection will grow.

Radiotherapy is a treatment option for patients with stage IA cervical cancer. The field can be modified to minimize treatment complications. We generally use radiotherapy for stage IA patients for older patients or other poor surgical candidates with multiple comorbidities.

Stage IB
Stage IB encompasses tumors that are larger than stage IA, meaning 5 mm or larger in measured stromal invasion and/or more than 7-mm lateral spread. Stage IB also includes all visible lesions, even if the invasion is superficial (<5 mm). Clinicians should be aware of low-grade squamous cancers that can be easily visualized without magnification and have very superficial invasion. In our judgment, these patients should be treated similarly to stage IA patients.

Stage IB1 patients have tumor limited to the cervix that is 4 cm or less in diameter. These patients have equally good outcomes with radical surgery or radiotherapy. A major factor in favor of radical surgery is younger age, especially premenopausal patients for whom ovarian preservation is an option. In addition, there is now increasing availability of ovum transfer and pregnancy surrogates. Other factors favoring radical surgery are smaller size, desire to preserve fertility, and absence of other comorbidities that escalate the risk of surgery. Factors that favor radiotherapy are the presence of indicators that would result in postoperative radiotherapy if surgery were the primary therapy. These include larger size, extensive LVSI, suspicious findings on preoperative imaging, high-risk histologic subtypes, and deep stromal invasion on imaging or examination that increases the risk of close margins.

The decision regarding radical surgery or radiotherapy should be made with the active involvement of the woman, gynecologic oncologist, and radiation oncologist. Both modalities are associated with the potential for significant short- and long-term complications. Some complications such as bladder atony, food intolerance, or loss of sexual function are not easy to measure and can persist for years following treatment. Long-term survival data are similar for well-selected patient populations. There are some data to suggest more long-term patient satisfaction with outcomes related to surgery than radiotherapy.

Most gynecologic oncologists and radiation oncologists recommend concurrent chemoradiation for patients with stage IB2 cervical cancer. Many reports demonstrate that up to 80% of stage IB2 patients who have undergone a radical hysterectomy will have clear indications for postoperative radiotherapy. Our experience is that postoperative radiotherapy results in greater toxicity than treatment with the cervix intact. The counterargument is that radical hysterectomy obviates the need for high-dose **brachytherapy** that is associated with the most severe and difficult to manage complications, notably pelvic fistulas. A number of innovations in treatment targeting techniques appear to be having a beneficial impact on reducing post-treatment fistula. Concurrent chemoradiation is our primary recommendation for stage IB2 patients.

Operative Therapy: Radical Hysterectomy and Pelvic Node Dissection
Radical hysterectomy and bilateral pelvic lymphadenectomy are effective for the treatment of stage IB and some early stage IIA cancers. It is important that the surgery removes the same volume of tissue that has received tumoricidal doses of radiation in patients for whom radiation is the sole therapy. The amount of tissue removed, particularly in the paracervical and parametrial areas near the ureter, depends on the extent and location

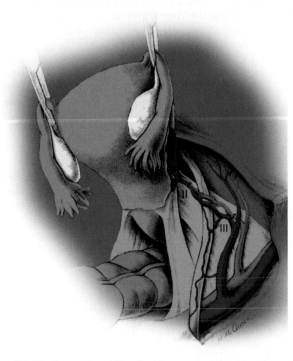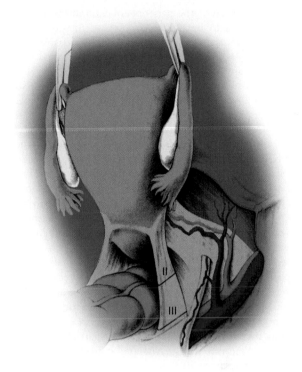

Figure 29-13 Classes I and II radical hysterectomy with points of dissection shown (see text).

of the tumor. Piver and colleagues have defined five classes to describe the extent of the operation. Class I guarantees the removal of the entire cervix and uterus. The ureter is not disturbed from its bed. In many cases, this is described as an **extrafascial hysterectomy**, the type used after preoperative radiation for treatment of a barrel-shaped cervix (see later). A class II operation (**Fig. 29-13**) removes more paracervical tissue than class I; the ureters are retracted laterally but are not dissected from their attachments distal to the uterine artery, and the uterosacral ligaments are ligated approximately halfway between the uterus and rectum. The operation is usually performed with pelvic lymphadenectomy and is often termed a *modified radical hysterectomy*. The operation is useful to treat small microscopic carcinomas of the cervix. Magrina and colleagues have used modified radical hysterectomy primarily for tumors smaller than 2 cm (median, 1.1 cm), with 5-year survival of 96%. This procedure may occasionally be used to treat small, central cervical recurrences of carcinoma that are diagnosed following radiation therapy of the primary tumor. For a class III operation, the uterine artery is ligated at its origin from the anterior division of the hypogastric artery and the uterosacrals are ligated deep in the pelvis near the rectum (see **Fig. 29-12**). This operation is usually termed a *radical hysterectomy* (Meigs-Wertheim hysterectomy) and is performed for stage IB and, rarely, for stage IIA carcinomas of the cervix.

Class IV and V operations are infrequently performed. A class IV procedure involves a complete dissection of the ureter from its bed and sacrifice of the superior vesical artery. A class V operation involves resection of the distal ureter, bladder, or both, with reimplantation of the ureter into the bladder (ureteroneocystotomy). Both are designed to remove small, central recurrent disease and would be attempted to avoid an anterior exenteration (see later). Extensive data are not available, but the latter two procedures appear to have high complication rates.

Preoperative preparation for a woman who is to undergo a radical hysterectomy includes the same basic considerations for anyone undergoing a major operative procedure. Graduated compression, below-the-knee leg stockings are used to reduce the risk of thromboembolism. Prophylactic antibiotics are also frequently prescribed. During the course of the operation, care is taken not to grasp the ureters with instruments such as forceps to avoid damaging the periureteral capillary blood supply.

An important complication of pelvic lymphadenectomy is lymphocyst formation. Most gynecologic oncologists have abandoned the use of closed suction drains in radical hysterectomy patients and leave the pelvic peritoneum open to allow lymph fluid to drain internally in the peritoneal cavity.

Ovarian function may be preserved in younger patients if there is little likelihood of postoperative radiation. If intraoperative findings suggest that radiotherapy will be given postoperatively, the ovaries may be transposed superior and lateral to preserve their function. This technique has some liabilities, including early loss of ovarian function and abdominal pain from ovarian cysts.

In stage I cases treated by radical hysterectomy and node dissection, the results obtained are related primarily to the status of the pelvic nodes, as well as the surgical resection margins around the primary tumor (ideally, > 1 cm). If the pelvic nodes are free of tumor, the 5-year survival rate can be expected to exceed 90%, whereas if the nodes are found to contain tumor, the 5-year survival rate drops to 45% to 50%. Lerner and coworkers have reported a 5-year survival rate (life table technique) of 93.4% for 108 patients using class III hysterectomy for stage IB carcinomas of the cervix. All but five of these tumors were smaller than 5 cm in diameter. Six patients experienced prolonged bladder dysfunction after operation. Only one postoperative ureterovaginal fistula developed, and there were no postoperative deaths, indicating that excellent results can be obtained with surgery, particularly if the patients are carefully selected. If the woman is found to have extensive spread of gross disease to the pelvic nodes, the studies of Potter and coworkers have suggested that it is preferable to cease the operation and complete radiation therapy to improve pelvic control of tumor. However, Hacker and associates have reported an estimated 5-year survival of 80% for 34 patients whose tumor-positive pelvic or para-aortic nodes were resected and the areas subsequently radiated. In a GOG study, Sedlis and coworkers evaluated disease-free survival for patients treated with radical hysterectomy who have negative lymph nodes and surgical margins but with intermediate risk factors, including more than one third stromal invasion, capillary lymphatic space involvement, adenocarcinoma, and large tumor diameter by randomizing patients to pelvic radiotherapy or observation. Survival was improved in those who received postoperative pelvic radiation; however, there were radiation complications, including bowel obstruction and death.

Numerous studies have been published evaluating low-dose preoperative radiation followed by radical hysterectomy and pelvic node dissection. The technique has been particularly widely used in Western Europe; Einhorn and colleagues evaluated the Swedish experience comparing complete treatment with full radiation therapy alone or preoperative partial radiation (two intracavitary radium treatments) and radical hysterectomy for patients younger than 40 years with stage IB or IIA carcinoma of the cervix. A significant ($P < .004$) improvement was noted in stage IB for the combined-therapy group as compared with radiation alone (5-year survival rate, 96% versus 81%). No significant difference was noted in stage IIA. Calais and associates used combined therapy for tumors smaller than 4 cm in diameter in 70 patients and reported a 10-year survival.

Nerve-sparing radical hysterectomy is a recent innovation described by Hockel and others. Bladder atony is a difficult to study outcome of radical hysterectomy. The incidence of complete bladder atony requiring self-catheterization or nerve stimulators is low, but milder forms are common. The severity of bladder atony is directly related to the trauma inflicted on the hypogastric nerves that may be traumatized during radical hysterectomy. The impact of the nerve-sparing approach on sexual function is not known.

Fertility-Sparing Surgery

In the 1980s, Dargent developed a combined laparoscopic and vaginal technique for removal of the pelvic lymph nodes, cervix, parametrium, and upper vagina. Dargent trained gynecologic oncologists from around the world to perform radical vaginal trachelectomy and laparoscopic pelvic lymphadenectomy. Long-term outcomes reported by Plante, Diaz, and others have confirmed that in well-selected patients, oncologic outcomes are identical to radical hysterectomy outcomes. First-trimester pregnancy loss rates are approximately the same for radical trachelectomy patients as for the general population. Second-trimester pregnancy loss is approximately doubled in trachelectomy patients compared with the general population presumably because of the loss of cervical stroma. Approximately two thirds of patients have a successful pregnancy following radical trachelectomy.

When fertility-sparing surgery was first described, the assumption was that it would be offered to only a small proportion of patients. Sonoda and colleagues have determined from a cohort of over 400 radical hysterectomy patients that approximately 50% of those younger than 40 years have low-risk histologic types and tumor size smaller than 2 cm, making them candidates for radical trachelectomy.

In spite of the contribution of radical vaginal surgery to fertility preservation, the technique has been difficult for gynecologic oncologists in the United States to master. Vaginal surgical skills are diminishing and there are no other indications for radical vaginal surgery. American gynecologic oncologists, unlike their counterparts in Canada and Europe, appear to have been discouraged by the long learning curve and have not invested the time to master the approach. Gynecologic oncologists in the United States have described abdominal radical trachelectomy as an alternative to the vaginal approach. Although smaller numbers have been published, it is anticipated that oncologic and fertility outcomes will be similar to the laparoscopic-vaginal approach. In addition, there are early reports of robotic radical trachelectomy that we anticipate will further advance use of the abdominal approach.

Minimally Invasive Surgery

Minimally invasive techniques for treatment of cervical cancer are attractive for several reasons. The tumor itself can be removed through the vagina so an abdominal incision is not needed for this purpose. Lymph nodes can be removed safely through laparoscopic ports as long as the nodes are not grossly involved with tumor. Minimally invasive surgery reduces postoperative adhesions. This is important, because these adhesions play a role in the severity of bowel complications if postoperative radiotherapy is given. Minimally invasive surgery is associated with shorter length of stay, less pain, few postoperative infections, fewer thromboembolic complications, and reduced blood loss compared with abdominal procedures.

Laparoscopic radical surgery has become more popular in North America because of faculty in major training programs who have embraced the concept and trained their associates. For gynecologic oncologists in practice, the long learning curve associated with laparoscopy has been an impediment to advancement.

The most recent minimally invasive technique, robotic laparoscopic surgery, offers new advantages. The robot more closely replicates the wristed motions that surgeons use during open cases, offers three-dimensional imaging, and completely eliminates the tremor of the surgeon and the assistant holding the camera. Many gynecologic oncologists who have not had the time or inclination to master traditional laparoscopic surgery can master robotics relatively quickly. Radical pelvic surgery (e.g., radical prostatectomy, hysterectomy) is an ideal application for robotic surgery and will continue to become increasing available in the United States.

Sentinel Node Biopsy

Cervical cancer, like most solid tumors, spreads primarily by lymphatic spread. Surgical management of solid tumors, as pioneered over 100 years ago by Halsted, is based on the resection of all regional lymph nodes and lymphatic channels connecting the lymph nodes to the primary tumor. Implicit in this approach is that all regional lymph nodes have the same risk of containing metastatic disease. Morton, working in patients with cutaneous melanoma, has demonstrated that there are sentinel lymph nodes that are the first nodes to receive lymphatic drainage from the primary tumor and are therefore the first site of metastases. Experience with thousands of melanoma and breast cancer patients has validated this concept, which has been successfully extended to other disease sites, notably vulvar cancer.

Cervical cancer is an excellent target for the sentinel lymph node concept because the tumor is easy to inject and the regional lymph nodes can be reached through on incision. Lymphatic drainage of the cervix is complex; however, most sentinel lymph nodes of the cervix are found along the external iliac artery or vein, obturator space, or parametrium. A number of investigators have reported their experience with sentinel lymph node biopsy in radical hysterectomy patients. So far, the procedure has shown great promise; however, the false-negative rates have been higher for cervical cancer patients than for those with, for example, vulvar cancer. Improving techniques and patient selection should correct this problem. It is likely that sentinel lymph node biopsy will ultimately be incorporated into the surgical management of cervical cancer.

Surgical Complications

Following radical hysterectomy, many patients experience long-term complications. Montz and associates have noted a 5% frequency of small bowel obstruction, which increases to 20% if radiation is used postoperatively. Fistulas from the urinary tract, particularly ureterovaginal fistulas, have been reported to occur in approximately 1% of cases. The low rate appears to result from the administration of antibiotics, prevention of retroperitoneal serosanguineous collections, and avoidance of direct manipulation of the ureter to avoid injury to the periureteral blood supply. Most gynecologic oncologists do not reperitonealize the pelvis, which allows direct drainage of lymphatic fluid to the peritoneal cavity, where it is reabsorbed.

Many women suffer postoperative bladder dysfunction. In part, this appears to be caused by disruption of the sympathetic nerve supply to the bladder. However, the dysfunction may be temporary. Low and associates have noted an increase in bladder pressure with a decrease in urethral pressure following radical hysterectomy. There was reduced bladder compliance with detrusor instability. The bladder can develop hypotonicity, and overdistention can then become a problem. If overdistention of the bladder and infection are avoided, progressive improvement of bladder function usually occurs. Forney has correlated the degree of bladder dysfunction after radical hysterectomy with the extent of resection of the cardinal ligament. Those who had a complete resection of cardinal ligaments could void satisfactorily at an average of 51 days compared with 20 days for those with only partial resection of the ligaments. All patients experienced a decrease in bladder sensation. In a few patients, the decrease in bladder sensation can be permanent. For patients in whom it is temporary, recovery usually occurs after continuous drainage of the bladder with an indwelling catheter. Westby and Asmussen have observed that by 1 year after surgery, a slight decrease in urethral pressure persists but that the decrease is not as great as that noted immediately after the operation. After 1 year, the postoperative changes and bladder function usually recover. In a 1999 study from Sweden, Bergmark and coworkers have noted compromised sexual activity, decreased lubrication, and shortened vagina in women treated for cervical cancer by surgery and/or radiation. During the consent process, patients should be informed regarding the potential impact of radical hysterectomy on their sexual function.

Lymphedema is another complication of radical pelvic surgery that can affect quality of life. The areas most affected are the mons, lower abdomen, and upper thighs. Lymphedema massage may help reduce this problem, but treatment options are limited and of only modest effectiveness.

Outcomes After Surgical Treatment

Reported 5-year survival rates for women with stage IB cervical cancer treated with radical hysterectomy and pelvic lymphadenectomy are approximately 80% to 90%. Patients with positive or close margins or positive lymph nodes have the highest risk of recurrence and poor outcome. In large prospective studies, 3-year disease-specific survival rates of 85.6% in patients with negative nodes and 50% to 74% in patients with positive nodes were reported. A randomized study has shown that postoperative chemoradiation improves survival in patients with positive lymph nodes and positive surgical margins.

Radiation Treatment

Most patients with carcinoma of the cervix are treated by radiation. The principles of external megavoltage treatment (**teletherapy**) and local implants (brachytherapy) are reviewed in Chapter 26. External beam radiation is administered in fractions, usually 180 cGy/day, 5 days/week, to destroy the tumor without causing permanent damage to normal tissues. This delivers uniform doses to the entire pelvis, including the regional pelvic nodes. The local implant delivers its highest energy locally to the cervix, surface of the vagina, and paravaginal and paracervical tissues. The radiation from the implant diminishes according to the inverse square law. The uterus and cervix serve as a receptacle for arranging and holding the intracavitary applicator stem (tandem) and accompanying vaginal applicators (ovoids) in a fixed and optimal position for delivering the desired radiation dosimetry (**Fletcher-Suit applicator**; see **Fig. 29-14**). Current low-dose rate treatment delivers approximately 40 cGy/hr to

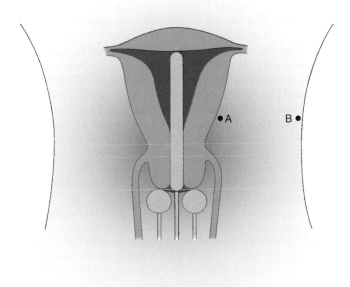

Figure 29-14 Points A and B with central stem (tandem) and two ovoids in place.

point A. Usually, the tandem and ovoids are inserted with the woman anesthetized and a pack is placed into the vagina to stabilize the apparatus and increase the distance from the mucosa of the bladder and rectum. After the position of the applicator has been confirmed to be satisfactory by radiographs, the radioactive source, such as cesium-137, is inserted (afterloading technique). Other types of applicators are available, but the principle of delivering intense radiation to the cervix and paracervical areas is the same. The goal is to increase the total dose of radiation to the maximum allowable to achieve tumor control without introducing a major risk of complications and injury to adjacent normal tissue. The specific protocols followed in various treatment centers differ; individualization for specific patients is often needed depending on the stage and size of the cervical tumor as well as the patient's local anatomy. In general, external therapy is given first to treat the regional pelvic nodes and shrink the central tumor mass, which then is more amenable for a local implant. In some patients, external therapy can lead to excessive shrinkage of the vaginal apex, making safe, effective implantation of local radiation sources difficult. This can be a problem, particularly in older or postmenopausal patients. Occasionally, in those patients, the implantation is done first, especially for smaller stage I tumors. Rotmensch and colleagues have also used intraoperative ultrasonography to provide optimal implant positioning in these difficult patients. In some cases, the central pelvis is shielded during external radiation therapy to allow for subsequent higher doses from the implant. Occasionally, interstitial therapy in the form of needles implanted into the area of the tumor is needed to achieve effective local tumor control. Although criteria differ, patients with stage III disease or poor vaginal anatomy are most often considered candidates for interstitial brachytherapy.

High-dose rate brachytherapy, given on an outpatient basis, has gained increased acceptance. A number of randomized and nonrandomized studies have suggested that survival rates and complications rates with high-dose rate brachytherapy are similar to those with traditional low-dose rate treatment. At least two studies from the United States have shown similar results with high- and low-dose rate treatment in early-stage disease; however, in stage IIIB disease, the survival rate was lower with the high-dose than with low-dose rate therapy.

In calculating the doses of radiation, two reference points, A and B, are used (**Fig. 29-14**). Point A is 2 cm above the external os and 2 cm lateral to the cervical canal. Point B is 5 cm lateral to the cervical canal and 3 cm lateral to point A, which places **point B** in the vicinity of the lateral pelvic wall. The total dose administered depends on tumor stage but, in general, at the pelvic wall, it is in the range of 50 to 65 Gy, with the higher doses used for high-stage disease. At point A, it varies, but approximately 80 Gy is given for small IB1 lesions and doses higher than 85 Gy for larger lesions. The normal cervix is particularly resistant to radiation and can tolerate doses as high as 200 to 250 Gy over 2 months, whereas the adjacent bladder, and in particular the rectum, are much more sensitive and their exposure in general should be limited at the point of maximal radiation to 80 Gy to the bladder and 70 Gy to the rectum, with overall average doses in the range of 65 to 70 Gy. The small bowel can be damaged at doses above 45 to 50 Gy, especially if adhesions limit intestinal mobility and a large volume is treated.

Recently, there has been increased interest in the use of image-based three-dimensional treatment planning for intracavitary and interstitial brachytherapy. Among the many potential advantages of image-based planning are its ability to provide a better sense of the actual doses delivered to critical structures and possibly a more solid basis for comparisons among institutions. Studies have used CT- and MRI-based images; at present, a large multi-institutional study of image-based brachytherapy is ongoing in Europe and worldwide.

Outcomes

Radical radiation therapy achieves excellent survival and pelvic disease control rates in patients with stage IB or IIA cervical cancer. Eifel and associates have reported 5-year disease-specific survival of 90%, 86%, and 67% in patients with stage IB tumors with cervical diameters less than 4 cm, 4.0 to 4.9 cm, and larger than 5 cm, respectively. In 1961, a report suggested that adjuvant hysterectomy improved local control in patients with stage IB disease with tumors larger than 6 cm; however, several studies since then have shown no improvement in local control but an increase in toxicity. One of these studies was a large GOG study in which patients were randomized to a trial of radiation, with or without extrafascial hysterectomy; results showed no difference in survival or local control but a higher complication rate. Mendenhall and coworkers have reported an 18% rate of major complication at 6 years for patients who underwent adjuvant hysterectomy compared with 7% for patients who received radiation therapy alone. Therefore, there is no clear evidence that adjuvant hysterectomy improves outcome in patients with early-stage disease and large tumor size. The 5-year survival for patients with stage IIA disease is similar to that of IB disease. For patients with more advanced disease, 5-year survival rates of 65% to 75%, 35% to 50%, and 15% to 20% have been reported for stage IIB, IIIB, and IV tumors, respectively. The addition of chemotherapy has further improved local control and survival for stage IB2 and higher (see later).

Chemoradiation

In 1999, prospective randomized trials involving concurrent cisplatin-containing chemotherapy to standard radiotherapy showed such improved survival that the trials were preliminarily halted to release the results, which changed clinical practice. In a recent GOG study, Rose and colleagues treated patients with advanced squamous cell, adenosquamous, or adenocarcinoma of the cervix (stages IIB, III, and/or IVA). The patients received external radiation therapy (40.8 to 51.0 Gy) followed by one or two brachytherapy implants. Total dosages to point B were 55 Gy for stage IIB cases and 60 Gy for stages III and IVA. The patients were randomized to receive one of three concomitant chemotherapy regimens—hydroxyurea, cisplatin, 5-fluorouracil, and hydroxyurea, or cisplatin alone. The best results were obtained with the cisplatin-containing regimens, with the least complications seen with weekly cisplatin (40 mg/m^2) alone. Progression-free survival at 24 months was an impressive 67% for this very high-risk group of patients.

In a further collaborative trial, Keys and associates have studied 369 women with bulky stage IB carcinoma (>4 cm) in diameter. They were randomized to receive radiation alone or with concomitant weekly cisplatin (40 mg/m^2). The total dosage to point B was 55 Gy. Patients with radiographic evidence of hydronephrosis or lymphadenopathy were excluded. Adjuvant extrafascial hysterectomy was performed 3 to 6 weeks after conclusion of the chemoradiation treatments. Acute severe toxicity, especially hematologic but also gastrointestinal (GI), was noted. However, the therapeutic results were markedly better in the chemoradiation group, with a 3-year 83% disease-free survival compared with 74% in the radiation group alone ($P = .008$). Recurrences and death were higher in the radiation-only group.

At the same time, the Radiation Therapy Oncology Group also conducted a trial comparing para-aortic–pelvic radiation therapy with concurrent chemotherapy and pelvic radiation in patients with stages IB to IVA tumors and also found a significant improvement in outcome for all stages of disease with concurrent chemotherapy compared with radiation therapy alone. Another trial studied concurrent chemotherapy with radiation therapy in patients who had undergone a **radical hysterectomy** for cervical cancer and were found to have pelvic lymph node metastases, positive margins, or parametrial involvement. In this trial, patients who received chemoradiation had a better disease-free survival rate than patients who received radiation therapy alone.

Only one large randomized trial has failed to demonstrate a significant advantage from concurrent cisplatin-based chemotherapy in cervical cancer patients. This trial, in Canada, was the smallest of six trials of concurrent cisplatin and radiation therapy.

In North America, the primary focus has been on cisplatin-based chemotherapy regimens, but international trials have evaluated others. In one trial by Wong, patients were randomized to receive radiation therapy, or radiation therapy with epirubicin administered every 4 weeks for five courses. The results showed significantly better rates of disease-free survival ($P = .03$) and overall survival ($P = .04$) from the use of chemotherapy. In another large trial from Thailand, patients were randomized into four arms—radiation therapy alone, radiation therapy with concurrent mitomycin and oral fluorouracil, radiation therapy with adjuvant fluorouracil, or radiation with concurrent and adjuvant chemotherapy. Patients in the two treatment groups that included concurrent chemotherapy had higher disease-free survival rates and lower rates of local recurrence than patients in the other two groups. More recently, Duenos-Gonzales presented a trial at the American Society of Clinical Oncology (ASCO, 2009) that studied cisplatin-radiation therapy compared with cisplatin-gemcitabine-radiation therapy followed by two courses of cisplatin-gemcitabine; patients who received gemcitabine had better overall survival and disease-free survival compared with patients who did not.

A meta-analysis review of 15 trials that included a comparison of chemotherapy plus radiation to radiation therapy alone found a 6% improvement in 5-year survival with chemoradiotherapy. A larger survival benefit was seen for the two trials in which chemotherapy was administered after chemoradiotherapy. There was a significant survival benefit for the group of trials that used platinum-based and non–platinum-based chemoradiotherapy but no evidence of a difference in the size of the benefit by radiotherapy or chemotherapy dose or scheduling was seen. Chemoradiotherapy also reduced local and distant recurrence and progression and improved disease-free survival.

Neoadjuvant Chemotherapy

Neoadjuvant chemotherapy may be given before surgery or before radical radiation therapy. Advantages of chemotherapy before surgery include the potential for reducing tumor volume, increasing resectability, and helping to control micrometastatic disease. Neoadjuvant chemotherapy may also have the potential to provide a viable alternative when access to radiotherapy is poor or if there are unavoidable delays in delivering radiotherapeutic treatment. In one study by Sardi and coworkers, 205 patients with stage IB1 were randomized to neoadjuvant chemotherapy plus radical hysterectomy or to radical hysterectomy alone. They reported that the patients who received neoadjuvant chemotherapy had more resectable tumors and better overall survival than patients who did not receive neoadjuvant chemotherapy. In the United States, the GOG closed a trial with 258 patients with stage IB2 cervical tumors who were randomized to neoadjuvant chemotherapy plus radical hysterectomy or to radical hysterectomy alone. They found no difference in the two arms in the rate of surgery performed (79% chemotherapy + surgery versus 54% surgery) in the surgical-pathologic findings, specifically in progression-free survival (56% chemotherapy + surgery versus 54% surgery) and overall survival (63% chemotherapy + surgery versus 61% surgery) at 5 years. A recent meta-analysis of six randomized trials of neoadjuvant chemotherapy plus surgery compared with surgery alone found that although progression-free survival was improved with neoadjuvant chemotherapy, there was no significant survival benefit, and distant recurrence and rates of resection only tended to favor the neoadjuvant chemotherapy. The authors observed heterogeneity in the trials but concluded that it remains unclear whether neoadjuvant chemotherapy consistently offers a benefit over surgery alone for women with early-stage or locally advanced cervical cancer. In the United States, neoadjuvant chemotherapy is rarely used; however, internationally, there is much interest in using neoadjuvant chemotherapy, especially in countries in which radiotherapy is not easily accessible.

The other use of neoadjuvant chemotherapy is prior to radiation therapy. Seven randomized trials have studied neoadjuvant chemotherapy plus radiation therapy compared with radical radiation therapy alone. Other randomized trials have studied neoadjuvant chemotherapy plus surgery compared with radical radiation therapy in locally advanced cervical cancer. A meta-analysis published in 2004 evaluated 21 of these trials; however, all the trials that were included in this analysis were carried out before 1999, when the concurrent chemotherapies were all published. Much heterogeneity was found in the trials, which made them difficult to analyze. However, it was concluded that the timing and dose intensity of cisplatin-based neoadjuvant chemotherapy appeared to have an important impact on whether it benefited women with locally advanced cervical cancer; further exploration was recommended. Presently, two trials of this issue are ongoing in Europe and India and in both trials the standard arm is concurrent chemoradiation.

Para-Aortic Node Involvement

Numerous small series of patients having documented para-aortic node involvement have demonstrated that some patients have long-term disease-free survival. Patients with microscopic involvement have a better survival duration than those with gross involvement; however, even patients with gross involvement have a 15% to 20% survival rate with aggressive management. Laparoscopy and laparotomy using the extraperitoneal approach allow the removal of positive nodes and sampling of other para-aortic nodes, which may enhance control with radiation therapy and help design the treatment field.

Patients with para-aortic lymph node involvement can be treated effectively with extended-field radiation. The superior boundary of the extended field is usually placed at the T12 vertebral body to cover the para-aortic nodes. Patients are treated with a combination of external beam radiation therapy and brachytherapy. The 5-year survival rates range from 25% to 50%. In a trial of biopsy-proven para-aortic node metastases, Varia and colleagues treated 96 patients with extended-field radiation and concomitant 5-fluorouracil and cisplatin at weeks 1 and 5. It was found that chemoradiation was feasible for this group, with a progression-free survival of 33% at 3 years. At present, the standard treatment for patients with positive para-aortic nodes is extended-field radiation therapy with concurrent weekly cisplatin.

Radiation Complications

Complications following radiation therapy are related to dose, volume treated, and sensitivity of the various tissues receiving radiation. The patient's habitus and presence of diseases that affect circulation, such as diabetes and high blood pressure, increase the risk, as does previous intra-abdominal surgery. Acute minor complications, such as diarrhea and nausea, subside after radiation therapy is completed. Complications usually develop in 1 to 2 years, but can occur as early as 6 months or as late as many years after radiation therapy has been completed. Scarring of normal tissues can lead to severe radiation fibrosis. The rare development of a second primary cancer after radiation for cervical cancer was reported by Kleinerman and associates from 13 population-based European registries. With 30 years of survival, there was approximately a doubling of the risk of a new primary in an irradiated pelvic organ, including the ovaries and bladder, as well as the vagina and vulva.

The treatment of radiation complications depends on the symptoms and location of the complication. Vaginal or cervical ulcerations occasionally occur, and local treatment with topical antibiotics and estrogen creams is usually satisfactory. Postradiation cystitis may manifest itself as urinary frequency or dysuria. After infection has been ruled out, symptomatic treatment is undertaken with drugs such as antispasmodics or urinary analgesics (e.g., phenazopyridine [Pyridium], 100 mg three times daily); these are prescribed until the symptoms clear. Occasionally, hemorrhagic cystitis develops, which may require hospitalization for continuous bladder irrigation or instillation of agents to control bleeding, such as silver nitrate or possibly fulguration of the bleeding points. In cases of hematuria, recurrent tumor should first be ruled out. Periureteral fibrosis can lead to ureteral obstruction and loss of kidney function. McIntyre and coworkers have studied 1784 patients with stage IB carcinomas who were treated by radiation therapy and found 29 cases of ureteral stenoses, which increased from a frequency of 1% at 5 years to 2.5% at 20 years. Although tumor recurrence was the most common cause of early ureteral obstruction, radiation fibrosis can be a rare but occasionally fatal late complication.

Bowel complications tend to be more frequent than urinary complications. Proctosigmoiditis can lead to diarrhea, severe pain on defecation, or GI bleeding. Conservative therapy with stool softeners and a low-roughage diet may suffice; occasionally, local corticosteroids (e.g., Cortisone enema) are of assistance. Fistulas or rectal ulcerations are occasionally seen in the area adjacent to the tip of the cervix, which is also the area maximally radiated during local vaginocervical implantation. If a fistula develops, or in cases of ulceration or severe bleeding and pain, a diverting colostomy is required. Serious small bowel complications may occur, leading to obstruction, fistula formation, or necrosis. The use of parenteral nutrition and IV hyperalimentation are excellent measures to help deal with these problems. Follow-up studies by Klee and colleagues have shown that bladder and bowel symptoms tend to be chronic in some patients, but long-term fatigue is also reported. In most patients, it regresses in a few months.

Compromise of sexual function because of inelastic vagina and decreased utilization was noted in the studies of Bergmark and associates. In a randomized trial of experimental psychoeducational intervention involving regular vaginal dilation, Robinson and coworkers have noted reduced fear of sexual activity post-treatment in the experimental group.

SPECIAL CONSIDERATIONS

Cervical Stump Tumors

Some patients undergo supracervical hysterectomy for nonmalignant disease. Carcinomas that subsequently develop in the cervical stump pose special problems because of the shortnessof the cervical canal and absence of the uterus, both of which curtail the effective use of brachytherapy, especially insertion of an intracervical tandem. There is also the risk that bowel adhesions to the apex of the vagina and cervix will increase the chances of radiation complications; a pretherapy barium study of the small and large bowel may be helpful to identify loops that adhere to the cervical apex. For patients with small stage IB tumors, an operative approach similar to radical hysterectomy can be considered. However, most patients are treated with radiation. External treatment is emphasized because of the difficulty of an optimal intracavitary implant. A transvaginal cone may also be used to supplement external pelvic therapy. Effective treatment of cervical stump carcinoma can be achieved; an overall 5-year survival rate of 45% in 173 patients was reported by Wolff and coworkers, and 60% for 70 patients was reported by Kovalic and colleagues. Stage for stage, the survival rates are comparable to those achieved for invasive carcinoma of the cervix but, because of the previous supracervical hysterectomy, there is an increased risk of complications. Results of chemoradiation studies of these tumors are not available but, based on data already presented, radiation combined with weekly cisplatin appears to be optimal.

Carcinoma of the Cervix Inadvertently Removed at Simple Hysterectomy

Unfortunately, the situation occasionally arises in which a woman undergoes a simple total hysterectomy and an invasive carcinoma of the cervix is found after operation. Patients with unsuspected invasive cervical carcinoma detected after simple hysterectomy have been classified into five groups according to the amount of disease and presentation: (1) microinvasive cancer; (2) tumor confined to the cervix with negative surgical margins; (3) positive surgical margins but no gross residual tumor; (4) gross residual tumor by clinical examination documented by biopsy; and (5) patients referred for treatment more than 6 months after hysterectomy (usually for recurrent disease).

The treatment plan is based on the amount of residual disease. Sometimes, the surgeon can subsequently perform a radical operation, removing the tissues that would normally be removed at radical hysterectomy, including the regional pelvic nodes. Such an approach has been used, particularly in younger patients, especially those with small tumors. A 5-year survival of 89% for 18 patients was reported by Chapman and associates. However, the woman is usually treated with some sort of radiation therapy. Patients with minimal or no known residual disease at most require brachytherapy to the vaginal apex; patients with gross disease at the specimen margin require full-intensity therapy. Patients with minimal or no gross residual disease (groups 1 to 3) have excellent 5-year survival rates (59% to 79%), whereas rates for patients with gross residual disease (groups 4 and 5) are poorer (in the range of only 41%). Chemoradiation is unproven in this setting, but may have value, especially for patients with gross or recurrent disease.

Carcinoma of the Cervix in Pregnancy

Rarely, an invasive carcinoma of the cervix is discovered in a pregnant woman. Within each stage, survival statistics are similar in pregnant and nonpregnant women. A concern has been that the delivery of a fetus through a cervix replaced by carcinoma might worsen the prognosis because of tumor dissemination, but there is no clear evidence to indicate that tumor dissemination is caused by the birth process. However, tumor recurrence in episiotomy sites following vaginal delivery has been reported by Cliby and coworkers. The major risk to the patient of delivery through a cervix containing invasive carcinoma is the risk of hemorrhage as a result of tearing of the tumor during cervical dilation and delivery.

A problem arising in pregnancy is whether a woman with an abnormal cytologic smear has intraepithelial neoplasia or invasive cancer. In general, if the cytologic and histologic findings of colposcopically directed biopsies are comparable and suggest intraepithelial neoplasia or carcinoma in situ, the woman is observed and delivered, with final evaluation and therapy completed approximately 6 weeks after delivery. Even if there is a question of microinvasion, a woman so diagnosed in the last trimester of pregnancy is usually followed and evaluated further after delivery. Cervical conization during pregnancy can lead to severe complications, particularly hemorrhage and loss of the fetus. If it is necessary to perform a conization or preferably a wedge resection of the cervix during pregnancy, it is probably best to perform this during the second trimester, when the risks of fetal loss and hemorrhage are minimal. For patients in whom invasive cancer is diagnosed, a therapeutic plan must be developed to deliver appropriate care, with regard also for the outcome of the pregnancy.

The therapy of carcinoma during pregnancy is influenced by the stage of the disease, time in pregnancy when the cancer is diagnosed, and beliefs and desires of the woman in terms of initiating therapy that can terminate the pregnancy, as opposed to postponing therapy until fetal viability is achieved. If carcinoma is diagnosed in the first trimester or early in the second trimester (before 20 weeks), treatment may be undertaken immediately because of the concern that a delay could lead to tumor progression or spread. However, Duggan and colleagues have found delays of 2 to 7 months in eight pregnant patients with stage I disease who demonstrated no adverse effects from the delay. If the woman has resectable tumor (stage IB or early IIA), effective treatment consists of radical hysterectomy and node dissection (class III). This procedure can usually be carried out without difficulty on a pregnant woman. Increased uterine motility and

edema of the pelvic tissue planes help simplify the procedure for the experienced surgeon, but pregnancy does increase the risk of blood loss. For higher stage tumors, therapy is begun with external beam radiation (teletherapy) and, usually in 4 to 6 weeks, this leads to spontaneous abortion. The dose of external therapy prescribed varies depending on the stage of the tumor, but approximately 40 to 50 Gy is given. Although the results of a published series are not available, it would appear preferable to augment the radiation with weekly cisplatin because the pregnancy in this case would be terminated. Following abortion, the uterus involutes and an implant (brachytherapy) is placed. If the pregnancy does not spontaneously abort, dilation and curettage, prostaglandin-assisted delivery or, rarely, hysterotomy may be necessary to empty the uterus before brachytherapy. Alternatively, if the initial tumor was small and has completely regressed, an extrafascial hysterectomy or modified radical hysterectomy may be performed.

For patients beyond the 20th week of gestation, therapy is often delayed until fetal viability. The health and maturity of the fetus are determined by appropriate ultrasound studies and amniotic fluid analysis to ensure fetal lung maturity. Delivery is usually accomplished by cesarean section; after this, therapy is completed by surgery or radiation with the usual considerations of tumor stage and size. Overall, treatment results in pregnant patients are similar to those in nonpregnant patients, stage for stage, as confirmed by van der Vange and associates. It should be noted that many published studies dealing with carcinoma of the cervix in pregnancy include cases treated as long as 1 year postpartum, which assumes that the carcinoma was present during pregnancy. Hacker and coworkers have summarized the results of 1249 cases reported in various series in the literature. Overall, a 5-year survival rate of 49.2% was recorded for pregnant patients compared with 51% for nonpregnant patients treated during the same period. Their statistics included not only patients treated during pregnancy, but also those treated up to 6 months after delivery, and the postpartum group had the poorest survival statistics. Survival was most closely related to stage, as expected, and those diagnosed during the first trimester had a better prognosis than those diagnosed during the third trimester.

RECURRENCE

Approximately one third of patients treated for cancer of the cervix will experience tumor recurrence, which is defined as the reappearance of tumor 6 months or more after therapy. Metastases can occur anywhere, but most are in the pelvis—centrally in the vagina or cervix, or laterally near the pelvic walls—or, less frequently, distally in the periaortic nodes, lung, liver, or bone. It should be noted that liver, lung, and distal bone metastases outside the pelvis likely result from hematogenous tumor spread.

The symptoms caused by recurrence depend on the site and extent of metastatic disease. Vaginal discharge and abnormal bleeding are often symptoms of an early central pelvic recurrence. Malaise, loss of appetite, and general symptoms associated with widespread metastatic disease are late manifestations of recurrence. Lateral pelvic recurrences often have a retroperitoneal component, which can lead to sciatic nerve irritation and cause severe pain around the distribution of the sciatic nerve in back of the leg, as well as loss of muscle strength, causing the woman to walk with a limp. Unilateral leg edema frequently accompanies such metastases, or leg swelling may occur from fibrosis of lymphatics following surgery or radiation. In addition, tumor recurrence can also cause ureteral obstruction, leading to unilateral or bilateral compromise of kidney function. Low back pain frequently occurs.

Patients treated for carcinoma of the cervix are examined according to the same schedule as patients with other malignancies—every 3 months the first 2 years, every 6 months from years 3 to 5, and yearly thereafter. More frequent examinations are done if abnormal symptoms or signs develop. Examination consists of vaginal and cervical cytology (Pap smear) as well as complete physical and pelvic examinations. Generally, chest radiographs are obtained annually, and IVP or abdominal pelvic CT is also performed annually, particularly during the first 2 years after treatment, when most recurrences will develop. Renal function tests may be indicated because ureteral fibrosis can occur more than 5 years after the completion of radiation therapy. A blood test for squamous cell carcinoma antigen has been studied as a modality to follow patients who have detectable levels of the antigen in their blood. Holloway and colleagues have noted elevated levels in 72 of 153 patients (53%) and found the test to be useful for following patients who initially had elevated levels. Once recurrent disease is suspected, verification is usually obtained by biopsy of an accessible mass or CT-directed thin-needle aspiration, depending on the location of the tumor recurrence.

PELVIC RECURRENCE

Approximately 50% of recurrences will develop in the pelvis. In addition to clinical assessment and CT, a vaginal ultrasound scan is often useful to document pelvic recurrence. Recurrences of adenocarcinoma are less frequent in the pelvis and are more likely to be at distant sites, such as the lung or supraclavicular areas. For patients who were initially treated by surgery, radiation is usually prescribed for pelvic recurrences; approximately 45- to 50-Gy whole-pelvis irradiation is given. Supplemental interstitial or intracavitary radiation is also prescribed, depending on the size and location of recurrence in the pelvis. As noted, chemoradiation is preferably used. Patients who have isolated central recurrences without pelvic wall fixation or regional metastasis can be cured in as many as 60% to 70% of cases. The prognosis is much poorer when the pelvic wall is involved; usually, 10% to 20% of patients survive 5 years after radiation therapy. For patients who were initially treated with radiation who have developed a localized pelvic recurrence, surgical eradication of the tumor should be considered because further effective radiation is not possible and limited surgical resection of the pelvic recurrence may not lead to a cure but will often cause severe complications of wound healing and intestinal and urinary fistulas. However, in rare, carefully selected patients initially treated with primary radiation therapy, radical hysterectomy may be a feasible alternative to exenterative surgery. Coleman and associates have reported on 50 patients who underwent a radical hysterectomy for persistent or recurrent disease and found 5- and 10-year survival rates of 72% and 60%, respectively, with complication rates of 64% for severe complications and 42% for permanent complications. The authors concluded that a radical hysterectomy was an alternative to exenteration in patients with small, centrally recurrent cervical cancer, but that it should be used only in carefully selected patients. If neither surgery nor radiation is a feasible alternative, palliative chemotherapy is considered.

Pelvic Exenteration

Exenterative therapy for central pelvic tumor recurrence is an extensive operative procedure used only if the preoperative evaluation suggests that the patient's condition can be cured by this procedure. Exenteration is not performed for palliation. Three types of procedures may be used. Anterior **pelvic exenteration** is removal of the bladder, uterus, cervix, and all or part of the vagina. Posterior pelvic exenteration is the removal of the anus and rectum and resection of the uterus, cervix, and all or part of the vagina. Total exenteration removes all the pelvic contents. Shepherd and coworkers have noted that patients older than 69 years, those who had a recurrence within 3 years, or those who had persistent disease or positive resection margins had a poorer prognosis for the procedure.

Before an exenterative operation is undertaken, the patient is thoroughly evaluated for any evidence of disease spread outside the pelvis. At operation, abdominal exploration is carried out to ensure that the tumor is resectable. Biopsy specimens of any enlarged lymph nodes or suspicious areas outside the pelvis are taken, and frozen-section studies are performed, including evaluation of the operative margins. Usually, total exenteration is performed.

Several surgical innovations have expanded the reconstruction options. The introduction of continent urinary diversion provides an alternative incontinent conduit. Continent conduits require the woman to catheterize the pouch every 4 hours, but no external appliance is required. Goldberg and colleagues have reported long-term dissatisfaction among women with continent conduits and, in our practice, we have been doing an increasing number of incontinent diversions.

Transverse rectus abdominis myocutaneous (TRAM) flaps have provided a welcomed alternative to gracilus flaps. TRAM flaps, even small ones, as described by Sood and associates, are reliable and provide patients with the option of intercourse.

The introduction of a continent urinary pouch has contributed to patient comfort; the operation has been well described by Penalver and coworkers. Generally, the urinary stoma is located in the abdomen on the right side and the intestinal stoma on the left side. The use of intestinal stapling devices sometimes allows preservation of the rectal sphincter and anal function and avoids a permanent colostomy. Long-term complications are usually ureteral stricture and/or difficulty catheterizing the intestinal reservoir.

Severe postoperative and intraoperative complications can occur with this extensive procedure and perioperative mortalities as high as 10% to 20% have been reported in the past. Infection and bowel obstruction are the major risks. However, current surgical techniques of preoperative bowel preparation, use of antibiotics, careful intraoperative fluid and volume monitoring, and use of parenteral nutrition have reduced the immediate postoperative mortality to less than 5%. The use of a peritoneal graft or an omental flap, created from the right or left side of the omentum and placed in the pelvis to protect the denuded pelvic floor, can help avoid bowel obstruction and reduce postoperative morbidity, as noted by Miller and colleagues. Occasionally, gracilis myocutaneous grafts are used to create a new vagina and bring a new blood supply to the previously irradiated pelvis, which aids in wound healing. Morley and associates have reported a 5-year survival rate of 61% in 100 patients aged 21 to 74 years. No patients with positive nodes in the operative specimen survived.

NONPELVIC RECURRENCE

Recurrences outside of the pelvis can be treated with radiation, surgery, or chemotherapy. Localized recurrences in areas not previously irradiated are occasionally treated by radiation. Resection of the metastasis is rarely done; it is usually restricted to a localized lesion that occurs 3 to 4 years after primary therapy on the assumption that such a solitary metastasis can be effectively treated with local resection. However, in general, distant metastases are usually manifestations of systemic disease and are not cured with local therapy.

CHEMOTHERAPY AS TREATMENT FOR RECURRENCE

Patients with advanced, recurrent, or persistent cervical cancer are the most difficult to treat and, for this patient population, chemotherapy offers the best hope. Many studies, including some by Bonomi, McGuire, and their coworkers, have attempted to identify active agents in this patient population, and most studies have established cisplatin as the most active agent. Several phase II studies have evaluated novel single agents or the combination of cisplatin with other agents, including mitolactol, ifosfamide, gemcitabine, topotecan, paclitaxel, and vinorelbine, and all have shown promising results. This has led to several phase III studies evaluating chemotherapy in patients with recurrent, advanced, or persistent cervical cancer.

The GOG has published results from four randomized phase III trials (protocols 110, 149, 169, and 179) trying to find the optimal platinum doublet to treat women with metastatic disease. The first of these trials to be published was GOG protocol 110, which compared single-agent cisplatin with cisplatin-mitolactol and cisplatin-ifosfamide. Despite the fact that overall response rates were 17.8% in the cisplatin-only arm, 21.1% in the cisplatin-mitolactol, and 31.1% in the cisplatin-ifosfamide arm ($P = .004$), there was no significant difference in overall survival and greater toxicity with the cisplatin-ifosfamide regimen. GOG protocol 149 demonstrated that the addition of bleomycin did not enhance the activity of the cisplatin-ifosfamide doublet, and GOG protocol 169 showed that the addition of paclitaxel to cisplatin or increasing the dose of cisplatin only improved response rate and prolonged progression-free survival but not overall survival.

The only trial that has been positive has been GOG protocol 179. In this trial, patients were randomized to single-agent cisplatin versus cisplatin and topotecan. There was a 2.9-month improvement in median survival in patients receiving the combination of cisplatin-topotecan versus cisplatin alone with no increase in toxicity, making this the new standard regimen in the setting of stage IVB or recurrent cervical cancer. A phase III trial that just closed, GOG protocol 204, compared cisplatin-paclitaxel with cisplatin-topotecan, cisplatin-gemcitabine, and cisplatin-vinorelbine in patients with advanced, recurrent, or persistent disease in an attempt to find the optimal platinum doublet. Results are still pending at this time. Despite all these efforts, survival rates are poor and newer agents are needed to move from palliation to cure.

KEY POINTS

- Carcinomas of the cervix are predominantly squamous cell carcinomas (85% to 90%), and approximately 10% to 15% are adenocarcinomas.
- Squamous cell carcinomas appear to have a viral and venereal association, particularly with HPV. In the United States, squamous cell carcinoma is more frequent in blacks than in whites.
- Cervical carcinoma is the third most frequent malignancy of the lower female genital tract, after endometrial and ovarian cancer, and the second most frequent cause of death, after ovarian cancer.
- Definitive diagnosis of microinvasive carcinoma is established only by means of cervical conization, not biopsy. The margins of the cone should be free of neoplastic epithelium before conservative therapy is undertaken
- Microinvasive carcinoma of the cervix can be effectively treated by total hysterectomy, with a 5-year survival rate of almost 100%, but recurrent neoplasia can develop after 5 years. However, a precise and reliable definition of microinvasion is controversial.
- Prognosis in squamous cell cancer of the cervix is related to tumor stage and lesion volume (size), depth of invasion, and spread to lymph nodes. Older patients tend to have a worse prognosis, and HPV-positive younger patients have a better prognosis.

- The prognosis of adenocarcinoma of the cervix is related to tumor stage, size, grade, and depth of invasion. Large adenocarcinomas tend to be poorly differentiated.
- Metastases to regional pelvic nodes in stage I squamous carcinomas correlate with lesion size, depth of invasion, and presence of capillary lymphatic space involvement, and correlate inversely with patient age.
- Cervical carcinomas are locally invasive tumors that spread primarily to the pelvic tissues and then to the pelvic and para-aortic lymph nodes. Less frequently, hematogenous spread to the liver, lung, and bone occurs.
- The risk of the spread of cervical carcinoma to pelvic nodes is approximately 15% for stage I, 29% for stage II, and 47% for stage III. For the para-aortic nodes, the figures are 6% for stage I, 19% for stage II, and 33% for stage III.
- Stage IB carcinomas of the cervix may be treated equally effectively by radical hysterectomy and pelvic node dissection or radiation. The 5-year survival rate is approximately 80%. If lymph nodes are free of tumor, the 5-year survival rate is approximately 90%; if the nodes contain metastatic tumor, the rate is 50%. Improved overall survival rates have been reported for patients with tumors smaller than 4 cm in diameter treated by preliminary brachytherapy followed by radical hysterectomy.
- Surgery is often used for treating stage IB and early-stage IIA carcinomas of the cervix, particularly for smaller tumors and for younger patients to preserve their ovarian function.

Surgery produces less scarring and vaginal fibrosis than radiation and is preferred for women with a pelvic mass, pelvic infection, or history of conditions such as inflammatory bowel disease, which increase the risk for radiation complications.

■ High-stage tumors are treated by chemoradiation. Current programs usually use cisplatin, 40 mg/m^2 weekly, during external treatment and with brachytherapy.

■ Urinary fistulas follow radical hysterectomy in approximately 1% of cases.

■ Most cancers of the cervix are treated by radiation therapy (teletherapy and brachytherapy). Radiation doses vary with tumor size and stage but are approximately 50 to 65 Gy at point B and 85 Gy at point A. Current practice is to combine radiation with simultaneous chemotherapy to optimize the results.

■ Improved cure rates of cervical cancers are obtained with increased doses, which also lead to an increased frequency of complications. Large increments in dose may increase complications without increasing cure rates.

■ Complications following radiation are related to dose and volume of tissue treated; these include radiation inflammation of the bladder or bowel, which may lead to pain, bleeding or, infrequently, fistula formation. The normal cervix is resistant to radiation, and the dose can be as high as 200 to 250 Gy over 2 months. The bladder and rectum can be injured at average doses in the range of 65 to 75 Gy. Overall, the rate of moderate to severe radiation complications for treatment of all stages is approximately 10%.

■ Worldwide 5-year survival rates reported for patients with carcinomas of the cervix are as follows: stage IA, 95%; stage IB, 80%; stage II, 70%; stage III, 50%; and stage IV, 20% with radiation therapy alone.

■ Pregnancy does not adversely affect the survival rate for women with carcinoma of the cervix, stage for stage.

■ Approximately one third of patients treated for cervical carcinoma develop tumor recurrence, and approximately 50% of these recurrences are located in the pelvis; most occur within 2 years.

■ Patients whose recurrences occur more than 3 years after primary therapy have a better prognosis than those with earlier recurrence.

■ Pelvic exenteration in carefully selected patients with central pelvic recurrence can lead to a 5-year survival rate of 50% or better.

■ Chemotherapy of recurrent squamous cell carcinoma of the cervix does not produce long-term cures, but response rates of approximately 50% (partial and complete) have been obtained with multiagent regimens that contain cisplatin.

■ Leg pain following the distribution of the sciatic nerve or unilateral leg swelling is often an indication of pelvic recurrence of carcinoma of the cervix.

REFERENCES CAN BE FOUND ON EXPERTCONSULT.com

30

Neoplastic Diseases of the Vulva
Lichen Sclerosus, Intraepithelial Neoplasia, Paget's Disease, and Carcinoma

Michael Frumovitz and Diane C. Bodurka

Cancer of the vulva accounts for approximately 5% of malignancies of the lower female genital tract, ranking it fourth in frequency after cancers of the endometrium, ovary, and cervix. Well-defined predisposing factors for the development of vulvar carcinoma have not been identified. In general, premalignant and malignant changes frequently arise at multifocal points on the vulva. Occasionally, invasive carcinoma arises from areas of **carcinoma in situ**, similar to the mechanism in cervical squamous cell carcinoma (see Chapter 29, Malignant Diseases of the Cervix). However, many cases of squamous cell carcinoma of the vulva appear to develop in the absence of premalignant changes in the vulvar epithelium. Human papillomavirus (HPV) has been noted in many young patients with carcinoma of the vulva. Other factors, such as granulomatous disease of the vulva, diabetes, hypertension, smoking, and obesity, have all been suggested as causative factors, but data do not provide consistent evidence regarding their association with vulvar carcinoma. Carcinoma of the vulva occurs with increasing frequency in those who have been treated for squamous cell carcinoma of the cervix or vagina, presumably as a result of the increased risk of carcinogenesis in the squamous epithelium of the lower genital tract in these patients. It appears that HPV DNA is involved in the development of a subset of vulvar carcinomas that tend to occur in younger patients, as noted by Crum and associates. Monk and colleagues have demonstrated that not only were the HPV DNA–associated carcinomas found in younger patients, but also the HPV-negative patients appear to have had a poor prognosis with tumors that were more likely to recur and lead to patient death. As demonstrated by Hording and coworkers, HPV-positive tumors tend to have a warty or basaloid appearance, whereas HPV-negative tumors tend to be keratinized. The former tend to be associated with premalignant vulvar changes (vulvar intraepithelial neoplasia [VIN]).

Most vulvar malignancies are squamous cell carcinomas. Although this is a disease of older women, Franklin and Rutledge have noted that 15% of cancers of the vulva in their series occurred in women younger than 40 years. The incidence of squamous cell carcinoma of the vulva increases progressively with age. Although more than 50% of patients with carcinoma of the vulva are older than 60 years at the time of diagnosis, Jones and colleagues have shown an increasing trend of squamous cell carcinomas of the vulva in women younger than 50 (**Fig. 30-1**). Although most patients with carcinoma of the vulva are older than 60, those with carcinoma in situ of the vulva are usually 10 to 15 years younger—that is, 40 to 55 years of age. Premalignant changes of the vulva have been seen with increasing frequency among younger patients, often in their 20s and 30s, possibly as a result of an increasing rate of multiple sexual contacts and increased exposure to venereal infections, particularly HPV, in this population. Carter and colleagues have reported a link between immunosuppression and invasive squamous cell carcinoma of the vulva in women younger than 40 years. Similar to cervical cancer, HPV-related infections would presumably progress through dysplasia to invasive cancer in these immunocompromised women. This chapter reviews the clinical and pathologic aspects of premalignant vulvar lesions and **vulvar atypias**. This is followed by consideration of the diagnosis, natural history, and management of invasive cancers of the vulva, which includes not only the squamous cell carcinomas but also the rarer melanomas and sarcomas.

VULVAR ATYPIAS

SPECIFIC CONDITIONS

Vulvar Atypias: Intraepithelial Neoplasia
Lichen sclerosus (**Fig. 30-2**) is a change in the vulvar skin that often appears whitish. Microscopically, the epithelium becomes markedly thinned, with a loss or blunting of the rete ridges. In some cases, there is also a thickening or hyperkeratosis of the surface layers (**Fig. 30-3**). Inflammation is usually present. Hart and associates have studied 107 patients with lichen sclerosus, and only one followed for 12 years eventually developed vulvar carcinoma. Five patients had vulvar carcinoma when lichen sclerosus was diagnosed. Twelve other patients subsequently developed malignancies at other sites, such as the cervix, colon, breast, ovary, and endometrium. In the past, patients with lichen sclerosus were thought not to be at increased risk for the development of vulvar carcinoma. A study by Carlson and colleagues has supported a small premalignant potential of lichen sclerosus. Their study, and a literature review, showed that a risk of lichen sclerosus and squamous cell carcinoma was 4.5%, with an average of 4 years latency between symptomatic lichen sclerosus and squamous cell carcinoma. The tumors that developed tended to be clitoral in location.

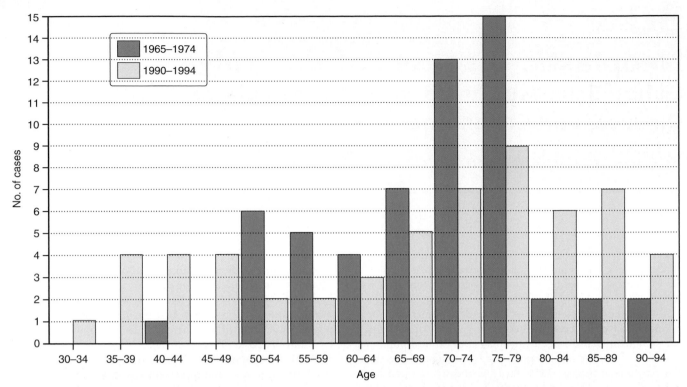

Figure 30-1 Age incidence curve for carcinoma of vulva in women from 2 different decades. (From Jones RW, Baranyai J, Stables S: Trends in squamous cell carcinoma of the vulva: The influence of vulvar intraepithelial neoplasia. Obstet Gynecol 90:448, 1997.)

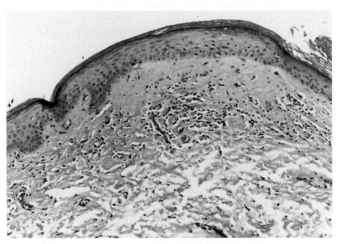

Figure 30-2 Lichen sclerosus et atrophicus. Homogeneous collagen in the papillary dermis is accompanied by a scattered lymphocytic infiltrate and atrophy of the epithelium (H&E, ×80). (Courtesy of Dr. Anthony Montag, Department of Pathology, University of Chicago, Chicago.)

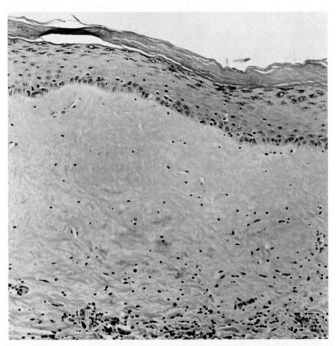

Figure 30-3 Lichen sclerosus. Hyperkeratosis is occasionally present. (From Friedrich EG, Wilkinson EJ: The vulva. In Blaustein A [ed]: Pathology of the Female Genital Tract. New York, Springer-Verlag, 1982.)

Squamous hyperplasia (formerly, hyperplastic dystrophy) involves the elongation and widening of the rete ridges, which may be confluent (**Fig. 30-4**). There may also be hyperkeratotic surface layers, and the tissue grossly is often whitish or reddish.

Atypical changes may appear in the vulvar epithelium. These are usually marked by a loss of the maturation process usually seen in squamous epithelium, as well as an increase in mitotic activity and nuclear-to-cytoplasmic ratio (**Fig. 30-5**). Mild dysplasia (atypia) is diagnosed if these changes involve the lower third of the epithelium, moderate dysplasia (atypia) if half to

two thirds of the epithelium is involved, and severe dysplasia (atypia) if more than two thirds of the epithelium is affected. Carcinoma in situ involves the full thickness of the epithelium. The term *VIN I* is used for mild atypia, *VIN II* for moderate atypia, and *VIN III* for severe atypia and carcinoma in situ. It is

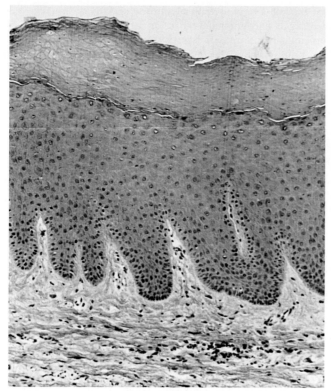

Figure 30-4 Squamous hyperplasia (formerly hyperplastic dystrophy), benign. Hyperkeratosis, acanthosis, and mild inflammation are present. (From Friedrich EG, Wilkinson EJ: The vulva. In Blaustein A [ed]: Pathology of the Female Genital Tract. New York, Springer-Verlag, 1982.)

sometimes difficult to distinguish between squamous hyperplasia and intraepithelial neoplasia. Crum has suggested that VIN usually contains nuclei that are fourfold or greater different in size, whereas differences in the size of nuclei in condyloma or non-neoplastic epithelia are threefold or less. Furthermore, abnormal mitoses are usually observed in VIN.

Carcinoma In Situ (Vulvar Intraepithelial Neoplasia III)

Carcinoma in situ is diagnosed if the full thickness of the epithelium is abnormal (**Fig. 30-6A**). Occasionally, the process may histologically resemble carcinoma in situ of the cervix and, in many lesions, there are multinucleated cells, abnormal mitoses, an increased density in cells, and an increase in the nuclear-to-cytoplasmic ratio.

Paget's Disease

Paget's disease is a rare intraepithelial disorder that occurs in the vulvar skin and histologically resembles Paget's disease in the breast. Paget cells are large pale cells (**Fig. 30-7**). The cells often occur in nests and infiltrate upward through the epithelium. Frequently, histologic abnormalities of the apocrine glands of the skin may be noted in these lesions. There has been an increased association of **Paget's disease of the vulva** with underlying invasive adenocarcinoma of the vulva, vagina, and anus, as well as distant sites, including the bladder, cervix, colon, stomach, and breast. Paget's disease of the vulva tends to spread, often in an occult fashion, and recurrences are frequent after treatment.

DIAGNOSIS

Clinical Presentation

Atypias of the vulva present with a variety of symptoms and signs. Irritation or itching is common, although some patients do not report these symptoms. The vulva often has a whitish change because of a thickened keratin layer. In the past, the term *leukoplakia* was used. This term has been discarded, in part because abnormal lesions of the vulva require biopsy to establish a correct diagnosis. When lichen sclerosus is present, there is usually a diffuse whitish change to the vulvar skin (**Fig. 30-8**). The vulvar skin often appears thin and there may be scarring and contracture. In addition, fissuring of the skin is often present, accompanied by excoriation secondary to itching. Areas of squamous hyperplasias (formerly called hyperplastic dystrophy without atypia) also appear as whitish lesions in general, but the tissues of the vulva usually appear thickened and the process tends to be more focal or multifocal than diffuse (**Fig. 30-9**).

Abnormal areas of vulvar atypia or VIN may also appear as white, red, or pigmented areas on the vulva. However, the clinical appearance of VIN is variable. Friedrich and colleagues have estimated that approximately one third of patients with carcinoma in situ will present with pigmented lesions, emphasizing the importance of a biopsy to establish the diagnosis. The lesions tend to be discrete and multifocal and occur more frequently in those who have had squamous cell neoplasia of the cervix. In addition, reddish nodules may also be foci of Paget's disease as well as of carcinoma in situ. Paget's disease often has a reddish eczematoid appearance. It should be reemphasized that these conditions cannot be accurately diagnosed from their clinical appearance, and biopsies are needed.

Diagnostic Methods

In general, cytologic evaluation (Pap smear) of the vulva has not proved helpful, in part because the vulvar skin is thick and keratinized and does not shed cells as readily as the epithelium of the vagina and cervix. However, in some cases, particularly if there is ulceration of the vulva, a cytologic smear can be helpful diagnostically (see Fig. 32-6B). A tongue depressor moistened with normal saline or tap water is scraped over the surface portion of the vulva to be sampled, and the specimen is placed on a glass slide and then fixed.

The toluidine blue test (1% toluidine blue applied for 1 minute, followed by 1% acetic acid) with biopsy of the retained blue-staining areas has generally been discarded because it appears to be so nonspecific.

Colposcopy of the vulva is difficult because the characteristic changes in vascular appearance and tissue patterns that are seen in the cervix are not present (see Chapter 28, Intraepithelial Neoplasia of the Lower Genital Tract). Nevertheless, the magnification of the colposcope may be used to help follow patients with VIN as well as identify the discrete whitish or pigmented areas that warrant biopsy. The colposcope is not used for routine vulvar examination but is primarily used for those who are being evaluated or followed for vulvar atypia or VIN. However, the addition of 3% acetic acid highlights whitish areas for biopsy.

Biopsy of the vulva can be conveniently accomplished with a **Keyes** dermal **punch biopsy** (**Fig. 30-10**). Usually, a 3- to 5-mm diameter punch is used. Each area in which a biopsy sample is to be obtained is usually infiltrated with local anesthesia using a fine 25-gauge needle. The punch is then rotated and downward pressure applied so that a disk of tissue is circumscribed. When the entire thickness of the skin has been incised, the specimen is elevated with forceps and removed with a sharp scissors. Occasionally, a larger biopsy is needed, in which case a larger field is anesthetized and a small scalpel or cervical punch biopsy

(see Fig. 28-14) is used to obtain the specimen. Usually, little bleeding is encountered and it can generally be controlled by applying silver nitrate or ferrous subsulfate (Monsel's solution). Depending on the size of the atypical area and the variety of atypical-appearing areas, one or multiple biopsies may be needed.

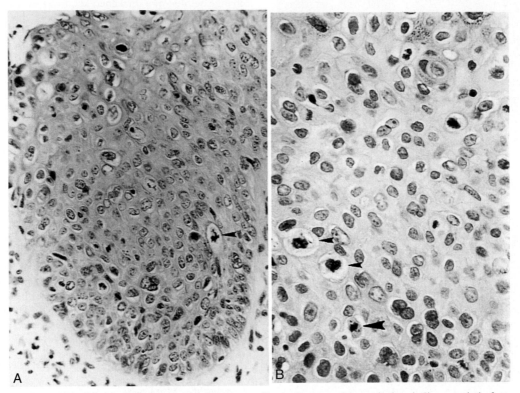

Figure 30-5 A, Vulvar intraepithelial neoplasia from which human papillomavirus type 16 was isolated. Characteristic features displayed here include abnormal mitoses (a two-group metaphase is denoted by the *arrowhead*), a full-thickness population of abnormal cells, and abnormal differentiation. Superficial cells contain perinuclear halos, which in contrast to condylomata are small and concentric. **B,** The higher power photomicrograph of vulvar intraepithelial neoplasia illustrates the marked variability in nuclear size and staining, with both enlarged nuclei and multinucleated cells. Coarsely clumped mitoses (*small arrowheads*) and a three-group metaphase (*large arrowhead*) are present. (From Crum CP: Pathology of the Vulva and Vagina. New York, Churchill Livingstone, 1987.)

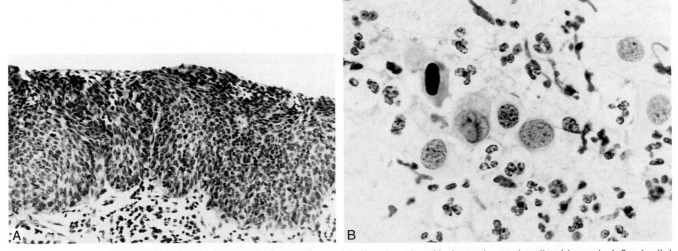

Figure 30-6 A, Carcinoma in situ, histology. The full thickness of the epithelium is replaced by hyperchromatic cells with poorly defined cellular borders (×80). **B,** Carcinoma in situ, cytology. Cells derived from carcinoma in situ of the vulva may exhibit varying sizes and shapes, as depicted in this photomicrograph. Note variation in nuclear pattern from one nucleus to another. Degenerated polymorphonuclear leukocytes are present in the background (×800).

Continued

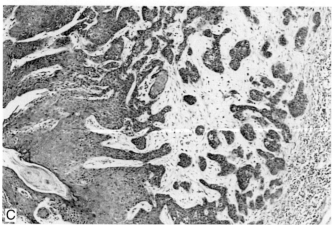

Figure 30.6—cont'd C, Invasive squamous carcinoma, histology. Tumor nests and cords infiltrate stroma. The squamous nature of the tumor is more apparent on surface (*left*), where cells have abundant dense cytoplasm. Keratin is also seen (×80).

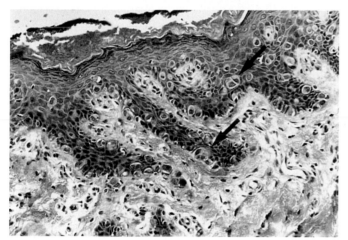

Figure 30-7 Vulvar epidermis with Paget's disease. Malignant cells (*arrows*) are seen infiltrating the epidermis and spreading along the dermal-epidermal junction (H&E, ×160). (Courtesy of Anthony Montag, MD, Department of Pathology, The University of Chicago.)

TREATMENT

Vulvar Atypias

Most vulvar atypias have pruritus as the major symptom, so the relief of itching is often the main concern of the woman. Once the correct diagnosis has been established by biopsy, appropriate therapy can be undertaken. Most whitish lesions will be benign, because lichen sclerosus is the most common condition encountered.

Topical testosterone can be used for atrophic conditions of the vulva, particularly lichen sclerosus. The most commonly used option for the treatment of lichen sclerosus is 0.05% clobetasol propionate ointment. This can be used anywhere from nightly to twice weekly for up to 12 weeks and then used to re-treat, as necessary. Although lichen sclerosus can be associated with the development of squamous cell carcinoma, some believe that the use of a potent steroid cream has a protective effect from malignant evolution.

For women who fail clobetasol, some advocate the use of steroid creams, although results from small clinical trials using

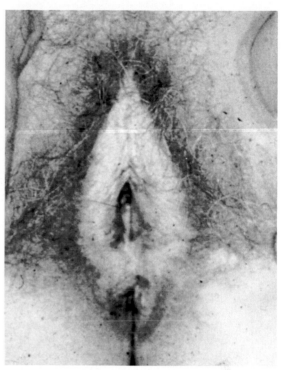

Figure 30-8 Vulva, lichen sclerosus. The tissue of the labia minora and perineum have a white, brittle, cigarette paper appearance. (From Kaufman RH, Gardner HL, Merrill JA: Diseases of the vulva and vagina. In Romney SL, Gray MJ, Little AB, et al [eds]: Gynecology and Obstetrics. New York, McGraw-Hill, 1980, pp .)

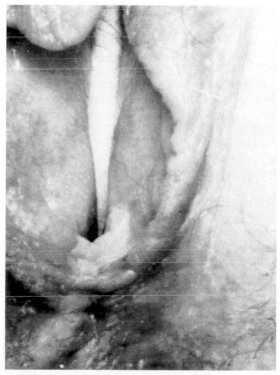

Figure 30-9 Vulva, hyperplastic dystrophy. A sharply demarcated, raised, white area is noted at lower tip of white pointer. (From Kaufman RH, Gardner HL, Merrill JA: Diseases of the vulva and vagina. In Romney SL, Gray MJ, Little AB, et al [eds]: Gynecology and Obstetrics. New York, McGraw-Hill, 1980 pp .)

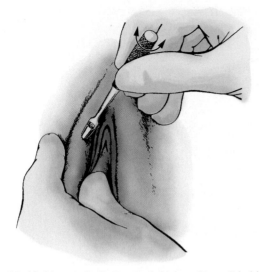

Figure 30-10 Diagnostic Keyes punch biopsy. (From Friedrich EG: Vulvar Disease, 2nd ed. Philadelphia, WB Saunders, 1983.)

testosterone and progesterone creams have been mixed. A preparation of 2% testosterone propionate in petrolatum can be used twice daily, with once-daily maintenance after the first week. Often, reducing the dosage of testosterone cream to twice weekly is a sufficient maintenance dose. Side effects, such as clitoral hypertrophy and increased hair growth, can occur. If there are undesirable side effects with testosterone, local progesterone cream is sometimes tried, with variable success. Those who have a beneficial response to testosterone should be continued on the medication indefinitely. The control of local irritation of the vulva is discussed in Chapter 18 (Benign Gynecologic Lesions). In addition to local measures to diminish irritation (e.g., cotton underclothes, avoidance of strong soaps and detergents, avoidance of synthetic undergarments), topical fluorinated corticosteroids are helpful to control itching. Frequently used preparations are 0.025% or 0.1% triamcinolone acetonide (Aristocort, Kenalog), fluocinolone acetonide (Synalar), and 0.01% or 0.1% betamethasone valerate. These are usually applied twice daily to control the itching, which is often relieved in 1 to 2 weeks. Unfortunately, the prolonged use of fluorinated topical steroids can lead to vulvar atrophy and contraction. Thus, once the symptoms of itching are controlled, the dose of topical corticosteroids is tapered off or, if long-term therapy is needed, a nonfluorinated compound such as 1.0% hydrocortisone is used to avoid vulvar contraction. Occasionally, 1% hydrocortisone is sufficient for initial therapy. In some cases, the corticosteroids are not successful, and numerous types of topical therapy need to be tried to control symptoms. Gentle soaps are helpful. Burow's solution (5% solution of aluminum acetate) is frequently used as a wet dressing to help control irritation and itching. Doak tar, 3%, in petrolatum (USP) or in 1% hydrocortisone ointment is useful for severe cases.

In some patients with lichen sclerosus, severe contracture of the vulva, particularly in the area of the posterior fourchette, will occur with concomitant scarring and tenderness. Intercourse may then become painful in these patients. Woodruff and co-workers have described a useful surgical technique to treat these vaginal outlet disorders by repair of the perineum. The contractured and fissured area in the posterior fourchette is excised, which results in an elliptic defect. This is then closed by undermining the distal 3 to 4 cm of the posterior vaginal mucosa and suturing the freed mucosa to the perineal skin (**Fig. 30-11**).

Vulvar Intraepithelial Neoplasia

Once the diagnosis of VIN has been established by biopsy, therapy is performed to eradicate the area containing the neoplasia. The clinician must be aware that the progress of vulvar atypia (mild dysplasia [VIN I]) to moderate dysplasia (VIN II) to severe dysplasia and carcinoma in situ (VIN III) and then to invasive carcinoma is not as well documented for vulvar neoplasia as it is for squamous cell neoplasia of the cervix. Moreover, vulvar neoplasia is frequently multifocal, requiring treatment of several areas. An additional complication is that some cases originally diagnosed as intraepithelial neoplasia have been reported to regress spontaneously.

In 1972, Friedrich reported bowenoid atypia (histologically similar to carcinoma in situ) in a pregnant woman who regressed spontaneously postpartum. Others also reported spontaneous regression of this lesion. These spontaneously regressing lesions tend to be discrete elevations in young women. Some may be explained by studies of the nuclear DNA content of vulvar atypias that suggest that not all lesions with this designation are premalignant. Fu and colleagues noted that only four of eight cases of vulvar atypia had an aneuploid (neoplastic) distribution. A polyploid distribution was noted in four of the cases, which is consistent with a benign process, whereas aneuploidy is consistent with intraepithelial neoplasia.

Although VIN has been diagnosed more commonly in younger women, the risk of progression to invasive cancer is higher for those who are older and for those who are immunosuppressed, such as women with AIDS or transplant recipients. Chafe and associates have studied 69 patients with a diagnosis of VIN treated by surgical excision. Unsuspected invasion was found in 13 patients. The median age was 36 years for those without invasive carcinoma, whereas the median age was 58 years ($P = .003$) for those with invasion found in the excision specimen, emphasizing the increased risk of invasion in the older patients. Furthermore, the risk of invasion was higher in those who had raised lesions with irregular surface patterns. Thus, patients who were older and those with irregular raised lesions had the greatest risk of unrecognized invasive carcinoma. A study by Modesitt and colleagues of 73 women, with a mean age of 45 years, has found an invasive carcinoma in 22% of VIN III excision specimens. Not surprisingly, the risk of recurrence was almost 50% if the margins were positive and only 17% if they were negative. A frequency of 20% invasive disease in 78 patients was also reported by Husseinzadeh and Recinto. Twelve of the 16 malignancies occurred in patients older than 40 years. The risk of progression from intraepithelial disease to invasive carcinoma appears to be less for vulvar cases than for cervical disease (see Chapter 28, Intraepithelial Neoplasia of the Lower Genital Tract).

Women with HIV-AIDS are also more likely to develop vulvar carcinoma in situ and invasive cancer than the general population. In a large population-based study, Chaturvedi and colleagues have found a relative risk (RR) of 1.59 for developing VIN III in the 28 to 60 months after the onset of AIDS and an RR of 4.91 for developing invasive carcinoma in this group.

Studies have suggested that the potential of VIN to develop into invasive cancer is low. Buscema and coworkers followed 102

Figure 30-11 Surgical correction of perineal scars. (From Woodruff JD, Julian CJ: Surgery of the vulva. In Ridley JH [ed]: Gynecologic Surgery: Errors, Safeguards, Salvage. Baltimore, Williams & Wilkins, 1974.)

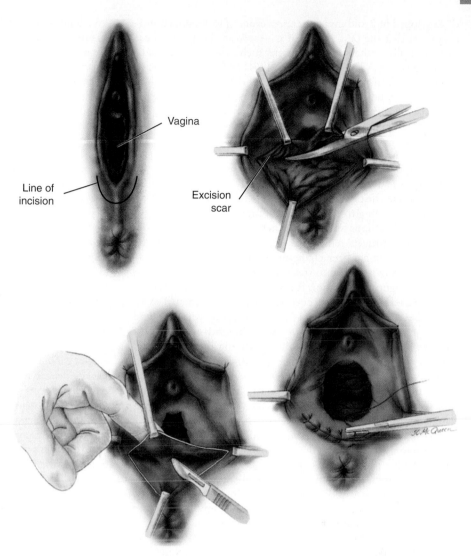

patients with vulvar carcinoma in situ for 1 to 15 years without treatment; 4 patients developed invasive disease, 2 of whom were immunosuppressed. Unfortunately, current techniques do not allow precise prediction of which lesions of VIN are at the greatest risk of progression to invasive disease. A population-based study from Norway has confirmed an increasing frequency of VIN III that nearly tripled from the mid-1970s to 1988 to 1991 but, during the same period, the age-adjusted frequency of invasive vulvar carcinomas remained almost constant. Iversen and Tretli have further noted an estimated conversion rate of VIN III to invasive carcinoma of approximately 3.4% for these in situ lesions. Jones and coworkers have noted spontaneous regression of VIN II and III pigmented lesions in young women (<30 years).

HPV types 6 and 11 have generally been recognized as being found most often in benign vulvar warts, whereas primarily HPV types 16, 18, 31, 33, and 35 are more frequently associated with intraepithelial neoplasia or invasive carcinoma (see Chapter 28, Intraepithelial Neoplasia of the Lower Genital Tract). The Centers for Disease Control and Prevention (CDC) has estimated that 80% of women aged 50 will have acquired a genital HPV infection at some point in their lives. Beutner and associates have predicted that as many as 1 million new cases of perineal warts

will occur annually in the United States. An additional complication is that HPV type 16 infection is not always accompanied by histologic evidence of VIN. Moreover, HPV types 6, 11, and 16 can be recovered from a single site, including those that show only condyloma as well as those that show carcinoma. Thus, a unique role for HPV types in VIN has not been elucidated. With current data, therapy should be based on histologic findings and not on the presence or absence of HPV infection or specific HPV types. Studies by Buscema and associates have suggested that HPV type 16 is frequently found in vulvar neoplasia and, as noted, HPV 16 has been frequently associated with some vulvar carcinomas.

Human Papillomavirus Therapy

The problem of the management of vulvar HPV infection is particularly complicated because it is extremely prevalent and the risk of progression from HPV infection to VIN is small. Planner and Hobbs have evaluated 148 women with cytologic evidence of vulvar HPV infection and found that two thirds of them had pruritus and dyspareunia. Results of the biopsy revealed that only 11 of the 148 women had VIN. Follow-up showed spontaneous regression of HPV infection in 56 patients, whereas VIN

III developed in 2 and invasive cancer eventually developed in 1. It appears that the best approach is to restrict therapy to those with clinically bothersome symptoms such as warts or to eradicate lesions with VIN, particularly VIN II and III. Cytologic or histologic evidence of an asymptomatic HPV infection, such as koilocytosis, is not an indication for therapy. Riva and colleagues have treated lower genital tract HPV infection with laser to include the cervix, vagina, and vulva; 25 patients had proved subclinical HPV infection, and their male partners were also evaluated and treated. All 25 patients suffered severe pain and many required hospitalization. At 3 months after therapy, 24 of 25 again had evidence of subclinical HPV infection and 22 had persistent histologic evidence of koilocytosis, indicating the futility of trying to eradicate HPV infection by this method.

Many VIN lesions tend to be posterior, predominantly in the perineal area. Surgical removal has been effectively used, but the type of operation has been changing. In the past, simple vulvectomy was widely practiced to treat carcinoma in situ of the vulva, but this disfiguring operation is now infrequently used, particularly because the disease is occurring in younger women. To improve the cosmetic result and sexual function, Rutledge and Sinclair introduced the method of **skinning vulvectomy**. This removes the superficial vulvar skin, preserving the clitoris, and replaces the removed skin with a split-thickness vulvar graft. In many cases, however, such extensive surgery is not needed. Often, the abnormal area of the vulva can be removed only with wide local excision. Of the patients in the series reported by Buscema and coworkers, 62 were treated with local excision; 68% showed no recurrence. For comparison, in 28 patients treated by vulvectomy, 70% showed no recurrence. The risk of recurrence is higher if neoplastic epithelium is found at the resection margin. Friedrich has noted a 10% risk of recurrence if the surgical margins are free of disease compared with a 50% risk if the surgical margins are involved with neoplasia. However, because recurrence may develop even if the resection margins are negative, long-term follow-up is mandatory.

The carbon dioxide laser has been used to treat VIN, usually to a depth of 1 to 3 mm, with a deeper depth being used for areas that contain hair. This results in eradication of the abnormal vulvar tissue and healing without scarring. Most patients require a single treatment but some require more, particularly those with large or multiple lesions. Usually, patients can be treated on an outpatient basis with local, general, or regional anesthesia. The laser is particularly useful for younger patients. It is essential to be certain that the woman does not have invasive disease before using the laser, so a biopsy of any suspicious lesions should be performed before laser ablation. The therapist should be experienced in the diagnosis and treatment of vulvar disease before using laser ablation. Older patients or those with raised lesions should be treated by surgical excision. Treatment is usually carried out to a depth of 3 to 4 mm, and healing is usually complete within 2 to 3 weeks. Leuchter and associates have treated 142 patients with carcinoma in situ of the vulva. Of the 42 treated by laser, 17% had recurrence; 4 of the 16 treated with vulvectomy (25%) and 15 of 45 treated by local excision (33%) also had recurrence. In view of the risk of unsuspected carcinoma in older patients, as noted by the studies of Chafe and colleagues, those older than 45 years and those with raised or irregular lesions should have an excision performed and the entire tissue submitted for histologic evaluation. Posterior lesions near the anus require particular attention because the anal canal is often involved and this abnormal tissue also needs to be removed.

5-Fluorouracil (5-FU) cream has been tried to treat carcinoma in situ of the vulva, but it causes severe burning and is generally not used. Investigators have explored using 5% imiquimod cream as primary treatment for VIN III, with promising results. Van Seters and coworkers have performed a randomized control study of 5% imiquimod topical cream versus placebo in 52 women with VIN II and III. Most women included in the study (96%) were positive for HPV prior to initiation of therapy. In the treatment group, 81% had at least a reduction in the size of the primary lesion by over 25% at 20 weeks and 35% had a complete response. In the placebo group, there were no patients with partial or complete responses. At 12 months after enrollment, 3 patients (6%), however, had progressed to **microinvasive vulvar carcinoma** (1 in treatment group, 2 in placebo group).

Therapeutic vaccines using HPV peptides have also been explored for the treatment of VIN III. Kenter and colleagues have combined long peptides from the E6 and E7 oncoproteins of HPV 16 into a vaccine and immunized 20 women with HPV 16–positive VIN III. At 12 months after last vaccination, 79% had a clinical response, with 47% achieving complete response. Of note, all the women who had a complete response by 12 months also remained disease-free at 24 months.

Paget's Disease of the Vulva

Paget's disease is generally seen in postmenopausal women and typically appears grossly as a diffuse erythematous eczematoid lesion that has usually been present for a prolonged time. Itching is a common problem. The disease is primarily seen in white women and the average age is approximately 65 years. The major importance of Paget's disease of the vulva is the frequent association with other invasive carcinomas. Squamous cell carcinoma of the vulva or cervix or an adenocarcinoma of the sweat glands of the vulva or Bartholin's gland carcinoma may be present. Cases of adenocarcinoma of the gastrointestinal (GI) tract and breast accompanying Paget's disease have also been reported. Once a diagnosis of Paget's disease of the vulva is made, it is important for the gynecologist to rule out the presence of breast and GI malignancy. In a review by Lee and associates, a total of 75 cases of Paget's disease of the vulva were identified; an underlying invasive carcinoma of the adnexal structures of the skin was reported in only 16 (22%) and a carcinoma in situ in 7 (9%). Of these patients, 22 (29%) had cancer at distant sites, including adenocarcinoma of the rectum, carcinoma of the breast, carcinoma of the urethra, basal cell carcinoma of the skin, and carcinoma of the cervix.

If no local or distant primary malignancy is uncovered, a wide excision of the affected area can be performed. It is important to remove the full thickness of the skin to the subcutaneous fat to ensure that all the skin adnexal structures are excised, because they may have a subclinical malignancy. Bergen and coworkers have evaluated 14 patients with Paget's disease of the vulva treated by surgery, usually vulvectomy, skinning vulvectomy with graft, or hemivulvectomy. With a median follow-up of 50 months, all patients were free of disease, although 2 with positive margins and 1 with negative margins required treatment for recurrence. Fishman and colleagues have studied 14 patients treated by various surgical procedures for Paget's disease. Frozen-section or gross visual inspection was used to judge the operative margins. In this series, visual estimation was as useful as frozen section insofar as the error rate for judging margins by the final pathology report was approximately 35%. In addition, 2 of 5 patients with positive margins had a recurrence after the initial operation compared with 3 of 9 with negative margins. This small series, therefore, suggests that gross visual inspection may be as useful as frozen section when judging the extent of surgical operation. Other small series evaluating Mohs micrographic surgery for treating vulvar extramammary disease have failed to reduce recurrence significantly. A conservative approach involving removal of gross Paget's disease with approximately a 1-cm margin appears to be the most appropriate, with the understanding that reexcision may be required for recurrence in the future. The full thickness of the vulvar skin to the adipose layer should be removed.

Even if resection margins are free of Paget's disease at the time of surgical excision, local recurrence remains a risk. Women who have been treated for Paget's disease of the vulva should have as part of their routine follow-up an annual examination of the breast, cytologic evaluation of the cervix and vulva, and screening for GI disease, at least by testing for occult blood in the stool. Progression of Paget's disease of the vulva to invasive adenocarcinoma has been rarely reported.

MALIGNANT CONDITIONS

SQUAMOUS CELL CARCINOMA

Squamous cell carcinomas comprise approximately 90% of primary vulvar malignancies, but a variety of other vulvar cancers are encountered; the manor types are listed in **Box 30-1**. Melanomas account for approximately 4% to 5% and the other types comprise the remainder.

Morphology and Staging

Grossly, vulvar carcinomas usually appear as raised, flat, ulcerated, plaquelike, or polypoid masses on the vulva (**Fig. 30-12A**). Biopsy sample of the lesion reveals the characteristic histologic appearance of squamous cell carcinoma (see **Fig. 30-6C**).

Four clinical stages are defined for carcinoma of the vulva according to the International Federation of Gynecology and Obstetrics (FIGO), similar to the system used for other gynecologic malignancies. In addition, many centers use the **TNM system** (tumor, nodes, metastases) for classification; T denotes the size and extent of the tumor, N the clinical status of the nodes, and M the presence or absence of metastatic disease.

In the clinical staging system, lymph node status was assessed clinically and incorporated into the stage. Enlarged or clinically suspicious lymph nodes were assigned a higher stage, regardless of disease status documented at surgery. Clinically negative nodes were assigned an earlier stage, which was upheld even if they were found to harbor metastasis after surgical removal and pathologic examination. Therefore, in 1988, the FIGO staging was modified to a **surgical staging of vulvar cancer** system to reflect lymph node status more accurately. In addition, a

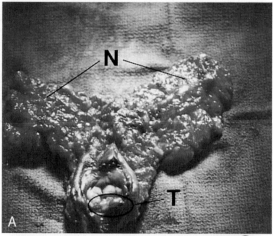

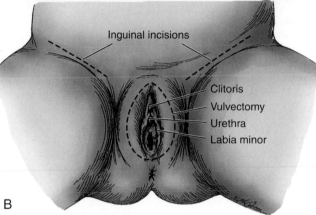

Figure 30-12 A, Radical vulvectomy specimen. **B,** Vulvectomy with operative incision lines shown. Note groin incisions.

location on the perineum is no longer assigned to stage III. This system, with the modifications introduced in 2009 for new definitions of stages I to III, is shown in **Box 30-2**.

Natural History, Spread, and Prognostic Factors

The vulvar area is rich in lymphatics, with numerous cross connections. The main lymphatic pathways are illustrated in **Figure 30-13**. Tumors located in the middle of either labium tend to drain initially to the ipsilateral inguinofemoral nodes, whereas perineal tumors can spread to the left or right side. Tumors in the clitoral or urethral areas can also spread to either side. From the inguinofemoral nodes, the lymphatic spread of tumor is cephalad to the deep pelvic iliac and obturator nodes. Although there has been concern in the past that tumors in the clitoral-urethral area would spread directly to the deep pelvic nodes, this rarely, if ever, occurs. The characteristics of lymph drainage of the vulva have been evaluated by Iverson and Aas, who injected technetium-99 m colloid subcutaneously into the anterior and posterior labia majora, anterior and posterior labia minora, clitoral area, and perineum. They then measured the radioactivity in the pelvic lymph nodes, which were surgically removed 5 hours later. More than 98% of the radioactivity was found in the ipsilateral node and less than 2% on the contralateral side. The anterior labial injections resulted in a 92% concentration of radioactivity in the ipsilateral side, with 8% on the contralateral side. The clitoral and perineal injections developed a bilateral nodal distribution of radioactivity in all the patients.

Box 30-1   Classification of Vulvar Atypias
Squamous cell hyperplasia (formerly hyperplastic dystrophy)
Lichen sclerosus
Intraepithelial neoplasia
VIN I: Mild dysplasia
VIN II: Moderate dysplasia
VIN III: Severe dysplasia–carcinoma in situ
Others
Paget's disease
Melanoma in situ (level 1)
VIN, Vulvar intraepithelial neoplasia.

Box 30-2 TNM and Staging Classifications of Carcinoma of the Vulva

TNM

T: Primary tumor

Tis: Preinvasive carcinoma (carcinoma in situ)

T1: Tumor confined to the vulva and/or perineum, ≤2 cm in diameter

T2: Tumor confined to the vulva and/or perineum, >2 cm in diameter

T3: Tumor of any size with adjacent spread to the urethra, vagina, anus, or all of these

T4: Tumor of any size infiltrating the bladder mucosa, rectal mucosa, or both, including the upper part of the urethral mucosa or fixed to the anus

N: Regional lymph nodes

N0: No nodes palpable

N1: Unilateral regional lymph node metastases

N2: Bilateral regional lymph node metastases

M: Distant metastases

M0: No clinical metastases

M1: Distant metastases (including pelvic lymph node metastases)

Staging (FIGO), Modified 2009

Stage I—T1/2, N0, M0: Tumor confined to vulva and/or perineum

 IA: Lesions ≤2 cm in size, confined to the vulva or perineum and with stromal invasion ≤1.0 mm; no nodal metastasis

 IB: Lesions >2 cm in size or with stromal invasion >1.0 mm, confined to the vulva or perineum, with negative nodes

Stage II—T3 N0 M0: Tumor of any size with extension to adjacent perineal structures (one third lower urethra, one third lower vagina, anus) with negative nodes

Stage III—T1-3 N1/2 M0: Tumor of any size with or without extension to adjacent perineal structures (one third lower urethra, one third lower vagina, anus), with positive inguinofemoral lymph nodes

 IIIA: (i) With one lymph node metastasis (≥5 mm) or (ii) one or two lymph node metastasis(es) (<5 mm)

 IIIB: (i) With two or more lymph node metastases (≥5 mm) or (ii) three or more lymph node metastases (<5 mm)

 IIIC : With positive nodes with extracapsular spread

Stage IV—any T, any N, M1: Tumor invades other regional (two thirds upper urethra, two thirds upper vagina), or distant structures

 IVA: Tumor invades any of the following: (i) upper urethral and/or vaginal mucosa, bladder mucosa, rectal mucosa, or fixed to pelvic bone; or (ii) fixed or ulcerated inguinofemoral lymph nodes

 IVB: Any distant metastasis including pelvic lymph nodes

FIGO, International Federation of Gynecology and Obstetrics; TNM, tumor-node-metastasis.

Adapted from FIGO Committee on Gynecologic Oncology, European Institute of Oncology, Milan, Italy: Revised FIGO staging for carcinoma of the vulva, cervix, and endometrium. Int J Gynecol Obstet 105:103, 2009.

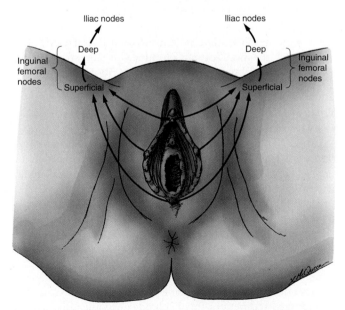

Figure 30-13 Vulvar lymph drainage is shown in this general schematic representation of major drainage channels of vulva.

It is of interest that two thirds of the patients with labial injections had a small amount of detectable radioactivity in the contralateral nodes. Thus, anastomoses of the lymphatics do exist, but a direct connection from the clitoris to the deep nodes was not demonstrated.

The prognosis of a woman with vulvar carcinoma is related to the stage of the disease (**Fig. 30-14**), lesion size, as well as the presence or absence of cancer in regional nodes. The worldwide actuarial 5-year survival results from the 25th FIGO Annual Report on the Results of Treatment of Gynaecologic Cancer were as follows: stage I, 76.9%; stage II, 54.8%; stage III, 30.8%; and stage IV, 8.3%. The presence of carcinoma in regional lymph nodes correlates with the size of the primary lesion, degree of tumor differentiation, and extent of involvement of vascular spaces by tumor. Tumor size is usually estimated by the greatest tumor diameter; for example, smaller than 2 cm or larger than 2 cm separates stage I from stage II disease.

The status of the regional lymph nodes is the most important factor prognostically and therapeutically. Numerous studies, including a multicenter collaborative investigation from the Gynecologic Oncology Group (GOG), have indicated that tumor stage, location on the vulva, microscopic differentiation, presence or absence of vascular space involvement, and tumor thickness are all important prognostic factors. In a GOG study of 588 patients reported by Homesley and colleagues, the risk of lymph node metastases was related to lesion size (19% for <2 cm and 42% for >2 cm). Additional independent predictors of positive nodes were as follows: (1) tumor grade; (2) suspicious, fixed, or ulcerated lymph nodes; (3) lymphovascular space involvement; (4) older age of the woman; and (5) tumor thickness. **Table 30-1** summarizes these factors.

Lymphovascular space invasion also appears to be a factor in vulvar tumors, as it is in cervical carcinoma (see Chapter 28, Intraepithelial Neoplasia of the Lower Genital Tract). In a small

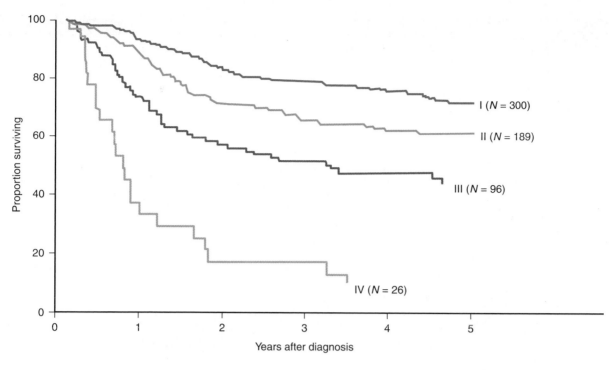

Strata	Patients (N)	Mean age (years)	Overall survival at					Hazards ratio[a] (95% Confidence intervals)
			1 year	2 year	3 year	4 year	5 year	
I	300	64.7	92.3%	82.3%	78.7%	75.7%	71.4%	Reference
II	189	67.4	86.5%	71.0%	65.8%	62.2%	61.3%	1.94 (1.36–2.75)
III	96	69.4	72.0%	57.2%	51.3%	47.5%	43.8%	3.84 (2.55–5.78)
IV	26	72.8	33.3%	16.7%	16.7%	8.3%	8.3%	12.2 (7.08–21.2)

[a]Hazards ratio and 95% confidence intervals obtained from a Cox model adjusted for country

Figure 30-14 Carcinoma of the vulva, patients treated from 1990 to 1992; survival by International Federation of Gynecology and Obstetrics stage (epidermoid invasive cancer only; N = 611). [a]Hazards ratio and 95% confidence intervals obtained from a Cox model adjusted for country. (From Pecorelli S, Creasman WT, Pettersson F, et al: FIGO Annual Report on the Results of Treatment in Gynaecological Cancer, vol 23. Milan, Italy, International Federation of Gynecology and Obstetrics, 1998.)

study of 22 patients, Rowley and associates have noted no metastases in 20 patients without lymphovascular space invasion and in 2 patients with lymphovascular space invasion.

Stage IA: Carcinoma of the Vulva (Early or Microinvasive Carcinoma)
Definition and Clinicopathologic Relationships
The term *microinvasive carcinoma of the vulva* typically refers to a lesion considered to be stage IA definition—that is, smaller than 2 cm, with less than 1 mm invasion—and is used to identify

early tumors unlikely to spread to regional nodes. However, varying clinicopathologic results are reported when this definition is used.

Part of the confusion is because of different reference points from which the depth of invasion is measured—that is, from the surface or basement membrane. Dvoretsky and coworkers have carefully analyzed the microscopic aspects of 36 cases of superficial vulvar carcinoma. Tumor penetration into the stroma was measured from the surface of the squamous epithelium (neoplastic thickness; **Fig. 30-15A**) and also from the tip of the adjacent

Table 30-1 Factors Related to Positive Inguinal Nodes (588 Cases)

GOG Grade	% Positive Nodes	Tumor Thickness (mm)	% Positive Nodes	Age (yr)	% Positive Nodes	LVSI	% Positive Nodes
1	2.8	≤1	2.6	<55	25.2	+	75
2	15.1	2	8.9	55-64	25.4	−	27
3	41.2	3	18.6	65-74	36.4		
4	59.7	4	30.9	>75	46		
		≥5	43				

GOG, Gynecologic Oncology Group; LVSI, lymphovascular space invasion.
Adapted from Homesley H, Bundy BN, Sedlis A, et al: Prognostic factors for groin node metastasis in squamous cell carcinoma of the vulva (a Gynecologic Oncology Group study). Gynecol Oncol 49:279, 1993.

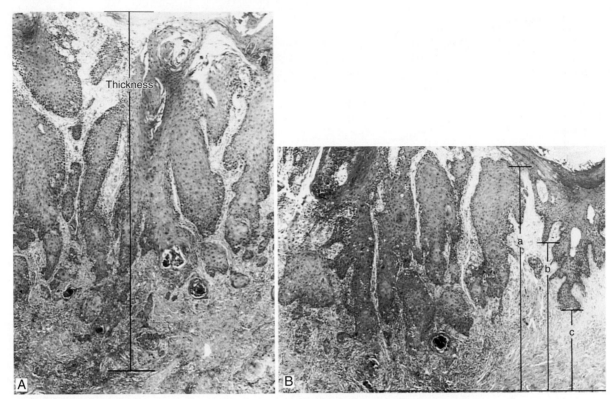

Figure 30-15 A, Measurement of neoplastic thickness in squamous cell carcinoma (×35). **B,** Superficially invasive squamous cell carcinoma. The reference point used to measure the depth of stromal invasion is demonstrated by line b. Note the striking variation in the measurement of stromal invasion, depending on which reference point is chosen (line a, b, or c; ×35). (From Dvoretsky PM, Bonfiglio TA, Helkamp BF, et al: The pathology of superficially invasive thin vulva squamous cell carcinoma. Int J Gynecol Pathol 3:331, 1984.)

epithelial ridge (stromal invasion; see **Fig. 30-15B**). Six of the 36 cases had spread to regional nodes and all had invaded more than 3 mm from the surface. Kneale and associates have pointed out that although there is almost no risk of metastases to regional nodes in stage IA lesions, late recurrence of these tumors can develop years after primary therapy; in a literature review, 8 cases of recurrence were reported in 88 cases of superficial vulvar carcinoma. All tumors were smaller than 2 cm diameter and invaded less than 1 mm into the stroma measured from the adjacent rete peg, which would correspond approximately to 3 mm measured from the surface because the vulvar epithelium is approximately 2 mm thick.

The presence of carcinoma in situ in the primary lesion decreases the risk of node involvement in these cases. Ross and Ehrman have noted that only 1 of 35 patients with adjacent carcinoma in situ had nodal metastases, and this tumor penetrated the stroma 1.7 mm. In contrast, 5 of 27 superficial stage I patients (2.1 to 5.0 mm penetration) without adjacent carcinoma in situ had positive nodes. Thus, spread to regional lymph nodes in stage IA carcinoma of the vulva is unlikely, particularly if the tumor is well differentiated (grade 1), invades less than 3 mm measured from the surface, or has a depth of invasion measured from the adjacent rete pegs of less than 1 mm and is without vascular space involvement. The presence of carcinoma in situ is a favorable factor. Less well-differentiated tumors or those with vascular involvement or confluence and with greater depths of invasion have an increased risk of lymph node involvement by cancer.

Treatment

Based on available evidence, it would appear prudent that most patients with stage IA carcinoma of the vulva by the criteria described earlier should be treated at least with a wide excision to give a margin of 1 to 2 cm. Depending on the location of the tumor, a hemivulvectomy may be needed. The lymph node dissection may be omitted or deferred, depending on the final pathologic evaluation of the tumor in the surgical specimen. For younger patients, especially with tumors that involve the labia or perineum at a distance from the clitoris, an operation that spares the clitoris should be used. Even if the criteria for stage IA is rigorously applied, a rare nodal metastasis may occur, as reported by Van der Velden and associates. However, a report by Magrina and coworkers on 40 patients with T1 lesions (less than 2 cm in diameter) and less than 1 mm invasion indicated that they could be effectively treated with wide excision. No nodal metastases were noted in this small group, and excision appeared to be as effective as a more radical operation in preventing recurrent disease.

INVASIVE CARCINOMA OF THE VULVA

Figure 30-12A shows a typical carcinoma of the vulva, which usually appears as a polyploid mass. The woman frequently reports a sore that has not healed. She may also report bleeding, but this does not usually occur early in the course of the disease. Unfortunately, the delay in diagnosis is common because older patients frequently fail to seek prompt medical attention and, often when they do, a biopsy is not initially performed. For example, some patients have their symptoms of irritation or itching treated with various medications to eradicate the symptoms. It is vital that a biopsy sample be taken of any vulvar lesion before undertaking therapy, as was emphasized earlier. A biopsy of a tumor such as that shown in **Figure 30-12*A*** can easily be obtained on an outpatient basis using local anesthesia and biopsy forceps such as a Kevorkian punch as illustrated in Chapter 28, Intraepithelial Neoplasia of the Lower Genital Tract.

Effective therapy of clinical stage I or II and early stage III vulvar carcinoma can be accomplished with a wide radical excision and inguinofemoral node dissection. Lesions located more than 2 cm from the midline typically need only an ipsilateral inguinofemoral lymphadenectomy, whereas midline lesions necessitate bilateral groin dissections. Because the deep pelvic nodes are almost never involved unless the inguinal nodes are also involved, only the inguinofemoral nodes are removed at the time of the primary operation and the deep pelvic nodes subsequently treated with external radiation if the superficial nodes are involved with tumor. The inguinofemoral node dissection is performed through separate inguinal incisions followed by the vulvectomy portion. **Figure 30-12*A*** shows the type of specimen that can be obtained through separate groin incisions. The operative incisions are shown in **Figure 30-12*B***. It appears that an adequate surgical dissection with decreased wound complications can be accomplished by this technique. It is advisable to use suction drainage in the inguinal area until all drainage is complete, which usually takes 7 to 10 days, and drains are also frequently used in the vulvar area. It is important that an adequate margin, usually 1 to 2 cm, be obtained around the primary tumor at the time of surgery. Grimshaw and colleagues have reported on 100 cases operated on through separate incisions and noted superb results with a corrected 5-year survival rate in stage I of 96.7% and stage II of 85%. Similar excellent results for separate skin incisions were reported by Farias-Eisner and

associates on 74 patients, with 5-year survival rates of 97% and 90% for stages I and II, respectively. Tumor recurrence has occurred rarely in the skin bridge over the symphysis when separate groin incisions are used, without an en bloc dissection of the vulva and intervening lymph tissue. Magrina and coworkers have noted comparable survival rates with fewer complications in those undergoing modified **radical vulvectomy** with inguinal incisions done separately.

In treating clinical stage I and stage II tumors of the vulva, the results of histologic evaluation of the inguinofemoral nodes are important. Many initially treat the superficial nodes above the cribriform fascia (**Fig. 30-16**). If these nodes are negative, the deep nodes are spared. The procedure can usually be accomplished with preservation of the saphenous vein, which was traditionally sacrificed. These modifications reduce the risk of leg edema. If the lymph nodes, particularly the upper femoral group, are involved with tumor, the deep pelvic nodes require treatment. Homesley and coworkers have reported improved survival for those who received radiation (4500 to 5000 rad) to the deep pelvic nodes in comparison with those who had a pelvic node dissection.

The results of therapy in clinical stages I and II disease relate not only to the stage of the disease but also to the status of the regional pelvic nodes. If the nodes do not contain metastatic tumor and the woman can be successfully treated by radical vulvectomy and bilateral node dissection, 5-year survival rates of approximately 95% have been reported. Iversen and associates, in a series of 424 patients, have noted lymph node metastasis in 10.5% of clinical stage I cases, 30% of clinical stage II, 66% of clinical stage III, and 100% of clinical stage IV. The number of positive nodes in the radical vulvectomy specimen correlates with the size of the primary tumor and also with the woman's survival. In a study of T1 and T2 tumors, Andrews and coworkers have noted that only unilateral inguinal node metastases occurred and, furthermore, the deep nodes were involved only if the superficial nodes were positive. However, there was a small

Figure 30-16 A, B, Injection of blue dye into vulvar lesion and identification of sentinel node in inguinofemoral triangle.

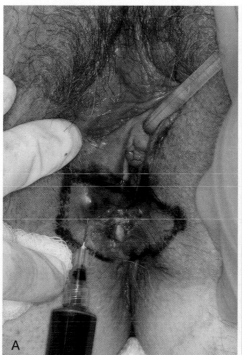
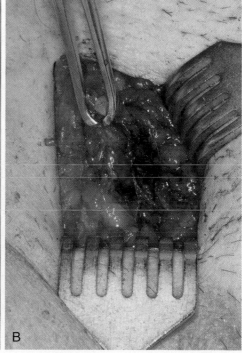

(2% to 3%) risk of contralateral node involvement of the larger T2 lesions. In a study of 113 patients, Hacker and colleagues have noted an actuarial 5-year survival rate of 96% for those with negative nodes, but there was a progressive decrease in the survival rate to 94% for those having one positive node, 80% for two positive nodes, and 12% for three or more positive nodes. In the various cases that have been studied, the deep pelvic nodes do not contain tumor unless the upper inguinofemoral nodes contain metastatic disease. The number of nodes involved and the size of the metastasis are both important. Hoffman and associates have noted that 14 of 15 patients with inguinal lymph node metastases smaller than 36 mm^2 survived free of disease at 5 years compared with 12 of 29 whose lymph node metastases measured more than 100 mm^2. These results should be taken into consideration when planning additional therapy for patients with positive nodes.

If tumor spread to the regional inguinofemoral nodes is identified, further treatment should be considered. If only one node is microscopically involved with tumor and the woman has undergone a complete lymph node dissection of the groin, no further therapy is usually needed, particularly if only a small volume is present. However, if one node is microscopically positive and the woman has undergone a superficial inguinofemoral lymph node dissection, many clinicians would be uncomfortable not treating the groin with adjuvant radiation therapy. If three or more nodes are involved, pelvic radiation as outlined is usually prescribed. For patients with only two nodes involved, the decision for further therapy will depend on the location of the nodes, extent of groin dissection performed, and size of the metastatic deposit of tumor, although most clinicians would opt for radiotherapy in such cases.

ADVANCED VULVAR TUMORS

Large tumors of the vulva, particularly those that encroach on the anal-rectal area or urethra, may require more extensive treatment than radical vulvectomy to achieve effective tumor control. In such cases, it may be necessary to remove the anus or urethra as part of a primary operative procedure, in which case diversion of the urinary or fecal stream is required (see discussion of exenterative surgery for carcinoma of the cervix in Chapter 29, Malignant Diseases of the Cervix).

For tumors that encroach on the urethra or anus, making procurement of negative margins improbable, multidisciplinary organ-sparing approaches may be used in an effort to reduce the morbidity of exenterative procedures. A useful therapeutic approach has been to treat large vulvar tumors with external radiation; then, after the tumor has been reduced in size, to remove the residual tumor surgically, usually by radical vulvectomy. External radiation is used to deliver approximately 4000 cGy to the tumor and 4500 cGy to the pelvis and inguinal nodes. The operation is usually performed approximately 5 weeks after the completion of radiation therapy. Although a large series of patients has not been treated by this technique, a sufficient number has been treated to demonstrate that marked tumor regression does occur. The primary cancer can be eradicated by a procedure that does not require diversion of the urine or feces. Boronow and associates initially summarized the treatment of 26 patients with primary carcinoma of the vaginal vulvar area with this technique and noted a 5-year survival rate of 80%. Rotmensch and colleagues have reported on 16 patients, 13 stage III and 3 stage IV, and achieved an overall 5-year survival rate of 45% with this technique, somewhat better than might be expected with stages III and IV (see Fig. 30-14). Recurrences are more likely if the resection margins were within 1 cm of the tumor.

Chemotherapy with radiation appears to offer a therapeutic advantage. Koh and coworkers have studied 20 patients with stages III and IV disease and 3 with recurrence, using 5-FU with radiation. In addition, some patients also received cisplatin with concurrent radiotherapy. Actuarial 3- and 5-year survival rates in this small group were 59% and 49%, respectively. Similar results with 5-FU and radiation, occasionally with the addition of cisplatin, were also reported by Russell and associates in 25 patients. Moore and colleagues have reported on a phase II GOG study and noted the need for a less extensive operation when chemotherapy with cisplatin and 5-FU were combined with preoperative radiation. Multiple chemoradiation programs are available, but a convenient outpatient regimen consists of weekly IV cisplatin with radiation, usually to 4500 cGy. Other complications reported include stenosis of the introitus, urethral stenosis, and rectovaginal fistula, but this technique is an effective alternative to primary exenteration for large vulvar vaginal carcinomas and is preferred in most treatment centers, although success with exenteration can occasionally be achieved, as noted by Miller and associates.

Radiation Therapy and Recurrences

In a few cases, the medical condition of the woman precludes surgery and radiation therapy may be used as the sole treatment. However, the vulvar skin is prone to radiation dermatitis fibrosis and ulceration, making irradiation as the sole form of therapy a less desirable treatment. Therefore, irradiation is seldom used as the sole treatment of carcinoma of the vulva. To manage recurrences, reoperation is often tried. Piura and colleagues have analyzed 73 patients whose disease recurred only on the vulva. Salvage was achieved with wide radical local excision, which appeared to be successful in 30 patients in whom the recurrence was only on the vulva.

As may be expected, the risk of recurring carcinoma rises as the stage of the disease increases. In an analysis of 224 patients with vulvar carcinoma, Podratz and associates noted a recurrence rate of 14% in stage I and 71% in stage IV. Local vulvar recurrences were the most common and occurred in 40 of 74 cases of recurrence (54%). The remaining recurrences were in the groin, pelvis, or distant sites. Radiation therapy or additional operations for local vulvar recurrences usually provide effective control and 5-year survival rates of approximately 50%. The risk of recurrence of the disease in the vulva requires careful attention to the surgical resection margins at the time of initial operation.

Combined chemotherapy and radiation has been used for primary treatment of late-stage advanced vulvar tumors, as noted. It has also been applied to recurrences, especially those near the anus and/or urethra. Radiation alone may also be used for vulvar recurrences, as reported by Perez and coworkers, although chemoradiation would appear to be a more effective choice.

Treatment of patients with disseminated disease requires chemotherapy but, unfortunately, no chemotherapeutic regimen has been successful for treatment of this disease. Squamous cell carcinomas of the female genital tract have generally not been responsive to cytotoxic chemotherapy; the protocols followed are similar to those described for recurrent squamous cell carcinomas of the cervix (see Chapter 29, Malignant Diseases of the Cervix).

Quality of Life and Vulvar Carcinoma

There have been few studies regarding quality of life in patients with vulvar cancer. Body image disturbance is significant and may account for decreased or absent sexual activity in women who have undergone vulvectomy. Interestingly, Green and colleagues have noted that the extent of surgery or type of vulvectomy performed does not correlate well with the degree of sexual dysfunction. They demonstrated a significant need to address sexual problems with all women undergoing any type of vulvectomy. The Functional Assessment of Cancer Therapy–Vulvar (FACT-V) is a valid and reliable instrument to assess quality of life in women with vulvar cancer. Perhaps this tool can be used to help assess quality of life and also facilitate vital communication about quality of life issues in women with this disease.

Lymphatic Mapping and Sentinel Lymph Node Biopsy

As noted, regional lymph node dissections are routinely performed in the surgical treatment of vulvar cancer because the status of regional lymph nodes is essential for therapeutic planning and overall prognosis. More than 80% of women with clinical stages I and II disease, however, will have no metastatic disease found in the lymph nodes, therefore making an extensive lymphadenectomy unnecessary while increasing postoperative morbidities, such as lymphedema and lymphocyst formation. Lymphatic mapping and sentinel lymph node biopsy, as used for the treatment of patients with melanoma and breast cancer, are appealing techniques for patients with vulvar cancer. The sentinel node(s) are those nodes that directly drain the primary tumor and are thought to predict the metastatic status of the upper echelon or nonsentinel nodes in the groin. If the sentinel node is negative, in theory, all the other groin nodes would also be negative and surgeons could abandon full groin dissections, thereby greatly reducing the associated morbidities of lymphocyst, lymphedema, and wound separation (see **Fig. 30-16**).

Van der Zee and colleagues have performed a prospective observational study in 403 women with clinical stage I squamous cell carcinoma of the vulva smaller than 4 cm. Women enrolled in this study underwent a sentinel node biopsy, with omission of complete inguinofemoral lymphadenectomy if no metastatic disease was found. Patients with negative sentinel nodes were triaged to no further therapy and observed for recurrence. With a median follow-up of 35 months, only six groin recurrences (2.3%) have been noted. In an accumulation of data from smaller studies on the subject, Frumovitz and colleagues reviewed the combined data on 279 patients with vulvar cancer who had undergone lymphatic mapping and sentinel lymph node identification. They found the overall sensitivity of the sentinel node for detecting metastatic disease in patients with vulvar cancer to be 97.7% and the false-negative rate for the procedure to be 2.3%. The overall negative predictive value was 99.3%. Although these numbers are promising, at this time, lymphatic mapping and sentinel lymph node biopsy are considered experimental, with the standard of care remaining full inguinofemoral node dissection.

OTHER VULVAR MALIGNANCIES

Bartholin's Gland Carcinoma

Bartholin's gland carcinomas are adenocarcinomas that comprise approximately 1% to 2% of vulvar carcinomas. An enlargement of Bartholin's gland in a postmenopausal woman should raise suspicion for this malignancy. These tumors are treated similarly to primary squamous cell carcinoma of the vulva; radical vulvectomy with bilateral inguinofemoral lymphadenectomy is the treatment of choice. If the regional lymph nodes are free of tumor, the prognosis is good. Rosenberg and associates have reported five cases of adenoid cystic carcinoma of Bartholin's gland, a variant of invasive adenocarcinoma, treated by surgery (usually hemivulvectomy) and postoperative radiation therapy. Four of the five patients were alive and disease-free 28 to 57 months after treatment.

Basal Cell Carcinoma

Basal cell carcinoma can arise in the vulva, as it can arise in the skin elsewhere in the body. It is rare and comprises approximately 2% of vulvar carcinomas. Therapy consists of wide local excision of the lesion, which is generally ulcerated. If the surgical resection margins are free of tumor, the disease is cured.

Verrucous Carcinoma

Verrucous carcinomas of the vulva are also rare. They are a special variant of squamous cell cancer, with distinctive histologic features. Clinically, they appear as a large condylomatous mass on the vulva. Histologically, they consist of mature squamous cells and extensive keratinization, with nests that invade the underlying vulvar tissue. It is often necessary to perform multiple biopsies of the condylomatous lesion to establish a diagnosis of malignancy. Radiation therapy is ineffective and can worsen the prognosis by causing anaplastic changes in the tumor, and is therefore contraindicated. The treatment of an authentic verrucous carcinoma is wide excision.

In 24 cases of verrucous carcinoma, Japaze and coworkers noted no lymph node metastases. Some of the primary tumors were as large as 10 cm in diameter. Recurrences developed in 9 patients, 5 of whom had previous radiation therapy. Wide local excision is effective therapy. Depending on the size and location of the tumor, simple vulvectomy may be needed, but a radical vulvectomy or inguinal node dissection is not indicated. The 17 patients treated surgically and reported by Japaze and colleagues had a 5-year survival rate of 94%. As noted by Crowther and associates, it is important to take a large biopsy specimen to establish the diagnosis. This is particularly important when dealing with a malignant-appearing tumor from a biopsy specimen that has been reported as benign, which can lead to incorrect therapy for condyloma acuminatum. Conversely, too shallow a biopsy may fail to show areas of squamous cell carcinoma that can coexist with verrucous carcinoma but, in the presence of areas of squamous cell carcinoma, local excision is inadequate therapy. Verrucous tumors with squamous cell carcinoma elements can metastasize to regional nodes; these tumors should not be treated as true verrucous carcinomas.

Melanoma

Melanoma is the most frequent nonsquamous cell malignancy of the vulva. It comprises approximately 5% of primary cancers of this area. As is true elsewhere in the body, melanomas arise from junctional or compound nevi. Pigmented lesions of the vulva are usually junctional nevi and all such lesions should be removed by excision.

Patients with malignant melanoma of the vulva vary widely in age, from the late teens to women in their 80s. The average

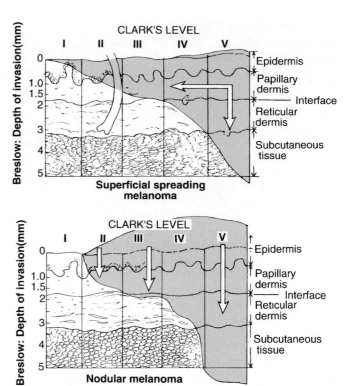

Figure 30-18 Level of invasion for superficial spreading melanoma and nodular melanoma. (From Podratz KC, Gaffey TA, Symmonds RE, et al: Melanoma of the vulva: An update. Gynecol Oncol 16:153, 1983.)

age is approximately 50 years. Clinically, melanomas appear as brown, black, or blue-black masses on the vulva. The lesion can be flat or ulcerated; occasionally, it is nodular, and small, darkly pigmented areas (satellite nodules) may surround the primary lesion. Some melanomas may be without pigment and can grossly resemble squamous cell carcinoma of the vulva. Most melanomas of the vulva occur on the labia minora or the clitoris (see **Fig. 30-16**).

Vulvar melanomas, if staged, use the same FIGO classification used for squamous carcinomas (**Box 30-3**). However, staging is not as useful a prognostic indicator as the depth of invasion. A staging system for vulvar melanoma analogous to that used by Clark for cutaneous melanomas has been adopted. Five levels (I to V) have been defined based on the Clark classification. **Figure 30-17** shows the depth of invasion for each level of superficial spreading melanoma and nodular melanoma, the two most common varieties of melanomas that occur on the vulva. Superficial spreading melanoma is more common and, fortunately, has a better prognosis, with a 5-year survival rate of 71% reported in the series by Podratz and associates. The 5-year survival for nodular melanoma, which is more invasive, was only 38%. The level of invasion correlates with survival, which varies from 100% for level II, to 83% for level IV, to 28% for level V.

Tumor thickness is also useful to evaluate the tumor. Breslow has reported that overall prognosis is excellent, and spread to a regional node is not likely for melanomas whose thickness is less than 0.76 mm, measured from the surface epithelium to the deepest point of penetration. Most of these lesions would

correspond to level I or II penetration by the modified Clark system. Stefanon and coworkers, in a study of 28 patients, noted no lymph node metastasis if melanoma thickness was less than 3 mm; the 5-year survival rate in this group was 50% compared with 25% for those whose melanomas were more than 3 mm thick. In a comprehensive long-term study of 219 Swedish women, Ragnarsson-Olding and coworkers have noted that tumor thickness and ulceration are prognostic factors. In addition, gross amelanosis and advanced age worsened the prognosis. They further noted that amelanotic tumors were seen in approximately 25% of patients and that overall, the vulvar melanomas were approximately 2.5 times more frequent than cutaneous melanomas. A preexisting nevus was not necessary; de novo melanoma development does appear to occur on the vulva, particularly in the glabrous (hairless) skin.

The standard therapy for vulvar melanoma is a wide excision of the primary tumor. Because the tumors are rare, a large clinical experience is not available. It was believed that melanoma of the vulva could metastasize to pelvic nodes, bypassing the inguinofemoral nodes, but it is now thought that there is no pelvic node involvement without previous inguinal node involvement. A further therapeutic consideration is that patients with melanoma whose pelvic nodes are involved with tumor usually do not survive the disease.

Excision margins have been extensively studied for cutaneous melanomas. Veronesi and colleagues have found that cutaneous melanomas smaller than 2 mm thick could be adequately treated with a 1-cm margin, which was as effective as a 3-cm margin for

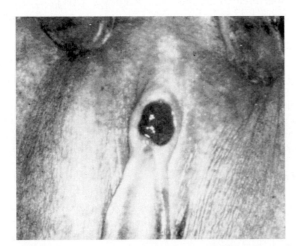

Figure 30-17 Nodular melanoma arising directly from glans clitoris. (Courtesy of Dr. J.M. Morris [deceased], Yale University School of Medicine, New Haven, CT.)

these thin lesions. Although comparable data do not exist for vulvar melanomas, evidence from studies of cutaneous melanomas has suggested that a 1-cm margin may be used for very thin vulvar melanomas. In a report of 36 melanoma cases, Rose and associates noted that wide excision was as effective as radical vulvectomy. They found that the prognosis was improved in younger patients, presumably because most of them had superficial spreading (good prognosis) rather than nodular (poor prognosis) melanomas. Although firm recommendations from available data are not possible, a reasonable approach would be to excise a melanoma with a 2-cm margin without node dissection for tumors that are smaller than 0.76 mm thick. An excision with a 2- to 3-cm margin combined with node dissection would be carried out for more advanced melanomas.

For lesions that correspond to **Clark's level** 1 or 2—that is, less than 0.76 mm thick—a wide local excision results in 5-year survival rates of approximately 100%. The prognosis is poor for patients with melanomas more than 3 mm thick. If the regional nodes are negative, the survival rate is greater than 60%, but decreases to less than 30% if the regional nodes are involved with tumor. Most series of malignant melanoma have reported overall survival rates of approximately 50%. Although metastases of melanoma to regional inguinal nodes are usually fatal, isolated prolonged survivals have been observed, as reported by Trimble and Tasseron and their associates, who noted in a series of 30 patients that 6 had positive nodes and 2 survived for longer than 5 years.

Distant metastases are frequently noted and no effective program of chemotherapy has been described. Regressions (but not cures) have been reported with various multiagent cytotoxic programs. Current efforts are devoted to developing an effective program of bioimmunotherapy.

Sarcoma

Sarcomas of the vulva are extremely rare, accounting for less than 3% of vulvar cancers. Leiomyosarcomas are the most common histologic subtype found, followed by liposarcomas, neurofibrosarcomas, angiosarcomas, and epithelioid sarcomas. The largest series of vulvar sarcomas in the literature have been 12 cases reported by DiSaia and associates. They found surgical removal of the primary tumor to be the treatment of choice. Chemotherapeutic considerations are the same as those for sarcomas of other sites in the female genital tract.

Granular Cell Myoblastomas

Granular cell myoblastoma is also an extremely rare tumor that is almost invariably benign but, morphologically, shows pleomorphism. Local excision is generally sufficient therapy. The tumor appears as a solitary, firm, nontender, slowly growing nodule in the subcutaneous tissue of the vulva.

KEY POINTS

- Squamous cell carcinomas comprise 90% of primary vulvar malignancies. More than 50% of patients are older than 60 years at the time of diagnosis.
- Cancer of the vulva accounts for approximately 4% of malignancies of the lower female genital tract and is less frequent than uterine, ovarian, and cervical cancers.
- Paget's disease generally occurs in postmenopausal women and is usually treated by wide excision. Invasive carcinomas at other sites should be ruled out.
- Prolonged use of fluorinated corticosteroids to treat itching accompanying vulvar dystrophy can lead to vulvar contraction.
- Topical testosterone is often beneficial to treat lichen sclerosus but is absorbed systemically and occasionally can produce masculinizing symptoms.
- Studies have indicated that symptomatic lichen sclerosus is a premalignant condition preceding carcinoma by a mean of 4.0 years. The tumors that develop tend to be clitoral in location and are in patients older than age 40 years.
- HPV vulvar infection is common. Intraepithelial neoplasia occurs much less frequently.
- HPV-positive tumors tend to occur in younger patients, and these tumors tend to have a better prognosis than HPV-negative tumors.
- A clear progression of dysplasia–carcinoma in situ (VIN I, II, and III) to invasive carcinoma in the vulva has not been clearly established. VIN may spontaneously regress. VIN III has an approximately 3.4% risk of progression to invasive carcinoma.

- Intraepithelial neoplasia of the vulva is usually treated by local excision. Laser therapy of the atypical area may be used for younger patients who do not have raised lesions.
- Vulvar carcinomas less than 2 cm in diameter and with a depth of invasion less than 1 mm (3-mm thickness) rarely metastasize to regional nodes.
- Unilateral vulvar tumors (>2 cm from midline) usually metastasize to ipsilateral inguinofemoral nodes only.
- Prognosis in vulvar cancer is primarily related to lesion size, lymph node status, and stage.
- The risk of lymph node groin metastases is related to tumor differentiation, lesion thickness, lymphovascular space involvement, patient age, and tumor size.
- The deep pelvic nodes do not become involved with metastatic vulvar cancer unless the inguinofemoral nodes are affected.
- The 5-year survival rate of vulvar carcinoma with negative nodes is more than 95%. With one positive node, the 5-year survival is approximately the same, 94%; with two nodes, it decreases to 80% and with three or more to 12%.
- The worldwide 5-year survival rate for carcinoma of the vulva by stage is stage I, 71.4%, stage II, 61.3%, stage III, 43.8%, and stage IV, 8.3%.
- Advanced vulvar tumors encroaching on the urethra and/or anus may be treated by preliminary radiation followed by wide radical excision rather than exenteration. Enhanced results have also been reported with the combined use of chemotherapy and radiation.

- Verrucous carcinomas are a variant of squamous cancer that do not metastasize to regional nodes. Radiation therapy is contraindicated and local surgical excision is the treatment of choice.
- Melanomas comprise 5% of vulvar cancers and are the most frequent nonsquamous cell malignancies.
- The overall 5-year survival of patients with vulvar melanoma is approximately 50%.

- Superficial spreading melanomas tend to occur in younger patients and have a better prognosis than nodular melanomas.
- Prognosis of vulvar melanoma is related to tumor invasion (Clark's level) and to tumor thickness.
- Basal cell carcinoma of the vulva is treated by wide local excision.

REFERENCES CAN BE FOUND ON EXPERTCONSULT.com

31

Malignant Diseases of the Vagina
Intraepithelial Neoplasia, Carcinoma, Sarcoma

Diane C. Bodurka and Michael Frumovitz

This chapter focuses on premalignant and malignant diseases of the vagina. Premalignant changes in the vagina occur less frequently than comparable lesions in the cervix and vulva. However, the histologic appearance of intraepithelial neoplasia of the vagina is similar to that described for the cervix (see Chapter 28). These changes are also similarly designated as dysplasia (mild, moderate, or severe) and carcinoma in situ. The term *VAIN* (*va*ginal *i*ntraepithelial *n*eoplasia) has been used to describe these histologic changes; the comparable categories are VAIN-1 (mild dysplasia), VAIN-2 (moderate dysplasia), and VAIN-3 (severe dysplasia to carcinoma in situ). VAIN-1 is classified as a low-grade squamous intraepithelial lesion, whereas VAIN-2 and VAIN-3 are grouped as high-grade squamous intraepithelial lesions. The cytologic and histologic features of these changes are illustrated in **Figure 31-1**.

VAIN occurs more commonly in patients previously treated for cervical intraepithelial neoplasia. The frequency of vaginal premalignancy in these patients is approximately 1% to 3%. Similarly, there is an increased risk of VAIN in those previously treated for squamous cell neoplasia of the vulva. The tendency to develop premalignant changes in the lower genital tract is known as a **field defect** and denotes the increased risk of squamous cell neoplasia arising anywhere in the lower genital tract in such individuals. The vast majority of VAIN is related to infection with human papilloma virus (HPV). Additional risk factors include HIV infection, cigarette smoking, previous radiation therapy of the genital tract, and immunosuppressive therapy. In situ and invasive vaginal neoplasia have many of the same risk factors as cervical cancer, including a strong association with HPV infection. Women who have previously been treated for anogenital cancer, particularly for cervical cancer, have a high relative risk of being diagnosed with vaginal cancer.

Primary cancer of the vagina is rare and constitutes less than 2% of gynecologic malignancies. Most vaginal malignancies are metastatic, primarily from the cervix and endometrium. Less commonly, ovarian and rectosigmoid carcinomas, as well as choriocarcinoma, metastasize to the vagina. The most common histologic type of primary vaginal cancer is squamous cell carcinoma, which is usually seen in women older than 60 years. Other types of carcinoma, including melanomas and adenocarcinomas, occur less commonly. Malignant transformation of endometriosis has been described in the vagina and rectovaginal septum. **Clear cell adenocarcinoma**, historically associated with young women exposed in utero to diethylstilbestrol (DES), may also occur in unexposed women. Primary vaginal sarcomas are rare and are usually a disease of children. **Table 31-1** summarizes the major primary malignancies of the vagina arranged according to the age at occurrence.

PREMALIGNANT DISEASE OF THE VAGINA

DETECTION AND DIAGNOSIS

Because premalignant disease of the vagina is generally asymptomatic, detection depends primarily on cytologic screening (see **Fig. 31-1B, D**). Usually, the changes will be observed in patients who have undergone previous therapy for intraepithelial disease of the cervix. This fact underscores the importance of continued examinations and Pap smears for women, even after hysterectomy for dysplastic conditions. VAIN usually occurs in the upper half of the vagina or along the vaginal cuff suture line. Once an abnormal smear from vaginal epithelium is identified, a biopsy is required for histologic identification (see **Fig. 31-1A, C**). A colposcopic examination is usually performed to identify the areas requiring biopsy. As in the case of cervical neoplasia, a repeat Pap smear is often taken before the colposcopic examination. Vaginal colposcopic techniques are similar to those described for the cervix. A large speculum is used to aid in visualizing the entire vaginal wall. Although the abnormal colposcopic findings resemble those of the cervix (see Chapter 28), full visualization of the entire vaginal wall is often difficult and time-consuming. A useful adjunct to colposcopy for identifying an area in which to perform a biopsy is to stain the vaginal epithelium with Lugol's solution and to take a biopsy sample from the nonstaining areas. The vaginal epithelium must be adequately estrogenized so that sufficient epithelial glycogen is present for the normal tissue to stain dark brown. The more rapidly dividing dysplastic epithelium uses up its glycogen and thus does not pick up the iodine stain. Vaginal estrogen cream used for 1 to 2 weeks before examination is helpful for evaluating postmenopausal women and those with atrophic vaginitis who present with cytologic atypia. The estrogen cream will not only increase epithelial glycogen, but also helps mature the squamous epithelium, reducing the number of parabasal cells at the surface. Parabasal cells, with their large nuclei, are a common cause of false-positive Pap tests in this age group.

A biopsy is performed with small instruments, such as the Kevorkian or Eppendorf punch biopsy forceps (**Fig. 31-2**) or similar instruments that are also used for the cervix. Occasionally, it is

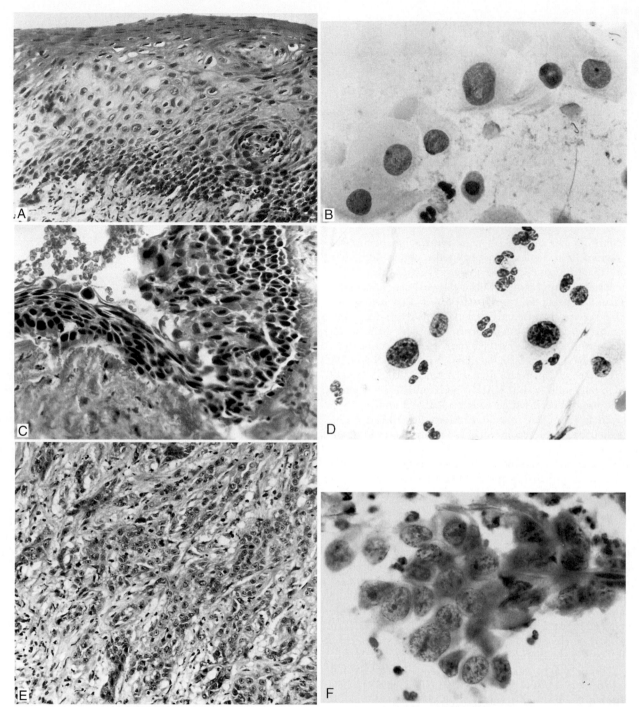

Figure 31-1 A, Section of a vagina showing dysplasia. The epithelium appears thickened and shows abnormal maturation. Immature hyperchromatic cells occupy the lower two to four layers. The middle and upper thirds of mucosa show evidence of cytoplasmic differentiation with well-defined cellular borders. Nuclei in these areas are enlarged and pleomorphic. Parakeratosis is apparent on the surface. Because immature cells are confined to the lower third of the mucosa, dysplasia is classified as mild (H&E stain, × 250). **B,** Cytologic specimen showing mild dysplasia. Note the sheet of dysplastic cells. Cells show well-defined cytoplasmic borders. Nuclei are enlarged, and the nuclear contour is smooth. Chromatin is uniformly and finely granular. Focal condensations of chromatin (chromocenters) are present in some nuclei. Nucleoli are not present (Pap stain, × 1000). **C,** Section showing severe dysplasia to carcinoma in situ. The entire epithelial thickness is occupied by hyperchromatic dysplastic cells. Marked nuclear variation and mitoses are seen. Because of occasional cells with squamous differentiation (spindle-shaped cells, cells with well-defined cytoplasmic borders) in superficial layers, this lesion is sometimes classified as severe dysplasia. In carcinoma in situ, immature cells replace the full thickness, and there is no evidence of squamous differentiation on the surface (H&E stain, × 400). **D,** Cytologic specimen showing carcinoma in situ. Several isolated immature cells with a high nuclei-to-cytoplasm ratio and poorly defined cytoplasmic borders can be seen. Chromatin is coarsely granular, and no nucleoli are present. In the background are several polymorphonuclear leukocytes and strings of mucus (Pap stain, × 1000). **E,** Section showing invasive squamous carcinoma. Cords and sheets of poorly differentiated tumor cells infiltrate the stroma. Nuclei are pleomorphic and nucleoli are distinct. The mitotic rate is high. Squamous differentiation (keratin pearl formation, single-cell keratinization) was present in other areas of tumor (H&E stain, × 200). **F,** Cytologic specimen showing invasive squamous cell carcinoma. Note aggregate of tumor cells. Cellular boundaries are poorly defined, and nuclear orientation is lacking. Chromatin is irregularly distributed and has areas of clumping and clearing. Note nucleoli in some cells, which were absent in cells of patients with dysplasia and carcinoma in situ (Pap stain, × 800).

Table 31-1 Common Primary Vaginal Cancers

Tumor Type	Predominant Age (yr)	Clinical Correlations
Endodermal sinus tumor (adenocarcinoma)	<2	Extremely rare, α-fetoprotein secretion, often fatal, multimodality therapy
Sarcoma botryoides	<8	Aggressive malignancy, multimodality therapy
Clear cell adenocarcinoma	>14	Associated with intrauterine exposure to diethylstilbestrol
Melanoma	>50	Very rare, poor survival
Squamous cell carcinoma	>50	Most common primary vaginal cancer

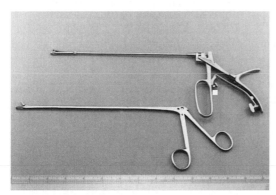

Figure 31-2 Eppendorf (*upper*) and Kevorkian (*lower*) punch biopsy instruments.

necessary to use a fine instrument, such as a nerve hook, to provide traction on the vaginal epithelium to obtain a biopsy sample. Most patients experience some discomfort during the biopsy. Local anesthesia is often helpful, although injection of the anesthetic may be as uncomfortable as the biopsy itself. Vaginal neoplasia is often multifocal. Although the process is most often located in the vaginal apex, it can occur anywhere along the vaginal canal, necessitating examination of the vagina in its entirety.

TREATMENT

There is limited information regarding the natural history of VAIN. The risk of progression to invasive cancer is thought to be low, approximately 9%. Those at highest risk of progression are women with high-risk strains of HPV, those with VAIN-3, cigarette smokers, and immunocompromised women. Significantly, Aho and colleagues have found that 28% of women undergoing evaluation for VAIN-3 have an underlying invasive carcinoma. This has led many to recommend surgical excision rather than destructive procedures for the treatment of VAIN-3.

The principles of managing VAIN are to rule out and prevent invasive disease and preserve vaginal function. As is true for cervical dysplasia, biopsy-proven VAIN-1, particularly those lesions associated with low-risk strains of HPV, can be observed, provided that the woman is compliant with follow-up. VAIN-2 and VAIN-3 are generally treated. Treatment options include CO_2 laser vaporization, topical 5-fluorouracil (5-FU) cream, and wide local excision. The choice of treatment depends largely on the number of lesions, their location, and the level of concern for possible invasion. Radiation therapy, although used in the past, often leads to scarring and fibrosis and is generally not recommended for the treatment of noninvasive disease. Because of the proximity of the bladder and rectum, cryotherapy is generally not used.

The main advantage of the CO_2 laser is that it vaporizes the abnormal tissue without shortening or narrowing the vagina, preserving vaginal function. Criteria for CO_2 laser vaporization include a lesion that is discrete and easily visible and proof that invasive cancer has been ruled out. The beam is directed colposcopically. Iodine staining of the vagina can help outline those areas requiring therapy. Treatment is occasionally performed on an outpatient basis with a local anesthetic and an analgesic. More frequently, general or regional anesthesia is required. The intensity of therapy is regulated by adjusting the wattage of the laser, most commonly 15 to 20 W carried to a depth of 1.5 to 2 mm. Care must be taken not to apply the laser too deeply because of the proximity of the bladder and bowel, particularly in older women whose vaginal epithelium may be quite thin. The woman will experience a discharge for 1 to 2 weeks after therapy. Healing usually requires a few weeks. The success rates of laser in treating VAIN vary in the literature, but generally are in the range of 60% to 85%. Regular follow-up every 4 months, including a Pap smear and colposcopy, is required during the first year and usually 6 to 12 months thereafter. The primary disadvantages of laser treatment are the lack of a pathologic specimen for evaluation of the adequacy of margins and the fact that the procedure can be tedious and difficult because of the many folds and crevices at the vaginal apex. It is often difficult to obtain a uniform depth of destruction in these areas.

Topical chemotherapy, 5% 5-FU cream, can be self-administered to cover the entire area at risk. It is most often used for widespread multifocal lesions of HPV-associated VAIN-1 or VAIN-2. Half of a vaginal applicator (approximately 5 g) is inserted into the vagina at bedtime for 7 days. Because the cream is irritating, some protective ointment such as zinc oxide should be applied to the vulva. If excess leakage occurs, less than half of an applicator should be used. In addition, the treatment should be discontinued before the 7-day course is completed if the woman notes excessive irritation. A cycle of therapy should be repeated in 3 to 4 weeks if intraepithelial neoplasia persists. In some cases, the application of 5-FU is continued for 10 to 14 days, in which case the nontherapy interval is increased to 2 or 3 months. In contrast, many postmenopausal women tolerate only small doses of 5-FU, presumably because of the relative thinness of the vaginal epithelium. In one study, one third of an applicator of 5% 5-FU was used weekly for 10 weeks. It was noted that 17 of 20 patients with vaginal condyloma were free of disease at 3 months. Three patients received a second cycle, and 16 of 18 were free of disease at 10 to 20 months. Success rates of 80% to 90% for patients with VAIN after multiple treatment cycles have been reported. The disadvantage of topical therapy with 5-FU cream is that patients must be highly motivated to complete therapy. 5-FU causes exfoliation and erosion of the vaginal mucosa and can be extremely painful. Only a small percentage of patients are able to complete a full course. Thus, use of this topical therapy is limited. Imiquimod has been evaluated for the treatment of **vaginal intraepithelial neoplasia**. Complete regression of neoplasia has been reported in 26% to

100% of patients, whereas 0% to 60% have partial regression. Recurrence of neoplasia was identified in 0% to 37% of the patients. The most commonly reported side effects were local burning and tenderness, although not severe enough to discontinue treatment. Because patients who experience disease partial regression will require less extensive excision, this treatment may prove to be a promising option.

Wide local excision (upper vaginectomy) is the treatment of choice for VAIN-3, especially for lesions occurring at the cuff after hysterectomy. Excision gives the surgeon the ability to excise the specimen to rule out invasion and ascertain margin adequacy. Excision also has a high success rate (84%). Upper vaginectomy, however, can result in vaginal shortening, which can be ameliorated by the use of topical estrogen cream and a vaginal dilator (or frequent intercourse) once healing is complete.

MALIGNANT DISEASE OF THE VAGINA

SYMPTOMS AND DIAGNOSIS

Primary vaginal cancers usually occur as squamous cell carcinomas in women older than 60 years. To be considered a primary vaginal tumor, the malignancy must arise in the vagina and not involve the external os of the cervix superiorly or the vulva inferiorly. If this occurs, the tumor is classified as cervical or vulvar.

Table 31-2 International Federation of Gynecology and Obstetrics Staging Classification for Vaginal Cancer

Stage	Characteristics
0	Carcinoma in situ
I	Carcinoma limited to vaginal wall
II	Carcinoma involves subvaginal tissue but has not extended to pelvic wall
III	Carcinoma extends to pelvic wall
IV	Carcinoma extends beyond true pelvis or involves mucosa of bladder or rectum (bullous edema as such does not assign a patient to stage IV)

This is also an important therapeutic consideration, insofar as the same management techniques apply to small tumors of the upper third of the vagina and cervical carcinomas. Tumors of the lower third of the vagina are treated similarly to vulvar cancers (see Chapter 32). **Table 31-2** lists the staging criteria for vaginal cancers according to the International Federation of Gynecology and Obstetrics (FIGO), which are illustrated in **Figure 31-3**.

Delay in the diagnosis of these cancers frequently occurs, in part because of their rarity and because of a lack of recognition that the abnormal symptoms may be caused by a malignancy. The most common symptom of vaginal cancer is abnormal

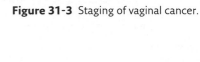
Figure 31-3 Staging of vaginal cancer.

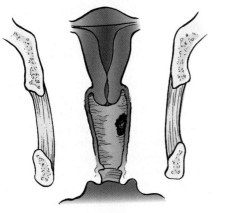
Stage I

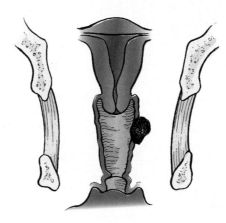
Stage II

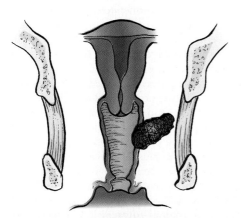
Stage III

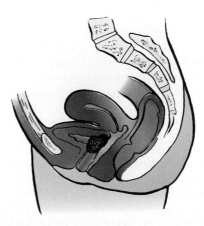
Stage IV

bleeding or discharge. Pain is usually a symptom of an advanced tumor. Urinary frequency is also reported occasionally, particularly in the case of anterior wall tumors, whereas constipation or tenesmus may be reported when the tumors involve the posterior vaginal wall. In general, the longer the delay in diagnosis, the worse the prognosis and the more difficult the therapy. Vaginal cancer is usually diagnosed by direct biopsy of the tumor mass (see **Fig. 31-1E**). Abnormal cytologic findings (see **Fig. 31-1F**) may prompt a thorough pelvic examination that will lead to diagnosis of vaginal cancer. It is important during the course of the pelvic examination to inspect and palpate the entire vagina and to rotate the speculum carefully to visualize the entire vagina, because a small tumor may occupy the anterior or posterior vaginal wall.

TUMORS OF THE ADULT VAGINA

Squamous Cell Carcinoma

Squamous cell carcinoma is the most common of the vaginal malignancies and accounts for 90% of primary vaginal cancers. Although reported in women in their 30s, the disease occurs primarily in women older than 60, and 20% are older than 80 years. Most squamous cell carcinomas occur in the upper third of the vagina, but primary tumors in the middle and lower thirds may also occur. Grossly, the tumor appears as a fungating, polypoid, or ulcerating mass, often accompanied by a foul smell and discharge related to a secondary infection. Microscopically (see **Fig. 31-1E**), the tumor demonstrates the classic findings of an invasive squamous cell carcinoma infiltrating the vaginal epithelium.

Treatment of these tumors is based on the size, **vaginal tumor stage**, and location of the lesion. Therapy is limited by the proximity of the bladder anteriorly and the rectum posteriorly. It is also influenced by the location of the tumor in the vagina, which determines the area of lymphatic spread (**Fig. 31-4**).

The lymphatics of the vagina envelop the mucosa and anastomose with lymphatic vessels in the muscularis. Those of the mid to upper vagina communicate superiorly with the lymphatics of the cervix and drain into the pelvic nodes of the obturator and internal and external iliac chains. In contrast, the lymphatics of the distal third of the vagina drain to the inguinal nodes and pelvic nodes, similar to the drainage of the vulva. The posterior wall lymphatics anastomose with the rectal lymphatic system and then to the nodes that drain the rectum, such as the inferior gluteal, sacral, and rectal nodes.

Treatment

Once the diagnosis of vaginal malignancy is established, a thorough bimanual and visual examination, documenting the size and location of the tumor and assessment of spread to adjacent structures (submucosa, vaginal sidewall, bladder, rectum), should be performed to determine the clinical stage. Cystoscopy and/or proctoscopy may be helpful, depending on clinical concern, to rule out bladder or rectal invasion. Distant spread may be evaluated by computed tomography (CT) of the abdomen, pelvis, and chest or positron emission tomography (PET).

Similar to cervical carcinoma, early-stage vaginal carcinoma, without lymph node involvement (stage I or II), may be treated with surgery or radiation. Young patients with early-stage disease and upper vaginal lesions may be treated with radical upper vaginectomy, parametrectomy, and pelvic lymphadenectomy.

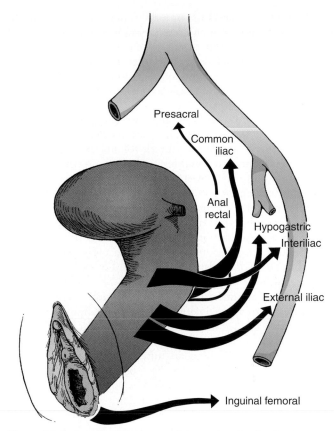

Figure 31-4 Lymphatic drainage of the vagina. Predominant pathways from various parts of the vagina are shown.

Radiation therapy is the most frequently used mode of treatment and can be used for early and advanced disease. Radiation is the most common therapy because most women with vaginal carcinoma are older, with a poorer surgical risk, and radiation is highly effective. **Pelvic exenteration** can be used primarily to treat advanced disease in the absence of lymph node metastasis, but is usually reserved for patients with localized recurrence after radiation. Cisplatin-based chemotherapy administered concurrently with radiation has been used with increasing frequency for squamous cell carcinomas of the vagina because of the well-documented improvements in outcomes for patients with squamous lesions of the cervix treated in this fashion. Although there have been no randomized prospective trials proving its effectiveness in this disease, the numerous similarities in pathophysiology between squamous lesions of the cervix and vagina would lead to the logical conclusion that concurrent chemotherapy with radiation will have increased efficacy over radiation alone in the treatment of vaginal carcinoma.

Stage I vaginal carcinoma may be treated with brachytherapy alone, without external beam therapy. Grigsby has recommended vaginal brachytherapy using vaginal cylinders, in one or two applications, delivering a dose of 65 to 80 Gy to the entire length of the vagina. For more advanced lesions, a combination of external beam and brachytherapy is used. External radiation therapy with megavoltage equipment is initially used to shrink the tumor. The size and extent of the radiation field will be determined by the presence or absence of nodal disease, as determined by the pretreatment PET or CT scan. The whole pelvis is generally treated to a dose of approximately 5040 cGy. This is followed by a local cesium or radium implant placed interstitially with needles or by intracavitary radiation using a vaginal cylinder or tandem and ovoids, if the cervix is still present. The brachytherapy will bring the total dose to between 7000 and 8500 cGy. The prognosis appears to improve if the interval from the end of external therapy to the initiation of brachytherapy is less than 28 days.

DiSaia and coworkers have reported using a fixed perineal template (Syed-Neblett applicator) to achieve reproducible isodose delivery to a large vaginal tumor volume. For lesions of the upper vagina after hysterectomy, a laparoscopy may be performed to remove any bowel loops from the vaginal apex. The omentum may be used to provide additional separation of the bowel from the vaginal apex. Paley and associates have reported using a retropubic approach in a small series of six patients to achieve direct visualization of needle placement. The treatment is individualized, depending on tumor size and stage. For larger lesions, the dose of the external component of radiation therapy is increased, with a concomitant reduction in the local vaginal component of treatment of the primary tumor. Usually, a total tumor dosage of approximately 7500 cGy is administered. Implants cannot be used in some patients with stage III or IV carcinoma; in such cases, only external therapy can be used, and a central boost is given after an initial 5000-cGy whole-pelvis treatment. Severe complications have been noted if the vaginal dose exceeds 9800 cGy. Kucera and Vavra, in a series of 434 patients treated with irradiation, noted that results were best for low-stage tumors, those in the upper third of the vagina, and when the tumor was well-differentiated. Kirkbride and colleagues have reported that stage, tumor size, and tumor grade are prognostic and that the tumor dose must reach at least 7000 cGy, consistent with other studies. Treatment time is also important; as noted by Lee and colleagues, it is preferable to complete the radiation therapy within 9 weeks.

Survival

Overall 5-year survival rates for patients with primary carcinoma of the vagina have been reported to be approximately 45%. The stage of the tumor is the most important predictor of prognosis. In one series of 89 patients treated with surgery and/or irradiation, the 5-year survival rates were 82% and 53%, respectively, for stage I and stage II disease. The use of concomitant chemotherapy with radiation can be expected to produce improved survival rates.

Clear Cell Adenocarcinoma

Clear cell adenocarcinomas in young women have been seen more frequently since 1970 as a result of the association of many of these cancers with intrauterine exposure to DES. Therapeutic considerations are similar to those for squamous cell carcinoma, taking into account the young age of the patients undergoing therapy. Cervical clear cell adenocarcinomas are treated in the same manner as primary cervical carcinomas. The results of therapy for vaginal and cervical clear cell adenocarcinoma in young women are discussed together in this section. These tumors are also staged according to the FIGO classification (see **Table 31-2**). Most (80%) have been diagnosed as stage I or II. The overall results of therapy, based on the stage of the tumor at the time of treatment, are shown in **Table 31-3**. The survival rate is related directly to the stage of the tumor, similar to other gynecologic malignancies at these sites.

Table 31-3 5- and 10-Year Survival Rates for 588 Patients with Clear Cell Adenocarcinoma of the Vagina and Cervix

Stage	5-Year Survival (%)	10-Year Survival (%)
I	91	85
IIA	80	67
IIB	56	47
II (vagina)	82	67
III	37	25
IV	0	0

Adapted from Registry Data, University of Chicago, Herbst A, Anderson D, Clear cell adenocarcinoma of the vagina and cervix secondary to intrauterine exposure to diethylstilbestrol, Seminars in Surgical Oncology 6:343-346 (1990).

In general, surgery is the primary treatment modality because of the young age of the patients. For stage I and early stage II tumors, radical hysterectomy with partial or complete vaginectomy, pelvic lymphadenectomy, and replacement of the vagina with split-thickness skin grafts has been the most common approach. In most cases, ovarian function is preserved. In addition, efforts have been made to preserve fertility in patients who have small tumors of the vagina by the use of local irradiation of the primary tumor and immediate adjacent tissues to spare the ovaries. Because metastases to regional pelvic nodes can occur, even with small stage I tumors, retroperitoneal lymph node dissections are usually performed before local therapy.

Local excision of the tumor can be performed before irradiation to facilitate local application. Senekjian and associates have noted that the survival of patients with small vaginal tumors treated by local excision and then local irradiation is comparable with that obtained with conventional extensive therapy. The best candidates are those with tumors smaller than 2 cm in diameter, a predominant tubulocystic pattern (**Fig. 31-5A**), and depth of invasion less than 3 mm. After wide local excision, the pelvic nodes are sampled to rule out tumor spread. If these are negative, local irradiation can then be given. Pregnancies have occurred in patients so treated. Larger tumors, however, are treated with full pelvic irradiation, in addition to an intracavitary implant. In a few cases, exenterative surgery has been successfully performed. This procedure is preferably applied to central recurrences after primary irradiation. Local vaginal excision as the sole therapy is not usually adequate for small tumors because the tumor frequently recurs.

Three predominant histologic patterns are found in patients with clear cell adenocarcinoma (see **Fig. 31-5**). In addition, a number of prognostic factors have been identified. The older patients (> 19 years) have been found to have a more favorable prognosis in comparison to younger patients (< 15 years). This difference is associated with a more favorable outcome for those with the tubulocystic pattern of clear cell adenocarcinoma, which is the most frequent histologic pattern found in older patients. In addition, smaller tumor diameter and superficial depth of invasion correlate with improved patient survival. Waggoner and coworkers have shown that patients with clear cell adenocarcinoma and a maternal history of DES use survive longer than those with a negative maternal DES history. If the regional pelvic nodes are free of tumor, the prognosis is also more favorable. It is more likely that the regional pelvic lymph nodes will be free of tumor if other factors are favorable.

Clear cell adenocarcinomas can spread locally, as well as via lymphatics and blood vessels. Metastases to regional pelvic nodes are found in approximately one sixth of stage I cases. The spread

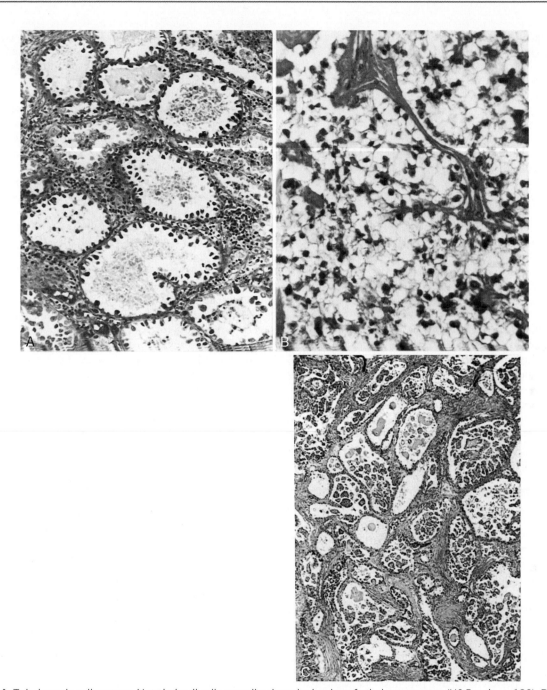

Figure 31-5 A, Tubulocystic cell pattern. Note hobnail cells extruding into the lumina of tubular structures (H&E stain, ×180). **B,** Solid pattern (H&E stain, ×300). **C,** Papillary pattern (H&E stain, ×50). (**A, B** from Scully RE, Robboy SJ, Herbst AL: Vaginal and cervical abnormalities, including clear cell adenocarcinoma, related to prenatal exposure to stilbestrol. Ann Clin Lab Sci 4:222, 1974; **C** from Scully RE, Robboy SJ, Welch WR: Pathology and pathogenesis of diethylstilbestrol-related disorders of the female genital tract. In Herbst AL [ed]: Intrauterine Exposure to Diethylstilbestrol in the Human. Washington DC, American College of Obstetricians and Gynecologists, 1978.)

to regional pelvic nodes becomes more frequent in higher stage tumors. Depending on the location of the tumor recurrence, therapy has consisted of additional radical surgery or extensive radiation in localized pelvic disease and systemic chemotherapy in cases of metastatic disease. Unfortunately, no single agent or combination of chemotherapeutic agents has emerged as an effective therapy. Prolonged follow-up is necessary for these patients because recurrences have been reported as long as 20 years after primary therapy, particularly in the lungs and supraclavicular areas. Data from the Registry on Hormonal Transplacental Carcinogenesis indicate that ovarian preservation with concomitant estrogen stimulation does not adversely affect survival in patients with clear cell adenocarcinoma.

Malignant Melanoma

Vaginal melanomas are rare and highly malignant. Only approximately 2% to 3% of primary vaginal cancers are melanomas. The most common presenting symptoms are vaginal discharge, bleeding, and a palpable mass. These lesions appear as darkly pigmented, irregular areas and may be flat, polyoid, or nodular.

The average age of affected women is 57 years. Vaginal melanomas tend to metastasize early, via the bloodstream and lymphatics, to the iliac and/or inguinal nodes, lungs, liver, brain, and bones. Patients with vaginal melanoma have a worse prognosis than those with vulvar melanoma, in part probably because of delay in diagnosis in comparison with vulvar carcinomas and in part because of their mucosal location, which seems to predispose to earlier metastasis.

Treatment usually consists of surgery with wide excision of the vagina and dissection of the regional nodes (pelvic, inguinal-femoral, or both), depending on the location of the lesion. Improved outcomes have been associated with the removal of all gross disease. Therapy is usually tailored to the extent of disease. Surgery, radiation, chemotherapy, and immunotherapy have all been described, but no single therapy or combination treatment is uniformly successful.

Local and distant recurrences are common, and the disease is usually fatal. Even with local control, distant failure is common in patients with melanoma. The overall 5-year survival rate is 8.4%, with an overall median survival of 20 months. Prognostic indicators include tumor size, mitotic index, and Breslow tumor thickness. Improved survival has been noted for patients whose tumors had fewer than six mitoses/10 high-power fields (HPF). Van Nostrand and associates have reported a 2-year survival for three of four patients with tumors smaller than 10 cm^2—that is, approximately 3.0 cm in diameter. However, Neven and coworkers have noted that among nine patients, all those with melanomas more than 2 mm thick died or had a recurrence regardless of therapy, emphasizing the importance of tumor thickness in melanoma prognosis.

Vaginal Adenocarcinomas Arising in Endometriosis

The malignant transformation of extraovarian endometriosis is rare, but has been reported with increasing frequency. The reason for this increase is not known. The rectovaginal septum is the most common extragonadal location. When these tumors occur in the vagina or rectovaginal septum, the typical clinical presentation is pain, vaginal bleeding, and/or a vaginal mass in a woman who has previously undergone extirpative surgery for endometriosis. Risk factors include unopposed estrogen and tamoxifen use. The most common histology is endometroid adenocarcinoma, followed by sarcomas (25%) and other tumors of müllerian differentiation. Treatment usually includes surgery plus radiation or chemotherapy. Leiserowitz and colleagues have reported a relatively favorable prognosis for women with endometriosis-related malignancies, with 70% alive at a mean follow-up of 31 months.

VAGINAL TUMORS OF INFANTS AND CHILDREN

Endodermal Sinus Tumor (Yolk Sac Tumor)

An **endodermal sinus tumor**, a type of adenocarcinoma, is a rare germ cell tumor that usually occurs in the ovary. The tumor secretes α-fetoprotein, which provides a useful tumor marker to monitor patients treated for these neoplasms. Approximately 69 cases of this unusual malignancy originating in the vagina of infants, predominantly those younger than 2 years, have been reported. The tumor is aggressive, and most patients have died. Young and Scully have reported 6 patients who were free of disease 2 to 9 years after surgery, irradiation, or both, with *v*incristine, *a*ctinomycin D, and *c*yclophosphamide (VAC)

chemotherapy. Copeland and colleagues have reported similar good results with combination chemotherapy and excision. Recently the combination of bleomycin, etoposide, and cisplatin (BEP) has also been used to treat this disease.

Sarcoma Botryoides (Embryonal Rhabdomyosarcoma)

Sarcoma botryoides is a rare sarcoma that is usually diagnosed in the vagina of a young girl. Rarely does it occur in a young child older than 8 years, although cases in adolescents have been reported. The most common symptom is abnormal vaginal bleeding, with an occasional mass at the introitus (**Fig. 31-6**). The tumor grossly will resemble a cluster of grapes forming multiple polypoid masses.

The tumors are believed to begin in the subepithelial layers of the vagina and expand rapidly to fill the vagina. These sarcomas are often multicentric. Histologically, they have a loose myxomatous stroma with malignant pleomorphic cells and occasional eosinophilic rhabdomyoblasts that often contain characteristic cross-striations (strap cells; **Fig. 31-7**).

These virulent tumors were treated in the past by radical surgery, such as pelvic exenteration. However, effective control with less radical surgery has been achieved with a multimodality approach consisting of multiagent chemotherapy (VAC), usually combined with surgery. Radiation therapy has also been used. Hays and associates have reported 21 patients with vaginal rhabdomyosarcomas who received chemotherapy. Seven relapsed, 5 of whom had residual disease after incomplete resection. One had disseminated disease. In 17 patients who received chemotherapy for 8 to 48 weeks, a delayed excision could be

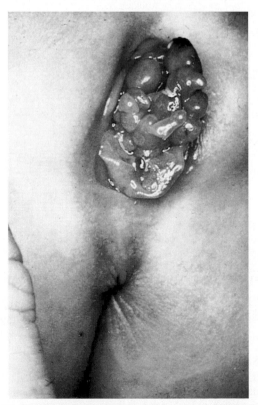

Figure 31-6 Sarcoma botryoides protruding through the vaginal introitus. (From Herbst AL: Cancer of the vagina. In Gusberg SB, Frick HC [eds]: Gynecologic Cancer, 5th ed. Baltimore, Williams & Wilkins, 1978.)

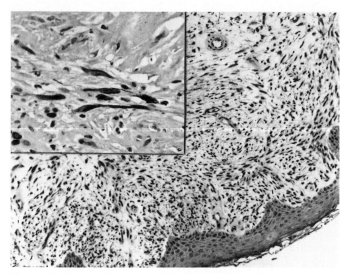

Figure 31-7 Vaginal mucosa with sarcoma botryoides showing condensation of malignant cells under the epithelium (H&E, ×100). *Insert,* Immunohistochemical stain for desmin illustrating strap cells (×240). (Courtesy of Dr. A. Montag, University of Chicago, Chicago.)

performed. Long-term survival data for a large number of patients are not available, but such a combined approach appears to result in effective treatment with less mutilating surgery. A multimodality approach, including chemotherapy, was used by Flamant and coworkers in 17 females with rhabdomyosarcoma of the vagina or vulva. At the time of their report, 15 appeared cured; 11 of 12 pubescent females have had menses, whereas 2 have successfully conceived and delivered healthy children. This was emphasized in a report from the Intergroup Rhabdomyosarcoma Study by Maurer and colleagues. They found VAC to be effective for disease confined to the vagina without nodal spread. Therapy was effective without irradiation for disease that was locally resected, suggesting that for these patients, chemotherapy plus surgery can be effective therapy.

Pseudosarcoma Botryoides

A rare, benign vaginal polyp that resembles sarcoma botryoides is found in the vagina of infants and pregnant women. Although large atypical cells may be present microscopically, strap cells are absent. Grossly, these polyps do not resemble the grapelike appearance of sarcoma botryoides. They are called **pseudosarcoma botryoides**. Treatment by local excision is effective.

KEY POINTS

- Predisposing factors associated with the development of vaginal intraepithelial neoplasia include infection with HPV, previous radiation therapy to the vagina, immunosuppressive therapy, and HIV infection.
- The tendency of intraepithelial squamous neoplasia to develop anywhere in the lower female genital tract is termed a *field defect* and describes the increased risk of premalignant changes occurring in the cervix, vagina, or vulva.
- Most cases of VAIN occur in the upper third of the vagina.
- VAIN can be treated by excision, laser, 5-FU, or imiquimod. Excision is often used for VAIN-3. Laser treatment is generally used for discrete lesions once invasion has been ruled out, and 5-FU and imiquimod cream are used to treat diffuse, multicentric, low-grade disease.
- The most common primary vaginal malignancy is squamous cell carcinoma (90%).
- Most cancers occurring in the vagina are metastatic.
- Vaginal cancers constitute less than 2% of gynecologic malignancies.
- Tumors of the upper vagina have a lymphatic drainage to the pelvis similar to cervical tumors. Tumors of the lower third of the vagina drain to the pelvic nodes and also to the inguinal nodes, similar to vulvar tumors.
- Radical surgery may be used to treat low-stage tumors, primarily of the upper vagina, in younger patients.
- Radiation therapy is the most frequently used modality for the treatment of squamous cell carcinoma of the vagina. Ideally, at least 7000 to 7500 cGy is administered in less than 9 weeks. Concurrent chemoradiation should strongly be considered.

- The overall 5-year survival rate of patients treated for squamous cell carcinoma of the vagina is approximately 45%.
- Clear cell adenocarcinoma is often associated with prenatal DES exposure. Prognosis is improved if the patient is older than 19 years, the tumor has a predominant tubulocystic tumor pattern, and the disease is low-stage. Those with a positive DES maternal history have a better prognosis.
- Local therapy for small, stage I clear cell adenocarcinomas of the vagina is best considered if the tumor is smaller than 2 cm in diameter, invades less than 3 mm, and is predominantly of the tubulocystic histologic type. Pelvic nodes should be sampled and be free of tumor.
- The overall 5-year survival rate of patients treated for clear cell adenocarcinoma is approximately 80%, partially because of the high proportion of low-stage cases.
- Vaginal melanomas are usually fatal. They occur primarily in patients older than 50 years.
- Endometrioid adenocarcinomas of the vagina may occur through the malignant transformation of endometriosis, often associated with the use of unopposed estrogen or tamoxifen.
- Endodermal sinus tumors occur in children younger than 2 years. They secrete α-fetoprotein and are usually treated by multiagent chemotherapy, followed by surgical excision.
- Sarcoma botryoides occurs primarily in children younger than 8 years. It is treated by a multimodality approach using multiagent chemotherapy with surgical removal and occasionally irradiation.

REFERENCES CAN BE FOUND ON EXPERTCONSULT.com

32

Neoplastic Diseases of the Uterus
Endometrial Hyperplasia, Endometrial Carcinoma, and Sarcoma: Diagnosis and Management

Pamela T. Soliman and Karen H. Lu

Endometrial carcinoma is the most common malignancy of the lower female genital tract in the United States. Approximately 42,000 new cases develop in the United States each year, according to recent figures (2009) from the American Cancer Society. This is approximately 1.3 times the frequency of ovarian cancer and almost four times the number of new cases of cervical cancer. However, 8,000 deaths occurred annually from uterine cancer, slightly more than for cervical cancer and much less than the estimated 14,000 for ovarian cancer. Overall, approximately 3 in 100 women in the United States will develop this disease during their lives.

This chapter reviews the clinical and pathologic features of **endometrial hyperplasias** and carcinomas, factors that contribute to the development of these diseases, and appropriate treatment methods. Sarcomas of the uterus and their clinical behavior and therapy are also discussed.

EPIDEMIOLOGY

Adenocarcinoma of the endometrium affects women primarily in their perimenopausal and postmenopausal years and is most frequently diagnosed in those between the ages of 50 and 65 years. However, these cancers can also develop in young women during their reproductive years. Approximately 5% of cases are diagnosed in women younger than 40 and approximately 10% to 15% in women younger than 50. Women diagnosed under the age of 50 years are also at risk for having a synchronous ovarian cancer. **Figure 32-1** plots a typical age-incidence curve for cancers of the endometrium. The curve rises sharply after age 45 and peaks between 55 and 60 years; there is then a gradual decrease.

Complex atypical hyperplasia results from increased estrogenic stimulation of the endometrium and is a precursor to endometrioid endometrial cancer. Some endometrial cancers develop without previous hyperplasia. These non–estrogen-related carcinomas including serous histology tend to be poorly differentiated and clinically more aggressive (see later).

A number of factors increase the risk of developing endometrial carcinoma (and hyperplasia) (**Box 32-1**). Obesity is a strong risk factor for endometrial cancer. Women who are obese (body mass index [BMI] > 30) have a two- to threefold increased risk. The association is believed to be caused in part by increased circulating estrogen levels that result from the conversion of androstenedione to estrone in the adipose tissue, decreased sex hormone-binding globulin, and other factors, including insulin resistance. Although more historical than clinically relevant, unopposed estrogen stimulation is strongly associated with endometrial cancer, increasing the risk by four to eight times for a woman using estrogen alone for menopausal replacement therapy. The risk increases with higher doses of estrogen (>0.625 mg conjugated estrogens), and more prolonged use but can be markedly reduced with the use of progestin (see Chapter 14, Menopause). Similarly, combination (progestin-containing) oral contraceptives decrease the risk. As noted by Grimes and Economy, combination oral contraceptives protect against endometrial cancer, with most studies showing a relative risk reduction to approximately 0.5. The protection begins after 1 year of use and lasts approximately 15 years after discontinuation. Other conditions leading to long-term estrogen stimulation of the endometrium, including the polycystic ovary syndrome (Stein-Leventhal syndrome) and the much more rare feminizing ovarian tumors, are also associated with increased risk of endometrial carcinoma.

Patients who receive the selective estrogen receptor modulator (SERM) tamoxifen are also at increased risk of developing endometrial carcinoma. In the National Surgical Adjuvant Bowel and Breast B-14 trial examining tamoxifen as adjuvant therapy in women with breast cancer, the risk of endometrial cancer was elevated 7.5-fold. This may be an overestimate because the risk of endometrial cancer in the control group was lower than expected. In the National Surgical Adjuvant Bowel and Breast P-1 trial examining tamoxifen as a chemopreventive agent, the risk of endometrial cancer was elevated 2.5-fold. Risk increased with duration of use. Most endometrial cancers that developed in tamoxifen users were of endometrioid histology and low **endometrial carcinoma grade** and **endometrial carcinoma stage**. However, high-grade endometrial cancers and sarcomas have also been reported in women taking tamoxifen. Screening strategies, including transvaginal ultrasound and office endometrial sampling, have been studied in this cohort. There is a high false-positive rate with transvaginal ultrasonography because tamoxifen causes subendometrial cyst formation, which makes the endometrial stripe appear abnormally thick. Barakat and colleagues have performed endometrial pipelle sampling on a large cohort of women taking tamoxifen.

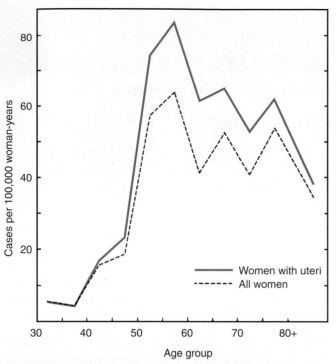

Figure 32-1 Incidence curve for carcinoma of the endometrium by age. (From Elwood JM, Cole P, Rothman KJ, Kaplan SD: Epidemiology of endometrial cancer. J Natl Cancer Inst 59:1055, 1977.)

Box 32-1   Endometrial Carcinoma Risk Factors

Increases the Risk
Unopposed estrogen stimulation
Unopposed menopausal estrogen replacement therapy (4-8×)
Menopause after 52 years (2.4×)
Obesity (2-5×)
Nulliparity (2-3×)
Diabetes (2.8×)
Feminizing ovarian tumors
Polycystic ovarian syndrome
Tamoxifen therapy for breast cancer

Diminishes the Risk
Ovulation
Progestin therapy
Combination oral contraceptives
Menopause before 49 years of age
Normal weight
Multiparity

They found very few cancers and concluded that women do not benefit from endometrial screening. Rather, women should be counseled that tamoxifen increases the risk of endometrial cancer, and all women on tamoxifen who have irregular vaginal bleeding (if premenopausal) or any vaginal bleeding (if postmenopausal) should undergo endometrial sampling or dilation and curettage (D&C).

Other factors increase the risk of endometrial cancer. Nulliparity is associated with a twofold increased risk in endometrial cancer. Diabetes increases the risk by 2.8-fold and has been found to be an independent risk factor. Hypertension is often related to obesity and diabetes and is not considered an independent risk factor. In regard to racial factors, the incidence of endometrial cancer among white women is approximately twice the rate in black women. However, studies of Hill and coworkers have demonstrated that black women tend to develop a much higher percentage of poorly differentiated tumors. The National Cancer Database report by Partridge and colleagues has confirmed that black patients with a low income present at an advanced stage and have a poor survival compared with non-Hispanic whites. The difference in survival between blacks and non-Hispanic whites does not appear to be based solely on access to care issues, and there are likely biologic differences that account for the disparity in survival.

Lynch syndrome, or hereditary nonpolyposis colorectal cancer syndrome (HNPCC), is an autosomal dominant hereditary cancer susceptibility syndrome caused by a germline defect in a DNA mismatch repair gene (*MLH1, MSH2,* or *MSH6*). Women with Lynch syndrome have a 40% to 60% lifetime risk for developing endometrial cancer, a 40% to 60% lifetime risk of developing colon cancer, and a 12% lifetime risk of developing ovarian cancer. This contrasts sharply with the general population risk of 3% for endometrial cancer, 5% for colon cancer, and 1.7% risk of ovarian cancer. Endometrial cancers in Lynch syndrome can be of any histology and grade. Broaddus and Lu have reported that although most are early stage, approximately 25% are high grade, high stage, or poor histology. Given that there are few longitudinal cohort studies, screening recommendations for gynecologic cancers are based on expert opinion; these include annual endometrial biopsy and transvaginal ultrasound to evaluate the ovaries. Colonoscopy every 1 to 2 years has been shown to decrease mortality from colon cancer in Lynch syndrome. Schmeler has reported on the efficacy of prophylactic hysterectomy and salpingo-oophorectomy to decrease endometrial and ovarian cancer risk, and women with Lynch syndrome should be offered this option after childbearing is complete. Lynch syndrome is likely to account for approximately 2% of all endometrial cancers. Women with endometrial cancer and a family history of colon, endometrial, or ovarian cancer should be referred for genetic evaluation and colonoscopy. In addition, women who have a personal history of endometrial and colon cancers have a significant risk for Lynch syndrome and should be referred. Although synchronous endometrial and ovarian cancers are fairly common, Soliman and colleagues have estimated the risk of Lynch syndrome in this cohort to be less than 10%.

Investigators have begun to define the molecular alterations present in endometrial cancer. PTEN mutations are frequently seen in endometrioid endometrial cancer and have also been seen in complex endometrial hyperplasia. Microsatellite instability occurs in approximately 25% to 30% of all endometrial cancers and is the result of a germline mutation in DNA mismatch repair proteins (MLH1, MSH2, or MSH6) or, more frequently, from the somatic methylation of the MLH1 promoter. In contrast to endometrioid endometrial cancers, **uterine papillary serous carcinomas** have a high frequency of p53 mutations. HER-2/neu amplification is seen in 10% to 20% of uterine papillary serous carcinomas and is likely associated with advanced stage and poor prognosis. Further studies will continue to elucidate our understanding of the molecular alterations of endometrial cancer.

ENDOMETRIAL HYPERPLASIA

The normal morphologic changes that occur in the endometrium during the menstrual cycle are reviewed in Chapter 4, Reproductive Endocrinology. Endometrial hyperplasia is believed to result from an excess of estrogen or an excess of estrogen relative to progestin, such as occurs with anovulation. Kurman and Norris have introduced terminology that has been adopted by the World Health Organization to describe endometrial hyperplasias and their premalignant potential. There are two important separate categories, atypical hyperplasia and hyperplasia without atypia. In these categories, two subgroups are recognized, **simple hyperplasia** and complex hyperplasia (**complex hyperplasia without atypia** and **complex atypical hyperplasia** (Table 32-1).

CATEGORIES

Simple Hyperplasia

This is a term that defines an endometrium with dilated glands that may contain some outpouching and abundant endometrial stroma (**Fig. 32-2**). The term *cystic hyperplasia* has been used to describe dilation of the endometrial glands, which often occurs in a hyperplastic endometrium in a menopausal or postmenopausal woman (cystic atrophy). It is considered to be weakly premalignant.

Complex Hyperplasia (Without Atypia)

In this condition, glands are crowded, with very little endometrial stroma and a very complex gland pattern and outpouching formations (**Fig. 32-3**). In traditional terminology, this is a

Table 32-1 World Health Organization Classification of Endometrial Hyperplasias

Simple hyperplasia
Complex hyperplasia
Atypical simple hyperplasia
Atypical complex hyperplasia

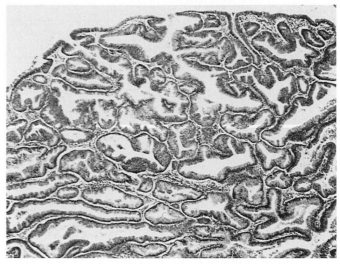

Figure 32-3 Complex hyperplasia characterized by crowded back-to-back glands with complex outlines. (From Kurman RJ, Kaminski PF, Norris HJ: Behavior of endometrial hyperplasia: A long-term study of "untreated" hyperplasias in 170 patients. Cancer 56:403, 1985.)

variant of adenomatous hyperplasia with moderate to severe degrees of architectural atypia but with no cytologic atypia. These hyperplasias have a low malignant potential.

Complex Atypical Hyperplasia

This term refers to hyperplasias that contain glands with cytologic atypia and are considered premalignant. There is an increase in the nuclear-to-cytoplasmic ratio, with irregularity in the size and shape of the nuclei (**Fig. 32-4**). Cytologic atypia occurs primarily with complex hyperplasia. Simple hyperplasia with atypia is rarely seen. Complex atypical hyperplasia has the greatest malignant potential.

A study from the Gynecologic Oncology Group has shed light on the difficulty of making the diagnosis of complex atypical hyperplasia. In this large prospective study, one third of cases

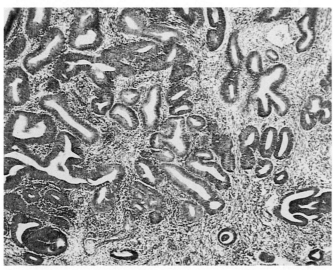

Figure 32-2 Benign simple hyperplasia. (From Kurman RJ, Kaminski PF, Norris HJ: Behavior of endometrial hyperplasia: A long-term study of "untreated" hyperplasias in 170 patients. Cancer 56:403, 1985.)

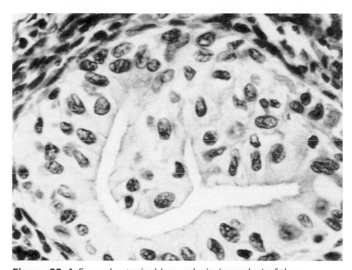

Figure 32-4 Severely atypical hyperplasia (complex) of the endometrium with marked irregularity of nuclei ($\times 720$). (From Welch WR, Scully RE: Precancerous lesions of the endometrium. Hum Pathol 8:503, 1977.)

Table 32-2 Endometrial Hyperplasia Follow-Up

Type	No. of Patients	Age Range (Mean)	Regressed*	Progressed to Carcinoma		Follow-Up (yr)
				No. of Cases	Mean (yr)	
Simple hyperplasia[†] pregnancies	93	17-71 (42)	74 (80%)	1	11	1-10
Complex hyperplasia[‡] pregnancies	29	20-67 (39)	23 (79%)	1	8.3	2-3
Atypical hyperplasia pregnancies	48	20-70 (40)	28 (58%)	11	4.1	1-3
Atypical simple hyperplasia	13		9	1		
Atypical complex hyperplasia	35		20	10		

*A total of 34 patients with simple hyperplasia, 7 with complex hyperplasia, and 15 with atypical hyperplasia had no further therapy.
[†]Benign proliferation of the glands.
[‡]Greater crowding of glands, no cytologic atypia present.
Adapted from Kurman RJ, Kaminski PF, Norris HJ: The behavior of endometrial hyperplasia. A long-term study of "untreated" hyperplasia in 170 patients. Cancer 56:403, 1985; and Kurman RJ, Norris HJ: Endometrial hyperplasia and related cellular changes. In Kurman RJ (ed): Blaustein's Pathology of the Female Genital Tract, 4th ed. New York, Springer-Verlag, 1994.

with a diagnosis of complex atypical hyperplasia were reproduced when evaluated by a gynecologic pathologist who was part of the study. However, one third of the cases were deemed to be less than complex atypical hyperplasia by the study pathologists and one third were greater than complex atypical hyperplasia—that is, they were considered endometrial cancers. Clinicians may benefit by consulting directly with the pathologist interpreting the endometrial histologic picture. The difficult distinction between various diagnostic categories makes this communication important.

NATURAL HISTORY

The rate at which endometrial hyperplasia progresses to endometrial carcinoma has not been accurately determined. Studies addressing this have been retrospective, based on samples obtained from D&C specimens at a single institution, and therefore are not necessarily generalizable. Kurman and associates have studied 170 patients with endometrial hyperplasia diagnosed by D&C at least 1 year before hysterectomy. **Table 32-2** shows the results of their study. Overall, complex atypical hyperplasias had the highest risk of progression to carcinoma. Simple hyperplasia had a 1% rate of progression to cancer, complex hyperplasia without atypia had a 3% rate of progression to cancer, and complex atypical hyperplasia had a 29% rate of progression to cancer. In addition to concern about progression to cancer, a Gynecologic Oncology Group (GOG) study has shown that 40% of women with complex atypical hyperplasia have endometrial cancer in their hysterectomy specimen. This high rate of cancer suggests that complex atypical hyperplasia may frequently be present with low-grade endometrial cancer and that endometrial sampling, whether by D&C or by office endometrial biopsy, may not identify an endometrial cancer when admixed with a complex atypical hyperplasia. Clearly, there is a spectrum of histology that makes a definitive diagnosis of complex atypical hyperplasia difficult; the clinician must be aware of this when planning treatment strategies.

DIAGNOSIS AND ENDOMETRIAL SAMPLING

Abnormal vaginal bleeding is the most frequent symptom of endometrial hyperplasia. In younger patients, hyperplasia may develop during anovulatory cycles and may even be detected after prolonged periods of oligomenorrhea or amenorrhea.

It can occur at any time during the reproductive years but is most common with abnormal bleeding in the perimenopausal period. Premenopausal women with irregular vaginal bleeding and postmenopausal women with any vaginal bleeding should be evaluated with an office endometrial sampling or a D&C. Office sampling instruments, such as a thin plastic pipelle, are introduced through the cervical os into the endometrial cavity and can provide accurate information. Many patients tolerate office endometrial sampling without an analgesic agent, but paracervical block can be an effective anesthetic aid, particularly in nulliparous women. Some patients benefit from an oral nonsteroidal anti-inflammatory drug (NSAID) taken approximately 30 minutes before biopsy.

Transvaginal ultrasonography has been evaluated as an adjunct for the diagnosis of endometrial hyperplasia and cancer. These studies have been performed in different populations, including asymptomatic postmenopausal women, women taking tamoxifen, and women presenting with postmenopausal bleeding. Langer and associates, in a study of 448 asymptomatic postmenopausal women, have found that a threshold of 5-mm endometrial thickness has only a 9% predictive value for detecting endometrial abnormalities. Its greater use was eliminating the diagnosis of neoplasia for those with thickness less than 5 mm (negative predictive value of 99%). These findings were confirmed in a literature review by Smith-Bindman and colleagues, who found that 96% of women with carcinoma had an abnormal ultrasound scan (endometrial thickness >5 mm). Conversely, 8% of postmenopausal women with an abnormal scan had no histologic abnormality, and the percentage grew to 23% for those on hormone replacement therapy. However, both these studies were conducted in postmenopausal asymptomatic women.

Cecchini and coworkers have performed biopsies on 108 postmenopausal patients on long-term tamoxifen with endometrial thickness more than 6 mm. One case of hyperplasia and one of carcinoma were found, and most patients had atrophic endometrium. The authors concluded that the false-positive rate of transvaginal ultrasonography in this population was too high to warrant its use as a screening modality; they recommended using irregular vaginal bleeding as an indication for endometrial sampling. Similarly, Love and associates have found that endometrial thickness is not necessarily a useful guide for biopsy in tamoxifen. The study by Barakat and colleagues found that routine screening with transvaginal ultrasonography was not of value, and they concluded that sampling should be done if the patient experiences bleeding.

In postmenopausal women with any vaginal bleeding, Gull and colleagues have found that an endometrial stripe less than 4 mm has a 100% negative predictive value. A finding of endometrial thickness less than 4 mm is a reasonable predictor of lack of endometrial pathology, even in a postmenopausal woman with bleeding. However, persistent vaginal bleeding should lead to endometrial sampling, regardless of the ultrasound findings.

Endometrial ablation is sometimes undertaken to control severe uterine bleeding (see Chapter 37, Abnormal Uterine Bleeding). However, pathologic evaluation of the endometrium should be performed before ablation to rule out an underlying endometrial hyperplasia or cancer.

TREATMENT

The therapy for endometrial hyperplasia depends on the woman's age and degree of atypia. For women with simple hyperplasia or complex hyperplasia without atypia, the risk of developing endometrial cancer is low, 1% and 3%, respectively. A diagnostic D&C can also be therapeutic, and progestins or combination oral contraceptive agents will likely be effective.

For complex atypical hyperplasia, the risk of developing endometrial cancer may be 29% and, as noted, a concurrent endometrial cancer may be present. Women who desire preservation of childbearing function are treated with high-dose progestin therapy, usually megestrol acetate 40 mg three or four times daily. The woman should have long-term follow-up and periodic sampling, the first at 3 months and at least every 6 months thereafter (**Fig. 32-5A**). In these patients, the risk factors that led to the development of complex atypical hyperplasia are likely to remain. Therefore, once the complex atypical hyperplasia is cleared, consideration should be given to periodic progestin treatment or oral contraception until the woman chooses to attempt pregnancy.

Studies have shown that younger patients with chronic anovulation and hyperplasia who desire children may also be treated by induction of ovulation with clomiphene citrate (Clomid) (see Chapter 41, Infertility). Weight reduction for very obese patients is also advised.

For older patients with complex atypical hyperplasia, the risk of carcinoma may be increased. Kurman and associates studied the uteri of patients after curettage had been performed, and atypical hyperplasia was found in the curettings. In their study, 11% of those younger than 35, 12% of those 36 to 54, and 28% of those older than 55 years with atypical hyperplasia were found to have carcinoma in their uterus. Thus, older patients with moderate or severe atypical hyperplasia generally require hysterectomy. In addition, those who fail progestin therapy, and especially those with severe cytologic atypia, should also be considered for hysterectomy (see **Fig. 32-5B**). If hysterectomy is not medically advisable, long-term high-dose progestin therapy can be used (megestrol acetate, 40 to 160 mg/day, or its equivalent, depending on the endometrial response). Current studies are being performed to evaluate the role of the progesterone-containing intrauterine device. Periodic sampling of the endometrium is also performed. **Figure 32-5** displays a flow chart guide to the management of endometrial hyperplasia. It is important to emphasize that the diagnoses are not distinct; these proliferative disorders are a continuum from mild abnormalities to malignant change.

ENDOMETRIAL CARCINOMA

SYMPTOMS, SIGNS, AND DIAGNOSIS

Postmenopausal bleeding and abnormal premenopausal and perimenopausal bleeding are the primary symptoms of endometrial carcinoma. The diagnosis of endometrial carcinoma is established by histologic examination of the endometrium. Initial diagnosis can frequently be made on an outpatient basis, with an office endometrial biopsy. If endometrial carcinoma is found, endocervical curettage may be performed to rule out invasion of the endocervix. A routine cytologic examination (Pap smear) from the exocervix, which screens for cervical neoplasia, detects endometrial carcinoma in only approximately 50% of cases.

If adequate outpatient evaluation cannot be obtained or if the diagnosis or cause of the abnormal bleeding is not clear from the tissue obtained, a hysteroscopy and fractional D&C should be performed. The endocervix is first sampled to rule out cervical involvement by endometrial cancer, hysteroscopy is done to visualize the endometrial cavity, and then a complete uterine curettage is performed.

HISTOLOGIC TYPES

The various types are listed in **Box 32-2**. **Figure 32-6** illustrates typical adenocarcinomas of the endometrium and demonstrates varying degrees of differentiation (G1, well differentiated; G2, intermediate differentiation; G3, poorly differentiated). Grading is determined by the percentage of solid components found in the tumor; grade 1 has less than 5% solid components, grade 2 has 6% to 50% solid components, and grade 3 has more than 50% solid components.

Squamous epithelium commonly coexists with the glandular elements of endometrial carcinoma. Previously, the term *adenoacanthoma* was used to describe a well-differentiated tumor and *adenosquamous carcinoma* to describe a poorly differentiated carcinoma with squamous elements. More recently, the term *adenocarcinoma with squamous elements* has been used with a description of the degree of differentiation of the glandular and squamous components. Zaino and colleagues, in a GOG study of 456 cases with squamous elements, have shown that prognosis is related to the grade of the glandular component and degree of myometrial invasion. They suggested the term *adenocarcinoma with squamous differentiation*, which has been generally adopted.

Uterine papillary serous carcinomas are a highly virulent and uncommon histologic subtype of endometrial carcinomas (5% to 10%). These tumors histologically resemble papillary serous carcinomas of the ovary (**Fig. 32-7**). Slomovitz and associates have evaluated 129 patients with uterine papillary serous carcinoma (UPSC) and found a high rate of extrauterine disease, even in cases without myometrial invasion. They recommended a thorough operative staging (see next section) in all cases of these tumors because of the high risk of extrauterine disease, even in cases admixed with other histologic types (endometrial and/or clear cell).

Clear cell carcinomas of the endometrium are less common (<5%). Histologically, they resemble clear cell adenocarcinomas of the ovary, cervix, and vagina. Clear cell tumors tend to develop in postmenopausal women and carry a prognosis much worse than typical endometrial adenocarcinomas. Survival rates

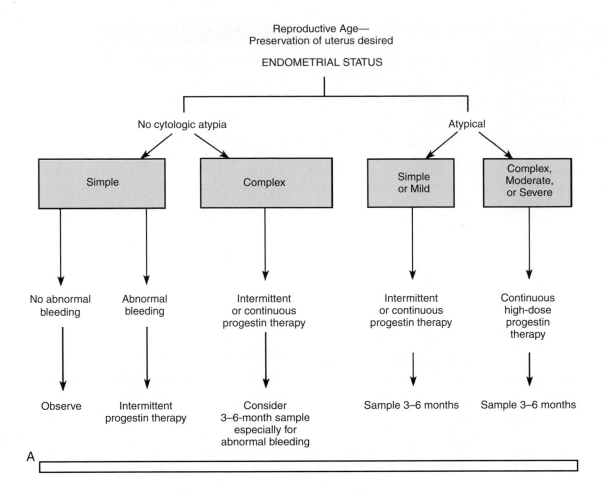

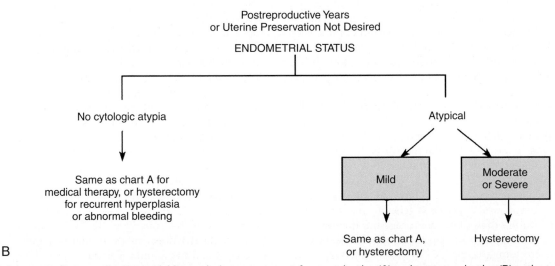

Figure 32-5 Schematic diagram of endometrial hyperplasia management for reproductive (**A**) and postreproductive (**B**) patients.

Box 32-2 Endometrial Primary Adenocarcinomas	
Typical endometrioid adenocarcinoma	Serous carcinoma
Adenocarcinoma with squamous elements*	Secretory carcinoma
	Mucinous carcinoma
Clear cell carcinoma	Squamous carcinoma

*Previously termed *adenoacanthoma* or *adenosquamous carcinoma*.

of 39% to 55% have been reported, much less than the 65% or better usually recorded for endometrial carcinoma. Abeler and Kjorstad have reviewed 97 cases and noted the best prognosis (90%) for those without myometrial invasion. Patients whose tumors had vascular invasion experienced a 15% 5-year survival. Carcangiu and Chambers have reviewed 29 cases and found 5-year survival rates for stages I and II of 72% and 59%, respectively.

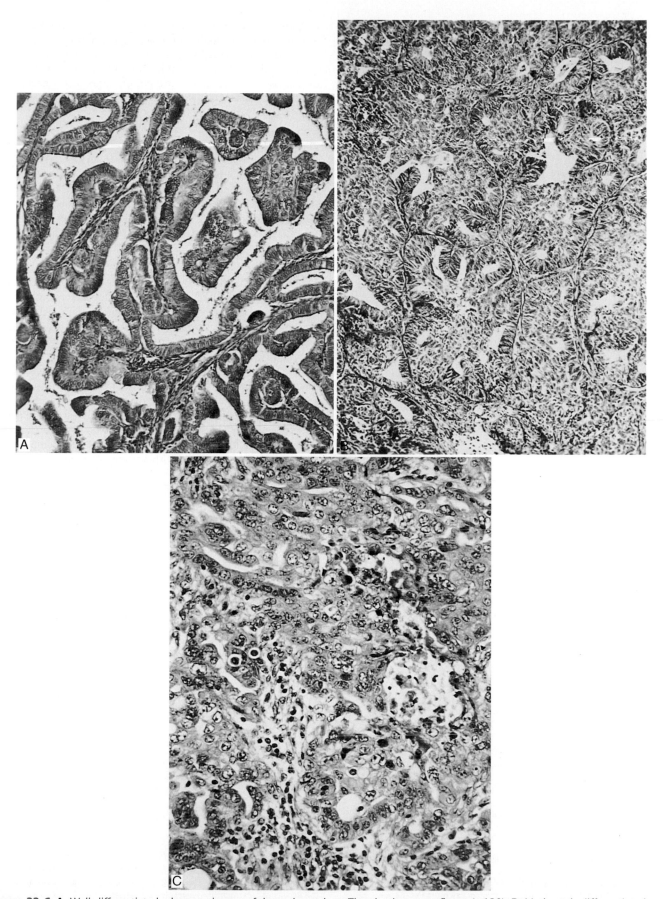

Figure 32-6 **A,** Well-differentiated adenocarcinoma of the endometrium. The glands are confluent (×130). **B,** Moderately differentiated adenocarcinoma of the endometrium. The glands are more solid, but some lumens remain (×100). **C,** Poorly differentiated adenocarcinoma of the endometrium. The epithelium shows solid proliferation with only a rare lumen (×100). (From Kurman RJ, Norris HJ: Endometrial neoplasia: Hyperplasia and carcinoma. In Blaustein A [ed]: Pathology of the Female Genital Tract, 2nd ed. New York, Springer-Verlag, 1982.)

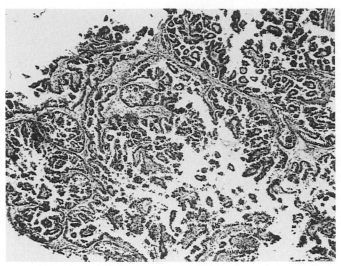

Figure 32-7 Serous carcinoma characterized by a complex papillary architecture resembling serous carcinoma of the ovary. (From Kurman RJ: Blaustein's Pathology of the Female Genital Tract, 3rd ed. New York, Springer-Verlag, 1987.)

STAGING

In 2009, a revised International Federation of Gynecology and Obstetrics (FIGO) surgical staging classification was introduced (**Table 32-3**). The surgical staging was modified to define clinically relevant risk strata better based on the FIGO Annual Report and other supporting publications.

PROGNOSTIC FACTORS

Many variables affect the behavior of endometrial adenocarcinomas. These can be conveniently divided into clinical and pathologic factors. The clinical determinants are patient age at

Table 32-3 Revised FIGO Staging for Endometrial Cancer (Adopted 2009)

Stage*	Characteristic
I	Tumor confined to the corpus uteri
IA	No or less than half myometrial invasion
IB	Invasion equal to or more than half of the myometrium
II	Tumor invades cervical stroma, but does not extend beyond the uterus[†]
III	Local and/or regional spread of the tumor
IIIA	Tumor invades serosa of the corpus uteri and/or the adnexae[‡]
IIIB	Vaginal and/or parametrial involvement#
IIIC	Metastases to pelvic and/or para-aortic lymph nodes[‡]
IIIC1	Positive pelvic nodes
IIIC2	Positive para-aortic lymph nodes with or without positive pelvic lymph nodes
IV	Tumor invades bladder and/or bowel mucosa, and/or distant metastasis
IVA	Tumor invasion of bladder and/or bowel mucosa
IVB	Distant metastases, including intra-abdominal and/or inguinal lymph nodes

*G1, G2, or G3.
[†]Endocervical glandular involvement only should be considered as stage I and no longer as stage II.
[‡]Positive cytology has to be reported separately without changing the stage.
Adapted from Pecorelli S: Revised FIGO staging for carcinoma of the vulva, cervix, and endometrium. Int J Gynaecol Obstet 105:103, 2009.

diagnosis, race, and clinical tumor stage. The pathologic determinants are tumor grade, histologic type, tumor size, depth of myometrial invasion, microscopic involvement of vascular spaces in the uterus by tumor, and spread of tumor outside the uterus to the retroperitoneal lymph nodes, peritoneal cavity, or uterine adnexa.

Clinical Factors

Older patients have tumors of a higher stage and grade when compared with younger patients. White patients have a higher survival rate than black patients, a finding partially explained by higher stage and higher grade tumors in black women. In addition, black women are more likely to develop UPSC. The 10-year survival of 136 black patients in the series of Aziz and coworkers was 40% compared with 72% for 135 white patients.

Pathologic Factors

Tumor stage is a well-recognized prognostic factor for endometrial carcinoma (**Table 32-4**). The results reflect a combination of clinical and operative staging because it was at the midpoint of the reporting period, 1988, when staging changed from a clinical to surgical staging system. Fortunately, most cases are diagnosed in stage I, which provides a favorable prognosis.

The histologic grade of the tumor is a major determinant of prognosis. Endometrial carcinomas are divided into three grades—grade 1, well differentiated; grade 2, intermediate differentiation; and grade 3, poorly differentiated. **Figure 32-8** shows the survival of 895 patients studied by the GOG that relates endometrial carcinoma survival to tumor grade and demonstrates the worsening of prognosis with advancing grade.

The histologic type of the endometrial carcinoma (**Fig. 32-9**) is also related to prognosis, with the best prognosis associated with endometrioid adenocarcinomas, as well as better differentiated tumors with or without squamous elements, and secretory carcinomas. Approximately 80% of all endometrial carcinomas fall into the favorable category. Poor prognostic histologic types are papillary serous carcinomas, clear cell carcinomas, and poorly differentiated carcinomas with or without squamous elements, as noted.

The degree of myometrial invasion correlates with the risk of tumor spread outside the uterus, but, in general, the higher grade and higher stage tumors have the deepest myometrial penetration (**Fig. 32-10**). The importance of tumor grade and myometrial invasion is also illustrated by a study of the relationship to their spread to the retroperitoneal pelvic and para-aortic lymph nodes. Studies of 142 patients by Schink and colleagues have indicated that tumor size is also prognostic. Only 4% of those with

Table 32-4 Carcinoma of the Corpus Uteri*

Stage	5-Year Survival Rate (%)
IA	90.9
IB	88.2
IC	81.0
II	71.6
III	51.4
IV	8.9

*Patients treated in 1990-1992, survival by 1988 FIGO surgical stage, N = 5562.
Adapted from Pecorelli S, Creasman WT, Pettersson F, et al: FIGO Annual Report on the Results of Treatment in Gynaecological Cancer, vol 23. Milan, Italy, International Federation of Gynecology and Obstetrics, 1998, pp 75-102.

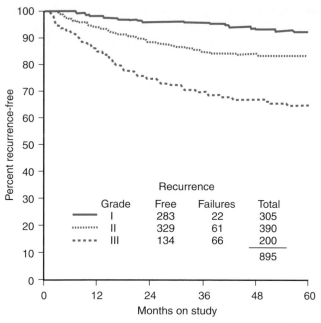

Figure 32-8 Recurrence-free interval by histologic grade. (Adapted from Morrow CP, Bundy BN, Kurman RJ, et al: Relationship between surgical-pathologic risk factors and outcome in clinical stage I and II carcinoma of the endometrium: A Gynecologic Oncology Group study. Gynecol Oncol 40:55, 1991.)

Grade	Recurrence Free	Failures	Total
I	283	22	305
II	329	61	390
III	134	66	200
			895

tumors 2 cm or smaller had lymph node metastases. The rate increased to 15% for those with tumors larger than 2 cm to 35% when the entire endometrial cavity was involved. **Table 32-5** summarizes the clinical and pathologic factors affecting outcome in early-stage tumors.

Peritoneal cytology has been studied as a prognostic factor and the results are conflicting. In a study of 567 surgical stage I cases, Turner and associates found that positive peritoneal cytology was an independent prognostic factor. In contrast, Grimshaw and coworkers evaluated 322 clinical stage I cases and found that positive peritoneal cytology was an adverse prognostic factor, but they did not find it to be an independent risk factor when other variables were considered. More recently, Kadar and associates and Lurain and colleagues have noted that positive peritoneal cytology is associated primarily with adverse features such as extrauterine disease and that therapy (see later) for positive peritoneal cytology as an isolated finding does not appear to improve survival. In the revised FIGO surgical staging (2009), positive cytology is no longer classified as stage IIIA.

Patterns of Spread of Endometrial Carcinoma

Plentl and Friedman have noted four major channels of lymphatic drainage from the uterus that serve as sites for extrauterine spread of tumor: (1) a small lymphatic branch along the round ligament that runs to the inguinal femoral nodes; (2) branches from the tubal and (3) ovarian pedicles (infundibulopelvic

Figure 32-9 Spread of endometrial carcinoma. The major pathways of tumor spread are illustrated (see text).

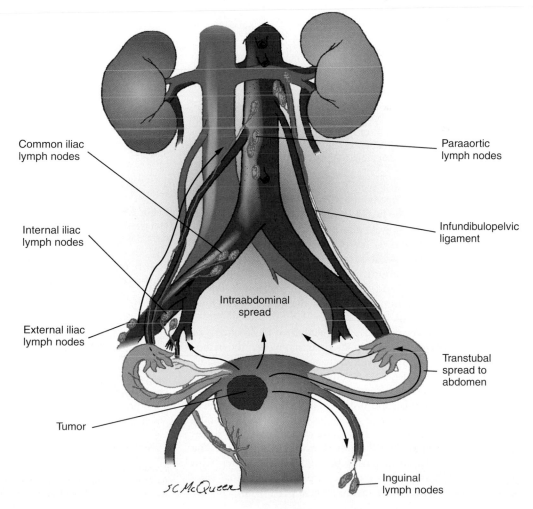

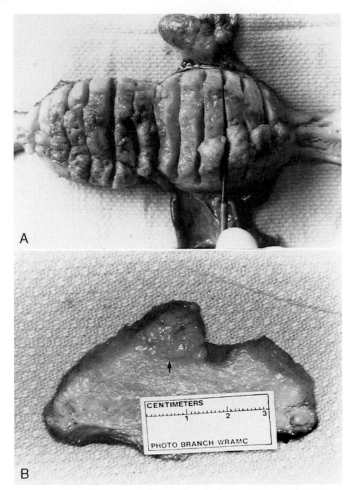

Figure 32-10 A, Technique for intraoperative assessment of the depth of myometrial invasion. **B**, Cross section of uterine wall demonstrating superficial myometrial invasion. The *arrow* shows the tumor-myometrial junction. (From Doering DL, Barnhill DR, Weiser EB, et al: Intraoperative evaluation of depth of myometrial invasion in stage I endometrial adenocarcinoma. Obstet Gynecol 74:930, 1989.)

Table 32-5 Surgical Stage I and II Tumors: Proportional Hazards Modeling of Relative Survival Time

Variable	Regression Coefficient	Relative Risk	Significance Test* (*P* value)
Endometrioid			
Grade 1	—	1.0	—
Grade 2	0.28	1.3	2.7 (0.1)
Grade 3	0.56	1.8	
Endometrioid with squamous differentiation			
Grade 1	0.20	1.2	
Grade 2	−0.01	1.0	0.3 (0.6)
Grade 3	0.22	0.8	
Villoglandular			
Grade 1	−4.91	0.01	
Grade 2	−0.59	0.5	10.4 (0.001)
Grade 3	3.73	41.9	
Myometrial invasion			
Endometrium only	—	1.0	
Superficial	0.39	0.5	
Middle	1.20	3.3	19.6 (0.0002)
Deep	1.53	4.6	
Age	0.17	—	
Age²	−0.000837	—	20.7 (0.0001)
45 (arbitrary reference)	—	1.0	
55	0.85	2.3	
65	1.52	4.6	
75	2.03	7.6	
Vascular space involvement	0.32	1.4	1.2 (0.3)

*Wald χ^2 test.
P value for grading is for overall grade within cell type.
Modified from Zaino RJ, Kurman RJ, Diana KL, Morrow CP: Pathologic models to predict outcome for women with endometrial adenocarcinoma. Cancer 77:1115, 1996.

ligaments), which are large lymphatics that drain into the para-aortic nodes; and (4) the broad ligament lymphatics that drain directly to the pelvic nodes. The pelvic and para-aortic node drainage sites (2, 3, and 4) are the most important clinically. In addition, direct peritoneal spread of tumor can occur through the uterine wall or via the lumen of the fallopian tube. Clinically, therefore, the clinician must assess the retroperitoneal nodes, peritoneal cavity, and uterine adnexa for the spread of endometrial carcinoma (see **Fig. 32-9**).

Extensive studies by the GOG have elucidated the frequency of lymph node metastases in endometrial carcinoma and the pathologic factors that modify this risk in stage I disease. Tumor grade, size of the uterus, and degree of myometrial invasion were studied. **Table 32-6** illustrates the frequency of lymph node metastases according to uterine size and tumor grade. There are differences in the proportion of positive nodes between stages IB and IA (pre-1988 staging) cases, as well as tumor grade. **Table 32-7** shows the effects of tumor grade and depth of myometrial invasion. The frequency of nodal involvement becomes much greater with higher grade tumors and with greater depth of myometrial invasion. The risk of lymph node involvement appears to be negligible

Table 32-6 Grade, Depth of Myometrial Invasion, and Node Metastasis: Stage I

Depth of Invasion	Pelvic		
	G1 (*n* = 180)	G2 (*n* = 288)	G3 (*n* = 153)
Pelvic			
Endometrium only (*n* = 86)	0 (0%)	1 (3%)	0 (0%)
Inner (*n* = 281)	3 (3%)	7 (5%)	5 (9%)
Middle (*n* = 115)	0 (0%)	6 (9%)	1 (4%)
Deep (*n* = 139)	2 (11%)	11 (19%)	23 (34%)
Aortic			
Endometrium only (*n* = 86)	0 (0%)	1 (3%)	0 (0%)
Inner (*n* = 281)	1 (1%)	5 (4%)	2 (4%)
Middle (*n* = 115)	1 (5%)	0 (0%)	0 (0%)
Deep (*n* = 139)	1 (6%)	8 (14%)	15 (23%)

G, grade.
Adapted from Creasman WT, Morrow CP, Bundy BN, et al: Surgical pathologic spread patterns of endometrial cancer. Cancer 60:2035, 1987.

Table 32-7 FIGO Staging and Nodal Metastasis

	Metastasis	
Staging	Pelvic	Aortic
IA G1 ($n = 101$)	2 (2%)	0 (0%)
G2 ($n = 169$)	13 (8%)	6 (4%)
G3 ($n = 76$)	8 (11%)	5 (7%)
IB G1 ($n = 79$)	3 (4%)	3 (4%)
G2 ($n = 119$)	12 (10%)	8 (7%)
G3 ($n = 77$)	20 (26%)	12 (16%)

FIGO, International Federation of Gynecology and Oncology; G, grade.
From Creasman WT, Morrow CP, Bundy BN, et al: Surgical pathologic spread patterns of endometrial cancer. Cancer 60:2035, 1987.

Table 32-8 Risk Factors for Nodal Metastases: Stage I

Factor	Pelvic	Aortic
Low risk—grade 1, endometrium only, no intraperitoneal spread	0/44 (0%)	0/44 (0%)
Moderate risk, grade 2 or 3, invasion to middle third	15/268 (6%)	6/268 (2%)
High risk—invasion to outer third	21/116 (18)	17/118 (15%)

Adapted from Creasman WT, Morrow CP, Bundy BN, et al: Surgical pathologic spread patterns of endometrial cancer. Cancer 60:2035, 1987.

for endometrial carcinoma involving only the endometrium. With invasion of the inner third of the myometrium, there is a negligible risk of node involvement for grade 1 and 2 cases. If the outer third of the myometrium is involved, the risk of nodal metastases is greatly increased. These data emphasize the importance of myometrial invasion and tumor spread, providing the basis for the FIGO Surgical Staging System. **Table 32-8** summarizes the risk of nodal metastases based on the GOG studies published by Creasman and colleagues. In a more recent GOG study cited previously, Morrow and coworkers noted that for patients without metastases at operation, the greatest risk of future recurrence was grade 3 histology. Furthermore, among 48 patients with histologically documented aortic node metastases, 47 were found to have positive pelvic nodes, adnexal metastases, or tumor invasion to the outer third of the myometrium, emphasizing the poor prognostic aspects of these three findings. Mariani and colleagues at the Mayo Clinic have found that tumor size can also be incorporated into a staging paradigm to identify patients at highest risk for nodal spread. They found that in grades 1 and 2 tumors with less than 50% invasion and tumor size smaller than 2 cm, the risk of lymph node involvement is almost zero.

Steroid Hormone Receptors

Steroid hormones affect the growth of target cells by binding with steroid receptors in the cell. The receptor steroid complex then interacts with DNA in the cell nucleus, stimulating the synthesis of messenger RNA, which acts in the cytoplasm to stimulate protein synthesis.

The steroid receptor level in endometrial carcinoma is lower than in normal endometrium. The highest levels of estrogen and progesterone receptors in tumors have been found in the well-differentiated (grade 1) tumors and the lowest in grade 3 tumors. Despite extensive research in this area, receptor status in endometrial carcinoma does not appear to have the same clinically relevant role as it does in cases of breast carcinoma.

EVALUATION

In addition to the usual routine preoperative evaluation, the woman should have a chest radiographic examination, and/or a chest and abdominal pelvic computed tomography (CT). However, a study by Connor and associates has noted that preoperative CT has only a 50% positive predictive value for nodal disease. Furthermore, postoperative CT monitoring did not appear to improve survival. The measurement of cancer antigen 125 (CA-125), generally used in cases of ovarian carcinoma, may occasionally be useful. Preoperatively, an elevated CA-125 level can often indicate extrauterine disease. It may be a particularly useful marker for those with serous carcinoma of the endometrium.

TREATMENT

Stage I

Surgery is the primary treatment modality for patients with endometrial carcinoma, except in patients with significant medical comorbidities. Complete surgical staging includes hysterectomy, bilateral salpingo-oophorectomy, pelvic cytology (washings), and pelvic and para-aortic lymph nodes. According to Orr and Chamberlin, the exceptions include women with significant medical comorbidities and young premenopausal women who desire future fertility, with grade 1 endometrial adenocarcinoma associated with endometrial hyperplasia.

Surgical staging allows accurate surgical and histologic assessment of the following: (1) tumor spread within the uterus; (2) degree of penetration into the myometrium; and (3) extrauterine spread to retroperitoneal nodes, adnexa, and/or the peritoneal cavity. This approach is used for cases that are staged according to the 2009 FIGO system (see **Table 32-3**).

The use of minimally invasive surgery in the treatment of early-stage endometrial cancer has continued to grow. The GOG has recently published a phase III randomized trial of surgical staging for endometrial carcinoma comparing the laparoscopic approach with the more traditional abdominal approach. The pathologic outcomes were the same and most patients in the laparoscopy arm were able to have the surgery completed. There were some benefits in the minimally invasive arm, including shorter hospital stay and improved quality of life in the postoperative period. Minimally invasive surgery can be used particularly for patients who are incompletely staged at the time of initial operation and require a second staging procedure.

For patients with significant medical comorbidities, radiation therapy alone can be used. However, radiation as the sole method of therapy yields inferior results, as Bickenbach and colleagues noted, with an 87% 5-year survival rate for patients with stage I carcinoma treated by surgery alone, in comparison with a 69% survival rate for those treated with radiation therapy alone. For those who cannot tolerate surgery or external beam therapy, treatment by intracavitary radiation alone offers some benefit. Lehoczky and associates have reported on 170 older patients treated with brachytherapy alone with uncorrected 5-year survival rates for stages IA and IB of 46% and 30%, respectively. For patients with grade 1 cancers, progesterone therapy could also be considered if patients are not medically fit for surgery or radiation therapy.

Occasionally, morbidly obese patients are encountered for whom an abdominal operation is very risky. Sood and coworkers have noted that for stage I patients with a preoperative CA-125 level less than 20 U/mL, the risk of extrauterine disease is only 3%, making vaginal hysterectomy a therapeutic option. Dotters has reported that a CA-125 level more than 35 U/mL usually predicts extrauterine disease, although approximately one third of patients needing full operative staging are not identified by an elevated CA-125 level for grade 1 or 2 cases, whereas for grade 3, the sensitivity increases to 88%. However, a few false-positive cases were noted, making the results a useful guide but not sufficiently precise to be the sole criterion for performing lymphadenectomy.

Stage I, Grade 1

The risk of spread of a grade 1 tumor to the pelvic nodes is extremely small (see **Table 32-7**). At the time of surgery, the abdomen is explored, peritoneal cytology is carried out, and an extrafascial total abdominal hysterectomy with bilateral salpingo-oophorectomy is performed. Pelvic and para-aortic lymph node dissection should be considered in cases with deep myometrial invasion. In patients with stage I, grade 1 tumors, postoperative radiation (vaginal brachytherapy and/or external beam irradiation) may be considered if there is deep myometrial invasion.

Stage I, Grades 2 and 3

Regardless of the surgeon's preference for the extent of surgical staging, all patients with grade 2 or 3 lesions should undergo complete surgical staging. Mariani and coworkers reported improved survival in patients at high risk of nodal disease who underwent para-aortic lymphadenectomy compared with those who did not have this procedure. The use of postoperative irradiation depends on the pathologic findings.

Three phase III randomized trials evaluating the use of adjuvant radiotherapy in patients with high-risk stage I endometrial cancer have shown no improvement in overall survival (see **Table 32-9**). In a Norwegian study comparing brachytherapy with brachytherapy plus pelvic radiation, local recurrences were decreased in the group of patients receiving pelvic radiation. In the PORTEC trial from The Netherlands, Creutzberg and colleagues reported on 714 patients with presumed stage I disease. Patients received full pelvic radiotherapy or observation. Although locoregional control was better in the treatment arm, there was no difference in overall survival. In a GOG trial, Keys and associates randomized almost 400 patients who underwent complete surgical staging to whole-pelvis radiation versus observation. Similar to the PORTEC trial, there was a decrease in local recurrences in the radiation arm, with no difference in overall survival. An ongoing GOG study is evaluating the role of vaginal brachytherapy and chemotherapy as adjuvant treatment in patients with high intermediate-risk disease.

Stage II

Three therapeutic options have been used for the treatment of stage II carcinoma of the endometrium that also involves the endocervix: (1) primary operation (radical hysterectomy and pelvic and para-aortic lymph node dissection); (2) primary radiation (intrauterine and vaginal implant and external irradiation), followed by an operation (extrafascial hysterectomy); and (3) simple hysterectomy, followed by external beam irradiation.

Radical hysterectomy and pelvic dissection have been used as effective therapy. Mariani and colleagues have reported on 57 patients with endocervical involvement at the time of diagnosis. Of these, 61% underwent radical hysterectomy and staging. There were no recurrences in the radical hysterectomy group if their nodes were negative at the time of surgery. Five year disease-related survival and recurrence-free survival in the radical hysterectomy patients was 76% and 71%, respectively.

Another option for patients with stage II carcinoma of the endometrium is treatment with a combination of radiation and extrafascial hysterectomy. The protocol includes external radiation (45 Gy) and a single brachytherapy implant, usually followed by extrafascial total abdominal hysterectomy, bilateral salpingo-oophorectomy, and para-aortic node sampling. Podczaski and coworkers have noted that those with gross cervical tumor have a poor prognosis and are likely to have extrauterine disease at operation. For patients with cervical involvement on biopsy but no gross tumor, Trimble and Jones have found radiation treatment by a single implant alone followed by a hysterectomy to be effective; they added external therapy depending on the nodal findings and myometrial invasion. Andersen has reported on 54 patients with stage II tumors and found a 70.6% survival rate in patients treated by abdominal hysterectomy followed by radiation.

Comparable outcomes have recently been reported using high dose rate brachytherapy approaches in stages I and II patients unable to undergo surgery. Nguyen and coworkers have reported a 3-year disease-free survival rate of 85% in 36 stage I patients treated with definitive radiation therapy. Nineteen patients were considered inoperable because of morbid obesity, and the remainder had significant medical problems precluding anesthesia. All patients were treated as outpatients with five weekly brachytherapy applications performed under conscious sedation. At a median follow-up of 32 months, the 3-year actuarial uterine control rate was 88%.

Adjuvant Systemic Therapy for Early-Stage Endometrioid Endometrial Cancer

In addition to radiation therapy, adjuvant chemotherapy is being explored for patients with endometrial cancer and high-risk features. Although the addition of postoperative radiation to high-risk patients reduces the local recurrence rate, distant metastasis

Table 32-9 Summary of Randomized Trials of Adjuvant Radiotherapy in Stage I Endometrial Carcinoma

Trial	Surgery	Randomization	Locoregional Recurrences	Survival
Norwegian, 1968-1974	TAH-BSO	Brachytherapy versus brachytherapy and pelvic RT	7% versus 2% at 5 yr; $P < .01$	89% versus 91% at 5 yr; $P = $ NS
PORTEC	TAH-BSO	Obs versus pelvic RT	14% versus 4% at 5 yr; $P < .001$	85% versus 81% at 5 yr; $P = .31$
GOG	TAH-BSO, nodes	Obs versus pelvic RT	12% versus 3% at 2 yr; $P < .01$	86% versus 92% at 4 yr; $P = .56$

continues to be problematic. In approximately 25% of patients with low-stage grade 3 lesions, the disease recurs at a distant site. In addition, 20% of clinical stage II patients and at least 30% of patients who present with extrauterine disease recur at distant sites, even after patients have received adjuvant pelvic radiation.

Adjuvant chemotherapy may also be useful in this group of patients. The Japanese GOG compared pelvic radiation with combination chemotherapy in high-risk, early-stage patients and found an improvement in progression-free and overall survival in the chemotherapy arm.

Stage I or II Uterine Papillary Serous Carcinoma

Several academic centers have tried to determine the best treatment for patients with early-stage UPSC. Even with minimal disease within the uterus, patients with UPSC often have extrauterine spread of disease. In a retrospective, multi-institutional study, Huh and associates reported on 60 patients with stage I UPSC who underwent comprehensive surgical staging. They found that recurrence rates were lower than previously reported and inferred that complete staging may provide a potential benefit. In their study, none of 7 patients who received chemotherapy had a recurrence. In a multi-institutional retrospective study of early-stage UPSC, Dietrich and colleagues have found that the combination of carboplatin and paclitaxel in the adjuvant setting is effective in improving survival and limiting recurrences. Further investigation is necessary.

Combined chemotherapy and radiation therapy may play a role in the management of patients with early-stage disease. Turner and associates have reported the application of vaginal irradiation at a high dose rate in combination with chemotherapy in surgical stage I patients. The 5-year survival rate was 94%, which is higher than that seen in most other studies for patients with stage I disease.

Stage III or IV Recurrent Endometrial Cancer

Because of the hematogenous and lymphatic spread of endometrial cancer, patients with recurrent or advanced disease often present with tumor outside the pelvis. Systemic therapy, therefore, plays an important role in the treatment of these patients. Hormonal and cytotoxic agents have activity in patients with advanced or recurrent endometrial cancer. In addition, there continues to be a role for radiation therapy to obtain local control or treat disease in the pelvis.

In stage III carcinoma, the disease has spread outside the uterus but remains confined to the pelvis or the retroperitoneal nodes. These tumors do not involve the mucosa of the rectum or bladder. They account for approximately 7% of all endometrial carcinomas and occur in women older than those with lower stage tumors and often medically less able to undergo an operation.

Patients with stage IIIA disease include those with disease spread to the adnexa and/or the serosa of the uterus. Stage IIIB involves the vagina and stage IIIC includes spread to the retroperitoneal lymph nodes. In the revised FIGO staging, stage IIIC has been further divided into those with positive pelvic nodes only (stage IIIC1) and those with positive para-aortic nodes (stage IIIC2). Patients with nonendometrioid histology or spread to the serosa or adnexa require adjuvant therapy (radiation, chemotherapy, or both). Approximately 3% of endometrial carcinomas are at stage IV, and many of these patients have tumor metastases outside the pelvis. If it is possible to carry out, optimal surgical debulking can be associated with prolonged survival. Bristow and coworkers have reported that the amount of residual disease after cytoreductive surgery, age, and performance status appear to be important determinants of survival in patients with stage IVB endometrial carcinoma.

Several chemotherapeutic agents or combinations have demonstrated activity in patients with endometrial cancer. Combination therapy is more effective than single-agent therapy in treating this disease. The challenge has been to combine agents to maximize efficacy while attempting to limit toxicity.

Doxorubicin was one of the first drugs identified with good activity against endometrial cancer. Single-agent doxorubicin has a response rate of approximately 25%, with a median duration of response of less than 1 year. Single-agent cisplatin also has demonstrated response rates between 20% and 42% when used as a first-line agent. The duration of response was again short (3 to 5 months). In several phase II studies, adding cisplatin to doxorubicin has resulted in response rates between 45% and 60%. In a GOG randomized phase III study, cisplatin and doxorubicin in combination had a higher response rate compared with single-agent doxorubicin (45% versus 27%), but there was no difference in overall survival. The European Organisation for Research and Treatment of Cancer (EORTC) has performed a similar trial comparing the same two regimens. Again, the combination arm had a higher response rate than the doxorubicin-alone treatment group. In this study, there was a modest survival advantage in those patients who received the combination regimen. The median overall survival in cisplatin- and doxorubicin-treated patients was 9 months compared with 7 months in patients who received doxorubicin alone ($P = 0.065$).

More recently, phase II studies of paclitaxel have found significant activity in chemotherapy-naïve patients with recurrent endometrial cancer, with a response rate of 36%. In patients who failed previous chemotherapy, paclitaxel also demonstrated activity, with a response rate up to 27%. The antitumor effect of single-agent paclitaxel has led to the incorporation of paclitaxel into combination therapy regimens. In a phase II study, the combination of cisplatin and paclitaxel demonstrated a 67% response rate. In a phase III study, the GOG found similar activity between the combination of cisplatin and doxorubicin versus doxorubicin and paclitaxel. Following this study, the GOG performed a phase III trial evaluating doxorubicin and cisplatin compared with doxorubicin, cisplatin, and paclitaxel (TAP) with granulocyte colony-stimulating factor. The TAP regimen yielded a superior response rate (57% versus. 34%; $P < .001$), longer progression-free survival (8.3 versus 5.3 months; $P < .001$), and longer overall survival (15.3 versus 12.3 months; $P = .037$). The results of this study have set the TAP regimen as the standard of care for the first-line treatment of advanced or recurrent endometrial cancer.

In an attempt to decrease the toxicity related to cisplatin therapy, carboplatin has been investigated. Single-agent carboplatin demonstrates modest activity in chemotherapy-naïve patients, with little or no activity in patients pretreated with chemotherapy. In a phase II study, the combination of paclitaxel and carboplatin was evaluated in patients with advanced and recurrent disease. In patients with advanced endometrioid endometrial cancer, there was a 78% response rate to this combination. The median failure-free survival time was 23 months and the 3-year overall survival rate was 62%. In patients with recurrent disease, the response rate was 56% and the median failure-free interval was 6 months.

The combination of carboplatin and paclitaxel has a more favorable toxicity profile than cisplatin and paclitaxel. Thus, many community physicians prefer this combination in the setting of advanced or recurrent endometrial cancer rather than the TAP regimen. The GOG recently completed accrual to a phase III randomized study comparing TAP with carboplatin and paclitaxel to address this question. In a phase III randomized trial, the GOG has recently reported that the combination of doxorubicin and cisplatin demonstrates improved progression-free and overall survival compared with whole-abdomen irradiation in patients with advanced disease.

Despite higher response rates, more effective cytotoxic agents with longer durations of response are needed. The alkylating agent ifosfamide has demonstrated a response rate of 24% in chemotherapy-naïve patients and a 0% to 15% response rate in patients pretreated with platinum agents. 5-Fluorouracil has demonstrated activity as a single agent and in combination with melphalan in the phase II setting. Oral etoposide has been shown to have some activity against chemotherapy-naïve patients with a tolerable toxicity profile, but this was not seen in patients who had received previous chemotherapy.

The prognosis is poor for patients who fail first-line chemotherapy. The response rates for second- and third-line agents are often less than 10% and the overall survival is less than 9 months. Paclitaxel may have better activity than other agents in this setting. In patients who have failed previous chemotherapy, paclitaxel has response rates up to 27%. In particular, in a cohort of patients who were refractory to platinum, paclitaxel was shown to have a 22% response rate. Preliminary data suggest that retreatment with a platinum-paclitaxel–based regimen may be effective for patients who previously responded to these agents.

For patients with an isolated recurrence in the pelvis, radiotherapy can be useful. Ackerman and coworkers have treated 21 patients with pelvic relapse and found that radiation achieved pelvic control of disease in 14 (67%). The best results were with recurrences in the vaginal mucosa. Similarly, Sears and colleagues have treated 45 patients with vaginal recurrence of endometrial cancer with radiation and achieved a 44% 5-year survival rate. As noted, Carey and associates salvaged 15 of 17 patients with vaginal recurrence initially treated by operation alone. The addition of chemotherapy at the time of radiation is currently being evaluated. In patients who have had previous irradiation, pelvic exenteration can be considered for those with an isolated central recurrence.

Chemotherapy for Advanced and Recurrent Uterine Papillary Serous Carcinoma

Most information available for patients with UPSC is from retrospective, nonrandomized case series. In addition, response rates to therapy often come from subset analyses of studies of all types of advanced or recurrent endometrial cancer, including phase III GOG studies. Levenback and associates have reported 20 patients with recurrent or advanced UPSC treated with cyclophosphamide, doxorubicin, and cisplatin. Of these patients, 58% were alive without disease after 24 months. However, this regimen was highly toxic. Price and coworkers have also evaluated cyclophosphamide, doxorubicin, and cisplatin in 19 patients with advanced disease and 11 patients with recurrent disease. Of the patients treated in the adjuvant setting for advanced disease, 58% were alive without evidence of disease, with a median follow-up of 24 months. In the patients with recurrent disease, the response rate was 27%.

In addition, all patients developed treatment-related toxicities. Most of these toxicities were hematologic. One treatment-related death was due to caused by cardiotoxicity.

Recently, more favorable results using paclitaxel with and without carboplatin have been demonstrated. In a phase II study evaluating carboplatin and paclitaxel, the response rate was 60% in 20 patients with high-stage UPSC. The progression-free survival time was 18 months and the 3-year overall survival rate was 39%. Two of 4 patients with recurrent UPSC demonstrated a response to carboplatin and paclitaxel. Zanotti and colleagues have evaluated 24 patients with measurable disease (progressive disease after initial surgery or recurrent disease). There was an 89% response rate in patients treated after initial surgery and a 64% response rate for patients with recurrent disease. At the University of Texas M.D. Anderson Cancer Center, single-agent paclitaxel demonstrated a 77% response rate in patients with recurrent disease. Despite this activity, the duration of response in these studies was less than 1 year. Other agents are under investigation for the treatment of UPSC.

HORMONE THERAPY

Progestins for Advanced or Recurrent Disease

For the past 50 years, progestational agents have been valuable in the armamentarium against endometrial cancer, particularly in patients with recurrent disease. Progestins are generally well tolerated. Side effects are usually minor and include weight gain, edema, thrombophlebitis, headache, and occasional hypertension. In patients with medical comorbidities, the use of hormonal agents may be preferable to cytotoxic chemotherapy. Initial clinical trials in patients with advanced or recurrent endometrial cancer have demonstrated response rates of 30% to 50%. Larger studies with more specific response criteria have demonstrated more modest response rates, usually between 11% and 24%. Podratz and colleagues have treated 155 patients with advanced or recurrent endometrial cancer with progestational agents. The objective response rate was 11%. Overall survival after the initiation of hormone therapy was 40% at 1 year, 19% at 2 years, and 8% at 5 years. In a GOG phase II study, patients who had no previous exposure to chemotherapy or hormonal agents were treated with megesterol acetate (800 mg/day). The overall response rate was 24%. Progression-free and overall survival were 2.5 and 7.6 months, respectively.

Current recommendations for progestin therapy include oral medroxyprogesterone acetate (Provera), IM medroxyprogesterone acetate (Depo-Provera), and megesterol acetate (Megace). Although there are no randomized studies that have directly compared different formulations of progestins, response rates are similar. In addition, although a dose-response effect of progestin therapy has been reported in breast cancer, there is no evidence of this effect in patients with endometrial cancer. In a randomized trial of oral medroxyprogesterone acetate, patients receiving the low-dose regimen (200 mg/day) had a higher response to therapy than those receiving the high-dose regimen (1000 mg/day).

There are a number of tumor characteristics that increase the likelihood of response to hormone therapy. These include low-grade tumors, the presence of steroid hormone receptors (i.e., progesterone receptor [PR] and estrogen receptor [ER]–positive), and a longer disease-free interval. The GOG has demonstrated a response rate of 8% in women whose tumors were PR-negative and 37% for women whose tumors were PR-positive. In addition, there was a 7% response rate in women with ER-negative tumors compared with a 26% response rate in women with ER-positive tumors. Patients with poorly differentiated tumors or hormone receptor-negative tumors have significantly lower response rates to progestin therapy.

Because of the low toxicity profile and modest efficacy, progestins should be considered for patients with recurrent endometrial cancer. In particular, all patients not eligible for clinical trials with well-differentiated hormone receptor–positive recurrent or advanced disease can be given a trial of progestin therapy. If the woman has an objective response, the progestin may be continued indefinitely until there is disease progression.

Selective Estrogen Receptor Modulators and Aromatase Inhibitors

SERMs with antiestrogenic effects in the uterus have been used to treat women with recurrent endometrial cancer. First-generation SERMs such as tamoxifen have mixed estrogenic agonist and antagonist activity. Early response rates for tamoxifen in advanced or recurrent endometrial cancer were between 20% and 36%. However, in a GOG phase II study of tamoxifen given at a dose of 20 mg twice daily, only 10% of patients demonstrated an objective response. Grade 1 and 2 tumors were more likely to respond to tamoxifen than grade 3 tumors.

Short-term administration of tamoxifen can cause an increase in PR levels in postmenopausal women with endometrial cancer. Studies with alternating tamoxifen and progestins have been performed to determine whether this upregulation increases the response to progestin therapy. Phase II trials of tamoxifen plus alternating cycles of progestin have demonstrated a 27% to 33% response rate. The Eastern Cooperative Oncology Group has found no difference in response rates between patients treated with progestin alone and those treated with progestin combined with tamoxifen.

Anastrozole, an oral nonsteroidal aromatase inhibitor, has been approved by the U.S. Food and Drug Administration (FDA) for postmenopausal women with progressive breast cancer following tamoxifen therapy. The aromatase level is elevated in the stroma of endometrial cancer. In a phase II trial by the GOG, anastrozole was found to have minimal activity (9% response rate) in an unselected population of patients with advanced or recurrent endometrial cancer. More than 25% of the patients in this study had nonendometrioid histologic subtypes, and only 22% of the patients had ER- and PR-positive tumors or demonstrated a response to previous therapy. In the subset of women with FIGO grades 1 and 2 tumors with endometrioid histology, the response rate was 30%.

SARCOMAS

Sarcomas comprise less than 5% of uterine malignancies and are much less frequent than endometrial carcinomas, particularly in Western countries. Numerous terms have been used to describe the many histologic types. One useful classification is based on determination of the resemblance of the sarcomatous elements to mesenchymal tissue normally found in the uterus (**homologous uterine sarcomas**) in contrast to tissues foreign to the uterus (**heterologous uterine sarcomas**). Homologous types include **leiomyosarcoma**, endometrial stromal sarcoma (ESS) and, rarely, angiosarcoma. Heterologous types include

---

Box 32-3   Modified Classification of Uterine Sarcomas

I. Pure sarcoma
  A. Homologous
    1. Smooth muscle tumors
      a. Leiomyosarcoma
      b. Leiomyoblastoma
      c. Metastasizing tumors with benign histologic appearance
        i. IV leiomyomatosis
        ii. Metastasizing uterine leiomyoma
        iii. Leiomyomatosis peritonealis disseminata
    2. Endometrial stromal sarcomas
      a. Low grade: Endolymphatic stromal myosis
      b. High grade: Endometrial stromal sarcoma
  B. Heterologous
    1. Rhabdomyosarcoma
    2. Chondrosarcoma
    3. Osteosarcoma
    4. Liposarcoma
  C. Other sarcomas
II. Carcinosarcoma—malignant mixed müllerian tumors
  A. Homologous (carcinosarcoma): Carcinoma + homologous sarcoma
  B. Heterologous: Carcinoma + heterologous sarcoma
III. Müllerian adenosarcoma
IV. Lymphoma

Adapted from Clement P, Scully RE: Pathology of uterine sarcomas. In Coppleson M (ed): Gynecologic Oncology. New York, Churchill Livingstone, 1981, p 591.

---

rhabdomyosarcoma, chondrosarcoma, osteosarcoma, and liposarcoma. These sarcomas may exist exclusively or may be admixed with epithelial adenocarcinoma, in which case the term *carcinosarcoma* (**malignant mixed müllerian tumor**) is applied. **Box 32-3** shows a morphologic classification for uterine sarcomas. A study by Zelmanowicz and colleagues has suggested that risk factors for these tumors are similar to those of endometrial carcinoma—that is, estrogens and obesity increase the risk and oral contraceptive use decreases the risk. No uniformly defined staging criteria exist for these tumors and the most widely used definitions are similar to those for endometrial carcinoma—stage I, confined to the corpus; stage II, corpus and cervix involved; stage III, spread outside the uterus but confined to the pelvis or retroperitoneal lymph nodes; and stage IV, spread outside the true pelvis or into the mucosa of the bladder or rectum. Similar to endometrial adenocarcinoma, operative stage is the most important predictor of survival.

LEIOMYOSARCOMA

Leiomyosarcomas represent 1% to 2% of uterine malignancies and approximately one third of uterine sarcomas (**Fig. 32-11**). Although the exact cause is unknown, leiomyosarcomas are not thought to arise from benign leiomyomas. Leibsohn and co-workers have noted that of 1423 patients who had hysterectomies for presumed leiomyomas with a uterine size comparable with a 12-week pregnancy or larger, the risk of sarcoma increased with age, from 0.4% for those in their 30s to 1.4% for those in their 50s. The determination of malignancy is made in part by ascertaining the number of mitoses/10 HPF (high-powered field) as well as the presence of cytologic atypia, abnormal mitotic figures, and nuclear pleomorphism (see **Fig. 32-11**). Vascular invasion and extrauterine spread of tumor are associated

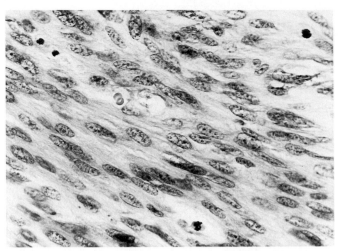

Figure 32-11 Leiomyosarcoma. Nuclear hyperchromatism and mitotic figures are present (×660), respectively. (From Clement PB, Scully RE: Pathology of uterine sarcomas. In Coppleson M [ed]: Gynecologic Oncology. Edinburgh, Churchill Livingstone, 1981.)

with worse prognoses. A finding of more than 5 mitoses/10 HPF with cytologic atypia leads to a diagnosis of leiomyosarcoma; when there are four or fewer mitoses/10 HPF, the tumors usually have a more benign clinical course. The prognosis worsens for tumors with more than 10 mitoses/10 HPF. The presence of bizarre cells may not necessarily establish the diagnosis because they can occasionally be seen in benign leiomyomas and in patients receiving progestational agents. Furthermore, it is important to note that an increase in mitotic count in leiomyomas occurs in pregnancy and during oral contraceptive use. This can occasionally cause confusion in the histologic diagnosis.

Usually, the woman has an enlarged pelvic mass, occasionally accompanied by pain or vaginal bleeding. Leiomyosarcomas are suspected if the uterus undergoes rapid enlargement, particularly in patients in the perimenopausal or postmenopausal age group. Approximately 85% of women diagnosed with a leiomyosarcoma have clinical stage I or II disease (i.e., disease limited to the uterus and cervix). The risk of lymph node involvement is very low. Primary treatment includes total hysterectomy, bilateral salpingo-oophorectomy, and staging. Despite the low incidence of high-stage disease, approximately 50% of patients will have a recurrence within 2 years. The recurrence in most of these patients is outside the pelvis.

The GOG has evaluated the role of adjuvant radiation therapy in patients ($n = 48$) with clinical stages I and II disease (**Table 32-9**). There was no difference in the progression-free interval, absolute 2-year survival rate, or site of first recurrence between patients who received pelvic radiation ($n = 11$) and those that did not ($n = 37$). This is not surprising, because most recurrences were outside the pelvis (83%). There was recurrence in 48% of patients and most of them had a recurrence within 17 months of diagnosis. In the adjuvant chemotherapy trial by the GOG, patients treated with doxorubicin (Adriamycin) had a recurrence less frequently than those in the observation arm (44% versus 61%); however, this difference was not statistically significant. There is no known benefit to adjuvant radiation or chemotherapy in women with leiomyosarcoma limited to the uterus.

Several studies have evaluated the treatment of advanced or recurrent leiomyosarcoma. Hannigan and colleagues used *v*incristine, *a*ctinomycin D, and *c*yclophosphamide (Cytoxan, VAC protocol) and noted a 13% complete response rate and 16% partial response rate in 74 patients with advanced metastatic uterine sarcomas. A large collaborative trial was conducted by the GOG and reported by Omura and associates. The best responses were obtained for patients with lung metastases who received doxorubicin and dacarbazine (DTIC). Current evidence suggests that a multidrug program offers the greatest response for these patients. Cisplatin, doxorubicin, paclitaxel (Taxol), ifosfamide, and etoposide (VP-16) all appear to have some effectiveness. Most recently, gemcitabine and docetaxel have been evaluated in a phase II study for patients with recurrent leiomyosarcoma. In this study, 34 patients with leiomyosarcoma were treated. The overall response rate was 53%; however, the duration of response was only 5.6 months.

ENDOMETRIAL STROMAL SARCOMA

Overall, stromal tumors comprise approximately 10% of uterine sarcomas. Their behavior correlates primarily with mitotic rate. Although these tumors were once divided into low grade and high grade, all ESSs are now considered low grade. If high-grade elements are present, these tumors would be classified as undifferentiated high-grade sarcomas. Undifferentiated sarcomas have a greater degree of anaplasia and lack the branching vasculature characteristic of ESSs. ESSs have a peak incidence in the fifth decade of life. There is no association with previous radiation nor are risk factors of endometrial carcinoma associated with the development of ESS. Histologically, ESS most resembles proliferative endometrial stroma. Prognosis depends on the extent of disease and ability to remove the entire tumor at the time of surgery. In general, ESSs are indolent, slowly progressing tumors.

Recurrent disease may be diagnosed as long as 30 years after diagnosis. ESS tends to recur locally in the pelvis or peritoneal cavity and frequently spreads to the lungs. In treating metastatic disease, it should be remembered that these tumors contain estrogen and progestin steroid hormone receptors and are often sensitive to hormone therapy. Complete resolution has been reported with megestrol acetate (Megace), medroxyprogesterone (Provera), letrozole (Femara), tamoxifen, and 17α-hydroxyprogesterone caproate (Delalutin).

There are reports of radiation in the treatment of pelvic recurrence, with resolution of all residual tumors, but extensive experience with radiation therapy is not available. Systemic chemotherapy with cytotoxic agents has not been reported to be effective, although good responses to doxorubicin have been seen.

UNDIFFERENTIATED SARCOMAS

These high-grade tumors behave aggressively and have a poor prognosis. They must be evaluated carefully because they are often confused with other large cell undifferentiated tumors (e.g., lymphoma, leukemia, high-grade endometrial cancer, carcinosarcoma).

Microscopically, more than 10 mitoses/10 HPF are present, and frequently 20 or more mitoses/10 HPF are present. Some series have reported 100% fatalities, although Vongtama and coworkers have reported survival of more than 60% for 24 patients with stage I and 1 patient with stage II disease. Recurrences are common in the pelvis, lung, and abdomen. If there has been no previous radiation treatment and the recurrence is confined to the pelvis, pelvic irradiation is usually prescribed. If there is disseminated disease, multiagent chemotherapy is used.

CARCINOSARCOMA (MALIGNANT MIXED MÜLLERIAN TUMORS)

As shown in **Box 32-3**, these tumors consist of carcinoma and sarcoma elements native to the uterus that may resemble the endometrial stroma of smooth muscle (homologous) or of sarcomatous tissues foreign to the uterus (heterologous). Spanos and colleagues have reviewed 188 patients with mixed mesodermal tumor and found the prognosis and pattern of survival to be similar for homologous and heterologous tumors. George and coworkers have shown that patients with these tumors have a markedly worse prognosis than patients with high-grade endometrial carcinomas. Unlike patients with endometrial stromal sarcoma or leiomyosarcoma, those with carcinosarcoma tend to be older and primarily postmenopausal, usually older than 62 years. Previous pelvic irradiation has been identified as an occasional predisposing factor and was experienced by 17 of 136 patients reviewed by Norris and Taylor. Heterologous and homologous tumors occur with approximately equivalent frequency. These tumors can spread locally into the myometrium and pelvis, or distally to the abdominal cavity, lungs and pleura, a pattern similar to the spread of endometrial carcinoma.

A common symptom is postmenopausal bleeding, often accompanied by an enlarged uterus. Occasionally, the diagnosis is made in tissue removed with D&C and the tumor may appear to be a polypoid excrescence from the cervix; diagnosis may also be made by vaginal ultrasound examination.

As is true for other sarcomas, the primary treatment is surgical removal of the uterus. The extent of the tumor and depth of myometrial invasion are important prognostic factors. Women with deep myometrial invasion are more likely to have spread to pelvic or para-aortic nodes. Patients with tumors confined to the uterus and little or no myometrial spread have the best prognosis. A comprehensive surgical staging procedure is recommended for all patients with this diagnosis. Nielsen and coworkers have reported a 5-year survival rate of 58% for these patients when the disease is confined to the uterus.

In a phase I and II study of ifosfamide and cisplatin as adjuvant therapy in patients with high-stage carcinosarcoma, the GOG found this combination to be tolerable. Progression-free and overall survival rates at 2 years were 69% and 82%, respectively. This study lacked appropriate controls so the impact of this regimen on improving survival could not be evaluated. For patients with advanced or recurrent disease, the GOG has evaluated ifosfamide versus ifosfamide and cisplatin in a phase III randomized study. The response rate to the combination therapy was superior (54% versus 36%); however, the toxicity was significantly higher. In addition, no significant difference in overall survival was seen. A follow-up study compared ifosfamide with ifosfamide plus paclitaxel in a phase III randomized study. Response rates in the combination arm were superior (45% versus 29%) but, more importantly, there was a significant difference in overall survival (13 versus 8 months).

MÜLLERIAN ADENOSARCOMA

Müllerian adenosarcoma is a rare low-grade malignancy composed of a sarcomatous stroma (homologous) and a proliferation of benign glandular elements that are intimately associated. It occurs predominantly in women older than 60 years. Total abdominal hysterectomy with bilateral salpingo-oophorectomy is the treatment of choice. Mitotic index and sarcomatous overgrowth are related to prognosis.

KEY POINTS

- Endometrial carcinoma is the most common malignancy of the female genital tract. In the United States, the lifetime risk of endometrial cancer is 3%.
- Most women who develop endometrial cancer are between 50 and 65 years of age.
- Women with Lynch syndrome (HNPCC syndrome) have a 40% to 60% lifetime risk of endometrial cancer, which is similar to their lifetime risk of colon cancer.
- Chronic unopposed estrogen stimulation of the endometrium leads to endometrial hyperplasia and, in some cases, adenocarcinoma. Other important predisposing factors include obesity, nulliparity, late menopause, and diabetes.
- The risk of a woman developing endometrial carcinoma is increased threefold if her BMI is greater than 30 kg/m^2.
- Tamoxifen use increases the risk of endometrial neoplasia two- to threefold.
- The primary symptom of endometrial carcinoma is postmenopausal bleeding. Women with abnormal bleeding should undergo endometrial sampling to rule out endometrial pathology.
- Cytologic atypia in endometrial hyperplasia is the most important factor in determining malignant potential.
- Simple hyperplasia will develop into endometrial cancer in 1% of patients, whereas complex hyperplasia will develop into cancer in 29% of patients.
- Studies have found that there is a 40% concurrent rate of endometrial cancer in patients with a preoperative diagnosis of complex atypical hyperplasia.
- Prognosis in endometrial carcinoma is related to tumor grade, tumor stage, histologic type, and degree of myometrial invasion.
- Older patients with atypical hyperplasia are at increased risk of malignant progression compared with younger patients.
- CT may miss as many as 50% of patients with nodal disease.
- A key determinant of the risk of nodal spread of endometrial carcinoma is the depth of myometrial invasion, which is often related to tumor grade.
- Well-differentiated (grade 1) endometrial carcinomas usually express steroid hormone receptors, whereas poorly differentiated (grade 3) tumors usually do not express these receptors.

- Uterine papillary serous carcinoma is an aggressive histologic subtype associated with metastatic disease even in the absence of myometrial invasion.
- Of recurrences of adenocarcinoma of the endometrium, 90% occur within 5 years.
- Overall survival rates for patients with adenocarcinoma of the endometrium by stage are as follows: stage I, 86%; stage II, 66%; stage III, 44%; stage IV, 16% (overall 72.7% 5-year survival rate combining clinical and operative staging systems).
- Histologic variants of endometrial carcinoma with a poor prognosis include uterine papillary serous carcinoma and clear cell carcinoma.
- Patients with uterine papillary serous or clear cell carcinoma of the endometrium should have a full staging laparotomy similar to that for ovarian carcinoma.
- The most frequent sites of distant metastasis of adenocarcinoma of the endometrium are the lung, retroperitoneal nodes, and abdomen.
- Primary treatment of endometrial cancer includes hysterectomy, bilateral salpingo-oophorectomy, pelvic cytology, bilateral pelvic and para-aortic lymphadenectomy, and resection of all disease. The exceptions include young premenopausal women with stage I, grade 1 endometrial carcinoma associated with endometrial hyperplasia and women with increased risk of mortality secondary to medical comorbidities.
- Postoperative adjuvant radiation has not been shown to improve overall survival.
- Patients with high-stage or recurrent disease should be treated with a multimodality approach, including chemotherapy, radiation, and/or hormone therapy.
- Uterine sarcomas comprise less than 5% of uterine malignancies.
- Uterine sarcomas are treated primarily by surgery, including removal of the uterus, tubes, and ovaries.
- Endometrial stromal sarcomas are low-grade sarcomas with an indolent course.
- Multiagent chemotherapeutic regimens are usually prescribed for metastatic sarcomas; complete responses are rare and usually temporary.

REFERENCES CAN BE FOUND ON
EXPERTCONSULT.com

33

Neoplastic Diseases of the Ovary
Screening, Benign and Malignant Epithelial and Germ Cell Neoplasms, Sex-Cord Stromal Tumors

Robert L. Coleman, Pedro T. Ramirez, and David M. Gershenson

Ovarian cancer is the second most common malignancy of the lower part of the female genital tract, occurring less frequently than cancers of the endometrium but more frequently than cancers of the cervix. However, it is the most frequent cause of death from gynecologic neoplasms in the United States. Cancer Statistics 2010 has reported that approximately 20,880 new cases of ovarian cancer will be diagnosed yearly in the United States, and there will be 13,850 deaths. A major contributing factor to the high death rate from the relatively few cases stems from the frequent detection of the disease after metastatic spread when symptoms direct clinical investigation or raise clinical concern. Surprisingly, most women diagnosed with ovarian cancer do report symptoms for months before diagnosis. As detailed later, only the severity and duration of symptoms differentially segregate cancer patients from noncancer patients. The incidence of ovarian cancer (**Fig. 33-1**) increases with age, becoming most marked beyond 50 years, with a gradual increase continuing to age 70 years followed by a decrease for those older than 80. Moreover, Yancik and associates have noted that those older than 65 are more likely to have their cancers diagnosed at an advanced stage, leading to a worse prognosis and poorer survival compared with those younger than 65 years.

Despite numerous epidemiologic investigations, a clear-cut cause of ovarian cancer has not been defined. A number of theories have been advanced. It is thought that these malignancies are related to frequent ovulation, and therefore women who ovulate regularly appear to be at higher risk. Included are those with a late menopause, history of nulliparity, or late childbearing. Conversely, women who have had several pregnancies or who have used oral contraceptives appear to have some protection against ovarian cancer. Casagrande and colleagues have related the development of ovarian cancer to ovulatory age—that is, the number of years during which the woman has ovulated. This number would be reduced by pregnancy, breast-feeding, or oral contraceptive use. Schildkraut and associates have correlated overexpression of mutant p53 protein in ovarian cancers with reproductive histories and found that overexpression was more likely in those who had high ovulatory cycle histories. In addition, talcum powder used on the perineum has been postulated to increase the risk but, as noted by Cramer and coworkers, it is a weak association. The use of oral contraceptives decreases the risk by approximately 50% after 5 years of use (approximately 10% to 12%/year). The protection increases with duration of use to 10 years and appears to last for approximately 15 years after discontinuation of use. Schlesselman has calculated a decrease of 369 ovarian cancer cases/100,000 women for 8 years of use. Given that the approximate occurrence of ovarian cancer cases in this group would be expected to be 1,400, such a decrease approximates 25%. Breast-feeding, pregnancy, tubal ligation and, to a lesser extent, hysterectomy with ovarian preservation also lower the risk of ovarian cancer. It has been suggested that ovulation-inducing drugs such as clomiphene citrate increase the risk of ovarian cancer, as noted by Whittemore and colleagues. Rossing and coworkers have reported an increase in risk from a population-based study that suggested that the risk is associated with prolonged use of clomiphene insofar as no association was noted with less than 1 year of use. The study was significant but had wide 95% confidence limits, and only 11 cancer cases occurred in the clomiphene group among 3,837 women studied in the infertility clinic. However, Venn and associates from Australia have not demonstrated an increase in ovarian cancer for those using fertility drugs for in vitro fertilization. Mahdavi and colleagues have assembled a review of cohort and case-control studies evaluating the relationship of fertility agents to ovarian cancer. In this report, little evidence supported the hypothesis that ovulation induction substantially increases cancer risk. Furthermore, a large population-based Danish cohort study also failed to demonstrate any increased risk of ovarian cancer among 54,362 women seeking consultation relating to fertility problems. Agents evaluated in this study were gonadotropins, clomiphene citrate, human chorionic gonadotropin, and gonadotropin-releasing hormone. Additionally, no associations were found between these agents and the number of cycles of use, parity, or length of follow-up. However, three reports specifically evaluating the association of these agents and the development of borderline tumor or low malignant potential tumors have suggest that a relationship may exist. The frequent presence of hormone receptors in these lesions, as well as the hyperestrogenic microenvironment, may support this observation.

Cramer and coworkers have found women with ovarian cancer to have a diet high in animal fat in compared with control subjects, and studies of Risch and associates have suggested that saturated fat increases the risk of ovarian cancer, whereas vegetable fiber may reduce it. **Table 33-1** shows the various factors that alter the risk of ovarian cancer. The familial or inherited aspects of the disease are considered subsequently.

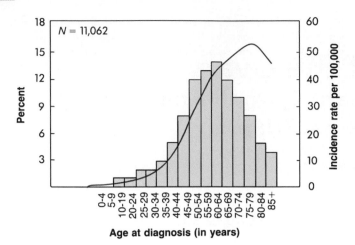

Figure 33-1 Ovarian cancer incidence rates by age, 1973 to 1982. (From Yancik R, Ries LG, Yates JW: An analysis of surveillance, epidemiology, and end results program data. Am J Obstet Gynecol 154:639, 1986.)

Table 33-1 Putative Associations of Increasing and Decreasing Risks of Ovarian Epithelial Carcinoma

Increases	Decreases
Age	Breast-feeding
Diet	Oral contraceptives
Family history	Pregnancy
Industrialized country	Tubal ligation and hysterectomy, with ovarian conservation
Infertility	
Nulliparity	
Ovulation	
Ovulatory drugs	
Talc (?)	

From Herbst AL: The epidemiology of ovarian carcinoma and the current status of tumor markers to detect disease. Am J Obstet Gynecol 170:1099, 1994.

There are geographic and racial differences in the distribution of ovarian cancers. These cancers occur most frequently in industrialized and affluent countries such as the United States and Western Europe and less frequently in Asia and Africa. The disease is more frequent among white than black women. Finally, patients with ovarian carcinoma have an increased risk of developing breast and endometrial cancer. Notwithstanding the familial syndromes, major factors appear to be related to the frequency of ovulation and residence in an industrialized country.

FAMILIAL OVARIAN CANCER

In a case-control study, Hartge and colleagues have shown that a familial history of breast cancer and a personal history of breast cancer are ovarian cancer risk factors. Lynch and associates have reported on families with these hereditary ovarian cancers and noted that they tend to occur at a younger age than in the general population. It appears that germline mutations of the *BRCA* tumor suppressor gene on chromosome 17q are responsible for a large proportion of hereditary cancers (see later). However, these

are a small proportion of all ovarian carcinomas. Risk alteration in these patients through oral contraceptive use is of uncertain impact. Narod and coworkers have suggested that it might be possible to reduce incident risk by their administration. However, Modan and colleagues have conducted a case-control study of Jewish women in whom *BRCA* founder mutational analysis was performed; they evaluated the risk of cancer development based by parity and oral contraceptive use. They were able to establish a protective effect by oral contraceptive use in the cohort, but subanalysis by carrier status demonstrated no effect in those harboring a *BRCA* founder mutation (odds ratio [OR] = 1.07; 95% confidence interval [CI], 0.63 to 1.83). Further studies are needed.

Hereditary ovarian cancers are uncommon, accounting for approximately 10% to 15% of all incident cases. However, identification of affected or unaffected women with significant familial risk is important, given their accelerated risk of ovarian and other cancers. In addition, these patients are frequently diagnosed at a younger age (median, 50 years), and unaffected individuals are able to consider prophylactic procedures that can affect their lifetime risk. The term *familial ovarian cancer* denotes an inherited trait that predisposes to ovarian cancer development. It has been widely studied and two definitions are important.

1. A first-degree relative is a mother, sister, or daughter of an affected individual.
2. A second-degree relative is a maternal or paternal aunt or grandmother.

As noted in the review by Kerlikowske and colleagues, previous studies suggested an increase from approximately 1.5% to 5% in the lifetime risk of ovarian cancer with one first-degree relative; with two or more, the risk reaches may exceed 7% to 12%. Because contemporary family size may preclude disease penetrance, careful attention to *BRCA*-associated cancers in either gender should be performed in a multigenerational history. Furthermore, the high association of fallopian tube cancer and underlying *BRCA* mutation has prompted some to call for routine *BRCA* testing in all such cases.

Most ovarian cancers develop sporadically. For the woman with a familial history of ovarian cancer (not the dominant genetic hereditary type), periodic surveillance with transvaginal ultrasonography 6 months after the age of 35 years has been suggested (see ultrasonography discussion later in this chapter). Unfortunately, such a strategy has not been shown to be worthwhile or cost-effective in disease prevention and may, on occasion, lead to additional tests or unnecessary procedures when a questionable ultrasound result is. The use of prophylactic oophorectomy in patients whose mothers had ovarian cancer has been a controversial topic. Kerlikowske and colleagues and Herbst have provided reasons opposing the widespread use of this practice. However, the use of prophylactic oophorectomy to reduce the risk of ovarian or peritoneal cancer in mutation carriers may have validity. Finch and associates have studied 1828 women enrolled in an international registry over an 11-year period ending in 2003. In this cohort, 575 (30%) had undergone oophorectomy before enrollment, 490 (27%) underwent the procedure after study entry, and 783 (43%) did not undergo the procedure. After a median follow-up of 3.5 years, 50 incident cases were identified, 18 in women undergoing oophorectomy and 32 in women with intact ovaries. The protective effect was 80% (hazard ratio [HR] = 0.2, 95% CI: 0.02 to 0.58; $P = .003$). It is reasonable that for patients with a significant family history in whom an operation such as hysterectomy is required, removal of both tubes and ovaries at the time of operation is appropriate. Similarly, mutation carriers who have finished childbearing may reduce their subsequent cancer risk by salpingo-oophorectomy. The recommendation for hysterectomy at this time is controversial but has been advocated by some to ensure complete removal of the fallopian tube (cornual segment). The woman must be aware that peritoneal carcinomatosis, a process resembling serous carcinoma of the ovary, can develop (rarely) despite the removal of both ovaries.

The following describes the classification and histology of the major **ovarian neoplasms**. Pertinent microscopic findings, clinical behavior, and appropriate therapy are presented.

CLASSIFICATION OF OVARIAN NEOPLASMS

The most widely used classification of ovarian neoplasms is that of the World Health Organization (WHO). This classification, along with frequency of occurrence of the primary ovarian neoplasms, is shown in **Table 33-2**.

Epithelial stromal tumors (common epithelial tumors) are the most frequent ovarian neoplasms. They are believed to arise from the surface (coelomic) epithelium. Germ cell tumors are the second most frequent and are the most common among young women. Histologically, they may be composed of extraembryonic elements or may have features that resemble any or all of the three embryonic layers (ectoderm, mesoderm, or endoderm). Germ cell tumors are the main cause of ovarian malignancy in young women, particularly those in their teens and early 20s. Sex cord–stromal tumors are the third most frequent and contain elements that recapitulate the constituents of the ovary or testis. These tumors may secrete sex steroid hormones or may be hormonally inactive. Lipid (lipoid) cell tumors are extremely rare and histologically resemble the adrenal gland. **Gonadoblastomas** consist of germ cells and sex cord–stromal elements. They occur in individuals with dysgenetic gonads, particularly when a Y chromosome is present. All these ovarian neoplasms are discussed later in this chapter.

Soft tissue tumors not specific to the ovary, such as a hemangioma or lipoma, are extremely rare and are categorized according to the criteria for soft tissue tumors arising elsewhere in the body. Unclassified tumors, as the name implies, cannot

be placed in any of the preceding categories. One example is **small cell carcinoma**, which is a highly virulent cancer affecting primarily young women (see later). Metastatic tumors to the ovary may arise elsewhere in the reproductive tract or from distant sites such as the bowel or stomach (**Krukenberg's tumors**). Tumor-like conditions refer to enlargements of the ovary, such as extensive edema, pregnancy luteoma, endometriomas, and follicular or luteal cysts, none of which are true neoplasms. With the exceptions of metastatic tumors and small cell carcinoma of the ovary, none of these are considered further in this chapter.

EPITHELIAL OVARIAN NEOPLASMS

According to Scully, two thirds of ovarian neoplasms are epithelial tumors; malignant epithelial tumors account for approximately 85% of ovarian cancers, probably arising from inclusion cysts lined with surface (coelomic) epithelium within the adjacent ovarian stroma. **Table 33-3** summarizes the five cell types that most commonly comprise epithelial ovarian tumors, indicating their relative frequency.

Epithelial tumors can be categorized as benign (**adenoma**), malignant (adenocarcinoma), or of an intermediate form, known as borderline tumor or tumor of low malignant potential. The term *papillary* or the prefix *cyst-* (as in cystadenoma) is used when the tumor has, respectively, papillae or cystic structures. The suffix *-fibroma* (as in **adenofibroma**) is added when the ovarian stroma predominates, with the exception of a Brenner tumor, which normally contains a large amount of ovarian stroma.

Low-grade (formerly well-differentiated) **serous tumors** (**Fig. 33-2A and B**) consist of ciliated epithelial cells that resemble those of the fallopian tube. Serous tumors (see **Fig. 33-2C**) are the most frequent ovarian epithelial tumors. The malignant forms account for 40% or more of ovarian cancers, benign forms (serous cystadenomas) occur primarily during the reproductive years, **borderline tumors** occur in women 30 to 50 years of age, and carcinomas typically occur in women older than 40 years. Molecular investigation of genetic changes associated with low-grade serous tumors support the reclassification of serous ovarian cancers into low- or high-grade binaries. Currently, a popular theory hypothesizes that high-grade serous carcinoma may arise from fallopian tube epithelium.

Mucinous tumors (**Fig. 33-3A and B**) consist of epithelial cells filled with mucin; most are benign. These cells resemble

Table 33-2 World Health Organization Classification: Frequency of Ovarian Neoplasms

Class	Approximate Frequency (%)
Epithelial stromal (common epithelial) tumors	65
Germ cell tumors	20-25
Sex cord–stromal tumors	6
Lipid (lipoid) cell tumors	<0.1
Gonadoblastoma	<0.1
Soft tissue tumors (not specific to ovary)	
Unclassified tumors	
Secondary (metastatic) tumors	
Tumor-like conditions (not true neoplasm)	

Table 33-3 Epithelial Ovarian Tumor Cell Types

Cell Type	Approximate Frequency (%)	
	All Ovarian Neoplasms	**Ovarian Cancers**
Serous	20-50	35-40
Mucinous	15-25	6-10
Endometrioid	5	15-25
Clear cell (mesonephroid)	<5	5
Brenner	2-3	Rare

Adapted from Scully RE: Tumors of the ovary and maldeveloped gonads. In Scully RE: Atlas of Tumor Pathology, fascicle 16, series 2. Washington, DC, Armed Forces Institute of Pathology, 1979.

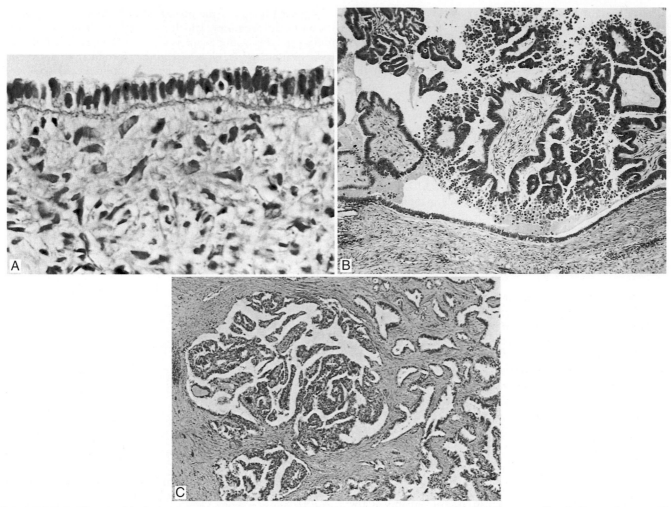

Figure 33-2 A, Ciliated epithelium of a well-differentiated serous tumor (×800.) **B**, Serous papillary cystadenoma of borderline malignancy. The epithelium resembles that of the fallopian tube, and a well-developed papillary pattern is present (×80.) **C**, Serous papillary adenocarcinoma (×50). The neoplastic epithelium invades the stroma. (**A** and **C** from Serov SF, Scully RE, Sobin LH: Histologic Typing of Ovarian Tumors. Geneva, World Health Organization, 1973. **B**, Courtesy of Dr. R. E. Scully.)

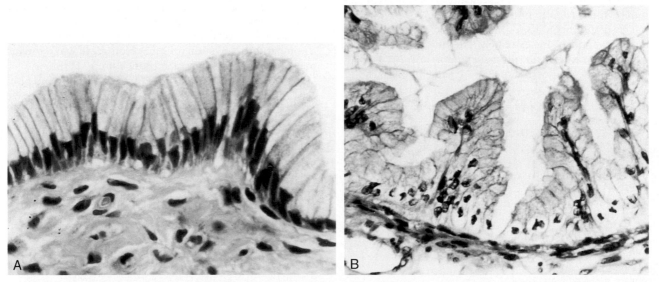

Figure 33-3 A, Mucinous cystadenoma (×800.) **B**, Mucinous borderline tumor. Epithelium resembles that of the endocervix.

Continued

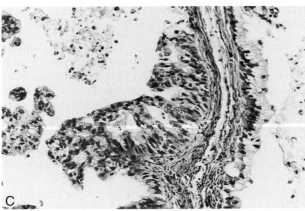

Figure 33.3—cont'd C, Mucinous carcinoma (×120). Incomplete stratification of cells and atypicality is present. (**A, C** from Serov SF, Scully RE, Sobin LH: Histologic Typing of Ovarian Tumors, Geneva, World Health Organization, 1973. **B,** Courtesy of Dr. R. E. Scully.)

cells of the endocervix or may mimic intestinal cells, which can pose a problem in the differential diagnosis of tumors that appear to originate from the ovary or intestine. Benign mucinous tumors are found primarily during the reproductive years, and mucinous carcinomas (see **Fig. 33-3C**) usually occur in those in the 30- to 60-year age range. Overall, they can account for approximately 25% of ovarian tumors and as many as 10% of ovarian cancers.

Endometrioid tumors (**Fig. 33-4**), as the name implies, consist of epithelial cells resembling those of the endometrium. In the ovary, these neoplasms are less frequent (approximately 5%) than serous or mucinous tumors, but the malignant variety accounts for approximately 20% of ovarian carcinomas. Endometrioid carcinomas usually occur in women in their 40s and 50s. They may be seen in conjunction with endometriosis and ovarian endometriomas, although an origin from endometriosis is rarely demonstrated. Most endometrioid carcinomas arise directly from the surface epithelium of the ovary, as do the other epithelial tumors.

Clear cell tumors (mesonephromas) contain cells with abundant glycogen (**Fig. 33-5A**) and so-called hobnail cells (see **Fig. 33-5B**), in which the nuclei of the cells protrude into the

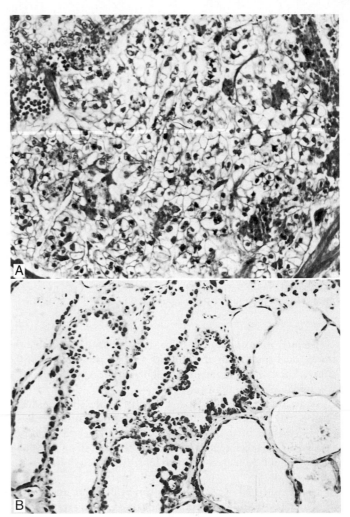

Figure 33-5 A, Clear cell adenocarcinoma (×200). A solid pattern of abundant polyhedral tumor cells containing abundant clear cytoplasm is present. **B,** Clear cell adenocarcinoma (×200). *Left:* Hobnail cells with scant cytoplasm; protruding nuclei line shows tubules. *Right:* Cysts lined by flattened tumor cells. (**A** from Barlow JF, Scully RE: "Mesonephroma" of ovary. Tumor of Mullerian nature related to the endometrioid carcinoma. Cancer 20:1405, 1967; **B** courtesy of Dr. R. E. Scully.)

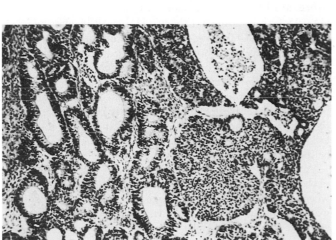

Figure 33-4 Endometrioid carcinoma. Tubular glands are lined by stratified endometrium (×80). (Courtesy of Dr. R.E. Scully.)

glandular lumen. Tumors with identical histologic features are found in the endometrium, cervix, and vagina, the latter two often associated with intrauterine diethylstilbestrol (DES) exposure. Molecular evaluation of these tumors suggests a homology to similar pathology occurring in the kidney, which may have therapeutic implications. Clear cell ovarian tumors are not related to DES exposure and comprise approximately 5% of ovarian cancers. They occur primarily in women 40 to 70 years of age and are highly aggressive.

The major cell types of ovarian epithelial tumors recapitulate the müllerian duct–derived epithelium of the female reproductive system (serous-endosalpinx, mucinous-endocervix, endometrioid-endometrium). This differentiation occurs even though the ovary is not derived directly from the müllerian ducts (see Chapter 2, Reproductive Genetics). The clear cell tumors also mimic this müllerian tendency, frequently being admixed with endometrioid carcinomas and with ovarian endometriomas.

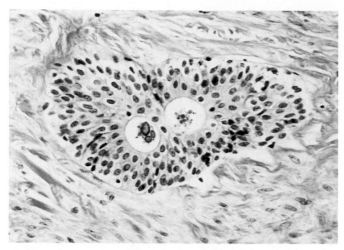

Figure 33-6 Brenner tumor (×350). Note the nest of transition-like epithelium containing spaces with eosinophilic material. (From Scully RE: Atlas of Tumor Pathology, fascicle 16, series 2. Washington, DC, Armed Forces Institute of Pathology, 1979.)

Brenner tumors (Fig. 33-6) consist of cells that resemble the transitional epithelium of the bladder and Walthard nests of the ovary. There is abundant stroma. These tumors constitute only 2% to 3% of all ovarian tumors.

In addition to the cell types shown in **Table 33-3**, epithelial tumors may be classified as undifferentiated if the tumor consists of poorly differentiated epithelial cells that are not characteristic of any particular cell type. They may be considered unclassifiable if they cannot be placed in any of the categories shown in this table.

Many epithelial ovarian tumors can be bilateral, and the risk of bilaterality is an important consideration in therapy, particularly when an ovarian tumor is discovered in a young woman of reproductive age. Widely varying percentages have been reported for bilaterality in ovarian tumors; the most widely quoted are summarized in **Table 33-4**. Malignant epithelial tumors tend to involve both ovaries more frequently than benign epithelial tumors. Serous tumors also tend to be bilateral more frequently than mucinous tumors.

Table 33-4 Bilaterality of Ovarian Tumors

Type of Tumor	Occurrence (%)
Epithelial Tumors	
Serous cystadenoma	10
Serous cystadenocarcinoma	33-66
Mucinous cystadenoma	5
Mucinous cystadenocarcinoma	10-20
Endometrioid carcinoma	13-30
Benign Brenner tumor	6
Germ Cell Tumors	
Benign cystic teratoma (dermoid)	12
Immature teratoma (malignant)	2-5
Dysgerminoma	5-10
Other malignant germ cell tumors	Rare
Sex Cord-Stromal Tumors	
Thecoma	Rare
Sertoli-Leydig cell tumor	Rare
Granulosa-theca cell tumor	Rare

BENIGN EPITHELIAL OVARIAN TUMORS: THE ADNEXAL MASS

As noted in Chapter 7 (History, Physical Examination, and Preventive Health Care), enlargement of the ovary beyond 5 cm is considered abnormal. However, age and menstrual status must also be considered before the appropriate course of action is chosen. A 5- to 8-cm ovarian mass in a woman with regular menses, even if she is in her 40s, is frequently a functioning ovarian **cyst**, such as a follicular or corpus luteum cyst. It will usually regress spontaneously during a subsequent menstrual cycle. Enlargements of this type in young patients in their 20s or early 30s do not automatically require immediate operative intervention and can be observed for two menstrual cycles. A potential exception would be a mass in a woman who is taking oral contraceptives. Because the principal mechanism of contraception is anovulation, the index of suspicion for neoplastic growth should be raised. However, contemporary oral contraceptives have lower sex steroid levels and may permit follicular development. Careful observation or immediate evaluation (see earlier) is warranted. Shushan and colleagues have reported ovarian cysts detected by ultrasonography in pre- and postmenopausal women taking tamoxifen for breast cancer. Unilocular 5- to 8-cm cysts are likely to be functional (see Chapter 18, Benign Gynecologic Lesions), whereas multilocular or partially solid tumors are more likely to be neoplastic. After the age of 40, the risk of malignancy rises. The ovary shrinks during menopause and normally is approximately 1.5 to 2.0 cm in size. A transvaginal ultrasound scan can reliably detect an ovary larger than 1.0 cm in diameter. Higgins and associates have estimated the upper limit of the volume of a postmenopausal ovary to be approximately 8 cm³ compared with 18 cm³ for the premenopausal ovary. Ten of their patients who exceeded these criteria and had solid or complex echo patterns had neoplastic tumors, and one carcinoma was discovered. An ultrasound examination, preferably with a vaginal probe, helps differentiate these adnexal masses (see later).

Occasionally, it is discovered that the adnexal mass is paraovarian. In a study of 168 paraovarian tumors, Stein and co-workers noted that only three (2%) were malignant. The three cysts all had solid components; the cysts were 8 to 12 cm size in patients 19 to 48 years of age.

Adnexal Mass and Ovarian Cancer

CA-125 (cancer antigen 125) was described by Bast and colleagues in the 1980s. It is expressed by approximately 80% of ovarian epithelial carcinomas but less frequently by mucinous tumors. The marker is increased in endometrial and tubal carcinoma, in addition to ovarian carcinoma, and in other malignancies, including those originating in the lung, breast, and pancreas. A level higher than 35 U/mL is generally considered to be increased. **Box 33-1** lists some of the benign conditions for which the CA-125 level also has frequently been found to be increased.

As can be seen, many of these are frequently found in women of childbearing age. This lack of specificity must be remembered when one is interpreting increased CA-125 levels in younger women with adnexal masses or when screening is being considered (see later). In addition, there are rare individuals who have no disease but are found to have levels of CA-125 as high as 200 to 300 U/mL as a consequence of developing idiopathic antibodies to mouse IgG.

Box 33-1 Cancer Antigen 125 Associations

Cancer	**Pelvic infection**
Ovarian, PP	Liver, heart, kidney failure
Uterine	Alcoholism
Colon	Peritonitis
Breast	Pancreatitis
Stomach	
Liver	**Condition**
	Pregnancy
Disease	Mild menstrual cycle
Leiomyomata	
Endometriosis	

One must also be cautious in the interpretation of an increased CA-125 level, particularly in a premenopausal woman with an adnexal mass. The specificity appears to be better for increased values in the postmenopausal woman. In a study of 182 patients, Vasilev and coworkers have noted that the CA-125 level is increased in 22% of cases of benign masses but, for postmenopausal patients, an increased level usually indicates malignancy. This was also shown in the CA-125 vaginal ultrasound study of 290 postmenopausal patients by Maggino and colleagues.

In addition to CA125 and transvaginal ultrasound, other biomarkers have been evaluated for their ability to preoperatively discriminate between benign disease and cancer. Currently, one test, OVA1, has been approved to aid this decision by providing a probability estimate of cancer based on a proprietary mathematical algorithm of five independent biomarkers: CA-125, β_2-microglobulin, transferrin, apolipoprotein A1, and transthyretin. OVA1 was the first blood test cleared by the U. S. Food and Drug Administration (FDA) to help evaluate the likelihood that a woman's ovarian mass is malignant or benign prior to a planned surgery. The OVA1 test, when performed in 516 women with adnexal masses deemed appropriate for surgical excision, improved the sensitivity of cancer versus noncancer discrimination in a double-blind clinical study from 72% to 92% when using the biomarker panel. Among gynecologic oncologists, the sensitivity increased from 86% to 99%. Although not approved for surveillance or diagnosis, the test may complement clinical decision making, particularly if a gynecologic oncologist is not available to perform appropriate staging should cancer be identified.

Evaluation of the Adnexal Mass

Ultrasound has helped define criteria to allow conservative follow-up and the risk of malignancy of some adnexal masses. Goldstein and associates have studied 42 postmenopausal patients whose ultrasound scans have shown unilocular cysts smaller than 5 cm in diameter; 28 were explored, and none had malignancy, and 14 were followed for as long as 6 years, with no change in ultrasound appearance. Finkler and colleagues have noted that the addition of a CA-125 serum assay to their ultrasound criteria in postmenopausal women increases the accuracy of preoperative evaluation. In a clinicopathologic study to define ultrasound criteria of malignancy, Granberg and associates studied the ovarian tumors in 1017 women. Of 296 with unilocular cysts, only one was malignant and had visible papillary formations on the cyst wall; 60% of these women were older than 40 years. In contrast, malignancy rates were 8% (20 of 229) for multilocular cysts, 65% (147 of 201) for multilocular solid tumors, and 39% (31 of 80) for solid ovarian masses.

In a follow-up study of 180 women, the authors noted that 45 of 45 unilocular cysts were benign. In an ultrasound study of cystic ovarian masses in women older than 50 years, Bailey and coworkers noted that unilocular cysts smaller than 10 cm in diameter are rarely malignant, whereas complex cysts or those with solid areas are at high risk of malignancy.

Several scoring systems have been proposed to try to determine the risk of an ovarian mass being malignant. They usually include the following:

1. Is the finding a simple (unilocular) or complex (multicystic or multilocular with solid components) cyst?
2. Are there papillary projections?
3. Are the cystic walls and/or septa regular and smooth?
4. What is the echogenicity (tissue characterization)?

These terms, definitions, and measurements have been standardized under a consensus opinion from the International Ovarian Tumor Analysis (IOTA) group and help refine the likelihood of malignancy. Shalev and coworkers have combined transvaginal ultrasonography and normal CA-125 values in 55 postmenopausal women with simple cystic or septate cystic ovarian masses; all 55 had benign disease. Although this was a small study, it suggests the potential of applying stringent ultrasound criteria with CA-125 evaluation of ovarian masses in postmenopausal women.

Others have advocated using transvaginal pulsed Doppler color-enhanced flow studies to differentiate benign from malignant masses. The resistance index, which measures resistance to flow in the vessels, has been used and presumably is low in the presence of neovascularization that is seen with malignant tumors. The vessels of neoangiogenesis are abnormal in their distribution, with disorganized branching and a loss of the muscularis layer, all of which contribute to the decreased resistance to flow. A resistance of 0.40 or less was found useful by Kurjak and coworkers in a study of 254 women. In contrast, Bromley and colleagues, in a study of 33 postmenopausal women, used a cutoff of 0.6, which did not greatly add to their specificities; they relied rely on morphologic criteria, e.g., solid elements, papillary projections) to diagnose malignancy.

Valentin and associates have evaluated the characteristics of 1066 adnexal masses; 266 were malignant (55 borderline ovarian tumors, 144 primary invasive epithelial cancers, 25 nonepithelial ovarian cancers, 42 metastatic cancers). A scoring system was used as well as information from color Doppler studies. They reported that borderline and stage I ovarian cancers shared similar morphology but had different characteristics from more advanced-stage tumors. They were larger, contained more papillary projections, and were more often multilocular, without solid components, but were less often purely solid and less likely to be associated with ascites. Significant variation was noted, however. Similarly, Twickler and colleagues described a scoring model to create an ovarian tumor index for women with adnexal disease. Of 244 women with follow-up, 214 had nonmalignant findings and 30 had cancer. In addition to age, transvaginal ultrasound variables, including ovarian volume, the Sassone morphology scale, and Doppler determination of angle-corrected systole, diastole, and time-averaged velocity, were evaluated. An ovarian tumor index was created from discriminant variables (continuous and weighted) correctly classifying the two cohorts. The area under the receiver operator characteristic curve (AUC) was highly significant (AUC = 0.91). Unfortunately, scoring systems such as these, developed from data produced by highly skilled and proficient sonographers, are difficult to generalize and, although promising, are highly operator-dependent. The IOTA group has temporally and externally validated the diagnostic performance of two logistic regression models containing clinical and ultrasound variables for malignancy identification. In this study, the prevalence of invasive cancer was 3%. The likelihood of cancer from a positive screen exceeded 6 for both models; a negative likelihood ratio was under 0.1, suggesting that the criteria may be of use for evaluating women with an adnexal masses.

It should be noted that there is a difference in using ultrasonography to screen for ovarian cancer as opposed to using different modalities of ultrasonography to characterize an ovarian mass as benign or malignant. For example, the addition of color Doppler sonography, which measures blood flow and direction of flow, and power Doppler sonography, which can detect slow flow in small vessels, can add useful information. These permit visualization of flow location (peripheral, central, or within a septum). Most malignant tumors have a central flow (75% to 100%) compared with only 5% to 40% of benign ovarian tumors. Schelling and colleagues have studied transvaginal B-mode and color Doppler sonography for the diagnosis of malignancy in 257 adnexal masses with unclear malignant status. They achieved 92% sensitivity and 94% specificity. The development of three-dimensional ultrasonography may allow more accurate volume assessments. In addition, color Doppler with three-dimensional ultrasonography may permit better detection of vessel irregularity, coiling, and branching. Another possibility is the use of contrast media to quantify and permit earlier detection of abnormal angiogenesis, as noted by Abramowicz. Contrast-enhanced (microbubble) power three-dimensional Doppler sonography has begun to be investigated to evaluate the efficacy of antiangiogenic biologic in serial scanning.

Ovarian Cancer Screening

Although ovarian cancer is characterized by advanced-stage disease at diagnosis and high mortality, early-stage disease is often curable. The greatest impact on these statistics, other than prevention, would be screening to identify early-stage disease. Three modalities, used individually or in combination, have been the common theme of this effort—physical examination, biomarkers (e.g., CA-125), proteomics-genomics (experimental) and sonography. For a disease to be amenable to screening, it should be sufficiently severe (high mortality) and have a natural history from latency to overt disease that is well characterized, and there should be a successful outcome if early disease is treated. The screening modality should have high positive and negative predictive values, and high sensitivity and specificity, and be acceptable to the population, cost-effective, and widely available. The screening population should be identifiable and, for those in whom early disease is identified, effective therapy should be available. Although ovarian cancer satisfies many of these mandates, it is rare in the general population and not readily characterized by an identifiable precursor, thus producing a high bar for any modality.

Of the three most commonly used modalities, the least sensitive and specific is physical examination. It is estimated that just one early ovarian cancer will be identified in 10,000 physical examinations. Although the easiest to implement, poor sensitivity limits this intervention as an effective strategy.

Biomarkers such as CA-125 are of great interest because they are easy to obtain and serial evaluation can be tracked. CA-125 has been used most consistently since being discovered as a reliable biomarker for epithelial nonmucinous ovarian cancer. Early, large, population-based studies highlighted its limitation as a sole strategy for ovarian cancer screening. Einhorn and associates have screened 5550 women and, in 1992, reported that only two stage I cancers in 175 women with elevated CA-125 values were identified. As noted, a differential effect would be expected between pre- and postmenopausal women. Using the modality in women with a pelvic mass (in whom prevalence is increased) has substantial effects on test characteristics but overlooks the obvious need for cancer identification before gross ovarian enlargement. This has led to the development of combined evaluation (sonography) described here.

Ultrasonography as an isolated modality has also been advocated for screening. Although more expensive and less amenable to population screening, it has become increasingly accurate in identifying early changes within the ovary, as noted. Campbell and coworkers screened 5479 patients and obtained 338 abnormal scans. Five early-stage ovarian cancers were identified. The positive predictive value was only 1.5%. Similarly, van Nagell screened 1300 patients and obtained 33 abnormal scans. Two early-stage ovarian cancers were identified. As with single-modality testing, sonography is too insensitive to be widely used for screening.

Population-based ovarian cancer screening programs have been difficult to recommend and implement because poor sensitivity and positive predictive value characteristics accompany expensive and inefficient testing methodology and triage algorithms. Menon and colleagues have approached this problem by evaluating a prospectively based algorithm in a population-based screening program in the United Kingdom. The population cohort used to evaluate this screening strategy involved 13,582 menopausal women 50 years or older with at least one ovary, of whom 6,532 randomized women completed a first screen; the remainder served as controls. The screening strategy was a staged process in which each CA-125 sample drawn underwent a calculation for risk of ovarian cancer (ROCA). The calculation was based on the woman's age and CA-125 value relative to her personal baseline. In this trial, an estimated risk of less than 1 in 2000 was considered normal, whereas a risk of more than 1 in 500 was considered increased; those in between were considered intermediate and required repeat testing. Those not considered normal were referred for a second stage of screening that incorporated a transvaginal ultrasound scan and repeat CA-125 testing. A transvaginal ultrasound scan was considered normal, abnormal, or equivocal based on ovarian volume and morphology. From the combination of CA-125 risk estimation and transvaginal ultrasound scan, a follow-up recommendation was made that could be a gynecologic oncology referral, repeat CA-125 testing, and/or transvaginal ultrasound scan or annual screening. In the screened group, almost 80% continued with annual screening; 91 (1.4%) were considered at increased risk. Among the intermediate group, repeat testing was normal in 92%, leaving 188 (2.9% of the initial population) to undergo second-stage evaluation. Of the 144 who stayed in the program, 95 were returned to annual screening based on CA-125 and transvaginal ultrasound scan findings, 6 were found to have nongynecologic malignancies, 43 were referred to a gynecologic oncologist, of whom 27 were returned to annual screening, and

16 women underwent surgery. From this group, five ovarian cancers were identified (four malignant epithelial and one borderline); the 11 remaining women had benign ovarian neoplasms. Compared with the authors' previous algorithm based on flat CA-125 values (normal = 30 U/mL), the new process referred less than 50% to secondary screening. It was concluded that this algorithm increases screening precision.

Two other prospective trials of general population screening deserve mention—the Prostate, Lung, Colorectal and Ovarian (PLCO) study and the United Kingdom Collaborative Trial of Ovarian Cancer Screening (UKCTOCS). The primary objective of the PLCO study is to evaluate the impact of annual screening with transvaginal ultrasound (TVUS) and CA-125 on ovarian cancer mortality. The study is following a cohort of over 34,000 largely postmenopausal women with intact ovaries prospectively with an algorithm indicating that an abnormal CA-125 level (≥ 35 U/mL) or an abnormality on TVUS is considered a positive screen. Follow-up procedures of a positive screen are not prespecified but have been tracked, as well as any surgical interventions resulting from these findings. Compliance over four rounds of screening has decreased slightly over the 3 years of postbaseline evaluation but remained above 75%. In contrast to CA-125, screen-positive TVUS decreased over the interval from 4.6% at baseline to 3.4% at year 3. Almost 90 ovarian cancers have been diagnosed so far; 60 were identified by screening abnormalities. Overall, the ratio of screen-positive ovarian cancers relative to benign disease decreased from 30:1 to almost 20:1. Of the ovarian cancers identified, 72% were advanced stage. The study continues to mature, with relatively good compliance. However, the impact of screening on the primary end point (mortality) is unknown.

The UKCTOCS was designed to assess the effect of ovarian cancer screening on mortality definitively, as well as comprehensively address the cost, acceptance, physical and psychosocial morbidity, and performance characteristics of multimodal screening and ultrasound-based screening. Between 2001 and 2005, a total of 202,638 postmenopausal women 50 to 74 years of age were randomly assigned to control (no screening), annual CA-125 screening (based on risk of ovarian cancer [ROC] algorithm) and second-line ultrasound testing (multimodal screening [MMS]) or annual transvaginal ultrasound (USS) alone in a 2:1:1 ratio. In the prevalence screen, 50,078 women (98.9%) underwent MMS and 48,230 (95.2%) underwent USS. Overall, 9% of the MMS cohort and 12% of the USS cohort required repeat testing. Surgery was undertaken in a small proportion of both cohorts but was significantly more likely following USS. Ovarian neoplasms, benign and malignant, were identified in both screening cohorts. The proportion of stage I and II cases was 48.3% and was balanced between the two screening algorithms. However, specificity was significantly higher for the MMS strategy (99.8%) relative to USS (98.2%). The performance of both screening modalities is encouraging and establishes feasibility (**Table 33-5**). The impact of stage migration following screening, as reflected in disease-specific mortality, is pending study completion, expected in 2014.

Successful prediction of cancer in the general public is limited by the low prevalence of disease. Creasman and DiSaia have estimated that if vaginal ultrasound scanning and CA-125 testing were performed annually on all women older than 45 years in the United States, the cost would exceed $10 billion annually.

Table 33-5 Screening Performance of Multimodal and Transvaginal Ultrasound in the UKCTOCS Prevalence Study

	Screening Modality	
Parameter	Multimodal Screening	Transvaginal Ultrasound
Repeat testing	9%	12%
Clinical evaluation	0.3%	3.9%
Surgery	0.2%	1.8%
Number of ovarian cancers	42	45
Borderline cancers	8	20
Stage I and II cancers (48.3% of cancers identified)	16	12
Sensitivity	89.5%	75%
Specificity	99.8%	98.2%
Positive predictive value	35.1%	2.8%

One strategy to improve the predictive index is to address a population in which prevalence is increased. A number of studies have been undertaken using transvaginal ultrasonography to screen for ovarian malignancy in higher risk women. Bourne and colleagues have screened 775 women who had at least one first-degree ($n = 677$) or second-degree ($n = 98$) relative with ovarian cancer. Overall, 43 women were referred for surgery with abnormal-appearing ovaries and 39 underwent surgery, with three stage IA ovarian carcinomas discovered (3.9 of 1000 screened); one of these was a borderline tumor. One screened patient was found to have peritoneal carcinomatosis 11 months after a normal screening study. The remainder had nonmalignant findings. DePriest and associates have screened 6470 asymptomatic postmenopausal women and defined abnormality as an ovary with a volume larger than 10 cm^3 and/or papillary projections in a cystic ovarian tumor. Ninety patients who had persistent findings by repeat ultrasound scanning at 4 to 6 weeks had an operation, with the finding of five early (stage IA; see later) and one advanced (stage IIIB) carcinomas. There were 37 serous cystadenomas and 20 assorted benign ovarian conditions. One woman with a normal scan was found to have peritoneal carcinomatosis 11 months later. These investigators noted that normal ovarian volume in a postmenopausal woman is smaller than 10 cm^3 and, in a premenopausal woman, is as much as 20 cm^3, as reported by Pavlik and colleagues.

Clinicopathologic studies of Bell and Scully, as well as ultrasound screening trials by Crayford and colleagues, have provided an explanation for the lack of success with ultrasound screening for detecting low-stage ovarian carcinomas. Bell and Scully have proposed the term *early de novo carcinoma* to explain their findings of 14 carefully studied cases. None of these patients had clinical evidence of ovarian carcinoma at the time of operation. All had microscopic foci of carcinoma in their ovaries, and three cases were detected only years later postoperatively, when the patients were discovered to have widespread carcinoma consistent with what was found in their ovaries on retrospective study. Crayford and colleagues have screened 5479 self-referred asymptomatic women by vaginal ultrasonography and removed all persistent ovarian cysts in an attempt to reduce the frequency of ovarian cancer. Of these, 88 patients had cysts removed. A slight nonsignificant increase in ovarian cancer deaths for this group was found 12 years after the conclusion of the study. Therefore, it appears that most ovarian carcinomas (particularly serous) arise from a tiny cancer of the surface of the ovary, from which it can spread rapidly before the ovary enlarges. Some ovarian tumors, such as endometrioid carcinoma, may have their origin in endometriosis. These carcinomas, as well as mucinous, tend to be detected more frequently at lower stages. Therefore, they appear more likely to have a cystic rather than a de novo origin. These observations strongly suggest that current strategies to use vaginal ultrasound screening to detect early ovarian carcinoma will have only limited success, as noted by Herbst.

Nonmalignant Neoplasms

Most nonmalignant epithelial ovarian tumors are asymptomatic unilateral adnexal masses that can be treated by oophorectomy or occasionally cystectomy (see later, Benign Cystic Teratomas [Dermoids]). In the past, some recommended bisecting the opposite ovary to rule out bilaterality in the case of benign epithelial ovarian tumors (see **Table 33-4**) but, in view of the risk of adhesions and infertility, as well as the availability of vaginal ultrasonography, this is no longer done. In a woman beyond her reproductive years, especially in the presence of a serous cystadenoma, which tends to be bilateral, hysterectomy and bilateral salpingo-oophorectomy are usually performed.

Mucinous tumors can become particularly large and reach sizes of 30 cm or larger. Possible complications of mucinous cystadenoma are perforation and rupture, which can lead to the deposit and growth of mucin-secreting epithelium in the peritoneal cavity (pseudomyxoma peritonei; see later).

Adenofibromas consist of fibrous and epithelial elements. The epithelial component may be serous, mucinous, clear cell, or endometrioid, the architectural subtypes of these benign ovarian tumors. Their appearance will depend on the predominant histologic features, epithelial or fibrous. These tumors are also managed by simple excision. Endometriomas are considered in Chapter 19 (Endometriosis).

Brenner tumors (see **Fig. 33-6**) are rare and often incidental findings when oophorectomy is performed for an indication other than ovarian enlargement. Usually, these tumors occur in women in their 40s and 50s, but younger and older patients have been found to have them. Brenner tumors are almost always benign and can usually be managed by oophorectomy. When the ovary is palpably enlarged, approximately 5% of Brenner tumors will prove to be malignant. These tumors often occur in perimenopausal and postmenopausal women, in which case, hysterectomy and bilateral salpingo-oophorectomy are indicated. Unfortunately, malignant Brenner tumors appear to have a poor prognosis despite this operative therapy, and an effective program of chemotherapy has not been developed.

The differential diagnosis for and approach to an adnexal mass in women of various ages are discussed in Chapter 7 (History, Physical Examination, and Preventive Health Care). Ovarian enlargement in the premenarchal female is usually the result of a germ cell tumor, which may be malignant but is usually benign (see later). During the reproductive years, ovarian neoplasms are usually benign. For the woman in her 20s or 30s, most ovarian enlargements can be approached surgically through a lower abdominal transverse (Pfannenstiel) incision or by laparoscopy. However, contingency plans in the setting of an unanticipated malignancy should be considered preoperatively and discussed with the woman. Larger masses usually require a vertical skin incision to ensure intact removal and safe dissection. Although the diagnosis of cancer can only be verified in tissue, patient characteristics (e.g., age, family history), preoperative

ovarian morphology (e.g., exophytic or endophytic masses, masses with large solid components, size) and biomarker studies (e.g., CA-125, HE4) may modulate risk assessment and thus the surgical approach.

The liberal use of intraoperative frozen-section assessment should be exercised, particularly in menopausal women. For women of reproductive age desiring fertility, if the diagnosis of malignancy is suspected but uncertain even after a frozen section is obtained, the operation should be terminated after removal of the ovarian tumor. A second procedure can be performed if malignancy is confirmed after detailed histologic study of the permanent sections. This is preferable to risking an unnecessary hysterectomy or bilateral salpingo-oophorectomy in a woman who desires to preserve childbearing function. Women in whom childbearing is not desired should undergo careful counseling to describe the potential need for a staging procedure in case a documented or suspected malignancy is identified from the frozen section.

CARCINOMAS

Diagnosis, Staging, Spread, Preoperative Evaluation, and Prognostic Factors

Ovarian carcinomas are usually diagnosed by detection of an adnexal mass on pelvic or abdominal examination. Occasionally, the diagnosis is made from a radiographic survey carried out for the evaluation of nonspecific gastrointestinal symptoms. Unfortunately, the diagnosis is frequently made only after the disease has spread beyond the ovary, as noted earlier when we described the de novo origin of these tumors. Scully has estimated that the risk of malignancy in a primary ovarian tumor increases to approximately 33% in a woman older than 45, whereas it is less than 1 in 15 for women who are 20 to 45 years of age. In general, more than 50% of ovarian carcinomas occur in women older than 50. In a hospital-based study of ovarian neoplasms in 861 women, Koonings and associates noted that the risk of malignancy was 13% in premenopausal women but rose to 45% in postmenopausal women. In their study, benign ovarian neoplasms were most common in those 20 to 29 years of age.

More than 90% of women diagnosed with ovarian cancer report symptoms before diagnosis. Unfortunately, these symptoms are vague and not specific for early-stage disease or even ovarian cancer. Goff and colleagues have conducted a prospective survey of women seeking medical care. The case patients were those about to undergo surgery for a known or suspected pelvic or ovarian mass; the controls were women presenting to one of two primary care clinics, in which approximately two thirds were being seen for a specific problem. The voluntary questionnaire instrument administered to both cohorts asked the respondents to score the severity, frequency, and duration of 20 symptoms generally reported by ovarian cancer patients. In both groups, recurring symptoms were common and nonspecific. Symptomatology in control patients was related to the purpose of their visit (general checkup versus specific complaint), underlying disease comorbidities, and menopausal status. Not surprisingly, women with the final diagnosis of ovarian cancer generally reported numerically more symptoms and of greater severity but of shorter duration of onset compared with the clinic controls or patients with benign ovarian tumors. Ovarian cancer patients were also statistically more likely to report increased

Table 33-6 Staging of Ovarian Carcinomas*

Stage	Characteristics
I	Growth limited to the ovaries.
IA	Growth limited to one ovary; no ascites present containing malignant cells; no tumor on the external surface; capsule intact
IB	Growth limited to both ovaries; no ascites present containing malignant cells; no tumor on the external surfaces; capsules intact
IC	Tumor stage IA or IB but with tumor on surface of one or both ovaries, or with capsule ruptured, or with ascites present containing malignant cells, or with positive peritoneal washings.
II	Growth involving one or both ovaries with pelvic extension
IIA	Extension and/or metastases to the uterus and/or tubes
IIB	Extension to other pelvic tissues
IIC	Tumor stage IIA or IIB, but with tumor on surface of one or both ovaries, or with capsule(s) ruptured, or with ascites present containing malignant cells, or with positive peritoneal washings
III	Tumor involving one or both ovaries with peritoneal implants outside the pelvis and/or positive retroperitoneal or inguinal nodes; superficial liver metastasis equals stage III; tumor limited to the true pelvis but with histologically proven malignant extension to small bowel or omentum
IIIA	Tumor grossly limited to the true pelvis, with negative nodes, but with histologically confirmed microscopic seeding of abdominal peritoneal surfaces
IIIB	Tumor of one or both ovaries with histologically confirmed implants of abdominal peritoneal surfaces, none >2 cm in diameter; nodes negative
IIIC	Abdominal implants >2 cm in diameter and/or positive retroperitoneal or inguinal nodes
IV	Growth involving one or both ovaries with distant metastases; if pleural effusion present, must be positive cytology to allot case to stage IV
IVA	Parenchymal liver metastasis equals stage IV.

*According to the International Federation of Gynecology and Obstetrics (FIGO); modified, 1985.

abdominal size, bloating, urinary urgency, and pelvic pain. Because the combination of increased abdominal size, bloating, and urinary urgency was reported five times more often and of greater severity in cancer patients than in controls, the authors recommended further clinical investigation when identified. The diagnosis is established by histologic examination of tumor tissue removed at operation. Occasionally, the initial diagnosis is suggested by malignant cells found in ascitic or pleural fluid obtained at paracentesis or thoracentesis, respectively.

The staging of ovarian cancer (**Table 33-6**) is designed according to the criteria of the International Federation of Gynecology and Obstetrics (**FIGO**). It is based on the results of operative exploration. Before surgical exploration for suspected ovarian carcinoma, the woman has a preoperative workup that is standard for a major abdominal operation (see Chapter 24, Preoperative Counseling and Management). Additional diagnostic studies may include a computed tomography (CT) scan of the abdomen to search for disease that would preclude a surgical intervention. Involvement of certain sites in the abdominal or pelvic cavity would be considered inoperable to achieve an optimal cytoreduction (<1 cm residual disease). These sites include

retroperitoneal suprarenal lymph node enlargement, mesenteric disease, porta hepatis disease, or bilateral parenchymal liver metastases.

A few studies have evaluated the role of combined positron emission tomography (PET) and CT in the treatment of primary epithelial ovarian cancer. Risum and associates have prospectively analyzed the diagnostic value of PET-CT for detecting a malignant tumor in 97 patients with no previous cancer history who presented with a pelvic mass. All the patients included in the study had PET-CT scans prior to surgery; the average serum CA-125 level was 784 U/mL. The sensitivity and specificity of PET-CT in diagnosing a malignant pelvic tumor were 100% and 92.5%, respectively.

Occasionally, a barium enema or colonoscopy is performed to evaluate pelvic and/or gastrointestinal symptoms. Consideration of gastrointestinal pathology is of importance for the potential of a primary colon carcinoma, which may present initially as an adnexal mass in the older woman. Approximately 4% of colon cancers will have metastatic involvement of the ovary at diagnosis. Determination of the serum carcinoembryonic antigen level may be useful in this setting and is recommended as part of the preoperative evaluation of a pelvic mass. An endoscopic or gastrointestinal radiographic examination is performed if there is evidence of gastrointestinal bleeding or the suggestion of any gastrointestinal pathology.

A CA-125 sample is obtained and, if the level increased at the time of operation, is useful for following the progress of the woman during and after treatment and for demonstrating the response to therapy or detecting tumor progression. Buller and associates have studied the regression slope for CA-125 during chemotherapy and found the slope of the regression curve to be predictive of therapeutic outcome. Other investigators have shown that patients whose CA-125 values decrease from increased to normal rapidly while undergoing primary chemotherapy have an improved prognosis over those whose values decrease more slowly. Markman has evaluated the survival impact of CA-125 levels reaching 50% of pretreatment baseline at 8 weeks after surgery and cisplatin-based chemotherapy. Survival was 21 months for those achieving this decrease versus only 10 months for those not achieving a 50% decrease. Clearly, this imperfect marker has prognostic significance in many situations. The serum inhibin level has been reported to be elevated in mucinous carcinomas and may serve as a marker, according to the studies of Henley and associates. Frias and coworkers have reported pretreatment levels of inhibin A to be a prognostic factor for survival in postmenopausal women with ovarian cancer. However, inhibin levels are not routinely determined in the woman with an epithelial ovarian malignancy.

Preoperatively, a program to cleanse the bowel is instituted in case intestinal resection is required. One protocol uses 4 liters of polyethylene glycol-electrolyte solution (GoLYTELY) given over 3 to 4 hours the evening before surgery. Neomycin sulfate, 1 g, with 1 g erythromycin base, may be given three times (3 PM, 7 PM, and 11 PM) on the day before surgery or IV broad-spectrum antibiotics may be given prophylactically just before the operation. Alternatively, magnesium citrate (16 oz) with oral bisacodyl (Dulcolax) tablets may be used. It is preferable to initiate bowel preparation early preoperatively so that liquid stool is evacuated before night sleep. However, mechanical cleansing of the bowel has engendered some controversy.

Venous thromboembolism prophylaxis is of particular importance in patients with ovarian cancer because a large tumor burden is associated with venous stasis and prolonged operation times. Treatment with variable compression leg support stockings and heparin (fractionated and unfractionated) appears to reduce the risk of thromboembolism in gynecologic oncology patients undergoing surgical tumor extirpation. A recent study by Einstein and colleagues has evaluated the usefulness of a dual prophylaxis protocol using sequential compression devices and heparin three times daily (or daily low-molecular-weight heparin) until discharge for patients with gynecologic malignancies. A dual prophylaxis protocol was shown to be associated with a significant reduction in the rate of venous thromboembolism without increasing bleeding complications.

Ovarian carcinomas infiltrate the peritoneal surfaces of the parietal and intestinal areas, as well as the undersurface of the diaphragm, particularly on the right side (Fig. 33-7). This is particularly important because tumors that appear at operation to be confined to the ovary may have small areas of diaphragmatic involvement as the sole site of extraovarian spread. As noted earlier, most ovarian carcinomas, particularly the serous type, appear to arise from microscopic ovarian sites and do not become clinically evident until there is widespread metastatic disease. Lymphatic dissemination is also a prominent part of disease spread (Fig. 33-8), and it is particularly important to note that the para-aortic nodes are at risk through lymphatics that run parallel to the ovarian vessels. Knapp and Friedman have noted that of 26 patients with ovarian cancer apparently limited to the ovary, 19% had para-aortic involvement, and all had poorly differentiated tumors. In a study of 180 patients, Burghardt and coworkers have observed that the proportion of positive nodes increases with higher stage tumors—24% in stage I, 50% in stage

II, and 73.5% in stages III and IV. A recent study conducted by Schmeler and colleagues has evaluated the prevalence of lymph node involvement in women with primary mucinous ovarian carcinomas. A total of 107 patients were identified. Of the patients with tumor grossly confined to the ovary at surgical exploration who underwent lymphadenectomy, none had metastatic disease to the pelvic or para-aortic lymph nodes. In addition, the authors found no significant differences in progression-free survival or overall survival between patients who underwent lymphadenectomy and those who did not.

The prognosis for patients with ovarian carcinoma is related to tumor stage, tumor grade, cell type, and amount of residual tumor after resection. Worldwide results for patients treated from 1990 to 1992 are summarized in **Table 33-7**. Recent data from the Survey Epidemiology and End Results (SEER) database are presented in **Table 33-8**.

Cell type has been reported to be an important factor in prognosis, as shown in **Figure 33-9**, which summarizes the 20-year survival rate of a group of patients. The most common invasive epithelial cancers, serous carcinomas, have the worst prognosis; prognosis may be better for mucinous and endometrioid tumors. A variant of papillary serous carcinoma termed *transitional cell carcinoma* is thought by some to be a rare but more chemosensitive tumor. However, this has not been established in multi-institutional studies. Endometrioid carcinoma may be associated with endometriosis and, according to McMeekin and colleagues, such cases more commonly occur in younger women and have a better prognosis than typical endometrioid carcinomas of the ovary. Clear cell cancers have a worse prognosis, but Kennedy and associates have noted that mitotic activity and tumor stage are important prognostic features of this tumor in their series. Tubulocystic pattern did not appear to affect prognosis, as

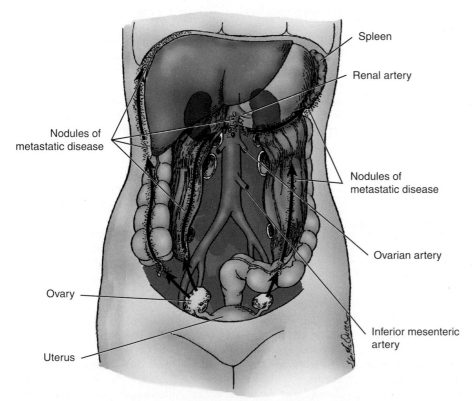

Figure 33-7 Peritoneal spread of ovarian cancer. Portions of the omentum, small intestine, and transverse colon have been resected. (From Knapp RC, Berkowitz RS, Leavitt T Jr: Natural history and detection of ovarian cancer. In Gynecology and Obstetrics, vol 4. Philadelphia, JB Lippincott, 1986, pp.)

Spleen

Renal artery

Nodules of metastatic disease

Nodules of metastatic disease

Ovarian artery

Ovary

Inferior mesenteric artery

Uterus

Figure 33-8 Lymph nodes draining ovaries. Primary routes of spread to the pelvic and para-aortic nodes are illustrated. (Adapted from Musumeci R, Banfi A, Bolis G, et al: Lymphangiography in patients with ovarian epithelial cancer: An evaluation of 289 consecutive cases. Cancer 40:1444, 1977.)

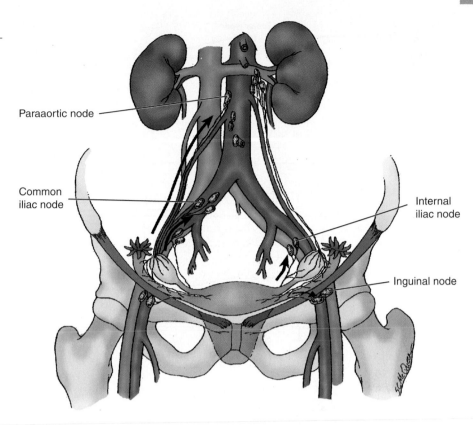

Table 33-7 Carcinoma of the Ovary: Survival by FIGO Stage*

Stage	No. of Patients	5-Yr Survival (%)
IA	342	86.9
IB	49	71.3
IC	352	79.2
IIA	64	66.6
IIB	92	55.1
IIC	136	57.0
IIIA	129	41.1
IIIB	137	24.9
IIIC	1193	23.4
IV	360	11.1

*For patients treated 1990-1992.
FIGO, International Federation of Gynecology and Obstetrics.
Adapted from Pecorelli S, Creasman WT, Pettersson F, et al: FIGO Annual Report on the Results of Treatment in Gynaecological Cancer, vol 23. Milan, Italy, International Federation of Gynecology and Obstetrics, 1998.

was suggested by the earlier studies of Aure and colleagues (see **Fig. 33-9**). Nonetheless, these are aggressive tumors with a propensity for recurrence, even in stage I. In a follow-up analysis, Kennedy and associates noted a survival probability of only 50% for stages I and II. It should be noted that stage and grade affect these observations. Serous tumors tend to be more poorly differentiated and discovered at a higher stage than mucinous tumors.

In some cases, patients are found to have small ovaries (<4 cm in diameter) and widespread papillary serous carcinoma in the abdomen. In such cases, the term *serous surface papillary carcinoma of the ovary* is applied. Fromm and coworkers have reported on 74 patients and found that survival is improved if the patients were treated postoperatively with combination chemotherapy (see later).

Another variety of serous carcinoma is **primary peritoneal carcinoma**. In these cases, the ovaries may be of normal size with

Table 33-8 Summary of Primary End Points in Randomized Phase III Studies

Outcome	Alberts et al (1996) (N = 546) IV	Alberts et al (1996) (N = 546) IP	Markman et al (2001) (N = 462) IV	Markman et al (2001) (N = 462) IP	Armstrong et al (2006) (N = 415) IV	Armstrong et al (2006) (N = 415) IP
Pathologic CR	36%	47%			41%	57%
P value	—					
PFS (mo)	—	—	22	28	18	24
P value		—		.01		.05
OS (mo)	41	49	52	63	50	66
P value		.02		.05		.03

CR, Complete response; OS, overall survival; PFS, progression-free survival.

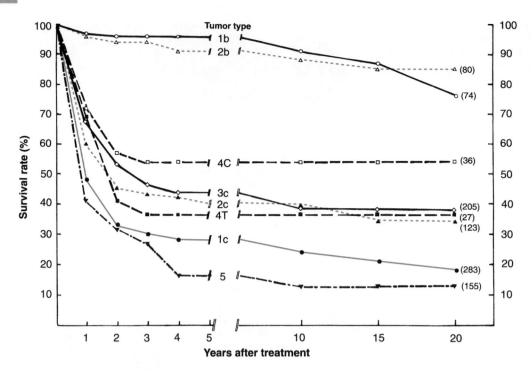

Figure 33-9 Survival rates for 983 patients with all stages of ovarian cancer by histologic type. *1b*, Serous, low malignant potential (74 cases); *2b*, mucinous, low malignant potential (80 cases); *1c*, serous carcinoma (283 cases); *2c*, mucinous carcinoma (123 cases); *3c*, endometrioid carcinoma (205 cases); *4c*, clear cell (36 cases); *4 T*, tubulocystic pattern of clear cell (27 cases); *5*, undifferentiated (155 cases). (Adapted from Aure JC, Hoeg K, Kolstad P: Clinical and histologic studies of ovarian carcinoma. Long-term follow-up of 990 cases. Obstet Gynecol 37:1, 1971.)

surface metastatic tumor deposits. There is widespread intra-abdominal spread of carcinoma of serous histology. These cases can be associated with *BRCA1* and *BRCA2* mutations, as shown by the studies of Karlan and colleagues. The cloning of the *BRCA1* gene has advanced our knowledge of the molecular genetics of ovarian cancer, but the role of this gene, which resides on chromosome 17q21, is not clear. It appears to be a tumor suppressor gene that is highly expressed in ovarian borderline carcinoma. Mutations in *BRCA1* are strongly associated with an increased risk of breast and ovarian cancer and a similar increase in risk occurs with mutations in *BRCA2* (**Table 33-9**). These mutations are seen in approximately 2% to 2.5% of Ashkenazi Jewish women, who appear to be an appropriate target group for testing whether breast cancer is diagnosed before age 50 in the woman or a close relative, according to Warner and associates. Prophylactic oophorectomy reduces the risk of ovarian cancer in those with a mutation, but does not eliminate the problem because of the potential for primary peritoneal carcinoma. The study of Rebbeck and colleagues of *BRCA1* mutation carriers has suggested that prophylactic oophorectomy may also reduce the subsequent risk of breast cancer. Boyd and coworkers have reported that stage for stage, the hereditary ovarian cancer group may have a better prognosis than those

with spontaneously occurring tumors. Lu and associates have noted a high proportion of microscopic carcinomas in apparently normal ovaries removed from patients with *BRCA* mutations, an observation consistent with the de novo origin of serous and poorly differentiated carcinomas.

In addition to stage, the grade of the tumor is a major determinant of patient prognosis. **Figure 33-10** demonstrates the survival of 442 patients with ovarian carcinoma by grade, with a markedly worse prognosis for poorly differentiated tumors (grade 3). The relationship between grade and survival also exists when the results are examined separately for each stage of disease.

The development of gene expression profiling has enabled a more precise evaluation of clinical behavior in some tumors. Bonome and coworkers have studied the gene expression of low malignant potential (LMP) serous neoplasms and invasive low-grade and high-grade serous tumors. A distinct and separate clustering was observed between LMP tumors and high-grade cancers. Low-grade serous tumors generally clustered with LMP neoplasms. High-grade tumors differentially expressed genes linked to cell proliferation, chromosomal instability, and epigenetic silencing. Based on these findings, high-grade epithelial cancers appear to have a distinct profile relative to LMP neoplasms. Low-grade serous tumors are remarkably similar to LMP serous neoplasms. These observations have ushered in the consideration of reclassifying invasive malignant cancers into two categories, low grade and high grade.

Studies of flow cytometry have indicated that the ploidy of the tumor is also prognostic, with aneuploidy being a negative prognostic factor. Klemi and colleagues have noted an independent prognostic association with the DNA index and S-phase fraction. A better prognosis was observed if the proportion of S-phase cells was less than 11% or if the DNA index (the relative DNA content of aneuploid cells compared with diploid) was less than 1.3. Genetic studies by Slamon and coworkers have shown that the HER-2/*neu* oncogene is amplified in ovarian and breast

Table 33-9 Carcinoma of the Ovary: Survival by SEER Registration for Patients Treated 1995-2001

Category	5-Year Survival (%)
Localized	94
Regional	69
Distant	9
All stages	45

SEER, Surveillance Epidemiology and End Results.
From Jemal A, Siegel R, Ward E, et al: Cancer statistics, 2006. CA Cancer J Clin 56:106, 2006.

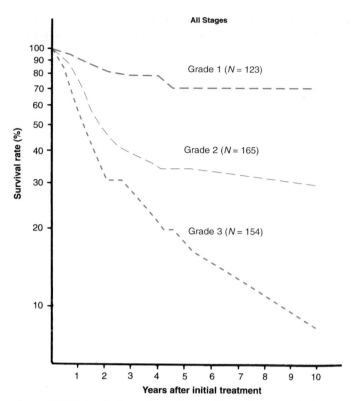

Figure 33-10 Survival rates for patients with ovarian cancer by tumor grade. Survival curves for the complete series according to the histologic degree of differentiation. All differences between curves are highly significant. (From Kosary CL: Ovarian carcinoma clinical trial. Semin Surg Oncol 10(1): 31-46, 1994.)

cancers. As noted in a review by Berchuck and associates, the overexpression of HER-2/*neu* was suspected to occur in approximately 30% of epithelial ovarian cancers and appears to be associated with a worse prognosis. However, a Gynecologic Oncology Group (GOG) study of trastuzumab (a monoclonal antibody to the extracellular domain of HER-2) in patients with recurrent ovarian cancer has suggested that the incident overexpression by fluorescence in situ hybridization is much lower. In this study, 837 samples were screened for immunohistochemistry overexpression (2+ or 3+) or fluorescence in situ hybridization positivity. Only 95 patients (11.4%) met criteria for therapy. It is likely that this prospective trial more accurately represents the incidence of this factor in ovarian cancer. The p53 tumor suppressor gene is mutated in approximately 50% of ovarian epithelial cancers studied, whereas the C-*myc* oncogene is overexpressed more commonly in serous cases and the K-*ras* oncogene has been identified more frequently in borderline ovarian cancers. The molecular genetic events surrounding ovarian carcinoma development and biologic behavior are incompletely understood.

The size of residual nodules and presence or absence of tumor after surgery has been related to the survival of patients treated for ovarian carcinoma. Chi and colleagues have analyzed survival by diameter of residual disease (grouped in five categories) to determine the optimal goal of primary cytoreduction for patients with stage IIIC epithelial ovarian cancer. The median overall survival (OS) by diameter of residual disease

were as follows: 106 months for no gross residual disease; 66 months for 0.5 cm or less; 48 months for 0.6 to 1.0 cm; 33 months for 1 to 2 cm; and 34 months for larger than 2 cm. Aure and colleagues have noted a 5-year survival rate of more than 30% for stage III tumors that were completely resected compared with 10% when resection was incomplete. The impact of cytoreduction for advanced-stage disease is discussed next.

TREATMENT

Borderline Ovarian Tumors: Ovarian Carcinomas of Low Malignant Potential

Approximately 20% of ovarian epithelial cancers are tumors of LMP and usually have an excellent prognosis, regardless of stage. Most studies have been confined to borderline tumors of the serous (see **Fig. 33-2B**) and mucinous (see **Fig. 33-3B**) varieties, which are the most common histologies; however, other epithelial types (see **Table 33-3**) can occur. The cells of these epithelial tumors do not invade the stroma of the ovary. It is extremely important that the ovarian tumor be thoroughly sampled by the pathologist to ensure that a borderline tumor is not mixed with invasive elements. Numerous studies have confirmed that borderline tumors have a slower growth rate than invasive ovarian carcinomas, manifested by prolonged survival (see **Fig. 33-9**).

Surgery is the primary treatment for women with borderline ovarian tumors. The principal objectives of surgery are as follows: (1) diagnosis; (2) fertility-sparing surgery for patients who have not completed childbearing or who are young and have only unilateral ovarian involvement; (3) surgical staging for apparent early-stage disease; and (4) **cytoreductive surgery** for the minority of patients who have obvious advanced-stage disease.

The typical scenario is surgery for an adnexal mass of unknown type. Once the mass is excised, frozen-section examination is a key element in assuring appropriate decision making. If the frozen section suggests a borderline ovarian tumor, considerations for fertility-sparing surgery include the woman's age, her desire for future childbearing, and the degree of involvement of the ovaries—unilateral versus bilateral disease. Options for fertility-sparing surgery include ovarian cystectomy and unilateral adnexectomy. Even with bilateral borderline ovarian tumors, bilateral ovarian cystectomies may be performed, depending on the extent of ovarian disease. Lim-Tan and associates have reported on 33 cases of stage I serous borderline tumors initially treated by cystectomy. Only 3 of 33 patients undergoing cystectomy had recurrence or persistence of borderline tumor and these patients had positive resection margins and/or multiple cysts present in the ovary, emphasizing the effectiveness of conservative operation. However, for most stage IA cases, unilateral adnexectomy is performed and, if the opposite ovary looks normal, no biopsy or wedge resection is done.

Surgical staging for borderline ovarian tumors remains somewhat controversial. The most compelling reason for surgical staging in a woman with borderline tumor on frozen-section examination is the risk of invasive carcinoma on final pathology. For women with pathologically confirmed borderline tumors, the incidence of lymph node involvement is only approximately 5%. Therefore, some investigators have recommended against routine pelvic and para-aortic lymphadenectomy. However, omental and peritoneal biopsies are recommended because peritoneal implants are usually small or microscopic.

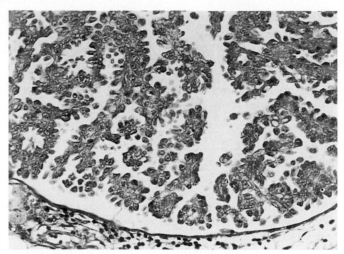

Figure 33-11 Noninvasive implant, epithelial type. Branching papillae and detached clusters of polygonal cells showing moderate cytologic atypicality are present (H&E, ×313). (From Bell DA, Weinstock MA, Scully RE: Peritoneal implants of ovarian serous borderline tumors. Histologic features and prognosis. Cancer 62:2212, 1988.)

For stage I serous borderline tumors, surgery alone is the standard of care because the cure rate associated with this treatment approaches 100% (see **Fig. 33-9**). On the other hand, approximately 30% of women will have peritoneal implants, which are classified as noninvasive (**Fig. 33-11**) or invasive (**Fig. 33-12**). For these women, the recurrence rate associated with noninvasive implants is 20% to 40% and the recurrence rate with invasive implants is 50% to 70%. Unfortunately, no studies to date have convincingly demonstrated any benefit to postoperative therapy for women with stages II to IV disease. Although no standard exists, some oncologists recommend postoperative treatment—paclitaxel-carboplatin chemotherapy or hormonal therapy—only for patients with invasive implants based on the very high risk of relapse.

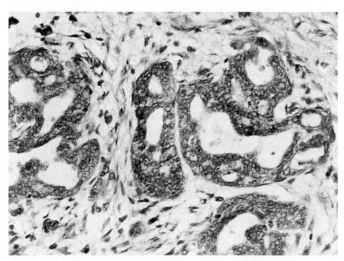

Figure 33-12 Invasive implant. Glands with an irregular contour lined by severely atypical epithelial cells with extensive intraglandular bridging are present (H&E, ×313). (From Bell DA, Weinstock MA, Scully RE: Peritoneal implants of ovarian serous borderline tumors: Histologic features and prognosis. Cancer 62:2212, 1988.)

For women with serous borderline tumors, evidence thus far indicates no significant prognostic influence of microinvasion or lymph node metastasis. The micropapillary pattern is associated with a higher risk of relapse, bilateral ovarian involvement, and invasive implants, but studies to date have not demonstrated a definite survival decrement associated with this variant.

Mucinous borderline tumors also are associated with an excellent prognosis (see **Fig. 33-9**). Hart and Norris have reviewed 97 patients with stage I tumors who were 9 to 70 years of age (median, 35 years). More than 10% of the tumors were discovered during pregnancy or in the immediate postpartum period. Follow-up data were available on 87 of the patients, and there were only three tumor-related deaths during the 5- to 10-year follow-up. The actuarial survival was 98% at 5 years and 96% at 10 years. This was also noted by Bostwick and colleagues, who reported on 109 borderline tumors, 33 of which were mucinous and all of which were stage I, contributing to the good prognosis.

Mucinous borderline tumors include two distinct subtypes, gastrointestinal and seromucinous or endocervical. In the seromucinous type, the association of endometriosis is high (≈40%). They also may have associated microinvasion and lymph node involvement. The prognosis associated with the seromucinous type is excellent. Conversely, the gastrointestinal type may rarely be associated with the condition known as **pseudomyxoma peritonei**, consisting of widespread growth of mucin-producing cells in the peritoneum. The result may be the accumulation of large amounts of mucinous material, which is sometimes associated with recurrent episodes of bowel obstruction. Studies by Young and coworkers have suggested that pseudomyxoma peritonei usually arises in the appendix. The review of Ronnett and coworkers supports a primary appendiceal origin for these tumors and, therefore, appendectomy is indicated for women with an intraoperative diagnosis of a mucinous ovarian tumor. The disease tends to recur and is frequently characterized by repeated laparotomy to relieve bowel obstruction. Chemotherapy and mucolytic agents have been tried but are usually not successful.

For women with newly diagnosed mucinous carcinomas of the ovary, stages II to IV, standard treatment with postoperative paclitaxel/carboplatin has been uniformly unsuccessful. Hence, in late 2010, GOG activated a randomized phase III trial of paclitaxel-carboplatin versus capecitabine-oxaliplatin, which is a regimen used extensively for colorectal cancer. This trial also includes a secondary randomization to bevacizumab or no bevacizumab, resulting in four different treatment groups. It is important to note that a high proportion of women who are diagnosed with advanced-stage mucinous carcinoma of the ovary actually have a gastrointestinal primary tumor metastatic to ovary. Immunohistochemistry testing for cytokeratin 7 and 20 and CDX-2 may be helpful in distinguishing these two origins.

Invasive Epithelial Carcinomas
The primary treatment of ovarian epithelial carcinoma is removal of all resectable gross disease. The woman's abdomen is explored through a vertical incision. If ascitic fluid is present, it is sent for cytologic evaluation; if ascites is not present, 200 to 400 mL of normal saline solution is used to obtain cytologic samples from the peritoneum by irrigating at least the pelvis, upper abdomen, and right and left paracolic gutters before any resection is done.

The diaphragm can be cytologically sampled by scraping the undersurface with a sterile tongue depressor and the sample placed on a glass slide and sprayed with a fixative. Biopsy or, preferably, excision of any suspicious nodules is performed. A total abdominal hysterectomy, bilateral salpingo-oophorectomy, and infracolic omentectomy are performed if technically possible. When there is no gross disease outside the pelvis, para-aortic and pelvic lymph node sampling is recommended, with care taken to remove enlarged nodes. Although the impact of systematic lymphadenectomy has been addressed in one randomized clinical trial by Benedetti-Panici and associates, without significant effect on overall survival, it is reasonable to explore these areas because inspection by palpation is notoriously inaccurate. Evidence suggests that if all gross disease can be resected, the duration of patient survival is enhanced. Although randomized clinical trials have not been performed to document this effect, a meta-analysis of 6885 patients gathered from 81 cohorts has suggested a linear relationship between the degree of cytoreduction and overall survival. In this report, Bristow and colleagues noted that for each 10% increase in cytoreduction, a 5.5% increase in survival was observed. The surgical procedures required to achieve maximal cytoreduction may be extensive and involve splenectomy, diaphragmatic stripping-resection, and posterior exenteration. It may occasionally be necessary to resect bowel to relieve impending obstruction or remove a tumor nodule, thereby eliminating all gross disease from the peritoneal cavity. Heintz and coworkers have noted that prognosis is improved for younger patients (<50 years), those with good initial performance status (Karnofsky score > 80), and those whose disease could be cytoreduced to less than 1.5 cm. Adverse factors were large before initial operation, ascites, and peritoneal carcinomatosis. In a small collaborative GOG study, Hoskins and colleagues have found that those who started with large-volume disease did worse than those who initially had small-volume disease; no survival advantage could be demonstrated for the debulking operation in the large-volume disease group. Chi and associates have noted that those with advanced disease and a preoperative CA-125 level higher than 500 U/mL had less than a 20% chance of an optimal surgical debulking (see later).

One exception to the required removal of the uterus and opposite ovary occurs in the case of well-differentiated (grade 1) ovarian tumors confined to one ovary (stage IA). DiSaia and coworkers have outlined criteria for preserving childbearing function in a young woman with stage IA, grade 1 ovarian epithelial carcinoma, as follows:

1. Tumor confined to one ovary
2. Tumor well differentiated (grade 1), with no invasion of capsule, lymphatics, or mesovarium
3. Peritoneal washings negative
4. Omental biopsy specimen negative
5. Young woman of childbearing years with a strong desire to preserve reproductive function

These criteria can be applied to all types of epithelial ovarian tumors but are more likely to be satisfied in the case of mucinous tumors, which are more frequently well differentiated and unilateral than serous carcinomas. Wedge resection of a normal-appearing contralateral ovary is unlikely to uncover an occult tumor. In these cases, it is reasonable to follow the woman closely with vaginal ultrasonography for any evidence of future ovarian enlargement.

Early-Stage Ovarian Carcinomas
Stage I

The standard therapy for all patients with early-stage ovarian cancer (EOC) includes hysterectomy (usually performed via celiotomy) with bilateral salpingo-oophorectomy. In patients interested in preserving fertility, unilateral salpingo-oophorectomy with preservation of the contralateral ovary and uterus is often feasible. In addition, all patients with early-stage disease should undergo pelvic washings, omental biopsy, cytologic sampling of the surface of the diaphragm, complete bilateral pelvic and para-aortic lymphadenectomy or lymph node sampling, and bilateral biopsies of the paracolic gutters and pelvic peritoneal surfaces. It is important to emphasize that careful assessment of the subdiaphragmatic areas and inspection of the entire peritoneum and the retroperitoneal para-aortic and pelvic nodes are important, particularly in view of the risk of diaphragmatic and nodal spread in higher-grade tumors that initially appear to be at stage I, particularly those on frozen section that appear to be less well differentiated than grade 1.

Le and colleagues have compared a group of patients who underwent minimal staging performed by a general gynecologist with a group of patients who underwent comprehensive staging performed by a gynecologic oncologist. They found the risk of recurrence to be increased for patients operated on by the general gynecologist. Another study by Mayer and associates has shown that patients operated on by a gynecologic oncologist had a 24% improvement in 5-year overall survival.

Rupture of Ovary. Occasionally, during removal, a stage I ovarian carcinoma is inadvertently ruptured (stage IC, **Table 33-6**). There are conflicting opinions as to the potential adverse effects on prognosis. In an analysis of 394 patients, Sjövall and associates found that rupture during surgery did not affect survival, whereas there was marked reduction in survival in that study among those whose ovarian rupture occurred *before* the operation. In general, the spilled fluid and all residual tumor should be removed promptly from the operative field after a rupture (see later discussion). Presumably higher grade and larger tumors are most prone to rupture.

A study by Dembo and colleagues of 519 stage I patients found that adverse factors were grade of tumor, dense pelvic adherence (no invasion but adhesion), or more than 250 mL of ascites. Patients without these features had a 98% 5-year survival rate. It appears that patients with stage I grade 3 tumors should have postoperative therapy, but data are unclear for stage I grade 2 patients.

Minimally Invasive Surgical Staging of Early-Stage Ovarian Cancer. An estimated 15% of women with EOC have early-stage disease at diagnosis. In these patients, comprehensive surgical staging is required to provide accurate prognostic information and plan treatment options. Frequently, the diagnosis of EOC is made incidentally during adnexal surgery for other indications. Because minimally invasive surgical procedures are becoming more common in gynecology and more in demand by the public at large, determining the feasibility and safety of these procedures for the staging of presumed early-stage EOC has become a necessity.

Laparoscopy often leads to a shorter hospital stay, less intraoperative blood loss, and a shorter recovery period than laparotomy. However, surgical staging for EOC requires meticulous inspection of the peritoneal cavity and careful dissection of lymph nodes, vessels, and other abdominal and pelvic structures.

Thus, to assess the feasibility of minimally invasive surgical staging, several issues must be considered, such as the frequency of complications, frequency of conversion to laparotomy, and recurrence rate following laparoscopic staging. Several recent studies have attempted to address these issues.

Tozzi and coworkers have retrospectively identified 24 patients with FIGO stage IA or IB ovarian or fallopian tube cancer who underwent comprehensive laparoscopic staging over a 7-year period. Initially, 42 patients were eligible to enter the study, but ultimately 18 were excluded because of conditions requiring conversion to laparotomy. Of the remaining 24 patients, 13 were undergoing primary staging and 11 were undergoing completion staging. Comprehensive surgical staging was performed according to FIGO guidelines. The authors encountered no intraoperative complications. The mean operating time was 176 minutes. The mean number of pelvic lymph nodes collected was 19.8 and the mean number of para-aortic lymph nodes collected was 19.6. One patient developed a postoperative complication (chylous ascites). At a median follow-up time of 46.4 months, the progression-free survival rate was 91.6% and the overall survival rate was 100%. However, 7 of 24 patients were found to have BOTs, which may have skewed the follow-up data in favor of improved survival. Although small, this study demonstrated that laparoscopic surgical staging of early-stage ovarian cancer is safe and feasible for primary and completion staging when staging guidelines are followed.

Shortly after this study, GOG reported their findings on the feasibility of completion laparoscopic staging for women with incompletely staged ovarian, fallopian tube, primary peritoneal, and uterine cancers; 73 patients had ovarian, fallopian tube, or primary peritoneal cancer and 17 patients required a laparotomy because of adhesions (13), complications (3), or macroscopic metastatic disease (1). Eleven patients were excluded on the basis of pathology, insufficient documentation of comprehensive staging, or patient refusal. In all, 58 patients underwent comprehensive minimally invasive surgical staging with a centralized review of surgical video or photographs for confirmation of staging adequacy. The authors found that women who underwent laparoscopy had significantly less estimated intraoperative blood loss and a shorter hospital stay than women who underwent laparotomy. The two groups had equivalent operative times and numbers of pelvic and para-aortic lymph nodes obtained. Despite the high rate of conversion to laparotomy, relatively high complication rate, and lack of follow-up data on disease progression and overall survival, the authors concluded that minimally invasive surgical staging is feasible for early-stage ovarian, fallopian tube, and primary peritoneal cancer. However, concerns remained about complications and long-term outcomes.

Colomer and colleagues have identified 20 patients who underwent laparoscopic staging for presumed EOC; 19 patients were successfully staged laparoscopically and there was one conversion to laparotomy because of lumbar vein injury. There were no other complications. Consistent with the literature, 4 of 17 patients (23.5%) who underwent primary surgery elsewhere had their disease upstaged following comprehensive surgical staging. During a median follow-up period of 24.7 months, there was only one recurrence in a woman whose disease was upstaged to stage IIIC, but who insisted on conservative surgery to preserve fertility. Nezhat and associates have performed a retrospective review of 36 patients who underwent laparoscopic staging for presumed early-stage ovarian and fallopian tube carcinoma from 1995 to 2007. Of the 36 patients, 20 were diagnosed with invasive EOC, 11 with BOTs, and 5 with nonepithelial tumors. There were no intraoperative complications but there were four postoperative complications (one partial small bowel obstruction managed conservatively, two lymphoceles, and one lymphocele cyst requiring drainage). The mean number of pelvic lymph nodes obtained was 14.8 and the mean number of para-aortic lymph nodes obtained was 12.2. Of the 9 patients who underwent completion staging, 7 (77.8%) had their disease upstaged. During a mean follow-up of 55.9 months, there were three recurrences in patients who underwent conservative surgery and the overall survival rate was 100%. Jung and coworkers have conducted a retrospective review to evaluate the feasibility and efficacy of laparoscopically assisted staging surgery for ovarian cancer in 24 patients with ovarian or fallopian tube cancer. There were no conversions to laparotomy and no intraoperative complications. The only postoperative complication was a port site metastasis. Ten patients (41.7%) had their disease upstaged. The mean number of pelvic lymph nodes obtained was 22.5 and the mean number of para-aortic lymph nodes obtained was 11. Interestingly, the mean hospital stay was 10.6 days, which was attributed to differences in practice patterns in Korea. Despite the small sample sizes and relatively short follow-up period in some of these studies, overall survival is excellent and recurrences are few. It appears that minimally invasive surgical staging of presumed EOC is safe and effective when performed by a trained gynecologic oncologist.

Adequacy of Minimally Invasive Surgery Compared with Laparotomy for Staging of Ovarian Neoplasms. Important concerns have been raised about laparoscopic staging for ovarian neoplasms, including concerns about the adequacy of the lymph node dissection, differences between laparoscopy and laparotomy in operative time, postoperative complications, and postoperative recovery. In a retrospective review of 20 laparoscopic staging cases and 30 laparotomy staging controls, Chi and colleagues have found no differences between the two groups in pelvic or para-aortic lymph node counts, omental specimen size, or complications. Although there were no complications in the laparoscopy group, there were three minor complications in the laparotomy group (two wound infections and one postoperative ileus). The laparoscopy group had a significantly longer operative time (321 versus 276 minutes; $P = .04$) but significantly less blood loss (235 versus 367 mL; $P = .003$) and a shorter hospital stay (3.1 versus 5.8 days; $P < .001$).

More recently, Park and associates conducted a retrospective review of 52 consecutive patients staged by laparoscopy (19) or laparotomy (33). They limited their study to patients with apparent EOC and excluded patients with BOTs. The laparoscopic group had a significantly shorter operative time, less blood loss, less need for blood transfusion, shorter postoperative course, faster return of bowel function, and shorter interval from surgery to adjuvant chemotherapy. There were no differences between the two groups in the number of total, para-aortic, or pelvic lymph nodes retrieved and the size of the omentum resected. During a median follow-up time of 17 months in the laparoscopy group and 23 months in the laparotomy group, there were no recurrences.

Data on the application of robotic surgery for ovarian cancer staging are scant. There are only case reports or series in the literature that have documented the experience with ovarian carcinoma and robot-assisted laparoscopy. A number of reports have included ovarian cancer in their case series analysis and reported on 1 to 64 patients, with no subgroup analysis.

Stage II

Stage II ovarian cancer is initially treated by removal of all gross disease, including the uterus, tubes, and ovaries, and an omentectomy (infracolic) is performed. The pelvic and para-aortic nodes are sampled.

Postoperative Management for Stages I and II

Recommendations for postoperative or adjuvant therapy generally have evolved around the identification of patients in whom a sufficient risk of recurrence is observed. The precision to make this assessment is low and has been based on morphologic features such as grade, histology, and presence of rupture and residuum. Historically, several modalities have been evaluated alone and in combination by prospective studies of unselected patients, including chemotherapy, radiation therapy, IP radiocolloids, and immunotherapy. Guthrie and coworkers have evaluated 656 patients treated for epithelial ovarian carcinomas that had been totally excised. Most carcinomas were stage I or II, and patients were randomly assigned to receive postoperative treatment of radiation therapy alone, chemotherapy alone, radiation therapy and chemotherapy, or no postoperative therapy. Follow-up was for at least 2 years. Approximately 20% of the tumors were borderline malignancies and the rest were invasive carcinomas. Perhaps surprisingly, the lowest frequency of death or recurrence was noted in the group receiving no postoperative therapy (2%), whereas in the other groups, the death or recurrence incidence was 14% to 17%. Thus, this study has shown no benefit for adjuvant therapy and highlights the need for careful case selection and pathologic review. In addition, because survivorship of low-stage cancer is better, long-term follow-up is necessary to tease out the merits of intervention.

Two large multicenter trials have been conducted and were combined for analytical purposes to address this issue. The International Collaborative Ovarian Neoplasm 1 (ICON1) and Adjuvant ChemoTherapy in Ovarian Neoplasm (ACTION) trials compared platinum-based chemotherapy with observation in patients after surgery with EOC. The two trials differed somewhat in patient eligibility with ICON1 predominantly enrolling postoperative stages I and II patients with limited staging and ACTION enrolling postoperative stage IA and IB, grades 2 and 3, stages IC to IIA, all grades, and clear cell tumor patients. Overall, 925 patients were collectively enrolled (477 in ICON1 and 448 in ACTION) and followed for a median 4 years. The overall survival rate at 5 years was 82% in the chemotherapy arm and 74% in the observation arm (HR, 0.67; 95% CI, 0.5 to 0.9; $P = .001$). Recurrence-free survival at 5 years was also significantly higher in the chemotherapy arm compared with observation (HR, 0.64; 95% CI, 0.5 to 0.82). In select patients, platinum-based therapy appears to improve survival and lower recurrence at 5 years over observation. In all, three randomized clinical trials have addressed platinum-based chemotherapy versus observation in EOC. These three trials were recently evaluated via meta-analysis to assess the role of adjuvant chemotherapy. As expected, the combined data mirror the results of the two larger studies with regard to the impact of adjuvant chemotherapy (HR, 0.71; 95% CI, 0.53 to 0.93) on 5-year survival. However, when subcategorized by surgical staging, this benefit

retained significance only in the group in whom nonoptimal staging was performed. These data highlight the importance of accurate surgical staging information when devising an appropriate postoperative treatment plan.

Young and colleagues have conducted two randomized studies of adjuvant therapy for patients with stage I disease. The first study showed that those with stage IA, grades 1 and 2, had 5-year survival rates more than 90% and did not benefit from adjuvant alkylating agent chemotherapy. The second study showed comparable results for adjuvant ^{32}P and platinum-based therapy for a higher risk cohort, including stage I, grade 3, as well as completely resected stage II cases. The assessable cohort included 229 randomized patients. The cumulative incidence of recurrence at 10 years was 29% lower for those receiving chemotherapy compared with ^{32}P (28% versus 35%; $P = .15$) but was not statistically significant. The recurrence risk in this cohort of patients was substantial—all stage I, 27%, and stage II, 44%. Inadequate distribution and small bowel perforation are cited as reasons that ^{32}P is less desirable as adjuvant therapy. Piver and associates have reported 93% 5-year survival for stage IC or stage I, grade 3, patients who received multiagent chemotherapy containing cisplatin. Vergote and coworkers have analyzed 313 patients treated with ^{32}P after the primary operation or second-look operation (see later). Bowel complications occurred in 22 (7%) and 13 required operation. Bolis and colleagues have reported two randomized trials comparing ^{32}P and chemotherapy with cisplatin, 50 mg/m^2, for six cycles. Stages IA and IB grades 2 to 3 and stages IC showed significantly reduced relapse rates in the cisplatin arms. Unfortunately, a survival advantage was not demonstrated, and those who had a recurrence after receiving chemotherapy did worse than those who received ^{32}P.

When indicated, the most frequently used modality is now chemotherapy, although the ideal regimen and number of courses needed are still debated. Bell and associates have reported the results of a GOG randomized study comparing three and six cycles of adjuvant paclitaxel and carboplatin for women with stages IA and IB, grade 3, all stage IC, clear cell tumor, and completely resected stage II epithelial ovarian cancer. The study was powered for a 50% or greater decrease in recurrence for six cycles of therapy. A total of 457 patients were recruited; 344 were alive a median of 6.8 years since entry. The overall treatment effect is a nonsignificant 24% reduction in recurrence for the six-cycle arm (HR, 0.76; 95% CI, 0.51 to 1.13; $P = .18$). The improved impact on estimated recurrence at 5 years was 5% and there was no difference in overall survival between the arms. Approximately one third of patients in both arms had stage II disease. Forest plot analysis by stage did not demonstrate any alteration in the study's conclusions in this cohort. Although no difference was observed in this trial, many investigators have questioned the pretreatment statistical goals and have continued to recommend six cycles of therapy in patients with early-stage disease requiring treatment. A post hoc analysis of the survival results by histology raises the hypothesis that six cycles of therapy may benefit patients with serous histology to a different degree than the others included in the trial. It also should be noted that the carboplatin dose used in this trial was AUC 7.5.

A follow-up study by the GOG (protocol 0175) has been recently reported addressing the role of maintenance therapy in this setting. Women with the same eligibility as GOG 157 were randomized to three cycles of paclitaxel and carboplatin (AUC 6) followed by normal surveillance or 24 infusions of low-dose

($40 \ mg/m^2$) weekly paclitaxel. The study was powered to address a 43% reduction in the risk of recurrence and enrolled 542 patients. The stage distribution was 71% stage I; 80% of patients randomized to the maintenance arm received all assigned therapy. Toxicity was similar between the two arms. The HRs for progression-free survival (PFS) and OS were 0.81 (95% CI, 0.56 to 1.15) and 0.78 (95% CI, 0.52 to 1.17), respectively. Subgroup analysis demonstrated no effect by stage, histology, or grade. There was remarkable consistency between the two GOG studies in the 5-year survival recorded by the three-cycle cohort. Although the optimal treatment is still not known, high-risk, early-stage patients clearly benefit from therapy.

Primary Cytoreductive Surgery

Most patients with ovarian cancer present with disease that has spread beyond the pelvis and into the upper abdomen. The routine recommendation for patients with advanced disease who are surgical candidates is to perform a total abdominal hysterectomy, bilateral salpingo-oophorectomy, complete omentectomy, and resection of all visible tumor. Bristow and colleagues have performed a meta-analysis of studies describing surgery in patients with advanced ovarian cancer. It was shown that the strongest predictor of improved median survival was the proportion of patients undergoing optimal cytoreductive surgery.

Aletti and associates have sought to estimate the effect of aggressive surgical resection on the survival of epithelial ovarian cancer patients. They found that the 5-year disease-specific survival rate was markedly better for patients operated on by surgeons who were most likely to use radical procedures than for patients operated on by surgeons who were least likely to use radical procedures (44% versus 17%; $P < .001$). Also, the rate of optimal resection was 84% for the surgeons most likely to use radical procedures compared with 51% for the surgeons least likely to use radical procedures, highlighting the value of extensive surgical effort.

Eisenkop and coworkers have applied a numeric ranking system to quantify the extent of disease at five intra-abdominal sites before cytoreduction. They used this system in patients with advanced epithelial ovarian cancer to investigate the effect of the extent of disease prior to surgery on survival, as well as the effect of the completeness of primary cytoreduction on survival. They found that the completeness of cytoreduction has a more significant influence on survival than the extent of metastatic disease present before surgery. They went on to suggest that the extent of an operative effort should be determined by the woman's medical status and her potential to tolerate an extensive operation, as well as by operator capability and experience, rather than by the location and extent of disease present at the initiation of cytoreductive surgery.

In a recent study, Zivanovic and colleagues have evaluated the impact of upper abdominal disease (UAD) cephalad to the greater omentum on surgical outcomes for 490 patients with stage IIIC ovarian, fallopian tube, and primary peritoneal cancers. Patients were divided into three groups according to the amount of disease in the upper abdomen. Group 1 was defined as no disease in the upper abdomen, group 2 as having tumors smaller than 1 cm, and group 3 as having bulky disease, larger than 1 cm. The authors found that optimal cytoreduction was achieved in 81%, 63%, and 39% of patients in groups 1, 2, and 3, respectively. In the largest study of postoperative tumor residuum and outcome, resection to no visible intraperitoneal disease was substantially related to progression-free and overall survival. The study population ($N = 3126$) was generated from three randomized phase III trials assessing primary chemotherapy regimens in advanced stage disease patients. Median overall survival was 99.1 months for patients with no postoperative tumor residua compared with 36.2 months for those with visible disease 1 cm or smaller and 29.6 months in those with more than 1 cm of tumor residua.

Diaphragmatic Stripping or Resection

At initial surgical exploration, diaphragmatic disease may be the largest volume metastatic disease. Unfortunately, the presence of diaphragmatic disease is one of the most common factors precluding optimal tumor reduction surgery. Large diaphragmatic metastases were cited as a significant barrier to optimal tumor-reductive surgery by 76% of the members of the Society of Gynecologic Oncologists in a study reported by Eisenkop and associates. In that same study, only 24% of those surveyed used diaphragm resection and 30% reported not being experienced with the procedure. Aletti and coworkers have evaluated the therapeutic value of diaphragmatic surgery in patients with advanced ovarian cancer and found that patients who underwent diaphragmatic surgery (stripping of the diaphragm peritoneum, full- or partial-thickness diaphragm resection, or excision of nodules) had an improved 5-year overall survival rate relative to patients who did not undergo diaphragmatic surgery (53% versus 15%, $P < 0.0001$).

Splenectomy

For optimal cytoreductive surgery, a splenectomy may be required if there is disease involving the hilum, capsule, or parenchyma of the spleen. Magtibay and colleagues have evaluated 112 patients who underwent splenectomy as part of primary or secondary cytoreductive surgery. They found that the most common indications for splenectomy were direct metastatic involvement (46%), facilitation of an en bloc resection of perisplenic disease (41%), and intraoperative trauma (13%). In that same study, the authors found that 65% of patients had hilar involvement, 52% capsular involvement, and 16% parenchymal metastases. Interestingly, patients with disease directly involving the splenic parenchyma did not have a worse prognosis than patients with disease involving the splenic hilum or capsule.

Hepatic Resection

The clinical significance of hepatic parenchymal metastasis on survival in patients with advanced ovarian cancer has been studied. Lim and coworkers have recently reported on a series of patients with hepatic parenchymal metastases. In this series, patients underwent wedge resection, segmentectomy, or hemihepatectomy as part of their tumor reductive surgery. The 5-year PFS and OS rates for patients with stage IIIC disease and patients with stage IV disease and hepatic parenchymal metastasis from peritoneal seeding were 25% and 23% and 55 and 51%, respectively. The authors advocated that complete hepatic resection should be attempted for patients with hepatic parenchymal metastasis.

Bowel Resection

Because ovarian cancer often presents with confluent tumor in the cul de sac, rectosigmoid resection—along with or en bloc with hysterectomy and bilateral salpingo-oophorectomy—is often necessary to achieve complete tumor resection in the pelvis. This results in high rates of optimal cytoreduction, with acceptable morbidity. An average of 26% of women with ovarian cancer undergo colon resection as part of their primary cytoreductive operation according to a study by Aletti and colleagues. Richardson and associates have noted that almost all women undergo primary colorectal anastomosis without a protective ostomy, with an average leak or fistula rate of 2.1% and a mortality rate of 0.8%. When metastatic ovarian cancer involves the transverse colon, it has been shown by Bristow and coworkers that a transverse colectomy can contribute significantly to a maximal ovarian cancer cytoreductive surgical effort, with acceptable morbidity. When the colonic involvement is multifocal, a subtotal colectomy with an ileorectostomy or cecorectostomy is usually an excellent option.

Retroperitoneal Lymphadenectomy

Whether systematic removal of retroperitoneal lymph nodes should be part of optimal cytoreductive surgery had been a topic of debate for many years. We now have evidence that systematic lymphadenectomy in patients with grossly uninvolved lymph nodes provides no benefit to the woman. A recent prospective randomized trial by Benedetti-Panici and colleagues has shown that systematic lymphadenectomy improves PFS but not OS in women with optimally debulked advanced ovarian cancer. In addition, the median operating time was longer (300 versus 210 minutes; $P < .001$) and the percentage of patients requiring blood transfusions was higher (72% versus 59%; $P = .006$) in the systematic lymphadenectomy arm. An ongoing randomized trial of systematic lymphadenectomy versus no further dissection is being conducted in stages II to IV patients in whom complete cytoreduction has been otherwise achieved at the point of primary cytoreduction. The primary end points of the LION (**L**ymphadenectomy **i**n **O**varian **N**eoplasms) study are OS, PFS, and quality of life.

Postoperative Therapy for Advanced Epithelial Carcinomas (Stages III and IV)

For historical interest, early adjuvant therapy attempts in advanced disease included single-agent and combination chemotherapy regimens based on the alkylating agents. A limited number of responses were observed, and treatment frequently continued for 1 to 3 years. With the discovery of cisplatin (and carboplatin, subsequently), several randomized trials were conducted comparing platinum and platinum combinations with nonplatinum regimens. These pivotal trials secured platinum as the agent of choice in primary adjuvant therapy, which continues to this day. In addition, several clinical trials have established that little additional benefit to treatment is observed beyond four cycles of therapy. Most recently, the development of the taxanes has documented the importance of this agent (see later). By convention, six to eight cycles of combination platinum- and taxane-based therapy are now recommended as adjuvant therapy for most patients with advanced disease.

The pivotal trial establishing the importance of paclitaxel in primary ovarian cancer management was reported by McGuire and associates on behalf of the GOG. They conducted a randomized trial comparing cisplatin, 75 mg/m^2, with cyclophosphamide, 750 mg/m^2, or paclitaxel, 135 mg/m^2, over 24 hours and demonstrated a survival advantage in the paclitaxel arm. All patients had residual tumors larger than 1 cm after the primary operation. Response rates were improved with paclitaxel relative to control in patients with measurable disease (73% versus 60%). The median PFS was 18 months in the paclitaxel arm compared with 13 months in the platinum arm ($P < .001$). OS was similarly improved (38 versus 24 months; HR = 0.6; 95% CI, 0.5 to 0.8; $P < .001$).

The results of this study were confirmed in similar randomized clinical trials conducted worldwide. The taxane-platinum combination was generally considered to be the recommended first-line therapy for ovarian cancer. The platinum analogue carboplatin was found to be less nephrotoxic and neurotoxic and easily administered without prehydration, thus shortening the time of infusion. After several randomized clinical studies demonstrating the equivalence of this agent to cisplatin in ovarian cancer, carboplatin was substituted for cisplatin in taxane-based regimens. In addition, paclitaxel infused over 3 hours was found likely to be equivalent to paclitaxel infused over 24 hours and, in combination with carboplatin, enabled the combination to be given on an outpatient basis. Phase III studies by Ozols and coworkers have shown that paclitaxel-carboplatin is a feasible outpatient regimen with less toxicity than paclitaxel-cisplatin and is associated with equivalent survival.

It should be noted that carboplatin is quantitatively excreted by the kidney and its effective serum concentration can be calculated from a formula based on the woman's glomerular filtration rate (GFR). This can be determined by various methods but is generally estimated by calculating the creatinine clearance. The Calvert formula is most commonly used and determines a total dose by this formula:

$$\text{Carboplatin, total dose} = \text{desired AUC} \times (\text{GFR} + 25)$$

AUC-based dosing is preferred for carboplatin because the AUC most accurately reflects observed dose-specific toxicity and is more reliable across patients than dosing based on the body mass index. A usual dose for carboplatin is calculated for AUC values of 5.0 to 7.5. Both paclitaxel and platinum compounds are neurotoxic, as noted by Warner, and this is often the dose-limiting toxicity. The taxane, docetaxel, was found to be potentially less neurotoxic than paclitaxel. Vasey and colleagues have reported a large phase III study comparing docetaxel and carboplatin with paclitaxel and carboplatin in patients with stages IC to IV ovarian cancer. Almost identical survival parameters were observed between the two agents. The docetaxel arm was significantly less neurotoxic; however, it was associated with more myelosuppression. Neurotoxicity, as evaluated by several objective measures, returned to parity several months after treatment. Granulocyte colony-stimulating factor is occasionally needed to reduce the duration of significant neutropenia in these regimens. A commonly used regimen is paclitaxel, 175 mg/m^2 over 3 hours, or docetaxel, 75 mg/m^2 over 1 hour, and carboplatin (AUC = 5 to 6) given as a 1-hour infusion every 3 weeks. Premedication is required for both taxanes to combat hypersensitivity reactions, which have been attributed to the taxane itself and the carrier vehicle required to make these agents water-soluble. In addition, steroid administration is necessary after treatment for docetaxel to combat fluid retention and effusion, a complication that may occur in as many as 25% of patients without prophylaxis.

Alterations in Frontline Treatment Strategies

Although the preferred sequence in primary advanced ovarian cancer management is surgery followed by chemotherapy, several authors have attempted to take advantage of the disease's intrinsic chemosensitivity to improve outcomes in patients with extensive disease. Two avenues have been pursued:

- **Neoadjuvant chemotherapy**, in which, following biopsy or limited surgery, chemotherapy is administered for a reduced number of cycles (usually three to four) and an operation is planned for removal of the primary tumor (if present) and residual metastases; and
- **Interval cytoreduction**, when an unsuccessful maximal attempt at cytoreduction is followed by a reduced number of chemotherapy cycles (usually three to four), followed by a second cytoreduction attempt.

Both strategies are followed by three to four cycles of chemotherapy after surgery. This latter strategy has been evaluated in randomized clinical trials with conflicting results; the former was evaluated in a recent randomized evaluation.

Neoadjuvant Chemotherapy

Neoadjuvant chemotherapy is practiced as an alternative for patients thought to have substantial operative risk or preoperative disease distribution that could preclude optimal cytoreduction. Several authors have noted the potential benefits to this strategy, including the opportunity to allow for an improvement in performance status, decreasing operative morbidity through less extensive surgery, and increasing the opportunity to achieve an optimal result. Each of these goals has been demonstrated in small, single-institution retrospective and prospective studies. For example, in a series of 85 women treated with either neoadjuvant chemotherapy ($n = 57$) or primary cytoreduction ($n = 28$), Morice and associates reported a significant decrease in major morbidity, defined as morbidity requiring a second operation (7% versus 36%; $P = .01$). Survival in this trial was similar between the cohorts, although with wide confidence limits.

Schwartz has reported on 59 women undergoing neoadjuvant chemotherapy and compared their surgical morbidity with 206 patients treated in the same time period by a standard approach. They found that patients in the former group have shorter intensive care unit stay and postoperative hospital stay compared with conventional patients. Both groups received platinum-based chemotherapy. Because patients in these small trials are selected for treatment based on presenting disease volumes or medical status, it has been difficult to determine whether there is a detriment to survival by this approach. Clearly, patients too infirm to be operated on gain from this approach because if they have chemoresistant disease, surgery would have little value and likely would hasten an adverse outcome. Conversely, patients able to undergo the procedure could have a poorer outcome because there could be further expansion of a large population of resistant clones by delaying cytoreductive disease.

Loizzi and coworkers have reported a case-control study of neoadjuvant chemotherapy in 60 patients (30 in each group). Patients were matched 1:1 based on date of diagnosis, histology, and stage. They documented that although the neoadjuvant cohort was older and represented a poorer performance status, these patients underwent optimal cytoreduction at a favorable rate (76% versus 60%) and, following platinum-based chemotherapy, had similar PFS and OS compared with the control cohort. A critical question to be answered in this methodology is one of biology, which can only be addressed in a prospective clinical study of potentially operable patients. Fortunately, two trials are ongoing to address this question, one of which was recently reported. In this prospective multi-institutional study, 668 evaluable patients were randomized to primary cytoreduction followed by six cycles of platinum-taxane chemotherapy or three cycles of neoadjuvant platinum-based therapy followed by interval cytoreduction and three additional cycles of therapy. Patients were diagnosed by biopsy before randomization. Only 10% of patients randomized to interval surgery did not undergo the procedure because of the uncommon event of primary platinum and taxane resistance. Optimal cytoreduction (to <1 cm or to no visible disease) was statistically higher in the neoadjuvant therapy arm. This arm was also associated with lower postoperative morbidity. However, no difference was observed in PFS (HR, 0.99; 95% CI, 0.87 to 1.13) or OS (HR, 0.98; 95% CI, 0.85 to 1.14). Low rates of primary optimal cytoreduction and relatively low absolute median survivals observed in this study have been raised as criticisms. Fortunately, confirmatory trials are underway.

Interval Cytoreduction

Cytoreductive surgery performed after an initial failed attempt or in patients who were initially not considered candidates for cytoreductive surgery is referred to as interval cytoreductive surgery. A prospective trial by van der Burg and colleagues was published in 1995 that evaluated the benefit of interval surgery after suboptimal primary cytoreduction. They compared patients treated with three cycles of cisplatin and cyclophosphamide, followed by interval cytoreduction and three additional cycles of the same chemotherapy ($n = 140$) with patients treated with the same chemotherapy without undergoing interval cytoreduction ($n = 138$). The results showed that patients who underwent interval surgery had a significant advantage in median survival time compared with patients who did not undergo interval surgery (26 versus 20 months, respectively; $P = .012$).

Rose and colleagues published a prospective trial in 2004 evaluating the role of interval cytoreduction. In this trial, GOG conducted a randomized phase III study involving 550 patients with stage III and IV EOC who had residual disease of more than 1 cm after an initial attempt at primary cytoreductive surgery. All patients received three cycles of initial chemotherapy in the form of cisplatin and paclitaxel. Eligible patients were randomly assigned to undergo interval cytoreductive surgery followed by chemotherapy ($n = 216$) or chemotherapy alone ($n = 208$). Protocol compliance was good; only 7% of the patients who were randomly assigned to undergo interval cytoreductive surgery did not undergo surgery. Among patients who were randomly assigned to receive chemotherapy alone, 3% had interval cytoreductive surgery. It was found that PFS did not significantly differ between the two groups (HR, 1.07; 95% CI, 0.87 to 1.31; $P = .54$). In addition, there was no significant difference in the relative risk (RR) of death for patients undergoing interval cytoreductive surgery compared with chemotherapy alone (RR, 0.99; 95% CI, 0.79 to 1.24; $P = 0.92$).

Additions to the Paclitaxel and Carboplatin Backbone

It has been postulated that agents with nonoverlapping cross resistance mechanisms or alternative mechanisms of action may be complementary opportunities in primary ovarian cancer patients

Figure 33-13 GOG-182 trial that randomized 4312 patients to one of 4 experimental arms against paclitaxel and carboplatin. (Adapted from Bookman MA, Brady MF, McGuire WP, et al: Evaluation of new platinum-based treatment regimens in advanced-stage ovarian cancer: A Phase III Trial of the Gynecologic Cancer Intergroup. J Clin Oncol 27:1419-1425, 2009.)

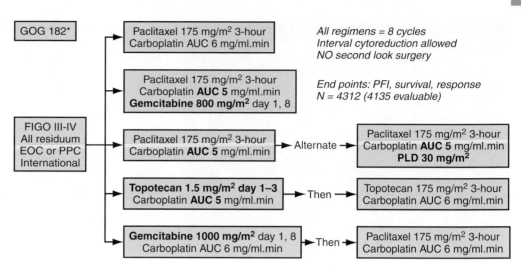

to improve the therapeutic index. Several trials have been recently completed, with mixed results. The prevalent strategy has been to add to platinum and taxane therapy or substitute another agent for paclitaxel. The largest trial reported to date is GOG-182, which randomized 4312 patients to one of four experimental arms against paclitaxel and carboplatin. Two of the experimental arms involved a three-drug strategy (adding gemcitabine or pegylated liposomal doxorubicin to paclitaxel and carboplatin, with the latter triplet given every other course) and two others substituted topotecan or gemcitabine for paclitaxel for four of the eight planned cycles in a sequential administration design (**Fig. 33-13**).

Although considered a highly successful trial in terms of global participation and recruitment, the trial failed to improve outcomes by any parameter (response, PFS, or OS). However, as anticipated, the three-drug regimens were more toxic. Two other trials, the MITO-2, which randomized patients to an experimental regimen with carboplatin and pegylated liposomal doxorubicin, and OVAR9, which randomized patients to an experimental arm of paclitaxel, carboplatin, and gemcitabine, also failed to demonstrate superiority to this strategy. It is unclear whether the addition or substitution of available cytotoxic agents in this setting will improve outcomes in primary disease, given the probability for overlapping toxicities.

Based on emerging efficacy data regarding angiogenesis inhibition on ovarian cancer response and prevention of progression, several trials were launched with the agent bevacizumab. GOG 218 included two experimental arms with bevacizumab—one arm also administered bevacizumab as a maintenance agent for 16 21-day cycles following primary therapy and the other experimental arm administered only placebo in maintenance. ICON7 is a two-armed trial in which bevacizumab is administered with chemotherapy at half the dose of GOG 218 (7.5 mg/kg), but for 12 cycles in maintenance after administration with paclitaxel and carboplatin for five or six cycles. The trials have important differences (**Table 33-10**). Both have reported meeting their primary end point, PFS, but OS data are immature. In GOG 218, the improvement in PFS over control paclitaxel and carboplatin was seen only for arm 3, in which bevacizumab was administered with chemotherapy and in the maintenance setting. There was no difference in PFS for arm 2 compared with control.

Table 33-10 Comparison of GOC-0218 and ICON7 Study Characteristics

	Trial	
Parameter	**GOG-0218**	**ICON7**
Setting and design	Double-blinded, placebo-controlled	Open-label
	Three-arm study	Two-arm study
	Bevacizumab for 16 cycles (maintenance)	Bevacizumab for 12 cycles
	Bevacizumab dose, 15 mg/kg/3 wks	Bevacizumab dose, 7.5 mg/kg/3 wks
Patient population	Stage III (suboptimal)	Stage I or IIA (grade 3/clear cell histology)
	Stage III (optimal, visual or palpable)	Stages IIB-IV (all)
	Stage IV	
Additional end point	OS analysis (formal testing at time of PFS)	Defined final OS analysis (end 2012)
	Independent radiology review (IRC)	No IRC

The HR for PFS arm 3 versus arm 1 was 0.717 ($P < .001$); the HR for PFS, arm 2 versus arm 1, was 0.908 ($P = .16$) and corresponded to median durations of 10.3, 11.2, and 14.1 months, respectively. The anticipated HR for ICON7 was 0.78, which was observed, but details of this study have not been released.

Additional studies of other molecules targeting one or more processes of angiogenesis as well as novel targets, such as the folate receptor, are being pursued in this setting.

Intraperitoneal Therapy

One promising but relatively old strategy that has been investigated is chemotherapy given by the IP route. Ovarian cancer appears to be IP-friendly because the distribution of disease is largely confined to this space, the pharmacokinetics of drug delivery are favorable, and the tumor is considered chemosensitive. Early experience with IP administration of chemotherapy has documented that it could be used to control ascites. Pharmacologic studies in the 1970s and 1980s demonstrated favorable profiles of relatively high direct drug exposure (high C_{max} and AUC) for a number of agents subsequently identified to be

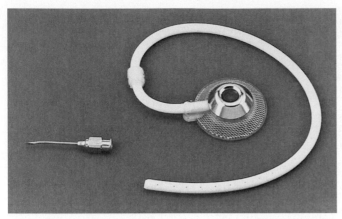

Figure 33-14 Peritoneal catheter with access port for infusion of drugs (Port-A-Cath, Pharmacia Deltec, St. Paul, MN.)

important for ovarian cancer treatment. In this regard, platinum (cisplatin and carboplatin) and taxanes (paclitaxel and docetaxel) have been shown to have superior pharmacokinetic profiles when delivered into the peritoneum directly compared with IV administration.

Currently, administration is done principally via an implantable vascular access device placed during surgery or subsequent minilaparotomy (**Fig. 33-14**). A number of phase I and II clinical studies have been performed in the past 4 decades to document safety of the strategy and suggest efficacy. This led to the performance and reporting of more than eight randomized clinical studies formally evaluating the efficacy of IP-based chemotherapy compared with IV-based chemotherapy in patients with advanced-stage ovarian cancer. A meta-analysis of these studies has been published and concluded that the route of administration "has the potential to improve cure rates from ovarian cancer." Similarly, the National Cancer Institute has issued a clinical announcement accompanying the publication of a large GOG study stating that the IV and IP regimen "conveys a significant survival benefit among women with optimally debulked epithelial ovarian cancer, compared to intravenous administration alone." In this latter study, patients with stage III epithelial ovarian cancer rendered optimal (defined as postsurgical disease residual < 1 cm) were eligible for randomization to standard IV cisplatin and paclitaxel (24-hour infusion) or to IV paclitaxel (135 mg/m^2 on day 1), IP cisplatin (100 mg/m^2 on day 2), and IP paclitaxel (60 mg/m^2 on day 8). This was the first phase III study to include IP paclitaxel in primary ovarian cancer therapy. Both cohorts were to undergo repeat cycles every 21 days for six total infusions. The primary end points were PFS and OS, and reassessment operations, if planned, were indicated at randomization.

This study was also the first to evaluate formally the impact of treatment on health-related quality of life. Assessment was made at baseline after the third cycle, after treatment completion, and 12 months after treatment completion. Overall, 415 eligible patients comprised the study population. Both PFS and OS were significantly improved in the intent to treat IP cohort (HR$_{PFS}$ = 0.80; 95% CI, 0.64 to 1.00; HR$_{Death}$ = 0.75; 95% CI, 0.58 to 0.97, respectively). The recorded median overall survival of 65.6 months is among the longest ever observed in an adjuvant therapy phase III ovarian cancer study. The results are even more impressive given that most (58%) randomized

IP patients did not complete all six cycles of their assigned therapy via IP administration. This was largely because of significant differences in hematologic and nonhematologic toxicities associated with the IP regimen. Leukopenia and thrombocytopenia were significantly more common in the IP arm, as were pain (11-fold increase), fatigue (fourfold increase), fever (2.5-fold increase), and metabolic (fourfold increase), renal (threefold increase), infection (2.5-fold increase), neurologic (twofold increase), and gastrointestinal (twofold increase) events, among others. In addition, almost one in five (40 of 205 patients) randomized IP patients experienced a catheter failure necessitating treatment discontinuation. A detailed assessment of IP catheter complications in this trial has been published. A clear profile for catheter malfunction risk was not identified, although timing and accompanying surgical procedures were closely scrutinized. In a reflection of these observed adverse events, health-related quality of life assessments were significantly lower throughout the trial but returned to parity 12 months after therapy. It was concluded that the IP regimen provides superior survival efficacy and is associated with significant but manageable toxicity. The authors encouraged the use of IP therapy in clinical practice. Unfortunately, toxicity concerns and a number of unanswered fundamental questions regarding efficacy (e.g., optimal agent, schedule, future trial designs) and the impact of alternative agents such as biologic therapies (e.g., vascular endothelial growth factor and epidermal growth factor targeting) have limited the general acceptance of this strategy in the clinical community without subsequent information. Clinical investigation with alternative agents such as docetaxel and carboplatin have completed phase I feasibility studies; phase III studies with the antiangiogenesis agent bevacizumab are currently ongoing.

Dose-Dense Chemotherapy

One additional strategy, dose-dense and dose-intense chemotherapy, has received attention based on positive results recently reported in primary ovarian cancer patients. The trial, conducted by the Japanese Gynecologic Oncology Group and published in 2009, randomized 631 patients to standard paclitaxel (180 mg/m^2) and carboplatin (AUC 6), or weekly paclitaxel (80 mg/m^2/wk) and carboplatin (AUC 6), for six to nine cycles. The dose density (measured in mg/m^2/wk) was 33% greater in the experimental arm. Despite just 62% of patients receiving six or more cycles of the dose-dense strategy (versus 73% in the control arm) the median PFS was 28.0 versus 17.2 months (HR, 0.714; P = .0015). OS, although early, also demonstrated a significant difference, with 3-year OS in the experimental arm at 72.1% versus 65.1% in the control arm (HR, 0.75; P = .03). This strategy is the subject of ongoing phase III studies with similar designs, addressing IP infusion, and with the addition of bevacizumab.

Evaluation of Chemotherapy Results

Chemotherapy is usually administered every 3 weeks. The patient is monitored with careful physical examination, blood tests to measure hematologic, liver, and kidney function, and radiographic studies, such as chest radiography, ultrasound or, usually, CT of the abdomen and pelvis. Granulocyte colony-stimulating factor is added as needed to combat neutropenia. Mild neutropenia after chemotherapy can be managed expectantly but, for the patient who develops severe neutropenia with fever and an absolute neutrophil count of less than 500 cells/mL, antibiotics are prescribed to prevent septic complications.

If tumor is suspected on CT scan, fine-needle biopsy can frequently document the presence of persistent or recurrent disease. A negative CT scan, however, does not guarantee complete clinical response. Goldhirsch and coworkers have noted that 5 of 26 patients with tumor nodules larger than 1 cm have negative CT scans, and the examination is most effective (80%) for detecting metastasis in retroperitoneal nodes. In 1989, Reuter and colleagues reported improved results of 8% false-negatives using newer equipment, with CT slices at 10- to 15-mm intervals. Patsner has reported that 24 of 60 patients with negative CT scans have a positive **second-look operation**, calling into question the value of this imaging study. Vaginal ultrasonography is particularly useful to assess the pelvis. CA-125 levels are used to monitor the course of the woman with carcinoma. As noted, Buller and colleagues have calculated that the CA-125 level follows an exponential regression curve in successfully treated patients. This provides the possibility of mathematically estimating the patient's response to chemotherapy early in treatment. Bridgewater and associates have reported that a greater than 50% decrease in the CA-125 level is a good sign of clinical response.

Second-Look Procedures

Second-look laparotomy was introduced in the late 1940s as a method of assessing disease status after primary therapy in patients with colon cancer. In the 1970s, the same procedure was introduced for the treatment of epithelial ovarian cancer. In the field of gynecologic oncology, the rationale for using second-look surgery was that the optimal duration of chemotherapy was unknown (at the time) and the second-look procedure allowed surgeons to decide the optimal duration of exposure to alkylating agents for their patients. The primary concern with prolonged exposure to alkylating agents was the potential for secondary malignancies. Ideally, a second-look procedure would be able to identify the presence or absence of disease, which would help guide subsequent management.

The goal of second-look surgery is to perform a comprehensive surgical reassessment in a woman who is clinically free of disease—that is, a woman with no evidence of disease on physical examination, no evidence of disease on imaging studies, and a normal serum CA125 level. The diagnostic validity of second-look surgery is dependent on random sampling of the abdominopelvic cavity peritoneum; second-look surgery is not intended to be a curative procedure. It is important to note that more than 50% of patients diagnosed with stage III epithelial ovarian cancer have clinical evidence of disease at the time of second-look surgery. In addition, even in patients who have no evidence of disease at the time of second-look surgery, the risk of recurrence is more than 50%.

Greer and coworkers have performed a nonrandomized comparison in patients undergoing second-look laparotomy or clinical follow-up after receiving six cycles of combination chemotherapy with paclitaxel plus cisplatin or carboplatin. The study evaluated patients entered on protocol GOG 158; all patients were required to undergo optimal cytoreduction surgery prior to trial entry. The researchers demonstrated that second-look surgery was not associated with longer survival (in the context of a nonrandomized study). Therefore, second-look surgery should only be performed in the setting of a clinical trial.

If a second-look laparotomy is performed, it is important to extensively sample the peritoneal surfaces and lymph nodes.

Particular attention is paid to areas that contained residual disease at the conclusion of the initial surgical procedure. Many patients with a negative second-look operation eventually develop recurrent disease. Early studies of a second-look laparotomy have shown that approximately half (range, 25% to 75%) of patients thought clinically and radiographically to be free of disease actually had persistent disease at a second-look operation. Walton and colleagues have shown that patients who initially have stage I or II disease rarely have positive second-look procedures; they recommend that the operation not be done for those with low-stage tumors, a result confirmed by Sonnendecker. Favorable factors for a negative second-look operation are low tumor grade, no residual disease after primary operation, young age (<55 years), and rapid regression to normal of increased CA-125 values during chemotherapy.

Maintenance Therapy

Unfortunately, many patients develop recurrent disease, even after a negative second-look operation. Rubin and associates have noted a high rate of recurrence (45%) in patients with a negative second-look laparotomy. Those initially with higher stage and higher grade tumors are more likely to recur after a negative second-look operation. However, those who were disease-free at 5 years are likely to remain disease-free at subsequent follow-up. Nonetheless, this high recurrence risk has prompted several authors to consider additional treatment at the identification of a complete response to primary treatment. This is often termed *maintenance* or *consolidation therapy*, although the former term is favored, given that the decision for treatment is based on the effect of primary therapy. Several randomized and nonrandomized clinical trials have been conducted in this arena, including hormones, vitamins, radiation therapy, chemotherapy, radioimmunoconjugates, immunotherapy, vaccines, gene therapy, biologic therapy, complementary medicines, and holistic approaches. Unfortunately, all have been negative in regard to improving overall survival. However, one randomized study did show an improvement in PFS. Markman and coworkers have studied whether 3 or 12 additional months of paclitaxel could influence time until progression in women who had achieved a complete clinical remission after primary treatment. The trial was designed to accrue 450 patients; however, at a planned interim analysis (after 277 patients were randomized), a statistically significant benefit for the longer treatment was demonstrated, which closed the trial to further accrual. The initial report demonstrated a 7-month improvement in median PFS (28 versus 21 months; $P = .0035$); a later report with long follow-up confirmed these earlier results (median PFS, 21 versus 14 months; $P = .006$). No effect on survival was demonstrated, however. As noted, the addition of a maintenance biologic agent such as bevacizumab improved PFS relative to placebo, but the effect on overall survival remains to be seen. Several additional biologic agents are entering phase III in this setting. Although the long-term administration of chemotherapy in this setting is impractical because of mounting toxicity, the agents targeting biologic processes raise the question of administration duration. Theoretically, the high percentage of recurrence, coupled with the cytostatic potential of these newer biologically targeted agents, suggests that prolonged administration could be advantageous. However, cost, toxicity, and potential adverse effects on tumor biology are relevant remaining questions, which rival those of overall survival.

Cancer Antigen125 Surveillance after Primary Therapy

Because patients with advanced ovarian cancer frequently have CA-125 values that pace tumor response and progression during therapy, a common practice for monitoring patients following therapy involves serial CA-125 level determinations. The supposition is that earlier identification of recurrent disease can be better controlled by earlier initiation of therapy. To formally address this hypothesis, the European Organisation for Research and Treatment of Cancer (EORTC) has conducted a randomized phase III trial in which women in complete clinical remission following primary surgery and chemotherapy were enrolled into a blinded surveillance program. Follow-up visits were scheduled every 3 months, when an examination was performed and blood was taken for CA-125 level assessment. All registrants were blinded to their CA-125 values during this time. However, when an individual's CA-125 level rose to twice the upper limit of normal, they were randomized 1:1 to unblinding of the result (early) or continued blinded surveillance (delayed). In this latter group, intervention was determined by the development of clinical or symptomatic relapse. Postprogression therapy was determined by local standards of care. The primary end point of the study was overall survival. In all, 1442 patients were registered, of whom 529 were randomly assigned to the treatment groups. Patients unblinded and made aware of their rising CA-125 values generally started treatment immediately, 4.8 months (median) before those in the delayed group. After a median follow-up of almost 57 months from randomization and 370 deaths, there was no difference in overall survival between the arms (HR, 0.98; 95% CI, 0.8 to 1.2). Median survival in the early treatment group was 25.7 months compared with 27.1 months in the delayed group. For patients receiving third-line therapy, the time differential to initiation was almost the same as the time differential to initiation of second-line therapy (median 4.6 months). Interestingly, a first deterioration in Global Health score occurred significantly sooner in the early treatment group. The authors concluded that no benefit in survival is gained by treatment dictated solely by asymptomatic rise in CA-125 level and challenge the practice of routine biomarker surveillance in this setting.

Although practice standards may individually change on the basis this new information, counseling patients to watchful waiting is a challenge in the setting of rising CA-125 level without measurable recurrent disease. An alternative approach in this setting has been the use of hormonal therapy, such as tamoxifen. GOG has recently completed a randomized clinical trial (GOG protocol 198) to address the impact of tamoxifen and thalidomide in women with significantly elevated CA-125 levels in the absence of measurable recurrent disease following primary therapy. Eligible patients had stage III or IV histologically confirmed epithelial ovarian, fallopian tube, or peritoneal primary cancer and a post-treatment CA-125 level exceeding twice the upper limit of normal in the absence of Response Evaluation Criteria In Solid Tumors (RECIST) 1.0 measurable disease. The primary end point of the trial was to compare PFS and OS between the two treatment arms and assess toxicity. At study closure, 139 women were randomized to oral thalidomide, 200 mg daily, with escalation to a maximum of 400 mg or tamoxifen, 20 mg orally twice daily. High-grade toxicities (grades 3 and 4) were experienced more frequently in the thalidomide arm (55% versus 3%), with randomized patients experiencing more constitutional, somnolence, and pulmonary toxicities.

There were more venous thromboembolism and gastrointestinal toxicities in the tamoxifen arm, but these were infrequent (<1.5%). The risk for progression was similar between the cohorts (HR, 1.31; 95% CI, 0.92 to 1.85) but the risk for death was significantly higher in the thalidomide arm (HR, 1.76; 95% CI, 1.16 to 2.68). Of interest, the time to measurable progression on tamoxifen was 4.5 months (versus 3.2 months for thalidomide), but mirrors the lead time to symptomatic progression in patients blinded to their rising CA-125 level observed in the EORTC trial (4.8 months). Appropriate therapy for patients with rising CA-125 levels in the absence of measurable disease has yet to be determined.

Recurrent Ovarian Cancer Management

Unfortunately, as many as 70% of patients who present with advanced staged disease, will exhibit recurrent or persistent disease after primary treatment. These women may have prolonged survival despite developing recurrence; however, they are rarely cured. Because of this, treatment is generally considered palliative and must balance efficacy with toxicity. The choice of therapy is largely empirical; the treatment plan usually involves several agents in sequence, depending on treatment history, observed and expected toxicity, and performance status. Surgery, chemotherapy, immunotherapy, radiation therapy, biotherapy, and hormone therapy are options, alone and in combination, in this cohort of patients. It is not uncommon for a woman to undergo five or more different chemotherapy regimens, including cycles of retreatment with one or more agents. This characteristic is reflective of the increasing number of agents available for use, short duration of response, and general health of those receiving therapy.

Although there are few specific treatment guidelines as to how recurrence should be approached, initial consideration is most often guided by the interval of time until recurrence is identified. Patients are categorized as potentially platinum-sensitive, -resistant, or -refractory based on the length of time from the completion of primary therapy until recurrence is identified. By convention, patients exhibiting a treatment-free interval of 6 months or longer are considered as having potentially platinum-sensitive disease. Those who achieved a complete response and were identified with recurrence under this benchmark are considered platinum-resistant and those who did not achieve a complete response or had disease progression during frontline therapy are considered platinum-refractory. In reality, the probability for subsequent chemotherapy response likely represents a continuum based on this interval of time. However, clinically, the arbitrary division is used frequently to make treatment decisions.

Platinum-Refractory Disease

Patients who fall into this designation have very difficult disease to treat because their objective response to almost all available agents is low and the duration of any individual therapy is short. The choice of therapy depends on the woman's wishes and comorbidities. Because expectations for response to standard agents are low, these women are good candidates for investigative clinical studies, in which new agents with alternative mechanisms of action or targets are being evaluated. Under these expectations, some patients may opt to continue active treatment, whereas others may choose supportive care.

Table 33-11 Clinical Efficacy of Cytotoxic Agents in Platinum-Resistant and Platinum-Sensitive Ovarian Cancer Toxicity

Agent	Response Rate (%)		Principal Toxicity
	Platinum-Resistant	Platinum-Sensitive	
PLD	14-20	28	PPE, mucositis
Topotecan	14-18	33	Myelosuppression
Hexamethy-Imelamine	10-18	27	Nausea, vomiting
Gemcitabine	16		Myelosuppression
Etoposide	27	35	Myelosuppression, leukemia
Ifosfamide	12		Hemorrhagic cystitis, CNS
Tamoxifen	10-15	10-15	Hot flashes, thromboembolic
Docetaxel	22-25	38	Myelosuppression
Paclitaxel	12-33	20-41	Myelosuppression
Vinorelbine	21	29	Myelosuppression

CNS, Central nervous system neurotoxicity; PLD, pegylated liposomal doxorubicin; PPE, palmar-plantar erythrodysthesia.

Platinum-Resistant Disease

Patients demonstrating an abbreviated initial response to front-line therapy represent cohorts who are unlikely to respond well to platinum retreatment. This is not to imply that some of these patients would not respond to retreatment with a platinum compound, just that the probability of response would be no greater than with any other agent and potentially lower. A current recommendation for most of these patients is to consider an alternative nonplatinum agent for the first treatment of recurrence. **Table 33-11** lists the potential agents for treating these patients, their respective response rates, and significant common toxicities. Patients achieving stable disease or better are usually treated until the agent no longer demonstrates a clinical benefit or toxicity precludes further infusion.

Platinum-Sensitive Disease

Patients in whom disease recurrence is identified more than 6 months after front-line treatment completion are considered potentially platinum-sensitive. These patients are good candidates for retreatment with platinum or a platinum-based combination regimen. In many cases, this combination is similar to that received in front-line treatment, paclitaxel and carboplatin. However, other two-drug and three-drug combinations have been investigated. A limited number of phase III studies have been conducted in this setting, but only one has demonstrated an overall survival advantage for the use of a taxane- and platinum-based regimen. The ICON4-AGO-OVAR 2.2 study randomized 802 women with recurrent ovarian cancer to paclitaxel and platinum or a nontaxane platinum regimen. Objective response was 66% in the taxane arm compared with 54% in the conventional arm ($P = 0.06$). PFS was significantly improved (12 versus 9 months; HR, 0.76; 95% CI, 0.66 to 0.89), as was OS (29 versus 24 months; HR, 0.82; 95% CI, 0.69 to 0.97). Approximately 75% of women in both groups had a treatment-free interval of at least 12 months and 64% were taxane-naïve at randomization. These are important factors when considering the study's conclusions. In all, six phase III clinical trials in platinum-sensitive patients have been completed. They differ substantially by agents investigated, sample size, use of measurable patients, prior exposure to paclitaxel and platinum in front-line therapy, and median progress-free interval prior to registration. Each of these factors has important consequences in regard to the data reported, making cross-trial comparisons among experimental groups hazardous. **Table 33-12** summarizes the key features of these trials. It is noteworthy that two of these efforts included the use of nonplatinum agents in potentially

Table 33-12 Phase III Trials in Patients with Platinum-Sensitive Recurrent Disease

Control	Experimental	No. of Patients	TTP/PFS (wk)	P	OS (wk)	P	Comments
Carboplatin	Carboplatin Epirubicin	190	65 versus 78	NS	109 versus 122	NS	TFI = 17 mo; grade 4 ANC, 45%; T RBC, 30%, Plt, 25%
Platinum*	Platinum Paclitaxel	802	43 versus 52; HR, 0.76	<.001	104 versus 130 HR, 0.82	0.023	TFI (75% > 12 mo); neuro 1% versus 20%; infection, 17%; hematologic, 46% versus 29%
Carboplatin	Carboplatin Gemcitabine	356	23 versus 35 HR, 0.72	<.001	75 versus 78	NS	TFI? (60% > 12 mo); RR: 31% versus 47% (0.0016) ANC, PLT more common in combination
Carboplatin, paclitaxel	Carboplatin PLD	976	41 versus 49 HR, 0.82	.001 (noninferiority) 0.005 (superiority)	PEND	—	TFI: Nonhematologic, 37% versus 29%; HSR, 19% versus 6%; grade 2-3 PPE, 2% versus 12%
Topotecan	Topotecan/ VP-16 Topotecan-gemcitabine (TG)	502	HR, 0.84 HR, 0.84	NS NS	HR, 1.13 HR, 1.07	NS NS	TFI? (64% > 12 mo) More hematologic toxicity, less alopecia in TG arm
PLD	PLD Trabectedin	672	25 versus 32 HR, 0.79	0.019	PEND, 6-12 mo	PLD	TFI? (32% > 12 mo); effect seen only in PS cohort; HFS less in combination; ANC, LFT

*This arm was mostly single agent platinum, however, platinum combinations were also allowed.

platinum-sensitive patients, according to the definition provided earlier. These are important trials to consider given the high rate of drug hypersensitivity (platinum or taxane), intolerance, and lack of a clear benefit between platinum-containing and non–platinum containing agents in patients with moderate platinum-sensitive disease, such as those recurring between 6 and 12 months after primary therapy. Currently, only the combination of gemcitabine and carboplatin is approved for use in patients with platinum-sensitive recurrent disease in the United States.

Secondary Cytoreduction

The recurrence rate in patients with advanced epithelial ovarian cancer ranges from 50% to 90%. Therefore, secondary cytoreductive surgery might be a viable treatment option for a select group of patients. Because patients with long treatment-free intervals have disease that is considered potentially chemotherapy-sensitive, investigators have evaluated the role of surgery in this setting as well. Although there is some inconsistency in the definition of **secondary cytoreduction** procedures, the specific intent in this setting is resection of disease at recurrence, with the intent of debulking. The treatment of recurrent epithelial ovarian cancer is variable and dependent on a number of important criteria, which are evaluated at the time of diagnosis of the recurrence. These include but are not limited to the time from completion of initial adjuvant therapy, site of disease, number of disease sites, and the woman's performance status. There is ample evidence in the literature that patients with platinum-resistant disease (recurrent disease within 6 months of completing platinum-based treatment) do not benefit from secondary cytoreductive surgery

No randomized trials have been conducted to identify a clinical benefit in this setting. However, several prospective and retrospective reports have suggested that only patients with extended treatment-free intervals and those who achieve a complete resection (no visible residual) benefit from the procedure. Tay and coworkers have conducted a multivariate analysis for survival on 46 women undergoing secondary cytoreduction for disease recurrence. They identified that only time to recurrence of 24 months or longer and resection to no visible residual as independent predictors of survival. The optimal resection rate in this study was 41%. Eisenkop and colleagues have conducted a prospective study of 106 patients identified with recurrence 6 months or longer from primary treatment. In this study, 82% of the patients were rendered free of visible tumor. In their multivariate analysis, four variables were found to be independent predictors of survival: disease-free interval, residual disease after secondary surgery, administration of chemotherapy before secondary surgery, and size of recurrent tumor. They concluded that complete resection can be obtained in most select patients and should be considered before the administration of second-line chemotherapy.

A study by Tebes and associates has sought to determine the impact of several preoperative characteristics on survival after secondary cytoreductive surgery in patients with recurrent EOC. The two preoperative factors that correlated with improved survival were a disease-free interval of longer than 12 months and residual disease after primary surgery of tumor smaller than 2 cm. The investigators also found that optimal resection to less than 1 cm of residual disease was achieved in 86% of patients who had a secondary cytoreduction. Small bowel and colon resection for cytoreduction was performed in 7% and 51% of patients, respectively. Operative complications occurred in 14% of patients and postoperative complications occurred in

21%. The median survival of patients with optimal cytoreduction was 30 months compared with 17 months for patients with residual disease of ≥ 1 cm or larger ($P < .05$).

The AGO study also reported their efforts in establishing (DESKTOP I trial) and validating (DESKTOP II trial) a panel of features that would reliably predict optimal (no visible disease) secondary surgical outcomes in women with platinum-sensitive disease. They found, as did others, that only complete surgical cytoreduction was associated with an improved OS and that this could be reliably achieved (>67% of the time) in patients who had a performance status of 0 or 1, were early stage, or had no visible tumor residuum following initial surgical cytoreduction and the absence of ascites.

Because patients with a high probability for response to platinum-based therapy are often considered candidates for secondary surgery, the impact of the surgical procedure on survival is a paramount question that heretofore has only been addressed in series biased to patients most likely to benefit from the procedure. Fortunately, two phase III trials are currently underway to address this question in patients with platinum-sensitive disease. GOG protocol 213 is evaluating the role of secondary cytoreductive surgery in patients with recurrent, platinum-sensitive ovarian cancer and the merit of adding an antiangiogenic agent (bevacizumab) to a combination of carboplatin and paclitaxel. In addition, this study will evaluate the usefulness of maintenance bevacizumab until progression relative to control. DESKTOP III is using the triage tool discussed earlier to identify patients likely to undergo complete surgical resection and randomizing them to surgery versus no surgery. Adjuvant therapy is not specified in this trial, but both are focused on overall survival as their primary end point.

Targeted Therapy

The processes that govern cell transformation and immortalization, tumor growth, and metastases for ovarian cancer are complex and nonuniform. Nonetheless, several critical targets have been identified that appear to be differentially expressed in tumors cells relative to normal cells. Novel agents that target disruption or inhibition of these specific processes have been incorporated into the care of ovarian cancer patients. The most developed of these are agents that disrupt the signals to engender new vessel growth and development or angiogenesis. This process appears critical for a tumor to continue its growth beyond 8 mm^3. A number of cytokines have been described that tip the balance to sustained angiogenesis, but the most potent is vascular endothelial growth factor (VEGF). Prognostically, VEGF expression has been documented in all **stages of ovarian cancer** and has been correlated with impaired survival. VEGF overexpression has also been directly associated with ascites formation. This clinical feature is the result VEGF-induced endothelial hyperpermeability. The compound furthest in development for the treatment for ovarian cancer is bevacizumab, which has been investigated for primary and recurrent ovarian cancers (see earlier). However, a number of agents targeting VEGF, its receptors, the epidermal growth factor receptor family, the phophatidylinositol-3-kinase (PI3K)/Akt/mTor pathway, and other cellular signaling pathways are also under investigation. In addition, new cytotoxics with alternative mechanisms of action, such as the tubulin poisons, new topoisomerase inhibitors, an agent that binds the minor groove of DNA (trabectedin) have been under phase III investigation.

Clearly, the spectrum of treatment likely available to women with this disease in the future will require some rational parameters for their use. Thus, detailed tumor profiling and tumor biomarkers will likely help customize treatment on an individual basis.

Poly (ADP-Ribose) Polymerase Inhibitors

Preclinical data have recently demonstrated the extreme sensitivity of *BRCA*-deficient cells to inhibition of the single-strand repair enzyme poly (ADP-ribose) polymerase (PARP). Inhibition of the PARPs leads to an accumulation of single-strand DNA breaks, which can lead to double-strand breaks at replication forks. Normally, these breaks are repaired through homologous recombination, in which the *BRCA* genes play a major role. However, synthetic lethality occurs when these genes themselves function improperly because of mutation or silencing. This has prompted the clinical development of a new class of novel therapeutics, the PARP inhibitors, which theoretically holds promise for patients whose tumors rely on PARP for continued cell growth.

To test this hypothesis and to evaluate the safety of the first drug in this class, olaparib, a phase I dose escalation clinical trial was conducted to examine the pharmacokinetic and pharmacodynamic effects in patients with cancers refractory to standard therapy. Given the mechanism of action of olaparib, the population was enriched for patients with *BRCA1* or *BRCA2* mutations. Overall, 60 patients were recruited to the trial, including 22 who carried a *BRCA1* or *BRCA2* mutation and one with a strong family history of *BRCA*-related cancer. The dose of olaparib ranged from 10 mg daily, administered for 2 or 3 weeks, to 600 mg twice daily, continuously. At the two highest dose levels, dose-limiting toxicities were observed. This led to a compromised dose of 200 mg twice daily, which was studied in a second cohort of *BRCA1* and *BRCA2* patients only. In general, the agent was well tolerated, with primary toxicities of somnolence, mood alteration, and fatigue. The toxicity profile was not increased in the *BRCA* subpopulation. Analysis of PARP function by pharmacodynamic studies has demonstrated rapid and high-level inhibition within the recommended dosing levels. In support of the hypothesis, objective antitumor activity (63% complete or partial response plus stable disease) was seen only in *BRCA* mutation carriers.

Olaparib has few side effects relative to conventional chemotherapy, inhibits PARP, and has antitumor activity only in patients with *BRCA* germline mutations. A recent phase II study in *BRCA* carriers has also been conducted, enrolling patients into two consecutive dosing cohorts. Overall, response rates were similar to those observed in the phase I study, with notable activity (>25%) in patients with platinum-resistant disease. Rates of discontinuation caused by adverse events were uncommon in both dosing cohorts. Currently, a number of PARP inhibitors are entering clinical investigation and are expanding eligibility to include patients whose tumors may harbor *BRCA* deficiency (so-called *BRCA*ness). Sophisticated technologies to identify patients with germline or somatic *BRCA* mutations in tumor tissue are being used in these trials and, if validated, may greatly expand the number of patients for whom PARP inhibitors may be helpful.

Complications and Other Considerations
Malignant Effusions

Pleural effusions are a common and devastating complication of advanced malignancies. Women with ovarian cancer frequently develop ascites, hydrothorax, or both, requiring repeated drainage by paracentesis or thoracentesis. In the vast majority of cases, malignant pleural effusion is associated with an incurable disease, with high morbidity and mortality. For the same reason, several studies have argued in favor of a palliative approach, rather than a conventional curative approach for treatment of this condition. Occasionally, sclerosing solutions are used in the thoracic cavity to prevent the reaccumulation of fluid, with resultant adherence of the pleural surfaces. New modalities, such as pleuroscopy and long-term indwelling pleural catheters, offer cost-effective outpatient or minimal hospital stay and less discomfort.

In a review by Musani and associates, it was reported that several mechanisms have been proposed to explain the development of malignant effusion. The inability of the parietal pleura to reabsorb pleural fluid because of the involvement of mediastinal lymph nodes by tumor is likely the most common cause of malignant pleural effusion. Therefore, tumors that involve the mediastinal lymph nodes, such as lung cancer, breast cancer, and lymphoma, are responsible for most malignant pleural effusions. Other possible mechanisms include direct tumor invasion, as is sometimes seen in lung cancer, chest wall neoplasms, breast cancer, and ovarian cancer, as well as hematogenous spread to the parietal pleura.

There are several options for therapy, such as thoracentesis, chemical pleurodesis with chest tubes, video-assisted thoracoscopy (VATS), pleuroperitoneal shunts, and chronic indwelling pleural catheters. The advantage of a thoracentesis largely relies on the rapid relief of symptoms; however, it is unfortunately often associated with reaccumulation of fluid, multiple procedures and hospital visits, and associated complications, such as pneumothorax or reexpansion pulmonary edema. The option of chemical pleurodesis offers the advantage that it is highly effective; however, this treatment may be associated with required hospitalization and high cost. The VATS procedure is also highly effective and can be a diagnostic procedure in addition to a therapeutic procedure. The disadvantages are its cost, invasiveness, and its contraindication for patients who cannot tolerate single-lung ventilation. A pleuroperitoneal shunt may be considered in patients who have recurrent reaccumulation of fluid and those who have failed pleurodesis. However, this approach is not practical for patients with advanced or recurrent ovarian cancer because disease in these patients often also causes significant ascites. The option of a chronic indwelling catheter is ideal for patients who have recurrent episodes of reaccumulation of the pleural effusion. This approach is minimally invasive, cost-effective, and successful. One of the major disadvantages is the risk for infection and the fact that the woman must be motivated to learn how to drain; otherwise, a family member or visiting nurse is required for home drainage.

A number of strategies have been studied in prospective trials. Most efficacious for problematic pleural effusion is pleurodesis with a sclerotic agent (e.g., talc slurry, antibiotic), decortication, or placement of an infusion catheter that can be operated by the woman. A systematic review has been conducted by Tan and coworkers. Symptomatic ascites can also be problematic because few sclerodesis or surgical decortication-type procedures are available for long-term care. It is also not uncommon for patients to develop implants of tumor in the subcutaneous tissues after aspiration. Numnum and colleagues have reported some success using bevacizumab as an adjuvant for this problem.

Malignant Bowel Obstruction

Intestinal obstruction is a common complication in patients with advanced epithelial ovarian cancer and is estimated to occur in 25% to 50% of patients. The onset of bowel obstruction is rarely an acute event. In cancer patients, compression of the bowel lumen develops slowly and often remains partial. Obstruction can result from partial or total occlusion of the bowel lumen or from alteration of the normal peristaltic motion. The initial symptoms are often abdominal cramps, nausea, vomiting, and abdominal distension that present periodically and resolve spontaneously.

Contrast radiography may help in defining the site and extent of the obstruction. Although barium may provide excellent radiographic definition, it is not absorbed well and may cause severe impaction. Diatrizoate meglumine and diatrizoate sodium solution (Gastrografin) is ideal for this type of contrast radiography because it offers similar radiographic definition and, in certain cases, may restore the intestinal transit. Abdominal CT is usually recommended because it can provide information about the location of the obstruction and the extent of disease. Surgical options may be offered to the woman, depending on a number of factors that dictate the success of surgical management. These include the site of obstruction, number of obstructions along the small or large bowel, number of prior chemotherapy regimens, prior episodes of bowel obstruction, nutritional status of the woman, and her overall functional status.

Pothuri and colleagues have reviewed a series of patients undergoing surgery for intestinal obstruction caused by recurrent epithelial ovarian cancer and found that the mean time from original diagnosis of epithelial ovarian cancer to obstruction was 2.8 years. Surgical correction (intestinal surgery performed to relieve the obstruction) was achieved in 84% of cases and successful palliation (the ability to tolerate a regular or low-residue diet by 60 days after surgery) was achieved in 71% of cases. The median survival in patients with successful palliation was 11.6 versus 3.9 months for all other patients. Major surgical morbidity was documented in 22% of patients. Interestingly, postoperative chemotherapy was administered to 79% of patients for whom surgical correction was possible. The authors noted that with respect to quality of life, it is important to consider that 56% of patients undergoing surgery for bowel obstruction had a colostomy or permanent gastrostomy tube. They also recommended that patients are not ideal surgical candidates if they have bulky carcinomatosis, rapidly progressive disease, multiple sites of obstruction, poor performance status, or heavy pretreatment with chemotherapy and radiation.

In patients who refuse palliative surgery or are considered poor surgical candidates, a percutaneous endoscopic gastrostomy (PEG) tube may offer symptomatic relief without the discomfort or complications of a nasogastric tube. The recent study by Pothuri and associates has shown that symptomatic relief (defined as the absence of nausea or vomiting) is achieved in 91% of patients with advanced epithelial ovarian cancer and bowel obstruction within 7 days of placement of a PEG tube. Only 13% of patients had resolution of obstruction and removal of the PEG tube after chemotherapy was administered. The median survival from the date of PEG tube placement was 8 weeks. The complication rate was 18% and the most common complication was leakage. This study also demonstrated that the administration of total parenteral nutrition after PEG tube placement was not associated with a survival benefit. It is important to note that PEG tube placement is feasible for patients with a tumor encasing the stomach, diffuse carcinomatosis, or ascites.

Another potential nonsurgical option for the management of bowel obstruction is the use of metallic stents. These stents are flexible and self-expanding and can be inserted using radiologic or endoscopic techniques. The most important reported complications include local pain, gastric ulceration, gastroesophageal reflux, bleeding, and bowel perforation. Metallic stents are contraindicated in patients with multiple obstructions and peritoneal carcinomatosis. The literature on the usefulness of metallic stents for bowel obstruction in patients with gynecologic cancers is limited.

Immunotherapy

Immunotherapy agents, such as *Corynebacterium parvum* and bacille Calmette–Guérin, have been administered to try to augment the immunologic response and promote tumor resistance in the host. These agents have also been used in combination with cytotoxic chemotherapy; preliminary improved results have been reported. IP immunotherapy approaches have been evaluated with agents such as interferon, lymphokine-activated killer cells, interleukin-2, and tumor necrosis factor. Berek and coworkers have conducted a phase I and II trial of IP cisplatin (60 mg/m^2) and interferon-α (25×10^6 IV) given every 4 weeks. Among 18 patients, there were three complete and four partial responses. Unfortunately, a randomized trial comparing interferon-α with no further treatment in women achieving complete response after primary chemotherapy has shown no benefit. A front-line study of adding interferon-γ to paclitaxel and carboplatin has been completed, with results pending.

The use of monoclonal antibodies as a form of site-directed therapy has been investigated. Epenetos and colleagues have used tumor-associated antigens linked to ^{131}I to treat recurrent ovarian carcinoma. After IP administration to 24 patients, responses were noted primarily in those with small-volume disease, with some responses lasting as long as 3 years evaluated by follow-up laparoscopy. Canevari and associates have noted responses in 3 of 26 patients treated with autologous T lymphocytes targeted with a bispecific monoclonal antibody. Berek and coworkers have reported a phase III study of oregovomab in women achieving a complete clinical response after primary therapy. This novel, murine-derived, immunotherapeutic agent targets the CA-125 antigen. In a placebo-controlled randomized trial, 145 women underwent infusion. The time to relapse was 13.3 months in the treatment arm and 10.3 months in the placebo arm ($P = .71$). Although no benefit was observed, an exploratory analysis identified a subgroup in which this therapy may have a better opportunity for efficacy.

Gene Therapy

The therapeutic impact of gene therapy in ovarian cancer has yet to be totally explored. Although the IP nature of this disease makes it well suited for this approach, various gene- or virus-based gene therapy programs have yielded mixed results at best. Several therapeutic models have been used in early investigations, including replacement of a tumor suppressor gene (e.g., *BRCA* and *P53*), suicide gene therapy, and inhibition of growth factor suppressors and regulators. As noted by Berchuck and Bast, there are a number of obstacles to developing this type of therapy to clinical usefulness. However, intensive investigation has been underway in a few centers to develop efficient and efficacious therapeutic programs.

Chemotherapy Sensitivity Assays

A chemotherapy sensitivity and resistance assay is a laboratory algorithm wherein a sample of human tumor is subjected, under experimental conditions, to various chemotherapeutic agents and concentrations to assess response (tumor survival). Two broad categories of assay intent separate the available technologies, those that evaluate the inhibition of cell growth and those that address chemotherapy-associated cell death. Although these appear similar, they are different in laboratory protocol and may produce vastly disparate results. In most cases, several agents alone and in combination are evaluated. Theoretically, the most active agent or combination could be picked (sensitivity assay) or eliminated (resistance assay) from an empirical program, offering a more precise decision tool. The hypothesis is that differential selection will improve outcome. Although the concept is simplistic and rational, the effects of chemotherapy response and survival are complex and sometimes counterintuitive. It is frequently noted that a limited sample of tissue obtained from the primary or a metastatic site, at primary diagnosis or in recurrence and after previous chemotherapy or radiation exposure, would not necessarily be representative of active disease at any one time. However, Tewari and colleagues have reviewed 119 synchronous and 334 metachronous ovarian primary, metastatic, and recurrent samples and found remarkable consistency in the tumor's drug resistance profile. However, efficacy requires clinical correlation. Loizzi and coworkers have reported a case-control study on 100 recurrent ovarian cancer patients treated by assay or empirical therapy. Overall response (65% versus 35%; $P = .02$), PFS (15 versus 7 months; $P = .0002$), and OS (38 versus 21 months; $P = .005$) were all improved using the assay. Similarly, however, inherent selection bias and treatment overlap necessitate validation by a randomized clinical trial. In 2004, the American Society of Clinical Oncology issued a statement based on an extensive review of global literature and concluded that this technology needs further investigation before widespread adoption. This still represents an area of active research.

Radiation Therapy

As presented earlier, radiation has been used for curative intent in women with early-stage cancer, with some success. Treatment planning involves a field that treats the entire abdomen as well as higher doses to the pelvis. Long-term efficacy must be balanced against uncommon toxicities of therapy, which include gastrointestinal stricture and fistulas and compromise of the bone marrow if chemotherapy is needed subsequently. The modality has also been used to treat recurrent disease. Cmelak and Kapp have treated 41 patients with platinum-refractory ovarian cancer who had undergone secondary cytoreduction. They treated the whole abdomen with 28 Gy and a pelvic boost to 48 Gy. For 28 patients with residual disease smaller than 1.5 cm, the 5-year survival rate was 53%, which is better than would be expected with chemotherapy. However, no large-scale trial data are available for this technique and, because of the risk of complications and lack of extensive data regarding its effectiveness, whole abdominal radiation has generally not been used in these cases. However, localized radiation can be of use in select patients with isolated recurrences or persistent disease after chemotherapy or to manage localized symptomatic disease, such as bone metastases. The development of intensity-modulated radiation therapy has widened the therapeutic index by reducing toxicity to surrounding unaffected tissues.

Summary

Therapy for epithelial ovarian carcinoma is based on the removal of all gross disease and sampling of areas at high risk of spread in the peritoneal cavity and retroperitoneal nodes. Postoperative therapy is used according to the stage and grade of the primary tumor. Multiagent platinum- and taxane-based chemotherapy is frequently used as adjunctive treatment for poorly differentiated tumors, such as stage I, grade 3, or for stage II cases without residual tumor.

For high-stage tumors and for patients with residual disease after initial operation, multiagent chemotherapy, usually paclitaxel and carboplatin, is used. It is accompanied by a number of short- and long-term toxic side effects, but initial response rates in stage III cases may exceed 90%. Five-year survival rates decrease to 30% or less. Long-term randomized trials and the development of new agents will be needed to improve rates of salvage and optimize therapy for epithelial ovarian carcinomas. Currently, second-line chemotherapy offers remission to some patients, but the best response rates are achieved with initial chemotherapy.

SMALL CELL CARCINOMA

Dickerson and colleagues have described a virulent type of ovarian malignancy that occurs in young women, usually between the ages of 15 and 30 years. Because of its histologic appearance, it has been designated a small cell carcinoma. The tumor is often but not always accompanied by hypercalcemia, as noted by Young and associates in an analysis of 150 cases. Most patients have died, although a few stage I survivors have been reported, some of whom have been treated with adjuvant multiagent chemotherapy. Reed has reported a patient with stage IC disease treated with cisplatin, etoposide, and bleomycin who survived 5 years. Benrubi and coworkers have treated a patient with stage II small cell carcinoma with debulking and multiagent chemotherapy followed by radiation; the woman was disease-free for 4 years at the time of the report. Other isolated stage I 5-year survivals have been reported with multiagent chemotherapy programs augmented with subsequent pelvic radiation. However, for advanced-stage disease, and even in most stage I cases, the course of the tumor has been fatal. Harrison and colleagues have reported the findings of the combined experience of the Gynecological Cancer Intergroup, which included 17 patients with small cell carcinoma of the ovary, hypercalcemic type. All patients were initially treated with surgery and platinum-based chemotherapy. Seven also received adjuvant radiotherapy with pelvic and para-aortic radiotherapy or pelvic and whole-abdomen radiotherapy. For 10 stage I patients, 6 received adjuvant radiotherapy, and 5 were alive and disease-free at the time of the report. All but one of the 7 patients with stage III or unknown stage had died.

MALIGNANT MIXED MÜLLERIAN TUMORS (CARCINOSARCOMAS)

These are extremely rare ovarian malignancies that histologically resemble comparable tumors in the uterus. Treatment involves operation for cytoreduction, as noted by Muntz and associates, with added therapy, usually in the form of multiagent chemotherapy.

Stage is a prognostic factor and those with advanced stages usually do not survive.

As noted by Hellstrom and coworkers, approximately 500 of these rare tumors have been reported. In their series of 36 of these cases over 20 years, the median survival was 16.6 months, with a 5-year actuarial survival rate of only 18%. Low-stage tumors and those treated with multiagent chemotherapy (cyclophosphamide, doxorubicin [Adriamycin], cisplatin) had an improved survival. Although there remains some question about the efficacy of postoperative platinum-based chemotherapy for treatment of these tumors, as noted by Bicher and colleagues, this approach continues to be the standard. The most commonly used regimens include the combination of cisplatin plus ifosfamide and the combination of paclitaxel and carboplatin.

GERM CELL TUMORS

These tumors are derived from the germ cells of the ovary. As a group, they are the second most frequent type of ovarian neoplasms and account for approximately 20% to 25% of all ovarian tumors. The classification of **germ cell tumors**, according to the WHO designation, is shown in **Box 33-2.**

The most frequent germ cell tumor is the benign cystic **teratoma** (**dermoid**); overall, only 2% to 3% of germ cell tumors are malignant. Of the malignant germ cell tumors, the most frequent is the **dysgerminoma**, which accounts for approximately 45% of

Box 33-2 Benign Conditions in which CA-125 Level Is Elevated
Endometriosis
Peritoneal inflammation, including pelvic inflammatory disease
Leiomyoma
Pregnancy
Hemorrhagic ovarian cysts
Liver disease

malignant germ cell tumors. Next in frequency are **immature teratomas** and then **endodermal sinus tumors**. In women younger than 30 years, germ cell tumors are the most frequent ovarian neoplasm, and approximately one third of the germ cell tumors found in those younger than 21 years are malignant.

The histogenesis of germ cell tumors has been extensively studied and summarized by Talerman. **Figure 33-15** shows the theoretical histogenesis of these tumors. They are thought to originate from the primitive germ cell and gradually differentiate to mimic the developmental tissues of embryonic origin (ectoderm, mesoderm, or endoderm) and extraembryonic tissues (yolk sac and trophoblast). Germ cell tumors that originate in the ovary have homologous counterparts in the testes—that is, dysgerminoma and seminoma. Germ cell tumors are usually unilateral, except for teratomas and dysgerminomas (see **Table 33-4**). The morphologic and clinical aspects of each of the various types of germ cell tumors are considered separately.

TERATOMAS

Teratomas consist of tissues that recapitulate the three layers of the developing embryo (ectoderm, mesoderm, and endoderm). One or more of the layers may be represented, and the tissues can be mature (benign) or immature (malignant). Chromosomal studies indicate that teratomas appear to arise from a single germ and have an XX karyotype. In the older literature, terms such as *malignant teratoma* and *teratocarcinoma* were used to denote the malignant variety of these tumors, but these terms have been replaced by the nomenclature shown in **Box 33-3.**

Benign Cystic Teratomas (Dermoids)

Benign cystic teratomas are the most common germ cell tumors and account for 25% of all ovarian neoplasms. They primarily occur during the reproductive years but may occur in postmenopausal women and in children. The risk of malignant transformation (see later) is markedly increased if these tumors are found

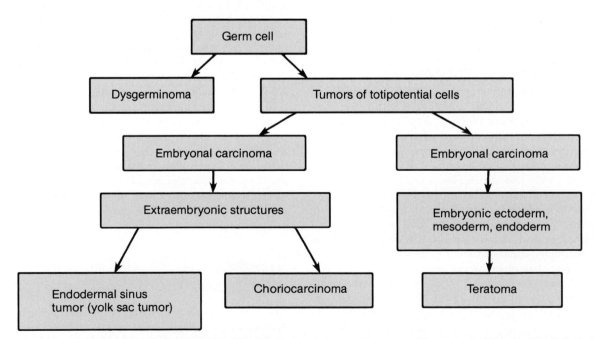

Figure 33-15 Histogenesis of germ cell tumors. (Adapted from Talerman A: Germ cell tumors of the ovary. In Blaustein A [ed]: Pathology of the Female Genital Tract. New York, Springer-Verlag, 1982, pp.)

Box 33-3 World Health Organization Classification of Germ Cell Tumors

Dysgerminoma
  Endodermal sinus tumor
  Embryonal carcinoma
  Polyembryoma
  Choriocarcinoma
  Teratomas
  Immature
  Mature
    Solid
    Cystic
  Dermoid cyst (mature cystic teratoma)

Dermoid cyst with malignant transformation
  Monodermal and highly specialized
    Struma ovarii
    Carcinoid
    Struma ovarii and carcinoid
    Others
  Mixed forms

in postmenopausal women. One of the interesting facets of teratomas is their ability to produce adult tissue, including skin, bone, teeth, hair, and dermal tissue. The presence of calcified bone or teeth allows the tumor to be diagnosed preoperatively by ultrasonography or radiography (**Fig. 33-16**).

Dermoids are usually unilateral, but 10% to 15% are bilateral. The outside wall of the tumor tends to be smooth, with a yellowish appearance caused by the sebaceous fatty material that fills the tumor. Hair is also a prominent feature once the cyst is opened (**Fig. 33-17**). Usually, the tumors are asymptomatic but can cause severe pain if there is torsion or if the sebaceous material perforates the cyst wall, leading to a reactive peritonitis. This rare complication is severe and can occur during pregnancy. Microscopically, a number of adult tissues are seen (**Fig. 33-18**).

Treatment of the reproductive-age woman or child consists of cystectomy or unilateral oophorectomy. In most cases, it should be possible to remove only the cyst and preserve normal ovarian tissue. The technique at open laparotomy is demonstrated in **Figure 33-19**. The opposite ovary should be inspected. If it is grossly normal, nothing further needs to be done. Current treatment involves preservation of the contralateral ovary without any biopsy if it grossly appears normal. In women beyond childbearing years, therapy for a dermoid usually consists of removal of the uterus, both tubes, and the ovaries.

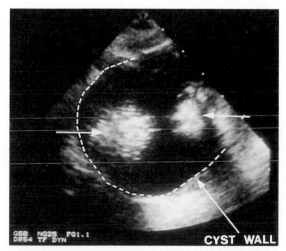

Figure 33-16 Transvaginal ultrasound image of an ovarian dermoid cyst. *Arrows* indicate balls of hair. (Courtesy of Dr. Zubie Sheikh, Department of Obstetrics and Gynecology, University of Chicago, Chicago.)

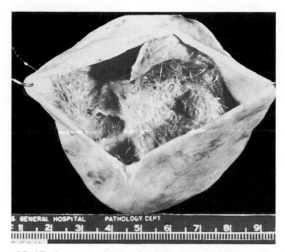

Figure 33-17 Gross specimen of a dermoid cyst that was filled with sebaceous material and hair. (Courtesy of Dr. R.E. Scully.)

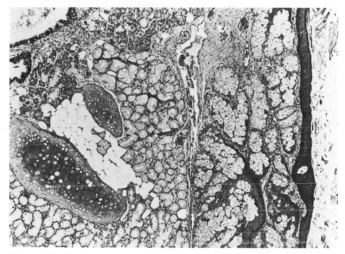

Figure 33-18 Photomicrograph of dermoid. Cartilage is shown *(right)* lined by epidermis and accompanying appendages *(left)* (×50). (From Serov SF, Scully RE, Sobin LH: Histologic Typing of Ovarian Tumors. Geneva, World Health Organization, 1973.)

Occasionally, teratomas may be solid and may consist only of adult tissues, leading to the diagnosis of a solid mature teratoma. These benign germ cell tumors are rare.

A cystic teratoma can undergo malignant degeneration, usually after menopause. Generally, it occurs in the squamous epithelial elements of the dermoid, producing a squamous cell carcinoma. It is a rare complication, estimated to occur in less than 2% of these tumors. If the malignant tissue has spread beyond the confines of the ovary, the prognosis is poor. In such cases, additional therapy for squamous cell carcinoma with radiation therapy, chemotherapy, or both is used.

Immature Teratomas

Immature teratomas are malignant and account for as many as 20% of the malignant ovarian tumors found in women younger than 20 years, but less than 1% of all ovarian cancers. They rarely occur in women after menopause. They consist of immature embryonic structures that can be admixed with mature elements. Approximately one third of immature teratomas express serum **α-fetoprotein**.

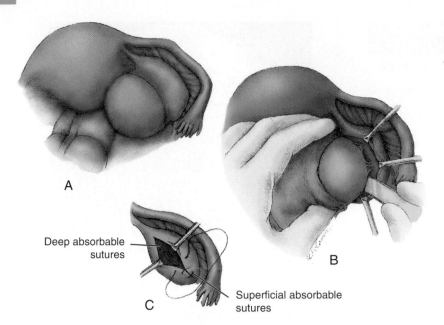

Figure 33-19 Shelling out of teratoma. **A,** Scalpel incision in ovary at intersection of dermoid and normal ovary. **B,** Dermoid being separated. Note how the upper part peels away. **C,** Reconstruction of normal ovary.

Deep absorbable sutures

Superficial absorbable sutures

The prognosis for patients with immature teratomas is related to the stage (FIGO) and grade of the tumor. The grade of the tumor is based on the degree of immaturity of the various tissues. Grade 3 tumors consist of the most immature tissues and often have a high proportion of immature neuroepithelium. **Figure 33-20** shows the survival of patients with immature teratomas by stage and grade before the advent of modern chemotherapy. Kurman and Norris have reported that patients with stage IA immature teratoma have a 10-year actuarial survival rate of 70% after unilateral salpingo-oophorectomy; this rate is comparable with that recorded after bilateral salpingo-oophorectomy.

OTHER GERM CELL TUMORS

Dysgerminomas

Dysgerminomas are the most common type of malignant germ cell tumors. They consist of primitive germ cells with stroma infiltrated by lymphocytes (**Fig. 33-21**). They are analogous to seminoma in the male testis and comprise approximately 1% of ovarian malignancies. Dysgerminomas occur primarily in women younger than 30 years. The tumor can be discovered during pregnancy. Some arise in dysgenetic gonads (see later). Unlike other malignant germ cell tumors, dysgerminomas are bilateral in approximately 10% of cases (see **Table 33-4**). Approximately 15% of dysgerminomas produce human chorionic gonadotropin related to areas of syncytiotrophoblast tissue.

Endodermal Sinus Tumors (Yolk Sac Tumors)

The endodermal sinus tumor, or yolk sac tumor, which comprises 10% of malignant germ cell tumors, in part resembles the yolk sac of the rodent placenta, thus recapitulating extraembryonic tissues (see **Fig. 33-15**). One typical histologic pattern is shown in **Figure 33-22**. The tumor secretes α-fetoprotein, which is a specific marker useful for identifying and following these tumors clinically. These rapidly growing tumors occur in females between 13 months and 45 years of age. A median age of 19 years at diagnosis was noted by Kurman and Norris. The yolk sac tumor is the prototype for α-fetoprotein production.

Choriocarcinomas

Nongestational choriocarcinoma is a highly malignant rare germ cell tumor resembling extraembryonic tissues. Like gestational choriocarcinoma (see Chapter 35, Gestational Trophoblastic Disease), it consists of malignant cytotrophoblasts and syncytiotrophoblast; human chorionic gonadotropin is a useful tumor marker. This tumor mostly develops in women younger than 20 years, primarily in the ovary. The disease was usually fatal in the past and does not appear to respond to single-agent chemotherapy (e.g., methotrexate, actinomycin D) with the same frequency as gestational trophoblastic disease. This lack of response may be caused in part by the occurrence of these tumors in combination with other malignant germ cell tumors (mixed germ cell tumor) and, occasionally, the other germ cell elements may not be histologically recognized.

Embryonal Carcinomas

An embryonal carcinoma is a rare malignant germ cell tumor composed of primitive embryonal cells. It occurs in young females between the ages of 4 and 28 years. Kurman and Norris have summarized 15 cases. Trophoblastic elements may be present; both human chorionic gonadotropin and α-fetoprotein have also been reported to be present.

Polyembryomas

Polyembryomas are exceedingly rare tumors that are usually found in the testes. They can occur in the ovary and consist of embryonal bodies that resemble early embryos. Trophoblastic elements with human chorionic gonadotropin and placental lactogen secretion have been reported.

Mixed Germ Cell Tumors

Mixed germ cell tumors are combinations of any of the germ cell tumors of the ovary described earlier. They can be bilateral if dysgerminoma elements are involved; otherwise, they are unilateral.

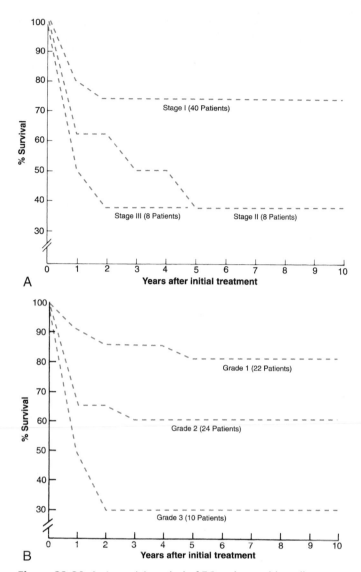

A

B

Figure 33-20 A, Actuarial survival of 56 patients with malignant teratoma by neoplasm stage. **B,** By neoplasm grade. (From Norris HJ, Zirkin JH, Benson WL: Immature [malignant] teratoma of the ovary: A clinical and pathologic study of 58 cases. Cancer 37:2359, 1976.)

TREATMENT OF MALIGNANT GERM CELL TUMORS

Current treatment modalities result in cure rates approaching 100% for patients with stage I malignant germ cell tumors and more than 75% for patients with advanced-stage disease (stages III and IV). Because most patients are young and most of these tumors are unilateral, fertility-sparing surgery consisting of unilateral salpingo-oophorectomy with preservation of the contralateral ovary and the uterus is appropriate. After unilateral adnexal excision, frozen-section examination should be performed to confirm the diagnosis preliminarily. Once a malignant ovarian germ cell tumor is documented, routine biopsy of a normal contralateral ovary should be avoided because such an intervention could lead to future infertility related to peritoneal adhesions or ovarian failure. If bilateral ovarian masses are encountered at surgery, a unilateral salpingo-oophorectomy of the more suspicious side is appropriate. If the opposite ovary contains tumor or is dysgenetic, bilateral salpingo-oophorectomy is generally indicated. In the case of bilateral ovarian dysgerminomas in

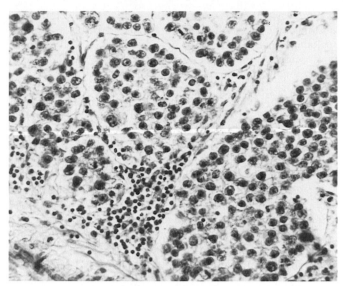

Figure 33-21 Dysgerminoma (×300). Dysgerminoma cells are demonstrated as well as infiltration of stroma by lymphocytes. (From Scully RE: Germ cell tumors of the ovary and fallopian tube. In Meigs JV, Sturgis SH [eds]: Progress in Gynecology, vol 4. New York, Grune & Stratton, 1963.)

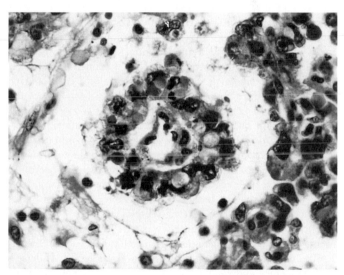

Figure 33-22 Schiller-Duvall body associated with numerous hyaline droplets in an endodermal sinus tumor (×350). (From Kurman RJ, Norris HJ: Malignant germ cells of the ovary. Hum Pathol 8:551, 1977.)

nondysgenetic ovaries, although not proven to be entirely safe, unilateral salpingo-oophorectomy and contralateral ovarian cystectomy may be considered in an effort to preserve fertility. Conversely, if a contralateral ovary contains a mature cystic teratoma, which is more likely because it is present in 10% to 15% of cases, ovarian cystectomy is indicated.

In general, if the tumor appears to be grossly confined to the ovary, comprehensive surgical staging is recommended, with cytologic washings, omentectomy, peritoneal biopsies, and bilateral pelvic and para-aortic lymphadenectomy. If obvious extraovarian metastases are present, the guiding principle is maximum cytoreductive surgery.

For most patients with malignant ovarian germ cell tumors, postoperative chemotherapy is indicated. Notable exceptions include patients with stage IA pure dysgerminoma and patients with stage IA, grade 1, immature teratoma; these patients have a high cure rate with surgery alone. The VAC regimen (*vi*ncristine, 1.5 mg/m^2 IV weekly for 8 to 12 weeks, and *a*ctinomycin D, 300 mcg/m^2/day for 5 days every 4 weeks, with *cy*clophosphamide [Cytoxan] 150 mg/m^2/day for 5 days every 4 weeks) was the first effective combination chemotherapy regimen for patients with malignant germ cell tumors. VAC was the most widely used regimen during the 1970s and early 1980s and produced a relatively high proportion of cures in stage I disease (82%) but, in patients with metastatic disease, the cure rate was less than 50%. During the VAC era, conversion of an immature teratoma to a mature teratoma under the influence of chemotherapy, so-called retroconversion, was observed.

By the late 1970s, based on the experience in testicular cancer, the combination of vinblastine, bleomycin, and cisplatin (VBP) was beginning to be used for malignant ovarian germ cell tumors, with superior outcomes compared with those achieved with the VAC regimen, particularly for patients with advanced-stage disease. By the mid-1980s, the VBP regimen was replaced by the combination of bleomycin, etoposide, and cisplatin (BEP) because of the latter's superior toxicity profile. The BEP regimen remains the standard today. Generally, most patients require three to four cycles of therapy. In 1990, Gershenson and colleagues reported that 25 of 26 patients treated with BEP for malignant germ cell tumors were in sustained remission. Subsequently, Williams and associates, reporting the GOG experience, noted that 89 of 93 patients (96%) with completely resected stage I, II, or III disease remained continuously disease-free.

Special note should be made regarding dysgerminoma. Historically, for patients with metastatic dysgerminoma, the traditional postoperative treatment was radiotherapy. Although dysgerminoma is exquisitely radiosensitive and survival rates with this treatment were excellent, most patients suffered loss of fertility. With the advent of successful combination chemotherapy, such as BEP, chemotherapy has almost exclusively supplanted radiotherapy, with a high rate of fertility preservation.

Although second-look surgery was part of standard management for patients with malignant germ cell tumors until the mid-1980s, reports from the University of Texas M.D. Anderson Cancer Center and the GOG called into question the value of this procedure. Gershenson and coworkers have reported their experience with second-look surgery, with negative findings in 52 of 53 patients; only 1 of the 52 negative patients relapsed and died of tumor. Subsequently, the GOG experience confirmed that the value of second-look surgery in patients with completely resected malignant germ cell tumors and incompletely resected malignant germ cell tumors not containing an immature teratoma element was negligible. For patients with incompletely resected malignant germ cell tumors with an immature teratoma element, however, second-look surgery appeared to have some impact. Advances in imaging technology may further minimize the need for second-look surgery, even in the latter group.

There has been a trend toward surveillance, with careful follow-up after surgery as an alternative to chemotherapy in select patients. Bonazzi and colleagues have treated 32 patients with operation alone for stage I or II, grade 1 or 2, tumors.

All patients with grade 3 or stage III tumors, or those with tumor recurrence, received cisplatin, etoposide, and bleomycin. Most patients underwent fertility-sparing surgery, and 10 received chemotherapy. All patients were free of disease with a median follow-up of 47 months, and five had delivered healthy infants. A Pediatric Oncology Group Study reported by Cushing and associates has indicated that patients younger than 15 years with a pure immature teratoma could be followed without chemotherapy; however, more than 90% of the tumors in their series were grade 1 or 2. In addition, a study by Billmire and coworkers has found that survival in 131 girls with malignant ovarian germ cell tumors is unaffected by less than comprehensive surgical staging.

The Children's Oncology Group has conducted a clinical trial in the pediatric population. This trial includes surveillance of the low-risk cohort, consisting of all patients with apparent stage I disease with close follow-up of serum markers and initiation of chemotherapy only if relapse occurs. In the intermediate-risk cohort, patients with stages II to IV disease receive a modified BEP regimen over 3 days instead of the standard 5-day regimen.

There is no standard surveillance for patients with malignant ovarian germ cell tumors after completion of primary therapy. For patients who have completed standard surgery plus chemotherapy, we generally recommend evaluation of serum tumor marker every 3 months for up to 2 years and then every 6 months until 5 years from diagnosis. Patients treated with fertility-sparing surgery should be closely followed with periodic transvaginal ultrasound and/or CT evaluations. Office visits, with a physical examination, are generally recommended every 3 months for the first 2 years and less frequently thereafter.

With the success of cure in a high proportion of young patients with malignant ovarian germ cell tumors has come an increasing focus on the late effects of therapy, particularly fertility preservation. In a report of 40 patients, Gershenson and colleagues noted that 27 had normal menses after multiagent chemotherapy for germ cell tumors, and 11 of 16 patients who attempted pregnancy were successful in bearing 22 children. Most of these patients received non–platinum-based chemotherapy. Peccatori and associates have reported on 139 patients with malignant germ cell tumors, 108 of whom had fertility-sparing operations. Multiagent platinum-containing chemotherapy was used, with a 96% survival rate and a mean follow-up of 55 months. In a GOG study, Williams and associates reported on 93 patients treated adjuvantly with cisplatin, etoposide, and bleomycin for three cycles. Of 93 patients, 91 were free of disease 4 to 90 months after treatment, although leukemia developed in one patient and lymphoma in a second patient. Brewer and coworkers have reported on 26 patients treated with BEP, with 25 alive and disease-free and a median follow-up of 89 months. They reported that 71% resumed normal menstrual function and 6 patients conceived. Three additional large studies from Australia, Italy, and the United States have provided further support for the concept of preservation of fertility in most treated with fertility-sparing surgery and chemotherapy. In a GOG matched control study of 132 survivors (all of whom were treated with surgery and platinum-based chemotherapy) and 137 controls, 71 (54%) survivors underwent fertility-sparing surgery. Of the fertile survivors, 87% reported having normal menstrual function and 24 survivors had 37 offspring after cancer therapy. However, compared with controls, cancer survivors had significantly greater reproductive concerns and less sexual pleasure.

Several nonrandomized studies have suggested that gonadotropin-releasing hormone agonist prophylaxis may be worthwhile to preserve ovarian function in young patients receiving chemotherapy. Blumenfeld and coworkers have administered gonadotropin-releasing hormone agonist during chemotherapy for nongynecologic tumors to women of reproductive age, and 15 of 16 surviving patients (93.7%) resumed menses and ovulation. However, randomized trials are needed to validate this approach.

SPECIALIZED GERM CELL TUMORS: STRUMA OVARII AND CARCINOIDS

Specialized ovarian germ cell tumors are rare; two types are commonly recognized (see **Box 33-3**), the **struma ovarii** and **carcinoids**. Struma ovarii are dermoids with thyroid tissue exclusively or with thyroid tissue as a major component. The thyroid tissue can be functional, leading to clinical hyperthyroidism. Most of these tumors are benign, but malignant changes are possible. Metastatic disease, if present, has been reported to be effectively treated with ^{131}I, as for primary thyroid carcinoma.

Carcinoids are ovarian teratomas that histologically resemble similar tumors in the gastrointestinal tract. Carcinoids are rare and are unilateral in the ovary. In approximately 30% of cases, a true carcinoid syndrome will develop, and 5-hydroxyindoleacetic acid can be detected and used to monitor the tumor postoperatively. These tumors occur primarily in older women and tend to grow slowly; the prognosis after hysterectomy and bilateral salpingo-oophorectomy is excellent. For a young woman desiring preservation of childbearing function, a stage IA carcinoid can be treated by unilateral salpingo-oophorectomy.

GONADOBLASTOMAS (GERM CELL SEX CORD-STROMAL TUMORS)

The term *gonadoblastoma* was introduced by Scully in 1953 to describe a tumor that consists of germ cell and sex cord–stromal elements. The germ cells usually resemble dysgerminoma, whereas the sex cord–stromal elements may consist of immature granulosa and Sertoli cells. Leydig cells and luteinized cells may be present. The tumor usually occurs in patients with abnormal (dysgenetic) gonads. Most patients have a female phenotype but may be virilized. These patients have a Y chromosome detected in their karyotype, and patients with gonadal dysgenesis and a Y chromosome are at risk of the development of gonadoblastoma or malignant germ cell tumors, predominantly dysgerminoma, which may occur in those as young as 6 months. Removal of these gonads is indicated when they are discovered. Both gonads should be removed and, if the presence of pure gonadoblastoma is confirmed, the prognosis is excellent because these tumors have not been reported to metastasize.

SEX CORD-STROMAL TUMORS

Sex cord–stromal tumors are derived from the sex cords of the ovary and the specialized stroma of the developing gonad. The elements can have a male or female differentiation and some of these tumors are hormonally active. This group accounts for approximately 6% of ovarian neoplasms and most hormonally functioning ovarian tumors. For the female derivatives, the sex cord component is the granulosa cell and the stromal component is the theca cell or fibroblast. For the male counterpart, the similar components are the Sertoli cell and Leydig cell. **Granulosa–theca cell tumors** and **Sertoli-Leydig cell tumors** tend to behave as low-grade malignancies. Their clinical and morphologic aspects considered separately.

GRANULOSA-THECA CELL TUMORS

Granulosa cell tumors consist primarily of granulosa cells and a varying proportion of theca cells, fibroblasts, or both. One characteristic microscopic pattern is shown in **Figure 33-23**, which demonstrates the so-called Call-Exner bodies, eosinophilic bodies surrounded by granulosa cells. Functional granulosa cell tumors are primarily estrogenic. Approximately 5% occur before puberty and they can be one cause of precocious puberty, but the tumors have been described in women of all ages. In postmenopausal women, these tumors can produce increased levels of blood estrogens, uterine bleeding, and occasionally endometrial carcinoma. It is estimated that approximately 5% of the granulosa cell tumors in adults are associated with endometrial carcinoma. In menstruating women, the functional granulosa cell tumor can produce abnormal menstrual patterns, menorrhagia, and even amenorrhea.

These tumors can become large and may present as a ruptured mass, leading to laparotomy for an acute abdomen with hemoperitoneum. Because of the low-grade malignant character of these tumors, recurrences are frequently more than 5 years after primary therapy. In general, prognosis does not correlate with the histologic pattern of the tumor. A total of 90% of granulosa cell tumors present as stage I. Advanced clinical stage, the presence of tumor rupture, a large primary tumor (>15 cm), and a high mitotic rate have been associated with a poorer prognosis. Overall 10-year survival rates of 90% have been reported. Studies by Klemi and colleagues and others have suggested that most

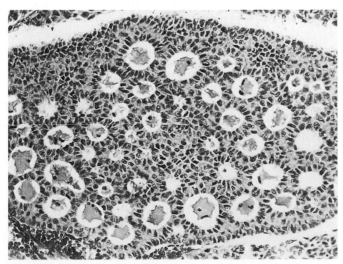

Figure 33-23 Granulosa cell tumor (×460). (From Scully RE, Morris J: Functioning ovarian tumors. In Meigs JV, Sturgis SH [eds]: Progress in Gynecology, Vol 3. New York, Grune & Stratton, 1957.)

granulosa cell tumors have a diploid pattern and a low (<60%) S-phase fraction when analyzed by flow cytometry. Those with an aneuploid pattern had a worse prognosis in the study of Klemi and associates. However, it is important to recognize that granulosa cell tumors can be confused histologically with poorly differentiated adenocarcinomas, and the latter would also have an aneuploid pattern as well as a poor prognosis. A variant found predominantly in females younger than 20 years is known as juvenile granulosa cell tumor. It was described by Young and coworkers and has an excellent prognosis, particularly if the tumor is confined to one ovary.

The primary therapeutic approach is the surgical removal of the tumor. Because these tumors are rarely bilateral (<5%), young patients with stage IA tumors can be treated by unilateral adnexectomy. Lack and colleagues have reported 10 cases of granulosa cell tumors in premenarchal female patients, all of whom were treated by unilateral salpingo-oophorectomy. Two tumors were ruptured. All 10 of the patients were alive with no evidence of disease 2 to 33 years after therapy. Evans and associates have noted a higher recurrence rate in women who were treated by unilateral salpingo-oophorectomy for stage IA cases compared with those treated with bilateral salpingo-oophorectomy. This finding has led to the recommendation that women of reproductive age treated for granulosa cell tumor by unilateral salpingo-oophorectomy have close follow-up. For women who have completed childbearing, abdominal hysterectomy and bilateral salpingo-oophorectomy are recommended. Regardless of the treatment of the pelvic organs, if a granulosa cell tumor is diagnosed on frozen-section examination, comprehensive surgical staging is recommended. Whether complete pelvic and para-aortic lymphadenectomy is indicated remains unresolved; there is some information that the incidence of lymph node metastases associated with this tumor type is low. A recent study by Brown and coworkers has evaluated the risk of lymph node metastasis in patients with sex cord–stromal tumors. A total of 262 patients were included in that study and, of these, 178 patients were diagnosed with granulosa cell tumors. It was noted that none of the patients who underwent lymphadenectomy had evidence of lymph node metastasis.

Tumor markers may be helpful for monitoring the clinical course of granulosa cell tumors. Studies by Lappohn and colleagues have suggested that the peptide hormone inhibin is secreted by some granulosa cell tumors and serum measurements could serve as a tumor marker. In addition, serum CA-125, serum estradiol, or serum testosterone levels may occasionally serve as markers that should be followed serially.

Historically, radiotherapy, the VAC regimen (see earlier), or the combination of cisplatin, doxorubicin, and cyclophosphamide have been used for the treatment of metastatic granulosa cell tumors, but none of these options are currently recommended for general application. Many questions remain regarding recommendations for postoperative treatment. For patients with stage IA granulosa cell tumors, surgery alone is recommended. The recommendation for those with stage IC disease remains controversial, but consideration can be given to adjuvant therapy based on the probable increased risk of relapse. Postoperative therapy is recommended for all patients with stages II to IV disease, as well as for those patients with recurrent tumor.

Because of the rarity of granulosa cell tumors, no standard regimen exists. The GOG has reported the largest series of women treated with the BEP regimen. Homesley and associates have reported on 57 eligible patients; 41 had recurrent disease and 16 had primary metastatic disease. Of these patients, 48 had granulosa cell tumors. Overall, 11 of 16 primary disease patients and 21 of 41 recurrent disease patients remained progression-free at a median follow-up of 3 years. However, toxicity was fairly severe, with two bleomycin-related deaths reported.

Brown and coworkers have reported the M.D. Anderson Cancer Center experience with taxane-based chemotherapy in a study of 44 patients with sex cord–stromal tumors of the ovary treated for primary metastatic or recurrent disease. The response rate for 30 patients treated with a taxane plus platinum for recurrent measurable disease was 42%. Thus, the combination of paclitaxel and carboplatin is also an option for these patients. Currently, GOG is conducting a randomized phase II study comparing BEP with the combination of paclitaxel and carboplatin for women with newly diagnosed or chemonaïve recurrent sex cord–stromal ovarian tumors.

Hormone therapy may also be considered for patients with metastatic granulosa cell tumors. Responses of these tumors to medroxyprogesterone acetate and gonadotropin-releasing hormone antagonists have been reported. Fishman and colleagues have treated six patients with recurrent or persistent granulosa cell tumors with leuprolide acetate; of five patients with assessable disease, two had partial responses and three had stable disease.

THECOMAS AND FIBROMAS

A **thecoma** is a benign tumor that consists entirely of stroma (theca) cells. It predominantly occurs in women in their perimenopausal and menopausal years. These tumors can be associated with estrogen production but not as frequently as granulosa cell tumors. Removal of the tumor alone is adequate treatment for women in their reproductive years. For older women, total abdominal hysterectomy and bilateral salpingo-oophorectomy are performed. Rarely, thecomas have been reported to be malignant, and these are most likely fibrosarcomas. A closely related tumor is the fibroma, which is the most common benign solid ovarian tumor and accounts for 4% of all ovarian tumors. Like the thecoma, it can occur at any age but is more common in older women; it does not secrete hormones. These tumors contain spindle cells and the tumors can grow to a large size. They are benign, and excision is adequate treatment. They are associated with ascites in approximately 40% of cases if the tumor is larger than 10 cm, according to Samanth and Black. They can also be responsible for hydrothorax with a benign ascites (Meigs' syndrome), which regresses following tumor removal.

SERTOLI-LEYDIG CELL TUMORS (ANDROBLASTOMAS)

Sertoli-Leydig cell tumors are very rare. Sertoli (sex cord) and Leydig (stromal) cells are present in varying amounts, and the tumor may consist almost entirely of Sertoli or Leydig cells (Fig. 33-24). These tumors tend to occur in young women of reproductive age and frequently are the cause of masculinization and hirsutism. The symptoms of virilization usually regress after tumor removal, but temporal hair recession and a deeper voice tend to remain. Rarely, they have also been reported to have estrogenic activity, leading to the same symptoms and signs as

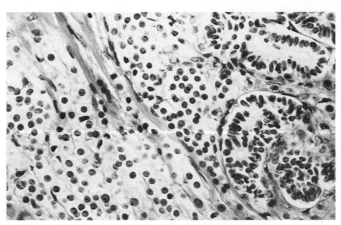

Figure 33-24 Sertoli-Leydig cell tumor. Tubules of Sertoli cells (*right*) and Leydig cells (*left*) are shown (×250). (Courtesy of Dr. R.E. Scully.)

those of granulosa cell tumors. The tumors tend to behave as low-grade malignancies and the 5-year survival rate can vary from 70% to 90%. Poorly differentiated types tend to have a poor prognosis, as do higher stage tumors. Young and Scully have reviewed 207 cases; 75% were in those 30 years of age or younger and less than 10% were older than 50 years. One third of patients had evidence of androgen excess. Both ovaries were involved in only three cases. The well-differentiated tumors behaved clinically as benign tumors, whereas recurrence or extra-uterine spread was noted occasionally in women with intermediate differentiation (11%) and frequently in those with poor differentiation (59%). Of 164 patients available for follow-up, 18% had metastasis or recurrence.

Treatment of metastatic Sertoli-Leydig cell tumors is similar to that for granulosa cell tumors. In addition, because the prognosis for patients with stage I poorly differentiated Sertoli-Leydig cell tumors is so poor, consideration should be give to adjuvant treatment. However, it should be emphasized that there are no therapeutic data in this setting and, if treatment is recommended, the optimal regimen remains unclear. The BEP regimen or the combination of paclitaxel and carboplatin may be considered for these patients.

OTHER SEX CORD–STROMAL TUMORS

Gynandroblastomas

Gynandroblastomas are rare sex cord–stromal tumors consisting of female (granulosa cells) and male (Sertoli cells) cell types. Theca or Leydig cells may also be present. Patients with this tumor typically present with androgenic manifestations, but stigmata associated with hyperestrogenism may also be observed. These tumors are usually unilateral and generally considered to be of low malignant potential.

Sex Cord Tumors with Annular Tubules

Sex cord tumors with annular tubules are unusual. As suggested by the name, there is a prominent tubular pattern. Features of both Sertoli and granulosa cell tumors are present. Young and colleagues have reviewed 74 cases; 27 were associated with mucocutaneous pigmentation and gastrointestinal tract polyposis (Peutz-Jeghers syndrome). The tumors may have estrogenic manifestations. Those associated with Peutz-Jeghers syndrome are benign and those not associated with this syndrome can be

malignant. It is of interest that 4 of these 74 cases were associated with a virulent form of cervical adenocarcinoma (adenoma malignum).

Leydig Cell and Hilus Cell Tumors

Leydig cell and hilus cell tumors are rare. They are composed of Leydig cells or cells of the ovarian hilus. Their cytoplasm contains hyaline bodies known as crystalloids of Reinke. They usually cause virilization and are benign. They tend to be small (<6 cm) and develop primarily in perimenopausal women.

LIPID (LIPOID) TUMORS

Lipid tumors are infrequently occurring ovarian tumors composed of large cells that resemble Leydig cells, luteinized cells, or cells that arise in the adrenal cortex. Approximately 100 tumors have been reported. These tumors usually cause virilization but have also been associated with excess cortisol production. There is not enough experience with them to delineate an effective form of treatment. However, metastases of lipid cell tumors have been reported.

METASTATIC OVARIAN TUMORS

Tumors from distant primary sites can metastasize to the ovary. Frequently, metastases are from primary tumors that originate elsewhere in the female reproductive tract, particularly from the endometrium and fallopian tube. Distant sites of origin occur most frequently from the breast and gastrointestinal tract. Metastatic tumors from the gastrointestinal tract to the ovary can be associated with sex hormone production, which usually leads to estrogenic manifestations. One special type of metastatic ovarian tumor is known as Krukenberg's tumor, which histologically consists of nests of mucin-filled signet ring cells in a cellular stroma (**Fig. 33-25**). The most common gastrointestinal tract origin for these tumors is the stomach, and the next frequent is the

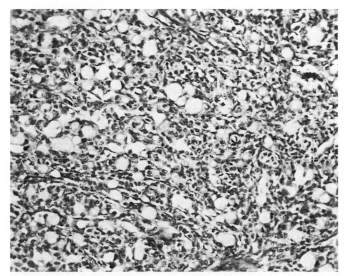

Figure 33-25 Krukenberg's tumor (×256). Mucin-filled signet-ring cells are present. (Courtesy of Dr. R.E. Scully.)

large intestine. However, breast metastases to the ovary can on occasion reveal the same histologic picture. A few cases of Krukenberg's tumors have been described, with no apparent distant primary malignancy, suggesting the rare possibility of a primary ovarian tumor with the histologic features of a Krukenberg's tumor. A primary gastrointestinal tract malignancy should be considered in older women with an adnexal mass, particularly if it is bilateral and solid. Pretherapy evaluation to rule out a gastrointestinal tract or breast primary tumor is indicated. The tumor should be removed when discovered, and the primary site should be treated. The prognosis is poor; it is rare for a woman to survive for 5 years or longer after treatment.

KEY POINTS

- Ovarian cancer is the leading cause of death from gynecologic cancer, but it occurs less frequently than endometrial cancers.
- Ovarian cancers of women older than 50 years are diagnosed at a more advanced stage, leading to a worse prognosis than for younger women.
- The risk of ovarian cancer is decreased by oral contraceptive use. Tubal ligation and hysterectomy also appear to decrease the risk.
- Most ovarian carcinomas are diagnosed in stage III or IV.
- Ovarian cancer risk rises from approximately 1.4% in general to 5% to 7% if the woman has one or two first- or second-degree relatives with ovarian cancer.
- Patients with ovarian cancer are at increased risk of developing breast cancer and endometrial cancer.
- It is important that the follow-up of ovarian cancer patients includes monitoring for breast cancer.
- Epithelial tumors are the most frequent ovarian neoplasm. They account for two thirds of all ovarian neoplasms and 85% of ovarian cancers.
- The major ovarian epithelial tumor cell types recapitulate müllerian-type epithelium (serous, endosalpinx; mucinous, endocervix; endometrioid, endometrium).
- Serous ovarian neoplasms are the most common type of epithelial tumors. Serous adenocarcinomas tend to be high grade, are the most virulent, and have the worst prognosis of epithelial adenocarcinomas. They are bilateral in 33% to 66% of cases.
- A cystic adnexal mass smaller than 8 cm in diameter in a menstruating female is most frequently functional.
- The normal postmenopausal ovary is approximately 1.5 to 2 cm in diameter.
- The risk of an ovarian tumor being malignant is approximately 33% in a woman older than 45, whereas it is less than 1 in 15 for those 20 to 45 years of age. More than 50% of ovarian cancers occur in women older than 50.
- There are three types of ovarian tumors with a serous histology: traditional serous adenocarcinoma, surface papillary tumors (ovary < 4 cm), and primary peritoneal carcinomas (serous carcinoma metastatic to the ovary, with normal ovarian size).
- Most ovarian carcinomas start from small microscopic foci and spread throughout the peritoneum before becoming clinically evident (de novo origin), especially serous and poorly differentiated tumors.
- Ovarian carcinomas having a cystic origin are primary mucinous or endometrioid, and are more likely to be discovered at a low stage.
- A vaginal ultrasound finding of a unilocular cyst of 5 cm or smaller in a perimenopausal woman can usually be followed without surgical intervention.
- Vaginal ultrasonography may detect early ovarian carcinoma but has not been proven to be a cost-effective screening technique.
- The primary distribution spread of epithelial carcinoma is transcoelomic to the visceral and parietal peritoneum, diaphragm, and retroperitoneal nodes.
- The risk of retroperitoneal node spread of epithelial carcinoma in apparent stage I cases is greatest for poorly differentiated tumors, for which the risk can reach 10% to 20%. The risk of retroperitoneal node spread increases in higher stage cases.
- The prognosis of a patient with ovarian epithelial carcinoma is related primarily to tumor stage and tumor grade, and to the amount of residual tumor remaining after primary resection.
- Laparoscopic staging of early ovarian cancers appears to be feasible and comprehensive, without compromising survival.
- The 5-year survival rate for patients with borderline epithelial ovarian carcinoma (grade 0) is close to 100% for stage I cases and more than 90% for all stages.
- The overall 5-year survival rate for patients with stage I ovarian carcinoma is 65%. For stage I, grade 1, the survival rate is reported to be more than 80%.
- Optimal surgical debulking (<1 cm residual nodules) appears to confer a survival advantage in cases of stages III and IV ovarian carcinoma.
- Interval cytoreduction has little additional effect on overall survival if a maximal attempt is made at primary surgery.
- Neoadjuvant chemotherapy can reduce surgical morbidity; a randomized trial has indicated that this strategy may be equivalent to standard treatment for advanced-stage patients with surgery followed by chemotherapy.
- IP chemotherapy appears to benefit patients with optimal cytoreduction more than conventional IV chemotherapy, but with greater toxicity.
- CT scanning for patients with ovarian cancer can be approximately 80% to 90% effective for detecting tumor in retroperitoneal nodes, but is much less successful in detecting intra-abdominal disease.
- Assessing the ovarian CA-125 level is useful to help monitor patients with ovarian carcinoma. Reaction to the antigen is positive in approximately 80% of cases.
- A rapid decrease in CA-125 values after treatment indicates a more favorable prognosis.
- The initial response rate of ovarian epithelial carcinomas multiagent chemotherapy is more than 90%, but the proportion of patients who survive decreases to approximately 30% in 5 years. Initial treatment is usually with platinum and taxane agents.

KEY POINTS—CONTINUED

- Approximately 50% of patients thought initially to be clinically free of disease are found to have gross or microscopic tumor at second-look laparotomy.
- The 5-year survival rate after a negative second-look operation is approximately 50%.
- Recurrent ovarian cancer is difficult to cure.
- Factors determining response to recurrent chemotherapy regimens include time to treatment progression, distribution and volume of disease, and performance status.
- Combination chemotherapy for platinum-sensitive recurrent disease improves response rates, with a less clear effect on survival.
- Secondary cytoreduction appears to benefit patients with limited recurrent disease who undergo complete tumor removal. The benefit may be most evident before chemotherapy for recurrence.
- Germ cell tumors are the second most common type of ovarian neoplasms and account for approximately 20% to 25% of all ovarian tumors.
- In women younger than 30 years, the most frequent ovarian neoplasm is a germ cell tumor; approximately one third of these germ cell tumors are malignant in those younger than 21. For women younger than 30 years, the most common ovarian neoplasm is the dermoid.
- The most common germ cell tumor is the benign cystic teratoma (dermoid). It is bilateral in 10% to 15% of the cases. Approximately 30% are calcified.
- Malignant germ cell tumors are usually unilateral except dysgerminomas, which are bilateral in approximately 10% to 15% of patients.
- Dysgerminomas are the most common malignant germ cell tumors and account for 1% to 2% of ovarian cancers.
- The prognosis for a patient with an immature teratoma is related to tumor grade and tumor stage. These tumors are the second most common type of malignant germ cell tumor.

- The 5-year survival rate of stage IA pure dysgerminoma treated by unilateral salpingo-oophorectomy is more than 90%.
- Pure dysgerminomas are radiocurable. However, multiagent chemotherapy, particularly with etoposide and platinum, with or without bleomycin, will frequently result in complete remission. Approximately two thirds of cases present as stage IA.
- Most patients with malignant ovarian germ cell tumors can be treated successfully with fertility-sparing surgery followed by BEP chemotherapy. Patients who do not require postoperative chemotherapy include those with stage IA dysgerminoma and stage IA, grade 1, immature teratoma. However, there has been a trend toward surveillance rather than chemotherapy for patients with stage I tumors of any histologic subtype.
- Multiagent chemotherapy has improved survival in patients with malignant germ cell tumors, preserving childbearing function in most cases. Standard chemotherapy consists of the BEP regimen.
- Gonadoblastomas are sex cord–stromal germ cell tumors that usually arise in dysgenetic gonads in patients with a Y chromosome; these are cured by removal.
- Granulosa cell tumors and Sertoli-Leydig tumors usually behave as low-grade malignancies, but there may be late recurrences.
- For patients with primary metastatic or recurrent sex cord–stromal tumors of the ovary, platinum-based chemotherapy is the treatment of choice. Commonly used regimens include BEP and paclitaxel-carboplatin.
- Some metastatic granulosa cell tumors may respond to hormone therapy, such as leuprolide acetate, tamoxifen, or aromatase inhibitors.
- Fibroma is the most common benign solid ovarian tumor.
- The most frequent sites of origin of tumors metastatic to the ovary are the lower reproductive tract, gastrointestinal tract, and breast.

REFERENCES CAN BE FOUND ON EXPERTCONSULT.com

34

Fallopian Tube and Primary Peritoneal Cancer
Causes, Diagnosis, Natural History, and Treatment

Kathleen M. Schmeler and David M. Gershenson

Fallopian tube and **primary peritoneal cancers** are similar but pathologically distinct entities from epithelial ovarian cancer. They have similar clinical characteristics, patterns of spread, response to treatment, and survival rates when compared with ovarian cancer. In addition, the most common histologic type for all three malignancies is high-grade papillary serous adenocarcinoma. However, fallopian tube and primary peritoneal cancers have distinct pathologic findings. This chapter reviews current information on fallopian tube and primary peritoneal cancer, with particular emphasis on diagnosis, natural history, and clinical management.

CAUSES

FALLOPIAN TUBE CANCER

Fallopian tube carcinoma is rare, comprising approximately 0.3% of gynecologic malignancies. The estimated incidence of fallopian tube cancer in the United States is 0.41/100,000 women. However, it has recently been suggested that many cases of ovarian carcinoma may actually arise from the epithelial lining of the fallopian tube fimbria, thereby grossly underestimating the incidence of primary fallopian tube carcinoma.

Similar to ovarian cancer, the primary risk factor for **fallopian tube cancer is** an inherited mutation in the **BRCA1 and BRCA2** tumor suppressor genes associated with hereditary breast and ovarian cancer syndromes. Previous reports have shown that approximately 15% to 45% of women with fallopian tube cancers have a *BRCA* mutation. A study by Levine and colleagues tested 29 patients with fallopian tube cancer and found that 17% had a germline *BRCA* mutation. In addition, a subsequent study by Cass and associates found a *BRCA* mutation in 12 of 28 patients (43%) with fallopian tube cancer.

However, in women without a *BRCA* mutation, the cause of fallopian tube carcinoma remains unclear. Similar to ovarian cancer, associated factors include infertility and low parity. Although previous reports have suggested an association between fallopian tube carcinoma and inflammatory conditions such as chronic pelvic inflammatory disease and fallopian tube tuberculosis, subsequent studies have failed to confirm this association.

PRIMARY PERITONEAL CANCER

Primary peritoneal carcinoma was first described in 1959 by Swerdlow. It is a malignancy that diffusely involves the peritoneal surfaces while sparing or minimally involving the ovaries. The exact incidence rates of primary peritoneal cancer are not available; however it is estimated that there is a 1:10 ratio of primary peritoneal cancer to ovarian cancer cases. Primary peritoneal cancer is histologically indistinguishable from epithelial ovarian cancer and has similar clinical characteristics, patterns of spread, response to treatment, and survival rates. Risk factors for primary peritoneal carcinoma are similar to those for ovarian and fallopian tube cancer, including *BRCA* mutation and low parity. However, primary peritoneal cancer has also been associated with older age at diagnosis and increased rate of obesity when compared with ovarian cancer.

The pathogenesis of primary peritoneal cancer is not well characterized. The germinal epithelium of the ovary and mesothelium of the peritoneum arise from the same embryonic origin, suggesting that primary peritoneal cancer may develop from a malignant transformation of these cells. However, another proposed theory is that there is a field effect, with the coelomic epithelium lining the abdominal cavity (peritoneum) and ovaries (germinal epithelium) manifesting a common response to an oncogenic stimulus. Molecular studies have been inconclusive in determining whether the tumor arises from the ovarian surface epithelium and spreads throughout the peritoneum, or if a multifocal malignant transformation process occurs.

SEROUS TUBAL INTRAEPITHELIAL CARCINOMA

It has recently been hypothesized that many cases of ovarian and primary peritoneal carcinoma may actually arise from the fallopian tube, thereby grossly underestimating the incidence of fallopian tube carcinoma. This hypothesis is supported by studies of women with *BRCA* mutations undergoing risk-reducing salpingo-oophorectomy (RRSO). Up to 10% of women undergoing RRSO are found to have occult serous cancers. A large number of these early cancers involve the fallopian tube as invasive fallopian tube carcinoma or as a precursor lesion known as **serous tubal intraepithelial carcinoma** (STIC). In most cases, the tumor involves the fimbriated end of the fallopian tube. These studies have suggested that the fallopian tube may be the primary source of ovarian and primary peritoneal serous carcinomas in women with *BRCA* mutations.

In addition, studies of unselected women with ovarian and primary peritoneal cancer have shown that a significant number of cases coexist with a STIC. Kindelberger and coworkers have reported that in 47% of 43 tumors classified as primary ovarian cancers, a STIC was present. Similarly, Carlson and colleagues have shown that 47% of 19 women with serous primary peritoneal cancers have a STIC in the fallopian tube. In both studies, *p53* mutational analysis showed the same mutations in the STIC and distant tumors, providing a genetic link between the two.

CLINICAL FINDINGS

FALLOPIAN TUBE CANCER

The mean age at diagnosis of fallopian tube carcinoma is 58 years, with a range of 26 to 85 years. However, in women with *BRCA*-associated fallopian tube carcinoma, the age at diagnosis is considerably younger. Cass and colleagues have reported the median age at diagnosis to be 57 years in *BRCA* mutation carriers compared with 65 years in sporadic cases. Fallopian tube cancer is more common among white women (age-adjusted incidence rate, 0.41), compared with black women (0.27), Hispanic women (0.27), and Asians and Pacific Islanders (0.25).

The presenting symptoms of fallopian tube carcinoma are largely related to the degree of obstruction of the distal tube. Many women are asymptomatic; however, the most commonly reported signs and symptoms include abnormal vaginal bleeding or serosanguineous vaginal discharge (35% to 60%), a palpable adnexal mass (10% to 60%), and crampy lower abdominal pain caused by tubal distention and forced peristalsis (20% to 50%). *Hydrops tubae profluens* is the term used to describe intermittent expulsion of clear or serosanguineous fluid from the vagina caused by contraction of a distended, distally occluded fallopian tube. The discharge may be followed by shrinkage or resolution of the adnexal mass. The triad of intermittent serosanguineous discharge, colicky pain, and a mass (**Latzko's triad**) is considered to be pathognomonic of fallopian tube cancer, but occurs in only approximately 15% of patients. In addition, approximately 10% to 40% of women with fallopian tube carcinoma have abnormal cervical cytology results, including adenocarcinoma or atypical glandular cells (AGUSs). Evaluation with a cancer antigen 125 (CA-125) level and transvaginal ultrasound to rule out ovarian and fallopian tube cancer should be considered in women with these cytologic findings who have a negative workup for endocervical and endometrial carcinoma.

PRIMARY PERITONEAL CANCER

Patients with primary peritoneal cancer tend to be older than women with ovarian or fallopian tube cancer, with the median age at diagnosis reported to range from 63 to 66 years. Similar to ovarian cancer, women with primary peritoneal cancer typically present with pain, abdominal distention, pressure, and/or gastrointestinal symptoms. A small proportion of patients are asymptomatic. Occasionally, primary peritoneal cancer is detected on a routine Pap test or during exploratory surgery for other reasons.

DIAGNOSIS

Similar to ovarian cancer, the diagnosis of fallopian tube or primary peritoneal cancer may be suspected based on imaging studies, CA-125 level, and/or symptoms, as well as physical examination findings. However, a definitive diagnosis is usually made at the time of surgery.

ULTRASOUND

The classic ultrasound findings for fallopian tube cancer include a fluid-filled, tubular or ovoid mass with internal papillations, mural nodules, and/or septations that is separate from the uterus and ovaries. In primary peritoneal and fallopian tube cancers, ascites and/or peritoneal implants may be present. With both malignancies, the ovaries are often normal in appearance.

OTHER IMAGING MODALITIES

Computed tomography (CT), magnetic resonance imaging (MRI), and positron emission tomography (PET) scans may provide additional information in women with suspected fallopian tube or primary peritoneal cancer. These studies can provide information regarding the extent of disease and sites of metastatic spread, allowing the physician to plan appropriate intervention and treatment.

CANCER ANTIGEN 125 LEVEL

The CA-125 level is elevated in more than 80% of women with fallopian tube and primary peritoneal cancer. Although the CA-125 value is useful for monitoring response to treatment or evaluating a woman in whom the disease is suspected, it is not recommended as a screening test.

STAGING

Both fallopian tube and primary peritoneal carcinomas are surgically staged. The International Federation of Gynecology and Obstetrics (FIGO) staging for fallopian tube cancer is shown in **Table 34-1**. The staging system is similar to that of epithelial ovarian carcinoma because of their similar patterns of spread, surgical approach, treatment, and prognosis. FIGO has not yet adopted a specific staging system for primary peritoneal cancer, and the ovarian cancer surgical staging system is typically applied to women with this disease.

PATHOLOGIC FINDINGS

FALLOPIAN TUBE CARCINOMA

Fallopian tube carcinomas arise in either tube with similar frequency and are bilateral in 3% to 8% of cases. The fimbriated end of the fallopian tube is grossly occluded in approximately 50% of patients, resulting in a dilated lumen filled with tumor and/or fluid (**Figs. 34-1 and 34-2**). Histologically, 80 to 90% of fallopian tube carcinomas are adenocarcinomas (**Figs. 34-3 and 34-4**). Most of these are serous carcinomas, followed by

Table 34-1 FIGO Staging of Fallopian Tube Cancer

Stage	Features
0	Carcinoma in situ (limited to tubal mucosa)
I	Growth limited to the fallopian tubes
IA	Growth limited to one tube with extension into the submucosa and/or muscularis, but not penetrating the serosal surface; no ascites
IB	Growth limited to both tubes with extension into the submucosa and/or muscularis, but not penetrating the serosal surface; no ascites
IC	Tumor stage IA or IB, but with tumor extension through or onto the tubal serosa or with ascites containing malignant cells or with positive peritoneal washings
II	Growth involving one or both fallopian tubes with pelvic extension
IIA	Extension and/or metastasis to the uterus and/or ovaries
IIB	Extension to other pelvic tissues
IIC	Tumor stage IIA or IIB and with ascites containing malignant cells or with positive peritoneal washings
III	Tumor involves one or both fallopian tubes with peritoneal implants outside the pelvis and/or positive retroperitoneal or inguinal nodes; superficial liver metastasis equals stage III; tumor appears limited to the true pelvis, but with histologically proven malignant extension to small bowel or omentum
IIIA	Tumor is grossly limited to true pelvis with negative nodes, but with histologically confirmed microscopic seeding of abdominal peritoneal surfaces
IIIB	Tumor involving one or both tubes with histologically confirmed implants of abdominal peritoneal surfaces, none > 2 cm in diameter; lymph nodes negative
IIIC	Abdominal implants > 2 cm in diameter and/or positive retroperitoneal or inguinal nodes
IV	Growth involving one or both fallopian tubes with distant metastases; if pleural effusion present, must be positive cytology to be stage IV; parenchymal liver metastases equal stage IV

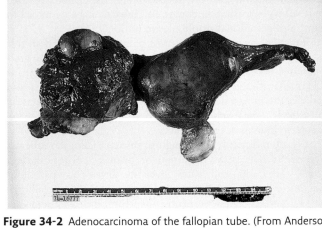

Figure 34-2 Adenocarcinoma of the fallopian tube. (From Anderson MC, Robboy SJ, Russell P: The fallopian tube. In Robboy SJ, Anderson MC, Russell P [eds]: Pathology of the Female Reproductive Tract. Edinburgh, Churchill Livingstone, 2002, pp .)

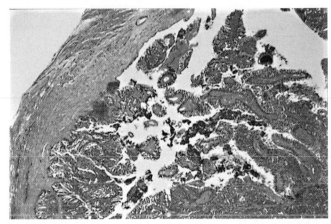

Figure 34-3 Microscopic appearance adenocarcinoma of fallopian tube confined to the endosalpinx, with minimal invasion into the muscular wall. (From Voet RL: Color Atlas of Obstetric and Gynecologic Pathology. St. Louis, Mosby-Wolfe, 1997.)

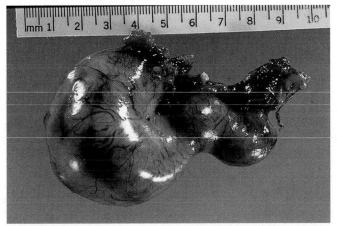

Figure 34-1 Adenocarcinoma of the fallopian tube revealing a dilated fallopian tube with an obstructed fimbriated end. (From Voet RL: Color Atlas of Obstetric and Gynecologic Pathology. St. Louis, Mosby-Wolfe, 1997.)

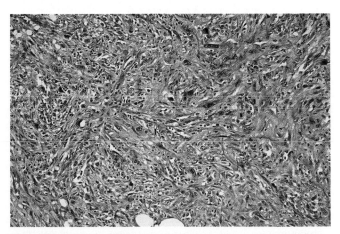

Figure 34-4 Poorly differentiated tubal carcinoma. (From Anderson MC, Robboy SJ, Russell P: The fallopian tube. In Robboy SJ, Anderson MC, Russell P (eds): Pathology of the Female Reproductive Tract. Edinburgh, Churchill Livingstone, 2002, pp .)

endometrioid and clear cell adenocarcinomas. Other rare histologic subtypes include sarcomas, carcinosarcomas, germ cell tumors, and gestational trophoblastic tumors.

Similar to ovarian cancer, most patients with fallopian tube cancer have grade 2 or 3 tumors, with less than 5% being grade 1 tumors. Previous reports have shown stage at diagnosis to be evenly distributed among localized disease, regional spread, and distant metastases. However, serous adenocarcinomas are more likely to be diagnosed at advanced stages and endometrioid adenocarcinomas at earlier stages.

It is often difficult to distinguish primary fallopian tube carcinoma from metastatic ovarian or primary peritoneal carcinoma. Hu and colleagues initially developed pathologic diagnostic criteria in 1950 for the diagnosis of primary fallopian tube carcinoma. These were subsequently modified by Sedlis and associates in 1978, and include the following:

1. The main tumor lies in the tube and arises from the endosalpinx.
2. The histologic pattern reproduces the papillary epithelium of tubal mucosa.
3. A transition can be demonstrated between the malignant and nonmalignant tubal epithelium.
4. The ovaries and uterus are normal or contain less tumor than the fallopian tube.

The patterns of spread of fallopian tube carcinoma are largely related to the degree of obstruction of the distal tube. If the fimbriated end of the tube is obstructed by tumor, previous injury, or infection, the by-products of tumor growth, such as blood and increased serous fluid, distend the tube and are discharged intermittently through the vagina. If the distal portion of the fallopian tube is patent, the malignancy spreads more easily out the distal end of the tube, resulting in tumor seeding of the peritoneal cavity, ascites, and omental caking. Intraperitoneal spread may also occur as the tumor grows through the muscular wall of the tube. The peritoneum is therefore the most frequent site of metastatic spread. However, lymphatic spread also occurs to the pelvic and para-aortic lymph nodes. Occult lymph node metastases have been reported in approximately 30% of patients with tumor that grossly appeared to be confined to the fallopian tube.

PRIMARY PERITONEAL CANCER

Primary peritoneal carcinoma tends to involve the abdominal and pelvic surfaces diffusely. The most common histologic type is papillary serous carcinoma but cases of endometrioid, clear cell, mucinous, and carcinosarcoma have been reported. Given the difficulty in distinguishing primary peritoneal carcinoma from ovarian carcinoma, the Gynecologic Oncology Group (GOG) has developed the following pathologic criteria for the diagnosis of primary peritoneal carcinoma:

1. Both ovaries must be physiologically normal in size or enlarged by a benign process.
2. Involvement in the extraovarian sites must be greater than involvement on the surface of either ovary.
3. Microscopically, the ovarian component must be one of the following:
   - Nonexistent
   - Confined to the ovarian surface epithelium with no evidence of cortical invasion

- Involving ovarian surface epithelium and underlying cortical stroma but with any given tumor size smaller than 5 × 5 mm
- Tumor smaller than 5 × 5 mm within the ovarian substance, with or without surface disease
4. The histologic and cytologic characteristics of the tumor must be predominantly of the serous type that is similar or identical to ovarian serous papillary adenocarcinoma, any grade.

TREATMENT

The treatment of fallopian tube and primary peritoneal cancer is similar to that of ovarian cancer. In most cases, surgery is initially performed. followed by chemotherapy.

SURGERY

Primary surgery for fallopian tube and primary peritoneal carcinomas generally includes collection of peritoneal washings or ascites, if present, followed by hysterectomy and bilateral salpingo-oophorectomy. A staging operation should be performed in patients with apparent early-stage disease. This includes omentectomy, pelvic and para-aortic lymph node dissection, and peritoneal biopsies. In cases of advanced disease, cytoreductive surgery with removal of as much visible tumor as possible should be performed. Similar to ovarian cancer, improved survival rates are associated with optimal cytoreduction for fallopian tube and primary peritoneal cancers. However, optimal cytoreduction may be more difficult to achieve in women with primary peritoneal cancer caused by widespread peritoneal disease without a predominant pelvic or ovarian mass.

CHEMOTHERAPY

The chemotherapeutic regimens used for fallopian tube and primary peritoneal cancers are the same as those used for ovarian cancer. Patients with advanced-stage disease are typically treated with a combination of carboplatin and paclitaxel. Many clinical trials for ovarian cancer include fallopian tube and primary peritoneal cancers because of their similar clinical and pathologic findings, as well as response to chemotherapeutic agents. Similar to ovarian cancer, neoadjuvant chemotherapy may be considered for patients with fallopian tube cancer and primary peritoneal cancer who have unresectable disease, a large tumor burden, or medical comorbidities precluding surgery.

RADIATION THERAPY

Similar to ovarian cancer, radiation therapy is not recommended for fallopian tube or primary peritoneal cancer. Because of the tendency of these cancers to spread throughout the abdominal cavity, external beam radiation therapy cannot be administered in therapeutic doses without causing excessive side effects, thereby minimizing its usefulness.

SURVEILLANCE

Surveillance following completion of treatment for fallopian tube and primary peritoneal cancer is identical that for to ovarian cancer. Follow-up visits are performed every 2 to 4 months for the first 2 years, every 3 to 6 months for the following 3 years, and then annually after 5 years. Visits include a physical examination with pelvic examination, as well as measurement of the CA-125 level if initially elevated. Imaging studies are not routinely performed unless clinically indicated because of the woman's symptoms, physical examination findings, or increasing CA-125 level. Pap tests are generally not indicated as part of surveillance for ovarian, fallopian tube, or primary peritoneal cancer.

PROGNOSIS

Similar to ovarian cancer, the prognosis for patients with fallopian tube cancer is strongly related to the stage of disease. The 5-year survival rates are 81% for stage I disease, 67% for stage II disease, 41% for stage III disease, and 33% for stage IV disease.

Other prognostic factors for early-stage disease include the degree of invasion of the fallopian tube wall, as well as the location of the tumor within the tube (fimbrial versus nonfimbrial). Similar to ovarian cancer, improved survival has been seen if the tumor can be completely removed at the time of surgery. In addition, patients with a *BRCA* mutation have been shown to have higher survival rates. Cass and colleagues have reported a median survival time of 68 months for patients with *BRCA*-associated fallopian tube cancer compared with 37 months for sporadic cases.

Most studies have reported a better survival for patients with advanced-stage fallopian tube cancer compared with primary ovarian cancer. In contrast, retrospective case-control studies have shown no difference in survival rates between patients with primary peritoneal cancer and patients with ovarian cancer. This favorable prognosis for patients with fallopian tube cancer may be the result of a higher rate of *BRCA* mutation carriers among women with fallopian tube cancer compared with ovarian and primary peritoneal cancers. However, if a subset of ovarian and primary peritoneal carcinomas actually arises from the fallopian tube, the prognosis for women with fallopian tube, primary peritoneal, and ovarian cancer may actually be similar.

KEY POINTS

- Fallopian tube and primary peritoneal cancers are similar but pathologically distinct entities from epithelial ovarian cancer.
- Fallopian tube and primary peritoneal cancers have similar clinical characteristics, patterns of spread, and response to treatment compared with ovarian cancer.
- The primary risk factor for fallopian tube and primary peritoneal cancer is an inherited mutation in the *BRCA1* or *BRCA2* tumor suppressor gene.
- The most common histologic subtype of fallopian tube and primary peritoneal carcinoma is high-grade papillary serous carcinoma.
- The treatment of fallopian tube and primary peritoneal cancer is identical to that for ovarian cancer and typically includes a combination of surgery and chemotherapy.
- Prognosis for ovarian and primary peritoneal cancer is most strongly related to the stage of disease and amount of residual tumor following the initial tumor reduction surgery.
- Fallopian tube cancer has been shown to have a better prognosis compared with ovarian and primary peritoneal cancer, but this may be because of a higher rate of *BRCA* mutation carriers in women with fallopian tube cancer.

REFERENCES CAN BE FOUND ON EXPERTCONSULT.com

35

Gestational Trophoblastic Disease
Hydatidiform Mole, Nonmetastatic and Metastatic Gestational Trophoblastic Tumor: Diagnosis and Management

Jacob McGee and Allan Covens

The most curable of all gynecologic malignancies, **gestational trophoblastic disease (GTD)**, represents an oncologic success story attributable primarily to early disease recognition, modern chemotherapy regimens, and accurate and reliable assessment of disease status with sensitive β-human chorionic gonadotropin (β-hCG) assays. Its importance as a disease process cannot be overstated to the general gynecologist, who is usually responsible for the initial diagnosis and management of GTD, as well as the timely referral to gynecologic oncology for further management in the setting of **gestational trophoblastic neoplasia (GTN)**. A structured approach to diagnosis and management will result in cure for most patients, even in the setting of advanced disease, without adversely affecting future fertility.

GTD describes a heterogeneous spectrum of diseases of abnormal trophoblastic proliferation ranging from benign to malignant, with varying predilections toward local invasion and distant metastasis. Historically, the various terminology and classification systems surrounding GTD have created confusion and complicated a thorough understanding of the disease. In 2000, the International Federation of Gynecology and Obstetrics (FIGO) released a new staging and risk factor scoring system for GTD, which has since become a common method for reporting the disease. GTD is classified according to histopathologic, cytogenetic, and clinical features, using the modified World Health Organization (WHO) classification of GTD. The various histologic categories of GTD include benign trophoblastic lesions (placental site nodule and exaggerated placental reaction), **hydatidiform mole (HM)**, which includes **complete hydatidiform mole (CHM)** and **partial hydatidiform mole (PHM)**, persistent and invasive mole, gestational **choriocarcinoma,** and placental trophoblastic tumor (**Table 35-1**). GTN is diagnosed based on clinical, laboratory, and histologic criteria, encompassing those diseases with tendencies to invade and metastasize (e.g., persistent or invasive mole, choriocarcinoma, **placental site trophoblastic neoplasia [PSTT]**).

HYDATIDIFORM MOLE

EPIDEMIOLOGY

Marked regional variations in the incidence of GTD are seen worldwide, but only recently has a more accurate estimation of the true incidence been possible. Prior estimates based on hospital data overestimated the incidence because deliveries (as opposed to pregnancies) were used in the denominator. With the introduction of census data, true denominators have added validity to reported incidence rates. Similarly, improvements in central reporting through tumor registries have increased the certainty of case ascertainment. Other factors leading to the improved accuracy of incidence estimations include standardized definitions of GTD variants, improvements in cytogenetics, and recognition of rare variants, such as PSTT.

Population-based studies suggest that the incidence of HM/ 1000 pregnancies is 0.81 to 2.0 in China, 0.6 to 1.1 in Europe and North America, and up to 2.0 in Japan. Reported rates from Africa range from 2.5 to 5.0. The highest rates are reported in Indonesia, 13/1000 pregnancies. The markedly higher incidence rates in Southeast Asia and Africa, although based on hospital data, suggest that the disease process is more common in these regions. Much of the geographic risk association may reflect the distribution of different ethnic groups.

RISK FACTORS

Age
Pregnancy occurring at extremes of maternal age (<15 and >40 years) is a well-established risk factor for HM, with incidence rates following a J-shaped distribution curve. Risk increases after age 35, and a five- to tenfold fold increase is seen in women conceiving after age 40, rising precipitously thereafter. This increase is accounted for by abnormal gametogenesis or abnormal fertilization with advanced maternal age. However, because of the decreased fecundity in this cohort, the overall effect on incidence rates is low. Teenagers have a 1.5- to twofold increased risk of GTD. The risk between maternal age and HM is best established for CHM, with studies showing no risk or only a small increase in PHM. Studies on the impact of advancing paternal age have been inconsistent.

Reproductive History
A reproductive history including HM is another risk factor, increasing the risk in future pregnancies by 5- to 40-fold that of the general population. Subsequent pregnancies have an approximate 1% risk, increasing to 25% when the number of previous HM is two or more. Bagshawe has shown that the risk following the first mole is 1 in 76 pregnancies, increasing to 1 in 6.5

Table 35-1 Modified World Health Organization Classification of Gestational Trophoblastic Disease

Molar lesions
Hydatidiform mole
Complete
Partial
Invasive mole
Nonmolar lesions
Choriocarcinoma
Placental site trophoblastic tumour
Epithelioid trophoblastic tumour
Miscellaneous trophoblastic lesions
Exaggerated placental site
Placental site nodule

pregnancies if more than one prior mole. Patients with recurrent molar pregnancies are also at increased risk for the malignant sequelae of GTN. The impact of parity and prior abortion on HM risk is unclear, with studies showing conflicting results.

Diet

Dietary risk factor analyses have shown conflicting results. Several case control studies have shown an increased risk of CHM with decreasing consumption of animal fat and beta-carotene (precursor to vitamin A). The hypothesis of a dietary link to GTD comes from the observation of the increased incidence of GTD in Southeast Asian countries at a time when dietary intake was poor. Other studies detailing food intake have failed to show a decreased incidence with increasing consumption of dietary protein or fat.

HISTOPATHOLOGY AND CYTOGENETIC FEATURES

During early embryonic differentiation, trophoblasts are derived from the outer blastocyst layer, with three distinct trophoblasts recognized—cytotrophoblasts, syncytiotrophoblasts, and intermediate trophoblasts. Cytotrophoblasts are the trophoblastic stem cells that differentiate along a villous and extravillous pathway. The villous trophoblast forms the interface between maternal and fetal tissues and is composed of cytotrophoblasts and syncytiotrophoblasts. This layer is responsible for molecular exchange across compartments and, in the case of syncytiotrophoblasts, production of the pregnancy-associated hormones β-hCG

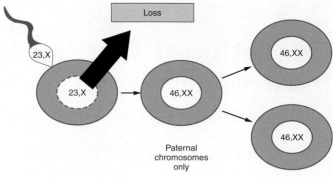

Figure 35-1 Paternal chromosomal origin of a complete classic mode (46,XX). *Left to right:* Entry of normal sperm with haploid set of 23,X into an egg whose 23,X haploid set is lost. The egg is taken over by paternal chromosomes, which duplicate (without cell division) to reach the requisite complement of 46. Observe that almost the same result can be obtained through fertilization by two sperm gaining entry into an empty egg (dispermy). (From Szulman AE, Surti UL: The syndromes of partial and complete molar gestation. Clin Obstet Gynecol 27:172-180, 1984.)

and human placental lactogen (HPL). Along the extravillous pathway, they differentiate into intermediate trophoblasts in the placental bed at the implantation site. This layer is responsible for establishing the maternal-fetal circulation and infiltrating the decidua and myometrium.

In HM, chromosomal abnormalities differentiate the disease, with complete and partial moles having distinct chromosomal profiles (**Figs. 35-1** and **35-2**). CHMs are completely derived from paternal origin, with greater than 90% having a 46, XX genotype, produced by fertilization of an empty (anuclear) ovum by a single haploid (23,X) sperm, which then duplicates in the ovum. A small percentage of CHMs have a 46,XY genotype, produced by dispermy, in which a 23,X sperm and a 23,Y sperm fertilize an empty ovum. Rarely, complete moles may be triploid or aneuploid. The mechanism for production of the empty ovum is unknown.

In contrast, PHMs are derived from paternal and maternal chromosomes, resulting in a triploid genotype. A haploid ovum is fertilized by two haploid spermatozoa, with 69,XXX or 69, XXY being the most common karyotypes. Although a triploid karyotype is usually seen in PHM, not all triploid pregnancies will show histologic changes consistent with a partial mole. In addition, PHM may present in conjunction with a viable fetus,

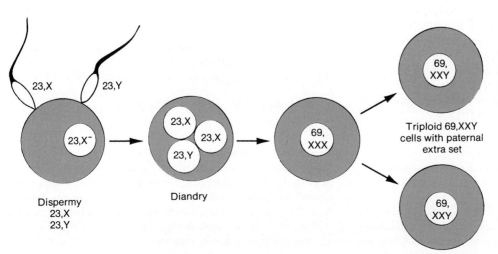

Figure 35-2 Triploid chromosomal origin of partial mole (69,XXY dispermy). Fertilization of an egg equipped with a normal 23,X complement by two independently produced sperm (dispermy) to give a total of 69 chromosomes. Observe that triploidy can also result through fertilization by sperm carrying father's total complement of 46,XY. (From Szulman AE, Surti UL: The syndromes of partial and complete molar gestation. Clin Obstet Gynecol 27:172-180, 1984.)

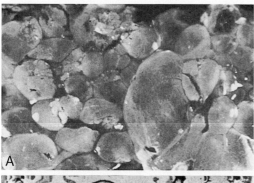

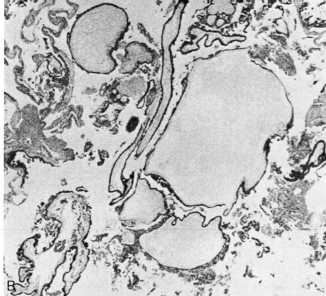

Figure 35-3 A, Hydatidiform mole. A few vesicles approach 1 cm in diameter. The background is formed by smaller vesicles. **B,** Hydatidiform mole aborted by suction curettage. A large intact vesicle is near the center. Many vesicles, however, have been ruptured and have collapsed. (From Bigelow B: Gestational trophoblast disease. In Blaustein A [ed]: Pathology of the Female Genital Tract, 2nd ed. New York, Springer-Verlag, 1982.)

Table 35-2 Features of Complete and Partial Hydatidiform Moles

Feature	Complete Moles	Partial Moles
Fetal or embryonic tissue	Absent	Present
Hydatidiform swelling of chronic villi	Diffuse	Focal
Trophoblastic hyperplasia	Diffuse	Focal
Trophoblastic stormal inclusions	Absent	Present
Genetic parentage	Paternal	Bipaternal
Karyotype	46,XX; 46,XY	69,XXY; 69,XYY
Persistent human chrionic gonadotropin	20% of cases	0.5% of cases

From Eifel PJ, Gershenson DM, Kavanagh JJ, Silva EG: Gynecologic Cancer. New York, Springer-Verlag, 2006, p 230.

at the molar implantation site; and (5) presence of trophoblastic scalloping and stromal inclusions.

Differentiation between CHM and PHM in early first-trimester abortions can be difficult because of less pronounced trophoblastic proliferation and only subtle hydropic swelling of the villi. Absence of the immunohistochemical nuclear stain p57 (a maternally expressed gene) suggests paternal origin and can be used to differentiate between CHM and PHM. A summary of the genetic and histopathologic differences between CHM and PHM is presented in **Table 35-2**.

CLINICAL FEATURES

Dramatic presentations of advanced HMs are currently less common in the developed world than in past decades, largely because of the increased use of ultrasonography and improvements in the sensitivity of β-hCG assays, leading to detection in early pregnancy. The average gestational age of diagnosis of CHM today is 9.6 weeks versus 17 weeks in the 1960s. Following a delayed menses, CHM typically presents in the first trimester as vaginal bleeding, with or without the passage of molar vesicles. Other classic signs of CHM include a large-for-date uterus, absence of fetal movement, anemia secondary to occult hemorrhage, gestational hypertension before 20 weeks' gestation, presence of theca lutein cysts, hyperemesis, hyperthyroidism, and respiratory distress from trophoblastic emboli to the lungs.

When uterine enlargement is more than 14 to 16 weeks, 25% of patients will have medical complications. Such complications are related to the high levels of β-hCG commonly seen in CHM and proportional to the volume of trophoblastic hyperplasia. β-hCG is homologous to thyrotropin-releasing hormone and the β-hCG isoforms seen in CHM may have a greater affinity for the thyrotropin-stimulating hormone receptor than normal β-hCG, causing excessive thyroid stimulation in some patients. Similarly, β-hCG is homologous to luteinizing hormone (LH), the purported mechanism whereby ovarian stimulation leads to the formation of theca lutein cysts in some patients.

Despite the possible medical complications associated with the disease, data from the New England Trophoblastic Disease Center have revealed the changing clinical presentation over time of HM (**Table 35-3**). Currently, patients are more likely to present without any symptoms than with anemia, preeclampsia, or hyperthyroidism. If medical complications are present, the woman should be stabilized, followed by evacuation of the HM as soon as possible.

showing signs of triploidy such as multiple congenital anomalies or severe growth retardation. Conditions that may be confused pathologically with PHM include Beckwith-Wiedemann syndrome, placental angiomatous malformation, twin gestation with complete mole and an existing fetus, early complete mole, and hydropic complete mole.

The histopathologic differences between CHM and PHM are well defined. The gross appearance of CHM may be impressive, with a large volume of grapelike vesicles made up of edematous enlarged villi (**Fig. 35-3**). Histopathologic characteristics include the following: (1) lack of fetal or embryonic tissues; (2) hydropic (edematous) villi; (3) diffuse trophoblastic hyperplasia; (4) marked atypia of trophoblasts at the implantation site; and (5) absence of trophoblastic stromal inclusions. In comparison, the gross appearance of PHM may only show subtle abnormalities, with generally a smaller volume of hydropic villi and the possible presence of a fetus or fetal tissue. The histopathologic features are the following: (1) presence of fetal or embryonic tissues; (2) less diffuse, focal hydropic swelling of villi; (3) focal trophoblastic hyperplasia; (4) less pronounced trophoblastic atypia

Table 35-3 Changing Clinical Presentation of Complete Hydatidiform Mole at the New England Trophoblastic Disease Center (%)

Symptom or Sign	1988-1993 (N = 74)	1965-1975 (N = 306)
Vaginal bleeding	84	97
Size greater than dates	28	51
Anemia	5	54
Preeclampsia	1.3	27
Hyperemesis	8	26
Hyperthyroidism	0	7
Respiratory distress	0	2
Asymptomatic	9	0

From Valena S-W, Bernstein M, Goldstein DP, Berkowitz R: The changing clinical presentation of complete molar pregnancy. Obstet Gynecol 86:775-779, 1995.

PHM usually presents incidentally following histopathologic examination of the products of conception from uterine evacuation of a suspected missed or therapeutic abortion. Medical complications such as gestational hypertension, hyperthyroidism, theca lutein cysts, and respiratory distress are rare with PHM. With a low clinical suspicion for PHM, underdiagnosis is a risk, reflecting the importance of a thorough histopathologic examination of curettage specimens as an important aspect of quality care.

DIAGNOSIS

The various symptoms associated with HM such as vaginal bleeding or a uterus large for dates often prompts ultrasound (US) examination to determine if a pregnancy is viable. US is the standard imaging modality for the diagnosis of a mole. A CHM has the appearance on US of an echogenic endometrial mass accompanying an enlarged uterus, the so-called snowstorm appearance (**Fig. 35-4**). As the molar pregnancy progresses into the second trimester, the anechoic spaces of the molar vesicles will become more evident. A transvaginal US may show the interface between molar tissue and endometrium and dilated

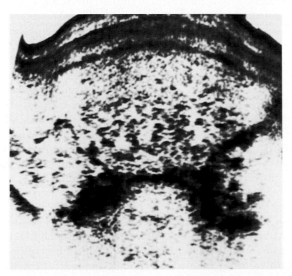

Figure 35-4 Ultrasound scan of uterus demonstrating snowstorm appearance of hydatidiform mole.

vesicles in the first trimester better, but risks worsening vaginal bleeding in the setting of metastatic disease to the vagina. Naumoff and colleagues have established criteria for diagnosis, including placental enlargement with multiple cysts, presence of a gestational sac, and underdeveloped fetal material for gestational age.

Although US may be the imaging modality of choice, Sebire and associates have reviewed 155 cases of histologically proven HM and have shown that only 34% of cases were diagnosed by US alone prior to histologic confirmation, reinforcing the importance of histology for diagnosis. The accuracy was higher for CHM (58%) than for PHM (17%).

Human Chorionic Gonadotropin

The anterior pituitary produces a series of glycoproteins that differ only in their beta subunits, including hCG, follicle-stimulating hormone, LH, and thyroid-stimulating hormone. Outside of pregnancy, an elevated β-hCG level signifies the following: (1) GTN, (2) nongestational tumors secreting hCG; (3) false-positives; and (4) menopause (secondary to LH elevation and cross reactivity of assays).

An unexpectedly elevated β-HCG level during pregnancy may suggest the diagnosis of CHM. β-hCG typically plateaus in pregnancy at approximately 10 weeks' gestation, with levels peaking at 100,000 IU/L and then falling thereafter. Gernst and coworkers have shown that 46% of patients with CHM managed over a 10-year period had pretreatment β-HCG levels higher than 100,000 IU/L. Conversely, Berkowitz and colleagues have shown in one series that PHM presented with an elevated β-HCG above 100,000 IU/L in only 2 of 30 cases.

TREATMENT

Preevacuation diagnosis of HM allows for optimal treatment planning, but the diagnosis of most patients will be made histologically after surgery. If HM is suspected preoperatively, a chest x-ray should be performed, because evacuation may transiently shower the lungs with trophoblastic emboli, complicating the interpretation of a postevacuation chest x-ray. A complete blood count, blood type with antibody screen, β-hCG level determination, and liver function testing should also be performed. Because RhD factor is expressed on the trophoblast, patients who are Rh-negative, with a Rh-positive or Rh unknown partner, should be treated with Rho(D) immune globulin postevacuation.

Suction Dilation and Curettage

The preferred method of uterine evacuation of HM is suction dilation and curettage (D&C) under general anesthetic. The cervix is serially dilated and then a large suction curette is advanced into the endometrial canal. After activating the suction device, a solution of crystalloid and oxytocin (20 IU/L) is infused to increase uterine tone; this is continued postoperatively to reduce bleeding. A gentle sharp curettage may be performed to complete the procedure. Care must be taken during D&C to avoid perforation of the enlarged soft uterus in HM.

Hysterectomy

For patients diagnosed with HM preoperatively for whom continued fertility is not an issue, hysterectomy with preservation of the adnexa is a treatment option. This decreases local (myometrial) persistence, but does not eliminate the risk of distant

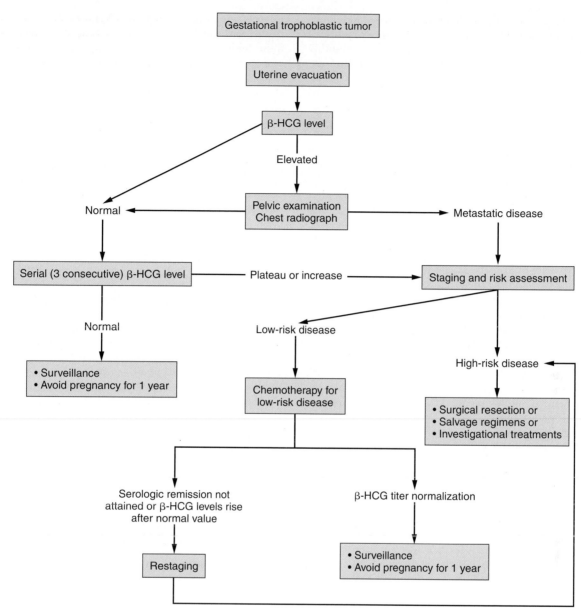

Figure 35-5 Treatment algorithm. This is a diagnostic and therapeutic approach to gestational trophoblastic disease as practiced at the University of Texas M.D. Anderson Cancer Center. HCG, Human chorionic gonadotropin. (Adapted from Eifel PJ, Gershenson DM, Kavanagh JJ, Silva EG: Gynecologic Cancer. New York, Springer-Verlag, 2006, p 235.)

metastases. For women older than 40 years with HM, hysterectomy is reasonable because of the risk of GTN developing in 37% of women older than 40 and 56% of women older than 50. Following hysterectomy, the risk of postmolar GTN is 3% to 5%, so continued β-hCG monitoring is still required.

Prophylactic Chemotherapy
Following surgical evacuation, postmolar GTN, usually in the form of a locally invasive mole, occurs in 15% to 20% of CHM cases (>50% when the woman is older than 50 years), and only rarely (<5%) following PHM. **Figure 35-5** outlines a treatment algorithm for GTD. If postevacuation follow-up is anticipated to be compromised, patients with high-risk CHM may be considered for treatment with prophylactic chemotherapy. In a nonrandomized clinical trial by Uberti and associates, prophylactic single-dose actinomycin D at the time of

surgical evacuation decreased the frequency of persistent HM in high-risk patients (determined at the time of evacuation) from 34.3% to 18.4% with, at worst, mild side effects reported in 21.5% of patients treated. In the prophylactic actinomycin D group, the relative risk for development of postmolar GTN was 0.54, and the number needed to treat (NNT) to prevent one case of GTN was 7. Although prophylactic chemotherapy is an option in high-risk patients, its routine use is not recommended because of the morbidity associated with even a single dose of chemotherapy, requirement for surveillance regardless, and ultimate high cure rates eventually achieved in GTN.

Surveillance Following Hydatidiform Mole Evacuation
Following evacuation of a HM, surveillance with serial β-hCG serum measurements are required to ensure a timely diagnosis of postmolar malignant GTN. Within 48 hours of evacuation, a

baseline β-hCG level should be obtained and then weekly until the level returns to normal (<5mIU/ml). Most cases of postmolar GTN will occur within 6 months of evacuation, so monthly β-hCG monitoring is recommended following normalization for a further 6 to 12 months.

Although 6 months observation is the minimum conventional period for observation, such a long duration of follow-up has been questioned, particularly in the setting of a woman with a narrow window of fertility because of advanced age. Wolfberg and coworkers have reviewed 1029 cases of CHM and found that when a β-hCG titer of less than 5 mIU/mL was used, no cases of invasive mole were encountered in patients who reached a negative titer. Thus, discontinuing surveillance after two negative β-hCG titers 1 week apart may spare patients unnecessary anxiety, limit resource expenditure, and obviate the problems of noncompliance inherent with prolonged follow-up. In a separate analysis, Wolfberg and associates found the risk of GTN to be 1.1% or less when the β-hCG dropped below 50 mIU/mL at any point during their follow-up. In another analysis of 320 patients who achieved one undetectable β-hCG titer, none developed relapse as GTN. In this cohort, the mean time to achieve nondetectable β-hCG levels was 5.8 weeks. Analysis of the Hydatidiform Mole Registry in Melbourne, Australia has revealed no cases of persistent disease in the setting of CHM if the β-hCG level normalizes within 8 weeks, and no cases with PHM if the β-hCG level normalizes. Despite these reports, the most recommended follow-up period continues to be 6 months.

During this period of surveillance, use of reliable contraception is strongly recommended to ensure that a rise in β-hCG level represents postmolar GTN and not a new pregnancy. One randomized controlled trial (RCT) has shown that use of the oral contraceptive pill (OCP) versus barrier methods of contraception results in 50% of the number of pregnancies during the surveillance period. In the past, there was concern that the OCP increased the risk of GTN, but two RCTs have shown no association between OCP use during postmolar surveillance and the incidence of GTN.

Prognostic factors associated with the development of GTN have only recently been identified. The timing of molar evacuation does not influence the development of GTN, with more advanced gestations not contributing an increased risk of invasive mole. As noted, advanced maternal age (>35 years) increases the risk of invasive mole, as does a history of HM. In addition, a β-hCG level higher than100,000 IU/liter on presentation may increase the risk of invasive mole. Other factors associated with persistent disease include uterine size large for date and bilateral ovarian enlargement (>8-cm theca lutein cysts) at the time of initial presentation. In addition, ultrasound (US) findings of uterine invasion may be predictive of the development of GTN. In a retrospective analysis, Garavaglia and coworkers have shown that the presence of hyperechoic lesions (nodules) within the myometrium or increased signal intensity suggesting hypervascularization at baseline ultrasound was associated with an odds ratio (OR) of 17.57 for the development of GTN (*P* < .001).

Quiescent Gestational Trophoblastic Disease

Following a hydatidiform mole, choriocarcinoma, or spontaneous abortion, the persistence of low levels (range, 1 to 212 IU/L) of β-hCG for 3 months or longer with no obvious increase or decrease in the β-hCG level trend is termed *quiescent gestational trophoblastic disease.* This process has been identified in patients treated with single-agent or multiagent chemotherapy, and in those undergoing repeat surgical procedures, with no disease evident on imaging despite persistent elevations of β-hCG level. With as many as 25% of these cases progressing to GTN-choriocarcinoma over a time frame ranging from 6 months to 10 years, it is best described as a premalignant condition. Cole and colleagues have shown that the incorporation of hyperglycosylated hCG (hCG-H), a marker of invasive cytotrophoblasts, will detect 100% of quiescent GTD cases that require no further treatment, and 96% of self-resolving HM cases that require ongoing surveillance, differentiating these from GTN-choriocarcinoma cases that require further treatment. This methodology, however, requires validation in a prospective fashion.

Phantom β-Human Chorionic Gonadotropin

Persistent low levels of β-hCG must be evaluated to rule out false-positive assay results or phantom hCG, a rare finding that is secondary to heterophilic antibodies or proteolytic enzymes that mimic hCG. The diagnosis is made when a serum β-hCG is positive but a corresponding urine β-hCG samples taken at the same time tests negative. Alternatively, despite serial dilutions of serum, the test result will usually remain positive if heterophilic antibodies are the cause. Finally, physicians can test against multiple β-hCG assays, when available; heterophilic antibodies may cause a positive result in one test and a negative result in another. The reason for the negative urine β-hCG test is that heterophilic antibodies are large glycoproteins unable to cross the glomeruli and thus are not excreted in the urine. These antibodies—typically derived from exposure to mouse, rabbit, goat or sheet antigens—are acquired through immunizations or time spent in agricultural settings, and persist over time.

GESTATIONAL TROPHOBLASTIC NEOPLASIA

This category includes invasive mole/postmolar GTN, choriocarcinoma, and placental site trophoblastic tumor.

CHARACTERISTICS

Histopathology and Cytogenetic Features

Invasive moles are HMs characterized by syncytiotrophoblast or cytotrophoblast hyperplasia, with the presence of villi. The presence of these villi extending into the myometrium constitutes invasion, and hence the name (epidemiology and cause of gestational trophoblastic diseases). Most of these tumors, as in HM, are diploid; anaplastic tumors are the exception.

The dominant histology in metastatic GTN is gestational choriocarcinoma following an HM or normal pregnancy. Reported age-standardized incidence rates range from 0.9/100,000 women years in Japan to 1.68/100,000 women years in Vietnam. The characteristic appearance of choriocarcinoma is sheets of cytotrophoblast and syncytiotrophoblast cells with absent chorionic villi. These cells invade adjacent tissues with a propensity for vascular infiltration. Choriocarcinomas are cytogenetically anaplastic. Primary gonadal (nongestational) choriocarcinomas can develop without pregnancy, with the same histologic appearance, and have significantly inferior outcomes compared with gestational choriocarcinoma.

The rarest form of GTN is PSTT. This tumor is comprised almost entirely of intermediate trophoblasts, lacking the syncytiotrophoblasts and cytotrophoblasts seen in other forms of GTD. PSTT has an infiltrative pattern, with nests or sheets of cells invading between myometrial cells and fibers. Immunohistochemical staining is positive in 50% to 100% for HPL and in less than 10% for β-hCG.

Clinical Features

Symptoms associated with invasive mole include irregular vaginal bleeding, uterine subinvolution, and theca lutein cysts. Most GTN is identified in patients undergoing surveillance following evacuation of HM on the basis of β-hCG criterion, as outlined by FIGO (**Table 35-4**). These include a plateau in β-hCG values (four over a 4-week period), a rising β-hCG value of 10% or more over a 2-week period, persistent β-hCG detectable for more than 6 months following evacuation for HM, or a histologic diagnosis of choriocarcinoma.

Following surgical evacuation of HM, β-hCG values decrease exponentially, with an expected initial steep decline followed by a slower decrease in β-hCG levels. Observing low levels of β-hCG for longer than 2 to 3 weeks is permitted, because delay will not adversely affect the woman's survival. This is particularly helpful for physicians faced with a plateau or increase of a low β-hCG level, for which continued observation as opposed to initiation of chemotherapy may be warranted.

Locally Invasive Gestational Trophoblastic Neoplasia

With invasive mole, myometrial invasion may involve local capillaries and veins, with persistent vaginal hemorrhage as the most commonly reported symptom. Also, uterine perforation with intraperitoneal hemorrhage, and infection secondary to tumor necrosis, may also occur. Although most of these tumors will regress spontaneously following evacuation, chemotherapy treatment may be initiated to prevent the serious morbidity, and even mortality, which might ensue (see later, Prophylactic Chemotherapy).

Malignant Gestational Trophoblastic Neoplasia

Most metastatic GTN results from choriocarcinoma. PSTTs are associated with metastases at the time of initial diagnosis in only 10% of cases. Both choriocarcinoma and PSTT may follow after any pregnancy event. Metastases result from hematogenous dissemination, with almost any site possible. These tumors tend to be hemorrhagic and necrotic. Local metastases may include the vagina, with distant metastasis to the lung, brain, liver, gastrointestinal (GI) tract and kidney having been seen. The lungs usually represent the first organ involved, followed by dissemination via the systemic circulation. Metastatic lesions are highly vascularized with thin-walled fragile vessels. Symptoms of metastatic GTN, such as hemoptysis or headache, may be related to hemorrhage at involved sites. When metastases are suspected, biopsy is contraindicated because of the potential risk of uncontrollable hemorrhage.

CLASSIFICATION AND STAGING

In 2000, a revised FIGO-WHO scoring system was adopted to attain uniformity in reporting, while indicating the extent of disease spread and risk factors important for predicting persistent disease and therefore appropriate chemotherapy treatment (**Table 35-5**). The stage of the disease relates to tumor spread, with stage I disease confined to the uterus, stage II disease including spread to the adnexa, vagina, and broad ligament, stage III disease defined by lung metastases, and stage IV disease including all other sites of metastases. A WHO score of 6 or lower is considered low risk and 7 or greater is considered high risk. Generally, stage relates to risk scoring, with stage I patients usually low risk and stage IV patients high risk. Prognostic factors included in the WHO scoring system are age, antecedent

Table 35-4 FIGO Criteria for Diagnosis of Gestational Trophoblastic Neoplasia

The International Federation of Gynecologists and Obstetricians (FIGO) standardized criterion for diagnosing gestational trophoblastic neoplasia GTN following a HM are: the following

1. Four β-hCG values plateauing (±10%) over a 3-week period (days 1, 7, 14, 21)
2. A rising β-hCG value of 10% or greater seen on three values measured over a 2-week period (days 1, 7, 14)
3. Persistence of detectable β-hCG for more than 6 months following evacuation of a HM
4. Histologic diagnosis of choriocarcinoma

Table 35-5 FIGO 2000 Classification for Gestational Trophoblastic Neoplasia

Staging	Features
Stage I	Disease confined to uterus
Stage II	GTN extends outside uterus, but limited to genital structures (adnexa, vagina, broad ligament)
Stage III	GTN extends to lungs, with or without known genital tract involvement
Stage IV	All other metastatic sites

Parameter	Scoring			
	0	1	2	4
Age (yr)	<40	≥40	—	—
Antecedent pregnancy	Mole	Abortion	Term	—
Interval from index pregnancy (mo)	<4	4 to <7	7 to <13	>13
Pretreatment β-hCG (IU/mL)	$<10^3$	10^3 to 10^4	10^4 to 10^5	$>10^5$
Largest tumor size (cm; including uterus)	—	3 to <5 cm	≥5 cm	—
No. of metastases	—	1 to 4	5 to 8	>8
Previous failed chemotherapy	—	—	Single drug	Two or more drugs

pregnancy, interval months from index pregnancy, pretreatment serum β-hCG levels, largest tumor size (cm), site of metastases, number of metastases, and previous failed chemotherapy.

DIAGNOSIS

Diagnosis of persistent disease via β-hCG monitoring should prompt a complete physical examination accompanied by quantitative β-hCG, CBC, and renal, liver, and thyroid function testing. As a diagnostic imaging test, US will rule out concurrent intrauterine pregnancy and provides superior visualization to computed tomography (CT) for discerning the interface between normal myometrium and trophoblastic tissue. Examination via Doppler US may show hypervascularity and areas of tumor necrosis. In addition, US will identify patients whose large-volume uterine disease is best treated surgically. Following US of the pelvis, FIGO recommends a chest x-ray as the test of choice to rule out lung metastases. If the chest x-ray is negative, CT of the thorax may demonstrate small-volume metastases, but the importance of these findings is unclear. In high-risk cases, up to 41% of patients will have findings identified on CT but not chest x-ray. Identification of lung metastases necessitates further imaging with CT or US of the abdomen, which includes assessment of the spleen, kidneys, GI tract, and liver. Use of IV contrast will identify metastases as round enhanced masses, which are usually multiple, heterogenous, and hypoechoic in appearance. An assessment of central nervous system (CNS) involvement, typically found at the gray-white matter junction, is best done with magnetic resonance imaging (MRI). MRI is also preferred for assessment of vaginal or parametrial lesions. The role of ^{18}F-fluorodeoxyglucose positron emission tomography (FDG-PET) in GTN is undefined, but its high sensitivity and specificity in other disease sites may make it a useful test when other modalities are equivocal; studies to date are limited to small case series. For patients with a negative chest x-ray and CT scan of thorax who are asymptomatic, further investigation is not required to assign a risk score, because high-risk sites of metastasis are rarely seen without evidence of pulmonary metastases.

TREATMENT

Low-Risk Gestational Trophoblastic Neoplasia

With the exception of PSTT, the management of malignant GTN is based more on clinical presentation than histologic diagnosis. Low-risk GTN includes localized and metastatic disease, and is defined by a prognostic score of 6 or lower. For these patients, clinicians can expect an excellent outcome with single-agent chemotherapy consisting of methotrexate or actinomycin D. While on chemotherapy, patients require monitoring of β-hCG level as well as hematologic and metabolic studies to gauge treatment toxicity. In addition, patients require reliable contraception, preferably with OCP, to prevent intercurrent pregnancies that would be adversely affected by the teratogenic chemotherapy and confuse the evaluation of β-hCG follow-up.

For patients with localized disease for whom fertility preservation is not an issue, hysterectomy may be undertaken to decrease the total number of chemotherapy cycles. Even with surgery, chemotherapy may still be required to treat occult disease. There have been no RCTs of combined hysterectomy and chemotherapy but, if chemotherapy has been given

preoperatively, it should be continued postoperatively until β-hCG levels are normal.

Some authors have advocated for a second D&C in the setting of localized GTN. The purpose of this debulking is to decrease the percentage of patients requiring chemotherapy and limit the treatment volume of chemotherapy in patients for whom a second curettage is not curative. Many believe that it is more than a debulking effect and may involve an inflammatory or immune response that contributes to the clinical response. There have been patients in whom no tumor was found on a second D&C and the woman's β-hCG level has decreased. The cohort analysis by von Tromel and associates have compared 85 patients who underwent a second D&C for persistent low-risk GTN with 209 patients who proceeded directly to chemotherapy. Of those treated surgically, 9.4% required no further treatment. The therapeutic effect of a second curettage was also seen, with a median of six cycles of chemotherapy seen in the control group versus five cycles in the D&C cohort ($P = .036$). Major complications were seen in 4.8% of patients in the D&C group, with two uterine perforations seen and patients experiencing blood loss of more than 1000 mL. Schlaerth and coworkers have demonstrated a similar magnitude of benefit with a second D&C, with cure achieved in 16% of patients and an 8% uterine perforation rate. The GOG has recently completed accrual to a phase II study exploring the response of a second D&C in patients with persistent low-risk nonmetastatic GTN.

A review of first-line therapies in low-risk GTN cases has identified 14 different treatment regimens. The most commonly used first-line treatments are methotrexate and actinomycin D, with various dosing schedules used. Methotrexate can be given on a 5-day schedule, once weekly, or every 2 weeks on an 8-day schedule, with or without folinic acid rescue,; actinomycin can be given on a 5-day schedule or every 2 weeks (pulsed actinomycin D). However, there are no RCTs comparing all these regimens.

Worldwide, the most common first-line agent (regimen) for low-risk disease is 8-day methotrexate alternating with folinic acid rescue because of factors such as established activity, low toxicity, and low cost. Methotrexate use requires normal liver and renal function because of hepatic metabolism followed by renal excretion of the drug. Depending on the regimen used, patients may experience cutaneous side effects, mucositis, serositis, GI toxicities, alopecia, and/or hematologic suppression. Actinomycin D side effects are increased with more dose-intense regimens. The 5-day regimen side effects include alopecia, nausea, and myelotoxicity. It is a vesicant, causing tissue necrosis if IV extravasation occurs. Effectiveness of pulse actinomycin D versus the 5-day regimen appear to be equivalent, with decreased toxicity, cost, and fewer patient visits with the pulsed regimen.

The use of methotrexate with folinic acid rescue has been reported by McNeish and associates in a series of 485 low-risk patients (using a Charing Cross scoring system of 0 to 8). Administration of methotrexate, 50 mg IM on days 1, 3, 5, and 7 with folinic acid, 7.5 mg PO on days 2, 4, 6, and 8 achieved a primary remission in 67% of women. The same regimen was used by Chalouhi and coworkers on 142 FIGO low-risk (0 to 6) patients, with 78% primary remission achieved and a mean time to β-hCG level normalization of 21 weeks. Three RCTs have compared weekly methotrexate at 30 mg/m[2] with pulsed dactinomycin (actinomycin D), 1.25 mg/m[2], showing an improved primary cure rate with pulsed actinomycin D (69-90%) versus methotrexate (48% to 53%) and fewer overall chemotherapy courses with actinomycin D (mean, 4 to 4.8) compared with methotrexate (mean, 6.5 to 6.8). Traditionally, chemotherapy treatment of low-risk disease has been given on a fixed time interval. The New England Trophoblastic Disease Center treats low-risk GTN on the basis of the β-hCG regression curve. Following administration of single-agent methotrexate, further doses are withheld provided that the β-hCG level falls progressively. Their indications for further chemotherapy include the following: (1) a β-hCG plateau for 3 or more consecutive weeks; and (2) failure of the β-hCG level to fall by 1 log within 18 days of the previous chemotherapy. A similar treatment strategy has been used by Chan and colleagues, with 45% of patients in their low-risk cohort achieving complete remission following a single dose of methotrexate.

Although most women with low-risk GTN will be cured with a first-line chemotherapy regimen, tumor resistance and relapse do occur. Resistance is defined as a β-hCG level increasing over two consecutive measurements or a β-hCG level plateauing or decreasing by less than 1 log over a 3-week period. In patients treated with single-agent methotrexate, resistance requiring a change to alternative first-line treatment can be expected in 10% to 31% of patients. The experience from the Charing Cross Hospital GTD database reveals that relapse after attaining a normal β-hCG level occurs in 2% of cases.

Table 35-6 provides an overview of management for low-risk GTN. Following normalization of the β-hCG level, chemotherapy is usually continued for an additional two cycles. The conventional period of observation with monthly β-hCG measurements before attempting pregnancy is 12 months, because most relapses will occur during this period. Irrespective of which first-line agent is used, cure rates approaching 100% can be achieved with diligent follow-up and salvage therapy for failures.

High-Risk Gestational Trophoblastic Neoplasia

In the developed world, high-risk GTN cases are uncommon. The timely involvement of specialist teams with experience in treating high-risk disease is key to achieving optimal outcomes.

Table 35-6 Management of Low-Risk Gestational Trophoblastic Neoplasia

Following metastatic evaluation and determination of low-risk disease:
1. Initiate single-agent methotrexate or dactinomycin; consider hysterectomy, if fertility is not desired.
Monitor hematologic, renal, and hepatic indices before each cycle of chemotherapy.
Monitor β-hCG levels while on treatment.
If severe toxicity or resistance develops, consider switching to the alternative single agent.
If resistance to the alternative agent develops:
2. Repeat the metastatic evaluation.
3. Consider hysterectomy if disease confined to uterus.
4. Multiagent therapy with EMA-CO (see treatment of high-risk GTN).

Remission is defined as three consecutive weekly β-hCG values in the normal range. Following the first normal β-hCG, continue with one or two cycles of maintenance or consolidation chemotherapy. Monitor β-hCG levels for 12 months, with reliable contraception used in this time period.
Adapted from Soper 2007.

Table 35-7 Chemotherapy Regimens for Intermediate- and High-Risk Gestational Trophoblastic Disease

Drug Regimen	Administration
EMA-CO (Preferred Regimen)—Course I (EMA)*	
Day 1	
Etoposide	100 mg/m^2 IV over 30 min
Methotrexate	100 mg/m^2 IV bolus
Methotrexate	200 mg/m^2 IV as 12-hr continuous infusion
Dactinomycin	0.5 mg IV bolus
Day 2	
Etoposide	100 mg/m^2 IV over 320 min
Folinic acid	15 mg IV/IM/PO every 6 hr for four doses
Dactinomycin	0.5 mg IV bolus
Course II (CO)	
Day 8	
Cyclophosphamide	600 mg/m^2 IV over 30 min
Vincristine	1 mg/m^2 IV bolus (up to 2 mg)

*Cytokine support may be used.
Adapted from Kantarjian HM, Wolf RA, Koller CA: M.D. Anderson Manual of Medical Oncology. New York, McGraw-Hill, 2006.

The use of multiagent combination chemotherapy reflects the increased risk of treatment failure with single agents as an individual's prognostic score increases to 7 or higher. Similar to low-risk disease, multiple treatment regimens exist, but no quality RCTs have been conducted comparing regimens. Direct comparison is further complicated by the various scoring systems used to classify the disease over time.

The greatest experience with combination treatment for high-risk GTN is with EMA-CO (Table 35-7). This intensive regimen consists of etoposide, methotrexate, and dactinomycin alternating with cyclophosphamide and vincristine. A number of case series, the largest from the Charing Cross group, have reported complete response rates of 78% to 80% using primary treatment with EMA-CO. In the Charing Cross cohort, 17% developed resistance to EMA-CO, but 70% of these were salvaged with the addition of platinum-based chemotherapy. Deaths from GTN occurred in 4% of patients, and two women developed acute myeloid leukemia following treatment with EMA-CO. Side effects include universal alopecia, stomatitis, and hematologic and gastrointestinal toxicities. Patients may require granulocyte colony-stimulating factor to prevent dose delays in the setting of neutropenia. The risk of secondary malignancies (e.g., acute myeloid leukemia, colon cancer, breast cancer), mainly related to cumulative etoposide dosing, is 50% greater than expected in a standardized nontreated cohort.

Although less than 5% of patients with low-risk disease will relapse following apparent remission, this increases to 25% in patients with high-risk disease. The approach to these patients is multimodality treatment, including surgical resection of chemotherapy resistance sites and salvage second-line (or third-line) chemotherapy. EMA-EP (substituting etoposide and cisplatin for cyclophosphamide and vincristine in EMA-CO) achieves complete response in 90% of recurrent patients, but alternative regimens, including TE-TP (taxol, etoposide, *cis*-platinum), BEP (bleomycin, etoposide, cisplatin), VIP (vinblastine, ifosfamide, cisplatin), and ICE (ifosfamide, carboplatin, etoposide) have also been used with success.

HIGH-RISK SITES OF METASTASES

Central Nervous System Metastases

Brain metastases portend a poor prognosis. Favorable outcomes have been achieved using a combination chemotherapy, with select craniotomy in some cases, with 30 of 35 patients in one series achieving complete response. Whole-brain radiotherapy to achieve hemostasis and tumor shrinkage has been used in conjunction with chemotherapy for patients with brain metastasis but, given the high success with chemotherapy and the deleterious long-term effects on overall function in survivors, including global intellectual impairment, chemotherapy is the preferred option. Many authors initiate steroid treatment and use one dose of single-agent methotrexate as a first regimen prior to EMA-CO to limit massive tumor necrosis, which might precipitate an intracranial bleed. Others have used a modified EMA-CO regimen, including intrathecal methotrexate in the CO portion of scheduling. However, given the vascular nature of these tumors, and the fact that they are not protected by the blood-brain barrier, intrathecal chemotherapy is probably unnecessary.

Pulmonary Metastases

Respiratory failure secondary to pulmonary metastases is a concern in patients with chest pain, cyanosis, anemia, and more than 50% lung field opacification. Cao and associates have reported on 62 patients who underwent lobectomy for pulmonary metastasis, with complete response (CR) seen in 89% of recurrent cases, 79% of drug-resistant cases, and 100% of cases in whom a satisfactory response to chemotherapy was seen in the setting of residual pulmonary lesion. They recommend operative treatment of pulmonary metastases for recurrent drug-resistant cases in patients with adequate performance status to tolerate surgery, no evidence of active tumor elsewhere, and pulmonary metastases limited to one lung.

Liver Metastases

Patients with liver metastases are at increased risk of hemorrhage with chemotherapy initiation. In addition to high-risk chemotherapy regimens, other treatment modalities described include radiation therapy, embolization, and surgical resection.

Vaginal Metastases

Patients with vaginal metastases are at high risk for hemorrhage. Embolization or surgery may be used to control acute bleeding.

TREATMENT OF PLACENTAL SITE TROPHOBLASTIC TUMOR

PSTTs are seen in 1% to 2% of trophoblastic tumors, with clinical behavior ranging from relatively benign to highly malignant. Metastases are seen in 10% of patients at the time of diagnosis and develop in a further 10% during post-treatment follow-up. Surgery is the cornerstone for the treatment of nonmetastatic PSTT, with hysterectomy sufficient provided that normal ovaries are present. For metastatic PSTT, surgery is followed by chemotherapy, with EMA-CO and EMA-EP use reported.

SURVEILLANCE FOLLOWING GESTATIONAL TROPHOBLASTIC NEOPLASIA

After β-hCG remission is achieved for three weekly cycles, patients with high-risk GTN require repeat testing every 2 weeks for 3 weeks, and then monthly for 1 year. Stage IV patients are encouraged to maintain monthly testing for 24 months. The risk of relapse beyond the first year is less than 1%. In patients who relapse, sustained remissions are achieved in more than 50%, suggesting value to prolonged β-hCG monitoring every 6 months, extending as long as 5 years.

The heterogeneity of β-hCG molecules in GTN is increased compared with that in normal gestation, with higher proportions of nicked β-hCG, β core fragment, and free β-hCG, stressing the requirement of an assay that detects both β-hCG as well as its fragments and metabolites. An assay with poor sensitivity may fail to detect low levels of β-hCG, leading to incorrect clinical decisions regarding treatment effect and disease persistence.

Reliable contraception in the post-GTN period is required, and the OCP is the method of choice. Cross reactivity of LH, and therefore false-positives, may occur with some assays. Patients treated with multiagent chemotherapy may have some degree of ovarian dysfunction, either transient or eventually premature ovarian failure, particularly those in their 30s or 40s.

RECURRENCE

Recurrences following remission relate to the initial stage of disease. Goldstein and coworkers have reported recurrences in 3% for stage I disease, 8% for stage II, 4% for stage III, and 9% for stage IV. The mean time from the last detectable β-hCG to recurrence was 6 months. For all stages I, II, and III patients, remissions were achieved with additional chemotherapy, whereas all stage IV patients who recurred died of their disease. Ngan and colleagues have found no relationship between time to relapse and mortality, with an overall survival of 78% in relapsed patients.

PREGNANCY FOLLOWING GESTATIONAL TROPHOBLASTIC NEOPLASIA

Following molar pregnancy or GTN, patients can expect normal reproductive outcomes. Garner and associates have summarized pregnancy outcomes following GTD from multiple centers. In a total of 2657 pregnancies following treatment for persistent GTN, 77% had live births, with 72% term deliveries, 5% preterm births, 1% stillbirths, 14% spontaneous abortions, and 2% of children born with congenital anomalies—pregnancy outcomes similar to those of the general population.

Following a molar pregnancy, however, there is an increased risk of subsequent molar pregnancy, increasing from roughly 1/1000 pregnancies to 1/100. Following two molar pregnancies, the risk in a subsequent pregnancy may be as high as 20%.

PSYCHOSOCIAL CONSIDERATIONS

Diagnosis and treatment for GTN may have long-lasting psychosocial sequelae for patients including sadness with a sense of loss following pregnancy, low self-esteem, sexual dysfunction, and anxiety about future pregnancies. Peterson and coworkers used validated questionnaires to assess quality of life in patients following treatment for molar pregnancy, finding that more than 50% showed psychological symptomatology suggestive of an underlying psychiatric disorder. They recommend a multidisciplinary approach to care to address the emotional and social aspects of a woman's well-being following treatment for GTN.

KEY POINTS

- Persistent abnormal bleeding following normal pregnancy, abortion, or ectopic pregnancy should lead to a consideration of the diagnosis of GTD. Pulmonary nodules present on chest x-ray after a normal pregnancy suggest GTD. β-hCG levels will be elevated in these situations.
- Investigation of a young woman with metastatic disease of unknown primary should include a β-hCG level measurement.
- Approximately 50% of cases of GTD follow molar pregnancy, 25% follow normal pregnancy, and 25% follow abortion or ectopic pregnancy.
- The major risk factors for molar pregnancy include maternal age (>40 and <20 years) and a history of prior HM.
- The risk of HM is approximately 0.75 to 1.0/1000 pregnancies in North America.
- The risk of a subsequent HM after a primary mole increases 5-40 fold.
- Complete moles are of paternal origin, are diploid, and carry a 20% risk of GTD sequelae.
- Partial moles are of maternal and paternal origin, are triploid, and are rarely (2 to 4%) followed by GTD. They nonetheless require follow-up for potential malignant sequelae, as done for a complete mole.
- The monitoring of trophoblastic disease and its follow-up is accomplished by measurement of the β-hCG level.
- The diagnosis of a molar pregnancy can be established with ultrasonography and may coexist with a normal pregnancy.
- Hydatidiform moles are effectively and safely evacuated from the uterus using suction D&C.
- Medical complications of HM are rare but may include anemia, gestational hypertension before 20 weeks, hyperthyroidism, hyperemesis gravidarum, cardiac failure and, rarely, pulmonary insufficiency.
- Patients are classified into low- or high-risk categories. Low-risk patients are treated with single-agent methotrexate or actinomycin D; high-risk patients receive combination chemotherapy, usually with EMA-CO.
- The cure rate of low-risk patients approaches 100%.
- Patients with high-risk metastatic GTN are successfully treated with chemotherapy in more than 70% of cases.
- Patients treated for GTD should not become pregnant for approximately 6 months after treatment to allow accurate follow-up of β-hCG levels.
- Fertility rates and pregnancy outcomes are similar in patients treated for GTD compared with those in the general population.
- Patients treated with the EMA-CO regimen have an increased rate of secondary malignancies, particularly hematologic malignancies.

REFERENCES CAN BE FOUND ON
EXPERTCONSULT.com

36

Primary and Secondary Dysmenorrhea, Premenstrual Syndrome, and Premenstrual Dysphoric Disorder
Etiology, Diagnosis, Management

Gretchen M. Lentz

Dysmenorrhea, premenstrual syndrome, and **premenstrual dysphoric disorder** afflict a large percentage of women in their reproductive years. These conditions have a negative effect on the quality of these women's lives and the lives of their families, and they are also responsible for a huge economic loss as a result of the cost of medications, medical care, and decreased productivity. This chapter will discuss current thinking with respect to the causes, pathophysiology, and management of these three conditions.

DYSMENORRHEA

Dysmenorrhea is defined as a severe, painful cramping sensation in the lower abdomen often accompanied by other biologic symptoms, including sweating, tachycardia, headaches, nausea, vomiting, diarrhea, and tremulousness, all occurring just before or during the menses. The term *primary dysmenorrhea* refers to pain with no obvious pathologic pelvic disease. We currently recognize that these patients are suffering from the effects of endogenous prostaglandins. The term *secondary dysmenorrhea,* on the other hand, is associated with pelvic conditions or pathology that causes pelvic pain in conjunction with the menses. Primary dysmenorrhea almost always first occurs in women younger than 20. Indeed, the woman will report pain as soon as she establishes ovulatory cycles. Secondary dysmenorrhea may, of course, occur in women younger than 20, but it is most often seen in women older than 20.

INCIDENCE AND EPIDEMIOLOGY

A number of studies have attempted to determine the prevalence of dysmenorrhea; a wide range (16% to 90%) has been reported. These studies have been performed on students, teenagers and their mothers, and individuals from various specific populations, such as industrial workers or college students. The best estimate of the prevalence of primary dysmenorrhea is approximately 75%. Andersch and Milsom have surveyed all the 19-year-old women in the city of Gothenburg, Sweden. A total of 90.9% of these women responded to a randomly distributed questionnaire, and 72.4% of these stated that they suffered from dysmenorrhea. In addition, 34.3% of the total population reported mild menstrual symptoms, 22.7% cited moderate symptoms that required analgesia, and 15.4% stated that they had severe dysmenorrhea that clearly inhibited their working ability and that could not be adequately assuaged by general analgesia (**Table 36-1**). A 2005 Canadian study of 1546 menstruating women reported that 60% had primary dysmenorrhea and 60% reported their pain as moderate or severe. Similarly, 17% missed school or work. Women who have vaginally delivered a child are less likely to have dysmenorrhea. Pregnancy itself without actual birth does not seem to alleviate dysmenorrhea, because women who have had ectopic pregnancies or spontaneous or voluntary terminations of pregnancy are not relieved of their symptoms. Oral contraceptive (OC) use was noted by Andersch and Milsom to reduce the prevalence and severity of dysmenorrhea significantly ($P = .01$). Fish intake, physical exercise, and being married or in a stable relationship also reduces the risk. Risk factors that have reported to increase the risk of dysmenorrhea include body mass index less than 20, premenstrual syndrome, pelvic inflammatory disease, sterilization, history of sexual assault, and heavy smoking.

Relationship to Menstruation and the Menstrual Cycle

Andersch and Milsom have demonstrated a significant positive correlation between the severity of dysmenorrhea and duration of menstrual flow, amount of menstrual flow, and early menarche. They showed no relationship with the actual duration of the menstrual cycle. In their series, 38.3% of patients reported that they had experienced dysmenorrhea for the first time during the first year after menarche and only 20.8% reported that dysmenorrhea had not occurred until 4 years after menarche.

Table 36-1 Severity of Primary Dysmenorrhea*

Severity	No. of Women	Percentage of Total
None	162	27.6
Mild[†]	201	34.3
Moderate[‡]	133	22.7
Severe[§]	90	15.4

*In a population of 586 19-year-old Swedish women.
[†]No systemic symptoms, medication rarely required, work rarely affected.
[‡]Few systemic symptoms, medication required, work moderately affected.
[§]Multiple symptoms, poor medication response, work inhibited.
Data from Andersch B, Milsom I: An epidemiologic study of young women with dysmenorrhea. Am J Obstet Gynecol 144:655, 1982.

Family History

Dysmenorrhea has been reported to be increased significantly in mothers and sisters of women with dysmenorrhea.

PRIMARY DYSMENORRHEA

Pathogenesis

The pathogenesis of dysmenorrhea shows there is a close association between elevated prostaglandin F2α (PGF2α) levels in the secretory endometrium and the symptoms of dysmenorrhea, including uterine hypercontractility, complaints of severe cramping, and other prostaglandin-induced symptoms. Arachidonic acid, the precursor to prostaglandin production, has been found in increased amounts in the endometrium during ovulatory cycles. Arachidonic acid is converted to PGF2α, PGE2, and leukotrienes, which are involved in increasing myometrial contractions. During menses, these contractions decrease uterine blood flow and cause ischemia and sensitization of pain fibers (**Fig. 36-1**). Endometrial concentrations of PGF2α and PGE2 correlate with the severity of dysmenorrhea; cyclooxygenase inhibitors decrease menstrual fluid prostaglandin levels and decrease pain. In small studies, ultrasound and magnetic resonance imaging (MRI) have correlated dysmenorrhea with myometrial changes and decreased blood flow. PGF2α and PGE2 affect other organs such as the bowel and result in nausea, vomiting, and diarrhea.

Diagnosis

Primary dysmenorrhea causes midline, crampy, lower abdominal pain, which begins with the onset of menstruation. The pain can be severe and can also involve the low back and thighs. The pain gradually resolves over 12 to 72 hours. Pain does not occur at times other than menses and only occurs in ovulatory cycles. Diarrhea, headache, fatigue, and malaise may be reported. The diagnosis is made largely by the history and physical examination. Women with primary dysmenorrhea have a normal pelvic examination. In adolescents experiencing dysmenorrhea in the first 6 months from menarche, consider an obstructing malformation of the genital tract in the differential diagnosis.

Treatment

Nonsteroidal anti-inflammatory drugs (NSAIDs) are prostaglandin synthetase inhibitors (PGSIs) and have been demonstrated to alleviate these symptoms of dysmenorrhea. These substances are nonsteroidal and anti-inflammatory. They are generally divided into two chemical groups—the arylcarboxylic acids, which include acetylsalicylic acid (aspirin) and fenamates

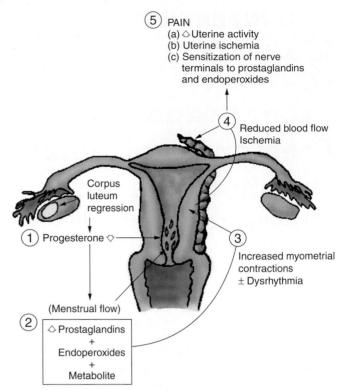

Figure 36-1 Mechanisms contributing to generation of pain in primary dysmenorrhea. (From Dawood MY: Nonsteroidal anti-inflammatory drugs and reproduction. Am J Obstet Gynecol 169:5, 1993.)

(mefenamic acid), and the arylalkanoic acids, including the arylpropionic acids (ibuprofen, naproxen, and ketoprofen) and the indoleacetic acids (indomethacin). The more specific cyclooxygenase (COX-2) inhibitors such as celecoxib have similarly been shown to alleviate the primary dysmenorrheal symptoms. COX-2 expression in the uterine glandular epithelium was maximal during menstruation in one trial of ovulatory women, suggesting a possible association with the cause. The increased expression of COX-2 was eliminated with continuous use of OCs, which are also an effective treatment (see later). The specific effects of these agents on the uterine musculature is reduction of contractility, as measured by reduction of intrauterine pressure.

In 1984, Owen reviewed the effectiveness of NSAIDs for the treatment of primary dysmenorrhea in 51 trials carried out in 1649 women. More than 72% of the women suffering from dysmenorrhea reported significant pain relief with NSAIDs, 18% reported minimal or no pain relief, and 15% showed a placebo response. Owen concluded that PGSI compounds were effective and safe for most women with primary dysmenorrhea. The fenamates seemed to be more effective in relieving pain than ibuprofen, indomethacin, or naproxen. All the compounds demonstrated minimal NSAID-associated side effects, with the exception of indomethacin. In trials with indomethacin, the dropout rate was higher, primarily because of symptoms involving the central nervous system (CNS) and gastrointestinal (GI) tract. Efficacy with the COX-2 inhibitors is similar, although several drugs in this class have been removed from the market because of serious adverse cardiovascular events.

Smith has demonstrated that the effectiveness of NSAIDs is related to tissue concentration. Using meclofenamate in 18

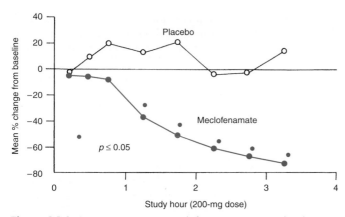

Figure 36-2 Average pressure, meclofenamate versus placebo. (Adapted from Smith RP: The dynamics of nonsteroidal anti-inflammatory therapy for primary dysmenorrhea. Obstet Gynecol 70:785, 1987.)

subjects who participated in a double-blind, placebo-controlled, crossover study, a parallel in time response curves was seen between the plasma levels of the drug and decrease in uterine contractility. **Figure 36-2** demonstrates the average intrauterine pressure relationships between placebo-treated and drug-treated patients over time. Intrauterine pressure declined 20% to 56% in these patients during meclofenamate therapy.

NSAIDs should be given the day prior to the expected menses or at the onset of menses. If one NSAID is ineffective, switching to a different class of NSAIDs may be helpful. NSAIDs should not be given to patients who have shown previous hypersensitivity to such drugs. They are also contraindicated for women who have had nasal polyps, angioedema, and bronchospasm related to aspirin or NSAIDs. In addition, these agents are contraindicated for individuals with a history of chronic ulceration or inflammatory reaction of the upper or lower GI tract and for those with preexisting chronic renal disease. During the use of these agents, autoimmune hemolytic anemia, rash, edema and fluid retention, and CNS symptoms, such as dizziness, headache, nervousness, and blurred vision, can occur. In up to 15% of users, a slight elevation of hepatic enzyme levels may also be found. **Table 36-2** lists some NSAIDs commonly used for the treatment of dysmenorrhea.

Table 36-2 Commonly Used Nonsteroidal Anti-inflammatory Drugs

Class	Brand Name	Generic Name	Usual Regimen (mg)*
Propronic acid	Motrin	Ibuprofen	400 (qid)-800 (tid)
	Naprosyn	Naproxen	250 (qid)-500 (bid)
	Anaprox	Naproxen sodium	275 (qid)-550 (bid)
	N/A	Ketoprofen	25-50 (tid)
Fenamic acid	Ponstel	Mefenamic acid	250 (qid)
Acetic acid	Indocin	Indomethacin	25 (tid)
	Voltaren	Diclofenac	75 (bid)
Cyclooxygenase-2 Inhibitors	Celebrex	Celecoxib	200 (bid)

*Maximum doses.

Other Therapy

Although NSAIDs are the standard therapy available for primary dysmenorrhea, other approaches are possible. OCs will relieve the symptoms of primary dysmenorrhea in approximately 90% of patients treated. This may be because OCs suppress ovulation and endometrial proliferation and the progestin component also blocks the production of the precursor to prostaglandin formation. The thinned endometrium from OCs then contains less arachidonic acid, which is the precursor to prostaglandins. If the woman also requires contraception, OC therapy may prove to be the treatment of choice. In small randomized controlled trials (RCTs), low-dose OCs (with 20 µg ethinyl estradiol) were effective in reducing dysmenorrhea in adolescents and adult women. Continuous OC administration compared with traditional monthly cyclic dosing has been shown to reduce the menstrual pain symptoms. Breakthrough bleeding can be an undesirable side effect, although a review of RCTs reported bleeding and discontinuation rates to be similar. The extended-cycle OCs available are also associated with less dysmenorrhea than monthly cyclic OCs. One study reported that the contraceptive vaginal ring reduces the incidence of dysmenorrhea from 17.4% to 5.9%. Depot medroxyprogesterone, a long-acting injectable contraceptive, has not been studied specifically for primary dysmenorrhea. Trials in contraceptive studies report a reduction in dysmenorrhea in adolescents. Because this often causes a thinned endometrium and light menses or amenorrhea, it theoretically should be effective.

The levonorgestrel-releasing intrauterine system (LNG-IUS) has been shown to reduce menstrual pain in women from 60% before use to 29% when studied 3 years after insertion. Levonorgestrel is a 19-nortestosterone derivative and affects the endometrial progesterone receptors, leading to an atrophic endometrial lining. A copper T380A IUD often increases dysmenorrhea. A randomized comparison of microwave endometrial ablation with transcervical resection of the endometrium for menorrhagia showed that both techniques reduced menstrual pain at the 5-year follow-up.

Because of its ability to block uterine contractility, nifedipine has been studied for dysmenorrhea. A dose of 20-40 mg orally can relieve pain. Moderate pain relief was noted in 36 of 40 women, but side effects of facial flushing, tachycardia, and headache can occur. With such effective first-line therapies, this is rarely needed. Narcotic analgesics may be necessary in treating patients with primary dysmenorrhea but should be used as last-line therapy when the desired therapeutic effect is not achieved with NSAIDs, OCs, or other hormonal treatment.

A meta-analysis of three trials has reported that transcutaneous electrical nerve stimulation (TENS) is more effective than placebo in relieving dysmenorrhea, although not as effective as analgesics. Milsom and colleagues, in Sweden, and Smith and Heltzel, in the United States, have noted that TENS relieves menstrual pain without reducing intrauterine pressure, suggesting that its mode of action may be in the CNS. High-frequency TENS provides more dysmenorrheal pain relief compared with placebo or low-frequency TENS. An abdominal patch delivering continuous topical heat was as effective as 400 mg of ibuprofen in reducing pain. There is limited evidence that acupuncture may be of benefit. Dietary and vitamin therapies may be beneficial but to date have not been studied in a rigorous fashion. A low-fat vegetarian diet decreased menstrual pain in one study, and vitamin E was more effective than placebo in reducing dysmenorrhea in adolescents. Although the evidence is weak, exercise may be of benefit. Vitamins B$_1$ and B$_6$, fish oil supplement, and a Japanese herbal combination have been helpful in reducing pain compared with placebo in small trials.

A 2005 meta-analysis of eight RCTs of surgical interruption of nerve pathways concluded that there was insufficient evidence to advise laparoscopic uterine nerve ablation (LUNA) or laparoscopic presacral neurectomy (LPSN) for primary dysmenorrhea.

SECONDARY DYSMENORRHEA: CAUSES AND MANAGEMENT

Many other conditions cause or are associated with dysmenorrhea. Pelvic disease should be considered in patients who do not respond to NSAIDs and OCs for presumed primary dysmenorrhea. The diagnosis should be considered when symptoms appear after many years of painless menses. These conditions may occur at any age and, in most cases, the pain experienced is secondary to the pathologic process of the condition or a specific result of it. These constitute the so-called secondary dysmenorrhea group of problems and include **cervical stenosis**, ectopic endometrial tissue, adenomyosis, fibroids, pelvic inflammation, pelvic congestion, congenital obstructive müllerian malformations, and conditioned behavior (**Box 36-1**).

Cervical Stenosis

Severe narrowing of the cervical canal, particularly at the level of the internal os, may impede menstrual flow, causing an increase in intrauterine pressure at the time of menses. In addition, retrograde menstrual flow through the fallopian tubes into the peritoneal cavity may take place. Thus, severe cervical stenosis may eventually be associated with pelvic endometriosis as well. The origin of cervical stenosis may be congenital or secondary to cervical injury, such as with electrocautery, cryocautery, or operative trauma (e.g., conization). The condition may also result from an inflammatory process caused by infection, the application of caustic substances, or hypoestrogenism. After any of these conditions, the cervical canal may narrow because of contraction of scar tissue.

Box 36-1   Causes of Secondary Dysmenorrhea

Gynecologic Pathology
Cervical stenosis
Endometriosis and adenomyosis
Pelvic infection and adhesions
Uterine polyps or fibroids
Ovarian cyst or mass
Pelvic congestion
Congenital obstructed müllerian malformations

Nongynecologic Disorders Causing Pelvic Pain
Conditioned behavior
Bowel disease
  Irritable bowel syndrome
  Inflammatory bowel disease
  Celiac sprue (?)
  Lactose intolerance (?)
Urinary tract disease
  Ureteral obstruction
  Interstitial cystitis
  Nephrolithiasis

The possibility of cervical stenosis should be considered if there is a history of scant menstrual flow and if severe cramping continues throughout the menstrual period. Hematometra or pyometra may occur.

The diagnosis is suspected when the external os appears scarred or when it is impossible to pass a cervical Pap smear brush or uterine sound through the internal os during the proliferative stage of the menstrual cycle. Diagnosis is generally documented by the inability to pass a thin probe of a few millimeters' diameter through the internal os or by a hysterosalpingogram, which demonstrates a thin, stringy-appearing canal. If hysteroscopy and dilation and curettage (D&C) are performed, finding the passage through the internal os with a thin probe is often difficult but can frequently be accomplished with patience. The woman should be anesthetized. Ultrasound guidance can be of great benefit to reduce the risk of making a false passage. Having the woman self-administer buccal or intravaginal misoprostol before the procedure has been done by our patients and can be helpful in relaxing the cervix, but this is not U.S. Food and Drug Administration (FDA)–approved nor has it been studied in large trials.

Treatment consists of dilating the cervix, which may be accomplished by D&C with progressive dilators or by the use of progressive *Laminaria* tents. Unfortunately, cervical stenosis often recurs after therapy, necessitating repeat procedures. Pregnancy and vaginal delivery often afford a more lasting cure.

Often, other problems obstructing the cervix can have a similar presentation. **Figure 36-3** shows anteroposterior and lateral views of a hysterogram in an 18-year-old nulliparous woman who had a 2-year history of severe disabling **dysmenorrhea** that usually required morphine therapy with each menstrual period. At hysteroscopy, she was found to have a tissue band across her internal os, at which site a large endocervical polyp had formed. Transecting the band and removing the polyp completely relieved the dysmenorrhea and she had no further symptoms after 3 years.

Ectopic Endometrial Tissue (Endometriosis)

Ectopic endometrial tissue or endometriosis (including endometriosis and adenomyosis) should be considered when there is a history of pain becoming more severe during menses. Frequently, dyspareunia and infertility are accompanying symptoms. Pertinent physical findings may include uterosacral ligament nodules, evidence for endometriosis in the vagina or cervix, and lateral displacement of the cervix.

Koike and colleagues, in an in vitro experiment using tissue slices, have found that the prostaglandin level in endometriosis implants is significantly higher than in normal endometrium, myometrium, leiomyomata, and normal ovarian tissue, and that adenomyosis implants produce larger amounts of 6-keto-PGF1 when the dysmenorrhea has been severe. They believe that prostaglandins in endometriosis increases painful menstruation. Treatment of endometriosis is discussed in Chapter 19.

Pelvic Inflammation

Pelvic infections secondary to gonorrhea, chlamydia, or other infections may cause pelvic inflammation or pelvic abscess and, with healing, may be associated with pelvic adhesions and tubal damage that might cause pelvic pain. Pelvic inflammatory disease (PID) can lead to chronic pelvic pain in up to 30% of women. This may often be aggravated during menses, causing

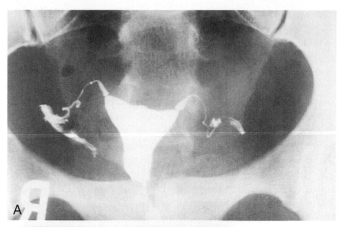

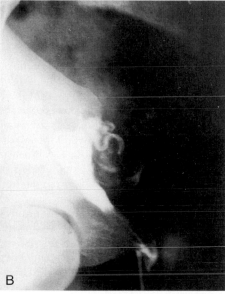

Figure 36-3 Hysterogram. Anteroposterior (**A**) view and lateral (**B**) views of an 18-year-old patient with severe disabling dysmenorrhea. At hysteroscopy, she was found to have a tissue band across the internal os and an endocervical polyp at this site. Removal of the polyp and transection of the band completely relieved the dysmenorrhea.

dysmenorrhea. Infections secondary to other conditions, such as appendicitis or intrauterine device (IUD) use, may also create a similar response. The pain may be secondary to the congestion and edema that occur normally at menses, which may subsequently be aggravated by the healed inflammatory areas and adhesions.

Pelvic Congestion Syndrome and Pelvic Venous Syndromes

Pelvic congestion syndrome, which was first described by Taylor in 1949, results from the engorgement of pelvic vasculature. Controversy exists regarding whether this is an actual disorder because it has been difficult to prove. However, we believe it exists, possibly secondary to past pregnancy or past inflammatory pelvic pathology. The pain is usually burning or throbbing in nature, worse at night, and worse after standing. Physical examination of the vagina and cervix usually reveals vasocongestion with evidence of some uterine enlargement and tenderness. Diagnosis is made by observation of the features noted and by laparoscopy, which not only rules out other causes of pelvic pain but also demonstrates congestion of the uterus and engorgement or varicosities of the broad ligament and pelvic sidewall veins. If laparoscopy is used for diagnosis, it is important to observe the broad ligament vasculature as the pressure of the carbon dioxide or nitrous oxide is released. At full pressure during the procedure, these vessels may be collapsed as the pneumoperitoneal pressure exceeds venous pressure, but the dilated veins will reappear as pressure is released.

More recently, other pelvic venous syndromes have been described that can cause pelvic pain and probably include what Taylor first described. Vulvar varices, hypogastric vein insufficiency, and gonadal venous insufficiency have been described in a review of 57 female patients ages 24 to 48 years. Symptoms included pelvic pain, dysuria, dysmenorrhea, and dyspareunia. These disorders are poorly understood and poorly studied so they often go undiagnosed. Diagnosis in this study was made by physical examination and a variety of radiologic investigations, including Doppler scans, duplex ultrasound scans, computed tomography (CT), MRI, and angiography. No standard therapeutic approach is available, so therapies range from ovarian hormone suppression, local sclerotherapy (for vulvar varices), and embolization of the hypogastric vein to resection of the gonadal vein to hysterectomy. A 2010 systematic review by Tu and coworkers has found 6 diagnostic and 22 treatment studies, but no consensus on diagnostic studies or treatment, although progestins and gonadotropin-releasing hormone (GnRH) agonists were effective in decreasing pain symptoms.

Women with chronic pelvic pain often have psychological issues, so careful evaluation of the patient's past and present social situation and referral for counseling may be appropriate.

CAUSATIVE FACTORS

Behavioral Influences

In individuals with strong family histories of dysmenorrhea, or when a careful history demonstrates a possibility for societal reward or control because of the symptoms of pain, a conditioned behavior should be considered. It is important to obtain a careful medical and social history and to rule out all other causes of acquired dysmenorrhea.

Treatment of women with conditioned behavior dysmenorrhea includes reeducation so that the pain is not considered a rewarding experience by the patient. Teaching the woman the cause of the problem, offering appropriate medical therapies, and consulting with trained mental health professionals may all be necessary.

Relation to Functional Bowel Disease

Crowell and coworkers have studied 383 women ages 20 to 40 using an NEO Personality Inventory on entry into the program, a Moos' Menstrual Distress Questionnaire, and a bowel symptom inventory every 3 months for 12 months. Dysmenorrhea was diagnosed in 19.8% of these women. Functional bowel disorder, defined as abdominal pain with altered bowel function, occurred in 61% of the women with dysmenorrhea but in only 20% of the others ($P < .05$). Bowel symptoms were significantly correlated with dysmenorrhea, even after controlling for the effects of neuroticism. Prostaglandin levels in vaginal fluid were elevated in patients with dysmenorrhea but did not consistently differentiate the diagnostic groups. It was concluded that there

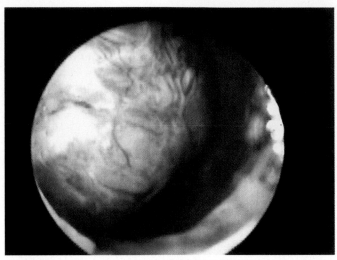

Figure 36-4 Submucous myoma blocking the internal os causing secondary dysmenorrhea.

was a strong covariance of menstrual and bowel symptoms, along with an overlap in their diagnosis, suggesting a common physiologic basis.

In a study of women with irritable bowel syndrome (IBS) and menstrual cycle symptoms, dysmenorrhea was twice as prevalent among women with IBS than controls (21% versus 10%; $P = .09$) although this was not statistically significant. Women with IBS on OCs had significantly less dysmenorrhea than women in the control group who were not on OCs (11% versus 28%, $P = .02$). One case report found an association of celiac sprue and dysmenorrhea, but little is known about this finding.

Other Causes

At times, dysmenorrhea may be related to unusual pathologic findings. These include small leiomyomas or polyps at the junction of the internal os and lower uterine segment (**Fig. 36-4**). Such a condition may produce a valvelike effect at the os at the time of menses. Frequently, myomas or polyps become engorged or edematous at the time of menses, accentuating the problem. Diagnosis is generally made by history and by saline infusion sonohysterography, hysterosalpingography, or hysteroscopy. Therapy consists of excising the pathologic tissue. In the case of a myoma, a myomectomy or hysterectomy may be necessary.

There are nongynecologic causes for pain during menses that should be considered in the differential diagnosis. These include appendicitis, lactose intolerance, celiac sprue, abdominal mass, and a number of urinary tract conditions (e.g., urinary tract infection, interstitial cystitis, nephrolithiasis, ureteral obstruction).

PREMENSTRUAL SYNDROME AND PREMENSTRUAL DYSPHORIC DISORDER

Premenstrual syndrome (PMS) is defined as a group of mild to moderate symptoms, physical and behavioral, that occur in the second half of the menstrual cycle and that may interfere with work and personal relationships. These are followed by a period entirely free of symptoms. Frank first described the condition in 1931 and attempted to relate symptoms of then so-called *premenstrual tension* with hormonal changes of the menstrual cycle.

The term *premenstrual syndrome* was first used by Dalton in 1953. The symptoms vary from woman to woman, and more than 150 symptoms have been linked with the disorder.

Premenstrual dysphoric disorder (PMDD) represents a more severe disorder, with marked behavioral and emotional symptoms. PMS differs from PMDD in severity of symptoms, and women with PMDD must have one severe affective symptom. These include markedly depressed mood or hopelessness, anxiety or tension, affective lability, and persistent anger, which occur regularly during the last week of the luteal phase in most menstrual cycles. A number of physical symptoms may also be present. PMDD also differs from PMS because there is substantial impairment in personal functioning. PMS and PMDD are similar in that the symptoms manifest in the luteal phase of the menstrual cycle and resolve during menses.

INCIDENCE AND EPIDEMIOLOGY

Although various reports place the prevalence of PMS at 30% to 80% of menstruating women, it is generally agreed that approximately 40% of women are significantly affected at one time or another. Most prevalence experts use severe symptoms of PMS to diagnosis PMDD and cite 1% to 7% of women between the ages of 18 and 48 years as having PMDD. Using the *Diagnostic and Statistical Manual of Mental Disorders,* 4th ed (DSM-IV) diagnostic criteria specific for PMDD, 5% to 6% of women is more accurate. The average age of onset is 26 years. Likely risk factors for PMS include family history of PMS in the mother, personal past or current psychiatric illness involving mood or anxiety disorders, history of alcohol abuse, and history of postpartum depression. Some studies have found that nulliparity, earlier menarche, higher alcohol and caffeine intake, more stress, and higher body mass index are risk factors for certain PMS symptoms. Recent studies have supported earlier reports that familial and stress factors play a role in the syndrome. Younger women may experience more severe symptoms of PMDD. Some racial and ethnic differences have been reported, but PMS appears consistently in all cultures studied. Data from a California HMO PMS severity study of 1194 women found that Hispanics reported greater severity of symptoms than whites and blacks, and Asian women reported less. Similar to PMS, PMDD prevalence is noted in many countries studied, including Croatia, Italy, Iceland, and Japan. A Japanese study found a 1.2% prevalence of PMDD, suggesting a cultural difference in prevalence or reporting.

In the Harvard Study of Moods and Cycles by Cohen and colleagues, a population-based, cross-sectional sample of 4164 premenopausal women was studied retrospectively regarding PMDD prevalence. A PMDD diagnosis was made in 6.4% of the women, and PMDD was associated with lower education, a history of major depression, and current smoking. This confirms the results of earlier studies reporting a significant lifetime comorbidity of PMDD and affective disorders. Past sexual abuse has been reported more frequently in women attending PMS clinics compared with women in the general population.

SYMPTOMS

In a review by O'Brien, a number of common somatic and affective symptoms were enumerated (**Box 36-2**). The most common somatic symptoms relate to abdominal bloating, breast

Box 36-2 Key Symptoms of Premenstrual Syndrome and Premenstrual Dysphoric Disorder*

Somatic Symptoms
Abdominal bloating, swelling, weight gain
Aches
Increased appetite, food cravings
Breast pain or tenderness
Headache
Dizziness, poor coordination, clumsiness
Cramps, change in bowel habits
Fatigue

Affective Symptoms
Depressed mood[+]
Irritability, persistent anger[+]
Mood lability, crying, social withdrawal[+]
Anxiety, tension[+]
Feeling hopeless or guilty
Poor impulse control or feeling out of control
Decreased interest, change in libido
Insomnia
Loss of concentration, confusion

*Severe PMS or PMDD is based on at least five symptoms, including one of four core psychological symptoms, with [+] being severe before menstruation starts and mild or absent after menstruation. Modified from the American Psychiatric Association: Diagnostic and Statistical Manual of Mental Disorders, 4th ed, text revision (DSM-IV-TR). Washington, DC, 2000, American Psychiatric Association, pp 771-774.

tenderness, and various pain constellations, such as headache. Psychological symptoms vary from fatigue, irritability, and tension to anxiety, labile mood, and depression. In Sternfeld and associates' severity of PMS symptoms study in an HMO population of 1194 women, consistency of symptoms was found over two consecutive cycles, especially for emotional symptoms.

Depression is a common complaint in the population in general and also in PMS-PMDD sufferers during the luteal phase. Mortola and coworkers have shown that 16 PMS patients had marked worsening of scores on the Profile of Mood States and Beck Depression Inventory during the luteal phase compared with 16 controls. However, 6 patients suffering from endogenous depression had scores threefold higher on both indices than PMS patients who were in the luteal phase. Also, the amplitude of cortisol secretion pulses was higher in the depressed patients than in the PMS patients or control patients. The data demonstrate that PMS patients have more episodes of depression during the luteal phase compared with controls, but these episodes are distinctly different from those suffered by patients with endogenous depression. The National Institute of Mental Health's STAR-D trial of clinically depressed women found that 64% of 433 subjects not on OCs reported worsening of their depressive symptoms before menses. Therefore, it can be challenging to differentiate women with PMS from women with depression and premenstrual exacerbations of depressive symptoms.

In addition, Rapkin and colleagues have demonstrated that PMS patients show no deficit in cognitive processing and performance, as well as no loss in ability to concentrate and sustain attention and motivation. No such alterations were seen in 10 PMS patients during the luteal phase. Their performance was similar to 9 controls when tested in these areas. In a later study,

this group studied 30 patients with PMS and 31 controls during the follicular and luteal phases. Despite feelings of inadequacy, patients showed no statistically significant differences from controls in tests for attention, memory, cognitive flexibility, and overall mental agility.

A PMS diagnosis not only affects quality of life, but also economic issues. Slight increases in direct costs (medical expenses) have been noted. Indirect costs to the employer in work absence and lost productivity amount to $4333/patient annually.

CAUSES

When Frank first described the syndrome, it was attributed to estrogen excess. Others have offered theories that the disorder is related to an imbalance of estrogen and progesterone, endogenous hormone allergy, hypoglycemia, vitamin B_6 deficiency, prolactin excess, fluid retention, inappropriate prostaglandin activity, elevated monoamine oxidase (MAO) levels, endorphin malfunction, and a number of psychological disturbances. In 1981, Reid and Yen reviewed the subject and concluded that PMS was a multifactorial psychoendocrine disorder. **Figure 36-5** shows a schematic of the proposed causes. Studies indicate that cyclic gonadal hormonal alterations and serotonergic neuronal mechanisms in the CNS may interact and be major causative factors for PMS in susceptible women. Evidence for this is indirect but includes successful clinical trials with selective serotonin reuptake inhibitors (SSRIs) and other neurotropic agents thought to affect the serotonin pump mechanism between CNS neurons. Other indirect evidence includes the fact that platelet tritium-labeled, imipramine-binding sites are thought to be reduced in patients suffering from depression and are believed to represent receptor sites that label for a presynaptic serotonin transporter on the presynaptic nerve terminal. In some studies, binding sites returned to normal several months after clinical remission of depression or during the response to psychotropic medications or electroconvulsive therapy. These platelet-binding sites have therefore been used as an indirect measure of the neuron receptor site. Steege and coworkers have demonstrated lower platelet tritium-labeled imipramine binding in women with late luteal phase dysphoric disorder (now called PMDD); they believe that this supported the hypothesis that such patients suffer from alterations of the central serotonergic systems. More recently, beta-endorphin and gamma-aminobutyric acid (GABA) neurotransmitters have been implicated. Estrogen has been found to modulate neurotransmitters such as GABA and dopamine, which may serve as inhibitory or excitatory agents in the brain.

That ovarian steroids and, in particular, ovulation and therefore progesterone production is important in this syndrome has been known for some time. Studies related to the relationship of estrogen and progesterone in the circulation and the severity of the symptoms have not been fruitful. There are no consistent differences between estrogen and progesterone levels in PMS sufferers and those in controls. These women may have an abnormal response to normal cyclic ovarian steroid changes. Although symptom relief has been noted in several studies using GnRH agonists to block ovulation completely, no relief was found in a study by Chan and colleagues, who blocked progesterone receptors with the progesterone antagonist RU-486. Rapkin and colleagues have evaluated the anxiolytic 3-α, 5-α reduced progesterone metabolite allopregnanediol during the luteal

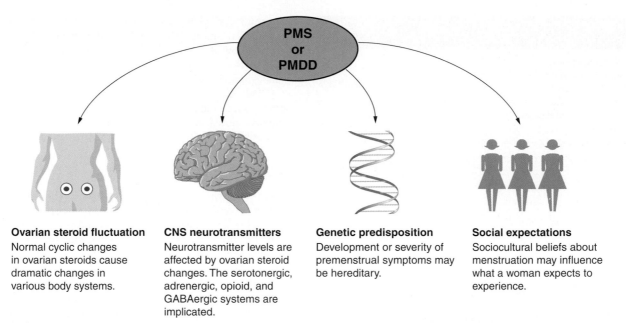

Figure 36-5 Proposed causes of PMS and PMDD. GABA, γ-Aminobutyric acid. (From Ling F, Mortola J, Pariser S, et al: Premenstrual Syndrome and Premenstrual Dysphoric Disorder: Scope, Diagnosis, and Treatment. Association of Professors of Gynecology and Obstetrics, Crofton, MD, 1998.)

phase of 35 women with PMS and 36 controls. Serum progesterone and allopregnanediol levels were measured on days 19 and 26 of the cycles as determined by luteinizing hormone (LH) kits. Allopregnanediol levels were significantly lower in the PMS patients than controls on day 26, but there were no significant differences with respect to progesterone itself. They concluded that because PMS patients had lower levels of this anxiolytic metabolite during the luteal phase, they could be at greater susceptibility for various mood symptoms such as anxiety, tension, and depression. Allopregnanediol enhances GABA-A receptor function. Chuong and associates have demonstrated that beta-endorphin levels throughout the periovulatory phase are lower in PMS patients than in controls, especially in postovulatory days 0 to 4. Similarly, Halbreich and coworkers have demonstrated that PMS patients treated with 200 mg/day of danazol for 90 days have complete relief of symptoms in 23 anovulatory cycles, but relief of symptoms occurred in only 6 of 32 ovulatory cycles. They concluded that the beneficial effect of danazol in the treatment of PMS was achieved only when the anovulatory state eliminated the hormonal cyclicity of the normal cycle and not because of action of drug per se. O'Brien and Abukhalil have advanced further evidence for this. They studied 100 women with PMS and premenstrual breast pain using a randomized, double-blind, placebo-controlled study of three menstrual cycles, using danazol, 200 mg/day, as the active drug. Treatment was given only during the luteal phase. Danazol did not effectively reduce the general symptoms of PMS, but did relieve mastalgia. Severe PMS has been shown to be relieved by total abdominal hysterectomy and bilateral salpingo-oophorectomy, even with hormone replacement therapy using an estrogen, but some women on cyclic estrogen and progesterone therapy postmenopausally continue to complain of PMS symptoms. A 2003 study by Roca and colleagues has suggested that women with PMS may have an abnormal response to progesterone. Women with PMS failed to show a normal increased luteal phase hypothalamic-pituitary-adrenal axis response to exercise stress testing compared with controls. This response is distinctly different in PMS patients compared with women with major depression.

Another potential causative factor is a genetic contribution. Twin studies have demonstrated a high heritability of PMS symptoms; the concordance rate is twice as high in monozygotic twins than in dizygotic twins.

Concerning other possible causes, most dietary and vitamin deficiency theories have been difficult to prove and have not been found to be a major cause of this syndrome. However, data from Bertone-Johnson and associates' case-control study involving the Nurses' Health Study II cohort has suggested that a high intake of calcium and vitamin D may reduce the risk of PMS, so further research is needed. Several studies have looked for prolactin excess because some of the women complain of breast tenderness, but no positive findings have been found. Although some of the symptomatology seems to relate to prostaglandin activity, and these symptoms are often reduced with treatment with NSAIDs, a direct cause and effect has not been established.

In summary, the cause of PMS and PMDD is associated with ovarian steroids and ovulation, which seems to produce alterations in neurohormones and neurotransmitters that lead to a reduction of serotonergic function during the luteal phase. The most effective evidence-based treatment for moderate to severe PMS and PMDD symptoms are SSRIs and agents that block ovulation. The temporal relationship between menstrual phase PMS and PMDD symptoms suggests a role of the reproductive hormones—not a direct linear role, but a more complex vulnerability to these cyclic hormonal shifts. Only 60% of women with PMDD respond to SSRI treatment, so serotonergic dysfunction may not be the only pathway involved. Beta-endorphin, GABA, the autonomic nervous system, and social expectations may all play a role in these complex disorders.

DIAGNOSIS

The diagnosis of PMS and PMDD is made by the history of two consecutive menstrual cycles demonstrating luteal phase symptoms of PMS and PMDD. The facts given by the woman may allow the physician to construct a specific, individualized, treatment regimen. It is important that the physician have a clear understanding of the woman's symptoms before undertaking therapy. After a complete history and physical examination, the physician should rule out any medical problems that could be influencing the symptomatology. The physician should then ask the woman to keep a diary of her symptoms throughout two menstrual cycles. Although she and her physician may focus on the second half of the menstrual cycle, the woman should be encouraged to keep track of all symptoms, regardless of the stage of the menstrual cycle. A number of validated tools with diary sheets and symptom checklists are available. The Daily Record of Severity of Problems (DRSP) or the Penn Daily Symptom Report (DSR) are examples. It can be useful to have the woman write the symptoms that she perceives in her own words using validated visual analogue scales rather than give her clues to specific response patterns. A full 2 months of tracking symptoms are necessary to compare follicular phase symptoms to luteal and menstrual phase data. At the end of two cycles, the physician should review the symptom diary with the woman and carefully discuss those symptoms that seem to be causing her the most difficulty. A change in the symptom severity score between 30% and 50% between the follicular and luteal phases is suggestive of PMS and PMDD. It can be challenging for women to complete a diary with 2 months of symptoms.

The American College of Obstetricians and Gynecologists (ACOG) Practice Bulletin establishes the key elements of the PMS diagnosis as symptoms characteristic of PMS, luteal phase symptoms confirmed by prospective menstrual cycle symptom charting, symptoms affecting the women's life, and exclusion of other diagnoses. It is important to differentiate PMS from other illnesses with similar symptomatology. Women with depression and anxiety disorders may present believing that they have PMS. A differentiating aspect is that PMS patients suffer their symptoms only during the luteal phase. Diagnosis can be difficult because women with depression and anxiety disorders can have premenstrual exacerbation of their symptoms, and PMS and PMDD can coexist with psychiatric disorders.

Many women who do not actually have PMS may be self-referred to a facility that treats this condition. In one study, Plouffe and coworkers carefully analyzed 100 consecutive women prospectively entering the uniform diagnostic and treatment protocol for PMS and found that 38 women had PMS; 24 had premenstrual magnification syndrome (i.e., other conditions that were magnified during the luteal phase), and 13 had affective or other psychiatric disorders. Only 44% of the women previously given a diagnosis of PMS were found to have this syndrome. Overall, in this study, 84% of the women with PMS and premenstrual magnification syndrome responded to treatment. A variety of currently accepted therapies were used.

No laboratory tests are available to make the diagnosis. Although it has been reported that many patients with PMS suffer thyroid hypofunction, a study by Nikolai and colleagues has demonstrated that there was no significant thyroid disease in 44 carefully studied PMS patients compared with 15 normal

---

Box 36-3 Considerations in the Differential Diagnosis of Premenstrual Dysphoric Disorder

Premenstrual syndrome
Endometriosis
Dysmenorrhea
Physical disorders with premenstrual exacerbations
Autoimmune disorders
Diabetes mellitus
Anemia
Hypothyroidism
Psychiatric disorders with luteal phase exacerbation
Depression
Anxiety
Dysthymic disorder
Bipolar disorder

---

controls. In addition, treating 22 with L-thyroxine and 22 with placebo led to no differences in relief of symptoms.

Other conditions to consider based on patient symptoms include anemia, diabetes, endometriosis, autoimmune disorders, chronic fatigue syndrome, collagen vascular disorders, and many psychiatric disorders (e.g., depression, anxiety, dysthymia, bipolar disorder).

The diagnosis of PMS is therefore made by symptom diary and by the elimination of other diagnoses. The diagnosis of PMDD is made following the DSM-IV criteria, which require 5 of 11 symptoms of PMS, including one affective symptom. Affective symptoms include feeling sad or hopeless or having self-deprecating thoughts, anxiety or tension, mood lability and crying, and persistent irritability, anger, and increased interpersonal conflicts. Prospective menstrual cycle charting is required for the diagnosis. **Box 36-3** lists physical and psychiatric disorders that should be considered in the differential diagnosis of PMDD.

TREATMENT

Diet, Exercise, and Lifestyle Changes

Although many individuals will suffer from symptomatology related to PMS, only approximately 3% to 8% are seriously affected. Reassuring women with mild PMS without serious coexisting gynecologic disorders that this is a common problem should be part of the counseling. Thus, the selection of medications and lifestyle changes should be tailored to the symptomatic needs of the patient. Lifestyle modifications can be recommended for 2 months while the woman completes the prospective diary for diagnosis.

Several dietary studies have been performed, but most were not rigorously controlled. Two trials have studied increasing complex carbohydrate intake, which reduced the severity of PMS mood symptoms. Complex carbohydrates may increase tryptophan availability and thereby increase serotonin. A study by Barnard and associates has suggested that a low-fat vegetarian diet improves dysmenorrhea duration and intensity and duration of premenstrual symptoms. Sex hormone-binding globulin (SHBG) concentrations increased with this vegetarian diet; SHBG binds and inactivates estrogens, which may possibly be a causative factor. Because food cravings or increased appetite, mood changes, sleep disturbances and irritability, and fluid retention are listed in the key 17 symptoms, symptom severity might be affected by reducing or eliminating sugar, alcohol, caffeine, salty foods, and red meat.

Patients should be encouraged to exercise 20 to 30 minutes at least three to four times per week for general health reasons. Small trials have suggested aerobic exercise to be beneficial for PMS sufferers, and one trial found high-intensity aerobic exercise to be superior to low-intensity aerobic exercise for PMS treatment. Avoiding stressful activities in the luteal phase and having enough sleep may also alleviate PMS and PMDD symptoms.

A multicenter RCT of 466 women has shown that 1200 mg of calcium/day for three cycles reduces PMS symptoms significantly compared with placebo (48% versus 30%; $P < .001$). This is a reasonable treatment to initiate because women need adequate calcium in their diet for bone health; it can be started while the woman completes the menstrual symptom charting. However, this trial had limitations in that other PMS treatments were allowed, and one other RCT showing benefits of calcium also had study limitations.

Vitamin B_6 deficiency in PMS patients has been suggested because vitamin B_6 is a coenzyme in the biosynthesis of dopamine and serotonin, and neurotransmitters have been implicated in the cause of PMS. One double-blind study by Abraham and Hargrove has demonstrated that vitamin B_6 administered at 200- to 800-mg doses daily prevents some of the symptoms of PMS, significantly better than placebo. They theorized that deficiencies of vitamin B_6 and magnesium could result in lower thresholds to stress and potential hormone imbalance. They believe that eventually the vitamin B_6 activity might lower brain serotonin levels. Although vitamin B_6 has been a conventional treatment, its effectiveness is still questioned. A review of nine RCTs of vitamin B_6 for the treatment PMS found no high-quality trials, although several suggested relief of PMS symptoms over placebo. The most recent double-blind placebo-controlled trial of 94 women with PMDD found a greater decrease in psychiatric symptoms with 80 mg of vitamin B_6. Vitamin B_6 (pyridoxine) supplement at the rate of 50 mg/day can be tried for mild PMS symptoms. Higher doses of pyridoxine should be administered with caution because neuropathy can occur in patients treated with as little as 100 to 200 mg/day. Other side effects, such as sensory deficit, paresthesia, numbness, ataxia, and muscle weakness, may occur.

There is inconclusive evidence from two RCTs that magnesium (200 to 400 mg/day) reduces PMS symptoms, although one trial showed a decrease in fluid retention. There does not appear to be any benefit of magnesium for psychiatric symptoms.

Many other complementary and alternative medicines (CAMs) have been studied. One of the better designed trials found that chasteberry extract (*Vitex agnus-castus*) reduced PMS symptoms 50% from baseline in 52% of women compared with 24% of women receiving placebo. Small RCTs supporting saffron and qi treatment have been carried out. Many other alternative therapies have been reported for PMS sufferers, including massage, biofeedback, yoga, acupuncture, chiropractic manipulation, evening primrose oil, and Chinese herbal medicines, but all have insufficient evidence to recommend them but are being studied. A systematic review of several trials has suggested that of all the alternative therapies, bright light therapy, which may increase serotonin, might be a reasonable option for PMDD. To date, calcium and vitamin B_6 are the most promising dietary treatments because the research on other CAMs is seriously flawed.

Cognitive Behavioral Therapy
Studies in the 1950s showed that 50% of patients improved with psychotherapy alone. However, Wyatt's review of seven RCTs found a significant reduction in PMS symptoms versus control treatments, but the effect was similar to the response rate of many placebo therapies. If patients have obvious psychiatric problems, as detected by history, psychotherapy should be added, but it is less effective as a primary therapy. Group psychoeducation in managing symptoms of PMS has been efficacious. Relaxation therapy may be of benefit for patients with significant stress and anxiety components.

Pharmacologic Agents
Diuretics
The physician may choose to add a diuretic to the regimen if the woman's complaints involve bloating, fluid retention, and perceived change in body habitus during the luteal phase of the cycle. A potassium-sparing diuretic should be selected, and the lowest dose possible to achieve symptomatic relief should be used. Although many patients report a feeling of fluid retention during the luteal phase, this has been difficult to demonstrate. Perceived swelling of the body is difficult to prove unless actual careful weight analysis is used. Faratian and colleagues have evaluated 148 menstrual cycles in 52 women and, in each cycle, various parameters were measured to determine an objective means of assessing the syndrome. These included daily mood assessment and measurement of body weight, plasma 17β-estradiol levels, and plasma progesterone levels. The abdominal girth was measured carefully in two dimensions: at the level of the umbilicus and then 10 cm below the umbilicus.

At the same time, the patient subjectively judged the dimensions. Mood scores showed a marked shifting during the premenstrual phase of each cycle. The symptoms of bloatedness were most marked during the premenstrual phase of the cycle. Despite these elevated scores for bloatedness, there was no increase in body weight or measured body dimension changes in any plane during this period. However, the woman's perception of body size increased and a discrepancy between the perceived body size and actual body size was noted. The authors divided their patients into those with predominantly somatic symptoms and those with predominantly psychological symptoms, and also studied a control group. No hormonal differences were noted in the three groups. Freeman and associates have studied transcapillary fluid balance in 10 women with well-defined PMS. The capillary filtration coefficient was measured by string gauge plethysmography. They noted that from the follicular to the luteal phase, interstitial colloid osmotic pressure on the leg was significantly reduced (mean, 3.6 mm Hg), whereas the interstitial colloid osmotic pressure on the thorax remained constant. The capillary filtration coefficient increased 30% from the follicular to the luteal phase. No change was observed in body weight. It was thought that these changes represented an instability of vascular regulation in women with PMS, which led support to the hypothesis that redistribution of fluid rather than water retention is responsible for the subjective symptom of bloatedness in PMS. This would explain why diuretics are beneficial to the patient. Spironolactone (100 mg/day) has been studied in four RCTs; three trials demonstrated moderate efficacy for breast tenderness and fluid retention and two found reduced irritability symptoms. Diuretics should be avoided in patients with chronic renal disease or in those who are suffering from diarrhea or other fluid loss.

Psychoactive Drugs

SSRIs have been shown to be extremely effective for treating PMS and have become first-line treatment for PMDD. Dimmock and coworkers' meta-analysis of 15 RCTs has shown SSRIs to be seven times more effective than placebo for treating PMS. Relief of physical and behavioral symptoms was noted. Medication dosages are generally lower than those used for depression. The onset of action can be rapid, within 1 to 2 days, unlike when SSRIs are used for depression (for dosing, see **Box 36-4**). If luteal phase treatment is not effective after 3 months, a trial of continuous SSRIs is warranted. SSRIs are effective in approximately 60% of PMS sufferers.

If one SSRI is ineffective, try other agents. Even for PMDD, using the psychoactive drugs in only the luteal phase of the menstrual cycle can be effective. However, Shah and colleagues' 2008 meta-analysis of 20 RCTs and 2964 women found that SSRIs are effective for treating PMS and PMDD (odds ratio [OR], 0.40; 95% confidence interval [CI], 0.31 to 0.51), but intermittent dosing was less effective (OR, 0.55) than continuous dosing (OR, 0.28). No SSRI was demonstrably better than another. Venlafaxine is a serotonin and norepinephrine reuptake inhibitor and has been studied in an RCT for PMDD. There was a significant reduction in symptoms; this medication may be helpful for patients who have side effects or no benefit on other SSRIs. After three cycles of SSRI treatment for PMDD, symptoms recurred with the first cycle after drug discontinuation, suggesting that prolonged therapy may be necessary. Although not FDA-approved, a Cochrane review has also revealed good evidence for the effectiveness of fluvoxamine, citalopram, and clomipramine. Serious adverse effects can occur and must be weighed against the severity of the woman's symptoms.

Approximately 15% of women on SSRIs have significant side effects, including sexual dysfunction (anorgasmia), sleep alterations, GI distress, including nausea, and CNS complaints such as headache and jitteriness. Some SSRIs can precipitate anxiety reactions, so caution should be used if anxiety symptoms predominate. Increased suicide rates have been observed with some SSRIs, so caution is needed if significant depressive symptoms are noted. This should be a low risk, given the low dose and intermittent luteal phase dosing.

In a carefully performed double-blind, placebo-controlled, crossover study of 19 patients suffering from PMS using alprazolam (Xanax), Smith and coworkers noted that the drug

significantly relieved the severity of premenstrual nervous tension, mood swings, irritability, anxiety, depression, fatigue, forgetfulness, crying, cravings for sweets, abdominal bloating, cramps, and headaches compared with the placebo. They prescribed alprazolam, 0.25 mg three times/day, on days 20 to 28 of each cycle, and then tapering to 0.25 mg twice daily on day 1 and 0.25 mg on day 2. Several RCTs have shown that doses higher than 0.75 mg/day are necessary to reduce PMS symptoms significantly. Alprazolam may be more effective for depressive and anxiety symptoms than other PMS complaints. However, approximately 50% of women complain of drowsiness and sedation on these doses. Patients with a strong tendency to habituation should not be treated with this regimen. Therefore, alprazolam is considered second-line treatment. Buspirone has less addictive potential than alprazolam and has been found in two RCTs to reduce symptoms. Continuous use of psychoactive drugs, such as tricyclics and lithium, has not yielded good PMS symptom relief.

Before using psychoactive drugs, it is extremely important to be sure of the diagnosis, because these drugs may not be effective and may actually be contraindicated in other psychiatric conditions that mimic PMS.

Progesterone and Estrogen

Although a common treatment previously, double-blind studies to date have not shown progestogens to be conclusively effective for PMS. Small RCTs have suggested small but significant reductions in some PMS symptoms. However, there is insufficient evidence to recommend progestogen therapy. Similarly, oral progesterone therapy has shown small but significant reduction in some PMS symptoms, but the improvement was not thought to be clinically important, especially given the much greater benefit of SSRIs.

Some relief of symptoms was noted in a double-blind, placebo-controlled, crossover study by Watson and coworkers using estradiol patches (200 μg every 3 days) and norethisterone 5 mg (days 19–26 of each cycle) when compared with placebo. The authors realized that they were suppressing ovulation and that this may have been the mechanism for obtaining symptom relief. Two other small RCTs have suggested improvement from estrogen for PMS, but the magnitude of benefit is unclear.

Oral Contraceptives

Early RCTs and descriptive studies using cyclic OCs have shown mixed results for the treatment of PMS, but OCs are likely beneficial because they inhibit ovulation. OCs mainly help physical symptoms such as breast pain, bloating, acne, and appetite. If used, monophasic OCs appear to be better. In Sulak and associates' retrospective review of 220 patients using an extended OC regimen and shortened hormone-free interval (3 to 4 days), 45% of patients chose this regimen for control of PMS symptoms and 40% for dysmenorrhea and pelvic pain symptoms. Continuous combined OCs should suppress ovulation and provide symptom relief. A 2005 review found that few studies have reported on premenstrual symptoms on continuous- or extended-use OCs, but relief was noted in headaches, tiredness, bloating, and menstrual pain. Finally, a prospective 2006 study by Coffee and colleagues has shown that an extended regimen of 30 μg of ethinyl estradiol with 3 mg of drosperinone for 168 days significantly reduces PMS symptoms compared with typical 21-day cyclic OCs. The FDA has approved a 20-μg ethinyl estradiol

Box 36-4 FDA-Approved Medications for Premenstrual Dysphoric Disorder	
Drug	**Starting Dose**
SSRIs	
Fluoxetine hydrochloride (Sarafem)	20 mg/day
Sertraline hydrochloride (Zoloft)	50 mg/day
Paroxetine hydrochloride (Paxil CR)	12.5 mg/day
Oral Contraceptive	
Ethinyl estradiol, drospirenone (YAZ)	One daily

and 3-mg drospirenone combination OC for the treatment of PMDD, although limiting use to women with PMDD who also need contraception was mentioned. Because of drospirenone's antimineral corticoid and antiandrogenic properties, it has been hypothesized to be more effective. A 2009 Cochrane systematic review supported its efficacy. One study directly compared a drospirenone containing combined OC with the intravaginal contraceptive ring and reported equivalent improvement in PMS symptoms.

Nonsteroidal Anti-inflammatory Drugs
For patients who complain of cramping or other systemic symptoms, such as aches, diarrhea, or heat intolerance, a trial with an NSAID may be useful. RCTs with mefenamic acid and naproxen have shown improvement in pain, mood, and somatic symptoms. It should be noted, however, that a toxic complication of NSAID use is nonoliguric renal failure. Because it is more likely to occur with NSAID use associated with severe dehydration, the agent should be discontinued if severe diarrhea is present and should not be used with diuretics.

Danazol
Sarno and associates have reported on the apparent effectiveness of danazol, 200 mg/day, days 20 to 28 of each menstrual cycle, for relieving PMS symptoms. Studying 14 patients in a double-blind, placebo-controlled protocol, they found significant relief of symptoms in 11 of the 14 patients compared with placebo. Because such a small dose given only during the luteal phase will not prevent pregnancy, and to avoid the potential of masculinizing a female fetus, patients should be cautioned to avoid this agent if pregnancy is contemplated. As noted, danazol may be effective because it causes anovulation in some subjects at this dose level. Another RCT of luteal phase danazol has shown only significant reduction in premenstrual mastalgia. Because of side effects (e.g., hirsutism, deepening of the voice, acne) and available treatments with more accurately known response rates, danazol is rarely recommended.

Bromocriptine
Bromocriptine may be used for patients with cyclic mastalgia and may be helpful for some other symptoms of PMS, although its use in any individual case will need to be evaluated. A dose of 2.5 to 5 mg/day during the luteal phase is appropriate.

GnRH Agonists
At least 10 RCTs have shown GnRH agonists (leuprolide, 3.75 mg IM monthly) to be effective for ovulation suppression and treatment of PMS and the physical symptoms of PMDD. GnRH agonists are less effective in treating the psychiatric symptoms of PMDD. However, they are expensive, can have marked side effects, and are limited in duration of use because of hypoestrogenism and osteoporosis. Using add-back estrogen and progesterone has been studied to offset the hypoestrogenic side effects without aggravating PMS and PMDD symptoms. The optimal add-back regimen is unclear from existing studies if GnRH agonists are to be used long term. Minimizing hormonal fluctuations with continuous estrogen and progesterone or minimizing the periods of exposure to progesterone seem prudent.

Surgical Treatment: Hysterectomy and Bilateral Oophorectomy
Casper and Hearn have reported complete relief of symptoms in 14 women with severe debilitating symptoms of PMS who had completed their families, had been shown to have relief of symptoms with ovarian-suppressing doses of danazol, and were now treated with total hysterectomy and bilateral oophorectomy followed by continuous low-dose estrogen replacement therapy. Casson and colleagues and Cronje have noted similar results. Although this approach is not offered as standard therapy for severe PMS, it may be a reasonable alternative for select patients for whom all other treatment regimens have failed. The use of a GnRH analogue for 3 to 6 months, with or without estrogen add-back, may be useful as therapy in severe cases or at least helpful when deciding who might benefit from surgical treatment. Hysterectomy without bilateral oophorectomy does not relieve symptoms. Bilateral oophorectomy without hysterectomy also seems to completely eradicate the symptoms of PMS. It is unknown whether endometrial ablation has the same effect.

The physician should be cautious when determining a treatment regimen for any individual patient and should attempt to verify the patient's symptoms and add medications only when relief has not been achieved. Medications that do not seem to be helping should be stopped. Because of the myriad of PMS symptoms, it is not surprising that individualization of treatment is essential. Many of the therapies mentioned, however, offer relief of most symptoms and hope for many sufferers.

KEY POINTS

- Primary dysmenorrhea almost always occurs before the age of 20 years. Secondary dysmenorrhea may occur at any time during the menstrual years.
- Approximately 75% of all women complain of primary dysmenorrhea. Approximately 15% have severe symptoms.
- NSAIDs are the treatment of choice for primary dysmenorrhea, with 72% of women suffering from dysmenorrhea reporting significant pain relief. NSAIDs reduced intrauterine pressure 20% to 56% during treatment of patients with dysmenorrhea in one study and blocked prostaglandin production and action.
- OCs reduce the prevalence and severity of dysmenorrhea. They can be used in long cycles for better relief. This is also

a reasonable first-line treatment, especially if contraception is desired.
- If dysmenorrhea symptoms are not relieved with NSAIDs or OCs or their combination, consider additional evaluation for pelvic pathology.
- Approximately 40% of all women suffer considerably from premenstrual syndrome (PMS), with 3% to 8% demonstrating severe symptoms (PMDD).
- PMS patients often suffer depression during the luteal phase but not as severe as the depression noted by patients with endogenous depression when measured by standard depression scales. It can be difficult to distinguish PMS from depression with luteal phase exacerbation.

KEY POINTS—CONTINUED

- The most useful diagnostic tool in caring for PMS and PMDD patients is a prospective symptom diary.
- Calcium and vitamin B_6 therapy can relieve PMS symptoms, as do medications including spironolactone and oral contraceptives.

- Therapy with psychoactive drugs, particularly the SSRIs given in relatively small doses during the luteal phase, may be helpful in relieving PMS and PMDD symptoms. Specific cautions for the use of these agents must be followed.

REFERENCES CAN BE FOUND ON EXPERTCONSULT.com

37

Abnormal Uterine Bleeding
Ovulatory and Anovulatory Dysfunctional Uterine Bleeding: Management of Acute and Chronic Excessive Bleeding

Roger A. Lobo

Abnormal uterine bleeding can take many forms—infrequent episodes, excessive flow, or prolonged duration of menses and **intermenstrual bleeding**. Alterations in the pattern or volume of blood flow of menses are among the most common health concerns of women. Infrequent uterine bleeding, defined as oligomenorrhea if the intervals between bleeding episodes vary from 35 days to 6 months, and amenorrhea, defined as no menses for at least 6 months, are discussed in Chapter 38 (Primary and Secondary Amenorrhea and Precocious Puberty). Excessive or prolonged bleeding will be discussed in this chapter. Several new therapeutic modalities are being successfully used to treat excessive uterine bleeding and will also be discussed here.

To define excessive abnormal uterine bleeding, it is necessary to define normal menstrual flow. The mean interval between menses is 28 days (± 7 days). Thus, if bleeding occurs at intervals of 21 days or less, it is abnormal. The mean duration of menstrual flow is 4 days. Few women with normal menses bleed more than 7 days, so bleeding for longer than 7 days is considered to be abnormally prolonged (menorrhagia). It is useful to document the duration and frequency of menstrual flow with the use of menstrual diary cards; however, it is difficult to determine the amount of menstrual blood loss (MBL) by subjective means. Several studies have shown that there is poor correlation between subjective judgment and objective measurement of MBL.

Although subjective methods are used in predicting blood loss, and some investigators have used a pictorial bleeding assessment chart, a more accurate method is the alkaline hematic method, which measures hematin. It has been shown that the average menstrual blood loss is 35 mL. Total volume, however, is twice this amount, being made up of endometrial tissue exudate. The amount of MBL increases with parity but not age in the absence of disease. A MBL of 80 mL or greater is defined as menorrhagia, which occurs in 9% to 14% of women.

CAUSES

The causes of abnormal bleeding can be divided into organic causes and dysfunctional (or hormonally related) abnormal bleeding. **Dysfunctional uterine bleeding (DUB)** is further divided into anovulatory bleeding and ovulatory bleeding.

ORGANIC CAUSES

The organic causes can be subdivided into systemic disease and reproductive tract disease.

Systemic Disease

Systemic diseases, particularly disorders of blood coagulation such as von Willebrand disease and prothrombin deficiency, may initially present as abnormal uterine bleeding. Other disorders that produce platelet deficiency, such as leukemia, severe sepsis, idiopathic thrombocytopenic purpura, and hypersplenism, can also cause excessive bleeding. Routine screening for coagulation defects is mainly indicated for the adolescent who has prolonged heavy menses beginning at menarche, unless otherwise indicated by clinical signs such as petechiae or ecchymosis. Claessens and Cowell have reported that coagulation disorders are found in approximately 20% of adolescent girls who require hospitalization for abnormal uterine bleeding. Coagulation defects are present in approximately 25% of those whose hemoglobin levels fall below 10 g/100 mL, in one third of those who require transfusions, and in 50% of those whose severe menorrhagia occurred at the time of the first menstrual period. A study by Falcone and associates has indicated that a coagulation disorder was found in only 5% of adolescents hospitalized for heavy bleeding. Both studies indicated that the likelihood of a blood disorder in adolescents with heavy menses is sufficiently high that all adolescents should be evaluated to determine whether a coagulopathy is present.

In the adult, abnormal bleeding may be encountered frequently in women receiving anticoagulation for a variety of medical disorders. Although the pattern of bleeding is usually menorrhagia, abnormal intracycle bleeding also occurs.

Any other chronic systemic diseases can result in abnormal bleeding. These include hepatitis, renal disease, and cardiac disease, as well as coronary vascular disorders. The mechanism of the abnormal bleeding is usually anovulation related to hypothalamic causes and/or problems with estrogen metabolism. In addition, a number of endocrine disorders may lead to abnormal bleeding. These include disorders of hormones such as thyroid, prolactin (PRL), and cortisol (see later discussion of anovulatory DUB).

REPRODUCTIVE TRACT DISEASE

The most common causes of abnormal uterine bleeding in women of reproductive age are accidents of pregnancy such as threatened, incomplete, or missed abortion and ectopic pregnancy. In addition, trophoblastic disease must be considered in the differential diagnosis of abnormal bleeding in any woman who has had a recent pregnancy. A sensitive β-human chorionic gonadotropin (β-hCG) assay should be performed as part of the diagnostic evaluation.

Any malignancy of the genital tract, particularly endometrial and cervical cancer, may present as abnormal bleeding. Less commonly, vaginal, vulvar, and fallopian tube cancer may produce abnormal bleeding. In addition, estrogen-producing ovarian tumors may become manifest by abnormal uterine bleeding. Thus, granulosa theca cell tumors may present with excessive uterine bleeding. Infection of the upper genital tract, particularly endometritis, may present as prolonged menses, although episodic intermenstrual spotting is a more common symptom. Endometriosis may also result in abnormal bleeding and frequently presents as premenstrual spotting. There are various explanations for this that relate to the location of the endometriosis implants.

Anatomic uterine abnormalities such as submucous myomas, endometrial polyps, and adenomyosis frequently produce symptoms of prolonged and excessive regular uterine bleeding. This is probably secondary to abnormal vasculature and blood flow, as well as increased inflammatory changes. Cervical lesions such as erosions, polyps, and cervicitis may cause irregular bleeding, particularly postcoital spotting. These lesions can usually be diagnosed by visualization of the cervix. In addition, traumatic vaginal lesions, severe vaginal infections, and foreign bodies have been associated with abnormal bleeding.

Foreign bodies in the uterus, such as an intrauterine device (IUD), frequently produce abnormal uterine bleeding. Other iatrogenic causes include oral and injectable steroids such as those used for contraception and hormonal replacement or for the management of dysmenorrhea, hirsutism, acne, or endometriosis. Tranquilizers and other psychotropic drugs may interfere with the neurotransmitters responsible for releasing and inhibiting hypothalamic hormones, thus causing anovulation and abnormal bleeding.

DYSFUNCTIONAL CAUSES

After organic, systemic, and iatrogenic causes for the abnormal bleeding have been ruled out, the diagnosis of DUB can be made. There are two types of DUB, anovulatory and ovulatory. The predominant cause of DUB in the postmenarchal and premenopausal years is anovulation secondary to alterations in neuroendocrinologic function. In women with anovulatory DUB, there is continuous estradiol production without corpus luteum formation and progesterone production. The steady state of estrogen stimulation leads to a continuously proliferating endometrium, which may outgrow its blood supply or lose nutrients with varying degrees of necrosis. In contrast to normal menstruation, uniform slough to the basalis layer does not occur, which produces excessive uterine blood flow

Anovulatory DUB occurs most commonly during the extremes of reproductive life—in the first few years after menarche and during perimenopause. In the adolescent, the cause of the anovulation is an immaturity of the hypothalamic-pituitary-ovarian (HPO) axis and failure of positive feedback of estradiol to cause a luteinizing hormone (LH) surge. In the perimenopausal woman, a lack of synchronization between the components of the HPO axis occurs as the woman approaches ovarian failure.

The pattern of anovulatory bleeding may be oligomenorrhea, **menometrorrhagia**, **metrorrhagia**, or **menorrhagia**. Why different patterns of bleeding occur within a distinct entity of anovulatory DUB is unclear but is probably related to variations in the integrity of the endometrium and its support structure. Up to 20% of women reporting normal menses may also be anovulating. However, the pattern of ovulatory DUB (see later) is mainly that of menorrhagia.

What are the causes of anovulatory DUB? Apart from the extremes of reproductive life, as noted, women in their reproductive years often have a cause for anovulatory bleeding. This is most frequently because of polycystic ovary syndrome (PCOS), which may be suggested by other symptoms and signs, such as acne, hirsutism, and increased body weight (see Chapter 40). If not PCOS, anovulation can result from hypothalamic dysfunction, which could have no known cause or be related to weight loss, severe exercise, stress, or drug use. In addition, abnormalities of other (nonreproductive) hormones can lead to anovulatory DUB. Strictly speaking, nonreproductive hormonal abnormalities are not considered to be DUB but are closely related. These cases of abnormal bleeding are discussed here because they lead to anovulatory bleeding. The most common hormones involved are thyroid hormone, prolactin, and cortisol.

Hypothyroidism, evidenced by an elevated thyroid stimulating hormone (TSH) level, can lead to anovulatory bleeding. Unexplained causes of ovulatory DUB (see later) may also be explained by subtle hypothyroidism. Hyperprolactinemia (PRL level > 20 ng/mL) can also lead to anovulatory bleeding, as can hypercortisolism. However, Cushing's syndrome is rare and may be considered only if other signs are present (e.g., obesity, moon facies, buffalo hump, striae, weakness). Accordingly, TSH and PRL assays should be part of the normal workup.

Ovulatory Dysfunctional Uterine Bleeding

Women who present with menorrhagia (without causes such as uterine lesions, polyps, fibroids) have ovulatory DUB. It is important to understand how menstrual bleeding ceases each month to appreciate what can go wrong in ovulatory DUB. The primary line of defense is a platelet plug. This is followed by uterine contractility, largely mediated by prostaglandin F2α (PGF2α). Thus, prolonged and heavy bleeding can occur with abnormalities of the platelet plug and/or inadequate uterine levels of PGF2α. It has been shown that in ovulatory DUB, some women have excessive uterine production of prostacyclin, a vasodilatory prostaglandin that opposes platelet adhesion and may also interfere with uterine contractility. Deficiency of uterine PGF2α or excessive production of PGE (another vasodilatory prostaglandin) may also explain ovulatory DUB. The ratio of PGF2α/PGE correlates inversely with menstrual blood loss (**Fig. 37-1**).

In addition to these, other uterine factors affecting blood flow, such as the endothelins and vascular endothelial growth factor, which controls blood vessel formation, may be abnormal in some women with ovulatory DUB.

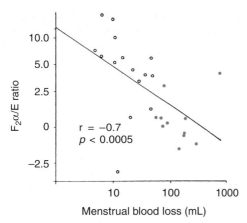

Figure 37-1 Correlation between ratio of endogenous concentrations of PGF2α and PGE and menstrual blood loss (MBL); normal secretory endometrium; persistent endometrium. (From Smith SK, Abel MH, Kelly RW, Baird DT: The synthesis of prostaglandins from persistent proliferative endometrium. J Clin Endocrinol Metab 55:284, 1982.)

DIAGNOSTIC APPROACH

When a woman presents with a complaint of abnormal bleeding, it is essential to take a thorough history regarding the frequency, duration, and amount of bleeding, as well as to inquire whether and when the menstrual pattern has changed. This history is extremely important for determining whether the menstrual abnormality is **polymenorrhea**, menorrhagia (hypermenorrhea), metrorrhagia, menometrorrhagia, or intermenstrual bleeding. History and physical examination provide clues about the diagnosis of PCOS and other disorders. Providing the woman with a calendar to record her bleeding episodes is a helpful way to characterize definitively the bleeding episodes. Because there is a poor correlation between a woman's estimate of the amount of blood flow and the measured loss, as well as great variation in the amount of blood and fluid absorbed by different types of sanitary napkins and tampons (and by the same type in different women), objective criteria should be used to determine if menorrhagia (blood loss > 80 mL) is present.

Because direct measurement of MBL is not generally possible, indirect assessment by measurement of hemoglobin concentration, serum iron levels, and serum ferritin levels is useful. The serum ferritin level provides a valid indirect assessment of iron stores in the bone marrow. Additional useful laboratory tests include a sensitive β-hCG level determination and a sensitive TSH assay, as well as PRL. If PCOS is suspected, androgen level measurements may be considered, but are not necessary. For adolescent girls, as well as older women with systemic disease, a coagulation profile should be obtained to rule out a coagulation defect. If the woman has regular cycles, it is important to determine whether she is ovulating. However, if bleeding is very irregular, it may be difficult to determine the phase of the cycle to document ovulatory function by means of serum progesterone level determination or other methods. Typically, ovulatory DUB displays a pattern of repetition with heavy bleeding. Endometrial biopsy may be indicated and, if obtained at the onset of bleeding, will show secretory changes. Transvaginal ultrasound can be helpful in ruling out pathology and helping to guide the need for endometrial biopsy. Women who are older (>35 years) and/or have a long history of excessive bleeding would benefit from an endometrial biopsy. It has been suggested that an endometrial lining of more than 8 mm has a greater sensitivity for picking up endometrial pathology. If bleeding has been prolonged and an ultrasound endometrial thickening is less than 4 mm, there is little benefit for a biopsy in this setting. A biopsy at the time of bleeding can also help determine whether the bleeding is caused by ovulatory function if it reveals a secretory endometrium.

Apart from obtaining a careful history and physical examination, blood testing (as noted earlier), ultrasound, and endometrial biopsy (if indicated), it is often valuable to assay the SHG level in women with menorrhagia. This is to rule out an intracavity lesion before ascribing the diagnosis to ovulatory DUB (**Fig. 37-2**).

Saline or sterile water, 10 to 15 mL, is usually introduced through the cervix with an insemination catheter, or with a special hysterosalpingography (HSG) catheter that has a balloon for inflation in the cervical canal, allowing continuous infusion. If this is not available, HSG may be ordered. Hysteroscopy is an excellent diagnostic technique and has the potential advantage of being able to treat the abnormality at the same time, for example, as removal of a polyp. However, it is not cost-effective as a diagnostic test if it cannot be carried out in an office setting.

Hysteroscopy can be performed in the office, with or without local anesthesia, and is clearly a more accurate diagnostic procedure than a dilation and curettage (D&C). A D&C is a blind technique and does not always detect focal lesions. In a comparison of hysteroscopy with endometrial biopsy and D&C in a group of 342 women, Gimpelson and Rappold found that hysteroscopy permitted the accurate diagnosis in 60 women in whom the diagnosis was not made by D&C. Most of these women had the diagnosis of submucous myomas and endometrial polyps made by hysteroscopy that was missed by D&C. March has reported that 25% of women with a presumptive diagnosis of DUB were found to have uterine lesions at the time of hysteroscopy.

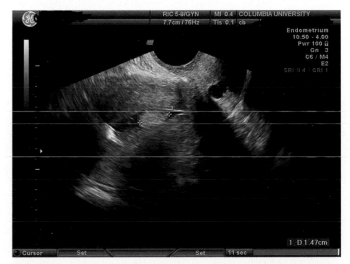

Figure 37-2 Saline sonography demonstrating a 1.4-cm diameter endometrial polyp in a woman with menorrhagia (Courtesy of Dr. J. Lerner, Columbia University Medical Center, New York.)

Apart from an SHG or similar technique to rule out lesions before a diagnosis of ovulatory DUB is made in some women presenting with menorrhagia, a subtle hypothyroidism can also be found. If this is found, it is strictly not ovulatory DUB. A third-generation ultrasensitive TSH assay should be performed and elevations should be assessed further. Finally, coagulation defects can also present in this setting.

Once thought to be extremely rare as a cause for abnormal bleeding, studies have found a fairly high prevalence of coagulation disorders in women presenting with menorrhagia. Most abnormalities are platelet-related. The single most common abnormality is a form of von Willebrand disease. It has been estimated that the prevalence of von Willebrand disease, the most common of these bleeding disorders, is 13% in women with menorrhagia. von Willebrand factor is responsible for proper platelet adhesion and protects against coagulant factor degradation. History is key before a comprehensive hematologic workup is undertaken. This includes a history of menorrhagia, family history of bleeding, epistaxis, bruising, gum bleeding, postpartum hemorrhage, and surgical bleeding. In the absence of these clues, a comprehensive workup is probably unnecessary at outset but should be considered in cases refractory to treatment. A hematologist should be consulted. Treatment involves a variety of options, including oral contraceptives for milder cases, levonorgestrel-releasing intrauterine system (Mirena IUS), tranexamic acid, 1 g every 6 hours during menses, or desmopressin (DDAVP) intranasally, one puff per nostril for the first 3 days of menses. All are discussed below.

TREATMENT

In the absence of an organic cause for excessive uterine bleeding, it is preferable to use medical instead of surgical treatment, especially if the woman desires to retain her uterus for future childbearing or will be undergoing natural menopause within a short time. There are several effective medical methods for the treatment of DUB. These include estrogens, progestogen (systemic or local), **nonsteroidal anti-inflammatory drugs (NSAIDs)**, antifibrinolytic agents, danazol, and gonadotropin-releasing hormone (GnRH) agonists. The type of treatment depends on whether it is used to stop an acute heavy bleeding episode or is given to reduce the amount of MBL in subsequent menstrual cycles. Before instituting long-term treatment, definitive diagnosis is required and should be made on the basis of hysteroscopy, sonohysterography, or directed endometrial biopsies, if indicated, with definitive treatment determined by the diagnosis.

This section is organized into treatment options for anovulatory DUB, ovulatory DUB, and the management of acute and heavy bleeding, which requires immediate action.

ANOVULATORY DYSFUNCTIONAL UTERINE BLEEDING

In adolescents, after ruling out coagulation disorders, the main direction of therapy is to temporize because with time and maturity of the HPO axis, the problem will be corrected. A cyclic progestogen—for example, medroxyprogesterone acetate, 10 mg for 10 days each month for a few months—is all that is needed to produce reliable and controlled menstrual cycles. This may be continued for up to 6 months with the situation

reevaluated thereafter. Alternatively, some clinics prefer to use an oral contraceptive (OC), although this may not be necessary and does not allow the HPO to mature on its own. If the problem persists beyond 6 months, OCs may be an option in that the condition may be more chronic.

In the perimenopausal woman who has dysregulation of the HPO axis, there is much variability and unpredictability of cycles because the HPO axis is in flux, moving toward ovarian failure. Although most of the bleeding in this setting is caused by anovulation, occasional ovulation can occur, with or without a normal luteal phase, which is highly variable and erratic. Here, it is more efficient to use a low-dose (20-μg) OC pill (OCP) in a nonsmoking woman. Progestogens used cyclically, although preventing endometrial tissue from building up because of anovulation, will help the endometrium but will not reliably control bleeding, because of the unpredictability of the hormonal situation.

During reproductive life, chronic anovulatory DUB, after a careful workup, is primarily caused by hypothalamic dysfunction leading to anovulation or PCOS. OCPs work well in this setting, although an alternative is cyclic progestogens, as noted. Some of these women may also wish to conceive, in which case ovulation induction is indicated.

OVULATORY DYSFUNCTIONAL UTERINE BLEEDING

For women with menorrhagia, for whom there is no known cause and anatomic lesions have been ruled out, the aim of therapy is to reduce the amount of excessive bleeding. As noted, some women with ovulatory DUB have abnormal prostaglandin production and some have alterations of endometrial blood flow.

Options for treatment to reduce blood loss include a more prolonged regimen of progestogens (3 weeks each month); shorter cyclic therapy does not work here. Doses in excess of 10 mg daily of medroxyprogesterone acetate (MPA) have been used, but large doses can cause side effects and weight gain when used for several months, and may not be necessary. OCPs will reduce the blood loss by 50% in women with ovulatory DUB. Another beneficial option is the use of the levonorgestrel IUS whereby menorrhagia can be substantially reduced (see later). It should be noted that in ovulatory DUB, although all obvious lesions have been ruled out, some anatomic abnormalities cannot be easily diagnosed. These include endometriosis and, in particular, adenomyosis, although this might be improved with imaging. Thus, other options also have to be considered for reducing blood loss.

Local Progestogen Exposure

The progesterone-releasing IUD has been found to be effective for the treatment of women with ovulatory DUB. Bergqvist and Rybo inserted this device into 12 women with ovulatory DUB and found their MBL declined from an average of 138 to 49 mL in 1 year, a 65% reduction in MBL (**Fig. 37-3**). This device needs to be reinserted annually because of the rapid diffusion of progesterone through polysiloxane; however, it is no longer available.

A levonorgestrel-releasing intrauterine system (LNG-IUS) has been developed that has an effective duration of action of more than 5 years. Milson and colleagues have studied the use of this IUS as treatment for menorrhagia and found that at the end of 3 months, it caused an average 80% reduction in

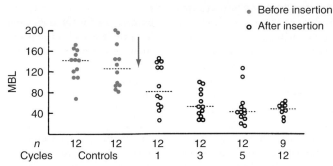

Figure 37-3 Menstrual blood loss (MBL) before and after insertion of progesterone IUD (Progestasert; *arrow*) in menorrhagic women. (Each *dot* marks a separate patient; the median value is marked with a *dotted line*.) (From Bergqvist A, Rybo G: Treatment of menorrhagia with intrauterine release of progesterone. Br J Obstet Gynaecol 90:255, 1983.)

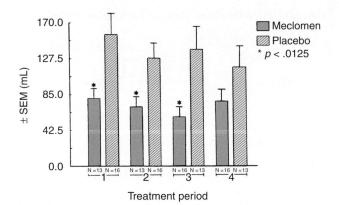

Figure 37-5 Menstrual blood loss (MBL) by treatment period and drug. (From Vargyas JM, Campeau JD, Mishell DA: Treatment of menorrhagia with meclofenamate sodium. Am J Obstet Gynecol 157:944, 1987.)

MBL, which increased to 100% at the end of 1 year. This reduction in MBL was significantly greater than that achieved with an antifibrinolytic agent or a prostaglandin synthetase inhibitor in studies by the same investigators (**Fig. 37-4**). Other studies have shown that the LNG-IUS reduces MBL by 74% to 97% and is effective in increasing hemoglobin levels, decreasing dysmenorrhea, and reducing blood loss caused by fibroids and adenomyosis. In addition, it has also been compared with hysterectomy for menorrhagia and had been considered to be a viable alternative.

Nonsteroidal Anti-inflammatory Drugs

NSAIDs are prostaglandin synthetase inhibitors that inhibit the biosynthesis of the cyclic endoperoxides, which convert arachidonic acid to prostaglandins. In addition, these agents block the action of prostaglandins by interfering directly at their receptor sites. To decrease bleeding of the endometrium, it would be ideal to block selectively the synthesis of prostacyclin alone, without decreasing thromboxane formation, because the latter increases platelet aggregation. Presently, there are no NSAIDs that possess this ability. All NSAIDs are cyclooxygenase inhibitors and thus

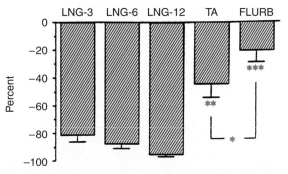

Figure 37-4 Reduction in menstrual blood loss (MBL) expressed as percentage of mean of two control cycles for each form of treatment. Significance of difference between treatment with levonorgestrel-releasing IUD (LNG-IUD) and tranexamic acid (TA) and flurbiprofen (FLURB), indicated by *double asterisks* (*P* < .01) and *triple asterisks* (*P* < .001), and between treatment with TA and FLURB indicated by a *single asterisk* (*P* < .05). (From Milson I, Andersson K, Andersch B, Rybo G: A comparison of flurbiprofen, tranexamic acid, and a levonorgestrel-releasing intrauterine contraceptive device in the treatment of idiopathic menorrhagia. Am J Obstet Gynecol 164:879, 1991.)

block the formation of both thromboxane and the prostacyclin pathway. Nevertheless, NSAIDs have been shown to reduce MBL, primarily in women who ovulate. However, the mechanisms whereby prostaglandin inhibitors reduce MBL are not yet completely understood, and their therapeutic action may take place through some as yet undiscovered mechanism. Several NSAIDs have been administered during menses to groups of women with menorrhagia and ovulatory DUB and have been found to reduce the mean MBL by approximately 20% to 50% (**Fig. 37-5**). Drugs used in various studies have included mefenamic acid (500 mg, three times daily), ibuprofen (400 mg, three times daily), meclofenamate sodium (100 mg, three times daily), and naproxen sodium (275 mg, every 6 hours after a loading dose of 550 mg), as well as other NSAIDs. These drugs are usually given for the first 3 days of menses or throughout the bleeding episode. They appear to have similar levels of effectiveness.

Not all women treated with these agents have reduction in blood flow, but those without a decrease usually had only a mildly increased amount of MBL. The greatest amount of MBL reduction occurs in women with the greatest pretreatment blood loss. Fraser and coworkers have reported that the treatment of menorrhagia with mefenamic acid in 36 women for longer than 1 year results in a significantly sustained reduction in amounts of MBL and a significant increase in serum ferritin levels. Thus, this can be used for long-term treatment because side effects, mainly gastrointestinal (GI), are mild with this intermittent therapy.

Although NSAIDs have been studied by themselves to treat women with MBL who ovulate, they can also be given in combination with OCs or progestins. With this combined approach, reduction in MBL can be achieved more effectively than with the use of any of these agents alone.

Antifibrinolytic Agents

ε-Aminocaproic acid (EACA), tranexamic acid (AMCA), and para-aminomethyl benzoic acid (PAMBA) are potent inhibitors of fibrinolysis and have therefore been used in the treatment of various hemorrhagic conditions. Nilsson and Rybo have compared the effect on blood loss of EACA, AMCA, and oral contraceptives in 215 women with menorrhagia. EACA was given in a dose of 18 g/day for 3 days and then 12, 9, 6, and 3 g daily on successive days. The total dose was always at least 48 g. AMCA was administered in a dose of 6 g/day for 3 days, followed by

Table 37-1 Mean Menstrual Blood Loss and Reduction with Treatment

	Mean Blood Loss (mL)		
Agent Used	Before Treatment	After Treatment	Decrease (%)
EACA	164	87	47
AMCA	182	84	54
Oral contraceptives	158	75	52
Methylergobaseimmaleate	164	164	0

AMCA, Tranexamic acid; EACA, ε-ammocaproic acid.
Adapted from Nilsson L, Rybo G: Treatment of menorrhagia. Am J Obstet Gynecol 110:713, 1971.

4, 3, 2, and 1 g/day on successive days. The total dose of AMCA was at least 22 g. There was a significant reduction in blood loss after treatment with EACA, AMCA, and OCs, and use of each of these agents resulted in approximately a 50% reduction in MBL (**Table 37-1**). Of interest was the finding that the greatest reduction in blood loss with antifibrinolytic therapy occurred in women who exhibited the greatest MBL. Preston and colleagues have compared the effects of 4 g of AMCA daily for 4 days each cycle with 10 mg of norethindrone for 7 days each cycle in a group of women with ovulatory menorrhagia with a mean MBL of 175 mL. AMCA reduced MBL by 45%, but there was a 20% increase with norethindrone. The side effects of this class of drugs, in decreasing order of frequency, are nausea, dizziness, diarrhea, headaches, abdominal pain, and allergic manifestations. These side effects are much more common with EACA than with AMCA. Other investigators have compared the use of AMCA with placebo in double-blind studies and have found no significant differences in the occurrence of side effects. Renal failure and pregnancy are contraindications to the use of antifibrinolytic agents.

Antifibrinolytic agents clearly produce a reduction in blood loss and may be used as therapy for women with menorrhagia who ovulate. However, their use is somewhat limited by side effects. These are mainly GI side effects and can be minimized by reducing the dose and limiting therapy to the first 3 days of bleeding. Furthermore, as with NSAIDs, they are best combined with another agent, such as oral contraceptives, for a greater effect on MBL reduction.

Androgenic Steroids (Danazol)

Danazol has been used by several investigators for the treatment of menorrhagia. Doses of 200 and 400 mg daily have been given over 12 weeks after careful pretreatment observation and evaluation. MBL was markedly reduced in these studies from more than 200 to less than 25 mL. Also, there was an increased interval between bleeding episodes (**Fig. 37-6**). The most common side effects of danazol treatment are weight gain and acne. Reduction of dosage from 400 to 200 mg daily decreased the side effects but did not alter the reduction in blood loss. Some women may ovulate when receiving this dose of danazol. Further reduction to 100 mg daily did not effectively reduce MBL in most women. Although danazol is effective, it is also expensive and has moderate side effects.

Dockeray and associates have treated 40 women with DUB, 50% with mefenamic acid (500 mg three times daily for 3 to 5 days of menses) and 50% with danazol (100 mg twice daily for 60 days). Danazol was more effective in reducing MBL, 60% compared with 20% for mefenamic acid. However, adverse side effects were more severe with danazol and occurred in 75% of patients, compared with side effects in only 30% of patients treated with mefenamic acid. A Cochrane review has noted that although nine randomized controlled trials (RCTs) were identified, studies have been generally underpowered. Nevertheless, danazol appears to be more effective than placebo, oral progestogens, oral contraceptives, and NSAIDs. However, compared with NSAIDs, the side effects of weight gain and skin problems were sevenfold and fourfold greater, respectively, when compared with progestogens.

Gonadotropin-Releasing Hormone Agonists

Although no large-scale studies have been performed, it is possible to inhibit ovarian steroid production with GnRH agonists. In a small study of four women, daily administration of a GnRH agonist for 3 months markedly reduced MBL from 100 to 200 mL per cycle to 0 to 30 mL per cycle. Unfortunately, after therapy was discontinued, blood loss returned to pretreatment levels (**Fig. 37-7**). Two other observational studies, one using sequential add-back in 20 women and another using goserelin in 60 women, have shown some benefit. Because of the expense and side effects of these agents, their use for menorrhagia caused

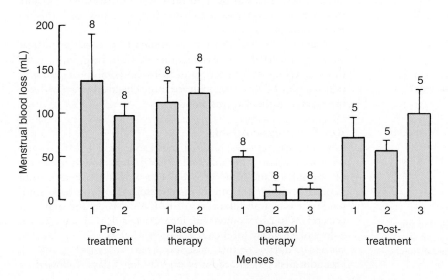

Figure 37-6 Mean (± standard error of the mean [SEM]) menstrual blood loss in eight patients with menorrhagia before treatment, with placebo therapy, with 200 mg danazol daily, and after treatment. Number of patients is shown above each histogram. (From Chimbria TH, Anderson ABM, Naish C, et al: Reduction of menstrual blood loss by danazol in unexplained menorrhagia: Lack of effect of placebo. Br J Obstet Gynaecol 87:1152, 1980.)

Figure 37-7 Alterations in measured monthly menstrual blood losses, number of days of menstrual bleeding, and hemoglobin (Hg) estimates before, during, and after therapy with intranasal luteinizing hormone-releasing hormone (LHRH) agonist. (From Shaw RW, Fraser HM: Use of a superactive luteinizing hormone-releasing hormone [LHRH] agonist in the treatment of menorrhagia. Br J Obstet Gynaecol 9:913, 1984.)

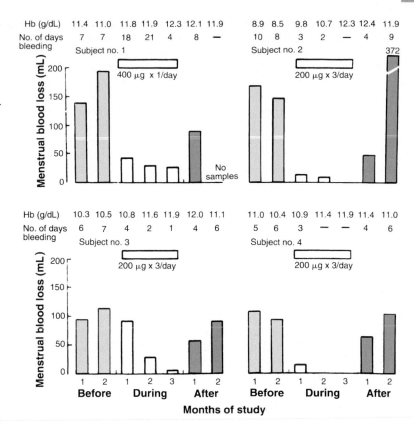

by ovulatory DUB is limited to women with severe MBL who fail to respond to other methods of medical management and wish to retain their childbearing capacity. Use of an estrogen and/or progestin (add-back therapy) together with the agonist will help prevent bone loss.

MANAGEMENT OF ACUTE BLEEDING

In women who are bleeding very heavily and are hemodynamically unstable, the quickest way to stop acute bleeding is with a curettage. This should also be the preferred approach for older women and those with medical risk factors for whom high-dose hormonal therapy might pose a great risk.

PHARMACOLOGIC AGENTS

To stop acute bleeding that does not require a curettage, the most effective regimen involves high-dose estrogen. This treatment, aimed at stopping acute bleeding, is diagnosis-independent and is merely a temporary measure.

Estrogens

The rationale for the therapeutic use of estrogen for the treatment of DUB is based on the fact that estrogen in pharmacologic doses causes rapid growth of the endometrium. This strategy is for the acute management of abnormal bleeding. The bleeding that results from most causes of DUB will respond to this therapy because a rapid growth of endometrial tissue occurs over the denuded and raw epithelial surfaces. This effect is independent of the cause of abnormal bleeding. To control an acute bleeding episode, the use of oral conjugated equine estrogen (CEE)

10 mg/day, in four divided doses, is a therapeutic regimen that has been found to be clinically useful. It is possible that in addition to the rapid growth mechanism of action, these large doses of CEE may alter platelet activity, thus promoting platelet adhesiveness. Livio and coworkers have reported that 6 hours after infusion of an average dose of 30 mg of CEE to individuals with a prolonged bleeding time caused by renal failure, the bleeding time was significantly shortened. In this study, measurements of various clotting factors were unchanged after CEE infusion. Acute bleeding from most causes is usually controlled, but if bleeding does not decrease within the first 24 hours, consideration must be given to an organic cause, e.g., accident of pregnancy should be considered, and curettage be considered.

IV administration of estrogen is also effective in the acute treatment of menorrhagia. DeVore and associates have reported that compared with women given a placebo, a significantly greater percentage of women had cessation of bleeding 2 hours after the second of two 25-mg doses of CEE was administered IV, 3 hours apart. There was no significant difference in cessation of bleeding between women administered estrogen and those given a placebo 3 hours after the first infusion. This study indicates that at least several hours are required to induce mitotic activity and growth of the endometrium, whether the estrogen is administered orally or parenterally. Thus, IV estrogen therapy accompanied by its rapid metabolic clearance does not appear to offer a significant advantage compared with the same dose of estrogen given orally. From a practical standpoint, if IV therapy is chosen, it usually requires that women remain in the office or clinical setting for 4 to 6 hours to receive at least a second dose.

Usually, estrogen therapy reduces the amount of uterine bleeding within the first 24 hours after treatment is initiated. However, because most women with an acute heavy bleeding episode bleed because of anovulation, progestin treatment is also required. Therefore, after bleeding has ceased, oral estrogen therapy is continued at the same dosage and a progestin, usually MPA, 10 mg once daily, is added. Both hormones are administered for another 7 to 10 days, after which treatment is stopped to allow withdrawal bleeding, which may have an increased amount of flow but is rarely prolonged. After the withdrawal bleeding episode, one of several other treatment modalities should be used. Before instituting long-term treatment, a definitive diagnosis should be made after reviewing the endometrial histology. Definitive treatment should be based on these findings. OCs are usually the best long-term treatment.

A more convenient method to stop acute bleeding than the sequential high-dose estrogen-progestin regimen is the use of a combination oral contraceptive containing both estrogen and progestin. Four tablets of an oral contraceptive containing 50 µg of estrogen taken every 24 hours in divided doses will usually provide sufficient estrogen to stop acute bleeding and simultaneously provide progestin. Treatment is continued for at least 1 week after the bleeding stops. This regimen is successful and convenient, and is thus the preferred method of some clinicians. However, in one study, it was found not to be as effective as the use of high doses of CEE. A theoretical reason for this difference might be that the combined use of estrogen and progestin does not cause as rapid endometrial growth as estrogen alone, because the progestin decreases the synthesis of estrogen receptors and increases estradiol dehydrogenase in the endometrial cell, thus inhibiting the growth-promoting action of estrogen.

It must be noted that high-dose estrogen, even for a short course, may be contraindicated for some women (e.g., those with prior thrombosis, certain rheumatologic diseases, estrogen-responsive cancer). In these cases, the options are therapy with progestogen alone given continuously or intermittently. Although invasive, curettage remains the fastest way to stop acute bleeding and should be used in women who are volume-depleted and severely anemic (hemodynamically unstable).

When ultrasound is available, it is more logical to use estrogen therapy if there is prolonged heavy bleeding in the setting of a thin endometrium (<5-mm stripe). Conversely, if the endometrium is thick (>10 to 12 mm), or if an anatomic finding is suspected, curettage should be considered. Also, unless bleeding is extremely heavy (where estrogen therapy is preferred), progestogens may be used initially, and will help by organizing the endometrium (see later). In the setting of a thickened irregular endometrium, if curettage is not performed, an endometrial biopsy should be obtained.

Progestogens

Progestogens not only stop endometrial growth but also support and organize the endometrium so that an organized slough occurs after their withdrawal. In the absence of progesterone, erratic unorganized breakdown of the endometrium occurs. With progestogen treatment, an organized slough to the basalis layer allows a rapid cessation of bleeding. In addition, progestogens stimulate arachidonic acid formation in the endometrium, increasing the PGF2α/PGE ratio. There is no evidence that progestogen will stop acute bleeding. After stabilization of the endometrium occurs (2 to 3 days), bleeding slows down and eventually stops. Therefore, as initial therapy, a regimen of progestogen only may be appropriate, but only for those with less significant acute bleeding who do not require immediate

cessation of bleeding. In general, progestogens, administered actively, do not stop bleeding but may slow it down as organization of the tissue occurs. Higher doses of norethindrone, however, which have been suggested to stop bleeding more acutely, may be efficacious on the basis of some conversion to ethinyl estradiol (thus mimicking the use of a low-dose OCP).

The mainstay of progestogen therapy is opposing the effects of estrogen in anovulatory women. For women with a history of bothersome menometrorrhagia, it is advisable to use intermittent progestogens for several months or an OC.

MPA, 10 mg/day for 10 days each month, is a successful therapeutic regimen that produces regular withdrawal bleeding in women with adequate amounts of endogenous estrogen to cause endometrial growth. 19-Norprogestogens, such as norethindrone or norethindrone acetate (2.5 to 5 mg) may be used in the same regimen. Although more androgenic progestogens are less favorable for metabolic parameters (e.g., high-density-lipoprotein [HDL] cholesterol, carbohydrate tolerance), short-term cyclic therapy is considered to be safe.

SURGICAL THERAPY

Dilation and Curettage

The performance of a D&C can be diagnostic and is therapeutic for the immediate management of severe bleeding. For women with markedly excessive uterine bleeding who may be hypovolemic, D&C is the quickest way to stop acute bleeding. Therefore, it is the treatment of choice in women who suffer from hypovolemia. D&C may be preferred as an approach to stop an acute bleeding episode in women older than 35 when the incidence of pathologic findings increases.

The use of D&C for the treatment of DUB has been reported to be curative only rarely. Temporary cure of the problem may occur in some women with chronic anovulation, because the curettage removes much of the hyperplastic endometrium; however, the underlying pathophysiologic cause is unchanged. D&C has not proved useful for the treatment of women who ovulate and have menorrhagia. Nilsson and Rybo have shown that more than 1 month after the D&C, there was no difference or an increase in MBL in women with menorrhagia who ovulate.

Therefore, D&C is only indicated for women with acute bleeding resulting in hypovolemia and for older women who are at higher risk of having endometrial neoplasia. All other women, after having an endometrial biopsy, sonohysteroscopy, or diagnostic hysteroscopy to rule out organic disease, are best treated with medical therapy, as outlined earlier, without D&C.

Endometrial Ablation

Abnormal bleeding may be treated by **endometrial ablation (EA)** if medical therapy is not effective. Exceptions are women who have very large uteri caused by fibroids or abnormal pathology, such as endometrial hyperplasia or cancer. A variety of methods are available and are an alternative to hysterectomy or to the use of the levonorgestrel IUS, which is also highly effective (see earlier).

Although the concept of EA was developed in 1937, the hysteroscopic technique was first used in 1981 with the introduction of the neodymium-yttrium-aluminum-garnet (Nd:YAG) laser. Laser-based approaches were largely replaced with resectoscopic techniques to resect, vaporize, or electrodessicate the endometrium. Currently, most commonly, various nonresectoscopic devices have been approved by the U.S. Food and Drug Administration (FDA) for this type of treatment.

Resectoscopic EA is usually carried out with a loop electrode, roller ball, or grooved or spiked electrode to vaporize the endometrium. Hysteroscopic surgical techniques have the advantage of dealing definitively with associated pathology (e.g., polyps, submucous fibroids) although they require greater surgical skill and have longer procedure times compared with nonresectoscopic methods.

Various nonresectoscopic methods are given in **Table 37-2**, which lists the success rates and limitations based on anatomy. Most systems, except the Hydro ThermAblator (Boston Scientific, Natick, MA) are carried out without hysteroscopic monitoring. Cryotherapy may be performed in approximately 10 minutes using a 4.5-mm disposable cryoprobe (HER option) which is moved from one uterine cornual recess to the other. The Hydro ThermAblator uses heated normal saline delivered through a 7.8-mm sheath. The uterus is distended and causes a closed circuit process, heating the saline to 90° C and maintaining this temperature for 10 minutes, followed by a 1-minute cooling process. The closed system is automated to shut down if there is 10 mL or more leakage of fluid via the cervix or fallopian tubes. Microwave endometrial ablation is carried out with an 8-mm reusable or disposable probe. Once the port is inserted into the fundus, transmission of endometrial tissue temperature is available, and the microwave system is activated when the tissue temperature is 30° C. Movement within the uterus of the microwave probe allows endometrial destruct to occur within 2 to 4 minutes.

The NovaSure radiofrequency electricity system (Hologic, Bedford, MA) uses a 7.2-mm probe with a bipolar gold mesh electrode that opens to conform to the shape of the uterus. A fixed volume of CO_2 is injected and monitored to confirm the integrity of the endometrial cavity. Suction is carried out during the application of radiofrequency energy to remove debris stream. The vaporization and desiccation is carried out over 80 to 90 seconds.

The Thermachoice system (Ethicon, Somerville, NJ) uses a balloon-tipped catheter (5.5 mm) through which heated 5% dextrose in water is injected up to a pressure of 160-HD 160-1BO mm Hg. A Controller unit heats the fluid and monitors the pressure and treatment time. Destruction of the endometrium is carried out in approximately 8 minutes.

Prior to any EA techniques, endometrial sampling is required as part of the workup evaluation of the woman with abnormal bleeding. The uterine cavity should be evaluated for size and presence of pathology that may limit come of the techniques.

With the possible exception of the use of the NovaSure system, a review by Sowter has confirmed the benefit of pretreatment with danazol or a GnRH agonist before an ablation. EA is more successful when a thin endometrial lining is present. Most systems typically treat to a depth of 4 to 6 mm. In the evaluation, it is important to note that there is no thinning of the myometrium from some other cause, such as prior surgery, particularly with the microwave method. The myometrium should be no less than 10 mm anywhere in the uterus. Most methods of EA, with the exception of the Her option, may be beneficial in treating submucous fibroids up to 3 cm in size, with the strongest data coming from the use of the microwave and Thermachoice systems (see **Table 37-2**). Complications are infrequent with EA if adherence occurs to the manufacturer's guidelines. Cervical lacerations and perforations occur more commonly with endometrial resection. Lower genital tract burns may occur, as well as endometritis ($\approx$1%) and there is a syndrome of tubal pain post-EA caused by trapping of endometria at the cornual recesses. This is less likely in women with a tubal ligation. If pregnancy occurs unexpectedly, there is a high incidence of poor outcomes, including prematurity and placenta accreta.

Most EA procedures can now be safely performed in an office setting with paracervical block and conscious sedation. Although amenorrhea may not always occur (only up to 55% of the time), bleeding is significantly improved for most women. Hysterectomy is thus avoided in 86% of women. Of note, the success is slightly worse in women with a retroverted uterus.

Hysterectomy

The decision to remove the uterus should be made on an individual basis and should usually be reserved for the woman with other indications for hysterectomy, such as leiomyoma or uterine prolapse. Hysterectomy should only be used to treat persistent ovulatory DUB after all medical therapy has failed and the amount of MBL has been documented to be excessive by direct measurement or abnormally low serum ferritin levels. With increasing use of EA to treat this problem, the use of hysterectomy as therapy for ovulatory DUB should decrease. It has been estimated that as many as 50% of women older than 40 years with menorrhagia without uterine lesions have been treated by hysterectomy and that 20% of all hysterectomies in women of reproductive age are performed for excessive uterine bleeding.

As noted, several reports have cited the benefits (and, for some women, the preference) of the LNG-IUS when hysterectomy or ablation is being considered. Uterine artery embolization is not particularly effective unless fibroids are the cause of excessive bleeding. If hysterectomy is chosen, many different options are available, including vaginal hysterectomy,

Table 37-2 Characteristics and Outcomes at 1 Year for Nonresectoscopic Endometrial Ablation

Option	Maximum Uterine Size (cm)	Use with Fibroids (<3 cm)	Amenorrhea (%)	Diary Success (%)*	Satisfaction[†]
Thermachoice III (balloon)	10	Yes	37	81	96
Her option (cryotherapy)	10	—	22	67	86
Hydro ThermAblator (heated fluid)	10.5	Yes	35	68	—
Microwave EA system	14	Yes	55	87	99
NovoSure (radiofrequency)	10	Yes	36	78	93

*Score < 75 using pictorial blood loss assessment chart (% patients)
[†]Similar rate of satisfaction as with levonorgestrel IUS but both significantly better than medical therapy.

laparoscopic-assisted vaginal hysterectomy (LAVH), laparoscopic or supracervical hysterectomy, laparoscopic total hysterectomy, and abdominal supracervical hysterectomy.

SUMMARY OF APPROACHES TO TREATMENT

Having reviewed the various options, an important perspective is to approach the woman according to her acute and chronic needs or short-term and long-term therapy. Acute bleeding, which necessitates immediate cessation of bleeding, requires the use of pharmacologic doses of estrogen or curettage; the latter is used more liberally in older women with risk factors or in those who are hemodynamically compromised. This approach is not dependent on whether the woman is anovulatory or ovulatory. Although estrogen will be temporarily helpful, even if there are abnormal anatomic findings, such as fibroids, it is preferable to perform curettage if pathology is suspected.

For less significant bleeding that warrants treatment, but not necessitating the immediate cessation of blood loss, high doses of progestogen alone may be used. Although this approach is used by many clinicians, there are no good data to support this approach.

After the acute episode it is imperative to know whether the woman is bleeding from an anovulatory or ovulatory dysfunctional state. Most women fall into the anovulatory category. In the adolescent, 10 mg of MPA, 10 days each month for at least 3 months, should be prescribed and observed carefully thereafter. In this group, additional diagnostic studies should be performed to detect possible defects in the coagulation process, particularly if bleeding is severe. For the woman of reproductive age, long-term therapy depends on whether she requires contraception, induction of ovulation, or treatment of DUB alone. In the latter case, oral OCs or MPA can be administered monthly for at least 6 months, whereas OCs and clomiphene citrate are used for the other indications. For the perimenopausal woman who characteristically has fluctuating amounts of circulating estrogen, use of cyclic progestogen alone is frequently not curative. In these women, abnormal bleeding is best treated by low-dose OCs.

The most difficult type of DUB to treat is chronic treatment of ovulatory women with menorrhagia. If anatomic abnormalities are absent, long-term treatment is necessary to reduce MBL. For these women, NSAIDs, progestins, oral contraceptives, danazol, and GnRH analogues are all useful therapeutic modalities. A combination of two or more of these agents is often required to obviate the need for endometrial ablation or hysterectomy. The LNG-IUS has become one of the most successful options.

KEY POINTS

- The mean amount of menstrual blood loss in one cycle in normal women was previously reported to be approximately 35 mL but may be as much as 60 mL, with an average loss of 13 mg of iron.
- Menorrhagia occurs in 9% to 14% of healthy women, and most have a normal duration of menses.
- DUB can be caused by anovulation but also occurs in women who ovulate.
- Diagnostic tests in women with menorrhagia include measurement of hemoglobin, serum iron, serum ferritin, β-hCG, TSH, and PRL levels, endometrial biopsy and hysteroscopy, sonohysterography, or hysterosalpingography.
- High doses of oral or IV estrogen will usually stop acute bleeding episodes in most cases of abnormal bleeding.
- Anovulatory DUB can be treated by cyclic use of progestins or oral contraceptives.

- Patients with ovulatory DUB are best treated with oral contraceptives, NSAIDs (antiprostaglandins), danazol, or progestins during the luteal phase or progesterone or progestins released locally from an IUD.
- NSAIDs administered during menses reduce MBL by 20% to 50% in women with ovulatory DUB.
- D&C should be used to stop the acute bleeding episode in patients with hypovolemia or those older than 35 years. D&C only treats the acute episode of excess uterine bleeding, not subsequent episodes.
- Various endometrial ablation techniques achieve a 22% to 55% amenorrhea success rate at 1 year but an 86% to 99% satisfaction rate.
- Within 4 years after endometrial ablation, approximately 25% of women so treated will have a hysterectomy.

REFERENCES CAN BE FOUND ON
EXPERTCONSULT.com

38

Primary and Secondary Amenorrhea and Precocious Puberty
Etiology, Diagnostic Evaluation, Management

Roger A. Lobo

Amenorrhea can be physiologic, when it occurs during pregnancy and the postpartum period (particularly when nursing), or pathologic, when it is produced by a variety of endocrinologic and anatomic disorders. In the latter circumstance, the failure to menstruate is a symptom of these various pathologic conditions. Thus, amenorrhea itself is not a pathologic entity and should not be used as a final diagnosis.

Although the absence of menses causes no harm to the body, it is abnormal in a woman who is not pregnant or postpartum and thus is a source of concern. For this reason, women usually seek medical assistance when the condition occurs.

Many individuals with ambiguous external genitalia resulting from various intersex problems are raised as females and never menstruate. The cause of the intersex problem is usually determined at birth or soon thereafter. Although women with **cryptomenorrhea** caused by anatomic disorders interfering with the outflow of menses, such as an imperforate hymen or transverse vaginal septum, have the symptom of amenorrhea, they are actually menstruating. These disorders are discussed in Chapter 11 (Congenital Abnormalities of the Female Reproductive Tract), so they will not be discussed here. Severe systemic diseases such as metastatic carcinoma and chronic renal failure can also cause amenorrhea; however, because amenorrhea is not the presenting symptom of these disorders, they will not be discussed in this chapter.

Primary amenorrhea is defined as the absence of menses in a woman who has never menstruated by the age of 16.5 years. Another definition includes girls who have not menstruated within 5 years of breast development. Breast development (thelarche) should occur by age 13 or otherwise requires evaluation. The incidence of primary amenorrhea is less than 0.1%. **Secondary amenorrhea** is defined as the absence of menses for an arbitrary period, usually longer than 6 to 12 months. The incidence of secondary amenorrhea of more than 6 months' duration in a survey of a general population of Swedish women of reproductive age was found to be 0.7%. The incidence was significantly higher in women younger than 25 years and those with a prior history of menstrual irregularity.

Outside the United States, it is common to see patients who have been categorized according to the World Health Organization (WHO) classification. WHO type I usually refers to women with low estrogen levels and low follicle-stimulating hormone (FSH) and prolactin (PRL) levels without CNS lesions; type II refers to a normal estrogen status with normal FSH and PRL levels; WHO type III refers to low estrogen levels and a high FSH level, denoting ovarian failure.

DELAYED MENARCHE

Before the onset of menses, the normal female goes through a progressive series of morphologic changes produced by the pubertal increase in estrogen and androgen production. In 1969, Marshall and Tanner defined five stages of breast development and pubic hair development (**Fig. 38-1**; **Table 38-1**). These changes sometimes are combined and called Tanner, or pubertal, stages 1 through 5. The first sign of puberty is usually the appearance of breast budding followed within a few months by the appearance of pubic hair.

Thereafter, the breasts enlarge, the external pelvic contour becomes rounder, and the most rapid rate of growth occurs (peak height velocity). These changes precede menarche. Thus, breast budding is the earliest sign of puberty and menarche the latest. The mean ages of occurrence of these events in American women are shown in **Table 38-2** and the mean intervals (with standard deviation [SD]) between initiation of breast budding and other pubertal events are shown in **Table 38-3**. The mean interval between breast budding and menarche is 2.3 years, with an SD of approximately 1 year. Some individuals can progress from breast budding to menarche in 18 months, and others may take 5 years. Thus, although the arbitrary age of primary amenorrhea is 16.5 years, if a woman 14 years of age or older presents to the clinician with absence of breast budding, a diagnostic evaluation should be performed. The absence of breast development is indicative of a lack of estradiol (E_2).

The mean time of onset of menarche was previously thought to occur when a critical body weight of approximately 48 kg (106 lb) was reached. However, it is now believed that body composition is more important than total body weight in determining the time of onset of puberty and menstruation. Thus, the ratio of fat to both total body weight and lean body weight is probably the most relevant factor that determines the time of onset of puberty and menstruation. Individuals who are moderately obese, between 20% and 30% above the ideal body weight, have an earlier onset of menarche than nonobese women. Malnutrition, such as occurs with **anorexia nervosa** or starvation, is known to delay the onset of puberty.

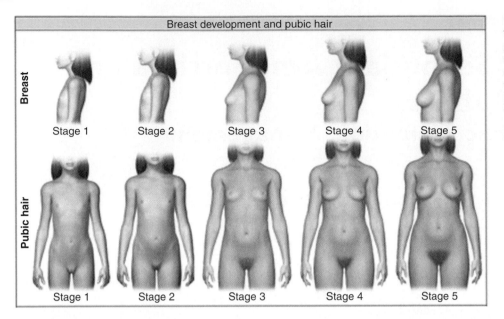

Figure 38-1 Pubertal rating according to Tanner stage. Breast development in girls is rated from 1 (prepubertal) to 5 (adult). Stage 2 breast development (appearance of the breast bud) marks the onset of gonadarche. For girls, pubic hair stages are rated from 1 (prepubertal to 5 (adult). Stage 2 marks the onset of adrenarche. (From Carel JC, Leger J. Clinical practice. Precocious puberty. N Engl J Med 358:2366, 2008.)

Table 38-1 Classification of Breast Growth and Pubic Hair Growth

Classification	Description
Breast Growth	
B1	Prepubertal: elevation of papilla only
B2	Breast budding
B3	Enlargement of breasts with glandular tissue, without separation of breast contours
B4	Secondary mound formed by areola
B5	Single contour of breast and areola
Pubic Hair Growth	
PH1	Prepubertal—no pubic hair
PH2	Labial hair present
PH3	Labial hair spreads over mons pubis
PH4	Slight lateral spread
PH5	Further lateral spread to form inverse triangle and reach medial thighs

Adapted from Roy S: Puberty. In Mishell DR Jr, Davajan V (eds): Infertility, Contraception and Reproductive Endocrinology, 4th ed. Blackwell Scientific, Malden, MA, 1997, pp 225-226.

Table 38-2 Mean Ages of Girls at the Onset of Pubertal Events (United States)

Event	Mean Age ± SD (yr)
Initiation of breast development (B2)	10.8 ± 1.10
Appearance of pubic hair (PH2)	11.0 ± 1.21
Menarche	12.9 ± 1.20

Adapted from Frisch RE, Revelle R: Height and weight in menarche and a hypothesis of menarche. Arch Dis Child 46:695, 1971.

Table 38-3 Pubertal Intervals

Interval	Mean Age ± SD (Years)
B2—peak height velocity	1.0 ± 0.77
B2—menarche	2.3 ± 1.03
B2-PH5	3.1 ± 1.04
B2-B5 (average duration of puberty)	4.5 ± 2.04

Adapted from Frisch RE, Revelle R: Height and weight in menarche and a hypothesis of menarche. Arch Dis Child 46:695, 1971.

One of the major links between body composition and the hypothalamic-pituitary-ovarian axis, and thus menstrual cyclicity, is the adipocyte hormone **leptin**. Leptin is produced by adipocytes and correlates well with body weight. Leptin is also important for feedback involving gonadotropin-releasing hormone (GnRH) and luteinizing hormone (LH) pulsatility, and also binds to specific receptor sites on the ovary and endometrium. Body weight and body fat content have been shown to be important for menstruation; a fatness nomogram is depicted in **Figure 38-2**. Well-nourished individuals with prepubertal strenuous exercise programs resulting in less total body fat have also been shown to have a delayed onset of puberty. Warren and colleagues have reported that ballet dancers, swimmers, and runners have menarche delayed to approximately age 15 years if they began exercising strenuously before menarche (**Fig. 38-3**). They also determined that stress is not the cause of the **delayed menarche** in these exercising girls, because girls of the same age with stressful musical careers did not have a delayed onset of menarche. Young women

with strenuous exercise programs have sufficient estrogen to produce some breast development and thus do not need extensive endocrinologic evaluation if concern arises about the lack of onset of menses. Frisch and coworkers have reported that for girls engaged in premenarchal athletic training, menarche is delayed 0.4 year for each year of training. Individuals who exercise strenuously should be counseled that they will usually have a delayed onset of menses, but it is not a health problem. They should be told that they will most likely have regular ovulatory cycles when they stop exercising or become older.

The metabolic features of amenorrheic athletes, who are considered to be in a state of negative energy balance, are fairly characteristic. These include elevated serum FSH, insulin-like growth factor-binding protein 1 (IGFBP-1), and lowered insulin insulin-like growth factor (IGF) levels.

Stress per se can lead to inhibition of the GnRH axis. This may be the key factor influencing amenorrhea in competitive athletes. The mechanism involves an increased secretion of

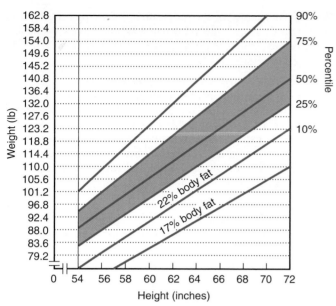

Figure 38-2 Fatness index nomogram. (Adapted from Frisch RE, Revelle R: Height and weight in menarche and a hypothesis of menarche. Arch Dis Child 46:695, 1971.)

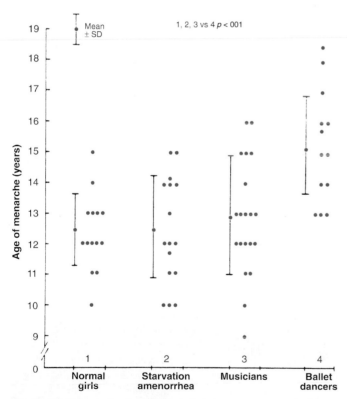

Figure 38-3 Ages of menarche in ballet dancers compared with those of three other groups. (From Warren MP: The effects of exercise on pubertal progression and reproductive function in girls. J Clin Endocrinol Metab 51:1150, 1980.)

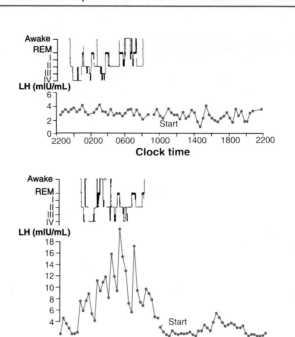

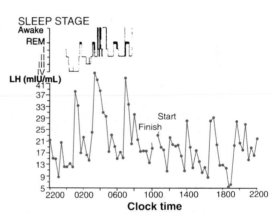

Figure 38-4 Plasma luteinizing hormone (LH) concentration measured every 20 minutes for 24 hours in normal prepubertal girl *(upper panel)*, early pubertal girl *(center panel)*, and normal late pubertal girl *(lower panel)*. In top and center panels, sleep histogram is shown above period of nocturnal sleep. Sleep stages are awake, rapid eye movement (REM), and stages I to IV by depth of line graph. Plasma LH concentrations are expressed as mIU/mL. (Adapted from Boyar RM, Katz J, Finkelstein JW, et al: Anorexia nervosa: Immaturity of the 24-hour luteinizing hormone secretory pattern. N Engl J Med 291:861, 1974.)

corticotropin-releasing hormone (CRH), releasing adrenocorticotropic hormone (ACTH) and cortisol. CRH itself is known to inhibit GnRH.

Before puberty, circulating levels of LH and FSH are low (FSH/LH ratio > 1) because the central nervous system (CNS)–hypothalamic axis is extremely sensitive to the negative feedback effects of low levels of circulating estrogen. As the critical weight or body composition is approached, the CNS–hypothalamic axis becomes less sensitive to the negative effect of estrogen and GnRH is secreted in greater amounts, causing an increase in LH and, to a lesser extent, FSH levels. The initial endocrinologic change associated with the onset of puberty is the occurrence of episodic pulses of LH occurring during sleep (**Fig. 38-4**). These pulses are absent before the onset of puberty. After menarche, the episodic secretions of LH occur during sleep and while awake. The last endocrinologic event of puberty is activation of the positive gonadotropin response to increasing levels of E_2, which results in the midcycle gonadotropic surge and ovulation.

PRIMARY AMENORRHEA

It is important that the clinician understand the sequential endocrinologic and morphologic chronologic changes taking place during normal puberty so as to make the differential diagnosis between delayed menarche and primary amenorrhea. Although the former condition requires only reassurance, the latter requires an endocrinologic evaluation.

CAUSES

Although numerous classifications have been used for the various causes of primary amenorrhea, it has been found most clinically useful to group them on the basis of whether secondary sexual characteristics (breasts) and female internal genitalia (uterus) are present or absent (**Box 38-1**). Thus, the findings on a physical examination can alert the clinician to possible causes and indicate which laboratory tests should be performed. In a series of 62 individuals reported by Maschchak and colleagues, the largest subgroup with primary amenorrhea (29) were those in whom breasts were absent but who had a uterus; the second largest subgroup (22) had both breasts and uterus; lack of a uterus together with breast development accounted for the third largest category (9); and those without breasts or a uterus were the least common

---

> **Box 38-1** Classification of Disorders with Primary Amenorrhea and Normal Female External Genitalia
>
> I. Absent breast development; uterus present
>   A. Gonadal failure
>   1. 45,X (Turner's syndrome)
>   2. 46,X, abnormal X (e.g., short- or long-arm deletion)
>   3. Mosaicism (e.g., X/XX, X/XX,XXX)
>   4. 46,XX or 46,XY pure gonadal dysgenesis
>   5. 17α-hydroxylase deficiency with 46,XX
>   B. Hypothalamic failure secondary to inadequate GnRH release
>   1. Insufficient GnRH secretion because of neurotransmitter defect
>   2. Inadequate GnRH synthesis (Kallman's syndrome)
>   3. Congenital anatomic defect in central nervous system
>   4. CNS neoplasm (craniopharyngioma)
>   C. Pituitary failure
>   1. Isolated gonadotrophin insufficiency (thalassemia major, retinitis pigmentosa)
>   2. Pituitary neoplasia (chromophobe adenoma)
>   3. Mumps, encephalitis
>   4. Newborn kernicterus
>   5. Prepubertal hypothyroidism
> II. Breast development; uterus absent
>   A. Androgen resistance (testicular feminization)
>   B. Congenital absence of uterus (uterovaginal agenesis)
> III. Absent breast development; uterus absent
>   A. 17,20-desmolase deficiency
>   B. Agonadism
>   C. 17α-hydroxylase deficiency with 46,XY karyotype
> IV. Breast development; uterus present
>   A. Hypothalamic cause
>   B. Pituitary cause
>   C. Ovarian cause
>   D. Uterine cause

CNS, Central nervous system; GnRH, gonadotropin-releasing hormone.

---

(2). This breakdown of the various accompanying conditions of primary amenorrhea reflects the referral pattern to the center and not necessarily the true incidence of each category.

Breasts Absent and Uterus Present

All individuals with no breast development and a uterus present have no ovarian estrogen production as a result of a gonadal disorder or a CNS hypothalamic-pituitary abnormality. The phenotype of individuals with either of these causes of low estrogen synthesis is similar. However, because the cause of the disorder and the prognosis for fertility differ, it is important to establish the specific diagnosis.

Gonadal Failure (Hypergonadotropic Hypogonadism)

Failure of gonadal development is the most common cause of primary amenorrhea, occurring in almost 50% of those with this symptom. **Gonadal failure** is most frequently caused by a chromosomal disorder or deletion of all or part of an X chromosome, but it is sometimes caused by a genetic defect and, rarely, 17α-hydroxylase deficiencies. The chromosomal disorders are usually caused by a random meiotic or mitotic abnormality (e.g., nondisjunction, anaphase lag) and thus are not inherited. However, if gonadal development is absent in the presence of a 46,XX or 46,XY karyotype (called **pure gonadal dysgenesis**), a gene disorder may be present, because it has been reported to occur in siblings. Reindollar and coworkers, in the largest single series of patients with primary amenorrhea, have reported that all individuals with gonadal failure and an X chromosome abnormality were shorter than 63 inches in height. Approximately one third also had major cardiovascular or renal anomalies.

Deletion of the entire X chromosome (as occurs in Turner's syndrome) or of the short arm (p) of the X chromosome results in short stature. Deletions of only the long arm (q) usually do not affect height. In place of the ovary a band of fibrous tissue called a **gonadal streak** is present (**Fig. 38-5**). Streaks are also present in individuals without gonads (pure gonadal dysgenesis). When ovarian follicles are absent, synthesis of ovarian steroids and inhibin does not occur. Breast development does not occur because of the very low circulating E_2 levels. Because the negative hypothalamic-pituitary action of estrogen and inhibin is not present, gonadotropin levels are markedly elevated, with FSH levels

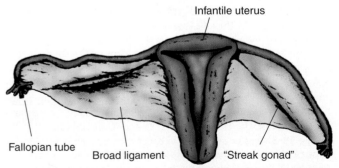

Figure 38-5 Internal genitalia of patient with gonadal dysgenesis (Turner's syndrome), featuring normal but infantile uterus, normal fallopian tubes, and pale, glistening streak gonads in both broad ligaments. (From Federman DD: Disorders of gonadal development: Gonadal dysgenesis [Turner syndrome]. In Federman DD [ed]: Abnormal Sexual Development: A Genetic and Endocrine Approach to Differential Diagnosis. Philadelphia, WB Saunders, 1967.)

being higher than LH. Estrogen is not necessary for müllerian duct development or wolffian duct regression, so the internal and external genitalia are phenotypically normal female.

An occasional individual with mosaicism, an abnormal X, pure gonadal dysgenesis (46,XX), or even Turner's syndrome may have a few follicles that develop under endogenous gonadotropin stimulation early in puberty and may synthesize enough estrogen to induce breast development and a few episodes of uterine bleeding, resulting early in **premature ovarian failure**; usually before age 25. Rarely, ovulation and pregnancy can occur.

Goldenberg and associates have reported that all individuals with primary amenorrhea and plasma FSH levels higher than 40 mIU/mL have no functioning ovarian follicles in the gonadal tissue. Thus, in women with primary amenorrhea, the diagnosis of gonadal failure can be established if the FSH levels are consistently elevated, without requiring ovarian tissue evaluation.

45,X Anomalies

Turner's syndrome occurs in approximately 1 per 2000 to 3000 live births but is much more frequent in abortuses. In addition to primary amenorrhea and absent breast development, these individuals have other somatic abnormalities, the most prevalent being short stature (<60 inches in height), webbing of the neck, a short fourth metacarpal, and cubitus valgus. Cardiac abnormality, renal abnormalities, and hypothyroidism are also more prevalent. The diagnosis is usually made before puberty (see Chapter 2, Reproductive Genetics).

A wide variety of chromosomal mosaics are associated with primary amenorrhea and normal female external genitalia, the most common being X/XX. In addition, individuals with X/XXX and X/XX/XXX mosaicism have primary amenorrhea. These individuals are generally taller and have fewer anatomic abnormalities than individuals with a 45,X karyotype. In addition, some of them may have a few gonadal follicles and approximately 20% have sufficient estrogen production to menstruate. Occasionally, ovulation may occur, as stated earlier. Isolated phenotypic features of Turner's syndrome may also occur in males and is known as Noonan's syndrome.

Structurally Abnormal X Chromosome

Although individuals with this disorder have a 46,XX karyotype, part of one X chromosome is structurally abnormal. If there is deletion of the long arm of the X chromosome (Xq), normal height has been reported to occur but, in Reindollar's series, these individuals were all relatively short. They have no somatic abnormalities. However, if there is deletion of the short arm of the X chromosome (Xp), the individual phenotypically resembles those with a 45,X karyotype (Turner's syndrome). A similar phenotype occurs in those with isochrome of the long arm of the X chromosome. Other X chromosome abnormalities include a ring X and minute fragmentation of the X chromosome.

Pure Gonadal Dysgenesis (46,XX and 46,XY with Gonadal Streaks; Gonadal Agenesis)

As noted, this abnormality is a genetic disorder and has been reported in siblings. Abnormalities in genes involved in gonadal development are expected to be involved. These individuals have normal stature and phenotype, absence of secondary sexual characteristics, and primary amenorrhea. Some of them have a few ovarian follicles, develop breasts, and may even menstruate

spontaneously for a few years. If a Y chromosome is present, with or without any clinical signs of androgenization, gonadectomy should be performed (see later).

17α-Hydroxylase Deficiency with 46,XX Karyotype

A rare gonadal cause of primary amenorrhea without breast development and normal female internal genitalia is deficiency of the enzyme 17α-hydroxylase (P450 C 17) in an individual with a 46,XX karyotype (it can also occur in genetic males 46,XY) who may present in a similar fashion. Only a few such individuals have been described in the literature, but it is important for the clinician to be aware of this entity because, in contrast to those described earlier, these individuals have hypernatremia and hypokalemia. Because of decreased cortisol, ACTH levels are elevated. The mineralocorticoid levels are also elevated, because 17α-hydroxylase is not necessary for the conversion of progesterone to deoxycortisol or corticosterone. Thus, there is excessive sodium retention and potassium excretion, leading to hypertension and hypokalemia. Serum progesterone levels are also elevated because progesterone is not converted to cortisol. In addition to sex steroid replacement, these individuals need cortisol administration. They usually have cystic ovaries and viable oocytes. Pregnancies have been documented following in vitro fertilization–embryo transfer (IVF-ET), despite low levels of endogenous sex steroids.

Genetic Disorders with Hyperandrogenism

Hyperandrogenism occurs in approximately 10% of women with gonadal dysgenesis. Most have a Y chromosome or fragment of a Y chromosome, but some may only have a DNA fragment that contains the testes-determining gene (probably *SRY*) without a full Y chromosome. Those with hypergonadotropic hypogonadism and a female phenotype who have any clinical manifestation of hyperandrogenism, such as hirsutism, should have a gonadectomy, even if a Y chromosome is not present, because gonadal neoplasms are frequent.

Central Nervous System–Hypothalamic–Pituitary Disorders

With CNS-hypothalamic-pituitary disorders, the low estrogen levels are caused by very low gonadotropin release. The cause of low gonadotropin production can be morphologic or endocrinologic.

Lesions

Any anatomic lesion of the hypothalamus or pituitary can be a cause of low gonadotropin production. These lesions can be congenital (e.g., stenosis of aqueduct, absence of sellar floor) or acquired (tumors). Many of these lesions, particularly pituitary adenomas, result in elevated prolactin levels (see Chapter 39, Hyperprolactinemia, Galactorrhea, and Pituitary Adenomas).

However, non–prolactin-secreting pituitary tumors (**chromophobe adenomas**), as well as craniopharyngiomas, may not be associated with hyperprolactinemia and can rarely be the cause of primary amenorrhea with low gonadotropin levels. Thus, all individuals with primary amenorrhea and low gonadotropin levels, with or without an elevated prolactin level, should have computed tomography (CT) scanning or magnetic resonance imaging (MRI) of the hypothalamic-pituitary region to rule out the presence of a lesion.

Inadequate Gonadotropin-Releasing Hormone Release (Hypogonadotropic Hypogonadism)

Those without a demonstrable lesion and a low gonadotropin level were previously thought to have primary pituitary failure (**hypogonadotropic hypogonadism**). However, when they are stimulated with GnRH, there is an increase in FSH and LH levels, indicating that the basic defect is either hypothalamic with insufficient GnRH synthesis or a CNS neurotransmitter defect, resulting in inadequate GnRH synthesis or release, or both. Although a single bolus of GnRH may not initially cause a rise in gonadotropin level in these individuals, after 4 days of GnRH administration they will have a rise in gonadotropin level after a single GnRH bolus. Because GnRH secretion occurs after migration of these specific cells from the olfactory lobe to the hypothesis during embryogenesis, anosmia may also occur in some patients with gonadotropin deficiency. This is caused by a specific defect of the *KAL* gene (Xp 22-3), which is responsible for neuronal migration. Other genetic defects resulting in gonadotropic deficiency may occur on the X chromosome or autosomes. Females with Kallman's syndrome and related forms of gonadotropic deficiency have normal height and an increase in growth of long bones, resulting in a greater wing span-to-height ratio. Men affected by gonadotropic deficiency have hypogonadism, an increased wing span-to-height ratio, and altered spatial orientation abilities. Anosmia in Kallman's syndrome needs to be tested for by blinded testing of certain characteristic smells, such as coffee, cocoa, or orange.

Isolated Gonadotropin Deficiency (Pituitary Disease)

Rarely, individuals with primary amenorrhea and low gonadotropin levels do not respond to GnRH, even after 4 days of administration. This is known as **isolated gonadotropin deficiency**. They almost always have an associated disorder such as thalassemia major (with iron deposits in the pituitary) or retinitis pigmentosa. Occasionally, this pituitary abnormality has been associated with prepubertal hypothyroidism, kernicterus, or mumps encephalitis.

Breast Development Present and Uterus Absent

Two disorders present with primary amenorrhea are associated with normal breast development and an absence of a uterus, androgen resistance and congenital absence of the uterus. The former is a genetically inherited disorder, whereas the latter is an accident of development and does not have an established pattern of inheritance.

Androgen Resistance

Androgen resistance syndrome, originally termed ***testicular feminization***, is a genetically transmitted disorder in which androgen receptor synthesis or action does not occur. It is rare, with an incidence of 1/60,000. The syndrome is caused by the absence of an X-chromosome gene responsible for the cytoplasmic or nuclear testosterone receptor function. It is an X-linked recessive or sex-linked autosomal dominant disorder, with transmission through the mother. These individuals have an XY karyotype and normally functioning male gonads that produce normal male levels of testosterone and dihydrotestosterone. However, because of a lack of receptors in target organs, there is lack of male differentiation of the external and internal genitalia. The external genitalia remain feminine, as occurs in the absence of sex steroids. Wolffian duct development, which normally occurs

as a result of testosterone stimulation, fails to take place. Because müllerian duct regression is induced by antimüllerian hormone (AMH), also called müllerian-inhibiting substance (MIS, a glycoprotein synthesized by the Sertoli cells of the fetal testes), this process occurs normally in these individuals because steroid receptors are unnecessary for the action of glycoproteins. Thus, people with this condition have no female or male internal genitalia, normal female external genitalia, and a short or absent vagina. Pubic and axillary hair is absent or scanty as a result of a lack of androgenic receptors, but breast development is normal or enhanced. It is known that testosterone is responsible for inhibiting breast proliferation. Thus, in androgen resistance, the absence of androgen action allows even low levels of estrogen to cause unabated breast stimulation. Estrogen levels here are in the normal male range.

Testes that are intra-abdominal or that occur in the inguinal canal have an increased risk of developing a malignancy (gonadoblastoma or dysgerminoma), with an incidence reported to be approximately 20%. However, these malignancies rarely occur before age 20. Therefore, it is usually recommended that the gonads be left in place until after puberty is completed to allow full breast development and epiphyseal closure to occur. After these events occur, which is typically around age 18, the gonads should be removed. It is recommended that those with androgen resistance be informed that they have an abnormal sex chromosome, without specifically mentioning a Y chromosome, because it is widely known that an XY karyotype indicates maleness. Currently, however, some families choose to have full disclosure and a complete understanding of the abnormality. In addition, because psychologically and phenotypically these individuals are female and have been raised as such, the term *gonads* should be used instead of testes. These individuals should also be informed that they can never become pregnant because they do not have a uterus and that their gonads (not testes) need to be removed after age 18 because of their high potential for malignancy.

Congenital Absence of the Uterus (Uterine Agenesis, Uterovaginal Agenesis, Rokitansky-Küster-Hauser Syndrome)

The *Hox* genes are important for uterine development, and mutations (e.g., in Hox-A13) have been found in genetic syndromes with uterine abnormalities (e.g., hand-foot-genital and Guttmacher syndromes) and also in cases of bicornuate uterus. To date, however, no abnormalities have been found in cases of congenital absence of the uterus.

This disorder is the second most frequent cause of primary amenorrhea. It occurs in 1 in 4000 to 5000 female births and accounts for approximately 15% of individuals with primary amenorrhea. Individuals with complete uterine agenesis have normal ovaries, with regular cyclic ovulation and normal endocrine function. Women with this disorder have normal breast and pubic and axillary hair development but have a shortened or absent vagina, in addition to absence of the uterus (**Fig. 38-6**). Congenital renal abnormalities occur in approximately one third of these individuals and skeletal abnormalities in approximately 12%. Cardiac and other congenital abnormalities also occur with increased frequency. Occasional defects in the bones of the middle ear can also occur, resulting in some degree of deafness. The overwhelming majority of these disorders are caused by an isolated developmental defect, but on occasion the condition is genetically inherited. It is usually easy to

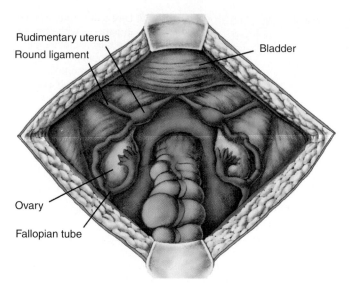

Figure 38-6 Congenital absence of vagina. Laparotomy revealed rudimentary uterus that showed evidence of failure of fusion of müllerian ducts. This is a common finding in this condition and indicates that disorder is more extensive than simple anomaly of vagina. (Adapted from Jones HW Jr, Scott WW [eds]: Hermaphroditism, Genital Anomalies and Related Endocrine Disorders, 2nd ed. Baltimore, Williams & Wilkins, 1971.)

Labels on figure: Rudimentary uterus; Round ligament; Bladder; Ovary; Fallopian tube

differentiate these individuals from those with androgen resistance by the presence of normal pubic hair, but some with incomplete androgen resistance have some pubic hair. Because women with congenital absence of the uterus are endocrinologically normal females, and those with androgen resistance are endocrinologically male, with male testosterone levels and an XY karyotype, the differential diagnosis is easily made.

Absent Breast and Uterine Development

Individuals with no breast or uterine development are rare. They usually have a male karyotype, elevated gonadotropin levels, and testosterone levels in the normal or below-normal female range. The differential diagnosis for this phenotype includes 17α-hydroxylase deficiency, 17,20-desmolase deficiency, and agonadism. Individuals with the first disorder have testes present but lack the enzyme necessary to synthesize sex steroids, and thus have female external genitalia. Because they have testes, AMH-MIS is produced and the female internal genitalia regress; with low testosterone levels, the male internal genitalia do not develop. Insufficient estrogen is synthesized to develop breasts. A similar lack of sex steroid synthesis occurs in males with a 17,20-desmolase deficiency. Individuals with agonadism, sometimes called the vanishing testes syndrome, have no gonads present, but because the female internal genitalia are also absent, it has been postulated that testicular AMH-MIS production occurred during fetal life but the gonadal tissue subsequently regressed.

Secondary Sex Characteristics and Female Internal Genitalia Present

This is the second largest category of individuals with primary amenorrhea, accounting for approximately one third of them. In the series reported by Maschchak and colleagues, approximately 25% of these individuals had hyperprolactinemia and

prolactinomas. The remaining women had profiles similar to those with secondary amenorrhea and thus should be subcategorized and treated similarly as women with secondary amenorrhea. Secondary amenorrhea is discussed later.

DIFFERENTIAL DIAGNOSIS AND MANAGEMENT

After a history is obtained and a physical examination performed, including measurement of height, span, and weight, those with primary amenorrhea can be grouped into one of the four general categories listed in **Box 38-1**, depending on the presence or absence of breasts and a uterus. If breasts are absent but a uterus is present, the diagnostic evaluation should differentiate between CNS-hypothalamic-pituitary disorders and failure of normal gonadal development. Although individuals with both these disorders have similar phenotypes because of low E$_2$ levels, a single serum FSH assay can differentiate between these two major diagnostic categories (**Fig. 38-7**). Women with hypergonadotropic hypogonadism (FSH > 30 mIU/mL), not those with hypogonadotropic hypogonadism, should have a peripheral white blood cell karyotype obtained to determine whether a Y chromosome is present. If a Y chromosome is present, the streak gonads should be excised, because the incidence of subsequent malignancy, mainly gonadoblastomas, is relatively high. If a Y chromosome is absent, it is unnecessary to remove the gonads unless there are signs of hyperandrogenism. It is also unnecessary to perform a karyotype on the gonadal tissue to detect possible mosaicism with a Y chromosome in the gonad unless there is some evidence of hyperandrogenism.

All women with an elevated FSH level and an XX karyotype should have electrolyte and serum progesterone levels measured to rule out 17α-hydroxylase deficiency. In addition to hypernatremia and hypokalemia, individuals with 17α-hydroxylase deficiency have an elevated serum progesterone level (>3 ng/mL), a low 17α-hydroxyprogesterone level (<0.2 ng/mL), and an elevated serum deoxycorticosterone level (>17 ng/100 mL), and usually have hypertension. Doses of conjugated equine estrogen (CEE) in the range of 0.625 mg or its equivalent are usually sufficient to cause breast proliferation. Those rare individuals with 17α-hydroxylase deficiency need to have adequate cortisol replacement in addition to sex steroid treatment.

Women with ovarian failure or hypergonadotropic hypogonadism who wish to become pregnant may undergo egg donation. As long as the uterus is normal, which is usually the case, high pregnancy rates above 50% per cycle may be expected.

If the FSH level is low, the underlying disorder is in the CNS-hypothalamic-pituitary region, and the serum PRL level should be determined. Even if the PRL level is not elevated, all women with hypogonadotropic hypogonadism should have a head CT scan or MRI to rule out a lesion. It is unnecessary to perform a karyotype, because all those with hypogonadotropic hypogonadism are expected to be 46,XX. The use of GnRH testing is optional but is usually clinically unnecessary unless GnRH is going to be used for ovulation induction. Ovulation can be induced in women with this disorder because their ovaries are normal. Initially, they should receive estrogen-progestogen treatment to induce breast development and cause epiphyseal closure. When fertility is desired, human menopausal gonadotropins or pulsatile GnRH should be administered. Clomiphene citrate will be ineffective because of low endogenous E$_2$ levels.

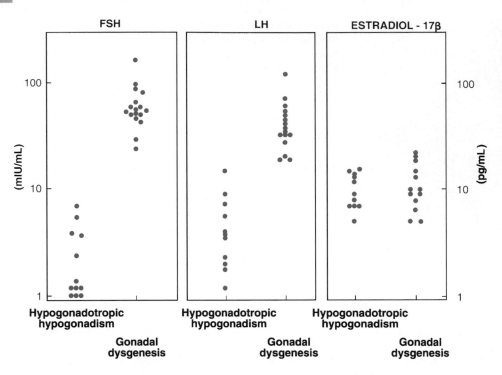

Figure 38-7 Levels of serum FSH, LH, and estradiol in patients with primary amenorrhea who have an intact uterus and no breast development. FSH, Follicle-stimulating hormone; LH, luteinizing hormone. (From Mashchak CA, Kletzky OA, Davajan V, et al: Clinical and laboratory evaluation of patients with primary amenorrhea. Obstet Gynecol 57:715, 1981.)

The differential diagnosis of androgen resistance from uterine agenesis can easily be made by the presence in the latter condition of normal body hair, ovulatory and premenstrual-type symptoms, biphasic basal temperature, and normal female testosterone level. Because women with uterine agenesis have normal female endocrine function, they do not need hormone therapy. A renal scan should be performed because of the high incidence of renal abnormalities. They may need surgical reconstruction of an absent vagina (McIndoe procedure), but progressive mechanical dilation with plastic dilators, as described by Frank, should be tried first, and is usually successful in motivated individuals. These women can now have their own genetic children. After ovarian stimulation and follicle aspiration, fertilized oocytes can be placed in the uterus of a surrogate recipient.

Individuals with androgen resistance have an XY karyotype and male levels of testosterone. After full breast development is attained and epiphyseal closure occurs, the gonads should be removed because of their malignant potential. Thereafter, estrogen replacement therapy should be administered. They do not need progestogen therapy in the absence of a uterus and lower doses of estrogen are sufficient (see Chapter 14, Menopause). The rare individuals without breast development and no internal genitalia should be referred to an endocrine center for the extensive evaluation necessary to establish the diagnosis. If gonads are present, they should be removed, because a Y chromosome is present. Hormone therapy should be administered to these individuals.

SECONDARY AMENORRHEA

CAUSES

The symptom of amenorrhea associated with hyperprolactinemia or excessive androgen or cortisol production will not be considered in this chapter because these disorders are discussed in

Chapters 39 (Hyperprolactinemia, Galactorrhea, and Pituitary Adenomas) and Chapter 40 (Hyperandrogenism). If amenorrhea is present without galactorrhea, hyperprolactinemia, or hirsutism, the symptom can result from disorders in the CNS-hypothalamic-pituitary axis, ovary, or uterus. In a review of 262 patients presenting with secondary amenorrhea during a 20-year period at a tertiary medical center, Reindollar and coworkers reported that 12% of cases resulted from a primary ovarian problem, 62% from a hypothalamic disorder, 16% from a pituitary problem (including prolactinomas), and 7% from a uterine disorder. The uterine cause of secondary amenorrhea is the only one in which normal endocrine function is present and will be discussed first.

Uterine Cause

Intrauterine adhesions (IUAs) **or synechiae** (Asherman's syndrome) can obliterate the endometrial cavity and produce secondary amenorrhea. Rarely, a missed abortion or endometrial tuberculosis can also cause endometrial destruction. The most frequent antecedent factor of IUAs is endometrial curettage associated with pregnancy—either evacuation of a live or dead fetus by mechanical means or postpartum or postabortal curettage. Curettage for a missed abortion results in a high incidence of IUA formation (30%). IUAs may also occur after diagnostic dilation and curettage (D&C) in a nonpregnant woman, so this procedure should be performed only when indicated and not routinely at the time of other surgical procedures (e.g., diagnostic laparoscopy). A less common cause of IUA is severe endometritis or fibrosis following a myomectomy, metroplasty, or cesarean delivery. This cause of amenorrhea should be considered most likely if a temporal relationship exists between the onset of symptoms and uterine curettage. The likelihood of the diagnosis is strengthened if sound cannot be passed into the uterine cavity.

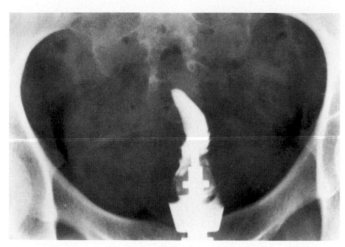

Figure 38-8 X-ray of patient with Asherman's syndrome. Patient (33 years, gravida 3, para 0, abortus 3) had been amenorrheic for 6 months after D&C for most recent therapeutic abortion (TAB). Filling of endocervical canal and nonvisualization of endometrial cavity are consistent with complete obliteration of cavity by adhesions or with obstruction at internal os level by adhesions in lower endometrial cavity. This appearance may also be seen with advanced endometrial tuberculosis. (From Richmond JA: Hysterosalpingography. In Mishell DR Jr, Davajan V [eds]: Infertility, Contraception and Reproductive Endocrinology, 4th ed. Malden, MA, Blackwell Scientific Publications, 1997.)

Confirmation of the diagnosis is usually made by hysterography (**Fig. 38-8**) or hysteroscopy. Although it has been suggested that sequential administration of estrogen-progestogen be used as the initial diagnostic procedure when IUA is suspected, withdrawal bleeding occurs following administration of the steroids in most women with IUA. Because of the lack of specificity of this test, steroid administration should not be performed prior to indirect or direct visualization of the uterine cavity.

Central Nervous System and Hypothalamic Causes

Lesions

The same anatomic lesions in the brain stem or hypothalamus that can produce primary amenorrhea by interfering with GnRH release can also cause secondary amenorrhea. Hypothalamic lesions include craniopharyngiomas, granulomatous disease (e.g., tuberculosis, sarcoidosis), and sequelae of encephalitis. When such uncommon lesions are present, circulating gonadotropin and E_2 levels are low, and withdrawal uterine bleeding will not occur after progestogen administration.

Drugs

Phenothiazine derivatives, certain antihypertensive agents, and other drugs listed in Chapter 39 (Hyperprolactinemia, Galactorrhea, and Pituitary Adenomas) can also produce amenorrhea without hyperprolactinemia, although usually the PRL level is elevated. Therefore, every individual with secondary amenorrhea should have a detailed medication history obtained, even if galactorrhea is not present. Oral contraceptive steroids inhibit ovulation by acting on the hypothalamus to suppress GnRH and directly on the pituitary to suppress FSH and LH. Occasionally, this hypothalamic-pituitary suppression persists for several months after oral contraceptives are discontinued, producing the syndrome termed *postpill amenorrhea*. This oral contraceptive-induced suppression should not last longer than 6 months. It has been reported that the incidence of amenorrhea persisting more than 6 months after discontinuation of oral contraceptives (0.8%) is approximately the same as the incidence of secondary amenorrhea in the general population (0.7%). Thus, the reason for amenorrhea persisting more than 6 months after discontinuation of oral contraceptives is probably unrelated to their use, except that the regular withdrawal bleeding produced by oral contraceptives masks the development of this symptom.

Stress and Exercise

Stressful situations, including a sudden change in environment (e.g., going away to school), death in the family, or divorce, can produce amenorrhea. A high percentage of women who had been placed in concentration camps or those sentenced for execution also became amenorrheic as a result of stress.

It is also now believed that the amenorrhea associated with strenuous exercise is also related to stress. Feicht and coworkers have reported that the incidence of secondary amenorrhea in runners has a positive correlation with the number of miles run per week (**Fig. 38-9**). In a comparison of amenorrheic and eumenorrheic athletes, they reported that physical parameters such as age, weight, lean body mass, and body fat were similar. The only significant difference between the two groups was the fact that the amenorrheic athletes ran more miles weekly. McArthur and associates have also reported there is no significant difference in the percentage of body fat in amenorrheic runners compared with runners who were menstruating. In a longitudinal study of competitive swimmers, it has been suggested that a stress-induced inhibition of the GnRH axis is characterized by higher levels of catechol estrogens and opioid peptides (particularly β-endorphin [β-EP]). Although Adashi and colleagues have shown that catechol estrogen infusion can suppress the release of GnRH and LH, and Reid and associates and others have demonstrated the inhibition of LH by β-EP, their levels are difficult and unreliable to measure in a clinical setting.

It is probable that emotionally stressful situations such as divorce or a sudden change in environment can also cause alterations in brain chemistry. When the stressful situation abates, whether emotional in origin or related to strenuous exercise, normal cyclic ovarian function and regular menses usually resume in a few months.

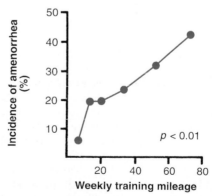

Figure 38-9 Correlation between training mileage and amenorrhea. Each point represents an average of 21 respondents. Statistical significance of relationship was obtained from point-biserial correlation (1 mile [1.6 km]). (From Feicht CB, Johnson TS, Martin BJ: Secondary amenorrhoea in athletes. Lancet 2:1145, 1978.)

Weight Loss

Both male and female animals who are malnourished have decreased reproductive capacity. Weight loss is also associated with amenorrhea in women and has been classified into two groups, the moderately underweight group includes individuals whose weight is 15% to 25% below ideal body weight and severely underweight women, whose weight loss is more than 25% of ideal body weight. Weight loss can occur from excessive dietary restrictions as well as malnutrition. Vigersky and colleagues have demonstrated that women with amenorrhea associated with simple weight loss have direct and indirect evidence of **hypothalamic dysfunction**, but pituitary and end-organ function is normal. Mason and Sagle have shown that in contrast to women with normal cycles, a group of women with weight loss amenorrhea had similar mean levels of LH as well as LH pulse amplitude, but decreased frequency of LH pulses. Thus, the amenorrhea associated with weight loss appears to be caused mainly by failure of normal GnRH release, with the lack of a pituitary response under extreme conditions. Hypoleptinemia as well as GH and thyroid dysfunction contribute to these findings.

A severe psychiatric disorder called anorexia nervosa is also associated with severe weight loss and amenorrhea. This condition is covered in Chapter 9, Emotional Aspects of Gynecology.

Polycystic Ovary Syndrome

Polycystic ovary syndrome (PCOS) is a heterogenous disorder that may present with prolonged periods of amenorrhea, although the more typical menstrual pattern is one of irregularity or oligomenorrhea. Women need not be overweight or obese, or have symptoms and signs of hyperandrogenism, which typically occurs. Although most women will have an elevated serum LH level, this level may be normal and measurement of LH is not required as a diagnostic criterion. Nevertheless, the diagnosis of PCOS may be confirmed by visualizing polycystic ovaries on ultrasound, particularly in the absence of classic findings such as hyperandrogenism. According to the European Society of Human Reproduction and Embryology–American Society for Reproductive Medicine (ESHRE-ASRM) criteria for the diagnosis of PCOS, women may be diagnosed as having PCOS with only the menstrual disturbance (in this case amenorrhea) and polycystic ovaries seen with ultrasound. This subject is discussed in detail in Chapter 40 (Hyperandrogenism).

Functional Hypothalamic Amenorrhea

There is a group of individuals with secondary amenorrhea who do not ingest drugs, do not engage in strenuous exercise, are not undergoing environmental stress, and have not lost weight. No pituitary, ovarian, or uterine abnormalities are present in these individuals. The general term ***functional hypothalamic amenorrhea*** (FHA) has been used to characterize this disorder. During normal ovulatory cycles, LH is secreted in a pulsatile manner that varies in frequency and amplitude at different times of the cycle, being more rapid in the follicular phase than in the luteal phase (**Fig. 38-10**). Women with amenorrhea caused by hypothalamic dysfunction do not exhibit these characteristic cyclic alterations in LH pulsatility. They have no pulses (**Fig. 38-11**) or have a persistent pattern of pulsatility that is normally found in only one portion of the ovulatory cycle, usually the slow frequency normally found in the luteal phase, despite having a steroid milieu similar to that in the follicular phase (**Fig. 38-12**). Because each LH pulse represents a response to a pulse of GnRH,

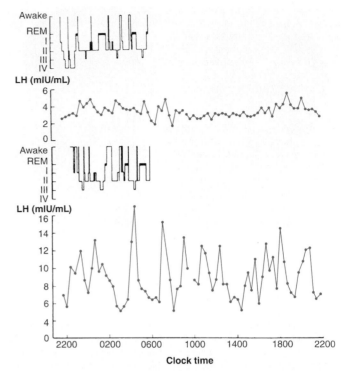

Figure 38-10 Plasma LH concentrations every 20 minutes for 24 hours during acute exacerbation of anorexia nervosa *(upper panel)* and after clinical remission with return of body weight to normal *(lower panel)*. (From Boyar RM, Katz J, Finkelstein JW, et al: Anorexia nervosa: Immaturity of the 24-hour luteinizing hormone secretory pattern. N Engl J Med 291:861, 1974.)

it appears that those with FHA have an abnormality in the normal cyclic variations of GnRH pulsatility, probably because of an abnormality in the CNS neurotransmitters and possibly produced by increased opioid activity. As reported by Ferin and colleagues, Quigley and coworkers, and Wildt and Leyendecker, administration of the opioid antagonists naloxone and naltrexone to women with FHA is followed by an increase in frequency of LH pulses, as well as by induction of ovulation.

Berga and associates have measured several pituitary hormones at frequent intervals in a 24-hour period in 10 women with FHA and 10 women with normal cycles. As also reported by others, they found a 53% reduction in LH pulse frequency among the women with FHA; however, the LH pulse amplitude was similar in the two groups. In addition to reduced secretion of LH, there was reduced secretion of FSH, PRL, and thyroid-stimulating hormone (TSH), as well as altered rhythms of growth hormone (GH) and cortisol with elevated cortisol levels. However, the pituitary response to releasing hormones was unchanged. Thus, a number of hormonal alterations occur in FHA as an adaptive central neuroendocrine event. Some data from Tschugguel and Berga have suggested that in stress-induced hypothalamic amenorrhea, hypnotherapy and cognitive behavior therapy may be able to restore ovarian activity. Although this is a difficult approach that is not easy to duplicate, it is a logical approach from a physiologic perspective. Also, this method may be beneficial in that chronic stress reduction is generally beneficial for general health and can prevent cardiovascular problems and immune compromise. In a controlled study over 20 weeks, normal ovarian activity was restored in approximately 80% of women (**Fig. 38-13**).

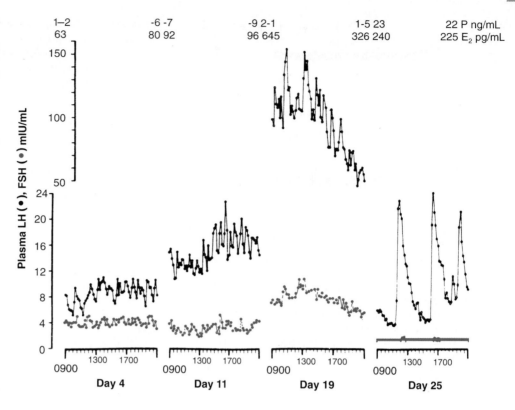

Figure 38-11 Serial measurements of plasma LH and FSH in two subjects sampled every 10 minutes at weekly intervals during cycles in which LH surge was observed on one of the sampling days. E₂, Estradiol; FSH, follicle-stimulating hormone; LH, luteinizing hormone; P, pregnanediol. (From Reame NE, Sauder SE, Kelch RP, et al: Pulsatile gonadotropin secretion during the human menstrual cycle: Evidence for altered frequency of gonadotropin-releasing hormone secretion. J Clin Endocrinol Metab 59:328, 1984.)

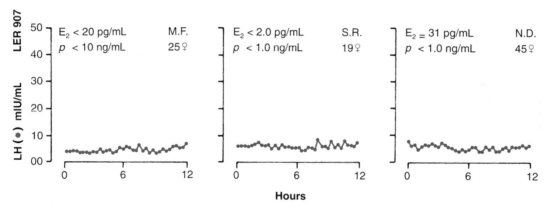

Figure 38-12 Pulsatile pattern of LH secretion in women with hypogonadotropic hypogonadism and hypothalamic amenorrhea. E₂, Estradiol; LH, luteinizing hormone; M.F., S.R., and N.D. are the three patient's initials. (From Crowley WF Jr, Filicori M, Spratt DI, et al: The physiology of gonadotropin-releasing hormone [GnRH] secretion in men and women. Rec Prog Hormone Res 41:473, 1985.)

When sufficient GnRH is produced to facilitate gonadotropin stimulation of the ovaries producing E_2 levels sufficient to proliferate the endometrium (30 to 40 pg/mL), the term *hypothalamic-pituitary dysfunction* is used to characterize this disorder. However, when the E_2 levels fall below 40 pg/mL, the term *hypothalamic-pituitary failure* has been used. There is not a marked distinction between women with dysfunction and failure, and this designation is merely a matter of severity of the hypothalamic suppression. Also, E_2 levels may fluctuate in this narrow range, and many clinical laboratories are not often able to measure these lower levels accurately. Accordingly, the functional or biologic estrogen status of these patients can be suggested by administering a progestogen. If endogenous E_2 has been sufficient to allow the endometrium to proliferate, then progestogen administration will result in withdrawal bleeding. This can also be determined by visualizing the endometrial stripe by ultrasound scan. If the thickness is less than 4 mm, hyperestrogenism is clearly present. The importance of knowing the estrogen status of these patients is that in the severe hypoestrogenism of hypothalamic failure, bone loss occurs in these young women at a very critical time.

Pituitary Causes (Hypoestrogenic Amenorrhea)
Neoplasms
Although most pituitary tumors secrete prolactin, some do not and may be associated with the onset of secondary amenorrhea without hyperprolactinemia. Chromophobe adenomas are the most common non–prolactin-secreting pituitary tumors;

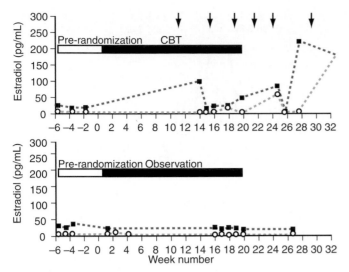

Figure 38-13 Estradiol (*dot*) and progesterone levels (*square*) in a woman with functional hypothalamic amenorrhea (FHA) who had return of ovulatory menstrual cycles while undergoing CBT (*top panel*) and estradiol and progesterone levels in a woman with FHA who remained anovulatory and amenorrheic during observation for 20 weeks (*bottom panel*). (From Berga, SL, Marcus MD, Loucks, et al: Recovery of ovarian activity in women with functional hypothalamic amenorrhea who were treated with cognitive behavior therapy. Fertil Steril 80:976, 2003.)

however, basophilic (ACTH-secreting) and acidophilic (GH-secreting) adenomas may be incapable of secreting prolactin. Individuals with the latter types of tumor, although having secondary amenorrhea, frequently have other symptoms produced by these lesions and present to the clinician with symptoms of acromegaly or Cushing's disease.

Non-neoplastic Lesions

Pituitary cells can also become damaged or necrotic as a result of anoxia, thrombosis, or hemorrhage. When pituitary cell destruction occurs as a result of a hypotensive episode during pregnancy, the disorder is called Sheehan's syndrome. When the disorder is unrelated to pregnancy, it is called Simmonds' disease. It is important to diagnose this cause of secondary amenorrhea because, in contrast to the hypothalamic disorders, pituitary damage can be associated with decreased secretion of other pituitary hormones, particularly ACTH and TSH, in addition to LH and FSH. Thus, these women may have secondary hypothyroidism or adrenal insufficiency that may seriously impair their health, in addition to their decreased estrogen levels.

Ovarian Causes (Hypergonadotropic Hypogonadism)

The ovaries may fail to secrete sufficient estrogen to produce endometrial growth if the follicles are damaged as a result of infection, interference with blood supply, or depletion of follicles caused by bilateral cystectomies. These women may become amenorrheic after a variable period of time has elapsed following medical treatment of a bilateral tubo-ovarian abscess, after bilateral cystectomy for benign ovarian neoplasms, or sometimes after a hysterectomy during which the vascular supply to the ovaries is compromised (also called cystic degeneration of the ovaries).

Occasionally, the ovaries cease to produce sufficient estrogen to stimulate endometrial growth several years before the age of

physiologic menopause. When this condition occurs before the age of 40, the term *premature ovarian failure* (POF) or *premature ovarian insufficiency* (POI) instead of premature menopause is best used to describe the clinical entity. Coulam and colleagues have estimated that as many as 1% of women younger than 40 years have hypergonadotropic amenorrhea, with the incidence steadily increasing from ages 15 to 39. Frequently, the condition of POI is transient before permanent ovarian failure occurs; occasionally, women with a diagnosis of POI may ovulate and conceive during this transition period. POI frequently occurs after gonadal irradiation or systemic chemotherapy and has also been reported in women with steroid hormonal enzyme deficiencies who menstruate temporarily and then have secondary amenorrhea.

Histologically, women with POI have two types of ovarian pathologic findings. In most of them, there is generalized sclerosis similar to the findings of a normal postmenopausal ovary (**Fig. 38-14**), whereas in up to 30%, numerous primordial follicles with no progression past the early antrum stage are seen (**Fig. 38-15**). The latter condition has been called the

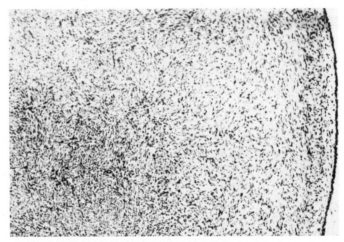

Figure 38-14 Representative section of ovary from patient with premature ovarian failure (POF). The cortex of the ovary is devoid of follicles. (From Tulandi T, Kinch RAH: Premature ovarian failure. Obstet Gynecol Surv 35:521, 1981.)

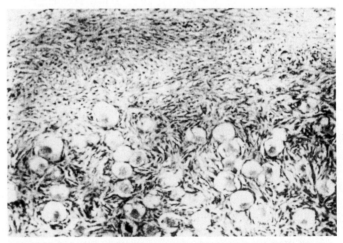

Figure 38-15 Representative section of ovary from patient with insensitive ovary syndrome. Numerous primordial follicles are seen. (From Tulandi T, Kinch RAH: Premature ovarian failure. Obstet Gynecol Surv 35:521, 1981.)

gonadotropin-resistant ovary syndrome, or ovarian hypofolliculogenesis, and is histologically different from the gonadal streak, in which no follicles are seen. Women with this condition may have primary amenorrhea, but usually sufficient estrogen is produced so that they menstruate for several months or even years. Many individuals with POI, particularly those with primordial follicles that appear normal, also have an autoimmune disease such as hypoparathyroidism, Hashimoto's thyroiditis, or Addison's disease. Many women with POI who do not have clinical evidence of an autoimmune disease have antibodies to gonadotropins as well as to several other endocrine organs, such as the thyroid and adrenal glands, suggesting an autoimmune origin.

Alper and Garner have estimated that approximately 30% to 50% of women with chromosomally normal POI without a history of irradiation or chemotherapy have an associated autoimmune disease, most commonly thyroid disease, which was present in 85% of the group with an autoimmune disorder. Using sophisticated immunofluorescence techniques, Mignot and coworkers demonstrated that 92% of women with POI have laboratory evidence of autosensitization. Approximately two thirds of these were positive for non–organ-specific antibodies, mainly antinuclear antibodies and rheumatoid factors, and 50% had organ-specific antibodies. Although most of these women had no evidence of autoimmune disease, it is recommended that immunologic screening be performed in young women with POF. In the absence of symptoms, such as weakness, lethargy, or pain, which may suggest systemic disease, it is probably sufficient to obtain a complete blood count (CBC) and sequential multiple analysis (SMA), as well as TSH and antithyroid antibody levels. If adrenal failure (e.g., weakness) is suspected, adrenal antibodies (against 21-hydroxylase) and cortisol may be obtained; rarely, an ACTH stimulation test is warranted. It may be sufficient to obtain a general screen for adrenal function by obtaining levels of DHEA-S. Nevertheless some data point to slightly lower (age specific) levels of dehydroepiandrosterone sulfate (DHEA-S) in women with POI. Although available clinically, measurements of antiovarian antibodies have not been properly validated.

DIAGNOSTIC EVALUATION AND MANAGEMENT

All women who consult a clinician for the symptom of secondary amenorrhea should have a diagnostic evaluation initiated at that visit, even though 6 months may not have elapsed since her last menstrual period. Amenorrhea is a source of concern to the woman, and it will relieve her concern if attempts are made to find the cause. The clinician should first take a detailed history and perform a physical examination to rule out pregnancy as a cause of the amenorrhea. In addition, he or she should determine whether there is the possibility of IUAs. Any instrumentation of the endometrial cavity, particularly temporally related to pregnancy, should alert the clinician to the possibility of IUAs. The initial diagnostic evaluation to determine whether IUAs are present is placement of a uterine sound into the uterine cavity, followed by a hysterography or hysteroscopy. The diagnosis can also be confirmed by detecting presumptive evidence of ovulation by means of a biphasic basal temperature or an elevated serum progesterone level. If IUAs are ruled out, the history should disclose whether medications are currently being used or if oral contraceptives have been recently discontinued. In addition, questions regarding diet, weight loss, stress, and strenuous exercise are pertinent. A history of hot flushes, decreasing breast size, and/or vaginal dryness, and physical examination, are helpful in estimating the degree of estrogen deficiency. If the history and physical examination fail to reveal the cause of the amenorrhea, a CBC, urinalysis, and serum chemistries should be carried out to rule out systemic disease. A sensitive TSH assay should also be performed to rule out the uncommon asymptomatic thyroid disorders that produce secondary amenorrhea and serum E_2, FSH, and prolactin levels should be measured (**Fig. 38-16**). If prolactin levels are elevated, a diagnostic evaluation for the cause of this problem should be undertaken (see Chapter 39, Hyperprolactinemia, Galactorrhea, and Pituitary Adenomas). Administration of injectable progesterone or oral progestogen is an indirect means of determining whether sufficient estrogen is present to produce endometrial growth that will slough after the progesterone levels fall (progesterone challenge test). However, it is preferable to order a sensitive E_2 assay, with organic solvent extraction, to determine the true estrogen status. As noted, the endometrial stripe is also beneficial.

Women with PCOS, moderate stress, exercise, weight loss, or hypothalamic-pituitary dysfunction will usually have E_2 levels of at least 30 to 40 pg/mL and withdrawal bleeding after progestogens usually occurs. Those with pituitary tumors, ovarian failure, severe dietary weight loss or anorexia nervosa, severe stress, or the rare hypothalamic lesion will usually have very low E_2 levels, typically in the postmenopausal range.

If a sensitive serum E_2 value is above 30 to 40 pg/mL, and ultrasound confirms the presence of polycystic ovaries, the diagnosis of PCOS may be considered (see Chapter 40, Hyperandrogenism). If there is no sonographic evidence of polycystic ovaries and the woman has a history of drug ingestion, stress, weight loss, or strenuous exercise, she should be told that hypothalamic-pituitary dysfunction is present and the exact cause cannot be determined with current technology because frequent LH sampling is costly and impractical. She should also be informed that hypothalamic-pituitary dysfunction is usually a self-limiting disorder and not a serious threat to health or a cause of untreatable infertility.

Women with low E_2 and low FSH levels have a CNS lesion or hypothalamic-pituitary failure. Women with low E_2 and elevated FSH levels (>30 mIU/mL) have POI. If severe weight loss, strenuous exercise, or severe stress is not present, and FSH and E_2 levels are low, CT or MRI of the hypothalamic-pituitary region should be performed to rule out a lesion, even if the prolactin level is normal. If a lesion is seen or if there is a history compatible with possible **pituitary destruction** (hypotension during pregnancy), a test of ACTH reserve should be performed. An **insulin tolerance test** in which hypoglycemia is induced should normally cause a cortisol increase of 6 μg/100 mL within 120 minutes, and is a satisfactory test of ACTH function. An alternative test is administration of CRH. If no lesion is identified, the term *hypothalamic-pituitary failure* may be used as a nonspecific diagnosis. Frequently, individuals with this diagnosis resume normal ovarian function without treatment.

If POI is diagnosed because of an elevated FSH level and no cause of ovarian destruction is elicited, the possibility of autoimmune disease should be considered, particularly in younger women. Therefore, antithyroid s and antinuclear antibody levels should be measured and other screening teats should be performed, as noted earlier. To rule out mosaicism or a dysgenetic gonad, including the possibility of a Y cell line, a karyotype

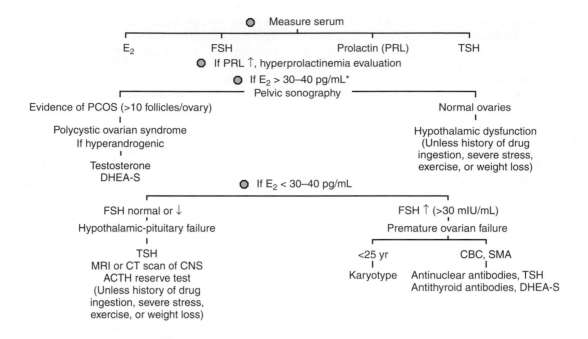

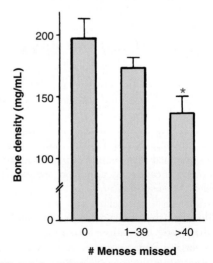

*The threshold level for E_2 is dependent on the normal follicular phase range of the laboratory but is typically 30–40 pg/mL.

Figure 38-16 Diagnostic evaluation of secondary amenorrhea. ACTH, Adrenocorticotropic hormone; CBC, complete blood count; CNS, central nervous system; CT, computed tomography; DHEA-S, dehydroeipandrosterone sulfate; E_2, estradiol; FSH, follicle-stimulating hormone; MRI, magnetic resonance imaging; PCOS, polycystic ovary syndrome; SMA, sequential multiple analysis; TSH, thyroid-stimulating hormone.

should be obtained in women with POF who are 25 years of age or younger. Biopsy of the gonads by laparoscopy or laparotomy is not indicated. Suppression of gonadotropin levels with estrogen, oral contraceptives, and GnRH analogues has been advocated to induce rebound ovulation following their withdrawal. Although gonadotropins are suppressed by these agents, these techniques are usually ineffective for inducing ovulation. If ovulation occurs following such treatment, it is a sporadic event and not a result of the therapy. Most cases of spontaneous pregnancy have occurred during estrogen replacement.

The appropriate treatment depends on the diagnosis and on whether conception is desired. Non–prolactin-secreting pituitary tumors should be surgically excised, if possible. Those who have lost weight should be advised to gain weight. If strenuous exercise results in low estrogen levels (<30 pg/mL), the amount of exercise should be reduced or estrogen supplementation administered to prevent possible development of osteoporosis. Several investigators have shown that amenorrheic and oligomenorrheic athletes with decreased E_2 levels have decreased density of trabecular bone in the lumbar spine (**Fig. 38-17**).

Klibanski and coworkers also have shown that women with low E_2 levels caused by hypothalamic amenorrhea, who have normal nutrition and activity levels, have a profound reduction in spinal bone mineral density. The reduction in bone loss is independent of whether the PRL level is elevated or not. Bone loss has been found to be similar in hyperprolactinemic amenorrheic women with low estrogen levels and women with normal prolactin and low estrogen levels (**Fig. 38-18**). A group of women with hyperprolactinemia and regular menses did not have bone loss. If women with PCOS or hypothalamic-pituitary dysfunction desire conception, clomiphene citrate administration is successful

in inducing ovulation. If pregnancy is not desired, monthly progestogen administration (medroxyprogesterone acetate, 10 mg/day, for the first 12 days of each month) should be given to reduce the increased risk of endometrial cancer associated with unopposed estrogen. If women with hypothalamic-pituitary failure desire fertility, ovulation can be induced with exogenous

Figure 38-17 Relationship between bone density and number of missed menses in collegiate women athletes. For each subject, number of missed menses was determined from her menarche to age 19. *Asterisk* indicates significantly different from control group. (From Lloyd T, Myers C, Buchanan JR, et al: Collegiate women athletes with irregular menses during adolescence have decreased bone density. Obstet Gynecol 72:639, 1988.)

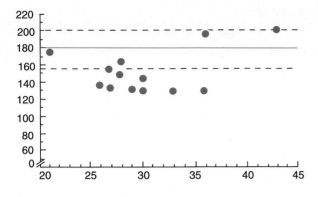

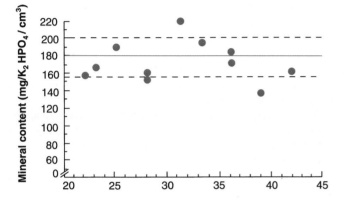

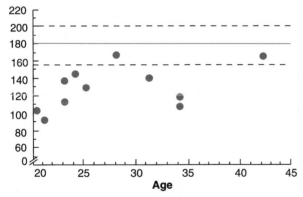

Figure 38-18 Spinal bone density in 13 women with hyperprolactinemic amenorrhea (*top panel*), 12 eumenorrheic hyperprolactinemic women (*middle panel*), and 11 women with hypothalamic amenorrhea (*bottom panel*). Mean (*solid lines*) and standard deviation (± SD, *dashed lines*) for 19 normal women are shown. (From Klibanski A, Biller BM, Rosenthal DI, et al: Effects of prolactin and estrogen deficiency in amenorrheic bone loss. J Clin Endocrinol Metab 67:124, 1988.)

gonadotropins or pulsatile GnRH. Clomiphene is not successful if the estrogen levels are low. If pregnancy is not desired, estrogen-progestogen replacement is indicated for all amenorrheic women with low E_2 levels, including those with POI, to reduce the risk of osteoporosis. Women with POI are also vulnerable to accelerated atherosclerosis. There is no increased cardiovascular risk in prescribing estrogen to these women. Women with POI may become pregnant with the use of donor oocytes and the priming of their endometrium with estrogen and progesterone for embryo transfer.

PRECOCIOUS PUBERTY

Puberty in the female is the process of biologic changes and physical development, after which sexual reproduction becomes possible. This is a time of accelerated linear skeletal growth and development of secondary sexual characteristics, such as breast development and the appearance of axillary and pubic hair. The usual sequence of the physiologic events of puberty begins with breast development and the subsequent appearance of pubic and axillary hair, followed by the period of maximal growth velocity and, finally, menarche. Menarche may occur before the appearance of axillary or pubic hair in 10% of normal females. Normal puberty occurs over a wide range of ages.

Precocious puberty is arbitrarily defined as the appearance of any signs of secondary sexual maturation at an early age. Puberty in girls is now recognized to be occurring earlier than in previous studies (**Table 38-4**). In an article by Kaplowitz and associates, it was suggested that girls with breast development or pubic hair should be evaluated when these signs occur before age 7 in whites and age 6 in black girls. Thus, evaluation of precocious puberty need not be performed for white girls older than 7 years and for black girls older than 6 years.

Precocious puberty is associated with a wide range of disorders. It should be emphasized that regardless of the cause, precocious puberty is a rare disorder. The incidence of this condition in the United States is estimated to be approximately 1 in 10,000 young girls. When it is diagnosed, the physician should undertake a detailed investigation of the cause of the condition so as not to overlook a potentially correctable pathologic lesion. The two primary concerns of parents of children with precocious puberty are the social stigma associated with the child being physically different from her peers and the diminished ultimate height caused by the premature closure of epiphyseal growth centers.

Puberty is a time of accelerated growth, skeletal maturation, and resulting epiphyseal closure. Although precocious puberty may occur early in a child's life, it usually develops in the normal sequence. Early in the course of the disease. the girls are taller and heavier than their chronologic peers who have not experienced the growth spurt (**Fig. 38-19**). However, although the patient is tall as a child, her eventual adult height will be shorter than normal because of premature closure of the epiphyses. Without therapy, approximately 50% of girls with precocious puberty will not reach a height of 5 feet.

TYPES OF DISORDERS

Precocious puberty is subdivided into GnRH-dependent (complete, true) and GnRH-independent (incomplete, pseudo) and isosexual and heterosexual disorders. These categories are of clinical value only after the eventual diagnosis has been established. The pathophysiology and corresponding categories of precocious puberty may change during the course of the disease; for example, congenital adrenal hyperplasia initially is GnRH-independent but subsequently, over many months, eventually becomes a GnRH-dependent form of precocious puberty. The pathophysiology of precocious puberty is divided into two distinct categories— a normal physiologic process involving GnRH secretion with an integrated hypothalamic–pituitary axis, which occurs at an abnormal time, or an abnormal physiologic process independent of an integrated hypothalamic-pituitary-ovarian axis.

Table 38-4 Prevalence of Breast and Pubic Hair Development in White and Black Girls*

Parameter	Age Range (yr)				
	5.00-5.99	6.00-6.99	7.00-7.99	8.00-8.99	9.00-9.99
Prevalence of breast development at Tanner stage 2 or higher (%)					
White girl	1.6	2.9	5.0	10.5	32.1
Black girl	2.4	6.4	15.4	37.8	62.6
Prevalence of pubic hair development at Tanner stage 2 or higher (%)					
White	0.4	1.4	2.8	7.7	20.0
African American	3.4	9.5	17.7	34.3	62.6

*Between 5 and 10 years of age.
From Kaplowitz PB, Oberfield SE: Reexamination of the age limit for determining when puberty is precocious in girls in the United States: Implications for evaluation and treatment. Drug and Therapeutics and Executive Committees of the Lawson Wilkins Pediatric Endocrine Society. Pediatrics 104:937, 1999.

GnRH-dependent precocious puberty involves premature maturation of the hypothalamic-pituitary-ovarian axis and includes normal menses, ovulation, and the possibility of pregnancy. GnRH-independent precocious puberty involves premature female sexual maturation, which may lead to estrogen-induced uterine stimulation and bleeding without any normal ovarian follicular activity. Both categories have increased circulating levels of estrogen. In the latter syndrome, however, secretion of estrogens is independent of hypothalamic-pituitary control. Depending on when the patient is first seen in relationship to

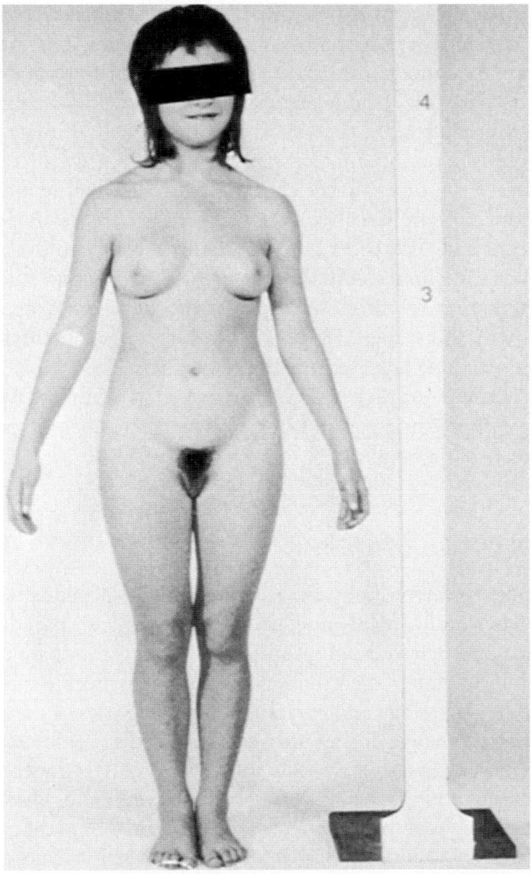

Figure 38-19 Child age 7 years with constitutional precocious puberty. Note increased height for age. (From Dewhurst CJ: Practical Pediatric and Adolescent Gynecology. New York, Marcel Dekker, 1980.)

the natural history of her disease, it may be necessary to observe her at regular intervals (for 2 to 3 years) to distinguish one syndrome from another (**Table 38-5**). Prolonged follow-up is sometimes necessary to rule out subtle, slow-growing lesions of the brain, ovary, or adrenal gland.

The vast majority of girls with precocious puberty (70%) develop a GnRH-dependent process. The exact cause of most cases of GnRH-dependent precocious puberty is unknown (constitutional); however, approximately 30% are secondary to CNS disease. Recently it has been realized that Kisspeptin, a hypothalamic peptide that stimulates the release of GnRH, is involved in the initiation of puberty. Two activating mutations of the Kisspeptin receptor have been described in girls with central precocious puberty. A definitive diagnosis is established more often for pseudoprecocious puberty, which is usually related to an ovarian or adrenal disorder. If the secondary sex characteristics are discordant with the genetic and phenotypic gender, the condition is termed *heterosexual precocious puberty*. This is premature virilization in a female child and includes development of masculine secondary sexual characteristics. The androgens that cause heterosexual precocious puberty usually come from the adrenal gland.

Premature Thelarche

Premature thelarche is defined as isolated unilateral or bilateral breast development as the only sign of secondary sexual maturation. It is not accompanied by other associated evidence of pubertal development, such as axillary or pubic hair or changes in vaginal epithelium. Breast hyperplasia is a normal physiologic phenomenon in the neonatal period and may persist up to 6 months of age. Premature thelarche usually occurs between 1 and 4 years of age. The breast buds enlarge to 2 to 4 cm and sometimes this process is asymmetrical. Nipple development is absent. This is a benign self-limiting condition that does not require treatment. Often, the breast enlargement spontaneously regresses. It is important to observe these children closely for other signs of precocious puberty. The cause of premature thelarche is not understood. Although it is postulated to be related to a slight increase in circulating estrogen levels, these levels are normally low to undetectable. This disorder may be associated with female infants who had extremely low birth weights. Evidence suggests that ovarian follicular activity may occur to explain this, which may be part of a continuum in cases of GnRH-dependent precocious puberty.

Table 38-5 Physical Findings Among Patients with Various Precocious Puberty Syndromes

Findings	Premature Thelarche	Premature Adrenarche	GnRH-Dependent and GnRH-Independent Syndromes			
			Idiopathic	McCune-Albright Syndrome	Central Nervous System Tumor	Hypothyroid
Breast enlargement	Yes	No	Yes	Yes	Yes	Yes
Pubic hair	No	Yes	Yes	Yes	Yes	Unusual
Vaginal bleeding	No	No	Yes	Yes	Yes	Yes
Virilizing signs	No	No	No	No	No	No
Bone age	Normal	Normal to minimally advanced	Advanced	Advanced	Advanced	Normal or retarded
Neurologic deficit	No	No	No	Yes	Yes	No
Abdominopelvic mass	No	No	Occ'l	No	No	Occ'l

Findings	Isosexual			Heterosexual		
	Ovarian Tumors	Adrenal Tumors	Factitious	Ovarian Tumors	Adrenal Tumors	Adrenal Hyperplasia
Breast enlargement	Yes	Yes	Yes	Yes	Yes	Yes
Pubic hair	Yes	Yes	Yes	Yes	Yes	Yes
Vaginal bleeding	Yes	Yes	Yes	Yes	Yes	Yes
Virilizing signs	No	Yes	No	Yes	Yes	Yes
Bone age	Advanced	Advanced	Advanced	Advanced	Advanced	Advanced
Neurologic deficit	No	No	No	No	No	No
Abdominopelvic mass	Usually	No	No	Occ'l	No	No

GnRH, gonadotropin-releasing hormone; Occ'l, occasional.
From Ross GT: Disorders of the ovary and female reproductive tract. In Wilson JD, Foster DW (eds): Williams Textbook of Endocrinology, 7th ed. Philadelphia, WB Saunders, 1985.

Premature Pubarche or Adrenarche

Premature pubarche is early isolated development of pubic hair without other signs of secondary sexual maturation. Premature adrenarche is isolated early development of axillary hair. Neither of these conditions is progressive and the girls do not have clitoral hypertrophy. However, it is important to differentiate premature pubarche from the virilization produced by congenital adrenal hyperplasia. Some children with premature pubarche have abnormal electroencephalograms (EEGs) without significant neurologic disease. The bone age should not be advanced in this disorder. The cause is poorly understood but is believed to be related to increased androgen production by the adrenal glands (DHEA and DHEAS). Similar to premature thelarche, the child should have periodic follow-up visits to confirm that the condition is not progressive. Many cases of premature adrenarche evolve into PCOS.

Gonadotropin-Releasing Hormone-Dependent Precocious Puberty

Idiopathic development is responsible for approximately 70% of the cases of GnRH-dependent precocious puberty. Some of these children are simply at the earliest limits of the normal distribution of the biologic curve (see **Table 38-4**). Most idiopathic cases are sporadic in distribution; however, some may be familial.

A high incidence of abnormal EEGs in children with idiopathic precocious puberty has raised the question of potential CNS disease. With the increasing use of high-resolution imaging techniques, such as brain CT scanning and MRI, the number of truly idiopathic cases is declining.

These girls have no genital abnormality except for early development. Occasionally, follicular cysts of the ovary may form secondary to increased pituitary gonadotropin levels (**Fig. 38-20**). In these cases, the cysts are the result, not the cause, of precocious puberty. Gonadotropin levels, sex steroid levels, and response of LH after administration of GnRH are similar to those in normal puberty. Most of the cases of premature maturation of the hypothalamic-pituitary-ovarian axis do not have a defined cause. The syndrome may appear as early as age 3 to 4 years. When observed for several decades, these women have normal menopausal ages. Emotional problems are a cause for concern because the young girls suffer from extreme social pressures. The intellectual, behavioral, and psychosocial development of girls with precocious puberty is appropriate for their chronologic age, but many are shy and withdraw from their peers.

A wide range of inflammatory, degenerative, neoplastic, or congenital defects that involve the CNS may produce GnRH-dependent precocious puberty. This occurs in at least 30% of cases and warrants a careful evaluation. Usually, symptoms of a neurologic disease, especially headaches and visual disturbances, precede the manifestations of precocious puberty. A most unusual neurologic symptom that may be associated with precocious puberty is seizures with inappropriate laughter (gelastic seizures). Anatomically, most CNS lesions are located near the hypothalamus in the region of the third ventricle, tuber cinereum, or mammillary bodies. Major CNS diseases associated with true precocious puberty include tuberculosis, encephalitis, trauma, secondary hydrocephalus, neurofibromatosis, granulomas, hamartomas of the hypothalamus, teratomas, craniopharyngiomas, cranial irradiation, and congenital brain defects, such as hydrocephalus and cysts in the area of the third ventricle. These children have markedly fluctuating estrogen levels and low gonadotropin concentrations that are independent of GnRH stimulation. These CNS space-occupying masses are most difficult to treat

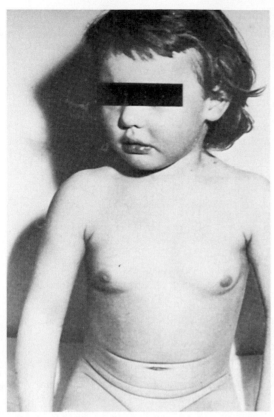

Figure 38-20 Precocious puberty in young girl. The child had large lower abdominal swelling, which at surgery was shown to be bilateral follicular cysts (result of premature ovarian stimulation and not cause of condition). (From Dewhurst CJ: Practical Pediatric and Adolescent Gynecology. New York, Marcel Dekker, 1980.)

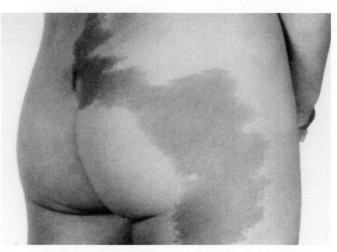

Figure 38-21 Large café-au-lait spot in child with precocious puberty as result of McCune-Albright syndrome. (From Dewhurst CJ: Practical Pediatric and Adolescent Gynecology. New York, Marcel Dekker, 1980.)

successfully by surgical means. The pathophysiology whereby CNS disease produces precocious puberty is poorly understood. It is known that hamartomas may secrete GnRH; this secretion is not subject to the normal physiologic inhibition that occurs during childhood.

Gonadotropin-Releasing Hormone-Independent Precocious Puberty

The most common cause of pseudoprecocious puberty is an estrogen-secreting ovarian tumor. Granulosa cell tumors are the most common type of ovarian tumors, accounting for approximately 60%. These tumors are usually larger than 8 cm in diameter when associated with precocious puberty; 80% can be palpated abdominally. Other ovarian tumors that may be associated with precocious puberty include thecomas, luteomas, teratomas, Sertoli-Leydig tumors, choriocarcinomas, and benign follicular cysts. Usually, thecomas and luteomas are much smaller than granulosa cell tumors and cannot be palpated. Overall, these tumors are rare during childhood, with only 5% of granulosa cell tumors and 1% of thecomas occurring before puberty. Infrequently, follicular cysts of the ovary may emerge spontaneously and secrete enough estrogen to be the cause, rather than the result, of precocious puberty. It is speculated that these benign cysts function in an autonomous fashion. The ability of many tumors, including teratomas, choriocarcinomas, and dysgerminomas, to secrete estrogen, human chorionic gonadotropin (hCG), α-fetoprotein, and other markers has been established.

McCune-Albright syndrome (MAS, polyostotic fibrous dysplasia) is a rare triad of café-au-lait spots, fibrous dysplasia, and cysts of the skull and long bones (**Fig. 38-21**). These patients also have facial asymmetry. Approximately 40% of girls with MAS have associated isosexual precocious puberty.

Adrenocortical neoplasms may produce isosexual or heterosexual precocious puberty. The relationship between congenital adrenal hyperplasia and puberty depends on the time of initial diagnosis and therapy. If the disease is diagnosed in the neonatal period and treated, normal puberty ensues. If the disease is untreated, the girl usually develops heterosexual precocious puberty (signs of androgen excess) from the adrenal androgens over time. However, if congenital adrenal hyperplasia is diagnosed late in childhood, isosexual precocious puberty may follow initial treatment of the adrenal disease.

Hypothyroidism is usually associated with delayed pubertal development. However, in rare cases, untreated hypothyroidism results in isosexual, GnRH-dependent, or GnRH-independent precocious puberty. The hypothyroidism associated with precocious puberty is caused by primary thyroid insufficiency, usually Hashimoto's thyroiditis, and not by a deficiency in pituitary TSH. The pathophysiology of this syndrome is a result of the diminished negative feedback of thyroxine, resulting in an increased production of TSH, which may be accompanied by an increase in production of gonadotropins. Interestingly, hypothyroidism is the only cause of precocious puberty in which the bone age is retarded. This syndrome is usually observed in girls between the ages of 6 and 8 years.

Iatrogenic or factitious precocious puberty results when a young female has used hormone cream or ingested adult medications such as oral estrogen or birth control pills. The secondary sexual characteristics regress after discontinuation of the medication.

DIAGNOSIS

The diagnostic workup of a young child with precocious puberty begins with a meticulous history and physical examination. The primary emphasis should be to rule out life-threatening

Table 38-6 Laboratory Findings in Disorders Producing Precocious Puberty

			Findings		
Disorder	**Gonadal Size**	**Basal FSH, LH**	**Estradiol or Testosterone**	**DHAS**	**GnRH Response**
Idiopathic	Increased	Increased	Increased	Increased	Pubertal
Cerebral	Increased	Increased	Increased	Increased	Pubertal
Gonadal	Unilaterally increased	Decreased	Increased	Increased	Flat
Albright	Increased	Decreased	Increased	Increased	Flat
Adrenal	Small	Decreased	Increased	Increased	Flat

Adapted from Speroff L, Glass RH, Kase NG: Clinical Gynecology Endocrinology and Infertility, 6th ed. Baltimore, Lippincott Williams & Wilkins, 1999, p 396.

neoplasms of the ovary, adrenal gland, or CNS. The secondary emphasis is to delineate the speed of the maturation process, because this is crucial in making decisions concerning therapy. The height of the girl and exact stage of pubertal development, including Tanner stage, should be recorded. Similar to other syndromes with a long list of causes, a number of tests, including imaging studies of the brain, serum estradiol level, FSH level, and thyroid function tests, may need to be carried out to establish the diagnosis (**Table 38-6**). With this acceleration of development, the sex steroid and adrenal androgen (DHEAS) levels are elevated, regardless of the cause. Acceleration of growth is one of the earliest clinical features of precocious puberty. Thus, bone age should be determined by hand-wrist films and compared with standards for a patient's age (**Fig. 38-22**). Usually, these films are repeated at 6-month intervals to evaluate the rate of skeletal maturation and the corresponding need for active treatment of the disease. Advancement of bone age more than 95% of the norm for the child's chronologic age indicates an estrogen effect.

Diseases of the CNS are suggested by symptoms such as headaches, seizures, trauma to the head, and encephalitis. These conditions are confirmed or excluded by a series of tests, including neurologic and ophthalmologic examinations, EEGs, and brain imaging.

Hypothalamic hamartomas can be categorized based on the tumor topology on MRI. This classification has been shown to correlate with the clinical manifestations of precocious puberty. Ultrasound, CT, or MRI of the abdomen and pelvis should be performed to evaluate enlargement of the ovaries (ovarian volume), uterus, or adrenal glands.

Serum levels of FSH, LH, prolactin, TSH, E_2, testosterone, DHEAS, hCG, androstenedione, 17-hydroxyprogesterone, triiodothyronine (T_3), and thyroxine (T_4) may be of value in establishing the differential diagnosis. Sometimes a GnRH stimulation test is diagnostic in differentiating incomplete from true precocious puberty, but does not specifically identify children with CNS lesions. The LH responses to gonadotropin stimulation after reaching a basal level are similar in cases of true

Figure 38-22 X-rays demonstrating bone age. **A,** Normal for 7 years of age. **B,** Advanced bone age in a girl 7 years of age who also shows other signs of isosexual precocity. (From Huffman JW: The Gynecology of Childhood and Adolescence, 2nd ed. Philadelphia, WB Saunders, 1981.)

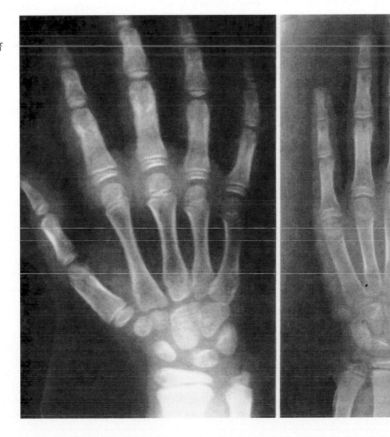

precocious puberty to the responses of a mature adult. In contrast, a child with precocious puberty secondary to a feminizing ovarian neoplasm does not have a significant elevation in LH level after exogenous GnRH. In summary, a stimulation test with exogenous GnRH is helpful for delineating the underlying pathophysiology.

TREATMENT

The treatment of precocious puberty depends on the cause, extent, and progression of precocious signs, and whether the cause may be removed operatively. For example, removal extirpation of a granulosa cell tumor and subtotal removal of a hypothalamic hamartoma are successful treatments because they remove the hormonal force. Because most cases involve premature maturation of the hypothalamic-pituitary-ovarian axis without a lesion, this discussion will focus on the medical management of this condition. Girls with menarche before age 8 years, progressive thelarche and pubarche, and bone age 2 years more than their chronologic age definitely should be treated. The goals of therapy are to reduce gonadotropin secretions and reduce or counteract the peripheral actions of the sex steroids, decrease the growth rate to normal, and slow skeletal maturation to allow development of maximal adult height.

The present drug of choice for GnRH-dependent precocious puberty is one of the potent GnRH agonists. These drugs are typically given by monthly or trimonthly injections or, rarely, intranasally. GnRH agonists are safe and effective treatments for children with the disease secondary to disturbances in the hypothalamic-pituitary-ovarian axis. Therapy should be initiated as soon as possible after the diagnosis is established so the child can achieve maximal adult height. The effect on adult height depends on the chronologic age at which therapy is initiated. Therapy is most effective in 4- to 6-year-olds. Continuous chronic administration of the drug is maintained until the median age of puberty. The optimal dosage of medication may be confirmed by determining that peripheral E_2 levels are in a normal prepubertal range. Medical treatment produces involution of secondary sexual characteristics, with amenorrhea and regression of breast development and amount of pubic hair. LH and FSH pulsations are abolished. Most importantly, the drug not only reverses the ovarian cycle but definitely changes the growth pattern. Growth velocity is usually decreased by approximately 50% (**Fig. 38-23**). In one series, the predicted adult height increased a mean of 6.5 cm in girls who were 6 years of age or younger when therapy was initiated.

A number of studies have documented that agonist therapy decreases gonadotropin levels within 1 week and decreases sex steroid levels to the prepubertal range within the first 2 weeks of therapy (**Fig. 38-24**). Serial ultrasound examinations have documented that the size of the ovaries and uterus regresses to normal prepubertal shape and size. The most common observed side effect to agonists was a cutaneous reaction at the site of injection. However, approximately one in four girls experienced recurrent and sometimes prolonged vaginal bleeding while receiving GnRH agonists. The effects of these drugs are reversible when the agonists are discontinued after normal height has been achieved. The effect on final adult height has not been clearly established.

It has been suggested that rare forms of GnRH-independent precocious puberty that do not respond to agonist therapy may

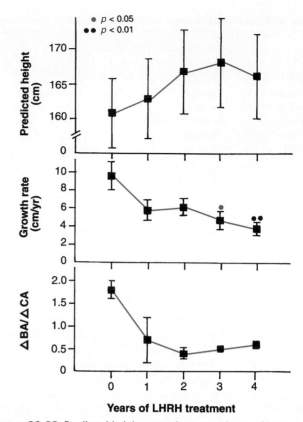

Figure 38-23 Predicted height, growth rate, and rate of bone age advancement in six children with central precocious puberty who received 4 years of therapy with the long-acting analogue of luteinizing hormone-releasing hormone (LHRH). *Asterisks* indicate significant differences compared with pretreatment value. ΔBA/ΔCA, Change in bone age/change in chronologic age. (Adapted from Comite F, Cassorla F, Barnes KM, et al: Luteinizing hormone-releasing hormone analogue therapy for central precocious puberty. Long-term effect on somatic growth, bone maturation, and predicted height. JAMA 255:2615, 1986.)

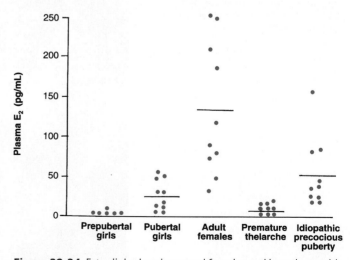

Figure 38-24 Estradiol values in normal females and in patients with premature thelarche and idiopathic precocious puberty. *Horizontal lines* depict mean levels. (Adapted from Escobar ME, Rivarola MA, Bergada C: Plasma concentration of oestradiol-17beta in premature thelarche and in different types of sexual precocity. Acta Endocrinol 81:351, 1976.)

be successfully treated using a GnRH antagonist. Here, there may be a direct antagonist effect on the ovary mediated through gonadotropin receptors. Small studies have suggested a minimal benefit from adding growth hormone to GnRH agonist therapy in girls with suboptimal growth. The initial observations of combination therapy have been encouraging, but the clinical data were from small series and of a preliminary nature.

McCune-Albright syndrome is caused by an activating mutation of a G protein that is coupled with gonadotropin receptors, resulting in the ovaries being stimulated autonomously. Girls may be treated with aromatase inhibitors, which prevent the conversion to biologically active estrogens. This treatment leads to diminished circulating estrogen levels, diminished frequency of menses, and decreased rate of growth and skeletal maturation.

The child with precocious puberty and her family need intensive counseling. The child will have the psychosocial and behavioral maturation of children of her chronologic age, not the age reflected by her physical appearance. She may be exposed to ridicule by her peers and to sexual exploitation. Thus, the child needs extensive sex education and help in anticipating and confronting various social experiences. Often, it is possible to dress the child in clothes that diminish the recognition of her advanced sexual maturation until the effects of her disease have been inhibited by drug therapy.

KEY POINTS

- The incidence of secondary amenorrhea of more than 6 months' duration in the general population is 0.7%.
- The incidence of amenorrhea lasting more than 6 months after discontinuation of oral contraceptives is 0.8%.
- The most important and probably most common cause of amenorrhea in adolescent girls is anorexia nervosa.
- An adolescent 13 years of age or older without any breast development has estrogen deficiency caused by a severe abnormality and needs diagnostic evaluation.
- Menarche is delayed approximately 0.4 year for each year of premenarchal athletic training.
- Gonadal failure is the most common cause of primary amenorrhea, accounting for almost 50% of patients with this syndrome.
- Individuals with gonadal failure and an X chromosome abnormality are shorter than 63 inches in height.
- The testes of individuals with androgen resistance have approximately a 20% chance of becoming malignant after the age of 20 years.
- Uterovaginal agenesis is the second most common cause of primary amenorrhea, with an incidence of approximately 15% of individuals with this symptom.
- Approximately one third of individuals with gonadal failure have major cardiovascular or renal abnormalities.
- Congenital renal abnormalities occur in approximately one third of women with congenital absence of the uterus.
- The differential diagnosis between estrogen deficiency caused by gonadal failure and hypogonadotropic hypogonadism is best established with measurement of serum the FSH level.
- The diagnosis of gonadal failure, or hypergonadotropic hypogonadism, can be established if the FSH level exceeds 30 mIU/mL.
- Individuals with gonadal failure should have a peripheral karyotype obtained to determine whether a Y chromosome is present. If it is present, or signs of hyperandrogenism are present, the gonads should be excised to prevent development of malignancy, mainly a gonadoblastoma.
- Individuals with primary amenorrhea and hypogonadotropic hypogonadism do not need karyotyping but need a cranial CT scan to rule out a CNS tumor.
- The most frequent cause of IUAs is curettage performed during pregnancy or shortly thereafter.
- The amenorrhea associated with strenuous exercise is related to stress, not weight loss, and is most probably caused by an increase in CNS opioids (β-endorphin) and catechol estrogens, both of which interfere with GnRH release.
- When women lose 15% below ideal body weight, amenorrhea can occur because of CNS-hypothalamic dysfunction. When weight loss decreases below 25% of ideal body weight, pituitary gonadotropin function can also become abnormal.
- Anorexia nervosa occurs in approximately 1 in 1000 white women. It is uncommon in men and women older than 25 years and rare in blacks and Asians.
- Individuals with anorexia nervosa have impaired peripheral conversion of T_4 to T_3, resulting in normal T_4 levels, decreased T_3 levels, and increased reverse T_3 levels.
- The normal cyclic pattern of LH pulsatility is not present in individuals with functional hypothalamic amenorrhea. Either no pulse or pulses of slow frequency, similar to those in the normal luteal phase, is usually observed.
- The GnRH alterations, as reflected in LH pulsatility in persons with severe weight loss and anorexia nervosa, are similar to those seen in normal prepubertal girls. When they gain weight, GnRH changes similar to those occurring during puberty take place.
- When uterine bleeding fails to occur after progestin is administered, E_2 levels are usually lower than 40 pg/mL.
- In contrast to hypothalamic disorders, pituitary causes of amenorrhea can be associated with ACTH and TSH deficiency.
- Individuals with premature ovarian failure have two different histologic findings, generalized sclerosis or primordial follicles scattered through the stroma.
- Women with premature ovarian failure or insufficiency may have antibodies to gonadotropins and other endocrine organs, indicating an autoimmune origin.
- A karyotype should be obtained in women with premature ovarian failure who is younger than 25 years but not in those who are older.
- Amenorrhea with low estrogen levels is associated with decreased density of trabecular bone.
- The most frequent cause of secondary amenorrhea is hypothalamic dysfunction.
- Physiologic development in females with precocious puberty usually follows the normal sequence of changes of secondary sexual characteristics.
- The two primary concerns of parents of children with precocious puberty are the social stigma associated with the

child being physically different from her peers and the diminished ultimate height caused by the premature closure of epiphyseal growth centers.

■ The exact cause of the majority of cases of GnRH-dependent (true or complete) precocious puberty is unknown; however, approximately 30% of cases are secondary to CNS disease.

■ A definitive diagnosis is established more often for GnRH-independent (pseudoprecocious or incomplete) puberty and is usually related to an ovarian or adrenal disorder.

■ Breast hyperplasia is a normal phenomenon in neonates and may persist up to 6 months of age.

■ The most common cause of GnRH-independent precocious puberty is a functioning ovarian tumor. Granulosa cell tumors are the most common type, accounting for approximately 60%.

■ The primary emphasis of the diagnostic workup of a child with precocious puberty should be to rule out life-threatening neoplasms of the ovary, adrenal glands, or CNS. The secondary emphasis is to delineate the speed of the maturation process, because this is crucial when making a decision about therapy.

■ The goals of therapy of precocious puberty are to reduce gonadotropin secretions and reduce or counteract the peripheral actions of sex steroids, decreasing the growth rate to normal and slowing skeletal maturation. This is best accomplished by the use of GnRH agonists.

■ The effect on adult height depends on the chronologic age at which GnRH therapy is initiated. The therapy is most effective in 4- to 6-year-olds.

■ The child with precocious puberty and her family need intensive counseling.

REFERENCES CAN BE FOUND ON EXPERTCONSULT.com

39

Hyperprolactinemia, Galactorrhea, and Pituitary Adenomas
Etiology, Differential Diagnosis, Natural History, Management

Roger A. Lobo

Prolactin (PRL) is a polypeptide hormone containing 198 amino acids and with a molecular weight (MW) of 22 kDa. It circulates in different molecular sizes—a monomeric (small) form (MW = 22 kDa), a polymeric (big) form (MW = 50 kDa), and an even larger polymeric (big-big) form (MW > 100 kDa). Big PRL is presumed to be a dimer and big-big PRL may represent an aggregation of monomeric molecules. The larger forms also contain added sugar moieties (glycosylation), which decreases biologic activity. The small form is biologically active and approximately 80% of the hormone is secreted in this form. Most immunoassays measure the small and large forms of PRL. The polymeric forms have reduced biologic activity and reduced binding to mammary tissue membranes. Women have been identified with high levels of PRL on routine immunoassay who are completely normal and have been found to have circulating polymeric forms on gel electrophoresis.

PRL is synthesized and stored in the pituitary gland in chromophobe cells called lactotrophs, which are located mainly in the lateral areas of the gland. PRL is encoded by its gene (10 kb) on chromosome 6. At the molecular level, it is stimulated and suppressed by a number of factors. The principal stimulating factor is thyroid-releasing hormone (TRH) and the major inhibiting factor is dopamine. Estrogen also enhances PRL secretion by enhancing the effects of TRH and inhibiting the effects of dopamine. A potential direct effect may also be mediated via galanin. The principal receptor with which dopamine interacts is D2, which is the target for various dopamine agonists used in the treatment of **hyperprolactinemia**.

In addition, PRL is synthesized in decidualized stroma of endometrial tissue. From these tissues, PRL is secreted into the circulation and, in the event of pregnancy, into the amniotic fluid. The control of decidual PRL is different from that of the pituitary and does not respond to dopamine. PRL is normally present in measurable amounts in serum, with mean levels of approximately 8 ng/mL in adult women. It circulates in an unbound form, has a 20-minute half-life, and is cleared by the liver and kidney. The main function of PRL is to stimulate the growth of mammary tissue as well as to produce and secrete milk into the alveoli; thus, it has mammogenic and lactogenic functions. Specific receptors for PRL are present in the plasma membrane of mammary cells, as well as in many other tissues.

PRL synthesis and release from the lactotrophs are controlled by central nervous system neurotransmitters, which act on the pituitary via the hypothalamus. The major control mechanism is inhibition, because pituitary stalk section results in increased PRL secretion. It appears that the major physiologic inhibitor of PRL release is the neurotransmitter dopamine, which acts directly on the pituitary gland. There are specific dopamine receptors on the lactotrophs, and dopamine inhibits PRL synthesis and release in pituitary cell cultures. Thus, dopamine appears to be the **prolactin-inhibiting factor** (PIF). Although a hypothalamic prolactin-releasing factor (PRF) has not been isolated, it is known that the neurotransmitter serotonin and thyrotropin-releasing factor stimulate PRL release. Because the latter stimulates PRL release only minimally unless infused, it appears that serotonin is a PRF or is responsible for its secretion. The rise in PRL levels during sleep appears to be controlled by serotonin.

PRL is secreted episodically and serum levels fluctuate throughout the day and throughout the menstrual cycle, with peak levels occurring at midcycle. Although changes in PRL levels are not as marked as the pulsatile episodes of luteinizing hormone (LH), estrogen stimulates PRL production and release. Under the influence of estrogen, PRL levels increase in females at the time of puberty.

During pregnancy, as estrogen levels increase, there is a concomitant hypertrophy and hyperplasia of the lactotrophs. The maternal increase in PRL levels occurs soon after implantation, concomitant with the increase in circulating estrogen. Circulating levels of PRL steadily increase throughout pregnancy, reaching approximately 200 ng/mL in the third trimester; the rise is directly related to the increase in circulating levels of estrogen. Despite the elevated PRL levels during pregnancy, lactation does not occur because estrogen inhibits the action of PRL on the breast, most likely blocking PRL's interaction with its receptor. A day or two following delivery of the placenta, estrogen and PRL levels decline rapidly and lactation is initiated. PRL levels reach basal levels in non-nursing women in 2 to 3 weeks. Although basal levels of circulating PRL decline to the nonpregnant range approximately 6 months after parturition in nursing women, following each act of suckling, PRL levels increase markedly and stimulate milk production for the next feeding.

Nipple and breast stimulation also increase PRL levels in the nonpregnant female, as does trauma to the chest wall. Other physiologic stimuli that increase PRL release are exercise, sleep, and stress. In addition, PRL levels normally rise following ingestion of the midday meal. Thus, PRL levels normally fluctuate throughout the day, with maximal levels observed during nighttime while asleep and a smaller increase occurring in the early afternoon. When the amount measured in the circulation in the nonpregnant woman exceeds a certain level, usually 20 to 25 ng/mL, the condition is called hyperprolactinemia. The optimal time to obtain a blood sample for assay to diagnose hyperprolactinemia is during the midmorning hours. Increases in PRL levels above the normal range can occur without a pathologic condition if the serum sample is drawn from a woman who has recently awakened, has exercised, or has had recent breast stimulation, such as breast palpation, during a physical examination.

The most frequent cause of slightly elevated PRL levels is stress, particularly the stress caused by visiting the physician's office. All women with initial PRL levels lower than 50 ng/mL should have subsequent samples drawn 60 minutes after resting in a quiet room to determine whether true pathologic hyperprolactinemia is present (**Fig. 39-1**).

Hyperprolactinemia can produce disorders of gonadotropin sex steroid function, resulting in menstrual cycle derangement (oligomenorrhea and amenorrhea) and anovulation, as well as inappropriate lactation, or **galactorrhea**. The mechanism whereby elevated PRL levels interfere with gonadotropin release appears to be related to abnormal gonadotropin-releasing hormone (GnRH) release. Women with hyperprolactinemia have abnormalities in the frequency and amplitude of LH pulsations, with a normal or increased gonadotropin response following GnRH infusion.

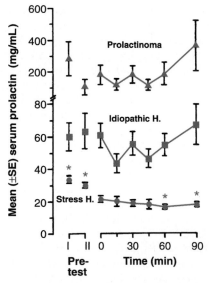

Figure 39-1 Serum prolactin levels (mean plus or minus standard error [±SE]) in women with prolactinoma ($N = 20$) and idiopathic ($N = 30$) and stress-related ($N = 20$) hyperprolactinemia before (pretest I and II) and during hyperprolactinemia test. Differences (*$P < .01$) are in relation to time zero values. (Mean prolactin values among groups were also significantly different [$P < .01$] at all times.) (From Muneyyirci-Delale O, Goldstein D, Reyes FI, et al: Diagnosis of stress-related hyperprolactinemia: Evaluation of the hyperprolactinemia rest test. NY State J Med 89:205, 1989.)

This abnormality of GnRH cyclicity thus inhibits gonadotropin release but not its synthesis. The reason for this abnormal secretion of GnRH is an inhibitory effect of dopamine and opioid peptides at the level of the hypothalamus. In addition, elevated PRL levels have been shown to interfere with the positive estrogen effect on midcycle LH release. It has also been shown that elevated levels of PRL directly inhibit basal and gonadotropin-stimulated ovarian secretion of estradiol and progesterone. However, this mechanism is probably not the primary cause of anovulation, because women with hyperprolactinemia can have ovulation induced with various agents, including pulsatile GnRH. Some women with moderate hyperprolactinemia, as determined by radioimmunoassay, have a greater than normal proportion of the big-big forms. Because of the reduced bioactivity of this form of PRL, they can have normal pituitary and ovarian function.

The clinician should measure serum PRL levels in all women with galactorrhea, as well as those with oligomenorrhea and amenorrhea not explained by another reason such as ovarian failure (elevated level of follicle-stimulating hormone [FSH]). Hyperprolactinemia has been reported to be present in 15% of all anovulatory women and 20% of women with amenorrhea of undetermined cause.

Because of possible clumping of PRL, if a tumor (adenoma) is suspected and values of PRL are only mildly elevated, the test should be done again in a diluted sample. This has been called the hook effect. Galactorrhea is defined as the nonpuerperal secretion of watery or milky fluid from the breast that contains neither pus nor blood. The fluid may appear spontaneously or after palpation. To determine whether galactorrhea is present, the clinician should palpate the breast, moving from the periphery toward the nipple in an attempt to express any secretion. The diagnosis of galactorrhea can be confirmed by observing multiple fat droplets in the fluid when examined under low-power magnification (**Fig. 39-2**). The incidence of galactorrhea in women with hyperprolactinemia has been reported to range from 30% to 80%, and these differences probably reflect variations in the techniques used to detect mammary excretion. Unless there has been continued breast stimulation after a pregnancy, the presence of galactorrhea serves as a biologic indicator that the PRL level is abnormally elevated.

CAUSES

Pathologic causes of hyperprolactinemia, in addition to a PRL-secreting pituitary adenoma (**prolactinoma**) and other pituitary tumors that produce acromegaly and Cushing's disease, include hypothalamic disease, various pharmacologic agents, hypothyroidism, chronic renal disease, or any chronic type of breast nerve stimulation, such as may occur with thoracic operation, herpes zoster, or chest trauma. **Box 39-1** lists the causes of hyperprolactinemia.

One of the most frequent causes of galactorrhea and hyperprolactinemia is the ingestion of pharmacologic agents, particularly tranquilizers, narcotics, and antihypertensive agents (**Box 39-2**). Of the tranquilizers, the phenothiazines and diazepam can produce hyperprolactinemia by depleting the hypothalamic circulation of dopamine or by blocking its binding sites and thus decreasing dopamine action.

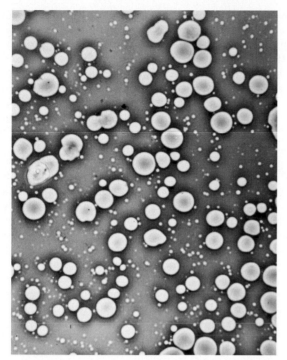

Figure 39-2 Fat droplets seen under microscope from a patient with galactorrhea. (From Kletzky OA, Davajan V: Hyperprolactinemia: Diagnosis and treatment. In Mishell DR, Davajan V, Lobo RA [eds]: Infertility, Contraception and Reproductive Endocrinology, 3rd ed. Cambridge, MA, Blackwell Scientific, 1991.)

Box 39-2 Pharmacologic Agents Affecting Prolactin Concentrations

Stimulators	Verapamil
Anesthetics, including cocaine	Dopamine receptor
Psychoactive drugs	antagonists
Phenothiazines	Metoclopramide
Tricyclic antidepressants	Antiemetics
Opiates	Sulpride
Chlordiazepoxide	Promazine
Amphetamines	Perphenazine
Diazepams	Others
Haloperidol	Cimetidine
Fluphenazine	Cyproheptiadine
Chlorpromazine	Protease inhibitors
SSRIs	Inhibitors
Hormones	L-Dopa
Estrogen	Dopamine
Oral-steroid contraceptives	Bromocriptine
Thyrotropin-releasing	Pergolide
hormone	Cabergoline
Antihypertensives	Depot bromocriptine
α-Methyldopa	SSRIs, selective serotonin
Reserpine	reuptake inhibitors

From Shoupe D, Mishell DR Jr: Hyperprolactinemia: Diagnosis and treatment. In Lobo RA, Mishell DR Jr, Paulson RJ, Shoupe D [eds]: Mishell's Textbook of Infertility, Contraception and Reproductive Endocrinology, 4th ed. Cambridge, MA, Blackwell Scientific, 1997.

Box 39-1 Causes of Hyperprolactinemia

Pituitary Disease	**Medications**
Prolactinomas	See Box 39-2.
Acromegaly	
Empty sella syndrome	**Neurogenic**
Lymphocytic hypophysitis	Chest wall lesions
Cushing's disease	Spinal cord lesions
	Breast stimulation
Hypothalamic Disease	
Craniopharyngiomas	**Other**
Meningiomas	Pregnancy
Dysgerminomas	Hypothyroidism
Nonsecreting pituitary	Chronic renal failure
adenomas	Cirrhosis
Other tumors	Pseudocyesis
Sarcoidosis	Adrenal insufficiency
Eosinophilic granuloma	Ectopic
Neuraxis irradiation	Polycystic ovary syndrome
Vascular	Idiopathic
Pituitary stalk section	

From Molitch ME: Prolactinoma. In Melmed S (ed): The Pituitary, 2nd ed. Malden, MA, Blackwell, 2002, pp 455-495.

The tricyclic antidepressants block dopamine uptake and propranolol, haloperidol, phentolamine, and cyproheptadine block hypothalamic dopamine receptors. The antihypertensive agent reserpine depletes catecholamines, and methyldopa blocks the conversion of tyrosine to dihydroxyphenylalanine (dopa). Ingestion of oral contraceptive steroids can also increase PRL levels, with a greater incidence of hyperprolactinemia occurring with higher estrogen formulations. Nevertheless, galactorrhea does not usually occur during oral contraceptive ingestion because the exogenous estrogen blocks the binding of PRL to its receptors.

Women who develop galactorrhea while ingesting oral contraceptives or any of the other drugs listed in **Box 39-2** should ideally discontinue the medication, and the PRL level should be measured 1 month thereafter to determine if the level has returned to normal. If the medication cannot be discontinued, the PRL level should be measured and, if elevated above 100 ng/mL, imaging of the sella turcica should be performed to determine whether a **macroadenoma** is present.

Primary hypothyroidism can also produce hyperprolactinemia and galactorrhea because of decreased negative feedback of thyroxine (T_4) on the hypothalamic-pituitary axis. The resulting increase in TRH stimulates PRL secretion and thyroid-stimulating hormone (TSH) secretion from the pituitary. Approximately 3% to 5% of individuals with hyperprolactinemia have hypothyroidism, so TSH, the most sensitive indicator of hypothyroidism, should be measured in all individuals with hyperprolactinemia. If the TSH level is elevated, triiodothyronine (T_3) and T_4 should be measured to confirm the diagnosis of primary hypothyroidism, because a TSH-secreting pituitary adenoma will occasionally be present. Treatment with appropriate thyroid replacement usually returns the TSH and PRL levels to normal within a short time.

Hyperprolactinemia can occur in those with abnormal renal disease resulting from decreased metabolic clearance and increased production rate. The cause of the latter is unknown.

Mild hyperprolactinemia (30 to 50 ng/mL) may occur in women with polycystic ovary syndrome (PCOS). This occurs in up to 30% of women and may be related to the chromic state of unopposed estrogen stimulation.

CENTRAL NERVOUS SYSTEM DISORDERS

Hypothalamic Causes

Diseases of the hypothalamus that produce alterations in the normal portal circulation of dopamine can result in hyperprolactinemia. These include **craniopharyngioma** and infiltration of the hypothalamus by sarcoidosis, histiocytosis, leukemia, or carcinoma. All these conditions are rare, with craniopharyngioma being the most common. These tumors arise from remnants of Rathke's pouch along the pituitary stalk. Grossly, they can be cystic, solid, or mixed, and calcification is usually visible on a radiograph. They are most frequently diagnosed during the second and third decades of life and usually result in impairment of secretion of several pituitary hormones.

Pituitary Causes

Various types of pituitary tumors, lactotroph hyperplasia, and the **empty sella syndrome** can be associated with hyperprolactinemia. It has been estimated that as many as 80% of all pituitary adenomas secrete PRL. The most common pituitary tumor associated with hyperprolactinemia is the prolactinoma, arbitrarily defined as a **microadenoma** if its diameter is less than 1 cm and as a macroadenoma if it is larger (**Fig. 39-3**). Hyperprolactinemia has been reported to occur in approximately 25% of those with acromegaly and 10% of those with Cushing's disease, indicating that these pituitary adenomas, which mainly secrete growth hormone (GH) and adrenocorticotropic hormone (ACTH), frequently also secrete PRL. Hyperplasia of lactotrophs has been reported to occur in approximately 8% of pituitary glands examined at autopsy. Individuals with hyperplasia of the lactotrophs cannot be distinguished from those having a microadenoma by any clinical, laboratory, or radiologic method. The diagnosis can be made only at the time of surgical exploration of the pituitary gland. Pituitary enlargement with suprasellar extension caused by lactotroph hyperplasia has been reported. *Functional hyperprolactinemia* is the term used for the clinical diagnosis of cases of elevated PRL levels without imaging evidence of an adenoma.

Another cause of hyperprolactinemia is the primary empty sella syndrome. The term *primary empty sella syndrome* describes a clinical situation in which an intrasellar extension of the subarachnoid space results in compression of the pituitary gland and an enlarged sella turcica. The cause is believed to result from a congenital or acquired (by radiation or surgery) defect in the sella diaphragm that allows the subarachnoid membrane to herniate into the sella turcica (**Fig. 39-4**). The syndrome is usually associated with normal pituitary function, except for hyperprolactinemia. Although some with primary empty sella syndrome have a coexistent prolactinoma, Gharib and colleagues have reported a series of 11 patients with an empty sella and hyperprolactinemia who had no histologic evidence of a prolactinoma or hyperplasia of the lactotrophs. They stated that approximately 5% of those with the empty sella have hyperprolactinemia, amenorrhea-galactorrhea, or both. It is theorized that with this syndrome, distortion of the infundibular stalk results in decreased levels of dopamine reaching the pituitary to inhibit PRL. Serum PRL levels are usually less than 100 ng/mL with the empty sella syndrome, and some women with this syndrome have normal PRL levels, with or without galactorrhea. Kleinberg and coworkers have reported that approximately 10% of all individuals with an enlarged sella turcica have the empty sella syndrome. The best modality for diagnosing this condition is magnetic resonance imaging (MRI). It is important to establish the diagnosis because the syndrome has a benign course.

PROLACTINOMAS

In an unselected series of 120 autopsies of individuals with no clinical evidence of pituitary disease, Burrow and associates found pituitary microadenomas to be present in 32 (27%). Molitch has noted that PRL incidentalomas occur in 11% of subjects at autopsy. It has also been reported that adenomas were found in 78 of 486 (16%) pituitary glands examined after unselected autopsies. In all series, PRL was found in approximately 50% of the glands, indicating that more than 10% of those in the general population have a prolactinoma.

Overall, approximately 50% of women with hyperprolactinemia have a prolactinoma. The incidence is higher when the PRL levels exceed 100 ng/mL, and almost all individuals with PRL levels greater than 200 ng/mL have a prolactinoma. The vast majority of prolactinomas in women are microadenomas. Kleinberg and coworkers have reported that 20% of those with galactorrhea and 35% of women with amenorrhea-galactorrhea have radiologic evidence of pituitary tumors.

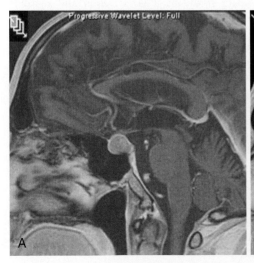

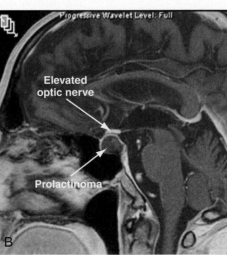

Figure 39-3 *Left,* MRI scan of the side view of the head (midway through the brain) showing a prolactinoma. *Right,* Same image, colorized, showing that the top part of the tumor (shown in red) elevates the optic nerve (actually, the optic chiasm) (From Conditions programs and conditions treated. UCLA Health System; Neurosurgery 3:31, 2010.)

Figure 39-4 Diagrammatic representation of empty sella syndrome. **A,** Normal anatomic relationship. **B-D,** Progression in development of empty sella syndrome. Note thinning of the floor and symmetrical enlargement of the sella turcica. (From Kletzky OA, Davajan V: Hyperprolactinemia: Diagnosis and treatment. In Mishell DR, Davajan V, Lobo RA [eds]: Infertility, Contraception and Reproductive Endocrinology, 3 rd ed. Cambridge, MA, Blackwell Scientific, 1991.)

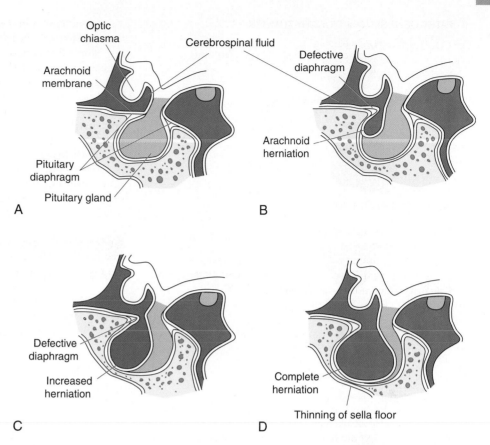

Tumors are also present in approximately 20% of women with hyperprolactinemia and menstrual irregularities without galactorrhea. The incidence of prolactinoma is greater in those with a more profound disturbance of normal hypothalamic-pituitary-ovarian function. Approximately 70% of women with hyperprolactinemia and galactorrhea, and secondary amenorrhea with low estrogen levels, have radiologic evidence of a pituitary adenoma. Evidence of a tumor occurs in only 20% to 30% of those with hyperprolactinemia and normal menses, oligomenorrhea, or secondary amenorrhea with normal estrogen status. No adenoma is found characteristically in individuals with normal menses, galactorrhea, and normal PRL levels. **Figure 39-5** depicts various possible causes of prolactinoma formation. In the past, it was firmly believed that adenomas or hyperplasia were the result of hypothalamic dopamine dysregulation, which was a functional defect or the result of altered blood supply. It is now believed that adenomas arise from single cell mutations, with clonal proliferation occurring subsequently. However, a search for mutations in oncogenes, the dopamine D2 or TRH receptor, signal transduction mechanisms, or transcription factors have not been rewarding to date. Prolactinomas that occur in 20% of patients with multiple endocrine neoplasia type 1 (MEN-1) may be caused by an inactivating mutation of the *MENIN* gene, although this special case is clearly different from the usual type of prolactinomas.

It is also important to note that prolactinomas may also secrete other hormones; GH is the most frequent combination. Also, up to 40% of GH-secreting adenomas also secrete PRL. Combinations of PRL and ACTH, PRL and TSH, and PRL and FSH have been described.

Long-term studies of individuals with microadenomas have demonstrated that enlargement is uncommon and that many of these tumors regress spontaneously. In a longitudinal retrospective study of women with hyperprolactinemia and a radiologic diagnosis of microadenoma, March and colleagues found that only 2 of 43 women had evidence of enlargement of the adenoma, with a mean duration of follow-up of 5 years. Of these 43 women, 3 had spontaneous regression of their hyperprolactinemia and resumption of normal menses. Koppelman and associates have reported similar results. Of 25 women with prolactinomas (18 with microadenomas and 7 with minimally enlarged sella) followed up for a mean duration of 11 years without treatment, only 1 woman had slight progression of a sella abnormality. None had visual field or other pituitary function changes, 7 resumed normal menses spontaneously, and galactorrhea spontaneously resolved in 6.

The results of these retrospective studies have been confirmed by two prospective studies of untreated microprolactinomas. In a 3- to 7-year prospective longitudinal study of 30 hyperprolactinemic women, Schlechte and coworkers found that of 13 women with initially abnormal radiographic findings, 4 became normal, 7 did not change, and 2 had evidence of tumor growth. Of 17 women with initially normal radiographic findings, 4 became minimally abnormal. None of the 30 developed a macroadenoma or pituitary hypofunction. In this study, as in the two retrospective studies reported earlier, more sensitive radiographic techniques (e.g., tomography, followed by computed tomography [CT]) were used as the study progressed and could account for the minimal evidence of tumor growth. Sisam and colleagues have overcome this problem by prospectively following a group

PATHOGENESIS OF PITUITARY TUMORS

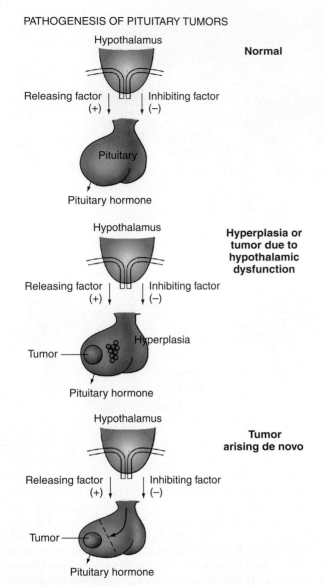

Figure 39-5 Possible mechanisms leading to the formation of a prolactinoma. *Top,* Normal regulation. *Middle,* Tumors could arise because of an increase in PRL-releasing factor (PRF) or a decrease in PRL-inhibiting factor (dopamine). *Bottom,* Tumors could arise de novo without hypothalamic influence. (From Molitch ME: Clinical features and epidemiology of prolactinomas in women. In Olefsky JM, Robbins RJ [eds]: Prolactinomas: Practical Diagnosis and Management. New York, Churchill Livingstone, 1986, pp 67-95.)

of 38 women with hyperprolactinemia and microprolactinomas by serial CT scans for a mean duration of 50 months. None of these women had evidence of tumor progression, even the 2 who had a marked increase in PRL levels. In this group, 9 (25%) had spontaneous improvement of their symptoms. Martin and co-workers have followed the natural history of 41 women with idiopathic hyperprolactinemia and amenorrhea-galactorrhea for up to 11 years. During this time, 9 women conceived spontaneously and 16 resumed spontaneous menses with cessation of galactorrhea. Only 1 woman developed a microadenoma. Thus, hyperprolactinemia with or without a microadenoma follows a benign clinical course in most women, and therapy is unnecessary unless pregnancy is desired or estrogen levels are low.

A combination of six studies in 139 women observed for at least 8 years without treatment has shown that the progression rate is only 6.5%. Several studies have reported that pregnancy is beneficial for women with functional hyperprolactinemia or PRL-secreting microadenomas. Following pregnancy, PRL levels decrease in approximately 50% of women. Crosignani and associates have reported that PRL levels normalized in approximately 30% of 176 hyperprolactinemic women after pregnancy. PRL levels decreased to normal in 36% of women with functional hyperprolactinemia and 17% of those with adenomas. Therefore, if women with hyperprolactinemia desire to become pregnant, they should be encouraged to do so, because pregnancy is likely to result in normal or lowered PRL levels.

DIAGNOSTIC TECHNIQUES

IMAGING STUDIES

Because most prolactinomas are microadenomas that do not cause enlargement of the sella turcica, the diagnosis usually cannot be made by ordinary anteroposterior and lateral coned X-ray examination of the sella turcica. With the development of more precise radiologic methods that can detect soft tissue pituitary abnormalities, it is now possible to detect even small adenomas.

Current recommended techniques are to obtain a CT scan with IV contrast or an MRI with gadolinium enhancement. The latter provides better soft tissue definition and the CT scan principally shows bony structural abnormalities. The MRI provides 1-mm resolution and thus should be able to detect all microadenomas. Stein and associates have compared results of CT and MRI in 22 individuals with suspected pituitary adenomas. MRI was found to be the superior diagnostic modality because of its greater soft tissue contrast (**Fig. 39-6**). In addition, MRI does not have the radiation exposure of a CT scan (23 rad; 0.03 Gy).

RECOMMENDED DIAGNOSTIC EVALUATION

It is recommended that PRL levels be measured in all women with galactorrhea, oligomenorrhea, or amenorrhea who do not have an elevated FSH level. These are also frequently measured in the workup of infertility. If the PRL level is elevated, a TSH assay should be performed to rule out the presence of primary hypothyroidism. If the TSH level is elevated, T_3 and T_4 should be measured to rule out the rare possibility of a TSH-secreting pituitary adenoma. If the TSH level is elevated and hypothyroidism is present, appropriate thyroid replacement should begin and the PRL level will usually return to normal. If the TSH level is normal and the woman has a normal PRL level with galactorrhea, no further tests are necessary if she has regular menses.

If PRL levels are elevated and the TSH level is normal, an MRI (preferably) or CT scan should be obtained to detect a microadenoma or macroadenoma. Macroadenomas are uncommon and rarely present with a PRL level less than 100 ng/mL. If the PRL level is more than 100 ng/mL or the woman complains of headaches or visual changes, the likelihood of a tumor extending beyond the sella turcica is increased. Microadenomas are a common cause of hyperprolactinemia, but rarely enlarge. Neither pregnancy, oral contraceptives, nor hormone replacement therapy stimulates the growth of these small tumors; therapy

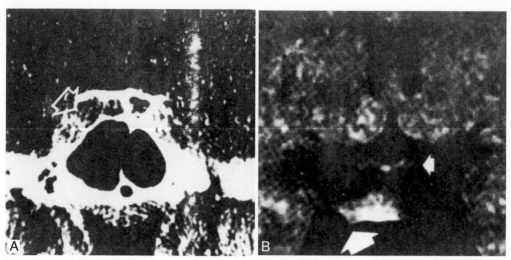

Figure 39-6 Comparison of results of CT and MRI evealuation of suspected pituitary adenomas. Images were selected to demonstrate pathology best and do not exactly correspond in level of section through the sella turcica. **A,** CT scan (coronal section) showing bony erosion of right sella turcica (*arrowhead*), with possible soft tissue extension into right cavernous sinus. Height of pituitary gland (not shown) is 9 mm. **B,** MRI (coronal section) showing soft tissue mass extending into right cavernous sinus near carotid artery (*large arrowhead*). Height of pituitary gland is 9 mm. Normal optic chiasm is seen (*small arrowhead*). (From Stein AL, Levenick MN, Kletzky OA: Computer tomography versus magnetic resonance imaging for the evaluation of suspected pituitary adenomas. Obstet Gynecol 73:996, 1989.)

is unnecessary unless ovulation induction is desired or hypoestrogenism is present.

Visual field determination and tests of ACTH level sand thyroid function are not necessary if a microadenoma is present, because these small tumors do not interfere with overall pituitary function and do not extend beyond the sella. However, these evaluations should be performed in those with macroadenomas because suprasellar extension of the tumor may exert pressure on the optic chiasm, resulting in bitemporal visual field defects and interference with vision. The size of these tumors may also affect other aspects of pituitary function. With a macroadenoma, other dynamic tests of pituitary function should be performed.

TREATMENT

EXPECTANT TREATMENT

Women with radiologic evidence of a microadenoma or functional hyperprolactinemia who do not wish to conceive may be followed without treatment by measuring PRL levels once annually. Many of these women have deficient estrogen, and low estrogen levels in combination with hyperprolactinemia have been shown to be associated with the early onset of osteoporosis. If the woman has low estrogen levels, exogenous estrogen should be administered. Replacement estrogen-progestin therapy, as is used for postmenopausal women, or oral contraceptives can be used. Corenblum and Donovan have reported that a group of women with functional hyperprolactinemia and PRL-secreting pituitary microadenomas who were treated with cyclic estrogen and progestin or oral contraceptives for several years did not have an increase in the size of the adenomas or a marked increase in PRL levels. Mean PRL levels actually declined with both treatment regimens. Testa has reported that 2 years of oral contraceptive use in a group of women with hyperprolactinemia with microadenoma does not alter the size of the adenoma. Because side effects and cost are less and compliance is better with

exogenous estrogen than with dopamine agonist therapy, it is not necessary to use unless ovulation and pregnancy are desired. Those with hyperprolactinemia, with or without microadenomas, who have adequate estrogen levels, as shown by the presence of oligomenorrhea or amenorrhea with follicular phase estradiol levels, who do not wish to conceive should be treated with periodic progestogen withdrawal (e.g., medroxyprogesterone acetate, 5 to 10 mg/day for 10 days each month) or with combination oral contraceptives to prevent endometrial hyperplasia.

MEDICAL TREATMENT

The initial treatment for women with macroadenomas, as well as for women with hyperprolactinemia who are anovulatory and wish to conceive, should be administration of a dopamine receptor agonist. **Bromocriptine**, pergolide, and **cabergoline** have been used with success for treating hyperprolactinemia.

Bromocriptine

The greatest amount of clinical experience has been with the use of bromocriptine. This semisynthetic ergot alkaloid was developed in 1967 to inhibit PRL secretion. It directly stimulates dopamine 2 receptors and, as a dopamine receptor agonist, it inhibits PRL secretion in vitro and in vivo. After ingestion, bromocriptine is rapidly absorbed, with blood levels reaching a peak 1 to 3 hours later. Serum PRL levels remain depressed for approximately 14 hours after ingestion of a single dose, after which time the drug is not detectable in the circulation. Therefore, the drug is usually given at least twice daily, with initial therapy being started at half of the 2.5-mg tablet to minimize side effects. The most frequent side effects are orthostatic hypotension, with an incidence of 15%, which can produce fainting and dizziness as well as nausea and vomiting. To minimize these symptoms, the initial dose should be taken in bed and with food at nighttime. Less frequent adverse symptoms include headache, nasal congestion, fatigue, constipation, and diarrhea. Most of these reactions are mild, occur early in the course of treatment, and are

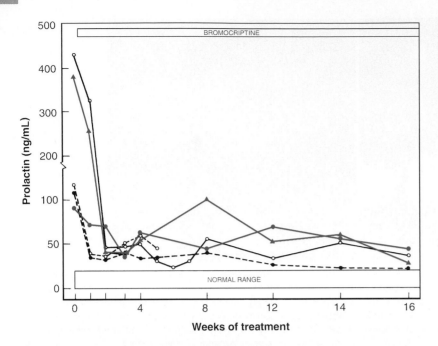

Figure 39-7 Mean serum prolactin response to bromocriptine therapy in five patients with radiographic evidence of pituitary adenoma and residual hyperprolactinemia. All five ovulated, and four conceived. (From Kletzky OA, Marrs RP, Davajan V: Management of patients with hyperprolactinemia and normal or abnormal tomograms. Am J Obstet Gynecol 147:528, 1983.)

transient. To reduce the adverse symptoms, the dose should be gradually increased every 1 to 2 weeks until PRL levels fall to normal. The therapeutic dose is usually titrated to normalize PRL (**Fig. 39-7**). Adverse effects such as nausea, vomiting, and nasal congestion occur in approximately 50% of women taking oral bromocriptine and may cause them to discontinue treatment. Vermesh and colleagues have reported that the drug is well absorbed vaginally, without side effects. Furthermore, when a single tablet is placed deep into the posterior vaginal fornix, therapeutic blood levels persist for more than 24 hours, during which time PRL levels remain suppressed. Ginsburg and coworkers have subsequently reported that this method of bromocriptine administration is well accepted, effective, and well tolerated in a group of 31 hyperprolactinemic women, 17 of whom could not tolerate oral bromocriptine. Minor side effects occurred in only 3 women. The tablet was digitally placed deep into the vagina nightly at bedtime. A single 2.5-mg dose reduced PRL concentrations in 90% of patients treated and brought the levels to normal in one third of the women. Higher doses did not appear to be more effective.

Bromocriptine is approved for the treatment of adverse symptoms associated with hyperprolactinemia, such as galactorrhea, as well as anovulatory infertility, with and without the presence of a PRL-secreting adenoma. In hyperprolactinemic women without adenomas, PRL levels return to normal in more than 90%, fertility is restored in 80%, and galactorrhea is eradicated in 60% of women with bromocriptine therapy. In women with hyperprolactinemia and a microadenoma, similar rates of success have been reported. Therefore, a dopamine agonist such as bromocriptine or cabergoline is the treatment of choice for women with PRL-secreting microadenomas who wish to ovulate or are bothered by galactorrhea.

Cabergoline

Cabergoline is a long-acting dopamine receptor agonist. This agent directly inhibits pituitary lactotrophs, thereby decreasing PRL secretion. It is given orally in doses of 0.25 to 1.0 mg twice weekly. The initial dose is half a 0.5-mg tablet twice a week. Peak plasma levels occur in 2 to 3 hours, and the drug has a half-life of 65 hours. Its slow elimination and long half-life produce a prolonged PRL-lowering effect. The initial dose is 0.25 mg twice weekly and the dosage may be increased at intervals of 4 weeks to achieve a satisfactory response. In a randomized trial with bromocriptine, cabergoline lowered PRL levels to normal in 83% of women, induced ovulation in 72%, and eliminated galactorrhea in 90%. The effectiveness of cabergoline was greater than that of bromocriptine. Adverse effects, particularly nausea, headaches, and dizziness, occurred with both agents but were less frequent, less severe, and of shorter duration with cabergoline. Therefore, cabergoline is better tolerated than bromocriptine and has higher continuation rates. Studies have suggested that cabergoline is more effective in lowering the PRL level than bromocriptine. Even in patients who had been treated previously with bromocriptine, cabergoline has been found to be effective (**Table 39-1**).

Cabergoline has been compared with other agents in regard to effectiveness for reducing tumor size (see **Table 39-1**). It may be concluded that in women who have never been treated, cabergoline is the agent of choice for reducing PRL levels and effecting tumor shrinkage. It is recommended that after serum PRL levels have remained normal for 6 months, cabergoline be discontinued to determine whether the PRL levels stay low without therapy. A potential concern with cabergoline and pergolide (now not available) is the development of cardiac valvular lesions. However, this has only been observed with large doses, as used for Parkinson's disease, and has not been reported with lower doses.

Outcomes

Although cabergoline is currently the dopamine agonist of choice, bromocriptine is preferred when use in pregnancy is contemplated because of its longer experience of use during pregnancy. If pregnancy occurs after ovulation is induced with bromocriptine, therapy is usually discontinued, although there is no evidence that the drug is teratogenic or adversely affects

Table 39-1 Comparison of Efficacy of Dopamine Agonists in Affecting Tumor Size Reduction*

Dopamine Agonist	No. of Cases	Tumor Size Reduction (%)			
		>50	25-50	<25	No Change
Bromocriptine	112	40.2	28.6	12.5	18.7
Pergolide	61	75.4	9.8	8.2	6.5
Quinagolide	105	48.1	20.2	17.3	14.4
Cabergoline	130	25.4	46.9	6.9	21.5

*It should be noted that in many of the studies of pergolide, quinagolide, and cabergoline, many patients had previously been found to be resistant to or intolerant of bromocriptine.

Adapted from Molitch ME: Prolactin in human reproduction. In Strauss JF III, Barbieri R (eds): Yen and Jaffe's Reproductive Endocrinology. Philadelphia, Elsevier, 2004, p 109.

pregnancy outcome. If pregnancy is not desired but bromocriptine is used to treat galactorrhea, therapy is usually continued for at least 12 months, after which it should be discontinued for a few weeks. Most women with microadenomas have recurrence of hyperprolactinemia, amenorrhea, and galactorrhea, although approximately 10% to 20% have permanent remission after discontinuing bromocriptine treatment.

Moriondo and associates have reported that after 1 year of bromocriptine treatment, 11% of women with microadenomas have persistent normalization of PRL levels, with return of regular menses after the drug is discontinued (**Fig. 39-8**). This incidence of permanent remission reached 22% after 2 years of treatment. A higher rate of permanent remission occurred in women treated with 10 mg/day than with lower dosages, but higher drug doses increase the incidence of adverse reactions and result in discontinuation of treatment. These investigators found that after bromocriptine was discontinued, there was a 40% reduction in mean PRL levels in all women treated, and approximately 60% had a more than 30% reduction from pretreatment PRL levels after the drug was discontinued.

Rasmussen and colleagues have reported the results of discontinuation of long-term (median, 2 years) bromocriptine therapy in 75 hyperprolactinemic women. In approximately 50% of the women, it was necessary to reinstate treatment because PRL

levels rose. However, in the other half, further treatment was unnecessary because mean PRL levels decreased more than 60% and returned to normal or were only slightly elevated. More than 50% of these 33 women resumed regular menses without further treatment. These data indicate that the remissions were drug-related and not spontaneous. Using CT before and during bromocriptine therapy, Bonneville and coworkers have found that approximately 75% of individuals with microadenomas have a reduction in tumor size during bromocriptine treatment and, in 40%, the tumor disappeared. To determine whether permanent remission has occurred, the PRL level should be measured approximately 6 weeks after discontinuation of treatment because the levels plateau at this time.

Recent data by Kharlip and coworkers have suggested that this recurrence rate (increase in PRL level) after cabergoline with microadenomas and macroadenomas was 50% to 60% within the first 18 months. There was no increase in tumor size with cessation of cabergoline. Although close follow-up is recommended, the Pituitary Society still recommends withdrawal from therapy in select patients.

Bromocriptine treatment has also been shown to reduce tumor mass in 80% to 90% of those with macroadenomas. In addition, visual disturbances, if present, are usually promptly relieved. Following subsequent surgical removal of these

Figure 39-8 Serum prolactin levels in four patients who had persistently normal prolactin levels after bromocriptine (BRC) treatment for 12 months. *P*, Pregnancy. (From Moriondo P, Travaglini P, Nissim M, et al: Bromocriptine treatment of microprolactinomas: Evidence of stable prolactin decrease after drug withdrawal. J Clin Endocrinol Metab 60:764, 1985.)

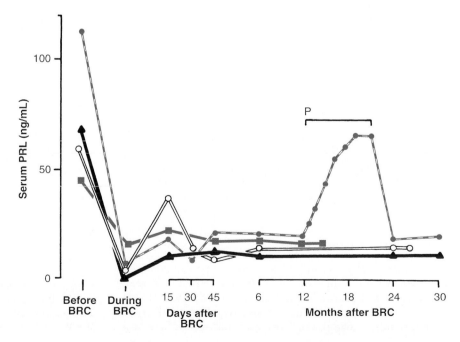

bromocriptine-treated tumors, histologic examination revealed a reduction of tumor cell size, with shrinkage of the cytoplasm being larger than the nucleus. In addition, there are modifications of cell structure and morphology as compared with tumors removed without prior medical treatment. The organelles responsible for PRL synthesis shrink, indicating that bromocriptine impairs PRL synthesis and release. The reduction in size of macroadenomas usually occurs rapidly, within a few weeks after starting treatment, but following withdrawal of drug the tumor size may increase just as rapidly. Thus, the drug should be withdrawn cautiously. In contrast to the frequent occurrence of pituitary insufficiency, including diabetes insipidus, after surgical or radiologic treatment of large tumors, bromocriptine treatment is not accompanied by any type of pituitary insufficiency.

Because permanent remission rarely occurs following withdrawal of bromocriptine treatment from individuals with large tumors, long-term treatment is usually necessary. The drug has been administered in some individuals for up to 12 years without problems and, once biochemical, radiologic, and clinical responses to treatment are established, they are generally maintained over a long-term period. Bromocriptine has also been successfully used to treat those with failure of, or recurrence after, surgical or irradiation therapy.

Molitch and associates have reported the results of a 1-year prospective multicenter study of the use of bromocriptine as primary therapy for PRL-secreting macroadenomas in 27 individuals. Bromocriptine dosage ranged from 5 to 12.5 mg daily, with 7.5 mg being the most frequent dose. PRL levels fell in all individuals and to 11% or less of pretreatment values in all but 1. Of this group, two thirds had PRL levels decrease to normal during treatment. Tumor shrinkage was observed in all individuals, reduced by more than 50% in half the patients and by approximately 50% in an additional 20% of the study group. Visual field impairment disappeared in 9 of 10 individuals with abnormalities. In two thirds of patients, reduction in tumor size occurred by 6 weeks, but in one third it was not evident until 6 months, indicating that there were rapid and slow responses of tumor to drug treatment. Therefore, at least a 6-month trial of medical therapy is warranted for those with a macroadenoma. Because of these excellent results, the poor initial results of operation, and the high recurrence rates, it was concluded that bromocriptine should be used as the initial management of those with PRL-secreting macroadenomas. After maximal shrinkage of tumor, medical therapy can be continued or operative treatment initiated. The cost of continuing bromocriptine treatment is considerable; it is inconvenient to take medication several times a day, and some people have unpleasant side effects with the higher dosages that may be necessary. Therefore, some prefer operative treatment. If they elect to have an operation, the drug should be continued until the time of operation to prevent tumor expansion. The rates of success after operation are no different in those who received or did not receive bromocriptine before surgery.

OPERATIVE APPROACHES

Trans-sphenoidal microsurgical resection of prolactinoma has been widely used for therapy, and numerous reports of large series of individuals treated by this technique have been published. In general, trans-sphenoidal operations have minimal risk, with a mortality of less than 0.5%. However, most deaths have been reported to occur after treatment of macroadenomas. The risk of temporary postoperative diabetes insipidus is 10% to 40%, but the risk of permanent diabetes insipidus and iatrogenic hypopituitarism is less than 2%. The initial cure rate, with normalization of PRL levels and return of ovulation, is relatively high for microadenomas (65% to 85%) but less so with macroadenomas (20% to 40%). Vision can return to normal in 85% of patients with loss of acuity and visual field defects.

The initial cure rate is related to the pretreatment PRL levels. Those tumors with PRL levels less than 100 ng/mL have an excellent prognosis (85%) and those with levels higher than 200 ng/mL have a poor prognosis (35%). Operative treatment of tumors in individuals older than 26 years with amenorrhea for longer than 6 months carries a poorer prognosis than tumors in younger women with a shorter duration of amenorrhea. Nevertheless, long-term follow-up of patients after operation has indicated that late recurrence of hyperprolactinemia is common. Serri and colleagues followed 28 women with microadenomas and 16 with macroadenomas for 6 years after operation. Although PRL levels normalized and menses resumed in 24 (85%) of those with microadenomas and 5 (31%) of those with macroadenomas who had a good initial postoperative response, hyperprolactinemia recurred in 50% of those with microadenoma and 4 of 5 with macroadenomas after a mean period of 4 and 2.5 years, respectively (**Fig. 39-9**). There was no significant difference in recurrence rates for those who conceived and those who did not. Rodman and coworkers have reported a lower postoperative recurrence rate (≈20% for both microadenomas and macroadenomas) following initial cure rates of 85% and 37%, respectively. The risk of recurrence in both series appeared to be related to the immediate postoperative PRL levels being higher in those with a PRL level higher than 10 ng/mL.

Overall, it can be concluded that after surgery, recurrence rates for microadenomas or macroadenomas are similar (21% and 19.8%, respectively). Long-term surgical cure rates are 58% for microadenomas but only 26% for macroadenomas using a normal PRL level as a criterion.

Because of the good results with medical therapy, surgery is recommended only for women with macroadenoma who fail

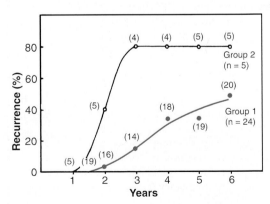

Figure 39-9 Cumulative recurrence rate in patients with microprolactinoma (group 1) or macroprolactinoma (group 2) after initially successful operation. Figures in parentheses indicate number of patients who were seen at each yearly interval. (From Serri O, Rasio E, Beauregard H, et al: Recurrence of hyperprolactinemia after selective transsphenoidal adenomectomy in women with prolactinoma. N Engl J Med 309:280, 1983.)

to respond to medical therapy or have poor compliance with this regimen. It is best to reduce the size of macroadenomas maximally with bromocriptine before surgical removal of these extrasellar tumors.

RADIATION THERAPY

External radiation with cobalt, proton beam, or heavy particle therapy and brachytherapy with yttrium-90 rods implanted in the pituitary have all been used to treat macroadenomas but are not the primary mode of treatment. More recently, the method of choice is probably the gamma knife and linear accelerator. Results have been inconsistent and damage to normal pituitary tissue may occur, leading to abnormal anterior pituitary function and diabetes insipidus. Damage to the optic nerves may also occur, which led to the more precise technique of the gamma knife. Thus, radiation therapy should be used only as adjunctive management following incomplete operative removal of large tumors.

PREGNANCY AND TREATMENT

Women with Hyperprolactinemia Who Wish to Conceive

Many women with hyperprolactinemia, with or without adenomas, wish to become pregnant. A small percentage of these women conceive spontaneously, but most require treatment to induce ovulation. Barbieri and Ryan have compiled a literature review of the pregnancy courses of 275 women with adenomas, most of whose conceptions had been induced by bromocriptine. They reported that of 215 women with microprolactinomas, less than 1% had changes in visual fields, radiologic evidence of tumor enlargement, or neurologic signs. Approximately 5% developed headaches during pregnancy. Of 60 women with macroprolactinomas, 20% developed adverse changes in their visual field and polytomographic or neurologic signs during pregnancy, and some of them required bromocriptine or operative treatment during pregnancy or shortly postpartum. Overall, although only 1.4% of women with microadenomas have symptoms during pregnancy, 24.4% of women with macroadenomas have symptoms. However, only approximately 3% of women with macroadenomas have symptoms if they are treated prior to pregnancy. Thus, excision of macroprolactinomas before pregnancy has been recommended in some cases. Nevertheless, because pituitary function is usually diminished after operation, induction of ovulation must be performed with complicated and expensive gonadotropin treatment. Bromocriptine treatment does not interfere with pituitary function and is thus the therapy of choice for women with macroadenomas who wish to conceive. Continuous bromocriptine treatment throughout pregnancy for women with macroadenomas has been recommended by some because, with this therapy, visual disturbances are rare. Despite a lowering of PRL levels, there is no effect on placental hormone production and pregnancy outcome does not appear to be affected.

Nevertheless, because bromocriptine crosses the placenta and suppresses fetal PRL levels, its long-term effects on the newborn are unknown. It is now advised that women with macroadenomas discontinue the drug after conception, as is the case for those with microadenomas, and have therapy reinitiated if and when symptoms of visual disturbance or severe headaches occur. Most women who conceive after bromocriptine treatment have ingested the drug for a few weeks after conception. In a review of 1410 such pregnancies compiled by Turkalj and associates, there was a spontaneous abortion rate of 11%, ectopic pregnancy rate of 0.7%, and twin pregnancy rate of 1.8%. The incidence of minor (2.5%) and major (1%) congenital defects was similar to pregnancy outcomes in untreated populations of women. The mean amount of drug ingested and duration of postconception treatment were similar in mothers who had normal children and those with defects. Thus, ingestion of bromocriptine during pregnancy does not appear to increase the risk of congenital abnormalities, spontaneous abortion, or multiple gestation. Postnatal surveillance of more than 200 children born in this series has revealed no adverse effects to date.

Ruiz-Velasco and Tolis have compiled the obstetric histories of almost 2000 pregnancies occurring in hyperprolactinemic women that have been reported in the literature. Most of these pregnancies were induced with bromocriptine. There was a full-term delivery rate of 85%, an abortion rate of 11%, a prematurity rate of 2%, and a multiple pregnancy rate of 1.2%. Although PRL levels increased during pregnancy, after delivery the levels returned to pretreatment values in approximately 85% of these women. A postpartum increase over pretreatment levels was uncommon (3%), and PRL levels returned to normal in 13%. Similarly, among women who had postpartum radiologic sellar examination, 84% showed no change, 9% improved, and 7% worsened. Thus, stopping treatment during pregnancy only occasionally results in tumor growth. It is advised that women with macroadenomas have a monthly visual field examination and neurologic testing during pregnancy, but this is probably unnecessary for women with microadenomas unless they develop symptoms of headache or visual disturbances.

Following delivery, breast-feeding may be initiated without adverse effects on the tumors. Godo and associates have reported that use of bromocriptine before conception and during pregnancy does not affect the incidence of persistent lactation following discontinuation of nursing. The incidence of menstrual abnormalities and degree of galactorrhea were usually similar to the state that existed before starting bromocriptine therapy. Therefore, following completion of nursing, as well as for women who do not breast-feed at all, bromocriptine should be ingested for 2 to 3 weeks and then discontinued. At that time, serum PRL level measurement should be performed and treatment reinstituted according to the findings.

Women with Hyperprolactinemia Who Do Not Wish to Conceive

For women who do not wish to conceive and for whom galactorrhea is not a problem, no therapy is necessary unless estrogen levels are low. Thus, to prevent osteoporosis in this clinical situation, estrogen-progestogen hormone replacement or oral contraceptives should be given, regardless of whether an adenoma is present. Long-term evaluation of all women with hyperprolactinemia should be carried out. Unless a macroadenoma is present, measurement of PRL levels once a year is advisable. Repeat imaging studies are unnecessary unless symptoms of headaches or visual disturbances occur or PRL levels increase substantially. If bromocriptine therapy is used, temporary discontinuation of medication every year is advisable, with PRL level measurement 6 weeks later. If the level is normal, repeat PRL measurements should be made semiannually. If the level is increased, therapy may be reinitiated. During medical treatment of macroadenomas, MRI or CT and visual field examination should be performed every 6 months to determine the effect of medication on the tumor. At these intervals, a decision can be made about whether to continue long-term bromocriptine treatment or to remove the tumor surgically.

KEY POINTS

- The main symptoms of hyperprolactinemia are galactorrhea and amenorrhea, the latter caused by alterations in normal GnRH release.
- Pathologic causes of hyperprolactinemia include pharmacologic agents (e.g., tranquilizers, narcotics, antihypertensive drugs), hypothyroidism, chronic renal disease, chronic neurostimulation of the breast, hypothalamic disease, and pituitary tumors (e.g., prolactinoma, acromegaly, Cushing's disease).
- Autopsy studies reveal that prolactinomas are present in approximately 10% of the population.
- Approximately 70% of women with hyperprolactinemia, galactorrhea, and amenorrhea with low estrogen levels will have a prolactinoma.
- Most macroadenomas enlarge with time; almost all microadenomas do not.
- The initial operative cure rate for microadenomas is approximately 80% and 30% for macroadenomas, but the long-term recurrence rate is at least 20% for each.

- In women with hyperprolactinemia and no macroadenoma, bromocriptine treatment returns PRL levels to normal in 90%, induces ovulatory cycles in 80%, and eradicates galactorrhea in 60%.
- When pregnancy occurs in women with microadenomas, less than 1% have visual field changes, tumor enlargement, or neurologic signs; approximately 20% of women with macroadenomas have these adverse side effects.
- Estrogen replacement therapy or oral contraceptives will not stimulate the growth of PRL-secreting microadenomas and can be used for treatment of hyperprolactinemia and hypoestrogenism.
- Surgical treatment of prolactinomas is recommended only for patients who fail to respond or do not comply with medical management.
- Cabergoline appears to be more effective and better tolerated than bromocriptine.

REFERENCES CAN BE FOUND ON
EXPERTCONSULT.com

40

Hyperandrogenism
Physiology, Etiology, Differential Diagnosis, Management

Roger A. Lobo

Hyperandrogenism in women is often referred to as androgen excess. Although most women with hyperandrogenism will have hyperandrogenemia (elevated androgen levels in blood) as well as skin manifestations (e.g., acne, **hirsutism**, or alopecia), many women exhibit only skin manifestations without demonstrable findings in blood, and women can have no clinical signs of hyperandrogenism despite hyperandrogenemia. This chapter will begin with a discussion of physiology, which will help explain this paradox.

The clinical signs associated with excessive androgen production in women are related to findings in skin and include acne, hirsutism, alopecia and, rarely, **virilization**. These skin disorders may be understood by understanding the **pilosebaceous unit**. The pilosebaceous unit is composed of a sebaceous component and pilary component from which the hair shaft arises. Abnormalities of the sebaceous component lead to acne and abnormalities of the pilary unit lead to excessive growth (hirsutism) or excessive shedding (alopecia). There are two types of hair; vellus hair is soft, fine, and unpigmented, whereas terminal hair is coarse, thick, pigmented, and undergoes cyclic changes. Anagen is the growth phase of hair. It is followed by the transitional catagen phase and, finally, by a resting, or telogen, phase, after which the hair sheds. Androgen is necessary to produce development of terminal hair and the duration of the anagen phase is directly related to the levels of circulating androgen.

There are several steroidogenic enzymes in the hair follicle but the activity level of the enzyme **5α-reductase** most directly influences the degree of androgenic effect on hair growth. With elevated levels of circulating androgen or increased activity of 5α-reductase, terminal hair appears where normally only vellus hair is present. With these alterations, the length of the anagen phase is prolonged and the hair becomes thicker. Excessive 5α-reductase activity also may lead to acne as well as scalp hair loss (alopecia).

The presence of hirsutism without other signs of virilization is associated with a relatively mild increase in androgen production or increased 5α-reductase activity, and circulating testosterone levels are normal or mildly to moderately elevated (<1.5 ng/mL). Hirsutism usually has a gradual onset and, if unaccompanied by signs of virilization, is not caused by a severe enzymatic defect or a neoplasm. The amount and location of hair growth found in women with hirsutism vary. In the milder forms, hair is found only on the upper lip and chin, whereas with increasing severity it appears on the cheeks, chest (intermammary), abdomen (superior to the umbilicus), inner aspects of the thighs, lower

back, and intergluteal areas. The severity of the hirsutism can be roughly quantified by the scoring system of Ferriman and Gallwey (**Fig. 40-1**; **Table 40-1**). Increased hair growth only on the extremities (**hypertrichosis**) should not be considered hirsutism, because terminal hair is normally found in this location in women. Women with hirsutism can have normal ovulatory menstrual cycles, oligomenorrhea, or amenorrhea.

Virilization is a relatively uncommon clinical finding and its presence is usually associated with markedly elevated levels of circulating testosterone (≥2 ng/mL). In contrast to the gradual development of hirsutism, signs of virilization usually occur over a relatively short period. These signs are caused by the masculinizing and defeminizing (antiestrogenic) actions of testosterone and include temporal balding, clitoral hypertrophy, decreased breast size, dryness of the vagina, and increased muscle mass. Women with virilization are almost always amenorrheic. The presence of androgen-secreting neoplasms should always be suspected in any woman who develops signs of virilization, particularly if the onset is rapid.

PHYSIOLOGY

Androgen production in women can be discussed in terms of three separate sources of production—the ovaries and adrenal glands, which are glandular sources, and the peripheral compartment, which comprises all extrasplanchnic and nonglandular areas of androgen production, specifically the skin and pilosebaceous unit noted earlier. The peripheral compartment modulates androgens produced by the ovaries and adrenals.

The major androgen produced by the ovaries is testosterone and that of the adrenal glands is **dehydroepiandrosterone sulfate (DHEAS)**. Measurement of the amount of these two steroids in the circulation provides clinically relevant information regarding the presence and source of increased androgen production. In addition to glandular production of androgens, conversion of androstenedione and DHEA to testosterone occurs in peripheral tissues.

The ovaries secrete only approximately 0.1 mg of testosterone/day, mainly from the thecal and stroma cells. Other androgens secreted by the ovary are androstenedione (1 to 2 mg/day) and DHEA (<1 mg/day). The adrenal glands, in addition to secreting large quantities of DHEAS (6 to 24 mg/day), secrete approximately the same daily amount of androstenedione (1 mg/day) as the ovaries and less than 1 mg of DHEA/day. The normal

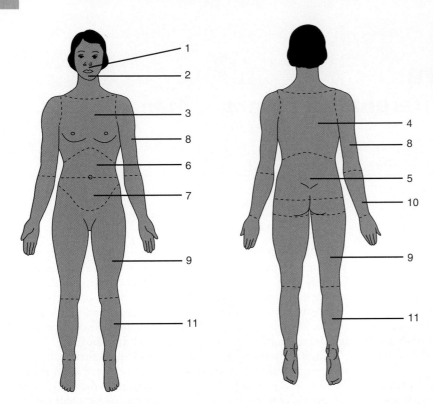

Figure 40-1 Demarcation of 11 sites used for numerically grading amount of hair growth-anterior and posterior views. (From Ferriman D, Gallwey JD: Clinical assessment of body hair growth in women. J Clin Endocrinol Metab 21:1440, 1961.)

adrenal gland secretes little testosterone, although some uncommon adrenal tumors may secrete testosterone directly.

Androstenedione and DHEA do not have strong androgenic activity but are peripherally converted at a slow rate to the biologically active androgen, testosterone. Only approximately 5% of androstenedione and a smaller percentage of DHEA are converted to testosterone. The total daily production of testosterone in women is normally approximately 0.35 mg. Of this, 0.1 mg comes from direct ovarian secretion, 0.2 mg from peripheral conversion of androstenedione, and 0.05 mg from peripheral conversion of DHEA (**Table 40-2**). Because the ovaries and adrenal gland secrete approximately equal amounts of androstenedione and DHEA, approximately two thirds (0.22 mg) of the daily testosterone produced in a woman originates from the ovaries. Thus, increased circulating levels of testosterone usually indicate abnormal ovarian androgen production. Normal circulating levels of these androgens in women of reproductive age are shown in **Table 40-3**. Only a small amount of testosterone is metabolized to testosterone glucuronide and then excreted in the urine. Testosterone, which is not a **17-ketosteroid** (17-KS), is mainly metabolized to androstenedione and then excreted as androsterone and etiocholanolone, both of which are 17-KSs. DHEA, DHEA-S, and androstenedione are excreted as DHEA, androsterone, and etiocholanolone, respectively, all of which are 17-KSs. The origin of the major amount of urinary 17-KS is the precursor androgen produced in the greatest amounts, DHEAS. Because DHEAS has a long half-life in serum, serum levels of DHEAS correlate well with amounts of 17-KS excreted in the urine. Urinary 17-KS levels were previously measured to assess adrenal androgenic activity but this test is rarely ordered today.

For practical purposes, circulatory levels of DHEAS reflect an adrenal source of production, and in women is more than 95% is adrenal-derived. Occasionally, in women who have increased production of ovarian DHEA, such as some with polycystic ovary syndrome (PCOS), the elevated levels of DHEAS might have an ovarian component because DHEA may be converted to DHEAS in the circulation. Another specific marker of adrenal androgen production, used for research purposes, is 11β-hydroxyandrostenedione, because only the adrenal has the ability to undergo 11-hydroxylation.

Most testosterone in the circulation (≈85%) is tightly bound to sex hormone-binding globulin (SHBG) and is believed to be biologically inactive. An additional 10% to 15% is loosely bound to albumin, with only approximately 1% to 2% not bound to any protein (**free testosterone**). Both the free and albumin-bound fractions (often called unbound) are biologically active. Serum testosterone can be measured as the total amount, the amount that is believed to be biologically active (unbound, or non-SHBG bound), and as the free form.

To exert a biologic effect, testosterone is metabolized peripherally in target tissues to the more potent androgen 5α-dihydrotestosterone (DHT) by the enzyme 5α-reductase. After further 3-keto reduction, DHT is converted to its distal metabolite, 5α-androstane-3α,17β-diol (3α-diol). 3α-Diol is conjugated to **5α-androstane-3α,17β-diol glucuronide (3α-diol-G)**, which is a stable, irreversible product of intracellular 5α-reductase activity (**Fig. 40-2**).

Even with normal circulatory levels of androgen, increased 5α-reductase activity in the pilosebaceous unit will result in increased androgenic activity, producing hirsutism (**Fig. 40-3**). We have measured 5α-reductase activity in skin biopsies and found the level of activity to be correlated well with the degree of hirsutism present. The degree of 5α-reductase activity can be measured in skin biopsies by a variety of methods. This technique is only used for investigational purposes; if necessary for diagnostic

Table 40-1 Definition of Hair Gradings at 11 Sites*

Site	Grade	Definition
Upper lip	1	Few hairs at outer margin
	2	Small mustache at outer margin
	3	Mustache extending halfway from outer margin
	4	Mustache extending to midline
Chin	1	Few scattered hairs
	2	Scattered hairs with small concentrations
	3, 4	Complete cover, light and heavy
Chest	1	Circumareolar hairs
	2	With midline hair in addition
	3	Fusion of these areas, with 75% cover
	4	Complete cover
Upper back	1	Few scattered hairs
	2	Rather more, still scattered
	3, 4	Complete cover, light and heavy
Lower back	1	Sacral tuft of hair
	2	With some lateral extension
	3	75% cover
	4	Complete cover
Upper abdomen	1	Few midline hairs
	2	Rather more, still midline
	3, 4	Half- and full cover
Lower abdomen	1	Few midline hairs
	2	Midline streak of hair
	3	Midline band of hair
	4	Inverted V-shaped growth
Arm	1	Sparse growth affecting not more than 25% of limb surface
	2	More than this; cover still incomplete
	3, 4	Complete cover, light and heavy
Forearm	1-4	Complete cover of dorsal surface; two grades of light and two of heavy growth
Thigh	1-4	As for arm
Leg	1-4	As for arm

*Grade 0 at all sites indicates absence of terminal hair.
From Ferriman D, Gallwey JD: Clinical assessment of body hair growth in women. J Clin Endocrinol Metab 21:1440, 1961.

reasons, 3α-diol-G levels can be directly measured in serum. We have found that the measurement of this metabolite is the most accurate indicator of the degree of peripheral androgen metabolism in women. Although serum levels of total testosterone are similar in normal and hirsute women, there are significant differences in the amounts of non–SHBG-bound testosterone as well as 3α-diol-G (**Fig. 40-4**). Non–SHBG-bound testosterone is elevated in approximately 60% to 70% of hirsute women, but the 3α-diol-G level is elevated in more than 80% of these women.

Table 40-2 Origin of Testosterone in Women

Origin	Amount (mg/day)
Ovarian secretion	0-1
Peripheral conversion	
Androstenedione → testosterone	0.2
Dehydroepiandrosterone → testosterone	0.05
Total testosterone production	0.35

From Lobo RA: Androgen excess. In Mishell DR Jr, Davajan V, Lobo RA (eds): Infertility, Contraception and Reproductive Endocrinology, 3rd ed. Cambridge, MA, Blackwell Scientific, 1991.

Table 40-3 Plasma Concentrations of Androgens During Menstrual Cycle Same

Steroid Hormone	Phase of Cycle	Plasma Concentration	
		Mean	Range
Androstenedione (ng/mL)	*	1.4	0.7-3.1
Testosterone (ng/mL)	*	0.35	0.15-0.55
Dehydroepiandrosterone (ng/mL)	*	4.2	2.7-7.8
Dehydroepiandrosterone sulfate (μg/mL)	*	1.6	0.8-3.4

*Unspecified; no major changes during menstrual cycle.
From Goebelsmann U: Steroid hormones. In Mishell DR Jr, Davajan V (eds): Infertility, Contraception and Reproductive Endocrinology, 2nd ed. Oradell, NJ, Medical Economics Books, 1986.

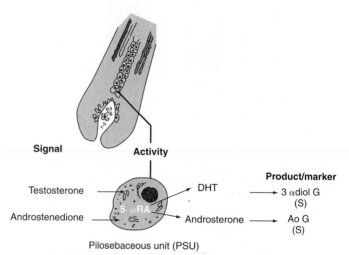

Figure 40-2 Peripheral androgen metabolism and markers of this activity. Ao G, Androsterone glucuronide; DHT, dihydrotestosterone; 3α-diol-G, 3α-androstanediol glucuronide; 5α- RA, 5α-reductase; (S), serum. (From Lobo RA: Androgen excess. In Mishell DR Jr, Davajan V, Lobo RA [eds]: Infertility, Contraception and Reproductive Endocrinology, 3rd ed. Cambridge, MA, Blackwell Scientific, 1991.)

Signal	Activity	Product
Normal	Normal 5α reductase	Normal DHT
Normal T	Increased 5α reductase	Increased DHT
Increased T	Normal 5α reductase	Increased DHT

Figure 40-3 Influence of androgen substrate (signal; e.g., testosterone or androstenedione) and 5α-reductase activity (in pilosebaceous units) on local production of biologically active androgens. T, Testosterone; DHT, dihydrotestosterone. (From Lobo RA: Androgen excess. In Mishell DR Jr, Davajan V, Lobo RA [eds]: Infertility, Contraception and Reproductive Endocrinology, 3rd ed. Cambridge, MA, Blackwell Scientific, 1991.)

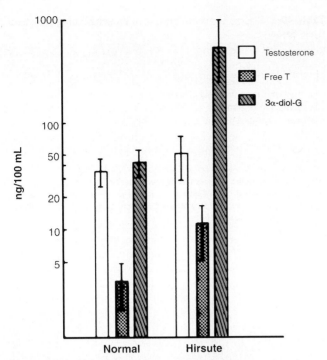

Figure 40-4 Plasma total testosterone, unbound testosterone (free T) and 5α-androstane-3α,17β-diol glucuronide (3α-diol-G) in normal and hirsute women. Note insignificant elevation with overlap for testosterone and free T testosterone and highly significant increase in 3α-diol-G without overlap between two groups of women. (From Horton R, Hawks D, Lobo RA: 3α,17β-androstanediol glucuronide in plasma: A marker of androgen action in idiopathic hirsutism. J Clin Invest 69:1203, 1982.)

Thus, increased levels of non–SHBG-bound testosterone indicate increased ovarian production. If levels of non–SHBG-bound testosterone are normal and levels of 3α-diol-G are elevated, testosterone production is not increased, but peripheral conversion of testosterone to its active metabolite (DHT) is increased above normal. Either of these processes can cause symptoms and signs of androgen excess. In summary, there are three markers of androgen production in serum, one for each compartment in which androgens are produced (**Table 40-4**). Interpretation of levels of 3α-diol-G is controversial because these levels are highly dependent on circulating levels of precursor androgens, such as testosterone and also androstenedione. A reasonable argument may be that if testosterone and DHEAS are normal but there is significant hirsutism, then measuring 3α-diol-G may not be necessary and one may merely assume a peripheral source of androgen excess.

Table 40-4 Markers of Androgen Production

Source	Marker
Ovary	Testosterone
Adrenal gland	DHEAS
Periphery	3α-diol-G

DHEAS, Dehydroepiandrosterone sulfate; 3α-diol-G (5α-androstane-3α,17β-diol glucuronide).
From Lobo RA: Androgen excess. In Mishell DR Jr, Davajan V, Lobo RA (eds): Infertility, Contraception and Reproductive Endocrinology, 3rd ed. Cambridge, MA, Blackwell Scientific, 1991.

CAUSES

There are 10 currently recognized causes of androgen excess in women. One frequent causative factor is administration of androgenic medication. In addition to testosterone itself, various anabolic steroids, 19-norprogestogens, and danazol have androgenic effects. Thus, a careful history of medication intake is important for all women with hirsutism.

Hirsutism or virilization can also be associated with some forms of abnormal gonadal development. With this cause, individuals have signs of external sexual ambiguity or primary amenorrhea, in addition to findings of androgen excess and a Y chromosome present in the gonad. These conditions are discussed further in Chapter 38 (Primary and Secondary Amenorrhea and Precocious Puberty).

Signs of androgen excess during pregnancy can be caused by increased ovarian testosterone production. This is usually caused by a luteoma of pregnancy or hyperreactio luteinalis. The former is a unilateral or bilateral solid ovarian enlargement; the latter is bilateral cystic ovarian enlargement. After pregnancy is completed, the excessive ovarian androgenic production resolves spontaneously and the androgenic signs regress.

A diagnosis of these three causes of androgen excess can usually easily be made by means of a careful history and physical examination. The remaining causes of androgen excess, together with the origin of hyperandrogenism, are listed in **Table 40-5**. Details of each of these causes will be described. Idiopathic hirsutism and PCOS are the most common disorders, together comprising over 90% of cases. PCOS is probably the most frequent disorder.

IDIOPATHIC HIRSUTISM (PERIPHERAL DISORDER OF ANDROGEN METABOLISM)

Idiopathic hirsutism is manifested by signs of hirsutism and regular menstrual cycles in conjunction with normal circulatory levels of androgens (both testosterone and DHEAS). Because this type of disorder is frequently present in several individuals in the same family, particularly those of Mediterranean descent, it has also been called familial, or constitutional, hirsutism. Because neither ovarian nor adrenal androgen production is increased, the cause of the androgen excess was not determined until rather recently— hence, the term *idiopathic hirsutism*. This is a common cause of hirsutism and is second in frequency only to PCOS. We have

Table 40-5 Differential Diagnosis of Hirsutism and Virilization*

Source	Diagnosis
Nonspecific	Exogenous, iatrogenic
	Abnormal gonadal or sexual development
Pregnancy	Androgen excess in pregnancy, luteoma or hyperreactio luteinalis
Periphery	Idiopathic hirsutism
Ovary	Polycystic ovary syndrome
	Stromal hyperthecosis
	Ovarian tumors
Adrenal gland	Adrenal tumors
	Cushing syndrome
	Adult-onset congenital adrenal hyperplasia

*Idiopathic hirsutism and polycystic ovary syndrome do not present with virilization.

found that approximately 80% of these women have increased levels of 3α-diol-G, indirectly indicating that the cause of hirsutism is largely because of increased 5α-reductase activity (5α-RA; **Fig. 40-5**). Also, we have directly measured the percentage conversion of testosterone to DHT in genital skin as an assessment of the 5α-RA level in the skin of women with idiopathic hirsutism. The amount of 5α-RA was increased in hirsute women as compared with normal women and correlated well with the degree of hirsutism and levels of serum 3α-diol-G. Thus, idiopathic hirsutism is actually a disorder of a peripheral compartment and is possibly genetically determined, although it is also possible that early exposure to androgens can program increased 5α-RA. Antiandrogens that block peripheral testosterone action or interfere with 5α-RA are effective therapeutic agents for this disorder. We have found that the symptomatic complaint of hirsutism is largely a disorder of the peripheral compartment, and the most effective treatments require peripheral blockade (see later).

POLYCYSTIC OVARY SYNDROME

Polycystic ovary syndrome was originally described in 1935 by Stein and Leventhal as a syndrome consisting of amenorrhea, hirsutism, and obesity in association with enlarged polycystic ovaries. The classic definition of PCOS includes women who are anovulatory and have irregular periods as well as hyperandrogenism, as determined by signs such as hirsutism or elevated blood levels of androgens, testosterone, or DHEAS. This should be in the absence of enzymatic disorders (e.g., 21-hydroxylase deficiency), Cushing's syndrome, or tumors.

Usually, in the United States, the diagnosis does not require findings on ultrasound (US) of characteristic polycystic ovaries.

This US-based definition has been referred to as the National Institutes of Health (NIH) consensus definition because it followed an NIH conference in 1989, but this was not a consensus conference and there was no true consensus among attendees. However, there have been two other definitions used for PCOS.

Because there was increasing evidence that some women with all the features of PCOS may be ovulatory and have regular menstrual cycles, a conference in Rotterdam came up with a new definition, which was published simultaneously in the journals *Human Reproduction* and *Fertility and Sterility* in 2004. This definition places an emphasis on finding polycystic ovaries on US as an important criterion. Other significant findings are the classic features of anovulation, menstrual irregularity, and hyperandrogenism. Women with PCOS may have all three findings, but it requires two of the three to make a diagnosis of PCOS. Thus, hyperandrogenic women with normal ovulatory cycles and polycystic ovaries on US may be diagnosed as having PCOS. We have found that approximately 95% of women who have classic symptoms (NIH criteria) of anovulation and hyperandrogenism have polycystic ovaries on US. Therefore it may be unnecessary to confirm the diagnosis by US in this setting.

Because hyperadrogenism is deemed to be an important feature of PCOS, the Androgen Excess and Polycystic Ovary Syndrome (AEPCOS) Society has offered a third definition of PCOS, which stresses hyperandrogenism as a key feature and then recognizes that women with PCOS can have polycystic ovaries on US or menstrual irregularity (anovulation). **Table 40-6** lists the three definitions with various phenotypes. **Figures 40-6** and **40-7** show the typical appearance of the polycystic ovary and US in a sagittal plane. The US diagnosis of polycystic ovaries has been made on the basis of finding

Table 40-6 Criteria for Diagnosis of Polycystic Ovary Syndrome

Study*	Criteria
NICHD 1990	Menstrual irregularity
	Hyperandrogenism (clinical or biochemical)
ESHRE-ASRM 2003	Menstrual irregularity
	Hyperandrogenism (clinical or biochemical)
	Polycystic ovaries on ultrasound (two of three required)
AEPCOS 2006	Hyperandrogenism (clinical or biochemical) and menstrual irregularity
	Polycystic ovaries on ultrasound (either or both of the latter two)

*All required the exclusion of other underlying hormonal disorders or tumors.

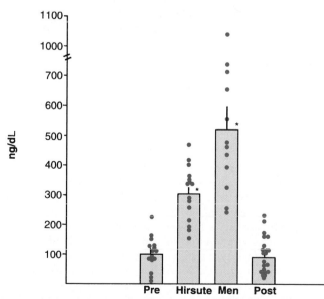

Figure 40-5 Serum 3β-diol-G in premenopausal nonhirsute women (Pre), hirsute women, normal men, and postmenopausal nonhirsute women (Post). The *asterisks* denote *P* < .05, as compared with Pre. (From Paulson RJ, Serafini PC, Catalino JA, Lobo RA: Measurements of 3α,17β-androstanediol glucuronide in serum and urine and the correlation with skin 5α-reductase activity. Fertil Steril 46:222, 1986.)

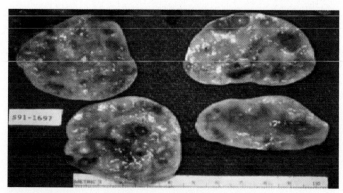

Figure 40-6 Surgical specimen of polycystic ovaries.

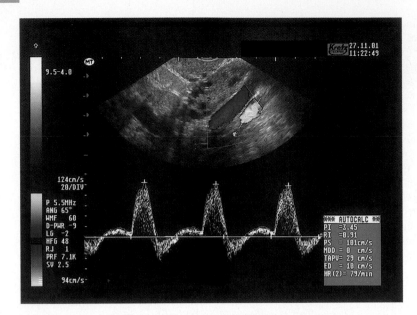

Figure 40-7 Typical color Doppler ultrasound of a polycystic ovary showing increased blood flow. (From Strauss JF, Barbieri RL [eds]: Yen and Jaffe's Reproductive Endocrinology, 6th ed. Philadelphia, WB Saunders, 2009, p 822.)

enlarged ovaries (>10 cm^3) and the presence of 10 or more peripherally oriented cystic structures (2 to 8 mm) surrounding a dense stroma. Since the Rotterdam conference, however, ovarian size alone has been though to be sufficient, with ovaries larger than 10 cm^3 being diagnostic; other evidence has suggested that this lower limit may be 7 cm^3.

It is also important to note that from 10% to 25% of the normal reproductive age population (no symptoms or signs of PCOS) may have polycystic ovaries found on US. These ovaries have been called polycystic-appearing ovaries (PAO) or polycystic ovarian morphology (PCOM) in the literature. This isolated finding should not be confused with the diagnosis of PCOS, but may be a risk factor for other features of PCOS (e.g., insulin resistance, cardiovascular risk factors) discussed later.

Using the classic definition of PCOS, which can also be heterogeneous in terms of the severity of the findings of menstrual irregularity and hyperandrogenism, approximately 3% to 7% of the reproductive age population will have PCOS. Thus, PCOS is an extremely common disorder; its diagnosis is important because of its consequences (see later section on consequences of PCOS).

Depending on the woman's country of origin, 30% to 70% of women with PCOS are overweight, although it is clear that thin women may also have PCOS. All symptoms of PCOS are worse in women who are overweight or obese. This relates most strongly to insulin resistance, which is a key factor of PCOS (see later). The degree of menstrual irregularity may also relate to the finding of insulin resistance.

Characteristic endocrinologic features include abnormal gonadotropin secretion caused by increased gonadotropin-releasing hormone (GnRH) pulse amplitude or increased pituitary sensitivity to GnRH. These abnormalities result in tonically elevated levels of luteinizing hormone (LH) in approximately two thirds of the women with this syndrome (**Fig. 40-8**). After a bolus of GnRH, there is usually an exaggerated response of LH, but not of follicle-stimulating hormone (FSH; **Fig. 40-9**). In addition, there are increased circulating levels of androgens produced by the ovaries and adrenal glands

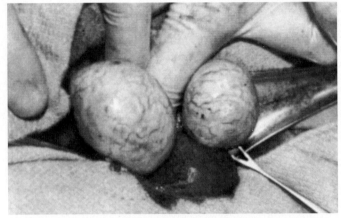

Figure 40-8 Gross characteristics of polycystic ovaries—bilateral enlarged ovaries with smooth and thickened capsule. (From Yen SSC: Chronic anovulation caused by peripheral endocrine disorders. In Yen SSC, Jaffe RB [eds]: Reproductive Endocrinology, 2nd ed. Philadelphia, WB Saunders, 1986.)

(**Fig. 40-10**), Serum testosterone levels usually range from 0.7 to 1.2 ng/mL and androstenedione levels are usually from 3 to 5 ng/mL. In addition, approximately 50% of women with this syndrome have elevated levels of DHEAS, suggesting adrenal androgen involvement. However, in some countries, this prevalence of putative adrenal involvement is lower. Evidence also exists for adrenal hyperactivity to stimulation in at least one third of women with PCOS. Although almost all women with PCOS have elevated levels of circulating androgens, we have found that the presence or absence of hirsutism depends on whether those androgens are converted peripherally by 5α-reductase to the more potent androgen DHT, as reflected by increased circulating levels of 3α-diol-G. Nonhirsute women with PCOS have elevated circulatory levels of testosterone, DHEAS, or both, but not 3α-diol-G. The tonically elevated levels of LH are usually above 15 mIU/mL.

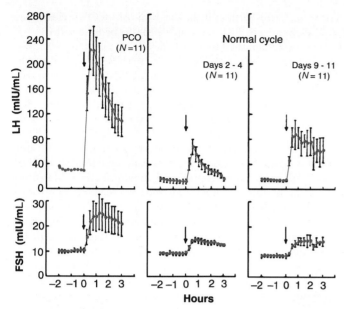

Figure 40-9 Comparison of quantitative luteinizing hormone (LH) and follicle-stimulating hormone (FSH) release in response to a single bolus of 150 µg of GnRH in patients with polycystic ovarian syndrome (PCOS) and in normal women during low-estrogen (early follicular) and high-estrogen (late follicular) phases of their cycles. (From Rebar R, Judd HL, Yen SSC, et al: Characterization of the inappropriate gonadotropin secretion in polycystic ovary syndrome. J Clin Invest 57:1320, 1976.)

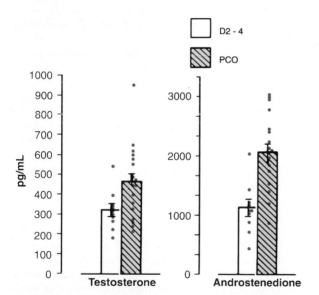

Figure 40-10 Mean (±SD) concentrations of testosterone and Δ⁴-androstenedione in 19 patients with polycystic ovarian syndrome (PCO) and 10 normal subjects between days 2 and 4 (D2-4) of their menstrual cycles. (From DeVane GW, Czekala NM, Judd HL, et al: Circulating gonadotropins, estrogens, and androgens in polycystic ovarian disease. Am J Obstet Gynecol 121:496, 1975.)

Because FSH levels in women with PCOS are normal or low, an elevated LH/FSH ratio has been used to diagnose PCOS. However, we have found that in women with a clinical diagnosis of PCOS, only 70% have an elevated level of immunoreactive LH or an immunologic LH/FSH ratio greater than 3. Although almost all women with PCOS had elevated serum levels of

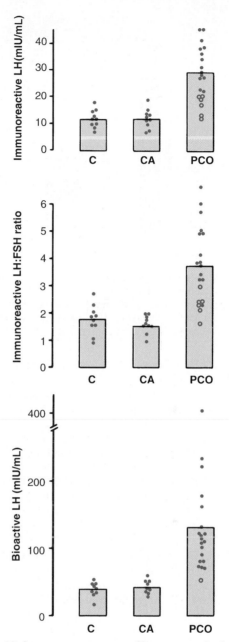

Figure 40-11 Serum measurements of immunoreactive luteinizing hormone (LH), immunoreactive LH-to- follicle-stimulating hormone (FSH) ratios, and bioactive LH in control subjects (C), women with chronic anovulation (CA), and women with PCOS (PCO). Boxes represent the mean ±3 SD of control levels. (From Lobo RA, Kletzky OA, Campeau JD, et al: Elevated bioactive luteinizing hormone in women with the polycystic ovary syndrome. Fertil Steril 39:674, 1983.)

biologically active LH (**Fig. 40-11**), use of LH or the LH/FSH ratio should not be part of the diagnostic evaluation of PCOS. Overweight and obese women with PCOS often have normal levels of LH, whereas thin women often exhibit this gonadotropic disturbance.

In addition to increased levels of circulatory androgens, we have found that women with PCOS have increased levels of biologically active (non–SHBG-bound) estradiol, although total circulating levels of estradiol are not increased (**Fig. 40-12**). The increased amount of non–SHBG-bound estradiol is caused by

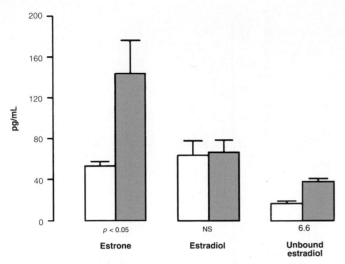

Figure 40-12 Serum estrogen concentrations in 13 normal women and 22 PCOS patients (*shaded areas*). (From Lobo RA, Granger L, Goebelsmann U, et al: Elevation in unbound serum estradiol as a possible mechanism for inappropriate gonadotropin secretion in women with PCOS. J Clin Endocrinol Metab 52:156, 1981.)

a decrease in SHBG levels, which is brought about by the increased levels of androgens and obesity, with high insulin levels present in many of these women. Estrone is also increased because of increased peripheral (adipose) conversion of androgen. The tonically increased levels of biologically active estradiol may stimulate increased GnRH pulsatility and produce tonically elevated LH levels and anovulation. In addition, the lowered SHBG level increases the biologically active fractions of androgens in the circulation. The importance of the decreased levels of SHBG is shown schematically in **Figure 40-13**. This relative hyperestrogenism (elevated levels of estrone and non–SHBG-bound estradiol), which is unopposed by progesterone because of anovulation, increases the risk of endometrial hyperplasia.

Approximately 20% to 30% of women with PCOS also have mildly elevated levels of prolactin (20 to 35 ng/mL), possibly related to the increased pulsatility of GnRH, to a relative dopamine deficiency, or to tonic stimulation from unopposed

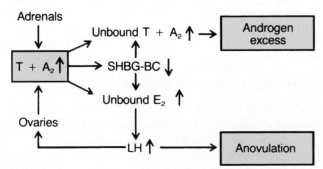

Figure 40-13 Scheme depicting the possible role of adrenal-derived androgen in initiating androgen excess and anovulation. A_2, Androstanediol; E_2, estradiol; LH, luteinizing hormone; SHBG-BC, sex hormone-binding globulin binding capacity; T, testosterone. (From Lobo RA, Goebelsmann U: Effect of androgen excess on inappropriate gonadotropin secretion as found in polycystic ovary syndrome. Am J Obstet Gynecol 142:394, 1982.)

estrogen. In this setting, if the diagnosis of PCOS is clear, these mild elevations in PRL level only need to be followed.

It is well established that some degree of insulin resistance occurs in most women with PCOS, even in those of normal weight. Insulin and insulin-like growth factor 1 (IGF-1) enhance ovarian androgen production by potentiating the stimulatory action of LH on ovarian androstenedione and testosterone secretion. High levels of insulin bind with the receptor for IGF-1 as a result of the significant homology of the IGF-1 receptor with the insulin receptor. The granulosa cells also produce IGF-1 and IGF-binding proteins (IGFBPs). This local production of IGF-1 and IGFBP may result in paracrine control and enhancement of LH stimulation and production of androgens by the theca cells in women with PCOS. Because IGFBP levels are lower in women with PCOS, this leads to increased bioavailable IGF-1, which increases stimulation of the theca cells in combination with LH to produce higher levels of androgen production. Insulin resistance and the resultant hyperinsulinemia stimulate ovarian androgen production. Insulin resistance (IR) in PCOS is primarily a peripheral insulin resistance, manifest primarily in muscle and adipose and minimally at the level of ovary or adrenal.

The cause of IR in PCOS is unknown; it is not caused by insulin receptor defects. Genetic and unknown other influences affect insulin signaling (post receptor). It has been shown that in PCOS there is increased serine phosphorylation, which is less efficient than the normal tyrosine phosphorylation. Most women with PCOS will be found to have euglycemia with peripheral IR; in more severe cases, there is also evidence of beta cell (secretory) dysfunction, which increases the risk of type 2 diabetes. In a prospective evaluation of 254 women with PCOS who had an oral glucose tolerance test, it was found that 31% had impaired glucose tolerance and 7.5% had undiagnosed diabetes. In nonobese women with PCOS, 10% had impaired glucose tolerance and 1.5% had diabetes. Norman and coworkers have shown that over a mean follow-up period of 6.2 years, 9% of women with PCOS in Australia progressed to having impaired glucose tolerance and 8% became diabetic. Thus, the negative effect of obesity and PCOS on insulin resistance is additive.

Fasting glucose levels are a poor predictor of diabetes in PCOS. It would appear prudent to perform an oral glucose tolerance test at the time of diagnosis in overweight women with PCOS, particularly before they attempt to conceive. Most recently, it has been suggested that measuring the level of hemoglobin A1C (HbA1C; normal <6%) is the most efficient means of ruling out glucose intolerance or frank diabetes. Various techniques have been used to diagnose IR in women with PCOS. These include more complicated but more accurate measures used only in a research setting, such as the clamp test and IV glucose tolerance test (**Table 40-7**). Using fasting glucose and insulin measurements and calculating the quantitative insulin sensitivity check index (QUICKI) or homeostasis model assessment of insulin resistance (HOMA) have been useful and correlate well with the more invasive techniques. However, it may not be necessary to compute these parameters in routine practice; clinicians should assume that overweight or obese women with PCOS are insulin-resistant and should be treated as such. In this setting, it is more important to rule out impaired glucose tolerance or diabetes, which cannot be assumed or discounted. **Figure 40-14** depicts the prevalence of abnormal testing parameters in women with PCOS.

Table 40-7 Measurements of Insulin Sensitivity

Test	Measurement	Normal Value*
Hyperinsulinemic Clamp	M/1 (mean glucose use/mean plasma insulin concentration)	$>1.12 \times 10^{-4}$
Homeostasis model assessment of insulin resistance (HOMAIR)	[Fasting insulin (μU/mL) $\times$ fasting glucose (mmol/L)]/22.5	<2.77
Glucose-to insulin ratio	Fasting glucose (mg/dL)/fasting insulin (μU/mL)	>4.5
Quantitative insulin sensitivity check index (QUICKI)	1/[log fasting insulin (μU/mL) + log + fasting glucose (mg/dL)]	>0.357
Fasting insulin	—	Assay-dependent

*Normal values may vary depending on the insulin assay used.

Pathophysiologic Considerations

It is clear that there is a genetic predisposition to PCOS. However, it is likely that several genes are involved. A susceptibility gene for PCOS has been suggested to lie in the region of 19p3.2, although this needs confirmation. Environmental factors are clearly involved as well, based on twin studies, in which PCOS is not always concordant on a genetic basis. Maternal exposure to androgen has been shown in a monkey model to contribute to the development of PCOS.

It has been long established that a vicious cycle propagates the disorder in PCOS, regardless of how it begins (**Fig. 40-15**). Thus, it was attractive to postulate that dopamine deficiency in the hypothalamus might give rise to the exaggerated LH responses in PCOS, and there are several similar hypotheses. However, it has been observed that morphologically identifiable polycystic ovaries are seen in children. This occurrence predicts puberty and other normal endocrinologic events, suggesting a central role for altered polycystic ovarian morphology in the disorder.

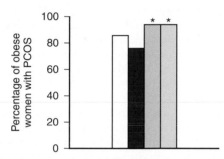

Figure 40-14 Percentage of 129 obese women with PCOS with insulin resistance (IR) based on fasting basal insulin (white), G/I ratio (red), HOMA (yellow), or QUICKI (light blue). *$P < .01$ compared with G/I ratio. HOMA, Homeostasis model assessment of insulin resistance; QUICKI, quantitative insulin sensitivity check index. (From Carmina E, Lobo RA: The use of fasting blood to assess the prevalence of insulin resistance in polycystic ovary syndrome [PCOS]. Fertil Steril 82:661, 2004.)

Acanthosis nigricans (AN) has been found in approximately 30% of hyperandrogenic women. Approximately 50% of the hyperandrogenic women who had PCOS and were obese had AN. Although it has been suggested that the presence of *hyperandrogenism*, *IR*, and *AN* constitute a special syndrome (the HAIR-AN syndrome), most investigators believe that many women with PCOS have some degree of AN, particularly when obese, and do not have another distinct endocrine disorder. The combination of increased insulin and IGF-1 enhances the development of AN.

Müllerian-inhibiting substance (MIS) or anti–müllerian hormone (AMH) is a glycoprotein produced by the granulosa cells of preantral follicules. Because of the larger number of preantral follicles in PCOS, the MIS or AMH level is significantly elevated in women with PCOS. Physiologically, AMH or MIS attenuates a sensitivity of FSH in stimulating granulosa cells. Because AMH or MIS reflects the number of preantral follicles, it serves as a useful measure of ovarian reserve and ovarian aging and decreases with age. This measurement, however, is not as predictive in PCOS in that levels are already higher than in normal women because of altered polycystic morphology.

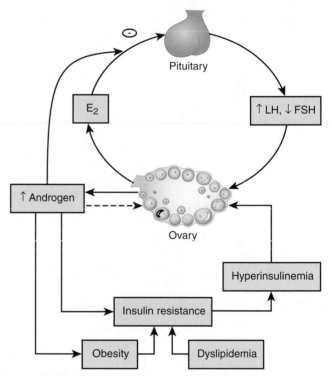

Figure 40-15 Pathophysiologic concept of polycystic ovary syndrome (PCOS). Increased luteinizing hormone (LH) secretion, together with enhanced theca cell responsiveness, drives the production of excess ovarian androgen. Increased androgen production may inhibit steroid negative feedback effects on hypothalamic gonadotropin-releasing hormone pulse generation to account for the rapid LH pulse frequency observed in women with PCOS. In addition, increased androgen levels are associated with android obesity, visceral fat deposition, and dyslipidemia, all of which may contribute to insulin resistance. Independently, hyperandrogenemia, obesity, and hyperinsulinemia may decrease sex hormone-binding globulin, thereby increasing bioactive testosterone. Finally, increased androgen may have direct effects on the ovary to increase follicle number and follicle size and possibly enhance granulosa cell responsiveness to follicle-stimulating hormone (FSH) E_2, Estradiol. (From Strauss JF, Barbieri RL [eds]: Yen and Jaffe's Reproductive Endocrinology, 6th ed. Philadelphia, WB Saunders, 2009, p 509.)

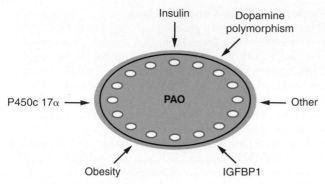

Figure 40-16 Pathophysiology of polycystic ovary syndrome (PCOS): The syndrome develops when one or more insults persist. IGFBG1, Insulin-like growth factor–binding protein 1; P450c 17α, cytochrome 450.

Furthermore not all women with isolated polycystic ovaries have PCOS. as stated earlier. Thus, a pathophysiologic model can be put together as follows. An ovary is polycystic in up to 20% of girls, according to data from Bridges and colleagues, so the ovary transitions early in life from normal to polycystic-appearing (PAO). This influence occurs in a specific way by genetic factors or environmental factors, or is induced by other endocrine disturbances (**Fig. 40-16**). The woman who develops PAO may have normal menses, normal androgen levels, and normal ovulatory function and parity. However, if subjected to various susceptibility factors or insults, with various degrees of severity, women with PAO may develop a full-blown syndrome (PCOS). The syndrome, if full-blown, will exhibit the full extent of hyperandrogenism and anovulation, with the most extreme form of this menstrual disturbance being amenorrhea. However, in this spectrum of disorders, the androgen disturbances may also be near-normal. Similarly, the menstrual disturbance may be mild (**Fig. 40-17**).

This model requires that normal homeostatic factors may be able to ward off stressors or insults in some women who can go through life without PCOS but have a PAO, which does not change morphologically. Alternatively, with varying degrees of success, a woman's homeostatic mechanisms may at any time, early or later in reproductive life, allow symptoms of PCOS to emerge with varying degrees of severity. Two of the major insults are thought to be weight gain and psychological stress.

Therefore, the typical teenager born with PAO may develop PCOS fairly quickly, but a PCOS picture may develop only later in life in some women, even after having children.

Consequences of Polycystic Ovary Syndrome

The importance of diagnosing PCOS is that there are known long-term consequences of the diagnosis warranting lifelong surveillance. **Figure 40-18** shows the ages at which various consequences may emerge. Although in the early reproductive years abnormal bleeding and infertility are common, concerns later in life relate to cardiovascular disease, diabetes mellitus, and ovarian cancer. The risk of ovarian cancer has been suggested to be increased twofold, a finding seen in women with general infertility. This risk is normalized with the use of oral contraceptives (OCs).

Women with PCOS have characteristic lipid and lipoprotein abnormalities (**Fig. 40-19**), including the presence of abnormal lipoprotein particles, which adds to a long list of abnormalities that tend to increase cardiovascular (CV) risk. **Table 40-8** depicts several CV risk factors, including the development of hypertension and diabetes as women approach menopause (**Fig. 40-20**). These risks pertain to women with more classic features of PCOS. particularly obesity. There is evidence that the milder phenotypes diagnosed using the Rotterdam criteria have less CV risk factors. **Figure 40-21** depicts a hypothetical scheme for increasing CV risk in women with PCOS with various phenotypes.

It is important to note, however, that there are no definitive data on whether PCOS increases CV mortality. Although the multiple risk factors present would suggest such a finding, retrospective analyses have shown no increase in mortality. However, a more recent study following a PM cohort presumed to have PCOS earlier in life has shown a lower CV event-free survival with time (greater CV mortality) in PCOS (**Fig. 40-22**). Although the conclusions are as yet unclear, women with PCOS should be counseled regarding CV risk factors and preventing hypertension, dyslipidemias, and diabetes by lifestyle modification and other means, as recently reviewed by the AEPCOS Society.

Obesity is one of the major factors leading to these risks and the development of metabolic syndrome, which is a precursor to many serious health concerns (e.g., coronary disease, stroke, diabetes). The prevalence of metabolic syndrome in the United States is approximately 60% in young (20 to 39 years) obese women with PCOS using Adult Treatment Panel III criteria (three of five of the following: waist circumference >88 cm; high-density

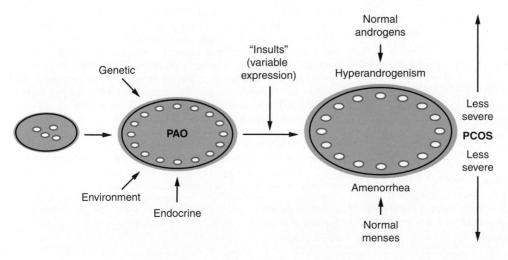

Figure 40-17 Pathophysiology of polycystic ovary syndrome (PCOS) showing differences in presentation. PAO, Polycystic-appearing ovaries.

Figure 40-18 Consequences of polycystic ovary syndrome (PCOS). ca, Cancer; CVD, cardiovascular disease; DM, diabetes mellitus.

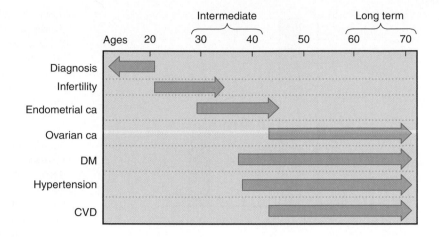

Figure 40-19 Lipid and lipoprotein profiles in 13 women with polycystic ovary syndrome (PCOS) versus control group when matched for percent ideal body weight. Differences are evident in all measures ($P < .01$). HDL, High-density lipoprotein; LDL, low-density lipoprotein. (From Wild RA, Bartholomew MJ: The influence of body weight on lipoprotein lipids in patients with polycystic ovary syndrome. Am J Obstet Gynecol 159:423, 1988.)

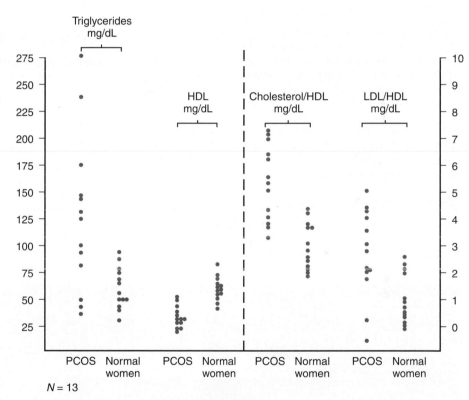

Table 40-8 Cardiovascular Risk Factors in Polycystic Ovary Syndrome

Risk Factor	Features
Traditional risk factors	Obesity, insulin resistance, dyslipidemia, abnormal homocysteine, C-reactive protein, plasminogen activator inhibitor-1, increase in inflammatory adipocytokines such as TNF-α, decrease in adiponectin; higher prevalence of diabetes, hypertension
Atherosclerosis	Coronary catheterization studies, increase in carotid intima-media thickness, coronary calcium
Endothelial dysfunction by blood flow studies	All increased in classic PCOS; less of a concern with milder phenotypes using Rotterdam criteria

TNF-α, Tumor necrosis factor-α.

lipoprotein <50 mg/dL; triglycerides >150 mg/dL; blood pressure >130/85 mm Hg; fasting blood sugar >110 mg/dL. In other countries in which obesity is less prevalent, the prevalence of metabolic syndrome in PCOS is still increased, but is much lower (5% to 9%). The constellation of risk factors comprising metabolic syndrome place women with PCOS at increased risk for CV disease and diabetes, but there is nothing specifically of more significance regarding metabolic syndrome in PCOS.

Isolated Polycystic Ovaries

We have found that normal ovulatory women with PAO or PCOM have a subtle form of ovarian hyperandrogenism when stimulated with GnRH-A or human chorionic gonadotropin (hCG). We have also found subtle changes in insulin sensitivity and altered lipoproteins. There may also be some reduction in

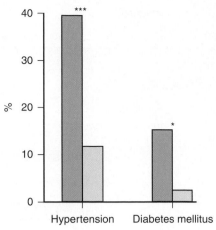

Figure 40-20 Prevalence of hypertension (medically treated) and manifest diabetes mellitus in 33 PCOS subjects and 132 referents. The *dark-shaded bars* indicate the polycystic ovary syndrome (PCOS) subjects. The *light-shaded bars* indicate the referents. Statistical comparisons were made between the women with PCOS and referents. Differences were considered significant at *$P = .05$ and ***$P = .001$. (From Dahlgren E, Janson PO, Johansson S, et al: Women with polycystic ovary syndrome wedge resected in 1956 to 1965: A long-term follow-up focusing on natural history and circulating hormones. Fertil Steril 57:505, 1992.)

fertility in these ovulatory women. Therefore, although many women with isolated PAO or PCOM may not have any problems, this finding may be considered as a risk factor for developing the consequences of PCOS.

STROMAL HYPERTHECOSIS

Stromal hyperthecosis is an uncommon benign ovarian disorder in which the ovaries are bilaterally enlarged to approximately 5 to 7 cm in diameter. Histologically, there are nests of luteinized theca cells within the stroma (**Fig. 40-23**). The capsules of these ovaries are thick, similar to those found in PCOS but, unlike PCOS, subcapsular cysts are uncommon. The theca cells produce large amounts of testosterone, as determined by retrograde ovarian vein catheterization. Like PCOS, this disorder has a gradual onset and is initially associated with anovulation or amenorrhea and hirsutism. However, unlike PCOS, with increasing age the ovaries secrete steadily increasing amounts of testosterone. Thus, when women with this disorder reach the fourth decade of life, the severity of the hirsutism increases and signs of **virilization**, such as temporal balding, clitoral enlargement, deepening of the voice, and decreased breast size, appear and gradually increase in severity. By this time, serum testosterone levels are usually higher than 2 ng/mL, similar to levels found in ovarian and adrenal testosterone-producing tumors. However, with the latter conditions, the symptoms of virilization appear and progress much more rapidly than with ovarian hyperthecosis, in which symptoms progress gradually over many years.

ANDROGEN-PRODUCING TUMORS

Ovarian Neoplasms

It is possible for almost every type of ovarian neoplasm to have stromal cells that secrete excessive amounts of testosterone and cause signs of androgen excess. Thus, on rare occasions, excess testosterone produced by benign and malignant cystadenomas, Brenner's tumors, and Krukenberg's tumors have caused hirsutism, virilization, or both. Certain germ cell tumors contain many testosterone-producing cells. The testosterone produced by two of these neoplasms, **Sertoli-Leydig cell tumors** and **hilus cell tumors**, almost always causes virilization. In addition, lipoid cell (adrenal rest) tumors can produce increased amounts of testosterone, DHEAS, or both. Rarely, granulosa/theca cell tumors can also produce testosterone in addition to increased levels of estradiol.

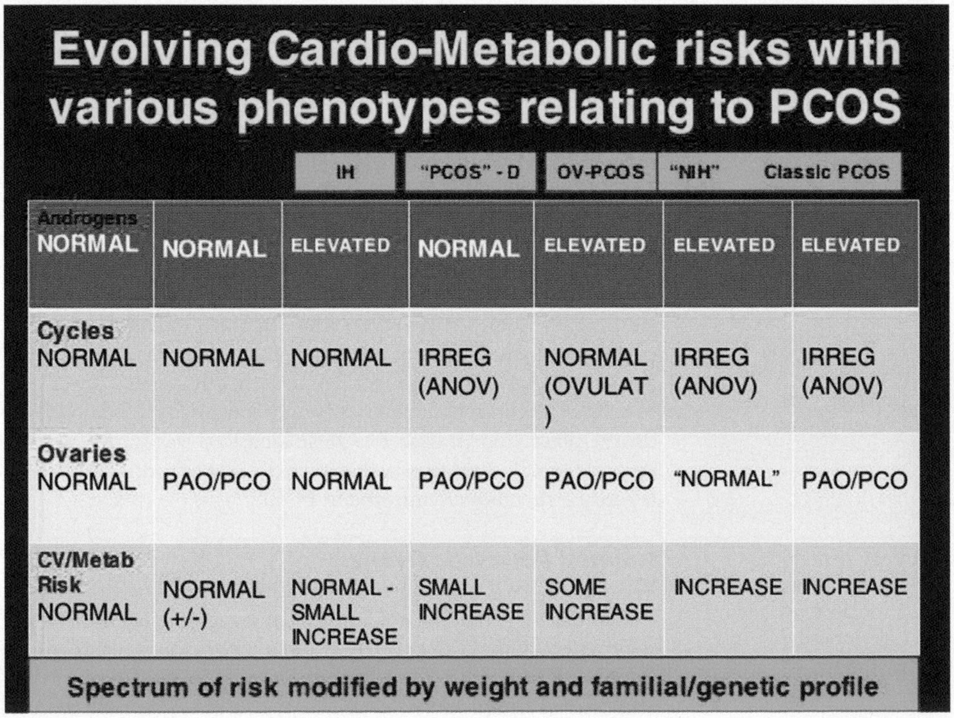

Figure 40-21 Evolving cardiometabolic risks with various phenotypes relating to PCOS. The spectrum of risk is modified by weight and familial and genetic profile. (From Jovanovic VP, Carmina E, Lobo RA: Not all women diagnosed with PCOS share the same cardiovascular risk profiles. Fertil Steril 94:826, 2010.)

Evolving Cardio-Metabolic risks with various phenotypes relating to PCOS

	IH	"PCOS"-D	OV-PCOS	"NIH"	Classic PCOS
Androgens NORMAL	NORMAL	ELEVATED	NORMAL	ELEVATED	ELEVATED	ELEVATED
Cycles NORMAL	NORMAL	NORMAL	IRREG (ANOV)	NORMAL (OVULAT)	IRREG (ANOV)	IRREG (ANOV)
Ovaries NORMAL	PAO/PCO	NORMAL	PAO/PCO	PAO/PCO	"NORMAL"	PAO/PCO
CV/Metab Risk NORMAL	NORMAL (+/-)	NORMAL - SMALL INCREASE	SMALL INCREASE	SOME INCREASE	INCREASE	INCREASE

Spectrum of risk modified by weight and familial/genetic profile

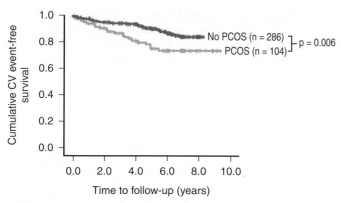

Figure 40-22 Cumulative unadjusted CV death or myocardial infarction (MI)–free survival in postmenopausal women with or without clinical features of PCOS (*P* = .006). (From Shaw LJ, Merz CNB, Azziz R, et al: Postmenopausal women with a history of irregular menses and elevated androgen measurements at high risk for worsening cardiovascular event-free survival: Results from the National Institutes of Health National Heart, Lung, and Blood Institute Sponsored Women's Ischemia Syndrome Evaluation. J Clin Endocrinol Metab 93:1276, 2008.)

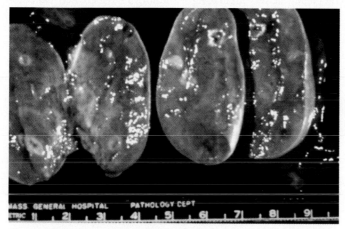

Figure 40-23 Surgical specimen of ovarian stromal hyperthecosis. Note fleshy appearance, without cystic activity.

Androgen-producing ovarian tumors usually produce rapidly progressive signs of virilization. Sertoli-Leydig cell tumors usually develop during the reproductive years (second to fourth decades) and, by the time they produce detectable signs of androgen excess, the tumor is almost always (>85% of the time) palpable during bimanual examination. These tumors are uncommon. Less than 1% of solid ovarian neoplasms are Sertoli-Leydig cell tumors. Hilus cell tumors usually occur after menopause. They are usually small and not palpable during bimanual examination; however, the history of rapid development of signs of virilization and the presence of markedly elevated levels of testosterone (more than 2.5 times the upper limits of the normal range), with normal levels of DHEAS, usually facilitate the diagnosis.

Adrenal Tumors

Almost all the androgen-producing adrenal tumors are adenomas or carcinomas that generate large amounts of the C19 steroids normally produced by the adrenal gland—DHEAS, DHEA, and androstenedione. Although these tumors do not usually secrete testosterone directly, testosterone is produced by extraglandular conversion of DHEA and androstenedione. Women with these tumors usually have markedly elevated serum levels of DHEAS (>8 µg/mL). Women with these laboratory findings and a history of rapid onset of signs of androgen excess should undergo a computed tomography (CT) scan or magnetic resonance imaging (MRI) of the adrenal glands to confirm the diagnosis. In addition to these uncommon tumors, a few testosterone-producing adrenal adenomas have been reported. The cellular patterns of these tumors resemble those of ovarian hilus cells, and the tumors secrete large amounts of testosterone. Because adrenal adenomas also secrete DHEAS, an adrenal adenoma is highly likely when DHEAS levels are greater than 8 µg/mL and testosterone levels are more than 1.5 ng/mL.

LATE-ONSET 21-HYDROXYLASE DEFICIENCY

Congenital adrenal hyperplasia (CAH) is an inherited disorder caused by an enzymatic defect (usually 21-hydroxylase [21-OHase] or, less often, 11β-hydroxylase), resulting in decreased cortisol biosynthesis. As a consequence, adrenocorticotropic hormone (ACTH) secretion increases and adrenal cortisol precursors produced proximal to the enzymatic block accumulate. These are converted mainly to 17-hydroxyprogesterone—androstenedione—and androstenedione in turn is converted to testosterone, which produces signs of androgen excess.

Because the enzymatic defects are congenital, the classic severe form (complete block) usually becomes clinically apparent in fetal life by producing masculinization of the female external genitalia. The severe form of CAH is the most common cause of sexual ambiguity in the newborn. The more attenuated (mild) block of 21-hydroxylase activity usually does not produce physical signs associated with increased androgen production until after puberty. Thus, this condition, known as **late-onset 21-hydroxylase deficiency (LOHD)** or late-onset congenital adrenal hyperplasia, is associated with the development of signs of hyperandrogenism in a woman in the second or early third decade of life.

Although the incidence of classic CAH is only 1 in 14,500 live births worldwide, Speiser and coworkers, using histocompatibility locus antigen (HLA)-B genotyping of families with LOHD-affected individuals, have concluded that the incidence of LOHD varies among different ethnic groups but, overall, is probably the most frequent autosomal genetic disorder in humans. The incidence of LOHD was estimated to be 0.1% in a diverse white population; in Yugoslavians, Hispanics, and Ashkenazi Jews, however, the incidence was 1.6%, 1.9%, and 3.7%, respectively (**Fig. 40-24**). Both classic CAH and LOHD are transmitted in an autosomal recessive manner at the *CYP21B* locus and are linked to the HLA-B locus.

The molecular basis of the disease is complex. The gene for CYP21 is located on 6p near the HLA complex. In proximity to this gene is a nonfunctional or pseudogene (CYP21P). Depending on the population, 20% to 25% of individuals with classic CAH have a deletion of the *CYP21* locus or a rearrangement between *CYP21* and *CYP21P*. Current molecular techniques of genotyping can pick up well over 95% of these abnormalities, with most cases being 1 of 10 common mutations. A spectrum of mutations results in the enzymatic defects and clinical presentations shown in **Table 40-9**.

LOHD is a phenotype that is symptomatic after adolescence and does not define the genotype. Affected individuals may be

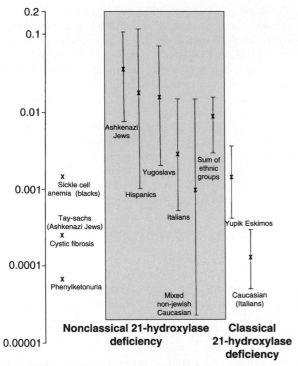

Figure 40-24 Relative frequencies of nonclassic 21-hydroxylase deficiency, classic 21-hydroxylase deficiency, and other autosomal recessive disorders. (From Speiser PW, Dupont B, Rubenstein P, et al: High frequency of nonclassical steroid 21-hydroxylase deficiency. Am J Hum Genet 37:650, 1985.)

homozygous for alleles, yielding mildly abnormal enzymatic activity, or compound heterozygotes with a combination of defective alleles. The so-called cryptic 21-hydroxylase deficiency, on the other hand, represents mild or asymptomatic individuals with biochemically identified defects that with the advent of molecular diagnostic techniques, have been redefined as belonging to several different clinical presentations.

New and associates have proposed a schema for identifying and classifying the clinical spectrum of disease shown in **Table 40-9**. Because there are three possible manifestations of

CYP21Y alleles (normal, mildly defective, or severely defective), there are six possible genotypes representing three clinical phenotypes (asymptomatic, LOHD, and classic CAH). Individuals with LOHD may be compound heterozygotes, with one mildly and one severely defective allele, or homozygous, with two mildly defective alleles. There is no perfect correlation between genotypes and phenotypes and, because the genetics are complex, with many possible abnormalities, particularly in diverse populations, it has been recommended that for clinical purposes, diagnosis and treatment of CAH should be based on biochemical findings. Carriers can be identified among family members who are heterozygous, with one normal allele. They have normal basal 17-hydroxyprogesterone levels, a mild degree of hirsutism, if present, and smaller increases of 17-hydroxyprogesterone after ACTH stimulation, usually between 3.5 and 10 ng/mL. Molecular genotyping is primarily used for prenatal testing when there is a known severe mutation to determine the risk of having a severely affected child.

LOHD is also usually associated with menstrual irregularity. It has been hypothesized that the mechanism for anovulation is similar to that which occurs with PCOS. The increased levels of androgen lower SHBG levels, thus increasing the amount of biologically active circulating estradiol. The increased estradiol stimulates tonic LH release, which increases ovarian androgen production and locally inhibits follicular growth and ovulation. Thus, women with this disorder present with postpubertal onset of hirsutism and oligomenorrhea or amenorrhea, similar to women with PCOS. However, women with LOHD, unlike those with PCOS, commonly have a history of prepubertal accelerated growth (at 6 to 8 years of age), with later decreased growth and a short ultimate height. A history of this growth pattern, a family history of postpubertal onset of hirsutism, and findings of mild virilization are indicators of the presence of CAH.

To differentiate LOHD from PCOS, measurement of basal (early morning) serum 17-hydroxyprogesterone levels should be performed. If basal levels are greater than 8 ng/mL, the diagnosis of LOHD is established. If 17-hydroxyprogesterone is above normal (2.5 to 3.3 ng/mL) but less than 8 ng/mL, an ACTH stimulation test should be performed. A baseline 17-hydroxyprogesterone level should be measured and 0.25 mg of synthetic ACTH infused as a single bolus. One hour, later another serum

Table 40-9 Genotypic Characterization of the Forms of 21-Hydroxylase Deficiency

Form of 21-Hydroxylase Deficiency	Clinical Phenotype	Hormonal Phenotype (in Response to ACTH)	Genotype
Classic (CAH)	Prenatal virilization, fully symptomatic	Marked elevation of precursors (serum 17-hydroxyprogesterone and Δ-androstenedione)	21-OH-def^severe / 21-OH-def^severe
Nonclassic (LOHD)	Symptomatic: later development of virilization; milder symptoms	Moderate elevation of precursors	21-OH-def^severe / 21-OH-def^mild
			21-OH-def^mild / 21-OH-def^mild
	Asymptomatic: no virilization or other symptoms		
Carrier	Asymptomatic	Precursor level greater than normal	21-OH-def^severe / 21-OHase (normal)
Normal	Asymptomatic	Lowest levels—some overlap seen with carriers	21-OH-def^mild / 21-OHase (normal)
			21-OHase (normal) / 21-OHase (normal)

From New MI, White PC, Pang S, et al: The adrenal hyperplasias. In Scriver CR, Beaudet AL, Sly S, Valle D (eds): Metabolic Basis of Inherited Diseases, 6th ed. New York, McGraw-Hill, 1989.

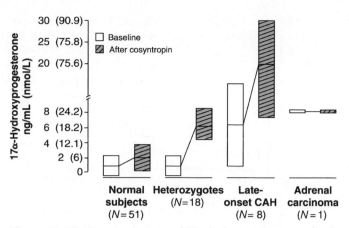

Figure 40-25 Means and ranges of 17α-hydroxyprogesterone levels before and after cosyntropin administered IM in normal subjects, suspected heterozygotes, patients with late-onset congenital adrenal hyperplasia (CAH), and one patient with adrenal carcinoma. (From Baskin HJ: Screening for late-onset congenital adrenal hyperplasia in hirsutism or amenorrhea. Arch Intern Med 147:847, 1987.)

sample of 17-hydroxyprogesterone should be measured. If the level increases more than 10 ng/mL, the diagnosis of LOHD is established (**Fig. 40-25**). Corticosteroid treatment is normally reserved for patients wishing to conceive to restore ovulatory function. In other women, treatment is more efficient and safer using OC pills, as in PCOS.

CUSHING'S SYNDROME

Excessive adrenal production of glucocorticoids caused by increased ACTH secretion (Cushing's disease) or adrenal tumors produces the signs and symptoms of Cushing's syndrome. These findings include hirsutism and menstrual irregularity in addition to the classic findings of central obesity, dorsal neck fat pads, abdominal striae, and muscle wasting and weakness. The latter catabolic effect of glucocorticoid excess differs from the anabolic effects of testosterone excess, but some women with PCOS may have other clinical findings similar to those found with Cushing's syndrome. In these cases, Cushing's syndrome can be easily excluded by performing an overnight dexamethasone suppression test. To perform this test, 1 mg of dexamethasone is ingested at 11 PM and the plasma cortisol level is measured the following morning, at 8 AM. If the cortisol level is less than 5 μg/100 mL, Cushing's syndrome is ruled out. If the cortisol level fails to suppress to this degree, the diagnosis of Cushing's syndrome is not established. It is necessary to perform a complete dexamethasone suppression test (Liddle's test) or measure the urinary free cortisol and plasma ACTH levels to determine whether Cushing's syndrome exists.

Depression and other conditions can cause failure to suppress with the dexamethasone screening test just described. Accordingly, many endocrinologists prefer to depend on measurement of the 24-hour urinary free cortisol level. A creatinine level is also measured to gauge completeness of collection. Values above 100 μg/24 hr are abnormal, and values greater than 240 μg are almost diagnostic of Cushing's syndrome. Cushing's syndrome may result from a pituitary tumor producing ACTH (Cushing's disease), an ectopic tumor in the body, adrenal neoplasms, or hyperplasia. Various algorithms have been developed for this differential diagnosis.

DIFFERENTIAL DIAGNOSIS

The differential diagnosis of the various causes of androgen excess can usually be made without difficulty by means of a complete history, careful physical examination, and measurement of serum of testosterone and DHEAS levels to determine whether there is an ovarian or adrenal source of excess androgen production.

Measurement of total testosterone, free testosterone, the **free androgen index**, and non–SHBG-bound testosterone (unbound testosterone) have all been advocated to assist in the diagnosis of hyperandrogenism. In a clinical setting, commercial assays for testosterone are insensitive and cannot discriminate reliably between normal and abnormal values, unless values are very high (tumor or male range). This is being addressed by several organizations, including the Endocrine Society, Centers for Disease Control and Prevention (CDC), AEPCOS Society, American Society for Reproductive Medicine (ASRM), and American Congress of Obstetricians and Gynecologists (ACOG), and standardized accurate assays will be available soon. It has been suggested that measurement of the free androgen index or non–SHBG-bound testosterone level is a more specific discriminator of hyperandrogenism than total testosterone. Clinically, however, an accurate measurement of total testosterone is all that is necessary. It is not clinically important whether a hirsute woman has a total testosterone level in the highest portion of the normal range or a mildly elevated level of non–SHBG-bound testosterone. Thus, to determine the magnitude of elevated androgens, as well as their source, measurement of total testosterone is more cost-effective than the other assays and provides the clinician with the information necessary to establish the diagnosis.

As noted, androgen excess caused by iatrogenic causes, sexual ambiguity, or pregnancy-associated ovarian tumors can usually be easily determined by the history and physical examination. Masculinizing ovarian or adrenal tumors are associated with rapidly progressive signs of hirsutism and virilization. Serum testosterone levels higher than 2 ng/mL, with normal DHEAS levels, indicate the probable presence of an ovarian tumor. The diagnosis can be confirmed by bimanual pelvic examination and ultrasonography, CT, or MRI. Women with a rapid progression of virilization and DHEAS levels greater than 8 μg/mL most likely have an androgen-producing adrenal adenoma; the diagnosis can be confirmed by CT or MRI. A long history of gradually increasing hirsutism, even if accompanied by virilization, is not consistent with the diagnosis of adrenal or ovarian tumors. The diagnosis of ovarian stromal hyperthecosis should be suspected for women with these signs and testosterone levels greater than 1.5 ng/mL. Women with physical findings consistent with Cushing's syndrome should have the diagnosis ruled out. PCOS, LOHD, and idiopathic hirsutism may be associated with a similar history and findings at physical examination. Menstrual irregularity, however, is uncommon in women with idiopathic hirsutism, and testosterone and DHEAS levels are normal. Women with LOHD commonly have a family history of androgen excess and often belong to an ethnic group with a higher gene frequency for an abnormality. The diagnosis of LOHD is established by measurement of 17-hydroxyprogesterone, either by testing of an early morning serum sample or following ACTH stimulation.

TREATMENT

SPECIFIC DISORDERS

Ovarian and Adrenal Tumors

Almost all Sertoli-Leydig cell tumors are unilateral. If the woman has not completed her family and these tumors are well differentiated and confined to one ovary, the tumors may be treated by unilateral salpingo-oophorectomy. Because most hilus cell tumors occur after menopause, they are best treated by bilateral salpingo-oophorectomy and total abdominal hysterectomy. Adrenal adenomas and carcinomas should also be treated by operative removal. Adrenal carcinomas frequently have metastasized to the liver by the time the androgenic signs have developed. Despite chemotherapy, the prognosis is poor after metastases have occurred. Stromal hyperthecosis is also best treated by bilateral salpingo-oophorectomy, together with total abdominal hysterectomy. After removal of the ovaries of women with stromal hyperthecosis or any of the androgen-producing tumors, the acne and oiliness of the skin disappear, breast size increases, and clitoral size decreases. The excess central hair becomes finer and grows less rapidly but does not disappear. Electrolysis can remove the facial hair and depilatories, bleaches, or shaving can be used to treat the body hair.

Late-Onset 21-Hydroxylase Deficiency

The treatment of women with LOHD depends on their primary complaint. The androgen excess and menstrual irregularity can be treated as for PCOS. However, if these women wish to conceive, it is preferable to use glucocorticoids such as hydrocortisone (15 to 20 mg), prednisone (5 to 7.5 mg), or dexamethasone (0.5 to 0.75 mg) in divided doses. Doses as low as 2.5 mg of prednisone or 0.25 mg dexamethasone may be used initially. The aim of treatment is to suppress androstenedione and bring 17-hydroxyprogesterone and progesterone levels into the normal range. Ovulation usually resumes rapidly.

Polycystic Ovary Syndrome

Before ovulation induction, it is necessary to normalize overt abnormalities in glucose tolerance and to encourage weight loss if the body mass index (BMI) is excessive (>28). Ovulation induction may be accomplished by a variety of agents including **metformin**, clomiphene, letrozole (and other aromatase inhibitors), gonadotropins, and pulsatile GnRH, as well as ovarian diathermy or drilling. Adjunctive measures include the use of dexamethasone, dopamine agonists, thiazolidinediones, and various combinations of these. In vitro fertilization (IVF; stimulated or unstimulated) may be indicated in difficult to manage cases or if other fertility factors are present.

Metformin had been used as a first-line treatment for infertility, although not all women with PCOS will respond. A Cochrane review has reported an odds ratio of 3.88 (95% confidence index [CI], 2.25 to 6.69) for restoration of ovulatory function. In a randomized trial of metformin (1700 mg/day versus clomiphene, 150 mg for 5 days), the cumulative pregnancy rate for metformin (68.9%) was significantly better than for clomiphene (34%; $P < .01$) and the abortion rate was lower with metformin (9.7% versus 37.5%; $P = .045$). However, more recent randomized trials with a focus on live births as an end point have suggested that clomiphene is superior to metformin for

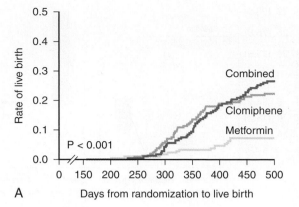

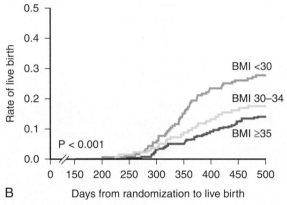

Figure 40-26 Kaplan-Meier curves for live birth, according to study group. (From Legro RL, Barnhart HX, Schlaff WD, et al. Clomiphene, metformin, or both for infertility in the polycystic ovary syndrome. N Engl J Med 356:551, 2007.)

first-line therapy (**Fig. 40-26**). Metformin should be used for overweight and obese women to achieve better metabolic control prior to pregnancy and for those who might have a more casual approach to their fertility, in that metformin takes longer to become effective and may not induce ovulation in some women. Even when metformin cannot induce ovulation, its continued use may be beneficial when combined with clomiphene or gonadotropins. An improvement in oocyte quality with metformin has been suggested, but the effect has not been proved. It may decrease the risk of ovarian hyperstimulation syndrome in women with PCOS undergoing IVF.

Clomiphene has been the mainstay for ovulation induction. Most pregnancies occur within the first few cycles. Accordingly, it is reasonable to use clomiphene, with or without metformin, as an initial approach, after obtaining a semen analysis, but not for more than three or four ovulatory cycles before a more comprehensive workup is undertaken. Letrozole (2.5 to 5 mg/day, 5 days) has proved to be efficacious as an alternative to clomiphene, and is particularly suited for women who have side effects with clomiphene. However, there are no long-term data to date. Low-dose gonadotropin therapy is highly effective as a second-line treatment, and there is no evidence that any one gonadotropin preparation is better than another.

Currently, pulsatile GnRH therapy is rarely used, primarily because its use is cumbersome and less effective in PCOS compared with its use for hypothalamic amenorrhea. Ovarian drilling (diathermy) is a reasonable second-line therapy, particularly in

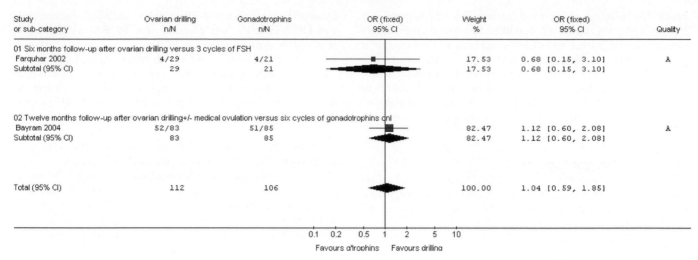

Footnotes: Test for heterogeneity: Chi² = 0.35, df = 1 (p = 0.55), I² = 0%
Test for overall effect: Z = 0.14 (p = 0.89)

A

Footnotes: Test for heterogeneity: Chi² = 0.35, df = 3 (p = 0.91), I² = 0%
Test for overall effect: Z = 2.89 (p = 0.91)

B

Figure 40-27 Results of a meta-analysis of RCTs of LOS versus gonatotropins for live birth rate **(A)** and multiple pregnancy rate **(B)**. (From Thessaloniki ESHRE/ASRM-Sponsored PCOS Consensus Workshop Group: Consensus on infertility treatment related to polycystic ovary syndrome. Hum Reprod 23:462, 2008.)

clomiphene failures and when gonadotropin therapy has proved difficult. In randomized trials against standard gonadotropin therapy, ovarian drilling resulted in similar pregnancy rates but with a lower rate of multiple pregnancies (**Fig. 40-27**).

As adjunctive treatment, thiazolidinediones have been found to be similar in effectiveness to metformin for ovulation induction. However, there is concern with their use because of the risk of teratogenicity.

Treatment of Manifestations
Skin Disorders
Hirsutism, acne, and alopecia are related to hyperandrogenism in women with PCOS. Although ovarian or adrenal androgen excess increases the likelihood of these complaints, enhancement of these effects because of increased 5α-reductase activity largely explains the abnormalities. Thus, successful strategy usually requires an antiandrogen added to ovarian suppressive therapy, usually with an OC. Clearly, women with PCOS who are

interested in pregnancy are not candidates for suppressive therapy or the use of antiandrogens.

Peripheral androgen blockade with antiandrogens is dose-related, and **spironolactone** and flutamide are the most frequently used agents, although finasteride, a specific 5α-2 inhibitor, also has efficacy. Cyproterone acetate (2 mg) is most frequently used in combination with ethinyl estradiol as an OC, although larger doses have been used as well. Flutamide, a pure androgen, should only be used in lower doses because of hepatic toxicity. This antiandrogen may have particular efficacy for androgenic alopecia, although there has been only limited success with any therapy for this disorder.

Use of a nonandrogenic progestogen (e.g., desogestrel, norgestimate, drospirenone) in an OC, in combination with spironolactone (100 to 200 mg), is suggested as first-line treatment. Adjuncts or other antiandrogens can be used, if necessary. In very severe cases, use of a GnRH agonist with estrogen or an OC add-back has been shown to be successful. However, this therapy is difficult to maintain long term. In the recently published

Endocrine Society guidelines for the treatment of hirsutism, it is suggested that OC use alone should be first-line therapy. However, in women with a significant complaint of hirsutism, it is probably more efficacious to combine an OC with an antiandrogen such as spironolactone. A more detailed discussion is presented later. Androgenic acne responds more quickly to treatment and is more successful than the treatment of hirsutism. Alopecia is least responsive to therapy, with responses rates only in the range of 30%.

Metabolic and Weight Concerns

The key management strategy should be directed at altering lifestyle variables. Exercise regimens, particularly when coordinated with a group of similar women, have been shown to be beneficial. Details of these approaches may be found elsewhere. However, this approach should be part of all therapies for PCOS, acknowledging that some thin and normal-weight women with PCOS probably already have a healthy lifestyle.

Metabolic syndrome (MBS), driven largely by weight in the United States, is usually treated by a combination of diet and metformin. Six- to 12-month therapy has been shown to reduce weight by 5% to 7%, as well as reduce insulin resistance and improve metabolic parameters. Recently, positive results also have been reported with the use of bariatric surgery as well in obese women with PCOS. This approach carries risks and should not be considered as first-line therapy.

Some data suggest that the use of antiandrogens (specifically flutamide) may also be efficacious for reducing body weight and visceral fat in women with PCOS. A combination of drospirenone and 17α-ethinylestradiol (EE$_2$) with flutamide and metformin has been used successfully in adolescents. However, this multidrug regimen has not been tested in an adult population. Although therapy for women with PCOS should be directed at a woman's specific complaint, improvement of lifestyle variables, including weight reduction and fitness, should be the mainstay of all treatments. Metformin has an important role for metabolic concerns, particularly when MBS is present, and may aid in cases of subfertility. For skin manifestations of androgen excess, as noted, treatment should include the combination of an OC with an antiandrogen.

A summary of various treatments for specific complaints in PCOS is provided in **Table 40-10**.

Idiopathic Hirsutism

Although hirsutism is a benign condition, it is frequently of great concern to the woman. Women with idiopathic hirsutism have normal circulating levels of testosterone and DHEAS. Almost all

Table 40-10 Treatment for Women with Polycystic Ovary Syndrome

Complaint	Treatment Options
Infertility	Metformin, clomiphene, letrozole, gonadotropins, ovarian cautery
Skin manifestations	Oral contraceptive + antiandrogen (spironolactone, flutamide, finestride), GnRH agonists
Dysfunctional bleeding	Cyclic progestogen; oral contraceptives
Weight, metabolic concerns	Diet/lifestyle management; metformin

those with symptomatic hirsutism who have normal testosterone and DHEAS levels have elevated skin 5α-RA, which may by reflected in elevated levels of 3α-diol-G. It is not necessary to measure 3α-diol-G in women with hirsutism without elevated circulating androgen levels, because the presence of hirsutism is itself evidence of increased peripheral androgen activity. An agent that inhibits peripheral androgen activity should be given to women with these findings.

Because of the length of the hair growth cycle, responses to treatment should not be expected to occur within the first 3 months of therapy. Objective methods of assessing changes of hair growth, such as photographs, are useful. With the use of various therapies, a successful response should occur in approximately 70% of women within 1 year of therapy. Remaining excess hair can be removed by electrolysis. Treatment should be continued for 4 years and then stopped to determine whether hirsutism recurs. If so, therapy can be reinitiated.

Many agents are available to inhibit the various sources of androgen production that may lead to hirsutism. OCs suppress LH and ovarian testosterone production by the inhibitory action of the progestational component. The estrogenic component in OCs increases SHBG levels in the circulation, which decreases free testosterone levels. The progestogens in the OCs also inhibit 5α-reductase activity in the skin. Women for whom OCs are contraindicated or produce side effects may be treated with medroxyprogesterone acetate. This agent also inhibits LH, which causes decreased testosterone production, although to a lesser extent than with combined OCs. Treatment with GnRH agonists is expensive and reserved for severe clinical manifestations of ovarian hyperandrogenism, not hirsutism alone.

Ketoconazole, which blocks adrenal and gonadal steroidogenesis by inhibiting cytochrome P450–dependent enzyme pathways, has been used in dosages of 200 mg, twice daily, to treat hyperandrogenism associated with PCOS and idiopathic hirsutism. This potent drug effectively decreases hair growth and acne, but major side effects and complications (including hepatitis) occur in most women so treated. These problems limit the use of ketoconazole to select women, who require careful monitoring. In these severe cases, it is probably preferable to use a GnRH agonist.

Spironolactone has been used and studied extensively and should be considered the treatment of choice in the United States for women with idiopathic hirsutism, as well as many with PCOS. In addition to being an androgen receptor blocker, it also decreases ovarian testosterone production and inhibits 5α-RA. Various dosages, from 50 to 200 mg daily, have been used. We have found that a dose of 200 mg/day of spironolactone is more effective than 100 mg/day. Barth and associates have found a clinically evident response of decreased hair after 3 months of spironolactone, 200 mg/day. After 1 year of treatment, a 15% to 25% reduction was seen in hair shaft diameter and linear growth rate at all body sites. With the higher dose of spironolactone, liver function test results and plasma electrolyte levels are usually unchanged, and side effects occur infrequently, except for irregular uterine bleeding. The latter can be controlled with concomitant use of OCs. Electrolytes and blood pressure should be monitored for the first few weeks of therapy to ensure that hypotension and hyperkalemia do not occur. Finasteride, a 5α-reductase inhibitor (5 mg/day), and flutamide, a nonsteroidal antiandrogen (250 to 500 mg/day) have also been used to treat hirsutism and have a level of effectiveness similar to that of spironolactone (100 mg/day). If flutamide is used, doses should be kept as low as possible and liver function tests should be performed regularly. None of these agents, however, has been approved for treatment in the United States. Antiandrogen therapy has been shown to be the most important modality for hirsutism treatment.

KEY POINTS

- The major androgen produced by the ovaries is testosterone and that of the adrenal glands is DHEAS.
- There are three markers of androgen production, one for each compartment in which androgens are produced. In the ovary, it is testosterone, in the adrenal gland, DHEA-S, and in the periphery, 3α-diol-G.
- Approximately 85% of testosterone is bound to SHBG and is biologically inactive, 10% to 15% is bound to albumin, and 1% to 2% is unbound. Both of the latter fractions are biologically active.
- Women with idiopathic hirsutism have increased 5α-RA.
- There are three criteria to diagnose PCOS; the diagnosis is based on clinical criteria, not laboratory values.
- The most frequently used diagnostic criteria for PCOS (called the Rotterdam criteria) require finding any two of the following: menstrual irregularity, hyperandrogenism, and/or polycystic ovaries on ultrasound.
- If untreated, women with PCOS have an increased risk of developing diabetes mellitus and hypertension after menopause.
- Women with ovarian neoplasms have testosterone levels more than 2.5 times the upper limits of the normal range.
- The diagnosis of LOHD is established if the basal (early morning) serum 17-hydroxyprogesterone levels are greater than 3 ng/mL or if the level 1 hour after infusion of 0.25 μg ACTH is more than 10 ng/mL.
- Metformin given to women with PCOS decreases glucose levels and may increase insulin sensitivity. It frequently causes ovulation to occur and increases the frequency of ovulation when clomiphene citrate is given to women with PCOS.
- Women with LOHD have a block in cortisol biosynthesis of 11β-hydroxylase or 21-hydroxylase, resulting in increased circulating levels of 17-hydroxyprogesterone.
- Because of the length of the hair growth cycle, response should not be expected until after 3 months of therapy. Successful responses should occur in approximately 70% of patients treated.
- The best treatment for hirsutism caused by increased peripheral androgen metabolism is the antiandrogen spironolactone.
- Women with PCOS who desire fertility should be treated with agents that stimulate ovulation, starting with metformin, clomiphene citrate and, if the condition is unresponsive, proceeding to gonadotropins. An alternative treatment for unresponsive patients is ovarian drilling.

> ### REFERENCES CAN BE FOUND ON EXPERTCONSULT.com

BIBLIOGRAPHY

Bridges NA, Cooke A, Healy MJ, et al: Standards for ovarian volume in childhood and puberty, *Fertil Steril* 60:456, 1993.

Carmina E, Lobo RA: The use of fasting blood to assess the prevalence of insulin resistance in polycystic ovary syndrome (PCOS), *Fertil Steril* 82:661, 2004.

Dahlgren E, Janson PO, Johansson S, et al: Women with polycystic ovary syndrome wedge resected in 1956 to 1965: A long-term follow-up focusing on natural history and circulating hormones, *Fertil Steril* 57:505, 1992.

Dunaif A, Graf M, Mandeli J, et al: Characterization of groups of hyperandrogenic women with acanthosis nigricans, impaired glucose tolerance, and/or hyperinsulinemia, *J Clin Endocrinol Metab* 65:499, 1987.

Gjønnaess H: Ovarian electrocautery in the treatment of women with polycystic ovary syndrome (PCOS): Factors affecting the results, *Acta Obstet Gynecol Scand* 73:407, 1994.

Gjønnaess H: Late endocrine effects of ovarian electrocautery in women with polycystic ovary syndrome, *Fertil Steril* 69:697, 1998.

Horton R, Hawks D, Lobo RA: 3 alpha,17beta-androstanediol glucuronide in plasma: A marker of androgen action in idiopathic hirsutism, *J Clin Invest* 69:1203, 1982.

Jovanovic VP, Carmina E, Lobo RA: Not all women diagnosed with PCOS share the same cardiovascular risk profiles, *Fertil Steril* 94:826, 2010.

Legro RL, Barnhart HX, Schlaff WD, et al: Clomiphene, metformin, or both for infertility in the polycystic ovary syndrome, *N Engl J Med* 356:551, 2007.

Legro RS, Kunselman AR, Dodson WC, et al: Prevalence and predictors of risk for type 2 diabetes mellitus and impaired glucose tolerance in polycystic ovary syndrome: A prospective controlled study in 254 affected women, *J Clin Endocrinol Metab* 84:165, 1999.

Lobo RA, Goebelsmann U: Adult manifestation of congenital adrenal hyperplasia due to incomplete 21-hydroxylase deficiency mimicking polycystic ovarian disease, *Am J Obstet Gynecol* 138:720, 1980.

Lobo RA, Goebelsmann U: Effect of androgen excess on inappropriate gonadotropin secretion as found in polycystic ovary syndrome, *Am J Obstet Gynecol* 142:394, 1982.

Lobo RA, Goebelsmann U, Horton R: Evidence for the importance of peripheral tissue events in the development of hirsutism in polycystic ovary syndrome, *J Clin Endocrinol Metab* 57:393, 1983.

Lobo RA, Shoupe D, Serafini P, et al: The effects of two doses of spironolactone on serum androgens and anagen hair in hirsute women, *Fertil Steril* 43:200, 1985.

Martin KA, Chang RJ, Ehrmann DA, et al: Evaluation and treatment of hirsutism in premenopausal women: An Endocrine Society Clinical Practice Guideline, *J Clin Endocrinol Metab* 93:1105, 2008.

Nestler JE, Jakubowicz DJ, Evans WS, et al: Effects of metformin on spontaneous and clomiphene-induced ovulation in the polycystic ovary syndrome, *N Engl J Med* 338:1876, 1998.

New MI, White PC, Pang S, et al: The adrenal hyperplasias. In Scriver CR, Beaudet AL, Sly S, Valle D, editors: *Metabolic Basis of Inherited Diseases*, ed 6, New York, 1989, McGraw-Hill.

Norman RJ, Davies MJ, Lord J, et al: The role of lifestyle modification in polycystic ovary syndrome, *Trends Endocrinol Metab* 13:251, 2002.

Polson DW, Adams J, Wadsworth J, et al: Polycystic ovaries: A common finding in normal women, *Lancet* 1:870, 1988.

Serafini P, Ablan R, Lobo RA: 5alpha-Reductase activity in the genital skin of hirsute women, *J Clin Endocrinol Metab* 60:349, 1985.

Shaw LJ, Merz CNB, Azziz R, et al: Postmenopausal women with a history of irregular menses and elevated androgen measurements at high risk for worsening cardiovascular event-free survival: Results from the National Institutes of Health-National Heart, Lung, and Blood Institute Sponsored Women's Ischemia Syndrome Evaluation, *J Clin Endocrinol Metab* 93:1276, 2008.

Speiser PW: Molecular diagnosis of CYP21 mutations in congenital adrenal hyperplasia: Implications for genetic counseling. Review, *Am J Pharmacogenomics* 1:101, 2001.

Speiser PW, Dupont B, Rubenstein P, et al: High frequency of nonclassical steroid 21-hydroxylase deficiency, *Am J Hum Genet* 37:650, 1985.

Urbanek M, Woodroffe A, Ewens KG, et al: Candidate gene region for polycystic ovary syndrome on chromosome 19p13.2, *J Clin Endocrinol Metab* 90:6623, 2005.

Wild RA, Bartholomew MJ: The influence of body weight on lipoprotein lipids in patients with polycystic ovary syndrome, *Am J Obstet Gynecol* 159:423, 1988.

Wild RA, Carmina E, Diamanti-Kandarakis E, et al: Assessment of cardiovascular risk and prevention of cardiovascular disease in women with the polycystic ovary syndrome: A position statement by the Androgen Excess and Polycystic Ovary Syndrome (AE-PCOS) Society, *J Clin Endocrinol Metab* 95:2038, 2010.

41

Infertility
Etiology, Diagnostic Evaluation, Management, Prognosis

Roger A. Lobo

The term ***infertility*** is generally used to indicate that a couple has a reduced capacity to conceive as compared with the mean capacity of the general population. In a group of normal fertile couples, the monthly conception rate, or **fecundability**, is approximately 20%. This figure is important for all couples seeking fertility to know, because it will alleviate unrealistic expectations of immediate success with various therapies, which can only approach 20%/cycle (with the exception of **in vitro fertilization–** embryo transfer [IVF-ET]). For most couples, the correct term should be *subfertility*, suggesting a decreased capacity for pregnancy but not an impossible feat.

The definition of infertility is the inability of a couple to conceive after 1 year of trying. This time line is relevant to help determine when an infertility investigation should begin. In women older than 35 years, this time line should be after 6 months of trying. Recently, the World Health Organization (WHO) has defined infertility as a disease. Clearly, infertility is a cause of major distress for couples and should be assessed thoroughly, and not neglected.

INCIDENCE

Results from the three U.S. National Surveys of Family Growth performed under the direction of U.S. government agencies have provided information about infertility in this country. Analyses of the data obtained from the surveys performed in 1982, 1988, and 1995 have indicated that the proportion of U.S. women ages 15 to 44 years with impaired fecundity increased from 8% in 1982 and 1988 to 10% in 1995, a 20% rise. It was estimated that the number of women with impaired fecundity in the United States increased from 4.6 to 6.2 million between 1982 and 1995, a 35% rise. Most of this increase occurred among nulliparous women in the oldest age group (35 to 44) because women of the Baby Boom generation were reaching this age. Many in this group had delayed their childbearing. According to data from the Centers for Disease Control and Prevention (CDC), in 2002 there were 7.3 million women in the United States with infertility, constituting 12% of the reproductive age population. The percentage of women seeking help for this problem is believed to be fairly constant (44% of women with impaired fertility).

INFERTILITY AND AGE

Data from both older and more recent studies have indicated that the percentage of infertile couples increases with increasing age of the female partner. Analysis of data from three national surveys in the United States has revealed that the percentage of presumably fertile married women not using contraception who failed to conceive after 1 year of trying steadily increased from ages 25 to 44 years (**Table 41-1**). Data from a study of presumably fertile nulliparous women married to husbands with **azoospermia** who underwent donor artificial insemination revealed that the percentage who conceived after 12 cycles of insemination declined substantially after age 30 (**Table 41-2**). This older, classic study used fresh semen; currently, only frozen donor sperm is used, which does not achieve as favorable pregnancy rates. Decreasing fecundability with age is even more pressing in this context. With IVF, recent data from SART in the United States has shown that the percentage of deliveries per oocyte retrieval procedure is 41.3% in women younger than 35, 22.2% by ages 38 to 40 ,and only 12.3% by ages 41 to 42 years.

In general terms, approximately one in seven couples are infertile if the wife is 30 to 34, one in five is infertile if she is 35 to 40, and one in four is infertile if she is 40 to 44 years of age. Another way to interpret these data is to state that as compared with women aged 20 to 24 years, fertility is reduced by 6% in the next 5 years, by 14% between ages 30 and 34, by 31% between ages 35 and 39, and to a much greater extent after age 40.

FECUNDABILITY: THE ABILITY TO CONCEIVE

Analysis of data from presumably fertile couples who stop using contraception to conceive has shown that approximately only 50% of the couples will conceive in 3 months, 75% will conceive in 6 months, and by 1 year approximately 90% will have conceived (**Fig. 41-1**). Statistical analysis of these data indicates that normal monthly fecundability is approximately 0.2.

This information is extremely important when analyzing data concerning the results of various treatment methods applied to a group of infertile couples. This group includes those with hypofertility from presumed causes (e.g., mild endometriosis) as well as those with idiopathic (unexplained) infertility. For example, it has been estimated that if the mean fecundability of the

Table 41-1 Married Women Who Are Infertile, by Age*

Age (yr)	Infertile (%)
20-24	7.0
25-29	8.9
30-34	14.6
35-39	21.9
40-44	28.7

*From three national U.S. surveys.
From Menken J, Trussell IJ, Larsen U: Age and infertility. Science 23:1389, 1986.

Table 41-2 Pregnancy Rates by Age at 1 Year in Normal Women with Azoospermatic Husbands After Donor Insemination

Age (yr)	Pregnancy Rate (%)
<25	73.0
26-30	74.1
31-35	61.5
36-40	55.8

From Schwartz D, Mayaux MJ: Female fecundity as a function of age: Results of artificial insemination in 2193 nulliparous women with azoospermic husbands. N Engl J Med 306:404, 1982.

Table 41-3 Incidence of Conception over Time among Nonsterile Couples with Mean Fecundability of 0.2

Months Without Conception	Couples Not Yet Having Conceived		Proportion (%) of Couples Who Will Conceive (within 12 mo)
	Proportion (%)	Mean Fecundability	
0	100.0	0.20	86.0
6	31.9	0.14	77.0
12	14.0	0.11	69.2
24	4.3	0.08	57.0
36	1.9	0.06	48.2
48	1.0	0.05	41.7
60	0.6	0.04	36.7

Adapted from Leridon H, Spira A: Problems in measuring the effectiveness of infertility therapy. Fertil Steril 41:580, 1984.

population is 0.2 (a 20% monthly rate), this rate decreases over time (**Table 41-3**). Analysis of these statistical tables reveals that after 2 years of trying to conceive, approximately 4% of these couples will not have done conceived. Their mean monthly fecundability is approximately 0.08, and 57% will conceive in the next year. Of the 2% still not pregnant at this time, 3 years after trying to conceive, the monthly fecundability drops to approximately 0.06, 0.05, and 0.04 in the next 3 years, respectively. Thus, in the fourth, fifth, and sixth years of attempting to conceive, 48%, 42%, and 37% of nonpregnant women should conceive without treatment.

Several studies have reported the incidence of spontaneous conception among infertile couples without a specifically diagnosed cause of infertility (**unexplained infertility**). A live birth rate of 873 infertile couples in several Canadian centers has been observed without treatment for 18 months; it steadily rose to more than 35% at 3 years and 45% after 7 years (**Fig. 41-2**).

Of the 562 couples in this group with unexplained infertility who received no treatment, one third had a live birth during the first 3 years of observation without treatment.

Thus, to determine that any method of treatment of infertility is superior to no treatment, the treatment results on the incidence of pregnancy over time need to be statistically analyzed. Ideally, these results should be compared with a nontreated control group. At the least, these pregnancy rates should be compared with the rates of the nontreated women with a normal diagnostic evaluation (see later). Various statistical formulas for performing these analyses based on life table analysis have been described. This statistical approach is necessary to determine whether treatment methods are beneficial, because data from uncontrolled studies can give a false impression of treatment effectiveness. These formulas provide mathematical techniques to determine the monthly probability of conception and the cumulative conception rate.

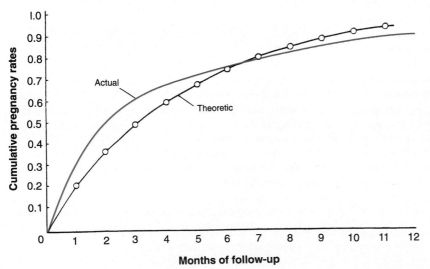

Figure 41-1 Curve of theoretical time to pregnancy in women with a monthly fecundability of 0.2 *(open circles)* and curve of actual time to pregnancy in fertile women discontinuing contraception *(solid line)*. (Open circle data from Hull MGR, Glazener CMA, Kelly NJ, et al: Population study of causes, treatment, and outcome of infertility. Br Med J 291:1693, 1985; solid line data from Murray DL, Reich L, Adashi EY: Oral clomiphene citrate and vaginal progesterone suppositories in the treatment of luteal phase dysfunction: A comparative study. Fertil Steril 51:35, 1989.)

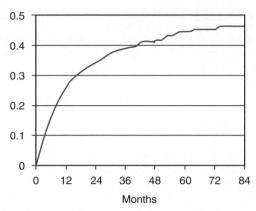

Figure 41-2 Cumulative rate of conceptions leading to live birth. Couples (873) who remained untreated throughout follow-up; cumulative rate of live birth conception at 36 months was 38.2% (95% CI, 34.2-42.3). (Adapted from Collins JA, Burrows EA, Willan AR. The prognosis for live birth among untreated infertile couples. Fertil Steril 64:22, 1995.)

CAUSES OF INFERTILITY

The exact incidence of the various factors causing infertility varies among different populations and cannot be precisely determined. Collins has reported that among 14,141 couples in 21 publications, ovulatory disorders occurred 27% of the time, male factors, 25%, tubal disorders, 22%, endometriosis, 5%; other, 4%, and unexplained factors, 17%. It has not been shown that other abnormalities, such as antisperm antibodies, luteal phase deficiency, subclinical genital infection, or subclinical endocrine abnormalities such as hypothyroidism or hyperprolactinemia in ovulatory women are true causes of infertility. No prospective randomized studies have demonstrated that treatment of these latter entities results in greater fecundability than without treatment. If any of these do cause infertility, they do so infrequently. With current techniques of investigation, it is impossible to diagnose the cause of infertility in up to 20% of couples, and they are considered to have unexplained infertility. After a rigorous investigation, other reports have suggested this figure to be as low as 10%. However, it is unclear if subtle abnormalities, as noted, have much to do with infertility. Also, most couples with unexplained infertility are hypofertile and some are able to conceive without treatment, although it may take several years and with a diminishing probability of this occurrence over time.

DIAGNOSTIC EVALUATION

The diagnostic evaluation of infertility should be thorough and completed as rapidly as possible. During the initial interview, the couple should be informed about normal human fecundability and how these probabilities decrease with increasing age of the female partner, older than 30 years, and duration of infertility for more than 3 years. The various tests in the diagnostic evaluation and why they are performed should be thoroughly explained. In addition, the sequence of performing these tests, their degree of discomfort, cost, and time in the cycle at which they should be performed should also be discussed. The available therapies and prognosis for treatment of the various causes of infertility should

also be included in the dialogue. The couple should be informed that after a complete diagnostic infertility evaluation, the cause for infertility cannot be determined in a large group of couples. For many couples, the reduced fecundability can be suggested to be age-related. Methods to increase the fecundity of couples with a normal diagnostic evaluation, such as **controlled ovarian hyperstimulation** and **intrauterine insemination**, as well as assisted reproductive techniques (ARTs), should also be covered.

Each couple should be instructed about the optimal time in the cycle for conception to occur and should be encouraged to have intercourse on the day before ovulation. Unless the husband has **oligozoospermia (oligospermia)**, daily intercourse for 3 consecutive days at midcycle should be encouraged. When ovulation is more precisely determined, as with luteinizing hormone (LH) monitoring (see later), intercourse should occur for 2 consecutive days around the LH surge. Because the egg disintegrates less than 1 day after it reaches the ampulla of the oviduct, it is best that sperm be present in this area when the egg arrives so that fertilization can occur. Because normal sperm retains its fertilizing ability for up to 72 hours, it is preferable to have sperm in the oviduct prior to the arrival of the oocyte.

A study was performed by Wilcox and coworkers of fertile couples who stopped contraception to conceive and recorded the cycle day when they had sexual intercourse. Hormone analysis was performed to determine the day of ovulation. None of the women became pregnant in the group of couples who had intercourse after ovulation occurred. The pregnancy rate was approximately 30% if intercourse occurred on the day of ovulation, as well as 1 and 2 days prior to ovulation. The pregnancy rate was approximately 10% if coitus occurred 3, 4, or 5 days before ovulation. No pregnancies occurred when intercourse took place 6 days or more before ovulation (**Fig. 41-3**). It is therefore considered optimal to perform insemination or have sexual intercourse on the day before ovulation.

Because peak levels of LH occur 1 day before ovulation, measurement of LH by urinary LH immunoassays is the best way to determine the optimal time to have intercourse or insemination. Tests that measure LH in a random daily urine specimen are

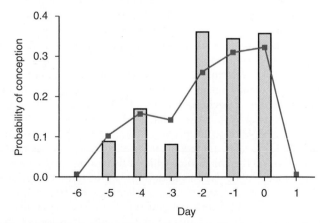

Figure 41-3 Probability of conception on specific days near the day of ovulation. The *bars* represent probabilities calculated from data on 129 menstrual cycles in which sexual intercourse was recorded to have occurred on only a single day during the 6-day interval ending on the day of ovulation (day 0). The *solid line* shows daily probabilities based on all 625 cycles, as estimated by the statistical model. (From Wilcox AJ, Weinberg CR, Baird DD: Timing of sexual intercourse in relation to ovulation. N Engl J Med 333:1517, 1995.)

usually more convenient for planning natural or artificial insemination than tests that detect LH in the first morning urine specimen. Ovulation most commonly occurs on the day following the detection of LH in a random specimen (12 to 24 hours later), and it occurs on the day when LH is detected in the first morning specimen, which contains urine formed during the prior night. Several types of commercial kits are available for determining peak LH, so women who find it difficult to determine a hormone change using one type can try another system or kit. Basal body temperature (BBT) charts are not as precise for determining ovulation, with ovulation occurring over a span of several days of the thermogenic shift.

In some cases, women produce less than adequate amounts of vaginal lubricant. Various vaginal lubricants and chemicals, as well as saliva, used to improve coital satisfaction may interfere with sperm transport. Some men experience midcycle impotence because of the pressure of performing intercourse on demand. In such cases, the intercourse schedule should be less rigorous. The couple should also be told that among fertile couples, there is only approximately a 20% chance of conceiving in each ovulatory cycle, even with optimally timed coitus, and that it takes time to become pregnant. Thus, the terms *time* and *timing* should be emphasized during the initial counseling session. Couples should also be advised to cease smoking cigarettes and drinking caffeinated beverages in excess. Cigarette smoking and caffeine consumption have been shown independently in several studies to decrease the chances of conception. The common practice of vaginal douching also reduces the chance of conception by approximately 30%.

All couples should have a complete history taken, including a sexual history, and a physical examination. After this initial evaluation, tests should be undertaken to determine if the woman is ovulating and has patent fallopian tubes and if a semen sample of the male partner is normal.

DOCUMENTATION OF OVULATION

Preliminary information that the woman is ovulatory is provided by a history of regular menstrual cycles. If the woman has regular menstrual cycles, a serum progesterone level should be measured in the midluteal phase to provide indirect evidence of ovulation as well as normal luteal function. Although serum progesterone levels vary in the normal luteal phase in a pulsatile manner, a serum progesterone level above 10 ng/mL is indicative of adequate luteal function. Progesterone levels of 10 ng/mL or higher are found during at least 1 day of the luteal phase of normal ovulatory cycles in which conception occurred. Measurement of the daily BBT provides indirect evidence that ovulation has taken place. The BBT graph also provides information about the approximate day of ovulation and duration of the luteal phase. The BBT should be taken shortly after awakening, only after at least 6 hours of sleep and prior to ambulating, with sublingual placement of a special thermometer with gradients between 96° and 100° F.

Women with oligomenorrhea (menses at intervals of 35 days or longer) or amenorrhea who wish to conceive should be treated with agents that induce ovulation, regardless of whether they have occasional ovulatory cycles. Therefore, for these women, direct or indirect measurement of progesterone is unnecessary until after therapy is initiated.

SEMEN ANALYSIS

While information about ovulation is being obtained, the male partner's reproductive system should be evaluated by means of **semen analysis**. The male partner should be advised to abstain from ejaculation for 2 to 3 days before collection of the semen sample, because frequent ejaculation lowers seminal volume and occasionally the sperm count in some men. It is best to collect the specimen in a clean (not necessarily sterile) wide-mouthed jar after masturbation. It is important that the entire specimen be collected, because the initial fraction contains the greatest density of sperm. Ideally, collection should take place in the location where the analysis will be performed. The degree of sperm motility should be determined as soon as possible after liquefaction, which usually occurs 15 to 20 minutes after ejaculation. Sperm motility begins to decline 2 hours after ejaculation and it is best to examine the specimen within this period. Semen should not be exposed to marked changes in temperature and, if collected at home during cold weather, the specimen should be kept warm during transport to the laboratory.

Parameters used to evaluate the semen include volume, viscosity, sperm density, sperm morphology, and sperm motility. The last parameter should be evaluated in terms of percentage of total motile sperm as well as quality of motility (rapidity of movement and amount of progressive motility). Sperm morphology is an extremely important parameter, which is correlated to fertilizing ability. Using strict criteria (Kruger), only approximately 4% or more of the sperm in an ejaculate may be considered normal. Recent WHO criteria have indicated decreased parameters of what constitutes a normal ejaculate as compared with older normal ranges. It should be remembered that the sperm analysis is a subjective test and that there is a fair degree of variability from test to test in the same man. Also, the semen profile reflects sperm production that occurred 3 months earlier, which is important to note if there were illness at that time. **Table 41-4** lists the parameters that are generally considered normal for a semen analysis, according to the latest WHO study. It is beyond our scope here to discuss fully the causes and diagnostic evaluation of semen abnormalities. In broad terms, the various causes of semen abnormalities are cited in **Table 41-5**.

When semen analyses were performed on a group of men whose wives had conceived within the past 4 months, approximately 75% had at least one abnormal characteristic and 25% had two abnormalities. These results confirm that there is normally a wide variability in the parameters used to characterize semen. Because the characteristics of semen may vary over time

Table 41-4 Lower Fifth Percentile Values in Fertile Men*

Parameter	Value
Semen volume (mL)	1.5
Sperm concentration (million/mL)	15
Total number (million/ejaculate)	39
Total motility (%)	40
Progressive motility (%)	32
Normal forms (%)	4

*With time to pregnancy ≤ 12 months.
Adapted from Cooper TG, Noonan E, von Eckardstein S, et al: World Health Organization reference values for human semen characteristics. Hum Reprod Update 16:231, 2010.

Table 41-5 Causes of Semen Abnormalities

Finding	Cause
Abnormal Count	
Azoospermia	Klinefelter's syndrome or other genetic disorder
	Sertoli-cell-only syndrome
	Seminiferous tubule or Leydig cell failure
	Hypogonadotropic hypogonadism
	Ductal obstruction, including Young's syndrome
	Varicocele
	Exogenous factors
Oligozoospermia	Genetic disorder
	Endocrinopathies, including androgen receptor defects
	Varicocele and other anatomic disorders
	Maturation arrest
	Hypospermatogenesis
	Exogenous factors
Abnormal Volume	
No ejaculate	Ductal obstruction
	Retrograde ejaculation
	Ejaculatory failure
	Hypogonadism
Low volume	Obstruction of ejaculatory ducts
	Absence of seminal vesicles and vas deferens
	Partial retrograde ejaculation
	Infection
High volume	Unknown factors
Abnormal motility	Immunologic factors
	Infection
	Varicocele
	Defects in sperm structure
	Metabolic or anatomic abnormalities of sperm
	Poor liquefaction of semen
Abnormal viscosity	Cause unknown
Abnormal morphology	Varicocele
	Stress
	Infection
	Exogenous factors
	Unknown factors
Extraneous cells	Infection or inflammation
	Shedding of immature sperm

From Bernstein GS, Siegel MS: Male factor in infertility. In Mishell DR Jr, Davajan V, Lobo RA (eds): Infertility, Contraception and Reproductive Endocrinology, 3rd ed. Cambridge, MA, Blackwell Scientific, 1991, p 629.

and undergo normal biologic variability, it is best to repeat the test on two or three occasions if an abnormality is found.

EVALUATION AND LABORATORY TESTS

Aspects of the woman's medical history that should be highlighted include the following: any pregnancy complications if previously pregnant; previous pelvic surgery of any type; significant dysmenorrhea; dyspareunia or sexual dysfunction; abnormal cervical cytology or procedures to treat cervical abnormalities; and use of medication, drugs, and tobacco. Family history should be explored for genetically related illnesses, birth defects and, most importantly, the history of age of menopause in female family members. Finally, any symptoms suggestive of

endocrine disorders should be solicited (e.g., weight changes, skin changes).

The physical examination should focus on extremes of body mass, skin changes, thyroid size, breast secretion, abnormal pain on abdominal or pelvic examination, and assessment of the vagina and cervix. In addition, if available, vaginal ultrasound performed at the same time may be extremely valuable in picking up abnormalities of the uterus (e.g., fibroids) endometrial thickness, pelvic masses, and ovarian morphology (e.g., polycystic appearance, unusually small). These may provide a guide for further testing.

In a healthy asymptomatic woman, only a complete blood count (CBC), blood type, Rh factor, and rubella status are needed, together with a Pap smear obtained within 12 months of the previous test. Cystic fibrosis screening is currently recommended for all women, as well as other genetic tests in certain populations. Infectious disease screening (for chlamydia and gonorrhea) is carried out routinely in most practices at the time of the Pap smear. Further infectious disease screening (e.g., syphilis, HIV, hepatitis) is warranted only on a selective basis and is required for all couples undergoing insemination or IVF.

In women older than 35 years, serum follicle-stimulating hormone (FSH) and estradiol (E_2) levels should be obtained on cycle day 2 or if three FSH values are abnormal (>10 mIU/mL), suggesting decreased ovarian reserve, which is the pool of viable oocytes remaining in the ovary. Levels over 20 mIU/mL are particularly bad prognostically. However, although FSH levels tend to fluctuate from cycle to cycle, once the FSH level has been elevated in a given cycle, the overall prognosis is reduced. E_2 levels, if elevated on days 2 and 3 (>70 pg/mL), do not allow for a valid interpretation of FSH values and may independently suggest a decreased prognosis regarding ovarian reserve.

Antimüllerian hormone (AMH) or müllerian-inhibiting substance (MIS) has become a valuable standard for assessing ovarian reserve. MIS, which is produced by the granulosa cells of small growing follicles, physiologically suppresses FSH stimulation of sustained follicular growth. MIS decreases with aging and, when levels reach 0.05 ng/mL (essentially undetectable levels), menopause occurs within 4 years. Levels are high in polycystic ovary syndrome (PCOS) and in women with cystic ovaries who are vulnerable to hyperstimulation; serum levels correlate with the number of oocytes retrieved in IVF cycles. In terms of ovarian reserve, higher levels (>2 ng/mL) suggest a larger cohort of small available follicles and low levels (<0.5 ng/mL) suggest a decreased ovarian reserve. Unlike FSH, MIS values are fairly constant and stable throughout the menstrual cycle, particularly in the low ranges. Higher values, however, exhibit more variability in the early to mid follicular phase. From a clinical perspective, assays for AMH and MIS have not been standardized, requiring each clinician to establish his or her own normative data and receiver operating characteristic (ROC) curves, as our group has done, reflecting the values quoted above.

Some specialists have suggested obtaining antibody titers for *Chlamydia trachomatis*, which if elevated may signify the possibility of tubal disease. It has been suggested that if the immunoglobulin G (IgG) antibody titer is greater than 1:32, 35% of patients have evidence of tubal damage. Whether this type of evaluation is routinely warranted as a focus for the infertility investigation continues to be debated. Routine measurement of thyroid-stimulating hormone (TSH) and prolactin in women with regular ovulatory cycles at the time of the initial visit may not be cost-effective but is routinely undertaken.

If an abnormality is found in one of the first two noninvasive diagnostic procedures (documentation of ovulation and semen analysis), it should be treated before proceeding with the more costly and invasive procedures, unless there is a history or findings suggestive of tubal disease. For example, if the woman has oligomenorrhea and does not ovulate each month, after a normal semen analysis is observed, ovulation should be induced with **clomiphene citrate** before performing the other diagnostic measures. The chance of having occult tubal disease in this setting depends on the patient population and various risk factors, but is no more than 5% in a general infertile population of anovulatory women. Provided that no other infertility factors are present, most anovulatory women (80%) conceive after induction of ovulation with therapeutic agents and half the couples will conceive during the first three ovulatory cycles.

If these initial diagnostic tests are normal, the more uncomfortable and costly **hysterosalpingography (HSG)** should be performed in the follicular phase of the next cycle.

Hysterosalpingography

It is best to schedule the HSG during the week following the end of menses to avoid irradiating a possible pregnancy. The HSG should be avoided if there has been a history of salpingitis in the recent past or if there is tenderness on pelvic examination. As noted, most practices routinely screen for chlamydia and gonorrhea during the initial examination. However, We still routinely advise using prophylactic antibiotics at the time of HSG. We prescribe doxycycline (100 mg twice daily for 3 days, starting 1 day before the procedure), but this recommendation is not universally followed. If a hydrosalpinx is seen with HSG, doxycycline should be continued for 1 week. The examination should be performed with use of a water-soluble contrast medium and image-intensified fluoroscopy. A water-soluble contrast medium enables better visualization of the tubal mucosal folds and vaginal markings than an oil-based medium. It is important to be able to evaluate the appearance of the intratubal architecture to determine the extent of damage to the tube. A meta-analysis, including four randomized trials, has indicated that a therapeutic benefit is more likely to occur when oil-soluble contrast media are used in an HSG performed for the diagnostic evaluation of infertility. The odds of pregnancy occurring after the procedure were twofold higher when oil-soluble media were used compared with water-soluble media. These results differ from those of a large randomized trial by Spring and colleagues that found no difference in pregnancy rates when the HSG was performed with oil-soluble or water-soluble contrast media. Thus, the therapeutic benefit of oil-soluble contrast media remains inconclusive.

Because oil-soluble contrast media have more complications than water-soluble media, including pain resulting from peritoneal irritation and formation of granulomas, it is probably best to perform routine HSGs with water-based media. The diagnostic HSG will not only determine whether the tubes are patent but also, if disease is present, will help determine the magnitude of the disease process and provide information about the lining of the oviduct, and uterine cavity in particular, that cannot be obtained by laparoscopic visualization. The procedure can also determine whether **salpingitis isthmica nodosa** is present in the interstitial portion of the oviduct. When an HSG shows lack of patency in one tube, this has been shown to be falsely positive approximately 50% of the time at laparoscopy. Therefore, it is not necessary to perform tubal reconstructive surgery on a woman with one patent tube. However, a diagnostic laparoscopy may be considered to detect the presence of peritubal adhesions. The finding of a normal endometrial cavity at the time of HSG obviates the need for hysteroscopy. If severe tubal disease, such as a large hydrosalpinx, is found at the time of HSG, based on success rates, it is preferable for the couple to undergo IVF-ET than for the woman to have tubal surgery. If the hydrosalpinx is large and clearly visible on ultrasound, it is preferable to perform laparoscopic salpingectomy prior to IVF-ET because the pregnancy rate with IVF-ET may be decreased by as much as 40%. When the extent of tubal disease is unclear or the couple prefers not to undergo IVF-ET, diagnostic laparoscopy should be carried out in the follicular phase of the cycle. In general, the goal should be to have all tubal reconstruction carried out laparoscopically (see later).

Postcoital Test

Although important from a physiologic standpoint (cervical mucus being important for sperm transport), the **postcoital test (PCT)** is now rarely indicated as a necessary part of the infertility investigation. It is a very subjective test. A normal PCT is one in which at least five motile sperm are visible in normal cervical mucus obtained from the upper canal just prior to ovulation. A suboptimal test can be the result of technique, timing of the test, and problems with cervical mucus and/or with sperm. Although a good PCT has been correlated with a better prognosis for pregnancy, sperm have been recovered at laparoscopy when there was a poor PCT. Moreover, because the suggested treatment for a poor PCT is intrauterine insemination after ovarian stimulation, this is the exact next step taken, even if the PCT is normal, in the setting of unexplained infertility. Occasionally, as may happen with an orthodox Jewish couple, a semen analysis cannot be obtained. Here, a PCT provides a surrogate for visualizing motile, normal-appearing sperm.

Laparoscopy

In the past, this was an obligatory final step in the infertility investigation when all other test results were normal. Data have shown that in 20% to 40% of cases, some minor abnormalities may be found (e.g., endometriosis, adhesions), which may have a bearing on fecundability, Obviously, if there is something suspicious on ultrasound or examination, there has been prior pelvic surgery or appendicitis, or there is pelvic pain and/or dyspareunia, the index of suspicion is increased. The probability that peritubal adhesions of sufficient severity to cause infertility will be found at the time of laparoscopy is less than 5% in a woman with no history of salpingitis or symptoms of dysmenorrhea, a normal bimanual pelvic examination, and normal antibody titers (if obtained). Provided the woman is younger than 40 years, is having ovulatory cycles, and there is an acceptable semen analysis, several cycles of controlled ovarian stimulation and intrauterine insemination may be undertaken before performing diagnostic laparoscopy or going directly to IVF-ET. At this juncture, a decision can be revisited about whether performing a laparoscopy should be considered, although many couples usually prefer to proceed with IVF-ET, particularly if they have insurance coverage for IVF.

The following additional laboratory procedures have been advocated by some to assist in determining the cause of the infertility: (1) measurement of serum TSH and prolactin levels in ovulatory women, if not already done; (2) luteal phase endometrial biopsy; (3) measurement of antisperm antibodies in the male and female partner; (4) bacteriologic cultures of the cervical mucus and semen; and (5) other sperm testing, such as hypoosmotic swelling, hamster egg penetration test, and DNA fragmentation.

If abnormalities are discovered in any of the initial three steps of the infertility evaluation, treatment has been found to increase the incidence of pregnancy significantly as compared with no treatment, particularly treatment of anovulation or total tubal obstruction. Treatment of abnormalities found in the diagnostic procedures just mentioned has not been documented to be more effective than withholding therapy. Therefore, the necessity and cost-effectiveness of performing these additional tests and correcting the abnormalities found by them have not been demonstrated. Until it is demonstrated conclusively that treatment of abnormalities diagnosed by these additional tests results in a significantly improved pregnancy rate compared with placebo or no treatment, the advisability of continuing the diagnostic evaluation beyond the initial three diagnostic steps remains unproven (see later).

Measurement of Thyroid-Stimulating Hormone and Prolactin in Ovulatory Women

If women with anovulation have hypothyroidism or hyperprolactinemia, treatment with thyroid replacement or dopamine agonists, respectively, have been shown to cause resumption of ovulation and enhanced fecundity. However, for women with regular ovulatory cycles who have mild hyperprolactinemia, it has been reported that pregnancy rates 1 year after the diagnostic evaluation without treatment were similar to those in ovulatory women without hyperprolactinemia. Several investigators have performed randomized clinical trials with bromocriptine and placebo that have shown that treatment with bromocriptine does not increase fecundity rates in ovulatory infertile women. It has been estimated that less than 1% of women with infertility and normal ovulatory cycles had elevated TSH levels. None of these women became pregnant when treated with thyroxine. Although the prevalence of slightly raised TSH levels has increased, because many consider values greater than 2.5 µU/mL to be slightly elevated (compared with >5 µU/mL), this finding does not change the arguments made earlier.

Luteal Deficiency

Although suggested for many years, it has never been established that lutea phase defects cause infertility. The diagnosis of luteal deficiency can be determined by finding serum progesterone levels consistently below 10 ng/mL 1 week before menses or finding consistent histologic evidence of a delay in development of the normal secretory endometrial pattern, indicating an inadequate effect of progesterone production on the endometrium. Using classic criteria to establish the diagnosis histologically, secretory endometrial development (usually obtained in the late luteal phase) must lag 3 days or more behind the expected pattern for the time of the cycle, as originally described by Noyes and associates. Furthermore, this finding must be consistent and found in at least two cycles. Dating needs to be calculated using indicators that will detect the day of ovulation, rather than by subtracting 14 days from the onset of the next menses.

Erroneous diagnosis of this entity also occurs because of the subjective interpretation of histologic dating criteria. There is at least a 10% disagreement of more than 2 days when the same observer dated the specimens on two separate occasions, and even more interobserver variability

As noted regarding the PCT, ovarian stimulation with intrauterine insemination (IUI) is often the first empirical treatment for unexplained infertility. This essentially treats the luteal inadequacy, if it exists, preempting the need for invasive and imprecise endometrial biopsies.

Immunologic Factors

Substantial evidence from animal studies has indicated that antibodies can be induced in females from antigens obtained from organs in the male reproductive tract, and that these antibodies interfere with normal reproduction. Both sperm-agglutinating and sperm-immobilizing antibodies have been found in the serum of some infertile women, but also in the serum of fertile control subjects. Agglutinating antibodies are found more frequently than immobilizing antibodies in most series and, in some reports, the incidence of sperm-agglutinating antibodies in infertile women is similar to that in the control group. Even with the finding of sperm agglutination or immobilization in serum, it has not been demonstrated that a similar degree of sperm inactivation occurs in the lower genital tract. Thus, there is no definitive evidence that sperm agglutination or immobilization in the serum of infertile women is the cause of their infertility. One of the reasons for this discrepancy is that both serum assays measure mainly IgM and IgG antibodies, whereas the antibodies locally produced in the genital tract are mainly IgA. Thus, some investigators have measured antisperm antibodies in cervical mucus and found a correlation between their presence and infertility. However, no data have shown that the finding of antibodies against sperm in the male or female partner is a cause of infertility. In addition, corticosteroid treatment of the male or female partner does not significantly increase the pregnancy rate compared with no therapy.

Autoimmunity to sperm in semen and serum has been found in some infertile men, particularly those who have had testicular infection, injury, or a surgical procedure such as vasectomy reversal. Men with these antibodies have been treated with corticosteroid therapy and sperm-washing techniques. Nevertheless, the effectiveness of such treatment remains to be established.

In 1993, four prospective studies reported the incidence of fertility occurring after a diagnostic infertility evaluation was performed in which the presence of antisperm antibodies was documented. These studies were performed in four different laboratories in three different countries. Several different techniques were used for the antibody tests. All four studies showed no correlation between the presence of antisperm antibodies in either member of the couple and the chance of conception. Pregnancy rates over time were similar in couples who had or did not have antisperm antibodies. Therefore, tests to detect these antibodies as part of the diagnostic infertility evaluation are not justified because their presence does not affect fecundity.

Infectious Factors

Some researchers have suggested that asymptomatic, or occult, infection of the upper female genital tract and male genital tract is a cause of infertility. As early as 1973, it was suggested that infection with what was then called T-mycoplasma in the male could interfere with normal sperm function, and infection of the female reproductive tract could interfere with normal sperm transport. The current name now used for these organisms is *Ureaplasma urealyticum*. Two other microorganisms found in the female genital tract are *Mycoplasma hominis* and *M. fermentans*. Although it has been reported that treatment of infertile couples with antibiotics, such as tetracycline or doxycycline, that eradicate these organisms result in high pregnancy rates, controlled studies have reported no difference in pregnancy rates between couples treated with antibiotics and those not treated. Harrison and colleagues have studied 88 infertile couples with no demonstrable cause of infertility. One third were treated with doxycycline, one third received placebo, and one third received no treatment. T-mycoplasma was isolated from approximately two thirds of the couples in each group and was eradicated only in the group treated with doxycycline. Nevertheless, conception rates were similar in each group (**Table 41-6**). Matthews and co-workers have performed a similar study and obtained similar results. Other investigators have suggested that asymptomatic *Chlamydia trachomatis* infection may also cause infertility, but the dosage of doxycycline used in these randomized studies would also have eradicated these organisms. Thus, there is no evidence that asymptomatic infection of the genital tract of the human male or female causes infertility.

Other Sperm Tests

The zona-free hamster egg penetration test originally described by Yanagimachi and associates was a test developed to predict the fertilizing ability of sperm and provides an additional, perhaps more sensitive, parameter for assessing sperm function than routine semen analysis. However, many variables factors affect the test results. It has been shown that this test does not correlate well with IVF of human eggs. The sensitivity and specificity of the **hamster egg penetration assay (sperm penetration assay)** is considered to be too low to justify its routine use as part of the infertility investigation.

Other functional tests of sperm, such as the hypo-osmotic swelling test, assess the integrity of the sperm cell membrane. However, there is no evidence that this adds additional information to the infertility investigation. More recently, DNA fragmentation in sperm by flow cytometry or direct microscopy has been determined. A higher rate of DNA fragments (DNA fragmentation index > 30%) indicates a poorer rate of fertilization and therefore suggests the need for IVF with **intracytoplasmic sperm injection (ICSI)**. There is no evidence that this

correlates with the success of IVF and so therefore cannot be advocated as a routine test.

PROGNOSIS

All infertile couples should be informed of the prognosis for pregnancy associated with treatment of their particular cause of infertility. The highest probability of conception with treatment other than with IVF-ET occurs among couples in whom anovulation is the only abnormality, with a substantially lower probability of pregnancy in couples with tubal disease or sperm abnormalities (**Fig. 41-4**). Although these data are older, this information from Hull still provides the best available comparisons. Among a group of infertile couples with unexplained infertility who were followed for 2 years without treatment after the evaluation was completed, it was found that the chances of becoming pregnant were greater in women younger than 35 years (≈75%) than in women older than 35 (50%; **Fig. 41-5**). The cumulative conception rate at the end of 2 years without therapy for those couples was much greater for those who had tried to conceive for less than 3 years before evaluation (≈75%) than those who had tried to conceive for more than 3 years (≈30%; **Fig. 41-6**). In three of the four studies of infertile couples who received no therapy mentioned earlier, more than 50% of the couples who eventually conceived did so in the first year after completing the infertility evaluation; the vast majority of those who conceived, which was greater than 50% of the entire group, who did conceive without treatment, did so within 2 years (see **Fig. 41-2**). Thus, infertile couples with no demonstrable cause of infertility have their best prognosis for conception without treatment for approximately 2 years after the initial infertility evaluation is completed, and a poor prognosis thereafter. To increase their chances of conception or to shorten the time interval until conception takes place, various treatment methods have been advocated.

For couples with unexplained infertility, IVF and **gamete intrafallopian transfer (GIFT)** afford the highest pregnancy rates. Although GIFT was considered to be more effective than IVF

Table 41-6 Controlled Studies of Outcome of Therapy of Couples with Unexplained Infertility and *Urea urealyticum* Infections

Study*	Treatment	No. of Couples	No. of Pregnancies	Conceptions (%)
Harrison et al	Doxycycline	30	5	17
	Placebo	28	4	14
	None	30	5	17
Matthews et al	Treated	51	10	20
	None	18	4	22

*From original source.
From Bernstein GS: Occult genital infection and infertility. In Mishell DR Jr, Davajan V, Lobo RA (eds): Infertility, Contraception and Reproductive Endocrinology, 3rd ed. Cambridge, MA, Blackwell Scientific, 1991.

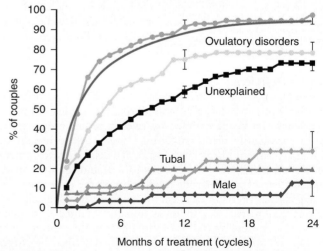

Figure 41-4 Effect of various treatments on fecundability—ovulatory, tubal, and male factors. (Adapted from Hull MGR, Glazener CMA, Kelly NJ, et al: Population study of causes, treatment, and outcome of infertility. Br Med J 291:1693, 1985.)

Figure 41-5 Cumulative rates of conception from first attendance at clinic in couples with unexplained infertility related to age of woman. Rates for each age group are shown as solid squares, <25 years; blue triangles, 25 to 29 years; solid triangles, 30 to 34 years; blue squares, >35 years. Standard errors of proportions are given at 6, 12, 18, and 24 months. (From Hull MGR, Glazener CMA, Kelly NJ, et al: Population study of causes, treatment, and outcome of infertility. Br Med J 291:1693, 1985.)

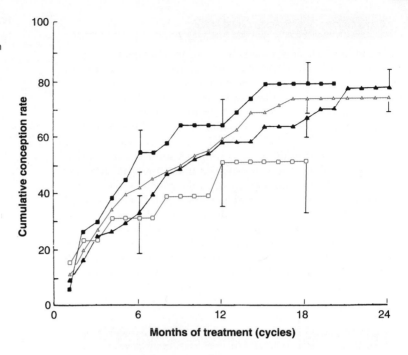

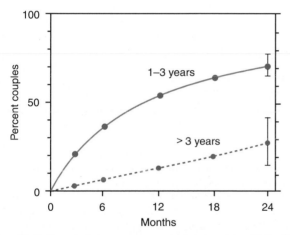

Figure 41-6 Cumulative pregnancy rates in unexplained infertility without treatment related to duration of infertility. (From Hull MGR: Effectiveness of infertility treatments: Choice and comparative analysis. Int J Gynaecol Obstet 47:99, 1994.)

Table 41-7 Aggregate Data for Each Treatment*

Treatment	No. of Studies	No. of Pregnancies Per Initiated Cycle (%)	Percentage of Quality-Adjusted Pregnancies Per Initiated Cycle
Control groups	11	64/3539 (1.8)	1.3
Control groups, randomized studies	6	23/597 (3.8)	4.1
IUI	9	15/378 (4)	3.8
CC	3	37/617 (6)	5.6
CC + IUI	5	21/315 (6.7)	8.3
HMG	13	139/1806 (7.7)	7.7
HMG + IUI	14	207/1133 (18)	17.1
IVF	9	378/683 (22.5)	20.7
GIFT	9	158/607 (26.0)	27.0

*Many studies appear in more than one row if they reported on more than one treatment.
CC, Clomiphene citrate; GIFT, gamete intrafallopian transfer; HMG, gonadotropins; IUI, intrauterine insemination; IVF, in vitro fertilization.
Adapted from Guzick DS, Sullivan MW, Adamson GD, et al: Efficacy of treatment for unexplained infertility. Fertil Steril 70:207, 1998.

taking into account patient selection, these therapies are equivalent. Because GIFT requires a laparoscopy, this procedure is rarely done at present. Noting that the normal cycle fecundability is in the range of 20% to 25%, IVF provides a cycle rate that is twice as high (see more detailed statistics later). In couples with unexplained infertility who undergo IVF, fertilization failure has been documented, explaining, at least in part, the inability to conceive naturally.

Controlled ovarian stimulation (COS) with clomiphene citrate or various gonadotropin preparations, followed by IUI, also increases pregnancy rates compared with no treatment during short time intervals. Data compiled by Guzick and colleagues from several studies have shown cycle fecundability lower than general (**Table 41-7**). This should be considered the conservative estimate when counseling patients about therapy. In a recent

randomized controlled trial by Reindollar (see later), the single-cycle rate for ovarian stimulation and IUI was approximately 10% and was similar with the use of clomiphene or gonadotropins.

After four to six cycles of COS and IUI in couples with unexplained fertility, the cumulative pregnancy rate should be approximately 50%. Because cycle fecundability and cumulative pregnancy rates are enhanced with COS and IUI, this combined therapy should be tried for several cycles prior to initiating IVF-ET. It should be noted that IUI alone has not been proved to be of benefit in unexplained infertility. However, in women older than 40 years or in couples with marked abnormalities in the semen analysis, IVF with intracytoplasmic sperm injection (ICSI) should be recommended.

OUTCOMES OF PREGNANCY

Several studies have reported the pregnancy outcomes of women with long-standing infertility who conceive after treatment. Ovulation-inducing drugs and reconstructive tubal surgery have independently been shown to be associated with an increased incidence of ectopic pregnancy compared with the normal population. Use of ovulation-inducing drugs alone, as well as when combined with IVF and GIFT, has been shown to increase the incidence of multiple gestations. Therefore, if conception occurs after treatment with ovulation induction or tubal reconstructive surgery, monitoring of early gestation with serial human chorionic gonadotropin (HCG) level measurements and ultrasonography assists in determining whether the pregnancy is intrauterine and how many gestational sacs are present. However, infertile couples who conceive do not have a higher rate of spontaneous abortion or perinatal mortality than normal couples. In older women, nevertheless, there is a higher loss rate because of aneuploidy.

TREATMENT OF THE CAUSES OF INFERTILITY

The management of the various causes of infertility will be presented here in the order generally followed in an infertility investigation.

ANOVULATION

Medical Treatment

Therapeutic agents currently available to induce ovulation are clomiphene citrate, urinary gonadotropins (HMG and other more FSH-enriched preparations), recombinant FSH, and recombinant LH. Adjunctive treatments include gonadotropin-releasing hormone (GnRH) agonist and antagonists, as well as HCG, which is used to trigger ovulation. There is also growing experience with the use of letrozole and metformin. In addition, as discussed in Chapter 39 (Hyperprolactinemia, Galactorrhea, and Pituitary Adenomas), if anovulation is caused by hyperprolactinemia, dopamine agonists are an effective means of inducing ovulation. As noted in Chapter 40 (Hyperandrogenism), ovulation may be induced by corticosteroid therapy in women with congenital adrenal hyperplasia.

Clomiphene Citrate

Clomiphene citrate (CC) is the usual first-line pharmacologic agent for treating women with oligomenorrhea and those with amenorrhea who have sufficient ovarian estrogen production. CC is a racemic mixture of en- and zu-clomiphene, which act as estrogen antagonists. The former has a shorter half-life and is more active than the zu-clomiphene isomer, which has a much longer half-life and is more estrogen agonistic than antagonistic. CC acts by competing with endogenous circulating estrogens for estrogen-binding sites on the hypothalamus, thereby blocking the negative feedback of endogenous estrogen. GnRH is then released in a normal manner, stimulating FSH and LH, which in turn cause oocyte maturation, with increased E_2 production. The drug is usually given daily for 5 days, beginning 3 to 5 days after the onset of spontaneous menses or withdrawal bleeding induced with a progestogen.

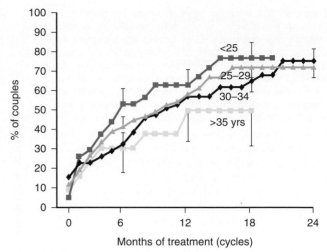

Figure 41-7 The effect of age on fecundability: 25-29 to more than 35 years. (From Hull MGR, Glazener CMA, Kelly NJ, et al: Population study of causes, treatment, and outcome of infertility. Br Med J 291:1984, 1985.)

During the days when the drug is ingested, serum levels of LH and FSH rise, accompanied by a steady increase in serum E_2 level (**Fig. 41-7**). After ingestion of CC is discontinued, E_2 levels continue to increase and the negative feedback on the hypothalamic-pituitary axis causes a decrease in FSH and LH levels, similar to the change seen in the late follicular phase of a normal ovulatory cycle. Approximately 5 to 9 days (mean, 7 days) after the last CC tablet has been ingested, the exponentially rising level of E_2 from the dominant follicle has a positive feedback effect on the pituitary or hypothalamus, producing a surge in LH and FSH levels, which usually results in ovulation and luteinization of the follicle.

Presumptive evidence of ovulation can be obtained by observation of a sustained rise in BBT or measurement of an elevation of serum progesterone level. It is best to obtain the serum sample for progesterone measurement approximately 2 weeks after the last CC tablet has been taken, because this will usually be in the middle of the luteal phase, approximately 1 week after ovulation. A rise in serum progesterone level above 3 ng/mL correlates well with the finding of secretory endometrium on an endometrial biopsy sample, but it has been reported that the maximal midluteal progesterone levels in CC-induced ovulatory conception cycles are consistently above 15 ng/mL. These levels are higher than the 10 ng/mL level, which is the minimum concentration of progesterone found in spontaneous ovulatory conception cycles because, following ovulation induction with CC, more than one follicle usually matures and undergoes luteinization.

Various treatment regimens have been advocated for the use of CC. Most start with an initial dosage of 50 mg/day for 5 days, beginning on the fifth day of spontaneous or induced menses. If presumptive evidence of ovulation occurs with this dosage, the same dosage of clomiphene citrate is taken in subsequent cycles until conception occurs. If ovulation fails to occur with the initial dosage, a sequential, graduated, increasing dosage regimen has proved to be effective, with a minimum of side effects. With this regime, if ovulation does not occur with the 50-mg dose, the dosage of drug is increased in the next treatment cycle to 100 mg/day for 5 days. If ovulation does not occur with

100 mg/day in subsequent cycles, the dosage is sequentially increased to 150 mg. In the past, we have used doses up to 250 mg, with and without HCG. In the 10 years' experience with this treatment regimen as reported by Gysler and associates, approximately half of the women who ovulated and half of those who conceived did so following treatment with the 50-mg/day regimen, and an additional 20% ovulated with the 100-mg/day dosage. However, approximately 25% of all women who ovulated or conceived did so following treatment with a higher dosage regimen, indicating the value of the individualized sequential treatment regimen. However, from a practical standpoint, it is unusual to use doses higher than 150 mg, particularly when adjuncts are available, such as metformin or switching to letrozole.

A more recently used regimen, the stair-step regimen, does not wait for menses after a failed response before moving to the next dose. Thus, if there is no follicular development on ultrasound 5 days after the last clomiphene tablet, the patient is immediately placed on 100 mg for 5 days and subsequently to 150 mg for 5 days in the same cycle if follicular development does not occur. Although preliminary retrospective reports have shown that this is a reasonable approach to hasten therapy, prospective randomized trials are still in progress.

With the dosage regimen of CC up to 250 mg, more than 90% of women with oligomenorrhea and 66% with secondary amenorrhea and normal estrogen status will have presumptive evidence of ovulation. Although only approximately 50% of patients who ovulate with this treatment will conceive, Gysler and associates have reported that 85% of those with no other causes of infertility conceive after such treatment. The fecundability during several months of treatment with CC, if no other causes of infertility are present, are similar to those of a normal fertile population. Using life table analysis, the monthly pregnancy rate (fecundability) of women treated with CC who had no other infertility factor was 22% compared with a rate of 25% for women discontinuing diaphragm use. The monthly fecundability remained constant throughout almost 1 year of treatment. Almost all the anovulatory women without other infertility factors in this series, as well as other women with correctable infertility factors, had conceived after 10 cycles of treatment. This rate is also similar to the use of gonadotropins (**Fig. 41-8**).

These data indicate that discontinuation of therapy is the major reason for the reported difference in ovulation and conception rates in anovulatory women treated with CC. However, despite these data, many investigators believe that pregnancy rates are lower with clomiphene than might be expected based on ovulation rates and other factors (in some women), such as cervical mucus and endometrial problems, explain this discrepancy. In anovulating women who respond to clomiphene, HSG should be performed if a pregnancy does not occur after 3 months. A semen analysis should be done before starting CC. When conception occurs after ovulation has been induced with CC, the incidence of multiple gestation is increased to approximately 8%, with almost all being twin gestations. However, when the drug is used in normally ovulating women with unexplained infertility, the rate increases to almost 20%. The incidence of clinical spontaneous abortion ranges between 15% and 20%, similar to the rate in the general population. The rates of ectopic gestation, intrauterine fetal death, and congenital malformation are also not significantly increased. Animal data have shown that if the drug is given in high dosages during the time of embryogenesis, there is an increased incidence of fetal

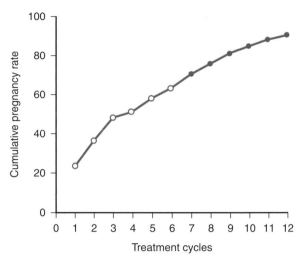

Figure 41-8 Cumulative pregnancy rate of 60% at 6 months with clomiphene. (From Messinis IE, Milingos SD: Current and future status of ovulation induction in polycystic ovary syndrome. Hum Reprod Update 3:235, 1997.)

anomalies. However, limited human data have indicated that if the drug is ingested during the first 6 weeks after conception has occurred, the incidence of fetal malformation, although higher (5.1%) than normal, is not significantly increased. Although no definitive data have shown that the drug is teratogenic in humans, it is best that the woman be reexamined before each course of treatment to be certain that she is not pregnant. It is also important to determine that the ovaries have not become enlarged, because formation of ovarian cysts is the major side effect of CC treatment. I obtain a baseline HCG level and perform an ultrasound scan before CC is prescribed.

If cysts are present, they will regress spontaneously without therapy, but if additional clomiphene citrate is given and further gonadotropin release is induced, stimulation and further enlargement of the cyst may occur. Clinically palpable ovarian cysts occur in approximately 5% of women treated with clomiphene citrate but in less than 1% of treatment cycles. The cysts usually range in size from 5 to 10 cm and do not require surgical excision, because they almost always regress spontaneously. Cysts can occur in any treatment cycle with any dosage, and the incidence is not increased with the higher dosages of drug. Recurrence of cyst formation with the same dosage is uncommon. Other side effects, which occur in less than 10% of women treated with this drug, include vasomotor flushes, blurring of vision, abdominal pain or bloating, urticaria, and a slight degree of hair loss.

Up to 10% of women treated with CC fail to ovulate with the highest dosage. Older data have suggested that this so-called resistance is not caused by the inability of the hypothalamic-pituitary axis to respond, but to the lack of the ovarian response to raised gonadotropin levels.

Some data suggest that in women with elevated levels of dehydroepiandrosterone sulfate (DHEAS), the use of low doses of dexamethasone may enhance the ovulation-inducing effect of clomiphene. This approach is less frequently used today. Other adjuncts that have been tested, but that lack validation, include adding a dopamine agonist such as bromocriptine and antiandrogens. Metformin and insulin sensitizers have also been used adjunctive treatment.

Metformin and Other Insulin Sensitizers

Metformin, a biguanine used to control blood sugar in diabetics, has a role in ovulation induction in women with PCOS. Although not a true insulin sensitizer, it decreases hepatic glucose production and has some minor peripheral action, leading to some decrease in insulin resistance. It also has a direct role in inhibiting ovarian androgen steroidogenesis and acts on the endometrium, which are probably the major mechanisms that help with ovulation and pregnancy.

Studies have confirmed the efficacy of metformin over placebo in inducing ovulation in women with PCOS. However, in direct comparisons with clomiphene, it was inferior to clomiphene in terms of live birth rates in women with PCOS. Therefore, although not necessarily a first-line choice in women with PCOS, it is clearly an adjunct and may be helpful in women who exhibit some degree of insulin resistance. Thus, it should be considered as a preliminary option in heavy or obese women and for those with impaired glucose tolerance or significant insulin resistance.

The typical dosage of metformin is 1500 mg/day. It is preferable to use long-acting tablets (XR or ES). in 500- and 750-mg tablet form, and to ingest them all at the same time at dinner. However, It should be initiated only at 500 mg and titrated up over several weeks. This is because of gastrointestinal effects (e.g., nausea, vomiting), which is the primary concern with metformin and that precludes its use in up to 20% of women.

Lactic acidosis is a rare complication that occurs primarily in older individuals. However, checking blood levels after 3 months of metformin is good practice, and women also should be reminded not to drink alcohol heavily, although the occasional drink is acceptable. Many endocrinologists advocate a dose of 2000 mg/day for heavier women.

When metformin alone is prescribed for anovulatory women who wish to conceive, the ovulation rate is approximately 60% in adherent women. In CC-resistant patients—those who fail to ovulate with 150 mg/day—although the data are mixed, approximately 25% of women will respond to CC with metformin. Metformin is a category B substance for pregnancy and has been continued through the first trimester and beyond in select patients (see Chapter 7, History, Physical Examination, and Preventive Health Care).

Rosiglitazone and Pioglitazone

In insulin-resistant patients with PCOS, the diabetic drugs (thiazolidinediones) may induce ovulation by improving the insulin hormone axis as well as through a direct effort on the ovary. These drugs have also been added to CC therapy. However, this should be reserved for short-term use under special circumstances because this class of drug is teratogenic. There is a small risk of hepatic enzyme changes and also a tendency for weight gain with long-term treatment.

Letrozole

Aromatase inhibitors are efficacious as primary agents for ovulation induction. Most of the experience is with letrozole. The mechanism of action is that of inhibition of E_2 production during the 5 days of administration, with a negative feedback causing an increase in FSH levels, much like the response to CC. Intraovarian androgen levels are also increased, which may enhance FSH sensitivity. Letrozole (2.5 or 5 mg; there is no good evidence for a dose difference) is administered for 5 days like clomiphene, beginning on cycle days 3 to 5.

Because letrozole is short-acting, the problems of thick cervical mucus or a thin endometrium associated with clomiphene have not been reported with letrozole. However, E_2 levels are usually lower at ovulation. Pregnancy rates are comparable to those with CC alone and there is a reduced incidence of multiple pregnancies because of its shorter half-life and lack of stimulation of gonadotropins beyond the early follicular phase (**Fig. 41-9**).

There is little information about the effects of letrozole in CC-resistant patients, but anecdotally it has been found to be effective in this regard in many women. Letrozole with gonadotropins has also been used for COS. A multicenter Canadian study has found no increase in congenital anomalies; their incidence is lower than with CC. However, letrozole is not U.S. Food and Drug Administration (FDA)–approved for ovulation induction and should be used with caution and informed consent. It is valuable as second-line therapy in CC failures and in women with side effects or poor responses to clomiphene.

Gonadotropins

Gonadotropin therapy is indicated for ovulation induction when estrogen levels are low. Low serum E_2 levels (usually < 30 pg/mL) or lack of withdrawal bleeding after progestogen administration signifies a state that will be unresponsive to oral therapies (clomiphene, letrozole) that are dependent on a negative feedback system. Apart from this indication in usually amenorrheic women, it is appropriate to use gonadotropins in clomiphene or letrozole failures, rather than on the basis of persistent anovulation or the inability to conceive after several (four to six) ovulatory cycles.

The original preparations of gonadotropin (HMG) were urinary extracts of postmenopausal urine. Although purified, they contained large amounts of protein contaminants. These preparations are less used today but are still available worldwide (Pergonal, Humegon). More recent preparations with additional purification have allowed them to be administered SC and IM, the only option for the older preparations. These preparations are titrated to provide an equal quantity of LH (75 IU) and FSH (75 IU) in one ampule.

Further modifications of these urinary products have eliminated most of the LH activity and provided a relatively pure FSH urinary preparation (Bravelle, Metrodin, containing 75 IU FSH/ampule). All nonrecombinant preparations, because they are extracted from human sources, have batch to batch variability in terms of biologic activity. Recombinant pure FSH preparations (from Chinese hamster ovarian cells) are currently available for SC administration (Gonal-F, Follistim, 75 IU FSH). Recombinant pure LH has also become available as a supplement (Luveris, 75 IU LH), although it is unclear if the addition of LH is really necessary in most cases.

Because each woman responds individually to the dosage of gonadotropins, even the same woman in different treatment cycles, it is essential to monitor treatment carefully with frequent measurements of estrogen levels and ovarian ultrasonography. Monitoring needs to take place frequently because there is little difference between the minimal degree of ovarian follicular development necessary to induce ovulation and the amount of follicular development that results in hyperstimulation. Close

Figure 41-9 Clomiphene citrate treatment. (From Casper RF, Mitwally MF: Review: Aromatase inhibitors for ovulation induction. J Clin Endocrinol Metab. 91:760, 2006.)

CLOMIPHENE CITRATE TREATMENT

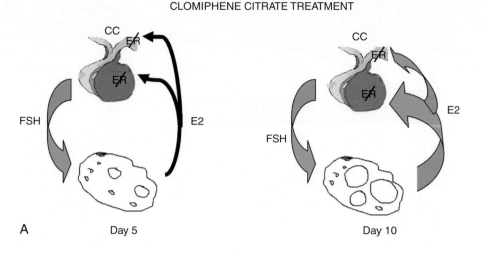

A   Day 5   Day 10

AROMATASE INHIBITOR TREATMENT

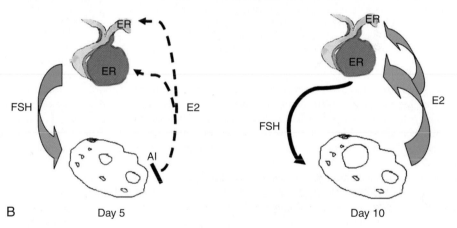

B   Day 5   Day 10

monitoring requires ultrasound to determine the number of follicles and the maturity status (ultrasound and E_2 level).

There is a different concept regarding induction of ovulation with gonadotropins when the problem is anovulation or when gonadotropins are used in the setting of unexplained infertility or for the purposes of IVF (see later). This concept is often lost by many practitioners, and leads to a high rate of hyperstimulation and multiple pregnancies. The goal of therapy in anovulatory women is to produce one mature follicle, sometimes two. In women with low estrogen status, cycle fecundability approaches the ideal ($\approx$20%/cycle) if there are no other infertility factors. It is a little lower, however, in women who are CC failures and/or have PCOS. In these patients, the risk of hyperstimulation is greatest and great care has to be used when monitoring these women.

By injecting gonadotropins, the physiology behind this approach is to increase the serum FSH level above a critical threshold level, which is an unknown at the outset. The window for this therapeutic threshold is fairly wide in normal and hypoestrogenic women, but is extremely narrow in PCOS, increasing the risk of hyperstimulation.

A starting dose of 150 IU with FSH is used (as a recombinant preparation of pure FSH or a combination of LH and FSH in a urinary preparation). The E_2 level is determined and ultrasound is performed after approximately 5 days, and then approximately every other day until a follicle reaches a diameter of at least 18 mm. The serum E_2 level should be at least in the range of 200 pg/mL for a mature follicle. At this point, 5000 to 10,000 IU of HCG is administered IM (or pure recombinant HCG, 250 µg SC) to trigger ovulation. Timed intercourse is usually advised if there is a normal semen analysis and good cervical mucus. Ovulation should occur between 36 and 48 hours after the trigger of HCG. Particularly in women with hypothalamic amenorrhea and low estrogen status, vaginal progesterone supplementation (100 mg/day) is usually prescribed, although this addition is not completely evidence-based.

In women with PCOS in whom the ovary is extremely sensitive to gonadotropin, a starting dose of only 50 to 75 IU is used. A slow step-up regimen is usually preferred, increasing the dose slowly only after 7 days (**Fig. 41-10**). Although there have been advocates for the use of a step-down approach (higher initial dose and then a rapid decrease), randomized trials in

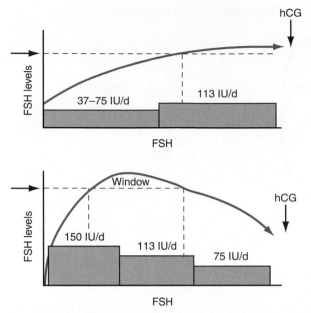

Figure 41-10 Schematic representation of serum follicle-stimulating hormone (FSH) levels and daily dose of exogenous FSH during low-dose step-up or step-down regimens for ovulation induction. (From Macklon NS, Bart CJM: Medical approaches to ovarian stimulation for infertility. In Strauss JF, Barbieri RL [eds]: Yen and Jaffe's Reproductive Endocrinology, 6th ed. Philadelphia, WB Saunders, 2009, p 701.)

PCOS have suggested the preference for using the traditional step-up approach, which has better outcomes.

The pregnancy rate per cycle should be similar to that following CC therapy ($\approx$20%). With sufficient duration of treatment and no other infertility factors, cumulative pregnancy rates should be greater than 90%. It has been reported that the cumulative pregnancy rate after nine cycles of gonadotropin therapy is approximately 77%. Although the incidence of spontaneous abortion after gonadotropin therapy is higher (25% to 35%) than the normal rate, cumulative pregnancy rates with

gonadotropins are influenced by age and the cause of anovulation. The pregnancy rates are highest for young women who are hypoestrogenic, with low to normal gonadotropin levels, as noted, and worse in older women and those with anovulation with normal estrogen status, such as CC-resistant women who have PCOS (**Fig. 41-11A and B**). The overall multiple pregnancy rate (usually twins) is in the range of 15%.

Ovarian Hyperstimulation Syndrome

Although enlarged ovaries are frequently encountered after gonadotropin administration, significant **ovarian hyperstimulation syndrome (OHSS)** occurs in approximately 0.5% of women receiving gonadotropins. OHSS can be life-threatening, causing massive fluid shifts, ascites, pleural effusion, electrolyte disturbances, and thromboembolism. The cause has not been completely elucidated but is related to the large cystic ovaries, high E_2 levels, and the ovarian elaboration of substances such as vascular endothelial growth factor (VEGF), which increase vascularity and vascular permeability. OHSS has been classified by several investigators into mild, moderate, and severe forms. A representative categorization may be found in **Table 41-8**. HCG triggers the syndrome, and blood levels of HCG continue to stimulate the ovaries in OHSS. Therefore, the syndrome is worse if pregnancy occurs and abates within 1 week in the absence of pregnancy. For this reason, if severe OHSS is anticipated, HCG injection should be withheld. In IVF cycles, the embryos may be frozen rather than replaced to avoid pregnancy.

Treatment of OHSS is largely supportive, with judicious use of fluids and prevention of thrombosis. Correction of electrolyte disturbances and maintenance of urine output are of greatest importance. Occasionally, admission for intensive care unit (ICU) monitoring is necessary.

Avoidance of excessive stimulation is the primary approach for preventing OHSS. Lowering or withholding the dose of HCG is also advisable. An alternative approach is to use a GnRH agonist instead of HCG to trigger ovulation because LH is much shorter acting and will clear from the circulation soon after ovulation, unlike HCG. An experimental approach being studied to

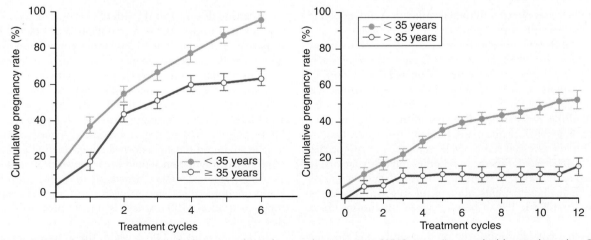

Figure 41-11 A, Cumulative pregnancy rates for hypogonadotropic anovulatory women (WHO group I) treated with gonadotropins. *Solid circles* represent the cumulative pregnancy rate in women younger than 35. *Open circles* represent the cumulative pregnancy rate in women older than 35 years. **B,** Cumulative pregnancy rates following gonadotropin treatment for anovulatory women who did not respond to clomiphene induction of ovulation (WHO group II). *Solid circles* represent the cumulative pregnancy rate in women younger than 35. *Open circles* represent the cumulative pregnancy rate in women older than 35 years. (From Lunenfeld B, Insler V: Human gonadotropins. In Wallach EE, Zacur HA [eds]: Reproductive Medicine and Surgery. St. Louis, Mosby, 1995, p 617.)

Table 41-8 Classification of Ovarian Hyperstimulation Syndrome

Mild
   Ovarian enlargement (5 cm or less)
   Abdominal discomfort
Moderate
   Ovarian enlargement (6-10 cm)
   Nausea or gastrointestinal symptoms
   Abdominal discomfort
   Normal laboratory evaluation
   Mild ascites, not clinically evident
Severe
   Symptoms as above and other symptoms, such as respiratory distress
   Ovarian enlargement
   Severe ascites (clinically evident)
   Hydrothorax
   Elevated hematocrit (>45%)
   Elevated WBC count (>15,000/μL)
   Elevated creatinine
   Electrolyte abnormalities (hyponatremia, hyperkalemia)
   Elevated liver function tests
Critical (As a Subcategory of Severe)
   Severe end-organ dysfunction
     Oliguria, creatinine >1.6 mg/dL
     Severe respiratory distress
   Thrombotic complications
   Infection
   Severe hemoconcentration
     Hematocrit >55%
     WBC count >25,000/μL

Modified from Navot D, Bergh PA, Laufer N: Ovarian hyperstimulation syndrome in novel reproductive technologies: Prevention and treatment. Fertil Steril 58:249-261, 1992.

treat OHSS is the use of a dopamine agonist such as cabergoline, which interferes with the action of VEGF.

The vast majority of studies and meta-analyses have not shown a statistically significant increased risk of ovarian or breast cancer in women receiving gonadotropin therapy.

Gonadotropin-Releasing Hormone

An alternative to the administration of HMG is GnRH treatment. Because continuous administration of GnRH will saturate the receptors and thus inhibit gonadotropin release to induce ovulation, GnRH needs to be administered in a pulsatile manner at intervals of 1 to 2 hours. GnRH is a peptide, so it cannot be administered orally; the two routes of administration in current use are the IV and SC routes. More drug must be administered by the SC route than by the IV route; however, the SC route avoids use of an IV catheter, with its accompanying problems. The success rates, however, are better with IV delivery. The medication is given by means of a small portable pump, which is usually worn attached to an article of clothing. Ovulation rates of approximately 75% to 85% per treatment cycle have been reported. However, this approach is cumbersome, requiring a continuous line and a portable pump 24 hours a day. Currently, it is not frequently used.

Other Therapeutic Modalities

Weight and Lifestyle Management

Particularly in women who are clomiphene-resistant, weight loss will often ameliorate the situation. In overweight women, it is important to ensure that abnormalities in glucose and lipid metabolism are normalized as much as possible, before induction of ovulation. There is evidence that lifestyle changes in diet and exercise may improve overall fitness and metabolic parameters, as well as ovulatory responses, even in the absence of true weight loss, although there could be a redistribution of body fat with lifestyle changes.

Ovarian Electrocauterization

At an ESRE/ASRH consensus meeting for the treatment of infertility in PCOS, it was concluded that a possible alternative to gonadotropin therapy in clomiphene-resistant women with PCOS is the use of ovarian electrocautery, which has similar efficacy (**Fig. 41-12**).

Laparoscopic electrical or laser-generated burn holes through the ovarian cortex have been associated with improving ovulation rates, as was described many years ago with ovarian wedge resection, which is no longer performed. The major advantage of this more invasive method of ovarian electrocauterization is that it decreases the risk of hyperstimulation and multiple pregnancies. In addition to a concern of surgical complications, excessive destruction of the ovarian cortex can lead to premature ovarian failure. Only a limited number of burn holes ($\approx$10) should be made.

Figure 41-12 compares the pregnancy rates after electrocauterization and gonadotropin therapy. It has been reported that the endocrine changes may persist for at least 10 years. A Cochrane review has also reported an overall term pregnancy rate of 50% after surgery and a low multiple pregnancy rate.

Nevertheless, ovulation induction in women with PCOS should still be a medical treatment, particularly with the use of adjuncts, if necessary. In my view, ovarian electrocauterization should be reserved for patients who have difficulties with gonadotropin stimulation (failure of dominant follicle selection or hyperstimulation risk).

MALE CAUSE OF INFERTILITY

All gynecologists who care for infertile couples should understand how to interpret a semen analysis and how to offer a prognosis for a disorder of abnormal semen. Although gynecologists usually do not perform a diagnostic evaluation or treat the man with a reproductive disorder, they should be able to provide counsel regarding the use of intrauterine insemination with the husband's or donor's semen, as well as with treatment by ICSI, **testicular sperm extraction (TESE)**, or microsurgical epididymal serum aspiration (MESA).

Male Partner Evaluation

If the semen analysis is abnormal and has been repeated, it is important that the man be evaluated by an andrologist, usually a urologist. Important medical conditions need to be ruled out, and occasionally an abnormality is found that can be treated. Blood should be obtained for hormone and other testing, as needed, and a careful urologic examination can diagnose problems such as testicular abnormalities and infection (**Fig. 41-13**). The more treatable conditions are hormonal abnormalities (apart from an elevated FSH level, signifying end-organ seminiferous failure), as well as infection. Varicocele repair remains somewhat controversial and the decision needs to be individualized based on the ages of the couple, other factors that may be involved, and whether the varicocele is symptomatic. Although

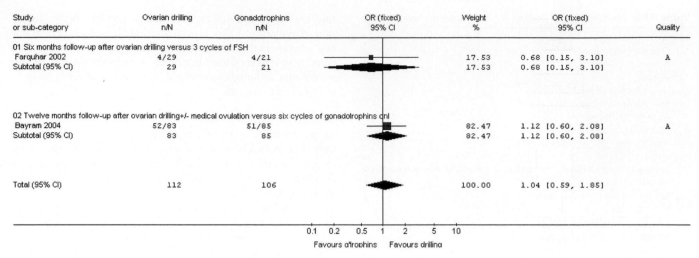

Footnotes: Test for heterogeneity: $Chi^2 = 0.35$, df = 1 (p = 0.55), $I^2 = 0\%$
Test for overall effect: Z = 0.14 (p = 0.89)

A

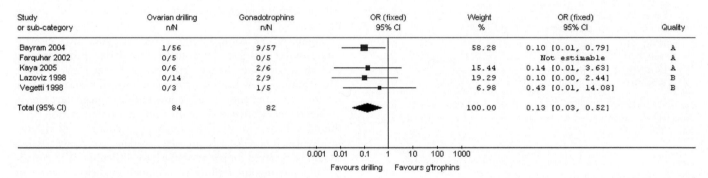

Footnotes: Test for heterogeneity: $Chi^2 = 0.35$, df = 3 (p = 0.91), $I^2 = 0\%$
Test for overall effect: Z = 2.89 (p = 0.91)

B

Figure 41-12 Results from the meta-analysis of the RCTs of LOS versus gonadotropins for live birth rate **(A)** and multiple pregnancy rate **(B)**. (From Thessaloniki ESHRE/ASRM-Sponsored PCOS Consensus Workshop Group: Consensus on infertility in PCOS. Fertil Steril; 89:505, 2008.)

a varicocele has been shown to correlate with poor motility and morphology, there is often a variable response to surgery. It is important to note that improvement may not be evident for 6 months, given that the cycle of spermatogenesis is approximately 3 months in length.

If the evaluation is nondiagnostic or if no treatment is possible or indicated, the best therapy should be directed at improving the ejaculate for intrauterine insemination or to carry out IVF with ICSI. A general algorithm for treatment is shown in **Figure 41-14**.

Intrauterine insemination has been used to treat oligospermia and abnormalities of semen volume or viscosity to enhance fecundability. The limitation of successful IUI is when there is significant oligospermia and/or motility problems (<5 million motile sperm available) or with very poor morphology.

The technique of IUI of sperm following their separation from the semen by centrifugation should be used to treat mild to moderate abnormalities in the semen analysis and unexplained infertility. This procedure is associated with higher pregnancy rates if combined with COS than when used in natural ovulatory cycles. IUI is also of benefit to women with variable

degrees of cervical stenosis. Ideally, insemination should take place on the day of, or 1 day before, ovulation. It is advisable to use a urinary LH enzyme-linked immunosorbent assay (ELISA) kit to determine the optimal date to perform insemination because the urinary LH peak occurs on the day prior to ovulation. Insemination should be scheduled for the morning after LH is initially detected in an afternoon urine specimen.

Separation of sperm from the seminal fluid by double centrifugation, the swim-up technique, or use of a density gradient should be performed before IUI. This enhances sperm motility and is thought to increase capacitation, membrane changes in sperm that facilitate fertilization) IUI of unwashed seminal fluid should not be used because it can produce severe uterine cramps as a result of prostaglandin release.

Until rather recently, if there were severe abnormalities in the semen analysis, the prognosis for fertility was less than that for any other cause of infertility (see **Fig. 41-4**), even with the use of IVF techniques. Attempts to enhance fertilization rates of aspirated oocytes with the technique of subzonal insemination of sperm were unsuccessful because fertilization rates remained low, approximately 15%. After Van Steirteghem and associates

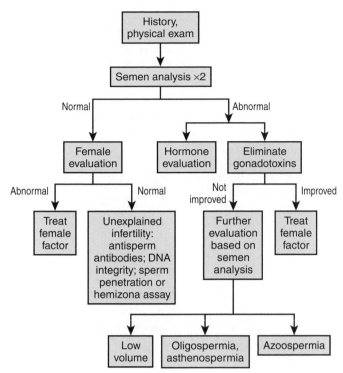

Figure 41-13 General algorithm for the diagnostic evaluation of male infertility. (From Turek PJ: Practical approach to the diagnosis and management of male infertility. Nat Clin Pract Urol 2:226,2005)

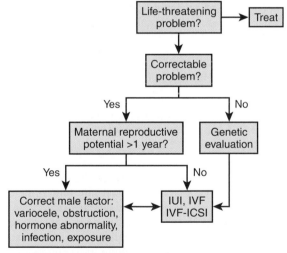

Figure 41-14 General algorithm for treatment of male infertility. ICSI, Intracytoplasmic sperm injections; IUI, intrauterine insemination; IVF, in vitro fertilization. (From Turek PJ: Practical approach to the diagnosis and management of male infertility. Nat Clin Pract Urol 2:226, 2005.)

developed the technique of ICSI, fertilization rates of oocytes injected with a single normal sperm obtained from men with severe abnormalities in their semen analysis were increased above 50%. Pregnancy rates per embryo transfer are now similar after ICSI compared with other indications for IVF. In several studies, it has been determined that fertilization rates of approximately 60% of the oocytes injected may be achieved with sperm from semen samples containing no motile sperm, few motile sperm, and high numbers of motile sperm. In addition, a fertilization

rate of approximately 60% was obtained whether the sperm were freshly obtained by masturbation, by electroejaculation, or were previously frozen. A fertilization rate of oocytes of almost 50% was also achieved when the sperm were aspirated directly from the epididymal fluid.

The excellent results obtained with ICSI by the group that originally described the technique have now been replicated in other centers. By using this technique, the pregnancy rate of couples whose male partner has an extremely low concentration of motile sperm in the semen samples ($<100,000$/mL) can reach a normal pregnancy rate for IVF, based on the age of the woman (see later). Studies of pregnancies resulting from ICSI and standard IVF have revealed a similar rate of pregnancy loss and multiple gestation. Therefore, ICSI is now the treatment of choice for all causes of male infertility, as well as for couples with no known cause of infertility for whom fertilization has failed with standard IVF procedures.

In the past, the finding of azoospermia in seminal fluid was considered an untreatable cause of infertility. After development of the techniques of ICSI as an adjunct to IVF, it was found that spermatozoa retrieved from the testes of azoospermic men could fertilize ova retrieved from their partner's ovaries. The clinical pregnancy rate is higher when testicular or epididymal sperm is retrieved from men with obstruction in their vas deferens (obstructive azoospermia) than when testicular sperm is retrieved from men with azoospermia without reproductive tract obstruction (nonobstructive azoospermia). Even if the sperm retrieved from the testes remains immotile, the pregnancy rate after ICSI is acceptable, 15% or higher. The likelihood of retrieval of spermatozoa from testicular tissue of men with azoospermia and normal FSH levels is almost 100%. Even if FSH levels are markedly elevated, there is at least a 50% likelihood that spermatozoa can be retrieved from the testes and used to perform an ICSI procedure. Thus, the presence of a combination of azoospermia and an elevated FSH level is not a contraindication for performing a TESE procedure, although it is advantageous to carry out a diagnostic TESE prior to an IVF cycle. Diligence is required with the aid of microscopy to select the best sperm for use in ICSI.

Although controversial, there is probably a slight but significant increase in chromosomal structural defects in children born after ICSI. In a study of 8319 live births, Van Steirteghem and coworkers have found a rate of sex chromosomal aneuploidy of 0.6% versus 0.2% and structural autosomal abnormalities in 0.4% versus 0.07%, as well as an increase in structural aberrations related to the infertile fathers. A Danish study has also suggested that although two reports have suggested abnormalities, 9 of 11 publications on this topic did not, suggesting that if there truly was an increased risk of chromosomal abnormalities after ICSI, the rate is low. Follow-up of the children, however, does suggest an increased rate of urogenital abnormalities, which may be related to the male subfertility. Counseling of patients before ICSI about these findings is important.

Some couples, particularly those whose male partner has azoospermia, may choose to use donor sperm insemination. If they choose this option, the attitudes of both partners regarding the use of donor semen and the stability of the marriage need to be thoroughly discussed before the procedure is performed. Donors from sperm banks are carefully screened for infectious diseases, and all semen samples are quarantined for at least 6 months because of the long time it takes for positive antibodies to HIV to appear after infection. A set of guidelines for semen donor insemination has been published by the American Society for Reproductive Medicine. These guidelines provide information regarding indications for donor insemination, as well as suggested procedures for selection and screening of possible semen donors.

Freezing of sperm is the only way that donor insemination should be done because of the time necessary to quarantine samples to rule out infectious diseases but freezing sperm affects fecundability. A cumulative pregnancy rate with insemination after 6 months of treatment is approximately 50% and a monthly fecundity rate of only 9% has been reported. However, the range is variable and may be as high as a fecundity rate of 18%, with a 45% cumulative pregnancy rate at 3 months. There is a known variability of semen quality after thaw, even in normal fertile sperm donors.

UTERINE CAUSES OF INFERTILITY

Intrauterine Adhesions

In addition to menstrual abnormalities and recurrent abortion, some women may not be able to conceive because of the presence of intrauterine adhesions (IUAs). As noted in Chapter 16 (Spontaneous and Recurrent Abortion), most women with IUAs have had a previous curettage of the uterine cavity, usually during or shortly following a pregnancy. If the only abnormal finding in the infertility investigation is the presence of IUAs, the prognosis for conception after hysteroscopic lysis of the adhesions is good. March and Israel have reported that of 69 infertile women with IUAs and no other infertility factors, 52 (75%) conceived after hysteroscopic treatment.

Leiomyoma

Congenital uterine defects rarely cause infertility and the uterine anomalies associated with maternal ingestion of diethylstilbestrol (DES) have not been shown in randomized studies to be a cause of infertility. It is also difficult to assess the effect of leiomyomas on conception, because many women with leiomyomas have no difficulty conceiving. However, depending on their location, fibroids may decrease the chance of conception and/or increase the miscarriage rate. Recent data indicate a global change in endometrial receptivity, even with intramural fibroids. If no other cause of infertility is found and myomas of moderate size and position are present, a myomectomy is justified. More recent data from the IVF literature point to a decreased pregnancy rate with submucous fibroids, larger intramural fibroids (≈4 cm), and those that distort the cavity. The overall pregnancy rate after myomectomy in women with no other causes of infertility has been found to be approximately 60%. However, no study has included a comparison group of infertile women with leiomyomas treated expectantly.

Tuberculosis

Although rare in the United States at present, genital tuberculosis should be kept in mind. If HSG reveals findings consistent with pelvic tuberculosis, endometrial biopsy and culture should be performed to confirm the diagnosis. The radiographic features of pelvic tuberculosis that are almost diagnostic include the following: (1) calcified lymph nodes or granulomas in the pelvis; (2) tubal obstruction in the distal isthmus or proximal ampulla, sometimes resulting in a pipe stem configuration of the tube proximal to the obstruction; (3) multiple strictures

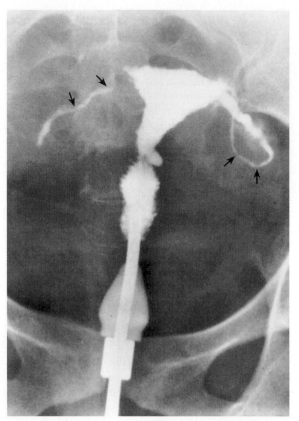

Figure 41-15 Tuberculous salpingitis in 37-year-old nulligravida with primary infertility for 15 years. Right tube is obstructed in the zone of transition between the isthmus and the ampulla. *Arrows* indicate multiple strictures in both tubes. Nodular contour of endometrial cavity may also be related to tuberculosis and is analogous to the pattern found in the ampulla in other cases. Small diverticulum near internal os probably represents adenomyosis. Diagnosis of tuberculosis was confirmed by endometrial culture. (From Richmond JA: Hysterosalpingography. In Mishell DR Jr, Davajan V, Lobo RA [eds]: Infertility, Contraception and Reproductive Endocrinology, 3rd ed. Cambridge, MA, Blackwell Scientific, 1991.)

along the course of the tube; (4) irregularity to the contour of the ampulla; and (5) deformity or obliteration of the endometrial cavity without a previous curettage (**Fig. 41-15**). Appropriate antituberculosis medication should be initiated, but women with pelvic tuberculosis should be considered sterile, because pregnancies after therapy are rare. Tubal reconstructive surgical procedures are therefore not indicated. If tuberculosis is present in the tube but not in the uterus, pregnancies have been reported following IVF.

Tubal Causes of Infertility

During the past 3 decades, the incidence of infertility caused by damage to the fallopian tube has increased because of an increased incidence of salpingitis. Obstructions occur at the distal or proximal portion of the tube and sometimes in both regions. Distal obstruction is much more common than proximal obstruction. The prognosis for fertility after surgical tubal reconstruction depends on the amount of damage to the tube, as well as the location of the obstruction. If there is extensive damage, the chances for conception after tubal reconstruction are unlikely. Women with extensive tubal disease have a greater chance of conceiving with an IVF procedure, so the extent and location of the intrinsic and extrinsic tubal disease should be ascertained by HSG and possibly laparoscopy in an effort to determine whether tubal reconstruction or IVF offers the better prognosis. As noted, if a large hydrosalpinx is seen at the time of HSG, it is best to suggest that the woman have IVF rather than undergo tubal reconstructive surgery. It is recommended that the hydrosalpinx be excised before IVF if it is large and visible by ultrasound. If proximal and distal obstructions of the tube exist, the damage to the tube is usually so extensive that the tube cannot function normally. Therefore, although it is possible to achieve tubal patency after surgical repair with proximal and distal blockage, subsequent intrauterine pregnancy is uncommon and surgical reconstruction should not be performed in such cases. In general, infertility surgery for tubal disease is a dying art—the pregnancy rates with IVF are far superior, and most women would prefer to avoid surgery as long as they have insurance coverage for IVF.

Distal Tubal Disease

HSG will determine whether the tubal obstruction is complete or partial, the size of the distal sacculation, and the appearance of the mucosal folds and rugal pattern of the endosalpinx (**Fig. 41-16**). Laparoscopy will assist in determining the size of the hydrosalpinx, amount of muscularis, and thickness of the wall of the tube after distention with dye. Laparoscopic examination will determine whether pelvic adhesions are present and the extent of these adhesions. Women with fimbrial obstruction are not a homogeneous group, and the prognosis for intrauterine pregnancy following distal tubal reconstruction is related to the extent of the disease process. Therefore, it is important to perform HSG and laparoscopy before surgical reconstruction to provide an individualized prognosis.

If the fimbriae of the distal end of the tube are relatively normal, with only partial occlusion by adhesions or fimbrial bridges, removal of these adhesions by means of a **fimbrioplasty**

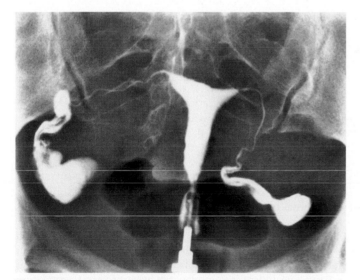

Figure 41-16 HSG showing bilateral hydrosalpinges with dilation, clubbing, and obstruction at fimbriated ends. Patient was 32-year-old woman with 10-year history of primary infertility. (From Richmond JA: Hysterosalpingography. In Mishell DR Jr, Davajan V, Lobo RA [eds]: Infertility, Contraception and Reproductive Endocrinology, 3rd ed. Cambridge, MA, Blackwell Scientific, 1991.)

procedure will result in higher conception rates (≈60%) than if the distal end is completely occluded and a cuff **salpingostomy** procedure is required. Overall conception rates following salpingostomy are in the 30% range, with a high percentage (≈25%) being tubal pregnancies. Although microsurgical techniques had been used for all tubal infertility surgery, all procedures are currently carried out via laparoscopy. The incidence of ectopic pregnancy after surgical reconstruction for distal tubal disease is directly related to the amount of tubal damage existing before the operative procedure.

The results of tubal reconstruction correlate with the degree of tubal damage according to the severity of five factors: (1) extent of adhesions; (2) nature of adhesions; (3) diameter of the hydrosalpinx; (4) appearance of the endosalpinx; and (5) thickness of the tubal wall. Using these criteria, prognostic categories have been identified: good, with a cumulative pregnancy rate of approximately 75%; intermediate, approximately 20%; and poor, less than 5%. In the good category, only 1 of 22 pregnancies may be ectopic, but in the intermediate group 50% of the pregnancies may be expected to be tubal. In the poor prognostic group, most of the pregnancies will be ectopic. Accordingly, in woman in whom there are fixed adhesions, with absent rugal folds and a thick, fixed tubal wall, distal tubal reconstructive surgery probably should not be performed.

The degree of distal tubal occlusion can be divided into four categories on the basis HSG findings (**Fig. 41-17**). Following microscopic tubal reconstruction, the cumulative pregnancy rate is directly related to the degree of occlusion. If the distal tubal ostium is completely normal but peritubal adhesions are present, lysis of these adhesions by **salpingolysis** have resulted in a 64% intrauterine pregnancy rate, similar to that obtained with a fimbrioplasty for partial obstruction. Approximately 50% of women who underwent salpingostomy for degree II occlusion conceived, with no ectopic pregnancies, but only approximately 25% of those with degree III or IV occlusions had subsequent intrauterine pregnancies and the ectopic pregnancy rate was approximately 10% (**Fig. 41-18; Table 41-9**). Thus, following operation for more extensive distal tubal disease, almost one third of the pregnancies that occurred were ectopic.

In all studies, the best prognostic factor was the thickness of the tubal wall. If there was a hydrosalpinx more than 2 cm in diameter, with a thick tubal wall, the prognosis for a term pregnancy following distal tubal reconstruction was extremely poor.

Rock and coworkers have classified women with distal fimbrial occlusion into three categories based on the extent of tubal disease (**Table 41-10**). A life table analysis of couples in these three categories with no other causes of infertility was performed after the female partner underwent neosalpingostomy. Of those women, 80% with mild tubal disease conceived, whereas only 31% of those with moderate disease and 16% of those with severe disease conceived (**Fig. 41-19**). The ectopic pregnancy rate was higher in the latter two categories. This information should be given to the woman when she is counseled and, if the prognosis for term pregnancy is poor, she should be advised to undergo IVF instead of surgical tubal reconstruction, as noted. Distal tubal reconstructive surgery should be carried out by operative laparoscopy. The results of a series of 65 consecutive distal tuboplasties, both fimbrioplasties and neosalpingostomies performed endoscopically, have shown that the intrauterine pregnancy rate is 26% after fimbrioplasty and 29% after neosalpingostomy, similar to the historical success rate after

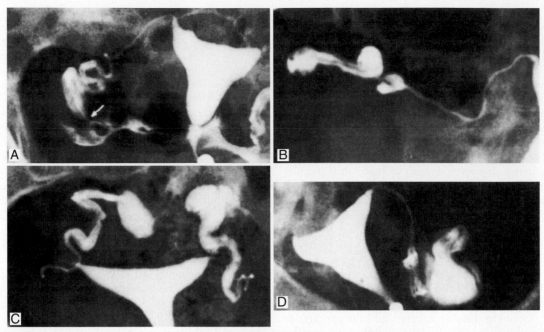

Figure 41-17 Classification of distal tubal occlusion based on degree of dilation seen on HSG. **A,** Degree I, conglutination of the fimbrial folds *(arrow)* with tubal patency. **B,** Degree II, complete distal occlusion with normal ampullary diameter. **C,** Degree III, complete distal occlusion with ampullary dilation of 15 to 25 mm in diameter. **D,** Degree IV, occlusion with ampullary distention greater than 25 mm. (From Donnez J, Casanas-Roux F: Prognostic factors of fimbrial microsurgery. Fertil Steril 46:200, 1986.)

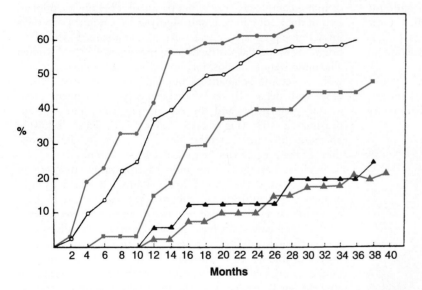

Figure 41-18 Cumulative pregnancy rates following microsurgical repair of these lesions are depicted. *Solid circles,* salpingolysis; *open circles,* fimbrioplasty; *squares,* salpingostomy (degree II); *black triangles,* salpingostomy (degree III); *blue triangles,* salpingostomy (degree IV). (From Donnez J, Casanas-Roux F: Prognostic factors of fimbrial microsurgery. Fertil Steril 46:200, 1986.)

microsurgery. The prognoses for fertility after salpingostomy is correlated more with the extent of disease than with the type of surgical procedure. Basically, it can be expected that one third of the patients will have intrauterine pregnancies within 2 to 3 years if they have mild or moderate disease.

Proximal Tubal Blockage

If no dye enters the tube during HSG, the diagnosis of proximal tubal blockage is likely. However, because spasm of the uterus during the procedure may occlude the intrauterine portion of the tube, the diagnosis cannot be confirmed. Here, at least half of the time, the tube will be found to be patent on subsequent

testing or at laparoscopy. Laparoscopy also allows examination of the distal portion of the tube, which cannot be visualized radiographically if there is proximal blockage.

Currently, it is common to attempt selective catheterization of the proximal portion of a tube at HSG under fluoroscopy if it does not fill with dye. Cannulation of the proximal portion is also possible under direct guidance at hysteroscopy. Cannulation to open the putative obstruction is possible as long as there is no gross disease visible, such as salpingitis isthmica nodosa (SIN). Proximal tubal blockage may be caused by debris or endometriosis, but a significant occlusion is usually explained by prior infection or SIN.

Table 41-9 Pregnancy Rate After Microsurgery and Ciliated Cell Percentage in Cases of Distal Tubal Occlusion

Type of Operation	No. of Patients	No. of Intrauterine Pregnancies	Ectopic Pregnancies
Fimbrioplasty Occlusion of degree I	132	79 (60%)	2 (2%)
Salpingostomy			
Occlusion of degree II	27	13 (48%)	0
Occlusion of degree III	16	4 (25%)	1 (6%)
Occlusion of degree IV	40	9 (22%)	5 (12%)
Total	83	26 (31%)	6 (7%)
Salpingolysis	42	27 (64%)	1 (2%)

Adapted from Donnez J, Casanas-Roux F: Prognostic factors influencing the pregnancy rate after microsurgical cornual anastomosis. Fertil Steril 46:1089, 1986.

Table 41-10 Classification of the Extent of Tubal Disease with Distal Fimbrial Obstruction

Mild
Absent or small hydrosalpinx <15 mm diameter
Inverted fimbriae easily recognized when patency is achieved
No significant peritubal or periovarian adhesions
Preoperative hysterogram reveals rugal pattern
Moderate
Hydrosalpinx = 15-30 mm in diameter
Fragments of fimbriae not readily identified
Periovarian or peritubular adhesions without fixation, minimal cul-de-sac adhesions
Absence of a rugal pattern on preoperative hysterogram
Severe
Large hydrosalpinx >30 mm diameter
No fimbriae
Dense pelvic or adnexal adhesions with fixation of the ovary and tube to the broad ligament, pelvic sidewall, omentum, or bowel
Obliteration of the cul-de-sac
Frozen pelvis (adhesion formation so dense that limits of organs are difficult to define)

From Rock JA, Katayama P, Martin EJ, et al: Factors influencing the success of salpingostomy techniques for distal fimbrial obstruction. Obstet Gynecol 52:591, 1978.

In the past, proximal obstructions were best handled by microsurgical cornual tubal reanastomosis, with pregnancy rates in the range of 50% and ectopic rates of only 10%. Although this approach may still be considered on a selective basis, most cases of obstruction not relieved by fluoroscopic or hysteroscopic selective cannulation are now treated by IVF.

Adjunctive Therapy

Adjunctive procedures for surgical tubal reconstruction previously included prophylactic antibiotics, intraperitoneal corticosteroids, postoperative hydrotubation, and placement of tubal stents. Prospective studies have not demonstrated postoperative hydrotubation to have any benefit, and tubal stents should not be used because they may cause mucosal damage. Data from the Nordic Adhesion Prevention Study Group have shown that intraperitoneal corticosteroids failed to reduce adhesion scores in infertility patients.

It is important to stress surgical technique, attention to hemostasis, and irrigation of blood and debris away from the surgical site with Ringer's lactate solution. The only barriers currently used with some efficacy are an absorbable adhesion barrier (Gynecare Interceed, Ethicon, Somerville, NJ), to be used only in areas that are dry and not bleeding, and barriers impregnated with hyaluronic acid (Seprafilm, Genzyme, Cambridge, MA). The latter can be used as a slurry at the end of laparoscopy. Gore-Tex requires suturing and removal; therefore, it is rarely used and is not applicable for tubal disease.

If pregnancy does not occur within 6 to 12 months after tubal reconstruction, HSG should be performed. If tubal obstruction has recurred, a repeat surgical procedure is not advised. In this setting, the pregnancy rates are less than 10%.

ENDOMETRIOSIS

Some investigators have estimated that as many as 40% of infertile women have endometriosis. If endometriosis is found at the time of laparoscopy, the extent of the disease should be documented The causes, diagnosis, and treatment of endometriosis are presented in detail in Chapter 19.

Although endometriosis is frequently encountered in an infertility population (20% to 40%), the diagnosis may be subtle and may only be realized if a laparoscopy is carried out. As noted,

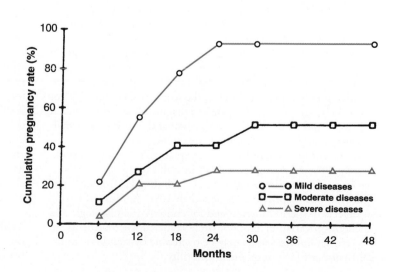

Figure 41-19 Life table analysis of pregnancy outcome after neosalpingostomy by extent of disease. (From Schlaff WD, Hassiakos DK, Damewood MD, Rock JA: Neosalpingostomy for distal tubal obstruction: Prognostic factors and impact of surgical technique. Fertil Steril 54:984, 1990.)

laparoscopy is often currently bypassed in the investigative workup. Thus, unless there is a strong component of pain as a presenting complaint, or an endometrioma is seen on ultrasound, the diagnosis may not be appreciated. The treatment for pain is somewhat different and has been reviewed in Chapter 19.

If laparoscopy is carried out and mild lesions are seen, it makes sense to ablate them surgically by electrocauterization or laser. Although this may not have a major therapeutic value, the current thinking is that peritoneal endometriosis may release substances that could impair fertilization at various levels.

A new classification of endometriosis has been developed, with fertility as the hard end point (see Chapter 19). The components of this classification scheme are based on structured factors that contribute to the infertility of endometriosis. In general, women with endometriosis have a reduced fecundity in relation to the extensiveness of the disease, and women with extensive disease usually have a mechanical (obstructive) cause of infertility as well.

Surgery in the setting of infertility is reserved for those patients with pain and if large endometriomas are present. Smaller, 2- to 4-cm endometriomas may be observed, particularly in older women, because of the concern of compromising ovarian reserve by ovarian cystectomy. Otherwise, women should be treated as if they have unexplained infertility (see later). Many women with unexplained infertility may have endometriosis that has not been diagnosed because laparoscopy was not performed. The lowered cycle of fecundity in endometriosis is similar to that of women with unexplained infertility ($\approx$4%). COS, generally with IUI, is the usual initial treatment. If pregnancy does not occur in three to six cycles, IVF is offered as the next step. When surgery has been offered as the primary treatment for moderate to severe disease, which is easily diagnosed, pregnancy rates of approximately 50% have been recorded with operative laparoscopy. This rate is similar to the rate after laparotomy.

IVF pregnancy rates are also reduced by approximately 20% in the presence of endometriosis, but because overall pregnancy rates are good, most patients are eventually successful. In select cases, prior suppression of known cases of endometriosis (e.g., using a GnRH agonist for 2 to 3 months) has been shown to improve IVF pregnancy rates.

UNEXPLAINED INFERTILITY

This diagnostic category is relatively arbitrary and is probably never truly unexplained. I categorize in this way if there is normal ovulation, pelvic examination with a normal uterus, and patent tubes on a hysterosalpingogram and a normal semen analysis. In the past, the diagnosis also required a normal laparoscopy. This is rarely carried out in a routine fashion unless there are clues to significant pelvic abnormalities in the workup. The rationale for omitting laparoscopy in the required diagnostic workup is that it is invasive and costly, and it is unlikely that the subtle abnormalities will change the outcome of treatment.

Using the broad definition of unexplained infertility, approximately 20% of all couples will fall into this category. If exhaustive meticulous testing is carried out, including laparoscopy, this figure has been reported to be less than 10%. Additional testing for defects in sperm function and for endometrial histologic and biochemical variables have not been validated for routine use in this setting. Subtle defects may be overcome by standard empirical treatment for unexplained infertility.

The routine empirical treatment of unexplained infertility is ovarian stimulation with clomiphene or gonadotropins, coupled with IUI. The efficiency of these procedures are age-dependent. In women in their 30s, the expected fecundity rate is approximately 9% and is not different with the use of clomiphene or gonadotropins, a conclusion that was not realized until recently, based on prospective data.

In 1998, Guzick and associates published a review of data from 45 published studies of various therapies of unexplained infertility, including mild endometriosis. After adjustment for study quality, pregnancy rates per initiated treatment cycle were 1.3% to 4.1% for no treatment, 8.3% for clomiphene citrate plus IUI, 17.1% for HMG plus IUI, and 20.7% for IVF (see **Table 41-7**). Although the pregnancy rate in this analysis of nonrandomized studies was higher with HMG plus IUI than with clomiphene citrate plus IUI, recent prospective data have shown that the rates are similar. In a prospective randomized trial comparing HMG plus IUI with HMG and intracervical insemination and intracervical or intrauterine insertion without HMG, the pregnancy rate per treatment cycle with HMG plus IUI was approximately twice as high as for the other three treatment regimens. One third of the couples treated with HMG plus IUI conceived after four treatment cycles (**Table 41-11**). Although these rates may seem low, the background rate for unexplained infertility is no more than 4%, so the fecundity is more than doubled. Unfortunately, even with monitoring, 20% to 30% of the pregnancies that occurred with the use of HMG were multiple gestations, with approximately 8% being higher order multiples (triplets or more).

Because of this, and the fact that treatment with clomiphene-IUI and gonadotropin-IUI are similar, a large prospective trial was carried out by Reindollar and colleagues to assess whether it was reasonable to skip gonadotropin-IUI therapy and proceed to IVF after three cycles of clomiphene-IUI (called fast track). The logical next step after clomiphene and/or gonadotropin-IUI therapy is still IVF. One of the concerns with unexplained infertility is that there may be failure to fertilize, even if there is normal ovulation and semen characteristics. IVF also has a higher cycle fecundity rate (see later). In the prospective trial, which also included a cost analysis, conventional therapy included 3 months of clomiphene-IUI followed by three cycles of gonadotropin-IUI and then up to six cycles of IVF. The other arm of this randomized trial omitted the gonadotropin-IUI step and proceeded directly to IVF after clomiphene-IUI. As shown in **Figure 41-20**, there was an increased pregnancy rate in the accelerated arm (100% to 156%; hazard ratio, 1.25). The median time to pregnancy was also shorter, 8 versus 11 months, and average charges per delivery were $9800 lower. Individual per cycle pregnancy rates for clomiphene-IUI, gonadotropin-IUI, and IVF were 7.6%, 9.8%, and 30%, respectively. The conclusion of these authors was that the gonadotropin-IUI step in the usual algorithm for unexplained infertility may be omitted. However, this remains an area of controversy and may not be applicable to couples who do not have insurance coverage for IVF, unlike in Massachusetts (where the study was carried out), where coverage is mandated.

Age is a significant factor in terms of efficacy of treatment. **Table 41-12** shows the results of a large retrospective study of the success of clomiphene-IUI. It is clear that in older women, because of reduced efficacy (after age 42, cumulative pregnancy

Table 41-11 Pregnancy Rates Per Couple

Treatment Group (%)	No. of Couples	Insemination Cycles	No. of Pregnancies	Pregnancy Rate/ Couple (%)*	No. of Pregnancies During Insemination Cycle (No. of Pregnancies/ No. of Insemination Cycles)†
Intracervical insemination	233	706	23	10	14/706 (2)
Intrauterine insemination	234	717	42	18	35/717 (5)
Superovulation and intracervical insemination	234	637	44	19	26/637 (4)
Superovulation and intrauterine insemination	231	618	77	33	54/618 (9)

*The results of tests of a χ^2 priori comparison, adjusted for center, are as follows: intracervical insemination as compared with superovulation and intracervical insemination, $P=.006$; intracervical insemination as compared with intrauterine insemination, $P=.01$; intracervical insemination as compared with superovulation and intrauterine insemination: $P<.001$; intrauterine insemination as compared with superovulation and intrauterine insemination, $P<.001$; superovulation and intracervical insemination as compared with superovulation and intrauterine insemination, $P<.001$. The P value that indicates statistical significance after the Bonferroni correction is .01.

†The results of χ^2 tests of a priori comparison, adjusted for center, are as follows: intracervical insemination as compared with superovulation and intracervical insemination, $P=.024$; intracervical insemination as compared with intrauterine insemination, $P=.003$; intracervical insemination as compared with superovulation and intrauterine insemination, $P<.001$; intrauterine insemination as compared with superovulation and intrauterine insemination, $P<.001$; superovulation and intracervical insemination as compared with superovulation and intrauterine insemination, $P=0.005$. The P value that indicates statistical significance after the Bonferroni correction is .01. Adapted from Guzick DS, for the National Cooperative Reproductive Medicine Network: Efficacy of superovulation and intrauterine insemination in the treatment of infertility. N Engl J Med 340:177, 1999.

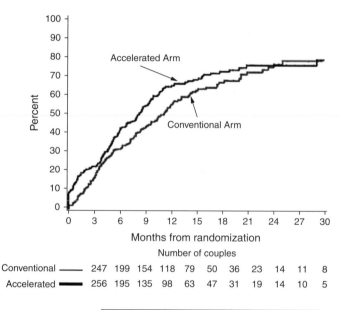

Number of couples

Conventional	247	199	154	118	79	50	36	23	14	11	8
Accelerated	256	195	135	98	63	47	31	19	14	10	5

Time Period (m)	Hazard Ratio	95% CI		P-value
≤3	1.52	1.02	2.28	0.04
>3 to 11	1.40	1.03	1.90	0.03
>11	0.60	0.34	1.06	0.08

Figure 41-20 Randomized clinical trial to evaluate optimal treatment for unexplained infertility: the fast track and standard treatment (FASTT) trial. (From Reindollar RH, Regan MM, Neumann PJ, et al: A randomized clinical trial to evaluate optimal treatment for unexplained infertility: The fast track and standard treatment (FASTT) trial. Fertil Steril 94:888, 2010.)

Table 41-12 Realistic Chances of Pregnancy with Intrauterine Insemination: Age Dependency*

Age of Woman (yr)	Pregnancy Rate per Cycle (%)
<35	≈10-11.5
35-37	≈8.2-9.2
38-40	≈6.5-7.3
40-41	≈3.6-4.3
>42†	≈0.8-1.0

*Large cohort of 4100 cycles of CC IUI.
†In women >42 years, cumulative pregnancy rates =1.8% (1 in 55).
From Dovey S, Sneeringer RM, Penzias AS: Clomiphene citrate and intrauterine insemination: Analysis of more than 100 cycles. Fertil Steril 90: 2281, 2008.

and AMH and visualize the ovaries for an antral follicle count. We have found that MIS and AMH are most predictive of decreased ovarian reserve; values under 0.4 ng/mL require a more aggressive therapeutic plan, regardless of age.

IN VITRO FERTILIZATION

In 2010, Bob Edwards was awarded the Nobel Prize for Physiology and Medicine for his pioneering work in making IVF a reality. IVF has revolutionized the field of reproduction. Not only has it opened up many avenues of research and understanding of basic human reproductive physiology, but its successful clinical use has allowed millions of couples to conceive who might otherwise have been unable to do so. IVF has also provided the ability to diagnose significant genetic defects before implantation and has led to the possibility of embryonic stem cell research. Although IVF–embryo transfer (ET) is usually the last step in the treatment algorithm for infertile couples, it has been used as primary therapy for certain indications, such as bilateral tubal occlusion and severe male factor. With the increased success rate of IVF-ET, which has developed gradually over the last 10 to 15 years, IVF-ET is now often chosen as the primary treatment for other causes of infertility as well.

The strategy behind successful IVF is the generation of good-quality embryos. IVF can be carried out in a natural cycle and was the method used when Steptoe and Edwards performed

rates over 3 to 9 months are approximately 1.8%), couples should consider going directly to IVF.

Cycle fecundity may be reduced substantially, even in women younger than 40 years who have a low ovarian reserve. Accordingly, it is important to measure day 3 FSH levels as well as MIS the first successful IVF procedure that led to the birth of Louise Brown. However, here usually only one oocyte and one embryo can be expected, and the success rate is lower than with conventional IVF, in which gonodotropins are administered to produce multiple follicles. Although unstimulated IVF remains an option on an individual basis, its use is currently limited because of the expectations of couples to become pregnant as quickly as possible.

Another option for IVF, without medication, is to aspirate immature eggs in a natural cycle, usually in anovulatory women with PCOS. In vitro maturation (IVM) of the oocytes is then carried out, followed by ICSI. There are some advantages of IVM for women with PCOS, in whom it is also easier to aspirate immature oocytes because of larger ovaries with multiple small follicles, such as eliminating the risk of hyperstimulation. However, the success rate for IVM, IVF, and ICSI is in the range of 25% in specialized centers, compared with an expected rate of 40% with conventional IVF-ET in PCOS.

There has been a debate about how much gonadotropin stimulation should be used for IVF-ET. It is accepted that excessive ovarian stimulation leads to the risk of hyperstimulation and a poor outcome, including the possibility of oocyte aneuploidy and a disordered endometrium. Nevertheless, obtaining an adequate number of mature oocytes leads to having more embryos available for transfer and possible cryopreservation.

Gonadotropin stimulation (75 IU to 600 IU of FSH) is administered for approximately 10 days. The traditional long cycle protocol begins with downregulation using a GnRH agonist for 2 weeks prior to gonadotropin administration. Increasingly, however, a GnRH antagonist is used to block spontaneous ovulation from occurring once follicular developments occur, and gonadotropins are begun on cycle day 2, without prior downregulation. Recent data support an equal efficacy of the two approaches. When at least three mature follicles are seen on ultrasound ($\approx$18 mm) with an appropriate rise of serum E_2, HCG is administered (5000 to 10,000 IU). Vaginal ultrasound aspiration of the follicles is typically carried out 34 to 36 hours later, when a semen sample is also obtained for natural insemination or ICSI.

The embryology laboratory environment is the key factor in the success of IVF. Typically, 3 days after aspiration, six to eight cell cleavage stage embryos are obtained. Increasingly, with sequential culture media, embryo culture is continued to days 5 to 6, when a blastocyst has developed (**Fig. 41-21**). Fertilized oocytes that can be cultured to day 5 are usually of better quality and afford a higher pregnancy rate. Embryo transfers are carried out with one of several specialized catheters (similar to those used for IUI) under ultrasound guidance. The decision regarding the number of embryos to transfer is key to optimizing success and reducing the chance of multiple pregnancies. The American Society for Reproductive Medicine (ASRM) has published firm guidelines to assist in this decision making process (**Table 41-13**). Implementation of these guidelines has proved to be successful in reducing the rate of high-order multiple pregnancies, although the rate of twins has not decreased substantially (average, 25%).

Excess embryos of good quality that are not transferred may be cryopreserved by the use of several validated techniques, typically slow cooling or vitrification. Recent studies have suggested an excellent success rate of pregnancy using cryopreserved embryos.

IVF-ET success rates are collected nationally by the Society for Assisted Reproductive Technology (SART) and the CDC. **Table 41-14** provides the latest published data. Consumers can look up clinic-specific pregnancy rates using the SART CORS database, available on line (www.sart.org).

A modification of IVF, called gamete intrafallopian transfer (GIFT), can be used if the infertile woman has functioning

Table 41-13 Recommended Limits on Numbers of Embryos to Transfer

	Age (yr)			
Prognosis	**35**	**35-37**	**38-40**	**41-42**
Cleavage stage embryos*				
Favorable[†]	1-2	2	3	5
All others	2	3	4	5
Blastocysts*				
Favorable[†]	1	2	2	3
All others	2	2	3	3

*See text for more complete explanations. Justification for transferring one additional embryo more than the recommended limit should be clearly documented in the patient's medical records.
[†]Favorable = first cycle of IVF, good embryo quality, excess embryos available for cryopreservation, or previous successful IVF cycle.
From Practice Committee of the American Society for Reproductive Medicine; Practice Committee of the Society for Assisted Reproductive Technology: Guidelines on number of embryos transferred. Fertil Steril 92:1518, 2009.

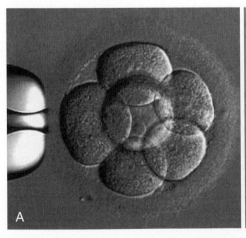
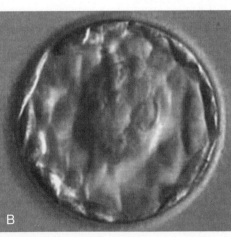

Figure 41-21 Day 3 good-quality embryo. **A,** Six- to eight-cell state. **B,** Expanded good-quality day 5 blastocyst.

Table 41-14 SART-CORS data for all clinics, 2008

Treatment Type	Procedure Frequency (%)		Diagnosis Frequency (%)			
IVF	>99	ICSI 64	Tubal factor	8	Other factor	8
GIFT	<1	Unstimulated 1	Ovulatory disfunction	6	Unknown factor	12
ZIFT	<1	PGD 4	Diminished ovarian reserve	14	Multiple factors	
			Endometriosis	4	Female only	12
			Uterine factor	1	Female and male	18
			Male factor	17		

	Age of Woman (yr)			
Fresh Embryos from Nondonor Oocytes	**<35**	**35-37**	**38-40**	**41-42**
No. of cycles	39,621	21,744	20,430	9,243
Percentage of cycles resulting in pregnancies	47.6	38.0	30.3	20.4
Percentage of cycles resulting in live births (reliability range)	41.3 (40.8-41.7)	31.1 (30.5-31.7)	22.2 (21.6-22.8)	12.3 (11.6-12.9)
Percentage of retrievals resulting in live births	44.5	34.9	26.1	14.9
Percentage of cycles with elective single embryo transfer	5.2	3.2	1.0	0.5
Implantation rate	34.1	24.8	16.7	9.3
Average no. of embryos transferred	2.2	2.4	2.7	3.1
Percentage of live births with twins	33.3	28.1	23.5	15.4
Percentage of live births with triplets or more	1.9	2.0	1.7	0.6

	Age of Woman (yr)			
Thawed Embryos from Nondonor Oocytes	**<35**	**35-37**	**38-40**	**41-42**
No. of transfers	10,303	5,382	3,639	1,194
Percentage of transfers resulting in live births	35.6	29.5	26.1	19.3
Average number of embryos transferred	2.2	2.1	2.3	2.3

Donor Oocyes (all ages)	**Fresh Embryos**	**Thawed Embryos**
No. of transfers	9,905	5,319
Percentage of transfers resulting in live births	55.0	32.7
Average number of embryos transferred	2.1	2.2

tubes. With this technique, both oocytes and sperm are placed into the tube through a catheter at the time of laparoscopy. Although IVF, embryo culturing, and embryo transfer into the uterus are avoided by this technique, ovarian hyperstimulation and laparoscopy are still required. Because this requires a laparoscopy, GIFT is rarely done at present in that pregnancy rates are similar to those of routine IVF-ET when matched for age and diagnosis. Modifications of GIFT include **pronuclear stage tubal transfer (PROST)**, or **zygote intrafallopian transfer (ZIFT)**, and **tubal embryo stage transfer (TEST)**. With ZIFT, the oocytes are fertilized in vitro and transferred 24 hours later. **Tubal embryo transfer (TET)** is similar to ZIFT except that the embryos are transferred 8 to 72 hours after fertilization. Again, because laparoscopy is required, these are rarely performed today.

What is important to couples is their overall chance of pregnancy. When a larger number of cycles have been studied over time, the overall optimistic chance of pregnancy after six cycles of IVF is 72% (95% confidence interval [CI], 70% to 74%). Optimistic means continuous treatment without any dropouts; the conservative cumulative pregnancy rate, which includes some drop outs, is 51% (CI, 49% to 52%; **Fig. 41-22**). However, this is very much influenced by age (**Fig. 41-23**).

Pregnancy rates over six cycles are fairly constant over time and may continue to increase at the same rate, although some data suggest a plateau effect after six cycles (**Fig. 41-24**). This latter point is unclear because there are few IVF patients (<10%) who exceed six cycles of treatment.

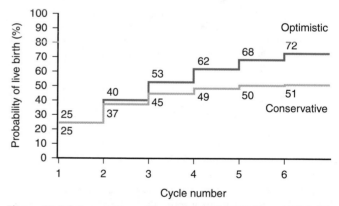

Figure 41-22 Expectations of live birth with IVF-ET. (From Malizia BA, Hacker MR, Penzias AS: Cumulative live-birth rates after in vitro fertilization. N Engl J Med.360:236, 2009.)

The major pregnancy concerns after IVF are related to multiples gestations resulting in prematurity and other sequelae. However, there are some pregnancy-related risks that occur, even with singletons (**Table 41-15**). Therefore, careful obstetric care is extremely important. Congenital risks of IVF may be slightly increased (3% to 4%) compared with a natural rate of birth defects in the normal population (2% to 3%), but this has not been confirmed definitively. There also are some potential risks with ICSI itself, as noted, and potentially some increase in imprinting disorders. The uncertainty surrounding these issues is that it is

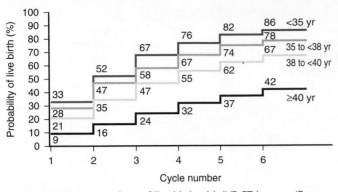

Figure 41-23 Expectations of live birth with IVF-ET by age. (From Malizia BA, Hacker MR, Penzias AS: Cumulative live-birth rates after in vitro fertilization. N Engl J Med. 360:236, 2009.)

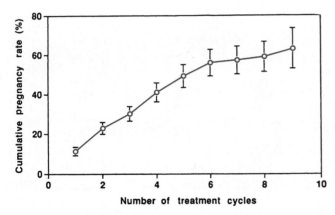

Figure 41-24 Overall cumulative pregnancy rate in IVF treatment (95% CI). (From Dor J, Seidman DS, Ben-Shlomo I, et al: Cumulative pregnancy rate following in-vitro fertilization: The significance of age and infertility aetiology. Hum Reprod 11:425, 1996.)

Table 41-15 Potential Risks in Singleton In Vitro Fertilization Pregnancies

Perinatal Risks	Absolute Risk in IVF Pregnancies (%)	Relative Risk (versus non-IVF pregnancies)
Preterm birth	11.5	2.0 (1.7-2.2)
Low birth weight (<2500 g)	9.5	1.8 (1.4-2.2)
Very low birth weight (<1500 g)	2.5	2.7 (2.3-3.1)
Small for gestational age	14.6	1.6 (1.3-2.0)
Neonatal ICU admission	17.8	1.6 (1.3-2.0)
Stillbirth	1.2	2.6 (1.8-3.6)
Neonatal mortality	0.6	2.0 (1.2-3.4)
Cerebral palsy	0.4	2.8 (1.3-5.8)
Genetic Risks		
Imprinting disorder	0.03	17.8 (1.8-432.9)
Major birth defect	4.3	1.5% (1.3-1.8)
Chromosomal abnormalities (after ICSI)		
Of a sex chromosome	0.6	3.0
Of another chromosome	0.4	5.7

In this table, the absolute risk is the percentage of IVF pregnancies in which the risk occurred. The relative risk is the risk in IVF versus the risk in non-IVF pregnancies; for example, a relative risk of 2.0 indicates that twice as many IVF pregnancies experience this risk as compared with non-IVF pregnancies. The numbers in parentheses (confidence interval) indicate the range in which the actual relative risk lies. Adapted from Reddy UM, Wapner RJ, Rebar RW, Tasca RJ: Infertility, assisted reproductive technology, and adverse pregnancy outcomes. Executive Summary of a National Institute of Child Health and Human Development Workshop. Obstet Gynecol 109:967, 2007.

likely that the infertile population also carries some risks (independent of IVF) when compared with the normal fertile population. There is also no evidence that IVF increases the risk of cancer.

Because of the risks of prematurity with high-order multiples, triplets, and more, couples may elect to undergo selective fetal reduction early in pregnancy. This is considered a safe procedure but carries an overall risk of pregnancy loss of approximately 1%.

Cryopreservation of embryos is now common and leads to an extended higher pregnancy rate. The results of thawed, good-quality embryos are almost equal to the rate of fresh cycles (see **Table 41-14**). There are no known increased fetal risks associated with embryo cryopreservation.

Cryopreservation of eggs is sometimes carried out, particularly in cancer patients prior to chemotherapy to preserve fertility. The oocyte, however, does not freeze and thaw as well as embryos, and therefore validated pregnancy rates and outcomes are based on limited data. Oocyte cryopreservation, therefore, is still considered experimental by the ASRM, although increasingly, even women without cancer are asking for this to be done. Essentially, the woman has to undergo IVF treatment but the treatment cycle stops after the eggs are retrieved.

Another controversial concern is preimplantation genetic screening. Here, an eight-cell embryo can be biopsied and tested for aneuploidy or a specific gene disorder. The latter technique is a validated way to detect known genetic diseases by testing with specific probes for these diseases. However, routine aneuploidy screening is still controversial and has not been shown to increase pregnancies by transferring only normal embryos. Recent data have suggested improved efficacy of genome-wide aneuploidy screening of a blastomeric biopsy on day 5 and cryopreservation prior to embryo transfer. This area is controversial and still in evolution.

COUNSELING AND EMOTIONAL SUPPORT

The diagnosis of infertility can be a devastating and life-altering event that affects many aspects of a woman's life. Infertility and its treatment can affect a woman and her spouse or partner medically, financially, socially, emotionally, and psychologically. Feelings of anxiety, depression, isolation, and helplessness are not uncommon in women undergoing infertility treatment. Strained and stressful relationships with spouses, partners, and other loved ones occur among patients undergoing infertility treatment as treatment gets underway and progresses.

It is important that every program address the emotional and social needs of couples undergoing treatment. Individual counseling and support groups, as well as patient information sessions, should be part of every infertility practice. National support groups such as the National Infertility Association (RESOLVE; www.resolve.org) and the American Fertility Association (www.theafa.org) are also available to provide assistance and information.

KEY POINTS

- Approximately 10% of all U.S. couples with women of reproductive age are infertile, approximately more than 7 million women; and the incidence of infertility steadily increases in women after age 30.
- Among fertile couples who have coitus in the week before ovulation, approximately 20% (monthly fecundability, 0.2) have a chance of developing a clinical pregnancy.
- In the United States, approximately 20% of cases of infertility are caused by anovulation, 30% to 40% by an abnormality of semen production, 30% to 40% by pelvic disease, and approximately 10% to 20% of cases are unexplained.
- Of all the causes of infertility, treatment of anovulation results in the greatest success with ovulation induction, if no other causes of infertility are present; conception rates over time are similar to those of a normal fertile population.
- When conception occurs after clomiphene treatment in anovulatory women, the incidence of multiple gestation is increased to approximately 8%, almost all of them being twin gestations. The incidences of clinical spontaneous abortion, ectopic gestation, intrauterine fetal death, and congenital malformation are not significantly increased.
- The prognosis for fertility after tubal reconstruction depends on the amount of damage to the tube as well as the location of the obstruction. If both proximal and distal obstructions of the tube exist, intrauterine pregnancy is uncommon, and operative reconstruction should not be performed with IVF being the best therapy.
- In women with unexplained infertility, the use of controlled ovarian stimulation (COS) and intrauterine insemination (IUI) yields monthly fecundity rates of approximately 10% and should be the initial treatment for unexplained infertility.
- For IVF with and without ICSI, the delivery rate per cycle in which ova are retrieved is as high as 50%, depending on the age of the woman. The rate of pregnancy following IVF is directly related to the number of embryos placed in the uterine cavity.
- Strict guidelines set forth by ASRM, which limit the number of embryos transferred, has reduced the rate of high-order multiple pregnancies in the United States.

REFERENCES CAN BE FOUND ON EXPERTCONSULT.com

Index

Note: Page numbers followed by "b" indicate boxes; "f" figures; "t" tables.